VOLUME II

TEXTBOOK
OF VETERINARY
INTERNAL MEDICINE
DISEASES OF THE DOG AND CAT

STEPHEN J. ETTINGER, D.V.M.

California Animal Hospital,
Los Angeles, California

Second Edition

W. B. SAUNDERS COMPANY
PHILADELPHIA/LONDON/TORONTO/MEXICO CITY/RIO DE JANEIRO/SYDNEY/TOKYO

W. B. Saunders Company: West Washington Square
Philadelphia, Pa. 19105

1 St. Anne's Road
Eastbourne, East Sussex BN21 3UN, England

1 Goldthorne Avenue
Toronto, Ontario M8Z 5T9, Canada

Cedro 512
Mexico 4, D.F., Mexico

Rua Coronel Cabrita, 8
Sao Cristovao Caixa Postal 21176
Rio de Janeiro, Brazil

9 Waltham Street
Artarmon, N.S.W. 2064, Australia

Ichibancho, Central Bldg., 22-1
Chiyoda-ku, Tokyo 102, Japan

Library of Congress Cataloging in Publication Data

Ettinger, Stephen J.

Textbook of veterinary internal medicine.

1. Dogs — Diseases.   2. Cats — Diseases.   3. Veterinary
medicine.   I. Title. [DNLM: 1. Cat diseases — Diagnosis.
2. Cat diseases — Therapy.   3. Dog diseases — Diagnosis.
4. Dog diseases — Therapy. SF 991 T355]

SF991.E88 1982   636.7'0896   81–40690

ISBN 0–7216–3423–0 (v. 1)   AACR2

ISBN 0–7216–3426–5 (v. 2)

ISBN 0–7216–3427–3 (2-vol. set)

Textbook of Veterinary Internal Medicine:
Diseases of the Dog and Cat

Volume I   ISBN   0-7216-3423-0
Volume II   ISBN   0-7216-3426-5
Complete Set   ISBN   0-7216-3427-3

Last digit is the print number: 9   8   7   6   5   4   3

Contents

SECTION III: SOCIAL AND ENVIRONMENTAL CONSIDERATIONS

SECTION IV: INFECTIOUS DISORDERS

SECTION V: THERAPEUTIC CONSIDERATIONS

SECTION VI: PRINCIPLES OF CANCER THERAPY

SECTION VII: DISEASES OF THE NERVOUS SYSTEM

SECTION VIII: DISEASES OF THE RESPIRATORY SYSTEM

SECTION IX: DISEASES OF THE CARDIOVASCULAR SYSTEM

SECTION X: THE ALIMENTARY SYSTEM, LIVER, AND PROSTATE

SECTION XI: THE ENDOCRINE SYSTEM

SECTION XII: THE REPRODUCTIVE SYSTEM

SECTION XIII: DISEASES OF THE URINARY SYSTEM

SECTION XIV: DISEASES OF THE BLOOD CELLS, LYMPH NODES, AND SPLEEN

SECTION XV: IMMUNOLOGIC DISEASES

SECTION XVI: JOINT AND SKELETAL DISORDERS

The Alimentary System, Liver, and Prostate

CHAPTER 55

Oral, Dental, Pharyngeal, and Salivary Gland Disorders

COLIN E. HARVEY,
JOAN A. O'BRIEN,
LOUIS E. ROSSMAN,
and NORMAN H. STOLLER

THE ORAL CAVITY

ANATOMY AND FUNCTION

The oral cavity is an open-ended tube that functions in prehension, mastication, imbibition of fluid, taste, and swallowing. Associated with the oropharyngeal tube and surrounding muscles and calcified tissues are the salivary glands.

The external opening of the oral cavity is bordered by the fleshy upper and lower lips. Between the external skin and the stratified squamous epithelium lining the lips and cheeks lie the muscles that cause changes in facial expression; these are innervated by the facial nerve (cranial nerve [C.N.] VII). The upper lips are separated rostrally by a midline fissure, the philtrum.

The fleshy, highly mobile tongue lies on the floor of the oral cavity. The root of the tongue is formed by muscles that arise from the hyoid bones, which are supplied by the hypoglossal nerves. The tongue is covered by stratified squamous epithelium. On the dorsal surface, specialized areas of epithelium form the taste buds, containing the gustatory nerve endings. The dorsal surface of the tongue of the cat also contains epithelial projections, which form horny spikes. The ordinary and special sensory nerve fibers from the tongue are carried in the lingual (mandibular branch, trigeminal nerve [C.N. V]), chorda tympani (facial nerve [C.N. VII]), and glossopharyngeal nerve (C.N. IX).

The palate forms the dorsal roof of the oral cavity, separating it from the nasal cavity. The stratified squamous epithelium that covers the rostral bony part of the palate is formed into horizontal folds. The caudal part of the palate is the soft palate, a muscular mobile structure that forms part of the nasopharyngeal closure mechanism during swallowing.

Dental Structures

The dental unit consists of the teeth, their supporting tissues, and the periodontium (the gingiva, the alveolar and supporting bony portion of the mandible and maxilla, the periodontal ligament, and the cemental surfaces of the teeth). The teeth vary in size, shape, and number of roots, depending upon location and function. A tooth consists of a mass of dentin surrounding the pulpal tissues. The root portion of the dentin is covered with cementum, the crown portion with enamel (Fig. 55–1).

In utero, the epithelium covering the maxilla and mandible differentiates to form the dental lamina, which gives rise to the tooth buds. The tooth bud becomes a cup-shaped dome, the enamel organ, which encapsulates invaginating mesenchymal tissue to form the dental papilla. Peripheral cells adjacent to the enamel organ differentiate into odontoblasts, which elaborate dentin. Once dentin is secreted, enamel formation starts. When enamel and dentin formation has reached the future cemento-enamel junction, root formation begins. An epithelial diaphragm directs dentin formation downward. As dentin is elaborated, the epithelial root sheath breaks up, creating the dormant epithelial cell rests of Malassez in the connective tissue. Throughout this development, the tooth bud is encased in a sac, which allows tooth formation to occur surrounded by bone. The sac condenses to become both the connective tissue of the periodontal ligament and the cells forming the thin cementum covering the dentin of the root.

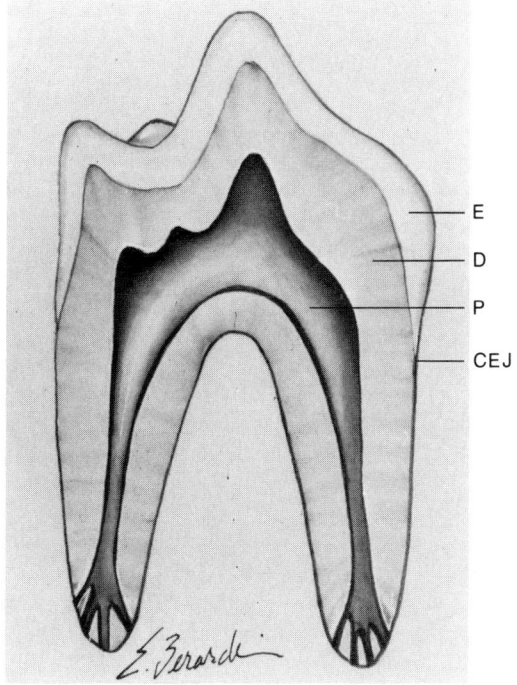

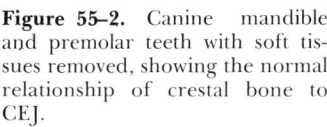

Figure 55–1. Diagram of the structure of a premolar tooth of a dog. CEJ, Cemento-enamel junction; D, dentin; E, enamel; P, pulp.

Enamel, the only portion of the tooth that is of ectodermal origin, is 95 per cent mineralized inorganic substance, mostly hydroxyapatite. It provides resistance to wear and protects the underlying dentinal tissue from caries. Enamel is not permeable except in regions where cracks or defects are present.

The internal wall of dentin follows the external outline of the pulp and is lined by odontoblasts: odontoblastic processes extend through the dentinal matrix to the periphery. Dentin, which is 75 per cent mineralized hydroxyapatite and 25 per cent organic collagen, is continuously synthesized throughout the life of the dental pulp, forming a uniform layer throughout the periphery of the pulp cavity. Dentin contains pain nerve endings that are stimulated by penetration or removal of enamel.

The dental pulp is a connective tissue organ occupying the root canal. Its primary function is the development of dentin: secondary functions are nutritive, sensory, and protective. It is a highly vascular organ, having a system of arteriovenous anastomoses that can divert blood from the capillary beds and increase drainage in case of inflammation. The pulp is contiguous with the periodontal ligament at the apex of the root. The dog has multiple apical foramina into each tooth, forming the apical delta (Newman, 1979).

Cementum is a thin, 50 per cent organic, bonelike tissue that covers the root surface. The periodontal ligament is attached to the tooth by means of collagenous Sharpey's fibers, which are embedded in it during cementum formation.

The alveolar process (the mandible and maxilla) consists of a mass of cancellous bone, the external surface of which is covered with cortical bone. The most coronal (toward the crown) aspect of the alveolar process is known as the alveolar crest (Figs. 55–2 and 55–3). Invaginations into the man-

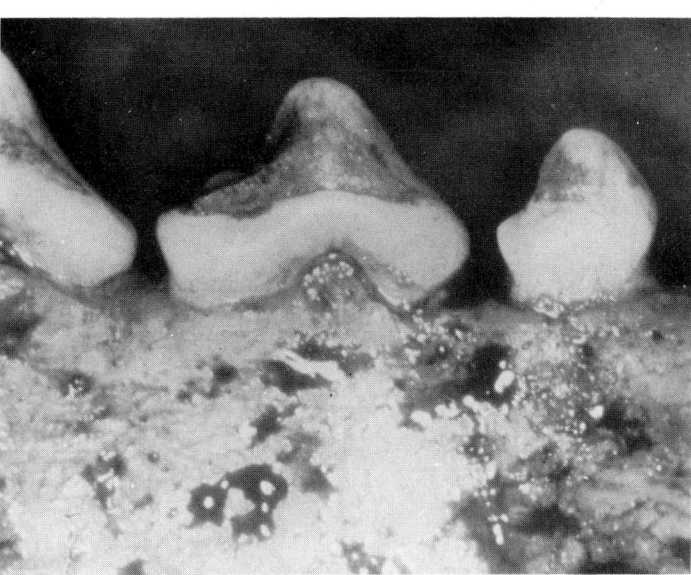

Figure 55–2. Canine mandible and premolar teeth with soft tissues removed, showing the normal relationship of crestal bone to CEJ.

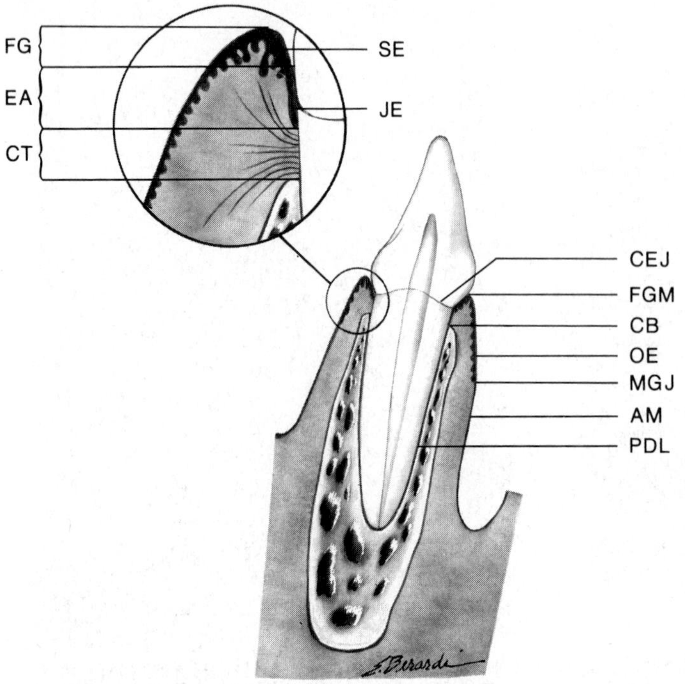

Figure 55–3. Diagram of a cross-section of the periodontium of the dog. AM, alveolar mucosa; CB, crestal bone; CEJ, cemento-enamel junction: CT, connective tissue attachment; EA, epithelial attachment; FGM, free gingival margin; JE, junctional epithelium; MGJ, mucogingival junction; OE, oral epithelium; SE, sulcular epithelium; PDL, periodontal ligament.

dible and maxilla form the sockets, which contain all but the most coronal one to two mm of the root. The sockets themselves are lined with cortical bone known as alveolar bone: the cancellous bone that surrounds the alveolar bone is known as the supporting bone. Connective tissue fibers (Sharpey's fibers) insert into the alveolar bone and anastamose with similar fibers that insert into the cementum. The connective tissue attachment between the tooth and bone is the periodontal ligament, whose function is to resist the stresses placed upon the teeth.

The gingiva is the keratinized squamous epithelium that covers the bone and attaches to the tooth (Fig. 55–4). The most coronal aspect of the gingiva is the free gingival margin (FGM), where the complex junction of gingiva to tooth structure occurs. The FGM approximately parallels the cemento-enamel junction (CEJ) and is located one to two mm coronal to it on the enamel surface of the crown. The junction of the gingiva with the nonkeratinized alveolar mucosa marks the most apical extent of the gingiva, the mucogingival junction (MGJ). The distance from the FGM to the MGJ is quite variable from breed to breed and from tooth to tooth: it is rarely less than one mm and may approach 10 to 20 mm.

The connective tissue underlying the gingiva is well vascularized, dense, nonelastic collagen, The deeper fibers of this connective tissue are confluent with the periosteum of the alveolar process. Connective tissue fibers (the gingival fiber apparatus) insert into the root surface, which is coronal to the alveolar crestal bone. Connective tissue fibers (transeptal fibers) also pass from the cementum of one tooth to the tooth adjacent to it. Around the circumference of each tooth is a one- to two-mm deep gingival sulcus between the gingiva and enamel surface. The gingiva within the sulcus is lined by the relatively nonkeratinized sulcular epithelium. Apical to the sulcular epithelium is the junctional epithelium that forms an attachment between the connective tissue of the gingiva and the tooth surface. The junctional epithelium is a nonkeratinized stratified squamous epithelium 15 to 30 cells thick at its most coronal extent, where it meets the sulcular epithelium and tapers down to one cell at its most apical extent at or just apical to the CEJ. Hemidesmosomes attach the junctional epithelium to a cuticle-like covering on the enamel.

Eruption of the Teeth. Cats and dogs are diphyodent (they have two succeeding generations of teeth), although they are edentulous at birth. The deciduous teeth are small and can be accommodated in the developing jaws, but as the animal grows, they are no longer adequate. As the tooth

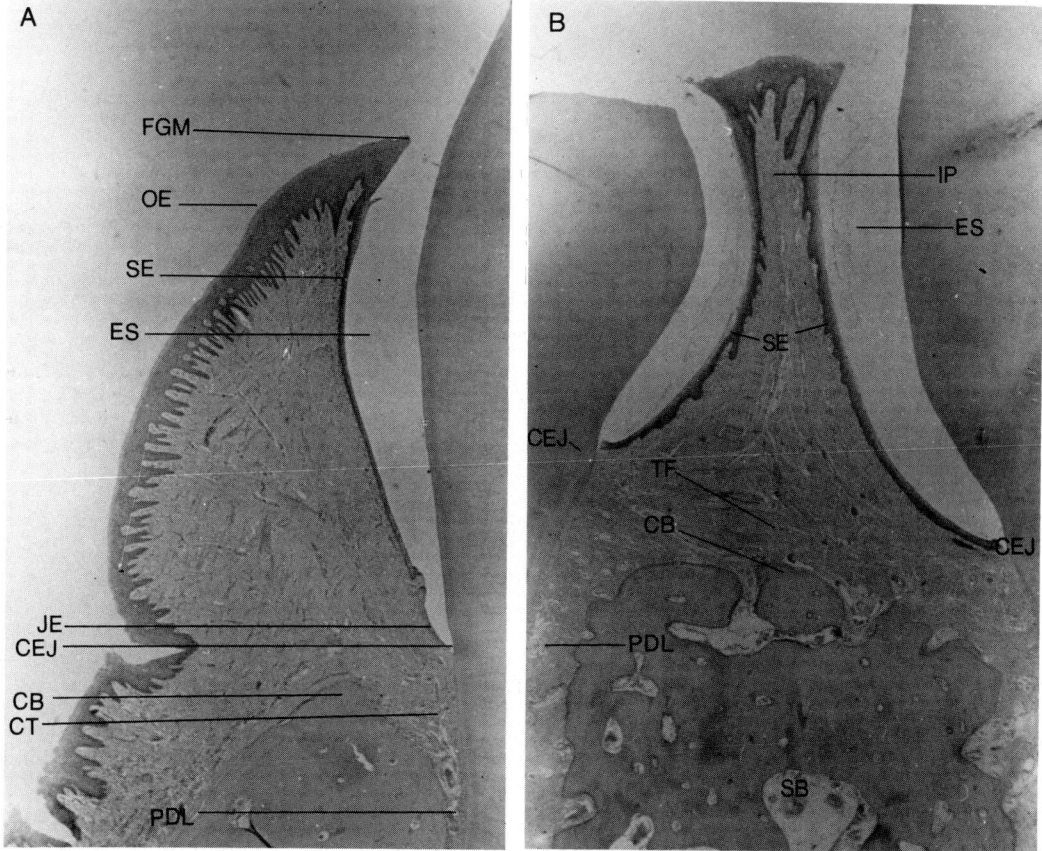

Figure 55–4. Histologic sections of the normal periodontium. *A*, Faciolingual section. *B*, Mesiodistal section. AB, alveolar bone; CB, crestal bone; CEJ, cemento-enamel junction; CT, connective tissue attachment; ES, enamel space; FGM, free gingival margin; IP, interdental papilla; JE, junctional epithelium; OE, oral epithelium; PDL, periodontal ligament; SB, supporting bone; SE, sulcular epithelium; TF, transeptal fibers.

erupts, the root forms apical to the CEJ. Once the tooth has erupted, mechanical forces result in maturation of the alveolus into the attachment apparatus, apical calcification occurs, and the root becomes fully formed. Apical resorption of the roots of deciduous teeth starts almost immediately as the developing permanent teeth start to form.

The deciduous teeth of the dog erupt between two weeks and eight weeks after birth. Dental formulas are shown in Table 55–1, and root arrangements are shown in Figure 55–5. From two to six months of age, shedding of the deciduous dentition occurs as the permanent teeth erupt. Eruption time appears to vary according to the breed of the dog. The larger the breed, the shorter the lifespan and the earlier the eruption sequence. Dogs seldom show signs of teething problems, except for a slight tenderness during the transition. The deciduous premolars act as molars during this period. The smaller jaw requires that the position of the functioning carnassial teeth is more rostral; shearing action is provided

Table 55–1. Dental Formulae of Dogs and Cats

	Dog	Cat
Deciduous dentition	3I, 1C, 3M 3I, 1C, 3M	3I, 1C, 3M 3I, 1C, 2M
Permanent dentition	3I, 1C, 4P, 2M 3I, 1C, 4P, 3M	3I, 1C, 3P, 1M 3I, 1C, 2P, 1M

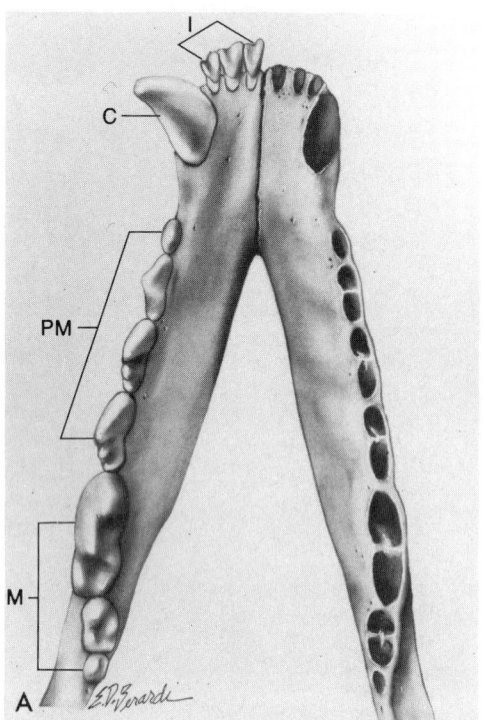
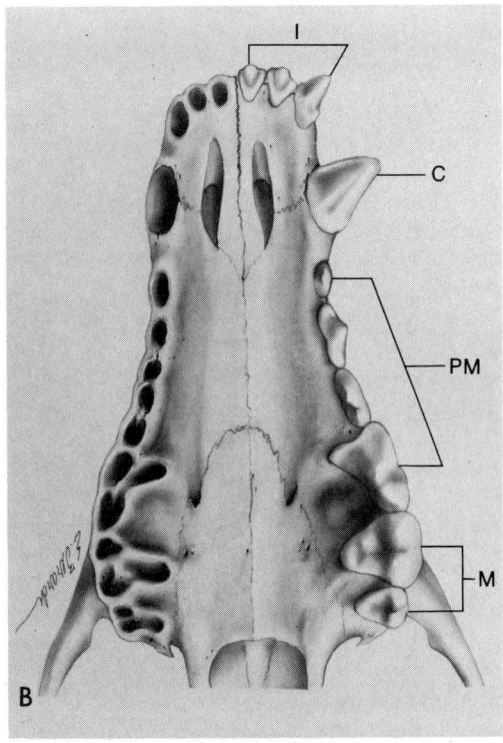

Figure 55–5. *A*, Drawing of a dog mandible showing tooth anatomy on the left side and the distribution of the tooth sockets on the right side. *B*, Drawing of a dog maxilla showing tooth anatomy on the right side and the distribution of the tooth sockets on the left. C, canine; I, incisors; M, molars; PM, premolars.

by the maxillary deciduous third premolar and the mandibular deciduous fourth premolar. Usually the deciduous tooth is shed before its successor erupts.

The cat's deciduous dentition starts to appear within two weeks of birth. All the deciduous teeth are present by about seven weeks. Dental formulas are shown in Table 55–1. The deciduous second premolars are the carnassial teeth. The permanent teeth erupt between three and six months of age.

In both the cat and dog, the mandible is smaller than the maxilla at birth, i.e., a retrognathic relationship. Mandibular growth occurs in a downward and forward direction and at a faster rate than the maxilla. The mature mandibular arch is larger than the maxillary arch; owing to the axial direction of the teeth, however, the maxillary teeth overlap the mandibular teeth.

Occlusion and Articulation. Breed selection has resulted in major variations in "normal" occlusion in the dog. The so-called "scissor bite" (see following discussion) most closely represents the occlusion of the primitive dog.

The deciduous incisors and canines of the dog closely resemble their permanent replacements, although they are somewhat smaller in size and more pointed. In the mandibular arch the deciduous first molar resembles the permanent first premolar, the deciduous second premolar resembles the permanent fourth premolar, and the deciduous third molar resembles the first molar. In the maxillary arch the deciduous first molar is a short single-cusped tooth, the deciduous second molar is similar to the permanent fourth premolar, and the deciduous third molar resembles the first permanent molar. Even in the short-faced breeds, there are generally spaces between the deciduous teeth. Since growth adds considerably more in arch length as opposed to arch width, the arch form in the puppy tends to appear much shorter than in the adult.

In the adult dog with the typical scissor bite, the arch form tends to be rather long and narrow. The widest portion of the maxillary arch occurs in the fourth premolar–first molar region, while the mandibular arch tends to be more "V"-like, with the widest part in the third molar region. The maxillary canine tooth is caudal to the mandibular canine, which fits between the maxillary canine and the maxillary lateral incisor (Fig. 55-6,B). The lingual aspect of the incisal portion of the mandibular canine contacts the gingiva in the space between the maxillary lateral incisor and canine teeth. The distal surface of the mandibular canine may come in contact with the medial aspect of the maxillary canine. The maxillary incisors slightly overlap the mandibular incisors (Fig. 55-6,A). The cusp tip of each of the mandibular premolars lies just medial to its maxillary counterpart. The maxillary first, second, and third premolars make no occlusal contact with the mandibular first, second, third, and fourth premolars. The large medial cusp of the mandibular first molar (the carnassial tooth) occludes just medial to the maxillary first molar (Fig. 55-6,C). The caudal cusp of the mandibular first molar occludes in the central fossa of the maxillary first molar, and the caudal cusps of the mandibular second molar occludes with the central fossa of the maxillary second molar.

Variations of the scissor bite are often seen in the incisor-canine area and also occur in the premolar-molar areas, but they are less obvious there. Some of the variations are due to the eruptive pattern of the teeth, while others are secondary to alterations in jaw size. When the mandibular incisors are caudal to the maxillary incisors, so that they do not occlude with one another, the occlusion is termed retrognathic ("overshot"). When the incisal edge of the mandibular incisor is even with or rostral to the maxillary incisors, the occlusion is said to be prognathic ("undershot"). Short-faced (brachycephalic) breeds are prognathic; in these animals the maxilla is considerably shorter than the mandible, and as a result, crowding of the teeth is common. Collies and similar long-nosed dogs are retrognathic.

In the cat, the maxillary incisors slightly overlap the mandibular incisors. The mandibular canine occludes rostral to the maxillary canine, there is a large diastema between the canine and premolar teeth, and the first premolar teeth do not occlude. Shearing action occurs between the mandibular molar and the maxillary third premolar carnassial teeth.

Breeds in which a short face is desirable in the cat (such as Persian) may predispose to an undershot incisor tooth relationship.

Temporomandibular Joint. The mandible is a movable, suspended, bony component that articulates with the skull at the temporomandibular joint (TMJ). The right and left condyles of the mandible articulate with the temporal bone in the glenoid fossa. Interposed between the fossa and the condyles is the cartilaginous meniscus. The jaws are closed by the masticatory muscles (masseter, temporal, and lateral and medial pterygoid), innervated by the mandibular branch of the trigeminal nerve (C.N. V),

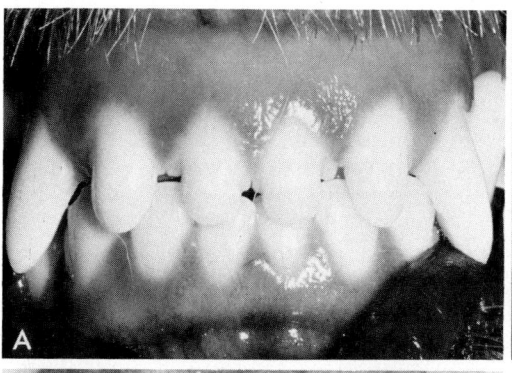
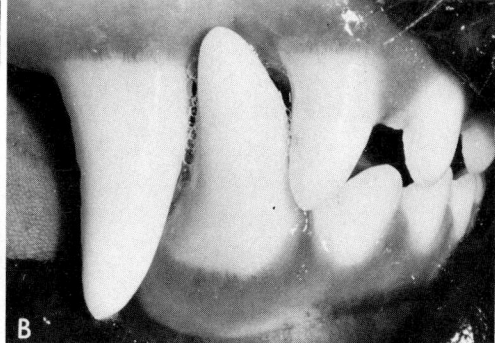
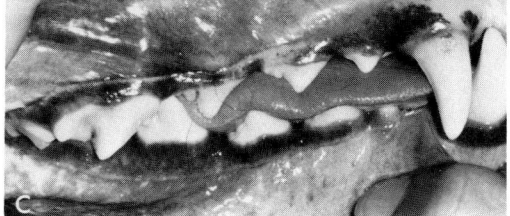

Figure 55–6. Normal occlusion in the dog. *A*, Incisor view. *B*, Canine — lateral incisor relationship. *C*, Canine — carnassial relationship.

and opened by the digastricus muscle (facial [C.N. VII] and trigeminal [C.N. V] nerves). The limits of TMJ movement are controlled by ligaments. Omnivorous animals classically have a high condyle, which permits anterior, posterior, and lateral movement. In the carnivorous dog and cat, which have shorter condyles with only limited lateral movement, the TMJ is limited largely to hingelike movement. The condyle is cylindrical and rotates in a transversely extended glenoid cavity. The skulls of both dogs and cats show a well-developed sagittal crest and flared zygomatic arches, indicative of powerful jaw muscles. The mass of these muscles coupled with the low position of the condyle reduces the frequency of dislocation of this joint in dogs and cats.

Oropharynx

The limits of the oropharynx are poorly defined in the dog because of the length and mobility of the soft palate and the absence of well-defined arches or pillars seen in other animals. The palatine tonsils are paired lymph nodes lying on the lateral wall of the oropharynx within crypts formed by folds of the pharyngeal wall (Fig. 55–7). They are elliptical in the dog, shorter and

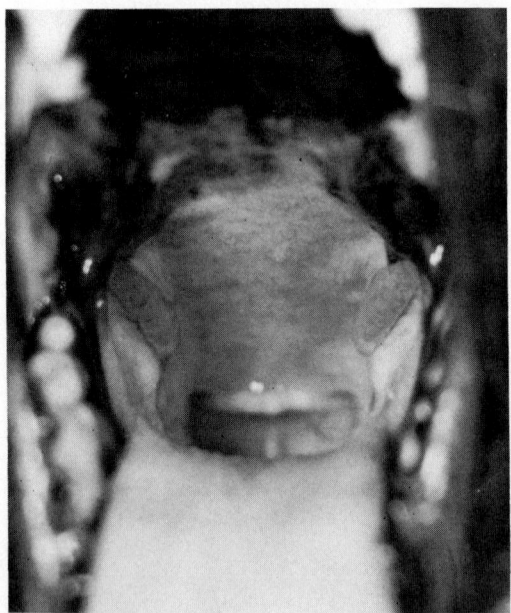

Figure 55–7. Pharynx of a normal dog. The tonsils are visible on the dorsolateral aspects of the oropharynx.

fatter in the cat. The tonsils of the dog are normally visible and in young dogs may stand out of their crypts. The tonsils of the cat are usually covered by the folds of epithelium forming the walls of the crypt.

Swallowing is a complex reflex action coordinating many muscles. The tongue is pulled caudally and dorsally, forcing the food or liquid bolus into the pharynx. The nasopharynx is constricted by the contraction of the muscles of the soft palate and the walls and roof of the nasopharynx. The epiglottis is moved caudally while the glottis is restricted by adduction of the arytenoid cartilages and vocal cords. The muscles of the pharyngeal wall contract and the cricopharyngeal muscle relaxes, allowing the bolus to be pushed into the esophagus. The glossopharyngeal, vagus, and hypoglossal nerves are the main motor nerves involved in swallowing.

HISTORY AND METHODS OF EXAMINATION

Many factors influence the oral cavity and must be considered when evaluating signs of disease; these include high temperature, moisture, mechanical irritation, and normal oral bacterial population. The most common clinical signs of oropharyngeal disease are inappetence, halitosis, pawing at the mouth, excessive salivation, and retching. Excessive salivation, initially seromucous in consistency, often progresses to ropey, tenacious saliva, becoming blood-streaked if ulceration develops. Some animals may look at or pick up food, but they either do not swallow or have difficulty in swallowing. A slowly enlarging mass may be the only finding in more chronic diseases.

Systemic diseases may cause clinical signs related primarily to the oropharynx; therefore, a careful complete physical examination is essential in all animals with oropharyngeal disease.

Physical Examination. In a cooperative animal most of the oropharynx can be readily inspected or palpated. Examination of the oropharynx should be conducted in a consistent, systematic manner. Inspection and palpation should include the gingiva, teeth, tongue, lingual frenulum and floor of the mouth, the entire buccal surface, and the hard and soft palate. The normal oral mucosa may be pink or partially pigmented

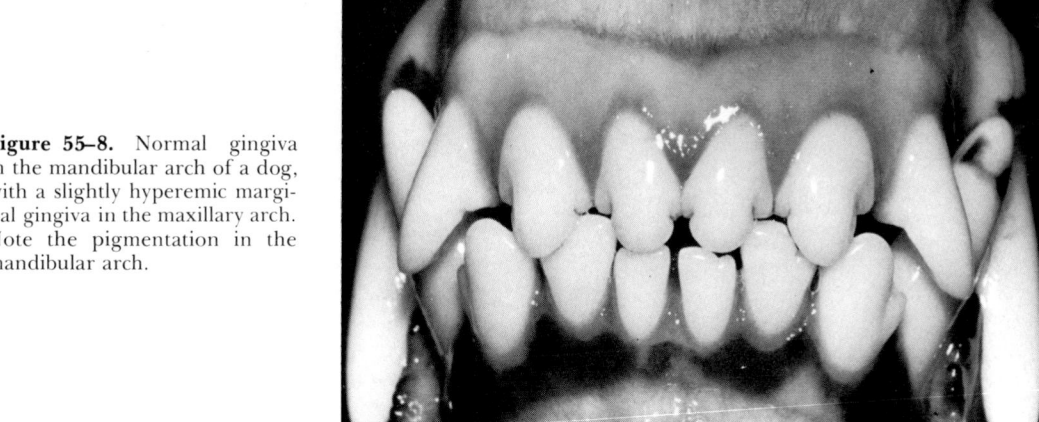

Figure 55–8. Normal gingiva in the mandibular arch of a dog, with a slightly hyperemic marginal gingiva in the maxillary arch. Note the pigmentation in the mandibular arch.

(especially in dark-colored breeds) and appears smooth and glistening, with little or no accumulation of secretions (Fig. 55–8). It is pliable when touched, and refill time is quick with no permanent blanching or hyperemia. Since response to touch varies with the animal's temperament, increased sensitivity is difficult to evaluate; however, a painful reaction should be obvious. It is preferable to examine the oral cavity while the animal is conscious to evaluate the function of the pertinent cranial nerves. Normally an animal will retch when the caudal pharynx is stimulated. Decreased sensitivity may be a manifestation of glossopharyngeal nerve dysfunction. In an uncooperative patient, observation of feeding, drinking, licking, and yawning must be supplemented by direct examination under anesthesia. A detailed dental examination requires a very cooperative patient or sedation. A dental explorer is used to examine crevices or other irregularities on the tooth surface for areas of softness: the use of the periodontal probe is described in the section on periodontal disease.

The breath of the normal dog and cat is not usually unpleasant; in the young puppy or kitten it has a characteristic milky smell. Alterations in the odor of the breath may indicate disease. In the ketoacidosis of severe diabetes and ethylene glycol poisoning, the breath may have a sweet, fruity smell. Foul-smelling breath may be caused by local disease (periodontal disease or stomatitis), or systemic disease (uremia, necrotic respiratory disease, or gastrointestinal disease). Food substances such as garlic cause halitosis. Patterns of dysphagia reported by the owner can be observed by offering the

animal a small amount of highly palatable food.

Biopsy. Biopsy of oropharyngeal masses is usually a simple, quick procedure, and histopathological examination can provide important information for treatment and prognosis. Cytologic examination of oral mucosal lesions is useful. Palpation of the cervical area, particularly lymph nodes, should be a routine part of the examination of the oropharynx.

A wide variety of bacteria as well as some fungal elements can be cultured from the oral cavity of a normal dog (Snow et al., 1969). *Pasteurella multocida* is present in the gingival area of 55 per cent of dogs and 80 per cent of cats; the strains isolated were generally sensitive to chloramphenicol and tetracycline, should treatment of an infected bite wound be necessary (Arnbjerg, 1978). Bacterial or fungal smears or cultures are thus of limited value unless the specimen is taken from an area of obvious disease.

Radiographic Examination. Lateral, ventrodorsal, and occlusal radiographs are useful to determine the presence of foreign bodies, and to investigate the extent of masses in the head and neck, particularly those involving the jaws. Definitive information on the nature and location of swallowing abnormalities can be obtained from fluoroscopic visualization of a barium swallow examination (Suter and Watrous, 1980).

Occlusal or oblique projection radiographs are particularly useful for examining dental structures. Dental pulp is considerably more radiolucent than dentin, which is less dense than the highly mineralized enamel covering the crown (Fig. 55–9). The cementum covering the root is not suffi-

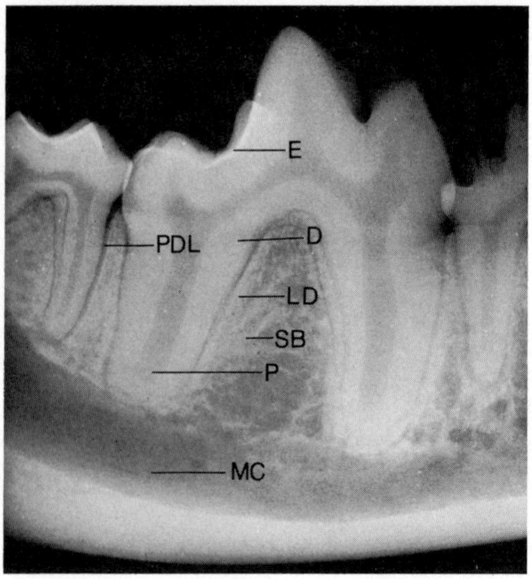

Figure 55–9. Radiograph of a normal tooth and mandible in a dog. D, dentin; E, enamel; LD, lamina dura; MC, mandibular canal; P, pulp; PDL, periodontal ligament; SB, supporting bone.

ciently different in density from the dentin to be differentiated radiographically. The sockets of the individual teeth are lined by the cortical alveolar bone (lamina dura), which is distinctly more radiopaque than the surrounding cancellous bone. Between the lamina dura and the root of the tooth is a radiolucent space approximately 0.1 to 0.2 mm wide, containing the periodontal ligament. Between the teeth is a mass of cancellous supporting bone. The alveolar crest (the most coronal aspect of the supporting bone) is cortical and appears as a radiopaque line which is perpendicular to the roots of the teeth and is confluent with the lamina dura.

Occasionally the roots of the teeth may be superimposed on the radiolucent mandibular canal. In the mandibular first and third premolar areas, the mental foramina can be seen; they may be confused with a periapical radiolucency but can be differentiated on an oblique projection radiograph. In radiographs of the maxillary arch, the nasal cavity and maxillary sinus recess can be seen in close proximity to the roots of the maxillary teeth. In young animals, the pulp cavity and apical foramina are large; as the animal matures these structures decrease in relative size. An excellent review of radiographic technique and interpretation of dental structures in the dog is available (Zontine, 1974).

DISEASES AFFECTING TOOTH STRUCTURE

CONGENITAL ANOMALIES

Anodontia

Anodontia is the congenital absence of teeth, which is common in dogs and may be inherited (Arnall, 1961). The most common area for anodontia in dogs is the premolar region. Incisors are commonly absent in the cat (Kratochvil, 1971). Complete anodontia occurs very occasionally in the dog and cat. Acquired tooth loss may be confused with anodontia and is much more common, particularly in older dogs. A tooth may occasionally be buried in the gingiva, mimicking anodontia. Anodontia and acquired tooth loss do not require treatment other than providing the animals' food in a form that can be prehended and swallowed.

Retained Deciduous Teeth

If the permanent tooth bud does not develop under the deciduous tooth, complete resorption of the roots will not occur and the deciduous tooth can be retained for the life of the animal. Retained deciduous teeth in the dog are most often seen with normal development of the permanent teeth. They occur most frequently in toy breeds and may cause displacement of the permanent teeth. Incisor and canine teeth are most commonly affected (Fig. 55–10,*A*). The retained deciduous tooth is usually rostral (incisor) or lateral (canine) to the erupting permanent tooth; it is narrower and has a sharper point. Extraction should be performed immediately if there is abnormal positioning of the permanent tooth or soft tissue damage resulting from impingement of the retained tooth (Fig. 55–10,*B*). The condition is seen occasionally in the cat.

Supernumerary Teeth

Additional permanent teeth may erupt into occlusion (Cuvier, 1871) and may result in crowding and rotation of teeth in the dog. This condition is common in the dog, particularly in spaniels, hounds, and greyhounds; the teeth most often involved are the premolars (Coyler, 1936). The distance between the teeth may allow the presence of supernumerary teeth without secondary

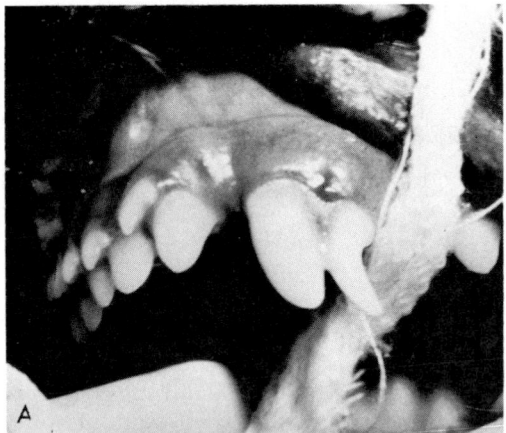

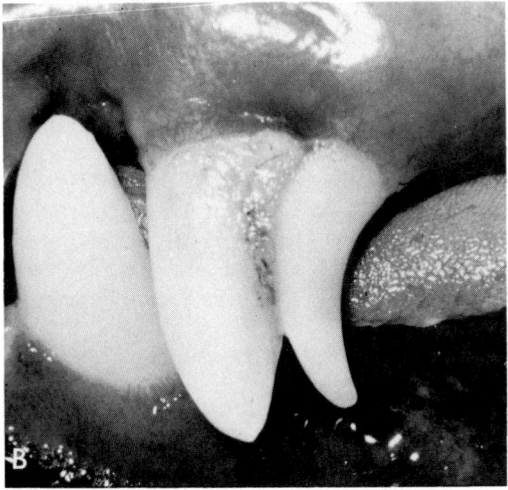

Figure 55–10. *A*, Retained incisor and canine teeth in the maxilla of a dog. *B*, Retained maxillary deciduous canine with accumulation of plaque and resultant soft tissue inflammation.

disease. The extra teeth should be extracted if there is crowding and periodontal health is jeopardized. Supernumerary teeth are also occasionally seen in the cat. Bizarre odontomas, with large numbers of formed

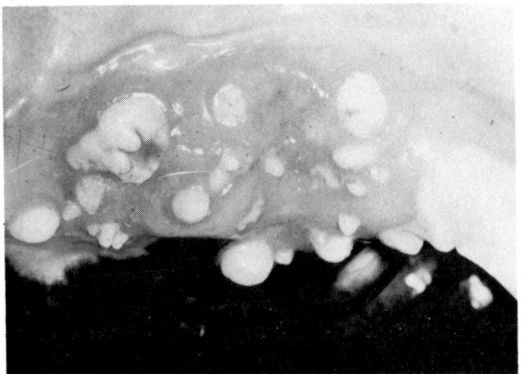

Figure 55–11. Multiple supernumary teeth arising from a complex odontoma in the maxilla of a dog.

or partly formed teeth (Fig. 55–11), are very rare; they may cause externally obvious distortion of the jaw.

Impaction

Teeth that do not erupt out of the alveolar bone or the soft tissue are considered impacted. If root formation is still progressing, uncovering these teeth surgically may allow them to erupt correctly, although this situation is rarely recognized in the dog or cat. If root formation is complete, no treatment is necessary. Extraction should be performed if partial impaction exists, so as to minimize the likelihood of periodontal abscess.

Abnormalities in the Shape of Teeth

Fusion of roots and abnormal crown shapes occur occasionally but are usually of no clinical significance. Dens in dente is a rare anomaly caused by invagination of the enamel organ into the dental papilla during tooth formation, forming a tooth within a tooth. There is communication between the oral environment and the enamel-lined cavity, visible directly or on radiographs as an irregular superimposed enamel density. If detected early, a restoration can be sealed into the opening so that infection will not enter the pulp cavity.

ACQUIRED DENTAL DISEASE

Enamel Hypoplasia

Enamel hypoplasia occurs as a result of disruption during enamel formation in utero or shortly after birth, usually caused by canine distemper infection (Dubielzig, 1979). The lesions appear as white opaque areas or brown-stained irregularities or depressions in the enamel of the crown (Fig. 55–12; see also Fig. 55–23,*A*). In those rare instances in which the enamel becomes soft owing to caries, it should be restored before pulpal disease occurs. Enamel hypoplasia is an acquired disease; as such, it is ethical to correct the esthetic abnormality by resin restoration in show animals (see Restorative Dentistry).

Tetracycline Staining

If tetracycline is administered during tooth development, the tetracycline bonds

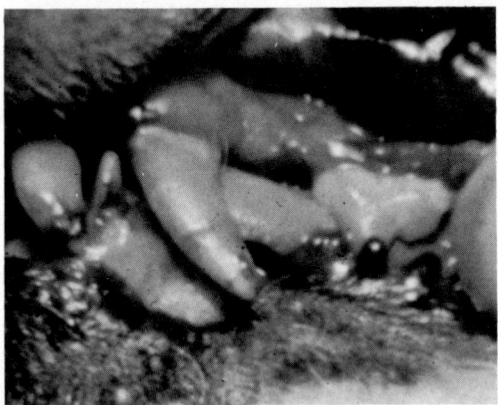

Figure 55–12. Enamel hypoplasia and tetracycline enamel staining in the permanent teeth of a dog.

with calcium in the dentin and enamel, creating a permanent discoloration of the teeth, which appear yellow-orange or brown (Fig. 55–12) (Bennett and Law, 1965). Tetracycline should not be administered before dogs and cats are five months old or to pregnant females, as maternal transfer has been demonstrated. There is no satisfactory bleaching technique available.

Dental Caries

Caries is the destruction of tooth structure caused by carbohydrate-fermenting bacteria, producing acids that attack the surfaces they contact. Caries, which is always initiated from the external environment, can be observed in the enamel, or if periodontal disease has caused recession, on an exposed root in the cementum (Fig. 55–13).

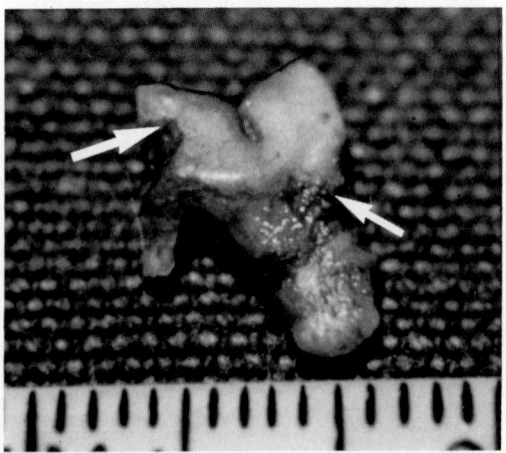

Figure 55–13. Caries lesions (arrows) at the cementoenamel junction of a tooth in a cat with periodontal disease.

Dental caries in dogs and cats is uncommon (Schneck, 1967), although not all surveys agree with this conclusion. The incidence is low because the diet is usually low in fermentable carbohydrates; the structure of the teeth is such that they are self-cleaning; the fissures of the crowns are often exposed to an abrasive diet, which keeps them clean; there are no true pits that permit retention of food and bacteria except in the maxillary molar teeth, which are the teeth most often carious; the interproximal spaces between teeth are not food traps, as is seen in species with higher caries indices; and the composition of saliva in dogs is not conducive to developing a cariogenic flora. The pH of saliva is alkaline, which tends to neutralize oral acids (Gardner et al., 1962).

Lewis (1965) attempted to develop caries in the dog. He drilled holes in the enamel surface, placed the animals on high sucrose diets, removed the major salivary glands, and injected lactobacilli into the oral cavity. This failed to produce carious lesions, however.

When seen in dogs and cats, caries occurs where plaque accumulates, usually in animals that are fed soft food diets that are high in fermentable carbohydrate concentration. Plaque accumulates in the gingival sulcus of animals with periodontal disease, allowing root caries to penetrate through the cementum into dentin, particularly in cats (Fig. 55–13). Halitosis, difficulty in eating, refusal of hard food, holding the head to one side, and teeth chattering are clinical signs associated with dental caries.

Careful clinical observation using a dental explorer can detect caries in its early stages. The lesion is usually dark-brown and soft, which differentiates it from exposed stained dentin. Enamel and dentin cannot repair themselves; the diseased tissue must be removed and restored with an appropriate filling material. The deeper caries extends into the dentin, the greater the inflammation in the dental pulp. Repair by the pulp can occur; however, persistent, deeper caries can directly infect the pulp, leading to necrosis and eventual abscess or cyst formation. At this point, endodontic therapy or extraction is indicated.

Trauma

Fracture. Dogs and cats are both prone to fracture of the teeth. Fractures were

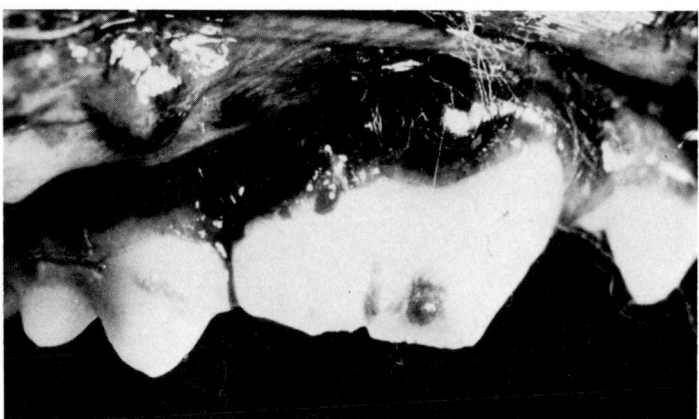

Figure 55–14. Fresh fracture of a maxillary carnassial tooth with pulp exposure.

observed in 27.4 per cent of dogs examined by Golden et al. (1981); the incisor teeth were most frequently involved, although canine or carnassial (Fig. 55–14 and 55–15) tooth fractures may be more noticeable by the owner. The causes are probably external trauma or activities such as stone chewing or catching. Enamel is a crystalline structure and is easily cleaved if struck. If the fracture is only of the enamel layer, no treatment is necessary. If the fracture extends into the dentin, inflammation occurs in the pulp and odontoblasts synthesize reparative dentin, insulating the pulp. If a fracture extends into the dental pulp, endodontic treatment or extraction is indicated to prevent endodontic disease and alveolar bone abscessation.

Avulsion. Partial or total avulsion of a tooth from the jaw results in disruption of the periodontal ligament and pulp tissue (Fig. 55–16). If the owner desires it for esthetic reasons, the tooth should be repositioned as quickly as possible to attempt to preserve the vitality of the periodontal ligament. If the tooth is firm after being replanted, no splint is necessary; an acid-etch composite splint is a useful technique for splinting loose teeth (see Restorative Dentistry). In those areas where vitality of the periodontal ligament is lost, ankylosis of the bone to the cementum may occur. The usual sequela of ankylosis is external resorption by osteoclasts, which invade the root surface from the alveolar bone.

If avulsion occurs in a tooth with an incompletely formed apical foramen, regeneration of pulpal tissue may occur; this can be monitored through radiographic examination. If avulsion occurs in a tooth with a mature root apex, endodontic therapy should be performed before repositioning the tooth.

Internal and External Resorption. Either of these two phenomena may occur if the pulp is traumatized and osteoclastic cells destroy the hard tooth structure. Internal resorption occurs at the expense of dentin inside the tooth; it can be stopped by removing the pulp tissue and performing endodontic therapy. External resorption occurs by action of osteoclasts in the alveolar bone. It can sometimes be stopped by endodontic therapy, but the prognosis is not as predictable because the aveolar bone may still supply osteoclasts. Loss of the tooth will eventually occur if external resorption continues. Calcium hydroxide is used in endodontic therapy to change the environmental pH and thus eliminate osteoclasts, with some success in preventing resorption.

Attrition. Attrition or occlusal wear is caused by feeding a coarse diet, or activities such as catching or carrying a stone or stick (Figs. 55–17 and 55–18). Wearing of

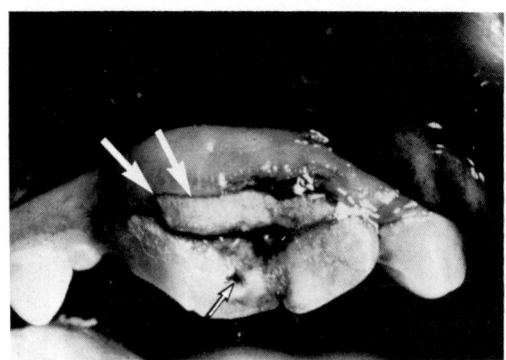

Figure 55–15. Fracture of a maxillary carnassial tooth, with exposure of the pulp cavity (single arrow) and a separate slab fracture of enamel (double arrow).

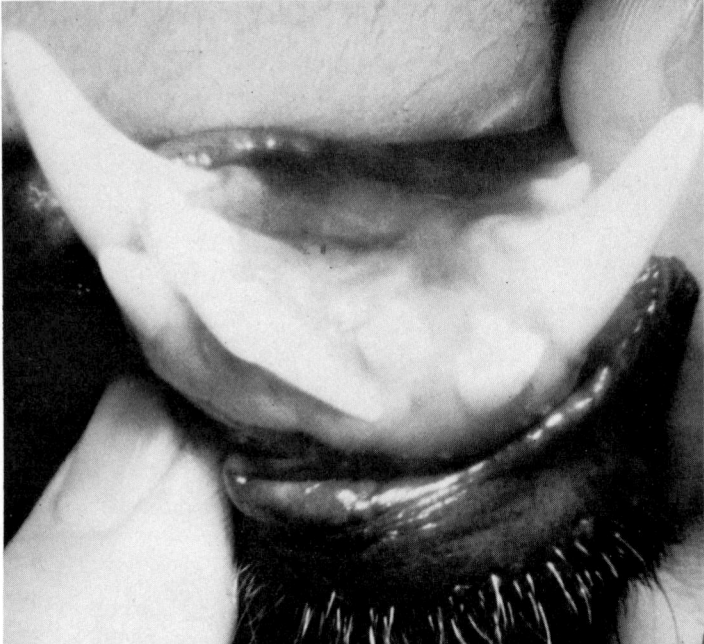

Figure 55–16. Effects of trauma to the mandible. Two incisor teeth are fractured, one is avulsed with the entire root exposed, and one is missing.

the incisal edges or biting surfaces of the teeth is physiologic to a certain point. It is commonly seen in the incisor teeth of dogs and cats (Golden et al., 1981). If the wear extends only into the dentin, no treatment is necessary. Wear occurs slowly enough to allow the pulp to establish reparative dentin, which is seen as a brown spot that does not accept the dental exploratory probe. If the tooth structure is worn away and vital pulp is exposed or if the pulp dies and abscess formation occurs (Fig. 55–19), extraction or endodontic therapy is indicated. Dogs that are kept in metal cages often chew on the bars; the external surface of the incisors or

canines of these dogs are often stained with metal, usually aluminum.

Carnassial Abscess (Malar Abscess, Facial Sinus)

Carnassial abscess is a soft fluctuant swelling or draining sinus on the side of the face just below the medial canthus of the eye. The fistula occasionally drains into the oral cavity. It is a common condition in middle-aged and old dogs, and is also seen in the cat. Clinical signs are usually confined to the swelling or draining fistula. The discharge is often not purulent. Carnassial abscess is also

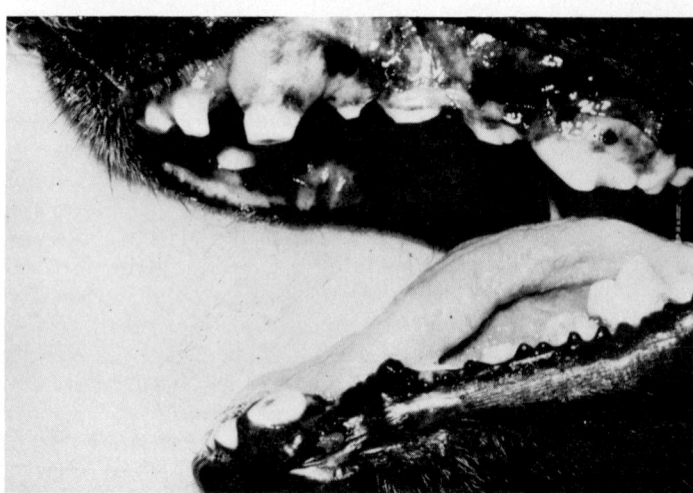

Figure 55–17. Severe attrition of the maxillary and mandibular incisor, canine, and premolar teeth in a dog. Brown stained reparative dentin is visible in both canine teeth.

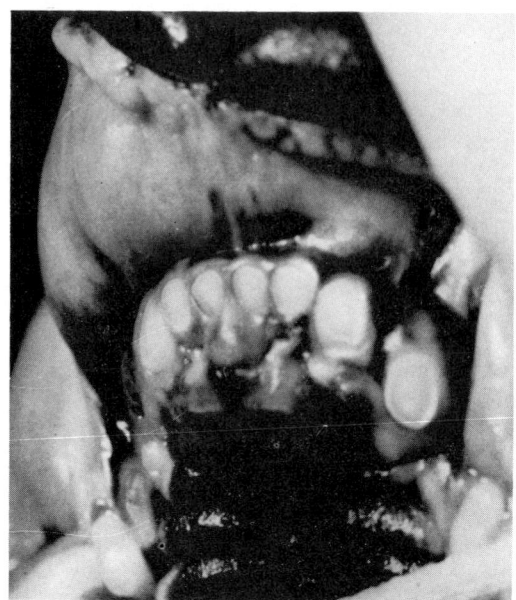

Figure 55–18. Extreme attrition of the maxillary incisor teeth in a dog caused by constant gnawing at hard surfaces.

seen, although much less frequently, in the mandible. The fistula drains onto the skin or into the oral cavity ventral to the lower carnassial tooth (Holmberg, 1979).

The swelling or fistula is caused by necrosis of the alveolar bone over one of the roots of the upper carnassial (fourth premolar)

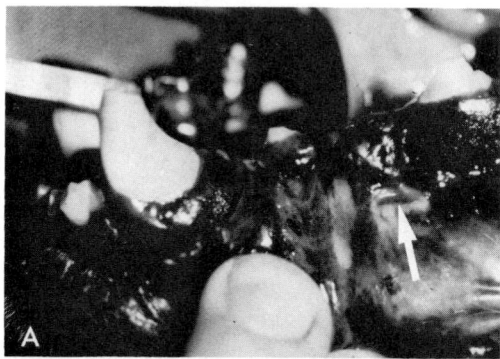
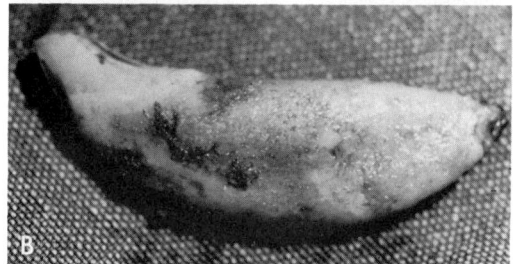

Figure 55–19. *A*, Fistula (arrow) from the root of a mandibular canine tooth with attritional exposure of the pulp cavity. *B*, Extracted canine tooth showing the size of the root relative to the crown.

tooth or lower carnassial (first molar) tooth. Intermittent concussion from chewing on sticks or bones, and periodontal disease are probably contributing factors; however, the carnassial tooth and surrounding gingiva may appear normal. Radiographs usually show a radiolucent area at the root, indicating a periodontal abscess or apical cyst (Fig. 55–20).

Treatment consists of either extraction of the carnassial tooth and establishment of drainage from the external lesion to the tooth socket, or endodontic treatment of the involved root. Recovery is usually uneventful, but occasionally complications occur owing to local extension of the inflammatory process, such as parotid duct injury, chronic maxillary osteomyelitis, or sinusitis.

Endodontic Disease

Endodontic disease results from crown fracture with pulpal exposure, carious erosion, or extension from periodontal disease, allowing infection to enter the pulp cavity. Pulpal exposure was seen in one or more teeth in ten per cent of dogs examined by Golden et al. (1981). With chronic diseases such as caries or periodontal disease, which stimulate the odontoblastic processes, the odontoblasts may have time to synthesize reparative dentin. When the pulp is exposed, an inflammatory process occurs, which, because the pulp is contained within a noncompliant tooth structure, usually causes pulpal necrosis. Bacteria remain and their toxins spread through the apical foramina. An inflammatory response occurs around the apex of the tooth in an attempt to localize the spread of the infections.

An acute periapical abscess is associated with liquefaction necrosis and severe pain. The polymorphonuclear leukocytes release lysosomal enzymes, pus is formed quickly, and pressure builds. The purulent debris must seek release through either the root canal or fistula; otherwise, it will create local swelling as pus enters other facial planes. If a fistula forms or drainage occurs through the root canal, a chronic state is attained. Endodontic therapy or extraction of the tooth will reverse this process.

An acute abscess may enter a quiescent stage, referred to as a chronic abscess or granuloma, which is recognized by tenderness or reluctance to eat, or may be asymptomatic. Dental radiographs demonstrate

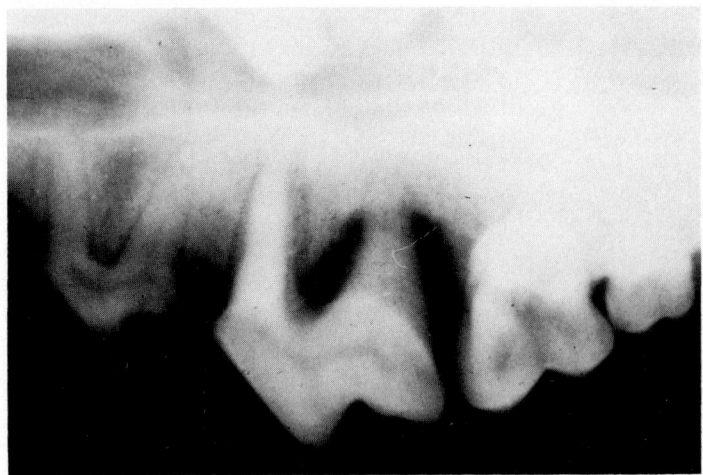

Figure 55–20. Radiograph showing extensive apical bone loss around the roots of a maxillary carnassial tooth in a dog with a carnassial abscess.

the encapsulated area of periapical radiolucency. Histologically, round cell infiltration can be observed with connective tissue encapsulation of the inflamed area. Extraction or endodontic therapy is the treatment of choice. If endodontic therapy is started, a change in the equilibrium between tissue resistance and infection may cause a painful acute abscess, which can usually be controlled by treatment with antibiotics.

An apical cyst may also form (Fig. 55–21). The epithelial cell rests of Malassez are activated to line the fluid-filled cavity in the bone. Extraction or endodontic therapy is the treatment of choice. If endodontic treatment cannot create an environment for the body to heal, surgical removal of the cyst is necessary.

Endodontic disease can lead to cellulitis, recognized by clinical signs of fever, malaise, and pain and edema in surrounding soft tissues. Systemic antibiotics (such as ampicillin, 20 mg/kg orally four times per day) should be started immediately, with drainage of the area of infection locally if practical.

Diagnosis of an inflamed or necrotic pulp is sometimes difficult. Dogs and cats appear to have a high pain threshold; they will often be unresponsive to situations that cause obvious pain in humans. They may first have pain with an exposed pulp, but this disappears when the pulp becomes necrotic. Classic signs of pulpal problems can be observed clinically if the nerve has just been exposed, or radiographically if the inflammation has reached the periapical area and developed into an abscess or cyst. The animal may become lethargic, favor one side of its mouth, stop eating, or stop performing normally. The tooth may appear discolored, loose, chipped, or cracked.

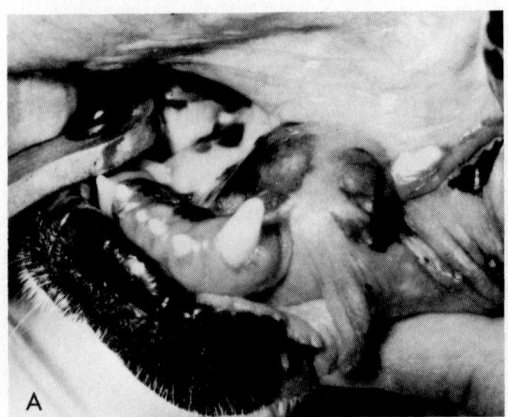
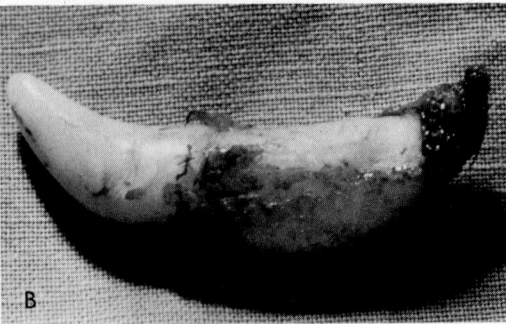

Figure 55–21. *A*, Cyst at the apex of a mandibular canine. The etiology is unknown, but the condition is most likely due to trauma and subsequent pulp death. *B*, The extracted canine with part of the cyst still attached to the root apex.

If the dentin is exposed, one should look for exposure of the root canal, which appears as a dark spot or area of hemorrhage in the center of the tooth. A fistula may be present, extending to the skin or oral mucosal surface. If no discoloration or void in the enamel is noted and radiographic observation demonstrates a radiolucent area, differential diagnosis should include superimposition of a normal anatomic landmark.

Endodontic Therapy. Endodontic therapy is indicated as an alternative to extraction where disease has penetrated the dental pulp cavity and is causing pain, fistulization, or spreading infection; or it may be used to prevent endodontic disease when the pulp cavity has been penetrated by trauma or external disease. The object is to remove the source of infection and seal off the root canal so that there is no tract from the oral environment to the bone. Infection already present in the alveolar bone is dealt with by normal body defense mechanisms.

A pulpotomy can be performed if treatment occurs immediately after traumatic exposure of the pulp. The dental pulp is removed in the coronal portion of the tooth, and a medicated dressing is placed over the tissue remaining in the root canal. Although it is not a predictable procedure (Seltzer and Bender, 1958), it is quick and can be performed under short-acting anesthesia or sedation. Calcium hydroxide is the material of choice to place over the remaining vital pulp tissue, and a sedative zinc oxide and eugenol dental cement is placed over the calcium hydroxide, followed by a permanent filling.

If a simple medicated dressing can be placed, or if replantation of an avulsed tooth can be done quickly, the tooth may be easily saved. More elaborate endodontic procedures must be carefully considered as an alternative to extraction for more chronic or severe disease, since dogs and cats can function well without their teeth. Probably the most common indication for endodontic therapy is fracture of the canine tooth in police or guard dogs. Maintaining function of these expensive dogs often requires intact canine teeth. Endodontic therapy will allow the carnassial tooth to be saved in dogs with carnassial abscess. Other patients in which extraction of teeth with acquired lesions may be contraindicated are show dogs and dogs whose owners desire to maintain their animals' dentition for esthetic reasons.

The techniques involved in performing endodontic therapy are adapted from those used for humans; general anesthesia is mandatory. The object is to cleanse the pulp cavity without irritation to the bone, using surgically clean technique to obtain an aseptic root canal (Ridgway and Zeilke, 1979) (Fig. 55–22).

Access to the root canal is made using a standard large dental round bur to create a hole through the crown. The access opening should approximate the diameter of the canal so that no overhanging margins of crown prevent instruments from reaching the canal walls. The single root of the canine tooth has the most direct and easiest access, although a large intact canine tooth may require an additional access cavity on the rostral surface of the lower part of the crown, because of the length and curve of the root canal. To gain access into the multi-rooted teeth, much of the crown must be destroyed because of the divergent roots, which limits the usefulness of endodontics for these teeth, although a successful technique has been described (Franceschini, 1974).

Careful cleansing of the root canal is performed with endodontic reamers (up to 40 mm for large canine teeth); copious irrigation, alternating solutions of sodium hypochlorite with hydrogen peroxide (which are effervescent), dissolve the proteinaceous material, decrease bacterial population, and help to eliminate much of the pulpal tissue. The canal is reamed and cleaned until the apical delta is reached, indicated by resistance to further reaming and confirmed by radiography. It is impossible to adequately clean the deltoid complex, which is left intact unless the root apex is radiolucent, in which case an apicoectomy is indicated. When clean dentin shavings are finally removed from the root canal, the canal is dried and is ready to be sealed. A hermetic seal is obtained by filling the canal with gutta percha points. The technique should be done in cooperation with an endodontist until some experience has been gained. If an abscess or cyst is suspected, antibiotics may be necessary. Silver amalgam is used to seal the access cavity against bacterial encroachment; a layer of composite polymers can be used to restore the external appearance, if necessary.

Blockage of the canal, severe curvatures, length of the root, and apical deltas are factors that may compromise complete cleansing of the root canal. Periapical surgery (apicoectomy) may be necessary if the root cannot be cleaned adequately via the crown, particularly if the pulpal tissue is necrotic. When performing an apicoectomy, the apices of roots of other teeth should be avoided. The alveolar bone over the length of the root can be easily seen. Most endodontic procedures in dogs are performed on canine teeth whose roots curve above the roots of the second premolar teeth.

The gingiva is reflected and the bone around the root apex is removed to reveal the apex of the root, which is removed with a dental handpiece. Only enough root must be removed so as to gain access to the canal. An amalgam restoration is then placed into the canal, effecting a seal against bacteria or their products from the root canal (Ross and Myers, 1970). Antibiotics are unnecessary following periapical surgery unless extensive soft tissue infection is present.

RESTORATIVE DENTISTRY

Restorative dentistry for veterinary patients has become a reality with the advent of composite polymers that bond to an etched enamel surface (Marvich, 1975; Bedford, 1977). The repair of minor fractures, abrasions, chipped enamel surfaces, and enamel hypoplasia can be accomplished with a minimal amount of equipment (Fig. 55–23). The composites can also be used to splint teeth that have been loosened as a

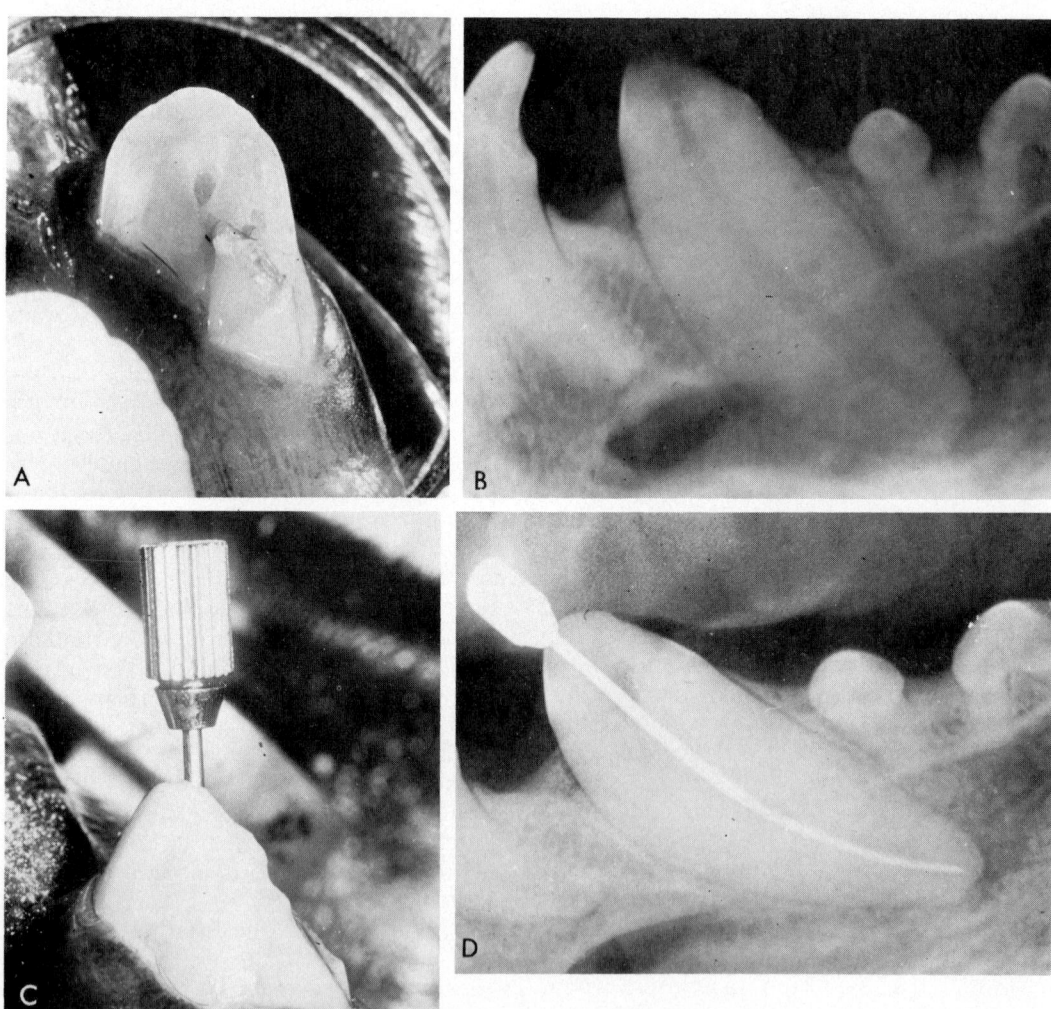

Figure 55–22. Endodontic treatment of a fractured mandibular canine tooth in a dog. *A*, Fractured tooth with an exposed pulp. *B*, Periapical radiograph — note the radiolucency at the tooth apex indicative of an abscess or granuloma. *C*, Endodontic reamer in place. *D*, Radiograph of the reamer to determine the tooth length.

Illustration continued on opposite page

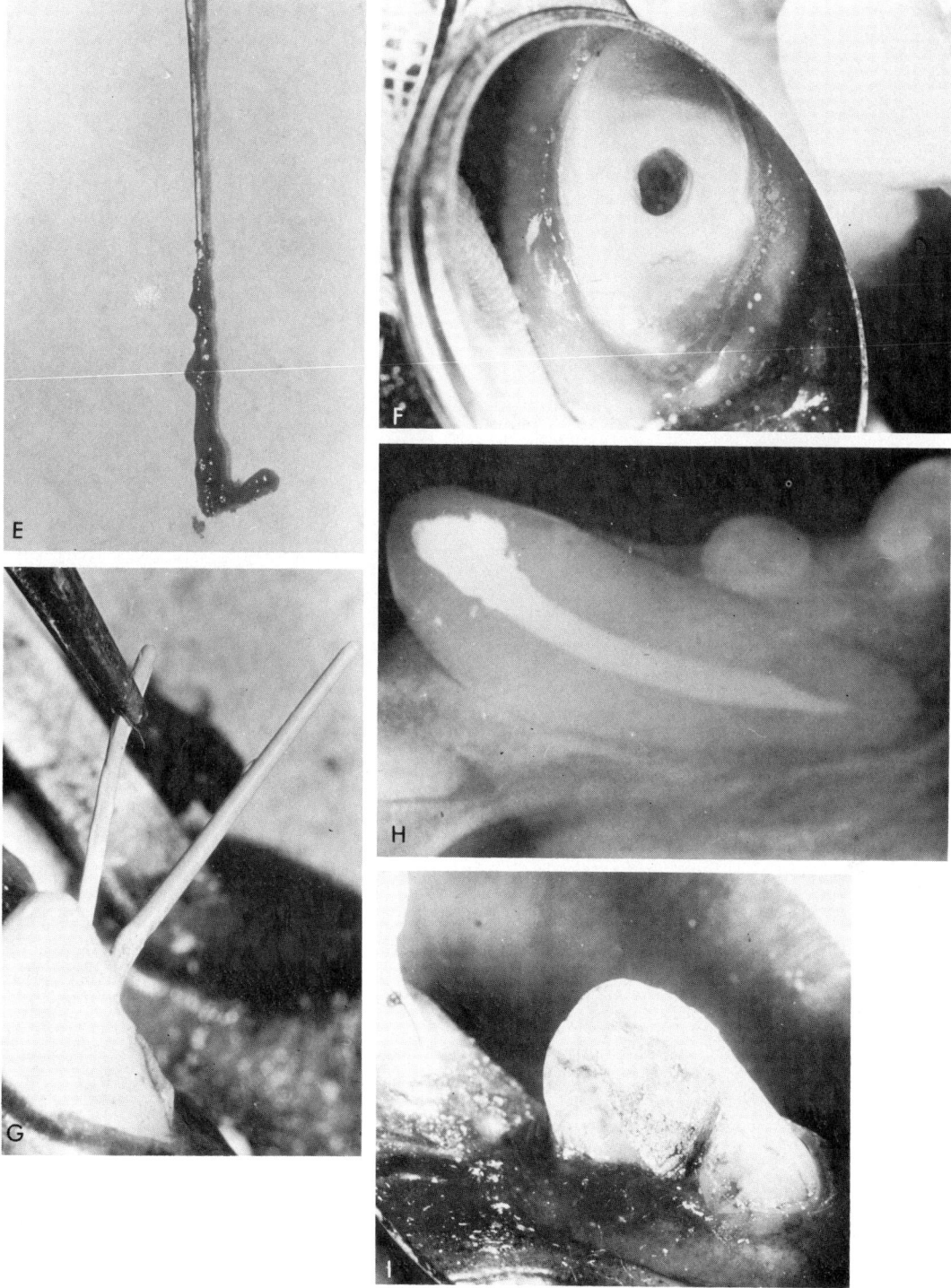

Figure 55–22 *Continued.* *E*, Pulpal tissue removed by the endodontic reamer. *F*, Instrumented canal ready to be filled. *G*, Gutta percha filling material. *H*, Radiograph of the filled root canal. *I*, Amalgam restoration of the pulp chamber.

result of trauma or periodontal disease; the loose teeth can be bonded together or to adjacent firm teeth to gain stability, particularly in the incisor region. The composites come in three basic forms: mixed pastes, mixed powder and liquid, and ultraviolet light–activated paste. The tooth to be restored is thoroughly cleaned and polished

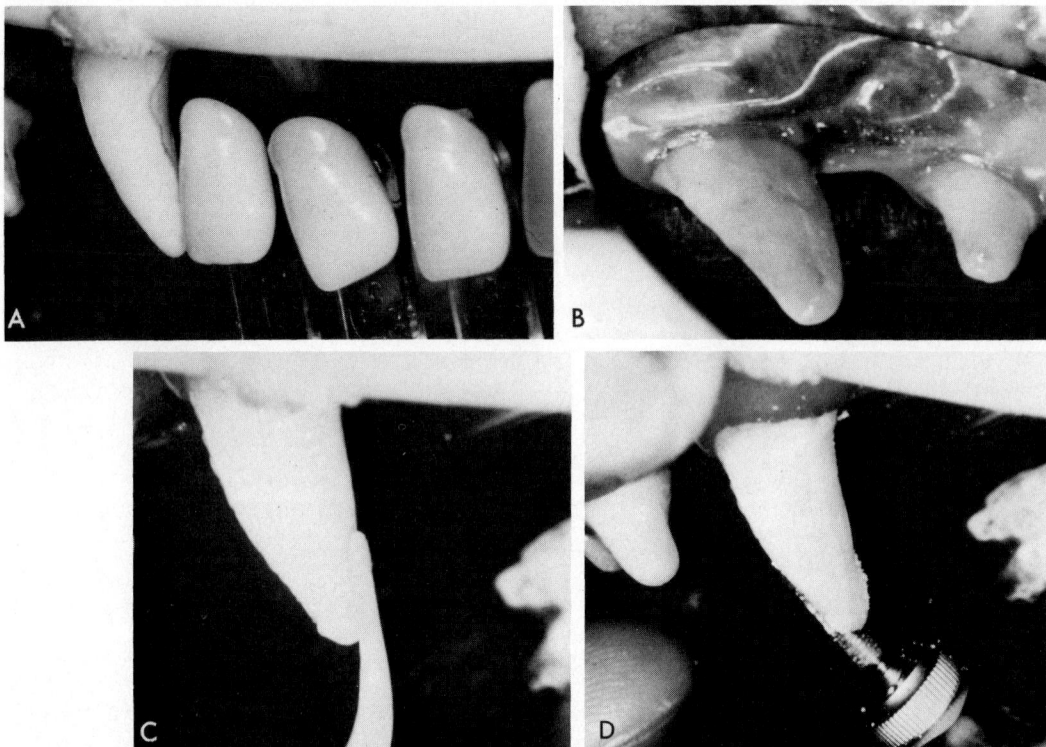

Figure 55–23. The restoration of a canine tooth with enamel hypoplasia using a composite restorative material. *A*, Shade selection. *B*, The hypoplastic area extends to the palatal aspect of the tooth. *C*, Application of the composite onto a clean acid-etched tooth surface. *D*, Finishing the restoration with a high-speed diamond tip.

with pumice, then etched with a solution of phosphoric acid for one to two minutes and washed with water. The tooth is then dried and the composite applied. The two-paste system and the powder-liquid system will cure within two to three minutes of being mixed. The light-activated paste does not cure until it is exposed to the ultraviolet light source, allowing the operator ample time to shape the restoration to the contours of the tooth. These materials can be used to restore the external appearance of a tooth that has undergone endodontic therapy in which a silver amalgam filling has been placed in the access cavity.

These materials come in a variety of shades. Although they are not recommended for use in areas that are subjected to occlusal stress, they perform well, especially if a broad base of enamel for bonding is available. The composites can also be reinforced with pins placed into the tooth. This technique requires a dental handpiece and appropriate drills (Peterson and Wightman, 1979).

When a tooth is severely fractured and its maintenance is important for either esthetic or functional purposes, the restoration of choice is a full crown, either cast gold or, if esthetics are a particular concern, porcelain veneer.

The restoration will require two procedures. Under general anesthesia, endodontic treatment can be performed if necessary, the tooth is prepared for the crown, an impression is taken, a shade selected, and a temporary crown fabricated. The temporary crown can be deleted if the tooth is nonvital. At a second procedure, under sedation, the finished crown is pinned and cemented in place. Large canine tooth restorations are subject to considerable force and may break subsequently; restoration with steel has been described.

Replacement of missing teeth is possible, although rarely indicated. In most cases some type of fixed restoration can be fabricated, although there are reports in the veterinary literature describing the successful use of removable partial dentures.

THE JAWS

The jaws are subject to conditions affecting bone in general, such as fractures resulting from trauma, neoplasms (although most neoplasms affecting the maxilla or mandible are soft tissue tumors invading bone), and disturbances in bone structure caused by nutritional deficiencies or metabolic disturbances. Bone weakness caused by renal secondary hyperparathyroidism is particularly evident in the maxilla and mandible, causing rubber jaw disease (see Hyperparathyroidism, Chapter 66).

Malocclusion

Normal occlusion was described earlier. Variations from the normal occlusal scheme for a particular dog or cat can be the result of a genetic defect or of various local factors. Local factors include deciduous teeth that have been retained, causing a displacement of the permanent teeth; malocclusion of the deciduous dentition that impedes the normal forward growth of the mandible; ectopic eruption of one or more of the permanent teeth; and trauma to the teeth or jaws during development. Malocclusion can also result from orthopaedic management of jaw fractures (Cechner, 1980). Correct characterization of jaw relationships requires observation of all the cuspal landmarks.

The correction of occlusal deformities to allow an animal to conform to breeding specifications for breeding or show purposes should only be performed if there is medical need for correction, or if one is convinced that the deformity is acquired. There is no satisfactory way of determining if a congenital defect is inherited in a partic- ular animal presented for correction. Radiographs may suggest the possibility of neonatal fracture.

Very few occlusal problems are detrimental to the well being of the animal. Although it is conceivable that severe crowding of the teeth can predispose to periodontal disease (Figs. 55–24, 55–25, 55–26), problems of this type can be managed initially by attempting to control plaque (see Periodontal Therapy). On occasion the position of a tooth may traumatize soft tissues in the opposite arch when the animal closes its mouth. Depending on the functional and esthetic significance of the tooth, it can be significantly reduced in size by grinding away tooth structure with a dental handpiece, it can be repositioned orthodontically, or it can be extracted.

Prevention of normal occlusion by impaction of a tooth in abnormal position against another tooth occurs in a wide variety of breeds of dogs. The teeth most frequently involved are the canine and lateral incisor teeth. Extraction or orthodontic therapy can be used to correct this condition. With the new dental materials that allow orthodontic brackets to bond directly to enamel surfaces, thus precluding the need for orthodontic bands, tooth movement is much more feasible in the small animal than it was five years ago. Within the framework of skeletal patterns there is almost no limit to what one can accomplish orthodontically. In general, movements that require a tooth to be tipped can be accomplished much more easily than movements that require a tooth to be moved

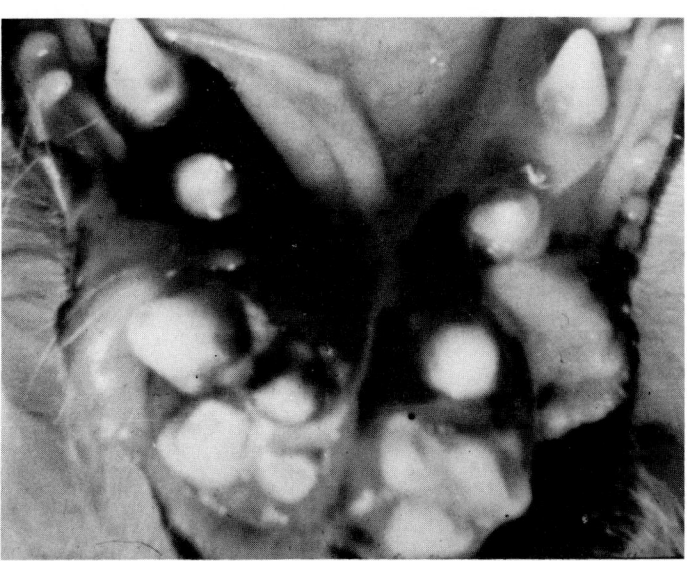

Figure 55–24. Crowding of the mandibular incisor teeth in a dog, contributing to an unhealthy periodontium.

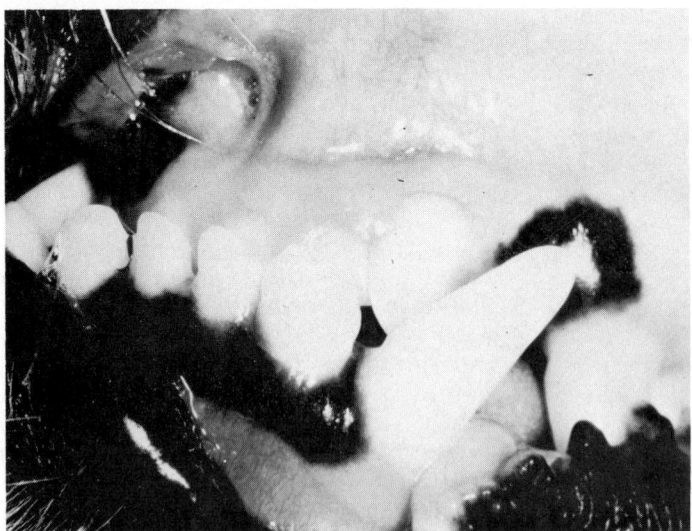

Figure 55–25. Prognathic (undershot) jaw relationship in a dog, causing impaction of the maxillary lateral incisor tooth against the mandibular canine tooth.

bodily. If orthodontics is attempted, it is imperative that the dentition be kept immaculately clean during therapy, since the combination of orthodontic pressures and periodontal inflammation can cause rapid periodontal breakdown (Graber, 1972).

Most occlusal therapy falls within the category of interceptive orthodontics: recognition and early management of retained deciduous teeth, malocclusions of the deciduous dentition that may preclude normal growth, and management of supernumerary teeth can prevent severe orthodontic problems. More severe lesions (Fig. 55–27) require orthopedic correction; appropriate techniques have been described (Rudy, 1975; Brass, 1976). Acrylic splints are particularly adaptable for repairing the mandible or maxilla (Latimer et al., 1977).

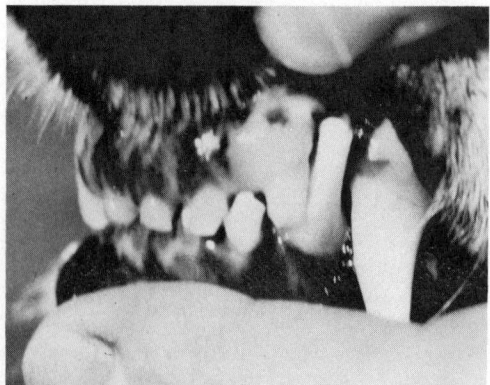

Figure 55–26. Malocclusion resulting in attrition of the maxillary lateral incisor and the mandibular canine teeth in a dog.

Mandibular Neuropraxia

Mandibular neuropraxia ("dropped jaw") is seen occasionally in the dog (Humphreys, 1974; Robins, 1976). It was first described, although incorrectly diagnosed, in 1824 by Cherry. These dogs present with the jaw hanging down symmetrically; the mouth can be closed easily by the owner or veterinarian but when released, the jaw drops to its former position. Tongue movement is normal, but because of the abnormal jaw position, swallowing is difficult. There is often a history of recent mechanical influences on the mouth, such as trauma or weight carrying. The condition is assumed to be due to abnormal stretching of the mandibular branch of the trigeminal nerve (C.N.V.), causing paralysis of the masticatory muscles. Full recovery occurs over a three-week period; the only treatment necessary is to place a loose bandage around the muzzle to support the jaw while allowing imbibition of food of a soupy consistency.

Temporomandibular Joint Abnormalities

Temporomandibular joint luxation due to trauma occurs infrequently in the dog. The animal has a dropped jaw that is painful on manipulation. The luxation is usually unilateral, causing asymmetry of position. An incorrect diagnosis of mandibular fracture may be made unless careful manipulation and radiographic examination are carried out. The luxation can usually be reduced under anesthesia by closing the jaws while placing a wooden rod across the

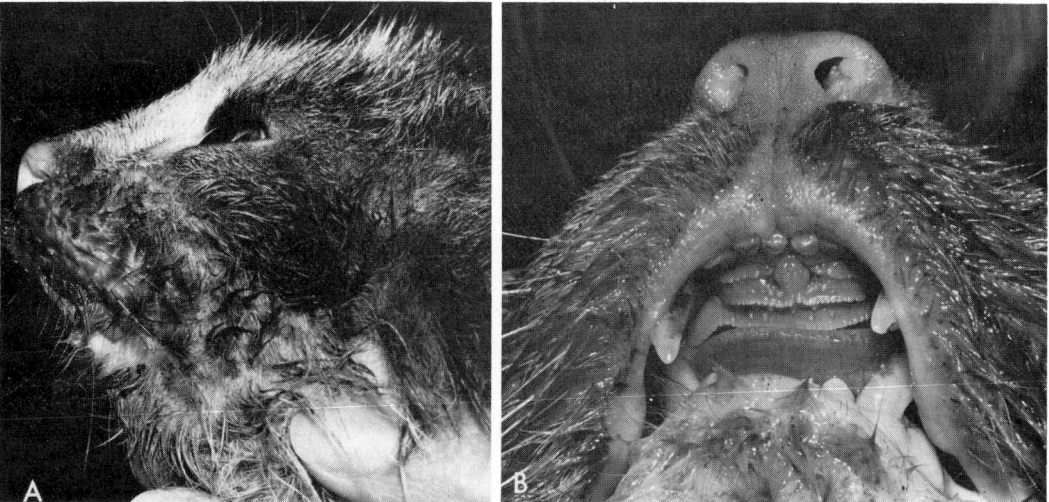

Figure 55–27. *A, B,* Cat with severe retrognathism causing constant drooling.

carnassial teeth (Knecht and Schiller, 1974).

Temporomandibular subluxation or dysplasia has been reported in young Irish setters and basset hounds, in which it has been observed in multiple members of a litter (Stewart et al., 1975; Robins and Grandage, 1977). When the mouth is opened fully, the coronoid process of the mandible on one side becomes locked lateral to the zygomatic arch. In some dogs, the locking condition corrects itself spontaneously. Treatment by resecting part of the ventral aspect of the zygomatic arch avoids further locking episodes. Mandibular condylectomy has been used as treatment for dogs with temporomandibular joint disease, with very good clinical results (Tomlinson, 1981).

Craniomandibular osteopathy (see Chapter 85) may become sufficiently severe as to prevent the jaws from opening normally. This condition, which classically occurs in young West Highland white terriers but is seen in other breeds also, is a proliferative disease of unknown cause affecting the bones of the base of the skull and mandible (Riser et al., 1967).

Temporomandibular joint disease is rare in the cat. Ticer and Spencer (1978) have described the radiographic findings in six cats with traumatic temporomandibular disease.

PERIODONTAL DISEASE

Periodontal disease is the general term used to denote diseases of the periodontium (gingiva, periodontal ligament, alveolar bone, and cemental surface of the tooth). It includes gingivitis (acute and chronic), periodontitis, and periodontal abscess.

There have been several studies that have examined the prevalence and severity of periodontal disease in the dog and cat (Rosenberg et al., 1966; Gad, 1968; Hull, 1974), and there is little doubt that the prevalence of periodontal disease approaches 95 per cent in animals over two years of age. Although in most cases the disease is confined to the soft tissues of the periodontium, loss of osseous support (periodontitis) is not uncommon. Periodontitis was found in 53 per cent of dogs and 14 per cent of cats examined by Golden et al. (1981). Hamp et al. (1975) found that 80 per cent of dogs showed periodontal bone loss. Certain breeds, such as poodles, had a higher incidence; others, such as German shepherd dogs, had a lower incidence.

The severity of periodontal disease correlates with the quantity of plaque and calculus present on the teeth as well as with the age of the animal (Golden et al., 1981). Plaque and calculus, however, have an independent effect on the severity of the disease (Gad, 1968). Calculus is not seen to any great extent in animals less than nine months of age. The initial deposits of calculus occur in the region of the parotid duct (the buccal surfaces of the maxillary molars) and on the lingual surfaces of the mandibular posterior teeth (Rosenberg et al., 1966).

A number of studies have shown a relationship between diet consistency and periodontal disease. For the most part these studies indicate that soft diets correlate positively with periodontal disease (Egelberg, 1965; Saxe et al., 1967; Golden et al., 1981).

GINGIVITIS

Clinical Manifestations. Gingivitis is manifested clinically by a change in the color of the marginal gingiva (when not masked by pigmentation). This reddening is usually accompanied by a blunting of the free gingival margin (FGM), so that the previously knifelike FGM becomes more bulky and rolled. In some animals the gingiva becomes hyperplastic and the FGM may be five to six mm coronal to its normal position, covering a substantial portion of the crown. Hyperplastic gingivitis is often associated with halitosis. The gentle insertion of a thin periodontal probe calibrated in millimeters into the sulcus indicates the depth from the FGM to the point where the probe stops in the inflamed subsulcular connective tissue; this dimension is normally one to three mm. The increase in depth noted in an animal with gingivitis reflects the coronal movement of the FGM. Loss of soft tissue integrity of the sulcular and junctional epithelium as well as the underlying connective tissue allows the probe to pass apical to the soft tissue attachment. Because the probe passes through the epithelial tissue it is not uncommon for blood to exude from the sulcus during probing. As a result of the underlying inflammation, thin clear gingival fluid often exudes from the sulcus. Purulent exudates may also be seen when pressure is applied to the gingiva.

Histopathology. The histopathologic changes that accompany early gingivitis are characteristic of an acute inflammatory reaction. There is loss of perivascular collagen, vasculitis, and an influx of lymphocytes and polymorphonuclear leukocytes into the connective tissues. The polymorphs actively migrate out through the junctional and sulcular epithelium into the sulcus. After approximately four days the inflammatory changes become more chronic. Fibroblasts decrease in number, and the gingival fiber apparatus loses its integrity as collagen breakdown occurs. By the end of two weeks the inflammatory infiltrate is predominantly plasma cells, and the junctional and sulcular epithelia lose integrity as the intercellular spaces widen. In some areas the sulcular epithelium may become ulcerated. Although the junctional epithelium loses its integrity, it does not detach from tooth surfaces (Page and Schroeder, 1976).

Etiology. Numerous experiments on dogs have demonstrated that dental plaque is the primary etiologic factor responsible for gingivitis. Plaque is found on the tooth surface, both subgingivally in the sulcus and

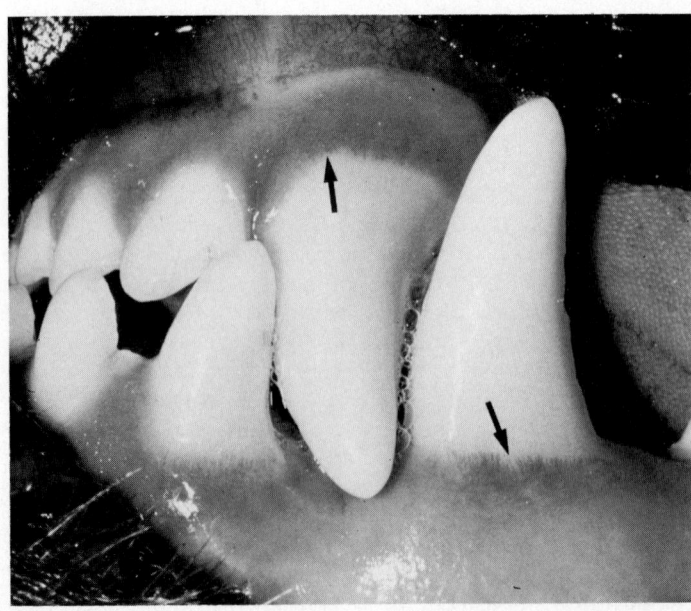

Figure 55–28. Early gingivitis in a dog. Note the slight color change in the marginal gingiva (arrows).

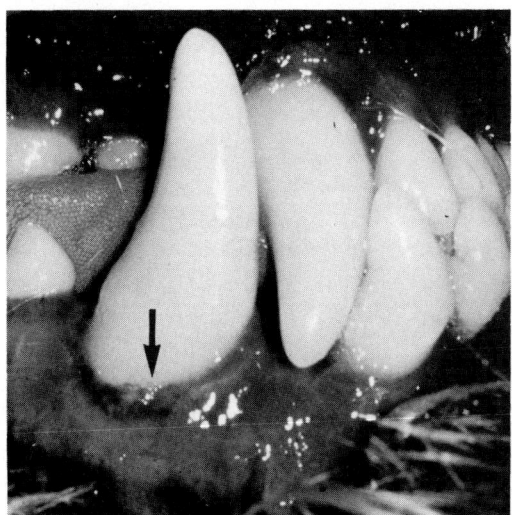

Figure 55–29. Established gingivitis. Note the color change (arrow) and rolled marginal gingiva.

supragingivally in the area coronal to the FGM (Lindhe et al., 1973; 1975).

Supragingival plaque formation begins with adhesion of bacteria to the tooth surface. The organisms adhere to an acid glycoprotein pellicle that precipitates from the saliva onto the enamel surfaces. The plaque mass increases in size through a combination of multiplication of the original organisms and the deposition of new organisms onto the plaque. Plaque consists of approximately 80 per cent water and 20 per cent organic and inorganic solids; approximately 80 per cent of the solid portion is bacteria. The organisms produce a matrix consisting

largely of polysaccharide protein complexes. Plaque is not a food residue. Diet does, however, play a significant role in the formation and maturation of the plaque. It has been well documented (Knasse and Brill, 1960; Carlson and Egelberg, 1965; Egelberg and Carlson, 1965) that soft diets induce more plaque formation and higher levels of gingivitis than do hard diets in dogs. The relative proportions of carbohydrates, protein, and fat do not quantitatively alter plaque formation. Egelberg (1965) has also demonstrated significant plaque formation in dogs fed through a tube.

The microbiology of plaque associated with gingivitis is complex. Various cocci, filaments, spirochetes, and rods are found, including facultative and anaerobic organisms. The specific organisms predominating in the dog are gram-negative anaerobes (Syed et al., 1980).

Plaque is a soft, colorless mass not readily seen by the naked eye unless it either is naturally stained by dietary constituents or is extremely thick. It can be demonstrated by various plaque-disclosing dyes, the most common of which are erythrosin (F.D. and C. Red #3) and fluorescein (D. and C. yellow #8). The latter requires a special light source to cause the dye to fluoresce; however, it is more specific for the bacterial components of the plaque than erythrosin (Lang and Loe, 1972).

The accumulation of plaque is enhanced by the presence of surface irregularities, the most common of which is calculus (Fig.

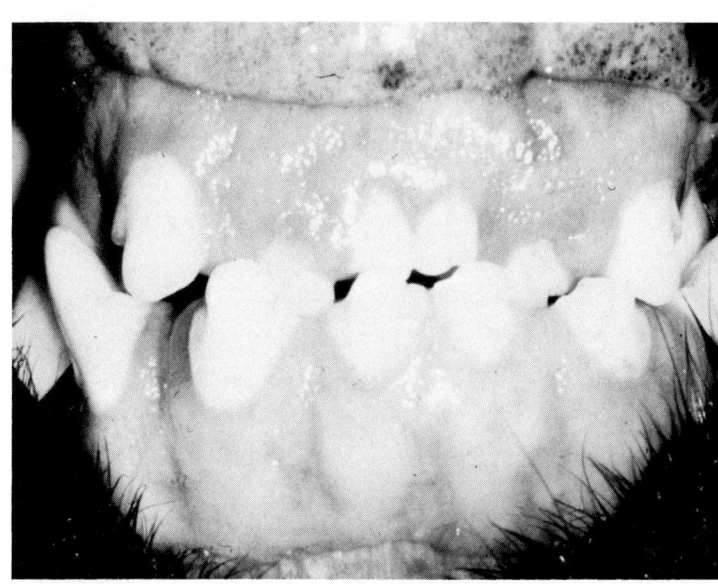

Figure 55–30. Mild hyperplastic gingivitis in a dog.

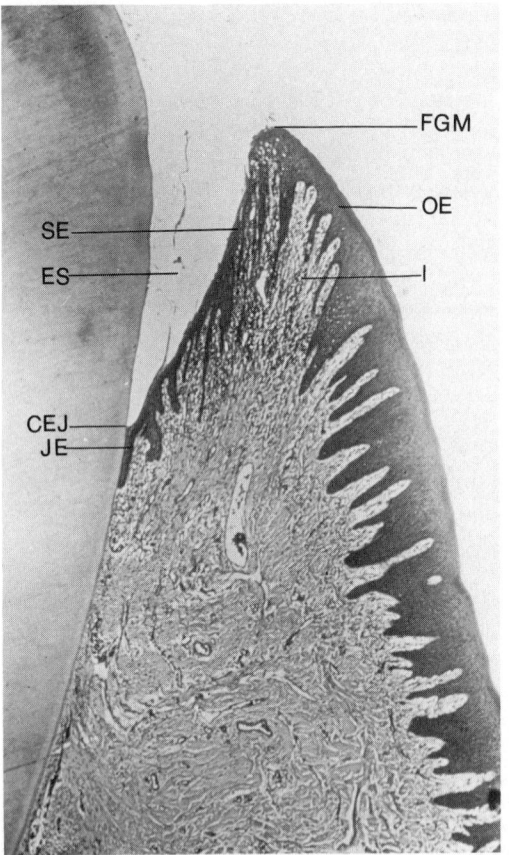

Figure 55-31. Histopathologic picture of gingivitis in a dog. CEJ, cemento-enamel junction; ES, enamel space; FGM, free gingival margin; I, inflammatory infiltrate; JE, junctional epithelium; OE, oral epithelium; SE, sulcular epithelium.

55–32), a mass of calcium salts precipitated from saliva. Calculus appears in both supragingival and subgingival locations and is most typically off-white, yellow, or brown. The plaque-retentive characteristics of cal-

culus are more important than its effect as a mechanical irritant. It has been shown that endotoxins from plaque may be found in calculus. In at least one study (Saxe et al., 1967) the formation of calculus in a colony of Beagle dogs was not found to be related to diet consistency. Hair or food impaction in the gingival sulcus and hypoplastic or other roughened surfaces on the enamel in the vicinity of the gingival margin exacerbate plaque retention and gingivitis (Fig. 55–33). When gingivitis has been present for a significant period of time, architectural changes in the gingiva, particularly gingival hyperplasia, also aid in the retention of plaque. Not only does the deepened pocket create an area for plaque to accumulate, but it has been suggested that the environment within the pocket is more supportive of some of the gram-negative pathogens that are associated with subsequent periodontal breakdown.

Primary viral infections, particularly leukemia virus (Barrett et al., 1975) and rhinotracheitis/calicivirus infection (Povey, 1976), can cause chronic, severe nonresponsive gingivitis in the cat (Fig. 55–34). The fluorescent antibody test for leukemia virus should be performed on all cats with a well-established gingivitis or generalized stomatitis. Gingival hyperplasia caused by sodium diphenylhydantoin (Dilantin, an anticonvulsant), which occurs in man, has been produced experimentally in the cat (Nuki and Cooper, 1972), and reported in the dog.

Treatment. The treatment of gingivitis is directed at the removal of bacterial plaque from the surfaces of the tooth on a consistent basis. All plaque-retentive features

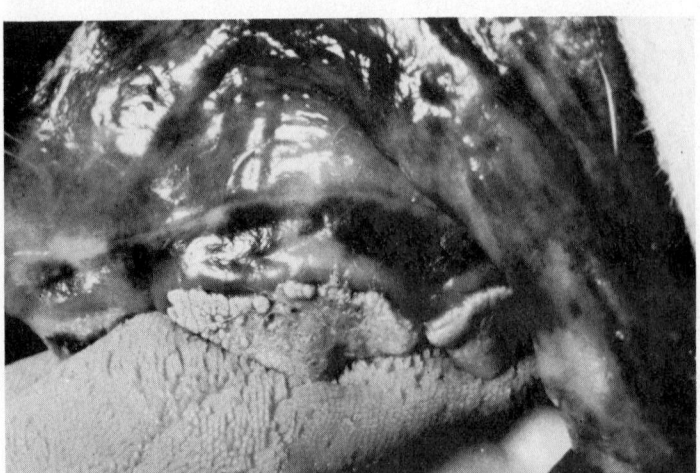

Figure 55-32. Calculus on the lateral aspect of a maxillary carnassial tooth in a dog. The soft tissue inflammation seen is the result of bacterial plaque on the calculus surface.

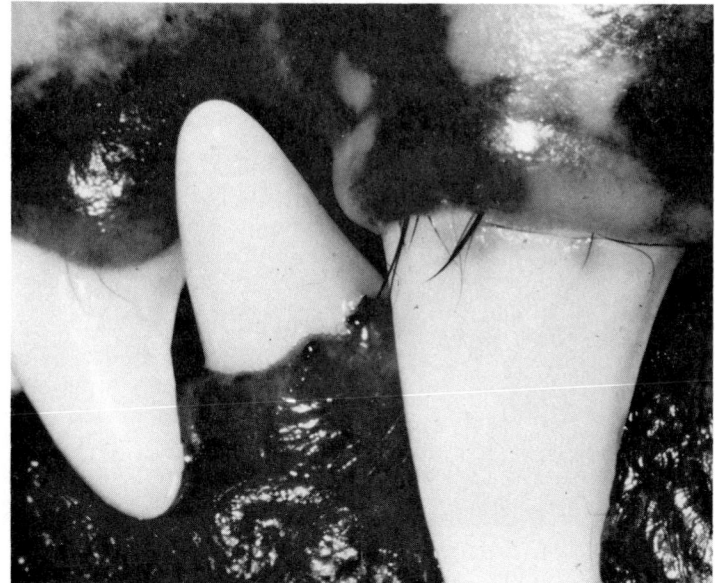

Figure 55–33. Hair impaction under the free gingival margin of a dog. The hair is acting as a matrix for calculus formation.

must be removed from the tooth surface to facilitate daily oral hygiene by the pet's owner. The removal of calculus without appropriate follow-up care will lead to a very transient result (Fig. 55–35). Treatment techniques are discussed under Periodontal Therapy.

The consistent removal of plaque from the tooth surfaces results in a predictable diminution of clinical signs. A solution of chlorhexidine gluconate applied to the teeth cures established gingivitis (Lindhe et al., 1970); however, teeth become stained, and plaque and gingivitis rapidly return when treatment is discontinued (Hill and Davies, 1972). Although various antibiotics have

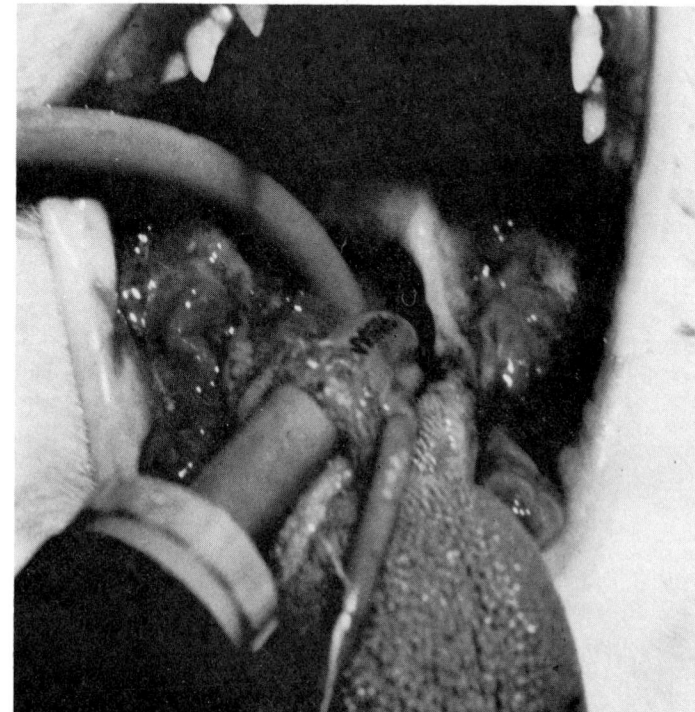

Figure 55–34. Extensive soft tissue proliferation at the commissures of the mouth in a cat with chronic nonresponsive gingivitis.

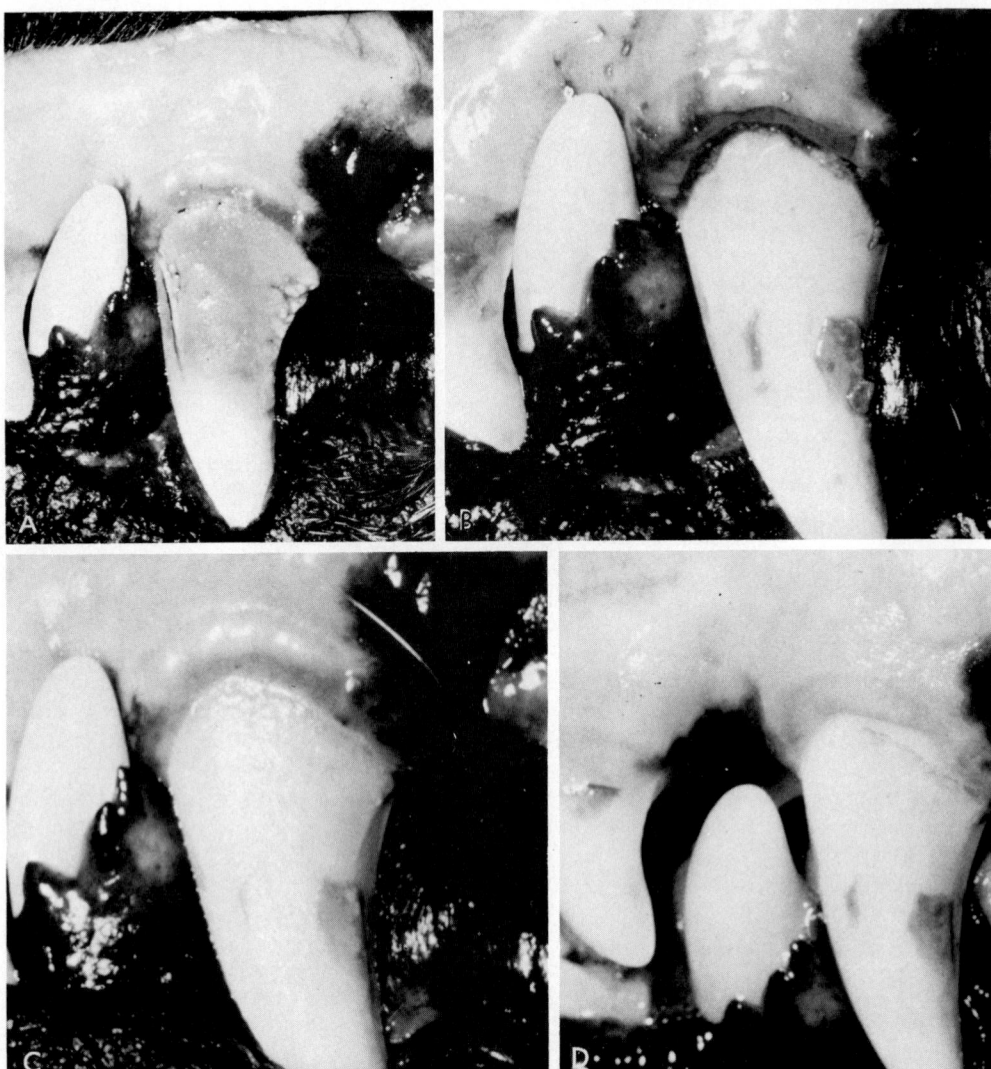

Figure 55–35. Canine and incisor teeth of an old dog with marginal gingivitis associated with plaque and calculus. *A*, Before treatment. *B*, Immediately after the removal of the gingival calculus. *C*, Three weeks after calculus removal. Note the persistent gingival inflammation and associated plaque. *D*, One week after instituting tooth brushing, the gingival inflammation has subsided.

also been shown to be effective in treating gingivitis, their long-term effects on the ecology of the oral cavity or on the intestinal ecology are unknown.

Necrotizing Ulcerative Gingivitis

Necrotizing ulcerative gingivitis (NUG) is an acute infection primarily involving the marginal tissues of the gingiva. It is characterized by ulcerations of the gingival tissues, usually starting in the interdental regions. The affected areas are typically covered by a grayish mass of necrotic tissue, bacteria, and other oral debris. The tissues bleed when touched. On occasion the disease process may affect the crestal bone. The animal's breath is extremely foul, the condition causes pain, and affected animals may experience difficulty eating (Kaplan and Jeffcoat, 1978).

Necrotizing ulcerative gingivitis has been reported to have occurred in 12 dogs aged 4 to 12 months in a colony of beagles (Van Camper et al., 1977). NUG has also been reported in cats (Calcott, 1975).

Although the etiology of this disease is not fully understood, two organisms, *Fusobacterium fusiforme* and *Borrelia vincentii,* have been associated with the disease in man. In addition to the bacteria, some host modifying factors seem to be necessary. The presence of elevated levels of 17-hydroxycorticosteroids in affected patients has been reported, possibly secondary to stress. Wouters (1977) attempted to inoculate bacterial plaque from an animal with NUG into six healthy one-year-old beagle dogs. Three of the beagles were first given corticosteroids. Only those dogs that received the corticosteroids contracted the disease.

The disease responds to the administration of penicillin. Generally a one-week regime of ampicillin (20 mg/kg orally four times per day) results in a dramatic improvement. Debridement of the necrotic tissue accompanied by plaque and calculus removal accelerates treatment. Healing often results in a gingival deformity that may be plaque retentive and predisposes to subsequent periodontal disease; follow-up gingival surgery may be indicated to correct the soft tissue deformity after the active disease is brought under control.

PERIODONTITIS

Clinical Manifestations. Periodontal disease does not progress beyond gingivitis in the majority of tooth surfaces in small animals. In some animals, however, there is a progression of the soft tissue inflammation into the deeper tissues of the peridontium (Page et al., 1981). The host factors and local factors that result in the progression of the disease are poorly understood. The loss of alveolar and supporting bone is accompanied by an apical migration of the gingival fiber apparatus, and the junctional epithelium. The loss of osseous support can occur either as a generalized horizontal loss involving all teeth on all surfaces or as isolated areas involving single teeth or even single surfaces of single teeth. Once initiated, the bone loss tends to be progressive. Typically, the soft tissues manifest the changes associated with gingivitis, with one notable exception: the free gingival margin (FGM) may recede in an apical direction as a result of the loss of osseous tissues. When this occurs the cemento-enamel junction (CEJ) and root surface will be visible. In more advanced cases when there is excessive bone loss, the furcation area (the area between the roots of a multirooted tooth) may be exposed to the oral environment (Figs. 55–36, 55–37, 55–38). Gingival recession does not always accompany the bone loss; hyperplasia of the gingiva may coexist with bone loss (Fig. 55–39). Thus, the clinical diagnosis of periodontitis cannot be based only on the position of the FGM relative to the CEJ; it is also necessary to use radiographs and/or the periodontal probe. When loss of crestal height is seen on the radiograph or when the tip of a periodontal probe can be passed two or more millimeters apical to the CEJ, the diagnosis of periodontitis can be made. The probe is inserted into the sulcus parallel to the long axis of the tooth, with its tip in contact with the tooth. Bleeding will invariably accompany probing in the animal with active periodontitis and purulent discharge may exude out of the pocket orifice. In cases with extreme bone loss, horizontal mobility of the teeth increases substantially. With the possible exception of maxillary and mandibular incisors and first, second, and third pre-molars in some of the smaller breeds, horizontal tooth mobility should not be seen

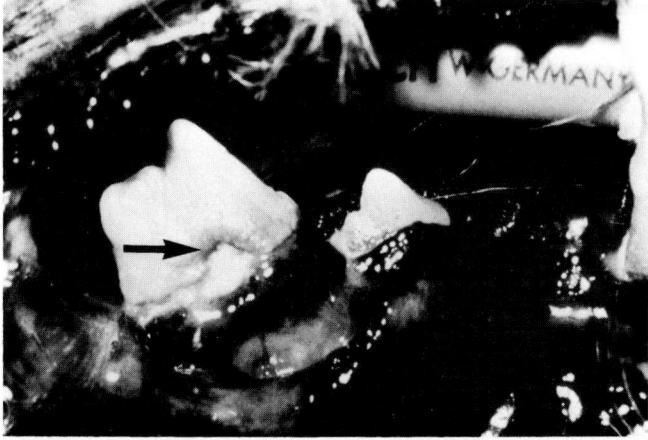

Figure 55–36. Mandibular carnassial tooth in a dog with gingival recession exposing the bifurcation (arrow).

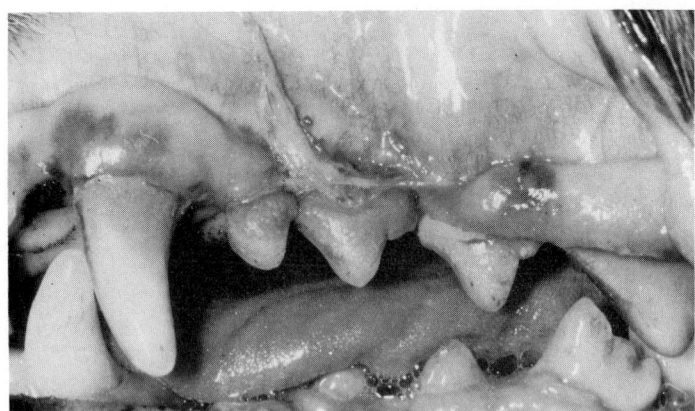

Figure 55–37. Hair impaction in the furcation area of a maxillary premolar of a dog.

in periodontally healthy dogs. As a result of the loss of osseous support, teeth frequently become mobile. The degree of mobility depends on root morphology, severity of the inflammatory process, and occlusal forces. The presence of mobility does not necessarily render the prognosis for a particular tooth as hopeless (Nyman et al., 1978).

A thorough history and physical examination is indicated for all animals with periodontal disease, as systemic disease may predispose to or manifest itself locally as periodontal disease.

Radiographic Manifestations. The earliest radiographic sign of periodontitis is loss of definition of crestal bone. In health, crestal bone appears as a radiopaque line that parallels and is one to two millimeters apical to an imaginary line drawn between the CEJ of two adjacent teeth. As periodontitis advances, an apical migration of the crestal bone is seen (Fig. 55–40). Radiolucent areas within the furcations of multirooted teeth also become apparent.

Histopathology. The gingival changes are the same as those in gingivitis. There is a chronic inflammatory reaction marked by a dense infiltrate of round cells; much of the gingival fiber apparatus is destroyed. Inflammatory cells are found in close proximity to the crestal bone, which may be actively resorbed by osteoclastic activity. The transeptal fibers, immediately coronal to the bone, are still present; the epithelial inflammatory infiltrate lies coronal to this connective tissue.

As the crestal bone resorbs, the transeptal fibers reattach at a more apical level on the root surface, which allows the junctional epithelium to move in an apical direction. The more coronal cells of the junctional epithelium detach from the tooth and become part of the sulcular epithelium, thus increasing the depth of the pocket. Bacterial plaque is seen in the pocket almost, but not quite, in contact with the most coronal cell of the junctional epithelium, although bacteria are not found within the periodontal

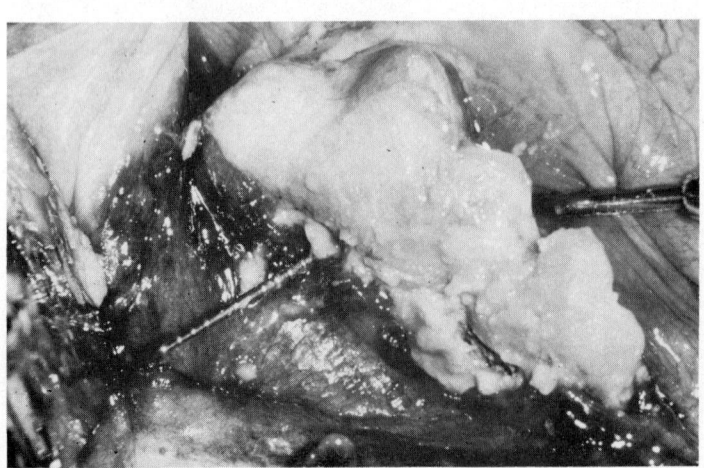

Figure 55–38. Extensive furcation involvement in a mandibular carnassial tooth. The periodontal probe can be passed from the medial to the lateral surface.

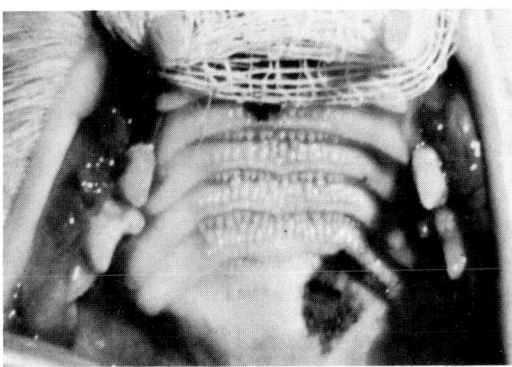

Figure 55–39. Extensive periodontal disease in a cat showing a combination of soft tissue hyperplasia and recession.

tissues. Calculus may or may not be present in the pocket. Necrosis is not seen in the soft or hard tissues of the periodontium affected by periodontitis. Page and Schroeder (1981) describe in detail the histopathology of naturally occurring periodontitis in dogs.

Etiology. It is now generally believed that periodontitis develops as a sequel to a persistent gingivitis. The factors that determine whether or not a gingivitis progresses to periodontitis have not been thoroughly elucidated. There is substantial although by no means conclusive evidence that the bacterial flora present in plaque is a determining factor.

It is still unknown precisely which organisms actually initiate the destruction of the periodontium. There are several bacteria that, when inoculated into the mouths of gnotobiotic rats, produce extensive alveolar

bone loss. Most of these organisms are found in high numbers in the plaque of human patients with active periodontitis. It has also been demonstrated in dogs that periodontitis could be produced by simply allowing plaque to accumulate on the tooth surface (Lindhe et al., 1975). The control animals, which were fed identical diets but had their teeth cleaned twice daily, did not manifest periodontitis at any time during the four years of the study. It also has been demonstrated that the flora associated with teeth that have periodontitis is distinctly different from the flora of teeth without periodontitis even within the same mouth (Heigl and Lindhe, 1979). The former have more spirochetes, motile rods, and in general, an anaerobic gram-negative flora. The flora associated with healthy areas tends to have relatively more cocci and filamentous organisms, with proportionally fewer spirochetes and motile rods.

As in gingivitis, any factor that allows for the retention of plaque on the tooth surface is likely to contribute to the demise of the periodontium. In addition to calculus and hair or food impaction, the formation of the deepened pocket is in itself a major plaque-retentive feature. As the pocket increases in depth, significant environmental change may occur that allows the more deleterious organisms to proliferate.

There are a number of investigators who feel that the primary etiologic factor is not bacterial but rather a calcium ion deficiency (Henrikson, 1968; Krook et al., 1972; Krook, 1976). Although nutrition almost

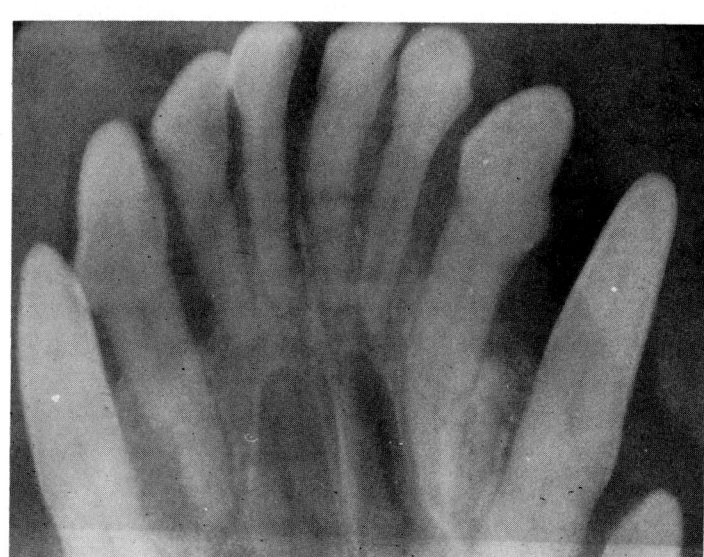

Figure 55–40. Radiograph of canine maxillary incisors showing generalized bone loss secondary to inflammatory periodontal disease.

certainly plays a role in the host's response to insult, in the case of periodontal disease the overwhelming evidence is that the initiating factor in the disease process is microbial.

Treatment. The treatment of periodontitis is directed toward the removal of bacterial plaque from the tooth surfaces; unless the disease is treated at its most incipient stage, however, it is almost impossible to control. Since plaque must be eliminated in the subgingival as well as the supragingival area, either the pocket must be cleaned on a more or less daily basis or the pocket must be surgically eliminated so that only supragingival areas need to be cleaned (Figs.

55–41 and 55–42). Although surgical pocket elimination is possible in some cases, it is technically difficult and time-consuming. Without proper postsurgical maintenance, the therapy will almost certainly fail. The animal's age, the type of posttreatment care the owner is willing to provide, and the willingness of the animal to accept treatment are factors to consider prior to treatment. By far the easiest and most predictable way to manage advanced periodontitis is to extract the involved teeth. When there is some overriding reason to keep the dentition intact (for example, in a show or guard dog), the most efficacious treatment is to thoroughly debride the tooth surfaces on a

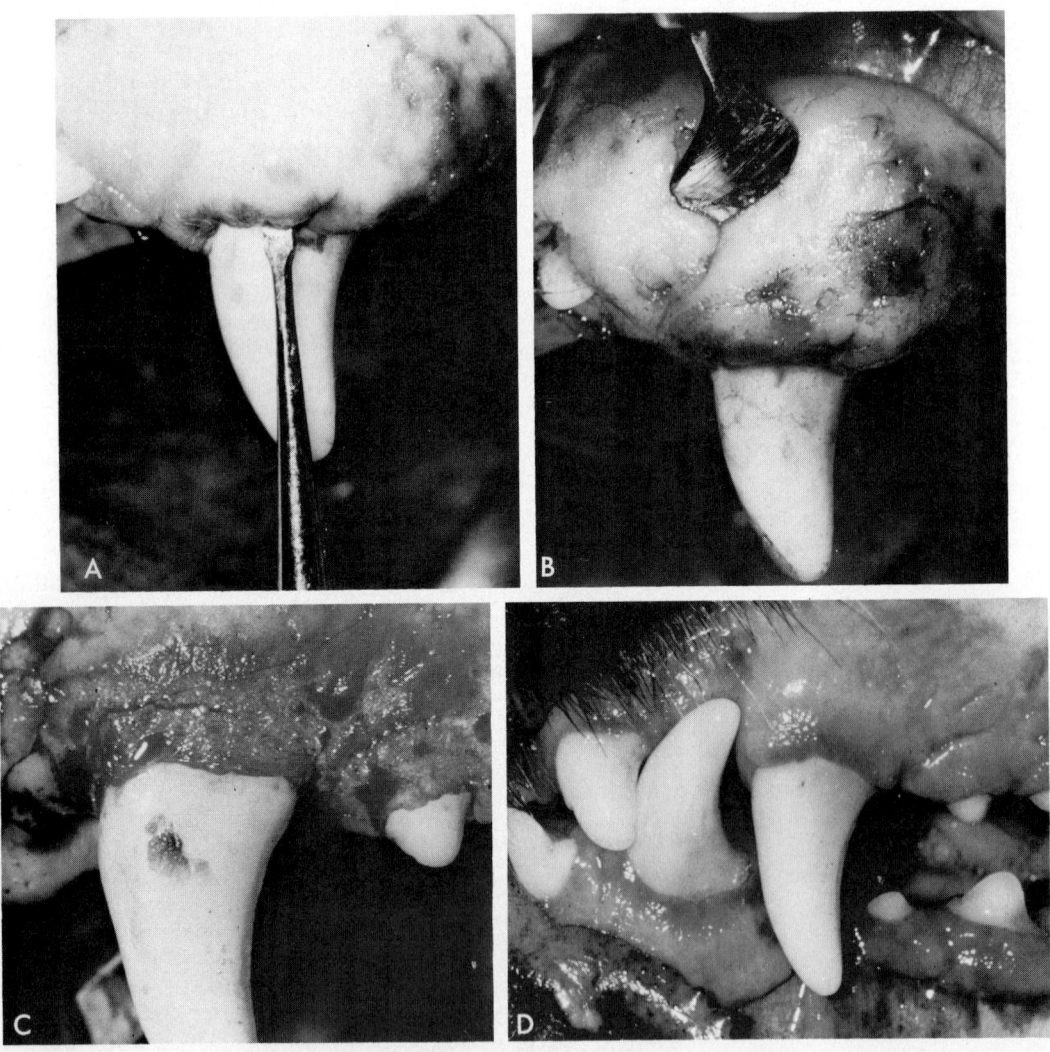

Figure 55–41. Gingivectomy for treatment of hyperplastic gingivitis in a dog. *A*, Maxillary canine tooth with dental instrument placed in the facial pocket. *B*, Gingivectomy knife in place for the excision of the free gingiva. *C*, The free gingiva has been excised. Note the piece of calculus which was not removed during the presurgical scaling. *D*, Postoperative healing (after four months). Note the marginal inflammation resulting from the reaccumulation of plaque.

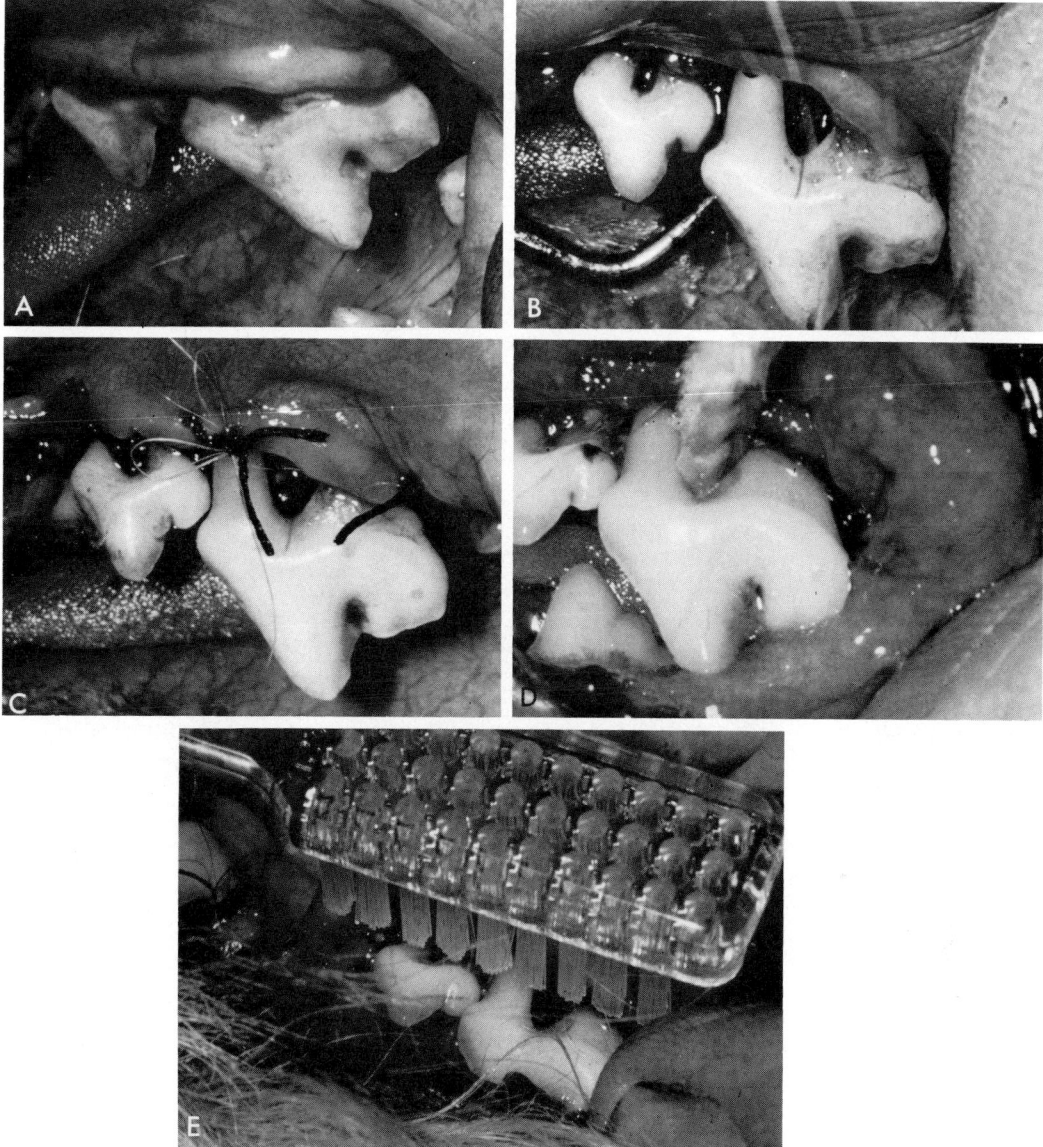

Figure 55–42. Apically positioned flap surgery in a dog with advanced periodontitis and furcation involvement of the maxillary 4th premolar. *A*, Pre-treatment. *B*, The free gingival margin has been moved in an apical direction to expose the furcation. *C*, The facial flap has been sutured to the platal flap. *D* and *E*, The furcation must be cleaned daily with pipe cleaners or a tooth brush. Although this treatment is feasible, it is often not practical. Prevention should be stressed.

regular basis every two to four months as needed, based on the severity of the problem. Debridement should consist of a thorough calculus and plaque removal as well as curettage of the inflamed pocket lining and the removal of the most superficial layer of cementum on the root surface within the pocket (see Periodontal Therapy). Although this treatment may not arrest the disease process, it may slow it enough to allow the teeth to remain in a relatively stable state. The long-term or intermittent use of antibi-

otics may be a useful adjunct. The better the follow-up care on the part of the patient's owner, the more successful the therapy. Follow-up care should include daily tooth brushing to increase the possibility of success. Switching to a totally dry food diet is also helpful.

Periodontal Abscess

Acute periodontal abscess is a localized, purulent inflammation in the periodontal tissues, generally appearing as a swelling within the gingival tissues. It may be firm or fluctuant, or if it has spontaneously drained, it may present as a mass of detached gingiva (Fig. 55–43). The gingival tissues in the area of the abscess are inflamed. In most cases a probe placed into the gingival crevice easily enters the abscess, causing pus to exude out of the crevice. At times the abscess is entirely within the gingiva and not easily entered through the pocket. Tooth mobility is usually markedly increased. Periodontal abscesses are most frequently associated with deep pockets, furcation areas, or occasionally relatively shallow pockets into which a foreign body has become lodged.

The radiographic appearance of the periodontal abscess can be quite variable. It appears as a discrete area of bone loss adjacent to the root, usually on the coronal half of the root, and it may involve the more apical areas.

There is some question as to whether carnassial abscess, which is usually associated with the maxillary fourth premolar or mandibular first molar teeth, is of periodontal or endodontic origin.

Although the acute abscess responds to antibiotic therapy, it generally recurs if more vigorous treatment is not rendered. If sufficient osseous support remains around the tooth, one can thoroughly debride the abscess either by flapping the gingival tissues away from the root or curetting the lesion through the gingival crevice. In most instances, however, bony destruction precludes salvaging the tooth, and extraction is indicated.

Periodontal Therapy

Oral Hygiene. A soft toothbrush with nylon bristles is the most practical implement for the daily removal of plaque. The teeth should be brushed with the toothbrush bristles aimed into the gingival sulcus, with the brush head at a 45-degree angle to the tooth surface. The brush is moved with a short back and forth motion. All of the facial, lingual, and palatal surfaces should be brushed. The brush should also be directed down at the occlusal surfaces of the tooth with a back and forth motion of the brush parallel to the interproximal areas. Although toothbrushing should be vigorous, it should not cause gingival abrasions. The owner should be advised that the presence of gingival bleeding during toothbrushing is evidence of gingival disease and that in most cases a week of conscientiously applied oral hygiene will cause the bleeding to stop. Although it is unnecessary to use a dentifrice for toothbrushing, a baking soda/peroxide combination has been advocated in humans with periodontitis (Keyes et al., 1978), and although its efficacy has not been proven in animals, it may be of some value. Once a dog or cat is affected by periodontitis to the extent that there is obvious pocket formation, recession, or furcation involvement, tooth brushing alone is probably inadequate.

In order for oral hygiene to be effective in the presence of periodontitis, the oral hygiene implement must overcome the architectural deformity created by the disease. Although dental floss, toothpicks, and rubber tips would be useful, their use is imprac-

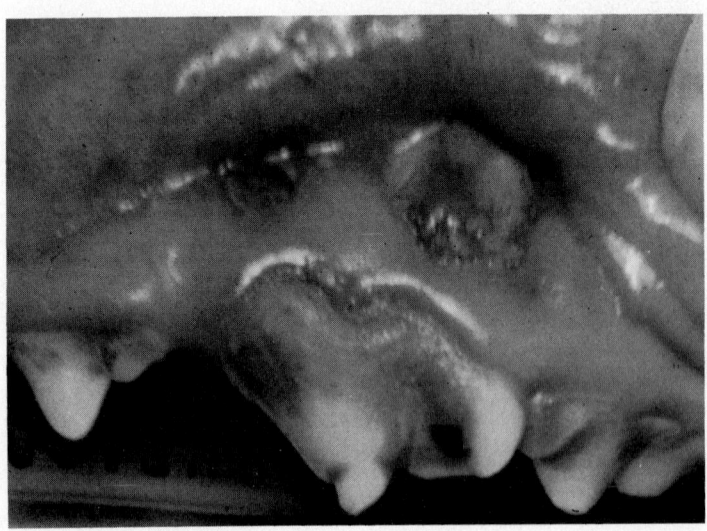

Figure 55–43. Gingival and bone loss caused by a periodontal abscess on the facial aspect of a maxillary carnassial tooth.

tical unless the animal is extremely cooperative and the owner is highly motivated (Dietrich, 1978).

Scaling and Root Planing. Once calculus has formed on the crown and roots of the tooth, it is no longer possible for toothbrushing to be effective. The teeth of the animal should be scaled. This can be accomplished either by an ultrasonic device that literally vibrates the calculus from the tooth surface, or by dental curettes and scalers. The tip of the ultrasonic device, which should be well cooled with a water spray, is gently moved over the tooth surfaces supra- and subgingivally (Lane, 1977). Ultrasonic dental scalers cause considerable spread of contamination (Zontine et al., 1969) and can cause bacteremia, particularly in dogs with gingivitis or periodontitis (Jackson et al., 1981). When using a dental curette, the tip should be placed apical to the calculus, with its face at a 45-75-degree angle to the long axis of the tooth. The curette is then pulled in a coronal direction, dislodging the calculus (Fig. 55–44). It is essential that the curette be extremely sharp. If calculus was removed from the root surface of the tooth, it is necessary to plane the cemental surface of

the tooth, which can also be accomplished with the curette. The purpose of root planing is to remove residual calculus as well as bacterial endotoxins that impregnate the superficial surface of the cementum. A jet of air in combination with a sharp dental explorer is useful in detecting calculus in the subgingival areas. After the teeth are scaled, they should be polished with a rotating rubber cup and mild abrasive. The value of scaling and root planing is extremely transient unless it is followed with daily oral hygiene and, preferably, a change to a hard food diet.

Curettage. The removal of the inflamed pocket lining and the soft tissue contents of infrabony pockets (which result from irregular resorption of bone) is useful in the control of active periodontal disease. A sharp curette in which the cutting edge is directed toward the sulcular and junctional epithelium and the osseous tissues is used to remove the inflamed tissue. This procedure can be accomplished at the same time as scaling and root planing.

Surgical Pocket Elimination. Some of the soft and hard tissue deformities (particularly gingival hyperplasia) created by periodontal disease are amenable to surgical treatment (Fig. 55–45). The successful management of periodontal disease requires that bacterial plaque be removed on a routine, preferably daily, basis. Even with a cooperative animal and owner, however, it is impossible to successfully remove plaque from subgingival areas on a daily basis in a dog or cat. The purpose of periodontal surgery is to eliminate the pocket, thus changing a subgingival area into a cleansable supragingival one.

The two basic procedures for eliminating pockets are gingivectomy and the apically positioned flap (Figs. 55–41 and 55–42), although the apically positioned flap is rarely indicated in dogs and cats. Pockets on the palatal aspect of the maxillary teeth are particularly difficult to manage because of the flatness of the palate in the dog and cat. It is beyond the scope of this chapter to describe these procedures in detail; they are described elsewhere (Carranza, 1979).

Extraction. Once periodontal disease has advanced to the point at which furcations have become involved or tooth mobility is excessive, the only practical modality for control of periodontitis is extraction of the involved teeth. This is not to say that

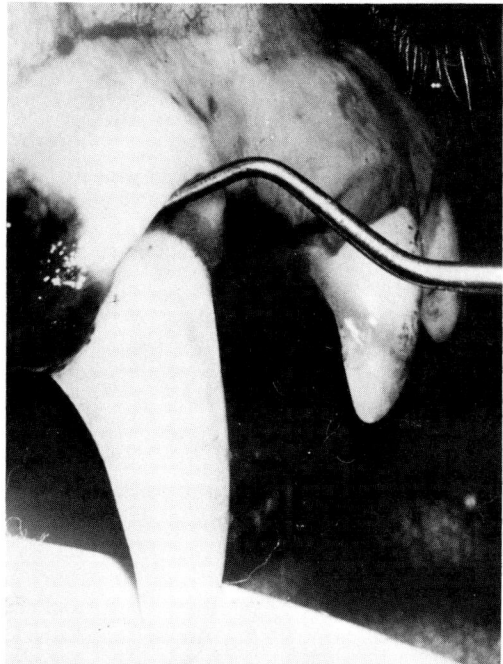

Figure 55–44. Use of the periodontal curette to remove calculus in a pocket apical to the free gingival margin.

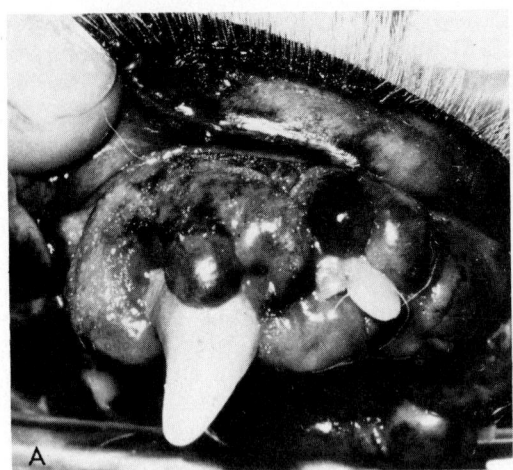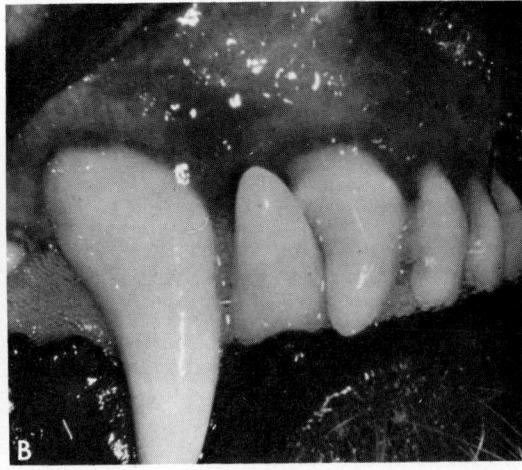

Figure 55–45. Extensive gingival hyperplasia in a miniature collie. *A*, Pretreatment. *B*, After surgical removal.

such teeth cannot be salvaged; however, the techniques involved and follow-up care necessary are impractical for use in small animals. Extraction is also a practical treatment for the earlier stages of periodontal disease if the owner is not concerned with the esthetics of the mouth. Tooth extraction techniques have been described in detail elsewhere (Annis, 1974).

Dental procedures involving the periodontium usually cause a bacteremia (Black et al., 1980), although in the normal dog this is rapidly cleared (Silver et al., 1975). Animals with valvular heart disease or animals with a predisposition to endocarditis should receive prophylactic antibiotic coverage (Withrow, 1979). Ampicillin is appropriate, given in high dosage immediately prior to and for 24 hours after the procedure. When the normal range of antibiotics has proven ineffective in treating gingivitis or periodontitis, metronidazole (30 mg/kg orally once each day for five to seven days) may be successful.

STOMATITIS

Stomatitis is inflammation of the oral mucosa. The clinician examining an animal with stomatitis must consider both the general health of the patient and local factors. Any circumstances that significantly alter the dynamic replication, maturation, and exfoliation of healthy mucosa favor the development of disease. Although the oral mucosa is subject to considerable trauma and can tolerate it well, swelling, dehydration, cell death, or replication caused by

disease will exaggerate the effect of normal trauma and produce injury (Ship and Galili, 1971). The saliva of carnivores is bactericidal because of the alkaline pH and lysozyme content; therefore, bacterial infection rarely becomes established unless other factors, infectious or physical, are present.

Diagnosis. A routine should be developed for the diagnosis of animals with stomatitis. When the animal is first presented, a complete history, including dietary information and thorough physical examination, is essential. Thorough examination of the oral cavity often requires sedation or anesthesia owing to the animal's temperament or to pain caused by the disease. The position, extent, symmetry, and nature of the lesions are of particular importance. Periodontal disease may be localized but is usually widespread along the gingival margins by the time that veterinary attention is sought. Usually the visible lesions are confined to the gingiva; however, ulcers are sometimes seen on the buccal mucosa that lies in contact with the diseased periodontium. Lesions caused by viruses or poisons are usually scattered over the mucosa. In cats, ulcers caused by feline viral rhinotracheitis or calicivirus infection are seen most commonly on the tongue, palate, or fauces. Single asymmetric lesions may be neoplastic (see Oropharyngeal Neoplasia). A disclosing solution should be used to demonstrate the extent of plaque. A calibrated periodontal probe and dental explorer are very useful for examining teeth and periodontium.

Initial laboratory examination should include a complete blood count, peripheral blood smear for FeLV fluorescent antibody test in cats, and creatinine and blood glucose determinations, particularly in older animals or in animals with polydypsia/polyuria. The next step will depend on the tentative clinical diagnosis. Observing the response to treatment is a frequent means of confirming the cause of stomatitis. Failure of the lesions to respond in the expected fashion should prompt further investigation. Cytologic examination or biopsy, histologic examination, and bacterial, fungal, or viral culture of the lesions are often helpful. Immunologic work-up may indicate an autoimmune or immune deficiency disease.

SYSTEMIC DISEASE CAUSING ORAL LESIONS

Oral changes caused by systemic diseases are important diagnostic aids to the clinician.

Uremia. The most common oral manifestation of systemic disease in the dog and cat is ulceration associated with severe uremia. Urea diffuses into all body secretions, including saliva. The irritation caused by ammonia resulting from bacterial action on urea, the dry mouth of the dehydrated uremic patient, and the clotting deficiencies that occur late in the disease all contribute to this syndrome. Local therapy can be soothing, but unless renal failure is reversed, the process is relentless. The rostral part of the tongue may undergo necrosis in dogs with acute renal failure or pancreatitis.

Diabetes. Oral infections are no more common in diabetic animals than in normal animals; however, they may be more severe, progressing rapidly to periodontitis or periodontal abscess. In an animal with nonresponsive stomatitis, the possibility of diabetes should be investigated. Meticulous attention to dental hygiene is necessary in diabetic patients. There is disagreement as to whether salivary flow rates are decreased in humans with diabetes; calcium ion and immunoglobulin G are found in higher concentration in saliva from diabetics (Conner et al., 1970; Marder et al., 1975). The relationship between these findings, the increased incidence and severity of periodontal disease in diabetics, and the xerostomia often associated with diabetes in humans is not yet clear. The mandibular salivary gland produces a tryptic inhibitor anti-insulin factor; resection of these glands in human diabetes improves but does not correct the diabetes. A mild xerostomia persists for up to three weeks (Godlowski and Withers, 1971).

Hematologic and Reticuloendothelial Diseases. Ulceration is uncommon, but petechiation of the palate or buccal mucosa, or blood oozing from the gums may be early signs of vitamin K deficiency (as in warfarin poisoning), thrombocytopenia, or other diseases that cause a clotting defect. Any disease depressing the function of the reticuloendothelial system can predispose to infection.

Deficiency Diseases. Documentation of specific vitamin-deficient states is now very rare. Classical niacin deficiency syndrome in the dog ("black tongue") is no longer seen as a clinical entity. In the rare animal with severe pica or a dietary idiosyncrasy that causes inadequate nutrition, replacement vitamin therapy may be justified.

Genetic Diseases. Stomatitis is a severe recurrent problem in silver-gray Collies afflicted with the simple recessive autosomal disease that causes cyclic neutropenia ("gray collie syndrome") (Cheville, 1968).

Poisons. All heavy metal compounds can cause oral inflammation and ulceration; thallium is the most common agent seen clinically. Warfarin and indanedione, used in rodent control, cause clotting deficiencies that may present as oral petechiation. Occasionally, other substances such as plants (e.g., Dieffenbachia) may cause oral disease when chewed by a dog or cat.

Immune System Abnormalities

Both immune deficiency disease and autoimmune disease can result in oral lesions. Immune deficiency diseases may allow local disease such as periodontal disease to worsen or secondary Candida sp. infection to become established. The severe T cell immunodeficiency often associated with nasal aspergillosis or penicillosis may present as oral disease by direct spread along the nasopalatine duct.

Immune system abnormalities should be included as a possible diagnosis in intractable or recurrent stomatitis. The lymphocyte transformation test is a useful screening test for immune deficiency diseases. Immune deficiency diseases are discussed in Chapters 81, 82, and 83.

Autoimmune Diseases. Several reports have been published recently detailing autoimmune disease affecting the oral cavity of the dog (Stannard et al., 1975; Hurvitz and Feldman, 1975; Scott, 1977; Bennett et al., 1980) and the cat (Brown and Hurvitz, 1979), indicating that the disease has been waiting for appropriate diagnostic tests to allow its recognition. The two forms of autoimmune disease that principally affect the oral cavity are pemphigus vulgaris and bullous pemphigoid. Both result from circulating autoantibodies to intercellular epidermal antigens, which cause acantholysis and intraepidermal bullae (pemphigus vulgaris) or epidermal connective tissue bullae (bullous pemphigoid).

PEMPHIGUS VULGARIS. This condition occurs in a wide range of age and breed of dogs. The oral mucosa, external nares, lips, eyelid margins, ears, anus, and prepuce or vulva are the most frequent sites of lesions. Oral lesions often appear as well-defined ulcers with scalloped edges. Diagnosis is based on careful histologic examination or direct immunofluorescence examination of a biopsy specimen. Treatment is covered in Chapter 82.

BULLOUS PEMPHIGOID. This condition appears to be somewhat less frequent than pemphigus vulgaris. Again, the oral mucosa is a frequent site, often with other mucocutaneous junction areas and sometimes more generalized skin lesions. Diagnosis and treatment are covered in Chapter 82.

LOCAL DISEASE CAUSING ORAL LESIONS

Periodontal disease is the most common condition affecting the mouth of the dog and cat, as discussed previously. Other causes are described here.

Infection

Viral Stomatitis. In the cat, both feline rhinotracheitis virus (FVR) and feline calicivirus (FCV) (synonym: feline picornavirus) can cause ulcerative stomatitis and gingivitis (Povey, 1976) (Fig. 55–46). Although FCV is more often responsible, the ulcerative lesions produced by FVR can be severe and extensive. Additional descriptions of these diseases are presented in Chapter 27.

Oral papillomatosis is a specific viral infection discussed under Oral Hyperplastic and Neoplastic Disease. Other viral diseases such as canine distemper or feline panleukopenia may cause stomatitis, although other organs are more severely affected.

Mycotic Infection. Moniliasis (infection with the yeast *Candida albicans*) is a rare cause of severe stomatitis in the dog and cat; it usually occurs in debilitated animals, animals that are immune-depressed, or those that have received long-term antibiotic or corticosteroid therapy. The classic white exudate covering the lesion ("thrush") is sometimes seen, although more often the lesions are irregular ulcerated areas surrounded by a zone of inflamed mucosa (Fig. 55–47). Diagnosis is by fungal culture of the lesion. Further description is presented in Chapter 26.

Oral Hyperplastic and Neoplastic Disease

The most common hyperplastic disease of the oral cavity is gingival hyperplasia caused by periodontal disease (Figs. 55–30 and 55–45). Tumors in the oropharynx of the dog and cat are usually accompanied by some degree of stomatitis, particularly when they enlarge and impinge on normal tissue or are traumatized during mastication. A sickening halitosis caused by bacterial activity in necrotic tissue or by food trapped in crevices is frequently a major reason for presentation of an animal with neoplastic disease. Malignant neoplasms are discussed under Oropharyngeal Neoplasia. The most common benign growths are epulis and oral papillomatosis.

Eosinophilic granuloma lesions may be seen in the palate, fauces, or tongue of cats. Diagnosis is by cytology or biopsy; treatment is as for labial granuloma. A similar condition has been reported as occurring on the tongue or palate of Siberian husky dogs (Fig. 55–49) (Madewell et al., 1980; Potter et al., 1980).

Epulis (Periodontal Fibrous Hyperplasia). Nonulcerated cauliflower-like growths at the gingival margin are frequently seen in the boxer and bulldog and, less commonly, in other breeds (Fig. 55–49). The lesions are not neoplastic, rarely causing clinical signs except when large enough to be damaged by the teeth of the other ipsilateral jaw. Treatment is rarely necessary; excessively large lesions may be removed by surgical excision or electrocautery. The pathology of epulides was reviewed by Dubielzig, Goldschmidt, and Brodey (1979).

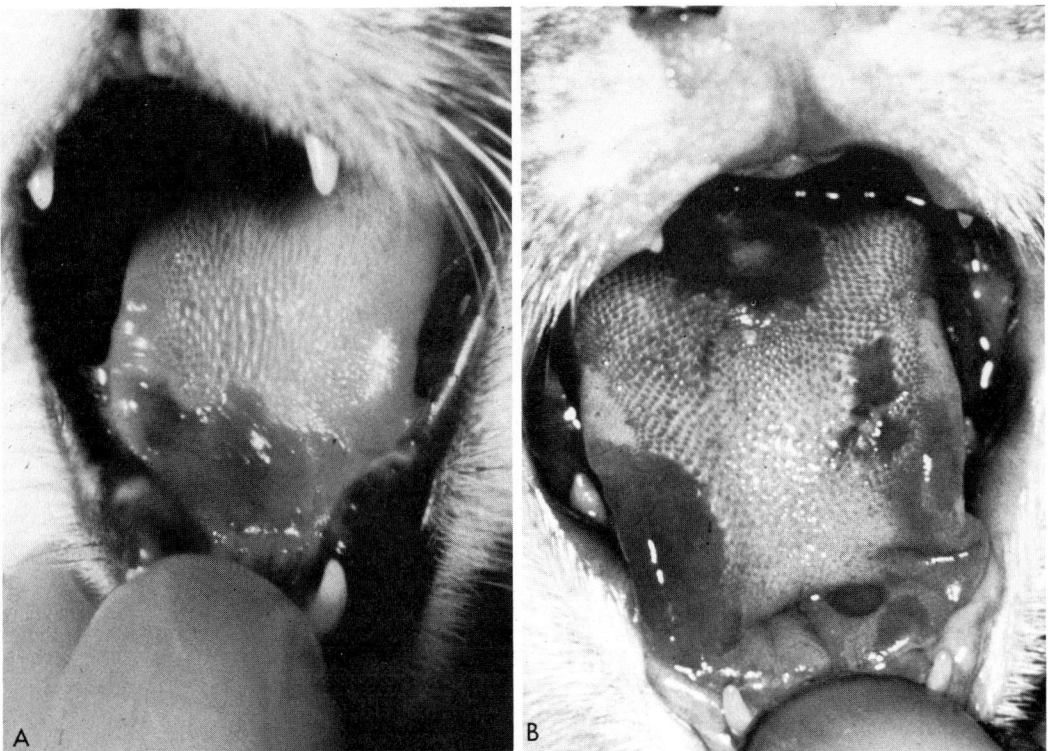

Figure 55–46. *A*, Glossal ulceration in a cat caused by feline calicivirus (FCV) infection. *B*, Severe glossal ulceration in a cat caused by feline viral rhinotracheitis (FVR) infection. (Courtesy of Dr. R. C. Povey.)

Oral Papillomatosis. This is a self-limiting viral disease usually seen in puppies and young dogs, consisting of wartlike growths that develop on the tongue and oral mucous membranes (DeMonbreun and Goodpasture, 1932). Clinical signs depend on the number and location of the lesions. In the severely affected animal there may be

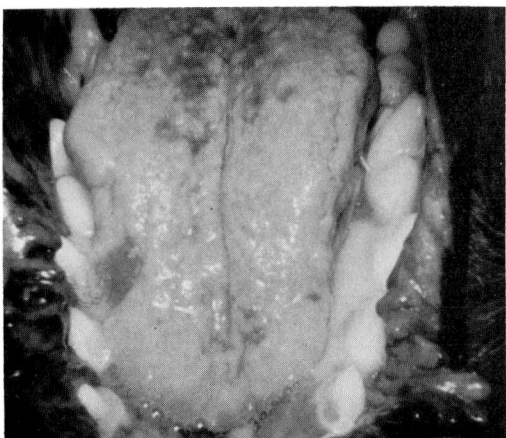

Figure 55–47. Tongue of a dog with moniliasis (*Candida albicans* infection). The tongue is almost completely covered by a thick white exudate.

dysphagia and drooling of saliva. Treatment should be supportive and conservative; definitive treatment is difficult to evaluate, since the disease is self-limiting (disappearing in 6 to 12 weeks). Surgical removal, which may initiate regression, should be reserved for dogs in which mechanical trauma causes injury. Although the disease is known to be viral in origin, the route of transmission is unknown. Immunity is life-long after the disease has been contracted.

Transmissible Venereal Cell Tumors. This tumor affects the mucosa of the genital organs of young, sexually mature animals. Oral lesions occasionally result from the animal's licking of the primary lesion and affect the lips, tongue, gingiva, or cheek. In most instances, these tumors regress spontaneously although occasional metastasis is seen. The tumors appear as lobulated, cauliflower-like sessile masses that are hyperemic and friable. Ulceration and necrosis develop later. The external genitalia should be examined. Surgical removal of lesions causing dysphagia is warranted, and treatment with cytotoxic drugs has been suggested.

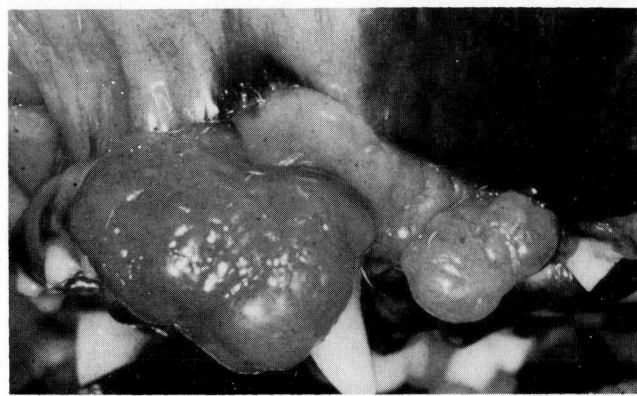

Figure 55–48. Maxilla of a boxer dog with epulis. A large, nonulcerated mass is partially covering the upper canine and several incisor teeth. A smaller epulis lesion is also present caudal to the canine tooth.

Chemical, Thermal, or Electric Burn Injury

Dogs or cats are occasionally presented after ingesting corrosive chemicals or chewing on electric cords. Corrosives damage the oral mucosa upon contact. If the initial communication with the owner is by telephone, he should be instructed to flush the animal's mouth copiously with water to prevent further damage. The active ingredients should be identified from the label, but it is unlikely that specific antidotes can be used early enough to be of value. Vinegar or lemon juice may be used if the chemical is an alkaline caustic (the most common caustics readily available in the home). Acids may be counteracted by sodium bicarbonate solution.

Animals that sustain electric burn injuries of the mouth should be examined carefully for signs of shock or pulmonary edema, and appropriate treatment commenced. Sustained sinus tachycardia is a complication of this problem that should not be overlooked.

Management of local injuries caused by chemical, thermal, or electric burns consists of gentle cleansing of the wounds with isotonic saline solution and careful debridement if the injury is severe. Management of specific injuries of the lips, palate, and tongue is discussed in a following section. Pharyngeal or esophageal scarring following ingestion of a caustic may require long-term steroid or surgical treatment.

Stomatitis of Unknown Origin

Occasionally, animals with severe ulcerative or necrotic stomatitis are seen in which the search for a cause is unrewarding. If the disease does not appear to be confined to or most severe at the periodontal tissues, arbi-

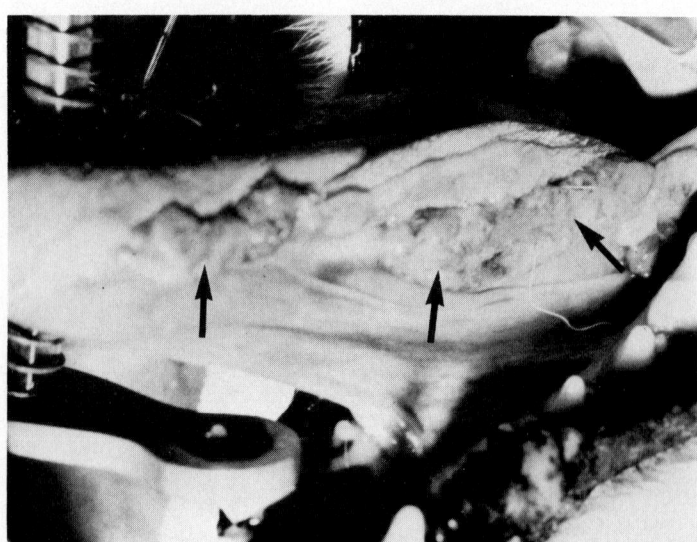

Figure 55–49. Eosinophilic granuloma lesions (arrows) on the tongue of a Siberian husky dog.

trary removal of teeth may worsen the disease. Prolonged, intermittent antibiotic and local therapy gives temporary relief, but signs of disease often reappear shortly after cessation of antibiotic therapy. Metronidazole (30 mg/kg orally once a day) used daily every other week is often helpful. Lesions that appear to consist of persistent, nonhealing granulation tissue may respond to oral prednisolone (1 mg/kg twice daily for two weeks). The use of levamisole as a nonspecific immune stimulant is effective in some cases of recurrent stomatitis in humans (Olson et al., 1976).

Local Therapy in Oral Diseases

In an uncooperative patient, analgesic troches and local gargles are not feasible. Local applications of potassium permanganate and gentian violet solution are time-honored remedies but rarely find client or patient acceptance. Gentle cleansing with cotton-wrapped applicators soaked in isotonic saline or sodium bicarbonate solution is soothing. Solutions of hydrogen peroxide and glycerin are helpful, but these can be used in only the most cooperative patient. An antibiotic-fungicidal agent combination (such as tetracycline–amphotericin B) applied locally three to four times per day may be helpful. A soft diet and rinsing of the mouth with salt solution after feeding reduce pain and bacterial growth in diseased tissue. Occasionally, chemical cautery (silver nitrate or phenol) is indicated for localized, chronic, nonresponsive oral ulceration.

LIPS AND CHEEKS

CONGENITAL ANOMALIES

Harelip occasionally occurs in the dog, often in association with cleft palate (Fig. 55–50) (Howard et al., 1976); repair is rarely attempted because of the ethical considerations of correction of congenital abnormalities. Harelip without associated cleft palate may be midline, bilateral, or unilateral, and rarely results in clinical signs other than the obvious deformity and a slight serous discharge from the nose.

Microcheilia (reduced oral fissure) reportedly occurs, particularly in schnauzers. Contraction of the muscles of the upper lip is seen in setters occasionally (Clifford and Clark, 1965).

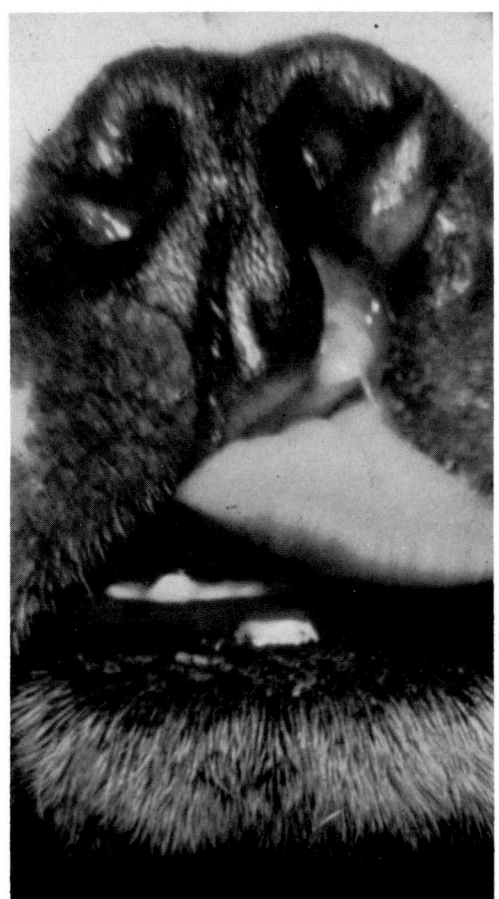

Figure 55–50. Nose and lips of a dog with congenital unilateral harelip.

ACQUIRED DISEASES

Injuries

The most common injuries of the lips are caused by fights or when the animal bites an electric cord. Avulsion of the lower lip from the mandible can result from blunt trauma.

Portions of lip that have been ripped from their normal attachment should be reattached as soon as possible to prevent contraction and fixation of the lip in an abnormal position, particularly in those animals in which the lower lip is separated from the mandible (Fig. 55–51). A wire tension suture looped around the lower canine teeth may be used to retain the avulsed skin in a normal position (Farrow, 1973). Subsequent reconstructive surgery to cover a denuded mandibular symphysis is difficult, because little loose skin is available

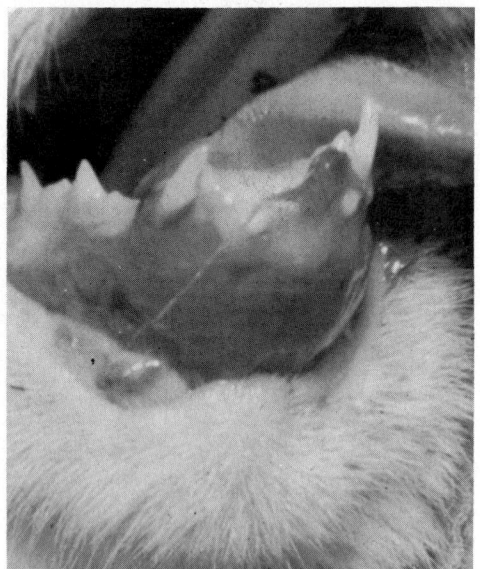

Figure 55–51. Mandible of a cat with an avulsed lower lip.

in the vicinity, which necessitates pedicle or tube grafts.

Electric cord burn injuries affecting the commissure of the lips may require subsequent surgical treatment if sloughing and cicatrization cause reduced jaw movement.

Cheilitis

Lip inflammation may be associated with inflammation of adjacent areas (Fig. 55–52) but rarely warrants treatment other than gentle cleansing. Inflammation caused by

contact with irritants such as plastic or plant material may produce a chronic cheilitis and associated dermatitis.

Firm nodules up to one cm in diameter, which are often multiple, may be felt in the lips of the dog and cat. Usually these nodules are chronically inflamed hair follicles or skin glands, or small abscesses caused by foreign body penetratiion. They may occasionally break open and discharge; treatment is rarely necessary.

Chronic Lip Fold Dermatitis

Spaniels and occasionally other breeds develop a chronic inflammation of the lower lip fold. Saliva runs down the fold, and chronic bacterial infection becomes established.

The clinical signs are a noxious odor, drooling from the lower lip, and pawing at the mouth. Diagnosis is made by inspection of the lip fold, since the odor can cause confusion with periodontal disease or uremic halitosis (Fig. 55–53).

Management consists of frequent gentle washing with an antibacterial soap and water; this is followed by application of an anti-inflammatory steroid cream. Clipping the hair around the lip fold is helpful. Surgical resection of the lip fold is curative in stubborn or recurrent cases.

Labial Granuloma

Labial granuloma (labial ulcer, eosinophilic granuloma) is a chronic granuloma-

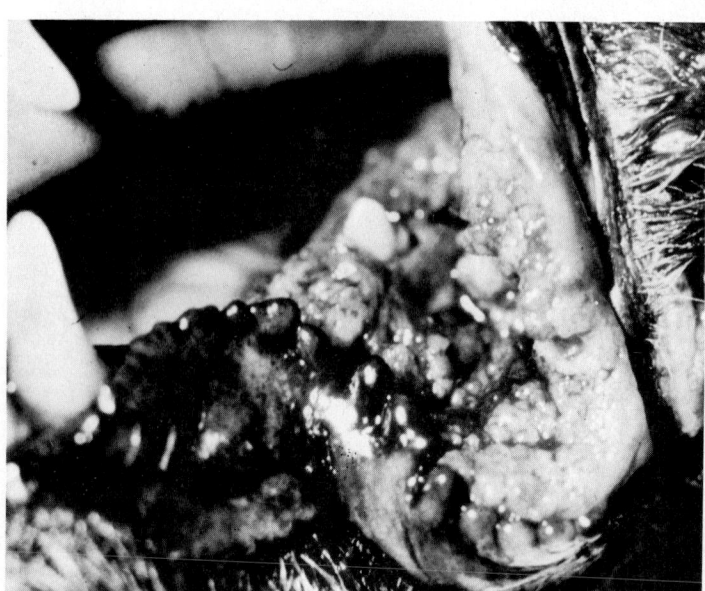

Figure 55–52. Extensive ulcerative and proliferative cheilitis secondary to severe periodontal disease in a dog.

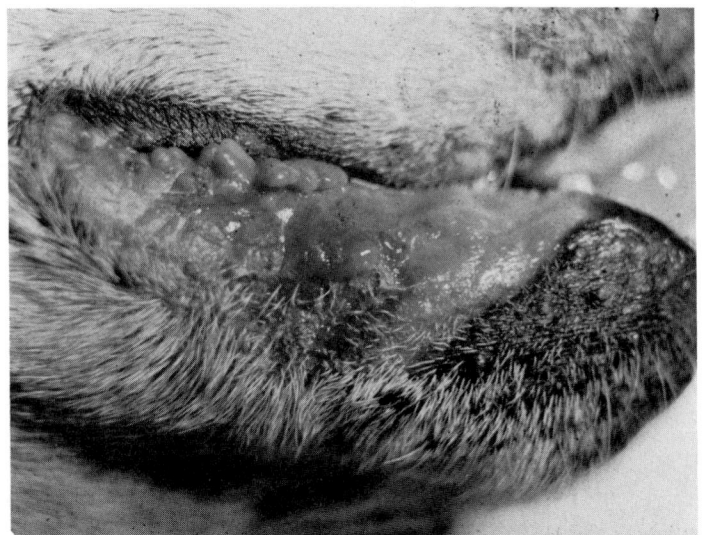

Figure 55–53. Lower lip of a dog with chronic lip-fold dermatitis.

tous lesion of the lip of the cat. The precipitating factor is unknown. Continued licking by the hard spines of the tongue aggravates the condition. The lesion is usually located in the midline or just to one side of the midline of the upper lip (Fig. 55–54). Licking may cause the lesion to spread to other areas, most often the skin of the hind limbs, although the base of the tongue, palate, and fauces of the oral cavity may also be affected. Diagnosis is made by inspection, scraping the lesion, cytologic examination, or biopsy and histopathologic examination.

Currently the most successful methods of treatment are administration of anti-inflammatory steroids and radiation. Steroids can be given systemically (prednisolone, 2 mg/kg divided twice per day and given orally until the lesions have disappeared; the dosage is then tapered off over two weeks), locally (intralesional injection of one to two ml of repository prednisolone), or in combination (Scott, 1975). The effective radiation dosage is 500 to 1000 Rads given as one or two applications (Roenigk, 1971). Alternative treatments that have been reported as successful include megestrol acetate (Ovaban, two to five mg every other day or twice weekly) and cryosurgery (Willemse and Lubberink, 1978). Recurrence is possible with any of these treatment methods.

Occasionally the disease erodes the external nares and part of the nasal bones and septum. Reconstruction following the arrest of the lesion is rarely feasible.

Neoplasms of the Lips and Cheeks

Neoplasms arising from the mucosal surface of the lips and cheeks are discussed under Oropharyngeal Neoplasia. Tumors of the skin and connective tissue of the cheek occasionally occur. Treatment and prognosis are based on histopathologic diagnosis.

TONGUE

CONGENITAL ANOMALIES

Abnormal narrowing of the tongue with inability to swallow has been attributed to a lethal simple recessive autosomal defect in

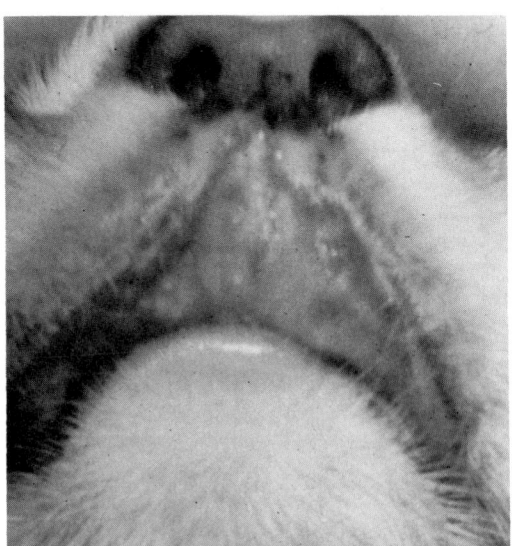

Figure 55–54. Upper lip of a cat with labial granuloma. The upper lip is ulcerated and thickened from the rhinarium to the lip margin.

the dog (Hutt and De Lahunta, 1971). The breed affected was not mentioned in the report. The condition (colloquially known as "bird tongue") causes the death of all affected pups a few days after birth. Lateral protrusion of the tongue has been reported in a King Charles spaniel (Dent, 1952) and was seen by the authors in a Great Pyrenees dog.

ACQUIRED DISEASES

Injuries

The most common tongue injuries are lacerations caused by licking sharp surfaces, ingesting caustics or foreign bodies, and biting electric cords (Figs. 55–55 through 55–57). Clinical signs of lacerations or foreign body penetration of the tongue are lingual swelling, drooling of blood-tinged saliva, and pawing at the mouth.

Clean lacerations should be sutured with surgical gut to control bleeding and appose cut edges. Jagged lacerations may require debridement prior to suturing. Foreign bodies, such as fishhooks, may require incision of the tongue to allow removal. If a piece of wood is embedded in the tongue, a careful check should be made to ensure that all splinters are removed. Animals with burn injuries caused by biting electric cords should be examined for signs of shock or pulmonary edema. The tongue lesion is cleaned and irrigated with isotonic saline, and broad-spectrum antibiotics are administered pending sloughing of necrotic tissue. When the necrotic section has sloughed, the tongue heals by granulation. Dogs manage

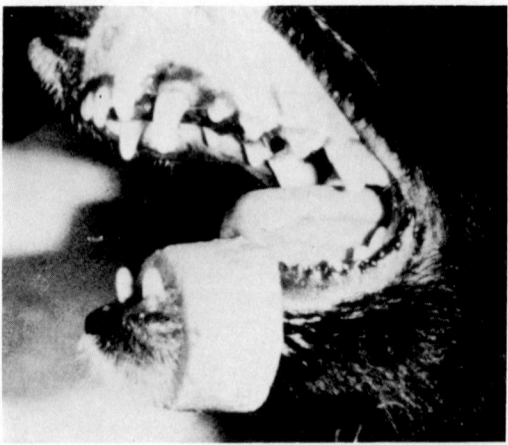

Figure 55–55. Oral foreign body. A section of bovine femur is trapped over the mandible and tongue.

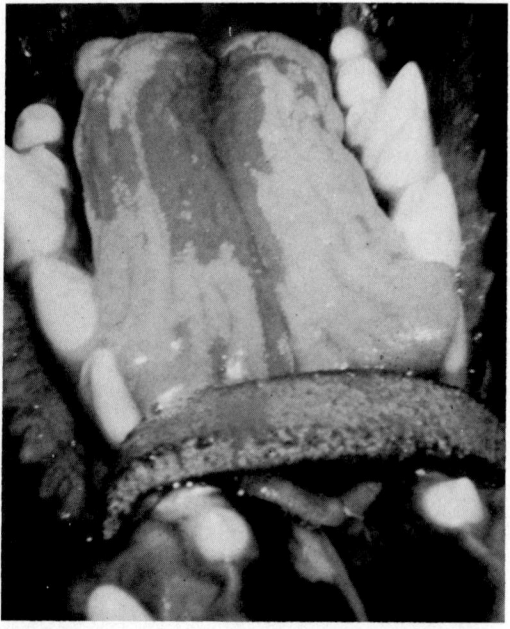

Figure 55–56. Tongue of a dog with superficial ulceration following lye ingestion.

well if the caudal two thirds of the tongue is intact. When more than the rostral third of the tongue sloughs, it is necessary to experiment with various types of food. Meatball-sized pieces that the dog can pick up and toss to the back of his mouth, or canned food mixed with water to a soupy consistency that the dog can suck, may be successful as management. Because of an inability to groom, a cat that has lost most of its tongue may represent a problem because of hair matting or soiling (Stauffer, 1973).

Another cause of injury is a linear foreign body such as string or thread that becomes caught around or beneath the tongue after both ends have been swallowed. The animal moves its tongue constantly trying to remove the offending object, causing the string to saw its way into the frenulum. The animal shows a characteristic head tucked down, tongue-moving posture. A circular foreign body (tracheal rings of food animals or rubber bands) can become caught around the tongue, occasionally causing swelling and subsequent necrosis of the tongue. Foreign bodies around or caught beneath the tongue should be removed; other treatment is usually unncessary. The granulomatous lesion seen in the frenulum caused by an embedded foreign body can be confused with a neoplasm (Fig. 55–58). since this is a classic site for squamous cell carcinoma in the cat.

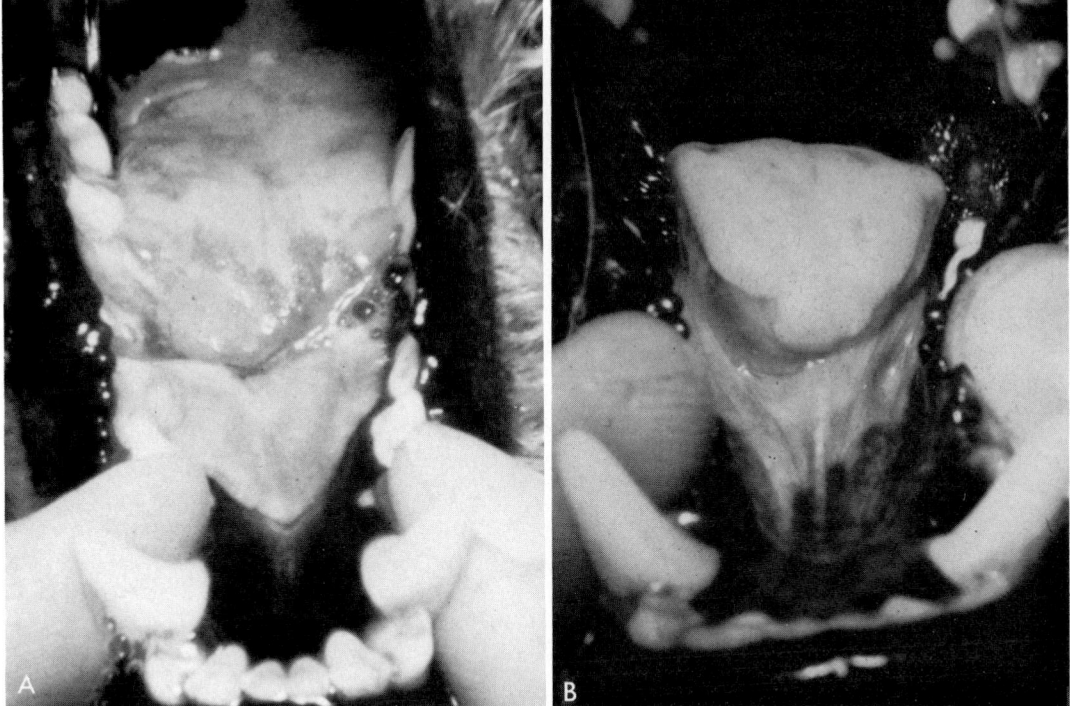

Figure 55–57. *A*, Tongue of a dog one day after biting an electric cord. The necrotic portion of the tongue is clearly demarcated. *B*, Eighteen days following the injury. The tongue is covered by epithelium. The dog was eating and drinking without difficulty.

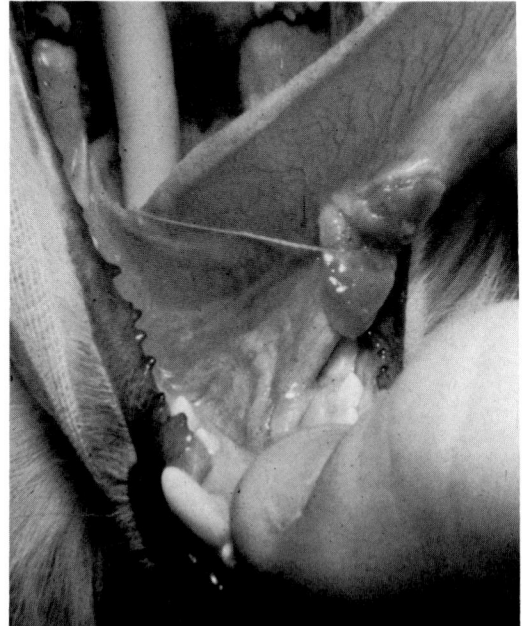

Figure 55–58. Tongue of a dog with thread caught around the tongue. The thread has sawn its way into the lingual frenulum.

Glossitis

Inflammation of the epithelium of the tongue can result from many causes (see Stomatitis). Sloughing of the rostral part of the tongue is seen occasionally in dogs with acute renal failure, pancreatitis, and leptospirosis; the mechanism causing the lesion is unknown. The lesions usually resolve if the primary disease can be corrected. Severe chronic renal failure causes a more intractable glossitis and glossal ulceration. An epizootic glossitis of military dogs in Southeast Asia has been reported; routine techniques for isolation of bacteria and viruses failed to suggest an etiologic agent (Stedham et al., 1973). Chronic exposure to sunlight caused a similar lesion in experimental dogs, both with and without photosensitizing medication to which clinically affected dogs may have been exposed (Jennings et al., 1974).

Occasionally, chronic inflammation of the deeper tissues of the tongue occurs and may be associated with embedded foreign material (Fig. 55–59) or chronic trauma from

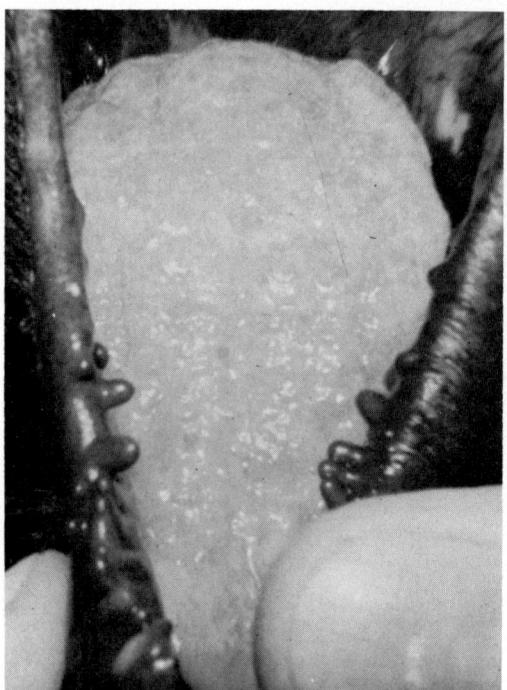

Figure 55–59. Tongue of a dog with glossitis resulting from chewing cockle burrs.

chewing on wood or metal surfaces. Secondary bacterial or fungal infections such as actinobacillosis may be superimposed. Polymyositis, which most often affects the muscles of mastication, occasionally affects the tongue. Calcinosis circumscripta occurs occasionally in the tongue of the dog (Douglas and Kelly, 1966) and has been associated with *Pasteurella multocida* infection (Arnbjerg, 1978).

Rows of hair follicles (either a single midline row or two rows symmetrically arranged to each side of the midline) that contain long fine hairs are occasionally seen as an incidental finding in the tongue of the dog. Rarely, a chronic granulomatous reaction may be associated with inflammation of hair follicles in the base of the tongue.

Lesions similar to labial granuloma of the cat can occasionally affect the tissues on one side of the base of the tongue in the cat or on the lateral edge or sublingual surface of Siberian husky dogs (Fig. 55–49) (Madewell et al., 1980; Potter et al., 1980). Diagnosis and treatment are the same as that for labial granuloma.

Interference with venous drainage caused by an abscess or neoplasm of the floor of the mouth results in edema of the lingual frenulum and sublingual tissue. This may be so severe as to resemble a ranula (salivary mucocele beneath the tongue; see Figure 55–60). Differentiation is based on the gray translucent appearance, retention of pressure marks, the finding of a causative lesion for the edema, and needle aspiration of mucus for the ranula.

Neoplasia of the Tongue

See Oropharyngeal Neoplasia.

DISEASES OF THE PHARYNX

Congenital Anomalies and Injuries

The occurrence, diagnosis, and management of congenital anomalies and injuries of the palate and pharynx are discussed in Chapter 39.

Pharyngitis

Primary pharyngitis is not common in the dog; it is usually part of a more widespread oral or systemic disease. Viral infections of cats can cause palatal ulceration with no other obvious signs of disease, although more frequently there will be sneezing and nasal discharge. Pharyngitis in the cat is usually seen as an increase in the number and size of blood vessels on the surface of the soft palate, although the presence of obvious vessels should not automatically be regarded as indicative of inflammation.

Localized pharyngeal irritation may be

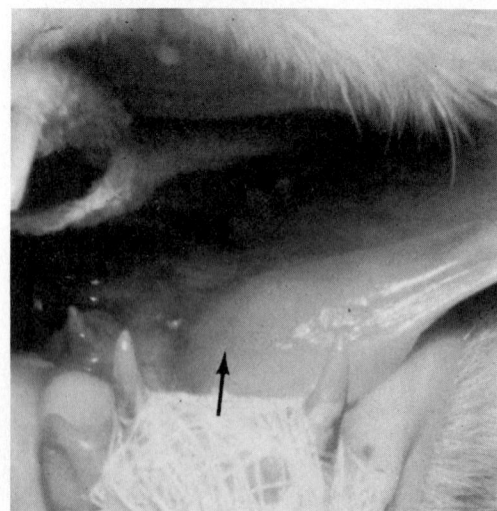

Figure 55–60. Mouth of a cat with abscessation of the lower jaw causing severe edema (arrow) of the sublingual tissues.

caused by a foreign body. Needles, pins, and bone spicules commonly lodge in the sub-epiglottal or pyriform fossa areas and may penetrate and migrate in soft tissue. Radiographic examination (two views) is necessary to pinpoint their location. Surgical removal of the foreign body combined with drainage of the associated abscess is curative.

Dysphagia

Difficulty in swallowing may be caused by localized diseases of the oropharynx and esophagus or by central cranial nerve disease. Clinical signs often associated with dysphagia are drooling, nasal discharge, and cough caused by airway aspiration of food or fluid.

The pain of severe inflammatory disease of the palate, pharynx, or tonsils causes dysphagia. The inflamed mucosa or tonsils are obvious on examination, and the dysphagia recedes as the animal responds to treatment for the inflammatory disease. Infiltrating tumors of the pharyngeal wall, particularly tonsillar squamous cell carcinoma, sometimes present because of dysphagia. Those diseases causing dysphagia that are insidious in onset or show no obvious cause on physical examination are a greater challenge to diagnosis and management (Kiuchi et al., 1969). Several neuromuscular conditions have been recognized in the dog as causing dysphagia; differentiation by fluoroscopic contrast swallowing study has been described by Suter and Watrous (1980). Similar information for the cat is unavailable.

Malfunction of the tongue can be caused by damaged hypoglossal nerves following bulla osteotomy or by sublingual salivary gland removal. Animals can usually manage well if food is provided in the form of meatballs that can be tossed to the back of the mouth.

Glossopharyngeal, vagal, and trigeminal neuropathy can cause a syndrome of dropped jaw, temporal and masseter muscle atrophy, drooling of saliva, and nasal regurgitation of fluid during drinking. The dog gags repeatedly during attempts at swallowing, and food often drops from the mouth. The pattern of dysphagia may suggest a diagnosis; however, careful neurologic examination and fluoroscopic visualization of a barium swallow is necessary to differentiate pharyngeal paralysis from crico-pharyngeal (upper esophageal sphincter) achalasia (described in Chapter 56). The etiology of this pharyngeal paralysis syndrome is unknown. Some animals recover spontaneously; in others, the neural dysfunction is progressive. Other possible causes of chronic dysphagia include temporomandibular joint disease, eosinophilic myositis, and pharyngeal space-occupying lesions or foreign bodies.

Supportive therapy maintains nutrition during the period of dysfunction. Feeding by nasogastric or pharyngostomy tube has been used, although often the owner can feed liquids by a syringe inserted into the buccal fold.

Retropharyngeal Abscess

Pharyngeal abscesses are common in the dog; evidence of external trauma is not usually found. Pins, needles, chicken bones, grass awns, and sticks are frequent causes (Fig. 55–61). Often the foreign body penetrates partially and is then expelled. Clinical signs are pyrexia, anorexia, and pain and swelling of the pharyngeal area (Fig. 55–62). If no foreign body is obvious on inspection and palpation of the mouth and pharynx, a therapeutic trial of systemic antibiotics is warranted. Should clinical signs persist or localized abscess occur, lateral and dorsoventral radiographs of the head should be taken to examine for the presence of a radiopaque foreign body. If a foreign body is seen on radiographs, it should be removed and the abscess drained. If no radiopaque foreign body is present, the abscess

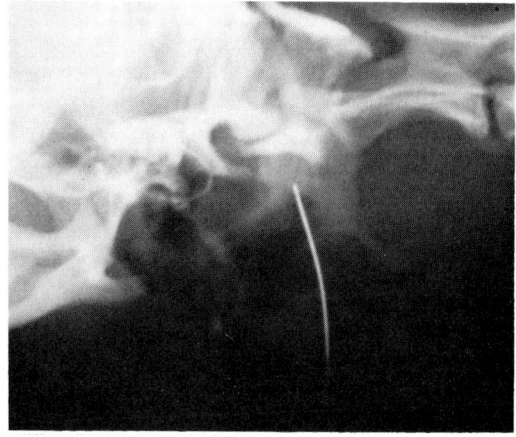

Figure 55–61. A sewing needle embedded in the pharyngeal soft tissues of a cat.

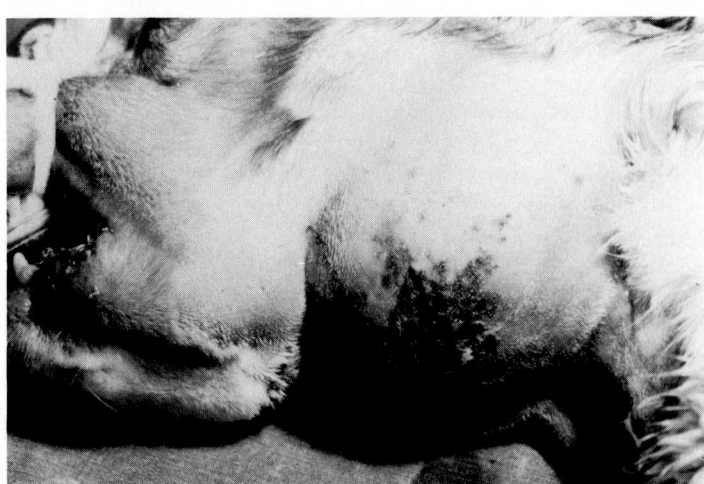

Figure 55–62. Retropharyngeal abscess, with necrosis of overlying skin and extensive edema of the mandibular and facial soft tissues rostral to the abscess.

cavity should be explored with a gloved finger in an effort to locate a nonradiopaque foreign body. A soft rubber drain is sutured in the abscess cavity and systemic antibiotics are continued. The drain is removed three to four days later. Recovery is usually uneventful. If the swelling recurs, the cavity should be laid open surgically and packed with antiseptic-soaked sponges until the wound closes by granulation-contraction.

Tonsillitis

Inflammation of the tonsils is common in the dog and, apparently, less frequent in the cat. Tonsillitis is usually bilateral, but in occasional cases, a foreign body such as a grass awn caught in the tonsillar crypt causes unilateral disease.

Clinically, tonsillitis patients can often be divided into two groups. One group consists of animals with concurrent, preexisting disease considered as predisposing to tonsillitis. Primary diseases causing secondary tonsillitis include those that cause chronic vomiting or regurgitation (megaesophagus, pylorospasm, gastric neoplasia), chronic productive cough (bronchitis or bronchiectasis), or chronic contamination of the nasopharynx (nasal disease causing a nasopharyngeal discharge, cleft palate, dysphagia due to pharyngeal dysfunction). The tonsillitis may be the most obvious clinical finding. Since there are many initiating causes, dogs and cats with a wide range of ages and breeds are affected.

The second group consists of animals with primary tonsillitis. Young, small breed dogs are most frequently affected. The ton-

sils form part of a ring of lymphoid tissue in the oropharynx that reacts to many stimuli. Dogs with primary tonsillitis retch, cough, and show malaise, fever, and inappetence. The clinical signs may be caused by inflammation of the pharyngeal mucosa, with or without tonsillar swelling. Treatment with antibiotics usually results in clinical improvement, although tonsillar swelling is often obvious on reexamination in five to seven days. Lymphocytic hyperplasia with lymphatic infiltration of the overlying epithelium is the most common histologic finding. Chronic or recurrent tonsillitis in young dogs is interpreted as part of the maturation of pharyngeal defense mechanisms (Kutschmann and Schafer, 1975). The most common bacteria associated with tonsillitis in the dog are *Escherichia coli; Staphylococcus aureus* and *S. albus;* hemolytic *Streptococcus*; and *Diplococcus, Proteus,* and *Pseudomonas spp*. (Dimic et al., 1972).

Diagnosis of tonsillitis is made by direct inspection of the tonsils. The owner should be questioned for signs of coexistant disease, which may be triggering the tonsillitis. The appearance of the tonsils in the dog varies considerably and may show little correlation with the animal's condition. Color is a more accurate indication of abnormality than size or prominence. Occasionally, the tonsils may be acutely inflamed but still be contained within the crypt; this is more likely to occur in the cat than in the dog. Acutely inflamed tonsils appear bright red, and inflammation of the surrounding mucosa may be obvious. Punctate hemorrhages may also be seen. Localized abscesses may be visible as white specks on the surface of the tonsil. The tonsil is friable and bleeds easily if touched. Other causes of tonsillar enlargement are squamous cell carcinoma and lymphosarcoma (see Tonsillar Neoplasia).

An inflamed, swollen tonsil is not an absolute indication for treatment. If the animal is showing clinical signs indicating pharyngeal irritation, broad spectrum antibiotics may be administered. Where pharyngeal irritation is severe, mild analgesics may offer relief.

Tonsillitis and pharyngitis may be recurrent in young dogs. Periodic attacks of retching usually cease when the dog matures. Tonsillectomy provides permanent relief from clinical signs caused by chronic, primary tonsillitis but is rarely necessary. General anesthesia and endotracheal intubation are essential. To prevent aspiration of blood, a moist gauze sponge should be placed in the pharynx around the endotracheal tube prior to removal of the tonsillar tissue by scissors or electrocautery. Individual bleeding vessels are ligated, or the edges of the tonsillar crypt are sutured with fine surgical gut. The animal should be allowed to recover slowly from anesthesia to permit further checks for bleeding.

Tonsillectomy is occasionally indicated in mature animals when the enlarged tonsils stand out in their crypts, causing mechanical interference with swallowing or airflow. This is most likely to be seen in dogs with a relatively narrow oropharynx, such as cocker spaniels or St. Bernards, or in dogs with upper airway disease when the superimposed mechanical obstruction due to the tonsillar enlargement may increase airway obstruction.

OROPHARYNGEAL NEOPLASIA

Neoplastic diseases of the mouth are important because of the high incidence (reported as 20/100,000 for the dog and 11/100,000 for the cat by Dorn et al., 1968) and the poor prognosis (Brodey, 1970). Male dogs are more at risk than females (Dorn and Priester, 1976).

The three most common malignant neoplasms of the dog's mouth are fibrosarcoma (Fig. 55–63), malignant melanoma (Fig. 55–64), and squamous cell carcinoma (Fig. 55–65). The clinical features of a series of 361 dogs are summarized in Table 55–2 (Todoroff and Brodey, 1979). The lesions usually appear both proliferative and ul-

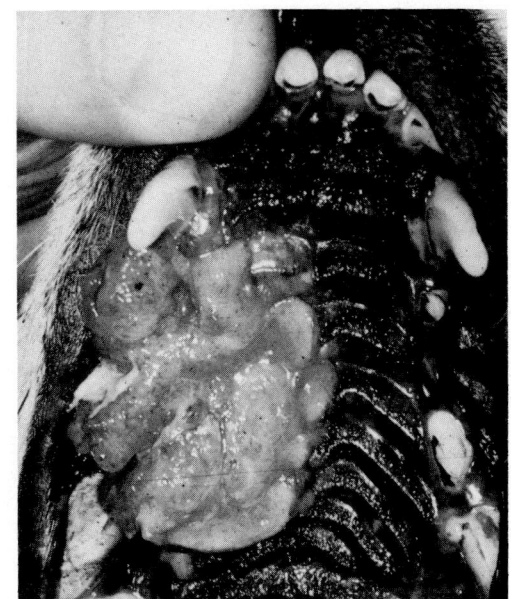

Figure 55–63. Hard palate of a dog with a large fibrosarcoma of the right gingival palate margin.

cerated, although destructive lesions with little tissue proliferation are also seen. Blood-tinged saliva and halitosis are the most common clinical signs. In many cases a diagnosis cannot be made from the gross appearance and position of an oral neoplasm in the dog. Malignant melanoma

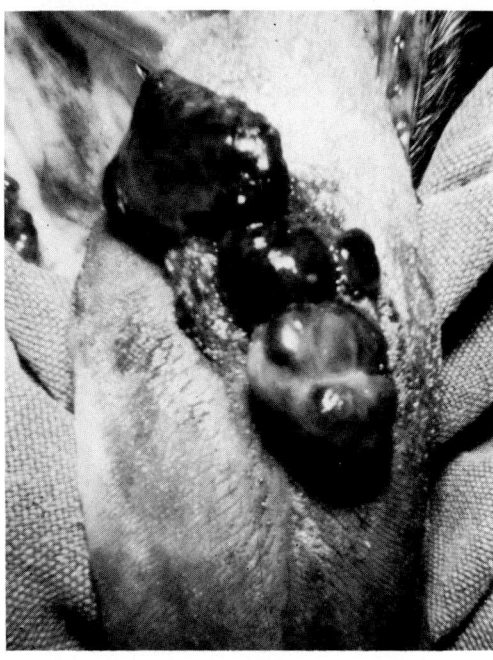

Figure 55–64. Tongue of a dog with melanoma of its dorsal surface.

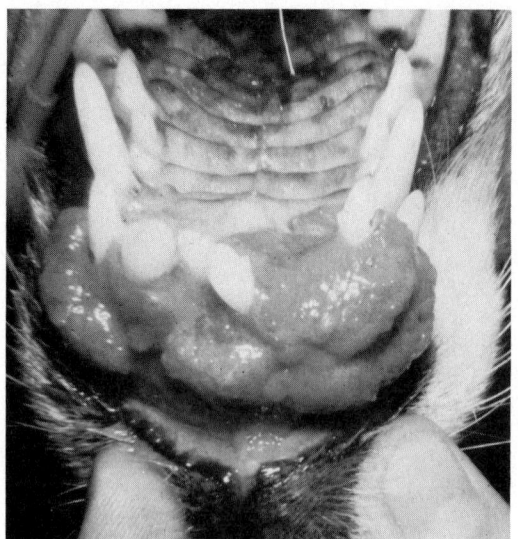

Figure 55–65. Upper jaw of a dog with an extensive squamous cell carcinoma of the incisive gingiva.

(which may be amelanotic) occurs with greater frequency in cocker spaniels, and German shepherd dogs more frequently develop fibrosarcoma than other breeds. In general, malignant oropharyngeal neoplasms occur in old dogs; the exception is fibrosarcoma, which occurs over a wide age range. Local invasion of bone is very frequent.

Because of the poor prognosis for common malignant lesions, confirmation of diagnosis by biopsy and histopathologic ex-

amination is essential. Thoracic radiographs should be examined prior to treatment. The most common oral tumor of the cat is squamous cell carcinoma. The sites most often affected are the gingiva and the tongue, especially in the area of the lingual frenulum. As with dogs, the prognosis is very poor.

Management of Oropharyngeal Neoplasms

After a histopathologic diagnosis has been established, treatment and prognosis should be discussed with the owner. Surgical treatment is rarely practical except as palliation, because malignant melanoma, fibrosarcoma, and squamous cell carcinoma all tend to invade surrounding tissue, including bone, and have a high recurrence rate after conservative surgical treatment. Radical surgical treatment is possible for rostral mandibular lesions; function following partial or complete horizontal ramus hemi-mandibulectomy is excellent. Complex orthopedic restoration techniques are not usually necessary; however, the tongue may tend to hang out of the mouth on the operated side.

Radiation therapy can successfully control some malignant oral soft tissue neoplasms (Fig. 55–66). The prognosis and treatment regimen depend on the type of tumor and its radiosensitivity, the type and tissue dose

Table 55–2. Clinical Features of Malignant Oral Neoplasms in the Dog

	Tonsillar Squamous Cell Carcinoma	Nontonsillar Squamous Cell Carcinoma	Fibrosarcoma	Malignant Melanoma
Age				
mean (years)	10	9	8	11
range (years)	3–17	1–14	6 mos–15	1–17
Male:Female Ratio	1.5:1	1:1	1.8:1	4.2:1
Site				
Lip		8%	4%	21%
Cheek		1%	–	8%
Gingiva		81%*	87%†	55%‡
Palate		1%	8%	11%
Tongue		8%	1%	3%
Tonsils	100%			
Extent of Disease§				
Local Only	23%	18%	65%	15%
Local and regional lymph nodes	35%	40%	12%	15%
Distant metastasis	42%	36%	23%	67%

*Mainly rostral to canine teeth
†Mainly between canine and carnassial teeth
‡Evenly distributed rostrocaudally
§At autopsy
Data from 361 cases seen at the University of Pennsylvania recorded by Todoroff and Brodey (1979)

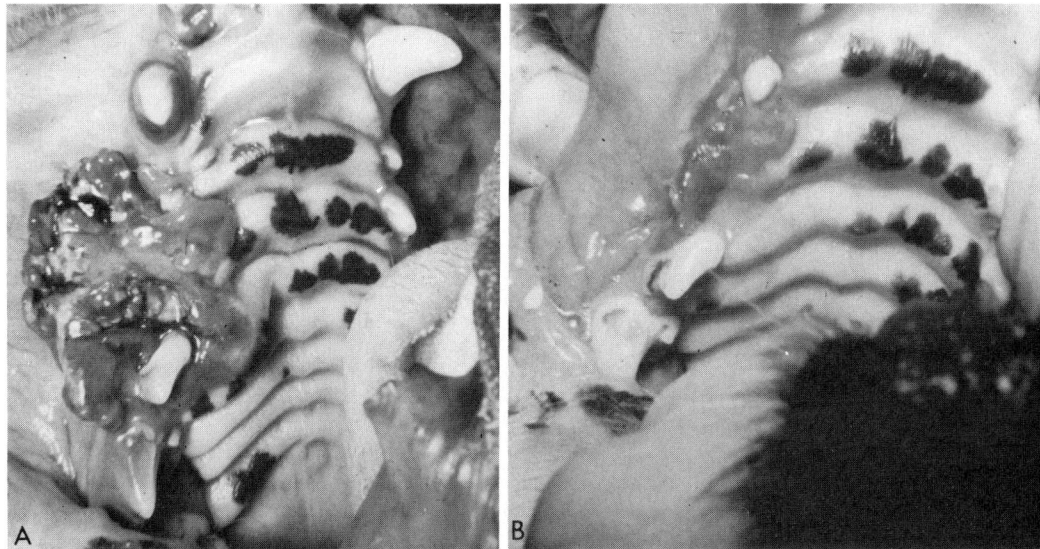

Figure 55–66. *A*, Palate and lip of a dog with undifferentiated sarcoma of the gingiva. *B*, The same lesion five months following radiation therapy (3800 Rads total dose). No recurrence was noted for at least 18 months following initial treatment. (Courtesy of Dr. D. N. Biery.)

of radiation used, and the amount of tumor infiltration of adjacent tissues such as bone. A veterinary radiologist should be consulted and the treatment conducted under his/her supervision. Technique and results are discussed in Chapter 31. Combination therapy (surgery/radiation/chemoimmunotherapy) is likely to produce the most satisfactory results. Several protocols are presently under investigation.

Neoplasia of the Tonsils

The most common tonsillar tumor of the dog and cat is squamous cell carcinoma (Fig. 55–67), a disease of old animals from an urban environment more often than a rural environment (Reif and Cohen 1971). It is usually discovered because of dysphagia or a mass in the retropharyngeal lymph nodes. The tonsillar lesion often appears as a unilateral, irregular, firm ulcerated mass. In most instances, treatment is not attempted because retropharyngeal or mandibular lymph node metastasis is obvious on palpation. Lung metastasis is also frequent (see Table 55–2). Prognosis is poor, even with surgery and radiation therapy in dogs with no visible or palpable metastatic lesions. The diagnosis can be confirmed by biopsy or cytologic examination of a specimen scraped from the surface of the tonsillar lesion. On postmortem examination, the tumor is often found in both tonsils, even if only grossly recognizable in one.

Lymphosarcoma of the tonsil occurs in middle-age or older dogs. The lesions, usually bilateral, appear as symmetric, smooth-surfaced, creamy-pink enlarged tonsils (Fig. 55–68). Treatment of lymphosarcoma is discussed in Chapter 30.

SALIVARY GLANDS

ANATOMY AND PHYSIOLOGY

The major salivary glands of the dog and cat are the paired parotid, mandibular, sub-

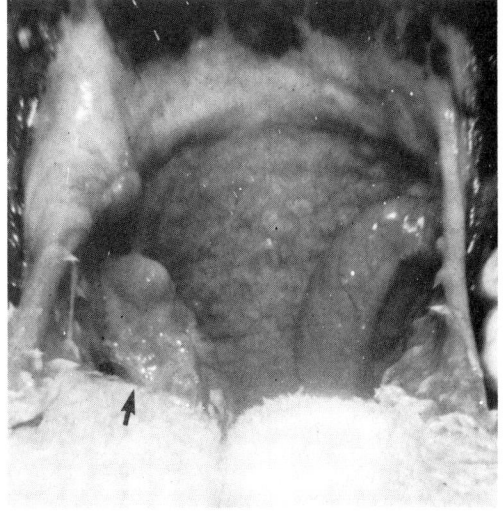

Figure 55–67. Pharynx of a dog with squamous cell carcinoma of the right tonsil (arrow), which is ulcerated and irregular. The left tonsil is enlarged and standing out of its crypt.

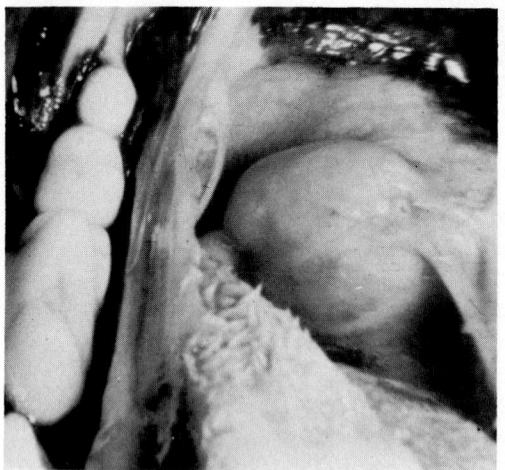

Figure 55-68. Pharynx of a dog with lymphosarcoma of the tonsils. A massive smooth-surfaced left tonsil is obvious. Part of the right tonsil is also visible.

lingual, and zygomatic (infraorbital) glands. The triangular parotid gland is a serous gland located below the horizontal ear canal. It is arranged in small lobules held together by connective tissue, so that the edges of the gland are irregular and poorly defined. The parotid duct runs from a branching collecting system in the gland to a prominent papilla on the mucosal surface of the cheek at the level of the upper carnassial (fourth premolar) tooth. The secretory nerve supply of the parotid gland is carried via the glossopharyngeal nerve and auriculotemporal branch of the trigeminal nerve.

The mandibular gland is a large, compact, ovoid structure lying within a strong fibrous capsule caudal and ventral to the parotid gland beneath the maxillary vein. The mandibular duct runs beside the sublingual gland on the floor of the mouth and opens on the lateral side of the small lingual caruncle at the base of the frenulum. The sublingual gland is divided into several loosely connected lobules that run from the rostral surface of the mandibular gland along the root of the tongue. The sublingual duct accompanies the mandibular duct, opening either on the lingual caruncle just caudal to the mandibular duct opening, or into the mandibular duct, forming a common opening into the mouth (Michel, 1956). The mandibular and sublingual glands are both mixed glands. The zygomatic gland is a mixed gland, irregularly ovoid in shape, and lies on the floor of the orbit ventrocaudal to the eye, medial to the zygomatic arch. Several ducts, of which the most

rostral is the largest, run ventrally and open on a fold of mucosa lateral to the last upper molar tooth. The oral cavity, particularly the cheeks, also contains scattered areas of glandular tissue.

The saliva of the dog and cat has no enzymatic activity of note. Saliva softens and lubricates the passage of food to the stomach but has no other apparent function in digestion. Saliva also functions in moistening the oral mucous membrane, which is of importance for heat loss in the dog: the rate of salivation increases dramatically in the dog as the ambient temperature rises (Blatt et al., 1972).

The role of the salivary glands, particularly the mandibular gland, in the control of blood glucose concentration and diabetes requires further clarification (Godlowski et al., 1971; Lawrence et al., 1976). See Diabetes in the section on Systemic Disease Causing Oral Lesions.

HISTORY AND METHODS OF EXAMINATION

Swelling is the most common sign of diseases of the salivary glands; it may be an accumulation of salivary secretions in an abnormal area or swelling of the salivary gland itself. "Excessive" salivation, or drooling, is usually caused by an animal's inability to swallow normally or by abnormal mouth conformation; rarely, hypersialosis is due to salivary gland abnormality or disease (Kelly et al., 1979; Harvey, 1980). Xerostomia (dry mouth) is uncommon because of the secretory capacity of the four major paired salivary glands, and the multiple minor areas of secretory tissue in the oropharynx.

The parotid and mandibular glands are easily palpable. In a cooperative or sedated animal, the sublingual gland can be palpated in the floor of the mouth, The zygomatic gland, located medial to the zygomatic arch, is not palpable unless grossly enlarged. Salivary gland function and duct patency can be evaluated by placing a drop of topical ophthalmic atropine solution on the tongue. In the normal animal, a copious flow of saliva ensues, particularly from the parotid papilla, from which a stream of saliva may be ejected rhythmically for one or two minutes. Pooling of saliva should also be seen in the floor of the mouth from the mandibular and sublingual glands.

Radiographic examination of the salivary glands and ducts may be performed by injecting a water-soluble radiopaque dye into the duct through a blunt-ended needle (Harvey, 1969). A dose of .25 ml/5 kg body weight of intravenous pyelogram contrast material allows good visualization of the ducts and glands in most dogs. Additional sialograms may be made five to seven minutes following each injection and radio-graph to allow absorption of the dye (Figs. 55–69 through 55–72).

DISEASES OF SALIVARY GLANDS

Drooling

Drooling is most often caused by reluctance or inability to swallow, resulting from

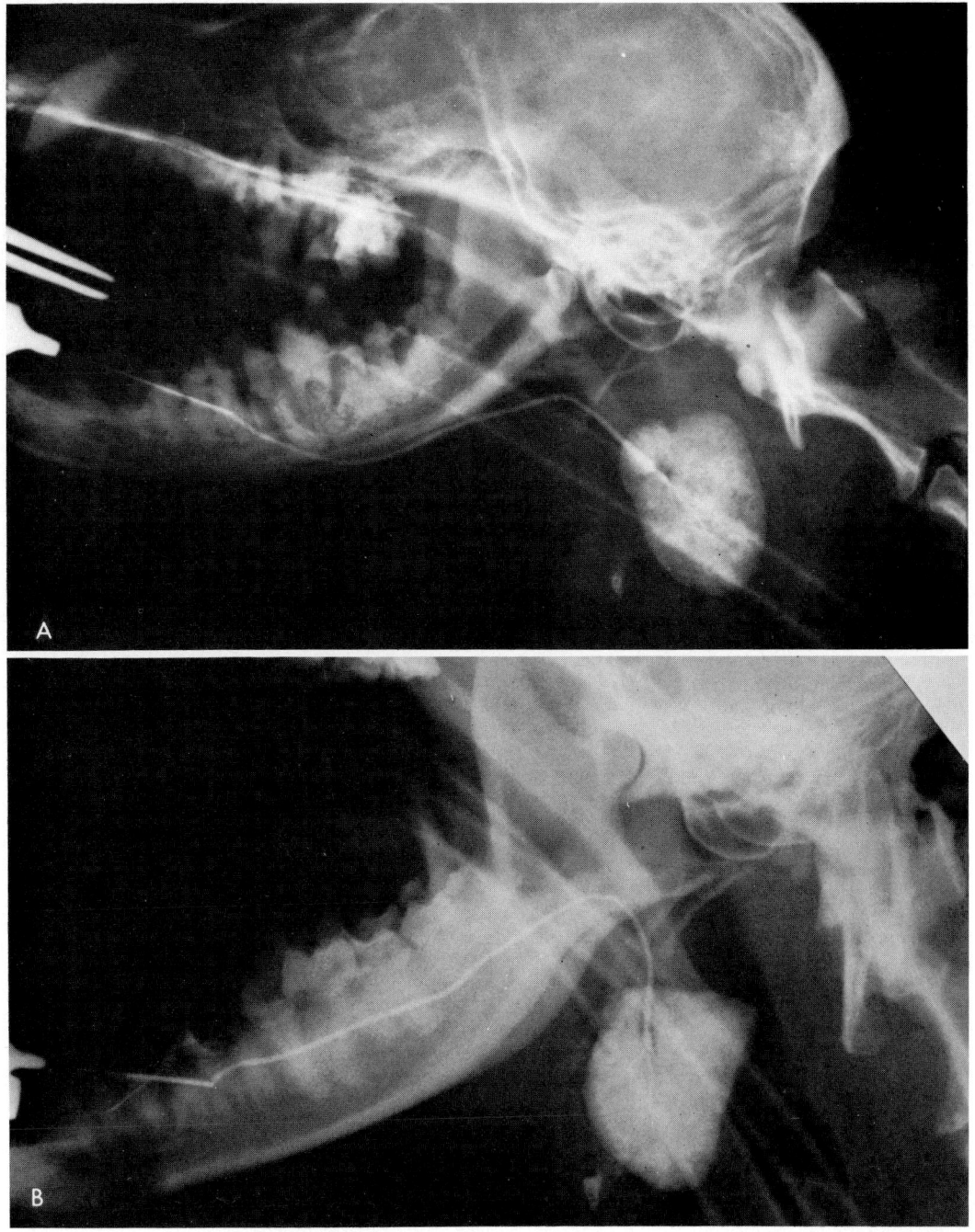

Figure 55–69. *A*, *B*, and *C*, Normal mandibular sialograms of dogs, showing the variation of gland and duct pattern.

Illustration continued on following page

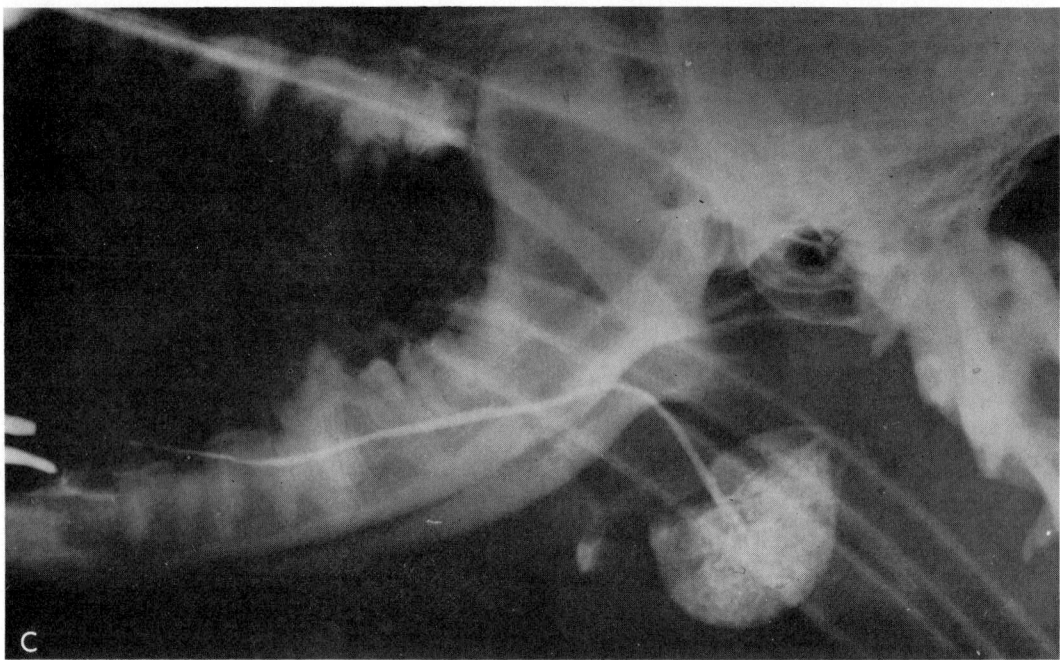

Figure 55–69. *Continued*

diseases causing painful oral or pharyngeal ulcers, and less often from neurologic disease or infiltrating disease of the oropharynx. These conditions can usually be diagnosed from the history and physical examination. Some dogs show constant or intermittent drooling from an early age. The giant breed dogs, particularly St. Bernards, are the worst offenders. These dogs do not have salivary gland abnormalities;

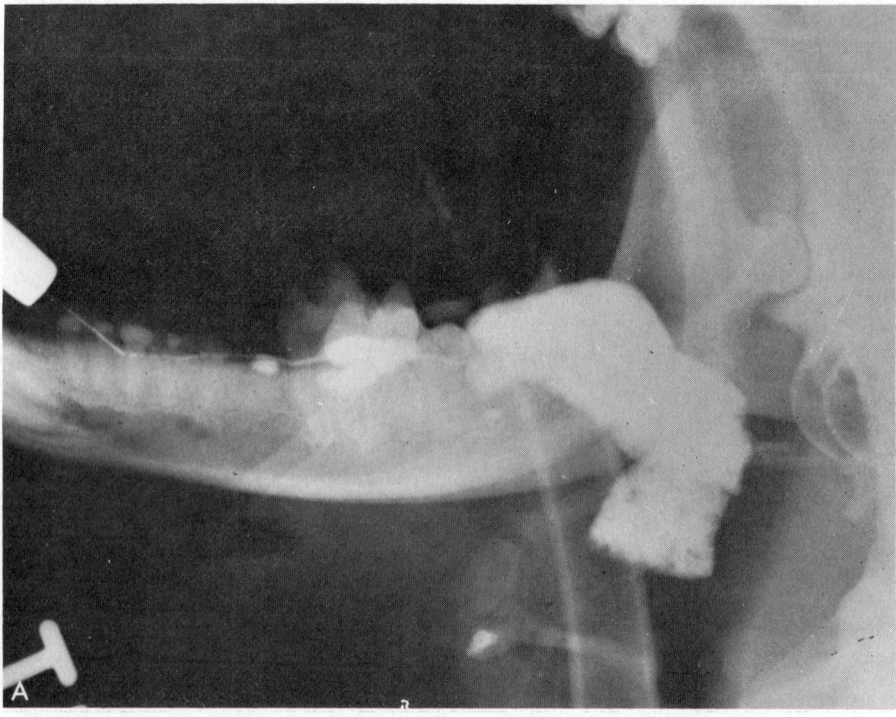

Figure 55–70. *A, B,* and *C,* Normal sublingual sialograms of dogs showing the variation of gland and duct pattern.

Illustration continued on opposite page

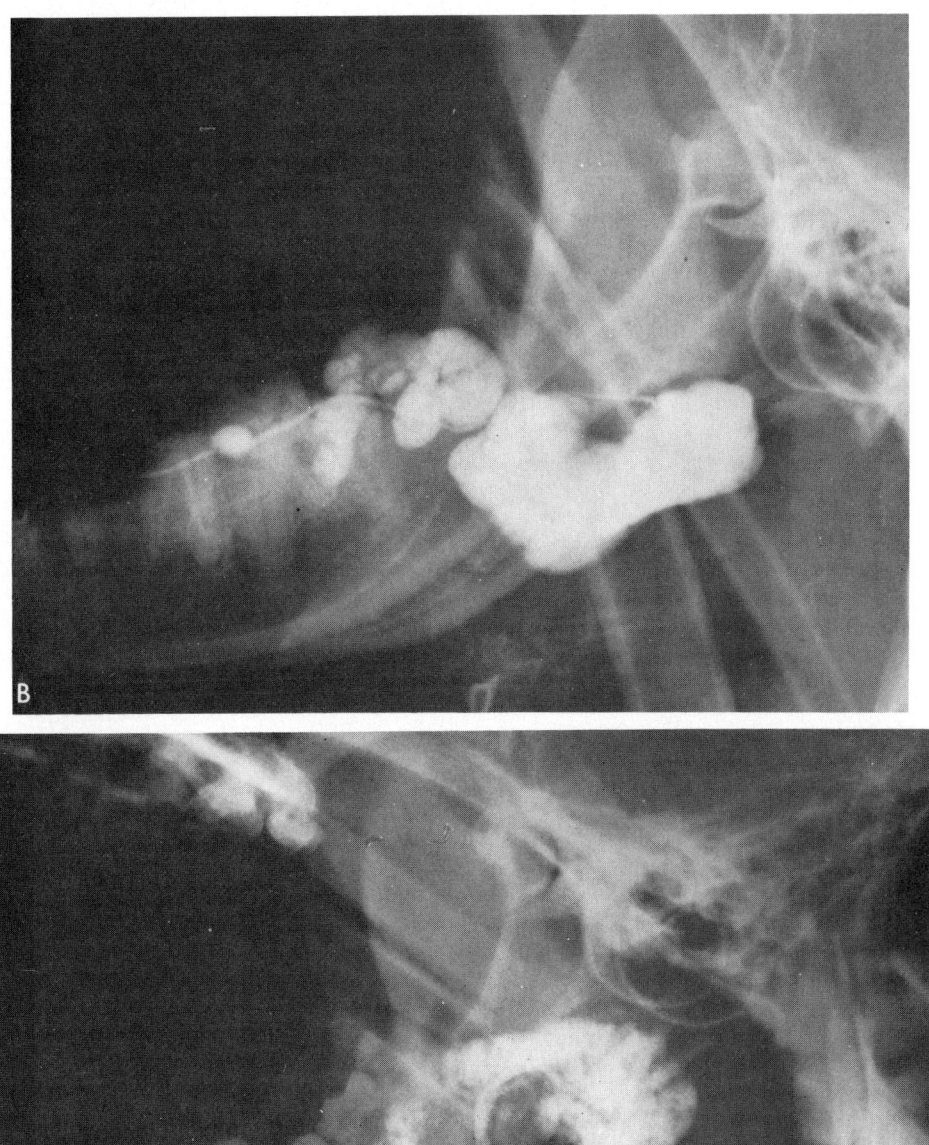

Figure 55-70. *Continued*

rather, the drooling and frothing seen is due to conformational abnormalities of the mouth and lips. Correction of the condition should not be performed on breeding or show animals. Treatment is directed at reducing the volume of saliva produced or rerouting the flow of saliva by surgical reconstruction. If the saliva is mucoid, hanging in ropes from the corners of the mouth, bilateral resection of the mandibular and sublingual salivary glands eliminates most of the excessive salivation. Lip reconstruction

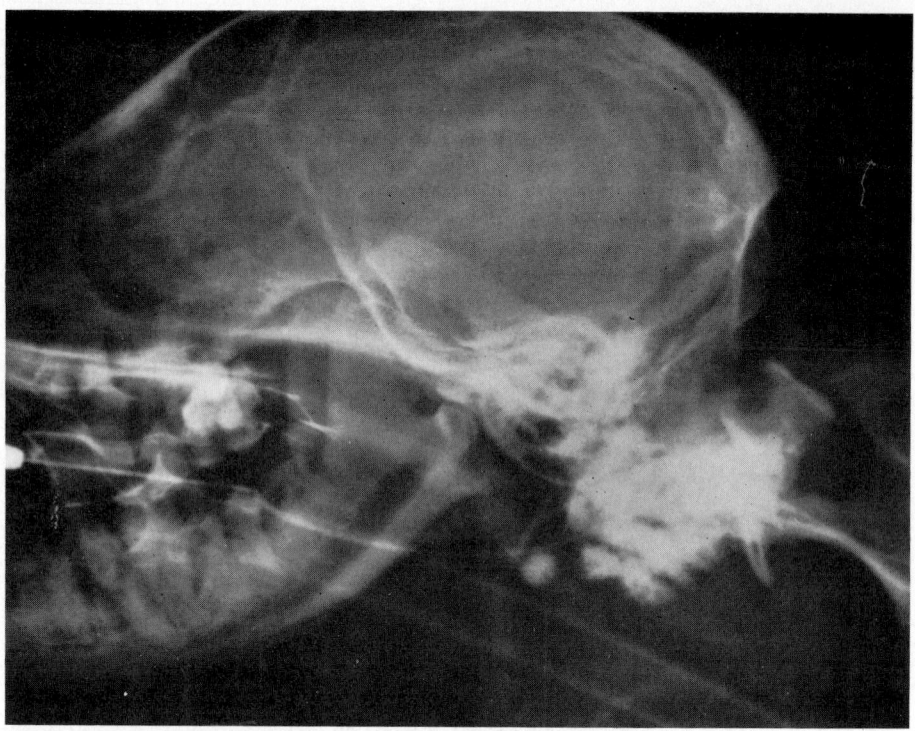

Figure 55–71. Normal parotid sialogram of a dog. There is some leakage of contrast medium around the duct opening.

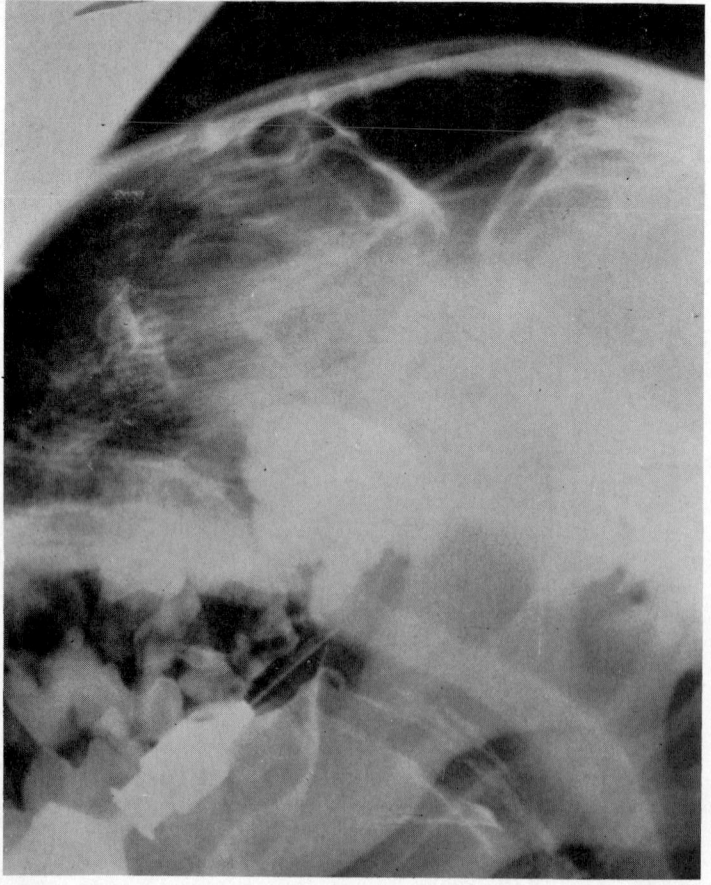

Figure 55–72. Normal zygomatic sialogram of a dog.

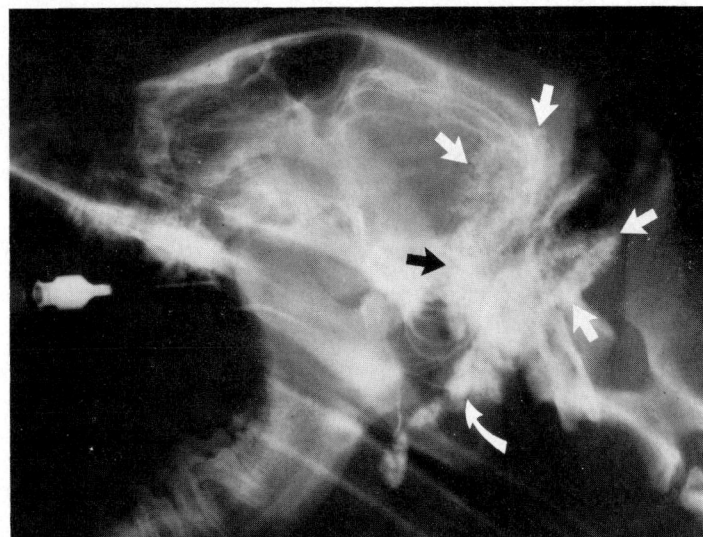

Figure 55–73. Sialogram of a dog with parotid gland enlargement (arrows) and hypersialosis.

to prevent drooling has been described by Stoll (1975). Parotid gland hyperplasia and hypersialosis has been reported in a chow (Fig. 55–73) (Harvey, 1980), and a dachshund (Bedford, 1980), and drooling of saliva was seen in four dogs, three of which were Jack Russell terriers, which were diagnosed as having mandibular gland infarction (Kelly et al., 1979).

Injuries

Injuries of the salivary gland are rarely recognized as acute conditions, and may resolve with no long-term effects in dogs (DeYoung et al., 1978). Salivary fistula or sialocele formation is caused by injury. Foreign bodies and sialoliths are rarely found in the salivary ducts of the dog or cat.

Parotid Gland and Duct Injury. The superficial location of the parotid gland and duct exposes these structures to injury by superficial blows, cuts, or bite wounds of the face. Surgical procedures such as vertical ear canal resection, external ear canal ablation, and treatment of bite wounds or abscesses are potential causes of parotid damage. Another potential cause of parotid duct injury is carnassial abscess or its treatment.

Severance of the parotid duct and a resulting sialocele or fistula are occasionally seen in the dog and cat (see Figs. 55–74 and 55–75) (Harvey, 1977). A previous history of trauma or surgical interference in the cheek is usually available. The fistula leads to a small skin opening oozing a clear serous fluid, which becomes more profuse while the animal is eating. Diagnosis is based on the position of the lesion, type of discharge, and the absence of saliva from the parotid papilla on the appropriate side when a drop of atropine is placed on the tongue.

The object of treatment is to reform or divert the duct or permanently obstruct the parotid flow proximal to the fistula. Parotid duct ligation is simple and effective. The parotid duct is located proximal to the fistula and the duct is ligated with nonabsorbable material, using two or three ligatures, placing the rostral one more tightly than the others so as to spread out the back pressure that follows ligation.

Intermittent blockage of the parotid duct by a carnassial abscess can cause permanent dilation and secondary infection, which result in a constant dribbling of mucopurulent discharge from the parotid papilla. As the condition progresses, the ductules within the gland and, later, the glandular tissue itself become involved. Diagnosis is made from a previous history of carnassial abscess and the appearance of the material milked from the parotid duct. Sialography confirms the dilation of the duct and indicates the extent of the disease (Fig. 55–76). Flushing the duct and installation of antibiotics provide temporary relief from signs of disease. After the carnassial abscess is treated, acute cases may require no further treatment. Ligation of the duct proximal to the dilation is the preferred treatment of dogs, with chronic disease limited to the main

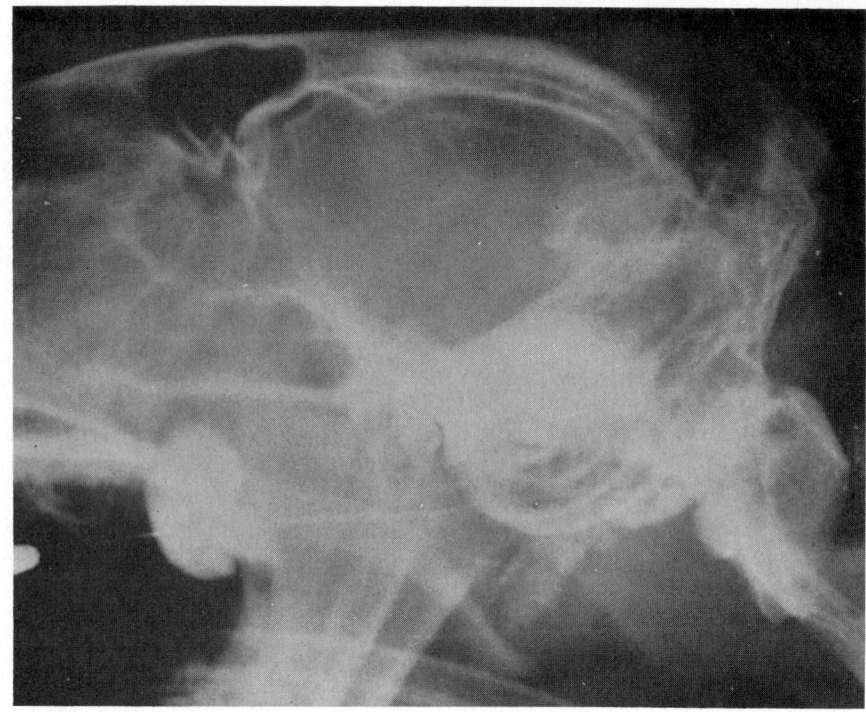

Figure 55–74. Parotid sialogram of a cat with a parotid sialocele following surgical treatment of a superficial abscess. The parotid duct and gland are poorly filled.

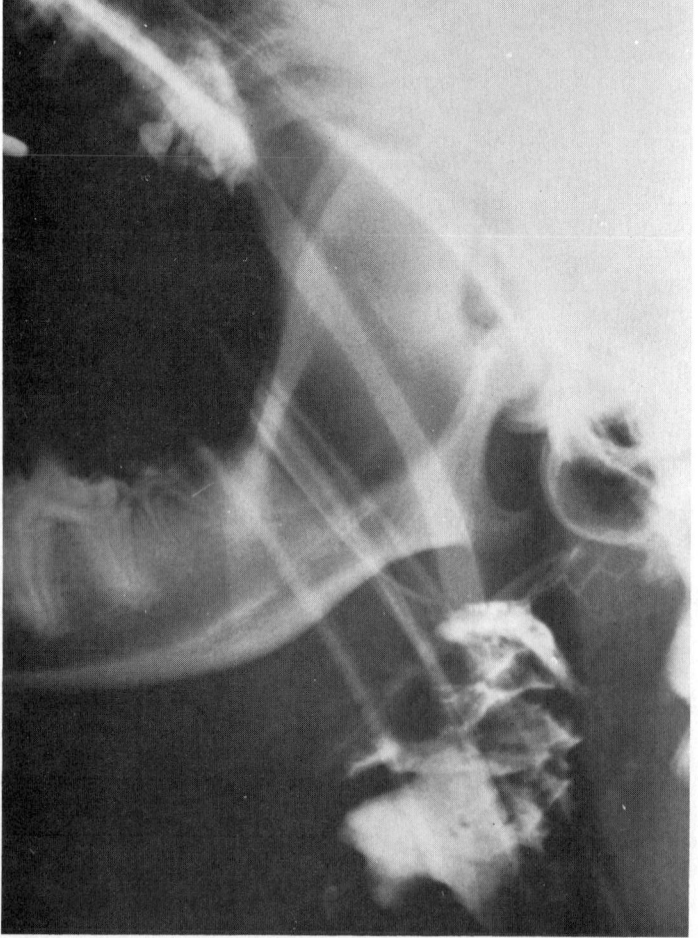

Figure 55–75. Parotid sialogram of a dog with a traumatic parotid fistula. The contrast material is leaking from the duct ventral to the tympanic bullae.

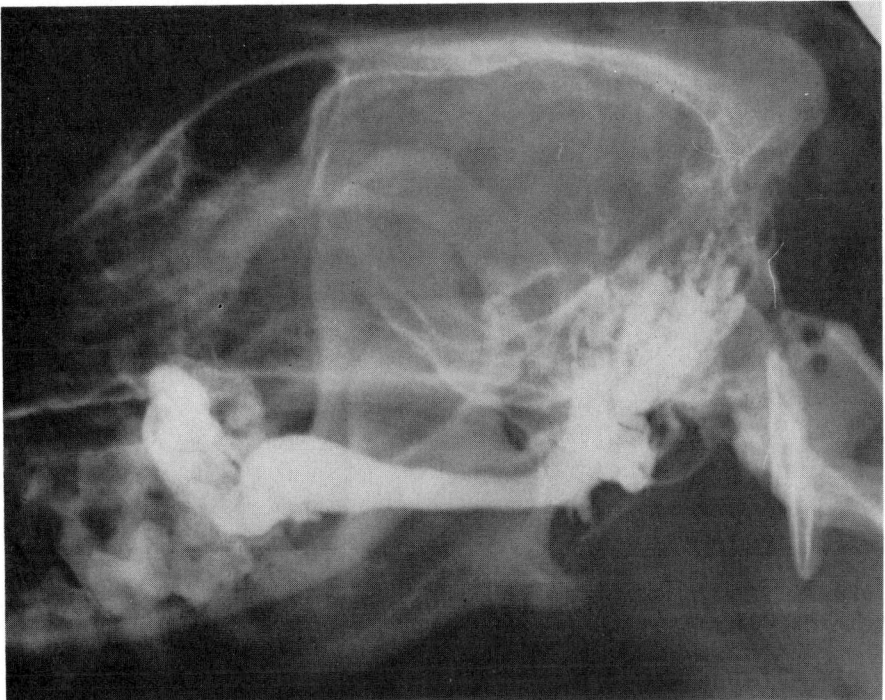

Figure 55–76. Parotid sialogram of a dog with parotid duct dilation following a carnassial tooth abscess.

parotid duct. Parotidectomy is the definitive treatment for intraglandular angiectasis.

Mandibular Gland and Duct Injury. Because the mandibular gland is contained within a firm fibrous capsule, long-term effects of trauma to this gland in the dog are rare (DeYoung et al., 1978). The mandibular duct is larger and thicker-walled than the accompanying sublingual duct.

Sublingual Gland and Duct Injury: Salivary Mucocele

Clinically, the most common condition of the salivary glands in the dog is salivary mucocele. The sublingual gland is most frequently involved. A salivary mucocele is a collection of salivary gland mucus in a nonepithelium-lined swelling. After damage to the salivary gland or duct, saliva leaks out and follows the path of least resistance. The most frequent sites for collection of the extravasated saliva are sublingual tissues on the floor of the mouth on one side of the tongue and the superficial connective tissues of the intermandibular or cranial cervical area. A less common site is the pharyngeal wall. The cause of the gland or duct damage is rarely known. Occasionally, a foreign body is found penetrating the gland in a dog with a mucocele; blunt trauma caused by sticks or bones that may be rammed into the mandible by chewing, squeezing the sublingual gland between, is another possible cause. Poodles and German shepherds have been reported as more frequently affected than other breeds (Knecht and Phares, 1971; Harvey, 1971). Harrison and Garret (1975) produced mucoceles in 12 of 27 cats by ligating the sublingual duct.

Clinical signs of a salivary mucocele depend on the position of the mucocele. A large sublingual swelling (commonly known as a ranula) is likely to be damaged by the teeth; this pushes the tongue to the opposite side, causing reluctance to eat and blood-tinged saliva. Usually the owner will have observed the lesion. A mucocele in the pharyngeal wall obstructs swallowing and respiration as it encroaches on the pharyngeal lumen.

A cervical salivary mucocele may commence with an acute period when the swelling is firm and somewhat painful; this is followed by reduction in swelling as the initial inflammatory reaction subsides. However, gradual enlargement of a soft, nonpainful mass is the most common presenting complaint.

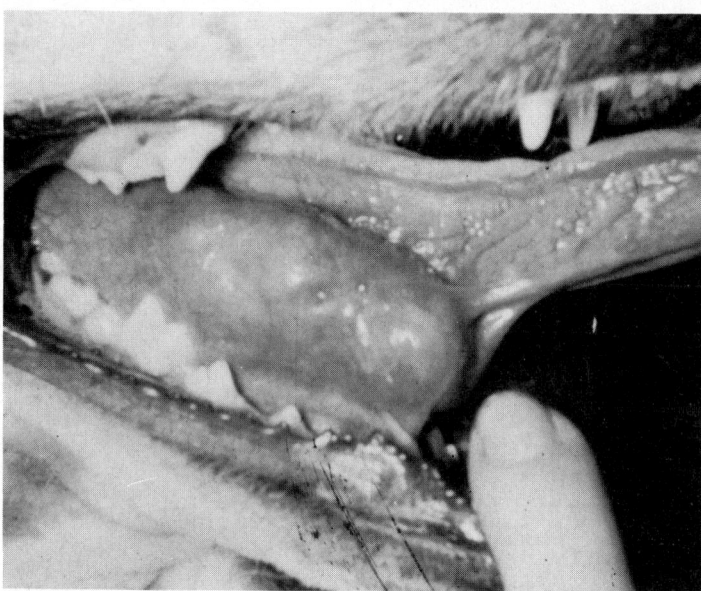

Figure 55-77. Mouth of a dog with a ranula (mucocele of the sublingual tissues).

Diagnosis of a salivary mucocele is based on palpation and aspiration of the mass, which may require sedation or anesthesia for a ranula or pharyngeal mucocele (Figs. 55–77 and 55–78). The material obtained by aspiration is clear or blood-tinged mucus. Some chronic cervical mucoceles contain nodules that are free within the swelling and that resemble calculi; these are folds of the inflammatory lining sloughed into the cavity. Confirmatory tests other than aspiration are rarely needed, because there are few instances of mucus-containing nonsalivary cysts in the pharyngeal area of the dog. Although sialography confirms salivary gland or duct leakage, it is more often used as an adjunct to management (Figs. 55–79 and 55–80). Histopathologic examination demonstrates the nonepithelial, nonsecretory nature of the wall of the cavity. The most common lesion with which salivary mucocele can be confused is retropharyngeal abscess. A chronic pharyngeal foreign body "abscess" may be sterile, and the fluid is serosanguineous.

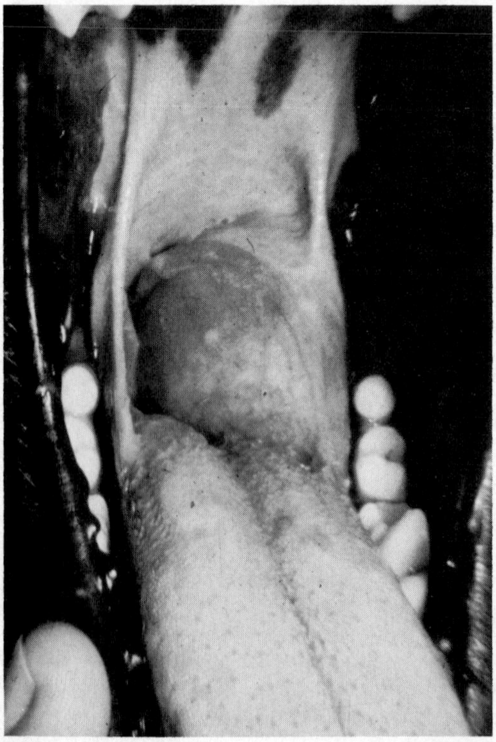

Management of Salivary Mucocele. A cervical salivary mucocele causes little problem to the dog after the initial inflammatory reaction has subsided, unless the mucocele becomes large enough to cause physical discomfort. Occasionally, salivary mucoceles will not recur after aspiration, presumably because scar tissue has sealed the gland or duct defect. Periodic aspiration as needed (usually every three to four months) to empty the mucocele may be sufficient treatment, particularly in an animal that is a poor surgical risk. Ranula (due to biting of the swelling) and pharyngeal mucocele (because of dysphagia or airway obstruction) can cause more severe problems.

Ranula can be treated by marsupialization, which is the creation of a fistula from

Figure 55-78. Pharynx of a dog with a pharyngeal mucocele of the left side.

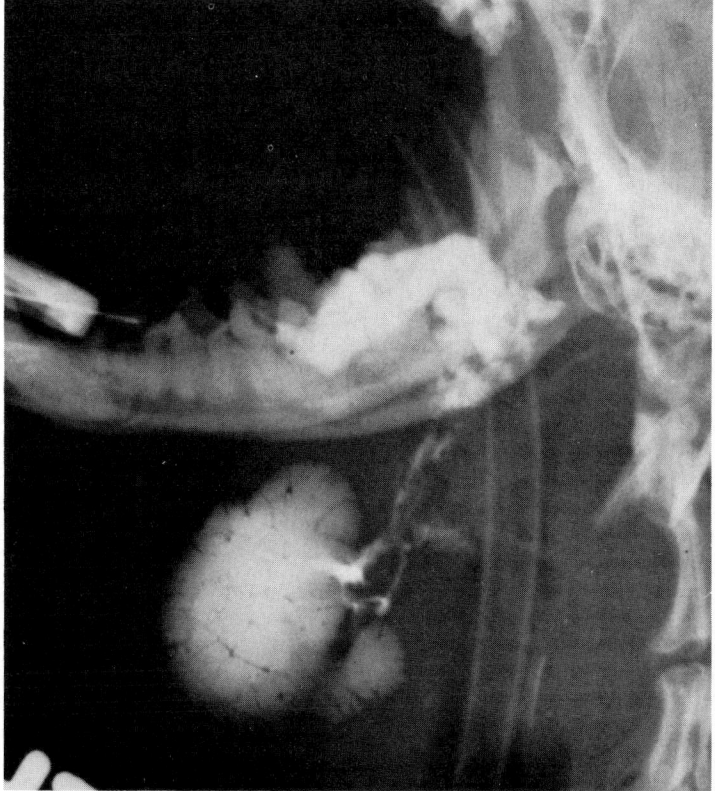

Figure 55–79. Sublingual sialogram of a dog with a salivary mucocele. The sublingual gland and mucocele are clearly visible.

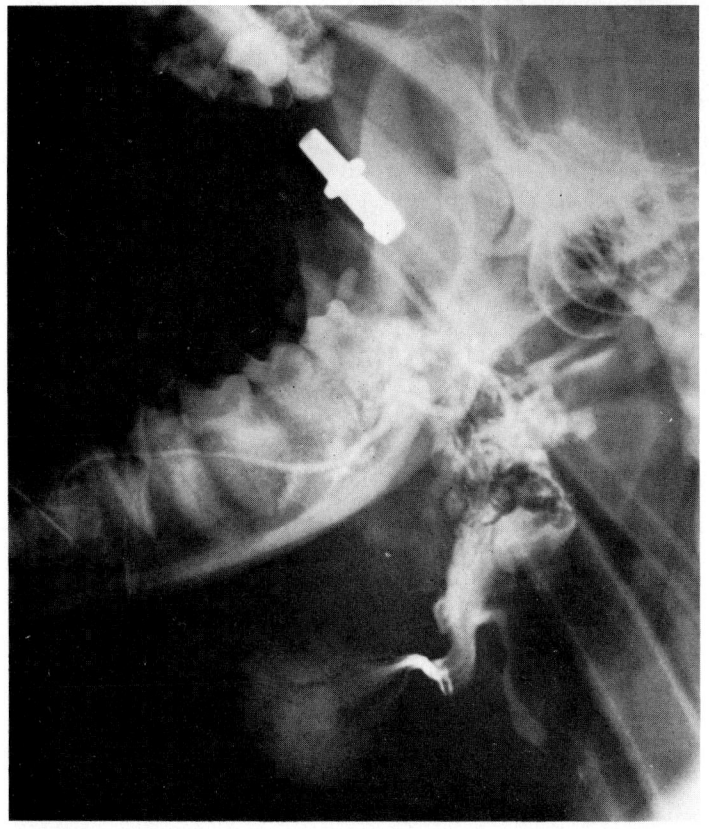

Figure 55–80. Sublingual sialogram of a dog with a salivary mucocele. The sublingual gland is not well outlined, although the area of leakage and mucocele are clearly visible.

the mucocele to the oral cavity. A section of the mucocele wall is removed with a scalpel or scissors. The inner cell layer of a ranula, as for any mucocele, is composed of inflammatory or connective tissue cells (fibroblasts or fibrocytes) except near the site of the original trauma, where there may be some overgrowth of duct or glandular epithelium. Because of the lack of an epithelial lining, there is little point in suturing the oral mucosa to the mucocele inner lining, and recurrence following marsupialization is frequent. Prescott (1968) has suggested the use of stainless steel sutures to maintain the patency of the fistula. Ranula can be treated satisfactorily by mandibular-sublingual gland removal.

A pharyngeal mucocele may present as an emergency because of airway obstruction. Needle aspiration alleviates such an obstruction temporarily. Marsupialization may be used, but a more satisfactory treatment to prevent recurrence is mandibular-sublingual salivary gland removal.

Resection of a cervical salivary mucocele is tedious. Recurrence is likely as the mucocele is merely the effect of damage to the sublingual gland or duct. Definitive treatment of cervical salivary mucocele is removal of the damaged salivary gland and drainage of the mucocele. Resection of redundant skin is rarely necessary. The gland most frequently affected is the sublingual gland. It is impractical to remove the sublingual gland without removing the mandibular gland because of the close apposition of the two. The glands are often spoken of as the mandibular-sublingual gland complex. Generally, it is obvious from the history or physical examination which side is involved. In instances where this is not the case, palpation and observation with the dog in dorsal recumbency under anesthesia may prove helpful. Sialography can determine the side involved, or the mandibular-sublingual gland complex can be removed from both sides. Mandibular and sublingual salivary gland resection has been described in detail elsewhere (Harvey, 1975). Following salivary gland removal, the mucocele is drained. When surgery has been performed and a mucocele recurs, the rostral part of the sublingual gland may not have been removed. Sialography delineates the remaining glandular tissue. The rostral part of the sublingual gland can be removed through an incision in the oral mucosa between the root of the tongue and the vertical ramus of the mandible. Salivary gland removal successfully prevents recurrence of the mucocele (Harvey, 1969; Glen, 1972).

Sublingual salivary mucocele in the cat has been described by Wallace et al. (1972). Treatment by mandibular and sublingual salivary gland removal was successful.

Zygomatic salivary cyst caused by trauma to the head of a dog has been described by Knecht et al. (1969) and has been seen on occasion by the authors. The presenting clinical sign is exophthalmos. Zygomatic salivary gland resection via zygomatic arch resection is curative.

Inflammatory Diseases of the Salivary Glands

Sialadenitis is rare in the dog and cat as a distinct clinical entity. Mild focal inflammatory changes are common incidental findings in salivary glands of dogs (Kelly et al., 1979). Parotid or mandibular gland swelling is occasionally recognized as part of a regional or systemic disease such as distemper. Swelling of the parotid and mandibular glands in dogs and cats associated with the paramyxovirus causing mumps in man was reviewed briefly by Chandler (1975).

Abscesses of the head and neck may involve the salivary glands. A syndrome of pyrexia, pain on opening the jaws, inflammation of the oral tissues lateral to the last upper molar tooth, and exophthalmos has been referred to as an abscess of the zygomatic salivary gland, although the condition is more likely to be a retrobulbar abscess secondary to a penetrating foreign body (Fig. 55–81). Treatment by draining the abscess through an incision in the inflamed oral mucosa combined with systemic antibiotics is effective.

Salivary Gland Neoplasia

Tumors of the salivary glands of the dog and cat are uncommon. The glands most often involved are the mandibular and parotid glands (Karbe and Schiefer, 1967; Head, 1976). The usual tumor type is adenocarcinoma. Affected animals are old (average age 10 to 12 years) and usually presented because of a slowly developing mass noted by the owner. Resection of the involved gland is curative for mandibular gland lesions if metastasis to the local lymph

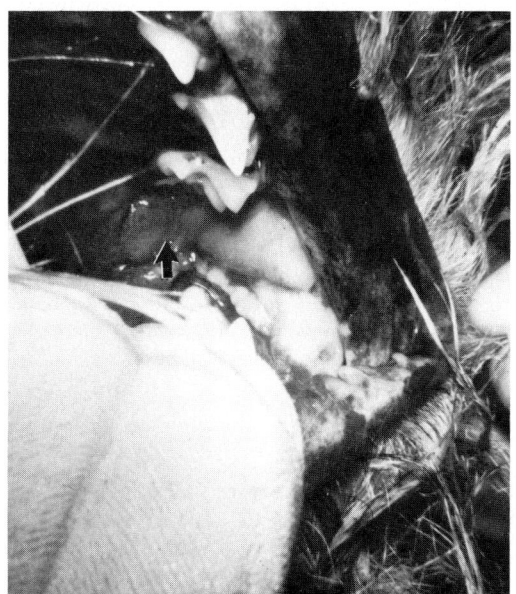

Figure 55–81. Mouth of a dog with a retrobulbar (zygomatic) abscess. The area of swollen, reddened oral mucosa is indicated by the arrow.

nodes or lungs has not occurred. Parotid gland lesions are more difficult to treat surgically because of the diffuse nature of the parotid gland and the many nerves and vessels that run close by or through the gland.

Tumors of the zygomatic gland occur occasionally, presenting with exophthalmos (Buyukmihci et al., 1975). A surgical ap-proach through the zygomatic arch allows resection of the zygomatic gland (Knecht, 1969; Harvey, 1977).

SUPERFICIAL MASSES IN THE PHARYNGEAL AREA

Animals are frequently presented with swellings in the pharyngeal area. The usual causes are retropharyngeal abscess and sali-vary mucocele. Other causes are lymphade-nopathy (primary lymphatic, metastatic, or benign) and tumors of the skin, thyroid glands, salivary glands, or carotid body.

Of less importance because of their rarity in the dog and cat are lesions such as bran-chial cleft and thyroglossal duct cysts (Karbe, 1965). In the dog, slowly developing mucus containing swellings of the pharyn-geal area should be considered as salivary in origin unless proved otherwise by histologic examination of the wall of the swelling. The rare, true branchial cyst in the dog can be satisfactorily treated by complete excision of the cyst (Karbe and Nielsen, 1965).

The role of radiology in the diagnosis of swellings in the oral and pharyngeal area was reviewed by Lee (1974). Foreign bodies and neoplastic infiltration of bone may be diagnosed radiographically. In other condi-tions, radiographs confirm the presence of the mass but are not usually helpful in differentiation of the cause.

REFERENCES

Amsterdam, A.: Periodontal prothesis. Alpha Omegan 67:9–52, 1974.

Annis, J. R.: Tooth extraction. *In* Archibald, J. (ed.): Canine Surgery. Am. Vet. Pub., Inc., Santa Barbara, 1974, p. 323.

Arnall, L.: Some aspects of dental development in the dog. Some common variations in dentition. J. Small Anim. Pract. 2:195–201, 1961.

Arnbjerg, J.: *Pasteurella multocida* from canine and feline teeth, with a case report of glossitis calcinosa in a dog caused by *P. multocida*. Nord. Vet. Med. 30:324–332, 1978.

Barrett, R. E., Post, J. E., and Schultz, R. D.: Chronic relapsing stomatitis in a cat associated with feline leukemia virus infection. Feline Pract. 5:34–38, 1975.

Bedford, P. G. C.: Unilateral parotid hypersialation in a dachshund. Vet. Rec. 107:557–558, 1980.

Bedford, P. G. C.: A repair technique for dental abrasion in the dog. Vet. Rec. 101:327, 1977.

Bender, I. B., and Seltzer, S.: The Dental Pulp. 2nd ed. J. B. Lippincott Co., Philadelphia, 1975.

Bennett, D., Lauder, I. M., Kirkham, D., and McQueen, A.: Bullous autoimmune skin disease in the dog. 1. Clinical and pathological assessment. 2. Immunopathological assessment. Vet. Rec. 106:497–503, 523–525, 1980.

Bennett, I., and Law, D.: Incorporation of tetracycline in developing dog enamel and dentin. J. Dent. Res. 44:788–793, 1965.

Berman, E.: The time and pattern of eruption of the permanent teeth of the cat. Lab. Anim. Sci. 24:929–931, 1974.

Black, A. P., Crichlow, A. M., and Saunders, J. R.: Bacteremia during ultrasonic teeth cleaning and extraction in the dog. J.A.A.H.A. 16:611–61, 1980.

Blatt, C. M., Taylor, C. R., and Habal, M. B.: Nose sweat: a function for Steno's gland in the dog. Fed. Proc. 31:2, 363, 1972.

Bohning, R. H., Jr., Dehoff, W. B., McElhinney, A., and Hofstra, P. C.: Pharyngostomy for maintenance of the anorectic animal. J.A.V.M.A. 156:5, 611, 1970.

Brass, W.: Zur Korrektur von Zahnstellungs – und Kieferanomalien des Hundes mit Dehungsplatten und durch kieferchirurgische Mafnahmen. Kleiner Praxis 21:79–82, 1976.

Brodey, R. S.: The biological behaviour of canine oral

and pharyngeal neoplasms. J. Small Anim. Pract. *11*:45, 1970.

Brown, N., and Hurvitz, A. L.: A mucocutaneous disease in a cat resembling human pemphigous. J.A.A.H.A. *15*:25–28, 1979.

Burwasser, P., and Hill, T. J.: The effect of hard and soft diets on the gingival tissues of dogs. J. Dent. Res. *18*:389–393, 1939.

Buyukmihci, N., Rubin, L. F., and Harvey, C. E.: Exophthalmos secondary to zygomatic adenocarcinoma in a dog. J.A.V.M.A. *167*:162–165, 1975.

Carlson, J., and Egelberg, J.: Local effect of diet on plaque formation and development of gingivitis in dogs. 2. Effect of high carbohydrate versus high protein-fat diets. Odont. Rev. *16*:42–49, 1965.

Carranza, F. A.: Glickmans' Clinical Periodontology. 5th ed. W. B. Saunders Co., Philadelphia, 1979.

Cechner, P. E.: Malocclusion in the dog caused by intramedullary pin fixation of mandibular fractures: two case reports. J.A.A.H.A., *16*:79–85, 1980.

Chandler, E. A.: Mumps in the dog. Vet. Rec. *96*:365–366, 1975.

Cherry: 1824, quoted in Blaine, D.: Canine Pathology. 4th ed. Longman Orme Co. London, 1841, p. 127.

Cheville, N. F.: The gray collie syndrome. J.A.V.M.A. *152*:6, 1968.

Clifford, D. H., and Clark, J. J.: Mouth, lips and tongue. *In* Archibald, J. (ed.): Canine Surgery. Am. Vet. Pub., Inc., Santa Barbara, 1965.

Conner, S., Iranpour, B., and Mills, J.: Alteration in parotid salivary flow in diabetes mellitus. Oral Surg., *30*:55–59, 1970.

Cotter, S. M., Hardey, W. D., and Essex, M.: Association of feline leukemia virus with lymphosarcoma and other disorders in the cat. J.A.V.M.A. *166*:449–454, 1975.

Coyler, F.: Variations and diseases of the teeth of animals. John Bale Sons and Danielsson, London, 1936.

Craig, R. G., O'Brien, W. J., and Powere, J. M.: Dental materials. Properties and manipulation. 2nd ed. C. V. Mosby Co., St. Louis, 1979.

Cuvier, M. F.: *In* Youatt, W. (Ed.): The Dog. Longmans Green and Co., London, 1871, p. 179.

Deitrich, U.: How to incorporate an effective preventive dentistry program into the veterinary practice. California Vet. *32*:16–17, 1978.

DeMonbreun, W. A., and Goodpasture, E. W.: Infectious oral papillomatosis of dogs. Am. J. Pathol. *8*:43, 1932.

Dent, R. St. C.: Operation for correction of lateral protrusion of the tongue in the dog. Vet. Rec. *19*:64, 1952.

DeYoung, D. W., Kealy, J. K., and Khige, J. P.: Attempts to produce salivary cysts in the dog. Am. J. Vet. Res. *39*:185–186, 1978.

Dimic, J., Andric, R., and Millivojevic, J.: Zur Frage der Pathologie und Therapie der tonsillener Kraukungen der Hunde. Kleinter Praxis *17*:77–81, 1972.

Dorn, C. R., and Priester, W. A.: Epidemiologic analysis of oral and pharyngeal cancer in dogs, cats, horses and cattle. J.A.V.M.A. *169*:1202–1206, 1976.

Dorn, C. R., Taylor, D., Schneider, R., Hibbard, H. H., and Klauber, M. R.: Survey of animal neoplasms in Alameda and Contra Costa Counties, California, II. Cancer morbidity in dogs and cats from Alameda County. J. Natl. Cancer Inst. *40*:307, 1968.

Douglas, S. W., and Kelly, D. F.: Calcinosis circum-scripta of the tongue. J. Small Anim. Pract., 7:441–443, 1966.

Dubielzig, R. R.: Effect of canine distemper virus on ameloblastic layer of developing tooth. Vet. Pathol. *16*:268–270, 1979.

Dubielzig, R. R., Goldschmidt, M. H., and Brodey, R. S.: The nomenclature of periodontal epulides in dogs. Vet. Pathol. *16*:209–214, 1979.

Egelberg, J.: Local effect of diet on plaque formation and development of gingivitis in dogs. I. Effect of hard and soft diets. Odont. Rev. *16*:31–41, 1965.

Egelberg, J.: Local effect of diet on plaque formation and development of gingivitis in dogs. III. Effect of frequency of meals and tube feeding. Odont. Rev. *16*:50–60, 1965.

Elzay, R. P., and Hughes, R. D.: Anodontia in a cat. J.A.V.M.A., *154*:667–670, 1969.

Farrow, C. S.: Surgical treatment of lower lip avulsion in the cat. VM SAC *68*:1418–1419, 1973.

Franceschini, G.: Traitement des fistules dentaries chez le chien par obturation des canaux. Rec. Med. Vet. *150*:675–685, 1974.

Gad, T.: Periodontal disease in dogs. I. Clinical investigation. J. Periodont. Res. *3*:268–272, 1968.

Gardner, A. F., Darke, B. H., and Keary, G. T.: Dental caries in domesticated dogs. J.A.V.M.A. *140*:433–436, 1962.

Gaskell, R. M., and Gruffydd-Jones, T. J.: Intractable feline stomatitis. Vet. Ann. *17*:195–199, 1975.

Getty, R.: Sisson and Grossman's The Anatomy of the Domestic Animals. W. B. Saunders Co., Philadelphia, 1975.

Glen, J. B.: Canine salivary mucoceles: results of sialographic examination and surgical treatment of 50 cases. J. Small Anim. Pract. *13*:515, 1972.

Godlowski, Z., and Withers, B. T.: Ablation of salivary glands as initial step in management of selected forms of diabetes mellitus. Laryngoscope *81*:1337–1358, 1971.

Golden, A., Harvey, C. E., and Stoller, N. H.: A survey of oral health in small animals. J.A.A.H.A. Accepted for publication, 1982.

Graber, T. M.: Orthodontics: Principles and Practice. 3rd. ed. W. B. Saunders Co., Philadelphia, 1972.

Grossman, L. I.: Endodontic Practice. 9th ed. Lea and Febiger, Philadelphia, 1978.

Hamp, S. E., Lindhe, J., and Loe, H.: Long-term effect of chlorhexidine on developing gingivitis in the beagle dog. J. Periodont. Res. *8*:63–70, 1973.

Hamp, S. E., et al.: Prevalence of periodontal disease in the dog. I. Clinical and roentgenographical observations. I.A.D.R. Abstract, *119*, 1975.

Harvey, C. E.: Hypersialosis and parotid gland enlargement in a dog. J. Small Anim. Pract. *22*:19–25, 1981.

Harvey, C. E.: Parotid salivary duct rupture and fistula in the dog and cat. J. Small Anim. Pract. *18*:163–168, 1977.

Harvey, C. E.: Exploration of the orbit. *In* Bistner, S. I., et al. (ed.): Atlas of Veterinary Ophthalmic Surgery. W. B. Saunders Co., Philadelphia, 1977.

Harvey, C. E.: Treatment of salivary mucoceles. *In* Bojrab, M. J. (ed.): Current Techniques in Small Animal Surgery. Lea and Febiger, Philadelphia, 1975.

Harvey, C. E.: Letter to the editor. J.A.V.M.A. *158*:1454, 1971.

Harvey, C. E.: Sialography in the dog. J. Am. Vet. Rad. Soc. *10*:18, 1969.

Harvey, C. E.: Canine salivary mucocele. J.A.A.H.A. 5:155, 1969.

Head, K. W.: Tumors of the upper alimentary tract. Bulletin, W.H.O. 53:145–166, 1976.

Heigl, L., and Lindhe, J.: The effect of metronidazole on the development of plaque and gingivitis in the beagle dog. J. Clin. Periodont. 6:197–209, 1979.

Henrikson, P. A.: Periodontal disease and calcium deficiency: an experimental study in the dog. Acta Odont. Scand. Supp. 50:26, 1968.

Hill, P. S., and Davies, R. M.: The effect of a chlorhexidine gel on tooth deposits in beagle dogs. J. Small Anim. Pract. 13:207–212, 1972.

Holmberg, D. C.: Abscessation of the mandibular carnassial tooth in the dog. J.A.A.H.A. 15:347, 1979.

Hoskins, J. D., Ouverson, A., Schlater, C., and Proctor, S. E.: Pemphigus vulgaris in the dog: a case report. J.A.A.H.A. 13:163–167, 1977.

Howard, D. R., Merkley, D. R., Lammerding, J. J., Ford, R. B., Bloomberg, M. S., and Davis, D. G.: Primary cleft palate (harelip) and closure repair in puppies. J.A.AH.A. 12:636–640, 1976.

Hull, P. S., Soames, J. V., and Davies, R. M.: Periodontal disease in a beagle dog colony. J. Comp. Pathol. 84: 143–150, 1974.

Humphreys, G. U.: Dropped jaw in dogs. Vet. Rec. 95: 222, 1974.

Hurvitz, A. L., and Feldman, E.: A disease of dogs resembling human pemphigus vulgaris: case reports. J.A.V.M.A. 166:585–560, 1975.

Hutt, F. B., and DeLahunta, A.: A lethal glossopharyngeal defect in the dog. J. Hered. 62:5, 1971.

Jennings, P. B., Lewis, G. E., Grumrine, H. H., Coppinger, T. S., and Stedham, M. A.: Glossitis of military working dogs in Vietnam: experimental production of tongue lesions. Am. J. Vet. Res. 35: 1295–1299, 1974.

Jackson, D. A., Huse, D. C., and Kissil, M. T.: Bacteremia following ultrasonic scaling in the dog. Presentation at Annual Meeting, A.C.V.S., February 1981.

Kaplan, M. L., and Jeffcoat, M. K.: Acute necrotizing ulcerative gingivitis. Canine Pract. 5:35–38, 1978.

Karbe, E., and Schiefer, B.: Primary salivary gland tumors in carnivores. Can. Vet. J. 8:212–215, 1967.

Karbe, E.: Lateral neck cysts in the dog. Am. J. Vet. Res. 26:112, 1965.

Karbe, E., and Nielsen, S. W.: Branchial cyst in a dog. J.A.V.M.A., 147:6, 1965.

Kelly, D. F., Lucke, V. M., Denny, H. R., and Lane, J. G.: Histology of salivary gland infarction in the dog. Vet. Pathol. 16:438–443, 1979.

Kelly, D. F., Lucke, V. M., Lane, J. G., Denny, H. R., and Longstaffe, J. A.: Salivary gland necrosis in dogs. Vet. Rec. 104:268, 1979.

Keyers, P. H., Wright, W. E., and Howard, S. A.: The use of phase contrast microscopy and chemotherapy in the diagnosis and treatment of periodontal lesions — an initial report. I. Quintessence Int. 1:51–75, 1978.

Kiuchi, S., Sasaki, J., Arai, T., and Suzuki, T.: Functional disorders of the pharynx and esophagus. Acta Otolaryngol. Supple. 256, 1–30, 1969.

Knecht, C. D.: Treatment of diseases of the zygomatic salivary gland. J.A.A.H.A. 6:1, 1970.

Knecht, C. D., and Phares, J.: Characterization of dogs with salivary cyst. J.A.V.M.A., 158:5, 1971.

Knecht, C. D., and Schiller, A. G.: Acquired lesions of the mandible. *In* Archibald, J. (ed.): Canine Surgery. Am. Vet. Pub., Inc., Santa Barbara, 1974.

Knecht, C. D., Slusher, R., and Guibor, E.: Zygomatic salivary cyst in a dog. J.A.V.M.A. 155:4, 1969.

Kratochvil, Z.: Oligodonty and polydonty in the domestic and wild cat. Acta Vet. Brno. 40:33–40, 1971.

Kraus, B., Jordan, R., and Abrams, L.: Dental Anatomy and Occlusion. Williams and Wilkins Co., Baltimore, 1969.

Krook, L.: Periodontal disease in dog and man. Adv. Vet. Sci. Comp. Med. 20:171–190, 1976.

Kutschman, K., and Schafer, R.: Zur Tonsillitis und Tonsillektomie beim Hund. Monat fur Veterinarmed 30:381–383, 1975,

Lane, J. G.: Small animal dentistry and the role of ultrasonic instruments in dental care. J. Small Anim. Pract. 18:787–802, 1977.

Lang, N., and Loe, H.: A fluorescent plaque disclosing agent. J. Periodont. Res. 7:59–67, 1972.

Latimer, K. S., Kemp, W. B., Taylor, L. A., and Barton, R. A.: Emergency stabilization of jaw fractures in dogs using acrylic splints. VM SAC 72:1029–1034, 1977.

Lawrence, A. M., Tan, S., Hojvat, S., Kirsteins, L., and Milton, J.: Salivary gland glucogen in man and animals. Metabolism 25:1405–1408, 1976.

Lee, R.: Radiographic examination of localized and diffuse tissue swellings in the mandibular and pharyngeal area. Vet. Clin. North Am. 4:723–740, 1974.

Lewis, T. M.: Resistance of dogs to dental caries: a two-year study. J. Dent. Res. 44:1254–1257, 1965.

Lindhe, J., and Schroeder, H. E.: Clinical stereologic analysis of the course of early gingivitis in dogs. J. Periodont. Res. 9:314–330, 1974.

Lindhe, J., Hamp, S. E., and Loe, H.: Plaque-induced periodontal disease in beagle dogs: a 4-year clinical, roentgenographical and histometrical study. J. Peridont. Res. 10:235–255, 1975.

Lindhe, J., Hamp, S. E., and Loe, H.: Experimental periodontitis in the beagle dog. J. Periodont. Res. 8:1–10, 1973.

Lindhe, J., Hamp, S. E., Loe, H., and Schott, R.: Influence of topical application of chlorhexidine on chronic gingivitis and gingival wound healing in the dog. Scand. J. Dent. Res. 78:471–478, 1970.

Loesche, W. J.: The bacteriology of dental decay and periodontal disease. Clin. Prevent. Dent. 2:18–24, 1980.

Lynch, M. A.: Burket's Oral Medicine. 7th ed. J. B. Lippincott Co., Philadelphia, 1977.

Madewell, B. R., Stannard, A. A., Pulley, L. T., and Nelson, V. G.: Oral eosinophilic granuloma in Siberian husky dogs. J.A.V.M.A. 177:701–703, 1980.

Marder, M. Z., Abelson, D. C., and Mandel, I. D.: Salivary alterations in diabetes mellitus. J. Periodont. 46:567–569, 1975.

Marvich, J. M.: Repair of enamel hypoplasia in the dog. VM SAC 70:697–699, 1975.

Matson, L., and Attström, R.: Development of experimental gingivitis in the juvenile and adult beagle dog. Test of a model for comparative studies. J. Clin. Periodon. 6:186–193, 1979.

Matsson, L., and Attström, R.: Histologic characteristics of experimental gingivitis in the juvenile and adult beagle dog. J. Clin. Periodon. 6:334–350, 1979.

McKeown, M.: The deciduous dentition in the dog — its form and function. Irish Vet. J. 25:169–173, 1971.

Michel, G.: Beitrag zur Topographie der Ausfuhrungsgange der gl. mandibularis und der gl. sublingualis major des Hundes. Berl. Muench. Tieraerztl. Wochenschr. 69:132–134, 1956.

Navia, J.: Animal models in dental research. University of Alabama Press, University, Ala., 1977.

Newman, P. M.: Canine Teeth. Letter to the Editor. J.A.V.M.A. 174:1075, 1979.

Nuki, K., and Cooper, S.: The role of inflammation in the pathogenesis of gingival enlargement during the administration of diphenylhydantoin sodium in cats. J. Periodon. Res. 7:102–110, 1972.

Nyman, S., Lindhe, J., and Ericsson, I.: The effect of progressive tooth mobility on destructive periodontitis in the dog. J. Clin. Periodontol. 5:213–225, 1978.

Olson, J. A., Nelms, D. C., Silverman, S., and Spitler, L. E.: Levamisole: a new treatment for recurrent aphthous stomatitis. Oral Surg., 41:588–600, 1976.

Orban, B. J.: Oral Embryology and Histology. C. V. Mosby Co., St. Louis, 1966

Page. R. C., and Schroeder, H. E.: Spontaneous chronic periodontitis in adult dogs: a clinical and histopathological survey. J. Periodon. 52:60–73, 1981.

Page, R. C., and Schroeder, H. E.: Pathogenesis of inflammatory periodontal disease: a summary of current work. Lab. Invest. 33:235–248, 1976.

Peterson, R. N., and Wightman, J. R.: Esthetic restoration of a fractured anterior tooth in a dog. VM SAC 74:683–686, 1979.

Potter, K. A., Tucker, R. D., and Carpenter, J. L.: Oral eosinophilic granuloma of Siberian huskies. J.A.A.H.A. 16:595–600, 1980.

Povey, R. C.: Viral diseases of cats: current concepts. Vet. Rec. 98:293, 1976.

Prescott, C. W.: Ranula in the dog: a surgical treatment. Aust. Vet. J. 44:382, 1968.

Reif, J. S., and Cohen, D.: The environmental distribution of canine respiratory tract neoplasms. Arch. Environ. Health 22:136, 1971.

Ridgway, R. L., and Zielke, D. R.: Nonsurgical endodontic technique for dogs. J.A.V.M.A., 174;82–85, 1979.

Riser, W. H., Parkes, L. J., and Shirer, J. F.: Canine craniomandibular osteopathy. J. Am. Vet. Rad. Soc. 8:23–31, 1967.

Robins, G. M.: Dropped jaw — mandibular neuropraxia in the dog. J. Small Anim. Pract. 17:753–758, 1976.

Robins, G., and Grandage, J.: Temporomandibular joint dysplasia and open mouth jaw locking in the dog. J.A.V.M.A. 171:1072–1076, 1977.

Roenigk, W. J.: Radiation Therapy. In Kirk, R. W. (ed.): Current Veterinary Therapy, IV. W. B. Saunders Co. Philadlephia, 1971.

Rosenberg, H. M., Rehfeld, C. E., and Emmering, T. E.: A method for the epidemiologic assessment of periodontal health. Disease state in a beagle hound colony. J. Periodon. 37:208–213, 1966.

Ross, D. C.: Occlusion in the Dog. Southwest. Vet. 28:247–250, 1975.

Ross, D. C.: Dental diagnostic and therapeutic techniques. J.A.V.M.A. 161:1462–1482, 1972.

Ross, D., and Myers, J.: Endodontic therapy for canine teeth in the dog. J.A.V.M.A., 157:1713–1718, 1970.

Ruben, M. P., McCoy, J., et al.: Effects of soft dietary consistency and protein deprivation on the periodontium of the dog. Oral Surg., 15:1061–1069, 1962.

Rudy, R. L.: Fractures of the maxilla and mandible. In Bojrab, M. J. (ed.): Current Techniques in Small Animal Surgery. Lea & Febiger. Philadelphia, 1975.

Saxe, R., Greene, J. C., and Vermillion, J. R.: Debris, calculus and periodontal disease in the beagle dog. Periodontics 5:217–225, 1967.

Schmeltzer, L., Carolan, R., and Ohta, R.: Use of conventional endodontic therapy in a case in veterinary medicine. J.A.D.A 100:218–219, 1980.

Schneck, G. W.: Caries in the dog. J.A.V.M.A. 150:1142–1143, 1967.

Scott, D. W.: Observations on the eosinophilic granuloma complex in cats. J.A.A.H.A. 11:261–270, 1975.

Scott, D. W.: Pemphigus vegetans in a dog. Cornell Vet. 67:374–384, 1977.

Seltzer, S., and Bender, I. B.: Some influences affecting repair of the exposed pulps of dogs teeth. J. Dent. Res. 37:678–687, 1958.

Ship, I. I., and Galili, D. A.: Systemic significance of mouth ulcers. Postgrad. Med. 49:1, 67, 1971.

Silver, J. G., Martin, L., and McBride, B. C.: Recovery and clearance rates of oral microorganisms following experimental bacteremias in the dog. Arch. Oral Biol. 20:675–679, 1975.

Snow, H. D., Donovan, M. L., Washington, J. O., and Fonkalsrud, E. W.: Canine respiratory disease in an animal facility. Arch. Surg., 99:126, 1969.

Soames, V., Entwisle, N., and Davies, M.: The progression of gingivitis to periodontitis in the beagle dog: histologic and morphometric investigation. J. Periodon. 47:435–439, 1976.

Stannard, A. A., Gribble, D. H., and Baker, B. B.: A mucocutaneous disease in the dog resembling pemphigus vulgaris in man. J.A.V.M.A. 166:575–582, 1975.

Stauffer, V. D.: Loss of the tongue in a cat. VM SAC 68:1266–1267, 1973.

Stedham, M. A., Jennings, P. B., Moe, J. B., Elwell, P. A., Perry, L. R., and Montgomery, C. A.: Glossitis of military working dogs in South Vietnam: history and clinical characteristics. J.A.V.M.A. 183:3, 1973.

Stewart, W. C., Baker, G. J., and Lee, R.: Temporomandibular subluxation in the dog: a case report. J. Small Anim. Pract. 16:345–349, 1975.

Stoll, S. G.: Cheiloplasty. In Bojrab, M. J. (ed.): Current Techniques in Small Animal Surgery. Lea & Febiger, Philadelphia, 1975.

Suter, P. F., and Watrous, B. J.: Oropharyngeal dysphagias in the dog: a cinefluorographic analysis of experimentally induced and spontaneously occurring swallowing disorders. Vet. Radiol. 21:24–39, 1980.

Svanberg, G.: Differences in plaque microbiota in periodontally healthy and diseased beagle dogs. I.A.D.R. Abs. 15, 1977.

Syed, S. A., Svanberg, M., and Svanberg, G.: The predominant cultivable dental plaque flora of beagle dogs with gingivitis. J. Periodon. Res. 15:123–136, 1980.

Ticer, J. W., and Spencer, C. P.: Injury of the feline temporomandibular joint: radiographic signs. J. Amer. Vet. Rad. Soc. 19:146–156, 1978.

Todoroff, R. J., and Brodey, R. S.: Oral and pharyngeal neoplasia in the dog: a retrospective study of 361 cases. J.A.V.M.A., 175:567–571, 1979.

Tomlinson, J.: Mandibular condylectomy. Presentation at Ann. Meeting. A.C.V.S., February 1981.

Van Campen, G. J.: The occurrence of acute necrotizing ulcerative gingivitis in a beagle dog colony. I.A.D.R. Abs. 12, 1977.

Wallace, L. J., Guffy, M. M., Gray, A. P., and Clifford, J. H.: Anterior cervical sialocele (salivary cyst) in a domestic cat. J.A.A.H.A. *8*:74, 1972.

Willemse, A., and Lubberink, A. A. M. E.: Eosinophilic ulcers in cats. Tijdschr. Diergeneeskd. *103*:1052–1056, 1978.

Withrow, J.: Dental extraction as a probable cause of septicemia in dog. J.A.A.H.A. *15*:345–346, 1979.

Wouters, S. L. S.: Experimentally induced acute necro-tizing ulcerative gingivitis in beagle dogs. I.A.D.R. Abs. *13*, 1977.

Zontine, W. J.: Dental radiographic technique and interpretation. Vet. Clin. North Am. *4*:741–762, 1974.

Zontine, W. J., Sims, S., and Donovan, M. L.: Bacterial contamination associated with ultrasonic dental procedures in dogs. J.A.A.H.A., *5*:150–154, 1969.

Zymet, C.: Periapical rarefaction associated with canine dental caries. J.A.V.M.A., *152*:483–486, 1968.

CHAPTER 56

BARBARA WATROUS

Esophageal Disease

INTRODUCTION

Alimentary tract disorders are a common clinical complaint confronting the veterinary practitioner. Esophageal diseases compose a low but significant proportion of these cases. A precise anamnesis, personal observation of eating behavior, and a good working knowledge of the normal swallowing process facilitate the acquisition of a definitive diagnosis of esophageal disease. It is essential to correlate well-defined signs with their respective clinical implications (Table 56–1). Localization of alimentary tract disorders is the first step in diagnosis. Conditions of the esophagus or oropharyngeal region must be distinguished from lesions of the gastrointestinal tract, which can be done with reasonable certainty based on the history and clinical signs. In contrast to gastrointestinal disturbances, oropharyngeal and esophageal disorders interrupt the swallowing process, resulting in dysphagia and regurgitation. Regurgitation, therefore, needs to be differentiated from vomiting. The distinction between regurgitation and vomition is often not made by the owner, however, leading the clinician to look at the wrong segment of the alimentary tract.

Regurgitation is characterized by passive, retrograde movement of ingested material, usually before it has reached the stomach. This movement is facilitated by gravity when the head and neck are held down and extended. The gag reflex associated with pharyngeal retention is often involved with neural afferents located in the pharyngeal mucosa. Regurgitation may occur immediately upon uptake of food or fluids or may be delayed several hours or more. The greater the interval between uptake of ingesta and regurgitation, the more likely the disorder is esophageal rather than oropharyngeal. Hypersalivation often accompanies regurgitation. Regurgitated food is mixed with or covered by mucus or saliva and often has a tubular shape. Ingesta being regurgitated after prolonged pharyngeal or esophageal retention may be fetid from bacterial fermentation, but it is neither liquefied by gastric digestion nor bile stained. A rare exception will be regurgitation of gastric contents associated with an incompetent gastroesophageal junction (lower esophageal sphincter, or LES). This event is recognized as normal in the human neonate (Hurvitz et al., 1979). It may also occur in diseases such as hiatal hernia or reflux esophagitis.

Vomition is an active process resulting from a sequence of neural reflexes centered in the medulla. The process is usually pre-

Table 56–1. Signs of Esophageal Disease

Signs	Definition	Clinical Implications
Dysphagia	Difficulty in swallowing.	May be due to motility disturbance, obstruction, or pain. If acute or persistent and progressive, suggests morphologic lesion. If episodic, suggests motility disturbance.
Regurgitation	Passive retrograde transport of food or liquid into oral or nasal cavity after swallowing attempt.	Disease associated with obstruction to or interference with bolus transport, often involving UES or LES. Timing may relate to level of lesion.
Inability to initiate swallow	Unable to prehend or organize bolus for transport.	Oral dysphagia; may be central or peripheral motor to tongue.
Odynophagia or esophageal colic	Pain on swallowing or radiating chest pain manifested as reluctance to eat; anorexia.	Most often with acute obstruction and vigorous esophageal contractions, esophagitis, esophageal perforation.
Laryngotracheal aspiration	Inspiration of oropharyngeal, esophageal, or gastric contents with pulmonary contamination.	Interference with reflex inhibition of respiration (Strombeck, 1979). Frequent consequence of oropharyngeal or esophageal dysphagia.

ceded by premonitory signs of hypersalivation, nausea implied by repeated licking of the lips and swallowing, irregular respiratory movements, and retching, and is accompanied by forceful abdominal contractions and extension of the head and neck. The result is oral transport of gastric or proximal small intestinal contents. This material may or may not be partially digested, bile stained, and with an acid pH.

Involvement of other organ systems, especially the respiratory tract, may mask an existing swallowing disorder. Several systemic or neuromuscular diseases may have esophageal involvement, which might be overlooked by the clinician. Recurrent unexplained pulmonary infection may be due to laryngotracheal aspiration associated with dysphagia or esophageal fistulation. Symptoms of coughing or gagging associated with swallowing, nocturnal cough, recurrent pneumonia, or diffuse interstitial pulmonary infiltrates with reduced exercise tolerance may occur as a complication of dysphagia.

Weight loss or inadequate growth rate may be a primary owner complaint. The inciting cause is usually inadequate caloric consumption. This may be due to the inability to consume an adequate quantity of food or a lack of desire to eat (anorexia). It is essential to differentiate the inability to swallow in an animal with persistent appetite from anorexia. Animals that are willing or eager to take up food but unable to get it into the stomach have oropharyngeal or esophageal problems. Anorexia, on the other hand, is usually due to systemic or gastrointestinal diseases. It is uncommonly due to esophageal problems, except in those cases in which it results from discomfort or pain (odynophagia or esophageal colic) associated with esophageal or pharyngeal problems complicated by spasm or inflammation.

A few dogs may exhibit unusual eating habits such as taking up food in unusual positions, dropping food from the mouth, chewing excessively, or tossing their heads while attempting to swallow. These habits have been recognized as compensatory maneuvers to overcome oropharyngeal swallowing disorders (Suter and Watrous, 1980). Pawing at the neck or submandibular area in an animal with swallowing problems is usually due to an oral or pharyngeal disorder rather than an esophageal problem.

The minimal data base for esophageal disease includes a general physical examination, with particular emphasis on gastrointestinal aspects and on associated neuromuscular functions, survey radiographs of the thorax *and* cervical area to include the entire esophagus, and a hemogram when pulmonary or systemic signs exist. In the specific examination for swallowing problems, one should try to differentiate between morphologic problems, such as foreign bodies or masses in the pharynx, and functional problems, such as esophageal hypomotility or inability to swallow. The examination should preferably progress from oral to caudal: namely, oral cavity, pharynx, upper esophageal sphincter (UES), esophageal body, and LES. A summary of the physical findings is provided in Table 56–2. An adequate oral and pharyngeal physical examination should rule out organic disorders of these regions and is discussed elsewhere (Chapter 55).

In suspected functional disorders it is advisable to study the eating behavior of the animal following the general physical examination. This permits the differentiation of oropharyngeal from esophageal swallowing problems (dysphagias, see p. 1223). At this time it is also advisable to check for neurologic deficits interfering with food uptake manifested as sloppy eating, random tongue activity, and inability to clean the muzzle.

NORMAL ANATOMY AND PHYSIOLOGY

The esophagus is a highly distensible musculomembranous tube, the primary function of which is to transport ingesta from the pharynx to the stomach. The esophagus is bounded cranially by the UES and ends caudally with a functional sphincter called the LES. These junctions reflexively relax to permit aboral passage of food or fluid boluses at precisely timed moments in the swallowing process and prevent reflux of luminal contents into the pharynx or esophagus.

UPPER ESOPHAGEAL SPHINCTER

The paired cricopharyngeal muscles serve as the upper, or cranial, esophageal sphincter (UES) with a portion of the thyropharyngeus and separates the cervical esophagus from the pharynx by an annular fold. The passage at rest is a high-pressure zone that normally relaxes in association with reflex pharyngeal peristaltic contraction and remains open only long enough to receive the bolus and pass it on to the cranial esophagus. The rapid closure of the UES prevents esophagopharyngeal reflux and subsequent laryngotracheal aspiration and also limits aerophagia during respiration.

ESOPHAGUS

The body of the esophagus is composed of four layers. These are the mucous lining of squamous epithelium, the loosely binding submucosa containing mucous glands, the inner circular and outer longitudinal muscular coats, and the outer fibrous layer or adventitia (Evans and Christensen, 1979). The canine muscular layer is characterized by striated skeletal muscle throughout its length. The muscle type changes to smooth muscle at the gastroesophageal junction.

Table 56–2. Summary of Physical Findings Associated With Esophageal Disease

Physical Finding	Significance
Evidence of weight loss	Dysphagia or anorexia due to discomfort on swallowing (odynophagia or esophageal colic).
Pulmonary disease; nasal discharge	Laryngotracheal aspiration; fistula between esophagus and tracheobronchial tree; nasal reflux.
Hypersalivation; +/− blood tinged	Dysphagia or odynophagia; esophageal foreign body, trauma, esophagitis. Stagnant food retention (pharyngeal or esophageal).
Change in bark, meow; muscle weakness	Neuromuscular disease (endocrine, autoimmune).
Incompressible cranial thorax; lymphadenopathy; cervical mass	Periesophageal mass with obstruction.
Heart murmur	Cardiomegaly, left atrial enlargement, with esophageal impingement; vascular ring.
Superficial or deep cervical wounds; thoracic or abdominal trauma	Esophageal trauma, hiatal hernia, diaphragmatic hernia.

The feline cervical esophagus is composed of striated muscle, whereas the terminal quarter section contains smooth muscle.

In the empty esophagus the lumen is obliterated by numerous longitudinal folds of mucosa drawn together by the underlying submucosa. The surface appears scale-like in the terminal thoracic esophagus of the cat, and when coated with barium sulfate, a herringbone or serrated pattern is seen radiographically (Kneller and Christensen, 1973) (Fig. 56–1,A).

LOWER ESOPHAGEAL SPHINCTER

The caudal or lower esophageal sphincter (LES) is located at the gastroesophageal junction, or cardia. This region serves as a functional sphincter in conjunction with several other anatomic structures. This structural complex includes (1) the mass of gastric rugal folds that converges at the gastroesophageal junction and continues a short way into the terminal esophagus, (2) a focal thickening of the inner smooth muscle found at the junction, (3) the right crus of the diaphragm, which provides a muscular sling, (4) the obliquely directed union of the terminal esophagus to the stomach (the angle of His) forming a valvelike closure as the gastric fundus enlarges, (5) the sling created by the deep oblique smooth muscle layer of the lesser curvature of the stomach, which supports the left side of the gastroesophageal junction, and (6) the physical compression exerted on the short intra-abdominal segment of terminal esophagus by the relative positive intra-abdominal pressure (Botha, 1958; and Watrous and Suter, 1979).

The UES lies dorsal to the cricoid cartilage, to which it is attached. The body of the esophagus follows a slightly leftward course through the cervical region with the trachea ventral and to the right. At the level of the first thoracic vertebra the esophagus lies lateral to the trachea. Through the cranial thoracic region it curves back to a dorsal location. At the level of the fourth rib the aortic arch crosses the esophagus on the left. The azygous vein crosses to the right of the esophagus at the level of the fifth to sixth ribs. These two vascular crossover points restrict the normal distensibility of the esophageal body. The esophagus passes dorsal to the left atrium and across the tracheal bifurcation and hilar lymph nodes to the esophageal hiatus. It passes through the right diaphragmatic crus and continues a short distance to empty obliquely into the gastric fundus (Popesko, 1971; Evans and Christensen, 1979).

NORMAL SWALLOWING

The normal swallowing sequence has been divided into three phases for detailed analysis, namely an oropharyngeal, an esophageal, and a gastroesophageal phase (Watrous and Suter, 1979). The oropharyngeal phase is subdivided into three stages of swallowing. The first or *oral stage* (Fig. 56–2, A) begins with the voluntary uptake of material by the interaction of the various muscles of mastication and the tongue. The muscles of the tongue and hyoid apparatus move the ingesta to the base of the tongue, where a bolus is gathered. The hyoid apparatus moves like a swing, drawing the larynx in an upward and rostral direction parallel with the movements of the tongue. At a precise moment, stimulated by pharyngeal contact, the pharynx undergoes a sequence of rapid, aborally directed reflex contractions, propelling the bolus towards the esophagus. This is the second or *pharyngeal stage* of the oropharyngeal phase (Fig. 56–2,B).

During the pharyngeal stage pharyngeal egresses to the nasopharynx, the oropharynx, and the larynx are closed. The oral cavity is closed by contraction of the tongue against the hard and soft palates. The dorsocaudal thrust of the tongue helps to propel the bolus aborally. The nasal cavity is closed by the contraction of the palatopharyngeal arches. The larynx is closed by apposition of the aryepiglottic folds and caudal tipping of the epiglottis over the glottis. The epiglottic movement is initiated by the dorsocranial movement of the larynx and is accompanied by reflex cessation of respiration.

The UES during rest is kept closed by tonic contraction (Mann and Shorter, 1964). In sequence with the cranial pharyngeal contraction, the cricopharyngeal muscle relaxes to receive the moving bolus, permits it to pass into the cranial esophagus, and initiates the third or *cricopharyngeal stage* (Fig. 56–2,C). The UES passage usually remains open for less than a second, with closure following the tail of the bolus. Few, if any,

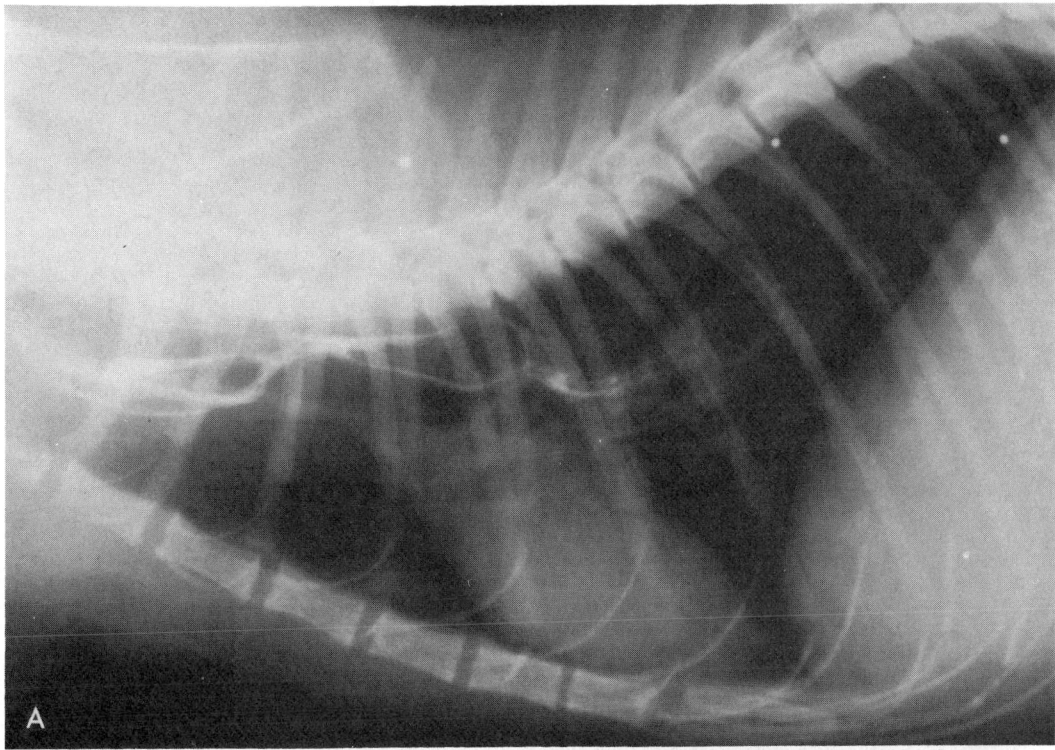

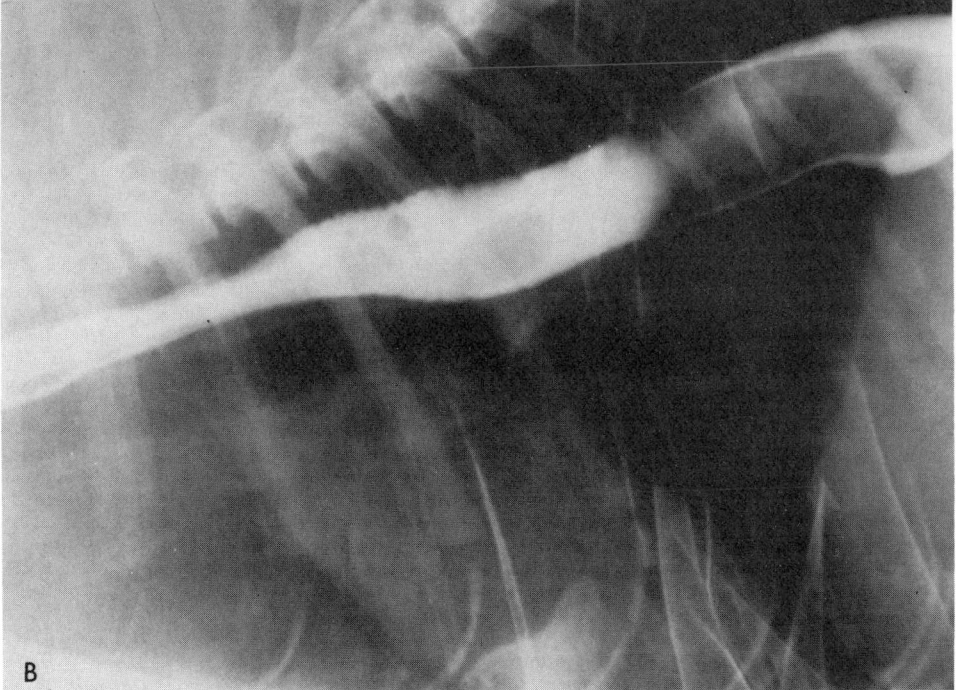

Figure 56–1. Lateral contrast and fluorographic spot radiographs of an adult tomcat with an acute history of frequent regurgitation during meals. *A,* The initial contrast radiograph suggested the presence of an esophageal stricture dorsal to the base of the heart. The esophagus appeared dilated proximal to this site. *B,* A subsequent fluorographic examination demonstrated intermittent relaxation of the esophagus at the narrowed site with normal bolus transport during these periods. Focal esophageal spasm was the subsequent diagnosis. (Note the luminal serrations of the terminal esophagus.)

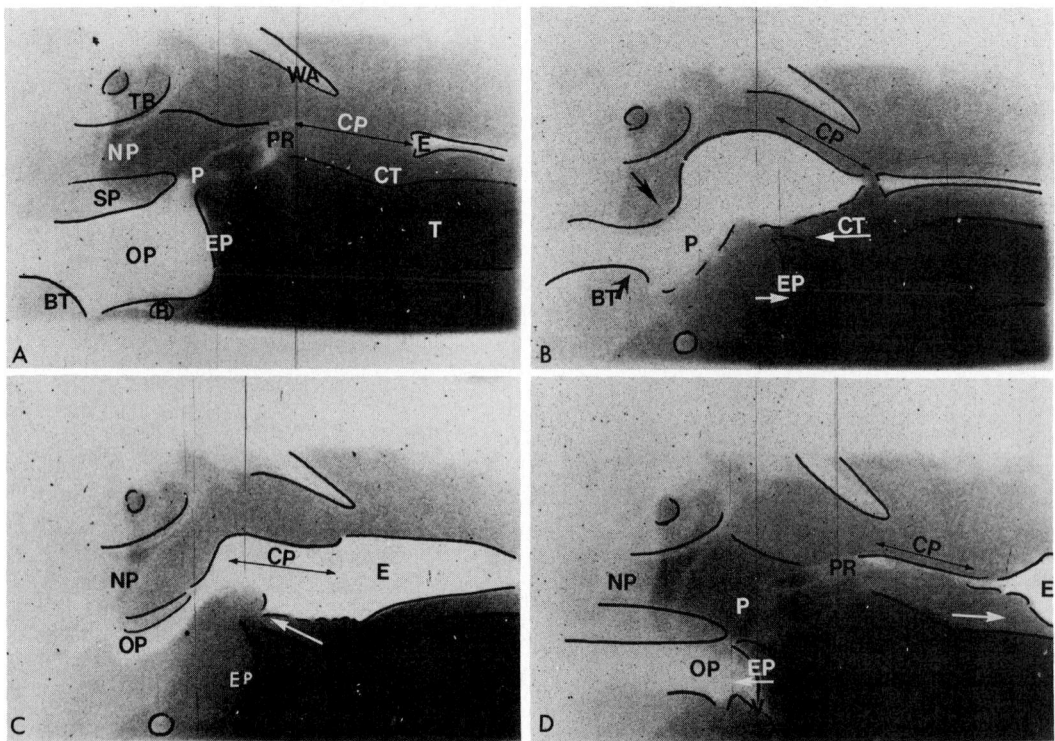

Figure 56–2. Single frames from a cinefluorographic examination of normal swallowing. *A, Oral stage* of oropharyngeal phase. A bolus of liquid contrast medium has been formed at the base of the tongue (BT). The pharynx (P) is air filled. The residue of contrast medium from the previous swallow coats the pharyngeal mucosa of the piriform recesses (PR). A small triangular shadow of contrast medium is seen in the cranial esophagus (E). TB, tympanic bulla; WA, wing of the atlas; B, basihyoid bone; CP, cricopharyngeal sphincter (UES); CT, cricothyroid junction; EP, epiglottis; NP, nasopharynx; OP, oropharynx; SP, soft palate; T, trachea; and V, valleculae. *B, Pharyngeal stage* of oropharyngeal phase. The liquid bolus has initiated a peristaltic contraction in the pharynx. The pharyngeal lumen is constricted cranially, and the base of the tongue has moved dorsocaudally. The cricopharyngeal passage has moved cranially and opened to engulf the bolus. The epiglottis has moved caudally about one cm with respect to the wing of the atlas and pulled back to cover the glottis. The cricotracheal junction and cranial esophagus have also moved cranially relative to the wing of the atlas. *C, Cricopharyngeal stage* of oropharyngeal phase. The cricopharyngeal passage is wide open to permit passage of the bolus into the proximal esophagus. The pharyngeal lumen is obliterated by contraction of the pharyngeal muscles. The egresses to the nasopharynx (NP), oropharynx (OP), and larynx (EP) are blocked. *D,* End of oropharyngeal phase; *Esophageal phase* begins. The pharynx has opened and is again air filled. The epiglottis has returned to its resting position. The residue of contrast medium is seen in the valleculae and coats the mucosa of the piriform recesses. No contrast medium remains in the pharynx proper. A primary peristaltic contraction is carrying the intraesophageal bolus (E) aborally. (From Watrous, B. J., and Suter, P. F.: Normal swallowing in the dog: A cineradiographic study. Vet. Rad., *20:99,* 1979.)

remnants of ingested material remain in the relaxing pharynx at the end of the oropharyngeal phase.

The dorsoventral diameter of the UES opening is proportional to the size and consistency of the bolus. The larger the bolus and the firmer or less malleable the material, the greater the opening. A small liquid bolus would only induce a small degree of opening. This is important in differentiating normal from abnormal function associated with cricopharyngeal dysphagia.

As the esophagus receives the bolus the

esophageal phase starts (Fig. 56–2, *D*). When the bolus is carried by an uninterrupted wave originating from the oropharyngeal phase, this is called a "primary peristaltic wave." The majority of normal swallows induce primary peristalsis; however, several factors may interfere. As commonly observed in sternally recumbent dogs during fluoroscopic examination of rapid swallowing sequences, no definable esophageal contraction occurs (Watrous and Suter, 1979), suggesting the presence of a refractory period for esophageal motility (Ingelfinger, 1958). Occasionally a solitary bolus may pause in the esophagus. This occurs most frequently with a liquid bolus in the proximal cervical esophagus and at the thoracic inlet. This bolus may subsequently be picked up by the primary peristalsis of a subsequent bolus or it may induce a "secondary peristaltic wave," which is generated by its presence in the esophagus. Table 56–3 summarizes the potential sequence of esophageal activity.

The *gastroesophageal phase,* during which the bolus passes into the stomach, is the final phase of the swallowing sequence. This phase overlaps the prior phases. The LES pressure drops during the late oropharyngeal phase long before the peak esophageal pressure wave reaches it (Mann and Shorter, 1964). The LES is thus relaxed well in advance of the arrival of the esophageal bolus. Occasionally gastroesophageal reflux is seen fluorographically. Reflux is not considered abnormal if the refluxed material is rapidly cleared by a new esophageal contraction. The passage of a bolus is followed by a rise in LES pressure above that of the gastric lumen. The closure of the passage prevents gastroesophageal reflux.

The function of the esophagus and its sphincters is influenced by neural, hormonal, myogenic, and mechanical factors. Certain drugs, foods, and other compounds are also modifiers of neuromuscular activity. Study of the extrinsic modifiers of the UES has been limited, but function would most likely parallel that of the esophageal skeletal musculature (Lund and Ardian, 1964; Christensen, 1976). Increase in LES tone occurs with administration of bethanechol (a cholinergic), neostigmine and edrophonium (anticholinesterases), phenylephrine and dopamine (alpha adrenergics), propranolol (a β-adrenergic blocking agent), Task and Proban (organophosphates), Lutalyse (prostaglandin $F_2\alpha$), high protein diets, gastric alkalinity, and gastric distention. Esophageal motility increases with the cholinergics and anticholinesterases, acidity, acute obstruction or distention, and Cushing's myotonia (in man). LES tone is de-creased by isoproterenol (a β-adrenergic), atropine (an anticholinergic), diazepam, morphine, esophageal distention, gastric acidity, hypoglycemia and hypothyroidism (in man), esophagitis, and high fat diets. Esophageal motility is also reduced by β adrenergics and anticholinergics as well as thyroid hormone disturbances, myasthenia gravis, and chronic esophageal obstruction (Hurwitz et al., 1979; Christensen, 1969; Christensen and Lund, 1976; Hall et al., 1975; Strombeck, 1979; Hoffer et al., 1980; Gaynor et al., 1980; Watrous and Suter, 1979; Freiman and Diamant, 1976; Eastwood, 1975; Snape and Cohen, 1976).

General anesthesia has a profound effect on esophageal function. During deep anesthesia the UES is flaccid and no gag reflex can be elicited. A dilated, air-filled esophagus may be seen during thoracic radiographic studies done under general anesthesia (Fig. 56–3). In superficial anesthesia the UES contracts during inspiration (Levitt et al., 1965). Acepromazine has been shown to alter response of the LES at levels of 0.2 to 0.4 mg/Kg (Gaynor et al., 1980). Lower doses used for minimal restraint, however, have not subjectively altered cinefluorographic studies of esophageal function (Watrous and Suter, 1979). Preanesthetic and anesthetic drugs and forceful respiration influence the tone of the LES and are contributing factors to gastroesophageal reflux under anesthesia.

EXAMINATION OF THE ESOPHAGUS AND ITS SPHINCTERS

RADIOGRAPHIC EVALUATION

The radiographic examination of the esophagus is an important adjunct to the evaluation of esophageal disorders. The radiographic procedures available can be divided into two groups, those that produce static images and those that produce dynamic images. Since the esophagus is a dynamic organ, its function is best evaluated by those radiographic procedures that allow observation of the actions and movements

Table 56–3. Summary of Potential Sequence of Esophageal Activity

1. Swallow ---------------------- primary peristaltic wave
2. Swallow ------- pause -------- secondary peristaltic wave
3. Swallow ------- pause -------- swallow -------- primary peristaltic wave
4. Swallow ------- pause -------- swallow ------- pause -------- secondary peristaltic wave

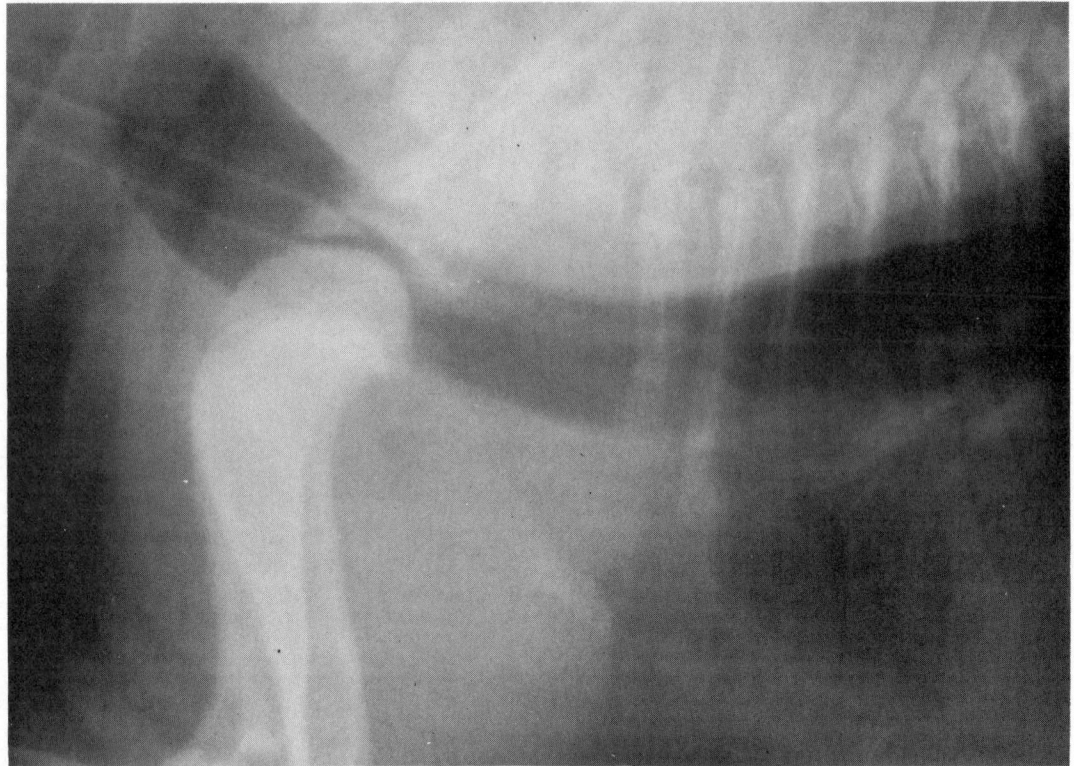

Figure 56–3. A lateral radiograph of a three-month-old male English bulldog under general anesthesia for evaluation of a hypoplastic trachea. The dilated, air-filled esophagus is secondary to the relaxant effects of the anesthetic agent (halothane) on the esophagus.

of the parts of the esophagus; unfortunately, the equipment necessary for these procedures is costly. Detection on standard radiographs is possible, however, since the morphology of the esophagus usually changes when esophageal dysfunction occurs. Nevertheless, one must be cautious in attempting to rule out esophageal dysfunction without performing a dynamic study.

Survey Radiographs

The esophagus is not normally seen on the survey radiographic evaluation of the neck and thorax. The visualization of its walls or lumen on survey radiographs is usually indicative of thoracic or esophageal pathology. If the periesophageal fascia or mediastinum is displaced by air (as may occur with subcutaneous emphysema of the neck or pneumomediastinum) the adventitia of the esophagus can be visualized. The empty esophagus surrounded by air may be seen on the lateral view as a linear soft tissue density with parallel walls originating from the base of the heart just dorsal to the

tracheal bifurcation and terminating a few centimeters dorsal to the posterior vena cava at the diaphragm. On the dorsoventral projection the esophagus will be missed owing to the superimposition of the spine and other mediastinal structures. The portions of the normal esophagus cranial to the base of the heart can rarely be identified on either view because of the confusing superimposition of vascular and muscular shadows.

If the esophagus is dilated and distended with air, food, or liquid material, it may be visualized along all or part of its length on the survey radiographs. In this instance, if the cervical esophagus is dilated it can often be visualized, originating at the UES dorsal to the trachea and then crossing somewhat ventral to the trachea at the thoracic inlet (Fig. 56–3). The flaccid thoracic esophagus may often be widely dilated with air, making its presence easily overlooked owing to the radiolucency of the surrounding lung field (Fig. 56–4,*A*). The uniformly dilated esophagus, although often discernible in the cranial thoracic and cervical areas, is usually most easily seen in the caudal thoracic area.

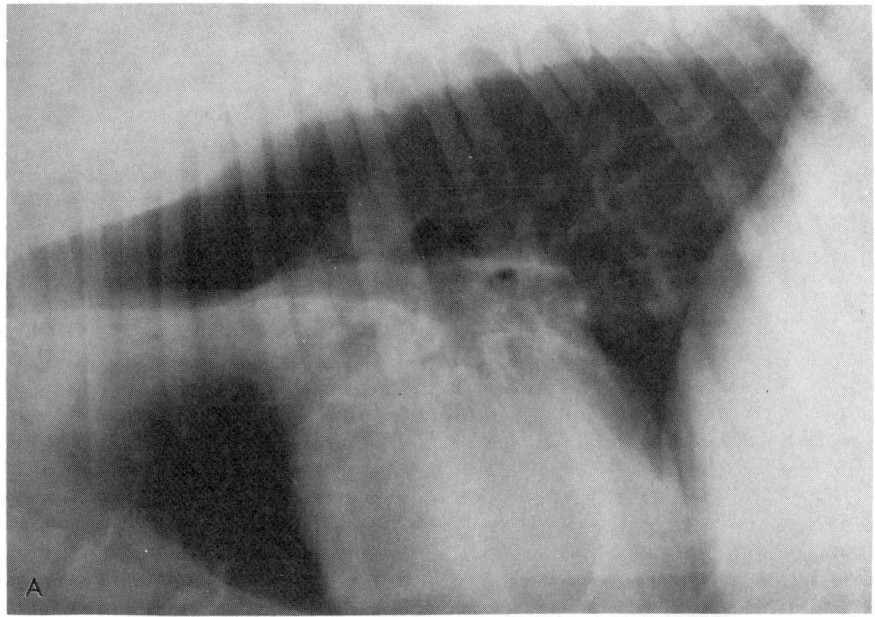

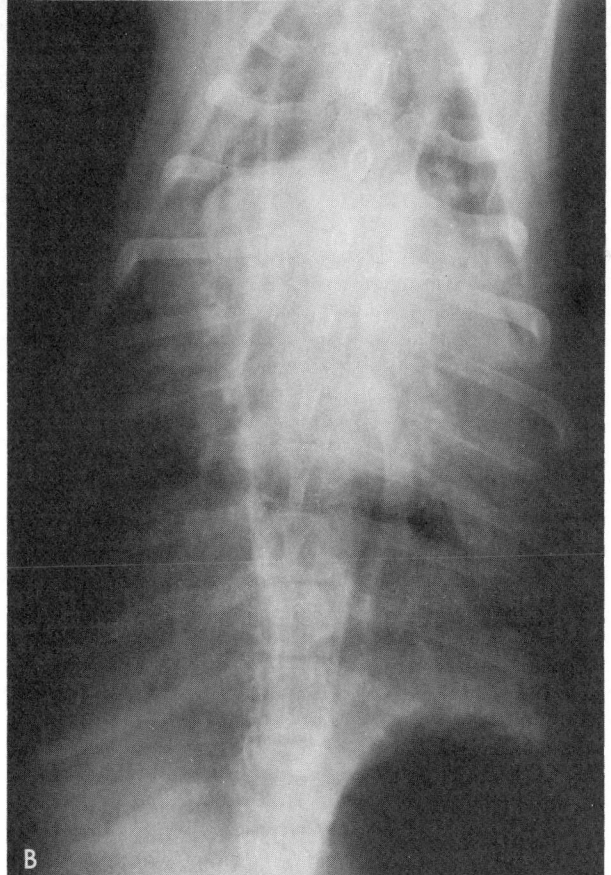

Figure 56–4. Lateral and dorsoventral survey radiographs of a nine-year-old male springer spaniel with idiopathic esophageal hypomotility (megaesophagus). He was presented for generalized extremity weakness and a one-year history of intermittent regurgitation. Clinicopathologic evaluation revealed only hypothyroidism. *A,* The dilated, air-filled esophagus is nearly invisible against the dorsal lungfield. *B,* The bilateral aspiration pneumonia is best seen in this view. The dilated esophagus is identified as a widened, air-filled shadow converging to a V at the hiatus.

Two thin soft-tissue stripes that converge to a "V" at the LES represent the walls of the dilated esophagus. The dorsal wall on the lateral view emerges from the soft tissues surrounding the midthoracic spine and curves ventrally towards the esophageal hiatus. It also has a characteristic indentation at the level of the sixth thoracic vertebra, which coincides with the normal location of the azygous vein. The ventral wall is often superimposed on the posterior vena cava. The dorsoventral or ventrodorsal view reveals a widened mediastinum identified as two parallel soft-tissue stripes on either side of the spine. At the hiatus they converge to a "V." A constriction in the midthoracic esophagus will be seen corresponding to the crossover points of the aorta and azygous vein (Fig. 56–4,B).

The Esophagram Using Static Images

When the history, clinical signs, physical exam, or survey radiographic findings indicate esophageal disease, further evaluation of the esophagus is usually necessary. The most common method employed is the standard esophagram. The esophagram involves the oral administration of a radiopaque contrast agent.

Barium sulfate paste suspensions are the most convenient for use in small animals when a morphologic disease is suspected. The heavy consistency of the paste prevents excessive spillage and provides for greater ease of administration. These preparations coat the pharynx and esophagus, allowing radiographs to be taken after passage of the bolus. If significant laryngotracheal aspiration is evident, however, the paste is not recommended, because of the greater difficulty in expelling it from the trachea. A liquid barium suspension is recommended for these cases. In functional disorders both liquid and food swallows are recommended to evaluate the differences in handling of these two consistencies.

The water soluble contrast agents are not recommended for routine evaluation of the esophagus because of their low viscosity and rapid dilution. Esophageal lacerations may be missed with water soluble preparations, and it has been shown that the reaction set up in the mediastinum by extravasated barium is no greater than that by normal oral microflora alone (Vessal et al., 1975). For cases of suspected esophageal perforation, a negative water soluble contrast examination should be followed by a barium liquid suspension examination.

Partial strictures of the esophagus may be missed if fluoroscopy is not available and standard contrast films alone are used. If stricture is suspected, the barium should be mixed with dry dog food, cotton balls, or marshmallows and readministered. The barium-coated bulky material will generally not pass a stricture area and can therefore be detected on a radiograph.

One should, however, be cautious when attempting to diagnose an esophageal stricture without the aid of fluoroscopy. A bolus can stall in the esophagus and be misinterpreted as a stricture (Fig. 56–1). If a stricture is suspected it is necessary to take multiple radiographs (separated by a few minutes) of the same bolus to determine if it is merely stalled or if in fact a stricture actually exists.

Fluoroscopic Examination

The fluoroscopic examination of the esophagus permits the evaluation of esophageal function as well as morphology. The relative strength, rate, and efficiency of contractions can be estimated. In addition, the coordination and function of the UES and LES can be evaluated. If fluoroscopy is available, the passage of the barium contrast medium should be observed fluoroscopically and spot films should be made before standard contrast radiographs are taken. This will insure the most complete examination of the esophagus and will preclude the need for many repeat radiographs.

The evaluation of esophageal function should include swallows of both liquid and solid boluses. The study should be initiated with recording of three to six complete swallows of liquid barium suspension and followed by a similar number of barium-coated food boluses to observe the possible differences in handling of the two consistencies.

OTHER PROCEDURES

If the esophagram is normal, then the esophagus is most probably not the cause of the clinical signs. Some pathologic conditions such as esophagitis can, however, be missed even after fluoroscopic examination. In these instances other methods need to be employed.

Esophagoscopy. This is the most sensitive method of evaluating lesions of the esophageal mucosa. Small or diffuse lesions of the mucosa may be missed radiographically. The use of modern fiberoptic endoscopes allows biopsy as well as visualization of lesions. Since esophagoscopy requires general anesthesia, it is recommended that it be conducted after a thorough radiographic evaluation to localize suspected areas of disease. Sufficient time should be allowed to pass after the radiographic examination, as barium retained in the esophagus will interfere with the endoscopic visualization of the esophagus.

Esophageal endoscopy may reveal numerous esophageal conditions, including esophagitis, esophageal foreign body, infiltrative disease, diverticulum, and chalasia of the gastroesophageal junction. The technique for esophagoscopy has been described (O'Brien, 1972). The endoscope is passed per os in the anesthetized animal dorsal to the larynx and through the UES. The lumen of the esophagus will be seen to be collapsed in a series of longitudinal folds. The mucosa appears a shiny pink color. Flushing the lumen with water and air to clear the viewing field will demonstrate the lumen to be easily distensible. The lumen of the esophagus assumes a slight dorsal direction at the thoracic inlet, and some resistance may be met here. The thoracic esophageal lumen will be seen to expand and collapse with the respiratory cycle. The lumen is less distensible at the crossover points for the aortic arch and the azygous vein. Pulsations may be seen as the esophagus passes the aorta and left atrium. The gastroesophageal junction is seen as a closed rosette. Bright red gastric mucosa may line the junction in some dogs. If resistance is met anywhere along the course a lumen finder should be used (O'Brien, 1972; Zimmer, 1980).

Manometry. Manometry involves the recording of pressures within the esophagus at rest and during the passage of a bolus. It is especially helpful in delineating dysfunction of the UES and LES. Although manometry has been performed in the dog (Schlegel and Code, 1958; Rogers et al., 1979; Gaynor et al., 1980), its success is dependent on a cooperative patient and its clinical usage is therefore restricted.

Nuclear Scintigraphy. This technique can also be used to evaluate esophageal transit. Prolonged fluoroscopic examination of the esophagus may produce undesirable exposure to the patient and surrounding personnel. By administering per os a small amount of radioactive particles (water labeled with ^{99m}Tc sulfur colloid), esophageal transit times as well as sphincter patency and reflux can be observed with a gamma camera (Malmud and Fisher, 1980).

MORPHOLOGIC DISEASES

ESOPHAGEAL FOREIGN BODIES

Ingestion of either nondigestable foreign materials or pieces of food too large to pass through the esophagus (often with sharp points or spicules on the surface) may lead to entrapment. Esophageal foreign bodies can cause complete, partial, or no obstruction. Areas of limited esophageal distention are most vulnerable to obstruction. They include the thoracic inlet, the base of the heart (owing to the proximity of the aortic arch, azygous vein, and left mainstem bronchus), and cranial to esophageal hiatus. The cranial esophagus is a frequent location for nonobstructive foreign bodies with points or spicules (Fig. 56–5). Esophageal foreign body obstruction is six times more common in dogs than in cats (Ryan and Greene, 1975). Cats occasionally ingest nonobstructive objects such as needles, fishhooks, or string. Objects commonly ingested by dogs include bones, rocks, sticks, fishhooks, strings, and large pieces of meat or gristle. The more angular the foreign body, the greater its size, and the longer the duration of the entrapment, the greater will be the esophageal injury.

The clinical signs may be different for complete or partial obstruction. With partial obstruction animals can survive for days or sometimes weeks by taking up liquids only instead of solids. Clinical signs in the acute phase include apparent discomfort, hypersalivation, and gagging with regurgitation of esophageal secretions. The animal may be reluctant to eat. Either partial or complete obstruction may occur, resulting in regurgitation of all ingested solids and possibly liquids. Gradual deterioration of condition over several weeks is common with respiratory complications or subsequent esophageal perforation. Esophageal laceration due to sharp or penetrating foreign bodies may be identified clinically by blood-tinged saliva or regurgitated material. When the ingested foreign body is very large, impingement on the adjacent respiratory tract may occur. Signs will be primarily

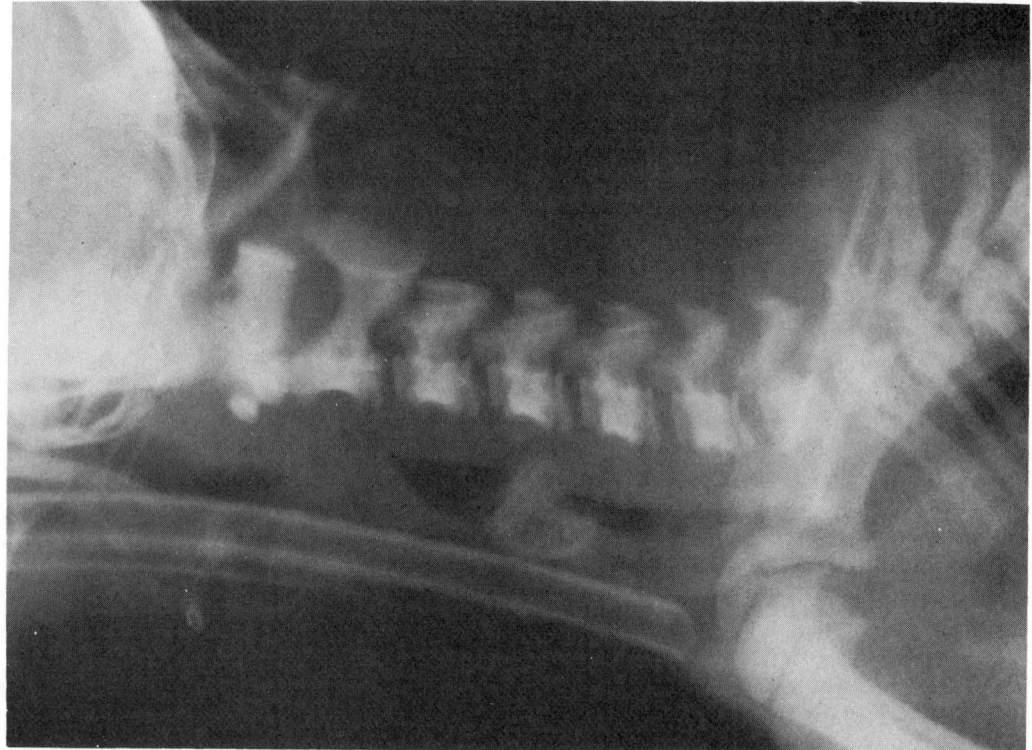

Figure 56–5. A lateral radiograph of a male poodle puppy that had been observed eating chicken at a picnic two days before presentation. Subsequent to the picnic he "vomited" everything he attempted to eat. A frequent location for large or sharp foreign bodies to lodge is in the cervical esophagus.

respiratory, with dyspnea or wheezing evident. Significant airway obstruction may lead to pulmonary edema and the mistaken conclusion of cardiovascular disease.

Diagnosis is made from a known history of foreign body ingestion by cognizant owners, by the clinician's high index of suspicion from the clinical signs, or by radiography and endoscopy. Radiodense foreign bodies are readily recognized. Some bony foreign bodies are semidense and not readily seen on radiographs because their high cartilage content and poor calcification result in a low radiodensity. Nonradiodense objects may be identified by entrapment of intraluminal air or esophageal fluid proximal to the object. Total obstruction or chronicity leads to greater accumulation of gaseous or liquid luminal contents as esophageal tone diminishes.

Contrast radiography will reveal foreign bodies as radiolucent filling defects surrounded by the pool of positive contrast media. Linear foreign bodies such as strings or yarn will not obstruct the flow of contrast media, but barium sulfate may adhere to their surfaces, thus allowing them to be seen. In order to avoid subsequent esopha-

geal perforation, contrast radiography should not be done if the foreign body is visible on the survey radiographs.

Laboratory findings will be normal unless complications such as esophageal perforation have occurred. In complete or chronic obstruction leukocytosis or stress response and an elevated hematocrit may be present.

Complications occur spontaneously with sharp objects, with chronic partial obstruction, and secondary to attempts by the owners or veterinarians to remove the foreign body. In many complications the esophageal wall has been damaged by pressure necrosis, infection, or both, and has become very friable. The signs of spontaneous esophageal perforation can be very misleading because the owner may only notice a sudden onset of severe depression and anorexia. In most animals the preceding history may be helpful.

Clinically, esophageal perforation is indicated by persistent regurgitation, hypersalivation, anorexia and depression, a rigid stance, leukocytosis, and often rapid onset of shock with signs of circulatory compromise. With chronic perforation the clinical signs are less specific and often overshadowed by the secondary inflammatory disease of mediastinitis, pleuritis, pericarditis, or necrotizing cellulitis. These complications result in depression, anorexia, dehydration, and fever. Radiographic examination is needed for the confirmation of the diagnosis.

Perforations in the acute phase are diagnosed when air is identified in the periesophageal tissues of the cervical region or in the mediastinum (pneumomediastinum) and axillae in the thoracic region. Chronic perforation is associated with cellulitis, exudation, and abscess formation in the cervical region. Fistulous tracts may develop. Mediastinitis and pleuritis result from thoracic esophageal perforation (Fig. 56–6). Spinal cord perforation has been caused by a migrating esophageal foreign body (Ryan and Greene, 1975).

Early in the disease process adequate communication with the periesophageal tissues may allow contrast media to demonstrate a perforation. As inflammatory tissue and adhesions develop, the chances for extravasation diminish. The other radiographic signs, however, remain supportive for loss of esophageal integrity (p. 1202). Strictures may also be a complication following foreign body removal (Fig. 56–7) (p. 1217). Esophagoscopy lends support to the diagnosis and may better define the status of the esophageal mucosa.

Treatment is aimed at immediate removal of the foreign body. If possible, this should be attempted by esophagoscopy and retraction by grasping forceps or by pushing the object aborally into the stomach. If more than *gentle* manipulation is required to move the foreign body, esophagotomy is necessary. Sharp objects (bones, hooks, and needles) and those present long enough to cause esophageal necrosis also mandate surgical extraction. The surgical approach involves a linear incision through a normal portion of the esophagus distal to the obstruction. The object is gently removed and closure is achieved. A two-layer pattern is most commonly proposed (Hoffer, 1978; Harvey, 1975). An everting simple interrupted or continuous suture pattern through the mucosa and submucosa is made using 3–0 to 5–0 nonabsorbable suture material such as silk. A second layer of simple interrupted sutures is placed in the muscular coats using 3–0 absorbable material

(Harvey, 1975). If preobstructive dilatation has occurred, the esophagotomy site is made in this region. When extensive necrosis requires resection, one to two cm of esophagus can be removed without concern for complications due to shortening. Greater damage may require esophagoplasty or esophageal patch grafting (Krahwinkel and Howard, 1975).

Glucagon has recently been advocated in man for esophageal obstruction by food boluses such as large pieces of meat. The hormone causes reduction in esophageal smooth muscle tone and may allow relief of esophageal spasm in acute obstruction so the bolus may pass (Glauser and Lilja, 1979). Owing to its greater smooth muscle content, the feline esophagus would theoretically be more amenable to this medical treatment.

ESOPHAGEAL AND PERIESOPHAGEAL MASSES

Neoplastic involvement of the esophagus is rare. Reports are scattered but include description of both benign and malignant processes of primary and metastatic origin. Branchiomas, branchial cleft cysts, papillomas, metastatic tonsillar carcinomas, and squamous cell carcinomas have been reported (Kliene, 1974; Moulton, 1978; Cotchin, 1951). A search of cases of esophageal neoplasia at the New York State Veterinary Medical College in the past five years uncovered a single case in a dog and one in a cat. Two cases of primary tumors and six metastatic tumors in the esophagus of dogs were diagnosed at the University of California Veterinary School in a ten-year study (Ridgeway and Suter, 1979).

Benign tumors of the canine esophagus are occasionally encountered at necropsy (King, 1980; Ridgeway and Suter, 1979). These are usually leiomyomas and may not be associated with significant clinical signs of esophageal dysfunction. Their relatively slow growth rate or lack of invasiveness may account for this. They are rarely encountered radiographically (Fig. 56–8).

Primary carcinomas may form as pedunculated luminal masses or annular mural constrictions. The occurrence of primary sarcomas is most commonly attributed to the helminth parasite *Spirocerca lupi*. The causal relationship is based on the characteristic location of the neoplasm in the tho-

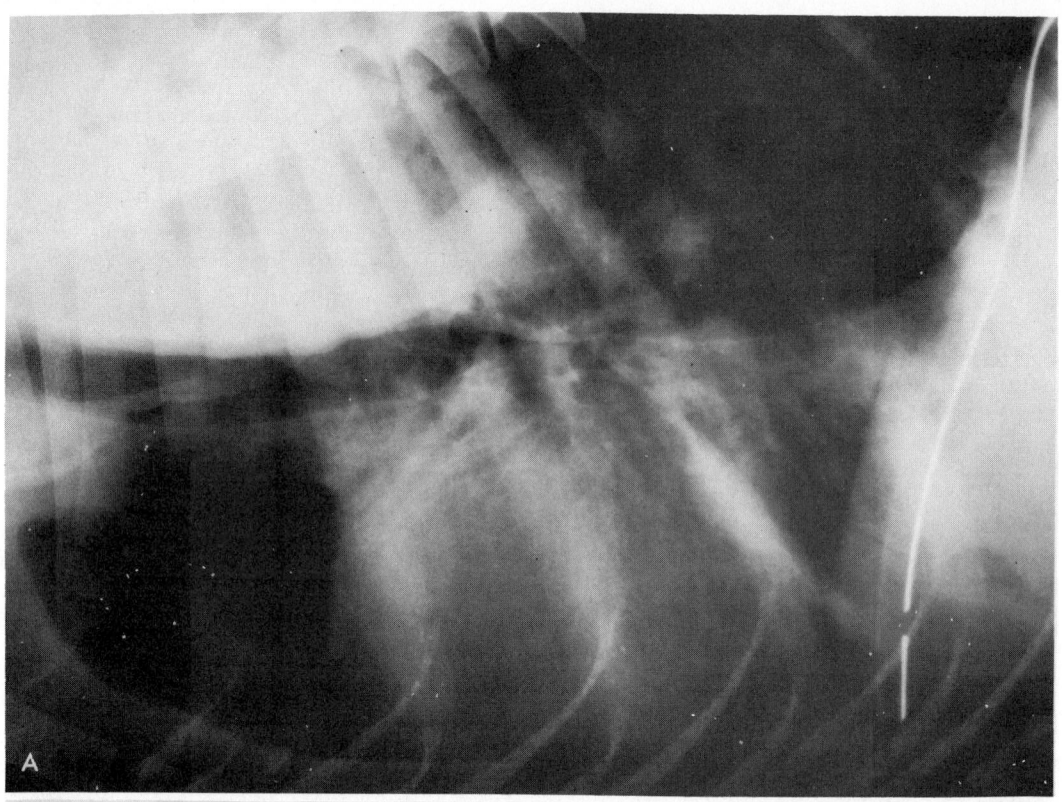

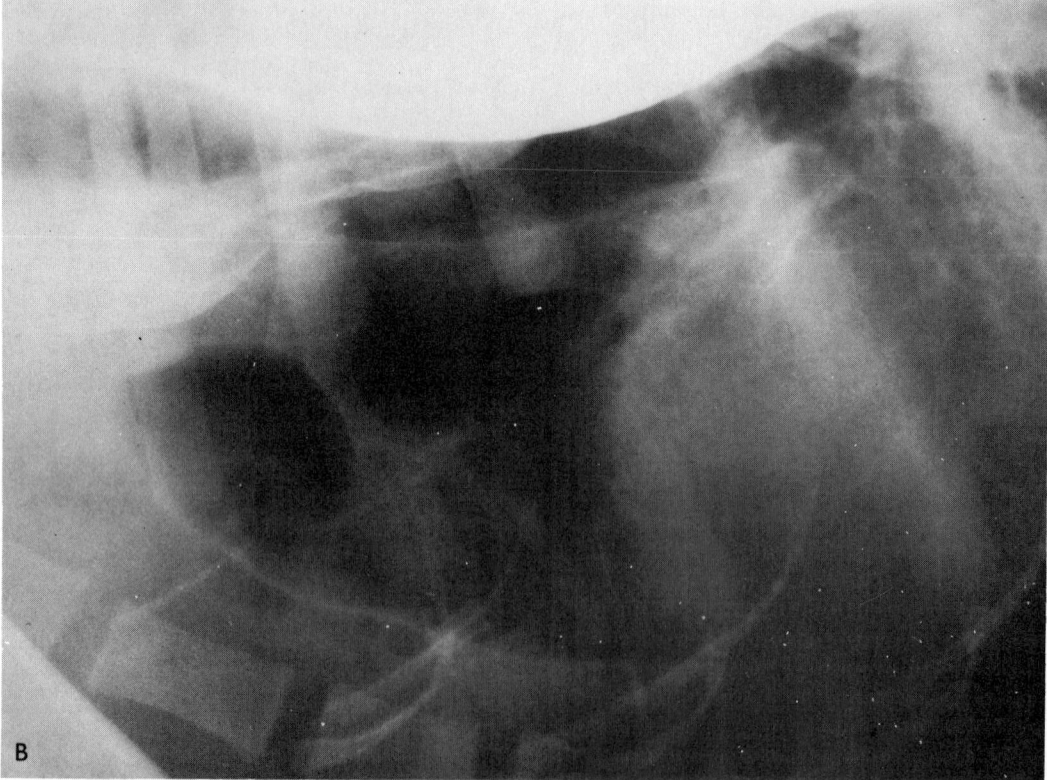

Figure 56–6. Lateral survey and contrast radiographs of a four-year-old castrated mongrel dog two days after a modified Heller's myotomy. The surgery was intended to treat the chronic congenital esophageal hypomotility and megaesophagus. *A,* Dehiscence resulted in esophageal leakage, pneumonia, and pleuritis with pleural effusion. *B,* An esophagram with Gastrografin demonstrates leakage of the aqueous organic iodine compound into the pleural space.

1204

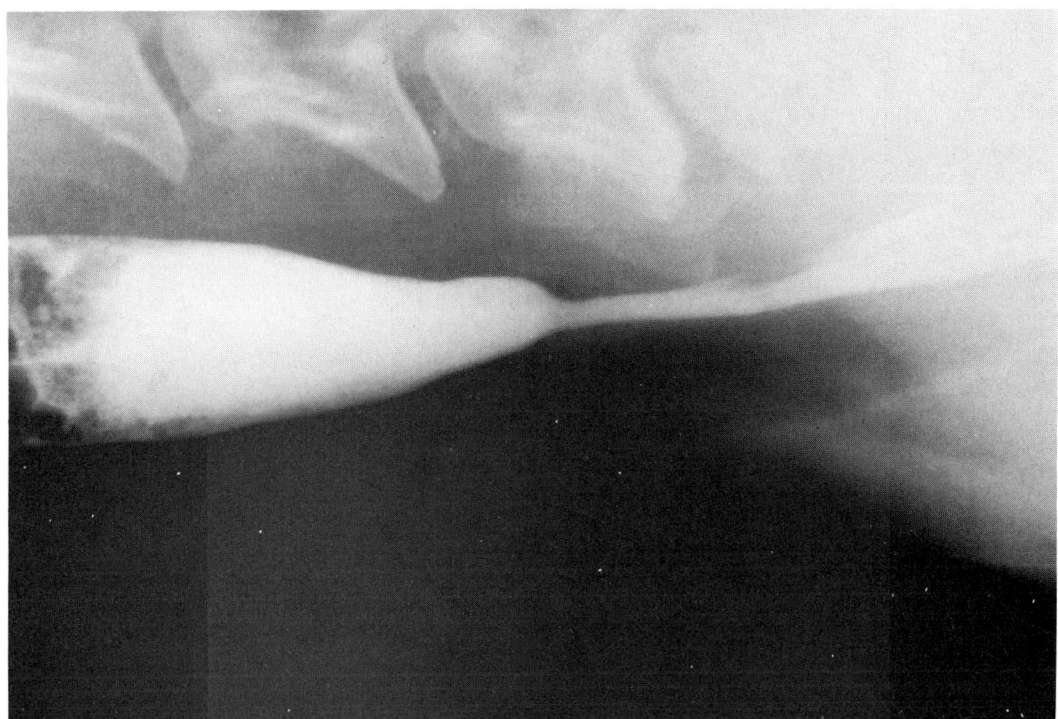

Figure 56–7. A lateral contrast radiograph centered just anterior to the thoracic inlet. This three-year-old male Doberman had had a prior history of an esophageal foreign body. The esophagus is now focally nondistensible owing to post-traumatic stricture formation.

racic esophagus between the aortic arch and hiatus, the presence of lesions indicative of existing or previous infection with *S. lupi* (spondylitis, aortic parasitic granulomas, scars or aneurysms, or esophageal granulomas), the frequent occurrence in hounds one to five years of age, the similarity in the morphologic appearance of the tumorous mass and *S. lupi* granulomas, and the geographic distribution in the southern and southeastern United States (Bailey, 1963). Metastatic extension to the esophagus occurs occasionally from thyroid carcinoma and primary pulmonary neoplasms (Brodey and Kelley, 1968) (Fig. 56–9). Extension of a gastric carcinoma has also been observed (Ridgeway and Suter, 1979).

Both esophageal and periesophageal abscesses and granulomas may occur. Abscessation most often is secondary to penetrating foreign bodies or migrating plant awns (Fig. 56–10). Granulomas may form in periesophageal lymph nodes as a part of disseminated disease, including infection by *Nocardia* and *Coccidioides*.

Both esophageal and periesophageal masses interfere with distention of the esophageal lumen during bolus transport, leading to progressive signs of dysphagia and regurgitation. Esophageal masses invade locally and distort the lumen. Periesophageal masses may invade or displace and obstruct the lumen (Fig. 56–11). If erosions are present, blood-tinged regurgitated secretions or occult blood in the stool may be observed. Hypertrophic osteopathy (hypertrophic pulmonary osteoarthropathy, Marie's disease) has been reported in cases of esophageal fibrosarcoma with and without pulmonary metastases (Bailey, 1963). Recurrent gastric dilatation may be encountered with masses involving the LES. The possibility of reduced LES tone (chalasia) due to disturbed sphincter function from diffuse invasion may allow reflux esophagitis to develop. With metastatic disease, signs of primary organ involvement may be manifested (dyspnea, cough, and enlargement of the cervical region for thyroid carcinoma; vomiting from gastric cancer; labored breathing from pulmonary neoplasia) (Ridgeway and Suter, 1979).

Survey radiographic findings may include entrapment of intraluminal esophageal air with possible dilatation oral to the obstruction, displacement of adjacent structures

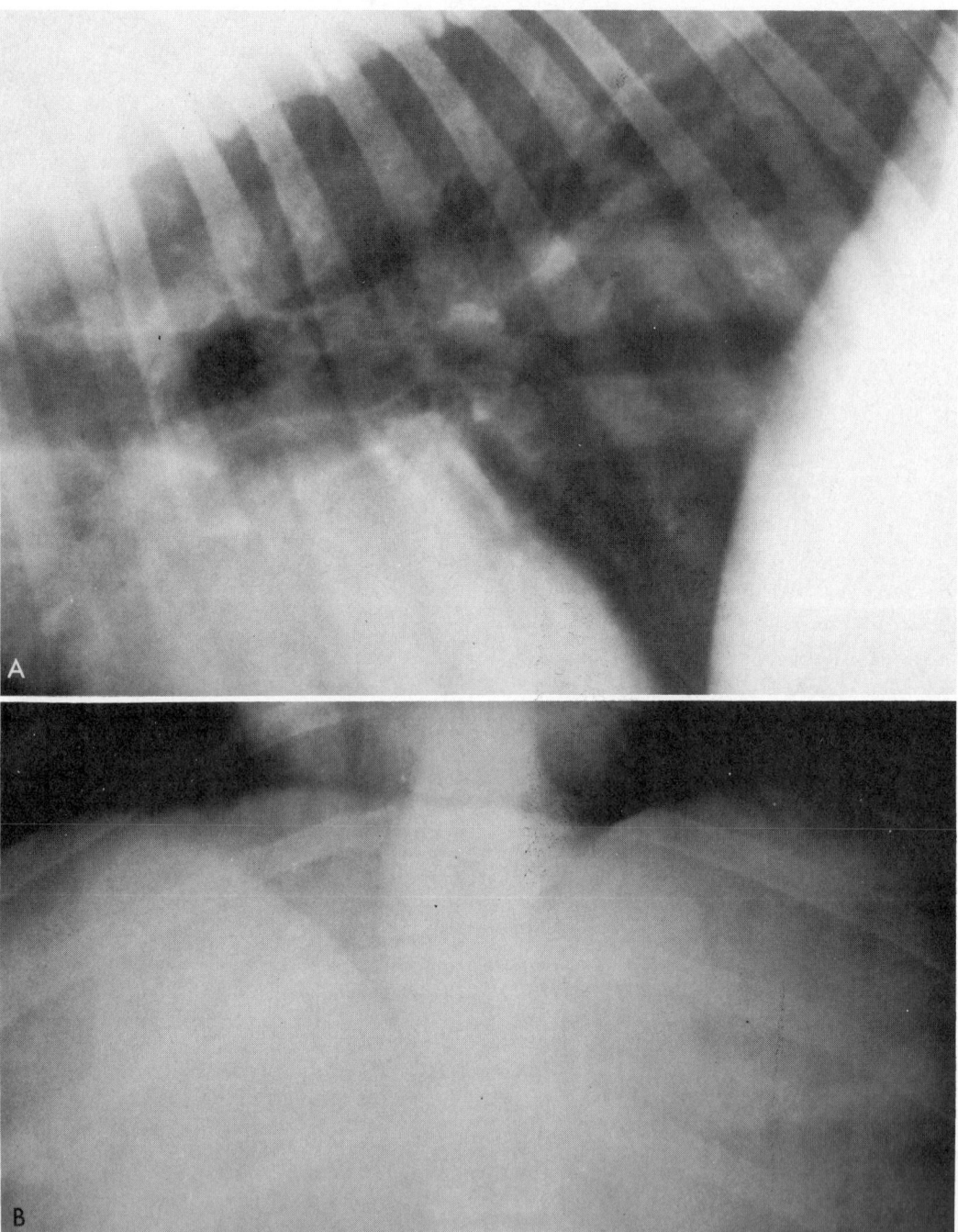

Figure 56–8. Lateral and dorsoventral radiographs. *A,* A soft tissue horizontal stripe can be seen between the descending aorta and the posterior vena cava in the caudal thorax. *B,* The caudal mediastinum widens between the two diaphragmatic crura corresponding to the same location on the lateral radiograph. This 12-year-old male Kerry blue terrier died of unrelated causes and was shown at necropsy to have an esophageal leiomyoma in the portion of the thoracic esophagus seen on the survey radiographs.

(larynx, trachea, or heart), and increase in soft tissue or mineral density in the mediastinum. The entrapped air may define an intraluminal mass, which must be differentiated from a swallowed foreign body, or outline an irregular mucosal contour. The trapped air is due to disturbed esophageal motility either from structural derangement and mural rigidity or from extensive invasion of the muscular coat of the esophagus.

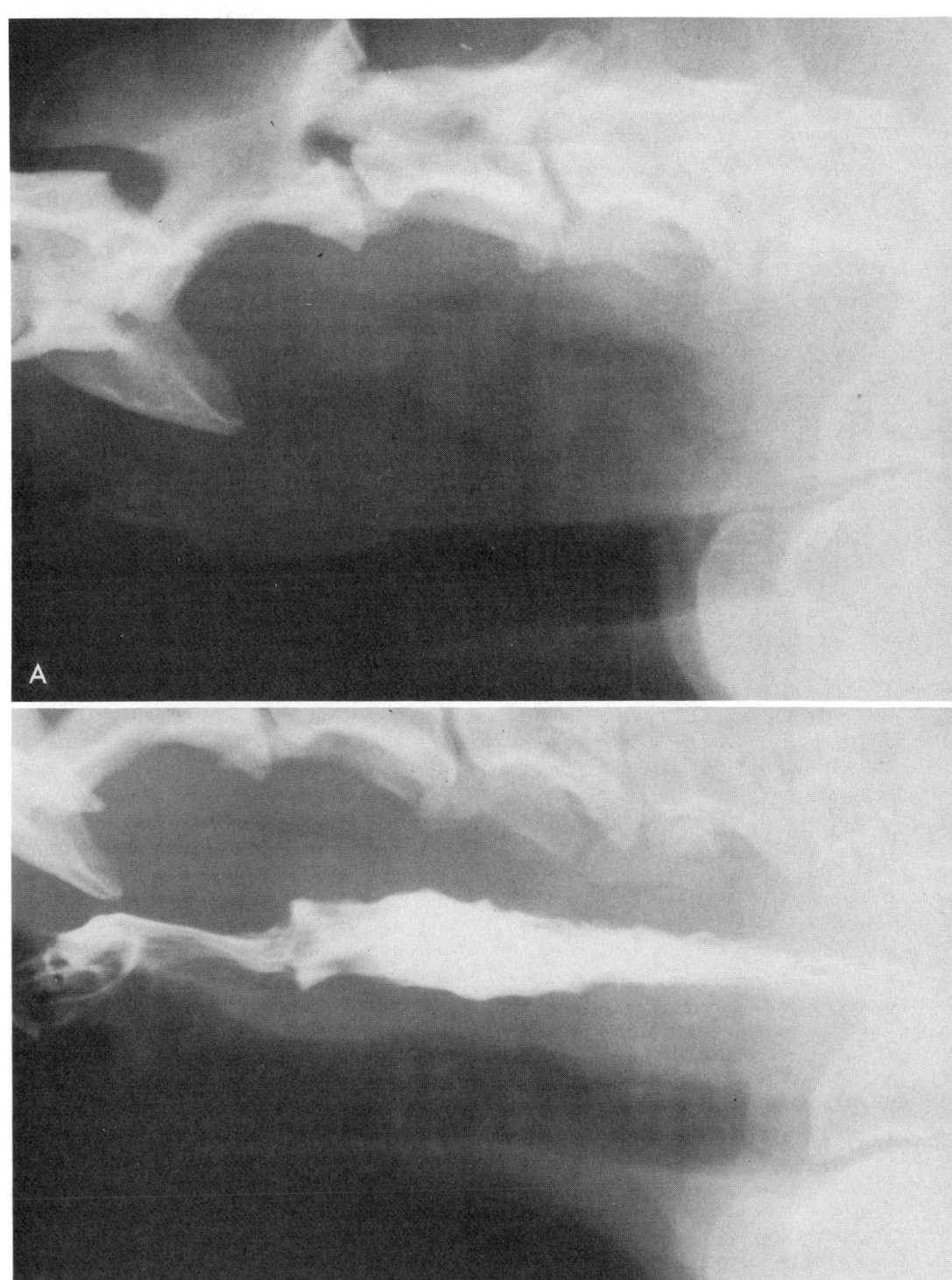

Figure 56–9. Lateral survey and contrast radiographs of a 12-year-old spayed female German shepherd dog with an enlarging mass in the cervical region and progressive signs of dysphagia. *A,* The retrotracheal soft tissues have increased, resulting in ventral displacement of the trachea. *B,* The barium reveals an irregular mucosal contour and focal dilatation of the esophagus, indicating diffuse mural invasion by the thyroid carcinoma.

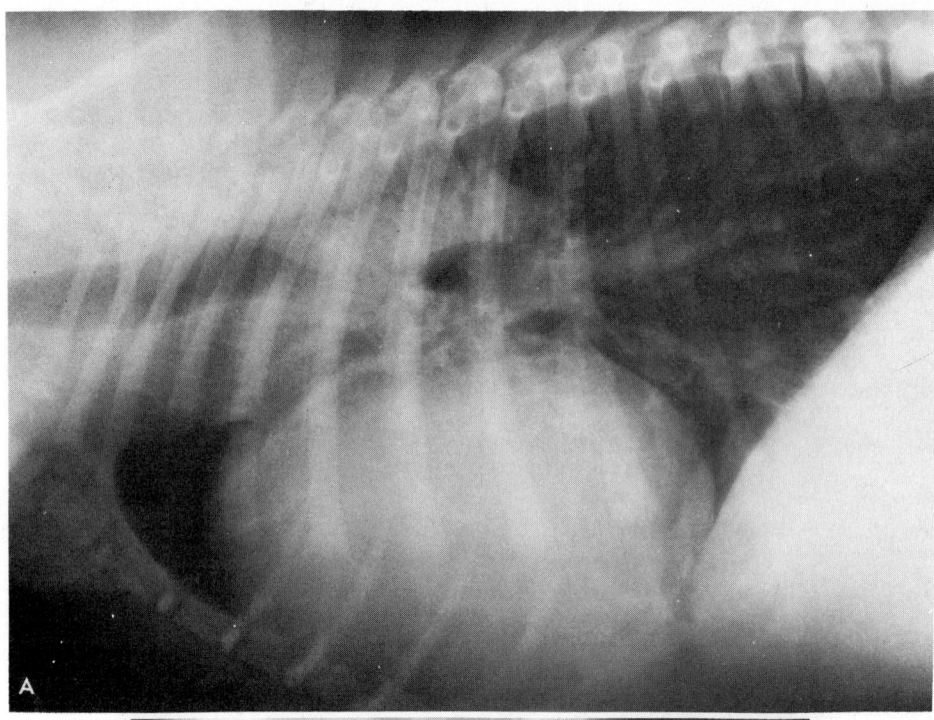

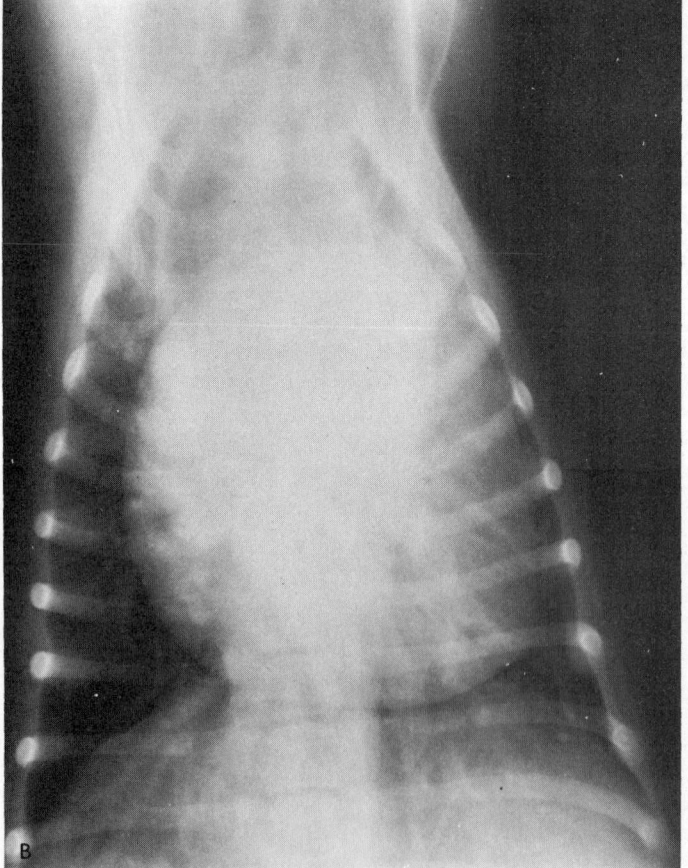

Figure 56–10. Survey and contrast radiographs of a three-month-old female English sheepdog presented with recurrent fever, bronchopneumonia, and occasional regurgitation. Note (*C*) the dorsal displacement of the esophagus on the lateral view, and (*D*) the widening with disruption of the normal mucosal pattern on the dorsoventral contrast radiograph. The involvement of the esophagus and the clinical signs are compatible with a periesophageal abscess. A perforation of the esophagus could not be found at necropsy. (Courtesy of Dr. Norman Ackerman.)

Illustration continued on opposite page

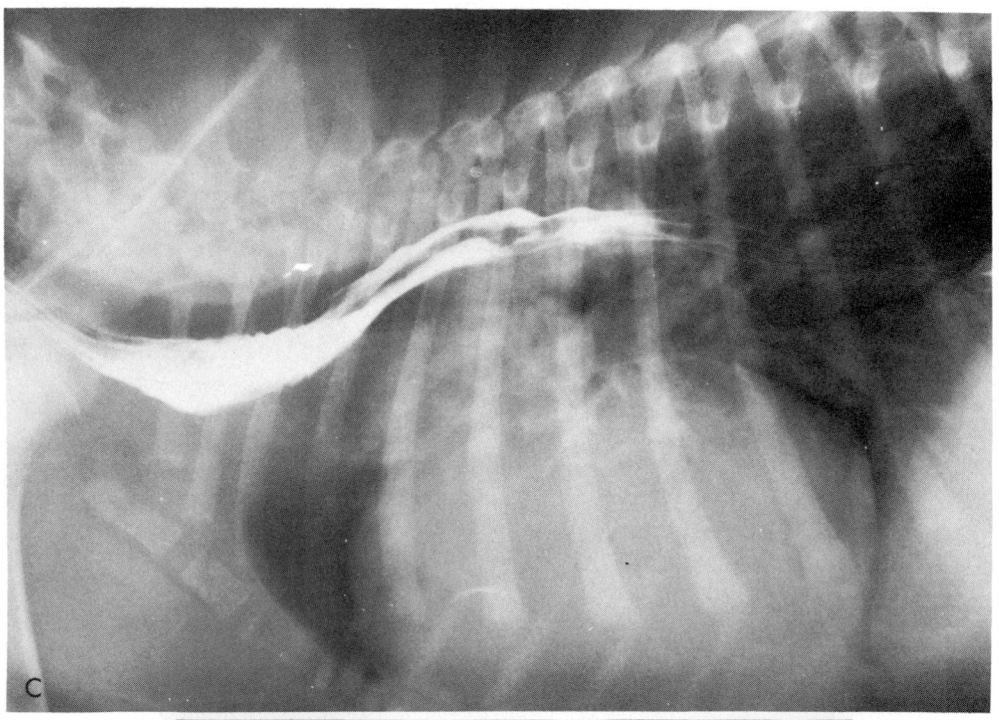

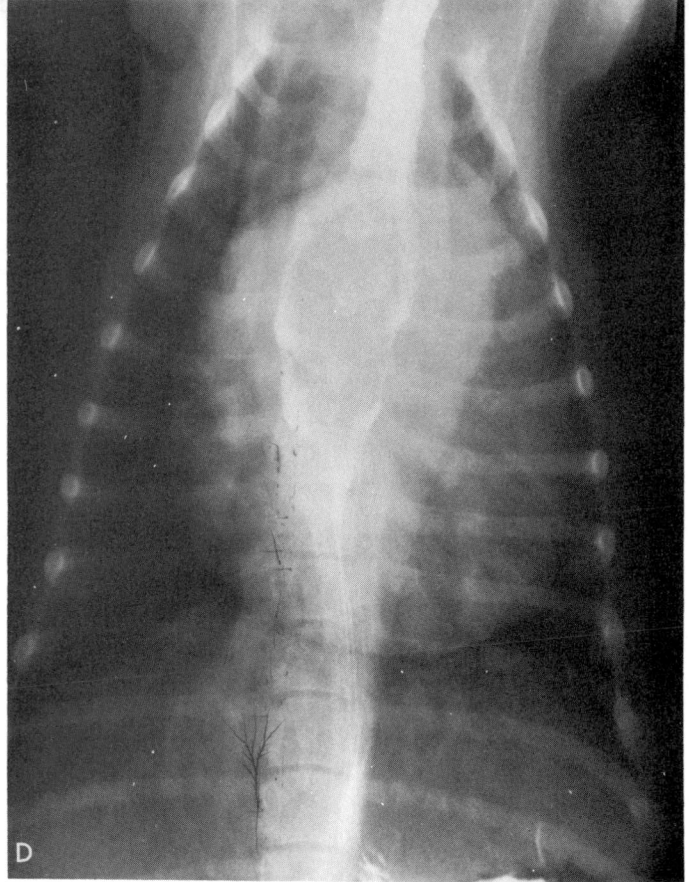

Figure 56–10. *Continued*

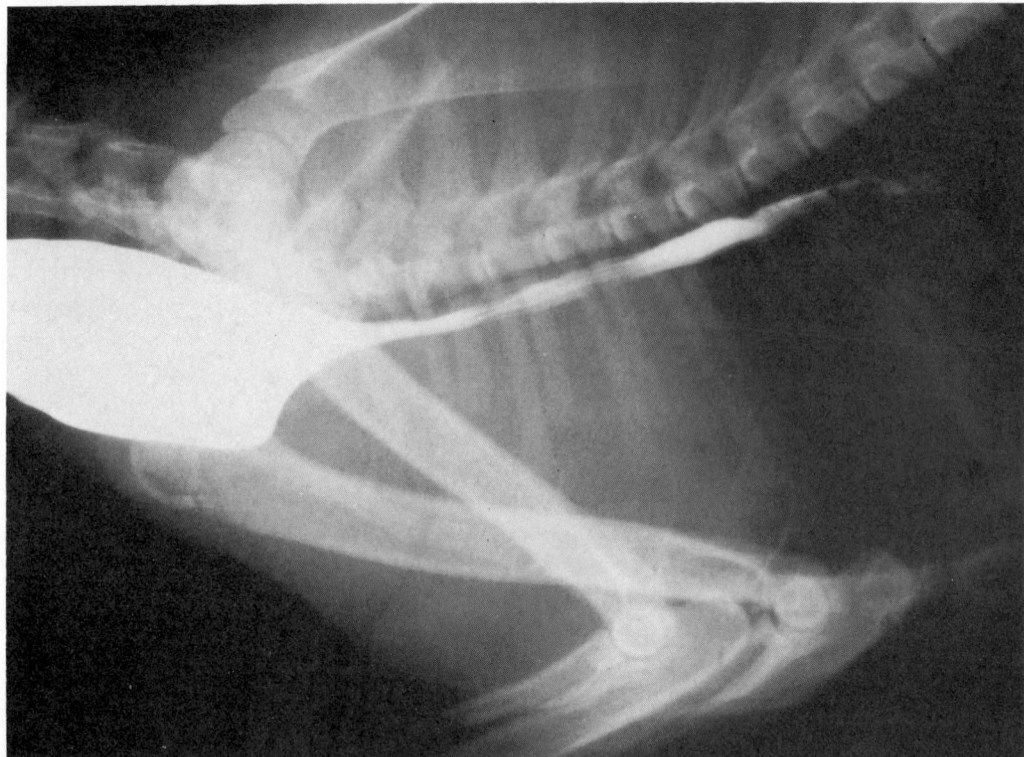

Figure 56–11. A lateral contrast radiograph of an immature female domestic shorthair cat with cranial mediastinal lymphosarcoma. Regurgitation and respiratory distress were presenting complaints. The esophageal lumen is greatly dilated proximal to the periesophageal lymphoid mass.

The thickened wall is rarely identified on survey radiographs. Infiltrating periesophageal masses may enlarge and displace the trachea, as well as the esophagus, sufficiently to be seen (Fig. 56–10). The identification of pulmonary metastases would lend support to suspected involvement of the esophagus.

Positive contrast radiography is often required to define the mural infiltration. Contrast radiographic findings include pooling of contrast cranial to a sudden or gradual luminal narrowing; prolonged contrast retention associated with a secondary motility disturbance; irregular, thickened, or missing mucosal folds; "staining" of the mucosal surface by adherent contrast media at sites of ulceration; and displacement of the esophageal body (Figs. 56–9, 56–10, and 56–11).

One case of metastatic bronchogenic carcinoma of the esophagus mimicked primary esophageal motor dysfunction because of its diffuse, invasive nature (Ridgeway and Suter, 1979).

Endoscopy may allow the mass to be visualized to verify the diagnosis and permit biopsy. Diffuse infiltration may be seen as a change in mucosal coloration, presence of erosion or ulceration, or lack of mural distensibility. The normal course of the esophageal lumen may deviate around periesophageal masses.

Treatment and prognosis are dependent upon the disease process. *Spirocerca lupi* granulomas respond to disophenol, diethylcarbamazine, and dithiazanine iodide (Stromback, 1979). Malignancy has a grave prognosis. Surgical excision may be possible if the tumor mass is small, but this is often not practical. Treatment of thyroid carcinoma by combination drug and radiation therapy has been advocated (Jeglum, 1980). Radiation-induced esophagitis, however, is a potential sequela. Lymph node enlargement with lymphosarcoma is often responsive to chemotherapy. Abscesses and granulomas may respond to appropriate antibiotic therapy.

VASCULAR RING ANOMALIES

Aberrant development of the major vessels arising from the embryonic aortic arches may result in a "vascular ring." This vascular arrangement may in turn entrap the esophagus, causing constriction. The most frequently encountered anomaly (the dextroaorta) is the development of the aortic arch from the embryonic right fourth arch instead of the left. The left sixth arch forms the ductus arteriosus, which provides a communication between the fetal pulmonary artery and the aorta *in utero.* When this closes in the neonate, the ligamentum arteriosum forms a dorsal constricting band, binding the esophagus between the dorsal and right-sided aortic arch, the dorsal and left-sided ligamentum arteriosum, and the pulmonary artery and heart base beneath. The embryology of the persistent right aortic arch is detailed by Wysong (1969) and Ettinger and Suter (1970). Other less common vascular anomalies include (1) double aortic arch due to persistence of both right and left fourth arches; (2) a dextroaorta and left subclavian artery, which crosses dorsally over the esophagus; and (3) a retroesophageal right subclavian artery with a normal aortic arch (Buergelt and Wheaton, 1970). Esophageal constriction by intercostal arteries has also been described (Bellenger and Warren, 1970).

Frequently, additional cardiac or vascular anomalies (such as a persistent left cranial vena cava) are present but may not be of physiologic significance. Rarely, when esophageal obstruction is associated with the ligamentum arteriosum, patency of the ductus is present and may be detected by auscultation of a machinery murmur. When a double aortic arch occurs, constriction is severe and will cause tracheal compression with subsequent respiratory signs. An anomalous right subclavian artery coexisted with a subaortic stenosis in one German shepherd dog (Carmichael et al., 1968).

The frequency of reports is greater in the dog than in the cat. Canine breeds predisposed to the congenital anomalies are German shepherds, Boston terriers and the Irish setters (Leipold, 1977; Patterson, 1968). Genetic transmission was shown in the German shepherd (Patterson, 1968). The occurrence is also reported in cats with no apparent predilection for sex or breed.

The clinical presentation is most often due to the acute onset of regurgitation at the time of weaning to solid foods. Occasionally signs associated with ingestion of maternal milk will occur in the neonate. These two groups account for over 90 per

cent of the cases and present before six months of age (Patterson, 1971). Rarely the signs will be intermittent or masked by recurrent pulmonary disease or suppressed by dietary management consisting of slurried meals instituted by the owners (Imhoff and Foster, 1963). In these cases the animals may present at a mature age. When noted, palpable pouches in the cervical region represent the dilated esophagus. Either impingement on the trachea by the dilated esophagus or aspiration pneumonia may cause dyspnea (Fig. 56–12). Poor growth and weight gain may occur.

The survey radiographic findings are often conclusive of a vascular ring anomaly. The esophagus will be seen as a dilated air- or fluid-filled sac or tubular structure in the cervical and cranial thoracic region that abruptly tapers over the base of the heart at the level of the sixth rib (Fig. 56–12,*A*). The degree of dilatation depends on the age of the animal and the length of time it has taken up solid food. When excessive, the esophageal enlargement causes ventral and right lateral displacement of the trachea. The heart may be small. Aspiration pneumonia is frequently present (Fig. 56–12,*B*).

A dorsoventral or ventrodorsal radiograph can confirm the diagnosis of a dextroaorta based upon the deviation of the esophagus and trachea relative to the aortic arch. In these cases the trachea fails to make the normal slight rightward bend between the thoracic inlet and bifurcation. The trachea is usually straight and may take a slight leftward path relative to midline. The esophagus drapes over the trachea, extending into both right and left hemithoraces. The normal bulge of the aortic arch to the left of the spine is absent.

A barium contrast swallow is recommended to confirm the presence of a stricture, determine the degree of dilatation, and rule out the possible presence of generalized esophageal dilatation due to concurrent congenital hypomotility (Fig. 56–13). Other esophageal diseases that need to be differentiated from a vascular ring anomaly include foreign body obstruction, intrinsic stricture, and diverticulum.

Treatment is aimed at early surgical correction of the stricturing band by ligation and transection of the compromising ligament or vessel. The esophagus should be freed from surrounding fibrous tissue to ensure correction of the stenosis. If a left cranial vena cava is present, the approach is

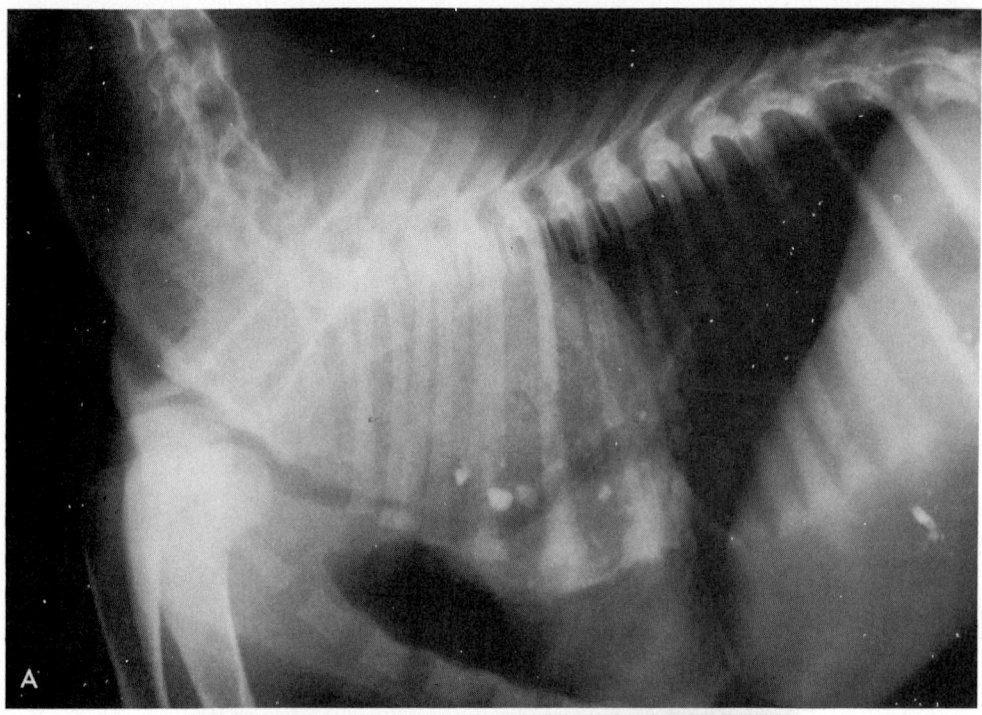

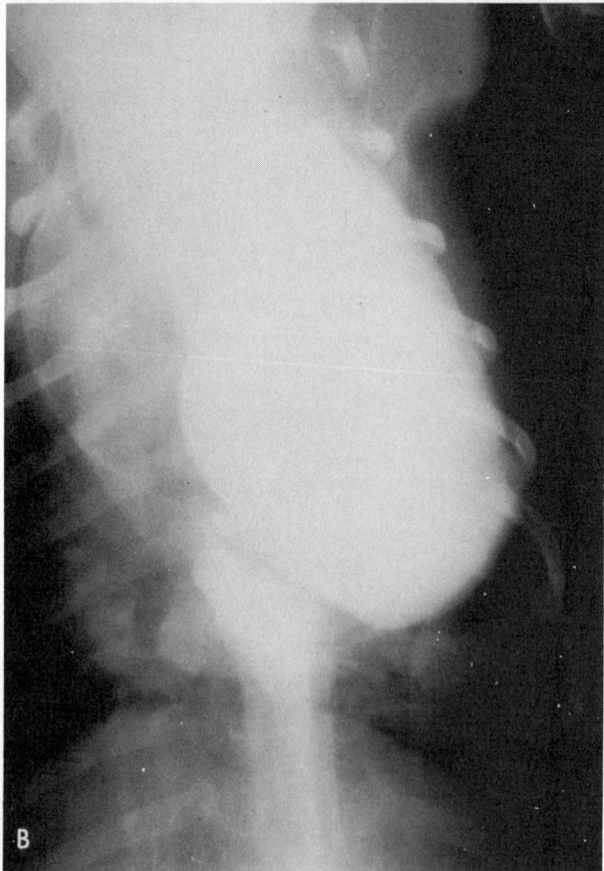

Figure 56–12. Lateral survey and dorsoventral contrast radiographs of an eight-week-old female Irish setter puppy that had regurgitated ingesta regularly since weaning. On physical examination, the cervical esophagus palpated to be thin and dilated. Increased respiratory sounds suggested the presence of aspiration pneumonia. *A,* A food-filled dilated esophagus extends from the UES to the base of the heart, indicating the presence of an obstruction due to a vascular ring anomaly. *B,* A contrast radiograph shows the dilated cranial thoracic esophagus extending to both sides of midline as it drapes over the trachea. The caudal thoracic esophagus shows a more normal conformation.

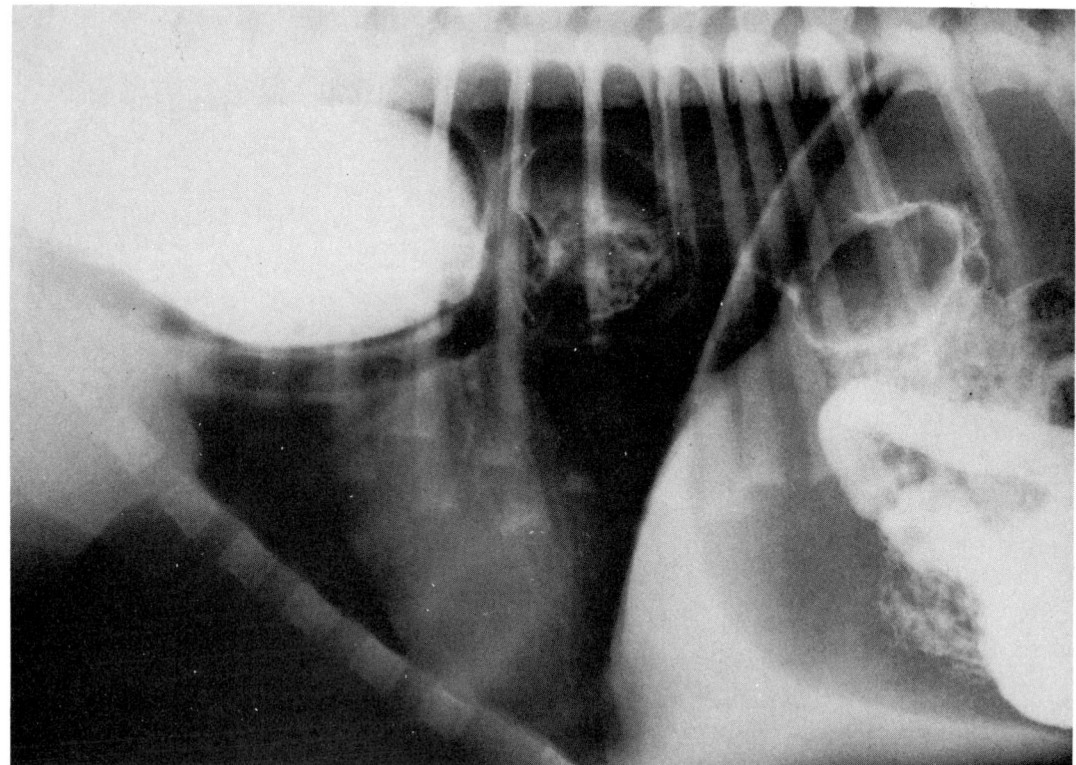

Figure 56–13. Lateral contrast radiograph of a ten-week-old male golden retriever with a persistent right aortic arch. It is important to recognize the dilated, air-filled caudal thoracic esophagus. This indicates the coexistence of congenital esophageal hypomotility. The prognosis for improvement following surgical correction of the vascular ring is worsened by the generalized megaesophagus.

hampered. The surgical technique is well described (Pyle, 1977; DeHoff, 1970). The finding of a markedly dilated cranial esophagus or generalized esophageal dilatation is cause for a poorer prognosis.

ESOPHAGEAL FISTULAE

Communication between the esophageal lumen and respiratory tract has been encountered rarely in the dog and cat. The fistulae may be esophagotracheal, esophagobronchial, or esophagopulmonary. Esophageal foreign bodies have been the only documented etiology. Potential causes include malignant esophageal disease, penetrating trauma to the esophagus, infectious or neoplastic pulmonary disease, preexisting esophageal diverticula, and periesophageal lymphadenopathy. Congenital occurrence has not been proven but might account for some neonatal deaths and has been suggested for one case that had signs since birth (Pozzi, 1973) and one that developed signs at two years of age (Stogdale et al., 1977).

Acquired fistulae develop from a process of gradual local esophageal necrosis leading to perforation and adhesion formation between the esophagus and adjacent airway. Local necrosis of the airway occurs secondarily, creating a communicating fistulous tract. When created by an esophageal foreign body the tract may be occluded until the foreign body is removed (Dodman and Baker, 1978).

Clinical signs usually pertain to the respiratory system. Coughing and choking are persistent and exacerbated by ingestion of fluids. Solids may be better tolerated owing to the small diameter of the communication. Regurgitation may occur, indicating significant esophageal disease. Moist rales may be auscultated over the consolidated region. Systemic signs of illness, including listlessness, weakness, and fever, may manifest the presence and degree of pneumonia or, with extension to the pleural space, pleuritis.

Survey radiographs may reveal a bronchopneumonia, indicating the presence of pulmonary contamination (Fig. 56–14,A and B). In the cat, consolidation of the left

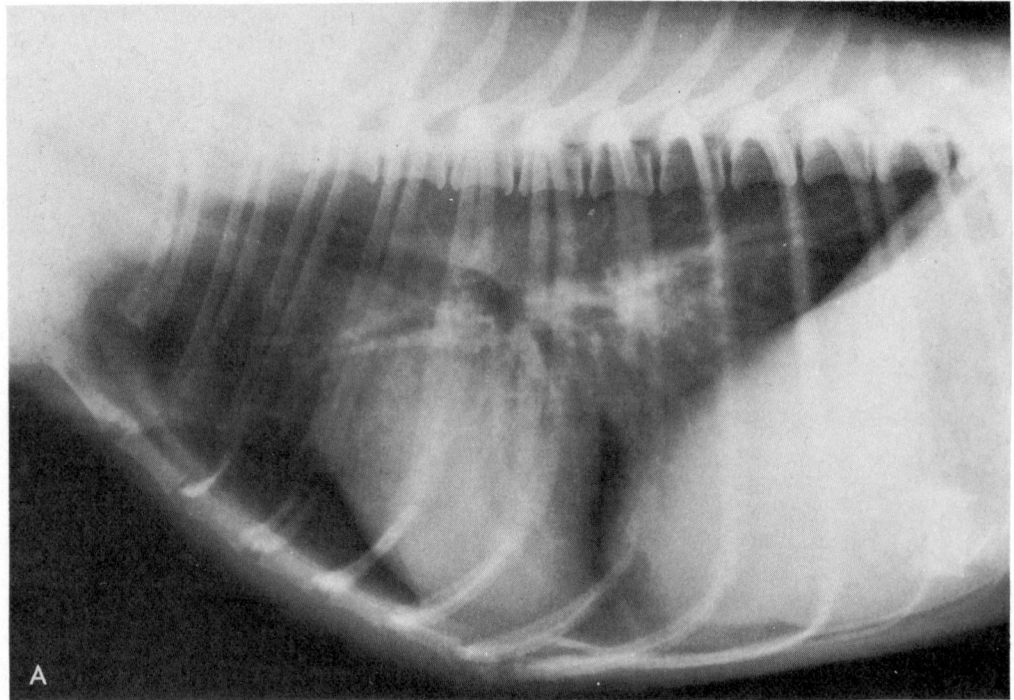

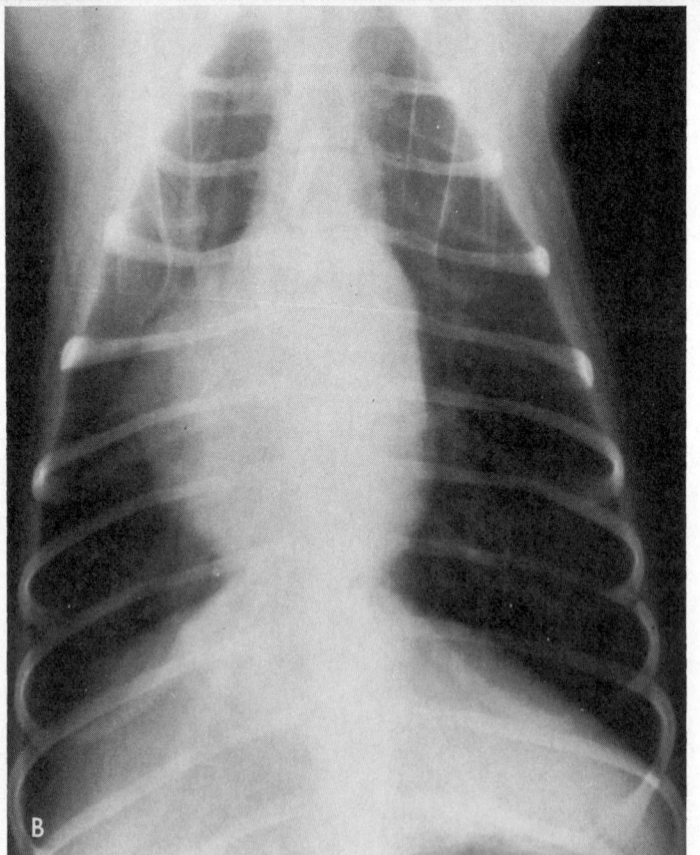

Figure 56–14. *A* and *B*, Survey radiographs of a two-year-old terrier cross with a history of coughing during and after eating. *C* and *D*, The esophagram shows simultaneous filling of the right bronchus and esophagus, indicating a bronchoesophageal fistula. (Courtesy of Dr. Richard Park.)

Illustration continued on opposite page

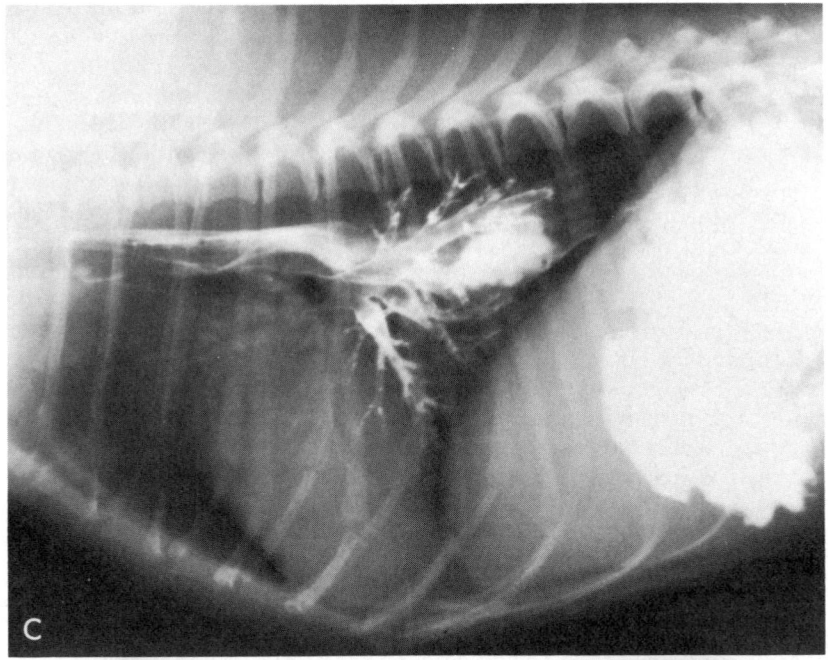

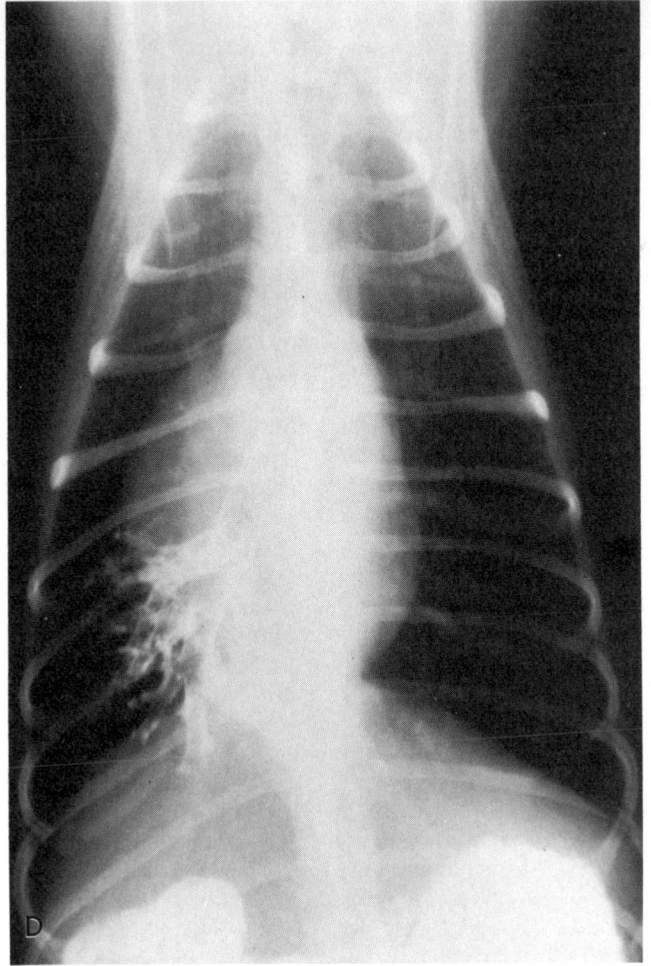

Figure 56–14 *Continued.*

middle lobe has been observed with a left esophagobronchial fistula (Reif, 1969). A right middle lobe pneumonia has been reported in dogs with esophagobronchial fistulae (Kleine, 1974; Thrall, 1973). The difference in location may relate to species differences in the path of the esophagus over the carina and mainstem bronchi (Thrall, 1973). A contrast radiographic examination will confirm the presence of esophageal perforation and locate the respiratory tract communication (Fig. 56–14, C and D). If pleural involvement is noted on the survey radiographs, an organic iodide compound approved for bronchography is recommended to minimize possible contamination of the pleural space by barium.

Endoscopy may or may not identify the site of esophageal fistulation. A focus of inflammation or laceration may be seen.

Esophageal fistulae must be differentiated from spontaneous bronchopneumonia, aspiration pneumonia secondary to a swallowing disorder, and pulmonary abscess or granuloma. Surgical correction of esophageal integrity is required. Lobectomy of the involved lobe with esophagobronchial and esophagopulmonary fistulae may be required to contain the pulmonary disease.

ESOPHAGEAL DIVERTICULA

An esophageal diverticulum is a focal dilatation in the wall that produces a pouch. Congenital diverticula are not well documented in small animals. Acquired forms are subdivided into pulsion and traction diverticula, based on their pathogenesis. Pulsion diverticula develop in association with a rise in intraluminal esophageal pressure and may arise from abnormal regional peristalsis (Lantz et al., 1976) or when normal peristalsis is obstructed by a stenosis (O'Brien, 1978). Pulsion diverticula secondary to foreign bodies or motility disturbances occur most often in the epiphrenic region (Pearson et al., 1978b; Lantz, 1976). Vascular ring stenosis may lead to a cranial thoracic diverticulum (O'Brien, 1978).

A traction diverticulum occurs as a result of periesophageal inflammation and fibrosis. Adhesion and contraction of the esophageal wall binds it to the adjacent tissues, causing a rigid focus in the normally distensible and movable tube. These arise most often in the cranial and midthoracic esopha-

gus. The clinical significance of both pulsion and traction diverticula is the same.

The outpouchings are not to be confused with the normal redundancy of the canine esophagus frequently seen in the brachycephalic breeds and when young normochondroid breeds are radiographed with their heads tucked under. The esophageal folding occurs in the thoracic inlet and allows for normal extension and flexion of the neck (O'Brien, 1978). Occasionally, however, clinically significant diverticula may be encountered in the brachycephalic dogs associated with esophageal deviation and compression by adjacent vascular structures in this location (Woods et al., 1978).

Small outpouchings are of little clinical significance per se and may exist for years, but the underlying esophageal disease may produce signs of dysphagia and regurgitation. With enlargement, the diverticula accumulate food, and gagging and retching with unsuccessful attempts at bringing up esophageal contents may be observed. Profound discomfort (odynophagia) with recurrent inappetence has also been a presenting complaint (Reed and Cobb, 1960). The stasis can cause obstruction of the lumen or inflammation, ulceration, and eventual perforation with its consequences. The medical history may include prior esophageal disorders, including foreign body, esophagitis, stricture, or esophageal motility disturbance.

The diverticula can be identified radiographically as either air- or food-filled masses in the path of the esophagus. A list of differential diagnoses includes an esophageal or periesophageal abscess, a necrotic tumor, or a pulmonary mass. A hiatal hernia or gastroesophageal intussusception can resemble an epiphrenic diverticulum.

Contrast radiography will demonstrate a focal dilated segment of the esophageal lumen that fills partially or completely with contrast media (Fig. 56–15). Cinefluorography or videofluorography might demonstrate an underlying esophageal motility disturbance, including significant gastroesophageal reflux, or a stenotic lumen caudal to the diverticulum. Endoscopy can confirm the morphologic problem and determine the presence of associated esophagitis. It can also facilitate the removal of entrapped debris.

Small luminal defects may be managed

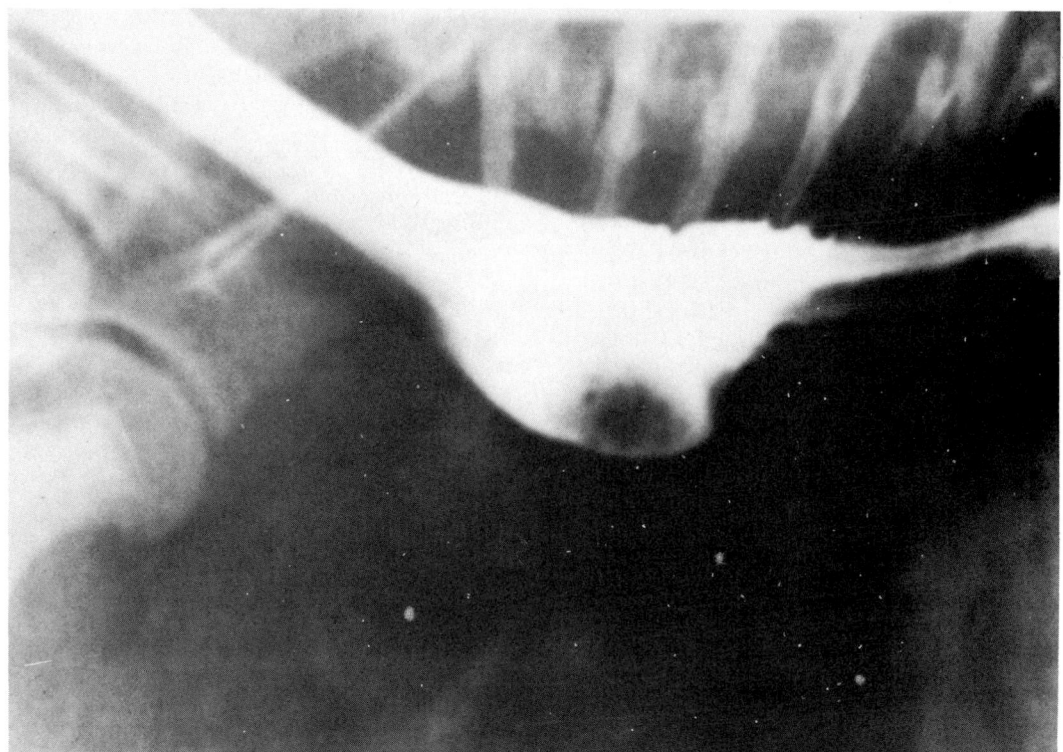

Figure 56–15. A lateral contrast radiograph of a five-month-old male bulldog with a cranial thoracic esophageal diverticulum and associated intermittent signs of regurgitation. The clinical signs gradually spontaneously resolved over several months.

by diet. Soft gruels and plenty of liquids will prevent excessive food accumulation in the pouch. Surgical excision and reconstruction of the esophageal wall are required for large diverticula.

ESOPHAGITIS, ESOPHAGEAL STENOSIS, AND PERFORATION

Inflammation of the esophagus can be a complication of transient or chronic insult to the esophageal lumen and is rarely caused by infectious agents. Nonmicrobial causes include ingestion of chemical irritants, thermal burns, acute and persistent vomiting, trauma from foreign bodies, and gastroesophageal reflux. The latter two causes will be discussed separately. Esophagitis caused by an infectious agent has been rarely reported. Immunosuppressed patients or those on long term antibiotics may be susceptible to *Candida* infection. Two cases of esophageal involvement by phycomycoses are described in a report of 17 cases (Ader, 1979). As in these cases, esophageal involvement most likely occurs in asso-

ciation with systemic disease that includes much of the gastrointestinal tract. Acute esophagitis with ulceration has been seen in some cats with upper respiratory infections, especially calicivirus (O'Brien, 1978). Thermal injuries happen when eager canine eaters bolt hot foods or when young puppies or kittens are fed gruels made with hot liquids. Caustic or thermal burns may be limited to the oral cavity, but if the inciting agent is swallowed, injury to the esophagus is imminent. Reflex reaction to the sensory stimulation of the esophageal mucosa leads to rapid regurgitation. The depth of tissue injury is proportional to the duration of contact. Severe injury, as reported in man, may lead to mucosal slough (Terracol and Sweet, 1958).

Esophagitis can be limited to mucosal damage or can involve submucosa and musculature. Superficial esophagitis is confined to mucosal involvement and is usually self-limiting when the inciting agent is removed. Clinical signs are minimal or absent. Deep or chronic esophagitis influences esophageal motility and can lead to complications such as ulceration, stricture formation, and rarely esophageal perforation with associated clinical signs.

Diagnosis of esophagitis is based on a known clinical history or high index of suspicion following a diagnostic workup. The clinical signs are dysphagia, reluctance to eat, hypersalivation, and regurgitation, often with specks of blood. Fever, depression, aspiration pneumonia, or shock occur in severe burns, particularly with esophageal perforation. A hemogram will be normal, except when complications occur.

Survey radiographic findings of esophagitis are often negative. Mild focal dilatation may lead to entrapment of air or fluid. A barium contrast examination may also be negative in mild cases, or in severe cases may outline an irregular mucosa and thickened folds due to erosion or ulceration and edema (Fig. 56–16). The contrast media becomes diluted when a large amount of fluid is present in the esophagus.

Dynamic radiographic studies are usually not required. If severe or widespread involvement is present, fluoroscopy may reveal abnormal esophageal motility. Caution must be maintained to prevent esophageal perforation during a contrast media examination.

Endoscopy may be required to make a definitive diagnosis by visualization of superficial mucosal changes including erythema, edema, and excess mucus. Biopsy may be indicated in questionable cases.

Treatment is aimed at removing the offending agent and symptomatic management of the esophagus and the systemic signs such as dehydration. If emesis or regurgitation has not occurred, it should not be induced. Toxic substances should be treated with oral administration of egg whites or vegetable oil. Gastric lavage should follow administration of milk of magnesia or magnesium oxide in the case of acid ingestion, or vinegar or one per cent acetic acid for alkali ingestion. Continued symptomatic treatment includes gastrointes-

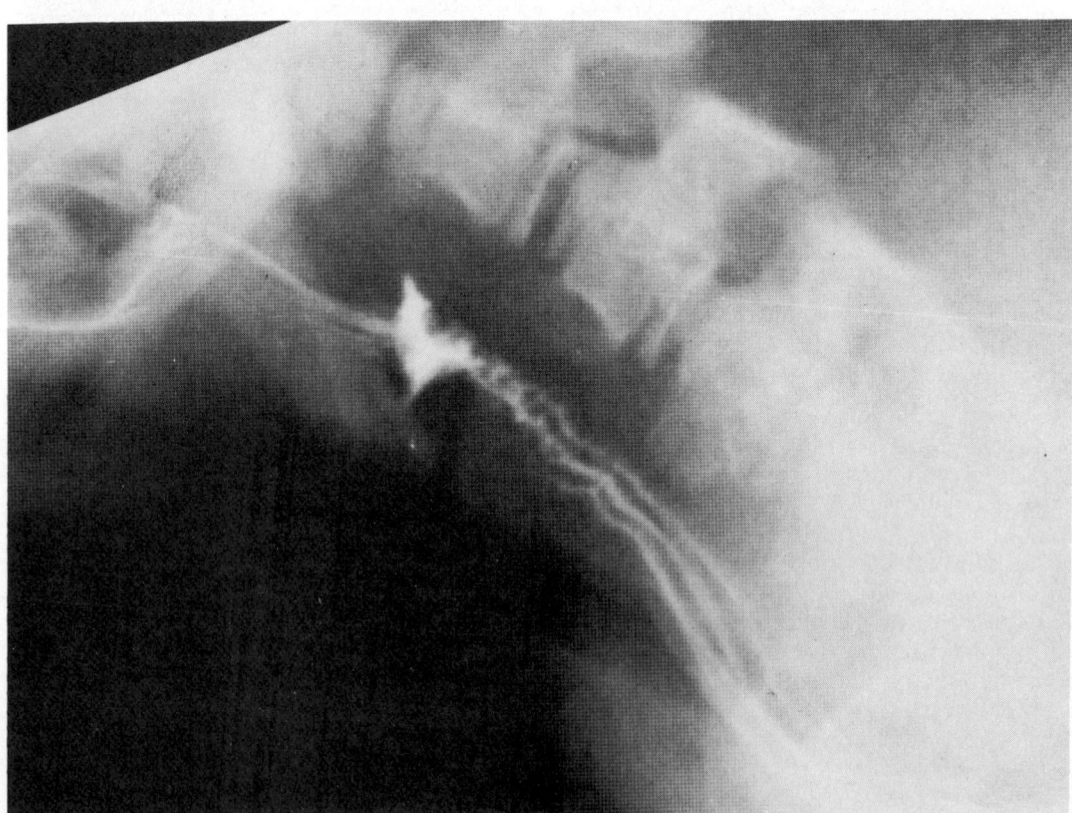

Figure 56–16. A lateral contrast radiograph of a six-week-old female Labrador retriever. Two of eight puppies in the litter were affected with signs of postprandial regurgitation of four days' duration. The litter's diet consisted of puppy kibble mixed with warmed milk. The irregular longitudinal folds of the proximal esophagus were indicative of esophagitis thought to be secondary to thermal injury.

tinal protectorants, an oral astringent (K permanganate), corticosteroids, and antibiotics (Atkins and Johnson, 1975). Oral alimentation should be postponed 24 to 72 hours, depending on the severity, and then reinstituted with a gruel for several days.

Complications are sequelae to ulceration and include stricture, perforation and secondary cellulitis, mediastinitis, pleuritis, or pulmonary-esophageal fistula formation. A clue to the development of esophageal stricture due to scarring is progressive dysphagia initially limited to solids, with difficulties with swallowing fluids developing later.

The most common cause of postinflammatory stricture is reflux of acid stomach content while the animal is under general anesthesia (Clifford et al., 1970; Wilson, 1977; Harvey, 1975; Pearson et al., 1978). Other likely causes include trauma from puncture wounds or following foreign body removal. Esophagitis following general anesthesia is often manifested by reluctance to eat and slow return to normalcy, with lethargy and vague discomfort. Regurgitation may be observed soon after recovery from anesthesia or delayed from eight to 14 days postoperatively (Harvey, 1975; Pearson et al., 1978).

Survey radiographic findings of stricture formation are often not present. The resultant esophageal dilatation containing gas or food material proximal to the stenosis develops with more severe strictures and with chronicity. Evidence of aspiration pneumonia may be present.

Esophagography of mild strictures using liquid barium may not reveal the lesion; however, severe strictures, especially with concurrent inflammation, show esophageal retention of contrast medium cranial and possibly caudal to the lesion. The contrast column tapers as it enters the stenotic lumen (Fig. 56–7). The column may be tortuous and irregular. The differential diagnosis includes obstruction by an intraluminal mass or foreign body or an extraluminal periesophageal mass. Intraluminal obstruction will be identified by an abruptly terminated or divergent contrast column cranial to the lesion as the contrast seeks to pass around the object. An extraluminal mass often displaces the narrowed contrast column.

To demonstrate a nondistensible lumen, increasing quantities of barium-impregnated solid pieces of food, cotton balls, marshmallows, or barium-filled livestock-sized gelatin capsules can be fed to the animal. Gastric tubes of varying diameter may also be passed until resistance is met. The animal can then be radiographed while liquid barium is administered through the tube.

Medical management of esophageal strictures is limited. Feeding of an adequate volume of gruel may maintain nutrition; however, bougienage (Harvey, 1975) or surgical intervention (Baker and Hoffer, 1966) is required in severe cases. The prognosis is guarded.

Esophageal perforation may be acute or insidious. Cervical esophageal perforations result in leakage of luminal contents into the loose periesophageal fascia, where chemical irritation stimulates inflammation. Accompanying sepsis further enhances the inflammatory response. Gradually an abscess may form or the cellulitis may extend along the deep fascial planes through the thoracic inlet to involve the mediastinum and/or pleural cavity. Thoracic esophageal perforations result in rapid contamination of the mediastinum and/or pleural cavity. Acute perforation with ensuing mediastinitis is usually a clinical emergency. Overwhelming infection and inflammation may lead to shock and death, although a more insidious process may occur with extension to the pleural space and subsequent pleuritis and pleural effusion. In these cases the clinical signs are milder, with regurgitation, hypersalivation, fever, malaise, anorexia, and generalized discomfort as the predominant features.

Radiographic findings of esophageal perforation may include deep soft-tissue gas around the cervical esophagus, soft tissue mass with or without displacement of the esophagus, widened mediastinum or mediastinal mass, pneumomediastinum, pneumothorax, variable amounts of intraluminal esophageal gas or fluid, and pleuritis (Fig. 56–6). When the survey radiographic findings are supportive of a suspected tear, further radiographic evaluation is not required.

Endoscopy may be used to help localize the perforation and ascertain the degree of esophageal involvement prior to surgical intervention. Thoracocentesis may produce a serosanguineous fluid with a high neutrophil content.

If the physical findings, clinical signs, or

radiographic interpretation are ambiguous, then an esophagram is recommended. A water soluble, organic iodine contrast medium such as Gastrografin is recommended to minimize contamination of the mediastinum and pleural cavity with a potentially irritating substance. If barium sulfate is inadvertently used and leaks from the esophageal perforation, adequate thoracic lavage will prevent the granulomatous response caused by the contrast media and esophageal contents (Vessal et al., 1975). Occasionally the water-soluble contrast media will fail to demonstrate a perforation either by not passing through the hole or by marked dilution in the thoracic effusion such that the contrast media is not identified radiographically (Fig. 56–6, B). In negative studies barium sulfate is then recommended.

Surgical intervention with debridement and primary closure of the esophageal lumen and drainage of the pleural space is required for treatment. The prognosis is poor.

DISEASES OF THE HIATUS

The esophagus passes through a perforation in the diaphragm to enter the abdominal cavity. The wall is tethered to this hiatus by a phrenoesophageal membrane that normally allows only minor cranial movement of the abdominal segment. This movement is observed during respiration and contraction of the outer longitudinal muscles of the esophagus, which cause shortening of the tube (Strombeck, 1979). A congenital or acquired abnormality of the esophageal hiatus may allow for a sliding hiatal hernia, a periesophageal hiatal hernia, a diaphragmatic hernia, or a gastroesophageal intussusception to occur. The differentiation of these disorders may be difficult owing to the similarity of clinical signs and survey radiographic findings.

A hiatal hernia allows for herniation of part or all of the abdominal esophagus, gastroesophageal junction, and stomach into the thoracic cavity. It may be self-reducing and cause only intermittent signs of regurgitation. The compromise in LES function may lead to gastroesophageal reflux, whereas gastric herniation could result in obstruction. Periesophageal hiatal hernias have been described (O'Brien, 1978) but are very rare.

Gastroesophageal intussusception or invagination occurs when all or part of the stomach telescopes into the esophageal lumen. Occasionally the spleen and pancreas are included. Infolding of gastric mucosa into the caudal esophageal lumen is observed regularly during the act of vomition (Smith et al., 1974) and may be an underlying factor in the development of gastroesophageal intussusception. Idiopathic megaesophagus may also be a predisposing condition (Pollack and Rhodes, 1970). Puppies of large breeds are most commonly affected, although the condition is uncommon.

Clinical signs of hiatal disease include dysphagia, regurgitation with possible hematemesis, dyspnea, and cachexia. The onset often follows a history of infrequent or recurrent regurgitation. The more acute the condition, the greater the discomfort exhibited by the animal. Abdominal pain may be manifest on palpation. The pH of regurgitated fluid may be low; obstruction to passage of a stomach tube is present. Death may occur.

Survey radiographs will reveal a focus of increased radiodensity and width to the caudal mediastinum. A short or long segment of gas-filled dilated thoracic esophagus may be seen proximal to the mass, which is continuous with the diaphragm. Frequently the fundic gas bubble is small or not seen. A barium contrast study is required to locate the gastroesophageal junction and gastric fundus.

With a hiatal hernia the LES, recognized as a focal narrowing of the barium contrast column, will be cranially displaced, with no identifiable abdominal esophageal segment. Variable amounts of the rugae-lined gastric fundus may be seen as an extension of the caudal esophagus in the thoracic cavity (Fig. 56–17). A periesophageal hernia will cause partial obstruction and displacement of the terminal esophagus laterally away from the herniated gastric fundus. On the dorsoventral contrast radiograph the fundus is identified by barium-coated gastric rugae and is lateral to the esophagus.

A gastroesophageal intussusception will be revealed by evidence of a mass lesion filling the terminal esophagus, which has a surface contour of rugal folds (Fig. 56–18). When the intussusception includes the spleen, its shadow will be absent on abdomi-

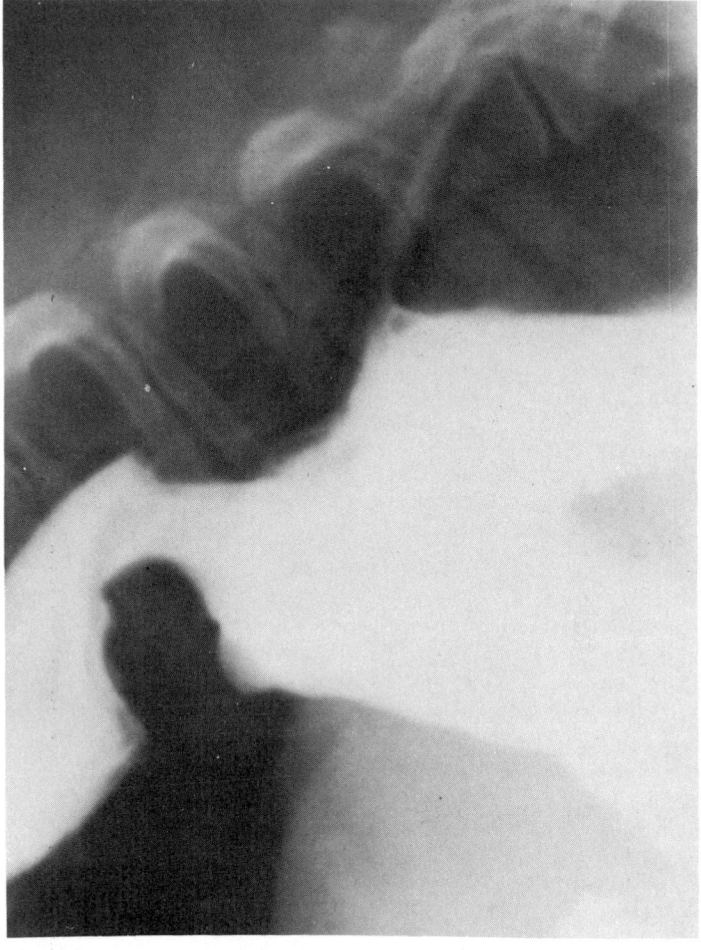

Figure 56–17. Lateral contrast radiograph of a ten-year-old neutered female beagle with a two-month history of gagging and regurgitation. The abdominal esophagus, gastroesophageal junction, and a portion of the gastric fundus are displaced cranial to the diaphragm. This hiatal hernia was surgically corrected.

nal radiographs. Surgical correction is required in all cases of persistent herniation or intussusception.

FUNCTIONAL DISORDERS OF SWALLOWING

Disorders of swallowing due to motility disturbances are caused by neurologic, neuromuscular junction, or muscular diseases. They can be acquired or congenital in origin and may be the primary disease or part of a systemic disease. The disorders arise from failure, spasticity, or incoordination of muscular contractions. Interruption of the coordinated interaction of the tongue, hyoid apparatus, soft palate, pharyngeal muscles, UES, esophagus, and/or LES will result in dysphagia. Classification of swallowing disorders by the region or regions of involvement has been described for the dog (Suter and Watrous, 1980; Watrous and Suter, 1979). The purposes for such a classification scheme are to localize the functional disorder; determine an appropriate treatment regimen, whether by medical management or surgery; predict a prognosis; and in some cases establish an etiology.

Accurate localization of the disorder often requires special examination techniques due to the ambiguity of the clinical signs and history. Survey radiographs and barium contrast studies serve to rule out gross morphologic abnormalities; however, due to the complexity and speed of the various phases of swallowing (in particular, the oropharyngeal phase), evaluation of the dynamics of the dysphagia are necessary. Videofluorography or cinefluorography allows a systematic analysis of function by enabling the clinician to slow down the swallowing process, evaluate it frame by frame, and review the recordings repeatedly. Manometry, electromyography, and endoscopy with biopsy may in some cases help to finalize the diagnosis.

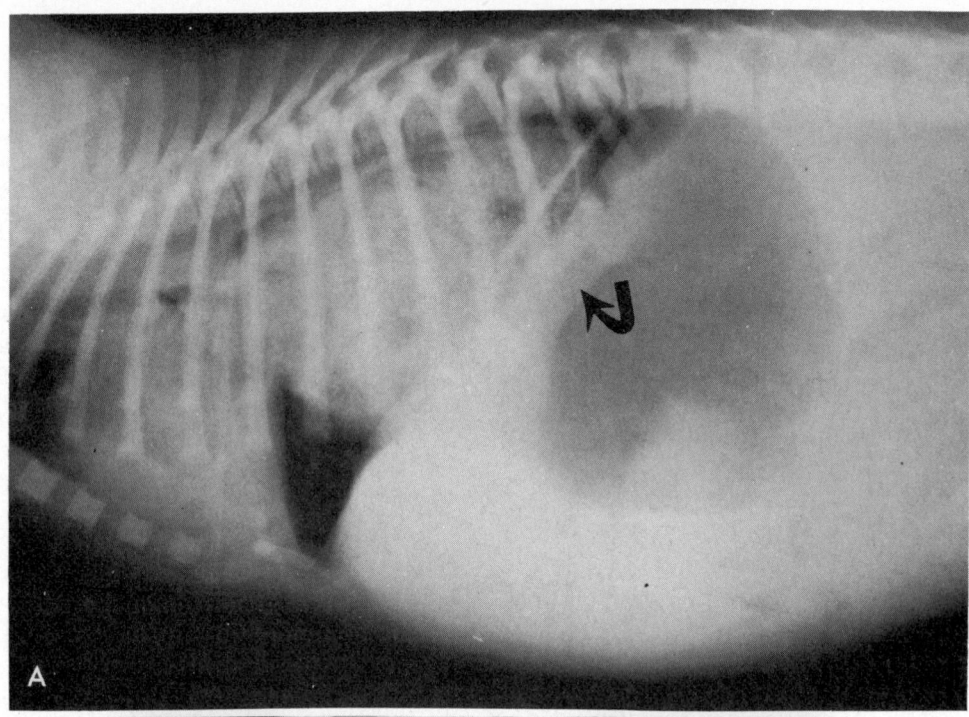

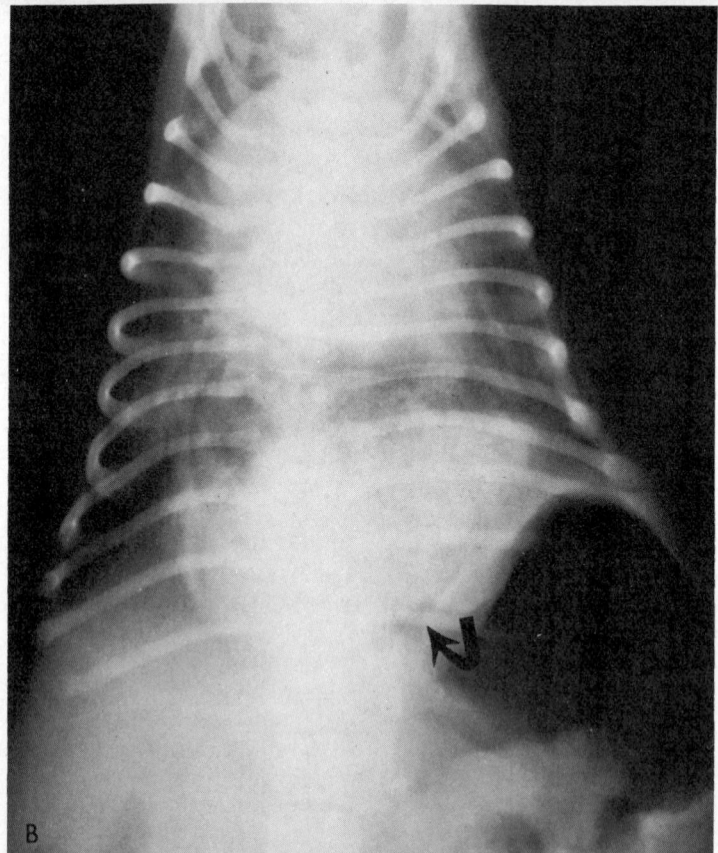

Figure 56–18. Lateral and dorsoventral radiographs of a six-week-old male beagle. The puppy was presented for dyspnea and cyanosis. Thoracic percussion revealed a water tissue density in the caudal half of the thorax. *A* and *B*, A nonhomogeneous "mass" is seen in the dorsal midline of the caudal thorax. The stomach is dilated with air. The curved arrows point to the site of gastric intussusception. *C,* The esophagram outlines the rugal folds covering the filling defect in the caudal thoracic esophagus, confirming the diagnosis of gastroesophageal intussusception.

Illustration continued on opposite page

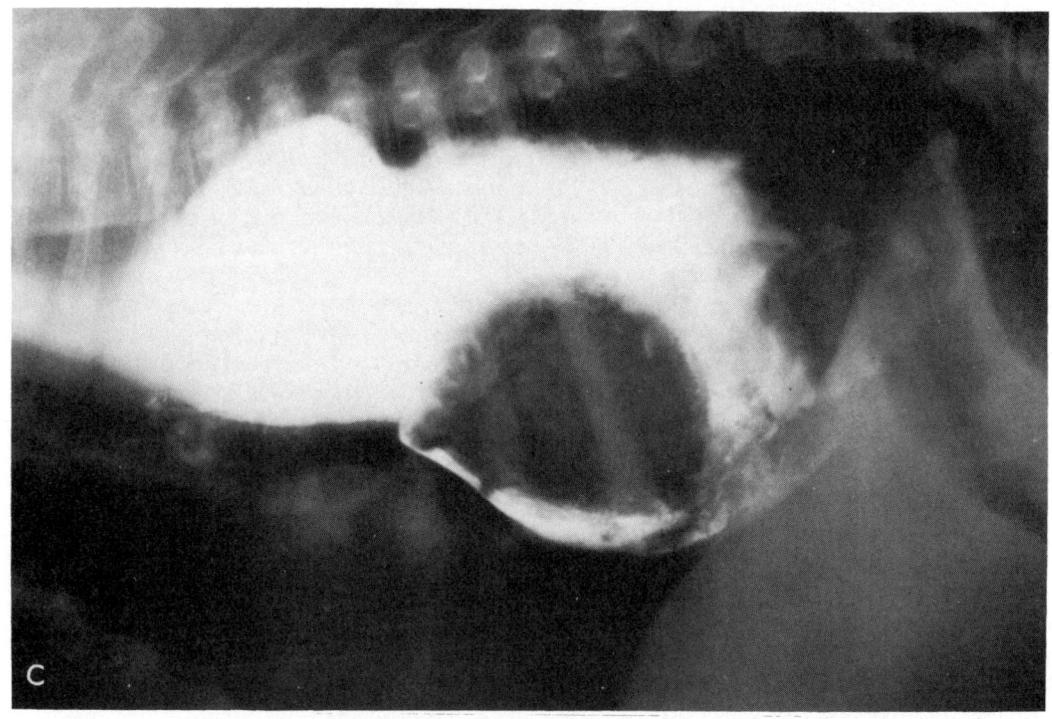

Figure 56–18 *Continued.*

OROPHARYNGEAL DYSPHAGIAS

Localization of signs relating to disorders of the oropharyngeal phase of swallowing has been discussed in the introduction to this chapter. *Oral stage* dysphagias have been reported in the dog (Suter and Watrous, 1980; Hoerlein, 1971). These have been due to hypoglossal nerve dysfunction resulting in loss of motor supply to the tongue and an inability to normally take up food or liquid. Hypoglossal nerve dysfunction has been associated with trauma, hydrocephalus, congenital defects, and suspected myasthenia gravis (Suter and Watrous, 1980; Hoerlein, 1971; Lorenz et al., 1972). Additional systemic muscular diseases reported rarely in the dog affecting the swallowing organs, including the tongue, are a muscular dystrophy–like myopathy (Griffiths and Duncan, 1973) and a familial myopathy of Irish terriers (Wentink et al., 1972). The condition has not been reported in the cat. A few cases have spontaneously recovered, others have been supported with elevated and hand feeding for a prolonged period. One dog was mistakenly diagnosed as having cricopharyngeal dysphagia and died from aspiration pneumonia following cricopharyngeal myotomy (Suter and Watrous, 1980).

Neuromuscular abnormalities of the tongue affect prehension of liquids and solids and the ability to organize a bolus at the base of the tongue. An animal with this problem is either unable to adequately take up food and hold it in its mouth or has acquired compensatory maneuvers to maintain nutrition and hydration. These include (1) submerging the muzzle deep into a pan of water to bypass the oral stage and initiate the pharyngeal stage of swallowing, (2) engulfing solids by tossing its head up and backwards to fling food into the oropharynx to initiate the pharyngeal stage, (3) chomping or excess chewing, during which food falls from the mouth, and (4) occasionally assuming an unusual posture during eating, such as the prone position. The tongue usually does not hang out of the mouth but fails to be retracted when grasped. These animals are unable to lick their nose. Hypersalivation is frequent. Coughing is occasionally encountered, but aspiration pneumonia is not. The presenting complaint may be only that of sloppy eating.

Survey radiographs are usually unremarkable but should be made to rule out structural abnormalities such as hyoid bone injuries. Contrast radiography is also of limited productiveness. Retention of contrast media may be seen in the oropharynx and valleculae (the deep ventral recesses on either side of midline of the oral surface of the epiglottis) following a swallow. The pharynx and esophagus are empty.

The motor deficit is best observed dynamically. Fluorography demonstrates pooling of contrast media throughout the oral cavity, with inadequate bolus formation at the base of the tongue. The tongue shows disorganized movements toward the hard and soft palate with inadequate stripping action. By instilling contrast at the base of the tongue with a tube, a large volume accumulates, spilling over into the pharynx, which will then initiate the pharyngeal stage accompanied by a weak tongue thrust and oropharyngeal reflux through the patent oral egress (Fig. 56–19).

Treatment of oral dysphagias is symptomatic. The compensatory maneuvers are often adequate to allow the animal to maintain nutrition and hydration. Hand feeding or feeding from an elevated platform also facilitates uptake of food. Although recovery from the deficit may not occur, the successful compensatory maneuvers adopted and the lack of respiratory complications permit a fair prognosis for longevity if systemic neuromuscular disease is not the underlying etiology for the deficit.

Pharyngeal Dysphagia. This condition is due to weakened pharyngeal contraction. The deficient aboral transport of the bolus across the pharynx and UES results in pharyngeal retention of ingested material. This may be associated with nasopharyngeal reflux and laryngotracheal aspiration. The dysfunction may be associated with oral and esophageal deficits. Histopathology has in most cases been unrewarding in establishing an etiology, but findings have included polyneuropathy, polymyositis, meningitis, brainstem hemorrhage, and idiopathic muscular degeneraton and necrosis (Suter and Watrous, 1980). Myasthenia gravis has also produced pharyngeal dysphagia.

Pharyngeal dysphagias usually mimic disorders of the cricopharyngeal (UES) sphincter. Uptake of liquids and solids is normal; however, repeated swallowing ef-

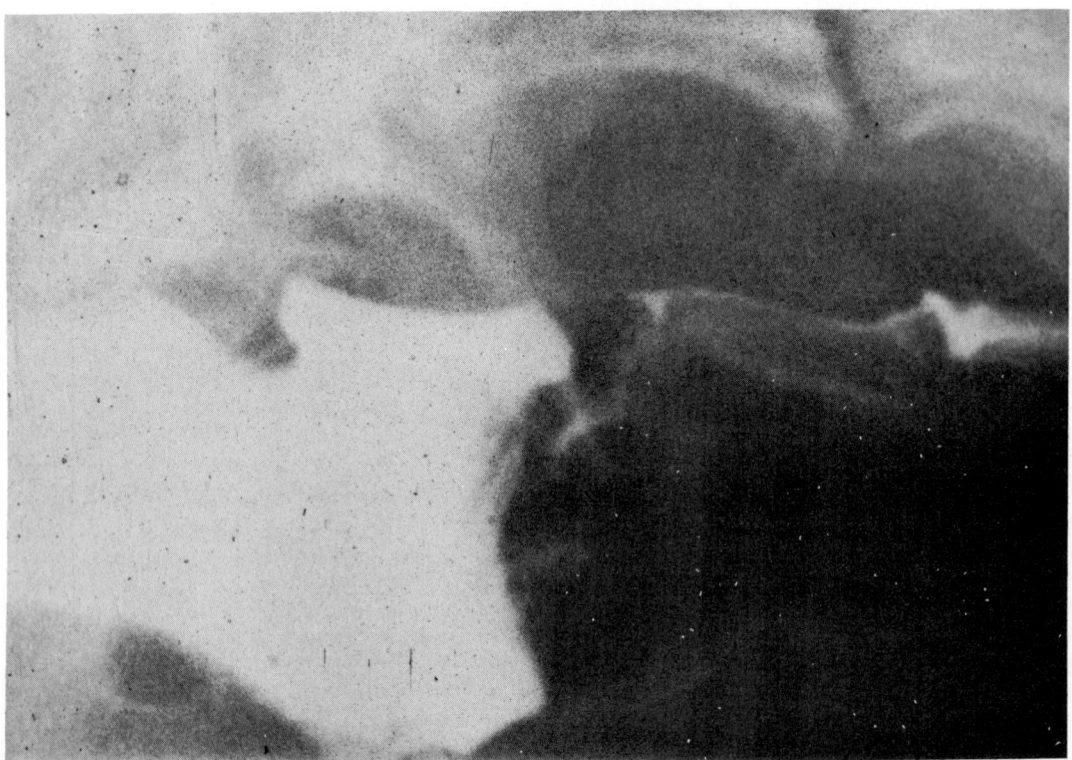

Figure 56–19. A lateral cine frame of a dog with a bilateral hypoglossal nerve deficit during the oral stage of swallowing. The dog was unable to ingest a sufficient volume of barium; therefore it was tube fed by depositing the liquid contrast media at the base of the tongue. The resultant bolus filled the oral cavity and pharynx and extended into the nasopharynx and hypopharynx. A normal pharyngeal stage would subsequently clear the pharynx but leave the oropharynx and valleculae filled with barium.

forts are observed, often with the head and neck tucked under in an exaggerated swallowing act. Differences in the ease of swallowing liquids and solids may be present. Saliva-coated food is often regurgitated or spit out only to be reingested until eventually swallowed. Pharyngeal retention of food may last for several hours and result in regurgitation of the bolus at times unrelated to eating. The retained food as well as the pharyngeal irritation may cause pharyngitis and oral fetor. Nasal reflux is frequent, owing to inadequate closure of the nasopharynx during the swallowing process. The gag reflex may be reduced. Respiratory complications, including aspiration pneumonia, are frequent. In severe cases the animals are debilitated and anorexic. The consequences of the swallowing disorder may be difficult to differentiate from an underlying neuromuscular disease with signs of muscle wasting and weakness.

Survey radiographs are usually unremarkable. Generalized neuromuscular disease may cause chalasia of the UES and megaesophagus. Contrast examinations will show significant retention of contrast media in the pharynx following a swallow. The oropharynx will be cleared. With resumption of respiration the glottis is exposed to pharyngeal contents and therefore laryngotracheal aspiration may be observed (Fig. 56–20).

Fluorography permits recognition of a weak pharyngeal contraction and a normal opening and closure of the UES and thus separates pharyngeal from cricopharyngeal dysphagia. The weak pharyngeal peristalsis may be seen to be assisted by a strong plunger-like thrust of the tongue that results in at least partial transport of the bolus through the UES. Nasal reflux is seen, owing to inadequate closure of the nasopharynx.

Treatment is symptomatic. Surgical intervention has shown disastrous consequences (Suter and Watrous, 1980). With myotomy of the UES, chalasia is created and esophagopharyngeal reflux occurs. This increases pharyngeal retention of ingesta and thus

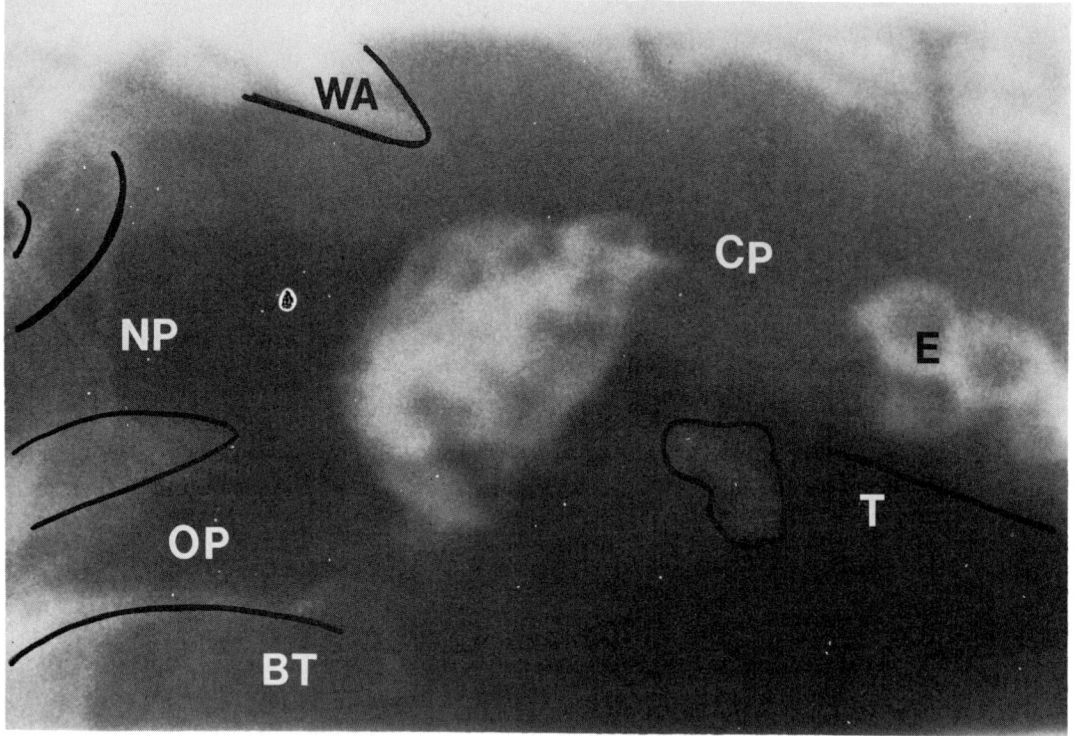

Figure 56–20. A lateral contrast cine frame during the early esophageal phase of swallowing. The barium coated food bolus has failed to be completely transported through the UES owing to a weak and ineffective pharyngeal contraction. Cricopharyngeal closure came at the same time that the weak pharyngeal stage died out. Laryngotracheal aspiration also occurred.

enhances laryngotracheal aspiration and pneumonia. The lack of adequate compensatory eating behavior or specific medical or surgical treatment and the high incidence of aspiration pneumonia make this a prognostically poor condition. Only myasthenia gravis and some of the inflammatory neuromuscular diseases may respond to specific therapy or time.

Cricopharyngeal Dysphagia. This condition may be due to nonopening (achalasia) or lack of coordination between opening or closure of the cricopharyngeal passage and pharyngeal contraction, or failure of the passage to close (chalasia). Failure of the UES to open prevents the vigorously contracting pharynx from delivering any of its contents to the esophagus. Cricopharyngeal achalasia has been repeatedly recognized in the dog but not in the cat. Observed muscle changes have included hypertrophy, inflammation with subsequent atrophy, fibrosis, and no change (Sokolovsky, 1967; Pearson, 1970; Rosin, 1972; Gourley and Leighton, 1972). A neurologic basis is likely.

Asynchrony between pharyngeal and cricopharyngeal relaxation may be due to premature opening or closure or delayed opening or closure. The result is similar to achalasia; the complete transport of the bolus is obstructed. Often small to large segments of the bolus may reach the esophagus through the opened UES. Clinical signs of cricopharyngeal dysphagia (both achalasia and the more frequently occurring incoordination) include a progressive to persistent dysphagia, in which ingestion of food is accompanied by frequent attempts at swallowing the same bolus. Often the head is held tucked under to enhance the force of swallowing by auxiliary neck muscles. Retained food will be spit out, picked up, and reswallowed. Occasionally, nasal reflux occurs with liquids. Coughing and gagging are frequent. Puppies are most commonly affected, and often onset is sudden and associated with weaning, suggesting a congenital origin. Their age at presentation, however, ranges from two months to ten years, indicating that some are acquired disorders. Poor growth rate and hair coat are observed in younger dogs. Severely affected animals may be emaciated and listless.

Survey radiographs are usually normal. A small triangle of air may be seen in the cranial esophagus but is not specific. Contrast radiographs following an attempted swallow of barium suspension reveals significant pharyngeal and cranial esophageal retention of contrast media; a distorted, identifiable UES bounded by the barium column; and probable demonstration of laryngotracheal aspiration and nasal reflux (Fig. 56–21). These findings are similar to pharyngeal dysphagia.

Fluoroscopically cricopharyngeal achalasia is manifested by consistent nonopening of the UES during a forceful contraction of the pharynx, which propels the bolus against the dorsocaudal wall of the pharynx and hypopharynx. Infrequently a small trickle of contrast media will pass through the narrow opening to pool in the cervical esophagus. With incoordination of the cricopharyngeal and pharyngeal function the UES is observed to open and close but at inappropriate times. As a consequence, part of the bolus reaches the esophagus but some is retained in the relaxing pharynx. Occasionally, complete transport of the bolus may occur. Laryngotracheal aspiration occurs when respiration resumes. A cough is usually initiated with rapid expulsion of the aspirated material. In some, no cough reflex occurs, suggesting that diminished laryngeal and tracheal sensitivity is present.

Out of 18 cases of oropharyngeal dysphagia presented to the University of California Veterinary Medical Teaching Hospital, eight were shown to have oral stage deficits, four had pharyngeal stage deficits, and only two had typical cricopharyngeal achalasia. Eight others demonstrated cricopharyngeal-pharyngeal incoordination. Ten of the 18 dogs underwent cricopharyngeal myotomy. Three subsequently died or were euthanized due to postoperative exacerbation of the laryngotracheal aspiration. Thus, it is important to differentiate these oropharyngeal dysphagias and to recognize all regions involved in order to institute the appropriate therapy. If either weak pharyngeal contraction or severely reduced cranial esophageal motility is present, cricopharyngeal myotomy is contraindicated. Signs of cricopharyngeal dysphagia, however, may be reduced or abolished by myotomy.

Cricopharyngeal Chalasia. This has been seen following cricopharyngeal myotomy and with generalized skeletal muscle weakness, including myasthenia gravis. Anesthesia will create incompetence of the

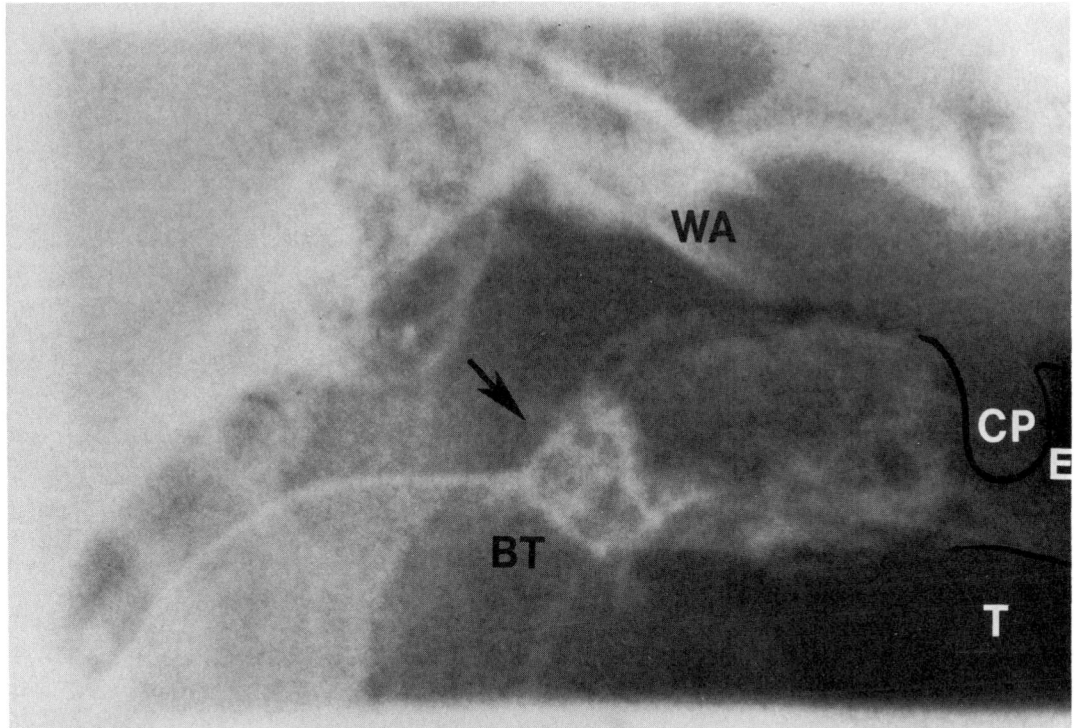

Figure 56–21. A lateral contrast cine frame during the pharyngeal and cricopharyngeal stages of swallowing. The pharynx is in vigorous contraction against a closing UES. The floor of this passage is open, allowing air and contrast to outline the distorted sphincter. This asynchrony between pharyngeal and cricopharyngeal stages occurs more commonly than true cricopharyngeal achalasia. A cricopharyngeal myotomy is palliative if pharyngeal function is good and laryngotracheal aspiration is minimal.

UES as well. The decreased tone of the sphincter results in recurrent esophagopharyngeal reflux.

Normally the cricopharyngeal passage is not visible on lateral survey radiographs. With chalasia the passage may be closed owing to sufficient tissue elasticity and residual muscle tone, but a small pocket of air is commonly present in the cranial esophagus, outlining the caudal margin of the UES. Often the passage is wide open and filled with air. Contrast examinations demonstrate a continuous column of barium extending from the pharynx into the cranial esophagus. UES chalasia is usually accompanied by esophageal dilatation when caused by a generalized neuromuscular disease (Fig. 56–22). Fluoroscopy will demonstrate esophagopharyngeal reflux and aerophagia.

If the UES chalasia is secondary to a treatable disease such as myasthenia gravis, the prognosis is fair. Swallowing may be facilitated by elevated feedings. When chalasia is present in conjunction with pharyngeal weakness, the dysphagia and secondary pulmonary contamination are severe and life threatening.

ESOPHAGEAL HYPOMOTILITY (MEGAESOPHAGUS)

Motor disturbances of the esophageal body result in abnormal or unsuccessful transport of ingesta between the pharynx and stomach. Numerous reports of these disturbances in veterinary literature have resulted in as many names, including esophageal hypomotility, atony or dysphagia, megaesophagus, esophageal dilatation, cardiospasm, achalasia, and idiopathic neuromuscular dysfunction. Some proponents of the term esophageal achalasia have based this on the acquired disorder of humans characterized by increased LES tone with failure to relax. Successful manometric evaluations have, however, been limited in animals and have indicated that some dogs actually have reduced LES tone (Clifford et al., 1975). Current literature favors the dysfunction to be a primary esophageal motor

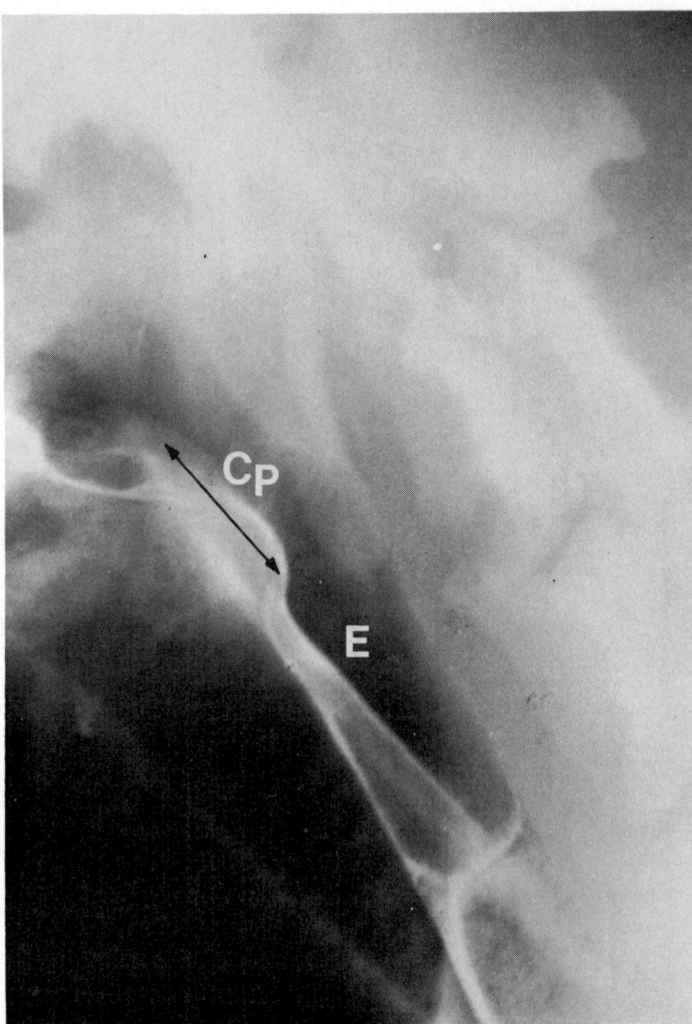

Figure 56–22. A lateral contrast radiograph of the pharynx and cranial cervical esophagus. The esophagus and UES are widely dilated (chalasia of the UES) due to the loss of muscular tone. This two-year-old male Brittany spaniel had myasthenia gravis that failed to respond to medical management.

disorder with or without secondary incoordination of the LES (Strombeck, 1978, 1979; Diamant et al., 1974).

Both congenital and acquired esophageal dysphagias have been seen in the dog and cat. There is evidence that *congenital esophageal hypomotility* is a hereditary disease in both the dog (Strating and Clifford, 1966) and cat (Clifford et al., 1971). The incidence is highest in Great Danes, followed by German shepherd dogs and Irish setters (Strombeck, 1979). Of the feline species Siamese and Siamese-related breeds are predisposed. The occurrence is also reported in many other breeds. The onset of dysphagia and regurgitation usually occurs around the time of weaning.

Acquired esophageal hypomotility may occur in any dog or cat at any age. In most instances the underlying etiology is undeter-

mined; however, dilatation due to hypomotility may be encountered in the dog with several systemic diseases affecting skeletal muscles, including myasthenia gravis, hypothyroidism, hypoadrenocorticism (Feldman and Tyrrell, 1977), immune mediated polyneuritis, and polymyositis of systemic lupus erythematosus (Krum et al., 1977; Kornegay et al., 1980), myotonia with myopathy (Griffiths and Duncan, 1973), trypanosomiasis (Marsden and Hagstrom, 1968), and "central-peripheral neuropathies" (Duncan and Griffiths, 1977). One report relates a high incidence of coexisting pylorospasm and megaesophagus in a group of vomiting cats. Surgical correction of the pyloric disease was associated with regression of the esophageal disease for no known reason (Pearson et al., 1974). Motor dysfunction has also occurred secondary to neoplastic invasion of the esophagus (Ridge-way and Suter, 1979) and in association with trauma, viral encephalitis (Osborne et al., 1967), and cachexia.

Signs of esophageal hypomotility include almost effortless regurgitation (when solids are ingested these return as mucus-coated tubular casts), weight loss, polyphagia, weakness, dehydration, impaired skeletal mineralization (Osborne et al., 1967), ballooning of the esophagus and gurgling sounds, and recurrent aspiration pneumonia. Oral fetor may be present due to stagnation of fermenting food retained in the dilated esophagus, causing esophagitis, and pharyngitis. Regurgitation may be seen immediately upon feeding or up to 12 or more hours later. The length of the interval between eating and regurgitation may relate to the degree of dilatation or activity of the animal. Usually both liquids and solids are poorly tolerated. Panting and evidence of discomfort may be observed following a meal.

Survey thoracic radiographs are almost always consistent in revealing a dilated esophageal body. The lumen usually contains air and can best be seen on the lateral radiograph as a pair of soft tissue stripes arising in the midthorax and converging toward the esophageal hiatus. Cranial to this the dorsal wall of the esophagus may merge with the longus coli muscle to outline a sharp margin. Ventral to this the ventral wall of the esophagus will silhouette with the dorsal wall of the air-filled trachea, creating a wide, soft tissue band called the "tracheal stripe." When the cervical esophageal segment is dilated, a saber-shaped radiolucent shadow is seen dorsal to the trachea and tapering towards the thoracic inlet (Fig. 56–4,A). A partially fluid-filled esophagus will present as a homogeneous gray shadow with a similar relationship to that described. With severe esophageal dilatation ventral displacement of the trachea and heart occurs. In the dorsoventral or ventrodorsal view the caudal thoracic esophagus is seen as a V-shaped pair of lines to either side of midline with the convergence at the hiatus. Aspiration pneumonia is a frequent finding and a hallmark of dysphagia (Fig. 56–4,B).

When the esophagus is not identified, contrast radiographs are required. A barium contrast examination also better defines the degree of esophageal dilatation, lack of function, and extent of involvement.

The study helps rule out vascular ring anomalies or other causes of focal obstruction that might lead to dilatation, and outlines the funnel shape of the terminal esophagus to rule out invasive processes that would cause irregular or asymmetric narrowing. If no contrast media enters the stomach following radiography, the animal's forequarters should be elevated for several minutes. A followup radiograph will determine whether the LES is opening either by reflex stimulation or by the weight of the esophageal contents. Relaxation of the LES is also stimulated by the oropharyngeal phase, which may be initiated by inducing the animal to swallow once while in the elevated position. Barium in the gastrointestinal tract implies that the LES is patent. Failure of the normal LES to relax and permit transit of esophageal contents is likely to be due to an incoordination between its relaxation and the poorly functioning terminal esophagus. The origin of the disease process that affects the skeletal muscle of the esophageal body is not likely to affect the smooth muscle and complex of structures that contribute to the LES.

Mild motor disturbances of the esophagus may not be identified by standard radiography. Segmental or early disease requires dynamic evaluation by fluoroscopy. With mild or focal deficits clinical signs are often intermittent. Standard radiography may reveal no or only focal dilatation, suggesting a morphologic disease such as stricture (Fig. 56–1). Fluoroscopic evaluation should include determination of the frequency of generation of a primary peristaltic wave following a swallow, presence of complete or partial transport of each bolus, rate and speed of generation of secondary peristalsis to transport a delayed bolus, difference in response to liquids and solids, coordination of opening and closure of the LES, and degree of gastroesophageal reflux. Swallows should be regularly followed by a primary peristalsis. Infrequent generation is correlated well with clinically apparent megaesophagus (Diamant et al., 1974). Loss of a portion of a bolus during transport indicates an abnormal reduction in esophageal force of contraction.

Manometry would enhance evaluation of peristaltic amplitude. Application in veterinary practice is limited, however.

For congenital esophageal hypomotility, proper dietary management in terms of frequent elevated feedings with foods of appropriate consistency for the particular animal (some handle bulky foods well, others tolerate slurries better) has been shown to result in spontaneous resolution of clinical signs in a number of cases identified at an early age. Esophagomyotomy and cardioplasty have been proposed for treatment but have met with variable success (Hofmyer, 1966; Clifford et al., 1967; Osborne et al., 1967). Related complications resulting in death are reported to be more common in surgically managed cases (Harvey et al., 1974).

The theory that congenital esophageal hypomotility is due to delayed neurologic development of esophageal innervation has been proposed (Sokolovsky, 1972; Diamant et al., 1973). With elevated feedings minimal stress and distention of the esophageal body occur until such time as normal function develops. If stasis of esophageal contents are allowed, however, gradual overdistention and atony result in megaesophagus. The earlier the dysfunction is recognized and the dietary management is instituted, the better the prognosis. Puppies diagnosed at the time of weaning and managed appropriately have a favorable prognosis. Puppies recognized later in age, around five to six months or older, have a guarded prognosis. Once severe megaesophagus occurs, recovery is unlikely. Aspiration pneumonia and poor nutrition limit the longevity of the animal.

With cases of acquired esophageal hypomotility, if the underlying etiology can be identified and successfully treated, then the esophageal motor disturbance may subside. Megaesophagus secondary to the functional deficit of myasthenia gravis has resolved in association with spontaneous recovery from this neuromuscular disease. However, the development of megaesophagus secondary to systemic disease has been correlated with a poorer response to therapy (Kornegay et al., 1980; Duncan and Griffiths, 1977). Esophagomyotomy may be advised for these cases (Hoffer et al., 1979). Acquired idiopathic esophageal hypomotility has a poor prognosis for recovery. Death is a consequence of aspiration pneumonia accompanied by cachexia.

GASTROESOPHAGEAL REFLUX

An incompetent LES permits reflux of acidic and enzymatic gastric contents into the esophagus. This chemical irritation causes peptic esophagitis. Reduced LES competence may be due to neuromuscular disease; structural abnormalities such as hiatal hernias, neoplasia, or esophagomyotomy; indwelling pharyngotomy tubes; esophagitis; and prolonged vomiting. Reduced pressure in LES (chalasia) has been determined to be present in some dogs with megaesophagus (Maksic and Small, 1964; Clifford et al., 1975). Inspiratory dyspnea has been shown to permit gastroesophageal reflux (Pearson et al., 1978). Certain drugs lower LES tone (see p. 1197).

The occurrence of gastroesophageal reflux, however, has been observed in the normal dog during cinefluorographic studies of swallowing (Watson, 1974; Watrous and Suter, 1979). Therefore, the determination of true pathology requires more than the radiographic recognition of existing reflux.

Clinical signs associated with abnormal reflux and esophagitis are variable and include regurgitation or vomition, sometimes blood-tinged; drooling; weight loss; and anorexia. The discomfort and pain associated with the esophagitis are a cause of the anorexia and may induce vomiting, aerophagia, and gastric bloating. The pH of the regurgitated ingesta will be low, indicating contact with gastric secretions. A history of recent anesthesia or medication may be of importance.

Survey radiographic evaluation of the esophagus is often normal, except in severe cases, but is an important diagnostic tool. Survey and contrast radiographs may demonstrate a hiatal hernia, esophageal mucosal irregularity or ulceration, focal or diffuse megaesophagus, LES chalasia or persistent gastroesophageal reflux of barium, or the complications of severe esophagitis, such as esophageal stricture or perforation. A negative study does not rule out clinical gastroesophageal reflux-induced esophagitis.

A fluoroscopic examination of swallowing may show the secondary effects of inflammation on motility. Spasticity and random peristaltic contractions may be seen with loss of portions of the bolus during transport. Observation of gastroesophageal reflux may be frequent or rare. Delay in return of the refluxed gastric material to the stomach is important. Application of abdominal compression during contrast fluoroscopy may or may not successfully produce reflux. The demonstration of persistent and recurrent reflux during dynamic studies of the esophagus warrant further examination.

Evaluation of esophageal pH and endoscopy with biopsy are required to confirm many cases of inflammation due to reflux. Prolonged low esophageal pH indicates the presence of reflux of gastric acid with poor esophageal clearance (Strombeck, 1979). Esophageal mucosal biopsy can be performed by endoscopy with general anesthesia or by biopsy capsule with suction in the awake animal (Strombeck, 1979). Histologic changes include cornification of the stratified squamous epithelium, hyperplasia of the mucosa, submucosal vascular congestion and hemorrhage, and increased submucosal inflammatory cellular elements (Geever,

1953). Endoscopy may reveal widened esophageal folds, an erythematous or hemorrhagic mucosa with erosions, ulcers, or pseudomembranous plaques, and reduced lumen distensibility. Manometry has been infrequently used but may prove valuable for determination of the presence of a low LES pressure.

Treatment of esophagitis by antacids and dietary control may improve LES tone. An increased gastric pH (such as with oral cimetidine) and frequent, small, high protein–low fat meals are factors that will increase sphincter pressure either directly or through hormonal modifiers. The use of glucocorticoids is advocated by some to reduce the inflammatory component.

REFERENCES

Ader, P. L.: Phycomycoses in fifteen dogs and two cats. J.A.V.M.A. *174*:1216, 1979.

Atkins, C. E., and Johnson, R. K.: Clinical toxicities of cats. Vet. Clin. North Am. 5:623, 1975.

Bailey, W. S.: Parasites and cancer — sarcoma in dogs associated with *Spirocerca lupi*. Ann. N.Y. Acad. Sci. *180*:890, 1963.

Baker, G. J., and Hoffer, R. E.: Surgical correction of esophageal stenosis in the dog. J.A.V.M.A. *148*:44, 1966.

Bellenger, C. R., and Warren, D. F.: Esophageal constrictions due to aberrant vessels in dogs. Mod. Vet. Pract. *51*:51, 1970.

Botha, G. S. M.: A note on the comparative anatomy of the cardio-oesophageal junction. Acta Anat. *34*:52, 1958.

Brodey, R. S., and Kelley, D. F.: Thyroid neoplasms in the dog — a clinicopathologic study of 57 cases. Cancer *22*:406, 1968.

Buergelt, C. D., and Wheaton, L. G.: Dextroaorta, atopic left subclavian artery and persistent left cephalic vena cava in a dog. J.A.V.M.A. *156*:1026, 1970.

Carmichael, J. A., Liu, S. K., Tashjian, R. S., Radford, G., and Lord, P.: A case of canine subaortic stenosis and aortic valvular insufficiency with particular reference to diagnostic technique. J. Small Anim. Pract. *9*:213, 1968.

Christensen, J.: Effects of drugs on esophageal motility. Arch. Intern. Med. *136*:532, 1976.

Christensen, J., and Lund, G. F.: Esophageal responses to distension and electrical stimulation. J. Clin Invest. *48*:408, 1969.

Clifford, D. H., Soifer, F. K., and Freeman, R. G.: Stricture and dilatation of the esophagus in the cat. J.A.V.M.A. *156*:1007, 1970.

Clifford, D. H., Soifer, F. K., Wilson, C. F., Waddell, E. D., and Guilloud, G. L.: Congenital achalasia of the esophagus in 4 cats of common ancestry. J.A.V.M.A. *158*:1554, 1971.

Clifford, D. H., Sokolovsky, V., and Rosin, E.: The esophagus. *In* Bojrab, M. J. (ed): Current Tech-

niques in Small Animal Surgery. Lea & Febiger, Philadelphia, 1975.

Clifford, D. H., Wilson, C. F., Waddell, E. D., and Thompson, H. L.: Esophagomyotomy (Heller's) for relief of esophageal achalasia in three dogs. J.A.V.M.A. *151*:1190, 1967.

Cotchin, E.: Neoplasms in small animals. Vet. Rec. *63*:67, 1951.

Crouch, J. E.: Text-Atlas of Cat Anatomy. Lea & Febiger, Philadelphia, 1969.

DeHoff, W. D.: Surgical correction of patent ductus arteriosus and vascular ring anomalies. *In* Ettinger, S. J., and Suter, P. F. (eds.): Canine Cardiology, W. B. Saunders Co., Philadelphia, 1970.

Diamant, N., Szczepanski, M., and Mui, H.: Idiopathic megaesophagus in the dog: Reasons for spontaneous improvement and a possible method of medical therapy. Can. Vet. J. *15*:66, 1974.

Dodman, N. H., and Baker, G. J.: Tracheooesophageal fistula as a complication of an oesophageal foreign body in the dog — a case report. J. Small Anim. Pract., *19*:291, 1978.

Duncan, I. D., and Griffiths, I. R.: Canine giant axonal neuropathy. Vet. Rec., *101*:438, 1977.

Eastwood, G. L., Castell, D. O., and Higgs, R. H.: Experimental esophagitis in cats impairs lower esophageal sphincter pressure. Gastroenterology *69*:146, 1975.

Ettinger, S. J., and Suter, P. F.: Congenital heart disease. *In* Canine Cardiology, W. B. Saunders Co., Philadelphia, 1970.

Evans, H. E., and Christensen, G. C.: Miller's Anatomy of the Dog. 2nd ed. W. B. Saunders Co., Philadelphia, 1979.

Feldman, E. C., and Tyrrell, J. B.: Hypoadrenocorticism. Vet. Clin. North Am., *7*:555, 1977.

Freiman, J. M., and Diamant, N. E.: Upper esophageal sphincter response to esophageal distension and acid, and its alteration with nerve blockade. Gastroenterology, *70*:970, 1976.

Gaynor, F., Hoffer, R. E., Nichols, M. F., Rosser, E., Moraff, H., Hahn, A. W., and MacCoy, D. M.:

Physiologic features of the canine esophagus: effects of tranquilization on esophageal motility. Am. J. Vet. Res. *41*:727, 1980.

Geever, E. D., and Merendino, K. A.: An evaluation of esophagitis in dogs following the Heller and Grondahl operations with and without vagotomy. Surgery *34*:742, 1953.

Glauser, J., Lilja, G. P., Greenfeld, B., and Ruiz, E.: IV glucagon in management of obstruction of the esophagus by food. J. Am. Coll. Emergency Phys., *8*:228, 1979.

Gourley, I. M., and Leighton, R. L.: Surgical treatment for cricopharyngeal achalasia in the dog. Pract. Vet. *44*:10, 1972.

Griffiths, I. R., and Duncan, I. D.: Myotonia in the dog: a report of four cases. Vet. Rec. *93*:184, 1973.

Griffiths, I. R., Duncan, I. D., McQueen, A., Quirk, C., and Miller, R.: Neuromuscular disease in dogs: some aspects of its investigation and diagnosis. J. Small Anim. Pract. *14*:533, 1973.

Hall, A. W., Moossa, A. R., Clark, J., Cooley, G. R., and Skinner, D. B.: The effects of premedication drugs on the lower oesophageal high pressure zone. Gut *16*:347, 1975.

Harvey, C. E., O'Brien, J. A., and Durie, V. R.: Megaesophagus in the dog: A clinical survey of 79 cases. J.A.V.M.A. *165*:433, 1974.

Harvey, H. J.: Iatrogenic esophageal stricture in the dog. J.A.V.M.A. *166*:1100, 1975.

Hoerlein, B. F.: Canine Neurology. 2nd ed. W. B. Saunders Co., Philadelphia, 1971.

Hoffer, R. E.: Surgical notes, senior course at Cornell Univ., 1978.

Hoffer, R. E., MacCoy, D. M., Gaynor, F., Moraff, H., Aron, D., Quick, C. B., and Law, K.: Physiologic features of the canine esophagus: effect of modified Heller's esophagomyotomy. Am. J. Vet. Res. *41*:723, 1980.

Hoffer, R. E., MacCoy, D. M., Quick, C. B., Barclay, S. M., and Rendano, V. T.: Management of acquired achalasia in dogs. J.A.V.M.A. *175*:814–817, 1979.

Hofmeyr, C. F. B.: An evaluation of cardioplasty for achalasia of the oesophagus in the dog. J. Small Anim. Pract. *7*:281, 1966.

Hurwitz, A. L., Duranceau, A., and Haddad, J. K.: Disorders of Esophageal Motility. W. B. Saunders Co., Philadelphia, 1979.

Imhoff, R. K., and Foster, W. J.: Persistent right aortic arch in a 10-year-old dog. J.A.V.M.A. *143*:599–600, 1963.

Ingelfinger, F. J.: Esophageal motility. Physiol Rev. *38*:533, 1958.

Janssens, J., Valembois, P., Vantrappen, G., Hellemans, J., and Pelemans, W.: Is the primary peristaltic contraction of the canine esophagus bolus-dependent? Gastroenterology *65*:750, 1973.

Jeglum, K. A.: Personal communication, West Chester, Penn, 1980.

King, J.: Ithaca, N.Y. Personal communication, 1980.

Kleine, L. J.: Radiologic examination of the esophagus in dogs and cats. Vet. Clin. North Am. *4*:663, 1974.

Kneller, S. K., and Lewis, R. E.: Contrast radiography of the normal cat esophagus. J.A.A.H.A. *9*:50, 1973.

Kornegay, J. N., Gorgacz, E. J., Dawe, D. L., Bowen, J. M., White, N. A., and DeBuysscher, E. V.: Polymyositis in dogs. J.A.V.M.A. *176*:431, 1980.

Krahwinkel, D. J., and Howard, D. R.: Reconstructive surgery. II. Esophageal patch grafting. A.A.H.A. Sci. Proc., Chicago, 1975, p. 441.

Krum, S. H., Cardinet, G. H., Anderson, B. C., and Holliday, T. A.: Polymyositis and polyarthritis associated with systemic lupus erythematosus in a dog. J.A.V.M.A. *170*:61, 1977.

Lantz, G. C., Bojrab, M. J., and Jones, B. D.: Epiphrenic esophageal diverticulectomy. J.A.A.H.A., *12*, 629, 1976.

Leipold, H. W.: Nature and causes of congenital defects of dogs. Vet. Clin. North. Am. *8*:47, 1977.

Levitt, M. N., Dedo, H. H., and Ogura, J. H.: The cricopharyngeus muscle, an electromyographic study in the dog. Laryngoscope, *75*:122, 1965.

Lorenz, M. D., DeLahunta, A., and Alstrom, D. H.: Neostigmine-responsive weakness in the dog, similar to myasthenia gravis. J.A.V.M.A. *161*:795, 1972.

Lund, W. S., and Ardian, G. M.: The motor nerve supply of the cricopharyngeal sphincter. Ann. Otol. Rhinol. Laryngol. *73*:599–617, 1964.

Maksic, D., and Small, E.: Diagnostic radiology of the canine esophagus. Part I. Vet. Med. *59*:397, 513, 1964.

Malmud, L. S., and Fisher, R. S.: Dynamic esophageal scintigraphy: esophageal clearance in patients with esophageal disorders. Appl. Radiol./NM: Mar/April 103, 1980.

Mann, C. V., and Shorter, R. G.: Structure of the canine esophagus and its sphincters. J. Surg. Res. *4*:160, 1964.

Marsden, P. D., and Hagstrom, J. W. C.: Experimental *Typanosoma cruzi* infection in beagle puppies. The effect of variations in the dose and source of infecting trypanosomes and the route in inoculation on the course of the infection. Trans. R. Soc. Trop. Med. Hyg., *62*:816, 1968.

Moulton, J. E.: Tumors in Domestic Animals. 2nd ed. University of California Press, Berkeley, 1978.

O'Brien, J. A.: Esophagoscopy. Vet. Clin. North Am. *2*:99, 1972.

O'Brien, T. R.: Radiographic Diagnosis of Abdominal Disorders in the Dog and Cat: Radiographic Interpretation—Clinical Signs—Pathophysiology. W. B. Saunders Co., Philadelphia, 1978.

Osborne, C. A., Clifford, D. H., and Jessen, C.: Hereditary esophageal achalasia in dogs. J.A.V.M.A. *151*:572, 1967.

Osweiler, G. D.: Sources and incidence of small animal poisoning. Vet. Clin. North Am. *5*:589, 1975.

Patterson, D. F.: Epidemiologic and genetic studies of congenital heart disease in the dog. Circ. Res., *23*:171, 1968.

Patterson, D. F.: Canine congenital heart disease; epidemiology and etiological hypothesis. J. Small Anim. Pract. *12*:263–287, 1971.

Pearson, H., Darke, P. G. C., Gibbs, C., Kelly, D. F., and Orr, C. M.: Reflux esophagitis and stricture formation after anesthesia: A review of seven cases in dogs and cats. J. Small Anim. Pract. *19*:507, 1978.

Pearson, H., Gibbs, C., and Kelly, D. F.: Oesophageal diverticulum formation in the dog. J. Small Anim. Pract. *19*:341, 1978.

Pearson, H., Gaskell, C. J., Gibbs, C., and Waterman, A.: Pyloric and oesophageal dysfunction in the cat. J. Small Anim. Pract. *15*:487, 1974.

Pearson, H.: Symposium on conditions of the canine oesophagus-foreign bodies in the oesophagus. J. Small Anim. Pract. *7*:107–116, 1966.

Pollack, S., and Rhodes, W. H.: Gastroesophageal intussusception in an Afghan hound: A case report. J.A.V.R.S. *11*:5, 1970.

Popesko, P.: Atlas of Topographical Anatomy of the Domestic Animals. W. B. Saunders Co., Philadelphia, 1971.

Pozzi, L.: Intrathoracic oesophageal diverticulum associated with an oesophagotracheal fistula in a dog. Radiographic findings. Atti Soc. Ital. Sci. Vet. *27*:371, 1973.

Pyle, R. L.: Common congenital heart defects: Persistent right aortic arch. In Kirk, R. (ed.): Current Veterinary Therapy VI, W. B. Saunders Co., Philadelphia, 1977.

Reed, J. H., and Cobb, L. M.: The diagnosis: Radiographic study and surgical relief of a case of esophageal diverticulum. Can. Vet. J., *1*:323, 1960.

Reif, J. S.: Solitary pulmonary lesions in small animals. J.A.V.M.A. *155*:377, 1969.

Ridgeway, R. L., and Suter, P. F.: Clinical and radiographic signs in primary and metastatic esophageal neoplasms of the dog. J.A.V.M.A. *174*:700, 1979.

Rogers, W. A., Fenner, W. R., and Sherding, R. G.: Electromyographic and esophagomanometric findings in clinically normal dogs and in dogs with idiopathic megaesophagus. J.A.V.M.A. *174*:181, 1979.

Rosin, E.: Surgery of the canine esophagus. Vet. Clin North Am. *2*:17, 1972.

Ryan, W. W., and Greene, R. W.: The conservative management of esophageal foreign bodies and their complications: a review of 66 cases in dogs and cats. J.A.A.H.A. *11*:243–249, 1975.

Schlegel, J. F., and Code, C. F.: Pressure characteristics of the esophagus and its sphincters in dogs. Am. J. Physiol. *193*:9, 1958.

Smith, D. M., Kirk, G. R., and Shepp, E.: Maturation of the emetic apparatus in the dog. Am. J. Vet. Res. *35*:1281, 1974.

Snape, W. J., and Cohen, S.: Hormonal control of esophageal function. Arch. Intern. Med. *136*:538, 1976.

Sokolovsky, V.: Achalasia and paralysis of the canine esophagus. J.A.V.M.A. *160*:943, 1972.

Sokolovsky, V.: Cricopharyngeal achalasia in a dog. J.A.V.M.A. *150*:281, 1967.

Stogdale, L., Steyn, D. G., and Thompson, B. C.: A congenital oesophagotracheal fistula in a 2-year-old dog. J. S. Afr. Vet. Med. Assoc. *48*:212, 1977.

Strating, A., and Clifford, D. H.: Canine achalasia with special reference to heredity. Southwest Vet. *19*:135, 1966.

Strombeck, D. R.: Pathophysiology of esophageal motility disorders in the dog and cat. Vet. Clin. North Am. *8*:229, 1978.

Strombeck, D. R.: Small Animal Gastroenterology. Stonegate Publishing, Davis, Ca., 1979.

Suter, P. F., and Watrous, B. J.: Oropharyngeal dysphagias in the dog: A cinefluorographic analysis of experimentally induced and spontaneously occurring swallowing disorders. I. Oral state and pharyngeal stage dysphagias. Vet. Radiol., *21*:24–39, 1980.

Terracol, J., and Sweet, R. H.: Diseases of the Esophagus. W. B. Saunders Co., Philadelphia, 1958.

Thrall, D. E.: Esophagobronchial fistula in a dog. J.A.V.R.S., *XIV*: 22, 1973.

Vessal, K., Montali, R. J., Larson, S. M., Chaffee, V., and James, A. E.: Evaluation of barium and gastrografin as contrast media for the diagnosis of esophageal ruptures or perforations. Am. J. Roentgenol. Radium Ther. Nucl. Med. *123*:307, 1975.

Watrous, B. J., and Suter, P. F.: Normal swallowing in the dog: A cineradiographic study. Vet. Radiol. *XX*:99, 1979.

Watrous, B. J., and Suter, P. F.: Oropharyngeal dysphagias in the dog: A cinefluorographic analysis of experimentally induced and spontaneously occurring swallowing disorders. II. Cricopharyngeal stage and mixed oropharyngeal dysphagias. Vet. Radiol., 1982, in press.

Watson, A. G.: Some aspects of the vagal innervation of the canine esophagus. An anatomical study. Master's thesis, Massey University, New Zealand, 1974.

Wentink, G. H., vanderLinde-Sipman, J. S., Meijer, A. E. F. H., Kamphuisen, H., vanVorstenbosch, C., Hartman, W. and Hendriks, H.: Myopathy with a possible recessive X-linked inheritance in a litter of Irish Terriers. Vet. Pathol. *9*:328, 1972.

Wilson, G. P.: Ulcerative esophagitis and esophageal stricture. J.A.A.H.A. *13*:180, 1977.

Woods, C. B., Rawling, C., Barbar, D., and Walker, M.: Esophageal deviation in four English bulldogs. J.A.V.M.A. *172*:934, 1978.

Wysong, R. L.: Embryology of persistent right aortic arch. Vet. Med. *64*:203, 1969.

Zimmer, J. F.: Personal communications, Ithaca, N.Y., 1980.

CHAPTER **57**

DAVID C. TWEDT
WAYNE E. WINGFIELD

Diseases of the Stomach

ANATOMY

GROSS ANATOMY

Position. As the fetus grows, the stomach increases in length, with the dorsal border growing more rapidly than the ventral wall and thus producing a convex *greater curvature* and a passively concave *lesser curvature*. The *fundus* arises as a local bulge near the cranial end and the stomach then begins to rotate 90 degrees to the right about its long axis. The greater curvature thus faces caudally, ventrally, and to the left. The lesser curvature faces cranially, dorsally, and to the right. The concave surface of the lesser curvature forms an acute angle, the *incisura angularis* (Fig. 57–1). This anatomic landmark is important in endoscopy and will interfere with visualization of the distal stomach unless flexible probes are passed around the angle. The papillary process of the liver lies in this angle.

The topographic anatomy of the stomach is divided into the following five regions: cardia, fundus, body, antrum, and pylorus. The *cardia* is the entrance of the intra-abdominal esophagus into the stomach. To the left and dorsal to the cardia lies the *fundus*. When filling with food the fundus fills first and displaces in a caudodorsal direction; further filling will then displace it caudoventrally.

The *body* is the second part of the stomach to fill and expand. It is the largest region of the stomach and is most capable of dilatation. Together with the cardia and fundus, the body represents the proximal storage portion of the stomach. This capacity for adaptation results with little change in the intragastric pressure and represents an important area for secretion of digestive juices.

A line drawn from the incisura angularis to the greater curvature represents the juncture between the body (proximal) and *antrum* (distal). This distal segment represents a region that functions in mechanical digestion and release of substances to regulate release of hydrochloric acid. The antrum is directed cranially and will expand with peristaltic contractions and the presence of foodstuffs (chyme).

At the junction between antrum and duodenum is an anatomic sphincter, the *pylorus*. This muscular structure contains the pyloric canal, which expels chyme into the duodenum and prevents reflux of duodenal contents. A layer of circular smooth muscle several times thicker than the outer longitudinal muscle layer is noted at the pylorus. There are actually two distinct loops of circular muscle; a right (oral or proximal) loop and a left (aboral or distal) loop. At the lesser curvature, both loops are united in a muscle torus and usually cover 0.5 to 1.5 cm of the gastric wall at the lesser curvature and are spread over 2 to 5 cm near the greater curvature. This musculature is thickest as it crosses the greater curvature.

Proximally, the circular muscle fibers form a weak cardioesophageal sphincter. This sphincter is augmented on the greater curvature by transversely running, inner oblique fibers. Oblique smooth muscle fibers cover the body of the stomach and lie adjacent to the submucosa.

An outer longitudinal coat of smooth muscle covers the circular muscle layer. Longitudinal smooth muscle fibers continue uninterruptedly from the esophagus to the duodenum only along the greater curvature. Most longitudinal fibers end before the duodenum.

Ligamentous Supports. Movement of the stomach is restricted. At the gastroesophageal junction, it is fixed where it passes through the diaphragm. Pyloric movement is restricted by the gastrohepatic ligament and common bile duct. Additional mesenteric attachments include the greater omen-

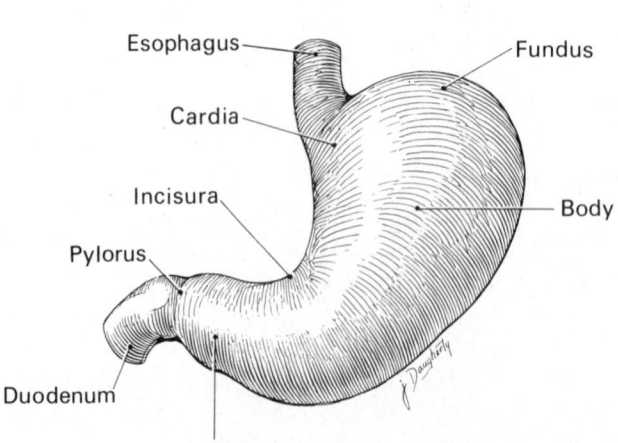

Figure 57–1 Diagram of the dog's stomach. The five regions of the stomach include the cardia, fundus, body, antrum, and pylorus.

tum and lesser omentum. The gastrosplenic ligament derives from the greater omentum and attaches the spleen to the greater curvature. The remainder of the double peritoneal sheet comprising the greater omentum attaches along the greater curvature of the stomach.

The lesser omentum loosely spans the lesser curvature of the stomach to the duodenum and porta of the liver. The portion of the lesser omentum passing from the liver to the stomach is the gastrohepatic ligament.

Blood Supply. The principal arterial supply to the stomach is derived from the celiac artery. This artery divides into the hepatic, left gastric, and splenic arteries, with each contributing arterial flow to the stomach (Table 57–1).

Satellite veins to the arteries of the stomach empty into either the gastroduodenal vein on the right or the splenic vein on the left. Both the splenic and gastroduodenal veins contribute to the portal vein just caudal to the hilus of the liver.

Lymphatic drainage from the stomach eventually enters the right or left hepatic lymph nodes. The left hepatic lymph node receives its drainage after passage through the splenic and gastric nodes. The right hepatic node receives drainage from the stomach after first having passed the duodenal node.

Nerves. The parasympathetic nerve supply to the stomach comes from the vagus nerves, which stimulate motility of the stomach and the secretion of acid, pepsin, and gastrin. Most of the fibers in the vagi are predominantly afferent.

Ventral vagus branches supply mainly the liver and stomach. Gastric supplies come to the pylorus and the ventral stomach wall. The dorsal vagus supplies the cardia of the stomach and then forms a plexus on its dorsal surface. Distribution of the dorsal vagus is primarily to the lesser curvature and pylorus. The distribution of the terminal gastric branches of the vagus nerves is segmental in nature (Polyak et al., 1971).

Sympathetic innervation of the stomach is both efferent and afferent and extends from the celiac plexus. In the dog's cardia, sympathetic α-receptors act excitatorily and β-receptors inhibitorily, whereas both receptors act inhibitorily in other parts of the stomach (Sakamoto, 1969).

MICROSCOPIC ANATOMY

The surface gastric mucosa is composed of mucus-secreting columnar epithelial cells. These lining cells extend into numerous invaginations in the mucosal surface, forming gastric pits. At the base of the gastric pits are mitotic foci, renewing the desquamated surface cells approximately once every one to three days (Baker, 1964). These cells produce a layer of mucus that lubricates and protects the gastric mucosa. This mucosal cell layer and mucous coat provides the basis of the gastric mucosal barrier that resists hydrochloric acid and digestive enzymes.

Three types of gastric glands are found in the stomach: cardiac glands, fundic glands (gastric glands), and pyloric glands (Banks, 1981). These open into the base of the gastric pits and extend deep into the mucosa (Fig. 57–2). The differences in the gland types permit histologic identification of three gland regions.

Table 57–1. Arterial Blood Supply to the Stomach

Arterial Branch of Celiac A.	Gastric Segment Supplied	Anastomotic Vessel
Hepatic A.		
R. gastric A.	Pylorus Pyloric antrum (lesser curvature)	L. gastric A.
R. gastroduodenal A.	Pylorus Pyloric antrum (greater curvature)	R. and L. gastric A. L. gastroepiploic A.
Left gastric A.	Fundus (lesser curvature) Caudal esophagus	R. gastric A.
Splenic A.		
L. gastroepiploic A.	Cardia Fundus Pyloric antrum (greater curvature)	R. gastroepiploic A.

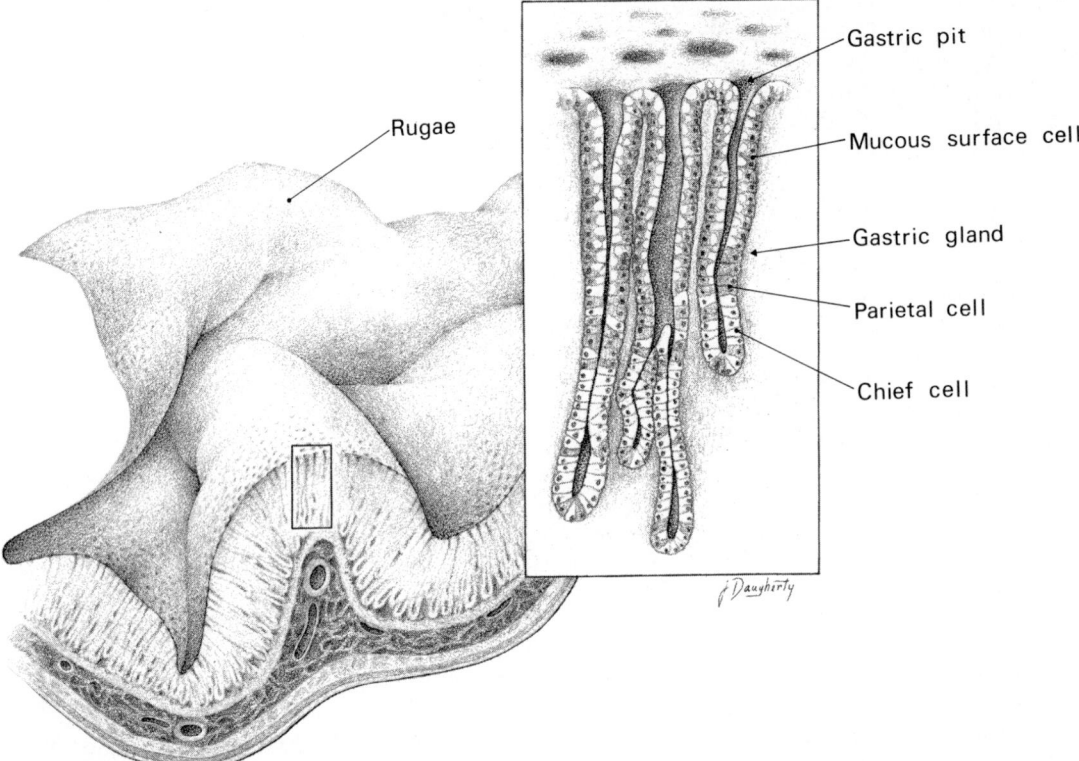

Figure 57–2. Cross-sectional anatomy of the dog's stomach, with a microscopic diagram of the gastric glands.

Cardiac Gland Region. The cardiac glands are found in a narrow zone around the cardia, are composed of mucous epithelial cells, and function in secreting mucus for lubrication.

Fundic Gland Region. The fundic gland region comprises the largest area, including the fundus and body of the stomach. These glands function in digestion by producing hydrochloric acid and pepsinogen. The four cell types comprising the fundic glands are chief cells, parietal cells, mucous cells, and argentaffin cells. The *chief cells* are in the highest concentration at the base of the gland and function in the production of pepsinogen. These cells appear basophilic, with many zymogen granules containing pepsinogen. The *parietal cells* (oxyntic cells) are scattered throughout the midportion of the gland, stain deeply eosinophilic, and are responsible for hydrochloric acid secretion. The cells are large and contain a complex series of invaginations or secretory canaliculi, which open toward the lumen of the gland. *Argentaffin cells* are one type of endocrine cell scattered throughout the gastric glands. These cells contain granules that hold serotonin, a potent vasoconstrictor

substance. The exact function of these cells is still unknown. The *mucous cells* are relatively few in number and are found in the neck region of the glands.

Pyloric Gland Region. The pyloric glands are found in the antral region of the stomach. The major cell type is the mucous cell. In the midgland region are many gastrin-containing cells (G-cells), which are pyramidal in shape and extend long processes into the gastric lumen to detect the nature and pH of the gastric contents. Upon stimulation, the hormone *gastrin,* a potent stimulator for hydrochloric acid secretions, is released.

Below the glands lies the lamina propria, the connective tissue portion of the gastric mucosal layer. The *muscularis mucosae,* the deepest layer of the mucosa, consists of a fine smooth muscle layer and is responsible for forming rugal folds or plicae. Between the mucosa and muscular layers is the submucosa, an elastic layer of areolar tissue containing small vessels, nerves, and lymphoid tissue. Scattered throughout both the lamina propria and submucosa are numerous mast cells, which act as one of the mediators of gastric acid secretion (Code,

1977). The thick muscular coat is composed of an outer longitudinal and an inner circular layer of smooth muscle fibers, with an additional oblique layer over the body of the stomach. The serosa, or outer coat, is thin and elastic and is continuous with the omentum.

PHYSIOLOGY

The stomach serves three important functions. First, it provides an adjustable reservoir by adapting quickly and markedly in volume with the intake of food, without the development of excessive intragastric pressure; second, gastric contents are mixed with gastric secretions; and third, the gastric contents are gradually passed into the intestinal tract for final digestion and absorption.

GASTRIC FILLING

The filling of the stomach is not an entirely passive process. To a small degree the empty stomach simply unfolds to accommodate a part of the ingested volume.

In order to maintain a rather constant intragastric pressure, the gastric smooth muscle contracts or relaxes with varying volumes. This ability to maintain basal intragastric pressure appears to be due in part to a centrally mediated reflex. The central reflex (esophageo-gastric vago-vagal relaxatory reflex) is initiated when there is an inhibition of tonic contraction of the proximal stomach in response to swallowing. A local reflex is also noted when distention by stomach contents produces reflex activation of the vagal relaxatory fibers. The gastric response to activation of the relaxatory fibers consists of a markedly prolonged relaxation, primarily affecting the body and fundic regions.

The capacity of the stomach varies from 0.5 to 8 liters in the dog. Greater ranges in relative size are noted in puppies than adult dogs (Evans et al., 1979). A capacity of 100 to 250 ml/kg of body weight has been reported by Neumayer and cited by Ellenberger et al. (1943).

GASTRIC SECRETION

Acid Secretion. The stomach secretes hydrochloric acid, other electrolytes, pepsinogen, gastrin, and mucus into the lumen. Gastrin and pepsinogen are also secreted by the stomach into the blood. These secretions are regulated by the cellular mass of the various mucosal secretory elements and by neural and hormonal stimulants and inhibitors.

HYDROCHLORIC ACID PRODUCTION. Parietal cells secrete hydrochloric acid into the gastric lumen. The hydrogen ion concentration in the gastric juices is three million times greater than that in the blood and tissues. The precise electrical and biochemical events that result in the secretion of hydrochloric acid are not understood, but the tremendous increase in hydrogen ion concentration represents a large gradient for the ion to be transported against, which concomitantly requires considerable energy. Secretion of one liter of hydrochloric acid at a concentration of 160 mEq/L requires 1500 calories of energy.

For each hydrogen ion secreted, a molecule of CO_2 derived from arterial blood or mucosal metabolism is converted to bicarbonate and ultimately enters the intestinal fluid. Parietal cells contain a high concentration of the enzyme carbonic anhydrase, which catalyzes this conversion. The metabolic alkalosis produced by active acid secretion is produced along with the *alkaline tide*. The amount of bicarbonate entering the blood during secretion is directly proportional to the amount of acid secreted (Fig. 57–3).

Agonists of gastric-acid secretion include the neurotransmitter acetylcholine, the gastrointestinal hormone gastrin, the biogenic amine histamine, digested protein, and a postulated intestinal-phase hormone called entero-oxyntin (Grossman, 1975).

A complex interaction between many neural and humoral factors dictate secretion at controlled rates and at the proper time. The mechanisms that control secretion have their effect at three different sequential times during digestion, namely, the cephalic phase, gastric phase, and intestinal phase.

The *cephalic phase* of gastric secretion is stimulated by the anticipation, sight, taste, smell, and passage of food through the oropharynx. Higher cortical areas of the brain mediate this phase through efferent vagal fibers. The vagal fibers terminate on gastrin-secreting G-cells, parietal cells, and chief cells. Thus, the vagus stimulates release of gastrin, hydrochloric acid, and pepsinogen.

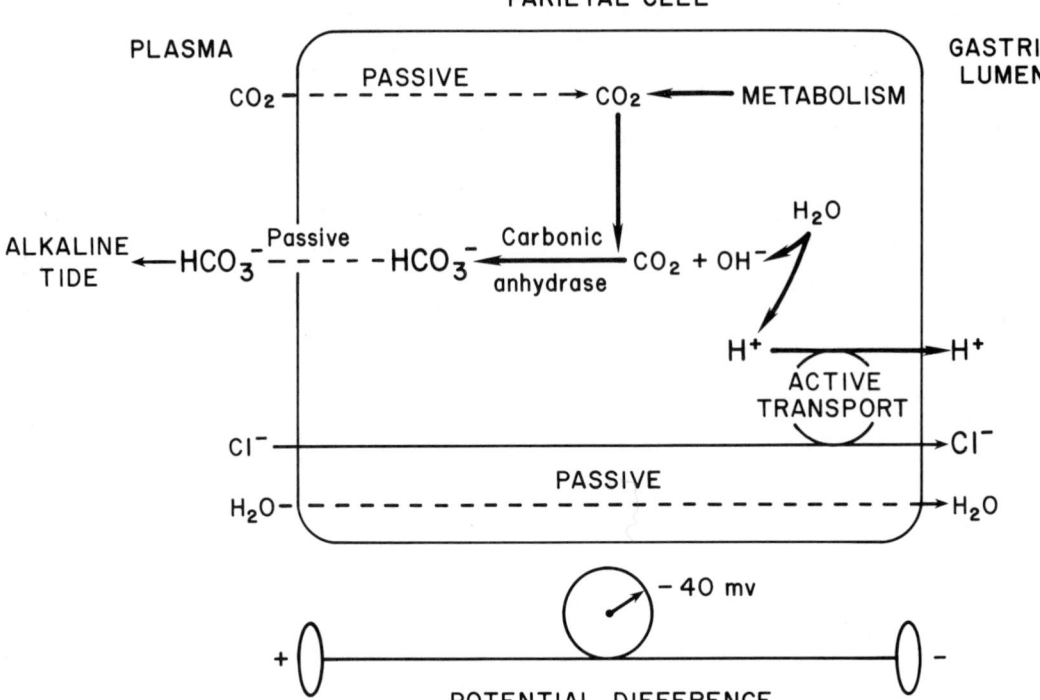

Figure 57–3. Hydrochloric acid secretion from the parietal cell and development of the alkaline tide. An electrical potential difference is maintained across the cell through chloride transport.

The *gastric phase* is the most important determinant of gastric secretion and is initiated via gastric distention and by digested proteins. Distention of either the parietal gland area (fundus and body) or the pyloric gland area results in activity of the G-cells and parietal cells, as do the cephalic vagal reflexes (Grossman, 1975).

The introduction of protein foods into the small intestine produces a distinct acid secretory response. In this *intestinal phase* three components can be discerned: direct stimulation of acid secretion, augmentation of maximal response to histamine and gastrin (Debras et al., 1975a), and release of antral gastrin by food in the intestine.

The role of histamine in gastric secretion is not completely understood. Usually, histamine is not present in the fluids of the body in any significant quantity. In dogs and cats, histamine is contained in eosinophils and mast cells of the gastric mucosa (Aures et al., 1968).

Some histamine escapes the gastric mucosa and enters the gastric juice. From this observation came the discovery of H_2-receptors and a correlation between histamine output and the output of gastric juice from the stomach of dogs during psychic and vagal stimulation. Histamine output occurs mainly during the early phases of gastric secretion (Code, 1975). The H_2-receptor is visualized to be on the basal membrane of the parietal cells. When occupied by histamine, and in the presence of acetylcholine, gastrin will act to stimulate maximal acid secretion. If all receptor sites are occupied, and then one site is blocked (i.e., atropine blocking acetylcholine or cimetidine, an H_2-receptor antagonist, blocking histamine), stimulation through the other receptors will result in less than maximum response (Fig. 57–4). Thus, the H_2-receptor on the parietal cell is a major controller of the cell's hydrogen ion production, and use of H_2-receptor antagonists makes them effective agents for control of gastric secretion.

Electrolyte Secretion. Chloride, potassium, and sodium are important electrolytes found in significant concentrations in gastric juices. As a result of these electrolytes, the mucosal surface of the stomach is electrically negative, when compared to the serosal surface. The specific cell responsible for generation of this negative potential has

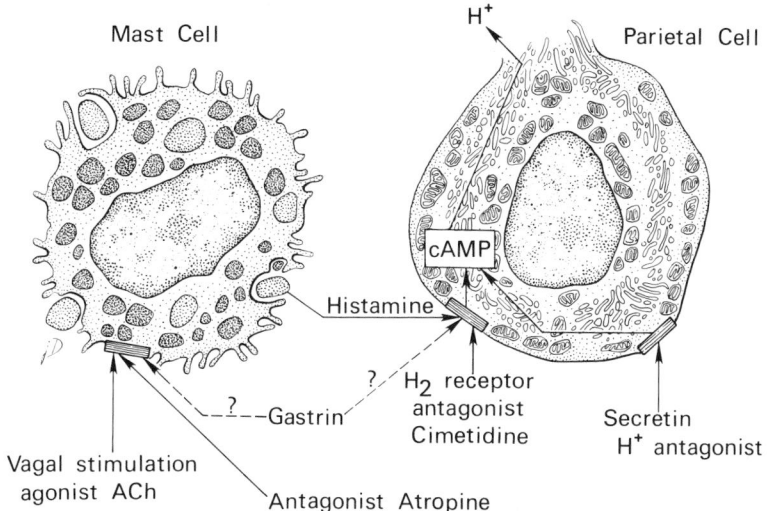

Figure 57–4. Relationship between H_2-receptors, histamine, and secretion of hydrochloric acid from the parietal cell. It is postulated that histamine may be the final mediator in parietal cell stimulation. Blockade of receptor sites will result in less than maximal acid secretion.

not been identified, but the potential appears to be generated primarily at the luminal cell border. The active transport of chloride ions from the intracellular space against both concentration and electrical gradients appears to be the principal source of the potential difference. During secretion of acid, proton (hydrogen ion) secretion is coupled with secretion of an equivalent additional amount of chloride ions; therefore, the potential does not change (see Fig. 57–3).

Sodium and hydrogen ion concentration in gastric juices vary inversely. The basal membrane of the epithelial cell is highly permeable to chloride and less permeable to sodium. As the intracellular concentrations of sodium and chloride are lower than extracellular fluid, both ions diffuse into the cell. Sodium is then actively pumped out of the cell.

Potassium concentration in gastric secretions is two to four times greater than that in plasma. As gastric secretion rates increase, the potassium in the juices increases, but after a prolonged period the potassium in gastric juices falls, presumably because intracellular potassium is depleted. Most potassium in the gastric juices is derived from intracellular stores. Depletion of these stores is often not reflected in a lowering of plasma potassium.

Pepsins. Pepsinogen is the inactive precursor to pepsin, the principal proteolytic enzyme of gastric juices. The chief cell in the fundic region stores most of the pepsinogens.

Pepsinogen is secreted into the gastric lumen, and its secretion is increased by the same stimulants of acid secretion, with the major exception that secretin inhibits acid secretion and *stimulates* pepsinogen. In the presence of an acid pH (hydrochloric acid), pepsinogens are autocatalytically converted to pepsins by the cleavage of several small peptides. Pepsin is active at an acid pH and irreversibly inactivated at a neutral or slightly alkaline pH. Thus, the proteolytic activity of pepsin ceases when chyme leaves the stomach and enters the more neutral duodenum.

Mucus. Gastric mucosal cells are coated with a gelatinous material called *gastric mucus,* which is composed of glycoproteins, proteins, and carbohydrates. Stimulation of mucus secretion occurs in response to local mucosal irritation and cholinergic stimulation. In cats, secretin and pentagastrin also stimulate mucus secretion (Vagne et al., 1973).

Mucus is assumed to provide lubrication to gastric contents and protection against physical irritants likely to produce surface injury. Mucus provides little impediment to the movement of water and electrolytes. No protection is afforded against gastric acid nor against the proteolytic activity of pepsin. Some of the components of mucus provide inhibition of pepsin activity, but they are not effective in the concentrations and pH ranges of the secreting stomach. Mucus has some buffering capacity, which provides some neutralization of acid, but this is negligible during active acid secretion.

Gastric Hormones. The primary physiologic processes of the digestive system are influenced by nervous and hormonal mechanisms. Gastrin, secretin, and cholecystokinin (CCK) have major activities in stimulating gastric acid secretion, pancreatic water and bicarbonate secretion, and gallbladder contraction and pancreatic enzyme secretion, respectively. In addition to the three commonly accepted gastrointestinal hormones, a virtual profusion of peptides has now been extracted from gastrointestinal mucosal tissues. There are still events for which physiologic evidence suggests hormonal mediation but for which the chemical messenger(s) have not been identified.

Gastrointestinal endocrines are produced by *amine-precursor-uptake decarboxylase (APUD) cells,* which originate in the neural crest of the embryo. All these hormones are polypeptides, have receptor sites in all tissues of the gastrointestinal tract, and effect motility and secretion.

Gastrointestinal hormones are released in response to neural reflexes, by other hormones, and by specific stimuli acting on the gastrointestinal mucosa. Both local neural reflexes and neural reflexes of the central nervous system have afferent and efferent fibers in the vagi.

Gastrin. Cells that synthesize gastrin peptides (G-cells) and release the hormones into the circulation when appropriately stimulated are numerous in the antrum of the stomach of the dog. In the canine duodenal bulb there are gastrin-containing cells, and none are found distal to the major duodenal papilla (Tobe et al., 1976). Distribution of G-cells in the cat is similar to that in the dog.

The regulation of circulating gastrin concentrations is best noted in terms of a basic feedback inhibition loop (Fig. 57–5). When the gastrin concentrations rise, the gastric parietal cells are stimulated to secrete acid. When the antral mucosa is bathed in acid, further release of gastrin is inhibited. Feeding is a most important regulator of gastrin release. Partially digested proteins, amino acids (Debas et al., 1974a), distention of the antrum (Debas et al, 1974b) or fundus (Debas et al., 1975b), and calcium are known to cause release of gastrin in the dog.

Gastrin will effect many secretory, absorptive, and smooth muscle activities of the digestive tract (Table 57–2). In the dog, serum gastrin levels increase to a peak of about 160 pg/ml after eating. The only actions of gastrin that will occur at this physiologic level include acid secretion, pepsin secretion, increased mucosal blood flow, and the trophic actions. The other actions require much higher doses. Gastrin is about half as potent as cholecystokinin for stimulation of pancreatic enzyme secretion in the dog.

The kidneys are a major site of removal of

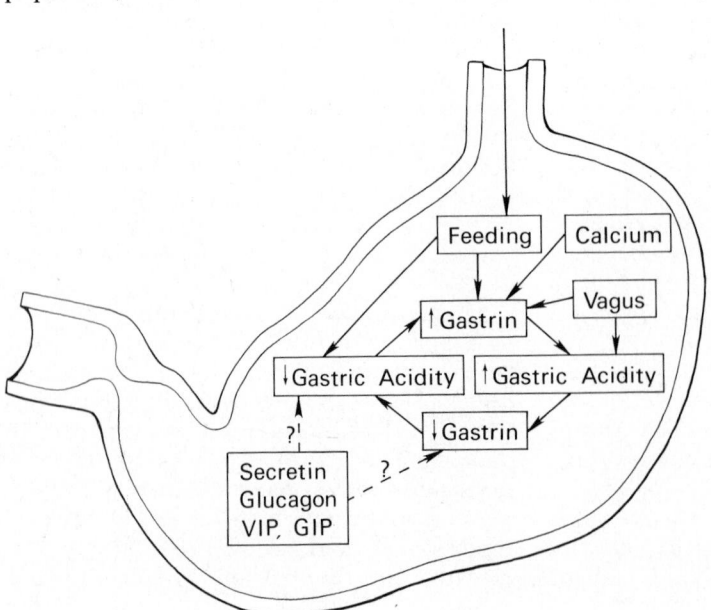

Figure 57–5. Regulation of circulating gastrin concentrations resulting from various feedback inhibition loops.

Table 57–2. Actions of Gastrin*

Action	Organs Affected
Stimulate water and electrolyte secretion	Stomach Pancreas Liver Small intestine Brunner's glands
Stimulate enzyme secretion	Stomach Pancreas Small intestine
Inhibition of water, electrolyte, and glucose absorption	Small intestine
Stimulation of smooth muscle	Lower esophageal sphincter Stomach Small intestine Colon Gallbladder
Inhibition of smooth muscle	Pyloric sphincter Ileocecal sphincter Sphincter of Oddi
Release of hormones	Insulin Calcitonin
Increase in blood flow	Small intestine Small intestine Pancreas
Trophic actions	Gastric mucosa Small bowel mucosa Pancreas

*After Walsh, J. H., and Grossman, M. I.: Gastrin. N. Engl. J. Med. *292* (25):1324, 1975.

gastrin from the circulation and of metabolism. Other organs also participate in the metabolism of gastrin, with the small intestine playing a role in metabolism. The liver plays a minor role in the inactivation of gastrin.

Secretin. The major action of secretin is to stimulate pancreatic secretion of water and bicarbonate. Hydrogen ions are secretagogues for secretin, but acid gastric chyme is rapidly neutralized upon entering the duodenum, and it is known that it requires large volumes of concentrated acid over long segments of the duodenum to stimulate a high postprandial bicarbonate secretion (Lee et al., 1976). Below pH 3, pancreatic output is related to the amount of titratable acid entering the gut (Meyer et al., 1970). Secretin is not released by vagal stimulation or irrigation of the duodenal mucosa with acetylcholine (Sum et al., 1969).

In the stomach, secretin influences secretion and motility (Table 57–3). Physiologic actions of secretin on the pancreas result in increased water and bicarbonate, trypsin, and insulin. There is increased volume and electrolyte output of bile by the liver, reduced gastric emptying in the stomach, reduced resting and gastrin-stimulated pressure of the lower sphincter of the esophagus, and decreased motility of the duodenum with secretin release (Rayford et al., 1976). Removal of secretin from the circulation results from renal excretion (Curtis et al., 1975).

Cholecystokinin. Fat in the small intestine was noted to release cholecystokinin, which causes active gallbladder contraction and stimulated pancreatic secretion (Table 57–4) (Rayford et al., 1976). Cholecystokinin distribution is limited to the mucosa of the small intestine. In rats, dogs, and baboons the maximal concentration is in the jejunum, with considerable quantities also located in the ileum and duodenum. Catabolism of cholecystokinin is through the kidney and probably through other tissues.

Newer Gastrointestinal Hormones. In addition to gastrin, secretin, and cholecystokinin, several peptides have recently been identified and physiologic phenomena observed, suggesting that other substances may be involved with the initiation and modulation of the digestive process. These possible hormones include vasoactive intestinal polypeptide (VIP), gastric inhibitor polypeptide (GIP), glucagon, bombesin, motilin, chymodenin, bulbogastrone, entero-oxyntin, and pancreatic polypeptide. To date there are many unanaswered questions regarding these and other gastrointestinal hormones (Rayford et al., 1976; Dockray, 1977; Straus, 1978; Walsh et al., 1979; Ambinder and Schuster, 1979).

Table 57–3. Effects of Secretin*

Effect	Action
Pyloric sphincter	Stimulates
Pepsin	Stimulates
Gastrin-stimulated acid secretion	Inhibits†
Food-stimulated gastrin release	Inhibits
Motility	Inhibits
Trophic actions of gastrin	Inhibits

*After Rayford, P. L., Miller, T. A., and Thompson, J. C.: Secretin, cholecystokinin and newer gastrointestinal hormones. N. Eng. J. Med. *294*:1093, 1976.
†Not in cats.

Table 57–4. Effects of Cholecystokinin*

Pancreatic Effect	Action
Enzyme secretion	Stimulates
Bicarbonate release	Stimulates
Insulin release	Stimulates
Trophic action	Stimulates

Gastrointestinal Effect	
Intestinal motility	Stimulates
Gastric contraction	Stimulates
Pyloric sphincter contraction	Stimulates
Brunner's glands	Stimulates
Increased blood flow in cranial mesenteric artery	Stimulates
Gastric motility	Inhibits
Absorption of fluid, sodium, potassium and chloride from jejunum and ileum	Inhibits
Contraction of sphincter surrounding minor pancreatic duct and common bile duct	Inhibits
Lower esophageal sphincter contraction	Inhibits

Hepatic Effect	
Hepatic bile flow	Stimulates
Gallbladder contraction	Stimulates

*After Rayford, et al.: Secretin, cholecystokinin, and newer gastrointestinal hormones. N. Engl. J. Med. 294:1093, 1976.

GASTRIC MOTILITY AND EMPTYING

The stomach receives and stores food, mixes it with gastric secretions, and then delivers the food to the duodenum. It empties liquids faster than solids and carbohydrates faster than fats. As a motor unit, the stomach has two functional areas, a proximal receptacle (fundus and body) and a distal pump (antrum) that mixes the gastric contents and delivers them to the duodenum. The pylorus is a low-pressure muscular sphincter that has little or no role in regulating gastric emptying of liquids but is important in preventing large food particles from entering the duodenum and in preventing reflux of duodenal contents (Stemper and Cooke, 1976).

The fundus is important in gastric motility and emptying. At this level an electrical potential is generated that spreads over the stomach and ends at the pylorus. This *electrical control activity* is an omnipresent event, occurring at a frequency of five cycles per minute in the dog. Whether or not the antrum contracts with each of these cycles depends upon a second electrical event called the *electrical response activity,* which will cause contraction of the antrum. Thus, the number of antral contractions does not always correspond to the contractions generated from the electrical control activity of the fundus.

Gastric electrical activity of the muscle and muscle contractions are influenced by a number of factors. These influences include cholinergic, adrenergic, and nonadrenergic inhibitory reflexes. Gastric hormones also influence this activity. Gastrin increases antral electrical and muscle contraction frequency, and secretin slows it. Cholecystokinin and gastrin will accelerate electrical response activity in the antrum, and secretin slows it. Motilin, a 22–amino acid polypeptide hormone from the upper small intestine, will stimulate the motility of the proximal stomach (Debas et al., 1977; Thomas et al., 1979).

Gastric emptying is influenced by the volume and composition of the meal (Cooke, 1975). The nutritive density (Kcal/ml), and not the initial volume, determines the rate of gastric emptying. It has been shown that with *isocaloric* amounts of fat, protein, and carbohydrates there will be equal slowing of gastric emptying (Hunt and Stubbs, 1975).

As the fundus and body fill with food they will relax, thus reducing intragastric pressure and decreasing the rate of emptying. If the gastric fundus possesses high motility, the food entering will increase intragastric pressure and accelerate emptying.

The pylorus and antrum (or both) constitute a discriminating mechanism that allows liquids to empty and acts to retain solids longer in the stomach. Dietary fats also leave the stomach slowly. This slow release of fats appears to be due to intragastric layering of the oil phase on the aqueous phase and also to a feedback inhibitory mechanism triggered in the intestine by fats (Malagelada, 1979).

Digestible and nondigestible solids empty by different gastric mechanisms. Digestible solids are reduced in size to fine particles by the grinding and mixing of the distal antrum. These particles are suspended in fluid and the liquid is emptied. The three crucial functions in the process are the grinding pressure waves of the distal antrum, the discriminatory mechanism that allows small suspended particles to leave with liquids and retains larger particles for further grinding in the stomach, and the propulsive forces (mostly fundic) that push the fluids into the duodenum.

Nondigestible solids trigger antral grinding contractions, but most of these particles are impervious to this mechanical grinding. The particles are only slightly reduced to a size that allows emptying. These particles are the last of the food to leave the stomach.

CLINICAL EVALUATION

History

The history, taken in a chronological order, will help the clinician localize the disease condition, decide on the severity of the disease, and determine whether further diagnostic tests or merely symptomatic therapy is required.

Vomiting is the principal clinical sign of gastric disease. It is, however, not synonymous with gastric disease and may be associated with other conditions not involving the stomach. When presented with the complaint of vomiting, it is imperative that the clinician obtain a description of the vomiting episode to adequately differentiate gastric disease from regurgitation associated with esophageal disease, or coughing and expulsion of phlegm associated with respiratory disease. The signs of vomiting are preceded by a period of nausea, with licking, salivation, or multiple attempts at swallowing. This is followed by retching or several forceful simultaneous diaphragmatic and abdominal contractions, and with the head lowered, expulsion of the gastric contents. Regurgitation is more passive, lacks retching, and results in the loss of undigested esophageal contents through gravity and increased intrathoracic pressure. Vomiting reported as a forceful or a projectile episode, often following shortly after eating, suggests a pyloric outflow obstruction. A gastric volvulus or dilatation results in frequent nonproductive retching, with a rapidly distending abdomen.

In addition to a complete description of the vomiting episodes, it is essential to determine in a chronological order the duration and frequency of the episodes, and their association with feeding or drinking. Acute gastritis will often have a sudden onset with numerous vomiting episodes, whereas in chronic gastritis the vomiting may be as infrequent as once every few days.

It is equally important to obtain a complete description of the amount, color, and the consistency of the vomitus, and whether or not it has changed since the onset of vomiting. If the vomitus consists of food, the degree of digestion is noted, thus suggesting the length of time it has remained in the stomach. The vomitus may contain mucus and fluid resulting from gastric and swallowed salivary secretions. Yellow- or green-stained vomitus indicates intestinal reflux of bile into the stomach. Fresh blood from gastric bleeding may be present as small, red flecks or as large blood clots. Blood that has remained in the stomach for some time soon becomes partially digested and appears to have a brown "coffee ground" consistency. The presence of blood in the vomitus generally signifies more serious gastric disease.

Other signs associated with gastric disease may include nausea, belching, polydipsia, or pica. Melena, or black tarry stools, occurs with high gastrointestinal bleeding and may imply gastric disease. Coughing may suggest an aspiration pneumonitis resulting from vomiting. Some owners may report increased bowel sounds or "growling" of the stomach. Animals with gastric pain may exhibit a position of relief ("praying position"), with the rear legs elevated (Thrall et al., 1978).

The history should include environmental factors such as the possible exposure to various toxins, garbage, or bones, which may precipitate a vomiting episode. Many drugs cause gastric disease, and medication being given should be recorded. The chewing and playing nature of young animals makes the possibility of foreign body ingestion a constant concern. Careful questioning for that possibility should always be included in the history.

PHYSICAL EXAMINATION

The physical examination of an animal with suspected gastric disease should include a complete review of all body systems with a careful notation of the animal's hydration, since serious fluid and electrolyte depletion may result in the vomiting animal.

Normally the stomach cannot be palpated, because it lies cradled within the rib cage. Palpation is only possible when the stomach is distended with gas or food and extends past the caudal ribs. Small dogs and cats are often easier to palpate, and in some cases the fingers can be pushed under the rib cage and the stomach palpated. Palpation of the cranial abdomen is often facilitated by elevating the front legs and letting the abdominal contents fall caudally.

Pain on palpation in the region of the stomach is an inconsistent finding with gastric disease. The gas-distended stomach of the gastric dilatation–volvulus syndrome can be ballotted and percussed as an air-filled density. Auscultation of the abdomen may reveal bowel sounds that occur from gastrointestinal motility caused by the movement of gas over fluid. The strongest and loudest bowel sounds generally originate from the stomach. An empty stomach will usually be silent but becomes vocal with fluid and gas (Politzer, 1976). Increased bowel sounds may occur in some conditions of gastric disease.

A physical examination of the gastrointestinal system is not complete without a rectal examination. The presence of melena suggests high gastrointestinal bleeding, possibly occurring from the stomach.

LABORATORY FINDINGS

There are few biochemical and hematologic alterations consistently associated with diseases of the stomach. Gastric lesions can occur secondary to other diseases, and laboratory testing is required to rule out these conditions. Acute gastric disease is usually self-limiting and often requires no laboratory support, while conditions such as the gastric dilatation–volvulus syndrome result in serious fluid, electrolyte, acid base, and biochemical abnormalities in which laboratory support is essential. Indications for laboratory testing are determined on the basis of the history, clinical findings, and past clinical experience. The dehydrated, debilitated, and critical patient or one with a chronic history should have laboratory support.

The minimum laboratory tests include the hematocrit (PCV) and total solids (total protein). These two simple tests give the approximate hydration state of the animal. With fluid loss resulting from vomiting and inadequate fluid intake, dehydration occurs and is reflected by a rise in the PCV and total solids. A normal PCV in a dehydrated animal with an elevated total solids suggests a pre-existing anemia.

A complete blood count (CBC) will also provide useful information. Most animals vomiting from gastric disease show a stress leukogram (mature neutrophilia, lymphopenia, and eosinopenia). A vomiting animal lacking a stress leukogram with a lymphocytosis and eosinophilia should suggest the possibility of adrenocortical insufficiency (Addison's disease). An increase in the total eosinophil count may also occur with gastrointestinal parasites, eosinophilic gastritis, or allergic conditions. Anemia from blood loss in gastric disease is characterized by regeneration with reticulocytosis, nucleated red blood cells, anisocytosis, and polychromasia. Chronic gastrointestinal blood loss eventually results in an iron deficiency anemia with microcytic hypochromic red blood cell indices. Biochemical profiles and urinalysis should be run to exclude systemic causes of gastric disease. Common conditions such as liver disease, uremia, and pancreatitis are easily ruled out on most biochemical profile screens.

Vomiting from gastric disease may result in electrolyte depletion and acid-base abnormalities. Substantial losses of water, chloride and sodium and, to a lesser degree, losses of hydrogen and potassium result through vomiting. Traditionally, vomiting has been associated with a metabolic alkalosis resulting from the loss of gastric acid. Clinically, the majority of the vomiting small animals with acid-base abnormalities have a *metabolic acidosis*. The acidosis occurs from the loss of fluid and electrolytes, resulting in contraction of the extracellular fluid volume with a minimal loss of acid. The normal empty stomach has a negligible basal acid secretion, and when hydrogen ions are actively secreted, there is a transient extracellular alkalosis. This is normally corrected by an equivalent loss of bicarbonate through the bile and pancreatic juices. In the vomiting state, an acid deficit does not occur, owing to the simultaneous loss of refluxed alkaline-rich duodenal fluid and to the reabsorption of hydrogen and chloride ions that may pass from the stomach into the intestine. Hypokalemia frequently results in conjunction with vomiting and occurs predominantly through urinary losses and to a lesser extent through losses in gastric juices.

Metabolic alkalosis can be precipitated by a net loss in hydrogen ions occurring from frequent and perfuse vomiting caused by a pyloric outflow obstruction. Gastric alkalosis is perpetuated through chloride depletion and contraction of the extracellular volume or hypokalemia (Dumler, 1981).

In the normal animal, most of the sodium

and bicarbonate entering the kidney is reabsorbed. When the plasma concentration of bicarbonate rises and the capacity for renal absorption is exceeded, the excess bicarbonate escapes in the urine, resulting in an increase in urine pH. Urinary bicarbonate excretion continues until homeostasis is again achieved. Metabolic alkalosis may, however, be perpetuated when renal bicarbonate absorption occurs concurrently with elevated plasma bicarbonate levels. This can result in a contracted extracellular volume and chloride depletion. With losses of salt and water the effective arterial blood volume contracts, which results in increased stimulation for proximal nephron reabsorption of sodium. Sodium is reabsorbed with the anion chloride; if chloride levels are reduced then another anion, bicarbonate, must be reabsorbed to maintain electrical neutrality. Thus, extracellular fluid depletion, especially when associated with hypochloremia from vomiting, results in inadequate bicarbonate excretion leading to or maintaining a state of metabolic alkalosis.

Potassium deficiency often occurs with metabolic alkalosis. The development of this deficiency may result from etiologic factors that caused hydrogen and chloride losses (i.e., vomiting), from renal wasting of potassium, and through increased aldosterone secretion when volume depletion is sufficient. Loss of cellular potassium will also cause a shift of extracellular hydrogen ions (derived from carbonic acid) into cells, which produces an increase in extracellular bicarbonate and thus perpetuation of the peripheral metabolic alkalosis.

Renal wasting of potassium results when there is a disparity between the availability of reabsorbable anion (chloride) in the glomerular filtrate and the simultaneous need to conserve body sodium (Fig. 57–6) (Sabatini et al., 1978). With these conditions, sodium-hydrogen exchange, as well as sodium-potassium exchange in the distal tubule, is accelerated. With a severe hypokalemia, sodium reabsorption will exchange only with hydrogen ions. When a metabolic alkalosis occurs in conjunction with renal bicarbonate reabsorption and a sodium-hydrogen exchange, a *paradoxical aciduria* will exist (Gardham, 1969).

The stool should be examined for evidence of gastrointestinal parasites and upper gastrointestinal bleeding. Obvious melena may be the consequence of severe gastric bleeding while mild hemorrhage is not evident grossly. The stool can be evaluated for occult blood by using Hematest tablets. Animals eating a meat protein diet will often show a false-positive occult test. The animal should be on a meat-free diet several days prior to the test.

Gastric Fluid Analysis. Analysis of gastric contents may offer further information in the evaluation of the animal with gastric disease. In addition to the gross physical examination of the vomitus, certain laboratory tests can be performed. Samples of the

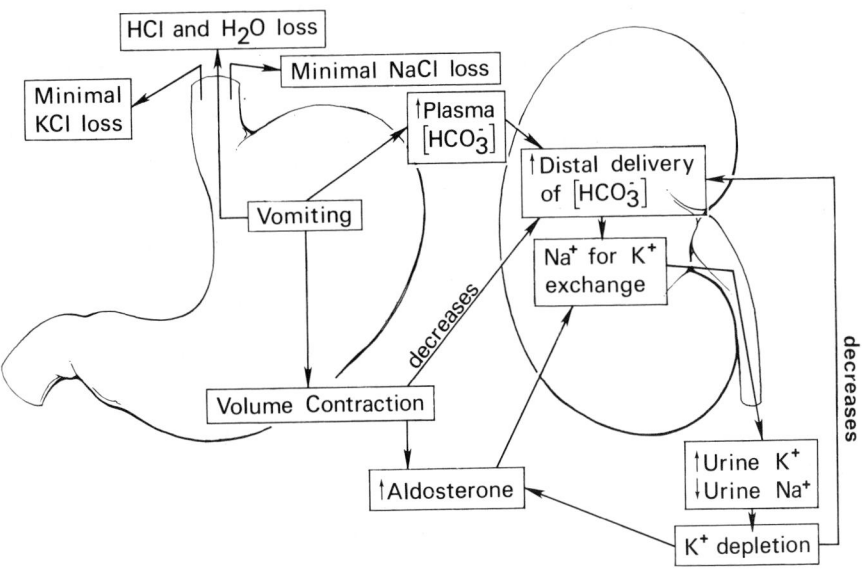

Figure 57–6. Pathophysiologic events present perpetuating metabolic alkalosis and renal potassium depletion.

vomitus or those collected by aspiration during endoscopy or by surgical placement of a gastric tube by pharyngostomy (Bohning, 1970) are analyzed.

The normal gastric contents of a fasted animal should be clear, with small amounts of mucus and saliva. The pH of the gastric fluid in the fasted animal will approach neutrality. With gastric acid stimulation, the pH of the gastric contents may fall to a level of 2 or less. Determining the pH of the vomitus serves as an indication of its origin. With regurgitation from esophageal disease, the pH will most often be alkaline. Bile-stained gastric juice occurring from duodenal reflux will raise the pH of the fluid.

Microscopic examination of the sediment of a centrifuged sample may reveal red blood cells, white blood cells, epithelial cells, bacteria, parasites, foreign material, or food particles. Owing to the acidity of the gastric juice, only the nuclear remnants of the cellular elements may remain. In cases of suspected neoplasia, a gastric lavage may retrieve neoplastic cells. Normal saline is instilled in the fasted stomach by means of a stomach tube and syringe. The solution is vigorously flushed back and forth prior to retrieval. The fluid is then collected and centrifuged, and the sediment is examined under the microscope for neoplastic cells.

RADIOLOGY

Radiology is an important diagnostic tool for evaluating the stomach. Gastric position, shape, intraluminal radiopaque foreign bodies, gastric wall abnormalities, and gastric emptying can be demonstrated radiographically.

When possible, animals should be fasted at least 12 hours before abdominal films are to be taken. Routine films are taken in two views (ventrodorsal and lateral). A radiograph taken in right lateral recumbency will usually show fluid in the pyloric antrum and gas in the gastric body, while a left lateral radiograph will usually demonstrate gas in the pyloric antrum. In certain instances, other views may be required to demonstrate suspected gastric abnormalities. The normal fasted stomach should be free from ingesta, containing only a small amount of fluid from salivary and gastric secretions with a variable amount of swallowed gas. The radiographic evidence of apparent gastric ingesta in a fasted animal should suggest a foreign body or gastric outflow obstruction.

Gastric size, shape, and location can usually be evaluated on routine abdominal radiographs. Changes in gastric position and shape are usually due to extragastric causes such as masses or organ enlargement, or from gastric wall lesions. The mucosal surface and the character of the rugal folds should be noted; however, this is difficult to assess on routine films. Complete evaluation of the luminal surfaces usually requires contrast and distention of the stomach.

Contrast studies are performed in animals with chronic signs of gastric disease and negative routine films, to confirm a suspected gastric lesion or foreign body, to identify gastric position, or to evaluate gastric emptying. Before contrast studies are performed, routine films and a minimal laboratory data base should be obtained.

Negative Contrast Study. A negative contrast study of the stomach is achieved using either air or carbon dioxide. A stomach tube is passed into the stomach and gas is introduced until the stomach is moderately distended. This contrast method is an inexpensive and easy means of outlining many suspected intraluminal gastric foreign bodies or for evaluating gastric wall thickness.

Double Contrast Study. Double contrast studies of the stomach involve using both a negative and positive contrast agent. This technique is useful in outlining gastric foreign bodies, gastric wall contour, and the mucosal surface. This technique is most beneficial when gastric foreign bodies absorb or are coated by the positive contrast agent. The technique involves giving the patient approximately one cc per kg body weight of a micropulverized barium sulfate (30 per cent W/V) (O'Brien, 1978). The animal is rolled so that the contrast material coats the mucosal surface, and a stomach tube is then reintroduced and the stomach distended with gas.

Positive Contrast Study. A positive contrast study is one employing a radiopaque contrast material. In most cases, barium sulfate is used. Commercially prepared micropulverized contrast agents (30 per cent W/V) give consistent homogeneous gastric filling. The suggested dosage, administered by stomach tube, is 8 to 12 cc/kg body weight in small dogs and cats and 5 to 7 cc/kg body weight for large dogs (Root and Morgan, 1969) given by stomach tube. Barium sulfate powder mixed with water or given in a gelatin capsule does not provide consistent homogenous gastric filling. Oral liquid organic iodine contrast agents have little use in the evaluation of the stomach. These solutions give poor mucosal coating, have a very rapid transit, and are used only when a stomach perforation is suspected. Due to osmotic pull of fluid into the bowel, the use of these hypertonic contrast agents is contraindicated in dehydrated or debilitated animals.

Positive contrast studies of the stomach are used to outline stomach position, foreign bodies, or lesions of the gastric wall. The mucosal and rugal pattern are best evaluated when the stomach is distended for a contrast or double contrast study. The rugal folds are absent in the fundus, longitudinal and parallel in the body, and small and spiral in the antral region. The normal mucosal-contrast interface is smooth and homogeneous. Inflammatory lesions with either increased mucus production or gastric wall inflammation and ulceration result in an irregular mucosal-contrast interface. Chronic gastritis may sometimes be demonstrated by rugal fold hypertrophy.

The demonstration of large gastric ulcers or masses involving the gastric wall requires careful radiographic technique and interpretation or they may go undetected. These lesions may be obscured by a dense barium mixture and often require other special techniques. Multiple views, including oblique positions, may help bring a lesion into view. When most of the contrast has left the stomach, air can be introduced for a double contrast study. By means of a simultaneous pneumoperitoneum, a mass or the amount of gastric wall thickening may be determined (Fig. 57–7).

Contrast studies crudely evaluate gastric motility and emptying. Being a dynamic process, fluoroscopy is the best means of evaluating gastric wall motility. Without fluoroscopy, multiple radiographs must be taken to observe changes in the gastric wall due to peristaltic contractions. A fixed, rigid, or nondistensible region of the stomach suggests a gastric wall lesion. Delayed gastric emptying results from gastric motility defects or from gastric outflow obstructions. Normally, the duodenum begins to fill in 5 to 15 minutes and the stomach empties in approximately one to four hours (Funkquist and Garmer, 1967). Total retention of the contrast in the stomach for longer than 30 minutes generally indicates some degree of pyloric occlusion (Gibbs and Pearson, 1973). The rate of gastric emptying can be altered by excitement, by nervous inhibition, or by various anticholinergic drugs or tranquilizers. If tranquilization is required, acetylpromazine maleate is reported to not affect gastric transit time (Zontine, 1973).

ENDOSCOPY

Endoscopy enables the clinician to visually examine the luminal surface of the stomach.

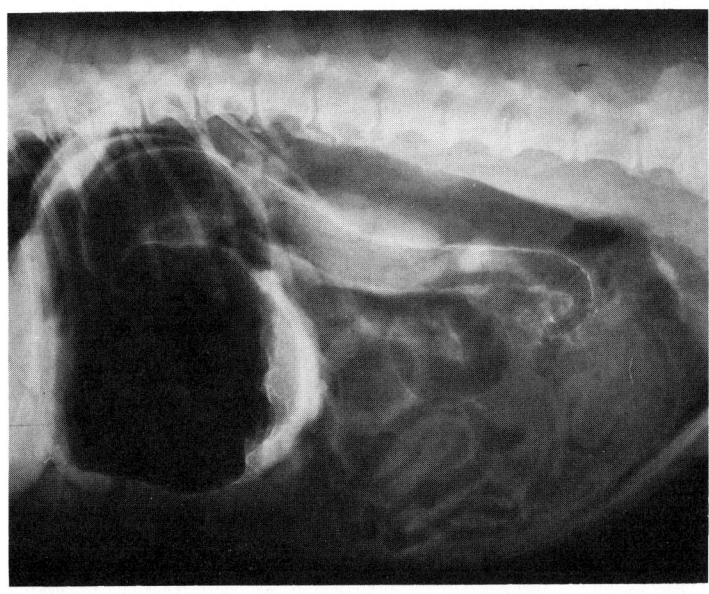

Figure 57–7. A double contrast study with a simultaneous pneumoperitoneum outlining a thickened caudal gastric wall due to a gastric adenocarcinoma.

Older, rigid endoscopes, either hollow tubes or solid optics, offered only limited value in the examination of the small animal stomach. They have been useful in aiding in the removal of various gastric foreign bodies.

With the development of flexible fiberoptics, examination of the gastrointestinal system has improved. The entire stomach can now be adequately visualized. Endoscopes used for examination of the stomach consist of a long, flexible insertion tube with a bending distal tip, an eyepiece, and control section. The distal tip of the endoscope is directed through either a two- or four-way control knob in the handpiece. In addition to the fiber bundles, two channels are present. One allows a variety of endoscopic tools to be passed and fluids to be suctioned. The other channel carries air for insufflation of the organ or for passing water to wash away mucus and other material from the viewing window. A separate light source with a pump for instillation of fluid and air and a separate suction apparatus are required. Biopsy forceps, cytology brushes, aspirating tubes, snares, and grasping forceps are available.

Most endoscopes are designed for human use, although less expensive veterinary endoscopes have been developed. Many veterinary endoscopists prefer a human pediatric endoscope (Fig. 57–8) (Johnson and Twedt, 1977). This endoscope has a working length of 110 cm and an outer diameter of nine

mm, making it versatile for small dogs and cats as well as for the giant breeds. Used or rebuilt endoscopes are less expensive and can be obtained from most manufacturers. Veterinary endoscopes presently available are cheaper, but their shorter length and larger outside diameter limit their use in some cases.

Indications. Endoscopy has added a new diagnostic modality but has not replaced other conventional diagnostic methods. An animal with signs suggestive of gastric disease (e.g., vomiting, hematemesis, or melena) is a candidate for a gastroscopy. The procedure should be preceded by adequate laboratory support and radiology. Endoscopy enables the clinician to visualize the luminal surface of the stomach and to evaluate for the presence of ulceration, hemorrhage, or tumors (Fig. 57–9). Endoscopy is also used when abnormal radiographic findings need to be confirmed or when radiology fails to demonstrate a lesion. During endoscopy the clinician can obtain a guided punch biopsy, brush cytology, or fluid aspiration, or can remove certain small foreign bodies (Johnson et al., 1976).

Technique. Animals are fasted 12 hours prior to the procedure. General anesthesia with tracheal intubation is required for most cases; heavy sedation is possible but increases the risk of damage to the endoscope. A mouth gag should always be used to protect the instrument. The animal is

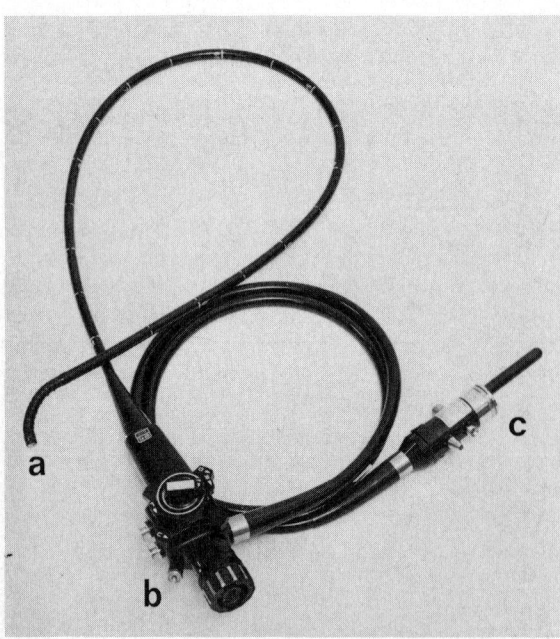

Figure 57–8. A gastrointestinal fiberoptic endoscope with viewing end (a), eyepiece and control section (b), and connector (c) for attachment to a light source (not shown).

placed in left lateral recumbency so that the antrum and pylorus are away from the table and thus less distorted. This position permits good visualization of the stomach and facilitates passage of the instrument into the antrum. As the endoscope is passed into the stomach, air is insufflated to distend the lumen. The distention will flatten the mucosal folds and aid in visualization of the mucosal surface. Location of the endoscope tip is known once the prominate incisura, a large fold demarcating the junction of the antrum and lesser curvature, is found. The cardia and fundus are visualized when the endoscope tip is retroflexed. To view the pylorus, the endoscope must be advanced into the antrum. With expertise, the scope can sometimes be passed through the pyloric sphincter into the proximal duodenum. This procedure is often aided by the use of intravenous glucagon, which has a hypotonic effect on the gastrointestinal tract, relaxing the pylorus.

The mucosal surface should be evaluated for changes in color or consistency. Submucosal hemorrhage or small mucosal ulcerations can be observed with gastritis (Fig. 57–9,*A*). Gastric tumors are often characterized by areas that lack distensibility, such as large protuberances or a large raised ulcer. Small polyps may be observed as incidental findings.

When a lesion is observed, biopsy forceps are passed through the endoscope and directed to the area to be biopsied. A cytology brush is used in a similar manner to obtain tissue. Small four-pronged grasping forceps or snares may be used to remove small gastric foreign bodies (Fig. 57–9,*B*).

Complications. The complications of gastroscopy are rare (Johnson, 1979). The major problem occurs with operator inexperience, in both the technical aspects and the ability to accurately interpret the findings. It is advantageous to gain experience with someone skilled in endoscopy. Anesthesia and overdistention of the stomach with air are always potential complications.

GASTRIC BIOPSY

Various types of biopsy capsules have been designed in which gastric biopsies may be obtained perorally. These instruments are relatively simple and noninvasive, and can easily be passed into the stomach to obtain a small mucosal section. All instruments work on the basic principle of a capsule attached to a long flexible tube. Suction is created when the operator, using a syringe and vacuum gauge, draws a piece of mucosa into a small hole in the capsule. A knife attached to a cable is pulled and cuts off the piece of tissue. The mucosal biopsy is then retained inside the capsule.

One type of capsule found suitable for gastric biopsy in small animals is a Sielaff's gastric biopsy probe (Fig. 57–10). Other instruments include the Quinton biopsy instrument and the Carrie gastrointestinal biopsy capsule. It is sometimes possible to obtain a Wood's gastric biopsy capsule from a human gastrointestinal unit, since these instruments have become outdated by modern endoscopic instruments and hydraulically-controlled multiple biopsy probes (Wood et al., 1949).

The animal to be biopsied should be held off food for 12 to 24 hours prior to the procedure. Sedation is generally not necessary. A mouth speculum is used, and the capsule and tube is introduced into the mouth and fed down the esophagus to the stomach. The position of the capsule is not known unless fluoroscopy is used simultaneously to direct the biopsy capsule or it is directed during endoscopy. If the dog is put in left lateral recumbency, the greater curvature is usually biopsied, while a right lateral recumbency usually retrieves lesser curvature and antral area. This biopsy technique is usually only feasible for diffuse mucosal lesions. Focal mucosal lesions or submucosal lesions are generally not obtained.

Few complications occur (Batt, 1979). The most serious potential complication would be gastric perforation or hemorrhage. The procedure should not be used in any animal with a bleeding disorder.

Surgical Biopsy. An exploratory celiotomy provides the best means of establishing a definitive diagnosis of gastric disease. Surgery provides the opportunity to palpate the stomach, examine the luminal surface, obtain a full thickness biopsy of the gastric wall, and remove gastric foreign bodies. Surgery is often required for the removal of gastric ulcers, polyps, and tumors and to correct gastric outflow obstructions. At the time of surgery the animal should be carefully evaluated for other intra-abdominal

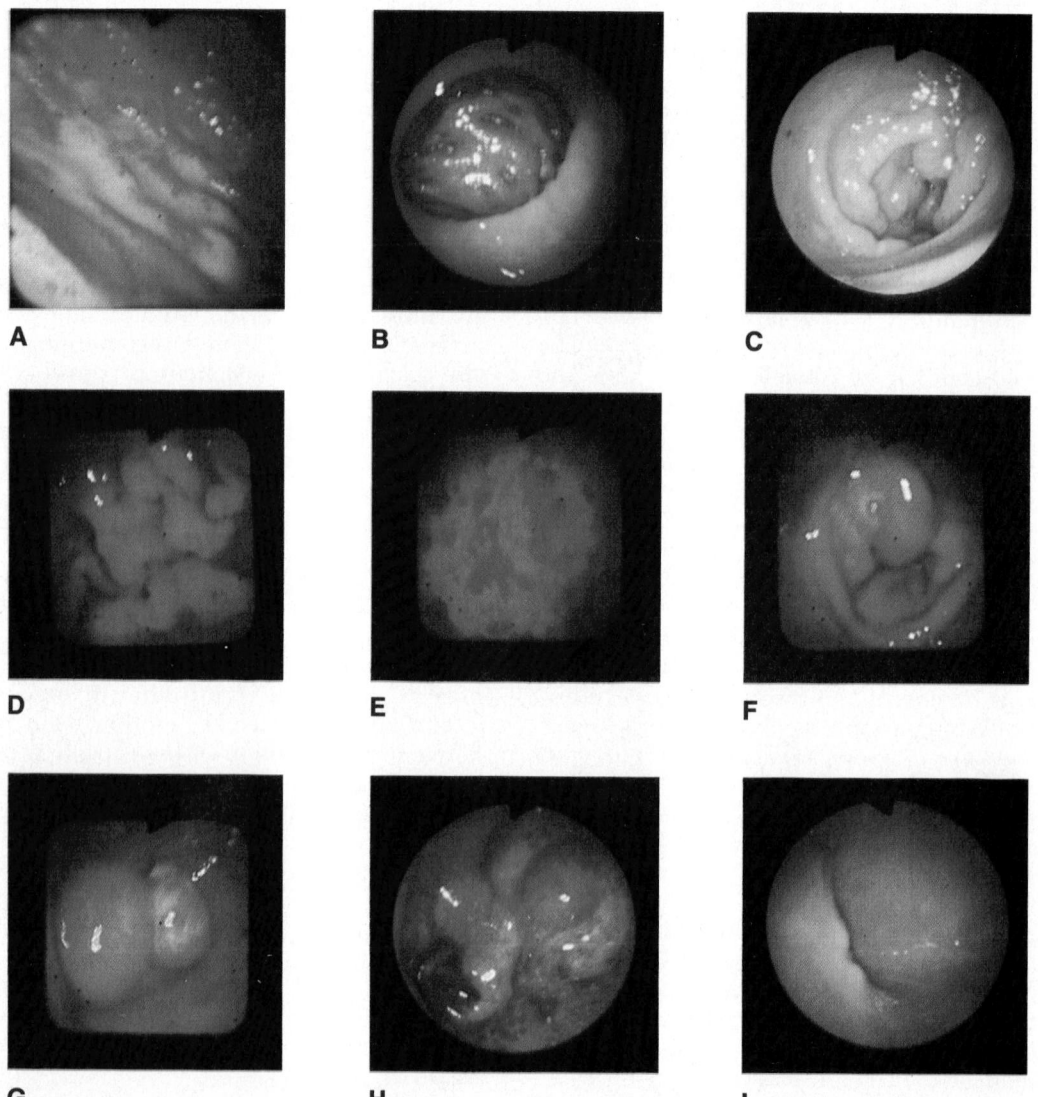

Figure 57–9. *A,* A view of the fundic region with a severe superficial gastritis characterized by a hyperemic gastric mucosa and increased mucous secretions. *B,* A peach pit gastric foreign body that resulted in a chronic superficial gastritis in a dog. *C,* An endoscopic view of the antrum. The pyloric canal is obscured by large rugal convolutions as a result of mucosal hypertrophy in a dog with systemic mastocytosis. *D,* A close-up view of the gastric mucosa with gastritis. Pictured are prominent hyperemic and edematous rugal folds with several small superficial erosions (arrows). *E,* An endoscopic view of the gastric mucosa of a dog with the history of acute hematemesis. Pictured is an acute superficial hemorrhagic gastritis. *F,* A view of the pylorus of a dog with pyloric hypertrophy and clinical outflow obstruction. The pylorus is accentuated by large folds of tissue around and extending into the pyloric canal (arrow). *G,* A bilobed polyp in the antrum just ahead of the pyloric canal, which caused a pyloric outflow obstruction. *H,* A leiomyoma in the antrum of a dog with an outflow obstruction. The lesion is arising from the muscle layers but protruding into the lumen. There are secondary superficial mucosal ulcerations. *I,* An endoscopic view of early gastric lymphosarcoma in a cat. The lesion is viewed as two light raised protrusions at the level of the incisura angularis (arrow) on the lesser curvature; behind is the antral canal.

Illustration continued on following page

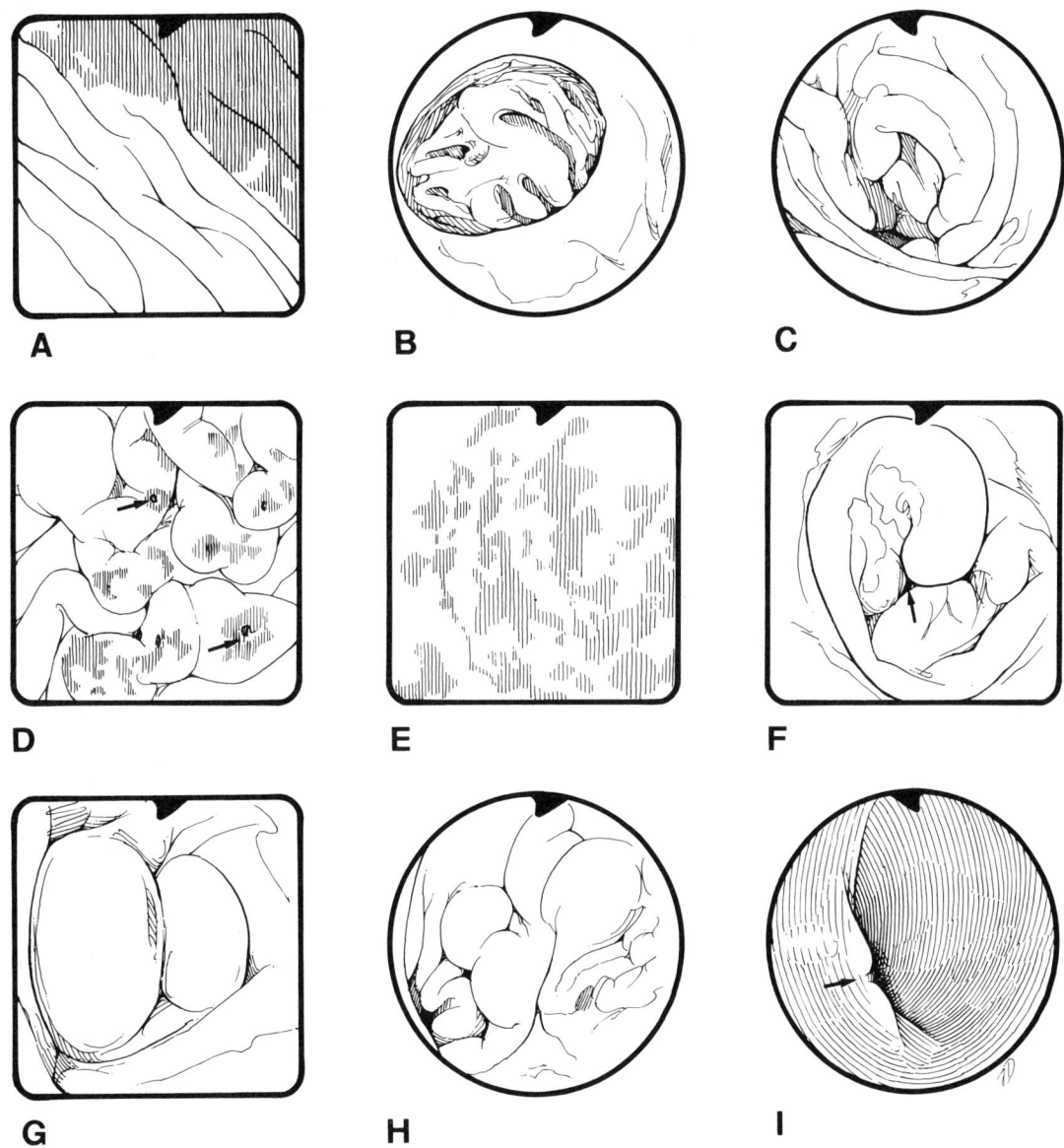

A   B   C

D   E   F

G   H   I

Figure 57–9. *Continued*

problems such as pancreatitis, enlarged regional lymph nodes, or small gastrin secreting tumors of the pancreas.

GASTRIC SECRETORY TESTING

A major function of the stomach is the secretion of hydrochloric acid. Disease states can occur with either an increase or a decrease in gastric acid secretion. Increased gastric acid secretion potentiates mucosal damage and may result in duodenal or gastric ulcers. A hyperacidic state occurs in the dog, owing to a gastrin-secreting tumor or to certain mast cell tumors. Other causes of increased acid production in animals with clinical gastric disease have not been reported and warrant investigation.

The collection of gastric secretions and the analysis of the acid content will help to recognize hyperacidic secretory states. Clinical gastric acid collection in the dog is best achieved by temporarily placing a gastric tube by pharyngostomy into the antral region of the stomach (Aagaard et al., 1972). Basal gastric acid output secretions (BOA) are collected in the fasted dog in 15 minute aliquots. The sample is pH meter titrated to

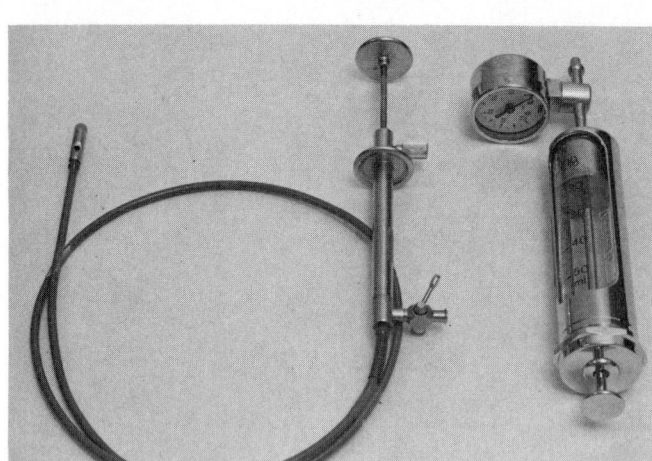

Figure 57–10. Gastric biopsy capsule with syringe and vacuum gauge.

a neutral pH and then expressed in millequivalents of hydrogen ion per 15-minute period (Isenberg, 1978). The basal acid output in the normal fasted dog is usually negligible. The potential acid-secreting ability of the stomach is directly proportional to the parietal cell mass (Marks et al., 1960). This maximal acid output (MAO) can be stimulated by various secretagogues such as histamine, betazole, or pentagastrin.

Antihistamines must be given with histamine to minimize the systemic effects of the drug. Antihistamines will block the H_1-receptors but have no effect on the H_2-receptors, which stimulate acid secretions. Betazole, an analog of histamine, has its main effect in stimulating acid production with little histamine-like action. Pentagastrin contains the C-terminal active site of natural gastrins and therefore acts as a physiologic gastric acid stimulator and is preferred for evaluating gastric secretory function. Pentagastrin, given at the rate of 6 mcg/kg body weight subcutaneously or intravenously, will cause a maximal acid secretion within one hour (Baron, 1979). In the normal dog a wide range of values are reported, depending on the methods used. Ranges of 3 to 12 mEq of hydrogen ion per 15 minutes are reported using pentagastrin stimulation (Hirschowitz and Gibson, 1978; Grossman and Konturek, 1974; Bilski and Kowalewski, 1978).

SYNDROMES OF MUCOSAL INJURY

MECHANISMS OF MUCOSAL DAMAGE

Gastric Mucosal Barrier. The parietal cells of the gastric mucosa produce hydro-chloric acid, often generating a luminal secretion with a pH as low as one. The unique ability of the stomach to withstand concentrated acid without cellular damage is referred to as the *gastric mucosal barrier* (Ivey, 1974). This barrier is resistant to the "back-diffusion" of hydrogen ions from the gastric lumen into the mucosa and the prevention of sodium loss into the lumen. The anatomic makeup of the barrier consists of two parts, the mucous layer lining the surface of the epithelial cells and the mucosal cells that comprise the epithelial membrane. The true function of the mucous layer is unclear, but it is believed to act predominantly in lubrication. Mucus has only a weak neutralizing and buffering capacity, and acid will readily diffuse through it. The gastric epithelial cells seem to be the most important anatomic barrier (Skillman and Silen, 1972).

The back diffusion of luminal acid into the mucosa is essential in the pathogenesis of gastric mucosal damage. Normally there is minimal leakage of secreted acid back into the mucosa. Such leakage occurs at a very slow rate and is rapidly removed by the vascular system (Cheung and Chang, 1977). The topical action of many endogenous and exogenous agents can alter this barrier, thereby increasing mucosal permeability to acid. With increased entry of acid, a chain of events ensues, beginning with the direct damage to the mucosa and followed by destruction of the subepithelium (Fig. 57–11). Mast cells present in the submucosa and lamina propria degranulate and release histamine upon contact with acid. The release of histamine stimulates parietal cell secretion of hydrochloric acid as well as local inflammation and edema. Acid may also

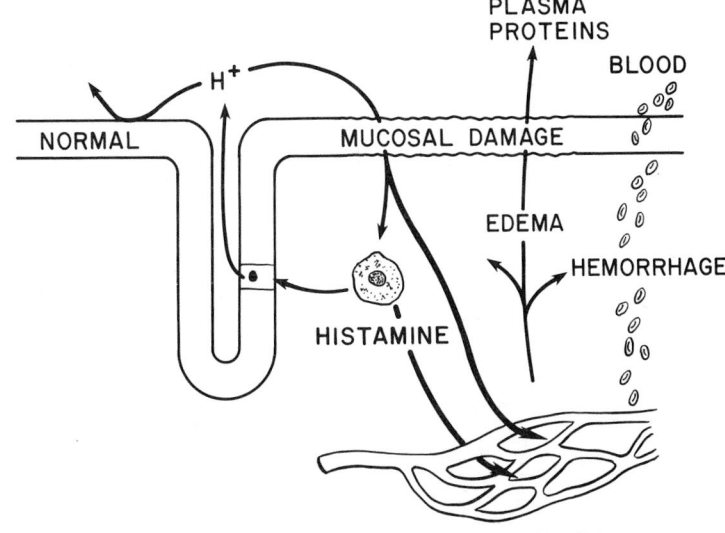

Figure 57–11. Mechanism of events resulting from damage to the gastric mucosal barrier and back-diffusion of acid into the gastric wall.

damage blood vessels and stimulate nerves of the stomach wall, leading to increased muscular contractions. When the gastric mucosal barrier is broken, acid enters the gastric wall and the luminal acid concentration decreases if gastric acid is measured by conventional means (see Gastric Secretory Testing).

Agents of Mucosal Damage. Normally, an electric potential difference of 40 to 60 millivolts exists across the gastric mucosa of the dog (Cooke, 1976). The production of hydrogen ions and the pumping of chloride into and sodium out of the lumen contribute to the potential difference. Only an intact gastric mucosal barrier can maintain such gradients of electrical and chemical activity. With the disruption of the barrier and back-diffusion of hydrogen ions, there is a simultaneous decrease in the potential difference. Experimentally, a decrease in the potential difference is used as a sensitive indicator of gastric mucosal damage. Various physiochemical agents have been shown to cause such changes.

Aspirin will consistently cause gastric lesions in the dog and cat (Kuo and Shanbor, 1976; Larsen, 1963). Aspirin damages the gastric epithelial cells by virtue of its lipid membrane solubility, which, upon entry into the cell, causes cellular damage. A dose of 100 mg/kg per day has been shown to consistently cause gastric lesions in the dog (Lev et al., 1972), while approximately half that dose is reported to cause gastric lesions in the cat (Herrgesell, 1976). Buffered aspirin

will also cause gastric lesions, while enteric coated aspirin produces fewer gastric lesions but has somewhat inconsistent drug absorption (Lanza et al., 1980). Other compounds entering the gastric mucosa by way of lipid solubility include bile acids, short-chain fatty acids, and certain detergents (such as digoxin).

Drugs such as phenylbutazone and indomethacin cause gastric mucosal lesions, though the specific mechanism is unclear. Indomethacin will cause severe gastric ulcers at a dose as low as one mg/kg body weight and, therefore, should not be used in dogs and cats (Ewing, 1972). Hypertonic agents can lower the transmucosal potential difference and cause gastric mucosal damage. Lesions also occur from such things as corrosive agents, heavy metal compounds, infectious agents, and various toxins. Finally, the physical presence of abrasive foreign agents in the gastric lumen may cause mucosal damage.

Corticosteroids alone do not alter the permeability of the gastric mucosa but will significantly enhance the effects of aspirin, bile acids, and other mucosal damaging agents. Corticosteroids decrease mucosal cell turnover, decrease mucous production, and increase gastrin levels and gastric acid production (Fenester, 1973).

Alterations in the blood flow of the gastric mucosal microcirculation will potentiate the formation of gastric mucosal lesions. Mucosal ischemia, without acid or cellular damage, does not break the barrier (Davenport and Barr, 1973). There is also evidence that ischemia results in a profound decrease in gastric mucosal energy and rapid cellular death (Moody and Cheung, 1976). A decreased blood flow to the gastric mucosa may result from a number of causes. Conditions such as hypotension, shock, and sepsis will alter the normal gastric microcirculation. Abnormal blood flow may occur with central nervous system lesions and is felt to result from an altered equilibrium between sympathetic and parasympathetic pathways. This happens most commonly in spinal cord lesions with a loss of sympathetic inhibitory influences, resulting in a paralytic vasodilatation and vagotonia in the vessels of the gastric wall. Parasympathetic overdrive also stimulates an increase in gastric acid and enzyme secretion.

Stress has been associated with gastric lesions by altering the gastric mucosa through a neuroendocrine mechanism. This results from a sympathetically mediated vasoconstriction in the vascular bed, promoting vascular stasis, and from the endogenous release of corticosteroids, vasoactive catecholamines, and serotonin (Skillman and Silen, 1972). (See Gastric Ulcers.)

The *reflux of bile and pancreatic enzymes* will result in increased permeability to hydrogen ions and damage to the mucosal barrier. Bile acids alter the barrier by virtue of their lipid solubility. Bile, gastric acid, and ischemia all work synergistically to destroy the gastric mucosal barrier. The importance of bile is emphasized in experimental studies of hemorrhagic shock wherein dogs in which the pylorus had been occluded, preventing duodenal reflux of bile, had a significantly lower incidence of gastric ulcerations (Guilbert et al., 1969).

Gastric lesions may result *secondary to metabolic diseases.* Renal failure results in the accumulation of uremic toxins that damage the gastric mucosa and vessels of the gastric wall (Cheville, 1979). Serum gastrin levels are also elevated during uremia due to reduced renal clearance (Gold et al., 1980). Gastric lesions may occur secondary to liver failure, though the exact mechanism is not completely known. Damage results in part from reduced mucosal blood flow, loss of the mucous barrier, and elevated gastrin levels. Systemic mastocytosis often causes gastric ulceration from the increased levels of histamine, which stimulate the parietal cells, resulting in increased gastric acid pro-

duction (Zontine et al., 1977). Gastric lesions have also been observed in some cases of adrenocortical insufficiency.

Acute Gastritis

Acute gastritis is a common disease entity occurring in small animals. Strictly defined, acute gastritis is inflammation and mucosal damage that has occurred in response to an insult to the gastric mucosa. Rarely do conditions of acute gastritis warrant biopsy and histologic confirmation; therefore, the diagnosis of acute gastritis is given when signs of gastric disease are acute and self-limiting.

Etiology. In most cases of acute gastritis, the etiology is never determined. In contrast to the reports of experimentally produced lesions, there is a paucity of published cases of spontaneously occurring acute gastritis. Acute gastritis has been associated with a multitude of factors, mainly related to the dietary indiscretions of dogs and cats. It is most often associated with ingestion of rancid or spoiled foodstuffs, which results in what is referred to as "garbage-can" intoxication. The actual incriminating agent is usually derived from the fermentation or putrifaction of food products, various bacterial enterotoxins, and mycotoxins (Harris, 1975).

The ingestion of *foreign material* such as food wrappings made of cellophane or aluminum, bones, plastic, rocks, and small toys will often damage the gastric mucosa by mechanical means. The incidence of ingested foreign bodies is more common in the young animal, possibly owing to their chewing habits and curious nature. Trichobezoars (hairballs) are frequently encountered in the stomachs of some long-haired cats and dogs. Certain drugs (e.g., aspirin, indomethocin, phenylbutazone, and corticosteroids) and chemicals are reported to cause gastritis in the dog and cat. Examples of chemical irritants include some heavy metals (e.g., lead), cleaning agents, fertilizers, and herbicides.

Many types of *plants and plant toxins* cause an acute gastritis, possibly the most common being associated with the ingestion of grass. The ingestion of grass and plants is probably a normal instinctive behavior; however, animals with gastric disease for some unknown reason, seem to ingest and frequently vomit plant material. Many common household plants will cause acute gastritis (Atkins and Johnson, 1975).

Infectious agents may cause acute gastritis. The incidence of bacteria-induced gastritis is low, because the gastric lumen generally contains few bacteria, owing to the acid environment. Viruses such as canine distemper, canine hepatitis, cornavirus, and parvovirus may cause gastric lesions as a portion of a more extensive disease condition. Mycotic infections of the stomach have been reported in the dog (Osborn and Wilson, 1969; Howard, 1966; Barsanti et al., 1975). Parasites generally do not produce gastric lesions or clinical signs. *Physaloptera spp.* are the most frequent gastric parasites, although ascarids and tapeworms may infrequently cause gastritis and vomiting. Spirochetes have been observed in the mucous layer and parietal cells of the stomachs of some dogs and cats and may be a factor in the cause of gastritis (Weber et al., 1958).

Acute gastritis may result from an *allergic reaction* to a previously sensitized antigen. Clinical conditions are often suggested as being simple food allergies. Other disease conditions including uremia, liver disease, neurologic disease, shock, sepsis, or even stress may play a role in the etiology of acute gastritis.

Pathophysiology. Acute lesions may be localized or diffuse. Necrosis of surface cells with extravasation of blood and plasma from the damaged vessels in the lamina propria produces superficial erosions, edema, and hemorrhage. There are variable amounts of polymorphonuclear (PMN) and lymphocytic infiltration. Occasionally, inflammation may extend to a purulent gastritis with necrosis and extensive PMN infiltration.

Diagnosis. A tentative diagnosis of acute gastritis is made on the basis of the history, clinical signs, and physical examination. Since acute gastritis is far more common than other causes of gastric disease, symptomatic therapy is usually initiated without extensive diagnostic procedures. A rapid and complete response to therapy confirms the diagnosis. Cases involving severely ill animals or those that fail to respond to symptomatic therapy require further diagnostic testing (see Clinical Evaluation).

Treatment. Most cases of acute gastritis respond to little or no therapy within 24 hours after the onset of signs. Such cases are usually treated on an outpatient basis. Those animals displaying severe clinical signs, evidence of dehydration, or failure to respond to previous conservative measures require further medical and laboratory support. The basic principles in the therapy of gastric disease include removing the initiating agent, providing proper conditions that promote mucosal repair, correcting secondary complications of gastritis (vomiting, abdominal pain, and infection), and correcting fluid, electrolyte, and acid-base abnormalities.

Dietary restriction should be the initial step in the therapy of acute gastritis. The ingestion of food or liquids results in gastric distention and increased gastric motility, and is a stimulus for further vomiting. Food results in further gastric acid production, stimulated through both the cephalic and gastric phases of gastric secretion (see Physiology). This results in greater back diffusion of hydrogen ions and mucosal damage. Food may also serve as an exogenous source of bacteria that could potentially invade the damaged gastric mucosa.

The animal with acute gastritis should be fasted (NPO) for a minimum of 12 hours. If no vomiting occurs during that time, the animal is offered frequent, small amounts of water or ice cubes, only enough to keep the mouth moist and to supply a modest fluid replacement. Only after a minimum of 24 hours following the onset of signs should the reintroduction of food be attempted. The animal is fed small amounts of a bland diet, and foods high in fat and protein are avoided. A diet consisting predominately of carbohydrates is used. Cooked rice or cooked cereals supplemented with such things as cottage cheese, lean boiled ground beef, or baby foods may be recommended. Commercial diets formulated for gastrointestinal disease (e.g., Prescription Diet I/D) may also be prescribed. If a favorable response is obtained with dietary management, the regular diet is gradually reintroduced over several days.

Parenteral fluids are only initiated when dehydration, electrolyte, or acid-base imbalances occur. The quantity of fluids given should be enough to supply daily maintenance needs (approximately 40 to 60 ml/kg/day), to correct existing dehydration, and to replace fluid losses that may occur with continued vomiting. Vomiting in acute gastritis generally results in volume depletion and losses of sodium, chloride, and potassium with a *metabolic acidosis.* An isotonic balanced electrolyte solution such as Ringer's lactate solution is usually given. Infrequently, in conditions of profuse vomiting or a gastric outflow obstruction, a severe hypochloremia, hypokalemia, and *metabolic alkalosis* may exist. Normal (0.9 per cent) saline is the fluid of choice for correcting metabolic alkalosis resulting from vomiting. Therapy with chlorides rectifies the deficit and allows for the renal excretion of bicarbonate (Finco, 1972). In either an acidotic or alkalotic state, potassium is usually depleted and requires additional supplementation with potassium chloride. The amount of potassium chloride supplemented is based on the existing serum potassium levels (Twedt, 1981).

Antiemetic drugs are given to control refractory vomiting when a pyloric obstruction or gastric foreign body has been ruled out. These drugs inhibit vomiting but do little for the primary treatment of gastritis. Antiemetic drugs act centrally to suppress either the chemoreceptor trigger zone (CTZ), the emetic center, or the vestibular apparatus (see Chapter 5).

Drugs that depress only the CTZ are generally not useful unless the gastritis is secondary to conditions such as uremia or other types of toxins that may directly stimulate the CTZ. The phenothiazine tranquilizers (e.g., chlorpromazine) have a broad spectrum pharmacologic effect, blocking the CTZ and vomiting center, as well as some anticholinergic action (Davis, 1980). These drugs are effective in blocking the viscera-stimulated vomiting that results from gastritis and should be used in those cases with repeated vomiting. The phenothiazines should not be used in a dehydrated or hypotensive animal, owing to their alpha adrenergic blocking action, which causes arteriolar vasodilatation.

Anticholinergic drugs reduce gastric motility and spasms, which are often among the factors that stimulate vomiting and pain occurring with acute gastritis. In addition to blocking the parasympathetic stimulation of smooth muscles of the gastric wall, they also block the cephalic and gastric phase stimulation of gastric acid secretion but do not block histamine- or gastrin-stimulated acid secretion. These drugs have the undesirable effect of reducing gastric emptying, which results in gastric distention and further gastric acid secretion. Overuse of these drugs may result in gastric hypotonia and an iatrogenic gastric outflow obstruction, which may result in continued vomiting. Anticholinergic drugs used in the therapy of gastric disease include atropine, methylscopolamine, isopropamide, and propantheline. These drugs are often combined with an antiemetic for veterinary use. Opiates (e.g., camphorated tincture of opium and diphenoxylate) are a class of drugs that have a similar action in decreasing gastric motility and emptying.

Oral protectants such as kaolin and pectolin compounds and *antibiotics* are generally not indicated in the treatment of acute gastritis. Protectants may bind certain bacteria or toxins but do not coat or protect the injured gastric mucosa. Any potential benefit is frequently outweighed by difficulty in owner administration and vomiting that may occur from gastric distention by these compounds. Similarly, antibiotics are not required unless a bacterial infection is suspected. Antibiotics for such a situation are best given parenterally.

Antacid therapy is not usually prescribed for simple cases of acute gastritis but reserved for refractory cases or for those that have serious gastric bleeding or ulcers (see Gastric Ulcers).

H_2-*receptor antagonists* (e.g., cimetidine) are effective in reducing gastric acid production in the dog and cat by blocking the histamine receptor of the parietal cells. These drugs have been indicated for the treatment of duodenal and gastric ulcers, in esophagitis from gastroesophageal reflux, for the prevention and treatment of acute gastric hemorrhage, and in syndromes resulting in gastric acid hypersecretion (Malagelada and Cortot, 1978). It may be useful in the treatment of some types of gastritis, Zollinger-Ellison syndrome, and gastric ulcers from mast cell tumors. A suggested dose based on experimental studies in the dog is 4 mg/Kg body weight four times daily. No toxicities have yet been noted at this dose level in the dog.

Other drugs, such as prostaglandin compounds, have been effective experimentally in reducing gastric acid secretion in the dog and may be clinically available in the future (Bontol and Cohen, 1979). Carbenoxolone, a drug that protects the gastric mucosa, and drugs with antipepsin activity may also prove clinically useful. Corticosteroids are not indicated for the treatment of acute gastritis as they potentiate the formation of gastric lesions; however, corticosteroids given to the dogs in septic shock will protect the gastric mucosa (Payne and Bowen, 1981).

Severe *gastric hemorrhage* should be treated as an emergency condition, with whole blood and fluids given to replace losses. Attempts are then directed at controlling bleeding through gastric lavage and local vasoconstriction (see Gastric Ulcers).

All *gastric foreign bodies* should be removed. The most accepted means is through a surgical gastrotomy. Surgery also offers the chance to examine the remaining gastrointestinal tract for other foreign bodies or abnormalities. A less invasive measure is endoscopy, since some gastric foreign bodies can be successfully removed using grasping forceps or snares under endoscopic control. Alternative methods include retrieving metallic foreign bodies with magnets or passing grasping forceps under fluoroscopic direction.

With ingestion of small objects (such as needles or pins) and no signs of gastric disease, one may elect to attempt natural passage of the foreign object. A high-fiber diet and lubricants are given under strict observation. The failure of passage in 48 hours requires removal of the foreign body. Administration of emetics to cause the animal to vomit the foreign body should be carried out with great caution and should be attempted only when the foreign body is small with smooth surfaces, so that it will not create a laceration, perforation, or esophageal obstruction. The animal should be fed cotton balls to coat the foreign object before initiation of vomiting. Small trichlobezoars are treated with vaseline or other petroleum products to lubricate passage through the gastrointestinal tract. Owners should not be advised to administer mineral oil, for the fear of an aspiration pneumonitis. Large, indurated trichobezoars require surgical removal.

CHRONIC GASTRITIS

Chronic gastritis is an infrequent clinical diagnosis. Gastric biopsies that correlate the clinical with histologic findings are rarely obtained; therefore, little is known regarding chronic gastric disease in small animals. Several distinct types of chronic gastritis have been reported to occur in the dog.

Etiology. The etiology of chronic gastritis is seldom determined. Most lesions probably occur as a result of a variety of extrinsic influences, particularly with repeated exposure, resulting in damage to the gastric mucosa. In addition, certain immune mechanisms or allergic conditions have been implicated as a cause of chronic gastritis in the dog.

Many chemicals, drugs, and physical agents will cause lesions of chronic gastritis. Most of these agents have similarly been incriminated as causes of acute gastritis, but repeated exposure may result in chronic lesions. The chronic ingestion of aspirin is an excellent example of an agent causing chronic gastritis. Gastric foreign bodies, if left in the stomach, will result in chronic gastric mucosal irritation and lesions of chronic gastritis. Atrophic gastritis has been produced experimentally in the dog by repeated immunization by gastric juices (Krohn and Finlayson, 1972), but naturally occurring immune-mediated gastric disease has not been documented. Hypertrophic gastritis may result from chronic mucosal inflammation or possibly from the trophic actions on the gastric mucosa by histamine or gastrin (see Zollinger-Ellison Syndrome).

Pathophysiology. *Chronic simple gastritis* is the most common form of chronic gastritis and is generally characterized by an excessive but variable inflammatory cell infiltrate and fibrosis of the mucosa and submucosa (Van Der Gaag, 1974). The inflammatory component consists of lymphocytes, plasma cells, and neutrophils. Superficial mucosal erosions, edema, and hemorrhage may be present. In this condition there is no obvious change in mucosal thickness. Long-standing irritation to the gastric mucosa may eventually cause a thickened mucosa, because of metaplasia, hyperplasia, or cyst formation (hypertrophic gastritis) (Kipnis, 1978), or a thin mucosa, because of atrophy of the gastric glands (atrophic gastritis).

Chronic atrophic gastritis is a diffuse lesion of the stomach involving particularly the body and fundus. Atrophy is evident by a thinner-than-normal mucosa, with a reduction in size and depth of the gastric glands. The chief and parietal cell numbers are reduced and often replaced by mucus-secreting cells. An inflammatory component is most always present.

Chronic atrophic gastritis is reported in the dog and is associated with achlorhydria (Ditchfield and Phillipson, 1960). Though not convincingly documented, it is reasonable that a hypochlorhydria would result from a reduction in the parietal cell mass. Further assumptions would suggest that serum gastrin levels would be abnormally elevated, owing to the loss of the negative feedback from acid secretion–inhibiting gastrin release. Atrophic gastritis is one predisposing factor for the development of gastric ulcers (Sorour, 1976).

Chronic hypertrophic gastritis is characterized by macroscopic thickening of the gastric mucosa with large rugal convolutions. These features result from mucosal hypertrophy and hyperplasia of gastric glands, inflammatory cell response, and cystic dilatation of mucous glands. These lesions may occur as either focal polypoid areas, often clinically resembling neoplasia (Kipnis, 1978), or as a diffuse hypertrophy of the rugae involving the majority of the stomach, as is described in a boxer (Van der Gaag et al., 1976). Giant hypertrophic gastritis, reported in basenjis (Van Kruiningen, 1977), presents as a protein-losing gastropathy.

Eosinophilic gastritis is a rare condition characterized as a diffuse eosinophilic and granulation tissue infiltration involving many or all layers of the stomach wall or less frequently, as discrete single or multiple granulomatous nodules (Hayden and Fleischman, 1977; Strombeck, 1979). Eosinophilic lymphadenitis and vasculitis are also said to occur in this condition. Hayden and Fleischman (1977) describe the gross lesions of diffuse eosinophilic gastritis as a scirrhous thickening of the gastric wall resembling gastric neoplasia.

The cause of the eosinophilic infiltration in the stomach is unknown but thought to be immunologically mediated, possibly allergic or parasitic in etiology. In a report of diffuse eosinophilic gastritis in a dog, microfilaria were observed in some histologic sections (Bishop et al., 1981). Dogs experimentally infected with *Toxocara canis* had focal eosinophilic gastritis, but the lesions rarely contained larva, and vasculitis was not found (Hayden and Van Kruinigen, 1975). This latter condition may be similar to the syndrome *eosinophilic gastroenteritis,* in which there is either a segmental or diffuse infiltration of eosinophils in the mucosa and submucosa of the stomach and/or intestine. Though the clinical presentation of the two conditions may be smaller, they differ significantly in their pathologic features.

Clinical Findings. The signs of chronic gastritis are ill-defined and often obscure, and may occur with periodic exacerbations. Many dogs show symptoms for several months before presentation, while others are asymptomatic. Vomiting is reported to be the most common sign observed in chronic gastritis, though it does not occur in every case (Van Der Gaag, 1974). Vomiting is usually infrequent and may or may not be associated with eating. Owners may describe periodic early morning vomiting of a bile-tinged fluid as the only sign. Frequent and severe vomiting occurs with gastric outflow obstructions or in advanced gastritis. With gastric mucosal ulceration, the vomitus may contain either digested or nondigested blood. Other signs of chronic gastritis may include a poor appetite, weight loss, abdominal pain, depression, and polydipsia. With gastric bleeding, anemia and melena may occur.

The physical examination is usually unrewarding but should be carefully performed to rule out conditions that may mimic chronic gastric disease.

Diagnosis. Routine laboratory screens are generally noncontributory but help exclude gastritis secondary to some other disease condition. Anemia, electrolyte imbalance, and dehydration may occur with chronic gastritis and will be reflected in the laboratory tests. The plasma proteins, both albumin and globulin, will be depressed in conditions resulting in a protein-losing gastropathy. A leukocytosis with an absolute eosinophilia occurs in most cases of eosinophilic gastritis. A presumptive diagnosis of eosinophilic gastritis can be made in animals with signs of chronic gastric disease, a peripheral eosinophilia, and a positive response to a trial dose of corticosteroids. At present, gastric acid analysis offers limited information, except in confirming suspected states of hypo- or hyperchlorhydria.

The diagnostic value of radiology was described earlier (see Radiology). Very few, if any, radiologic signs are pathognomonic for lesions of chronic gastritis. Contrast studies may demonstrate a paucity of rugal folds in atrophic gastritis, large rugal folds in hypertrophic gastritis, granulomatous nodules or a thickened gastric wall in eosinophilic gastritis, gastric ulcers, or delayed gastric emptying.

Gastroscopy is a useful tool in the diagnosis of chronic gastritis (Fung et al., 1979).

In some types of gastritis, the mucosa may appear normal through the endoscope while in severe cases mucosal erosions, hemorrhage, or large ulcers are readily observable. Atrophic gastritis results in easy visualization of the submucosal vessels through the thinner-than-normal mucosa. Large, prominent mucosal folds, especially in the antral region, may occur with hypertrophic gastritis, gastric edema, or neoplasia (Fig. 57–9,C).

Gastric biopsies are required for a definitive diagnosis of chronic gastritis.

Treatment. The primary aim in the therapy of chronic gastritis should be the removal of the etiologic agent. The elimination of the chronic ingestion of drugs or known toxic agents and the removal of gastric foreign bodies is obvious. With the elimination of the causative agent, the prognosis is good. The etiology of most cases is never determined, and the therapy must be directed in a logical but often "trial and error" approach. The prognosis in such cases is quite variable. There have been no reported clinical studies evaluating the effectiveness of therapies for chronic gastritis in the dog and cat.

Dietary controls should be attempted in the therapy of chronic gastritis in which the etiologic agent is suspected to have been ingested. Using dietary elimination and a positive response to dietary control confirms those suspicions. Strombeck (1979) reports that dogs with eosinophilic gastritis placed on controlled diets show clinical improvement and resolution of previous peripheral eosinophilia. Diets high in antigenic proteins (meat diets) or those with many supplements should be avoided. Multiple small feedings of a bland, predominately carbohydrate diet may be beneficial. Prescription diets developed for (allergic) gastrointestinal disease (e.g., Prescription diets D/D) may also be useful.

Corticosteroids are indicated to control chronic gastritis resulting from an immune mechanism or those conditions suggestive of an immune response when a biopsy sample shows a predominance of lymphocyte and plasma cell infiltration or in cases of eosinophilic gastritis (Strombeck, 1979). Corticosteroids will stimulate regeneration of gastric parietal cells and may be beneficial in the treatment in some cases of atrophic gastritis (Jeffries, 1978). Corticosteroids do, however, enhance the ulcerogenic potential of mucosal lesions. The immunosuppressant azathioprine prevents experimentally produced immune gastropathy in dogs and may be clinically useful in treating immune-mediated etiologies (Davenport, 1976).

Cimetidine, which is used to inhibit gastric acid secretion, may play an important role in the therapy of chronic gastritis with hyperchlorhydria. Some dogs with chronic simple gastritis and mild mucosal atrophy have shown a positive response with this drug. Antacids may be equally beneficial in these cases. Long-term anticholinergic therapy should be avoided, for it may result in a hypotonic stomach and continued vomiting.

Surgical resection is required for the removal of areas of focal hypertrophic gastritis, granulomas, or large gastric ulcers. A partial gastrectomy is indicated when a protein-losing gastropathy occurs with chronic hypertrophic gastritis. If gastric lesions result in delayed gastric outflow, either a pyloromyotomy or a pyloroplasty is necessary.

GASTRIC ULCERS

Ulcers of the gastric mucosa are now more frequently diagnosed in the dog and cat than in previous years. This is probably due to increased professional awareness, increased drug and surgical therapy, and pursuit of clinical diagnosis through necropsy.

Gastric ulcers are usually peptic. By definition, the presence of gastric acid and pepsin is a prerequisite for development of "peptic" ulcers. Peptic ulcers are usually benign, acute or chronic, circumscribed mucosal defects that extend through the muscularis mucosae and have a firm, raised margin.

Peptic ulcers occur in adult dogs ranging from 2½ to 12 years of age. Females have a higher incidence than males and there is no breed predilection (Murray et al., 1972).

Etiology. Gastric ulceration in the dog may result from any of the agents causing acute or chronic gastritis. In addition to these agents, stress and mastocytosis are important etiologic factors.

Stress ulceration results in the development of multiple erosions in the gastric, duodenal, or colonic mucosa of acutely ill patients. The lesions are usually superficial to the muscularis mucosae and are thus usually only *erosions*, but occasionally a penetrating ulcer is noted, surrounded by erosions. Stress ulceration is infrequently reported in the dog but, when present, may have a significant mortality (Hoerlein and Spano, 1975; Ader, 1979; Toombs et al., 1980).

In systemic mastocytosis, histamine produced by mast cells is released in large quantities and is associated with gastric lesions. Gastric ulcers secondary to mast-cell neoplasms in dogs (Howard et al., 1969; Carrig and Seawright, 1968), cats (Seawright and Grono, 1964), and oxen (Trautwein and Stober, 1965) have been reported. In the dog, the concentration of histamine in mast-cell tumors varies considerably and has been found to equal up to 3000 μg of histamine base per gram of wet tissue (Howard and Kenyon, 1965). Lesions in the dog's stomach are most frequent with mastocytomas (Howard et al., 1969).

The mechanism of induction of the gastroduodenal lesions with mastocytomas is not completely understood. Interestingly, heparin has been shown to prevent mucosal ulceration in the stomach of guinea pigs (Watt et al., 1966) and dogs (Howard et al., 1969). Thus, in dogs there may be a pronounced histamine intoxication without a concomitant heparinemia. The mast cell contains both compounds in abundance; it therefore must follow that in mastocytomas either the heparin is not released in significant amounts or it may be bound or rapidly metabolized following liberation. In canine mastocytoma the neoplastic cells are anaplastic and contain little cytoplasmic metachromasia, indicating the lack of heparin (Howard et al., 1969).

Mucosal lesions in mastocytoma are partially associated with mucosal ischemia and intravascular thrombosis. Small vascular thrombi were observed in 8 of 24 stomachs of dogs with mastocytoma (Howard et al., 1969).

Pathophysiology. Most peptic ulcers occur in the intermediate zone between the body and fundus (where acid is secreted) and the proximal duodenum. Between these two sites lies the pylorus, separating the stomach (with a mucosa highly adapted to withstand acid) from the duodenum (with a mucosa adapted to withstand bile and pancreatic juice).

Luminal acid is generally accepted as essential for the pathogenesis of gastric ulceration. Other factors that affect gastric-mucosal resistance to injury include mucosal permeability and blood flow, secretory state,

acid-base balance, and the presence of pepsin (Kivibakso and Silen, 1979). Nutritional status is also important (Smale et al., 1980). These factors have been discussed in the previous gastritis sections.

Stress ulceration most frequently involves the body of the stomach. The mechanism of this ulceration is not entirely known but is usually attributed to mucosal ischemia, which in most clinical circumstances is due to an episode of hypotension. The focal mucosal necrosis may also result from an energy deficit, which is particularly severe in the body of the stomach because of its primarily aerobic energy metabolism (Menguy and Masters, 1974). Gastric acid secretion will fall during acute stress and then recover as the patient improves. The foci of ischemic necrosis then undergo acid peptic digestion with bleeding, before healing by cell migration from the crypts.

As mentioned previously, hydrogen ions are a requisite for the genesis of erosive gastritis. Interestingly, in all species except the rabbit, stress does not lead to a break in the mucosal cation barrier (Moody et al., 1976).

The precise role of stress in the genesis of acute erosions remains obscure. Central or autonomic neural pathways (Davis and Brooks, 1963; Reed et al., 1971), neurohumoral influences, and the release of histamine from mast cells have been suggested.

Clinical Findings. Vomiting is the most frequent clinical sign of gastric ulcers. The vomitus may be tinged with partially digested blood ("coffee ground" appearance) or with fresh blood and clots, in severe ulcers. Melena, a variable appetite, and weight loss are often reported. With severe blood loss the patient may show anemia and with vomiting, dehydration and a secondary polydipsia may be noted. Some dogs may be asymptomatic with gastric ulcers, while others are encountered following perforation, which rapidly results in death.

Diagnosis. Abdominal pain is the most frequently encountered finding on physical examination. The location of the stomach prevents actual palpation, but abdominal splinting should include gastric ulceration in the rule-outs. Anemia, hematemesis, and melena are all useful in assessing the patient for ulceration. The presence of cutaneous mastocytomas may result in significant gastric disease, as discussed above.

A regenerative anemia is one parameter

associated with peptic ulcer. In 16 of 22 cases of peptic ulceration in dogs, liver disease was also noted. The pathological changes in the liver range from severe disease to fatty and degenerative changes (Murray et al., 1972). Lead poisoning may also result in gastric ulcers (Sass, 1970).

Gastric ulcers, mucosal niches, craters, or fissures of varying sizes will be demonstrated by contrast radiography. Superficial stress erosions cannot usually be seen by a barium contrast examination.

Endoscopy affords the best objective evidence of gastric ulcers. With acute ulcers, the mucosal lesions may be bleeding, have an inflammatory appearance around their periphery, and usually have no evidence of fibrin in the ulcer crater. Chronic ulcers may show little inflammatory response and have a fibrin-filled crater and wrinkled mucosa peripheral to the ulcer (Fig. 57–12). With stress ulceration, early in the post-stress period, focal areas of pallor and cyanosis are seen. Later, discrete areas of extravasation of red blood cells may be observed. Numerous small, well-delineated punctate lesions can be identified along the crests of the rugae within the proximal stomach (Fig. 57–9,D and E). These lesions are usually only a few millimeters in size.

Exploratory gastrotomy can be a useful diagnostic tool in gastric ulceration. Gastric ulceration can occur in association with benign and malignant neoplasms of the stomach. Cytology and histopathology should be included in all cases of gastric ulceration.

Treatment. Secretion of gastric acid perpetuates mucosal lesions and is required for new lesions to occur. Treatment is intended either to decrease hydrogen ion and peptic activity or to increase the ability of the gut to deal with and resist the effects of these agents. Two pharmacologic agents that are practical and useful in the management of gastric ulceration are *antacids* and the newer *histamine analogs* such as cimetidine.

Antacids function to reduce the total amount of available hydrogen ions, as well as to irreversibly inactivate pepsin if the gastric contents can be brought above pH 6 within the stomach. A third effect of antacids on gastric juice is to diminish peptic activity as the pH is raised above the range for optimal proteolysis.

Antacids must be given frequently, as infrequent antacid administration may result in a *rebound hypersecretion* of acid. The rebound effect is most frequently noted when antacids are given two to three times a day, rather than being continuously administered.

The rate of gastric emptying is a major determinant of antacid effectiveness. Thus, with the exponential emptying characteristic of the stomach, the administration of a given quantitity of antacid in large, infrequent doses is less likely to provide sustained buffering. Aluminum-containing antacids will delay gastric emptying in some species (Hurwitz et al., 1976).

Various preparations are available, but no antacid is free of hazard. Sodium bicarbonate may produce sodium overload and systemic alkalosis. Magnesium preparations may lead to severe diarrhea and are hazardous to renal failure patients. Calcium carbonate may lead to hypercalcemia, renal impairment, and stimulation of gastric secretion. Aluminum hydroxide may lead to phosphate depletion, with consequent mus-

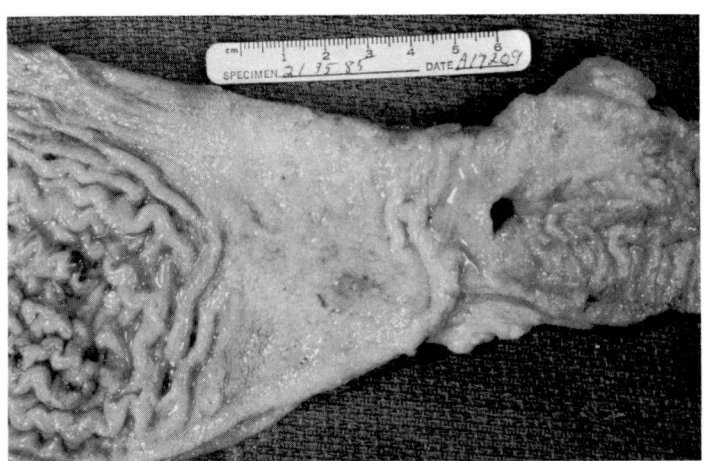

Figure 57–12. Perforated peptic ulcer in the proximal duodenum occurring in a dog with a gastrinoma (Zollinger-Ellison syndrome). Also shown is hypertrophy of the gastric mucosa and small gastric erosions.

cle weakness, bone resorption, and hypercalciuria (Morrissey and Barreras, 1974). Milk is not considered an antacid.

Clinical assessment of histamine analog drugs like cimetidine is lacking in the veterinary patient, although it has been reported to be effective in one dog with gastric ulceration (Schulman, 1979). Cimetidine dosage for the dog is 4 mg/kg body weight four times daily. Experimental usage of this drug in research dogs showed an insignificant effect on healing of experimentally induced gastric ulcers, but it enhanced the healing of duodenal ulcers (Okabe, 1978).

With acute gastrointestinal bleeding (i.e., stress ulceration), an H_2-receptor antagonist like cimetidine is less effective than are antacids in providing adequate prophylaxis. This ineffectiveness results because this agent impairs the secretory state of the mucosa — decreasing intracellular buffering capacity — and inadequately reduces intraluminal acidity (Priebe et al., 1980). Antacids may be more beneficial because they do not affect the secretory state of the mucosa and thus do not affect its buffering capacity, and they also reduce intraluminal acid in a more reliable fashion.

With severe gastric blood loss, intragastric lavage with ice water is indicated. Levarterenol (norepinephrine) may be added to the ice water solution at a rate of 8 mg/500 ml (Palmer, 1975). This potent α-adrenergic vasoconstrictive agent is almost completely destroyed in one passage through the normal liver. The lavage is instilled into the stomach and left for 30 minutes; then the lavage repeated to assess whether or not gastric bleeding has ceased.

Occasionally, surgical therapy is required for gastric ulceration. A partial gastrectomy is generally required for removal of the ulcer. This technique, along with pyloromyotomy and vagotomy, has been successfully used in the dog (Damiano, 1967). With peritonitis secondary to perforation of a gastric ulcer, immediate surgery is indicated.

GASTRIC RETENTION

Retention of gastric contents is often associated with pyloric dysfunction or motility disorders of the stomach or both. The pylorus is an anatomic scapegoat because of its location at the distal end of the stomach and because it impedes emptying and prevents duodenal reflux.

Etiology. Pyloric dysfunction may result from intrinsic, extrinsic, or obturative lesions. The intrinsic lesion of the pylorus results either from a hypertrophy of the circular muscle fibers or from intrinsic pyloric neoplasia. Extrinsic pyloric lesions include hepatic and pancreatic abscesses, neoplasia, and inflammatory lesions. Histoplasmosis may provide intrinsic or extrinsic lesions. Foreign bodies, gastric and/or duodenal ulcers, antral mucosal hypertrophy, and antral polyps result in obturative pyloric lesions.

Acute stress, trauma, psychogenic causes, and inflammatory disease reduce motility in the digestive tract. Reducing the motility in the stomach results in retention of gastric contents. Inhibition of gastric motility is generally associated with stimulation of the sympathetic nervous system. Drugs, hypokalemia, recurring gastric dilatation, and chronic obstruction of the pylorus are also factors leading to gastric hypomotility and retention.

Pylorospasm has been described as an abnormal contraction of the pyloric musculature in order to close the sphincter. Although the pyloric sphincter in the dog does have a high pressure zone (Brink et al., 1965), its effect on gastric emptying is minor (Stemper and Cooke, 1975). In fact, because of the anatomic continuity of the antrum and pylorus, these two function as a single muscle unit (Stemper and Cooke, 1975). As noted previously, the grinding and emptying of solids are primarily a function of the gastric antrum, whereas emptying of liquids depends on tonic activity in the fundus. In fact, the retardation of gastric evacuation is due to decreased antral propulsive peristalsis (Quigley et al., 1943).

Pathophysiology. Pyloric stenosis may result from the excessive secretion of gastrointestinal hormones. With antral distention, the G-cells are stimulated to release gastrin, and this ultimately leads to a decrease in gastric pH. Gastrin has a potent trophic effect on gastric smooth muscle. Gastrin injections given to pregnant bitches cause a 28 per cent incidence of pups born with pyloric stenosis. The circular muscle is hypertrophied, as in spontaneous disease (Dodge, 1970). This report was recently refuted when it was noted that human gastrin does not cross the placenta of the dog and also that human maternal and cord-blood gastrin levels may vary independently (Janik et al., 1978).

Pyloric stenosis may also be associated with neurogenic dysfunction. The overall number of myenteric ganglion cells and nerve fiber tracts are reduced in the pyloric region, and the circular muscle of the pylorus is hypertrophied (Belding and Kernoham, 1953). A nonorganic stenosis accompanied by antral dilatation and muscular hypertrophy can be produced by selective destruction of the intramural ganglia of the pylorus (Okamoto et al., 1967).

Partial obstruction to gastric outflow results in gastric hypersecretion in the dog. An obvious consequence of this outflow obstruction is gastric distention. With chronic distention, gastric mucosal hyperplasia arises as a consequence of increased secretory cell mitosis (Crean et al., 1969; Kaye, 1971).

From the preceding it is possible to suggest that gastric retention either is present at birth or develops with age. With gastric retention comes the worsening of outflow obstruction from the trophic actions of gastrin on smooth muscle and mucosa. Gastric dilatation results from chronic outflow obstruction, leading to a loss of motility of the antrum. No loss of motor function is noted, nor is there always constriction of the pylorus, suggesting there is poor filling of the antrum with each contraction and thus greater gastric retention and less rapid gastric emptying (Fig. 57–13).

Clinical Findings. Vomiting at fairly regular intervals following ingestion of solid foods, with accompanying gastric distention, is the primary sign of gastric retention. The vomitus is usually undigested food and is rarely bile stained. Chronic vomiting generally is associated with some weight loss and dehydration.

Projectile vomiting is often associated with gastric retention and involves the abrupt occurrence of vomitus without the warning of increased salivation and retching. In most instances the vomitus is thrown for a considerable distance and readily empties the stomach.

Brachycephalic breeds have a high incidence of gastric retention, as do Siamese cats (Pearson et al., 1974). No specific sex incidence is reported for the dog or cat. Two female kittens with pyloric stenosis have been reported, suggesting the possible inheritable nature of the disease (Twaddle, 1971).

Diagnosis. There are no specific findings on physical examination of an animal with gastric retention. Observation of emesis may be useful. Vomiting of undigested or only partially digested food when the stomach should be empty is diagnostic of gastric retention. Normally the stomach should be completely empty within six to eight hours after eating. After vomiting, the animal will usually readily resume feeding, only to vomit again at variable intervals.

Laboratory assessment usually shows hematologic changes of dehydration. With severe gastric outlet obstruction and vomiting there may be a metabolic alkalosis.

Since there are smaller concentrations of bicarbonate being delivered to the distal nephron because of enhanced proximal bicarbonate reabsorption, urinary sodium and bicarbonate decrease. This results in a

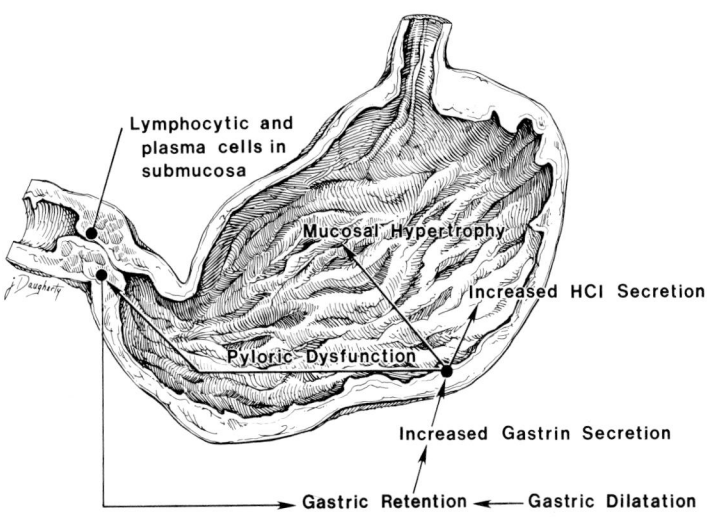

Figure 57–13. Gastric dilatation will result from chronic outflow obstruction occurring from a perpetuating scheme of hormonal, anatomic, and pathological changes.

Lymphocytic and plasma cells in submucosa

Mucosal Hypertrophy

Increased HCl Secretion

Pyloric Dysfunction

Increased Gastrin Secretion

Gastric Retention ←— Gastric Dilatation

paradoxical aciduria in the presence of a metabolic alkalosis (see Fig. 57–6).

RADIOGRAPHY. Radiography affords the most definitive method of diagnosing gastric retention. The presence of gastric distention with food and/or air long after ingesta should be in the intestine is diagnostic of gastric retention (Gibbs and Pearson, 1973). In the cat, an increased gastric volume, with the fundus and body becoming elongated craniocaudally but remaining on the left side of the midline, and the mucosal folds being stretched and having a smooth appearance, is seen with gastric retention (Pearson et al., 1974). The pyloric antrum is often enlarged in size and the pyloric canal narrow and elongated.

Contrast radiography is helpful in assessing the rate of gastric emptying. The term "gastric emptying time" in radiography is usually regarded as the time required for the stomach to begin to empty — but not to empty completely. Less than thirty minutes is reported to be normal gastric emptying time. Normally barium is retained for five to fifteen minutes. The presence of barium within the stomach for more than 12 to 24 hours is abnormal and should be considered a sign of gastric retention. The stress of chemical (Zontine, 1973) or manual restraint may delay gastric emptying.

Fluoroscopy with contrast material is useful for assessing gastric motility. Many times the peristaltic waves are of normal rate and intensity, but these only result in a dilatation of the antrum, with little barium passing through the pyloric canal. Filling defects within the antrum or pylorus may also be identified.

The usefulness of gastroscopy in the canine patient with hypertrophy of the pyloric musculature is not documented (Fig. 57–9,F). One report suggests that the pyloric orifice is fixed or narrowed and that peristaltic waves result in the incomplete closure of the orifice (Zimmer, 1977). It is well to remember that the pyloric orifice of the dog is usually partially open. With the presence of foreign bodies, ulcers, neoplasms, inflammation, or granulomatous changes, biopsies may be taken for diagnosis and prognosis.

Treatment. Obstruction to gastric outflow is generally managed surgically. Intrinsic hypertrophy of the pylorus is successfully managed with pyloromyotomy or pyloroplasty (Archibald, 1954; Archibald et al., 1960; Lawther, 1961; Twaddle, 1970,

1971). With either technique, the surgeon must extend the incision well on to the antrum as well as on to the duodenum in order to alleviate the area of hypertrophied muscle.

Obturative lesions must be carefully assessed. With severe mucosal damage and ulceration it may be necessary to surgically excise the affected area. Occasionally the severity of the lesion necessitates elaborate surgical dismemberment of the pylorus, as in gastroduodenostomy (Butler, 1969) or gastrojejunostomy. Surgery on the pylorus in normal dogs has little effect on the emptying of solids and causes a slight acceleration of emptying of liquids (Hinder and Bremner, 1978).

Motility disorders of the stomach have received no attention in veterinary medicine. Therapy has been directed to the control of symptoms, mainly by use of centrally acting antiemetics. Gastric stimulation with a cholinergic agent such as bethanechol (Urecholine) has also been tried.

Surgery for gastroparesis has not been objectively studied in veterinary patients. Guidelines similar to those used in man may be useful in assessing veterinary patients with gastric emptying disorders involving decreased motility. Only patients with objective abnormalities in gastric motor function and stasis whose symptoms cannot be controlled by medical therapy are considered, and some attempt should be made to verify that other motor disturbances of the digestive tract are absent (Malagelada, 1979).

ZOLLINGER-ELLISON SYNDROME

The Zollinger-Ellison syndrome, or gastrinoma, is characterized by a *gastrin-secreting tumor* of the pancreas, resulting in hypergastrinemia, gastric acid hypersecretion, and upper gastrointestinal ulceration (Zollinger, 1975). Cases resembling Zollinger-Ellison syndrome have been reported in the dog (Jones et al., 1976; Straus et al., 1977a; Happe et al., 1980).

Etiology. The Zollinger-Ellison syndrome in the dog involves a functional non-beta islet cell tumor of the pancreas that produces gastrin. These tumors are believed to derive from the delta (D) cells, which normally comprise approximately five to ten per cent of the cells in the islets of Langerhans.

Pathophysiology. Gastrinomas release a

biologically active gastrin, resulting in a hypergastrinemic state. Elevated serum gastrin levels stimulate parietal cell secretion, which leads to increased hydrochloric acid secretion (hyperchlorhydria). Further, gastrin has a trophic effect on the gastric mucosa, causing mucosal hypertrophy. The increased gastric acid secretion causes gastric mucosal damage, often resulting in large peptic ulcers in the stomach or proximal duodenum (see Fig. 57–12). Esophagitis occurs from the gastric reflux of the highly concentrated acid secretions. Diarrhea may develop with steatorrhea caused by the inactivation of pancreatic lipase and the precipitation of bile salts in the abnormally acidic upper intestine. The gastric secretions are also irritating to the intestinal mucosa, causing inflammatory changes, and high circulating levels of gastrin may contribute to the diarrhea by altering intestinal absorption of water and electrolytes (McGuigan, 1978). Hypocalcemia may be produced by elevated gastrin levels; this in turn stimulates hyperplasia of the C-cells of the thyroid and elevates calcitonin levels. Elevated secretin levels are reported in one dog with a gastrinoma thought to result from the excessive secretion stimulated by an abnormally acid duodenum (Straus and Yalow, 1977b).

Clinical Findings. The majority of dogs with a gastrin-secreting tumor are middle aged or older, with signs of chronic vomiting and weight loss. The vomiting often consists of large volumes of gastric secretions and may contain fresh or digested blood. Gastric or duodenal ulcers may result in blood loss and melena, and if an ulcer perforates, the animal will present with signs of peritonitis. Depression, anorexia, polydipsia, and diarrhea have also been reported.

Diagnosis. The diagnosis of Zollinger-Ellison syndrome should be considered in any animal with persistent vomiting, diarrhea, and upper gastrointestinal ulceration that is only partially responsive or nonresponsive to conservative therapy. Laboratory findings of hypochloremia and hypokalemia with a metabolic alkalosis may occur with a Zollinger-Ellison syndrome (Straus et al., 1977a). Abnormal liver-specific enzymes may result from hepatic metastasis, and hypocalcemia from gastrin-stimulated calcitonin secretion. Steatorrhea often develops and is demonstrated with a positive fecal Sudan stain.

Finding certain contrast radiographic abnormalities may assist in the diagnosis of Zollinger-Ellison syndrome. The gastric rugal folds will be increased and extremely prominent, usually occurring with an ulcer in the stomach or proximal duodenum. The stomach usually contains large amounts of secreted fluid, which often tends to flocculate the contrast media. There may also be some irregularity in the wall of the proximal intestine occurring from an acid-induced enteritis.

Endoscopy is the best means for evaluating the esophagus, stomach, and proximal duodenum for inflammation and ulceration found in a Zollinger-Ellison syndrome (Regan and Malagelada, 1978). Endoscopic examination may find inflammation of the distal esophagus due to reflux and vomiting of the acidic gastric contents. The gastric mucosal folds will be prominent, both in number and size. The mucosal surface is often hyperemic, and there may be small superficial ulcerations. The endoscopist may note an increased amount of fluid in the stomach of a fasted animal. There may be a large, one- to two-cm ulcer in the pyloric antral region or in the proximal duodenum. Biopsies will reveal inflammation of the esophageal mucosa, gastric mucosal hypertrophy, and chronic gastritis.

At present, the most reliable means for establishing the diagnosis of the Zollinger-Ellison syndrome, short of surgery and biopsy, is demonstrating hyperchlorhydria in conjunction with increased serum concentrations of gastrin. Until gastrin levels and secretory testing are evaluated in other clinical gastric diseases in the dog, only a presumptive diagnosis can be made.

Gastric secretory testing is performed as previously described. The normal dog has a negligible basal acid output, while fasting levels of 3 to 15 mEq of hydrogen ion per hour have been measured in dogs with gastrinomas (Straus et al., 1977a; Happe et al., 1980). This collection is then followed by measuring the maximal acid output. In a dog with Zollinger-Ellison syndrome, the acid output is generally already near maximum and therefore, with stimulation, does not show a large rise in acid output, as does the acid output of a normal dog.

The reported fasting basal plasma gastrin levels in dogs with gastrinomas are approximately 2 to 40 times greater than normal control values. Since gastrin levels may be elevated in other disease conditions, further diagnostic tests are run to characterize a Zollinger-Ellison syndrome. Both secretin and calcium are known to stimulate the release of gastrin from these tumors and are useful in provocative diagnostic testing. An intravenous infusion of calcium (calcium gluconate, 2 mg/kg body weight) results in a significant rise in serum gastrin levels in cases of Zollinger-Ellison syndrome but causes little if any rise in normal animals. An intravenous injection of secretin (4 U/kg body weight) will lower serum gastrin levels in normal animals, but in gastrinomas the levels may rise or remain the same (Fig. 57–14). Secretin generally inhibits gastrin release; the mechanism resulting in elevated levels in a gastrin-secreting tumor is unknown (McGuigan and Wolfe, 1980).

Discovery of a gastrin-secreting pancreatic non-beta islet cell tumor during exploratory surgery offers the definitive diagnosis. Most of these pancreatic tumors are one to a few centimeters in diameter. The regional lymph nodes and liver should be carefully examined for metastatic lesions, and large gastric or duodenal ulcers should be resected. It is important to emphasize that any cases involving chronic gastritis or gastric ulcerations undergoing surgery should include a careful examination of the pancreas for a gastrinoma.

Treatment. The treatment of choice is surgery. Surgery not only offers a definitive diagnosis but affords an opportunity to remove the primary pancreatic tumor and to evaluate possible metastasis. Surgery may also be required to remove large peptic ulcers. Medical therapy is frequently unsuccessful because of the high incidence of metastasis of these tumors. Therefore, patients with this syndrome are usually treated with a total gastrectomy, which removes the target organ, the stomach (McCarthy, 1980).

With the development of H_2-receptor blocking agents (cimetidine), which inhibit gastrin stimulated gastric acid secretion, beneficial results may be obtained in the medical treatment of canine gastrinomas. Successful medical management of human Zollinger-Ellison syndrome using a combination of cimetidine and an anticholinergic is reported but has yet to be evaluated in the dog (Richardson and Walsh, 1976).

The prognoses of the reported cases of canine Zollinger-Ellison syndrome have

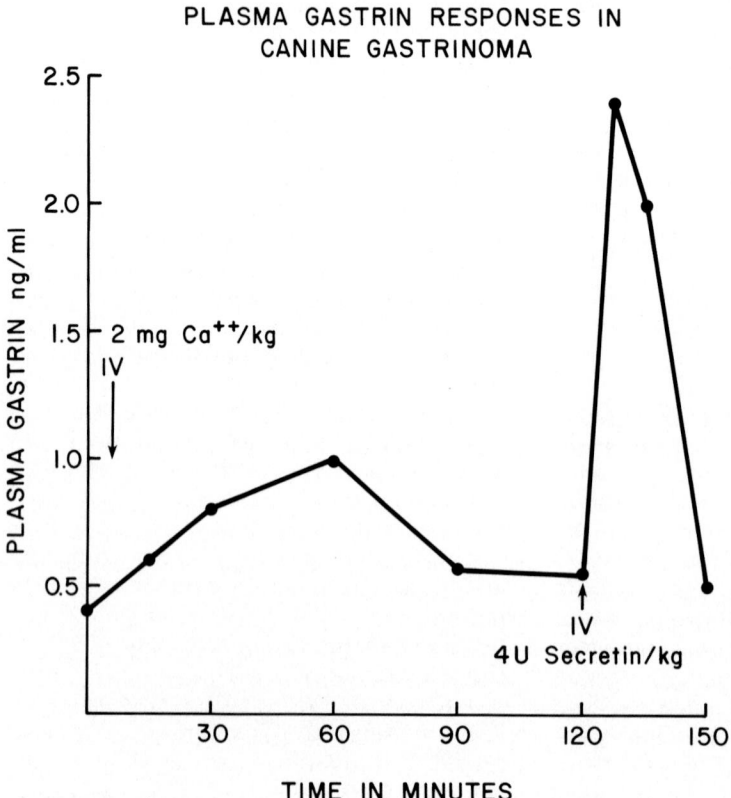

PLASMA GASTRIN RESPONSES IN CANINE GASTRINOMA

Figure 57–14. Plasma gastrin responses to administration of calcium and secretin in a dog with proven Zollinger-Ellison syndrome (From Straus, E., et al.: Gastroenterology 72:380, 1977. By permission.)

been poor, with the major clinical threat being the physiologic effects of the gastrin release rather than the biologic effects of the tumor. All but one dog had evidence of metastasis and all dogs eventually died from complications of the disease. With surgery in conjunction with the use of H₂-blockers and anticholinergic drugs, the prognosis should improve. Other endocrinopathies occur in conjunction with the Zollinger-Ellison syndrome in man and should be investigated in the dog. Straus (1977b) reports a gastrinoma also secreting ACTH in a dog showing simultaneous signs related to hyperadrenocorticism.

GASTRIC NEOPLASIA

The occurrence of benign and malignant gastric neoplasia in the dog and cat is low. Adenocarcinoma is the most common neoplasm reported in the canine stomach, accounting for one per cent of all malignant neoplasms and comprising from 42 to 72 per cent of all gastric malignancies (Patnaik et al., 1978). The incidence of gastric neoplasia in the cat is unknown, but it occurs far less frequently than that found in the dog. In reports of gastrointestinal neoplasms in the cat, the stomach was the least affected organ (Brody, 1966), with lymphosarcomas being the most frequent feline gastric neoplasia (Tyler, 1977).

The signs of gastric neoplasia, regardless of cell type, are usually the result of either altered motility of the gastric wall or gastric outflow blockage. The most common signs include persistent vomiting and weight loss.

BENIGN TUMORS

Benign Adenomatous Polyps. These polyps occur as pedunculated or polypoid nodules of mucosal proliferation that protrude above the gastric surface. Though there are a few reported cases of adenomatous polyps in the dog and cat (Murray et al., 1972; Hayden and Nielsen, 1973), the incidence of nonclinical polyps may actually be higher. Most occur as either single or multiple solitary nodules ranging from a few millimeters to centimeters in size; however, diffuse, multiple polyps invading the entire gastric mucosa have been reported (Happe et al., 1977; Conroy, 1969). Gastric adenomatous polyps are often incidental

findings during endoscopy or at necropsy. They generally cause no clinical signs unless they are diffuse or arise to occlude the pyloric antrum and gastric outflow (Fig. 57-9,G). The etiology is unknown but felt to occur secondary to chronic gastric mucosal damage. It is suggested that adenomatous polyps have a premalignant tendency, though this is not proven in the dog.

Leiomyomas. Leiomyomas are the second most common gastric tumor found in older dogs (average age 15 years) (Patnaik and Hurvitz, 1977). These tumors vary in size and arise from the muscle layers of the gastric wall. Most are found incidentally at necropsy, are distributed randomly, and involve different segments of the muscular layer. Ulceration is infrequent, and the tumor exerts its effect by mass involvement, altering either motility or pyloric outflow (Fig. 57-9,H).

MALIGNANT TUMORS

Adenocarcinoma is the most common malignant tumor in the stomach of the dog; however, it is exceedingly rare in the cat. The average age of dogs diagnosed with gastric adenocarcinoma is eight years (Lingman et al., 1971), with males more commonly affected than females. Grossly, these gastric tumors appear as raised plaques with a central ulcer, as polypoid lesions projecting into the lumen, or as a very firm, diffusely infiltrating mass invading the stomach wall. This latter type is often referred to as a scirrhous carcinoma or linitis plastica (leather bottle stomach) because of the rigid nondistensible consistency of the stomach wall (Pollock and Wagner, 1973). Most tumors have superficial mucosal ulcerations, and more than half originate in the pyloric antral area.

Patnaik and Hurvitz (1977) describe two main histologic types of adenocarcinoma, diffuse and intestinal, with several subtypes in each group. The most common and most malignant is the diffuse type, lacking a distinct glandular structure. In some unknown way, the neoplastic cells of this type stimulate mesenchymal elements and bring about a tremendous fibrous connective tissue component of the tumor (Lauren, 1965). The other histologic group, the intestinal type, has a glandular structure. This type often presents as a raised mass in the gastric wall. Regardless of the histologic type, metastasis is frequent, extending to regional lymph nodes, liver, lungs, and adrenals.

Primary sarcomas of the stomach occur most frequently as *lymphosarcomas* and are the most common gastric tumor in the stomach of the cat. The majority of the cats with these tumors are FeLV negative. The tumors occur either as raised masses or as a diffuse infiltration in the gastric wall, with various sized ulcers in the gastric mucosa. Other, less frequent malignant tumors of the stomach include *leiomyosarcomas* and *fibrosarcomas*. Rarely, metastatic tumors result from adenocarcinomas (of mammary glands, GI tract, liver, or pancreas), lymphosarcomas, or hemangiosarcomas.

Clinical Findings. The most consistent sign of gastric neoplasia is vomiting. The vomiting may vary in both the frequency and onset after eating, with the severity of signs often related to the amount of gastric wall involvement or pyloric outflow obstruction. With a complete pyloric obstruction the vomiting may become projectile. Hematemesis and melena occur, with mucosal ulceration and bleeding. Malignant gastric neoplasia often results in anorexia, chronic debilitation, and weight loss. The average duration of clinical signs for most dogs in one report ranges from two weeks to three months (Sautler and Hanlon, 1975).

Diagnosis. Gastric neoplasia should always be suspected in the older animal displaying chronic vomiting. Abdominal palpation is generally unrewarding, although occasionally a gastric mass may be palpated. Gastric pain is inconsistent unless rare perforation of the tumor has resulted in peritonitis. Anemia with melena is a frequent finding with chronic bleeding lesions. Ascites, jaundice, or respiratory distress may result from metastasis to other areas.

In addition to routine laboratory support, radiology should be the first step in the diagnosis of gastric neoplasia. Plain films are usually nondiagnostic but in extensive involvement may demonstrate a mass or thickened gastric wall. All require contrast studies to definitively demonstrate a gastric lesion (see Gastric Radiology). In many cases a double contrast study best outlines lesions of the gastric wall. Certain characteristic radiographic findings are suggestive of gastric neoplasia. These include thickening and rigidity to gastric wall as viewed on multiple radiographs, distortion of the gastric lumen and derangement of the rugal folds, filling defects, ulcers, and a marked delay in gastric emptying. Because gastric neoplasia often alters motility and pyloric emptying, fluoroscopy is beneficial in evaluating some lesions. Lesions invading the gastric wall without a mass effect may not be appreciated without fluoroscopy.

Endoscopy is used to confirm suspected gastric lesions observed with radiology. A skilled endoscopist can often appreciate lesions not demonstrated on gastric contrast studies (Laufer et al., 1971). Polyps, ulcerations, or raised masses protruding into the luminal surface are easily observed (Fig. 57–9,*I*). Gastric neoplasia without mass or mucosal involvement is more difficult to appreciate. The operator must be aware of areas that have lost distensibility or normal rugal fold patterns. Gastric adenocarcinomas of the linitis plastica type with predominately submucosal involvement are often missed on endoscopic examination. When lesions are observed, biopsy forceps or cytology brushes can be directed under endoscopic control for obtaining samples with good results.

Gastric lavage and cytology may retrieve diagnostic cells of gastric neoplasia; however, there have been no reported cases using this technique in the available veterinary literature.

Surgery offers the best diagnostic method for evaluating gastric neoplasia. The surgeon is able to palpate the stomach wall for inconsistencies, perform a gastrotomy and evaluate the mucosal surface and pyloric canal diameter, and obtain a full-thickness biopsy of the gastric wall. Surgery also allows evaluation of the regional lymph nodes, liver, and adjacent organs for evidence of metastasis.

Treatment. The current treatment of choice for most gastric neoplasia is surgical removal. Partial gastrectomy or segmental resection is usually indicated. Since the majority of the gastric neoplasms involve the pyloric antral area, resection of the pylorus may be required. In such cases, surgical anastomosis of the remaining stomach to the intestines (gastroduodenostomy or gastrojejunostomy) is required; this procedure is not without complications, however. Palliative surgery in malignant gastric neoplasia may justifiably increase survival times by several months (Douglas et al., 1970; McDonald, 1978). Chemotherapy is suggested for lymphosarcomas following surgical removal of single or multiple solitary masses and has resulted in a good response in some cases (MacEwen, 1980). Therapy for sarcomas is outlined in Chapter 30 and involves the use of vincristine, cyclophosphamide, and prednisone combinations. Those sarcomas in which there is diffuse infiltration of the gastric wall and which are not surgical candidates show a poor response to chemotherapy. Chemotherapy may also be used as an adjunct to surgical removal of other malignant gastric tumor types (Moertel, 1978).

The prognosis for malignant gastric neoplasia is generally poor, owing to the advanced nature of the disease at the time of diagnosis, surgical complications of gastric resection, and frequent metastasis.

ACUTE GASTRIC DILATATION-VOLVULUS

Overeating by immature animals, and occasionally adults, results in gastric distention. This gluttony is often relieved with vomiting. Of more serious consequence is the acute gastric dilatation of mature, large breed dogs, which results in a rotation of the stomach. Dilatation produces a torsion of the gastroesophageal junction. The greater curvature moves ventrally with gastric distention. With their deep chest conformation, an eventual laxity of the gastrohepatic ligament results. With this laxity the pylorus is freed to move dorsally, cranially, and to the left, resulting in a volvulus of the stomach.

Gastric dilatation-volvulus (GDV) is a serious, life-threatening syndrome. Gastric gas and fluid accumulate and cannot pass via the esophagus nor the duodenum. This distention of the stomach results in additional fluid generation and complicates fluid and electrolyte losses. If not promptly relieved, death may rapidly ensue.

Incidence. Large breed, deep chested dogs are most frequently affected with GDV. To date, 28 breeds have been reported (Todoroff, 1979). Among these breeds are dachshunds, Pekingese, and others not conforming to the generalization of a large breed, deep chested dog. Domestic cats have also been reported with GDV (Key, 1977). Other species with GDV are reviewed by Van Kruiningen (1974). Most dogs with GDV are mature, middle aged or older dogs

(Todoroff, 1979). Males predominate over females by 2:1 (Betts et al., 1974).

Etiology. Gastric dilatation precedes volvulus. In order for GDV to occur there must be a source of gas and an obstruction to the relief of this distention. Gastric distention with gas results in both postprandial and fasting stomachs. Aerophagia appears to be the source of gas (Caywood et al., 1977). In two studies, gastric gas analysis resulted in gas concentrations consistent with atmospheric air and an absence of significant concentrations of either hydrogen or methane (Van Kruiningen et al., 1974; Caywood et al., 1977). There were increased carbon dioxide concentrations in both studies, which likely resulted from a reaction of salivary bicarbonate and gastric hydrochloric acid.

Bacterial fermentation is not important in the formation of gas in the normal empty stomach. Only after feeding do bacterial numbers increase to 10^5 per gram of contents. The sources of these bacteria are the oral cavity and the diet. *Clostridium perfringens* has been found in the stomach of dead dogs and was thought to be a source of gas in GDV (Van Kruiningen, 1974). More recently it was reported there was no difference in clostridial incidence between the stomach of healthy dogs and dogs with GDV (Warner and Van Kruiningen, 1978). Due to the acuteness of GDV and the inconsistent ability to isolate gas forming bacteria, it is unlikely bacteria are responsible for the gas of GDV.

Endogenously produced carbon dioxide may result from the interaction of bicarbonate secretions and gastric hydrochloric acid. Salivary secretions have high levels of bicarbonate and may represent one source of this gas. With increases in the intragastric pressure, the pyloric region of the stomach undergoes abnormal excitation, resulting in antiperistaltic waves (Nogoaka, 1968). These antiperistaltic waves may regurgitate pancreatic bicarbonate secretions and provide an additional source for carbon dioxide production.

The role of the diet in GDV is unclear. Animals being fed free choice or selectively, meat or cereal, soybean containing or soybean-free, and small quantities or large quantities are seen with GDV (Cott et al., 1976). Attempts at reproducing GDV with dietary manipulation have been unsuccessful. If there is a relationship between diet and GDV, it is probably associated with anatomic changes and resultant development of laxity of the gastrohepatic ligament, allowing eventual rotation of the stomach.

Gastric retention may also be an etiologic factor in GDV. Pyloric dysfunction and delayed gastric emptying are reported in dogs with GDV (Funkquist and Garmer, 1967).

Pathophysiology. Following gaseous distention, the stomach is unable to relieve itself. This may be due to an abnormal gastroesophageal angulation interfering with belching or vomiting; compression of the duodenum by the dilated stomach, preventing passage of gas into the small bowel; or a disturbed extrinsic innervation of the stomach.

As the stomach dilates, the gastrosplenic ligament causes the spleen to move passively. Thus, any movement of the greater curvature also moves the spleen. Eventually the splenic vessels come to lie ventrally across the esophagus and become partially obstructed, leading to venous congestion and a secondary splenomegaly. Rotation of the spleen also is important in the development of an area of gastric necrosis (Baronofsky and Wangensteen, 1945). The site is seemingly always on the greater curvature of the fundus at a site where the vasa brevi anastomose with the left epigastric arteries. Torsion of the splenic pedicle may occur independently or in association with gastric volvulus.

Also, as the stomach dilates it exerts pressure upon the caudal vena cava (Wingfield et al., 1975b). The vessel is partially occluded, and blood is shunted via the ventral vertebral sinuses and azygos vein to the cranial vena cava. Rotation of the stomach actively occludes the portal vein, leading to venous congestion of abdominal splanchnic viscera. This occlusion promotes the onset of severe shock.

As intragastric pressures increase, the peristaltic activity decreases with the onset of ischemic hypoxia. Severe damage to the ganglion cells of Auerbach's plexus may result and contribute to the large, atonic stomach frequently noted at surgery. If the hypoxia is corrected within three and one half to four hours, the neurologic insult is reversible.

Arterial pressures to the stomach are maintained even with gastric dilatation, while venous drainage is compromised and intravascular venous stasis arises. Gastric

mucosal injury results and may lead to subepithelial hemorrhage and edema. Erosions and ulcers may arise in the gastric mucosa.

With continued gastric distention, the systemic arterial pressures fall while the caudal vena caval pressure rises. Blood becomes sequestered in organs draining to the caudal vena cava. With the sequestration, oxyhemoglobin desaturation results in blood collected from the caudal vena cava and right atrium (Merkely et al., 1976).

The decreased venous return to the right atrium results in a decreased cardiac output. Neurogenic stimulation of the splanchnic sympathetics by the distended stomach may also result in hypotension. The consequences of this hypotension and decreased circulating blood volume are manifest by a low velocity of flow. At low velocity, blood tends to increase in viscosity and the ability to perfuse tissues decreases (Matheson, 1969). This sludging also promotes disseminated intravascular coagulation in gastric volvulus (Lees et al., 1977).

Portal venous occlusion may initiate septic shock in dogs with GDV. When the portal vein is experimentally occluded, a high mortality is noted in the dog (Boyce, 1935; Johnstone, 1957). This mortality is caused by hypovolemia, a neurogenic enhancement of the shock state, or a failure of the capacity of the reticuloendothelial system to neutralize endotoxins. Gram-negative bacteria within the gut release their endotoxins with portal venous occlusion (Olkay et al., 1974). This endotoxin enters the circulatory system either via the peritoneal surface (Cyevas and Fine, 1972) or via the lymphatic channels (Gans, 1974; Olkay et al., 1974).

The encroachment of the dilated stomach on the thoracic space initially decreases tidal volume and increases respiratory rate in order to maintain minute volume. Lung compliance decreases with gastric dilatation (Bryne and Cahill, 1961) and may result in a compromised ventilation-perfusion ratio (Peters, 1968).

Clinical Findings. Young animals presented with gastric dilatation rarely have tympany upon percussion of the abdomen. The animal will often be lethargic and reluctant to move, and make a grunting sound with respiratory effort. Attempts to palpate the abdomen are met with abdominal splinting and increased respiratory grunting. In most instances the animal makes no effort to retch or vomit.

Dogs with acute gastric dilatation have

cranial abdominal distention with tympany. The abdomen is tensed with palpation. Increased respiratory efforts, hyperpnea, and open-mouthed panting are frequently seen. Observing the dog as it stands will generally show an asymmetry to the abdomen, when looking from dorsal to ventral, concentrated on the animal's right side.

Abdominal palpation may provide evidence of splenomegaly. The spleen may orient from cranial to caudal along the ventral midline of the abdomen.

Retching with an inability to vomit is an important clinical finding in GDV. The retching may become quite violent, with no productive vomitus. With increasing efforts to retch, the abdomen further distends with gas via aerophagia.

As gastric distention progresses, the clinical signs of shock are manifested. A weak femoral pulse, tachycardia, and prolonged capillary refill time of the mucous membranes are commonly noted. Increased venous pressures can be observed by lying the dog in a lateral recumbency and observing the saphenous vein. As the leg of normal animals is slowly raised, this vein will disappear as the leg reaches the level of the dog's right atrium; in dogs with GDV, the leg may be extended well above the right atrial level before it collapses.

Passage of an orogastric tube was once believed to be important in ruling out volvulus of the stomach. This technique is *not a diagnostic test* for GDV. Even though a gastric tube may be passed, this does *NOT* rule out volvulus.

With increasing time of gastric distention, the shock state of the animal progresses. Pathophysiologic changes proceed and may rapidly lead to death (Wingfield et al., 1976). Animals may be presented to the hospital unable to rise, in severe shock, and moribund.

Diagnosis. Definitive diagnosis of gastric volvulus is through abdominal radiography. Because enforced manipulation for positioning increases the stress and risk of the patient, radiography is performed *after* the initial shock therapy and gastric decompression. A lateral projection as well as dorsal recumbency is necessary for assessment of gastric positioning. Barium administration is occasionally used.

The radiographic course of events after successful gastric decompression shows great variation between cases. Sometimes the stomach returns to a normal position immediately or within hours. In other cases the stomach remains malpositioned for days or weeks without functional disturbance (Funkquist, 1979).

As the stomach dilates, the pylorus moves caudodorsally and the greater curvature lies along the ventral abdominal wall. Gradually the pylorus moves dorsally, cranially, and toward the left. The spleen follows the greater curvature toward the right side. A large gas and/or fluid filled stomach is generally seen. A soft-tissue density will often separate the fundus from the pylorus (Kneller, 1976).

Treatment. Gastric decompression is achieved most quickly by passing a stomach tube or by gastrocentesis (trocarization). A colt-sized, moderately stiff stomach tube can frequently be passed, and the gastric contents removed by lavage. In the event a stomach tube cannot be passed, the stomach may be trocarized with a 12- to 16-gauge needle to achieve decompression. Partial relief of gastric gas will often allow passage of the orogastric tube.

Gastrostomy may be employed as a decompressive procedure. Use of this technique at one institution reduced the mortality of GDV from 68 per cent (Pass and Johnston, 1973) to 33 per cent (Walshaw and Johnston, 1976). An assessment of tissue viability is possible with gastrostomy. A definitive surgical procedure is required to anatomically realign the stomach and spleen. The gastrostomy must be closed first.

Improved cardiovascular function results following gastric decompression. This is further enhanced with rapid volume replacement intravenously, with isotonic fluids. Surprisingly, clinical patients with GDV have not proved to be in the severe acidosis state of experimental dogs (Wingfield et al., 1982). At present, bicarbonate therapy is no longer condoned in routine treatment of GDV.

A transient hyperkalemia results from gastric decompression (Wingfield et al., 1975a). Of greater consequence is the total body hypokalemia that results. Intravenous replacement of potassium is found to decrease the incidence of postoperative cardiac dysrhythmias and patient muscle weakness.

It is important to gather baseline laboratory parameters prior to large volume fluid replacement. A simple packed cell volume (PCV) and total solids (TS) will provide information useful in assessing fluid replacement. A complete blood count (CBC) and blood glucose are useful in assessing the presence of septic shock. A leukopenia (3000/mm³), a significant left-shift, and hypoglycemia (<60 mg/dl) suggest septicemia.

Corticosteroids are routinely used in the management of shock (Rawlings et al., 1976). Their beneficial effects are attributed to competitive inhibition of endotoxin, stabilization of lysosomal membranes, improved cell metabolism, antagonism of vasoactive substances released in shock, and improved cardiac performance. Fluid therapy should *always* precede corticosteroid therapy.

Antibiotics of a broad-spectrum are useful in controlling bacterial numbers pre- and postoperatively. Currently, bactericidal drugs are favored for lessening the severity of endotoxemia.

Surgical Therapy. Surgical procedures in GDV involve the anatomic repositioning of the stomach and spleen, pyloric surgery to improve gastric emptying, and techniques to adhere the stomach to the abdominal wall in order to prevent recurrence of gastric volvulus.

Anatomic realignment includes the careful assessment of the stomach for areas of necrosis. With necrosis or questioned viability the affected area is excised. Thrombi within splenic vessels are occasionally noted. These thrombi prevent the spleen from returning to normal size and require splenectomy. It is important to note that splenectomy will *not* prevent recurrence of GDV (Wingfield et al., 1975c).

Pyloromyotomy or pyloroplasty is used to relieve gastric retention or gastric obstruction. This surgery will alter terminal antral contractions and disrupt antral retropulsion of solid particles.

Numerous operative techniques have been attempted to prevent recurrence of GDV. These include gastropexy (Wingfield and Hoffer, 1975), gastrocolopexy (Christie and Smith, 1976), "permanent" gastropexy (Betts et al., 1976), and tube gastrostomy (Parks and Greene, 1976). Currently the tube gastrostomy is favored. Tube gastrostomy provides an adhesion between the stomach and abdominal wall when the Foley catheter is removed after five to seven days. This tube is also useful for postoperative gastric decompression and in medicating the stomach. Use of a rib gastropexy shows promise as a prophylaxis in GDV without use of the Foley catheter (Fallah et al., 1982).

Complications. Postoperative complications are associated with shock, hypokalemia, cardiac dysrhythmias (Muir and Lipowitz, 1978), and gastrostomy complications. Fluid therapy and patient monitoring are important in the recognition and treatment of possible complications. Owing to the gastritis of GDV, nothing per os is offered for 24 to 48 hours. During this interval it is important to maintain electrolyte balance and fluid needs.

Supraventricular dysrhythmias include atrial premature contractions and atrial fibrillation. Ventricular premature contractions, paroxysmal ventricular tachycardia, ventricular tachycardia, and multifocal ventricular tachycardia are noted postoperatively. These dysrhythmias are often resistant to therapy with intravenous lidocaine or intravenous or oral procainamide hydrochloride in reestablishing sinus rhythm. With potassium replacement these dysrhythmias are less frequently encountered.

Gastrostomy complications result from premature removal of the Foley catheter or leakage. Peritonitis will result when the tube is in place for less than five days. This usually requires an immediate laparotomy and medical management of the peritonitis.

Occasionally, leakage occurs about the Foley catheter. This leakage may produce either a peritonitis or cellulitis with subcutaneous leakage. Most frequently, this complication has been experienced when the gastrostomy is placed too ventrally upon the abdominal wall. This tube should exit just ventral to the 13th rib in order to lessen tension upon the gastrostomy due to the deep abdomen of affected breeds.

Prevention. In that the cause of GDV is unknown, it is difficult to advocate preventive measures. As mentioned above, no specific foodstuff, homemade nor commercial, can prevent GDV.

Application of various principles of gastric emptying may be useful. It is important to feed frequent, small quantities to decrease gastric distention. Moistening dry foods and prohibiting postprandial exercise or excitement may help. Most large breed dogs are fed dry foodstuffs because they provide more calories on a weight to volume basis. Dry foodstuffs generally provide about 1500 kcal per pound, while semimoist and canned foods only yield about 500 kcal per pound. The presence of soybeans as a protein source does not result in a high incidence of GDV.

The presence of fat in the diet will generally delay emptying of the stomach. Alternatively, by increasing the fat content it is possible to decrease the volume of food to satisfy caloric demands of the dog.

Antifoaming antacids are not useful in GDV, since a frothy bloat does not exist in the dog.

REFERENCES

Aagaard, P., Fischerman, K., and Funding, J.: Augmented histamine test in dogs. Methods of aspiration technique. Scand. J. Gastroenterol. 7:279, 1972.

Ader, P.: Penetrating gastric ulceration in a dog. J.A.V.M.A. 175(7):710, 1979.

Ambinder, R. F., and Schuster, M. M.: Endorphins: new gut peptides with a familiar face. Gastroenterology 77:1132, 1979.

Archibald, R. M., and Milton, A. R.: Surgical relief of pyloric stenosis in the dog. Can. J. Comp. Med. 18:394, 1954.

Archibald, J. A., Cawley, A. J., and Reed, J. H.: Surgical technic for correcting pyloric stenosis. Mod. Vet. Pract. 41:28, 1960.

Atkins, C. E., and Johnson, R. K.: Clinical toxicities of cats. Vet. Clin. North Am. 5:623, 1975.

Aures, D., Hakanson, R., Owman, C., et al.: Cellular stores of histamine and monoamines in the dog stomach. Life Sci. 7:1147, 1968.

Baker, B. L.: Cell replacement in the stomach. Gastroenterology 46:202, 1964.

Banks, W. J.: Digestive System. Applied Veterinary Histology. Williams and Wilkins Co., Baltimore, 1981, p 373.

Baron, J. H.: Maximal stimuli. Clinical Tests of Gastric Secretion. Oxford University Press, New York, 1979, p 25.

Baronofsky, I., and Wangensteen, O. H.: Obstruction of splenic vein increases weight of the stomach and predisposes to erosion and ulcer. Proc. Soc. Exp. Biol. Med. 59:234, 1945.

Barsanti, J. A., Attleberger, M. N., and Henderson, R. A.: Phycomycosis in a dog. J.A.V.M.A. 167:293, 1975.

Batt, R. M.: Technique for single and multiple peroral jejunal biopsy in the dog. J. Small Anim. Pract. 20:259, 1979.

Belding, H. H., III, and Kernohan, J. W.: A morphologic study for the myenteric plexus and musculature of the pylorus with special reference to the changes in hypertrophic pyloric stenosis. Surg. Gynecol. Obstet. 97:322, 1953.

Betts, C. W., Wingfield, W. E., and Green, R. W.: A retrospective study of gastric dilatation-torsion in the dog. J. Small Anim. Pract. 15:727, 1974.

Betts, C. W., Wingfield, W. E., and Rosin, E.: "Permanent" gastropexy — as a prophylactic measure against gastric volvulus. J.A.A.H.A. 12:177, 1976.

Bilski, R., Kowalewski, K., and Secord, D. C.: The effect of L-amino acids given intravenously on gastric secretion stimulated by pentagastrin in dogs. Digestion 18:240, 1978.

Bishop, L., Sheffield, W. D., and Strandberg, J. D.: Eosinophilic gastritis in a dog associated with microfilaria. Manuscript in preparation, 1982.

Bohning, R. J., Jr., DeHoff, W. E., McElkinney, A., and

Hofstra, P. C.: Pharyngostomy for maintenance of the anorectic animal. J.A.V.M.A. 156:611, 1970.

Bolton, J. P., and Cohen, M. M.: The effect of prostaglandin E₂, 15-methyl prostaglandin E₂, and metiamide on established canine gastric mucosal barrier damage. Surgery 8:333, 1979.

Boyce, F. F., Lambert, R., and McFetridge, E. M.: Occlusion of the portal vein. J. Lab. Clin. Med. 20:935, 1935.

Brink, B. M., Schlegel, J. F., and Code, C. F.: The pressure profile of the gastroduodenal junctional zone in dogs. Gut 6:163, 1965.

Brody, R. S.: Alimentary tract neoplasms in the cat: a clinicopathologic survey of 46 cases. Am. J. Vet. Res. 27:74, 1966.

Butler, H. C.: Gastroduodenostomy in the dog. J.A.V.M.A. 155:1347, 1969.

Carrig, C. B., and Seawright, A. A.: Mastocytosis with gastrointestinal ulceration in a dog. Aust. Vet. J. 44:503, 1968.

Caywood, D. H., Teagne, D., Jackson, D. A., Levitt, M. D., and Bond, J. H., Jr.: Gastric gas analysis in the canine gastric dilatation-volvulus syndrome. J.A.A.H.A. 13:459, 1977.

Cheung, L. H., and Chang, N.: The role of gastric mucosal blood flow and H⁺ back-diffusion in the pathogenesis of acute gastric erosions. J. Surg. Res. 22:357, 1977.

Cheville, N. F.: Uremic gastropathy in the dog. Vet. Pathol. 16:292, 1979.

Christie, L. R., and Smith, C. W.: Gastrocolopexy for prevention of recurrent gastric volvulus. J.A.A.H.A. 12:173, 1976.

Code, C. F.: Reflections of histamine, gastric secretion, and the H₂ receptor. N. Engl. J. Med. 296(25):1459, 1975.

Conroy, J. D.: Multiple gastric adenomatous polyps in a dog. J. Comp. Pathol. 79:465, 1969.

Cooke, A. R.: Gastric damage by drugs and the role of the mucosal barrier. Aust. N. Z. J. Med. 6:26, 1976.

Cooke, A. R.: Control of gastric emptying and motility. Gastroenterology 68:804, 1975.

Cott, B., Shelton, M., and DeYoung, D. W.: Preliminary report on AGD/V questionaire. Pure-Bred Dogs Am Kennel Gazette April:76, 1976.

Cream, G. P., Hogg, D. F., and Rumsey, R. D. E.: Hyperplasia of the gastric mucosa produced by duodenal obstruction. Gastroenterology 56(2):193, 1969.

Curtis, P. J., Rayford, P. L., and Thompson, J. C.: Renal extraction of circulating secretin in dogs. Physiologist 18:181, 1975.

Cyevas, P., and Fine, J.: Route of absorption of endotoxin from the intestine in nonseptic shock. J. Reticuloendothel Soc. 11:535, 1972.

Damiano, S.: Chronic follicular hypertrophic gastritis in a dog. Acta. Med. Vet. *13*:363, 1967.

Davenport, H. W.: Prevention and suppression by Azathioprine of venom-induced protein-losing gastropathy in dogs. Proc. Natl. Acad. Sci. *73*:968, 1976.

Davenport, H. W., and Barr, L. L.: Failure of ischemia to break the dog's gastric mucosal barrier. Gastroenterology *65*:619, 1973.

Davis, L. E.: Clinical pharmacology of the gastrointestinal tract. *In* Anderson, N. V. (ed.): Veterinary Gastroenterology. Lea and Febiger, Philadelphia, 1980, p. 277.

Davis, R. A., and Brooks, F. P.: Experimental peptic ulcer associated with lesions on stimulation of the central nervous system. Surg. Gynecol. Obstet. *116*:307, 1963.

Debas, H. T., Konturek, S. J., Walsh, J. H., et al.: Proof of a pyloro-oxyntic reflex for stimulation of acid secretion. Gastroenterology *66*:526, 1974b.

Debas, H. T., Slaff, G. F., and Grossman, M. I.: Intestinal phase of gastric acid secretion: Augmentation of maximal response of Heidenhain pouch to gastrin and histamine. Gastroenterology *68*:691, 1975a.

Debas, H. T., Walsh, J. H., and Grossman, M. I.: Evidence for oxynto-pyloric reflex for release of antral gastrin. Gastroenterology *68*:687, 1975b.

Debas, H. T., Yamagishi, T., and Dryburgh, J. R.: Motilin enhances gastric emptying of liquids in dogs. Gastroenterology *73*:777, 1977.

Debra, H. T., Crendes, A., Walsh, J. H., et al.: Release of Antral Gastrin. *In* Chey, W. P., and Brooks, S. P., (ed.): Endocrinology of the Gut. Charles B. Slack, Inc., Thorofare, New Jersey, 1974a, p. 222.

Ditchfield, J., and Phillipson, M. H.: Achlorhydria in dogs, with report of a case complicated by avitaminosis C. Can. Vet. J. *1*:396, 1960.

Dockray, G. J.: Molecular evaluation of gut hormones: Application of comparative studies on the regulation of digestion. Gastroenterology *72*:344, 1977.

Dodge, J. A.: Production of duodenal ulcers and hypertrophic pyloric stenosis by administration of pentagastrin to pregnant and newborn dogs. Nature *225*:284, 1970.

Douglas, S. W., Hall, L. W., and Walker, R. G.: The surgical relief of gastric lesions in the dog: Report of seven cases. Vet. Rec. *86*:743, 1970.

Dumler, F.: Primary metabolic alkalosis. Am. Fam. Physician *23*:193, 1981.

Ellenberger, W., and Baum, H.: Handbuck der Vergleichender Anatonie der Haustiere. Springer-Verlag, Berlin, 1943.

Evans, H. E., and Christensen, G. C.: Anatomy of the Dog. W. B. Saunders Co., Philadelphia, 1979, p. 476.

Ewing, G. O.: Indomethacin — associated gastrointestinal hemorrhage in a dog. J.A.V.M.A. (6):1665, 1972.

Fallah, A., et al. Rib gastropexy in the treatment of gastric dilatation-volvulus. J. Vet. Surg. *11*(1): In Press, 1982.

Fenester, L. F.: The ulcerogenic potential of glucocorticoids and possible prophylactic measures. Med. Clin. North Am. *57*:1289, 1973.

Finco, D. R.: Fluid therapy for profuse vomiting. J.A.A.H.A. *8*:200, 1972.

Fung, W. P., Papadimitriou, J. M., and Matz, L. R.: Endoscopic, histological, and ultrastructural correlations in chronic gastritis. Am. J. Gastroenterol. *71*:269, 1979.

Funkquist, B.: Gastric torsion in the dog. I. Radiological picture during nonsurgical treatment related to the pathological anatomy and to the further clinical course. J. Small Anim. Pract. *20*:73, 1979.

Funkquist, B., and Garmer, L.: Pathogenetic and therapeutic aspects of torsion of the canine stomach. J. Small Anim. Pract. *8*:523, 1967.

Gans, H.: The escape of endotoxin from the intestine. Surg. Gynecol. Obstet. *139*:395, 1974.

Gardham, J. R. C.: Pyloric stenosis: An experimental study of alkalosis and the paradox of acid urine in dogs. Br. J. Surg. *56*:628, 1969 (Abst).

Gibbs, C., and Pearson, H.: The radiological diagnosis of gastrointestinal obstruction in the dog. J. Small Anim. Pract. *14*:61, 1973.

Gold, C. H., Morley, J. E., Viljoen, M., Tim, L. O., de Formseca, M., and Kalk, W. J.: Gastric acid secretion and serum gastrin levels in patients with chronic renal failure on regular hemodialysis. Nephron *25*:92, 1980.

Grossman, M. I.: The chemicals that activate the "On" switches of the oxyntic cell. Mayo Clin. Proc. *50*:515, 1975.

Grossman, M. I., and Konturek, S. J.: Inhibition of acid secretion in dog by metiamide, a histamine antagonist acting on H_2 receptors. Gastroenterology *66*:517, 1974.

Guilbert, J., Bounous, G., and Gurd, F. N.: Role of intestinal chyme in pathogenesis of gastric ulceration following experimental hemorrhagic shock. J. Trauma *9*:723, 1969.

Happe, R. P., Van Der Gaag, I., Lamers, C. R. H. W., Van Toorenburg, J., Rehfeld, J. F., and Larsson, L. I.: Zollinger-Ellison syndrome in three dogs. Vet. Pathol. *17*:177, 1980.

Happe, R. P., Van Der Gaag, I., Wolvekamp, W. T. H. C., and Van Toorenburg, J.: Multiple polyps of the gastric mucosa in two dogs. J. Small Anim. Pract. *18*:179, 1977.

Harris, W. F.: Clinical toxicities of dogs. Vet. Clin. North Am. *5*:605, 1975.

Hayden, D. W., and Fleischman, R. W.: Scirrhous eosinophilic gastritis in dogs with gastric arteritis. Vet. Pathol. *14*:441, 1977.

Hayden, D. W., and Van Kruiningen, H. I.: Experimentally induced canine toxocariasis: Laboratory examinations and pathologic changes, with emphasis on the gastrointestinal tract. Am. J. Vet. Res. *36*:1605, 1975.

Hayden, D. W., and Nielsen, S. W.: Canine alimentary neoplasia. Zentralbl. Veterinaermed. *20*:1, 1973.

Herrgesell, J. D.: Aspirin poisoning in the cat. J.A.V.M.A. *151*:452, 1967.

Hinder, R. A., and Bremmer, C. G.: Relative role of pyloroplasty size, truncal vagotomy, and milk meal volume in canine gastric emptying. Am. J. Dig. Dis. *23*:210, 1978.

Hirschowitz, B. I., and Gibson, R. G.: The effect of cimetidine on stimulated gastric secretion and serum gastrin in the dog. Am. J. Gastroenterol. *70*:437, 1978.

Hoerlein, B. F., and Spano, J. S.: Non-neurological complications following decompressive spinal cord surgery. Arch. Am. Coll. Vet. Surg. *IV*:11–16, 1975.

Howard, E. B.: Acute mycotic gastritis in a dog. VM SAC *61*:549, 1966.

Howard, E. B., and Kenyon, A. J.: Canine mastocytoma: Altered alpha-globulin distribution. Am. J. Vet. Res. 26:1132, 1965.

Howard, E. B., Sawa, T. R., Nielsen, S. W., and Kenyon, A. J.: Mastocytoma and gastroduodenal ulceration. Pathol. Vet. 6:146, 1969.

Hunt, J. N., and Stubbs, D. F.: The volume and energy content of meals as determinants of gastric emptying. J. Physiol. (London) 245:209, 1975.

Hurwitz, A., Robinson, R. G., Vats, T. S., Whittier, F., and Herrin, W. F.: Effects of antacids on gastric emptying. Gastroenterology 71:268, 1976.

Isenberg, J. I.: Gastric secretory testing. In Sleisenger, M. H., and Fordtran, J. S. (eds.), Gastrointestinal Disease. 2nd ed. W. B. Saunders Co., Philadelphia, 1978, p. 714.

Ivey, K. J.: Gastritis. Med. Clin. North Am. 58:1289, 1974.

Janick, J. S., Akbar, A. M., Burrington, J. D., and Burke, G.: The role of gastrin in congenital hypertrophic pyloric stenosis. J. Ped. Surg. 13:151, 1978.

Jeffries, G. H.: Gastritis. In Sleisenger, M. H., and Fordtran, J. S. (eds.): Gastrointestinal Disease. 2nd ed. W. B. Saunders Co., Philadelphia, 1978, p. 733.

Johnson, G. F.: Gastroscopy. In Anderson, N. V. (ed.): Veterinary Gastroenterology. Lea and Febiger, Philadelphia, 1979, p. 84.

Johnson, G. F., and Twedt, D. C.: Endoscopy and laparoscopy in the diagnosis and management of neoplasia in small animals. Vet. Clin. North Am. 7:77, 1977.

Johnson, G. F., Jones, B., and Twedt, D. C.: Esophagogastric endoscopy in small animal medicine. Gastrointes. Endosc. 22:226, 1976. (Abst.)

Johnstone, F. R. C.: Acute ligation of the portal vein. Surgery 41:958, 1957.

Jones, B. R., Nicholls, M. R., and Badman, R.: Peptic ulceration in a dog associated with an islet cell carcinoma of the pancreas and an elevated plasma gastrin level. J. Small Anim. Pract. 17:593, 1976.

Kaye, M. D.: The effect of partial pyloric obstruction on gastric secretion and stomach size in the rat. Dig. Dis. Sci. 16(3):217, 1971.

Key, D. M.: Dilatation and torsion of the stomach in a cat. Feline Pract. 7(1):38, 1977.

Kipnis, R. M.: Focal cystic hypertrophic gastropathy in a dog. J.A.V.M.A. 173:182, 1978.

Kivilakso, E., and Silen, W.: Pathogenesis of experimental gastric-mucosal injury. N. Engl. J. Med. 301:364, 1979.

Kneller, S. K.: Radiographic interpretation of the gastric dilatation-volvulus complex in the dog. J.A.A.H.A. 12:154, 1976.

Krohn, K. J. E., and Finlayson, D. C.: Interrelations of humoral and cellular immune responses in experimental canine gastritis. Clin. Exp. Immunol. 14:237, 1973.

Kuo, Y. J., and Shanbour, L. L.: Mechanism of action of aspirin on canine gastric mucosa. Am. J. Physiol. 230:762, 1976.

Lanza, F. A., Royer, G. L., and Nelson, R. S.: Endoscopic evaluation of the effects of aspirin, buffered aspirin, and enteric-coated aspirin on gastric and duodenal mucosa. N. Engl. J. Med. 303:136, 1980.

Larsen, E. J.: Toxicity of low doses of aspirin in the cat. J.A.V.M.A. 143:837, 1963.

Laufer, M. D., Mullers, J. E., and Hamilton, J.: The diagnostic accuracy of barium studies of the stomach and duodenum-correlation with endoscopy. Radiology 115:569, 1972.

Laurin, P.: The two histologic main types of gastric carcinoma: diffuse and so-called intestinal type carcinoma. An attempt at histo-clinical classification. Acta Pathol. Microbiol. Scand. 64:31, 1965.

Lawther, W. A.: Pyloric stenosis in a puppy. Aust. Vet. J. 37:317, 1961.

Lee, K. Y., Tai, H. H., and Chey, W. Y.: Plasma secretion and gastrin responses to a meat-meal and duodenal acidification in dogs. Am. J. Physiol. 230:784, 1976.

Lees, G. E., Leighton, R. L., and Hart, R.: Management of gastric dilatation-volvulus and disseminated intravascular coagulation in a dog: A case report. J.A.A.H.A. 13:463, 1977.

Lev, R., Siegel, H. I., and Glass, G. B.: Effects of salicylates on the canine stomach: a morphological and histochemical study. Gastroenterology 62:970, 1972.

Lingeman, C. H., Garner, F. M., and Taylor, D. O. N.: Spontaneous gastric adenocarcinomas of dogs: a review. J. Natl. Cancer Inst. 47:137, 1977.

MacEwen, E. G.: Canine Lymphosarcoma. In Kirk, R. W. (ed.): Current Veterinary Therapy VII. W. B. Saunders Co., Philadelphia, 1980, p. 419.

Malagelada, J. R.: Physiologic basis and clinical significance of gastric emptying disorders. Dig. Dis. Sci. 24(9):657, 1979.

Malagelada, J. R., and Cortot, A.: H_2-receptor antagonist in perspective. Mayo Clin. Proc. 53:184, 1978.

Marks, I. N., Kemarov, S. A., and Shay, H.: Maximal secretory response to histamine and its relation to parietal cell mass in the dog. Am. J. Physiol. 199:579, 1960.

Matheson, N. A.: Factors in tissue perfusion. The microcirculation in shock. Postgrad. Med. 45:530, 1969.

McCarthy, D. M.: The place of surgery in the Zollinger-Ellison syndrome. N. Engl. J. Med. 302:1344, 1980.

McDonald, A. E.: Primary gastric carcinoma of the dog: Review and case report. Vet. Surg. 7:70, 1978.

McGuigan, J. E.: The Zollinger-Ellison syndrome. In Sleisenger, M. H., and Fordtran, J. S. (eds.): Gastrointestinal Disease. 2nd ed. W. B. Saunders Co., Philadelphia, 1978, p. 860.

McGuigan, J. E., and Wolfe, M. W.: Secretin injection test in the diagnosis of gastrinoma. Gastroenterology 79:1324, 1980.

Menguy, R., and Masters, Y. F.: Gastric mucosal energy metabolism and "stress" ulceration. Am. Surg. 180:538, 1974.

Merkely, D. F., Howard, D. R., Eyster, G. E., Krahwinkel, D. J., Sawyer, D. C., and Krehbiel, J. D.: Experimentally induced acute gastric dilatation in the dog: Cardiopulmonary effects. J.A.A.H.A. 12:143, 1976.

Meyer, J. H., Way, L. W., and Grossman, M. I.: Pancreatic bicarbonate response to various acids in the duodenum of the dog. Am. J. Physiol. 219:964, 1970.

Moertel, C. G.: Current concepts in cancer: Chemotherapy of gastrointestinal cancer. N. Engl. J. Med. 299:1049, 1978.

Moody, F. G., and Cheung, L. Y.: Stress ulcers: Their pathogenesis, diagnosis, and treatment. Surg. Clin. North Am. 56:1469, 1976.

Moody, F. G., Cheung, L. Y., Simons, M. A., and Zalewsky, C.: Stress and the acute gastric mucosal lesion. Dig. Dis. Sci. 21(2):148, 1976.

Morrissey, J. F., and Barreras, R. F.: Antacid therapy. N. Engl. J. Med. 290(10):550, 1974.

Muir, W. W., and Lipowitz, A. J.: Cardiac dysrhythmias associated with gastric dilatation-volvulus in the dog. J.A.V.M.A. 172:683, 1978.

Murray, M., McKeating, F. J., Baker, G. J., and Lauder, I. M.: Primary gastric neoplasia in the dog: a clinico-pathological study. Vet. Rec. 91:474, 1972.

Murray, M., Robinson, P. B., McKeating, F. J., and Sauder, I. M.: Peptic ulceration in the dog: A clinico-pathological study. Vet. Rec. 91(19):441, 1972.

Nogoaka, K.: Electromyography study on the mechanism of delayed gastric emptying after vagotomy in dogs. Tokaku J. Exp. Med 95:1, 1968.

O'Brien, T. R.: Stomach. In O'Brien, T. R. (ed.): Radiographic Diagnosis of Abdominal Disorders in the Dog and Cat. W. B. Saunders Co., Philadelphia, 1978, p. 204.

Okabe, S., Takeuchi, K., Murata, T., and Urushidni, T.: Effects of cimetidine on healing of chronic gastric and duodenal ulcers in dogs. Dig. Dis. Sci. 23(2):166, 1978.

Okamoto, E., Iwasaki, T., Kakutani, T., and Uera, T.: Selective destruction of the myenteric plexus: Its relation to Hirschsprung's disease, achalasia of the esophagus and hypertrophic pyloric stenosis. J. Ped. Surg. 2(5):444, 1967.

Olkay, I., Kitaham, A., Miller, R. H., Drapanas, T., Trejo, R. A., and Diluzio, N. R.: Reticuloendothelial dysfunction and endotoxemia following portal vein occlusion. Surgery 75:64, 1974.

Osborne, A. D., and Wilson, M. R.: Mycotic gastritis in a dog. Vet. Rec. 85:487, 1969.

Palmer, E. D.: Upper gastrointestinal hemorrhage. J.A.M.A. 231:605, 1975.

Parks, J. L., and Greene, R. W.: Tube gastrostomy for the treatment of gastric volvulus. J.A.A.H.A. 12:168, 1976.

Pass, M. A., and Johnston, D. E.: Treatment of gastric dilation and torsion in the dog. Gastric decompression by gastrostomy under local analgesia. J. Small Anim. Pract. 14:131, 1973.

Patnalk, A. K., and Hurvitz, A. I.: Neoplasms of the Digestive Tract in the Dog. In Kirk, R. W. (ed.): Current Veterinary Therapy VI. W. B. Saunders Co., Philadelphia, 1977, p. 938.

Patnalk, A. K., Hurvitz, A. I., and Johnson, G. E.: Canine gastric adenocarcinoma. Vet. Pathol. 15:600, 1978.

Payne, J. G., and Bowen, J. C.: Hypoxia of canine gastric mucosa caused by Escherichia coli sepsis and prevented by methyl prednisolone therapy. Gastroenterology 80:84, 1981.

Pearson, H., Gaskell, C. I., Gibbs, C., and Waterman, A.: Pyloric and esophageal dysfunction in the cat. J. Small Anim. Pract. 15:487, 1974.

Peters, R. M.: Physiologic review — coordination of ventilation and perfusion. Ann. Thorac. Surg. 6:570, 1968.

Politzer, J. P., Devroede, G., Vasseur, C., Gerard, J., and Thibault, R.: The genesis of bowel sounds. Influence of viscus and gastrointestinal content. Gastroenterology 71:282, 1976.

Pollock, S., and Wagner, B. M.: Gastric adenocarcinoma or linitis plastica in a dog. VM/SAC 68:139, 1973.

Polyak, R. I., Gresew, V. V., and Fisher, A. A.: Parasympathetic innervation of the stomach. Bull. Exp. Biol. Med. 71(4):373, 1971.

Priebe, H. J., Skillman, J. J., Bushnell, L. S., Long, P.

C., and Silen, W.: Antacid versus cimetidine in preventing acute gastrointestinal bleeding. N. Engl. J. Med. 302:426, 1980.

Quigley, J. P., Bauor, H. J., Read, M. R., and Brofman, B. L.: Evidence that body irritations or emotions retard gastric evacuation, not by producing pylorospasm but by depressing gastric motility. J. Clin. Invest. 22:839, 1943.

Rawlings, C. A., Wingfield, W. E., and Betts, C. W.: Shock therapy and anesthetic management of gastric dilatation-volvulus. J.A.A.H.A. 12:158, 1976.

Rayford, P. L., Miller, T. A., and Thompson, J. C.: Secretin, cholecystokinin and newer gastrointestinal hormones. N. Engl. J. Med. 294:1093, 1976.

Reed, J. D., Sanders, D. J., and Thorpe, V.: New stimulation on gastric acid secretion and mucosal blood flow in the anesthetized cat. J. Physiol. 214:1, 1971.

Regan, P. T., and Malagelada, J. R.: A reappraisal of clinical, roentgenographic and endoscopic features of the Zollinger-Ellison syndrome. Mayo Clin. Proc. 53:19, 1978.

Richardson, C. T., and Walsh, J. H.: The value of histamine H_2-receptor antagonist in the management of patients with the Zollinger-Ellison syndrome. N. Engl. J. Med. 294:133, 1976.

Root, C. R., and Morgan, J. P.: Contrast radiography of the upper gastrointestinal tract in the dog. J. Small Anim. Pract. 10:279, 1969.

Sakamoto, H.: A pharmacological study on the autonomic innervation of cardia, corpus and pylorus in the dog stomach. Fukuoka Acto. Med. 60(7):561, 1969.

Sass, B.: Perforating gastric ulcer associated with lead poisoning in a dog. J.A.V.M.A. 157:76, 1970.

Sautler, J. H., and Hanlon, G. F.: Gastric neoplasms in the dog: A report of 20 cases. J.A.V.M.A. 166:691, 1975.

Schulman, J.: Control of gastric ulcers in a dog using cimetidine. Canine Pract. 6(6):42, 1979.

Seawright, A. A., and Grono, L. R.: Malignant mast cell tumor in a cat with perforating duodenal ulcer. J. Pathol. Bact. 87:107, 1964.

Skillman, J. J., and Slen, W.: Gastric mucosal barrier. Surg. Annu. 4:213, 1972.

Smale, B. F., Mullen, J. L., and Rosato, E. F.: Experimental gastric mucosal injury. N. Engl. J. Med. 302:61, 1980.

Sorour, V. E.: The relationship between atrophic gastritis and gastric ulcer. Suid-Afrikaanse Tydskrif vir Chirurgie 14:47, 1976.

Stemper, T. J., and Cooke, A. R.: Effect of a fixed pyloric opening on gastric emptying in the cat and dog. Am. J. Physiol. 230:813, 1976.

Stemper, T. J., and Cooke, A. R.: Gastric emptying and its relationship to antral contractile activity. Gastroenterology 69:649, 1975.

Straus, E.: The explosion of gastrointestinal hormones. Med. Clin. North Am. 62:21, 1978.

Straus, E., Johnson, G. F., and Yalow, R. S.: Canine Zollinger-Ellison syndrome. Gastroenterology 72:380, 1977a.

Straus, E., and Yalow, R. S.: Hypersecretinemia associated with marked basal hyperchlorhydria in man and dog. Gastroenterology 72:992, 1977b.

Strombeck, D. R.: Chronic Gastritis, Gastric Retention and Gastric Neoplasms. In Small Animal Gastroenterology. Stonegate Publishing. Davis, CA, 1979, p. 110.

Sum, P. T., Schippier, H. L., and Preshaw, R. M.:

Canine gastric and pancreatic secretion during intestinal distention and intestinal perfusion with choline derivatives. Can. J. Physiol. Pharmacol. *47*:115, 1969.

Thomas, P. A., Kelly, K. A., and Go, V. L. W.: Does motilin regulate canine interdigestive gastric motility? Dig. Dis. Sci. *24*(8):577, 1979.

Thrall, D. E., Bovee, K. C., and Biery, D. N.: Demonstration of a position of relief in dogs with lesions of the stomach or small bowel. J.A.A.H.A. M*14*:343, 1978.

Tobe, T., Chen, S. T., Henmi, K., and Fukuchi, K.: Distribution of gastrin in canine, cat, and human digestive organs. Am. J. Surg. *132*:581, 1976.

Todorff, R. J.: Gastric dilatation-volvulus. Compend. Cont. Ed. *1*:142, 1979.

Toombs, J. P., Caywood, D. D., Lipowitz, A. J., and Stevens, J.B.: Colonic perforation following neurosurgical procedures and corticosteroid therapy in four dogs. J.A.V.M.A. *177*(1):68, 1980.

Trautwein, G., and Stöber, M.: Leukämische Mastzellenreticulose beim Rind. Ein Beitrag zum klinischen und histopathologischen Bild der nichtlymphatischen Leukose des Rindes. Zbl. Veterinaermed. *12*:211, 1965.

Twaddle, A. A.: Congenital pyloric stenosis in two kittens corrected by pyloroplasty. N. Z. Vet. J. *19*:26, 1971.

Twaddle, A. A.: Pyloric stenosis in three cats and its correction by pyloroplasty. N. Z. Vet. J. *18*:15, 1970.

Twedt, D. C.: Jaundice, hepatic trauma, and hepatic encephalopathy. Vet. Clin. North Am. *11*:121, 1981.

Tyler, D. E.: Gastric neoplasia in the dog and cat. Arch. Am. Coll. Vet. Surg. *6*:47, 1977. (Abst.).

Vagne, M., and Fargier, M. C.: Effect of pentagastrin and secretin on gastric mucus secretion in conscious cats. Gastroenterology *65*:757, 1973.

Van Der Gaag, I., Happe, R. P., and Wolvekamp, W. Th. C.: A boxer dog with chronic hypertrophic gastritis resembling Menetrier's disease in man. Vet. Pathol. *13*:172, 1976.

Van Der Gaag, I., Happe, R. P., and Wolvekamp, W. Th. C.: Investigation of the dog stomach. Netherlands Small Anim. Vet. Assoc. Proc. *5*:60, 1974.

Van Kruiningen, H. J.: Giant hypertrophic gastritis of basenji dogs. Vet. Pathol. *14*:19, 1977.

Van Kruiningen, H. J., Gregoire, K., and Meuten, D. J.: Acute gastric dilatation: A review of comparative aspects, by species, and a study in dogs and monkeys. J.A.A.H.A. *10*(3):294, 1974.

Walsh, J. H., and Grossman, M. I.: Gastrin. N. Engl. J. Med. *292*:1324–1377, 1975.

Walsh, J. H., Tompkins, R. K., Taylor, I. L., Lechago, J., and Hansky, I.: Gastrointestinal hormones in clinical disease: Recent developments. Ann. Intern. Med. *90*:817, 1979.

Walshaw, R., and Johnston, D. E.: Treatment of gastric dilatation-volvulus by gastric decompression and patient stabilization before major surgery. J.A.A.H.A. *12*:162, 1976.

Warner, N. S., and Van Kruiningen, H. J.: The incidence of clostridia in the canine stomach and their relationship to acute gastric dilatation. J.A.A.H.A. *14*:618, 1978.

Watt, J., Eagleton, G. B., and Marcus, R.: The effect of heparin on gastric secretion stimulated by histamine or ametrazole hydrochloride. J. Pharm. Pharmacol. *18*:615, 1966.

Weber, A. F., Osman, H., and Sautter, J. H.: Some observations concerning the presence of spirilla in the fundic glands of dogs and cats. Am. J. Vet. Res. *19*:677, 1958.

Wingfield, W. E., and Hoffer, R. E.: Gastric Dilatation-Torsion Complex in the Dog. *In* Bojrab, M. J. (ed.): Current Techniques in Small Animal Surgery. Lea and Febiger, Philadelphia, 1975, p. 112.

Wingfield, W. E., Cornelius, L. M., and DeYoung, D. W.: Experimental acute gastric dilation and torsion in the dog. I. Changes in biochemical and acid-base parameter. J. Small Anim. Pract. *16*:41, 1975a.

Wingfield, W. E., Cornelius, L. M., Ackerman, N., and DeYoung, D. W.: Experimental acute gastric dilation and torsion in the dog. 2. Venous angiographic alterations seen in gastric dilation. J. Small Anim. Pract. *16*:55, 1975b.

Wingfield, W. E., Betts, C. W., and Greene, R. W.: Operative techniques and recurrence rates associated with gastric volvulus in the dog. J. Small Anim. Pract. *16*:427, 1975c.

Wingfield, W. E., Betts, C. W., and Rawlings, C. A.: Pathophysiology associated with gastric dilatation-volvulus in the dog. J.A.A.H.A. *12*:136, 1976.

Wingfield, W. E., Twedt, D. C., Moore, R. W., et al.: Acid-base and electrolyte values in dogs with acute gastric dilatation-volvulus. J.A.V.M.A. *180*(9): In press, 1982.

Wood, I. J., Doig, R. K., Motteram, R., and Hughes, A.: Gastric biopsy: report on fifty-five biopsies using a new flexible gastric biopsy instrument. Lancet *1*:18, 1949.

Zimmer, J. F.: Gastrointestinal fiberoptic endoscopy. *In* Kirk, R. W. (ed.): Current Veterinary Therapy VI. W.B. Saunders Co., Philadelphia, 1977, p. 987.

Zollinger, R. M.: Islet cell tumors of the pancreas and alimentary tract. Am. J. Surg. *129*:102, 1975.

Zontine, W. J., Meierhenry, E. F., and Hicks, R. F.: Perforated duodenal ulcer associated with mastocytoma in dog: A case report. J. Am. Vet. Rad. Soc. *18*:162, 1977.

CHAPTER 58

Diseases of the Small Bowel

ROBERT G. SHERDING

STRUCTURE AND FUNCTION OF THE SMALL INTESTINE

ANATOMY

The structure of the small intestine provides maximal surface area for optimal performance of the intestinal functions of digestion, absorption, and secretion. The interface between mucosal surface and luminal content, where these functions take place, is increased by (1) the looped and folded, hollow tubular structure of the small bowel; (2) a mucosal lining that is folded and has fingerlike mucosal projections called villi; and (3) the covering of the mucosal surface of the villi, with a single layer of specialized epithelial cells that possess microvilli on their luminal membrane (brush border).

The small intestine of the dog and cat consists of three parts: the duodenum, the shortest and most proximal portion, which receives the openings of the stomach, common bile duct, and pancreatic ducts and lies largely to the right of midline; the jejunum, the longest portion, which consists of up to eight loops of gut that occupy most of the mid-abdomen and are covered by the omentum; and the ileum, the terminal portion, which opens into the ascending colon at the ileum osteum.

The arterial supply of the small bowel is provided largely via the cranial mesenteric artery, although the duodenum also receives arterial supply via the gastroduodenal artery, which originates from the common hepatic branch of the celiac artery. Venous drainage is into the portal vein via the cranial and caudal mesenteric veins and, for a portion of the duodenum, via the gastroduodenal vein. Intestinal lymphatics generally parallel the intestinal arteries and veins. Intestinal lymph drains via intestinal lymphatics into mesenteric lymph nodes, then into large intestinal lymphatic trunks that converge to become the cisterna chyli (the dilated caudal portion of the thoracic duct); finally it is transported by the thoracic duct into the venous circulation (Anderson and Anderson, 1980).

The small intestine is innervated by the autonomic nervous system. Extrinsic parasympathetic and sympathetic supply are via the vagus and splanchnic nerves, respectively. Intrinsic neural control of intestinal function is largely through an intramural network of neurons and nerve fibers called the myenteric and submucosal plexuses.

The layers of the intestinal wall, listed from inside (lumen) to outside (serosa), are the columnar epithelium of the mucosal surface, the basement membrane, the lamina propria, the muscularis mucosae, the submucosa, circular and longitudinal muscle layers, and the serosa. The luminal surface or microvillous border of the epithelium is coated with a glycoprotein substance called the glycocalyx. A one-cell thick layer of epithelium covers the intestinal villi and lines the "valleys" or crypts between the villi. There are four basic types of intestinal epithelial cells: (1) the columnar cell or enterocyte, which is the most populous cell and is specialized for digestion and absorption; (2) the goblet cell, which secretes mucus; (3) the Paneth cell, whose function is unclear but is probably secretory in nature; and (4) the enteroendocrine cell, which secretes hormones in response to chemical stimuli (Eastwood, 1977).

Constant turnover of intestinal epithelium is characterized by a balance between cell production in the crypts and cell loss at the villous tips. Only the undifferentiated crypt cells can replicate. Thus, the immature epithelial cells within the crypts proliferate continuously to supply new epithelial cells, which migrate out onto the villi, to be eventually extruded into the gut lumen from the villous tip (Fig. 58–1). As the villous epithelial cells migrate, they mature and differentiate, becoming specialized for digestion and absorption. This process of replication, migration, and differentiation of intestinal epithelium is sometimes called epithelial renewal and under normal conditions spans from two to six days. Epithelial renewal time varies with the villous length in different segments of the bowel and varies between species. Epithelial renewal is accelerated by intestinal disease or surgical resection of a portion of the bowel, and is prolonged by factors such as food withdrawal, uremia, radiation, and chemotherapeutic agents that inhibit DNA synthesis (Eastwood, 1977; Williamson and Chir, 1978). In addition, cell renewal is faster in conventionally-reared animals that have a normal microflora than in germ-free animals (Eastwood, 1977; Hirsh, 1980).

Although the crypt-villus model is somewhat of an oversimplification, it is useful in understanding the morphogenesis of lesions and functional changes in certain diarrheal diseases, especially infections caused by the epitheliotropic viruses that have a predilection for different parts of the crypt-villus epithelium (Moon, 1978) (Fig. 58–2). Normally, absorption by the differentiated digestive-absorptive cells of the intestinal villi exceeds secretion by the immature proliferative-secretory cells of the intestinal crypts, resulting in net absorption by the crypt-villus unit. Enteroviruses that selectively destroy villous epithelium (coronaviruses and rotaviruses) will cause villous atrophy, malabsorption, and crypt hyperplasia, resulting in net secretion by the crypt-villus unit and diarrhea. In general,

the severity of the diarrhea will parallel the extent of villous destruction. This contrasts with viruses that selectively destroy crypt epithelium, such as parvoviruses. These virus infections initially destroy the crypts while leaving intact villi; however, without crypt cells to proliferate and replace villous cells as they are lost by normal turnover, complete mucosal collapse or denuding eventually occurs. Because of the extensive loss of epithelium, diarrhea is severe and mucosal regeneration is slow.

Another component of the small intestinal microanatomy that deserves special mention is the lymphoid tissue associated with the gut. Immunocompetent cells (lymphocytes and plasma cells) are widely distributed throughout the length of the small bowel. They are located in between mucosal epithelial cells, scattered diffusely throughout the lamina propria beneath the epithelium, located at various sites along the GI tract as structured collections of cells called lymphoid nodules and as unique aggregates of lymphoid nodules called Peyer's patches (Hirsh, 1980). These immunocytes participate in the local immune response to antigens that contact the animal via the gastrointestinal mucosal surface largely through the production of immunoglobulin A (IgA), the major Ig in intestinal secretions (Walker and Isselbacher, 1977), but also through the production of other Ig types and through cell-mediated immunity. It is of interest to note that animals reared in a germ-free environment, thereby lacking bacterial colonization of their mucosa, have many fewer lymphocytes and plasma cells in their lamina propria than do conventional animals. Thus, the constant contact of the normal microflora (and their antigens) with the mu-

Figure 58–1. The crypt-villus unit of the intestinal mucosa consists of immature proliferative-secretory cells, which line the crypts, and mature digestive-absorptive cells, which populate the villi. The crypt cells proliferate to continuously supply new cells that migrate out onto the villi, where they differentiate into cells specialized for digestion and absorption as they migrate and are finally extruded into the gut lumen from the villous tip. Villous absorption exceeds crypt secretion, resulting in net absorption by the crypt-villus unit.

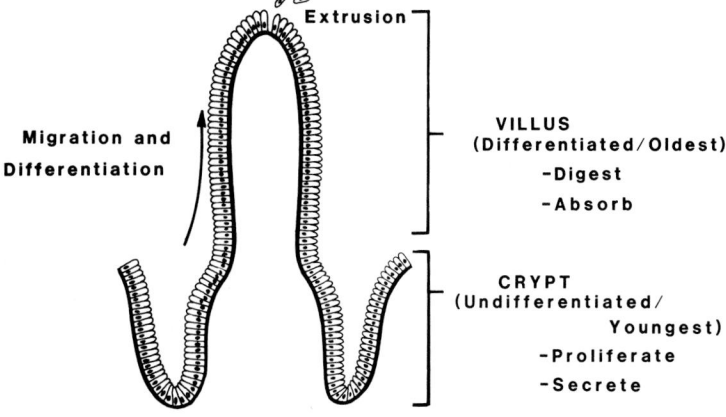

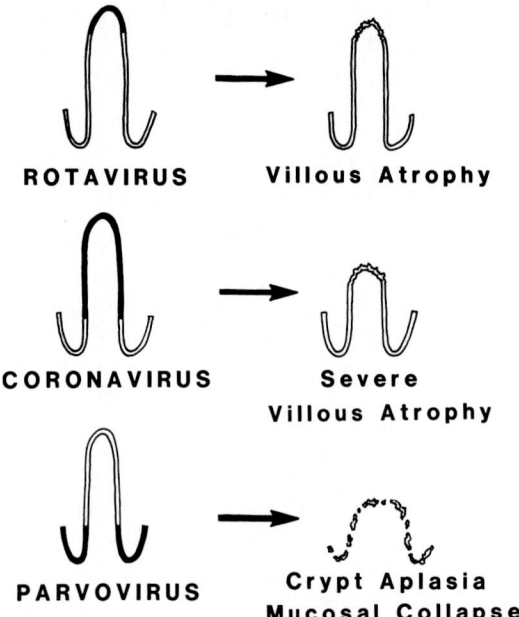

Figure 58–2. Enteric viruses have predilections for different parts of the crypt-villus epithelium. Villus-selective viruses (rotavirus, coronavirus) cause villous atrophy, leading to malabsorption and crypt hyperplasia; crypt-selective viruses (parvovirus) cause crypt aplasia, leading to mucosal collapse.

cosa of the normal animal apparently stimulates a physiologic inflammation (Eastwood, 1977). In addition to lymphoid cells, other cells that participate in immune responses are scattered throughout the small intestine, including macrophages, eosinophils, neutrophils, and mast cells.

ASSIMILATION

The primary function of the small intestine is to assimilate nutrients by the processes of digestion and absorption. Enzymes that are secreted into the gut lumen and associated with the mucosal brush border break down ingested material, and the products of digestion are then transferred from the gut lumen into the blood, where they become available for systemic use as metabolic substances. For the purpose of this discussion, the three major classes of nutrient — fat, carbohydrate, and protein — will each be discussed in terms of three sequential phases of digestion and absorption, the luminal phase, the mucosal phase, and the delivery phase (Fig. 58–3).

Fat

The assimilation of fat is extremely efficient. Under most circumstances, over 95

per cent of ingested fat is assimilated, and fecal fat excretion in the dog remains relatively constant over a wide dietary intake range. A large portion of the fat that is normally found in feces comes from desquamated colonic cells, colonic secretions, and bacterial synthesis, rather than from dietary fat. Long-chain triglycerides made up of three long-chain fatty acids (16 to 18 carbons) on a glycerol backbone are the primary component of dietary fat, although a smaller portion of dietary fat consists of medium-chain triglycerides (fatty acids of 6 to 12 carbons).

The luminal phase of fat digestion includes emulsification, hydrolysis, and micellarization, with participation by pancreatic lipase and biliary secretions (Gray, 1978; Riley and Glickman, 1979). The stomach does not contribute to the breakdown of fat, but it does perform a reservoir function insofar as gastric emptying, under neuro-hormonal influence, regulates the rate of fat entry into the duodenum. The first step of intraluminal fat digestion is the release of the hormone cholecystokinin (CCK) from the duodenum. This hormone stimulates enzyme-rich pancreatic secretion, which includes pancreatic lipase. Simultaneously, CCK causes contraction of the gallbladder and relaxation of the sphincter of Oddi, releasing bile into the duodenum. Hence, in a well-orchestrated chain of events, the duodenum is the recipient of fat (ingesta), lipase, and bile salts.

Duodenal triglycerides are insoluble in the intraluminal water, and lipase hydrolyzes lipid mainly at the oil-water interface. The surface area of this interface, and therefore the activity of lipase, is enhanced by intraluminal fat emulsification. Since bile salts promote emulsification because of their detergent action, they facilitate the action of pancreatic lipase. Lipolysis, however, can proceed in the absence of bile salts. In the hydrolysis of long-chain triglyceride, lipase preferentially splits off two α-fatty acids, leaving a single β-fatty acid attached to glycerol as a β-monoglyceride.

The free fatty acids and monoglycerides that result from the hydrolysis of fat undergo the final luminal step in fat assimilation, called micellarization. Insoluble fatty acids and monoglycerides are rapidly brought into solution — i.e., "solubilized" — by formation of macromolecular aggregates with bile salts, called micelles. Bile salts are amphipathic molecules, containing polar (hy-

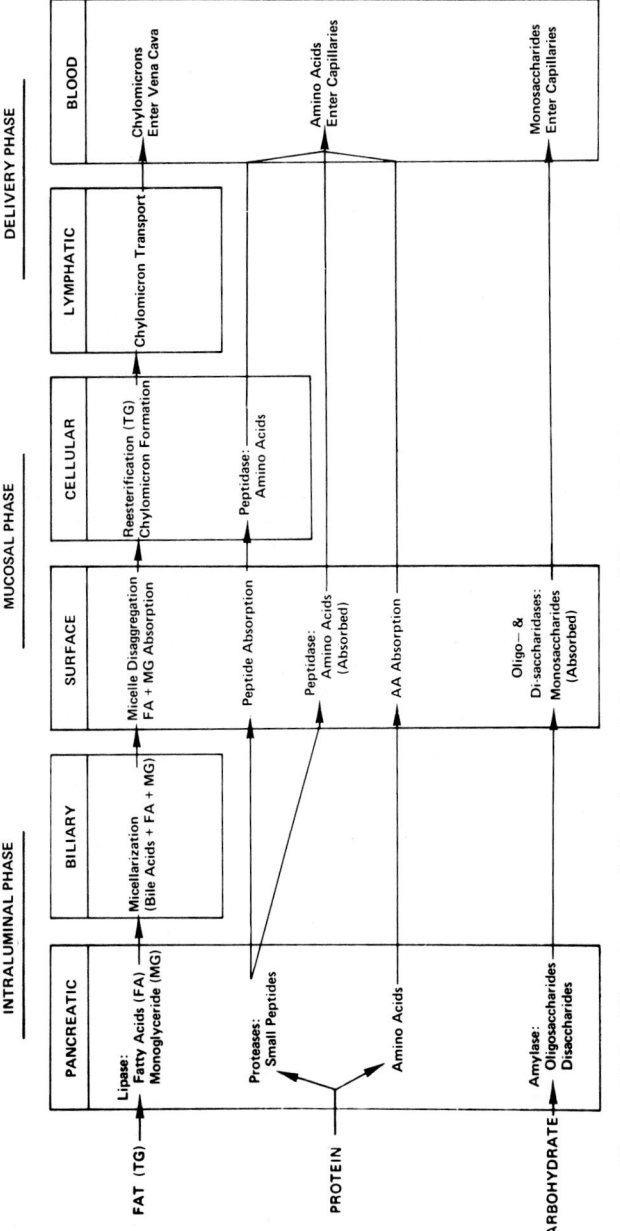

Figure 58–3. The phases of digestion and absorption of fat, carbohydrate, and protein. Note the greater complexity of fat assimilation, which includes biliary and lymphatic steps.

drophilic) and nonpolar (hydrophobic) regions. When a critical concentration of bile salts is attained, they aggregate into a small sphere with the water soluble (polar) end facing out toward luminal water and the fat soluble (nonpolar) end toward the center of the sphere. Fatty acids and monoglycerides, as well as fat soluble vitamins (A, D, E, K) are incorporated into the center of this sphere and are maintained in micellar solution for presentation to the intestinal epithelial cell for absorption.

The first step in the mucosal phase of fat assimilation is disaggregation of the micelle at the mucosal surface. The released fatty acids and monoglycerides passively diffuse into the epithelial cell. The released bile salts remain in the lumen until reaching the terminal ileum, where 95 per cent of the bile salts are then reabsorbed by active transport, recirculated to the liver, and resecreted in bile (enterohepatic circulation). Once inside the cell, free fatty acids and monoglycerides are enzymatically reesterified into triglyceride. To enable transport out of the cell, this newly formed triglyceride is then aggregated with lipoprotein, cholesterol, and phospholipid to form large transport particles called chylomicrons.

Finally, in the delivery phase, these chylomicrons exit from the base of the intestinal epithelial cell into the lamina propria and enter the central lacteal of the villus by a poorly understood mechanism. The pumping action of the villous smooth muscle propels chylomicron-laden lymph into draining lymphatics, which transport the chylomicrons to the thoracic duct and into the venous circulation.

The aforementioned sequence of events occurs in the assimilation of long-chain triglyceride (LCT), the major component of dietary fat. However, triglyceride composed of fatty acids of shorter chain length, i.e., medium-chain triglyceride (MCT), is digested and absorbed differently and more efficiently (Gray, 1978). The differences are noteworthy, because MCT is commercially available for dietary management of malabsorption syndromes and certain other disorders. Pancreatic lipase is more active against MCT than against LCT, and it is able to split off all three fatty acids, leaving minimal monoglyceride. The resulting medium-chain fatty acids (MCFA) form micelles more readily than LCFA, although micellarization is probably not necessary, since MCFA are more water soluble. Furthermore, an estimated 30 per cent of an oral MCT dose can be absorbed intact without any prior lipolysis. Once absorbed into the epithelial cell, MCFA are not reesterified or formed into chylomicrons, as LCFA are, but instead leave the cell as fatty acids. Finally, and most importantly, the removal phase of MCFA is by direct entry into the capillary venous system of the villus for transport to the liver via the portal vein, thereby entirely bypassing lymphatic transport.

A thorough knowledge of the physiology of fat assimilation is pertinent to the clinician's understanding of the pathogenesis of steatorrhea, since disruption of the fat assimilation sequence at any step can potentially result in steatorrhea (Riley and Glickman, 1979). Of the three classes of nutrient, fat seems to be the most susceptible to deranged assimilation, since its assimilation is the most complex and specialized, requiring the most steps. Fat is the only nutrient that requires micellarization (bile salt dependent) and lymphatic transport. Also, enterocytes on the apex of the villus tip, the portion of the crypt-villus unit most susceptible to mucosal injury, are the most specialized for assimilation of fat (Shiau et al., 1980). Therefore, fecal fat excretion (readily quantitated by fecal fat analysis) is an important clinical indicator of the functional status of the small bowel, steatorrhea often appearing in maldigestive and malabsorptive states. The mechanisms of steatorrhea and their relationship to the fat assimilation sequence are illustrated in Figure 58–4.

Carbohydrate

Dietary carbohydrate consists of disaccharides (sucrose, lactose), which are digested at the brush border surface membrane of intestinal epithelial cells, and polysaccharides (starch, glycogen), which are first hydrolyzed within the lumen by pancreatic amylase to oligosaccharides and then further digested at the brush border surface (Gray, 1975; Noon et al., 1977). In response to the entry of ingesta into the duodenum, the release of CCK stimulates amylase secretion from the pancreas. Intraluminal digestion of starch by pancreatic amylase is extremely rapid (within minutes) and efficient, yielding a mixture of oligosac-

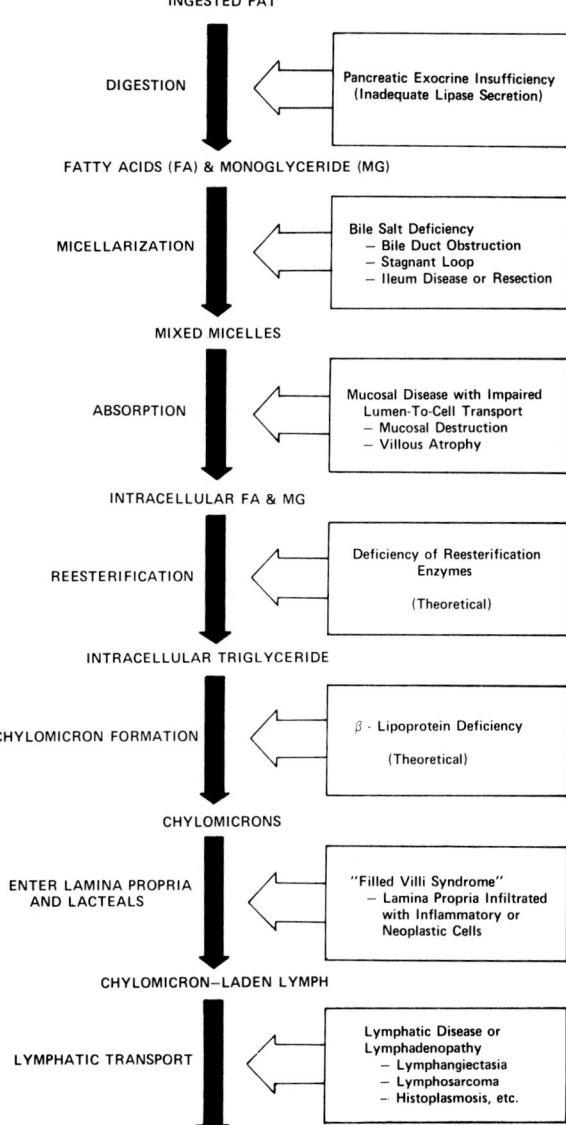

FAT ASSIMILATION   MECHANISMS OF STEATORRHEA

INGESTED FAT

DIGESTION → Pancreatic Exocrine Insufficiency (Inadequate Lipase Secretion)

FATTY ACIDS (FA) & MONOGLYCERIDE (MG)

MICELLARIZATION → Bile Salt Deficiency
— Bile Duct Obstruction
— Stagnant Loop
— Ileum Disease or Resection

MIXED MICELLES

ABSORPTION → Mucosal Disease with Impaired Lumen-To-Cell Transport
— Mucosal Destruction
— Villous Atrophy

INTRACELLULAR FA & MG

REESTERIFICATION → Deficiency of Reesterification Enzymes
(Theoretical)

INTRACELLULAR TRIGLYCERIDE

CHYLOMICRON FORMATION → β - Lipoprotein Deficiency
(Theoretical)

CHYLOMICRONS

ENTER LAMINA PROPRIA AND LACTEALS → "Filled Villi Syndrome"
— Lamina Propria Infiltrated with Inflammatory or Neoplastic Cells

CHYLOMICRON–LADEN LYMPH

LYMPHATIC TRANSPORT → Lymphatic Disease or Lymphadenopathy
— Lymphangiectasia
— Lymphosarcoma
— Histoplasmosis, etc.

BLOOD

Figure 58–4. The mechanisms of steatorrhea and their relationship to the fat assimilation sequence.

charides (maltose, maltotriose, and α-dextrins).

The intestinal epithelial cell functions in the digestion as well as the absorption of carbohydrate. Hydrolytic enzymes called oligosaccharidases (e.g., maltase, isomaltase, sucrase, lactase, amyloglucosidase) are located in the brush border surface membrane of these cells. The oligosaccharide products from the intraluminal digestion of starch, plus the ingested disaccharides sucrose and lactose, are rapidly hydrolyzed to their constituent monosaccharides by these brush border enzymes at the lumen-cell interface. The resulting monosaccharides — glucose, galactose, and fructose — are then absorbed by active transport mechanisms.

Glucose and galactose are actively transported across the brush border into the intestinal epithelial cell by a protein-carrier–mediated process that requires energy and couples their entry with Na^+ entry. Fructose, the other monosaccharide, is absorbed by facilitated diffusion, involving a specific carrier mechanism that does not require Na^+. Once inside the cell, monosaccharides are released from their carriers and exit the cell. They diffuse down a concentration gradient through the lamina propria and into the capillaries of the portal venous system.

In general, the breakdown of carbohydrate into an absorbable form (monosaccharide) is rapid and efficient. It is the active transport of monosaccharide into the cell that is the rate-limiting step for carbohydrate assimilation. Lactose, however, may be an exception. Evidence suggests that the rate-limiting step in the assimilation of lactose is its hydrolysis by brush border lactase, rather than its absorption into the cell. Lactose intolerance may explain the apparent frequency of milk-induced diarrhea.

The clinical settings in which malassimilation of carbohydrate are observed include (1) impaired digestion of starch (amylorrhea) caused by deficiency of amylase, most commonly found in dogs with complete exocrine pancreatic insufficiency and generalized maldigestion (see Chapter 61); (2) generalized carbohydrate malabsorption because of impaired brush border hydrolysis of oligosaccharides together with impaired absorption of monosaccharides, usually resulting from severe diffuse mucosal disease (for example, villous atrophy); and (3) malabsorption of dietary lactose (milk intolerance) resulting from a deficiency of brush border lactase relative to the quantity of milk ingested. Congenital deficiencies of specific brush border enzymes and monosaccharide carrier proteins are rare causes of carbohydrate malabsorption in man but have not yet been described in dogs or cats (Batt, 1980).

Protein

Protein digestion is initiated in the stomach by pepsin but is limited. In the absence of pepsin activity protein digestion proceeds normally. Most intraluminal protein digestion occurs in the duodenum and upper jejunum under the influence of pancreatic proteases. These proteases are secreted as inactive proenzymes in response to the CCK that is released when ingesta enters the duodenum, and also in response to vagal activity. One of these proenzymes, trypsinogen, is converted to active trypsin by a duodenal brush border enzyme called enterokinase. The active trypsin in turn activates the other proteases and autocatalyzes

further trypsinogen activation. The optimum pH for pancreatic protease activity is 7, so the low duodenal pH created by the entry of gastric acid is efficiently buffered by the secretion of bicarbonate-rich pancreatic juice in response to the hormone secretin.

The intraluminal phase of protein digestion is the result of the sequential action of endo- and exopeptidases, each proteolytic enzyme having optimal activity against specific peptide bonds. Trypsin, elastase, and chymotrypsin are endopeptidases that split internal peptide bonds in the protein molecule, resulting in small peptides. Carboxypeptidase A and B are exopeptidases that act only on terminal peptide bonds, resulting in small peptides and some amino acids. There is an overabundance of pancreatic proteases secreted normally in response to a meal, such that the intestinal cell phase rather than the intraluminal phase is the rate-limiting step in overall protein assimilation. It has been estimated that pancreatic protease secretion has to decrease to less than ten per cent of normal before noticeable protein maldigestion occurs.

In the mucosal phase of protein assimilation, small peptides resulting from intraluminal digestion are hydrolyzed to amino acids at the brush border surface, and in some cases, within the cell itself. The peptidases involved are found within the brush border membrane of the intestinal epithelial cell, as well as inside the cell, and the enzymes found in these two locations appear to be distinctly different. The resulting amino acids are absorbed into and transported across the cell by an active, Na^+-dependent, protein-carrier–mediated mechanism. Four different such mechanisms are known, each for a specific group of amino acids. Amino acids then diffuse across the basolateral membranes of the cell and into the capillaries for portal venous delivery (Freeman et al., 1979; Sleisenger and Kim, 1979).

The aforementioned processes of protein assimilation may be impaired in the dog and cat by diseases of the exocrine pancreas or the small intestine. Severe exocrine pancreatic insufficiency, when proteolytic enzyme output drops below ten per cent of normal, may cause severe protein maldigestion, usually accompanied by fat and starch maldigestion, as mentioned previously (see also Chapter 61). Diseases of the intestinal mucosa may lead to defective protein assimilation by causing impaired mucosal digestion of peptides and reduced absorption of amino acids and small peptides. Furthermore, some intestinal diseases are accompanied by excessive loss of endogenous protein (protein-losing enteropathy).

ENTEROSYSTEMIC CYCLES

The clinician gains a useful perspective on the overall intestinal handling of water, bile salts, protein, and fat by considering these substances in the context of an enterosystemic cycle. A substance has an enterosystemic cycle if it is secreted or lost from a proximal location and then is recovered (reabsorbed) farther downstream for recycling and systemic reutilization. Hence, an enterosystemic cycle is a conserving mechanism that prevents depletion of the recycled substance. The enterohepatic recirculation of bile salts has already been mentioned.

In the case of water and ions, the small intestine is both a secretory and absorptive organ. Large volumes of isotonic fluid in the form of secretions enter the lumen of the small intestine every day, but efficient distal recovery (reabsorption) of most of this fluid is necessary to prevent excessive loss in the feces and rapid depletion of extracellular fluid volume. This has been called the enterosystemic cycle of water (Phillips, 1972).

Large quantities of endogenous protein and fat from secretions and extruded cells enter the GI lumen. The quantity of endogenous protein entering the lumen each day exceeds protein ingested as food. Most of this protein and fat is digested, reabsorbed, and reutilized systemically.

INTESTINAL MOVEMENT OF WATER AND SOLUTE

Diarrhea, regardless of etiology, is basically the passage of feces containing an excess of water, resulting from abnormal intestinal handling of water and solute. Therefore, to understand the pathophysiology of diarrhea, the concepts of normal intestinal movement of water and solute will be considered. Large volumes of fluid, which are derived largely from endogenous secretions and, to a lesser extent, ingested fluids, enter the lumen of the small bowel to become the absorptive load (Phillips, 1972; Moon,

1978). The greatest volume of this fluid is absorbed in the jejunum. By the time the luminal fluid load reaches the colon, it is much reduced in volume. This small residual fluid load is acted on very efficiently by the colon, so that the end result is formed feces rather than liquid.

Continuous fluxes of water and solute across the intestinal mucosa occur simultaneously in opposing directions: absorptive fluxes in a lumen-to-blood direction, and secretory fluxes in a blood-to-lumen direction (Moon, 1978; Argenzio and Whipp, 1980). For the formation of normal feces, absorptive fluxes should exceed secretory fluxes, so that the overall net transmucosal flux is one of net absorption. Even though this net flux is relatively small, it represents the sum of massive, but opposing, fluid shifts. A small percentage change in these large fluid shifts, e.g., slightly increased secretory flux or decreased absorptive flux, is all that is needed to cause massive outpouring of fluid into the intestinal lumen, resulting in diarrhea. Thus, it is not surprising that animals with severe diarrhea may succumb to dehydration, electrolyte imbalance, and shock.

At the cellular level, transepithelial movement of water and solute may occur through transcellular or intercellular pathways and involve active or passive processes (Moon, 1978; Whipp, 1978; Argenzio and Whipp, 1980). Water transport is passive secondary to osmotic and hydrostatic pressure gradients that are mainly generated by solute transfer. In the transcellular pathway, solute is transported through the epithelial cell itself, usually by active transport mechanisms that involve membrane pumps (basolateral membrane sodium pump) or membrane carriers (brush border carriers). The other major pathway, the intercellular or shunt pathway, is quantitatively the most important mechanism and involves passive diffusion through aqueous channels or pores in the tight junctions between epithelial cells under the influence of electrochemical, osmotic, and hydrostatic pressure gradients.

MOTOR FUNCTION

Motor function of the small intestine consists of mixing and propulsive movements that provide for optimal contact of bowel content (ingesta) with secretions and the absorptive surface (Davenport, 1977; Christensen, 1978; Meshkinpour, 1979). Two basic types of motor activity are recognized in the small intestine, segmentation and peristalsis. Segmentation contractions are localized, circumferential constrictions of the lumen, spaced a few centimeters apart, which divide the content into segments, producing a mixing action. The frequency of these contractions is characteristic of a species, being 18 to 22/min in the dog and 28 to 30/min in the cat (Davenport, 1977). Peristalsis, on the other hand, is an advancing wave of contraction that propels bowel content downstream. During the interdigestive state in dogs fasted over 12 hours, there is a unique motility pattern characterized by recurring intense annular contractions that start at the stomach and sweep downstream along the entire length of small bowel. This interdigestive motility is thought to cleanse the GI tract in preparation for the next meal (Itoh et al., 1978).

The major determinants of the patterns of small bowel contractions are the inherent myoelectric properties of smooth muscle and its slow waves of depolarization (basal electrical rhythm). Motor function is modulated, however, by neural factors; the autonomic nervous system regulates motility through intrinsic (intramural) and extrinsic innervation. In general, parasympathetic influence (cholinergic) via the vagus nerve is an excitatory influence and sympathetic influence (adrenergic) via the splanchnic nerves is an inhibitory influence on intestinal smooth muscle. Sensory input is from mechanoreceptors that respond to pressure, movement, and stretch (volume) stimuli, or from chemoreceptors that respond to osmotic stimuli, pH, and digestion products. Gastrointestinal hormones can also affect motility.

ENDOCRINE FUNCTION

The gastrointestinal tract contains a variety of endocrine cells, scattered sparsely among the mucosal cells, collectively called APUD cells because of their distinctive biochemical property of *A*mine *P*recursor *U*ptake and *D*ecarboxylation. APUD cells are also found in the pancreatic islets. Polypeptide hormone products from alimentary endocrine cells include gastrin, secretin, cholecystokinin (CCK), enteroglucagon, vasoactive intestinal polypeptide (VIP), gas-

tric inhibitory polypeptide (GIP), somatostatin, motilin, and others, all of which have an effect on gastroenteropancreatic function. It is apparent from this list, that the alimentary tract should be considered an endocrine organ as well as a digestive organ. Also, recent evidence suggests that some of these GI peptides may not act as classic circulating hormones but instead are released locally to act on adjacent tissues (paracrine function). Furthermore, the localization of some of these peptides to neural structures within the gut wall suggests a neurotransmitter-like (neurocrine) function. It is beyond the scope of this chapter to discuss the complex functions and interrelationships of each of these hormones; however, numerous reviews on the subject are available (Walsh, 1978).

IMMUNE FUNCTION

The small intestine, like the lung, is in the seemingly precarious state of being separated from a potentially hostile external environment by an epithelial barrier that is only one cell thick (Strombeck, 1979; Hirsh, 1980). Intestinal lymphoid tissue plays a major "watchdog" role in maintaining local immunity of the mucosal surface, as well as contributing to the overall scheme of the body's immune system. Intestinal secretory antibodies, most of which are IgA, originate from plasma cells located in the lamina propria beneath the mucosal surface, and play an essential role in the maintenance of the epithelial surface as a barrier to penetration of harmful microorganisms, enterotoxins, and antigens (allergens) from the lumen Walker and Isselbacher, 1977; Doe, 1979). These IgA-secreting plasma cells are first sensitized to intestinal antigens as immunoblasts in Peyer's patches, then after proliferating and hemolymphatic circulation, they return to the intestinal mucosa (homing response) to reside in the lamina propria.

Local cell-mediated immunity also plays a role in gut defenses (Welliver and Ogra, 1978). Other nonimmunologic host defense mechanisms include normal alimentary secretions, peristalsis, and the native microflora that provide a barrier against the colonization of the gut by pathogens (Welliver and Ogra, 1978; Hirsh, 1980). Insufficiency or impairment of intestinal immune function may be important in a number of clinical disorders. On the other hand, an aberrant intestinal immune response has been postulated, but is unproven, for certain inflammatory diseases, e.g., eosinophilic enteritis and lymphocytic-plasmacytic enteritis, in which the lamina propria distends with cells that are known to be primary or secondary participants in immune reactions (lymphocytes, plasma cells, eosinophils).

MECHANISMS OF DIARRHEA

The mechanisms of diarrhea in intestinal disease may be categorized as decreased absorption (osmotic diarrhea), hypersecretion (secretory diarrhea), increased permeability (exudative diarrhea), and abnormal motility (transit time) (Moon, 1978; Argenzio and Whipp, 1980). This well-established classification scheme is based on separations that are somewhat artificial and simplistic, insofar as the pathogenesis of most diarrheal diseases is probably a complex integration of several mechanisms. The mechanistic approach, however, puts the pathophysiology of diarrhea into a perspective that is useful in the diagnosis and treatment of intestinal disease.

OSMOTIC DIARRHEA

Osmotic diarrhea occurs when poor absorption results in an accumulation of nonabsorbable solutes in the gut lumen, where they retain water by their osmotic activity (Phillips, 1972; Moon, 1978; Argenzio and Whipp, 1980). This excess luminal solute and water causes bowel distention and is then expelled as bulky, fluid diarrhea. The unabsorbed solutes are largely derived from malassimilated dietary constituents, especially carbohydrates. Unabsorbed carbohydrates are hydrolyzed by colonic bacteria to small organic acids, adding to the osmotically active molecules that retain water in the lumen, as well as acidifying the colonic content. Malassimilated fat exerts minimal osmotic effect because it is water insoluble; however, steatorrhea may induce diarrhea by another mechanism. Unabsorbed fatty acids are hydroxylated by colonic bacteria to hydroxy fatty acids, which alter water and electrolyte transport in the large intestine to produce secretory diarrhea (Phillips, 1972; Ammon and Phillips, 1973).

Clinically, osmotic diarrhea is most often the result of malassimilation from primary digestive failure (maldigestion) or primary absorptive failure (intestinal malabsorption). In maldigestion, even though absorptive capacity remains normal, material presented to absorptive cells is not in an absorbable form because it has not been digested. This occurs in pancreatic exocrine insufficiency. In intestinal malabsorption, on the other hand, the primary defect is impaired absorptive capacity and brush border activity caused by intrinsic intestinal disease, such as diffuse inflammatory, neoplastic, or villous atrophy disorders (Moon, 1978). Osmotic diarrhea from malassimilation usually improves or ceases during fasting, and the osmolality of fecal fluid exceeds the sum of fecal electrolyte concentrations (osmol gap), implicating the accumulation of an unabsorbed solute.

Another example of the osmotic mechanism is the catharsis produced by laxatives that contain poorly absorbed substances (magnesium sulfate, sodium phosphate, lactulose) that osmotically retain water in the bowel lumen.

SECRETORY DIARRHEA

Secretory diarrhea occurs when the small or large bowel mucosa is stimulated to secrete fluid independent of changes in absorptive capacity, mucosal permeability, or exogenously generated osmotic gradients (Moon, 1978). The net intestinal efflux of fluid and electrolytes in secretory diarrhea is usually from an exaggeration of normal intestinal transport mechanisms. If secretions exceed absorptive capacity, then the net secretion is expelled as diarrhea.

The intestinal secretions are usually isotonic and similar to extracellular fluid, although the composition may be altered during transit. Stools contain excess water, electrolytes, and bicarbonate. Therefore, the consequences of secretory diarrhea are isotonic dehydration, electrolyte depletion, and acidosis. In pure secretory diarrhea, fecal osmolality is almost entirely accounted for by the concentration of Na^+, K^+, and their accompanying anions.

Stimuli that provoke intestinal secretion of fluid are numerous and diverse, and probably contribute to the pathogenesis of a wide variety of acute and chronic diarrheal diseases. These secretagogues include bacterial enterotoxins, gastrointestinal hormones, prostaglandins, serotonin, parasympathetic stimulation, dihydroxy bile acids, hydroxylated fatty acids, and certain laxatives (Moon, 1978; Argenzio and Whipp, 1980).

The mechanisms by which many of these secretagogues influence intestinal secretion are poorly understood. Nevertheless, some secretagogues, most notably certain bacterial enterotoxins and hormones, have been shown to activate adenyl cyclase, resulting in increased mucosal cyclic adenosine monophosphate (cAMP) followed by cAMP-mediated hypersecretion. In human patients with pancreatic and nonpancreatic endocrine tumors, a watery secretory-type diarrhea is often encountered, which is attributed to humoral substances elaborated by the tumor. Similar observations have been made in dogs with thyroid medullary carcinoma and Zollinger-Ellison syndrome.

Stimulation of intestinal secretion may occur secondary to malabsorptive states, when unabsorbed fatty acids or unabsorbed bile acids reach the colon in excessive quantities and are acted upon by colonic bacteria. Within the colon, both hydroxylated fatty acids and dihydroxy bile acids stimulate cAMP-mediated secretion of water and electrolytes (Phillips, 1972; Bright-Asare and Binder, 1973; Binder et al., 1975; Cline et al., 1976). These mechanisms probably contribute to the diarrhea of fat malabsorption (steatorrhea) and in part to the diarrhea that accompanies ileal disease or resection (bile salt malabsorption) (Phillips, 1972; Mekhjian et al., 1971). Furthermore, it has been suggested that bile salts may also act as secretagogues in the small bowel, when bacterial overgrowth causes bile acid deconjugation within the jejunum. Ricinoleic acid, the active component of castor oil, is chemically similar to hydroxy fatty acid and induces catharsis, at least in part, by a similar mechanism (Phillips, 1972).

PERMEABILITY OR EXUDATIVE DIARRHEA

Permeability or exudative diarrhea occurs when increased mucosal permeability, usually accompanied by increased transmucosal hydrostatic pressure, causes a net loss of protein-rich fluid into the intestinal lumen by passive leakage, a process sometimes called filtration-secretion (Duffy et al., 1978). Because this mechanism becomes most clinically important when permeability is altered enough to allow exudation of

plasma proteins, it is often called exudative diarrhea, and it is characterized by the outpouring of plasma proteins, blood, or mucus from sites of the inflammation, ulceration, or infiltration of the gut (Phillips, 1972; Moon, 1978).

In the normal intestine, permeability of mucosal epithelium may be represented as pores in the mucosal membrane (Moon, 1978). The size of these pores will determine the size of the molecule that can leak through the mucosa. A large increase in pore size due to disease of the gut may permit leakage of plasma proteins and may lead to the syndrome of protein-losing enteropathy. With entire breakdown of the mucosal barrier, permeability may increase over 10,000-fold, allowing the leakage of erythrocytes and leading to hemorrhagic exudate (Moon, 1978).

The passive transmucosal leakage of fluid, electrolytes, and protein from blood to lumen is dependent upon not only the size of the pores in the mucosal membrane, but also on the mucosal interstitial fluid or hydraulic pressure, which is the driving force for this movement (Duffy et al., 1978; Argenzio and Whipp, 1980). Any factor that affects mucosal interstitial fluid dynamics, especially factors that increase net transcapillary filtration, may cause the accumulation of mucosal interstitial fluid and elevate mucosal hydrostatic tissue pressure. This increases mucosal permeability and fluid leakage, resulting in permeability diarrhea and, if plasma protein leakage is severe enough, the syndrome of protein-losing enteropathy. Clinical situations in which this occurs are mucosal inflammation, with increased capillary permeability and arteriolar dilatation; increased portal venous pressure (portal hypertension or right-sided congestive heart failure); circumstances that elevate capillary hydrostatic pressure; obstruction to lymph flow due to intestinal diseases that involve lymphatics (lymphangiectasia, lymphosarcoma, or histoplasmosis); decreased plasma protein oncotic pressure associated with hypoalbuminemic states; and volume expansion.

DIARRHEA CAUSED BY ABNORMAL INTESTINAL MOTILITY OR TRANSIT TIME

Intestinal hypermotility due to a primary increase in intensity, frequency, or rate of progression of peristalsis could accelerate bowel transit to such a degree that diarrhea would theoretically result from insufficient mucosal contact time for digestion and absorption. But in fact, hypermotility by itself rarely, if ever, plays a primary role in the pathogenesis of diarrheal disease (Moon, 1978; Argenzio and Whipp, 1980). Furthermore, the complex relationship between transit and absorption is unclear. Motility may, however, be increased secondary to increased volume and fluidity of intestinal content caused by one of the other previously mentioned mechanisms of diarrhea. Motility may also be stimulated by gastrointestinal surgery, drugs, hormones, and enterotoxins, but the effects exerted by these agents are considered to be relatively minor (Phillips, 1972; Argenzio and Whipp, 1980). In contrast to the dubious role of hypermotility and rapid transit in the pathogenesis of diarrhea, prolonged transit may cause diarrhea by encouraging stasis and allowing bacterial overgrowth in the small bowel (stagnant loop syndrome) (Argenzio and Whipp, 1980).

DIAGNOSIS

Diarrhea, an increase in the frequency, fluidity, or volume of feces, is the most consistent clinical manifestation of intestinal disease in small animals. Therefore, the clinical approach to diarrhea as the classic sign of intestinal disease will be emphasized.

The diagnosis of intestinal disease can be approached in stages:

Stage 1: exclusion of dietary problems, parasitism, or systemic disorders and anatomic localization of the lesions to small or large bowel using the history, physical exam, stool characteristics, and preliminary laboratory tests.

Stage 2: functional characterization of dogs with chronic small bowel diarrhea by determining whether digestive or absorptive functions are defective through studies that first identify steatorrhea or malassimilation, and then differentiate maldigestion from malabsorption.

Stage 3: definitive etiologic or histopathologic diagnosis through an extended data base consisting of more sophisticated laboratory tests, radiographs, biopsies (laparotomy for the small bowel, proctoscopy for the large bowel), and response to therapy.

Many animals with acute diarrhea are re-solved in the first stage of this scheme and do not require any in-depth workup, while the etiology of chronic diarrhea is often elusive, necessitating a more in-depth approach to diagnosis. Tables 58–1, 58–2, and 58–3 list the diagnostics available for small bowel diarrhea.

HISTORY AND PHYSICAL EXAM

The initial step in the diagnosis of problem diarrhea in the dog and cat is the anatomic localization of the lesion to large or small bowel by history, physical examination, and stool characteristics (frequency, volume, consistency, color, odor, and composition) (Table 58–4). This distinction is an important one, because it determines the direction of further workup. Small bowel diarrhea is associated with diseases of the small intestines or the accessory digestive glands whose secretions function within the small intestinal lumen (pancreas, enzymes; liver, bile salts).

Small bowel disease may be associated with maldigestion or malabsorption. Characteristics include passage of large quantities of voluminous, malodorous, unformed, steatorrheic feces; excessive intestinal gas (flatus); and weight loss despite adequate or even increased food intake. Sometimes small intestinal disease is characterized by profuse, watery diarrhea. By contrast, large bowel disease is characterized by

---

Table 58–1. Diagnostic Aids for Intestinal Disease

1. CBC, serum proteins, serum chemistries
2. Fecal examinations (see Table 58–2)
   a. Parasite examinations
   b. Stool microscopy
   c. Chemical determinations
   d. Fecal cultures
3. Tests for malassimilation (see Table 58–3)
4. Radiography—plain and barium
5. Serology—for histoplasmosis
6. Virology—for enteric viruses
7. Endoscopy (duodenoscopy): visualize lesions, mucosal biopsies, intestinal aspirates
8. Specialized assays
   a. Assays of mucosal brush border enzymes
   b. Radioimmunoassay of GI hormones
   c. Radiolabeled macromolecule excretion (for protein-losing enteropathy)
9. Pancreatic secretory function test (CCK-secretin response test)
10. Intestinal biopsy (by laparotomy, endoscopy, peroral suction biopsy capsule)
11. Response to therapy

Table 58–2. Fecal Examinations Used for Diagnosis of Intestinal Disease

1. Gross inspection (volume, weight, consistency, color, composition, odor)
2. Fecal parasite exam
   a. Flotation (metazoa)
   b. Visualization of proglottids (tapeworms)
   c. Sedimentation/Baerman (Strongyloides)
   d. For protozoa
      1) Saline smear
      2) Stains (for Giardia, NMB or iodine; for trichomonads, Wright's)
      3) $ZnSO_4$ for Giardia cysts
      4) Formalin-fixed
3. Stool microscopy
   a. Saline—for protozoa
   b. Sudan—direct, indirect (steatorrhea)
   c. Lugol's iodine—starch (amylorrhea), protozoa
   d. NMB, Wright's—creatorrhea, exudates, protozoa
4. Chemical determinations on feces
   a. Proteolytic (trypsin) activity—pancreatic exocrine insufficiency
   b. Water content
   c. Fat content—steatorrhea (malassimilation)
   d. Nitrogen content—azotorrhea (malassimilation)
   e. pH (carbohydrate malassimilation)
   f. Electrolytes (osmotic vs. secretory diarrhea)
   g. Osmolality (osmotic vs. secretory diarrhea)
   h. Tests for occult blood
5. Fecal cultures (bacterial, fungal)

tenesmus and urgency, with frequent passage of small volumes of bloody-mucoid feces (discussed in Chapter 59). Melena, vomiting, emaciation, and generalized malaise may also be seen in certain diseases of the small bowel.

Along with the history and stool charac-

Table 58–3. Tests for Malassimilation

1. Fat
   a. Sudan-stained fecal smears
   b. Plasma turbidity test
   *c. Fecal fat analysis (quantitative)
   d. Triolein-oleic acid
   e. Vitamin A absorption
2. Carbohydrate
   a. Iodine-stained fecal smears
   *b. D-Xylose absorption
   c. Glucose absorption
   d. Starch tolerance (digestion)
   e. Lactose tolerance
3. Protein
   a. Fecal stains for creatorrhea
   b. Proteolytic (trypsin) activity in feces
   *c. BT-PABA test
   d. Fecal nitrogen output
4. Vitamin B_{12} absorption (Schilling)

*Preferred tests in each category,

teristics, the physical examination may yield some helpful information in the diagnosis of small intestinal disease. Abdominal palpation of intestinal loops may reveal neoplastic masses, diffuse thickening of the bowel wall (infiltrative diseases), painful intestinal loops, intussusceptions, intestinal foreign bodies, aggregation and plication of loops indicative of linear intestinal foreign body, and gas or fluid distention of the bowel. Enlarged mesenteric lymph nodes are palpated in some intestinal disorders, especially those with inflammatory and neoplastic lesions. Abdominal palpation should also include a careful evaluation of other abdominal structures for abnormalities that could cause or result from intestinal disease. The state of malnutrition that accompanies malassimilation often leads to emaciation and a dull, unthrifty haircoat. Greasy, oily perineal hair is suggestive of steatorrhea. Mucous membrane pallor may suggest enteric blood loss. Abnormal fluid homeostasis, characterized by edema, ascites, or pleural effusion, may result from hypoproteinemia due to protein-losing enteropathy.

THE INITIAL DATA BASE

The initial data base should include a CBC, total plasma protein to detect hypoproteinemia, and to rule out parasitism, fecal flotations for metazoan ova and direct saline fecal smears for protozoa. On the CBC, an eosinophilia may suggest endoparasitism or eosinophilic enteritis, rarely hypoadrenocorticism; a regenerative neutrophilia may suggest infectious, inflammatory, or necrotic intestinal disease; a degenerative or toxic neutropenia may suggest parvoviral infection, acute septicemia or endotoxemia, or overwhelming bacterial peritonitis accompanying bowel perforation; a lymphopenia may accompany intestinal lymphangiectasia from persistent loss of lymphocytes into the gut lumen; an increased packed cell volume (PCV) and hemoglobin value are indicative of hemoconcentration from fluid loss; and finally, anemia may result from enteric blood loss, or from depressed erythropoiesis due to chronic malnutrition or chronic inflammation. Total plasma protein is useful for screening for hypoproteinemia associated with protein-losing enteropathy. Albumin and globulin determinations or serum

Table 58–4. Clinical Differentiation of Small Bowel Disease from Large Bowel Disease

Sign	Small Bowel	Large Bowel
Frequency of defecation	Normal or slightly increased	Very frequent
Fecal volume	Large quantity of bulky or watery feces	Small quantities often
Urgency	Absent	Usually present
Tenesmus	Absent	Usually present
Mucus in feces	Usually absent	Abundant
Blood in feces	Dark black (digested)	Red (fresh)
Steatorrhea (malassimilation)	May be present	Absent
Weight loss and emaciation	May be present	Rare
Vomiting	May be present	Uncommon
Generalized "malaise"	May be present	Rare

protein electrophoresis may be desirable.

The importance of a careful search for parasites through fecal examinations cannot be overemphasized; endoparasitism can mimic virtually any of the more complex small and large bowel disorders, and in many practice areas parasites are the most frequent cause of diarrhea. Feces should be visually inspected for tapeworm proglottids, and several conventional flotations should be performed to identify metazoan ova. Under circumstances where *Strongyloides stercoralis* infection is suspected, a direct smear, sedimentation, or Baerman technique can be used to look for larvae in the feces. Protozoan parasites, including *Giardia canis, Trichomonas spp., Entamoeba histolytica,* and *Balantidium coli,* can be identified microscopically in a drop of fresh feces suspended in one or two drops of isotonic saline. The distinguishing characteristics of each of these protozoa will be discussed later. *Giardia* may be stained with Lugol's iodine or new methylene blue to facilitate identification, while trichomonads are rendered more visible with Wright's stain. *Giardia* cysts, which may be more abundant in feces than the motile trophozoites, may be identified by using $ZnSO_4$ flotation solution. Cysts will stain light brown for easier identification if Lugol's iodine is added to the flotation mixture. Feces can also be fixed with formalin-based fixative, stained, and examined for protozoa (Yang and Scholten, 1977).

In addition to this initial data base, a biochemical profile and urinalysis should be considered to exclude metabolic or extraintestinal disorders that could cause or result from diarrhea. For example, underlying systemic disease, such as uremia (increased BUN, creatinine) or hypoadrenocorticism (hyperkalemia and hyponatremia) may be discovered, or the consequences of fecal loss of fluid, electrolytes, and bicarbonate can be assessed so that proper therapy can be initiated.

SIMPLE QUALITATIVE SCREENING TESTS FOR MALASSIMILATION

Once chronic small bowel diarrhea is suspected, efforts are directed toward identifying and characterizing malassimilation. The physiologic processes of digestion, absorption, and delivery, which are required for normal nutrient assimilation, may be malfunctioning in small intestinal disease. Stool microscopy, the plasma turbidity fat absorption test, and the x-ray film or gelatin tube digestion test for fecal trypsin are simple, in-office qualitative screening tests used to initially identify malassimilation. Since these are only screening tests, they should be performed several times before valid conclusions are made.

Stool microscopy includes preparations of direct and indirect Sudan stain, Lugol's iodine stain, and new methylene blue or Wright's stain (Lorenz, 1976). Saline smears for protozoa identification are usually done at the same time and have already been discussed. Feces for these evaluations should be fresh, either tested within 15 minutes of defecation or obtained directly from the rectum digitally or with a loop or swab. In each test one to two drops of feces and one to two drops of stain are mixed well on a microscope slide, coverslipped, and examined. The direct Sudan III or IV preparation stains excessive undigested (neutral) fat in the feces as refractile orange droplets, indicating steatorrhea due to maldigestion (Fig. 58–5). This preparation is strongly positive in dogs with exocrine pancreatic insufficiency (EPI). Numerous orange lipid droplets on an indirect Sudan preparation (one to two drops each of feces, 36 per cent acetic acid, and Sudan III or IV mixed and heated twice to boiling on a slide) in an animal with a negative direct Sudan preparation, suggests steatorrhea (excessive fecal fatty acids) due to malabsorption of digested fat rather than maldigestion (Drummey et al., 1961; Luk and Hendrix, 1978). Lugol's two per cent iodine solution stains excessive undigested starch in the feces (amylorrhea) as dark blue-black granules. Feces containing an excess of undigested starch suggests maldigestion due to EPI. As previously mentioned, *Giardia* trophozoites and cysts are stained light brown with Lugol's. New methylene blue (NMB) or Wright's stain is used to identify undigested striated muscle fibers in the feces (azotorrhea or creatorrhea), provided a meat source is part of the animal's diet, again suggesting maldigestion due to EPI. A positive control for each of these preparations can be obtained by staining canned, meat-base dog food along with patient feces, while normal feces from another animal can serve as a negative control.

Cytology stains, such as NMB or Wright's,

can also be used to examine feces for leukocytes, which appear in inflammatory bowel diseases when there is disruption of distal intestinal or colonic mucosa (Harris et al., 1972; Pickering et al., 1977). Similarly, exfoliative cytology of colonic mucosal scrapings or swabbings taken during proctoscopy or directly from the rectum may also reveal colonic mucosal disease. Cytology may, in some cases, provide a definitive diagnosis. In endemic areas, for example, intestinal histoplasmosis may be diagnosed by finding the organisms within macrophages obtained by colonic scraping (Fig. 58–6). When lesions are confined to the small intestine, fecal leukocytes are usually absent and colonic scrapings are normal.

The plasma turbidity test is a simple screening test for maldigestion or malabsorption of fat and is based on the principle that lipemia (plasma turbidity) should be observed two or three hours after a fatty meal if digestion and absorption of that fat was effective (Anderson and Low, 1965; Lorenz, 1976). Following a 12-hour fast, a presample of plasma is taken, then three ml/kg of vegetable oil or Lipomul are administered orally, and two- and three-hour plasma samples are compared with the presample for turbidity. Lack of turbidity suggests malassimilation, although delayed gastric emptying is always a possibility. In animals with EPI, failure to obtain turbidity because of fat maldigestion can be corrected by repeating the test with the addition of pancreatic enzymes (Viokase-V powder, one tsp), whereas turbidity is absent with or without enzymes in absorptive failure. By measuring the lipemia with spectrophotom-

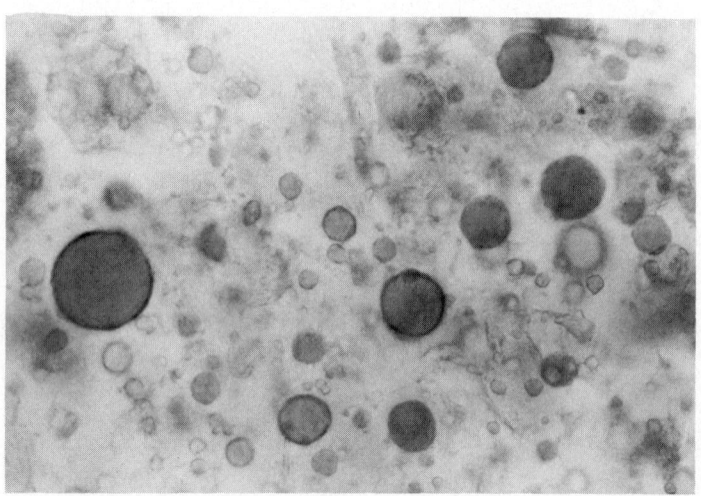

Figure 58–5. Refractile orange fat droplets in the Sudan-stained feces of an animal with steatorrhea.

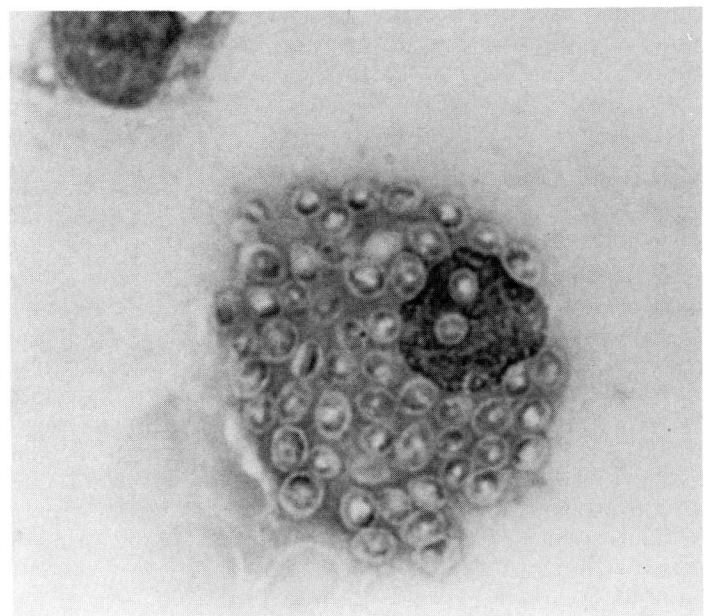

Figure 58–6. Numerous *Histoplasma capsulatum* organisms within the cytoplasm of a macrophage. The specimen was obtained by colonic scraping of a dog with chronic diarrhea due to *Histoplasma* enterocolitis (Wright's stain).

etry (Brobst and Funk, 1972), or by analyzing the rise in plasma polyunsaturated fatty acid concentration after feeding linseed oil (Sateri, 1975), there is little additional sensitivity over simple visual analysis of turbidity to warrant the increased complexity.

The x-ray film and gelatin tube digestion tests are qualitative tests for proteolytic (trypsin) activity of feces that are used in the diagnosis of EPI (see Chapter 61). Quantitative analysis of fecal trypsin has also been used (Burrows et al., 1979).

DIGESTION AND ABSORPTION TESTS

Digestion-absorption tests are generally more complex and sophisticated than screening tests, and are designed to evaluate specific aspects of pancreatic and intestinal function, as related to the assimilation of fat, carbohydrate, and protein. These tests are indicated if the results of other tests have been equivocal in identifying malassimilation or differentiating malabsorption from EPI (Table 58–3).

In the author's opinion, when all factors are considered, the most useful tests in this category are the quantitative fecal fat determination, the D-xylose absorption test, and the BT-PABA digestion test. For completeness, however, other tests will be mentioned as well. For the purposes of this discussion, the function tests will be categorized on the basis of the nutrient whose assimilation the test is evaluating.

Fat is the nutrient most susceptible to malassimilation. The role of Sudan-stained fecal smears and the plasma turbidity test in the initial detection of impaired fat assimilation have already been discussed. The most sensitive and reliable test for overall evaluation of fat assimilation is the quantitative analysis of fecal fat excretion for documentation of steatorrhea. Other, less useful tests of fat assimilation are the vitamin A absorption test and the ^{131}I-labeled triolein–oleic acid absorption test.

Quantitative analysis of fecal fat content is a reliable method of detecting the degree of steatorrhea and malassimilation, although it does not differentiate EPI from intestinal malabsorption (Lorenz, 1976; Burrows et al., 1979). The test is available through commercial laboratories, but it is somewhat cumbersome and expensive to perform. The procedure involves collection of feces (preferably for 72 hours to minimize sampling error) after the animal's diet has been standardized for three days. The feces are collected into a preweighed paint can, then weighed and sent to a lab for lipid analysis. Daily fecal fat output varies with body size and dietary fat intake, and has been expressed as output in grams/day, output in grams/day/unit of body weight, and per cent assimilation of ingested fat using a fat balance procedure. Normal values are variously reported as (1) less than 5 gm/day in dogs (Hayden and Van Kruiningen, 1976), without diet or body weight specification; (2) 0.24 ± 0.01 gm/kg/day in dogs, with > 0.3

gm/kg/day indicative of steatorrhea (Merritt et al., 1979); (3) 0.35 ± 0.23 gm/kg/day or 1.33 ± 0.8 gm/day in cats, with > 3.5 gm/day indicative of malassimilation (Lewis et al., 1979); and (4) net fat assimilation in dogs of > 94 to 96 per cent of consumed fat (Hill, 1972a), or 97 per cent assimilation on a meat-based diet versus 90 per cent assimilation on a cereal-based diet (Merritt et al., 1979). Dogs with EPI have been found to have fecal fat excretion of 2.08 ± 0.36 gm/kg/day and fecal fat assimilation of 41 to 78 per cent, while dogs with malabsorption excreted 1.14 ± 0.11 gm/kg/day and had 78 to 89 per cent assimilation (Burrows et al., 1979; Hill, 1972a).

The vitamin A absorption test has been used to measure intestinal lipid absorption in the presence of adequate bile salts and pancreatic enzymes (Hayden and Van Kruiningen, 1976). After a 12-hour fast, a presample of serum is collected and 200,000 units of vitamin A, as cod liver oil concentrate, are given orally. Serum vitamin A concentration is measured in the presample and in samples taken at two, four, six, eight, and 24 hours, and a three- to fivefold increase of serum vitamin A above the fasting concentration at six to eight hours is considered normal. Because of inconsistent results and lack of sensitivity and specificity, this test has limited usefulness.

Radiolabeled triglyceride (^{131}I-triolein) and fatty acid (^{131}I-oleic acid) have been administered on separate days and their absorption curves compared, to distinguish between fat maldigestion and fat malabsorption in the dog (Kaneko et al., 1965; Kallfelz et al., 1968). Plasma radioactivity following oral administration of each radiolabeled substance is measured as an indicator of absorption of that substance. If steatorrhea is due to pancreatic insufficiency, oleic acid absorption will be normal, but that of triolein, which requires lipolysis prior to absorption, will be reduced. In intestinal malabsorption, the absorption of both substances will be reduced. The need for radioisotope handling and analysis greatly limits the availability and usefulness of this procedure.

Aside from initial screening of feces for undigested starch with Lugol's iodine stain, four absorption-digestion tests are available for the assessment of carbohydrate assimilation: the D-xylose absorption test, the glucose absorption test, the starch digestion (tolerance) test, and the lactose digestion (tolerance) test. In this group, the preferred test for detection of absorptive failure is the D-xylose absorption test. D-xylose is a pentose monosaccharide that is absorbed by both passive and active mechanisms; once absorbed, it is relatively inert, unaffected by insulin, and excreted mainly by the kidney. After a 12-hour fast, plasma xylose concentration is determined before and at 30, 60, 90, and 120 minutes (just 60 and 90 minute samples are satisfactory for routine diagnostic use) after the oral administration of 0.5 gm D-xylose/kg body weight, given as a five to ten per cent solution (with water). Normal dogs should have a peak xylose level greater than 45 mg/dl at 60 to 90 minutes, indicative of normal absorption, whereas dogs with malabsorption should have a flat D-xylose curve (Hill et al., 1970; Hill, 1972a; Lorenz, 1976). The peak value in healthy dogs, in the author's experience, may be considerably higher than published normal values would suggest, often exceeding 60 mg/dl (Fig. 58–7). False results with the D-xylose test include a factitiously low peak due to delayed gastric emptying, intraluminal bacterial metabolism of xylose in states with bacterial overgrowth, or sequestration of xylose in ascitic fluid, whereas a falsely elevated peak may result from decreased urinary xylose excretion because of renal failure. As the preferred test for intestinal absorptive function, the D-xylose absorption test can be conveniently combined with a test of pancreatic digestive function, the BT-PABA digestion test, for the simultaneous evaluation of pancreatic digestion and intestinal absorption (Rogers et al., 1980).

The glucose absorption test also measures the intestinal absorption of carbohydrate (monosaccharide); however, its disadvantage compared with D-xylose is that once absorbed, serum concentration is affected by insulin and body metabolism. Nevertheless, glucose is considerably cheaper and easier to measure. After a 12-hour fast and a baseline serum glucose determination, 2 gm dextrose/kg body weight are given orally as a 12½ per cent solution, and samples are taken at 15, 30, 60, 90, and 120 minutes. Normally, serum glucose concentration will rise about 50 mg/dl above resting level in 30 minutes and then return within two hours. Although a lower and later peak is expected in intestinal malabsorption, there is much

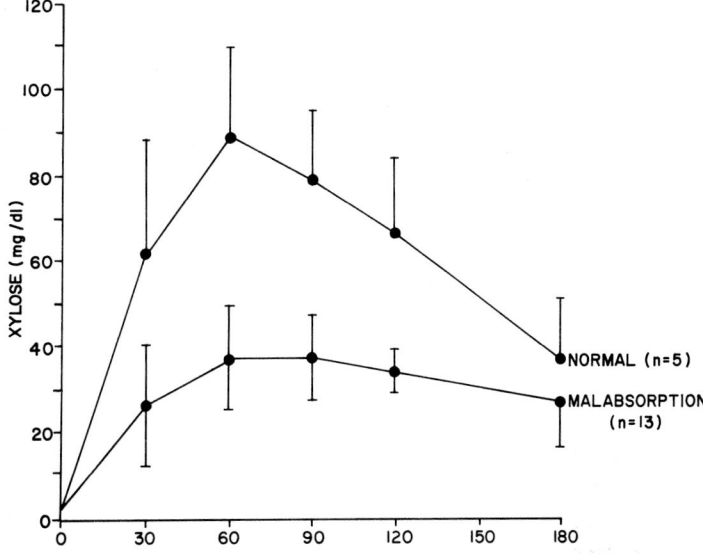

Figure 58–7. D-Xylose absorption curve in clinically normal dogs and 13 dogs with malabsorption (brackets = standard deviation).

overlap between normal and abnormal curves (Hill and Kidder, 1972).

The starch digestion test is based on measuring the rise in serum glucose following an oral starch dose, as a means of determining pancreatic amylase activity (Hill; 1972b). It is a relatively insensitive test, requiring almost complete pancreatic exocrine dysfunction before becoming abnormal. Therefore, the same information is probably obtainable by the previously mentioned screening examination of iodine-stained feces for undigested starch.

A lactose tolerance test has been used to evaluate brush border disaccharidase (lactase) activity (Hill, 1972a). The principle is similar to the starch tolerance test: lactose is given orally (2 gm/kg as 12½ per cent solution), and changes in serum glucose are measured. Again, glucose absorptive capacity must be determined to be normal before an abnormal test can be attributed to lactose maldigestion.

Tests of protein assimilation include stool microscopy for undigested muscle fibers and the film or gel digestion test for fecal trypsin activity, which have already been discussed. Excessive fecal output of nitrogen is a measurable indicator of protein malassimilation (pancreatic insufficiency, intestinal malabsorption) or excessive loss of protein into the gut, but it is not in routine use (Merritt and Reed, 1980). Tests to detect excessive enteric loss of endogenous protein (protein-losing enteropathy) will be discussed later.

Recently, an oral peptide–PABA digestion test has shown promise as a useful and reliable pancreatic function test for demonstrating deficient secretion of the protease chymotrypsin (diagnosing EPI) (Strombeck, 1978; Batt et al., 1979a; Stradley et al., 1979; Rogers et al., 1980). The key to this test is a synthetic chymotrypsin-labile peptide, N-benzoyl-L-tryosyl-paraaminobenzoic acid (BT-PABA). When given orally to the dog with normal exocrine pancreatic function, BT-PABA is cleaved by chymotrypsin to yield free PABA, which is subsequently absorbed into the blood. Once in the blood, PABA is excreted into the urine. The content of PABA in urine collected for six hours after oral administration of peptide-PABA (Strombeck, 1978) or the PABA levels in plasma 60 to 90 minutes after administration (Rogers et al., 1980) can be used to evaluate exocrine pancreatic function. Because they secrete very little chymotrypsin, dogs with EPI develop a negligible rise in the plasma level of PABA and excrete less than 15 per cent of orally administered PABA in six hours. The BT-PABA digestion test has been combined with the D-xylose absorption test for simultaneous evaluation of exocrine pancreatic function and intestinal absorptive function in dogs (Stradley et al, 1979; Rogers et al., 1980).

A vitamin B_{12} absorption (Schilling) test is used in human medicine when achlorhydria, intrinsic factor deficiency, or small intestinal disease (especially ileal disease or "stagnant loop" with bacterial overgrowth) is suspected. The procedure has been applied to dogs experimentally but has not yet found clinical application in small animal medicine (Merritt, 1980).

TESTS FOR INFECTIOUS DISEASES

Specific testing for infectious causes of intestinal disease includes bacterial and fungal cultures of feces, serologic testing for systemic mycoses, and virologic tests for specific enteroviruses. Considering that less than one per cent of enteric organisms are aerobic, the limitations of conventional aerobic bacterial culture of feces becomes apparent. Nonetheless, pathogenic organisms such as *Salmonella spp., Shigella spp., Campylobacter spp.,* and pathogenic strains of *Escherichia coli* can be isolated from feces using sophisticated microbiologic identification techniques. The clinical features of these bacterial infections will be discussed later. Feces can also be cultured for fungal organisms, such as *Histoplasma capsulatum* or *Candida spp.;* however, isolation attempts often fail. Serodiagnosis of systemic mycoses, especially histoplasmosis, is usually more rewarding. The agar gel precipitin (immunodiffusion) and complement fixation tests for systemic mycoses are preferred (see Chapter 26).

With the emerging importance of intestinal virus infections, there has been increasing use of the virology laboratory for diagnosis. Coronavirus, parvovirus, rotavirus, and astrovirus particles have been identified in diarrheic canine and feline feces with the use of electron microscopy (Appel et al., 1979a). Virus isolation and immunofluorescent-antibody techniques have also been used to detect enteric viruses. For canine parvovirus, a fecal hemagglutination (HA) test and a serum hemagglutination inhibition (HI) test have been developed (Carmichael et al., 1980). The diagnosis of these viruses is discussed further later in this chapter.

OTHER FECAL TESTS

Additional determinations that can be performed on feces include fecal electrolytes, osmolality, pH, and occult blood. The first three differentiate osmotic and secretory diarrhea. In osmotic diarrhea, because osmotically-active substances are retained in the gut lumen and feces, there is an osmol gap such that the calculated osmolality using fecal electrolytes (sum of Na^+ and K^+ concentrations multiplied by two) is much less than the actual measured osmolality of the fecal fluid. In purely secretory diarrhea, fecal osmolality is almost entirely accounted for by the fecal concentration of Na^+, K^+, and their anions, so that: $[Na^+ + K^+] \times 2$ approximates the actual fecal osmolality. The fecal pH in osmotic diarrhea is usually low because carbohydrate malabsorption acidifies colonic content (Krejs and Fordtran, 1978).

The commercial tests for detection of occult blood (Occultest, Hemoccult) are based on the peroxidase activity of blood releasing oxygen from hydrogen peroxide and thus oxidizing the chemicals orthotoluidine and benzidine to colored products (Strombeck, 1979). Guaiac has also been used as an indicator chemical but is less sensitive. Because of the sensitivity of these tests, it has been recommended that diets should not contain red meat for three days before testing for occult blood to avoid false positive results. The main indication to test feces for occult blood is when GI bleeding is suspected on the basis of hematologic changes (blood loss anemia) but cannot be demonstrated by grossly visible melena.

GASTROINTESTINAL RADIOGRAPHY

In the animal with diarrhea, radiography is usually performed for completeness so that the few causes of diarrhea that show radiographic changes will not be overlooked. An upper GI barium series should be considered when other tests fail to determine a cause for chronic diarrhea. Although it is generally of low diagnostic yield in most chronic diarrhea cases, upper GI barium studies have been helpful in detecting certain intestinal neoplastic, granulomatous, and chronic inflammatory diseases (Figs. 58–8 and 58–9). Other tests should be completed first, inasmuch as barium interferes with fecal cultures, finding protozoa on fecal smears, absorption tests, and proctoscopy. A thorough discussion of the radiographic diagnosis of canine and feline intestinal disorders is found elsewhere (O'Brien, 1978).

In the animal suspected of having a mechanical or obstructive disorder (foreign

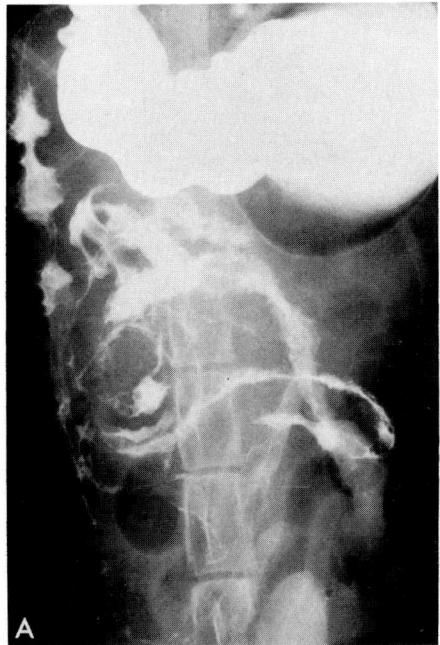

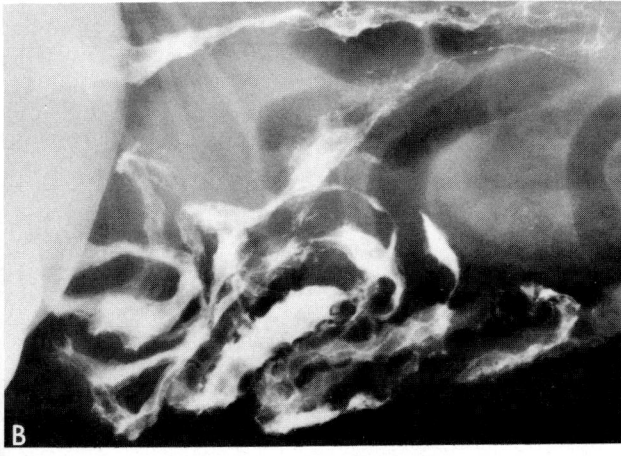

Figure 58–8. One hour after barium administration, ventrodorsal (*A*) and lateral (*B*) radiographs of the abdomen in this dog with chronic diarrhea showed diffuse mucosal irregularity and nodular infiltration throughout the duodenum and jejunum. These radiographic abnormalities prompted a small bowel biopsy, which confirmed diffuse intestinal lymphosarcoma.

body or intussusception), radiography often provides the diagnosis or at least sufficient information to support surgical intervention (Fig. 58–10).

GASTROINTESTINAL FIBEROPTIC ENDOSCOPY

Fiberoptic endoscopy (duodenoscopy) can be used for the visual inspection of the duodenum, duodenal aspiration (for culture, isolation of *Giardia,* and pancreatic response testing), and mucosal biopsy (Johnson et al., 1978; Johnson, 1980). Duodenoscopy in small animals is performed with the Olympus GIF-P or GIF-P$_2$ endoscope and an Olympus CLE halogen cold light source. The equipment expense and expertise required for duodenoscopy preclude its routine use except by referral

centers and veterinarians with special interest in gastrointestinal medicine. Animals are prepared, restrained, and positioned as described for gastroscopy in Chapter 57. The most challenging part of the procedure is advancing the endoscope tip through the pylorus. This may be facilitated by avoiding prior overdistention or manipulation of the stomach, both of which may increase pyloric tone. If advancement through the pylorus meets with difficulty, the pylorus may be relaxed with intravenous glucagon at 0.05 mg/kg body weight (not to exceed total dose of one mg) (Johnson, 1980). During the procedure, the animal's cardiovascular status should be carefully monitored for excessive vagal activity induced by the manipulation.

Accessory instruments can include polyethylene tubing for use through the endo-

Figure 58–9. Infiltrative disorders of the gut, such as chronic inflammatory diseases, may be detected radiographically. The barium study on this dog with chronic malabsorption due to lymphocytic-plasmacytic enteritis showed diffuse mucosal irregularity and ulceration.

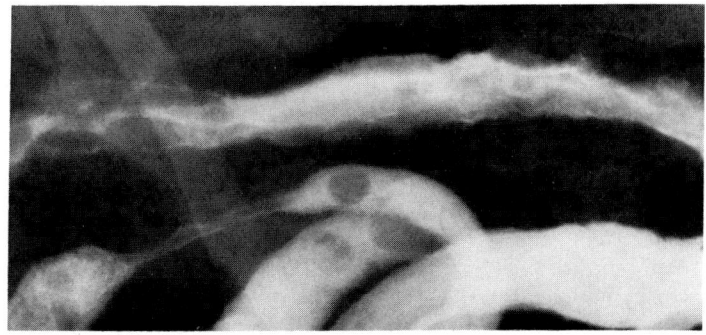

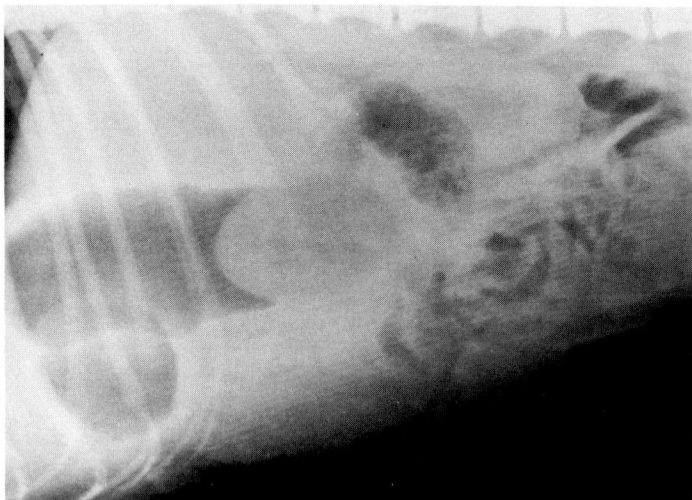

Figure 58–10. The radiographic delineation of a gas-distended gut loop associated with an egg-shaped intraluminal object in this vomiting dog suggested intestinal foreign body obstruction and provided the information needed to support surgical intervention. A foam rubber ball was removed from the small bowel.

scope biopsy channel for aspirations, endoscopic biopsy brush for cytology specimens, endoscopic biopsy forceps for passing down the endoscope biopsy channel for directed mucosal biopsy, and Quinton or Crosby-Kluger suction biopsy capsule for passage alongside the endoscope for biopsy of diffuse mucosal lesions.

MISCELLANEOUS SPECIALIZED TESTS

Other specialized tests are occasionally used at specialized facilities for the diagnosis of specific gastrointestinal disorders. Radiolabeled macromolecules may be used to document leakage of plasma proteins into the bowel. In the dog, ^{51}Cr-labeled albumin at a dose of 1.47 μCi/kg, IV, has been shown to be effective for this purpose (Finco et al., 1973). The normal dog excretes < two per cent of an IV dose into the feces in three days, whereas the dog with protein-losing enteropathy will lose a greater amount of the radiolabeled protein. The disadvantages of handling and analyzing radioactive material limit the usefulness of this procedure.

Another specialized procedure is the assay of specific mucosal enzymes in intestinal mucosal biopsies, especially the brush border enzymes (disaccharidases). Values for numerous mucosal enzymes have been determined for healthy canine jejunal mucosa obtained via peroral suction biopsy (Batt and Peters, 1978). Presently these assays are largely used in research; however, future clinical applications seem likely. Mucosal enzyme assays have been performed on dogs with EPI (Batt et al., 1979b).

Much of the knowledge regarding GI endocrinology obtained through radioimmunoassay (RIA) has been learned from the canine model; thus, normal values for many GI hormones are available for the dog. Although these assays are currently only available through specialized medical research centers, RIA of plasma gastrin, for example, has aided in the diagnosis of canine gastrinoma (Zollinger-Ellison syndrome) (Straus et al., 1977).

Specialized testing is available for measuring pancreatic secretory function. The most direct method for assessing exocrine function of the pancreas is by analysis of pancreatic secretion obtained by a pancreatic duct cannula or duodenal probe after intravenous infusion of the pancreatic stimulatory hormones, cholecystokinin (CCK) and secretin (Sateri, 1975; Arvanitakis and Cooke, 1978). Information can be obtained regarding the volume, bicarbonate content, and enzyme content of stimulated pancreatic secretion, all of which may be impaired in the dog with EPI. Under most circumstances, however, this approach is too impractical for clinical application.

INTESTINAL BIOPSY

Definitive diagnosis of intestinal malabsorptive diseases is usually best accomplished by exploratory laparotomy, with inspection and biopsy of the small bowel and the mesenteric lymph nodes. Biopsies should be taken even if there are no lesions visible by gross inspection. Other abdominal organs, especially the pancreas, liver, and colon, should also be evaluated during laparotomy. Duodenal aspirates or duodenal mucosal impression smears may be examined for *Giardia* or cultured for bacteria. It should be noted that healing of surgical wounds may be impaired in animals with severe hypoproteinemia. In cases in which diffuse mucosal lesions are suspected, alternatives to laparotomy with full-thickness intestinal biopsy are mucosal biopsy via duodenoscopy (Johnson, 1980) or peroral mucosal biopsy with a suction biopsy capsule (Batt et al., 1976; Batt et al., 1979c).

It should be emphasized that colonoscopic biopsy of the colon may be useful in the diagnosis of certain generalized enteric diseases (enterocolitis), such as inflammatory disease (eosinophilic enterocolitis), protothecosis, histoplasmosis, and diffuse intestinal lymphosarcoma, which can affect both small and large bowel. Colon biopsy can be diagnostic, even though the majority of signs may be of small bowel origin. Thus, when diseases of this nature are suspected, a colonoscopic biopsy of the colon may be as diagnostic as a surgical biopsy of the small intestine taken via laparotomy, yet it is easier and of much less risk to the animal (see Chapter 59 for discussion of colonoscopy).

RESPONSE TO THERAPY

Response to therapy is a valid means of confirming certain diagnoses, when backed up with sufficient supportive evidence. Trial and error test diets, for example, are commonly used to exclude dietary intolerance to certain food, most notably for milk intolerance. In EPI, the diagnosis is usually confirmed by response to pancreatic enzyme replacement. Response to antibacterial therapy is often a practical method for confirming a bacterial overgrowth phenomenon. Other examples are mentioned later as specific intestinal disorders are discussed.

ACUTE DIARRHEA

ACUTE DIARRHEA IN PERSPECTIVE

The categorization of diarrhea as acute or chronic is a clinically useful method of classification. Chronic diarrheas may be thought of as protracted or recurrent diarrheal illnesses that require an in-depth approach to diagnosis. Acute diarrheas have an abrupt onset and a short clinical course

that ranges from transient and self-limiting to fulminating and explosive. In acute diarrhea, the elaborate gastrointestinal function testing used for chronic diarrhea is usually not necessary. It should be emphasized that for some enteric diseases, such as parasitism, this categorization is somewhat arbitrary, because such diseases may be acute or chronic depending on the animal and individual circumstances.

It is convenient to further separate acute diarrhea into (1) nonfatal, self-limiting acute diarrhea, (2) acute diarrhea resulting from a systemic or extraintestinal disorder, and (3) severe, fulminating, potentially life-threatening acute diarrhea. The clinician must be able to recognize and distinguish these different categories in order to facilitate decisions regarding the need for hospitalization as opposed to outpatient management; simple conservative medical treatment of self-limiting diarrhea versus intensive emergency treatment, particularly of fluid, electrolyte, and acid-base imbalances that are consequences of severe diarrhea; nonspecific antidiarrheal therapy versus specific therapeutic measures; treatment of an underlying nonenteric disorder, the diarrhea being of only secondary importance; and possible surgical intervention.

Causes of Acute Diarrhea

Common causes of nonfatal or self-limiting acute diarrhea include simple (uncomplicated) parasitism, dietary indiscretions or intolerances, and drug or toxin-induced diarrhea. Intestinal parasites, which are discussed in detail later in this section, are diagnosed by fecal examination (flotations, direct smears), visual inspection of feces (tapeworm proglottids, roundworms), or a presumptive history, and are treated with specific parasiticides. Dietary causes of diarrhea are numerous. These include intestinal overload from overeating, ingestion of spoiled foods from scavenging of decomposing garbage or carrion, ingestion of indigestible and abrasive foreign material (e.g., bones, stones, hair, plants, wood, cloth, plastic), intolerance of lactose ingested as milk, and miscellaneous food intolerances, such as fatty or spicy foods. These causes of diarrhea are often identified by careful history-taking or by institution of a controlled diet. Dietary diarrheas are self-limiting with dietary restriction, i.e., prevention of dietary indiscretion or elimination of the offending dietary substance. Food allergy as a cause of diarrhea is poorly defined in small animals and has been used to loosely refer to nonspecific food intolerances (Povar, 1947; Knowles, 1966; Michaux, 1966).

Nonfatal acute diarrhea in small animals is also commonly caused by chemicals, either as a side effect from therapeutic drugs or as an effect from environmental (exogenous) toxins. The potential to induce diarrhea by an adverse effect on normal microflora is a common property of most antibacterial drugs. In addition, an individual sensitivity or intolerance to almost any other therapeutic agent administered to an animal may be manifested as diarrhea. Some examples of drugs that commonly cause diarrhea are corticosteroids, nonsteroidal antiinflammatory agents (aspirin, indomethacin), digitalis and many other cardiac drugs, dithiazanine (Dizan), magnesium-containing antacids, antiparasitic drugs, and most anticancer drugs. Drug-induced diarrhea usually resolves after discontinuing the offending drug or reducing its dosage.

Various exogenous toxins cause a diarrhea that is usually self-limiting with nonspecific therapy and elimination of the toxin. Examples of diarrheogenic toxins are lead, arsenic, organophosphates (including dips and flea collars), other chemical dips, lawn and garden products (herbicides, fungicides, insecticides), house plants, and contaminated stagnant or run-off water. Vomiting with or preceding chemical-induced diarrhea is common. Some of these chemicals also produce dramatic extraintestinal signs (e.g., neurologic dysfunction in lead or organophosphate poisoning) and therefore are discussed elsewhere in this book. Generally, toxin-induced diarrhea is suspected on the basis of exposure history, clinical signs, and exclusion of other causes of acute diarrhea.

Acute diarrheas that occur secondary to systemic disorders, especially infectious diseases (canine distemper, leptospirosis) or metabolic diseases (uremia, hypoadrenocorticism), require no specific workup for the diarrhea component. Since this category of diarrhea is a manifestation of an obvious extraintestinal disease, therapy is aimed at that underlying disease, the diarrhea only warranting symptomatic treatment.

The category of severe, fulminating acute diarrhea that is potentially life-threatening is most often caused by (1) infectious diseases, especially enteric viruses, but occasionally bacteria such as *Salmonella spp.*; (2) severe intestinal parasitism, particularly in neonates; (3) hemorrhagic gastroenteritis syndrome (HGE); and (4) mechanical disorders with intestinal obstruction (intestinal foreign body, intussusception, and volvulus). Mechanical disorders are discussed under Intestinal Obstruction at the end of the chapter. The diagnosis of fulminating viral enteritis is usually suspected on clinical signs and exposure history, and confirmed by virologic-serologic testing. HGE is recognized by clinical signs plus the demonstration of profound hemoconcentration on a CBC. Radiography is generally helpful in mechanical-obstructive diseases.

Diagnosis of Acute Diarrhea

This is usually based on information obtained by history and physical examination, often without detailed diagnostic workup. A review of the animal's vaccination status, diet, current medications, and possible exposure to toxins or infectious diseases is essential. Parasites should always be considered a possible cause of acute diarrhea until proven otherwise. Diagnostic efforts should also be directed toward detection of underlying nonenteric diseases that could be a cause of acute diarrhea. Acute diarrheas recognized as nonfulminating or non–life-threatening are common, especially in the young animal, and are usually managed on an outpatient basis with symptomatic therapy, sometimes in the absence of a definitive etiology. Diagnostic evaluations that should be considered in acute diarrhea are fecal identification of parasites, fecal cultures for *Salmonella*, and radiography for detection of GI obstruction. Specific virologic tests are increasingly being used to diagnose enteric viral infections. Particularly helpful to successful treatment in the serious acute diarrheas are initial evaluation and continual monitoring of fluid, electrolyte, and acid-base status by means of analysis of hematocrit, total plasma protein, serum electrolytes, and blood gases.

Nonspecific, Symptomatic Treatment of Acute Diarrhea

Many animals with acute diarrhea improve spontaneously in a day or two without any treatment, suggesting that treatment may not always be indicated. General treatment measures to be considered (Table 58–5) include maintenance of fluid, electrolyte, and acid-base homeostasis; symptomatic antidiarrheal therapy with drugs that affect GI motility; symptomatic antidiarrheal therapy with drugs that act locally within the lumen (protectorants); dietary restriction; and antibacterial drugs (DuPont, 1978; Strombeck, 1979).

Since the cause of death in severe, acute diarrhea is usually dehydration and intravascular volume contraction, replacement of fluid and electrolytes is an essential aspect of therapy. Parenteral fluid therapy is appropriate in most cases. Orally-administered glucose (or sucrose) electrolyte solutions have been used successfully to treat dehydrating diarrhea in humans, based on the observation that glucose facilitates the intestinal absorption of sodium and water. These oral glucose solutions are espe-

Table 58–5. **Symptomatic Treatment of Acute Diarrhea**

1. Maintenance of fluid, electrolyte, acid-base homeostasis
   a. Parenteral fluid therapy
   b. Oral glucose-electrolyte solutions (Pedialyte, Gatorade)
2. Drugs that alter intestinal motility
   a. Opiates
      1) Diphenoxylate (Lomotil)
      2) Loperamide (Imodium)
      3) Paregoric
   b. Anticholinergics-Antispasmodics (less effective than opiates)
3. Drugs that act locally in the lumen (adsorbents/protectorants—efficacy unproven)
   a. Kaolin-pectin (1–2 ml/kg, q.i.d.)
   b. Aluminum hydroxide (10–30 ml, q.i.d.)
   c. Magnesium trisilicate (10–30 ml, q.i.d.)
   d. Bismuth (10–30 ml, q.i.d.)
   e. Activated charcoal (0.3–5.0 gm, t.i.d.)
   f. Barium sulfate
4. Bismuth subsalicylate (Pepto-Bismol, 10–30 ml, q.i.d.) (proposed actions: protectorant, antisecretory, antienterotoxin, antiprostaglandin, antibacterial)
5. Dietary restriction
   a. Initially withhold food (12 to 24 hr. GI rest)
   b. Then give small, bland, low-fat meals
      1) i/d or r/d Prescription Diets
      2) Boiled rice, tapioca, potatoes, or macaroni combined with cooked lean meat, eggs, or cottage cheese
6. Antibiotics
   a. Used only for bacterial diarrhea
   b. Alteration of normal flora may be detrimental

cially useful in secretory diarrheas in which the absorptive capacity of the intestinal mucosa remains intact. By exploiting the intact absorptive capacity of the gut, enhanced absorption of fluid and electrolytes counterbalances losses from hypersecretion (Palmer et al., 1977; DuPont, 1978; Moon, 1978). A commercially prepared oral glucose-electrolyte solution (Pedialyte) is available for the treatment of infant diarrhea and should be evaluated for oral diarrhea replacement therapy in small animals.

To understand how drugs affect motility, it should be remembered that intestinal motor activity consists of two basic types, propulsive (peristalsis) and nonpropulsive (segmentation) movements. Increased propulsive activity is not a prerequisite for diarrhea. In fact, in some diarrheal states, loss of nonpropulsive motility resulting in a flaccid intestine is thought to be more important (Strombeck, 1979). This open pipe effect offers very little resistance to flow, so that there is unimpeded movement of bowel content through the intestine. The ideal motility modifier should theoretically decrease propulsive activity and increase the resistance to flow by stimulating nonpropulsive activity. Unfortunately, drugs such as anticholinergics, which are commonly used in antidiarrheal therapy, reduce peristalsis at the expense of segmentation. These agents cause a generalized reduction of motility, so that the flow of intestinal content is uninhibited. This may limit the usefulness of anticholinergics as motility modifiers. In contrast, narcotic analgesics, such as paregoric, diphenoxylate, and loperamide (and other members of the opiate family, such as codeine, morphine, meperidine), are motility modifiers that are effective in treating diarrhea, because they delay bowel transit by increasing nonpropulsive contractions and muscular tone of the gut while decreasing propulsive activity (Plant and Miller, 1926; Vaughan Williams, 1954; Galambos et al., 1976; Pelemans and Vantrappen, 1976). Opiates may have an adverse effect on diarrhea caused by invasive bacteria such as *Salmonella,* and thus the use of these agents should be restricted when such pathogens are suspected (DuPont and Hornick, 1973; DuPont, 1978).

The antidiarrheal action of opiates may be more than just motility modification. Opiate drugs have been observed to reduce intestinal fluid accumulation, stool frequency, and stool weight (volume). Recently, evidence has suggested that opiates influence water and electrolyte transport by the intestine, leading to speculation that such a mechanism may contribute to the antidiarrheal activity of opiates. This would agree with the current concept of the pathophysiology of diarrhea in which the most important role is played by the mucosa (water and electrolyte transport) and not the muscle (motility) (McKay et al., 1981; Powell, 1981).

Protectorants are often used as locally-acting symptomatic antidiarrheal therapy because of their ability to adsorb bacteria and toxins and their protective coating action on inflamed or ulcerated mucosal surfaces. Examples of protectorants include kaolin-pectin, bismuth, magnesium trisilicate, aluminum hydroxide, activated charcoal, and barium sulfate. Documentation of the efficacy of these agents as antidiarrheals is limited. They are widely accepted as among the safest of therapeutic agents; recently, however, it has been cautioned that kaolin-pectin may increase fecal salt loss during diarrhea (McClung et al., 1980).

A commercial preparation of bismuth subsalicylate (Pepto-Bismol) has been shown to provide effective antidiarrheal therapy for certain enterotoxigenic E. coli infections in man (traveler's diarrhea), presumably by inhibiting the intestinal secretion of fluid and electrolytes (DuPont, 1978). In addition to its antisecretory effect, bismuth subsalicylate may prevent mucosal attachment or colonization by bacteria (DuPont et al., 1980), and it relieves the symptoms of viral gastroenteritis (Steinhoff et al., 1980). Suggested mechanisms of action include antienterotoxin, antibacterial, antiprostaglandin (by the salicylate moiety), and neuromuscular effects. Further evaluation will likely establish a role for bismuth subsalicylate in the treatment of diarrhea in small animals.

The initial aim of dietary management of acute diarrhea is to rest the GI tract by withholding food for 24 hours or more. When feeding is resumed, small bland meals are fed frequently to facilitate assimilation, and the diet should consist of mainly protein and carbohydrate with minimal fat. Well-tolerated foods include boiled rice or potatoes combined with cooked lean meat, eggs, or cottage cheese. The diet is gradually converted to regular commercial pet food once the diarrhea resolves.

Antibacterials are often used empirically in the treatment of diarrhea for purposes of eliminating pathogens or microflora that might be invading the mucosa. The benefits of antibacterial therapy must be weighed against the potentially adverse effects on normal intestinal microflora. The use and risks of antibiotics in the animal with diarrhea are discussed further under Bacterial Diarrhea. A preparation of *Lactobacillus* has been used in the treatment of diarrhea to recolonize the intestine with a flora that will ferment carbohydrate and acidify the lumen to deter enteropathogens. The efficacy of this agent in altering the microflora or relieving diarrhea has not been substantiated (DuPont, 1978).

BACTERIAL DIARRHEA

The normal flora consists of hundreds of different species of bacteria that inhabit the GI tract in a symbiotic relationship with the animal (Strombeck, 1979; Hirsh, 1980). Each location along the GI tract has its own stable population of microorganisms; the numbers and types of bacteria, however, vary from site to site. At birth, the GI tract is sterile, but shortly thereafter a microflora becomes established in the newborn (Smith, 1965). The most abundant enteric microorganisms in the dog and cat are *Bacteroides spp.*, *Escherichia coli*, *Clostridium perfringens*, enterococci, lactobacilli, and *Fusobacterium spp.* The normal canine small intestine contains up to 10^6 or 10^7 microbes per gram of contents, whereas the colon contains about 10^{11} organisms per gram of feces. Anaerobes outnumber aerobes by 1000 to 1 (Strombeck, 1979).

Factors that influence or regulate this stable microflora include diet, bacterial interactions (including mutual competition for nutrients and the effects of bacterial metabolic byproducts on other bacteria), luminal pH, amount of available oxygen within the lumen, and host factors (gastric acid, bile salts, intestinal motility, and characteristics of the mucosal surface) (Strombeck, 1979; Hirsh, 1980).

The normal microflora act as an important defense barrier against pathogens by preventing colonization through competition for mucosal attachment sites, or by creating an environment that is hostile for pathogens. Hence, it follows that any disruption of the normal host-flora ecosystem weakens this defense barrier and may provide easier access for pathogens. The microflora can be adversely affected by several mechanisms, and alteration of the flora can be a cause or consequence of intestinal disease. Diarrhea itself can disrupt the normal flora (Gorbach et al., 1970). Malnutrition and stress may alter the microflora and allow intestinal colonization by pathogens (Strombeck, 1979). The cleansing action of normal intestinal motility prevents the overmultiplication of bacteria in any section of gut, so a consequence of impaired motility (gut stasis) is the overgrowth of colonic-type flora in the cranial small intestine (Drasar and Shiner, 1969) (discussed later in the chapter). Antimicrobial agents can be especially detrimental to the normal microflora, enabling intestinal colonization by pathogens. In addition, antibacterials usually suppress some strains of intestinal bacteria more than others, so that nonsusceptible microorganisms are given a competitive edge for mucosal attachment sites and their numbers increase disproportionately. Bacterial or fungal overgrowth may then result in serious illness (Hirsh, 1980). These effects have important implications for the indiscriminate use of antibacterials in treating diarrhea. During most diarrheas the microflora is probably compromised, and antibiotics may interfere with the return of the flora to normal, encourage the development of resistant strains, and facilitate secondary opportunistic invasion by enteropathogens or overproliferated normal flora (Strombeck, 1979; Hirsh, 1980).

Bacteria that attach to the mucosal surface, multiply there, and cause disease are called enteropathogenic. Enteropathogenic bacteria produce intestinal disease either by invading the epithelium (invasive bacteria) or by remaining attached to the epithelium without penetrating it and liberating an enterotoxin (noninvasive or enterotoxigenic bacteria). In addition, some invasive strains may produce systemic infection (septicemia), as well as intestinal infection, by invading the submucosa and entering lymphatics and the blood stream. Bacteria capable of invading the mucosal barrier include *Salmonella spp.*, *shigella spp.*, *Campylobacter*, and invasive *E. coli*. Numerous other pathogenic bacteria are known to produce diarrhea through the release of toxins, including toxigenic *E. coli*, *Clostridium spp.*, *Klebsiella spp.*, *Salmonella spp.*, *Vibrio cholerae*, staphylo-

cocci, and probably others. Many of these enterotoxigenic bacteria produce diarrhea by a secretory mechanism that is mediated by the adenyl cyclase–cAMP mechanism.

The role of enteropathogenic bacteria in canine and feline diarrhea is poorly understood. Potential bacterial enteropathogens harbored by dogs and cats, not all of which have been definitely linked with clinical disease, include enteropathogenic *E. coli*, *Salmonella spp.*, *Yersinia enterocolitica*, *Campylobacter jejuni*, *Bacillus piliformis* (Tyzzer's disease), *Clostridium spp.*, staphylococci, and *Shigella spp.* (Table 58–6). Some of these agents are also human pathogens, and there is considerable interest in the dog as a reservoir for human infection, particularly for *Salmonella*, *Yersinia*, and *Campylobacter*. Hopefully, the recognition and understanding of bacterial diarrheas in small animals will improve with the further development and availability of sophisticated microbiologic techniques.

Escherichia coli

The significance of *E. coli* as a primary intestinal pathogen in small animals is especially unclear, because *E. coli* is a component of the normal resident flora of both the small and large bowel. Therefore, isolation of *E. coli* from the feces or intestine of the dog or cat is not in itself significant. To

Table 58–6. Enteric Pathogens of Dogs and Cats

Viral
  Coronavirus
  Parvovirus
  Rotavirus
  Astrovirus and others*
Bacterial
  Enteropathogenic *E. coli**
  Salmonella spp.
  Yersinia enterocolitica
  Campylobacter jejuni
  Bacillus piliformis (Tyzzer's disease)
  *Clostridium spp.**
Rickettsial (Salmon Poisoning)
  Neorickettsia helminthoeca
  Elokomin fluke fever agent
Mycotic
  Histoplasma capsulatum
  Aspergillus spp.
  Candida albicans
  Phycomycetes
Other — Prototheca (algae)

*Pathogenicity in dogs and cats is likely but not yet proven.

determine pathogenicity, sophisticated inoculation studies should be performed to differentiate invasive or enterotoxigenic *E. coli* from nonpathogenic *E. coli*. Serotyping is also used, but is considered to be a less reliable method of indicating enteropathogenicity (Echeverria et al., 1976). In inoculation studies, invasive *E. coli* are identified by their ability to induce conjunctivitis within 24 hours after application to the eye of a guinea pig (Sereny test) (Formal et al., 1978), while enterotoxigenic E. coli are identified by the effect of their toxins on inoculated tissue cultures (*in vitro* assay) or gut loops (or other similar *in vivo* assays) (Thorne and Gorbach, 1978; Merritt and Reed, 1980). Also, radioimmunoassay (RIA) and enzyme-linked immunosorbent assay (ELISA) have been used to detect enterotoxin. Unfortunately, definitive studies such as these have not been reported on isolates from naturally-occurring cases of diarrhea in small animals, although the enterotoxin of *E. coli* isolated from a human patient with secretory diarrhea was shown to stimulate adenyl cyclase activity and fluid secretion by canine jejunum (Guerrant et al., 1973). Nevertheless, some authors regard *E. coli* as the most common bacterial cause of diarrhea in dogs, causing profuse watery or sometimes bloody acute diarrhea, especially in young animals (Anderson, 1975; Buckner, 1979). In early studies, hemolytic strains of *E. coli* were considered potential pathogens that could be frequently isolated from normal dogs as well as from cases of fatal hemorrhagic gastroenteritis (Osborne, 1967). In one report, an endemic coliform enteritis in a highly inbred basenji colony was described (Fox et al., 1965).

Salmonella

Salmonella spp. are frequently isolated from the feces of normal dogs and cats, but clinical signs of salmonellosis are uncommon, indicating a prevalent asymptomatic carrier state. Numerous culture surveys of *Salmonella* infection in apparently healthy dogs in the U.S. and foreign countries have been reported; the prevalence in the U.S. canine population has been estimated at ten per cent, but fecal carrier rates in some areas reach 15 to 20 per cent or higher (Morse and Duncan, 1975). Isolation prevalence in cats has generally been lower, ranging from 0.5 per cent to 13.6 per cent (Shimi

and Barin, 1977; Fox, 1980). Many different serotypes have been isolated from the dog and cat. The public health significance of *Salmonella* infection in pets is emphasized by documented reports of animal-to-human transmission (Kaufman, 1966; Morse and Duncan, 1975; Morse et al., 1976). Salmonellosis is transmitted by the fecal-oral route and through contaminated food.

Clinical salmonellosis, when it does occur, causes clinical signs of acute diarrhea (sometimes containing blood or mucus), vomiting, fever, anorexia, depression, abdominal pain, and progressive dehydration. If the infection is limited to mucosal invasion, the lesions are disrupted and inflammation of the mucosa (acute enterocolitis) is often accompanied by mesenteric lymphadenitis. In overwhelming Salmonella infection, acute enterocolitis and rapidly fatal bacteremia may develop, resulting in widespread lesions of septicemia and disseminated intravascular coagulation (DIC) (Krum et al., 1977). Although *Salmonella spp.* are thought of as highly invasive enteric pathogens, evidence suggests that they also produce diarrhea through a secretory mechanism, mediated by prostaglandins or toxins (Giannella et al., 1975).

The clinical disease occurs primarily in young or debilitated animals. Susceptibility is increased by overcrowded or unsanitary kennel conditions, any stressful event (such as shipment or surgery), immunosuppression, or the use of oral antibiotics that upset the normal microflora (Merritt, 1980). Occasionally epizootics of clinical salmonellosis are seen. One such outbreak of *S. typhimurium* affecting cats admitted to a veterinary hospital was associated with a morbidity of 32 per cent and high mortality (61 per cent) (Timoney, 1978). A similar epizootic of *S. agona* affected dogs in the author's institutional practice, with the highest morbidity and mortality occurring in postsurgical animals and dogs in the intensive care unit. This prevalence in debilitated and heavily stressed animals emphasizes the opportunistic nature of the disease.

The use of antibacterials in the treatment of salmonellosis is a confusing and controversial issue (Strombeck, 1979; Merritt, 1980). *Salmonella* invasion confined to the mucosa produces a self-limiting gastroenteritis, the course of which is not likely to be affected by antibacterials. This is possible because the organisms reside within macrophages, where they are somewhat out of reach of antibiotics. In addition, antibacterials may prolong the shedding of organisms and increase the chances of a prolonged carrier state. The use of orally-administered nonabsorbable antibiotics is especially discouraged (Merritt, 1980). Antibiotics are also not reliably effective in eliminating the *Salmonella* carrier state. Notwithstanding these limitations, if *Salmonella* invasion severely disrupts mucosal integrity, causing severe dehydrating diarrheal illness, and especially if bacteremia is suspected or impending, antibacterials should be given. The choice of an antibacterial should be based on culture and sensitivity testing; however, chloramphenicol, gentamicin, and trimethoprim-sulfa are often effective. In severe cases, fluid and electrolyte replacement and nutritional management are important.

Yersinia

Yersinia enterocolitica, a gram-negative rod (previously called *Pasteurella pseudotuberculosis* and *Bacterium enterocoliticum*) has been recognized worldwide with increasing frequency as a cause of acute or chronic enterocolitis with diarrhea (dysentery) and fever in humans (Vantrappen et al., 1977), and has been isolated from dogs and cats (Pedersen, 1976; Kaneko et al., 1977; Yanagawa et al., 1978; Pedersen and Winblad, 1979; Wooley et al., 1980). *Yersinia* infection of dogs may be a public health problem (Wilson et al., 1976). Specialized isolation methods are needed to culture the organism from feces. *Yersinia* is usually susceptible to tetracycline, chloramphenicol, streptomycin, and kanamycin; however, culture and antibiotic sensitivity testing is recommended.

Campylobacter

Campylobacter jejuni, motile, fastidious, microaerophilic bacteria (gram-negative curved or spiral rods), which have emerged as important enteric pathogens in humans (Skirrow, 1977; Price et al., 1979; Willoughby et al., 1979; Blaser et al., 1980a), have been isolated from normal dogs and cats, from dogs with diarrhea, and from a dog with fatal hemorrhagic gastroenteritis (Skirrow, 1977; Blaser et al., 1978; Hastings, 1978; Hosie et al., 1979; Slee, 1979; Blaser, 1980b; Fleming, 1980, Bruce et al., 1980).

In addition, dogs and cats, especially puppies with diarrhea, are implicated as sources of human infection (Blaser et al., 1980b). Isolation rates have varied widely from study to study but range from less than five per cent to as high as 75 per cent in puppies, 50 per cent in mature dogs, and ten per cent in cats, with the highest prevalence in young animals with diarrhea (Bruce et al., 1980). The organism is tissue invasive, causing acute enterocolitis and sometimes bacteremia. At the author's institution, *Campylobacter* has also been found as a secondary invader in dogs with canine parvovirus infection and salmonellosis, similar to findings in kenneled dogs with diarrhea studied in Great Britain (Fleming, 1980). The diagnosis of campylobacteriosis depends upon isolation of the organism from feces, using a special selective media (Skirrow, 1977). Erythromycin is often used in treating human infection, and often sensitivity tests also show susceptibility to clindamycin, gentamicin, and chloramphenicol.

Bacillus piliformis

Tyzzer's disease, caused by a pleomorphic, gram-negative, spore-forming bacillus called *Bacillus piliformis,* is a rare but fatal disease characterized by chronic hemorrhagic or necrotizing enterocolitis with diarrhea and multifocal hepatic necrosis (Kovatch and Zebarth, 1973; Kubokawa, 1973; Poonacha and Smith, 1976, Qureshi et al., 1976). Tyzzer's disease affects young puppies and kittens most often, but not exclusively. In puppies, the disease may complicate canine distemper or parasitism; in the cat, the signs and lesions are very similar to feline panleukopenia. Rodents are the principal reservoir of *Bacillus piliformis.* Diagnosis of the disease is difficult, since the organism cannot be cultured on the usual artificial media. Instead, typical intracellular (obligate) filamentous bacilli are demonstrated at the margins of necrotic foci within liver and intestine by special stains such as methenamine silver, Giemsa, and PAS.

Clostridia

Pseudomembranous colitis, a severe form of colitis in man, has been attributed to an overgrowth of toxin-producing *Clostridium spp.,* especially *Clostridium difficile,* in the colon subsequent to antimicrobial-induced suppression of the normal flora (especially by clindamycin, lincomycin, ampicillin, and cephalosporins) (Bartlett et al., 1978). The infection is usually treated orally with vancomycin, although metronidazole, bacitracin, and tetracycline also may be effective (George et al., 1980). A similar clindamycin-associated pseudomembranous colitis in the dog was recently described (Burrows, 1980). Further study is likely to establish a role for toxin-producing *Clostridia* in antibiotic-associated diarrheas of small animals.

Peracute, necrotizing hemorrhagic enteritis that was fatal in two dogs was attributed to large numbers of *Clostridium perfringens (welchii)* found in the intestinal mucosa at necropsy (Prescott et al., 1978). Comparison was made with clostridial toxin-induced enteropathies of food-producing animals. *C. perfringens* is part of the normal microflora in the dog.

Other Bacteria

Staphylococcal food poisoning in man is caused by ingestion of an enterotoxin produced by staphylococci. This may also be a cause of vomiting and diarrhea in the dog (Anderson, 1975). In Japan, canine enterotoxigenic staphylococci were isolated from the bowel of 26 (5.8 per cent) of 451 dogs (Kato et al., 1978).

Shigella spp. are invasive enteropathogenic bacteria that cause a *Salmonella*-like dysentery in primates. Although occasionally isolated from canine feces (Butler and Herd, 1965), clinical disease or diarrhea has not been linked to *Shigella* in small animals

Other bacteria such as *Proteus spp.* and spirochetes were once thought to cause diarrhea in the dog (Craige, 1948). *Proteus spp.*, however, are normal inhabitants of the canine bowel and appear to lack enteropathogenicity. Spirochetes are now known to be normal inhabitants of colonic crypts (Pindak et al., 1965; Turek and Meyer, 1977; Turek and Meyer, 1978). Diarrhea of any cause apparently dislodges spirochetes from the crypts and increases their numbers in the feces (Strombeck, 1979). However, there is no direct evidence that spirochetes themselves cause diarrhea.

VIRAL DIARRHEA

During the last decade, numerous viruses have been discovered in canine and feline feces by either virus cultivation in cell culture or electron microscopy (EM). Since several of these viruses are frequently found in normal feces as well as in feces from animals with diarrhea, their role as potential pathogens that cause gastroenteritis needs to be determined (see Table 58–6).

In the dog, these viruses include the "minute virus" isolated from normal dogs in 1970 by Binn et al. (now known to be a parvovirus that is distinct from the enteritis-producing parvovirus), canine coronavirus (Keenan et al., 1976), canine parvovirus (cause of parvoviral enteritis) (Appel et al., 1978), canine rotavirus (England and Poston, 1980), astrovirus (Williams, 1980), paramyxo-like virus, adenovirus, and picornavirus (Appel et al., 1979a). In addition, human "ECHO" and coxsackie-viruses have been isolated from canine feces (Pindak, 1964; Lundgren et al., 1968). Of these, canine coronavirus, parvovirus, and possibly rotavirus and astrovirus are presently known to be clinically important causes of viral enteritis and diarrhea in the dog. Canine distemper virus can also cause diarrhea.

In the cat, the most clinically important primary enteric virus is the parvovirus, feline panleukopenia virus (FPV). Diarrhea in the cat has also been attributed to enteric coronavirus (Pedersen et al., 1981), rotavirus (Snodgrass, 1979), and astrovirus (Hoshino et al., 1981). In addition to these, other viruses of uncertain importance as enteric pathogens that were found by EM screening of 185 feline fecal samples includes calicivirus, reovirus Type III, and noncultivable enteric picornaviridae-like virus (Hoshino et al., 1981). Also in the cat, the intestine may be involved as part of generalized viral infection due to either feline leukemia virus (FeLV) or feline infectious peritonitis (FIP coronavirus). A panleukopenia-like syndrome characterized by severe enterocolitis has been associated with FeLV infection (although the virus may not be a direct cause of the lesion), while in FIP, pyogranulomatous enteritis or serositis may occur (Fig. 58–11). Canine and feline viral diseases are discussed in detail in Chapter 27; however, pertinent aspects of those with primary intestinal involvement will be briefly described here.

Canine Coronavirus

Canine coronavirus (CCV) is an acute contagious enteritis of dogs caused by an epitheliotropic enteric virus that induces

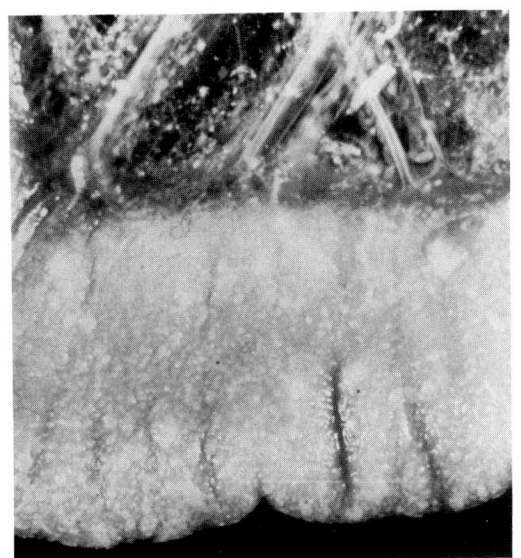

Figure 58–11. Pyogranulomatous serositis and enteritis in a kitten with feline infectious peritonitis (FIP). Notice the granular fibrinous deposits on the serosa and mesentery.

villous destruction, atrophy, and fusion, leading to malabsorption and diarrhea (Keenan et al., 1976; Appel et al., 1978; Appel et al., 1979a; Pollock, 1979). Clinical features of CCV are anorexia and depression followed by vomiting and diarrhea. Vomiting may precede diarrhea by a few hours or begin simultaneously with diarrhea. The diarrhea may be mushy or watery, may be yellowish-orange in color or overtly bloody, may contain mucus, and usually has a very offensive fetid odor. Most dogs infected with CCV are afebrile.

The incubation period is 24 to 72 hours experimentally, and virus shedding may persist for a few weeks after recovery. Deaths are uncommon, although fatalities have been reported. Young puppies may die within 48 hours of first developing signs. Most animals, however, recover in seven to ten days, or earlier with treatment. Some dogs show persistent refractory diarrhea for three to four weeks.

The diagnosis of CCV is based on clinical signs, exposure history, the absence of leukopenia (to help distinguish CCV from CPV), demonstration of virus in feces (electron microscopy, virus isolation, immunofluorescent testing), or serologic testing (indirect fluorescent antibody test [IFA], serum neutralizing antibody). Treatment of CCV consists of fluid therapy and symptomatic treatment.

Feline Coronavirus

Recently, a feline enteric coronavirus was described that is antigenically related to, but distinctly different from, the FIP coronavirus and the canine coronavirus (Pedersen et al., 1981). The virus is shed in the feces of many asymptomatic, seropositive cats, and may be ubiquitous in the cat population. Thus, inapparent infection is frequent; in catteries, however, infection may cause enteritis and diarrhea, especially in kittens 6 to 12 weeks of age. Like enteric coronaviruses in other species, the feline enteric coronavirus induces villous atrophy because of an affinity for the villous tip epithelium.

Canine Parvovirus

Canine parvovirus (CPV) is an acute, highly contagious enteritis of dogs caused by an epitheliotropic enteric virus with an affinity for rapidly dividing cells (intestinal, bone marrow, lymphoid), thereby causing leukopenia and intestinal crypt aplasia that leads to intestinal mucosal collapse and profuse diarrhea (Appel et al., 1978; Appel et al., 1979a; Appel et al., 1979b; McCandlish et al., 1979; Pollock, 1979). All ages are affected, but highest incidence and mortality are in puppies. Transmission is by the fecal-oral route, and fomites probably play an important role. Epizootic outbreaks of CPV have been documented in many parts of the world, including many parts of the United States.

Clinical Signs. Clinical signs include severe vomiting (which is often noticed first) and intractable fluid diarrhea, both of which may be profuse and hemorrhagic, anorexia, depression, and rapidly progressive dehydration. Most dogs with CPV are febrile. Some animals lack GI signs initially and just show depression or collapse. Sudden, shock-like deaths have occurred within 24 hours of onset of signs. Death is usually attributable to dehydration and shock or overwhelming bacterial infection (septicemia) from leukopenia. Mild or inapparent infections that result in seroconversion are probably common. Parvoviral myocarditis, usually without GI involvement, is seen in pups 4 to 12 weeks of age and is characterized by a sudden onset of acute heart failure with death in minutes to hours following signs of dyspnea, crying, or acute collapse (see Chapter 50 for details) (Hayes et al., 1979; Jezyk et al., 1979; Carpenter et al., 1980; Mulvey et al., 1980).

Complications during the course of parvovirus enteritis are frequent. These have included hypoglycemia, which may be due to sepsis (Miller et al., 1980), hepatic disease, DIC, anemia due to intestinal blood loss, hypoproteinemia attributed to enteric loss of protein, intestinal intussusception, and secondary bacterial infections (subcutaneous injection site abscesses, endocarditis, thrombophlebitis, pneumonia, urinary tract infection, and intestinal campylobacteriosis or salmonellosis).

Diagnosis. The diagnosis of CPV is usually suspected on the basis of clinical signs, exposure history (such as a confirmed outbreak in the area), and hematologic abnormalities. During the first few days of clinical signs, most dogs develop a severe leukopenia, especially granulocytopenia, usually with 500 to 2000 WBC/mm³, sometimes even less. It appears that the lower the WBC, the more guarded the prognosis should be. Some dogs have a normal WBC at presentation, but in many of these the WBC is found to drop one or two days later (Jacobs et al., 1980). A rise in WBC is a useful indicator of impending recovery. Rebound leukocytosis is common during convalescence. The hematocrit in CPV enteritis is usually normal or decreased, which helps to clinically differentiate CPV from the syndrome of hemorrhagic gastroenteritis (HGE), in which profound hemoconcentration usually causes elevation of the hematocrit.

Several methods have been used to confirm CPV infection, the most useful and readily available ones being the fecal hemagglutination (HA) test for demonstration of fecal excretion of virus, and the serum hemagglutination inhibition (HI) test for serodiagnosis of anti-CPV antibodies (Fig. 58–12) (Carmichael et al., 1980). Serum neutralization and indirect fluorescent antibody techniques have also been used to measure antibody titers but are more cumbersome than the HI titer and give comparable results. The fecal HA test is based on the hemagglutinating activity of feces, since CPV has the biologic property of agglutinating pig RBC's, and each gram of feces from an infected dog typically contains > 10^9 virus particles during the acute phase of the disease. Thus, a diagnostic fecal HA titer is usually ≥ 1:64, and blocking of virus-specific HA by anti-CPV antiserum authenticates a positive HA test by ruling out nonspecific or false agglutination. The serum HI antibody titer rises very early in infected dogs (within four to seven days post-exposure), usually to levels of 1:1280 to 1:5120 or higher, and remains positive for

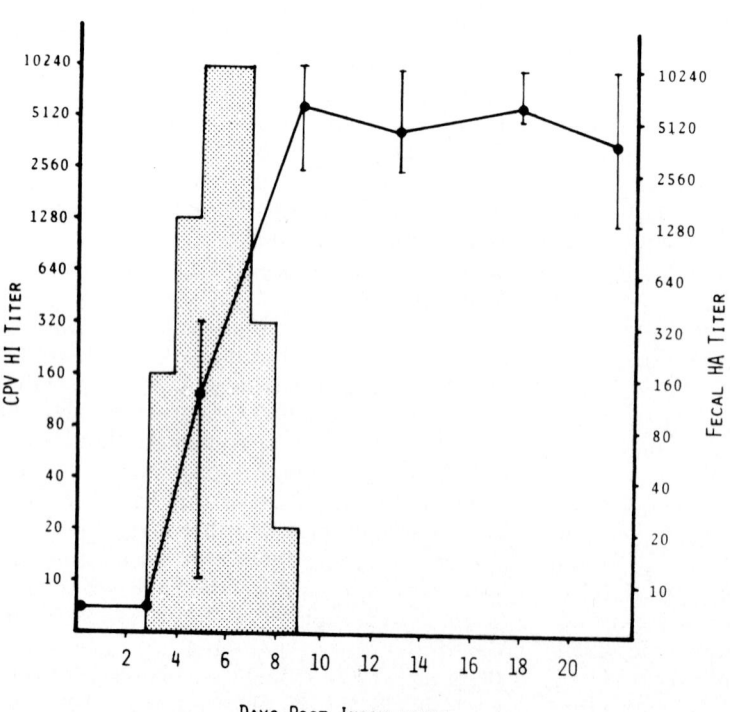

Figure 58–12. The CPV HI antibody and fecal HA responses after oral infection with CPV. Shaded portion represents the period of fecal viral shedding as measured by fecal HA test (right axis), while the solid line represents the mean HI antibody titer (left axis). (Carmichael, L. E., et al.; Am. J. Vet. Res. *41*:784–791, 1980, reprinted with permission.)

more than one year. Therefore, a high antibody titer is useful for diagnosing current or past infection; however, it may also result from prior vaccination. Demonstration that anti-CPV antibodies are mostly IgM may allow serodiagnosis of active infection. Other methods of detection of CPV include demonstration of the virus in feces by EM or virus isolation, and demonstration of the virus in tissues by immunofluorescent antibody testing.

Treatment. The cornerstone of treatment of CPV enteritis is vigorous fluid and electrolyte replacement therapy. Parenteral antibiotics are indicated because of the frequency of bacterial complications associated with granulocytopenia. Because of the depletion of granulocytes, bactericidal antibiotics are preferred over bacteriostatic ones. In dogs that develop hypoglycemia, an IV bolus of 50 per cent dextrose is given, followed by supplementation of IV fluids with dextrose for prevention. Corticosteroids can be used initially if needed to treat refractory shock but otherwise are not routinely used. Nonspecific antiemetic and antidiarrheal therapy is often helpful. In animals that develop severe blood loss anemia or hypoproteinemia, blood transfusions or plasma infusions are beneficial. Nothing is given per os until vomiting has ceased for at least 24 hours and diarrhea is improving and free of blood. When feeding is resumed, small bland meals are used. The success or failure of treatment often depends on the quality and intensity of general nursing care.

Because CPV and feline panleukopenia virus (FPV) are antigenically related, both killed and modified live FPV vaccines have been used successfully to immunize dogs against CPV. Killed and modified live CPV vaccines are also available (Appel et al., 1980). Elimination of CPV from infected premises is difficult, since the virus is so resistant to inactivation; however, isolation of acutely ill dogs and disinfection with dilute (1:30) chlorine bleach are recommended.

Feline Panleukopenia Virus

Feline panleukopenia virus (FPV) is a severe, highly contagious parvovirus infection of cats with a predilection for rapidly dividing cells, particularly for intestinal crypt epithelium resulting in enteritis, for hematopoietic tissue resulting in panleukopenia, and for lymphoid tissue resulting in lymphoid depletion. The clinical picture of FPV is similar to CPV, including anorexia, profound depression, vomiting, diarrhea, fever, and dehydration. The incidence and mortality is highest in kittens. Infection probably occurs by ingestion or inhalation of the virus, and the extreme resistance of FPV to inactivation potentiates its transmission on fomites.

The pathogenesis of the intestinal lesions in FPV infection has been extensively studied (Csiza et al., 1971a; Csiza et al., 1971b; Rohovsky and Fowler, 1971; Larsen et al., 1976; Carlson et al., 1977; Carlson and Scott, 1977; Kahn, 1978; Shindel et al., 1978). In the course of FPV infection, the virus reaches the intestinal crypt epithelium hematogenously, and the crypt cells are destroyed. Without crypt cells available to proliferate and replace villous cells as they migrate and are extruded, the villi shorten and extensive mucosal disruption occurs. Severe damage to the intestinal absorptive surface results in diarrhea and dehydration. Colonic lesions similar to the small intestinal lesions also occur, although they tend to be more focal and less severe (Shindel et al., 1978).

The observation that the lesions of experimentally induced FPV in germ-free cats are much milder than in conventional cats, has focused attention on the role of the resident microflora in the disease. The severity of the crypt lesion in FPV appears to be dependent on the rate of crypt cell proliferation (mitotic activity). Since the gut of the germ-free animal is devoid of microorganisms, there is an absence of physiologic inflammation and the crypt mitotic activity is greatly depressed. Decreased mitotic activity results in relative insusceptibility of the germ-free cat's mucosa to FPV (Carlson et al., 1977; Carlson and Scott, 1977; Kahn, 1978). Hence, in natural FPV infection, the bacterial flora is not directly responsible for the epithelial damage; rather, bacteria provide the conditions for viral-induced damage through their stimulatory effect on mitotic activity of crypt epithelium.

FPV is usually clinically diagnosed on the basis of signs and the hematologic findings of panleukopenia (usually less than 2000 WBC/mm^3, not uncommonly less than 500/mm^3) in a susceptible (unvaccinated) cat. The treatment is similar to that discussed for CPV, mainly supportive or symptomatic treatment such as fluid replacement, antibiotics, antiemetics, antidiarrheals, and dietary management. Initially, a guarded prognosis should be given, but cessation of vomiting and diarrhea, rebound leukocytosis, and return of appetite are usually indicative of recovery. Widespread prevention of FPV has been facilitated by the availability of highly effective immunizing agents.

Canine and Feline Rotaviruses

Rotavirus infections have been recognized as important causes of neonatal diarrhea in many mammalian and avian species (Woode and Crouche, 1978). Rotavirus-like particles have been identified by EM and subsequently isolated from diarrheic feces of dogs and cats (Eugster and Sidwa, 1979; Snodgrass, 1979; England and Poston, 1980). In addition, antibodies to rotavirus have been demonstrated in dogs (Panel Report, 1978) and in 26 of 94 cats (28 per cent) (Snodgrass, 1979). The importance of this viral agent in canine and feline diarrhea needs to be determined. In other species, including man, rotaviruses cause potentially fatal diarrhea in the young but often only subclinical infection in adults. The virus appears to replicate exclusively in enterocytes, and the pathogenesis of diarrhea is thought to depend on shortening (blunting) of villi with accelerated migration of secretory crypt cells. The villi are then populated with mainly immature secretory cells rather than normal absorptive cells, which leads to net secretion of sodium and water and fluid diarrhea (Middleton, 1978). The clinical disease-producing potential of rotaviruses may depend on the presence of other viral or bacterial enteropathogens (Moon et al., 1978).

Canine and Feline Astroviruses

Astrovirus particles have been observed by EM in diarrheal feces from a litter of beagle pups (Williams, 1980) and in the feces of a four-month-old kitten with diarrhea (Hoshino et al., 1981). Astroviruses cause mild gastroenteritis in many species, including man, and are thought to infect the mature villous epithelial cell. Asymptomatic fecal excretion of virus had also been observed. The importance of astroviruses in canine and feline gastroenteritis needs to be established.

MYCOTIC DIARRHEA

Mycotic infections of the small bowel are rare; however, fungi are opportunists that capitalize on predisposing factors such as lowered host resistance, malnutrition, antecedent debilitating illness, or prolonged therapy with antimicrobials or corticosteroids (Merritt, 1980). Mycotic diarrhea may be an acute, dysentery-like diarrhea, or a chronic diarrhea accompanied by chronic emaciation. Multisystemic involvement is frequent. The causes of mycotic intestinal disease are *Candida albicans,* Phycomycetes, *Aspergillus spp.,* and *Histoplasma capsulatum* (see Table 58–6) (Smith, 1968; Merritt, 1980) (see also Chapter 26).

Candidiasis is a rare yeast infection of the mucosal surface that is diagnosed by culture or by the finding of yeast bodies in a fecal smear, and is treated with oral nystatin or IV amphotericin B. Phycomycosis (also called mucormycosis) refers to a group of mycotic infections caused by ubiquitous, spore-forming molds (Ader, 1979). These fungi are tissue-invasive, and the GI tract is the most common site of infection. Intestinal thickening due to granulomatous inflammation may palpate as a large, firm abdominal mass and cause luminal narrowing (Fig. 58–13). Phycomycosis is diagnosed by demonstrating broad, nonseptate hyphae invading tissue obtained by biopsy (Fig. 58–14) or at necropsy, and less readily by culture. Intestinal aspergillosis is similar and characterized by diffuse infiltration of the intestinal submucosa with branching septate hyphae. Both phycomycosis and aspergillosis have a poor response to therapy and are usually fatal.

Intestinal histoplasmosis usually causes a diffuse granulomatous inflammation of the bowel wall and chronic malabsorption. It is discussed in Chapter 26 and under Chronic Diarrhea.

MISCELLANEOUS INFECTIONS
(Table 58–6)

Salmon Poisoning

Salmon poisoning is a systemic rickettsial infection (*Neorickettsia helminthoeca,* Elokomin fluke fever agent) of dogs in the Pacific

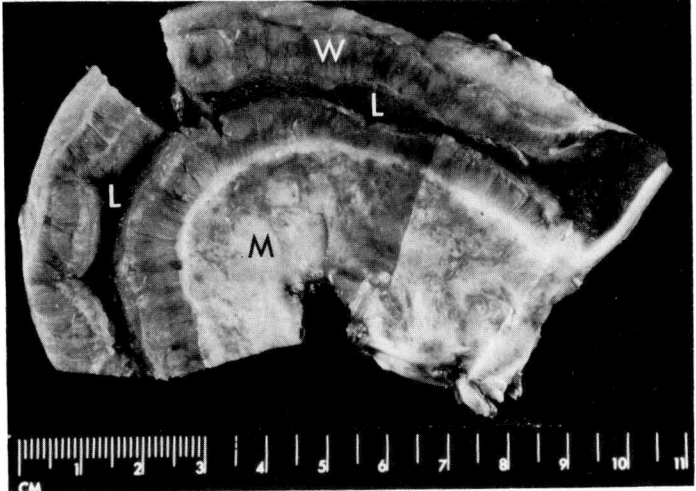

Figure 58–13. Longitudinal section of a resected segment of bowel from a dog with chronic diarrhea and weight loss due to phycomycosis. Note the extensive granulomatous thickening of the bowel wall (W), narrowed lumen (L), and extensive involvement of the mesentery (M).

Northwest, associated with the ingestion of fish containing infected metacercariae of the fluke *Nanophyetus salmincola* (Farrell, 1974). Following an incubation period of five to seven days after ingestion of infected fish, a severe hemorrhagic gastroenteritis develops, characterized by high fever, vomiting, diarrhea, anorexia, depression, dehydration, and lymphadenopathy. The mortality rate is high (50 to 90 per cent) in untreated cases. The diagnosis is suspected when these clinical signs are seen in a dog from an endemic area and confirmed by examination of feces for characteristic fluke eggs by a wash-sedimentation method, or by detection of rickettsial bodies in lymph node aspirates. Therapy includes tetracycline as a specific antirickettsial agent and general supportive treatment.

Protothecosis

Prototheca are rare pathogenic unicellular algae that can invade the small and large bowel and cause hemorrhagic, necrotizing, ulcerative enterocolitis with chronic diarrhea, weight loss, and extraintestinal dissemination (see Chapter 59 for details).

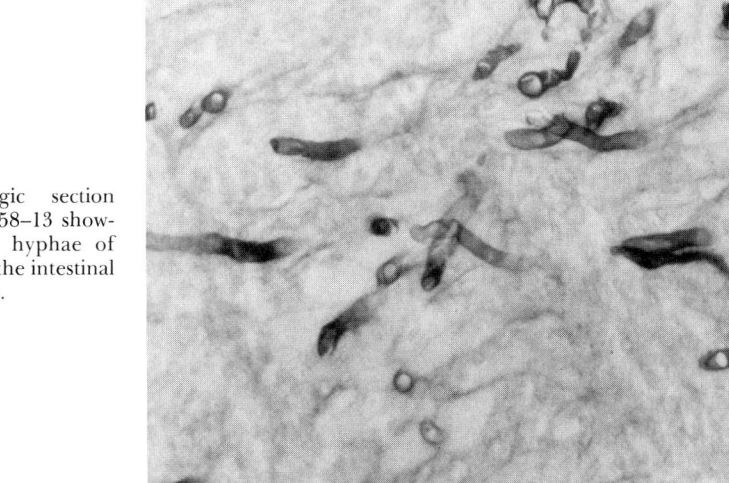

Figure 58–14. Histologic section of the lesion in Figure 58–13 showing broad, nonseptate hyphae of phycomycetes invading the intestinal submucosa (Silver stain).

PARASITIC DISEASES

The most consistent clinical features of intestinal parasitism are diarrhea, weight loss, and unthriftiness, although asymptomatic infections are also common. Young, growing animals are generally more frequently and severely parasitized, but endoparasitism should never be overlooked as a possible cause of acute or chronic diarrhea in dogs and cats of all ages. Other intestinal disorders, such as viral or bacterial diarrhea, are often complicated by the presence of endoparasites.

As mentioned previously, because the shedding of eggs, larvae, trophozoites, or proglottids in the feces can be intermittent, it is important that fecal examinations are performed several times before an animal with diarrheal illness is regarded as free of intestinal parasites. Methods of parasite identification may include gross inspection of the stool for tapeworm proglottids or ascarids; standard fecal flotation for parasite ova; fresh saline smears of feces for ova, larvae, or protozoan trophozoites; and sedimentation or Baerman techniques for larvae of *Strongyloides stercoralis*.

Small intestinal metozoan parasites that commonly affect dogs and cats include ascarids, hookworms, tapeworms, and *Strongyloides stercoralis* (in the dog). Rarely, intestinal trematodes affect the dog. The whipworm *(Trichuris vulpis)* is an important pathogen that mainly affects the large bowel; it is therefore discussed in Chapter 59. Protozoan parasites of importance include Coccidia, *Toxoplasma, Giardia,* trichomonads, *Entamoeba,* and *Balantidium,* the last two being more important as large bowel pathogens. Parasites are listed in Table 58–7.

Some basic differences between canine and feline intestinal parasite infections should be mentioned. Helminths are generally less of a problem in the cat than in the dog, largely because the cat's fastidious habit of burying its feces reduces the risk of widespread environmental contamination with ova. Feline hookworms are not voracious bloodsuckers, so infection is milder than in the hookworm infested dog. Ascarids are less of a problem in the cat, since prenatal infection does not occur. On the other hand, the cat is of tremendous public health concern with regard to the protozoal disease toxoplasmosis, insofar as the cat appears to be the primary host for

Table 58–7. Intestinal Parasites of Dogs and Cats

Helminths
Ascarids: *Toxocara canis, T. cati,* and *Toxascaris leonina*
Hookworms: *Ancylostoma caninum, A. tubaeforme, A. braziliense,* and *Uncinaria stenocephala*
Whipworms: *Trichuris vulpis*
Cestodes (tapeworms): *Dipylidium caninum, Taenia spp.,* and others
Strongyloides stercoralis
Others: *Trichinella spiralis,* trematodes
Protozoa
Coccidia: *Isospora, Sarcocystis, Besnoitia, Hammondia, Toxoplasma*
Giardia canis and *duodenalis*
Trichomonas spp.
Entamoeba histolytica
Balantidium coli

Toxoplasma gondii and the only shedder of oocysts.

Ascarids

Ascarid nematodes are the most common parasites of dogs and cats worldwide. The ascarids of the dog are *Toxocara canis* and the less common *Toxascaris leonina,* while those in the cat are *Toxocara cati* and *T. leonina* (Glickman, 1979; Schantz, 1979; Roberson, 1980).

Clinical signs of ascariasis are most often seen with heavy infections in young puppies and kittens, where the adult worms in the small intestine may cause abdominal discomfort, whimpering and groaning, potbellied appearance, dull haircoat, unthriftiness, stunted growth, and diarrhea. Worms are frequently passed in vomitus or diarrhea (Fig. 58–15). Occasionally, large tangled masses of worms occlude the lumen in young pups and cause death from intestinal obstruction, intussusception, or intestinal perforation (Fig. 58–16). In the neonatal pup, the migration of large numbers of *T. canis* larvae through the lungs can cause severe damage and fatal pneumonia. In young animals with light infections and in adults, infection is most commonly asymptomatic or merely evidenced by loss of body condition.

Ascarid infection occurs by four routes: (1) prenatal infection as a result of transplacental migration, which occurs only with *T. canis*; (2) milk-borne infection as a result of transmammary migration, which occurs with both *T. canis* and *T. cati*; (3) infection by

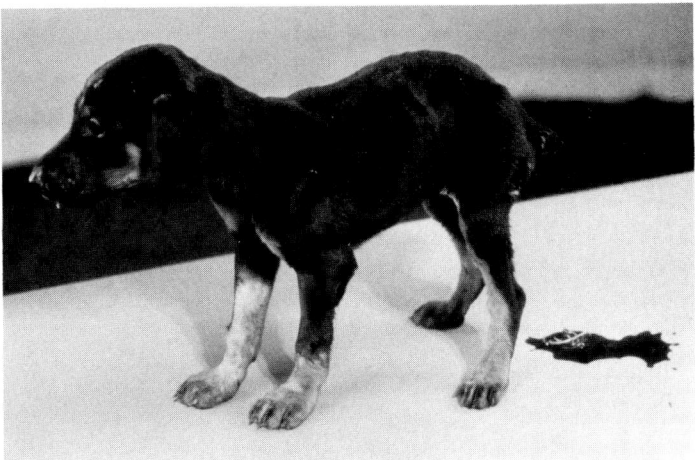

Figure 58–15. A parasitized puppy passing ascarids in diarrheic feces.

ingestion of infective eggs, which occurs with all three ascarids, *T. canis, T. cati,* and *T. leonina;* and (4) infection by ingestion of a paratenic (transport) host *(T. canis, T. cati)* or intermediate host *(T. leonina).* In addition, there are three types of migration patterns that occur once an animal is infected: liver-lung migration *(T. canis, T. cati),* migration within the wall of the GI tract (all three ascarids), and somatic tissue migration *(T. canis, T. cati).*

Since *T. canis* is the most common intestinal parasite in small animals, and since it may be transmitted by all four routes, its life cycle will be discussed in detail. It appears that the neonatal pup (< five weeks) and the whelping bitch lack resistance to *T. canis.* In the U.S., virtually 100 per cent of pups are infected with *T. canis;* most are born infected because of transplacental migration of the bitch's somatic larvae into the fetus (prenatal infection). The prenatally infected pup is born with the third stage larvae (L3) of *T. canis* within its lungs. These L3 are coughed up, swallowed, and then develop into mature egg-producing adult worms in the small intestine within three weeks after birth. Many pups, therefore, begin passing large numbers of eggs in their feces at about three weeks of age and continue to shed eggs for most of early puppyhood (four to six months) if untreated. Neonatal puppies may also become infected with L3 contained in the dam's milk for the first month of lactation. These larvae develop to adults in the gut without going through a migrating phase.

Dogs of all ages may be infected by the ingestion of embryonated (infective) eggs from their environment, mainly from the soil. In pups less than five weeks old, this results in liver-lung migration followed by intestinal ascarid infection. In older dogs, however, there is an age-related resistance that causes instead a somatic migration and subsequent arrest of *T. canis* larvae (L3) in somatic tissues such as muscles, kidneys, eye, and brain. It is these larvae arrested in somatic tissues that are reactivated at about 42 days of gestation in the pregnant bitch; they then migrate to the placenta or mammary gland to produce prenatal or milk-borne infection of the pup.

In contrast to *T. canis* in pups, prenatal infection is not known to occur with *T. cati* in cats. The other routes of infection do occur in the cat, however. The ingestion of paratenic hosts (mice, birds, and insects) is

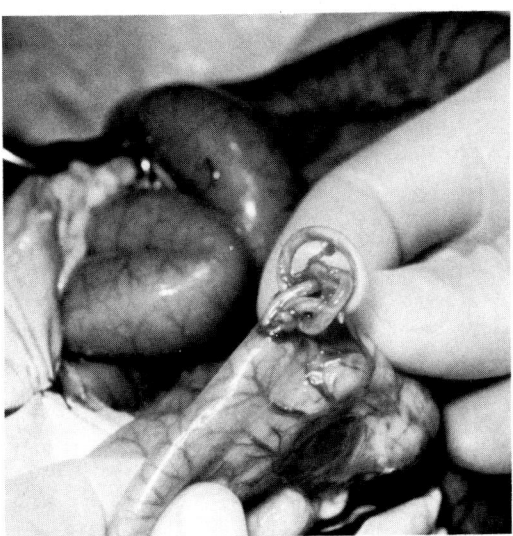

Figure 58–16. This tangled mass of ascarids protruding from an enterotomy incision was associated with an intussusception.

not a very important source of infection of *T. canis* in the dog, although it occurs; in the adult cat, however, this route is a major source of *T. cati* infection. Infection of *T. cati* in the cat is followed by all three forms of migration; liver-lung migration and migration within the wall of the GI tract result in adult worms in the small intestine, while somatic migration, similar to that for *T. canis*, may culminate in milk-borne (but not transplacental) infection of nursing kittens. This is the major source of ascariasis in kittens.

T. leonina infection in dogs and cats is less common than *T. canis* or *T. cati*. Infection occurs by ingestion of embryonated eggs or by an intermediate host such as the mouse. Migration is confined to the intestinal wall.

Numerous effective anthelmintics of adult ascarids are available (see Table 58–8). Since most pups are born infected with *T. canis*, it is recommended that treatment be started at two weeks of age, before eggs are first passed in the feces, and then continued at four, six, and eight weeks to kill all worms derived from prenatal infection, milk-borne infection, and ingestion of embryonated eggs. Pyrantel pamoate has been convenient for this purpose because it is well-tolerated in puppies and also effective in controlling hookworms. Treatment of the nursing bitch should also be part of the roundworm control program. Currently, there is no approved drug available for killing larvae in somatic tissues.

Because of toxocaral visceral larva migrans (VLM), a serious disease of humans (especially children) produced by the invasion of visceral tissues by migrating *T. canis*, *T. canis*-infected pups are considered public health hazards (Schantz, 1979). Human fatalities from VLM have been reported. In addition to the prevalence of prenatal *T. canis* infection in pups, two other features of the parasite increase its potential as a public health problem. First, *T. canis* is a prolific egg layer; each adult female worm may shed 200,000 ova per day. Second, once these eggs embryonate in three to four weeks and become infective for dogs or humans, their resistance to inactivation enables them to remain viable in the soil for months or years.

Hookworms

The most common hookworm in the dog is *Ancylostoma caninum*, a voracious blood-sucker (Miller, 1971; Migasena et al., 1972a; Roberson and Cornelius, 1980). The common hookworm in the cat, *Ancylostoma tubaeforme*, is more of a tissue feeder than a bloodsucker and is far less pathogenic than *A. caninum* in dogs. Two other less common hookworms, *Ancylostoma braziliense* and *Uncinaria stenocephala*, occur in both dogs and cats and are only mildly pathogenic, because they are not as hematophagous. *A. braziliense* is most prevalent in the southern United States and in tropical or subtropical regions, whereas *U. stenocephala* is a "cold weather" hookworm and is most prevalent in Canada (Miller, 1971).

The pathogenicity of the hookworm is directly related to its bloodsucking activity and capacity for causing intestinal blood loss (Miller, 1966a; 1966b). The most pathogenic hookworm, *A. caninum*, may cause a daily blood loss per adult worm of 0.01 to 0.2 ml; by comparison, daily blood loss from *A. braziliense* (0.001 ml per adult) or *U. stenocephala* (0.0003 ml per adult) is relatively insignificant. Hence, an important consequence of severe *A. caninum* infection is blood loss anemia.

The clinical signs of ancylostomiasis in the dog include tarry (melena) or bloody diarrhea accompanied by pallor, weakness, emaciation, and dehydration. In heavily infected young pups, severe acute GI hemorrhage and rapidly progressive blood loss anemia may result in death. In others, chronic blood loss from chronic infection eventually causes iron deficiency anemia, and erythrocytes show hypochromasia and microcytosis (Miller, 1971). One study has shown impaired intestinal absorption of fat, carbohydrate, and amino acids in dogs with severe ancylostomiasis (Migasena et al., 1972b). Infections with the other species of hookworm, and light *A. caninum* infections, especially in partially resistant older dogs, are often asymptomatic.

Hookworm infection can occur by five routes: prenatal, milk-borne, ingestion of infective larvae (L3), skin penetration by infective larvae, and ingestion of paratenic hosts (Miller, 1971). It is thought that ingestion of larvae or active penetration of the skin by larvae are the most common routes of infection, and in contrast to *T. canis*, *A. caninum* infects neonatal pups more frequently by the milk-borne route than prenatally. Oral ingestion (including milk-borne ingestion) is followed mainly by direct development in the intestine, while larvae pene-

Table 58–8. Anthelmintics

Drug	Dosage	Ascarids	Hookworms	Whipworms	Tapeworms	Strongyloides	Comments
					Efficiency (%)		
Albendazole (Valbazen)*	25 mg/kg PO × 3 to 5 days	100	100	100	0 Dipylidium 100 Taenia	—	Do not use with Styquin; may cause rare acute deaths and transient hypospermia.
Bunamidine HCl (Scolaban)	25 to 50 mg/kg PO	—	—	—	56 to 90 Dipylidium 100 Taenia	—	Not in pups <8 wks, heartworm+ dogs, or breeders; fatal with Scolaban; pain at injection site.
Butamisole (Styquin)	2.4 mg/kg SC	—	85	99	—	—	Not in debilitated, heartworm+, or anticholinesterase-treated animals
Dichlorvos (Task)	27 to 33 mg/kg (pellets) PO 11 mg/kg (tablets) PO	95	95	90	—	—	Fourfold overdose is fatal.
Disophenol (DNP)	10 mg/kg, SC	—	95	—	—	—	Currently unavailable.
Fenbendazole (Panacur)*	50 to 100 mg/kg PO × 3 days	99	98	100	—	Possibly Effective	Very safe.
Glycobiarsol (Milibus-V)	220 mg/kg PO × 5 days	—	—	90	—	—	May cause vomiting. Hepatic necrosis in a small percentage.
Ivermectin*	Needs to be determined	100	100	100	—	—	
Mebendazole (Telmintic)	22 mg/kg PO × 3 to 5 days	95	95	95	0 Dipylidium 100 Taenia	Possibly Effective	May cause vomiting and ataxia; currently unavailable.
Niclosamide (Yomesan)	100 to 157 mg/kg PO	—	—	—	18 to 56 Dipylidium 80 Taenia	—	
Phthalofyne (Whipcide)	250 mg/kg IV	—	—	90	·	—	
Piperazine	100 mg/kg PO	85	—	—	—	—	
Praziquantel (Droncit)	5 mg/kg SC	—	—	—	100 Dipylidium 100 Taenia	—	Very safe; drug of choice for tapes.
Pyrantel pamoate (Nemex)	5 mg/kg PO	95	95	—	—	—	Safe in nursing pups.
Thenium closylate (Canopar)	500 mg (dogs >5 kg) PO	—	89	—	—	—	May cause vomiting; do not use in nursing pups or dogs <5 kg.
Thiabendazole*	25 to 50 mg/kg PO × 3 days	—	—	—	—	95	

*Not approved for use in the dog or cat.

trating the skin migrate by somatic or circulatory transport to the lung before reaching the intestine. Prenatal or milk-borne infection occurs in pups from bitches that have migrating somatic larvae from past infection. With all routes of infection, eggs are passed in feces after two to three weeks. The strongyloid-type hookworm eggs rapidly hatch into infectious free-living larvae that survive well for three to four months in warm, moist environments but are killed by drying, direct sunlight, or cold winter conditions. Acute, pruritic dermatitis is occasionally associated with the active penetration of skin by hookworm larvae.

Anthelmintics effective against hookworms include pyrantel pamoate (safest in young pups), dichlorvos, mebendazole, thenium, disophenol, butamisole, and others (see Table 58–8). Severely anemic animals should also receive whole blood transfusions, iron supplementation, and supportive therapy. In areas where *A. caninum* is a frequent problem, bitches and puppies should be routinely treated. Because of prenatal and milk-borne infection, treatment of pups can be started at two weeks of age, along with treatment for *T. canis*. Pyrantel pamoate suspension (Nemex) is an excellent choice for nursing pups because it is well tolerated and active against both hookworms and ascarids. Parasite control is aided by good sanitation and impervious flooring in kennels and dog runs. A vaccine containing irradiated hookworm larvae was once used for hookworm prevention, but it is no longer available (Miller, 1971; Steves et al., 1973).

Strongyloides

Strongyloides stercoralis is a tiny (two mm) rhabditoid nematode that burrows in the mucosa of the proximal small bowel, causing mucosal destruction and hemorrhagic diarrhea (Anderson and Low, 1975). Strongyloidiasis is mainly a problem in puppies in warm, humid tropical regions, and fatalities are common. Infection of dogs with third-stage larvae is by the oral or cutaneous route, and adult worms develop in the small intestine following migration in the circulation and lung. Verminous pneumonia may result from migration. Parthenogenetic female adults produce eggs that hatch within the gut lumen, so that first-stage (rhabdoid) larvae are passed in the feces. These larvae may develop into either infectious third-stage (filariform) larvae or into free-living adults. The diagnosis depends on finding motile first-stage larvae, 0.8 to 1.6 mm long and 30 to 80 μ wide, in fresh feces. Recently, a *Strongyloides* infection was described in a dog that was shedding both larvae and unusually large ova in fresh feces (Malone et al., 1980). *S. stercoralis* larvae must be distinguished from larvae of *Filaroides spp.*, or in old fecal samples from hookworm larvae that have hatched from ova in the feces. Treatment includes thiabendazole, mebendazole, dithiazanine, and possibly fenbendazole.

Another *Strongyloides*, *S. tumefaciens*, sometimes parasitizes the large intestine of cats in the southern United States. It is usually an asymptomatic infection but may cause mucosal and submucosal nodular lesions in the colon with signs of chronic diarrhea and debilitation (Malone et al., 1977).

Tapeworms

Tapeworms (cestodes) that parasitize the small bowel of dogs and cats are relatively harmless, rarely causing more than a subtle decline in body condition. The most common tapeworm is *Dipylidium caninum* (Roberson, 1980). Fleas and lice are intermediate hosts. The proglottids of *D. caninum* are highly motile and may cause anal pruritus as they crawl on the perineum, and crawling proglottids are often detected in the stool or on the perineum by observant owners. Several species of *Taenia* can be acquired by dogs and cats (most commonly *T. pisiformis* in the dog, *T. taeniaformis* in the cat) from ingestion of cysticerci-infected tissues from intermediate hosts, e.g., rabbits, rodents, sheep, and ungulates. *D. caninum* proglottids are distinguished from *Taenia* by their barrel shape and double genital pore. Also, a proglottid can be squashed in a drop of water between a slide and coverslip to find the characteristic *D. caninum* egg capsules that contain up to 20 eggs. Other cestode infections that rarely occur in the dog include *Echinococcus spp.*, *Multiceps spp.*, and *Mesocestoides spp.* Praziquantel and bunamidine HCl are the most effective all-around drugs for cestodiasis, although others are available (see Table 58–8). Flea and lice control are important for preventing *D. caninum* reinfection, while control of predation and scavenging help prevent infection with other cestodes.

Other Metazoan Parasites

Transient hemorrhagic enteritis with bloody diarrhea was observed in a cat with trichinosis (Holzworth and Georgi, 1974). Numerous adult *Trichinella spiralis* nematodes (1.5 to 4.0 mm) were found in the sediment of a centrifuged fecal suspension, and migrating larvae (100 μ) were identified in the blood with a modified Knott's test. The illness was self-limiting without treatment, but eosinophilia persisted for three months. The source of infection was undetermined, but predation of an infected rodent was considered most likely.

Trematodes occasionally parasitize the small intestine. The intestinal fluke *Nanophyetus salmincola* is endemic to the Pacific Northwest and acquired from eating raw fish. The fluke itself is unimportant; however, it is the vector of the fatal rickettsial disease of dogs called salmon poisoning discussed earlier. Asymptomatic infection of the jejunum of a dog by the fluke *Alaria arisaemoides* (alariasis) has been reported (Hayden, 1969).

Parasitic shistosomiasis caused by *Heterobilharzia americana* in a dog was characterized by extensive schistosome egg deposition in the intestinal wall and liver, accompanied by granulomatous inflammation (Pierce, 1963).

PROTOZOAN PARASITES

Coccidia

Canine and feline coccidia belong to five genera, *Isospora, Sarcocystis, Besnoitia, Hammondia,* and *Toxoplasma* (Dubey, 1976). With the exception of *Toxoplasma gondii* and certain species of *Isospora,* most coccidia infections are self-limiting and asymptomatic. It is currently unclear why most coccidia are relatively nonpathogenic experimentally in dogs and cats, while in clinical situations, especially in kittens and puppies, they appear to be associated with fluid diarrhea (sometimes bloody or mucoid), vomiting, depression, weight loss, and fever. Coccidiosis may cause malabsorption. One isolate (*Isospora ohioensis*) was shown to cause necrosis, desquamation, and atrophy of the tips of villi (Dubey, 1978).

Infection is usually acquired by ingestion of oocysts from a contaminated environment or by ingesting the infected cyst-containing tissues (meat) of an intermediate host (usually herbivores). Clinical disease most commonly is seen in weanling age animals, associated with high-stress conditions such as shipping or weaning, and high-density housing such as pet shops, kennels, and catteries. The diagnosis of coccidiosis is made by detection and identification of oocysts in fresh feces. Many normal dogs and cats harbor coccidia. Therefore, the finding of oocysts in a healthy animal with formed feces does not necessarily warrant treatment. If clinical signs are attributed to coccidiosis, however, treatment with intestinal sulfas, sulfadimethoxine, nitrofurazone, or amprolium is recommended. Coccidiosis and toxoplasmosis are discussed further in Chapter 27.

Giardia

Giardia spp. are pear-shaped, binucleated, flagellated protozoa that reside mainly in the proximal small intestine. The parasite has two forms, the trophozoite and the cyst. Motile trophozoites are found either attached to the microvillous border of the mucosal epithelium by means of ventral, cup-shaped suction discs, or free within the intraluminal mucus. They can be seen in diarrheic feces, but usually not in formed stool. The infective stage, the nonmotile cyst, is usually found in formed feces and is thought to be an encysted trophozoite that has transformed into a cyst during transit through the terminal small bowel and colon. Giardiasis in the dog is usually caused by *G. canis* (Barlough, 1979) and in the cat by *G. duodenalis* (Brightman and Slonka, 1976).

The most consistent clinical sign of giardiasis is diarrhea, which may be acute or chronic, and self-limiting, intermittent, or continuous. Asymptomatic infections are found, especially in mature animals. Most clinically apparent infections are in young animals, and dogs are affected more often than cats. Acute giardiasis is manifested by a sudden onset of explosive, watery, foul-smelling diarrhea with depression and anorexia. The signs may mimic other acute enteritides, such as viral enteritis. Chronic giardiasis is characterized by chronic malabsorption with intermittent or protracted diarrhea (usually soft, mushy stools), steatorrhea, weight loss, and failure to thrive.

The pathogenesis of diarrhea and clinical illness due to *Giardia spp.* is not completely understood. Pathogenicity probably results from the interplay of several mechanisms. This is emphasized by the lack of correlation between the severity of illness, morphologic mucosal damage (if any), and number of *Giardia* present in human infections. Malabsorption probably plays an important role (Brasitus, 1979; Hartong et al., 1979). Impaired absorption of carbohydrate (D-xylose, lactose), fat, vitamin A, and vitamin B_{12}, as well as deficiency of brush border enzymes have been demonstrated. Mechanical irritation or damage to mucosal microvilli from the sucking disc of the trophozoite, which has been observed with scanning EM, may impair microvillous digestive and absorptive functions (Wolfe, 1978). In some patients, more severe lesions are seen, including epithelial damage, blunted villi, and mononuclear inflammatory infiltrate of the lamina propria. Mucosal and submucosal invasion by *Giardia* has been shown but is thought to be rare. Contrastingly, in some patients reversible deficiency of brush border enzymes can be demonstrated, even in the absence of histologic mucosal damage, suggesting biochemical dysfunction of the enterocyte (Wolfe, 1978; Hartong et al., 1979).

Bile salt deconjugation, with or without bacterial overgrowth, may also contribute to malabsorption in giardiasis. The severity of infection, or appearance of blood and mucus in the feces, is possibly affected by concomitant enteric viral, bacterial, or parasitic infection. Puppies and kittens with giardiasis are frequently coinfected with helminths or other protozoa. Immune deficiency states predispose to giardiasis in humans, an association that needs to be explored in animal cases.

The source of *Giardia* infection is the ingestion of food or water contaminated with cysts. Since wild animals are potential reservoirs of *Giardia spp.*, infection by drinking from contaminated streams and ponds is feasible.

The diagnosis of giardiasis should be considered in dogs or cats with unexplained diarrhea or malabsorption, and is usually established by finding cysts or trophozoites in fecal specimens. Cysts (oval, 9 to $13\mu \times 7$ to 9μ) stain well with Lugol's two per cent iodine and may be found in direct fecal smears or by zinc sulfate or sodium dichromate flotation. Formalin-ether sedimenta-

tion can also be used. Trophozoites (pear-shaped, 12 to $17\mu \times 7$ to 10μ) are found in freshly-passed diarrheic feces stained with iodine or suspended in saline. Since there is a periodicity of cyst excretion, multiple fecal samples should be examined, preferably a minimum of three on alternative days. Barium, antibiotics, antacids, antidiarrheals, laxatives, and enemas may mask the presence of *Giardia* for about a week.

If parasites cannot be demonstrated by fecal examination, then trophozoites may be found in duodenal aspirates or intestinal biopsy specimens. However, since recovery is rapid with appropriate treatment, the author prefers diagnosing "occult" giardiasis by response to a therapeutic trial of metronidazole rather than by these more expensive and invasive procedures.

Three drugs are considered to be effective for eliminating *Giardia spp.*, metronidazole (Flagyl), quinacrine HCl (Atabrine), and furazolidone (Furoxone). In dogs and cats, metronidazole (30 mg/kg twice daily for five days; or 60 mg/kg, once daily for five days) and quinacrine HCl (50 to 100 mg twice daily for three days then repeat in three days) have been most often recommended. Response to therapy is usually rapid and complete. The use of a high-protein diet may also be beneficial.

Trichomonads

Trichomonas spp. are motile, flagellated protozoa that have been found in both normal and diarrheic dogs and cats (Greene and Thorson, 1954; Burrows and Lillis, 1967; Burrows and Hunt, 1970). The pathogenicity of this organism is not well-established in dogs and cats, but trichomoniasis is often associated with watery diarrhea. The incidence is highest in puppies and is especially associated with unsanitary kennel conditions and coinfection with other parasites. The diagnosis is established by finding motile, pear-shaped flagellates with a characteristic undulating membrane and constant turning or rolling motion in diarrheic feces suspended in saline. Trichomonads lack a cyst stage. The treatment is metronidazole.

Other Protozoa

Amebiasis, caused by *Entamoeba histolytica*, and balantidiasis, caused by *Balantidium coli*, are characterized by bloody-mucoid diarrhea (colitis). Both diseases are diagnosed by identification of the protozoa in fresh saline fecal smears and are treated with metronidazole. Since these are primarily large bowel pathogens, the details are discussed in Chapter 59.

CANINE HEMORRHAGIC GASTROENTERITIS

Hemorrhagic gastroenteritis (HGE) is a syndrome of unknown etiology characterized by sudden onset of vomition, severe bloody diarrhea, and marked hemoconcentration (Hill, 1973; Bernstein, 1977; Burrows, 1977; Strombeck, 1979). Rapidity of onset and the clinical signs are similar to experimental endotoxic shock and allergic or anaphylactic reactions to bacterial endotoxin in dogs; however, there is no direct evidence yet for such a mechanism in HGE (Hill, 1973). One author has suggested an immune-mediated pathogenesis, resembling experimentally induced models of immune-mediated colitis in dogs (Strombeck, 1979). HGE is not truly an inflammatory disease; usually lesions of inflammation are lacking, suggesting a functional gut change that causes altered mucosal permeability or secretion. A role for *Clostridia spp.* has also been suggested.

The disease affects all ages, but especially young adults two to four years of age. Although any breed may be affected, a predilection for toy and miniature breeds, particularly schnauzers and poodles, has been demonstrated. No sex predilection has been found.

Clinical signs of HGE include sudden onset of emesis (which may precede diarrhea by a few hours and contain blood), severe bloody diarrhea with a fetid odor, depression, and decreased capillary refill time. Precipitating factors for the crisis are rarely ascertained from the history. If untreated, HGE will cause death from circulatory failure and shock in a matter of hours. If treated, however, mortality is low. The majority of dogs experience single episodes, but others experience periodic episodes throughout their lifetime.

The single most helpful diagnostic parameter is the hematocrit, which should be performed on all dogs showing explosive hemorrhagic diarrhea. The diagnosis of HGE is based on finding marked elevation of hematocrit (often greater than 60 per cent, sometimes up to 80 per cent) without comparable loss of skin turgor in a dog with an acute onset of vomiting and fetid bloody diarrhea. Hemoconcentration is attributed to rapid fluid loss into the gut, probably from increased capillary permeability, and to splenic contraction. In the dog with HGE, WBC count, blood chemistries, and abdominal radiographs are usually unremarkable. DIC has been reported in a few dogs (Burrows, 1977). These cases may represent a separate disease entity, and are noteworthy insofar as DIC experimentally induced by endotoxin in dogs causes severe hemorrhagic necrosis of the intestinal mucosa (Kondo et al., 1978).

HGE is treated as a medical emergency; prompt vigorous fluid therapy usually prevents mortality. A balanced multiple electrolyte solution is given intravenously, preferably by means of an indwelling IV catheter. Initially, 90 ml/kg body weight of the solution are infused rapidly, or until capillary refill time is normal and hematocrit drops below 50 per cent; then, 40 to 65 ml/kg or more are given over the next 24 hours as needed to maintain hematocrit at less than 50 per cent. If shock appears refractory to IV fluids, then a shock dose of corticosteroid should be considered. Nonspecific antidiarrheal and antiemetic therapy may also be used. If fluid therapy is vigorous enough, then within a few hours the hematocrit should stabilize, shock should abate, and the animal should be less depressed. Bloody diarrhea usually ceases in 12 to 48 hours, followed by one to two days of dark tarry stools and then normal solid stools. Food and water are withheld for at least the first 24 hours, but once vomiting and bloody liquid stools have been absent for 24 hours, then small amounts of bland food can be fed. Failure to respond to this regimen in 24 to 48 hours should suggest that other diseases that may mimic HGE be considered (parvovirus, GI foreign body, intussusception, volvulus, and others).

CHRONIC DIARRHEA

OVERVIEW

Chronic diarrhea in small animals is considerably less common than acute diarrhea. Nevertheless, chronic diarrheal disorders as a group are generally challenging diagnostic problems that often require in-depth knowledge and expertise in gastrointestinal medicine. In relation to chronic diarrhea, broadly descriptive terms, such as malabsorption syndrome, protein-losing enteropathy, and chronic inflammatory small bowel disease, are frequently used to refer to chronic enteropathies or their functional consequences. These descriptive categories are closely interrelated, and commonly a single chronic small bowel disease may fit into two or all three of these categorizations.

Malabsorption syndrome includes chronic enteropathies that cause a generalized failure of digestion and absorption (most consistently involving fat), resulting in chronic diarrhea and weight loss (Hill, 1972a; Hill and Kelly, 1974; Olsen, 1979). The pathophysiology of malabsorption has been discussed earlier in this chapter. The most common causes of intestinal malabsorption syndrome are diffuse mucosal or bowel wall diseases, including chronic inflammatory bowel disease (eosinophilic enteritis, lymphocytic-plasmacytic enteritis, granulomatous enteritis), intestinal histoplasmosis, lymphangiectasia, idiopathic villous atrophy, and diffuse-type intestinal lymphosarcoma (Table 58–9) (Hill, 1972a; Hill and Kelly, 1974). A definitive etiology for many of these disorders is lacking. Malabsorption may also be a consequence of parasitic infections such as giardiasis (Brasitus, 1979), bacterial overgrowth (Isaacs and

Kim, 1979; Hoenig, 1980), or massive bowel resection (Joy and Patterson, 1978; Weser et al., 1979). Protein-losing enteropathy may accompany intestinal malabsorption. Diagnostic criteria that establish the presence of intestinal malabsorption syndrome include (1) steatorrhea (indirect Sudan-stained feces positive for split fat, increased 24- or 72-hour fecal fat excretion, decreased fat assimilation), (2) flat D-xylose absorption curve, and (3) normal pancreatic function tests. Intestinal biopsy is often necessary to determine the cause of malabsorption (Hill and Kelly, 1974; Brandborg, 1979).

Protein-losing enteropathy (PLE) refers to a group of chronic enteropathies that share in common the excessive loss of plasma proteins into the gut lumen and feces, usually resulting in panhypoproteinemia (Waldmann, 1976). The intestinal lymphatic lesion of lymphangiectasia, with or without an accompanying inflammatory cell infiltration, is often referred to as primary PLE, while other chronic enteropathies, many of which have already been listed as causes of malabsorption, are often considered to be secondary causes of PLE. In addition, PLE may result from extraintestinal diseases that increase intestinal capillary or lymphatic hydrostatic pressure, such as congestive heart failure.

Chronic inflammatory small bowel disease

Table 58–9. Diagnosis and Treatment of Chronic Intestinal Malabsorptive Diseases

Disorder	Diagnosis	Treatment*
1. Chronic inflammatory small bowel disease		
a. Eosinophilic enteritis†	Eosinophilia, biopsy	Corticosteroids
b. Lymphocytic-plasmacytic enteritis†	Biopsy	Corticosteroids
c. Granulomatous Enteritis†	Radiography, biopsy	Corticosteroids, surgical resection
2. Lymphangiectasia† (primary and secondary)	Lymphopenia, biopsy	Diet (MCT), corticosteroids (±)
3. Villous atrophy		
a. Gluten enteropathy	Response to gluten-free diet, biopsy	Gluten-free diet
b. Idiopathic	Biopsy	Diet, corticosteroids (±) antibiotics (±)
4. Histoplasmosis†	Serology, cytology, biopsy	Amphotericin-B
5. Lymphosarcoma†	Biopsy	Chemotherapy (anti-neoplastic drugs)
6. Bacterial overgrowth ("stagnant loop")	Culture intestinal aspirate, response to antibiotics	Antibiotics
7. Parasitism (Giardia)	Fecal examinations, response to parasiticides	Parasiticides (metronidazole)
8. Lactase deficiency	Response to lactose-free diet	Eliminate milk from diet

*In addition to these specific treatments, the nonspecific measures from Table 58–10, such as diet, are also used.

†Diseases that are also frequent causes of canine protein-losing enteropathy.

refers to a diverse group of disorders of unknown etiology that are characterized by distention of the intestinal lamina propria and sometimes deeper layers of the bowel wall with inflammatory cells. Classification of these disorders is based on the predominant inflammatory cell in the infiltrate: eosinophilic, lymphocytic-plasmacytic, or granulomatous enteritis. Some cases show mixed inflammatory cell infiltration that renders classification difficult. Although an etiology for these diseases has not been determined, they are often steroid-responsive. These diseases may cause either malabsorption syndrome or PLE, and sometimes both.

NONSPECIFIC THERAPY OF MALABSORPTION

There are some measures that are useful for nonspecific medical management of malabsorption and chronic diarrhea (Table 58–10). Dietary restriction, modification, or supplementation form the foundations for this therapy (Regan and DiMagno, 1979). Specific treatment, when available, will be discussed separately with each disease (Table 58–9).

The diet of the animal with malabsorp-

Table 58–10. Nonspecific Medical Management of Intestinal Malabsorption

1. Frequent small feedings (3 to 4/day)
2. Dietary modification
   a. High-protein, fat-restricted diet with minimal lactose (such as r/d or rice and uncreamed cottage cheese)
   b. MCT to replace calories lost by removal of fat (LCT) from the diet (up to 30 ml MCT oil/lb of food)
   c. Vitamin-mineral supplements (fat soluble vitamins — A, D, E, K; folate, B_{12}, calcium)
3. Special nutritional supplementation (in selected cases)
   a. Parenteral (IV) hyperalimentation
   b. Enteral hyperalimentation (liquid elemental diets)
4. Eradicate concomitant parasite infections
5. Antibiotics — broad spectrum with anaerobic coverage (when bacterial overgrowth is a cause or complication of malabsorption)
6. Corticosteroids (used in those idiopathic chronic enteropathies thought to have an immune pathogenesis)
7. Pancreatic enzyme supplementation (Viokase) (transient exocrine pancreatic insufficiency with acinar atrophy may be seen with severe malabsorption)

tion should be high in protein, low in fat, and low in lactose. Since unabsorbed protein (fecal nitrogen) is not considered detrimental, protein restriction is unnecessary (Regan and Di Magno, 1979). In fact, prevention of protein malnutrition by providing high quantities of good biologic quality protein may facilitate intestinal adaptation to or recovery from intestinal disease. Restriction of dietary fat (long-chain triglyceride), on the other hand, may provide some amelioration of diarrhea by reducing steatorrhea. Medium-chain triglyceride (MCT) can be used to replace calories lost by removal of fat from the diet. Normal dietary fat is long-chain triglyceride (LCT) and is consistently malassimilated in malabsorption and intestinal lymphatic disorders (lymphangiectasia). The usefulness of MCT supplementation is based on the premise that MCT is hydrolyzed more efficiently and rapidly than LCT, and then is absorbed directly into the portal venous system, bypassing lymphatic transport (Regan and Di Magno, 1979). Commercially available MCT is derived from coconut oil and can be mixed in with low-fat foods (such as r/d Prescription Diet or homemade diet of rice and uncreamed cottage cheese) in gradually increasing amounts up to 30 ml per pound of food.

Carbohydrate restriction is generally not needed, except that lactose content of the diet should be limited because brush border lactase may be deficient. If dairy products are desired as a protein source, ¼ cup of cottage cheese provides nearly as much protein (7.5 gm) as one cup of whole milk (8.0 gm), but considerably less lactose (1.5 gm compared to 11.8 gm) (Regan and Di Magno, 1979). Daily food intake should be divided into three to four small feedings to avoid overload of intestinal digestive-absorptive capacity.

Vitamin supplementation of the diet, especially with fat-soluble vitamins (A, D, E, K) is indicated. In human patients with malabsorption, subclinical deficiencies of all vitamins and minerals are common, and clinically important deficiencies of fat-soluble vitamins, folic acid, vitamin B_{12}, and occasionally calcium are found (Reagan and Di Magno, 1979). Reduced serum and RBC levels of folate and B_{12} have been found in dogs with villous atrophy (Batt et al., 1979c).

Two modalities of nutritional support for

treatment or prevention of malnutrition associated with gastrointestinal disease have found widespread use in human patients: parenteral (intravenous) hyperalimentation and supplemental feedings with liquid elemental diets (enteral hyperalimentation) (Regan and Di Magno, 1979). Parenteral therapy is used for temporary in-hospital maintenance of nutrition when there is almost complete inability to use the gut, while awaiting for bowel adaptation to occur (Fischer, 1979; Sheldon, 1979). Elemental diets are used as an enteral alternative to IV feeding or in the transition from IV to oral feeding, especially during the recovery or adaptation phase of bowel resection (Heymsfield et al., 1979; Koretz and Meyer, 1980). Commercial elemental diets consist of liquid mixtures of amino acids, dextrins, glucose, electrolytes, small amounts of fat, trace minerals, and vitamins (no lactose), and may be administered by oral instillation, gastric intubation, indwelling pharyngostomy tube, or by direct infusion into the small intestine via an enterostomy catheter. The expense and technical expertise required for parenteral hyperalimentation have limited its usefulness in small animals. Elemental diets are too expensive to use routinely, but they have been helpful in selected cases.

In some cases, an empirical trial of broad-spectrum antibiotic, with emphasis on those that are effective against anaerobes, may be considered, since bacterial overgrowth can cause or complicate malabsorption (Regan and Di Magno, 1979). In addition, concomitant parasite infections should be eradicated in any animal with malabsorption. Finally, the use of pancreatic enzyme supplementation (Viokase) may be indicated in malabsorption. It has been shown in animals and humans that severe protein malnutrition (as occurs in malabsorption and PLE) may cause reversible impairment of pancreatic exocrine function, as well as acinar cell atrophy (Freeman et al., 1979).

CHRONIC INFLAMMATORY SMALL BOWEL DISEASE

Eosinophilic Gastroenteritis

Eosinophilic gastroenteritis (EGE) is a well-documented but poorly understood disease that is characterized by diffuse or segmental infiltration of one or more layers of the bowel wall with eosinophils, usually accompanied by a peripheral eosinophilia (Hall, 1967; Easley, 1972; Legendre and Krehbiel, 1973; Hayden and Van Kruiningen, 1973; Strombeck, 1979). Since any portion of the GI tract may be affected, the signs may include any combination of the following: vomiting due to eosinophilic gastritis (see Chapter 57), chronic small bowel-type diarrhea due to eosinophilic enteritis, and chronic large bowel diarrhea due to eosinophilic colitis (see Chapter 59). The regional lymph nodes may also be infiltrated. Diffuse involvement of the mucosa and submucosa may result in malabsorption, diarrhea, protein-losing enteropathy, and sometimes bloody stools, especially when mucosal ulcers are present. The course is often one of recurring diarrheal illness and progressive weight loss. Occasionally, eosinophilic granulomas cause segmental tumor-like masses in the gut wall that partially obstruct the lumen (Strombeck, 1979).

Eosinophilic gastroenteritis is considered to have an allergic or immunologic basis, yet elimination diets and intradermal allergy testing have been unsuccessful in implicating allergy to specific food antigens in most cases. Some human patients have been found to have high IgE antibody levels to specific food substances (Cello, 1979). There is evidence in dogs that at least in some cases the lesion may be associated with the visceral migration of *T. canis* larvae (Hayden and Van Kruiningen, 1973; Hayden and Van Kruiningen, 1975).

The diagnosis of EGE is based on finding a peripheral eosinophilia (although not present in all cases), rigorous exclusion of parasites (and perhaps food allergy), characteristic infiltration of the bowel wall with eosinophils on a biopsy, and response to corticosteroids. Even though enteritis signs may predominate, the colon or stomach may be affected, so that endoscopic biopsy of either site may yield a diagnosis without the necessity of a laparotomy. Ancillary findings may include detection of thick, rigid intestinal loops on abdominal palpation, thickened loops and mucosal irregularity on barium GI radiography, hypoproteinemia, and abnormal GI function tests.

Eosinophilic gastroenteritis responds well to oral prednisolone treatment. Initially, two to three mg/kg are given daily in divided doses until the disease has been controlled for one to two weeks, then the dose is gradually tapered over two to three weeks. In some dogs the drug can be withdrawn after several weeks, while in others long-term alternate-day maintenance treatments are necessary to prevent recurrence.

Since visceral larva migrans (VLM) has been implicated as at least one cause of this disease in dogs (Hayden and Van Kruiningen, 1973), there may be a role for the use of drugs effective against migrating *T. canis* larvae. Although no drugs currently approved for use in the dog are effective against VLM, thiabendazole, levamisole, and other newer and safer experimental broad-spectrum anthelmintics with potential activity against migratory larvae need to be evaluated in this disease.

A syndrome of eosinophilic enteritis and marked eosinophilia was recently described in six cats with signs of vomiting, diarrhea (which was sometimes bloody), anorexia, and weight loss (Hendrick, 1981). All six cats had diffuse or segmental thickening of the small intestine from mucosal and submucosal eosinophilic infiltration accompanied by fibrosis, sometimes affecting the stomach and colon as well. No evidence of parasites was found. In contrast to canine EGE, where lesions tend to be confined to the GI tract and mesenteric lymph nodes, some cats had disseminated eosinophilic infiltration of other organs, especially liver, spleen, and nonenteric lymph nodes. Poor

response to steroids and fatal outcome were also unique features of the disease.

Lymphocytic-Plasmacytic Enteritis

Some dogs with chronic watery diarrhea, with or without malabsorption or PLE, are found on intestinal biopsy to have a diffuse lymphocytic-plasmacytic infiltration of the lamina propria of unknown cause (Van Kruiningen and Hayden, 1972; Anderson, 1975; Merritt, 1980) (Fig. 58–17). The fact that the offending cells are immunocytes and that the disease is steroid-responsive suggests an immune pathogenesis, such as chronic local immune response to antigens ingested as food, produced within the lumen, or derived from parasites or infectious agents (Van Kruiningen and Hayden, 1972), or possibly an immune complex mechanism (Merritt, 1980). Also, the possibility that this lesion is a nonspecific response to chronic enteric inflammation cannot be excluded. Lymphocytic-plasmacytic infiltrate may also accompany other chronic enteropathies, such as lymphangiectasia or villous atrophy, but the pathogenetic significance of this is unclear. The treatment includes a corticosteroid regimen similar to that discussed for eosinophilic gastroenteritis, and the nonspecific dietary measures discussed for malabsorption. Consideration should also be given to exclusion of occult giardiasis with an empirical course of metronidazole therapy. The antibiotic tylosin

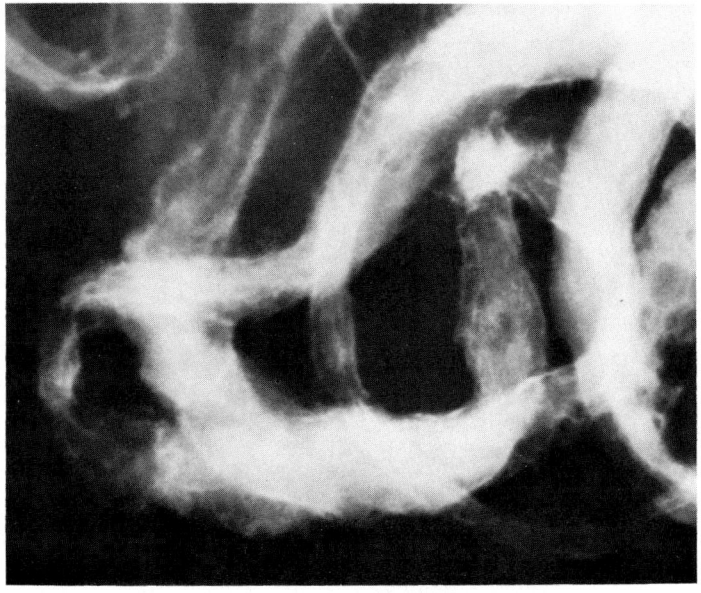

Figure 58–17. Barium radiography in this eight-year-old male Alaskan malamute with chronic watery diarrhea and protein-losing enteropathy demonstrated diffuse mucosal irregularity, which was suggestive of an infiltrative bowel disorder. Intestinal biopsy showed diffuse lymphocytic-plasmacytic enteritis.

has reportedly been efficacious in some cases (Van Kruiningen, 1976).

Granulomatous Enteritis

Chronic inflammatory bowel disease is occasionally manifested as a segmental (regional) masslike thickening of the bowel wall, usually confined to the ileum and colon, with histologic features of granulomatous inflammation (Strande et al., 1954; Merritt, 1980). The lesion, however, is variable and may have a significant eosinophilic or lymphocytic-plasmacytic component that makes distinction from the other inflammatory bowel diseases difficult. Furthermore, although a thickened, granulomatous section of bowel is present, diffuse mixed inflammation of the lamina propria of the remainder of the small intestine may be found. Granulomatous enteritis usually causes chronic diarrhea and weight loss, may often be delineated on barium radiographs, and is confirmed by biopsy. It may also be associated with PLE and hypoproteinemia. Radiographically, the granulomatous gut wall may cause segmental narrowing of the lumen with partial obstruction that can be confused with intestinal neoplasia (Fig. 58–18). Treatment has been mainly

with corticosteroids, with mixed success, and occasionally by surgical resection of segmental lesions. This disease is often compared with a human enteropathy called regional enteritis (Merritt, 1980).

PROTEIN-LOSING ENTEROPATHY AND LYMPHANGIECTASIA

Protein-losing enteropathy (PLE) refers to the excessive loss of serum proteins into the gut resulting in hypoproteinemia (Waldmann, 1976). It has been associated with a variety of GI disorders, including many of the diseases that also cause malabsorption (Table 58–9) (Tams and Twedt, 1981). The most clinically important mechanisms of enteric protein loss are defective intestinal lymphatic drainage with leakage of protein-rich lymph fluid into the lumen and protein leakage from exudation and increased mucosal permeability associated with inflammation or ulceration of the mucosa. Both lymphatic involvement and mucosal disruption may account for PLE in diseases such as lymphangiectasia, lymphosarcoma, or intestinal histoplasmosis. Excessive loss of protein into the gut may also be a consequence of elevated central venous pressure (CVP) due to cardiac dysfunction, especially con-

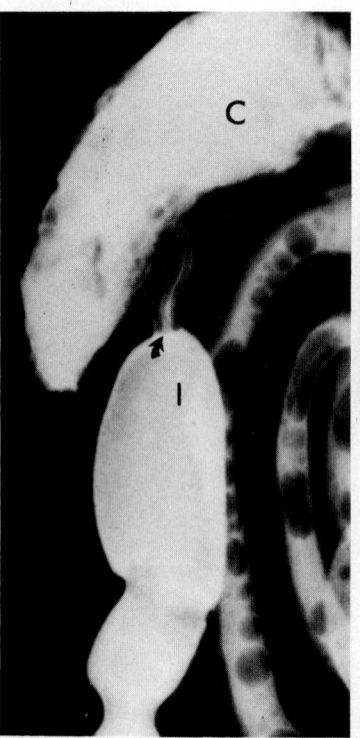
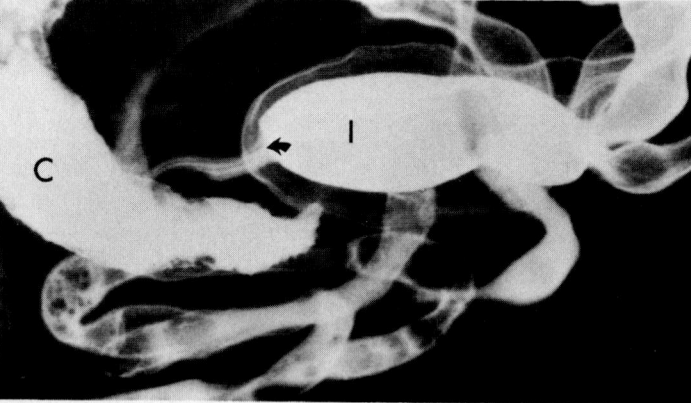

Figure 58–18. Ventrodorsal *(A)* and lateral *(B)* barium radiographs of this 13-year-old female (spayed) DSH revealed a circumferential constrictive lesion involving the terminal ileum (arrow). Notice the abrupt narrowing of the lumen of the ileum just before it enters the colon (C), and the dilatation of the ileum (I), proximal to the stenosis. The tentative diagnosis was neoplasia (adenocarcinoma); however, histopathologic sections of the surgically resected segment revealed granulomatous ileitis. The same lesion was found several months later when surgery was again performed because of recurrence of regional thickening and stenosis of the terminal ileum. Since the second surgery, remission has been maintained for over a year with alternate-day corticosteroids.

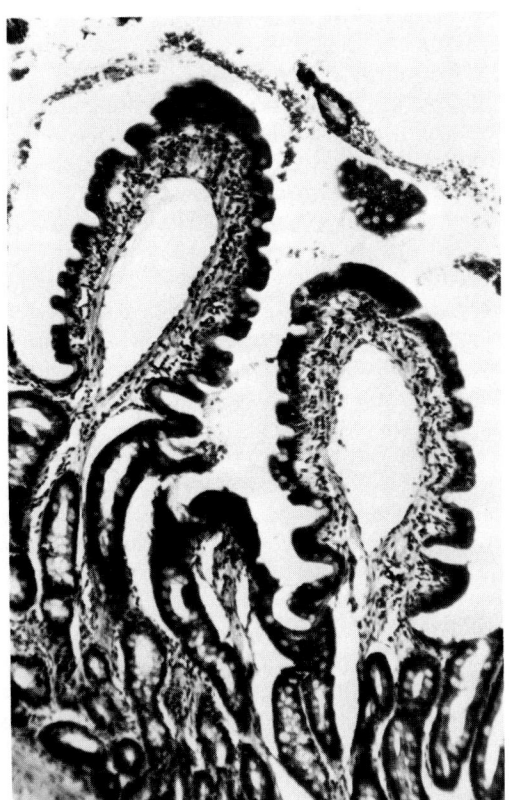

Figure 58–19. The hallmark lesion of lymphangiectasia is a ballooning distortion of villi due to marked dilatation of lacteals, as demonstrated by this mucosal biopsy from a seven-year-old male Yorkshire terrier with protein-losing enteropathy (albumin, 0.9 gm/dl; globulin, 1.6 gm/dl).

strictive pericarditis. In PLE, essentially all serum proteins (albumin, globulins, and others) are affected by excess leakage into the gut. When the rate of albumin loss

exceeds the rate of synthesis, hypoalbuminemia develops. This causes decreased plasma colloid osmotic pressure and altered body fluid hemodynamics, which may lead to widespread edema and body cavity effusion.

The most common lesion in canine PLE is intestinal lymphangiectasia, an obstructive disorder of lymphatics of unknown etiology that is characterized by marked dilatation of intestinal mucosal and submucosal lymphatics (Campbell et al., 1968; Finco et al., 1973; Flesja and Yri, 1977; Barton et al., 1978; Olson and Zimmer, 1978; Breitschwerdt et al., 1980). Congenital and acquired forms probably occur. In lymphangiectasia, defective intestinal lymph drainage and lymphatic dilatation lead to rupture and leakage of lymph fluid from dilated lacteals. The constituents of lymph fluid — protein, lymphocytes, and lipid — are lost into the lumen. The consequences of this are panhypoproteinemia, lymphocytopenia, hypocholesterolemia, and steatorrhea.

The typical lesion of lymphangiectasia appears as a ballooning distortion of villi owing to dilatation of lacteals (Fig. 58–19). Because of this abnormal villous architecture, the surface texture of the small bowel mucosa may grossly have a "shag carpet" appearance. A weblike network of milky-white dilated lymphatic channels may be seen in the mesentery and on the serosal surface (Fig. 58–20). Lymphangiectasia is often accompanied by a mononuclear inflammatory cell infiltrate in the lamina propria and obstructive granulomatous lesions in and around lymphatics (Fig. 58–21). Li-

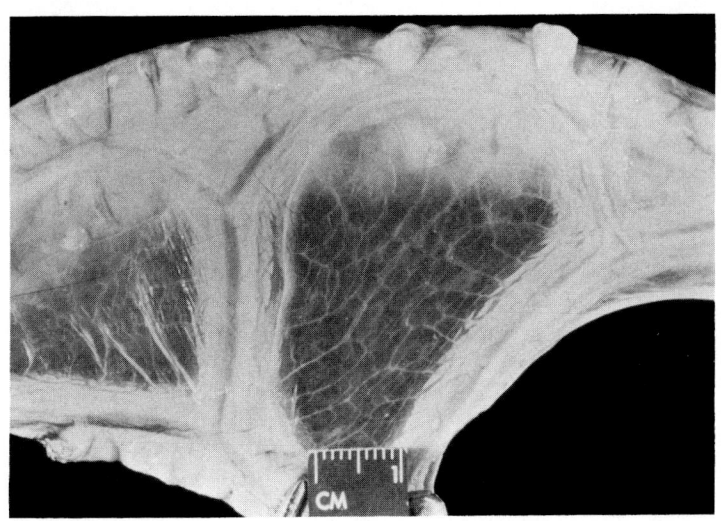

Figure 58–20. A weblike network of dilated lymphatic channels is seen in the mesentery of a dog with lymphangiectasia. Also, notice the nodular lesions (lipogranulomas) at the mesenteric border of the intestine.

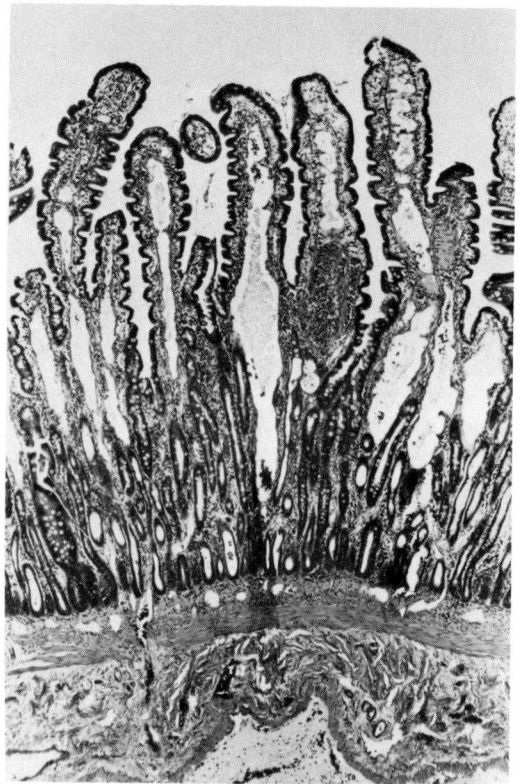

Figure 58–21. Intestinal biopsy from a seven-year-old female Yorkshire terrier with PLE. Accompanying the dilated lacteals (lymphangiectasia) is a diffuse mononuclear cell infiltration of the lamina propria and submucosa. In the center of the picture, a granulomatous lesion appears to be obstructing the central lacteal of a villus.

pogranulomas may be grossly visible during laparotomy as yellow-white nodules (Fig. 58–22) or granular, foamy deposits (Fig. 58–23) along the mesenteric border of the gut and associated with lymphatics (Fig.

58–24). The pathogenesis of these lesions needs to be determined.

The clinical signs of canine PLE are chronic, intermittent diarrhea of a watery to semisolid consistency; weight loss or emaciation; and evidence of altered fluid homeostasis (hypoalbuminemia), seen as pitting subcutaneous edema, ascites (abdominal distention), or hydrothorax (dyspnea). It is possible for the animal with PLE to pass normal-appearing feces and be free of any other GI signs. Generalized intestinal malabsorption may or may not accompany PLE; however, in lymphangiectasia steatorrhea can usually be demonstrated, since the transport of fat as chylomicrons in lymph (delivery phase) may be impaired. Familial PLE has been described in the Lundehund and basenji, suggesting a genetic etiology in some cases (Flesja and Yri, 1977; Breitschwerdt et al., 1980). The author has observed a high incidence of lymphangiectasia in the Yorkshire terrier.

The diagnostic features of canine PLE include (1) panhypoproteinemia, including hypoalbuminemia and hypogammaglobulinemia (Table 58–11) (hyperglobulinemia was found in hereditary PLE syndrome of basenjis); (2) steatorrhea and abnormal carbohydrate absorption tests (D-xylose) may be found but are inconsistent; (3) lymphopenia, due to loss of lymph into the gut; (4) hypocholesterolemia, due to loss of chylomicron-laden lymph into the gut; (5) hypocalcemia (Table 58–11), due to decreased protein-bound fraction associated with hypoalbuminemia, unabsorbable calcium–fatty acid soaps and calcium-protein complexes formed in intestinal lumen, and vitamin D

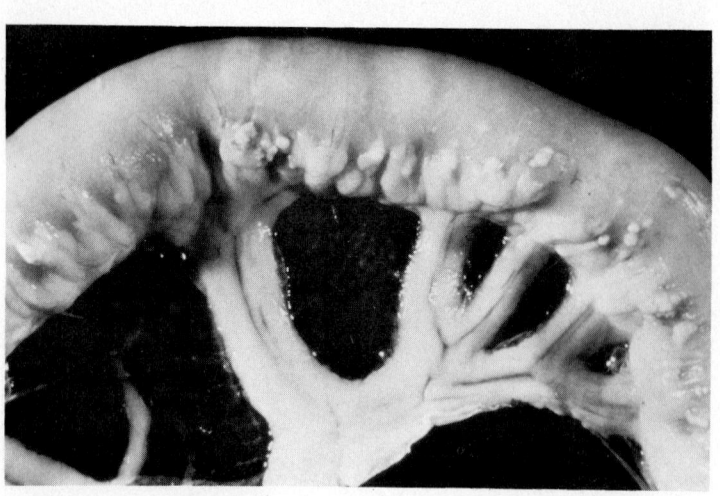

Figure 58–22. Lipogranulomas are visible as white nodules along the mesenteric border of the intestine and associated with lymphatics in a dog with PLE due to lymphangiectasia.

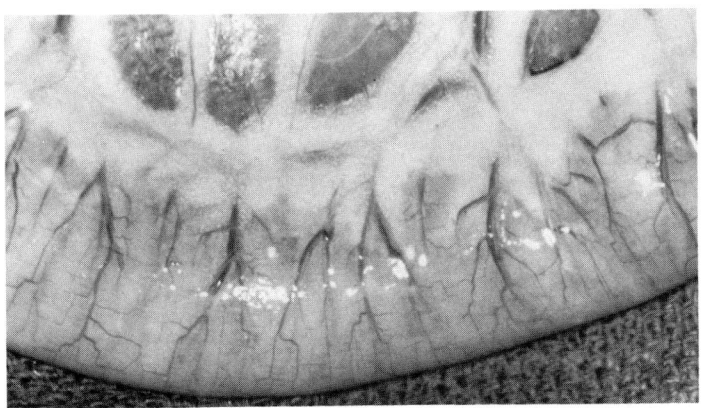

Figure 58–23. Granulomatous mesenteric lesions may appear as foamy granular deposits in some cases of lymphangiectasia.

malabsorption; (6) radiographs — confirmation of ascites or pleural effusion; (7) body cavity fluid analysis — transudate or chylous effusion; (8) normal cardiac evaluation (auscultation, thoracic radiographs, ECG, CVP); (9) excessive fecal excretion of radiolabeled macromolecules (^{51}Cr-labeled albumin) given IV and (10) characteristic lesions on a small bowel biopsy.

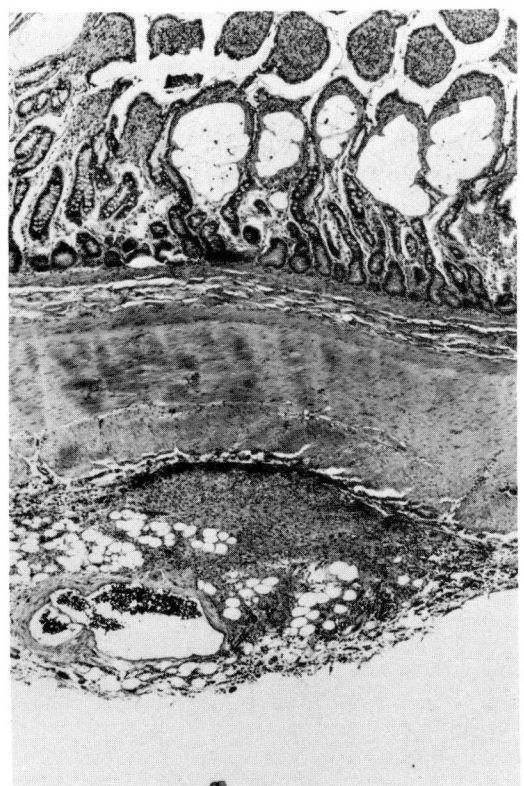

Figure 58–24. Full-thickness biopsy from a dog with PLE showing villous lesion of lymphangiectasia on the mucosal side, and a lipogranuloma associated with the lymphatics on the serosal (mesenteric) side.

Treatment of canine PLE should include use of a long-chain triglyceride-free diet such as r/d Prescription Diet or a homemade diet (such as boiled rice and uncreamed cottage cheese) with MCT oil added as a source of calories and the principal source of fat (30 ml/lb of food), and with vitamin-mineral supplementation. MCT is also available as part of complete, powdered elemental diets (such as Portagen), which can be added to low-fat food. Because an inflammatory lesion usually accompanies the lesions of lymphangiectasia, anti-inflammatory doses of corticosteroids and antibiotics can be used empirically. Treatment can often control clinical signs, restore serum protein levels, and eliminate effusions for several months (Fig. 58–25). Some animals, however, fail to respond and eventually succumb to severe protein-calorie depletion.

IDIOPATHIC VILLOUS ATROPHY

A syndrome of chronic diarrhea and malabsorption associated with blunt or flattened mucosal villi (villous atrophy) of undetermined cause has been seen in the dog, often accompanied by an increased number of lymphocytes and plasma cells in the lamina propria (Vernon, 1962; Kaneko et al., 1965; Merritt, 1980). In addition to this idiopathic variety, other conditions may produce a similar villous atrophy lesion in dogs, including the villus-selective enteric viruses, parasitic infections (especially *Giardia*), chronic diffuse inflammatory disease, intestinal lymphosarcoma, and possibly gluten-induced enteropathy (Strombeck, 1979). In some dogs with villous atrophy and malabsorption, biochemical and ultrastructural studies of mucosal lesions suggest

Table 58–11. Lab Data from 15 Dogs with Protein-Losing Enteropathy

Signalment	Total Protein (g/dl)	Albumin (g/dl)	Globulin (g/dl)	Calcium (mg/dl)	Cholesterol (mg/dl)	Lymphocytes (cells/mm^3)	Intestinal Biopsy
Normals	(6–8)	(2.3–3.4)	(2.7–4.4)	(8.8–11.3)	(125–250)	(1200–5200)	
1. Yorkshire terrier, F, 7 y	4.5	1.3	3.2	6.8	252	672	Lymphangiectasia
2. Yorkshire terrier, FS, 7 y	2.5	0.9	1.6	5.4	61	852	Lymphangiectasia
3. Yorkshire terrier, M, 3 y	2.8	1.2	1.6	5.1	—	384	Lymphangiectasia
4. Yorkshire terrier, M, 7 y	2.5	0.9	1.6	6.4	90	672	Lymphangiectasia
5. German shorthair pointer, M, 1 y	4.8	1.8	3.0	7.9	80	615	Lymphangiectasia
6. Rottweiler, M, 2 y	2.5	0.9	1.6	7.9	—	2576	Lymphangiectasia
7. Scottish terrier, FS, 5 y	3.8	1.8	2.0	8.5	—	615	Lymphangiectasia
8. Dachshund, FS, 5 y	4.5	1.2	3.3	5.9	—	119	Lymphangiectasia
9. Cocker spaniel, FS, 10 y	2.7	0.9	1.8	4.4	136	663	Lymphangiectasia
10. English setter, M, 1½ y	2.5	0.9	1.6	7.0	60	2847	Lymphangiectasia
11. Mix, MC, 6 y	4.8	2.1	2.7	7.9	121	3140	Lymphosarcoma
12. Doberman pinscher, MC, 5 y	4.4	1.9	2.5	7.9	148	1617	Lymphosarcoma
13. Cocker spaniel, M, 8 y	6.2	1.4	4.8	8.3	126	816	Eosinophilic enteritis
14. German shepherd, M, 3 y	5.9	1.6	4.3	8.4	152	2700	Granulomatous enteritis
15. Doberman pinscher, M, 3 y	3.1	—	—	7.4	—	1070	Histoplasmosis (serologic diagnosis)
Mean	3.8	1.3	2.5	7.0	123	1290	
Number	13/15	14/14	8/14	15/15	5/10	10/15	
Below normal (%)	87%	100%	57%	100%	50%	67%	

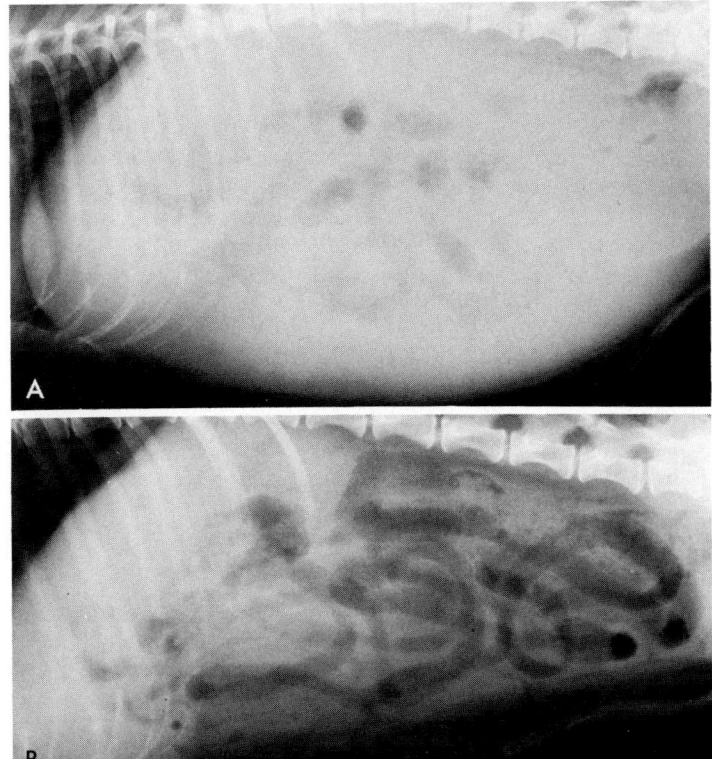

Figure 58–25. Although the lesions of lymphangiectasia may be irreversible, medical management based on dietary restriction of long chain fatty acids can elevate plasma protein levels and control effusions. Abdominal radiographs of a dog with lymphangiectasia and an initial albumin of 0.9 g/dl were taken before *(A)* and during *(B)* treatment to show resolution of abdominal effusion in response to therapy.

a canine enteropathy that resembles tropical sprue, a villous atrophy disorder of humans considered to be caused by an as yet unidentified infectious agent (Batt et al., 1979c).

In humans, villous atrophy (celiac sprue) has been attributed to hypersensitivity (immune or cytotoxin-mediated) to gluten, a protein contained in certain cereal grains, including wheat, rye, barley, buckwheat, and oats (Falchuk, 1979). The signs and lesions of this gluten enteropathy resolve after eliminating gluten from the diet. A comparable gluten sensitivity has also been implicated in some cases of canine villous atrophy (Strombeck, 1979); however, in others a specific etiology is not found and they are labeled idiopathic. Diet manipulation is used to confirm gluten enteropathy. A controlled, gluten-free diet should result in remission; then, when gluten is provocatively reintroduced into the diet, diarrhea and villous atrophy reoccur.

The role of gluten in canine malabsorption syndromes needs to be clarified; nevertheless, initial treatment of villous atrophy should include trial elimination of gluten-containing cereal grains from the diet. Most commercial dog foods contain gluten. However, gluten-free diets that are available

include d/d and i/d Prescription Diets; Science Maximum Stress and Canine Growth Diets; and IAMS Chunks, Plus, or Eukanuba. Alternatively, since rice and corn do not contain gluten, homemade diets based on these grains and lean meat may be fed. When gluten exclusion does not alleviate the condition, one should look for other underlying causes of villous atrophy. In some cases, favorable results are obtained by empirical treatment with parasiticides (especially metronidazole for occult giardiasis), antibiotics (for bacteria that may cause or complicate the disease), or corticosteroids (for immunosuppression, since villous atrophy, including gluten enteropathy, may have an immune basis). In addition, other nonspecific dietary guidelines previously mentioned for malabsorption also apply, such as high-protein, low-fat, low-carbohydrate (lactose) diet supplemented with vitamins, calcium, and possibly MCT. It should be noted that in some cases the lesion of villous atrophy is irreversible.

INTESTINAL HISTOPLASMOSIS

Histoplasma capsulatum is a chronic systemic fungal infection that usually invades the body via the respiratory tract and has a predilection for the reticuloendothelial tissues. The disease may disseminate widely in some dogs and cats, occasionally causing severe diffuse granulomatous inflammation of the bowel wall and mesenteric lymph nodes (Robinson and McVicker, 1952; Mahaffey et al., 1977; Stickle and Hribernik, 1978; Ford, 1980). The bowel wall may become thickened, distorted, and corrugated (Fig. 58–26). This severely disrupts intestinal function, and animals with intestinal histoplasmosis often manifest malabsorption with profuse, intractable steatorrheic diarrhea, and emaciation (Fig. 58–27). In addition, intestinal histoplasmosis may be a cause of PLE. The large bowel may be affected simultaneously or separately, resulting in bloody mucoid diarrhea (colitis).

Signs of systemic illness are common, including fever, pallor, anorexia, depression, lymphadenopathy, and evidence of involvement of other organs (granulomatous pneumonia, hepatosplenomegaly, and chorioretinitis). The details of diagnosis and treatment of histoplasmosis are discussed in Chapter 26. In the intestinal form, the diagnosis is generally established by serologic tests or by identifying the organisms in feces, colonic scrapings or biopsies, or small intestinal biopsies. Amphotericin B has been used for treatment.

INTESTINAL LYMPHOSARCOMA

Malabsorption, with or without PLE, commonly occurs in both dogs and cats with diffuse lymphosarcoma of the bowel wall.

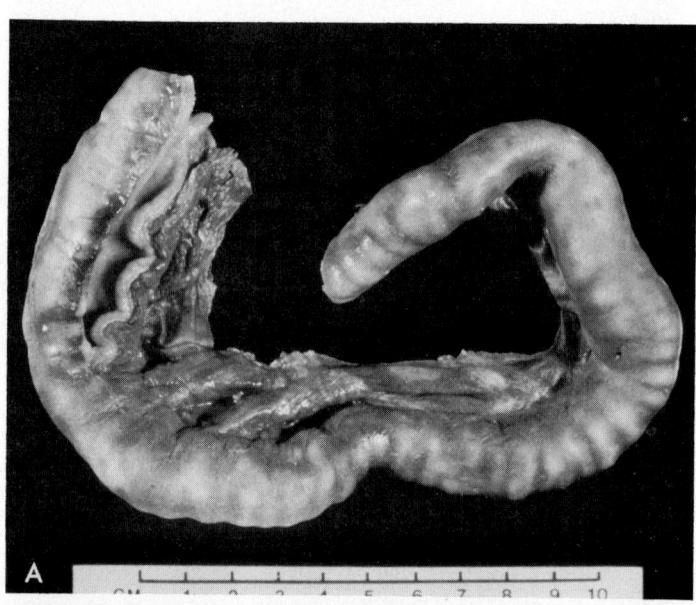

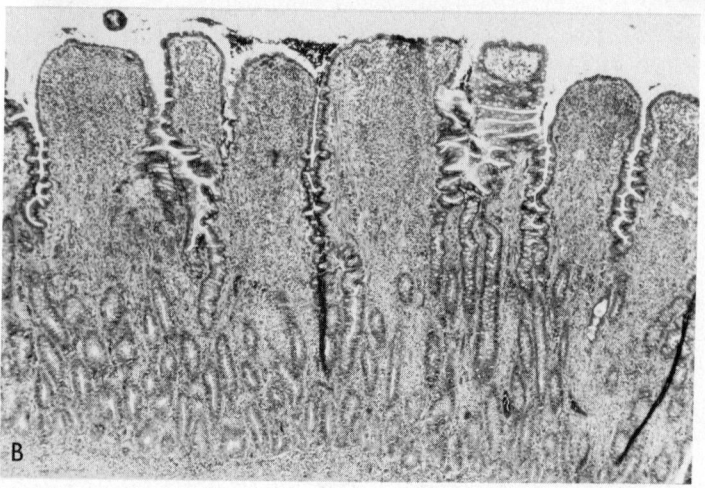

Figure 58–26. Thickened, corrugated segment of small intestine from a dog with histoplasmosis (A). The lesion was characterized by extensive distortion and thickening of the villi and deeper layers with granulomatous inflammation (B).

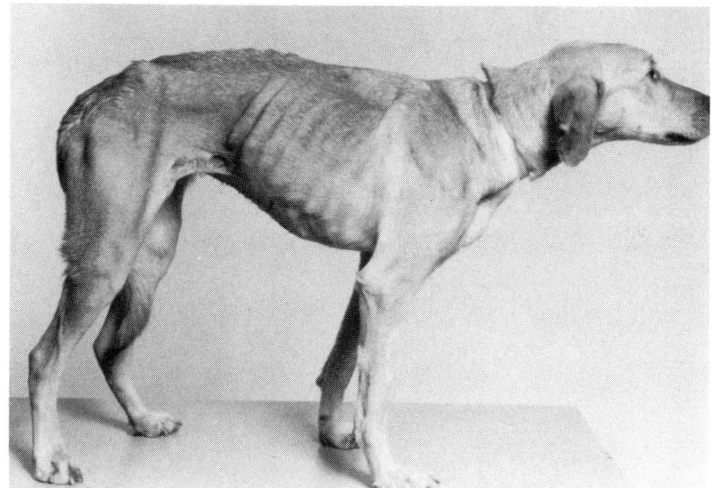

Figure 58–27. Intestinal histoplasmosis caused malabsorption, chronic diarrhea, and weight loss in this dog. The bowel lesions are depicted in Figure 58–26.

Severe morphologic changes that contribute to the malabsorption of intestinal lymphosarcoma include villous atrophy, "filled villi" from infiltration of the lamina propria, bowel wall disfigurement from infiltration of the submucosa, and lymphatic obstruction associated with mesenteric lymphadenopathy (Fig. 58–28). Radiographic abnormalities may be found (Fig. 58–29), and intestinal biopsy is diagnostic. Chemotherapy strategies are discussed in Chapter 30.

BACTERIAL OVERGROWTH

Bacterial overgrowth in the small intestine, an important cause of malabsorption in man, has been reported in the dog (Hoenig, 1980) and probably occurs more often in animals than is recognized. Factors that predispose to overgrowth include partial anatomic obstructions that create a so-called stagnant or blind loop, stasis from loss of motility that normally has a cleansing action in preventing bacterial overgrowth, and decreased gastric acid secretion. Bacterial deconjugation of bile salts and resulting steatorrhea are important in the pathogenesis of overgrowth diarrhea (Isaacs and Kim, 1979). Mucosal damage and the use of host nutrients by bacteria may also be contributing factors. Definitive diagnosis depends upon quantitative aerobic and anaerobic cultures of aspirated small intestinal fluid obtained by intestinal intubation or laparotomy. On a more practical basis, the diagnosis may be supported by the reversal of clinical signs and absorptive defects (such as a flat D-xylose curve and steatorrhea) with antibacterial therapy. Broad-spectrum antibiotics that give anaerobic coverage, such as

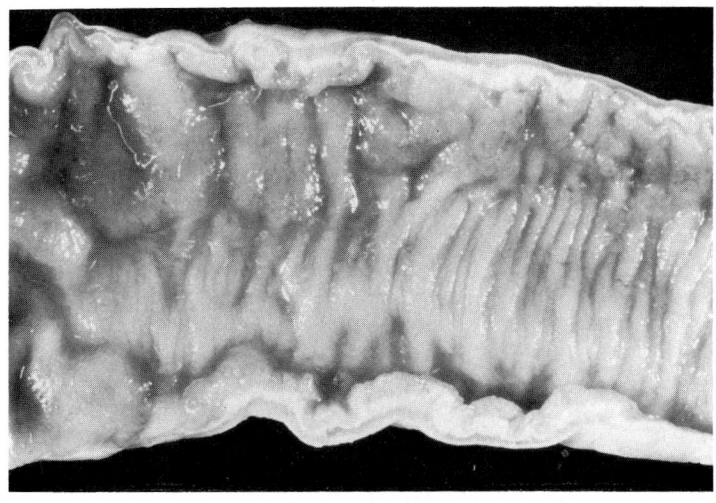

Figure 58–28. Opened section of intestine from a dog with diffuse intestinal lymphosarcoma. Notice the thickened gut wall and puffy, infiltrated-appearing mucosal lining.

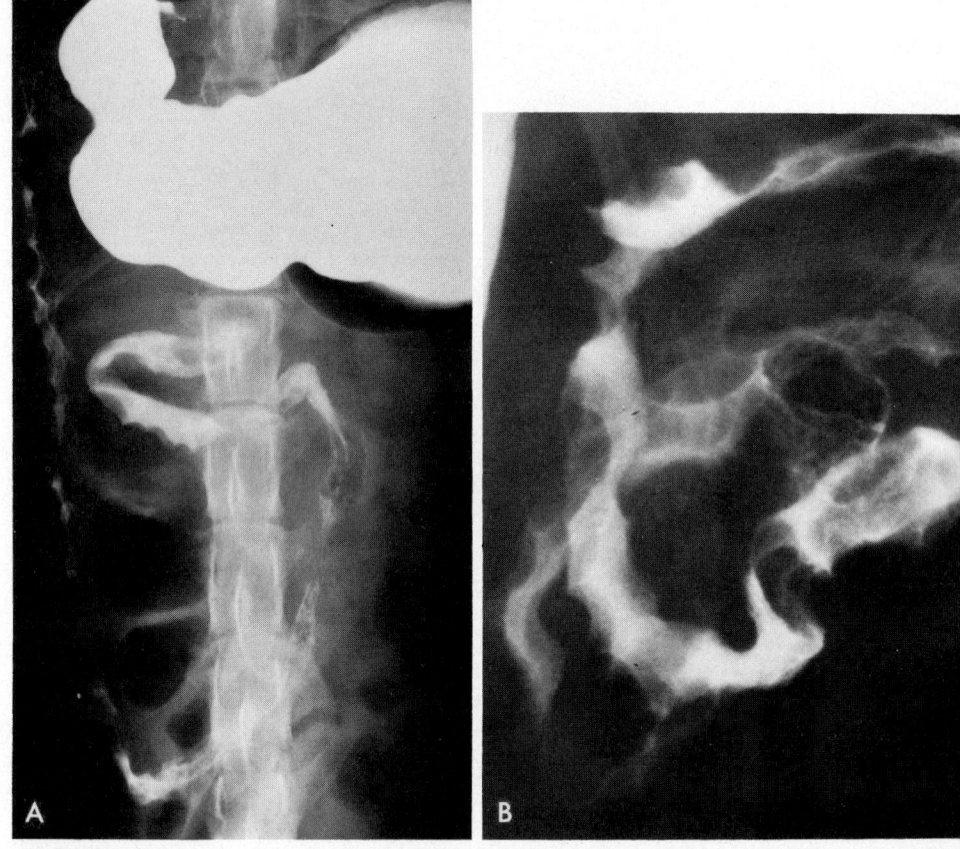

Figure 58–29. Ventrodorsal *(A)* and close-up lateral *(B)* barium radiographs of a dog with diffuse intestinal lymphosarcoma. Notice the nodular distortion and infiltration of the gut wall causing luminal filling defects and narrowing.

tetracycline or chloramphenicol, are recommended. Others to consider are ampicillin, clindamycin, metronidazole, lincomycin, erythromycin, or tylosin. Treatment should include vitamin supplementation (especially B_{12}) and surgical correction of predisposing anatomic defects when possible.

THYROID-RELATED DIARRHEA

Chronic diarrhea has been described in association with thyroid lesions in dogs and cats. In one report, a medullary carcinoma of the thyroid was associated with watery diarrhea of three months duration (Leav et al., 1976). The diarrhea resolved two days after tumor excision. This case may represent a diarrheic syndrome similar to that described in humans with medullary thyroid carcinoma, in which secretory diarrhea is attributed to humoral substances secreted by the tumor that stimulate adenyl cyclase, such as serotonin and prostaglandins (Steinfeld et al., 1973). In cats with hyperthyroid-

ism due to functioning thyroid tumors (Fig. 58–30), chronic passage of voluminous, soft steatorrheic stools is seen in association with weight loss despite polyphagia (Holzworth et al., 1980). In thyrotoxicosis, the effects of excess thyroid hormone on motility and intestinal fluid transport, as well as excessive food intake (overload), may be responsible for the diarrhea.

DUODENAL ULCER

Duodenal ulcers are rarely seen spontaneously in dogs and cats, and usually cause signs of vomiting (hematemesis), melena, weight loss, and abdominal pain (Murray et al., 1972) (Fig. 58–31). Blood-loss anemia and perforation are potential complications. Gastroduodenal ulceration is found in dogs and cats with mast cell tumors and disseminated mastocytosis, presumably resulting from chronic stimulation of gastric acid hypersecretion by histamine released from the mast cells (Howard et al., 1969). In addition,

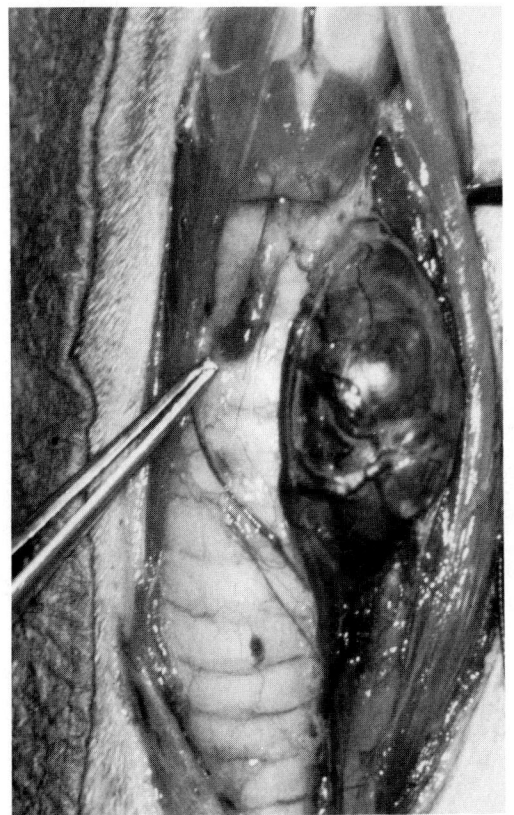

Figure 58–30. Thyroid gland neoplasm in a cat with chronic diarrhea and weight loss associated with hyperthyroidism (thyrotoxicosis).

perforation of mast cell-associated duodenal ulcer has been reported in both dogs and cats (Seawright and Grano, 1964; Carrig and Seawright, 1968; Zontine et al., 1977). An unexplained association between liver disease and peptic ulcer in dogs has been found (Murray et al., 1972). Gastroduodenal ulceration in dogs can also result from ulcerogenic drugs such as corticosteroids, aspirin, and indomethacin (Ewing, 1972). Finally, duodenal ulceration from gastric hypersecretion has been described in association with gastrin-producing pancreatic islet cell tumors (gastrinoma) in dogs (canine Zollinger-Ellison syndrome) (Jones et al., 1976; Straus et al., 1977; Happe et al., 1980).

INTESTINAL NEOPLASIA

Lymphosarcoma and adenocarcinoma are the most common GI tumors of dogs and cats (Brodey, 1966; Lingemann and Garner, 1972; Patnaik et al., 1976; Patnaik et al., 1977). Less frequent neoplasms include leiomyoma, leiomyosarcoma, fibrosarcoma, mastocytoma, and carcinoid tumors (Patnaik et al., 1980). The clinical signs of GI neoplasia are typically vague, and the onset is slow and insidious. The clinical course is usually progressive in parallel with tumor growth. Anorexia and weight loss may be the only early signs, but often diarrhea, vomiting, dehydration, and anemia develop. Abdominal effusion may also occur.

Intestinal lymphosarcoma (LSA) affects any age animal and has two morphologic types, the diffuse type and the nodular type. In diffuse LSA, extensive infiltration of the lamina propria and submucosa with neoplastic lymphocytes may cause malabsorption, steatorrhea, diarrhea, and weight loss.

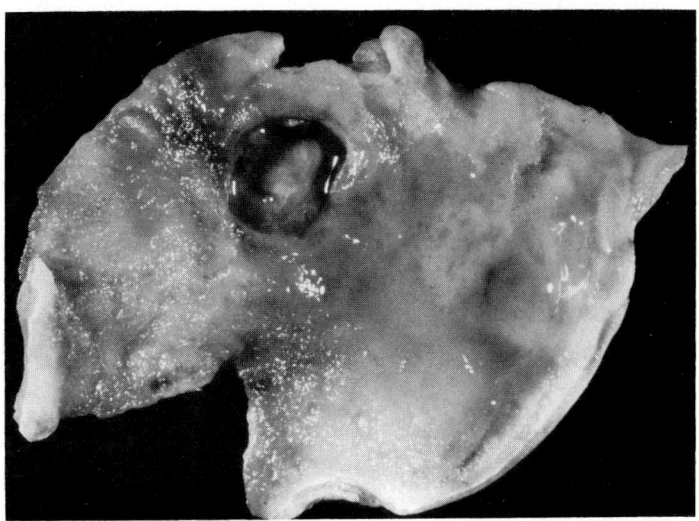

Figure 58–31. Duodenal ulcers in dogs are typically well-circumscribed oval lesions. This ulcer extended through the mucosa and submucosa down to the circular muscle layer.

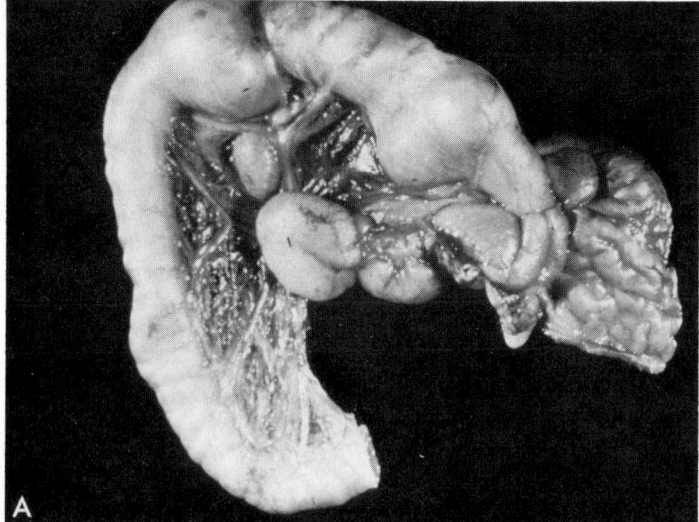

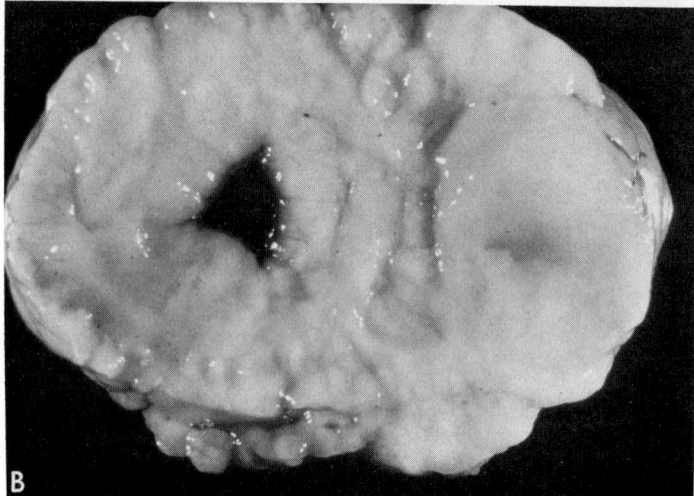

Figure 58–32. A typical segmental-nodular type intestinal lymphosarcoma (*A*) at the ileocecocolic junction and with involvement of the regional lymph nodes. Cross-section of the neoplasm (*B*) shows narrowing of the lumen, resulting in partial intestinal obstruction.

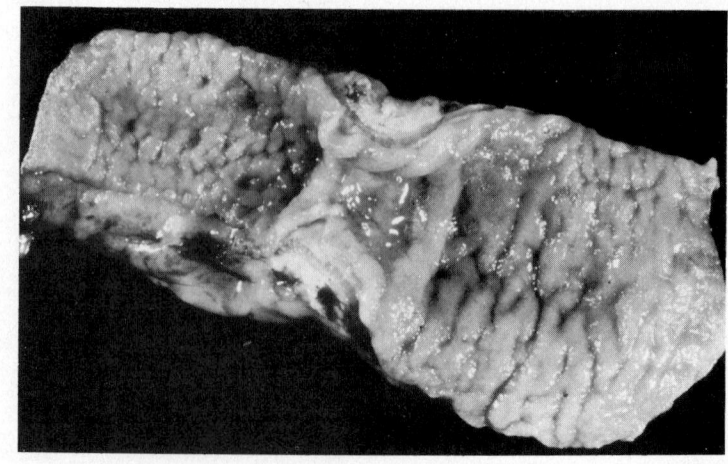

Figure 58–33. Opened segment of intestine showing an annular constricting adenocarcinoma that caused intestinal obstruction.

In the nodular type, a segmental thickening of the bowel, most often in the ileocecocolic region, may cause luminal narrowing and partial intestinal obstruction (Fig. 58–32). Metastasis to regional lymph nodes in either type is common.

The adenocarcinoma affects mainly older animals (in cats, incidence is also higher in males and in Siamese), and it may cause a segmental thickening within the bowel wall with the effect of an expanding mass, or it may grow inward toward the lumen (especially in cats), producing an annular fibrous constricting band with minimal outward enlargement (Patnaik et al., 1976) (Fig. 58–33). This stenotic type produces partial obstruction and is easily confused with a stricture on barium radiography and even at surgery. Mucosal ulceration is frequent, sometimes resulting in melena and blood loss anemia. Local invasion of the mesentery, omentum, and regional lymph nodes is common. More widespread metastasis may also occur. In the cat, adenocarcinomas most commonly occur in the ileum (Lingemann and Garner, 1972; Patnaik et al., 1976), while canine adenocarcinomas occur more frequently in the large intestine and duodenum (Patnaik et al., 1977; Patnaik et al., 1980).

The diagnosis of intestinal neoplasia may be suspected from clinical signs and abdominal palpation. Nodular LSA, outwardly expanding adenocarcinomas, and most of the less common tumors can be palpated as firm, irregular abdominal masses. Diffuse-type LSA palpates as a thickened gut loop, whereas stricture-like adenocarcinomas may not be palpable at all. With any GI neoplasm, mesenteric lymphadenopathy (metastasis) may be palpable. Radiography, particularly the barium study, is helpful in delineating tumor masses, partial obstruction, constrictive lesions (adenocarcinoma), mucosal defects, or wall thickening (Fig. 58–34). Definitive diagnosis is usually made by surgical excision or biopsy of the affected segment of bowel. Generally, the prognosis for LSA and adenocarcinoma is poor in that the surgical margins or regional lymph nodes are usually invaded; however, survival of 28 months after resection of an intestinal adenocarcinoma has been reported in a cat (Patnaik et al., 1981). Chemotherapy is available for LSA.

INTESTINAL OBSTRUCTION

Intestinal obstruction in dogs and cats may be caused by foreign body, intussusception, volvulus, incarceration of bowel in a hernia (includes abdominal hernias of all types, diaphragmatic hernia, and internal

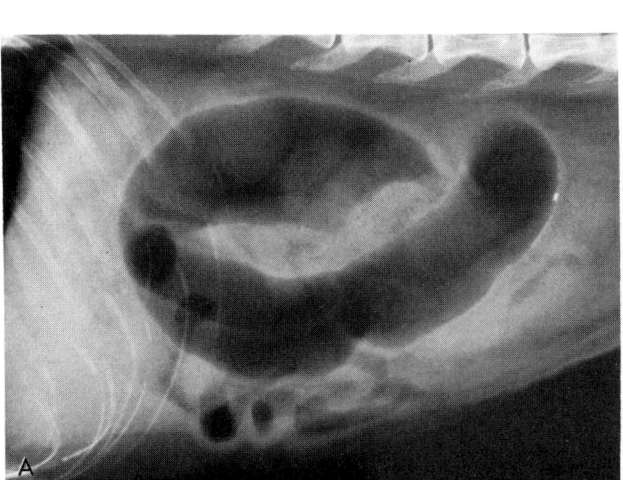
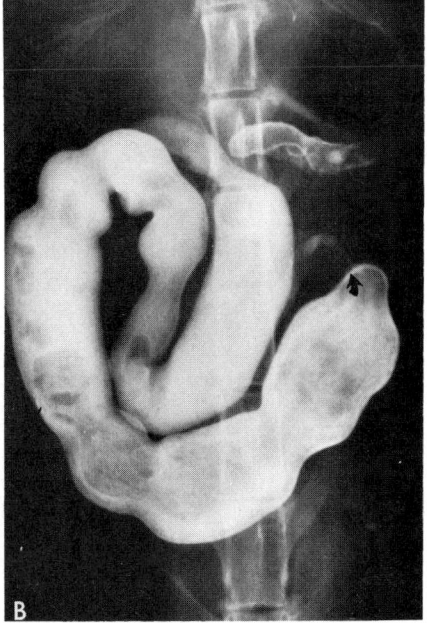

Figure 58–34. Lateral radiograph of the abdomen (*A*) of an eight-year-old female Siamese with chronic anorexia and weight-loss, showing a gas-distended loop of intestine. A ventrodorsal barium radiograph (*B*) delineates the narrowed lumen at the site of obstruction (arrow) and dilatation proximal to it. Exploratory laparotomy revealed an annular stricture-like lesion in the ileum that was an adenocarcinoma.

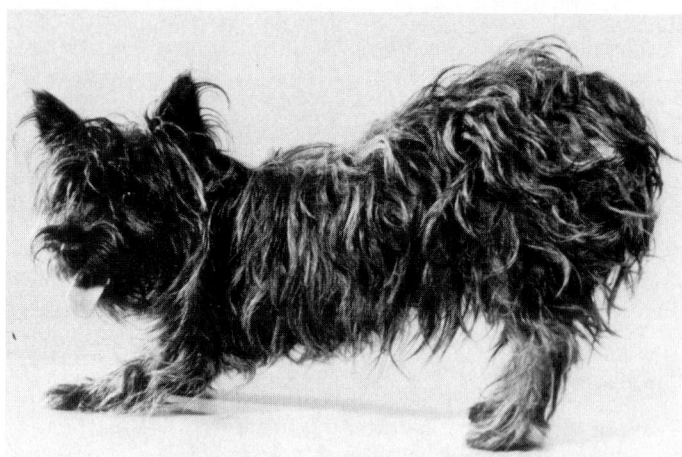

Figure 58–35. The abdominal pain of intestinal obstruction is sometimes manifested as a distinctive "praying" posture, also called the "position of relief." This dog was found to have an intussusception.

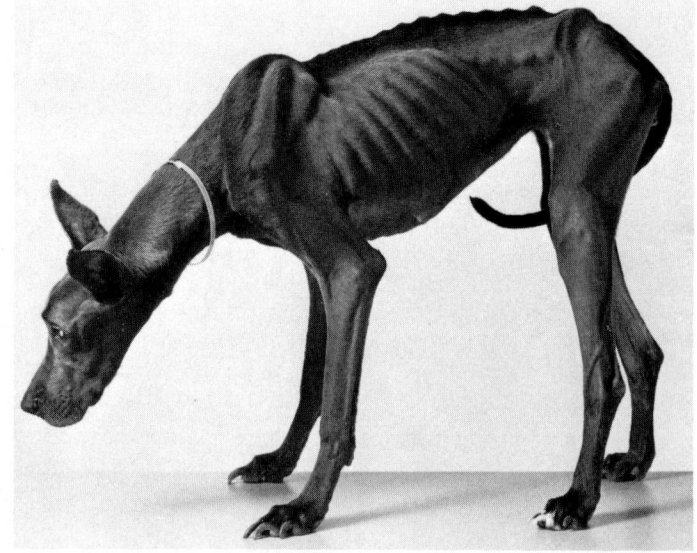

Figure 58–36. Incomplete intestinal obstruction may have a chronic course characterized by prolonged anorexia and progessive starvation. This severely emaciated Great Dane had panty hose removed from its small bowel.

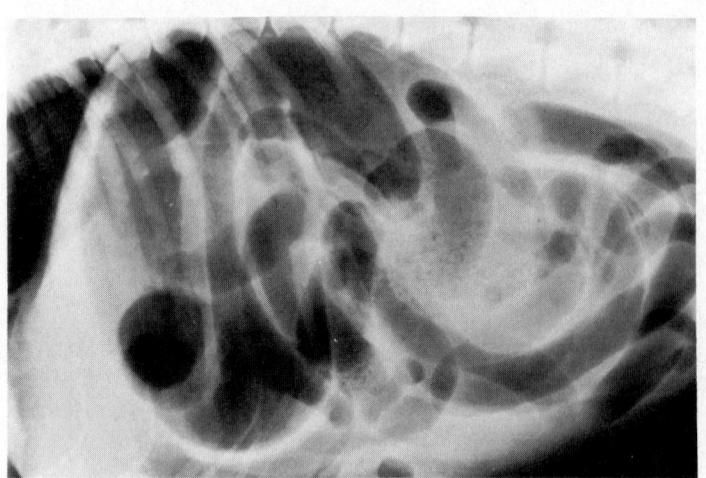

Figure 58–37. Lateral radiograph of the abdomen showing gas-distended bowel suggestive of intestinal obstruction. Intestinal volvulus was found by exploratory laparotomy.

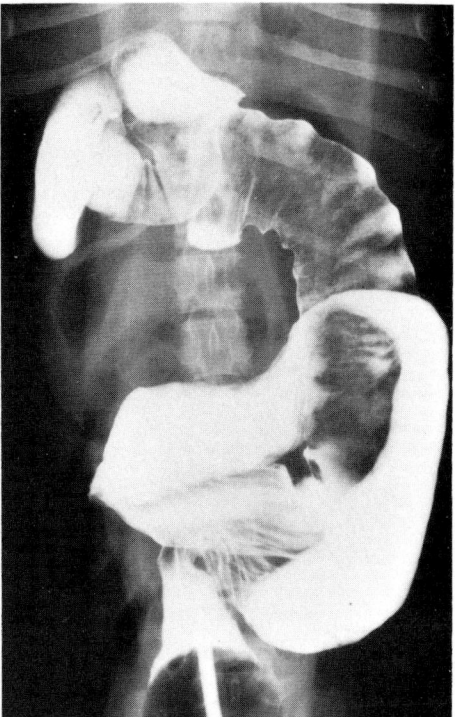

Figure 58–38. Barium enema radiography showing a coiled intraluminal filling defect within the colon indicative of ileocolonic intussusception.

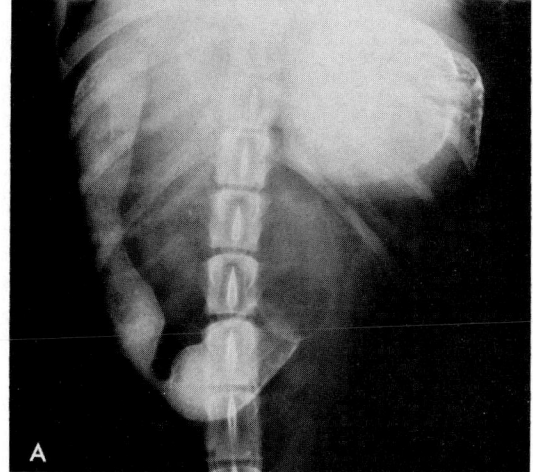

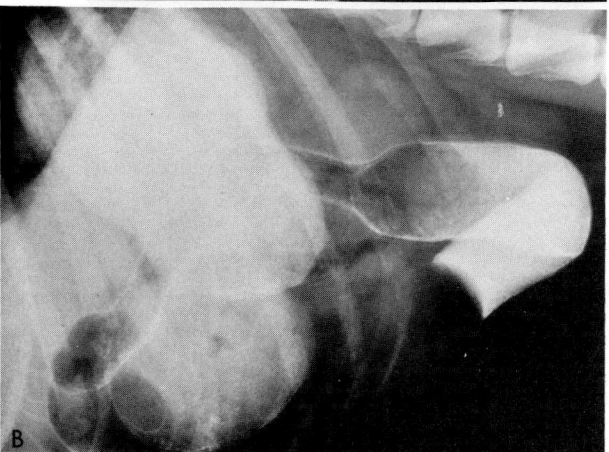

Figure 58–39. Ventrodorsal *(A)* and lateral *(B)* barium radiographs showing obstructed passage of contrast material by a radiolucent spherical foreign body within the lumen. A rubber ball was removed surgically.

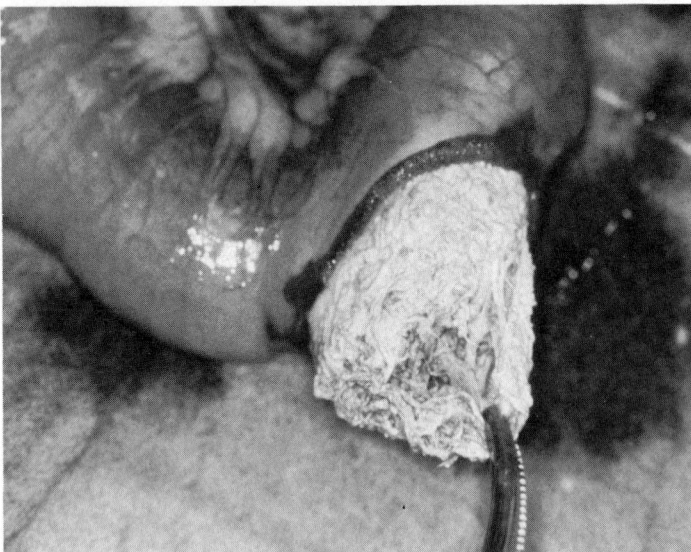

Figure 58–40. A cloth intestinal foreign body is removed through an enterotomy incision.

herniation of gut loops through a tear in the mesentery), adhesions or stricture (post-trauma or postsurgery), intramural abscess or granuloma, congenital malformation (stenosis or atresia), and intestinal neoplasm (Hornbuckle and Kleine, 1977). The clinical manifestations and consequences of obstruction depend on its location, completeness, and duration, as well as the vascular integrity of the affected bowel segment. Vomiting, anorexia, and depression are the most consistent clinical signs. Others include abdominal distension, diarrhea, and abdominal pain, evidenced by restlessness, panting, or abnormal body posture (Thrall et al., 1978) (Fig. 58–35).

Generally, the more proximal and complete the obstruction, the more intense and fulminating the signs will be, and the greater the likelihood of dehydration, electrolyte imbalance, and shock. Proximal duodenal obstructions cause, in effect, gastric outlet occlusion leading to persistent vomiting, loss of gastric secretions (HCl), and metabolic alkalosis. Obstructions at more distal sites cause varying degrees of metabolic acidosis. Distal and incomplete obstructions can be insidious with vague, inter-

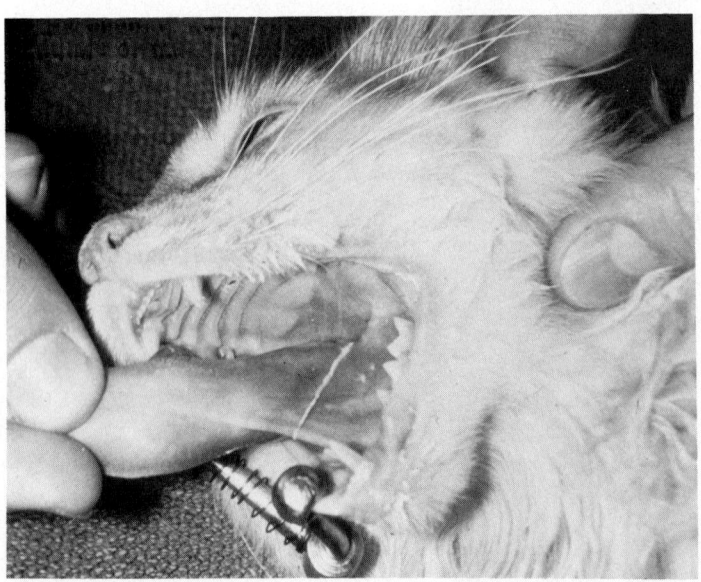

Figure 58–41. Linear intestinal foreign bodies such as thread are often looped around the base of the tongue in cats and can be detected by careful examination under the tongue. The free end of the thread is swallowed and passes into the intestine, where it causes plication.

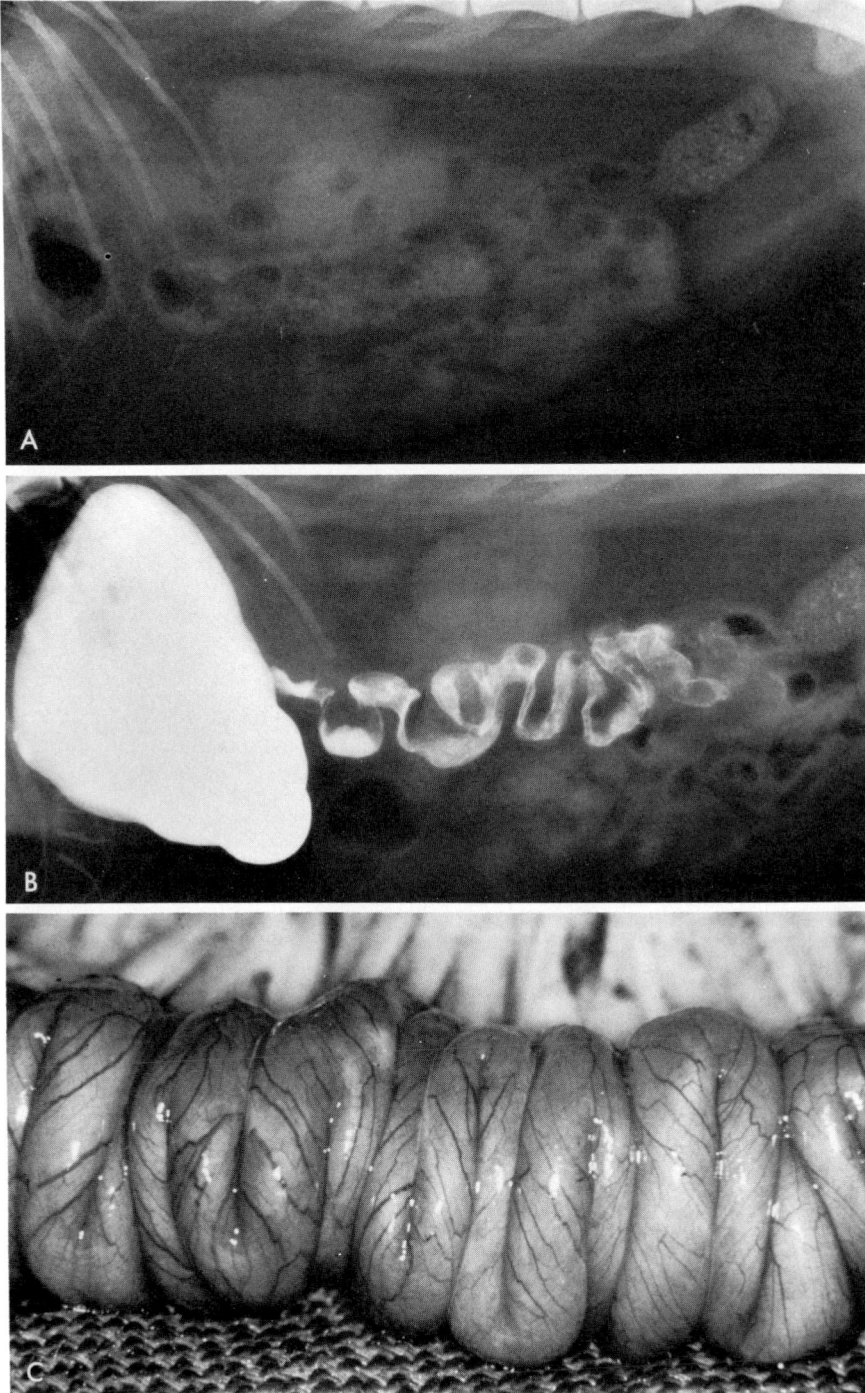

Figure 58–42. A lateral abdominal radiograph of a one-year-old male DSH with anorexia, vomiting, and abdominal pain shows aggregation and bunching of gut loops into the mid-abdomen and eccentrically located gas bubbles in the lumen *(A)*. These findings suggest radiolucent linear foreign body. The diagnosis is confirmed by a barium study showing characteristic intestinal plication *(B)*. The plication caused by the linear foreign body is seen at surgery *(C)*.

mittent signs of chronic anorexia and occasional vomiting that span several days or even weeks, leading to progressive starvation (Fig. 58–36).

Intestinal obstructions can also be simple or strangulated. Simple obstructions occlude the lumen without significant loss of vascular integrity, while strangulation involves vascular compromise of the obstructed bowel segment. This occurs most often with intussusception, volvulus, or incarcerated hernia. The sequence of events following strangulation are edema and engorgement of the affected loop, tissue hypoxia and infarction of the bowel wall, accumulation of gut bacteria and toxins in the peritoneal fluid, and rapidly progressive toxemia and shock, culminating in death.

The diagnosis of obstruction may be established by palpation of a foreign body, intussusception ("sausage loop"), or gas- and fluid-distended loops of bowel proximal to the obstruction. Radiography can usually confirm the presence of obstruction and often delineates the cause, especially when contrast studies are used. Radiographic findings that suggest obstruction include gas or fluid distension of the bowel (Fig. 58–37), delayed transit of contrast material, fixation or displacement of gut loops, luminal filling defects (Fig. 58–38), or the presence of

foreign objects within the lumen (Fig. 58–39) (Hornbuckle and Kleine, 1977). Almost any object that the curious or indiscriminant animal takes into its mouth may become a GI foreign body if swallowed; common examples are bones, toys, cloth (Fig. 58–40), metallic objects, stones, peach pits, acorns, rubber nipples, or rubber balls. Cats commonly acquire radiolucent linear intestinal foreign bodies (such as thread, string, cloth, fishing line, dental floss, decorative tinsel) that cause aggregation and plication of the bowel and a distinctive radiographic pattern (Figs. 58–41 and 58–42).

Intestinal obstructions are treated surgically. Close attention is given to supportive care, especially to maintenance of fluid, electrolyte, and acid-base homeostasis before, during, and after surgery. Complications of intestinal obstruction are necrosis or perforation of the bowel, peritonitis, and endotoxic shock.

REFERENCES

Ader, P. L.: Phycomycosis in fifteen dogs and two cats. J.A.V.M.A. *174*:1216–1223, 1979.

Ammon, H. V., and Phillips, S. F.: Inhibition of colonic water and electrolyte absorption by fatty acids in man. Gastroenterology *65*:744–749, 1973.

Anderson, N. V.: Disorders of the Small Intestine. *In* Ettinger, S. J. (ed.): Textbook of Veterinary Internal Medicine. W. B. Saunders Co., Philadelphia, 1975, pp. 1150–1191.

Anderson, N. V., and Low, D. G.: Juvenile atrophy of the canine pancreas. Anim. Hosp. *1*:101–109, 1965.

Anderson, W. D., and Anderson, B. G.: Comparative Anatomy. *In* Anderson, N. V. (ed.): Veterinary Gastroenterology. Lea and Febiger, Philadelphia, 1980, pp. 127–171.

Appel, M. J. G., Carmichael, L. E., McGregor, D. D., and Pollock, R. V. H.: Canine parvovirus vaccination. Mod. Vet. Pract. *61*:983–985, 1980.

Appel, M. J. G., Meunier, P., Greisen, H., et al.: Enteric viral infections of dogs. Gaines 29th Veterinary Symposium, 1979a, pp. 3–8.

Appel, M. J. G., Scott, F. W., and Carmichael, L. E.: Isolation and immunization studies of a canine parvo-like virus from dogs with haemorrhagic enteritis. Vet. Rec. *105*:156–159, 1979b.

Appel, M. J. G., Cooper, B. J., Greisen, H., and Carmichael, L. E.: Status report: Canine viral enteritis. J.A.V.M.A. *173*:1516–1518, 1978.

Argenzio, R. A., and Whipp, S. C.: Pathophysiology of Diarrhea. *In* Anderson, N. V. (ed.): Veterinary Gastroenterology. Lea and Febiger, Philadelphia, 1980, pp. 220–232.

Arvanitakis, C., and Cooke, A. R.: Diagnostic tests of exocrine pancreatic function and disease. Gastroenterology *74*:932–948, 1978.

Barlough, J. E.: Canine giardiasis: A review. J. Small Anim. Pract. *20*:613–623, 1979.

Bartlett, J. G., Chang, T.-W., Gurwith, M., et al.: Antibiotic-associated pseudomembranous colitis due to toxin-producing clostridia. N. Engl. J. Med. *298*:531–534, 1978.

Barton, C. L., Smith, C., Troy, J., et al.: The diagnosis and clinicopathological features of canine protein-losing enteropathy. J.A.A.H.A. *14*:85–91, 1978.

Batt, R. M.: The molecular basis of malabsorption. J. Small Anim. Pract. *21*:555–569, 1980.

Batt, R. M.: Techniques for single and multiple peroral jejunal biopsy in the dog. J. Small Anim. Pract. *20*:259–268, 1979.

Batt, R. M., and Peters, T. J.: Subcellular fractionation studies on peroral jejunal biopsies from the dog. Res. Vet. Sci. *25*:94–100, 1978.

Batt, R. M., Bush, B. M., and Peters, T. J.: A new test for the diagnosis of exocrine pancreatic insufficiency in the dog. J. Small Anim. Pract. *20*:185–192, 1979a.

Batt, R. M., Bush, B. M., and Peters, T. J.: Biochemical changes in the jejunal mucosa of dogs with naturally occurring exocrine pancreatic insufficiency. Gut *20*:709–715, 1979b.

Batt, R. M., Bush, B. M., and Peters, T. J.: Morphologic and biochemical studies of a naturally occurring enteropathy in the dog resembling chronic tropical sprue in man. (Abstr.) Gastroenterology *76*:1096, 1979c.

Batt, R. M., Jones, P. E., and Peters, T. J.: Peroral jejunal biopsy in the dog. Vet. Rec. *99*:337, 1976.

Bernstein, M.: Hemorrhagic Gastroenteritis. *In* Kirk, R. W. (ed.): Current Veterinary Therapy VI. W. B. Saunders Co., Philadelphia, 1977, pp. 951–952.

Binder, H. J., Filbur, C., and Volpe, B. T.: Bile salt alteration of colonic electrolyte transport: role of cyclic adenosine monophosphate. Gastroenterology *68*:503–508, 1975.

Binn, L. N., Lazar, E. C., Eddy, G. A., and Kajima, M.: Recovery and characterization of a minute virus of canines. Infect. Immun. *1*:503–508, 1970.

Blaser, M. J., Parsons, R. B., and Wang, W.-L. L.: Acute colitis caused by *Campylobacter fetus ss. jejuni.* Gastroenterology 78:448–453, 1980a.

Blaser, M. J., LaForce, F. M., Wilson, N. A., et al.: Reservoirs for human campylobacteriosis. J. Infect. Dis. *141*:665–669, 1980b.

Blaser, M., Cravens, J., Powers, B. W., and Wang, W. L.: Campylobacter enteritis associated with canine infection. Lancet *2*:979–980, 1978.

Brandborg, L. L.: Histologic diagnosis of diseases of malabsorption. Am. J. Med. *67*:999–1006, 1979.

Brasitus, T. A.: Parasites and malabsorption. Am. J. Med. 67:1058–1065, 1979.

Breitschwerdt, E. B., Halliwell, W. H., Foley, C. W., et al.: A hereditary diarrhetic syndrome in the basenji characterized by malabsorption, protein losing enteropathy, and hypergammaglobulinemia. J.A.A.H.A. *16*:551–560, 1980.

Bright-Asare, P., and Binder, H. J.: Stimulation of colonic secretion of water and electrolytes by hydroxy fatty acids. Gastroenterology *64*:81–88, 1973.

Brightman, A. H., and Slonka, G. F.: A review of five clinical cases of giardiasis in cats. J.A.A.H.A. *12*:492–497, 1976.

Brobst, D. F., and Funk, A.: Simplified test of fat absorption in dogs. J.A.V.M.A. *161*:1412–1417, 1972.

Brodey, R. S.: Alimentary tract neoplasms in the cat. A clinicopathological survey of 46 cases. Am. J. Vet. Res. *27*:74–80, 1966.

Bruce, D., Zochowski, W., and Fleming, G. A.: Campylobacter infections in cats and dogs. Vet. Rec. *107*:200–201, 1980.

Buckner, R. G.: The Small Intestine. *In* Catcott, E. J. (ed.): Canine Medicine, Vol. 1, 4th edition. Santa Barbara, American Veterinary Publications, Inc., 1979, pp. 336–351.

Burrows, C. F.: Diseases of the Colon, Rectum, and Anus of the Dog and Cat. *In* Anderson, N. V. (ed.): Veterinary Gastroenterology, Lea and Febiger, Philadelphia, 1980, pp. 523–592.

Burrows, C. F.: Canine hemorrhagic gastroenteritis. J.A.A.H.A. *13*:451–458, 1977.

Burrows, C. F., Merritt, A. M., and Chiapella, A. M.: Determination of fecal fat and trypsin output in the evaluation of chronic canine diarrhea. J.A.V.M.A. *174*:62–66, 1979.

Burrows, R. B., and Hunt, G. R.: Intestinal protozoan infections in cats. J.A.V.M.A. *157*:2065–2067, 1970.

Burrows, R. B., and Lillis, W. G.: Intestinal protozoan infections in dogs. J.A.V.M.A. *150*:880–883, 1967.

Butler, C. W., and Herd, B. R.: Human enteric pathogens in dogs in central Alaska. J. Infect. Dis. *115*:233–236, 1965.

Campbell, R. S. F., Brobst, D., and Bisgard, G.: Intestinal lymphangiectasia in a dog. J.A.V.M.A. *153*:1050–1054, 1968.

Carlson, J. H., and Scott, F. W.: Feline panleukopenia. II. The relationship of intestinal mucosal cell proliferation rates to viral infection and development of lesions. Vet. Pathol. *14*:173–181, 1977.

Carlson, J. H., Scott, F. W., and Duncan, J. R.: Feline panleukopenia. I. Pathogenesis in germfree and specific pathogen-free cats. Vet. Pathol. *14*:79–88, 1977.

Carmichael, L. E., Joubert, J. C., and Pollock, R. V. H.: Hemagglutination by canine parvovirus: Serologic studies and diagnostic applications. Am. J. Vet. Res. *41*:784–791, 1980.

Carpenter, J. L., Roberts, R. M., Harpster, N. K., and King, N. W.: Intestinal and cardiopulmonary forms of parvovirus infection in a litter of pups. J.A.V.M.A. *176*:1269–1273, 1980.

Carrig, C. B., and Seawright, A. A.: Mastocytosis with gastrointestinal ulceration in a dog. Aust. Vet. J. *44*:503–507, 1968.

Cello, J. P.: Eosinophilic gastroenteritis — a complex disease entity. Am. J. Med. *67*:1097–1104, 1979.

Christensen, J.: Movements of the Small Intestine. *In* Sleisenger, M. H. and Fordtran, J. S. (ed.): Gastrointestinal Disease, Vol. II, 2nd ed. W. B. Saunders Co., Philadelphia, 1978, pp. 1002–1010.

Cline, W. S., Lorenzsonn, V., Benz, L., et al.: The effects of sodium ricinoleate on small intestinal function and structure. J. Clin. Invest. *58*:380–390, 1976.

Craige, J. E.: Proteus group organisms infecting dogs. J.A.V.M.A. *113*:154–156, 1948.

Csiza, C. K., Scott, F. W., deLahunta, A., et al.: Pathogenesis of feline panleukopenia virus in susceptible newborn kittens. I. Clinical signs, hematology, serology, and virology. Infect. Immun. *3*:833–837, 1971a.

Csiza, C. K., deLahunta, A., Scott, F. W., et al.: Pathogenesis of feline panleukopenia virus in susceptible newborn kittens. II. Pathology and immunofluorescence. Infect. Immun. *3*:838–846, 1971b.

Davenport, H. W.: Motility of the Small Intestine. *In* Physiology of the Digestive Tract, 4th ed. Chicago, Year Book Med. Publishers, Inc., 1977, pp. 58–71.

Doe, W. F.: An overview of intestinal immunity and malabsorption. Am. J. Med. *67*:1077–1084, 1979.

Drasar, B. S., and Shiner, M.: Studies on the intestinal flora. II. Bacterial flora of the small intestine in patients with gastrointestinal disorders. Gut *10*:812–819, 1969.

Drummey, G. D., Benson, J. A., and Jones, C. M.: Microscopical examinations of the stool for steatorrhea. N. Engl. J. Med. *264*:85–87, 1961.

Dubey, J. P.: Pathogenicity of *Isospora ohioensis* infection in dogs. J.A.V.M.A. *173*:192–197, 1978.

Dubey, J. P.: A review of Sarcocystis of domestic animals and of other coccidia of cats and dogs. J.A.V.M.A. *169*:1061–1078, 1976.

Duffy, P. A., Granger, D. N., and Taylor, A. E.: Intestinal secretion induced by volume expansion in the dog. Gastroenterology *75*:413–418, 1978.

DuPont, H. L.: Interventions in diarrheas of infants and young children. J.A.V.M.A. *173*:649–653, 1978.

DuPont, H. L., and Hornick, R. B.: Adverse effects of lomotil therapy in shigellosis. J.A.M.A. *226*:1525–1528, 1973.

DuPont, H. L., Sullivan, P., Evans, D. G., et al.: Prevention of traveler's diarrhea (emporiatric enteritis). Prophylactic administration of subsalicylate bismuth. J.A.M.A. *243*:237–241, 1980.

Easley, J. R.: Gastroenteritis and associated eosinophilia in a dog. J.A.V.M.A. *161*:1030–1032, 1972.

Eastwood, G. L.: Gastrointestinal epithelial renewal. Gastroenterology *72*:962–975, 1977.

Echeverria, P. D., Chang, C. P., and Smith, D.: Entero-toxigenicity and invasive capacity of "enteropatho-genic" serotypes of *Escherichia coli*. J. Pediatr. 89:8–10, 1976.

England, J. J., and Poston, R. P.: Electron microscopic identification and subsequent isolation of a rotavirus from a dog with fatal neonatal diarrhea. Am. J. Vet. Res. 41:782–783, 1980.

Eugster, A. K., and Sidwa, T.: Rotaviruses in diarrheic feces of a dog. Vet. Med. Small Anim. Clin. 74:817–819, 1979.

Ewing, G. O.: Indomethacin-associated gastrointestinal hemorrhage in a dog. J.A.V.M.A. 161:1665–1668, 1972.

Falchuk, Z. M.: Update on gluten-sensitive enterop-athy. Am. J. Med. 67:1085–1096, 1979.

Farrell, R. K.: Canine Rickettsiosis. *In* Kirk, R. W. (ed.): Current Veterinary Therapy V. W. B. Saunders Co., Philadelphia, 1974, pp. 985–987.

Finco, D. R., Duncan, J. R., Schall, W. D., et al.: Chronic enteric disease and hypoproteinemia in nine dogs. J.A.V.M.A. 163:262–271, 1973.

Fischer, J. E.: Hyperalimentation. Med. Clin. North Am. 63:973–983, 1979.

Fleming, M. P.: Incidence of campylobacter infection in dogs. Vet. Rec. 107:202, 1980.

Flesja, K., and Yri, T.: Protein-losing enteropathy in the Lundehund. J. Small Anim. Pract. 18:11–23, 1977.

Ford, R. B.: Canine histoplasmosis. Compend. Cont. Ed. 2:637–642, 1980.

Formal, S. B., O'Brien, A., Gemski, P., et al.: Invasive *Escherichia coli*. J.A.V.M.A. 173:596–598, 1978.

Fox, I. W., Hoag, W. G., and Strout, J.: Breed suscepti-bility, pathogenicity, and epidemiology of endemic coliform enteritis in the dog. Lab. Anim. Care 15:194–200, 1965.

Fox, J. G.: Feline Salmonellosis. *In* Kirk, R. W. (ed.): Current Veterinary Therapy VII. W. B. Saunders Co., Philadelphia, 1980, pp. 1305–1307.

Freeman, H. J., Kim, Y. S., and Sleisenger, M. H.: Protein digestion and absorption in man: normal mechanisms and protein-energy malnutrition. Am. J. Med. 67:1030–1036, 1979.

Galambos, J. R., Hersh, T., Schroder, S., et al.: Lopera-mide: A new antidiarrheal agent in the treatment of chronic diarrhea. Gastroenterology 70:1026–1029, 1976.

George, W. L., Rolfe, R. D., and Finegold, S. M.: Treatment and prevention of antimicrobial agent-induced colitis and diarrhea. Gastroenterology 79:366–372, 1980.

Giannella, R. A., Gots, R. E., Charney, A. N., et al.: Pathogenesis of salmonella-mediated intestinal fluid secretion. Gastroenterology 69:1238–1245, 1975.

Glickman, L. T., Schantz, P. M., and Cypess, R. H.: Canine and human toxocariasis: Review of transmis-sion, pathogenesis, and clinical disease. J.A.V.M.A. 175:1265–1269, 1979.

Gorbach, S. L., Neale, G., Levitan, R., et al.: Alterations in intestinal microflora during experimental diarr-hoea. Gut 11:1–6, 1970.

Gray, G. M.: Mechanisms of Digestion and Absorption of Food. *In* Sleisenger, M. H., and Fordtran, J. S. (ed.): Gastrointestinal Disease, Vol. I, 2nd ed. W. B. Saunders Co., Philadelphia, 1978, pp. 241–250.

Gray, G. M.: Carbohydrate digestion and absorption. N. Engl. J. Med. 292:1225–1230, 1975.

Greene, J. E., and Thorson, R. E.: Canine intestinal

protozoa as related to enteritis. 4th Gaines Veteri-nary Symposium, 1954, pp. 6–9.

Guerrant, R. L., Ganguly, U., Casper, A. G. T., et al.: Effect of *Escherichia coli* on fluid transport across canine small bowel. Mechanism and time-course with enterotoxin and whole bacterial cells. J. Clin. Invest. 52:1707–1714, 1973.

Hall, C. L.: Three clinical cases of eosinophilic enteritis. Southwest Vet. 21:41–42, 1967.

Happe, R. P., VanDerGaag, I., Lamer, C. B. H. W., et al.: Zollinger-Ellison syndrome in three dogs. Vet. Pathol. 17:177–186, 1980.

Harris, J. C., DuPont, H. L., and Hornic, R. B.: Fecal leukocytes in diarrheal illness. Ann. Intern. Med. 76:697–703, 1972.

Hartong, W. A., Gourley, W. K., and Arvanitakis, C.: Giardiasis: Clinical spectrum and functional-structural abnormalities of the small intestinal muco-sa. Gastroenterology 77:61–69, 1979.

Hastings, D. H.: Campylobacter enteritis in pets. Lan-cet 2:1249–1250, 1978.

Hayden, D. W.: Alariasis in a dog. J.A.V.M.A. 155:889–891, 1969.

Hayden, D. W., and Van Kruiningen, H. J.: Control values for evaluating gastrointestinal function in the dog. J.A.A.H.A. 12:31–36, 1976.

Hayden, D. W., and Van Kruiningen, H. J.: Ex-perimentally induced canine toxocariasis: Laborato-ry examinations and pathologic changes, with em-phasis on the gastrointestinal tract. Am. J. Vet. Res. 36:1605–1614, 1975.

Hayden, D. W., and Van Kruiningen, H. J.: Eosino-philic gastroenteritis in German shepherd dogs and its relationship to visceral larva migrans. J.A.V.M.A. 162:379–384, 1973.

Hayes, M. A., Russell, R. G., and Babiuk, L. A.: Sudden death in young dogs with myocarditis caused by parvovirus. J.A.V.M.A. 174:1197–1203, 1979.

Hendrick, M.: A spectrum of hypereosinophilic syn-dromes exemplified by six cats with eosinophilic enteritis. Vet. Pathol. 18:188–200, 1981.

Heymsfield, S. B., Bethel, R. A., Ansley, J. D., et al.: Enteral hyperalimentation: An alternative to central venous hyperalimentation. Ann. Intern. Med. 90:63–71, 1979.

Hill, F. W. G.: Acute Intestinal Haemorrhage Syn-drome in Dogs. *In* Grunsell, G. S. G., and Hill, F. W. G. (ed.) Vet Annual. John Wright, Bristol, England, 1973, pp. 98–101.

Hill, F. W. G.: Malabsorption syndrome in the dog: A study of thirty-eight cases. J. Small Anim. Pract. 13:575–591, 1972a.

Hill, F. W. G.: A starch tolerance test in canine pancre-atic malabsorption. Vet. Rec. 91:169–171, 1972b.

Hill, F. W. G., and Kelly, D. F.: Naturally occurring intestinal malabsorption in the dog. Dig. Dis. 19:649–665, 1974.

Hill, F. W. G., and Kidder, D. E.: The oral glucose tolerance test in canine pancreatic malabsorption. Br. Vet. J. 128:207–214, 1972.

Hill, F. W. G., Kidder, D. E., and Frew, J.: A xylose absorption test for the dog. Vet. Rec. 87:250–255, 1970.

Hirsh, D. W.: Microflora, Mucosa, and Immunity. *In* Anderson, N. V. (ed.): Veterinary Gastroenterology, Lea and Febiger, Philadelphia, 1980, pp. 199–219.

Hoenig, M.: Intestinal malabsorption attributed to bac-terial overgrowth in a dog. J.A.V.M.A. 176:533–535, 1980.

Holzworth, J., and Georgi, J. R.: Trichinosis in a cat. J.A.V.M.A. *165*:186–191, 1974.

Holzworth, J., Theran, P., Carpenter, J. L., et al.: Hyperthyroidism in the cat: Ten cases. J.A.V.M.A. *176*:345–353, 1980.

Hornbuckle, W. D., and Kleine, L. J.: Obstruction of the Small Intestine. In Kirk, R. W. (ed.): Current Veterinary Therapy VI. W. B. Saunders Co., Philadelphia, 1977, pp. 952–958.

Hoshino, Y., Baldwin, C. A., and Scott, F. W.: New insights in gastrointestinal viruses. Cornell Feline Health News *2*:2–4, 1981.

Hosie, B. D., Nicolson, T. B., and Henderson, D. B.: Campylobacter infections in normal and diarrheic dogs. Vet. Rec. *105*:80, 1979.

Howard, E. B., Sawa, T. R., Nielsen, S. W., and Kenyon, A. J.: Mastocytoma and gastroduodenal ulceration. Pathol. Vet. *6*:146–158, 1969.

Isaacs, P. E. T., and Kim, Y. S.: The contaminated small bowel syndrome. Am. J. Med. *67*:1049–1057, 1979.

Itoh, Z., Takeuchi, S., Aizawa, I., and Takayanagi, R.: Characteristic motor activity of the gastrointestinal tract in fasted conscious dogs measured by implanted force transducers. Am. J. Dig. Dis. *23*:229–238, 1978.

Jacobs, R. M., Weiser, M. G., and Hall, R. L.: Clinicopathologic features of canine parvoviral enteritis. J.A.A.H.A. *16*:809–814, 1980.

Jezyk, P. F., Haskins, M. E., and Jones, C. L.: Myocarditis of probable viral origin in pups of weaning age. J.A.V.M.A. *174*:1204–1207, 1979.

Johnson, G. F.: Duodenoscopy. In Anderson, N. V. (ed.): Veterinary Gastroenterology, Lea and Febiger, Philadelphia, 1980, pp. 89–92.

Johnson, G. F., Jones, B., Twedt, D. C., and Patnaik, A. K.: Gastrointestinal fiberoptic endoscopy in small animal medicine. 28th Gaines Vet Symposium, 1978, pp. 27–31.

Jones, B. R., Nicholls, M. R., and Badman, R.: Peptic ulceration in a dog associated with an islet cell carcinoma of the pancreas and an elevated plasma gastrin level. J. Small Anim. Pract. *17*:593–598, 1976.

Joy, C. L., and Patterson, J. M.: Short bowel syndrome following surgical correction of a double intussusception in a dog. Can. Vet. J. *19*:254–259, 1978.

Kahn, D. E.: Pathogenesis of feline panleukopenia. J.A.V.M.A. *173*:628–630, 1978.

Kallfelz, F. A., Norrdin, R. W., and Neal, T. M.: Intestinal absorption of oleic acid ^{131}I and triolein ^{131}I in the differential diagnosis of malabsorption syndrome and pancreatic dysfunction in the dog. J.A.V.M.A. *153*:43–46, 1968.

Kaneko, J. J., Moulton, J. E., Brodey, R. S., et al.: Malabsorption syndrome resembling nontropical sprue in dogs. J.A.V.M.A. *146*:463–473, 1965.

Kaneko, K., Hamada, S., and Kato, E.: Occurrence of Yersinia enterocolitica in dogs. Jpn. J. Vet. Sci. *39*:407–414, 1977.

Kato, E., Kaji, Y., and Kaneko, K.: Enterotoxigenic staphylococci of canine origin. Am. J. Vet. Res. *39*:1771–1773, 1978.

Kaufmann, A. F.: Pets and salmonella infection. J.A.V.M.A. *149*:1655–1661, 1966.

Keenan, K. P., Jervis, H. R., Marchwicki, R. H., and Binn, L. N.: Intestinal infection of neonatal dogs with canine coronavirus I-71: studies by virologic, histologic, histochemical, and immunofluorescent techniques. Am. J. Vet. Res. *37*:247–256, 1976.

Knowles, J. O.: Provocative exposure for the diagnosis and treatment of certain canine allergies. J.A.V.M.A. *149*:1303–1306, 1966.

Kondo, M., Yoshikawa, T., Takemura, S., et al.: Hemorrhagic necrosis of the intestinal mucosa associated with disseminated intravascular coagulation. Digestion *17*:38–45, 1978.

Koretz, R. L., and Meyer, J. H.: Elemental diets: facts and fantasies. Gastroenterology *78*:393–410, 1980.

Kovatch, R. M., and Zebarth, G.: Naturally occurring Tyzzer's disease in a cat. J.A.V.M.A. *162*:136–138, 1973.

Krejs, G. J., and Fordtran, J. S.: Physiology and Pathophysiology of Ion and Water Movement in the Human Intestine. In Sleisenger, M. H., and Fordtran, J. S. (ed.): Gastrointestinal Medicine, Vol. I, 2nd ed. W. B. Saunders, Co., Philadelphia, 1978, pp. 297–335.

Krum, S. H., Stevens, D. R., and Hirsch, D. C.: *Salmonella arizonae* bacteremia in a cat. J.A.V.M.A. *170*:42–44, 1977.

Kubokawa, K.: Two cases of feline Tyzzer's disease. Jpn. J. Exp. Med. *43*:413–422, 1973.

Larsen, S., Flagstad, A., and Aalbaek, B.: Experimental feline panleucopenia in the conventional cat. Vet. Pathol. *13*:216–240, 1976.

Leav, I., Schiller, A. L., Rijnberk, A., et al.: Adenomas and carcinomas of the canine and feline thyroid. Am. J. Pathol. *83*:61–94, 1976.

Legendre, A. M., and Krehbiel, J. D.: Eosinophilic enteritis in a Chesapeake Bay Retriever. J.A.V.M.A. *163*:258–259, 1973.

Lewis, L. D., Boulay, J. P., and Chow, F. H. C.: Fat excretion and assimilation by the cat. Feline Pract. *9*:46–49, 1979.

Lingemann, C. H., and Garner, F. M.: Comparative study of intestinal adenocarcinomas of animals and man. J. Natl. Cancer Inst. *48*:325–346, 1972.

Lorenz, M. D.: Laboratory diagnosis of gastrointestinal disease and pancreatic insufficiency. Vet. Clin. North Am. *6*:663–670, 1976.

Luk, G. D., and Hendrix, T. R.: Microscopic examination of stool as a screening test for steatorrhea (abstr.). Gastroenterology *74*:1134, 1978.

Lundgren, D. L., Clapper, W. E., and Sanchez, A.: Isolation of human enteroviruses from beagle dogs. Proc. Soc. Exp. Biol. Med. *128*:463, 1968.

Mahaffey, E., Gabbert, N., Johnson, D., and Guffy, M.: Disseminated histoplasmosis in three cats. J.A.A.H.A. *13*:46–51, 1977.

Malone, J. B., Breitschwerdt, E. B., Little, M. D., et al.: *Strongyloides stercoralis*-like infection in a dog. J.A.V.M.A. *176*:130–133, 1980.

Malone, J. B., Butterfield, A. B., Williams, J. C., and Stuart, B. S.: *Strongyloides tumefaciens* in cats. J.A.V.M.A. *171*:278–280, 1977.

McCandlish, I. A. P., Thompson, H., Cornwell, H. J. C., et al.: Isolation of a parvovirus from dogs in Britain. Vet. Rec. *105*:167–168, 1979.

McClung, H. J., Beck, R. D., and Powers, P.: The effect of a kaolin-pectin adsorbent on stool losses of sodium, potassium, and fat during a lactose-tolerance diarrhea in rats. J. Pediatr. *96*:769–771, 1980.

McKay, J. S., Linaker, B. D., and Turnberg, L. A.: Influence of opiates on ion transport across rabbit ileal mucosa. Gastroenterology *80*:279–284, 1981.

Mekhjian, H. S., Phillips, S. F., and Hofmann, A. F.: Colonic secretion of water and electrolytes induced by bile acids: perfusion studies in man. J. Clin. Invest. *50*:1569–1577, 1971.

Merritt, A. M.: Small Intestinal Diseases. *In* Anderson, N. V. (ed.): Veterinary Gastroenterology, Lea and Febiger, Philadelphia, 1980, pp. 463–522.

Merritt, A. M., and Reed, J. H.: Gastrointestinal Function Testing. *In* Anderson, N. V. (ed.): Veterinary Gastroenterology, Lea and Febiger, Philadelphia, 1980, pp. 247–262.

Merritt, A. M., Burrows, C. F., Cowgill, L., and Streett, W.: Fecal fat and trypsin in dogs fed a meat-base or cereal-base diet. J.A.V.M.A. *174*:59–61, 1979.

Meshkinpour, H.: State of the art. Intestinal motility: Current concepts. Am. J. Gastroenterol. *71*:101–106, 1979.

Michaux, H. R.: A mutton and rice diet for treating chronic diarrhea in the dog. J.A.V.M.A. *149*:296–297, 1966.

Middleton, P. J.: Pathogenesis of rotaviral infection. J.A.V.M.A. *173*:544–546, 1978.

Migasena, S., Gilles, H. M., and Maegraith, B. G.: Studies in *Ancylostoma caninum* infection in dogs. II: Anatomical changes in the gastrointestinal tract. Ann. Trop. Med. Parasitol. *66*:203–207, 1972a.

Migasena, S., Gilles, H. M., and Maegraith, B. G.: Studies in *Ancylostoma caninum* infection in dogs. I: Absorption from the small intestine of amino-acids, carbohydrates, and fat. Ann. Trop. Med. Parasitol. *66*:107–128, 1972b.

Miller, S. I., Wallace, R. J., Jr., Musher, D. M., et al.: Hypoglycemia as a manifestation of sepsis. Am. J. Med. *68*:649–654, 1980.

Miller, T. A.: Vaccination against the canine hookworm diseases. Adv. Parasitol. *9*:153–183, 1971.

Miller, T. A.: Blood loss during hookworm infection, determined by erythrocyte labeling with radioactive ^{51}chromium. I. Infection of dogs with normal and with x-irradiated *Ancylostoma caninum*. J. Parasitol. *52*:844–855, 1966a.

Miller, T. A.: Blood loss during hookworm infection, determined by erythrocyte labeling with radioactive ^{51}chromium. II: Pathogenesis of *Ancylostoma braziliense* infection in dogs and cats. J. Parasitol. *52*:856–865, 1966b.

Moon, H. W.: Mechanisms in the pathogenesis of diarrhea: A review. J.A.V.M.A. *172*:443–448, 1978.

Moon, H. W., McClurkin, A. W., Isaacson, R. E., et al.: Pathogenic relationships of rotavirus, *Escherichia coli*, and other agents in mixed infections in calves. J.A.V.M.A. *173*:577–584, 1978.

Morse, E. V., and Duncan, M. A.: Canine salmonellosis: Prevalence, epizootiology, signs, and public health significance. J.A.V.M.A. *167*:817–820, 1975.

Morse, E. V., Duncan, M. A., Estep, D. A., et al.: Canine salmonellosis: A review and report of dog to child transmission of Salmonella enteritidis. Am. J. Public Health *66*:82–84, 1976.

Mulvey, J. J., Bech-Nielsen, S., Haskins, M. E., et al.: Myocarditis induced by parvoviral infection in weanling pups in the United States. J.A.V.M.A. *177*:695–698, 1980.

Murray, M., Robinson, P. B., McKeating, F. J., et al.: Peptic ulceration in the dog: A clinico-pathological study. Vet. Rec. *91*:441–447, 1972.

Noon, K. F., Rogul, M., Brendle, J. J., and Keefe, F. J.: Detection and definition of canine intestinal carbohydrases, using a standardized method. Am. J. Vet. Res. *38*:1063–1067, 1977.

O'Brien, T. R.: Radiographic Diagnosis of Abdominal Disorders in the Dog and Cat: Radiographic Interpretation. Clinical Signs. Pathophysiology. W. B. Saunders Co., Philadelphia, 1978.

Olsen, H. A.: A pathophysiologic approach to diagnosis of malabsorption. Am. J. Med. *67*:1007–1013, 1979.

Olson, N. C., and Zimmer, J. F.: Protein-losing enteropathy secondary to intestinal lymphangiectasia in a dog. J.A.V.M.A. *173*:271–274, 1978.

Osborne, A. D.: Bacteriological and pathological aspects of diarrhea in the dog. J. Small Anim. Prac. *8*:117–122, 1967.

Palmer, D. L., Koster, F. T., Islam, A. F. M. R., et al.: Comparison of sucrose and glucose in the oral electrolyte therapy of cholera and other severe diarrheas. N. Engl. J. Med. *297*:1107–1110, 1977.

Panel report on the colloquium on selected diarrheal diseases of the young. J.A.V.M.A. *173*:515–518, 1978.

Patnaik, A. K., Johnson, G. F., Greene, R. W., et al.: Surgical resection of intestinal adenocarcinoma in a cat with survival of 28 months. J.A.V.M.A. *178*:479–481, 1981.

Patnaik, A. K., Hurvitz, A. I., and Johnson, G. F.: Canine intestinal adenocarcinoma and carcinoid. Vet. Pathol. *17*:149–163, 1980.

Patnaik, A. K., Hurvitz, A. I., and Johnson, G. F.: Canine gastrointestinal neoplasms. Vet. Pathol. *14*:547–555, 1977.

Patnaik, A. K., Liu, S.-K., and Johnson, G. F.: Feline intestinal adenocarcinoma. A clinicopathologic study of 22 cases. Vet. Pathol. *13*:1–10, 1976.

Pederson, K. B.: Isolation of *Yersinia enterocolitica* from Danish swine and dogs. Acta Pathol. Microbiol. Scand. [B]84:317–318, 1976.

Pederson, K. B., and Winblad, S.: Studies on *Yersinia enterocolitica* isolated from swine and dogs. Acta Pathol. Microbiol. Scand. [B]87:137–140, 1979.

Pederson, N. C., Boyle, J. F., Floyd, K., et al.: An enteric coronavirus infection of cats and its relationship to feline infectious peritonitis. Am. J. Vet. Res. *42*:368–377, 1981.

Pelemans, W., and Vantrappen, G.: A double-blind crossover comparison of loperamide with diphenoxylate in the symptomatic treatment of chronic diarrhea. Gastroenterology *70*:1030–1034, 1976.

Phillips, S. F.: Diarrhea: a current view of the pathophysiology. Gastroenterology *63*:495–518, 1972.

Pickering, L. K., DuPont, H. L., Olarte, J., et al.: Fecal leukocytes in enteric infections. Am. J. Clin. Pathol. *68*:562–565, 1977.

Pierce, K. R.: *Heterobilharzia americana* infection in a dog. J.A.V.M.A. *143*:496–499, 1963.

Pindak, F. F., and Clapper, W. E.: Isolation of enteric cytopathogenic human orphan virus type 6 from dogs. Am. J. Vet. Res. *25*:52–54, 1964.

Pindak, F. F., Clapper, W. E., and Sherrod, J. H.: Incidence and distribution of spirochetes in the digestive tract of dogs. Am. J. Vet. Res. *26*:1391–1402, 1965.

Plant, O. H., and Miller, G. H.: Effects of morphine and some other opium alkaloids on the muscular activity of the alimentary canal. I: Action on the small intestine in unanesthetized dogs and man. J. Pharmacol. Exp. Ther. *27*:361–383, 1926.

Pollock, R. V., and Carmichael, L. E.: Canine viral enteritis. Recent developments. Mod. Vet. Pract. *60*:375–380, 1979.

Poonacha, K. B., and Smith, H. L.: Naturally occurring Tyzzer's disease as a complication of distemper and mycotic pneumonia in a dog. J.A.V.M.A. *169*:419–420, 1976.

Povar, R.: Food allergy in dogs (a preliminary report). J.A.V.M.A. *111*:61–63, 1947.

Powell, D. W.: Muscle or mucosa: The site of action of antidiarrheal opiates? Gastroenterology *80*:406–408, 1981.

Prescott, J. F., Johnson, J. A., and Patterson, J. M.: Haemorrhagic gastroenteritis in the dog associated with *Clostridium welchii*. Vet. Rec. *103*:116–117, 1978.

Price, A. B., Jewkes, J., and Sanderson, P. J.: Acute diarrhea: Campylobacter colitis and the role of rectal biopsy. J. Clin. Pathol. *32*:990–997, 1979.

Qureshi, S. R., Carlton, W. W., and Olander, H. J.: Tyzzer's disease in a dog. J.A.V.M.A. *168*:602–604, 1976.

Regan, P. T., and DiMagno, E. P.: The medical management of malabsorption. Mayo Clin. Proc. *54*:267–274, 1979.

Riley, J. W., and Glickman, R. M.: Fat malabsorption: Advances in our understanding. Am. J. Med. *67*:980–988, 1979.

Roberson, E. L., and Cornelius, L. M.: Gastrointestinal Parasitism. *In* Kirk, R. W. (ed.): Current Veterinary Therapy VII. W. B. Saunders Co., Philadelphia, 1980, pp. 935–948.

Robinson, V. B., and McVickar, D. L.: Pathology of spontaneous histoplasmosis. A study of twenty-one cases. Am. J. Vet. Res. *13*:214–219, 1952.

Rogers, W. A., Stradley, R. P., Sherding, R. G., et al.: Simultaneous evaluation of pancreatic exocrine function and intestinal absorptive function in dogs with chronic diarrhea. J.A.V.M.A. *177*:1128–1131, 1980.

Rohovsky, M. W., and Fowler, E. H.: Lesions of experimental feline panleukopenia. J.A.V.M.A. *158*:872–875, 1971.

Sateri, H.: Investigations on the exocrine pancreatic function in dogs suffering from chronic exocrine pancreatic insufficiency. Acta Vet. Scand. (Suppl)*53*:1–86, 1975.

Schantz, P. M., and Glickman, L. T.: Canine and human toxocariasis: The public health problem and the veterinarian's role in prevention. J.A.V.M.A. *175*:1270–1273, 1979.

Seawright, A. A., and Grono, L. R.: Malignant mast cell tumor in a cat with perforating duodenal ulcer. J. Pathol. Bacteriol. *87*:107–111, 1964.

Sheldon, G. F.: Role of parenteral nutrition in patients with short bowel syndrome. Am. J. Med. *67*:1021–1029, 1979.

Shiau, Y.-F., Boyle, J. T., Umstetter, C., and Koldovsky, O.: Apical distribution of fatty acid esterification capacity along the villus-crypt unit of rat jejunum. Gastroenterology *79*:47–53, 1980.

Shimi, A., and Barin, A.: Salmonella in cats. J. Comp. Pathol. *87*:315–318, 1977.

Shindel, N. M., Van Kruiningen, H. J., and Scott, F. W.: The colitis of feline panleukopenia. J.A.A.H.A. *14*:738–747, 1978.

Skirrow, M. B.: Campylobacter enteritis: A "new" disease. Br. Med. J. *2*:9–11, 1977.

Slee, A.: Hemorrhagic gastroenteritis in a dog. Vet. Rec. *104*:14, 1979.

Sleisenger, M. H., and Kim, Y. S.: Protein digestion and absorption. N. Engl. J. Med. *300*:659–663, 1979.

Smith, H. W.: The development of the flora of the alimentary tract in young animals. J. Pathol. Bacteriol. *90*:495–513, 1965.

Smith, J. M. B.: Mycoses of the alimentary tract of animals. N.Z. Vet. J. *16*:89–100, 1968.

Snodgrass, D. R.: A rotavirus from kittens. Vet. Rec. *104*:70, 1979.

Steinfeld, C. M., Moertel, C. G., and Woolner, L. B.: Diarrhea and medullary carcinoma of the thyroid. Cancer *31*:1237–1239, 1973.

Steinhoff, M. C., Douglas, R. G. Jr., Greenberg, H. B., et al.: Bismuth subsalicylate therapy of viral gastroenteritis. Gastroenterology *78*:1495–1499, 1980.

Steves, F. E., Baker, J. D., Hein, V. D., et al.: Efficacy of a hookworm (*Ancylostoma caninum*) vaccine for dogs. J.A.V.M.A. *163*:231–234, 1973.

Stickle, J. E., and Hribernik, T. N.: Clinicopathological observations in disseminated histoplasmosis in dogs. J.A.A.H.A. *14*:105–110, 1978.

Stradley, R. P., Stern, R. J., and Heinhold, N. B.: A method for the simultaneous evaluation of exocrine pancreatic function and intestinal absorptive function in dogs. Am. J. Vet. Res. *40*:1201–1205, 1979.

Strande, A., Sommers, S. C., and Petrak, M.: Regional enterocolitis in Cocker Spaniel dogs. Arch. Pathol. *57*:357–362, 1954.

Straus, E., Johnson, G. F., and Yalow, R. S.: Canine Zollinger-Ellison syndrome. Gastroenterology *72*:380–381, 1977.

Strombeck, D. R.: Small Animal Gastroenterology. Stonegate Publishing, Davis, California, 1979.

Strombeck, D. R.: New method for evaluation of chymotrypsin deficiency in dogs. J.A.V.M.A. *173*:1319–1323, 1978.

Tams, T. R., and Twedt, D. C.: Canine protein-losing gastroenteropathy syndrome. Compend. Contin. Ed. *3*:105–114, 1981.

Thorne, G. M., and Gorbach, S. L.: Enterotoxigenic *Escherichia coli*: detection and importance in diarrheal disease of children. J.A.V.M.A. *173*:592–595, 1978.

Thrall, D. E., Bovee, K. C., and Biery, D. N.: Demonstration of a "Position of Relief" in dogs with lesions of the stomach or small bowel. J.A.A.H.A. *14*:343–347, 1978.

Timoney, J. F., Neibert, H. C., and Scott, F. W.: Feline salmonellosis: A nosocomial outbreak and experimental studies. Cornell Vet. *68*:211–219, 1978.

Turek, J. J., and Meyer, R. C.: Studies on a canine intestinal spirochete: Scanning electron microscopy of canine colonic mucosa. Infect. Immun. *20*:853–855, 1978.

Turek, J. J., and Meyer, R. C.: Studies on a canine intestinal spirochete. I: Its isolation, cultivation and ultrastructure. Can. J. Comp. Med. *41*:332–337, 1977.

Van Kruiningen, H. J.: Clinical efficacy of tylosin in canine inflammatory bowel disease. J.A.A.H.A. *12*:498–501, 1976.

Van Kruiningen, H. J., and Hayden, D. W.: Interpreting problem diarrheas of dogs. Vet. Clin. North Am. *2*:29–47, 1972.

Vantrappen, G., Agg, H. O., Ponette, E., et al.: Yersinia enteritis and enterocolitis: Gastroenterological aspects. Gastroenterology *72*:220–227, 1977.

Vaughan, Williams, E. M.: The mode of action of drugs upon intestinal motility. Pharmacol. Rev. *6*:159–170, 1954.

Vernon, D. F., Jr.: Idiopathic sprue in a dog. J.A.V.M.A *140*:1062–1067, 1962.

Waldmann, T. A.: Protein-Losing Enteropathy. *In* Bockus, H. L. (ed.): Gastroenterology, 3rd ed. W. B. Saunders Co., Philadelphia, 1976, pp. 361–385.

Walker, W. A., and Isselbacher, K. J.: Intestinal antibodies. N. Engl. J. Med. *297*:767–773, 1977.

Walsh, J. H.: Gastrointestinal Peptide Hormones and Other Biologically Active Peptides. *In* Sleisenger, M. H., and Fordtran, J. S. (ed.): Gastrointestinal Disease, Vol. 1, 2nd ed. W. B. Saunders Co., Philadelphia, 1978, pp. 107–155.

Welliver, R. C., and Ogra, P. L.: Importance of local immunity in enteric infection. J.A.V.M.A. 173:560–564, 1978.

Weser, E., Fletcher, J. T., and Urban, E.: Short bowel syndrome. Gastroenterology 77:572–579, 1979.

Whipp, S. C.: Physiology of diarrhea: Small intestines. J.A.V.M.A. 173:662–666, 1978.

Williams, F. P.: Astrovirus-like, coronavirus-like, and parvovirus-like particles detected in the diarrheic stools of beagle pups. Arch. Virol. 66:215–226, 1980.

Williamson, R. C. N., and Chir, M.: Intestinal adaptation (Part 2). Mechanisms of control. N. Engl. J. Med. 298:1443–1450, 1978.

Willoughby, C. P., Piris, J., and Truelove, S. C.: Campylobacter colitis. J. Clin. Pathol. 32:986–989, 1979.

Wilson, H.D., McCormick, J. B., and Freeley, J. C.: Yersinia enterocolitica infection in a 4 month old infant associated with infection in household dogs. J. Pediatr. 89:767–769, 1976.

Wolfe, M. S.: Current concepts in parasitology. Giardiasis. N. Engl. J. Med. 298:319–321, 1978.

Woode, G. N., and Crouch, C. F.: Naturally occurring and experimentally induced rotaviral infections of domestic and laboratory animals. J.A.V.M.A. 173:522–526, 1978.

Wooley, R. E., Shotts, E. B., Jr., and McConnel, J. W.: Isolation of Yersinia enterocolitica from selected animal species. Am. J. Vet. Res. 41:1667–1668, 1980.

Yanagawa, Y., Maruyama, T., and Sakai, S.: Isolation of Yersinia enterocolitica and Yersinia pseudotuberculosis from apparently healthy dogs and cats. Microbiol. Immunol. 22:643–646, 1978.

Yang, J., and Scholten, T.: A fixative for intestinal parasites permitting the use of concentration and permanent staining procedures. Am. J. Clin. Pathol. 67:300–304, 1977.

Zontine, W. J., Meierhenry, E. F., and Hicks, R. F.: Perforated duodenal ulcer associated with mastocytoma in a dog: A case report. J. Am. Vet. Radiol. Soc. 18:162–165, 1977.

CHAPTER 59

Diseases of the Large Bowel

MICHAEL D. LORENZ

Although the colon of carnivorous animals is comparatively simple in anatomy and function, this organ is the site of frequent small animal problems. Knowledge of the physiology and pathophysiology has been obtained from experimental studies on the dog colon that were applied to the human. Important anatomic and pathophysiologic differences do exist between human and animal colons, however, and these will be stressed when appropriate.

SIGNS OF COLONIC DISEASE

The cardinal sign of colonic disease is tenesmus. The patient strains and makes frequent attempts to defecate. A small amount of fecal matter is passed. Irritation of the rectum and anus, which accompanies many colonic diseases, is responsible for constant stimulation of the defecation reflex. The amount of feces passed with colonic diseases is variable. Initially, the patient may pass a fairly normal stool volume. This episode is followed by repeated straining. A scant amount of feces is passed each time. Tenesmus is less common if the disease involves only the ascending colon. The feces may be liquid or semi-solid in consistency and usually will contain visible amounts of red blood and large quantities of mucus. With colonic irritation or ulceration, the intestinal glands become hyperactive and goblet cells respond by secreting large quantities of mucus, presumably to coat and lubricate the irritated colonic mucosa. Red blood cells released from ulcerated areas in the colonic mucosa are apparently not hemolyzed and appear intact in the feces. Because most digestion and absorption of nutrients occurs in the small intestine, colonic disorders usually do not result in weight loss. Certain large bowel disorders such as histiocytic ulcerative colitis are associated with weight loss in long-standing cases and may be very severe in terminal cases. Vomiting occurs occasionally with colonic disorders. The mechanism responsible for this event is unknown, although a reversed gastrocolic reflex has been proposed. Excess flatulence usually indicates a small bowel disorder that results in poor intestinal digestion or absorption of fermentable substances. Fermentation of these substrates by colonic bacteria produces excessive gas, which produces flatulence. Flatulence may also occur with constipation disorders that directly result from disease of the colon, rectum, anus, or perineal structures. Table 59–1 compares the differential diagnosis of small and large bowel diarrhea. Further information concerning the small bowel can be found in Chapter 58, Diseases of the Small Bowel.

EXAMINATION OF THE COLON

The colon can be directly examined by abdominal and rectal palpation and by proctoscopy. Indirect examination can be achieved by special radiographic techniques or by fecal examinations. Significant information can be obtained by proctoscopy coupled with histologic examination of tissue taken through the proctoscope with a biopsy instrument. These techniques allow the clinician to rapidly determine the cause of the disorder and the prognosis.

PALPATION

Abdominal Palpation. Although the descending colon can be easily palpated through the abdomen, this procedure usually adds little to the documentation of diseases involving the colonic wall. Palpation of the ascending and transverse colon of the dog is difficult because closely associated structures confuse identification of these colonic segments. Foreign objects within the colon may be palpated through the abdomen. The cecum may be identified by palpation but is easily lost in the closely associated intestinal mass. Occasionally, inversion of the cecum may be indicated by palpation of a firm, painful linear structure near the ileocolic junction. Other diseases involving the colon, such as fecal impaction, can be easily identified by palpation of the distal colon. The abdomen of a cat can be thoroughly palpated and is much easier to palpate than that of a dog. The small volume of the feline abdomen allows the experienced clinician to identify most abdominal organs, including all segments of the colon and cecum; abnormal thickening of the colonic wall, large strictures, and tumors may be identified. In both dogs and cats, the presence of pain or discomfort should be noted during abdominal palpation of the colon. Colonic pain is relatively nonspecific and has low priority as a diagnostic sign.

Digital Palpation of the Rectum. Examination of the rectum and colon by digital palpation is possible except in small dogs and cats, but is limited to the anus and

Table 59–1. Differential Diagnosis of Small and Large Bowel Diarrhea

Sign	Small Bowel	Large Bowel
Number of stools per day	3 to 5 movements	Frequent movements
Stool quantity	Large amounts of watery or bulky feces	Small amounts of semiformed feces
Tenesmus	Usually absent	Present
Gross stool characteristics		
Blood	Dark black if present	Red (fresh)
Mucus	Absent	Present
Fat	May be present	Absent
Rectal exam	Usually normal	Mucus, fresh blood, thickened mucosa, stricture, or tumors may be found. Pain is usually produced.

rectum. Many diseases involving the distal colon also produce lesions in the rectum that can be identified by digital examination. The rectum should be examined for strictures; rough, corrugated, or thickened mucosal folds; tumors or masses; and foreign bodies. Any painful response by the patient should be noted. The tone and strength of the perineal reflex should be characterized. The gloved finger should be inspected for the presence of blood, mucus, or other exudates, and this material should be examined under the microscope for cytologic elements and protozoa.

FECAL EXAMINATIONS

Fecal examinations should include several flotations, direct smears in physiologic saline solution for protozoa, and cytologic examination with new methylene blue stain. In addition, fecal cultures for bacteria, fungi, and algae should be submitted to the laboratory if salmonellosis, histoplasmosis, or *Prototheca* is suspected. Twenty-four-hour fecal fat excretion and fecal trypsin analyses, which are useful as diagnostic tests in small bowel diseases, are *not* indicated for colonic diseases. Cytologic examination of feces may help to establish the presence of mucosal or transmural colonic disease. This procedure is rapidly accomplished by staining thin fecal smears with new methylene blue and examining them with light microscopy. Mucosal diseases are characterized by the presence of erythrocytes and numerous leukocytes. Transmural diseases more typically produce erythrocytes, but rarely leukocytes, in the feces (Van Kruiningen, 1972).

PROCTOSCOPY

Proctoscopy, when combined with colonic biopsy, is uniformly successful in establishing a diagnosis and prognosis in most colonic diseases. The procedure is relatively simple, quick, and safe for the patient and is the single most important means of establishing a diagnosis of inflammatory colonic disease (Zetzel, 1971). It requires two or more fiberoptic tubes of varying lengths and diameters. Fiberoptic proctoscopes that have circular illumination at the end of the tube are superior to instruments with a focal light source, because circular illumination affords even light in the colon and tends to prevent annoying blackouts caused by

mucus or feces that accumulate at the end of the tube. Focal light sources are easily blacked out by minimal amounts of mucus or feces. For small dogs and cats, a pediatric proctoscope 1.2 cm in diameter by 15 cm in length is satisfactory. For larger dogs, an adult sigmoidoscope 2.0 cm in diameter by 25 to 30 cm in length is used. With the longer instruments, the investigator can inspect all of the rectum and most of the distal colon. Shorter instruments are available, but they limit examination to the rectum. The construction of the tube should allow insufflation of air into the colon. This, held under pressure, distends the colonic folds and allows the investigator to view the entire colonic wall. Good proctoscopes are equipped with a magnifying lens in the viewing end, which also serves as a sealed door to prevent the escape of air from the colon. Most tubes can be disassembled from the primary light source and insufflation bulb for autoclaving or gas sterilization.

In preparation for proctoscopy, patients should be fasted at least 12 hours and preferably 24 hours. An enema should be given the evening before the procedure, and a low enema should be given one to two hours prior to examination. Deep sedation or light general anesthesia is usually required. Cats can be routinely examined under ketamine anesthesia, while dogs are best examined under thiamyl sodium anesthesia. If the procedure is prolonged, anesthesia can be maintained with an inhalant agent. Preanesthetic medications such as atropine sulfate are advised if the patient is to be intubated.

The patient is examined in dorsal or lateral recumbency. The caudal end of the dog should be slightly higher than the head to allow residual fluid in the colon to gravitate away from the site of investigation. The proctoscope tube is well lubricated and gently rotated as it is advanced into the colon. After the tube has been inserted to the maximum length tolerated by the patient, the probe is removed and the colon is fully distended with air. The tube is slowly withdrawn as the colonic wall is thoroughly inspected.

The normal canine colonic mucosa distends evenly with air; all folds in the mucosa are easily flattened. The mucosal surface is pink, smooth, and glistening. Solitary lymph nodules are easily identified. The presence of mucosal ulcers and their shape and suspected depth should be recorded, as well as the presence and extent of strictures, fistulae, and mucosal friability. Occasionally, *Trichuris vulpis* is observed attached to the mucosa of the proximal descending colon. The shape of tumors and their association with strictures should also be noted.

Mucosal diseases produce superficial ulcers and a glistening granularity of the mucosal surface. The mucosa may be quite friable and bleed easily when rubbed with the end of the proctoscope. The colon distends evenly with air, and strictures are absent. The colon maintains its normal length. Transmural diseases are likely to produce deep ulcers with rough edges. The mucosal surface is firm, corrugated, and very friable. The colon may distend poorly with air, and infrequently, strictures and fistulae may be observed. Occasionally the colon is shortened.

Colonic Biopsy. The colon wall can be easily biopsied at the time of colonoscopy. Although colonic biopsy can be accomplished with a multipurpose suction biopsy instrument (Van Kruiningen, 1972), a less expensive standard rectal biopsy punch (approximately 30 cm long) can be used for this purpose. With this instrument, the clinician can biopsy any suspicious lesion under direct vision through the proctoscope.

A small piece of mucosa and submucosa is carefully pinched from the margin of the lesion. The biopsy is retrieved from the colon in the jaws of the biopsy instrument and is immediately fixed in formalin. For immediate cytologic examinations, impression smears may be made just prior to fixation. The patient is fasted for 12 hours after the biopsy and then is started on a low bulk diet for three to five days.

Complications. The most feared sequela to colonoscopy and biopsy is perforation of the colon wall, with associated hemorrhage and peritonitis. The incidence of this complication is low if the investigator is gentle and experienced. Occasionally, the pathologist will report the presence of serosa in the colonic section. Fortunately, most of these cases do not develop complications. A retroperitoneal abscess that requires drainage and extended antibiotic therapy is a very rare complication.

The splenic flexure prevents examination of the transverse colon by standard proctoscopic methods. Flexible fiberoptic colonoscopes have been developed that allow examination of the entire colon and ileocecocolic region. Biopsy and suction attachments are available and are used to collect tissue and cytologic specimens from all areas of the colon. Although quite expensive, the equipment works well in dogs. Pediatric scopes are used in small dogs and cats. Good biopsy specimens may be somewhat difficult to procure until the operator gains experience with the equipment.

RADIOGRAPHIC TECHNIQUES

The transverse and ascending colons are best examined by radiology, exploratory laparotomy, or colonoscopy. The author takes standard ventrodorsal and lateral radiographs of the posterior abdomen following proctoscopy. The insufflation of air during proctoscopy creates a negative contrast study of the colon, and lesions such as polyps, strictures, tumors, and cecal inversion may be visualized with this technique.

Barium Enema. Examination of the colon by barium enema is indicated when fecal examinations and proctoscopy fail to establish a diagnosis. Barium enema studies are also indicated when the clinician suspects diseases of the ileocecocolic area and proximal colonic segments. A superior technique combines radiographs of the barium-filled colon with postevacuation radiographs. This procedure provides good double contrast studies of all segments of the colon and cecum, and clearly defines such abnormalities as ulcers, strictures, and intraluminal masses or tumors. Thickened, irregular, mucosal folds are best evaluated on postevacuation radiographs (Lawson et al., 1970).

The patient should be prepared for a barium enema study by withholding food for 24 hours and cleansing the bowel with mild enemas. Deep sedation or light general anesthesia is usually required for restraint unless the patient is quite cooperative or debilitated. A Bardex balloon catheter is used to fill and hold barium in the colon. The colon is gently filled by gravity flow with 25 to 30 per cent barium sulfate suspension warmed to body temperature. Five to seven ml/lb body weight will usually fill the colon to the ilecoceal sphincter (Guffey, 1972). Standard radiographs are then taken. Patients that have recently experienced colonic biopsy should not be submitted for barium enema examinations until the biopsy sites are nearly healed; at least seven to ten days should elapse between biopsy and barium examination of the colon.

INFLAMMATORY DISEASE OF THE CECUM AND COLON

The large bowel disorders have been classified by Van Kruiningen (1972) as mucosal or transmural, depending upon the presence or absence of involvement of deeper layers of the gut. Mucosal diseases produce inflammation of the epithelial colon glands, lamina propria, and superficial parts of the submucosa. Colons so involved show little change in length, pliability, and diameter. Mucosal diseases respond favorably to medical therapy; transmural diseases of the colon produce extensive lesions that result in grossly altered colons, secondary systemic complications, and poor response to medical therapy (Van Kruiningen, 1972). Inflammation is deep and may involve all layers down to and including the subserosa, as well as regional lymph nodes.

ACUTE COLITIS

Acute inflammation of the canine colon usually produces lesions in the mucosa and only rarely involves the deeper layers. The most common causes of acute colitis are parasites and foreign body irritations. Less common causes are primary bacterial infections, such as salmonellosis, and the poorly documented syndrome of food-induced allergic colitis. Male dogs suffering from prostatic enlargement due to infection, hyperplasia, or cysts show clinical signs similar to those of acute colitis. Acute colitis is an uncommon disease in cats.

TRICHURIS TYPHLITIS AND COLITIS

Etiology. *Trichuris vulpis* is a common cause of acute colitis in the dog. The parasite usually invades the cecum and proximal colon, but occasionally it parasitizes the distal colon. The anterior portion of the parasite's body is quite thin and is usually embedded in the mucosa (Fig. 59–1). The posterior end is thicker and contains the reproductive organs. The female parasite passes brown, football-shaped eggs. Infective larvae develop in the eggs in 10 to 12 days and emerge from the egg shortly after

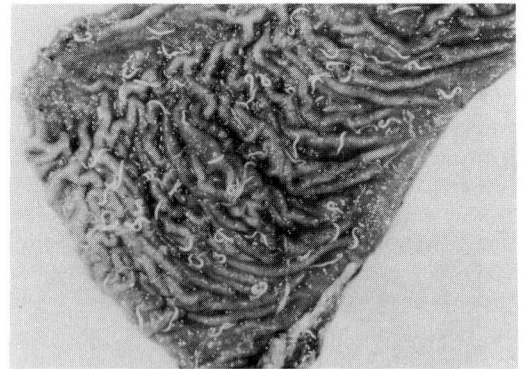

Figure 59–1. Adult *T. vulpis* attached to the descending colon of a dog. Most dogs with this heavy burden of parasites will have the typical ova in their feces. Diagnosis of occult trichuriasis is made by finding the adult parasite via endoscopic examination of the colon. (Courtesy of Dr. Ed Roberson, UGA.)

ingestion by the host. The infective larvae penetrate the mucosa of the small intestine and invade the intestinal crypts. They mature in these crypts for eight to ten days and then move on to the cecum, where they complete their maturation. The adult parasites attach to the mucosa, and the females begin producing ova 70 to 85 days after infection.

Clinical Signs. Light infestation produces minimal clinical signs. Moderate and severe infestations produce signs referable to colonic disease. Inflammation is confined largely to the cecum and proximal colon; however, in severe cases, the distal colon may be involved. In younger dogs or in long-standing cases, the hemorrhagic diarrhea may cause severe weight loss, dehydration, and anemia. Death may result from severe infestations and in cases complicated by other intestinal parasites such as hookworms. Signs referable to inflammation of the cecum are vague and difficult to document. Biting at the flank is an uncommon sign and is largely overemphasized in veterinary literature. Careful palpation of the abdomen may reveal pain or tenderness in the area of the cecum if it is palpable. The most outstanding sign of inflammation of the cecum is bloody or mucoid diarrhea.

Diagnosis. The diagnosis of trichuriasis is best made by diligent and persistent fecal examinations. Because stages of active whipworm infestation may occur when few or no ova can be demonstrated (occult trichuriasis), it is extremely important to check several fecal specimens for whipworm ova by flotation. Examination of material collected from the mucosal folds of the rectum may reveal ova, even though fecal flotations are repeatedly negative. During proctoscopy, the author has found whipworms in the descending colon of dogs whose fecal examinations were repeatedly negative for parasite ova.

Treatment. Medical therapy to kill the parasite cures most cases of trichuriasis because the mucosal involvement is superficial. Antibiotic therapy is seldom needed. Antispasmodics and local protectants such as Kaopectate or milk of bismuth provide temporary control of the diarrhea. Several drugs are effective in killing the parasite. Glycobiarsol (Milibis V), 45 mg/kg/day for five consecutive days, is effective in most dogs. No fasting is necessary prior to therapy; however, vomiting is a common side effect. Vomiting can be minimized by lightly feeding the dog before treatment. Resistant *T. vulpis* have been observed. Dichlorvos (Task), 33 mg/kg, remains an effective agent against *T. vulpis*. It is convenient to administer; however, it must be given to dogs free of adult *Dirofilaria immitis* or to dogs on heartworm prophylaxis. Mebendazol (Telmintic), 22 mg/kg daily for five days, is also effective and can be given without regard for heartworm status of the patient. The five-day course of therapy is inconvenient for many clients. Butamizole (Styquin), 2.4 mg/kg SQ, has been recently introduced but is painful when injected. It should not be used simultaneously with bunamidine HCl (Scolaban) or in heartworm-positive dogs. Fenbendazole, an experimental drug in dogs, has shown promise as an effective antihelmintic when administered at a dosage of 50 mg/kg/day for three days. Dogs should be retreated 21 days and three months after the original therapy.

Effective management of trichuriasis involves not only proper diagnosis and therapy but also sanitation of the kennel. Daily removal of feces is beneficial in preventing reinfestation. Concrete runs are easier to clean than dirt or gravel kennels. Maintaining and raising dogs on wire is also very effective in controlling infestation with *Trichuris vulpis*.

ACUTE BACTERIAL COLITIS

Etiology. This acute inflammatory disease of the colon is a common sequela to garbage ingestion or the passage of abrasive foreign bodies through the colon. Small intestinal disease frequently accompanies the large bowel signs. The passage of bone chips through the colon commonly abrades the mucosal lining, and this mechanical irritation results in signs of acute colitis. Secondary bacterial agents that may play a role in the pathogenesis of the acute inflammation have been poorly defined. The presence of spirochetes in fecal suspensions from affected dogs has created considerable concern that these bacteria are the causative agent. However, their significance is still uncertain. Other possibilities include clostridial bacteria and other normal gut inhabitants, such as *E. coli,* which act as opportunists on the irritated mucosa. The bacterial agent *Salmonella typhimurium* may produce disease of the colon as part of a syndrome involving the small intestine, liver, and mesenteric nodes. This disease (primarily an enterocolitis) is especially severe and significant in puppies. In addition to *S. typhimurium, S. enteritidis* and *S. dublin* have also been isolated (Thompson and Wright, 1969). *Salmonella* organisms have also been isolated from clinically normal dogs (Brown and Lorenz, 1973). The role of *Salmonella* organisms in the pathogenesis of many canine intestinal problems is still questionable. (See Chapter 27 for a discussion of *Salmonella* infections.)

Clinical Signs. The clinical signs of acute colitis are often associated with a recent episode of acute vomiting. The patient often has a history of scavenging, which suggests garbage ingestion. Direct smear of the feces may reveal a mixed population of extremely motile bacteria. Rectal examination is indicated. Often, remnants of bone chips, sticks, or aluminum foil suggest foreign body irritation as the initial cause of the clinical signs. In the case of a puppy recently purchased from a pet shop or "puppy mill," the clinican should be alert to the possibility of acute salmonellosis.

Diagnosis. Proctoscopic examination reveals small punctate ulcers in the mucosa. The ulcerated mucosa may have a hyperemic and granular appearance. The margin of the ulcers may bleed if rubbed with the proctoscope tube. The mucosal folds distend evenly and are not usually thickened; no strictures are observed. Mucus is excessive and may cling to the margin of the ulcers. A barium enema is not indicated in most cases, but fecal flotations are indicated to rule out concomitant parasitism. Fecal cultures should be taken to document all cases of suspected salmonellosis because of the public health importance of *S. typhimurium.* (see Chapter 27.)

Treatment. Treatment of acute colitis should be directed at the primary cause, if it can be established. In many cases, the underlying cause is not apparent and symptomatic therapy is indicated to correct dehydration and electrolyte imbalances, and to prevent further fluid losses by control of the diarrhea.

In the initial management of acute colitis, multiple fecal samples should be evaluated for parasites (fecal flotation, direct fecal smears, phenol-formalin fixed feces). In *Salmonella* endemic areas, one-gram stool samples or rectal swabs should be submitted for bacterial culture and antibiotic sensitivity tests. Food should be withheld for 24 hours and oral glucose-electrolyte solutions given to maintain hydration. Dehydration may be present and parenteral administration of lactated Ringer's solution may be necessary for 24 to 48 hours. After 24 hours, food is slowly returned to the patient. A bland low residue diet such as boiled lean hamburger or chicken with cooked white rice may be beneficial, particularly if the colonic mucosa has been severely ulcerated.

If given in large volumes every four hours, intestinal protectants and binding agents such as kaolin-pectin, aluminum hydroxide gel, or bismuth subsalicylate may be beneficial, particularly if colonic hypersecretion is involved in the pathogenesis of the diarrhea. In the dosages routinely used, these agents are probably ineffective. A dosage of 4 to 6 ml/kg every four hours is recommended.

If bacterial infection other than *Salmonella* is suspected, tetracycline (15 mg/kg tid) or chloramphenicol (30 mg/kg tid) may be given for seven to ten days. Antibiotic therapy for the treatment of enteric *Salmonella* infections may actually prolong the clinical course and carrier state. Antibiotic therapy is definitely indicated when systemic signs of salmonellosis accompany the enteric signs. Specific antibiotics are administered, based on sensitivity results; prior to receiving this information, however, gentamycin (2 mg/kg three times daily SQ or IM) or trimethoprim sulfadiazine (Tribressin, Septra) therapy will likely be effective. Ampicillin and chloramphenicol may be effective; however, isolates of *Salmonella* organisms in our hospital during the past two years have been resistant to these antimicrobial agents. *Salmonella* enteric infections are best managed by isolation of the patient, oral glucose-electrolyte solutions (Gatorade, Pedilyte), and parenteral fluids. Motility altering drugs such as diphenoxylate hydrochloride (Lomotil) (1.0 to 2.5 mg every six hours) or paragoric should be used sparingly. Antibiotics are used in cases with systemic illness. Enteric antibiotics (poorly absorbed sulfonamides, oral aminoglycosides) are not effective. Trimethoprim-sulfadiazine (Tribressin) may hold some promise as a drug effective for treating the chronic *Salmonella* carrier.

Opiates prolong fecal transit time by stimulating segmental peristalsis of the gut and may help correct the diarrhea and prevent further fluid loss. In addition, these drugs may decrease colonic distension, abdominal cramping, and tenesmus. Diphenoxylate hydrochloride, 1.0 to 2.5 mg every six hours, is the most effective of the drugs available and is usually given for two to three days. Anticholinergic antispasmodics, although oftentimes used to decrease intestinal motility, may not be indicated inasmuch as hypermotility may not be a contributing factor in the pathogenesis of large bowel diarrhea. In fact, these drugs may actually hasten fecal transit time by inhibiting segmental peristaltic contractions (contractions that effectively retard movement of luminal contents). Atropine-like antispasmodic agents are indicated if severe tenesmus has produced a rectal prolapse. Even in this situation, these drugs should be given in moderation and for short periods of time. Propantheline bromide (Pro-Banthine) has antiparasympathetic activity and decreases intestinal secretion and spasm. Although primarily indicated to decrease gastrointestinal secretions, this drug may also be beneficial in the treatment of acute colitis because of its effect in relieving colonic spasm. A dosage of 7.5 to 15 mg every six hours is recommended.

PSEUDOMEMBRANOUS COLITIS

Diarrhea and colitis have been associated with antimicrobial therapy in man and laboratory animals. The severity of diarrhea varies from a mild, self-limited process to a fulminant necrotizing or pseudomembranous colitis (PMC) (George et al., 1979). To the author's knowledge, this syndrome has been suspected but has not been thoroughly documented in dogs and cats.

Etiology. This disease is caused by antimicrobial agents such as penicillin, ampicillin, cephalexin, cephalothin, cotrimoxazole, lincomycin, and clindamycin. Apparently, these drugs suppress the growth of certain normal intestinal or colonic bacteria that inhibit replication of bacteria capable of producing colonic cytotoxins. *Clostridium difficile* is a bacteria that produces fecal toxins capable of inducing severe colonic cytotoxicity. This cytotoxicity can be blocked by the administration of polyvalent gas gangrene antitoxin. In addition, the disease can be prevented if antibiotics that inhibit *C. difficile* are given prior to development of clinical signs.

Clinical Signs. In man, clinical signs are those of acute to chronic watery, nonbloody diarrhea. Abdominal pain, cramps, and leukocytosis are common. Signs usually develop 12 to 14 days after the start of antibiotic therapy. Signs in guinea pigs, hamsters, and rabbits may develop acutely (within 72 hours) following antibiotic therapy. Severe depression, anorexia, and diarrhea that rapidly progresses to death are typical signs.

Diagnosis. This syndrome should be suspected when colonic signs suddenly develop in animals on antibiotic therapy with the agents previously listed. In man, colonoscopy reveals small whitish-yellow plaques that may coalesce to form a pseudomembrane (George et al., 1979). A confirmed diagnosis is based upon demonstration of a fecal cytotoxin that can be neutralized by specific clostridial antitoxin. Recovery of a toxigenic bacterium from the feces is also highly suggestive of this disease.

Treatment. The offending antibiotic should be discontinued, and vancomycin, which tends to inhibit the growth of cytotoxic clostridial organisms, is given orally. The value of constipating agents such as diphenoxylate hydrochloride is questionable. Other drugs used in humans include cholestyramine and specific antitoxins; again, their value is unknown.

AMEBIASIS

Etiology. Acute colitis can be caused by the protozoan agent *Entamoeba histolytica.* The parasite inhabits the large intestine, where conditions are favorable for its growth. The organism may be present as a commensal agent in the lumen or may invade the intestinal wall, causing symptoms of acute colitis. Spontaneous infections of the canine colon have been infrequently reported in the veterinary literature (Eyles et al., 1953; Jordan, 1967; Burrows and Hillis, 1967). Unlike the human patients suffering from this disease, the canine patients appear to be resistant to systemic infection. Only one case of systemic amebiasis associated with canine distemper has been reported (Thorson et al., 1956).

Entamoeba histolytica exists in two major forms, a relatively resistant cyst and a trophozoite that survives poorly outside the body. In man, transmission of amebiasis is by the resistant cysts (Marsden, 1971); however, this mode of transmission has not been well documented for the dog. Most investigators report that cysts are rarely found in feces from affected dogs (Jordan, 1967). The feeding of a liver diet to infected dogs stimulates cyst production by an unknown mechanism (Faust and Kagy, 1934). Trophozoites are found in low numbers in the feces of naturally infected dogs and have been used to experimentally transmit the disease in dogs (Jordan, 1967). The trophozoites measure 10 to 40 μ and the cysts measure 10 to 20 μ.

Amebae thrive under conditions of low oxygen tension, and therefore, conditions in the colon are suitable for amebae growth because bacterial multiplication lowers the oxidation reduction potential (Marsden, 1971). The exact function of bacteria in determining the pathogenicity of *E. histolytica* is unclear. In studies with germ-free animals, sterile amebae have shown different degrees of invasiveness when monocontaminated with different bacterial species (Marsden, 1971). The presence of coincident helminth infections in dogs may be a factor that favors the invasion by *E. histolytica.* In one study of spontaneous and experimental cases of canine amebiasis, concomitant infection with *Ancylostoma caninum* and *Trichuris vulpis* was common (Jordan, 1967). The nature of this relationship has not been documented.

The incidence of canine amebiasis appears to be quite low (Swartzwelder and Avant, 1952; Eyles et al., 1953). *Entamoeba histolytica* is quite difficult to isolate or culture from the canine colon, and this factor may have contributed to the apparent low incidence of the disease in past surveys.

Clinical Signs. Clinical signs of amebiasis develop within 7 to 14 days in dogs experimentally infected with trophozoites by the oral route. The method of natural canine infection is unknown, although the ingestion of infected human feces (Gaefar, 1968) or fresh infected canine feces (Jordan, 1967) has been suggested. Jordan (1967) has classified the clinical signs of amebiasis as follows: (1) *mild:* diarrhea with some blood, recovery is spontaneous; (2) *chronic:* mucoid feces, occasionally diarrhea. The disorder may become subclinical or recur in the acute form; (3) *subacute:* bloody diarrhea, becoming chronic or acute; (4) *acute:* fulminating dysentery, terminating in death; (5) *systemic:* dysentery, terminating in death.

Clinical signs result from colonization of the colonic wall by the trophozoites. Foci of mucosal ulceration develop from involvement or destruction of the epithelium. Patchy infiltration of inflammatory cells in the submucosa and lamina propria can be found. Clinical cases are usually presented in the acute stages of the disease. Hemorrhagic dysentery is a common sign and may be so severe that there is continual oozing of blood from the anus (Jordan, 1967). Death may occur within three to seven days unless good supportive care is given. In other cases there may be repeated episodes of bloody mucoid diarrhea, and in some of these cases, there may be spontaneous recovery.

Diagnosis. Trophozoites are most readily found in the bloody mucus of the feces (Jordan, 1967) (Fig. 59–2). Few trophozoites are found in canine fecal specimens, however. Therefore, direct saline solution smears are likely to be negative even though active infection is present. Preserving the specimen in polyvinyl alcohol and then staining the sediment with iron-alum hematoxylin improves the recovery of trophozoites from fresh canine feces. In one study, culture of fresh feces on Nelson's medium was superior to other procedures for the isolation and subsequent identification of *E. histolytica* (Eyles et al., 1953).

Proctoscopic examination may reveal a very hyperemic mucosa with small erosions (two to three mm) or friable-edged ulcers. The appearance of the colonic mucosa may be slightly inflamed in subacute or chronic

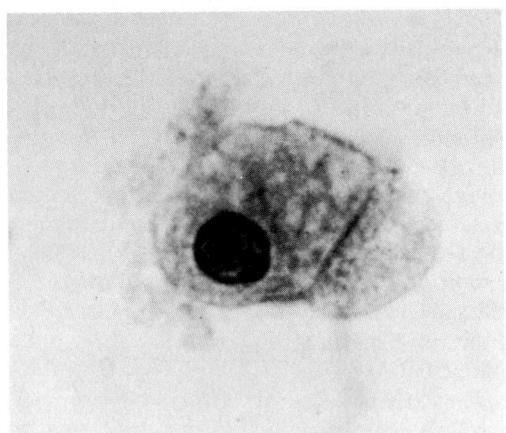

Figure 59–2. Trophozoite of *E. histolytica* found in dog feces. (Courtesy of Dr. Ed Roberson, UGA.)

cases. Intestinal biopsy is reported to be diagnostic of amebiasis (Van Kruiningen, 1972).

Therapy. Documentation of reliable therapy for *E. histolytica* in dogs is scarce. In one study, the use of Anamoeba (a combination of bacitracin and iodochlorhydroxyquin) produced sporadic results (Jordan, 1967). Emetine and dehydroemetine are effective drugs for invasive bowel amebiasis in man. Perhaps the drug most applicable to veterinary practice is metronidazole (Flagyl). This compound is both a luminal and a tissue amebacide. Metronidazole has reportedly been given orally to adult dogs in dosages of 45 mg/lb per day for 30 days without toxic side effects (Buckner and Ewing, 1971).

Since the resistant cysts are not passed in the feces and trophozoites survive poorly outside the host, it is unlikely that dogs with amebiasis pose a public health threat. Therefore, unless close or intimate contact occurs between the patient and people, it is unlikely that the dog represents an important source of infection to man.

CHRONIC INFLAMMATORY DISEASES OF THE COLON

Chronic inflammatory diseases of the colon have been well documented in the dog. These diseases have been rarely reported in the cat and apparently occur infrequently. Recently, a case of histiocytic colitis was reported in a five-year-old spayed female Persian cross-bred cat (Van Kruiningen and Dobbins, 1979).

HISTIOCYTIC ULCERATIVE COLITIS OF BOXER DOGS

Etiology. Histiocytic ulcerative colitis of the boxer dog (also known as granulomatous colitis, histiocytic colitis, and boxer colitis) is a chronic disease of unknown origin. Some investigators consider this disease to be a variant form of ulcerative colitis (Ewing and Gomez, 1973). In the boxer, the disease is most frequently found in dogs under two years of age (Van Kruiningen et al., 1965; Koch and Skelley, 1967; Starnes, 1969; Ewing and Gomez, 1973). Some signs of the disease are similar to those of ulcerative colitis, Whipple's disease, and granulomatous colitis of man. Although the etiology of these human diseases is not completely established, several factors are associated with their occurrence, and these same factors may occur in dogs affected with chronic colitis. Human ulcerative colitis and granulomatous colitis may be different manifestations of the same cause. The proposed causes of these two diseases are similar.

Early studies in man revealed an association of chronic colitis following bacterial infections of the colon, such as bacillary dysentery. However, the infrequency of ulcerative colitis in more than one member of a family, the absence of consistent bacteriologic confirmation, and the failure of therapeutic agents to eradicate *Shigella* suggest that these microorganisms play a minor role in the etiology of ulcerative colitis (Zetzel, 1971). Other bacteria, such as *Bacterium necrophorum,* have not been established as etiologic agents, even though they are abundantly present in stools from human cases. The presence of blood and pus in the feces may favor growth of these organisms, and this factor may explain their presence in feces from human cases of ulcerative colitis.

Whipple's disease is a chronic enteropathy involving the human jejunum, which results in malabsorption. The jejunum is infiltrated by PAS-positive histiocytes that are also indicative of histiocytic ulcerative colitis. Electron microscopic studies have revealed bacilliform bodies that may be infectious agents in and near these histiocytes. Studies suggest that a tetracycline-susceptible pleomorphic organism is involved in the cause of Whipple's disease (Haubrich et al., 1960).

An infectious agent has been suspected as the cause of histiocytic ulcerative colitis because the disease has a tendency to occur in several dogs from the same kennel, the disease is mildly responsive to antibiotic therapy, and large numbers of macrophages are present in the submucosa of the colonic wall (Van Kruiningen et al., 1965). Histologic studies, special stains, and cultures have consistently failed to demonstrate the presence of significant bacteria, viruses, protozoa, or yeasts. Bacterial cultures have yielded *Proteus* spp., *Aerobacter aerogenes,* nonhemolytic Clostridia, and *Bacteroides* spp. (Van Kruiningen et al., 1965). All of these bacteria are considered normal flora of the canine colon. Occasionally, *Salmonella* spp. are isolated, but their recovery from dogs with histiocytic ulcerative colitis is no more frequent than from normal dogs (Ewing and Gomez, 1973). Van Kruiningen (1972) describes the presence of lipid-rich coccoid structures, 100 to 500 mμ in diameter, in the colonic histocytes. These structures were interpreted as being infectious agents, perhaps psittacoid agents. Cockrell and Krehbiel (1972) suggest that these coccoid structures are membrane-bound cytoplasmic granules that are PAS-positive in light microscope studies. These researchers also found unusual tubular granules, varying in length from 200 to 450 mμ, which occurred in both nuclear and cytoplasmic regions of the histiocyte. These particles are morphologically dissimilar to known animal viruses or rickettsia agents. Their significance is currently unknown.

A relationship between psychological trauma and human ulcerative colitis is based on observations that stressful life situations may be reflected in disturbances of the motor, secretory, and vascular responses of the colon (Zetzel, 1971). It is extremely difficult to document emotional or psychic abnormalities in the dog. The function of psychological factors in the cause of chronic colitis in the dog is unknown and nearly impossible to document. Most affected dogs are of good temperament and not easily excited.

The prevalence of histiocytic ulcerative colitis in the boxer breed suggests a genetic predisposition for this disease. Many affected dogs can be traced to two ancestral animals instrumental in development of the boxer breed in the United States; however, most of the affected dogs were raised in the same kennel, so a common environmental factor must also be considered. Both genetic and environmental factors may work together to cause the disease (Ewing and Gomez, 1973).

The occasional dramatic remission of signs in human ulcerative colitis following the omission of certain foods from the person's diet suggests food allergy as a possible cause of the disease. However, canine histiocytic ulcerative colitis is histologically dissimilar to food allergy enteritis, and hypoallergenic diets have failed to improve the signs of histiocytic ulcerative colitis in canine patients.

Colon antibodies that crossreact with *E. coli* have been found in the serum of some human patients with ulcerative colitis. A mechanism may exist whereby these antigenic bacteria provoke the production of specific antibodies directed against the epithelial cells of the colon. Delayed hypersensitivity reactions against colon epithelial cells have also been documented in human ulcerative colitis, but similar immunologic studies are lacking for the dog. Table 59–2 summarizes the proposed causes of canine histiocytic ulcerative colitis.

Gross Pathology. Histiocytic ulcerative colitis usually affects the descending colon and rectum. In more advanced cases, the cecum and proximal colon may also be affected, but less severely than the rectum and descending colon. The earliest gross lesions are punctate reddened foci in the mucosa of the rectum and colon. Slightly more advanced lesions are circular to linear in morphology, one to five mm in size. These foci are reddened and depressed (Russell et al., 1971). More chronic lesions include severe mucosal ulceration, with the mucosal surface appearing irregularly reddened and granular. Small islands of normal epithelium may be surrounded by ulcerated mucosa. The colon and rectum may be shortened and the wall thickened. The colonic wall may have a corrugated or cobblestone appearance. Upon cut surface, the submucosa is usually irregularly thickened and firm. The muscle layers may be thicker than normal and often compressed (Van Kruiningen et al., 1965). As the disease worsens, small ulcers become large and coalesce with one another to form large denuded segments of colon. Rarely, scar tissue and strictures in the colonic wall are observed.

Lymph nodes that drain the rectum, colon, and cecum are enlarged in chronic cases of histiocytic ulcerative colitis. Initially, lymphoid hyperplasia is responsible for the increased size; later, the nodes are infiltrated by PAS-positive histiocytes. Generalized lymphadenopathy also occurs, and PAS-positive histiocytes are occasionally found in the peripheral lymph nodes.

Leiomyometaplasia of the small intestine is an infrequent gross finding. The significance of this lesion is unknown. Vitamin E deficiency has been suggested as the cause (Van Kruiningen et al., 1965).

Histopathology. The pathogenesis of mucosal ulceration in histiocytic ulcerative colitis is debatable. Mucosal ulceration may be a primary lesion due to epithelial degeneration (Russell et al., 1971), or it may be a lesion secondary to disruption by histiocytes that infiltrate and distend the submucosa (Van Kruiningen et al., 1965). This uncertainty apparently stems from histologic studies made at different stages of the disease.

Table 59–2. Proposed Causes of Histiocytic Ulcerative Colitis

Cause	Supportive Evidence
Infectious agent	Multiple occurrence in kennels, mild response to antibiotics; histiocyte response in submucosa; bacilliform structures in the histiocytes.
Genetic	Many affected dogs are descendants of the same ancestors; predisposition for boxers.
Psychological	Studies in man.
Immunologically mediated	Studies in man; mild response or remissions with corticosteroids.
Food allergy	None

The earliest histologic lesion discernible by light microscopy is focal, acute inflammation with degeneration of the luminal surface epithelium (Russell et al., 1971). The mucosa becomes hypercellular; the lamina propria is infiltrated with lymphoreticulum cells, plasma cells, mast cells, and some neutrophils. Focal degeneration of the luminal surface epithelium, and to a lesser extent of the adjacent crypt epithelium, develops early in the lesion (Russell et al., 1971). Microabscess or crypt abscess is rarely found.

The most conspicuous ultrastructural alterations within the epithelium in early lesions include dilatation of the epithelial intercellular spaces, degenerative changes within epithelial cells, effacement of the basement membrane, and migration of neutrophils between the epithelial cells (Gomez et al., 1977). Evidence for an infectious cause of these early changes was not found. Bacteria were identified in some lesions, but only after mucosal ulceration had occurred. This finding suggests that microorganisms are probably secondary invaders.

The most characteristic microscopic lesion in chronic histiocytic ulcerative colitis is the invasion of the mucosa and submucosa by several layers of PAS-positive histiocytes. A theory offered by Van Kruiningen (1975) is that the infiltration of histiocytes creates the luminal ulcerations by compression or disruption of the surface epithelium. This theory does not explain epithelial changes, including ulceration, that occur before histiocyte invasion can be documented. However, it is certainly reasonable to assume that this mechanism adds to the severity of mucosal ulceration and the retardation of healing characteristic in chronic cases.

The ultrastructure of the PAS-positive histiocytes has been studied in an attempt to discern the pathogenesis of this lesion. Van Kruiningen (1975) concluded that structures within PAS-macrophages represented the phagocytosis and digestion of a lipid-rich coccoid and coccobacillary organisms. A later study also suggested that the PAS-positive histiocytes were engorged with numerous digestive vacuoles that mainly contained phospholipid membranes (Gomez et al., 1977). This study suggested that these PAS-positive cells arise from active phagocytic macrophages found in the surface-oriented mucosal lesions. There was *no* consistent morphologic evidence of a specific infectious agent.

Clinical Signs. Histiocytic ulcerative colitis occurs most commonly in young boxer dogs. In one study, 78.9 per cent of affected boxer dogs developed clinical signs before two years of age, whereas only 5.3 per cent of boxer dogs developed colitis after four years of age (Ewing and Gomez, 1973). There is no sex predisposition for this disease.

Chronic hemorrhagic diarrhea characterizes histiocytic ulcerative colitis. The patient is usually afebrile and in good body condition. The patient exhibits all of the signs previously described for colonic diseases. Affected dogs make repeated attempts to defecate and pass small volumes of feces of varying consistency. Stools passed may be formed or very liquid, and blood and mucus are grossly evident in the feces of most patients. Blood may be unevenly streaked in the fecal matter or may compose the entire stool. Tenesmus is usually present, inasmuch as histiocytic ulcerative colitis affects the rectum in most cases. Tenesmus may not always indicate stricture formation in the rectum but invariably occurs if strictures are present.

Loss of body weight is uncommon and quite variable in affected dogs. In some cases, this loss of weight is related to inappetence; however, some dogs experience weight loss and develop an unthrifty appearance even though they continue to eat well. The cause of this weight loss is unknown, but loss of protein and other nutrients through the ulcerated mucosa may partially explain the weight loss and unthrifty coat.

Vomiting occurs in one third of the cases and may be one of the early signs in a few cases. In one study, a high incidence of vomiting was associated with anorectic dogs (Ewing and Gomez, 1973). The mechanism for emesis in colitis is unknown, but as described previously, it may result from a reversed gastrocolic reflex mediated through the hypothalamus. Pain, except upon defecation, is uncommon. Abdominal palpation may reveal pain in the posterior abdomen, but localization to the colon is difficult. Pain upon rectal examination is common. The clinician may also palpate a roughened, corrugated rectal mucosa. Rectal strictures are rarely palpated.

Pallor of the mucous membranes and fever are uncommon. Peripheral lymphadenopathy occurs in very chronic cases. Perforation of the colonic wall is a rare complication in canine patients with histiocytic ulcerative colitis. Long-term studies to determine the incidence of colonic neoplasia in affected dogs are lacking.

Diagnosis. The outstanding diagnostic procedure for confirmation of histiocytic ulcerative colitis is proctoscopy with concomitant biopsy of the colon or rectal wall. Proctoscopic findings are variable, depending upon the degree and duration of involvement. In mild cases, the colon is reddened and edematous. In more advanced cases, the muscosal folds are thickened and distend poorly with air. The mucosa may be friable, and hemorrhage commonly occurs from the trauma of proctoscopy. Gross ulceration with severe hemorrhage is common. Mucosal ulcers vary in size from small punctate erosions to large ulcerative areas that may surround islands of normal mucosa. The most chronic changes grossly evident at proctoscopy are localized strictures and contracture of the colonic wall. Biopsy, made at the time of proctoscopy, will confirm the diagnosis.

Fecal examinations are necessary in order to eliminate the possibility of parasitism. The feces of dogs affected with histiocytic ulcerative colitis contain both erythrocytes and leukocytes; however, the presence of these cells does not confirm the diagnosis of histiocytic ulcerative colitis inasmuch as several colonic diseases may produce similar cytologic findings in the feces.

Hemograms are normal in most cases of histiocytic ulcerative colitis. Slight leukocytosis and anemia are present only in long-standing cases.

Roentgenographic studies are usually abnormal. Radiographic abnormalities, as documented by barium enema, do not occur as early as the clinical signs and confirmatory proctoscopic findings. Proctoscopic findings of the distal colon and rectum usually indicate a more severe disease state than that revealed by barium enema studies (Lawson et al., 1970). Fine mucosal serrations and thickened mucosal folds are frequent abnormalities found by barium enema in the descending colon and rectum. Deep ulcers are less commonly found and are usually associated with severe involvement of the

Table 59–3. Ways in Which Some Common Human Bowel Diseases Resemble and Differ from Canine Histiocytic Ulcerative Colitis

Human Disease	Similarities to Canine Diseases	Differences from Canine Diseases
Ulcerative colitis	Most cases have gross blood in the feces, and rectal involvement is common; infrequent involvement of the terminal ileum; diffuse colonic disease with no skin lesions; uncommon perianal fistula; subserosa rarely diseased.	Absences of PAS-positive macrophages; presence of crypt abscesses; less involvement in lamina propria and submucosa.
Granulomatous colitis	Severe involvement of the lamina propria and submucosa; similar morphology of colonic ulcers; eccentric thickening of the colon wall.	Absence of rectal bleeding in over 50% of the cases; rectal involvement uncommon; disease of the ileum is common; diffuse colonic involvement is rare; subserosa commonly diseased; no PAS-positive macrophages; rectal and perianal fistulae are common.
Whipple's disease	PAS-positive macrophages; disease of the regional lymph nodes; peripheral lymphadenopathy; bacilliform bodies in macrophages; involvement of the lamina propria is common.	Largely confined to the jejunum and ileum; rare mucosal ulceration; characteristic lymphatic dilatation and lipogranulomatous inflammation.

colon. Major deformities include colonic spasm in mild to moderate cases and shortening or stricture of the colon in moderate to severe cases. The colon may appear narrow, owing to fibrosis and strictures.

Barium enema is indicated in those cases that have negative proctoscopic findings. Barium enema can provide a positive diagnosis in cases that have lesions limited to the ascending and transverse colon. The combination of proctoscopy with barium enema allows the clinician to thoroughly evaluate a patient with suspected histiocytic ulcerative colitis.

Treatment. Treatment of canine histiocytic ulcerative colitis is discussed in the section dealing with therapy of chronic ulcerative colitis.

Discussion. Canine histiocytic ulcerative colitis has been compared to several diseases of the human colon and small intestine (Van Kruiningen et al., 1965; Koch and Skelley, 1967; Sanders and Langham, 1968; Ewing and Gomez, 1973). Table 59–3 summarizes the similarities and differences between canine cases of histiocytic ulcerative colitis and human intestinal diseases. As can be readily noted, canine histiocytic ulcerative colitis is not identical to any human disease of the small or large intestine.

IDIOPATHIC ULCERATIVE COLITIS OF DOGS

Canine idiopathic ulcerative colitis has not been as extensively studied as histiocytic ulcerative colitis of boxer dogs. Evidently, this disease is most common in breeds other than the boxer. Ewing and Gomez (1973) report that the disease is slightly more common (57.9 per cent) in nonboxer dogs over two years of age. In these dogs, 27.6 per cent developed signs after four years of age, compared with only 5.3 per cent of boxers of similar age. Van Kruiningen (1972) reports several cases of colitis in purebreed dogs similar to regional enteritis and mucosal colitis in man.

The basic lesion of this disease is similar to that of histiocytic ulcerative colitis, with one notable exception. PAS-positive histiocytes are not found in the lamina propria or submucosa. Figure 59–3 shows the radiographic abnormalities of idiopathic ulcerative colitis.

The reader is referred to the section on histiocytic ulcerative colitis for a discussion

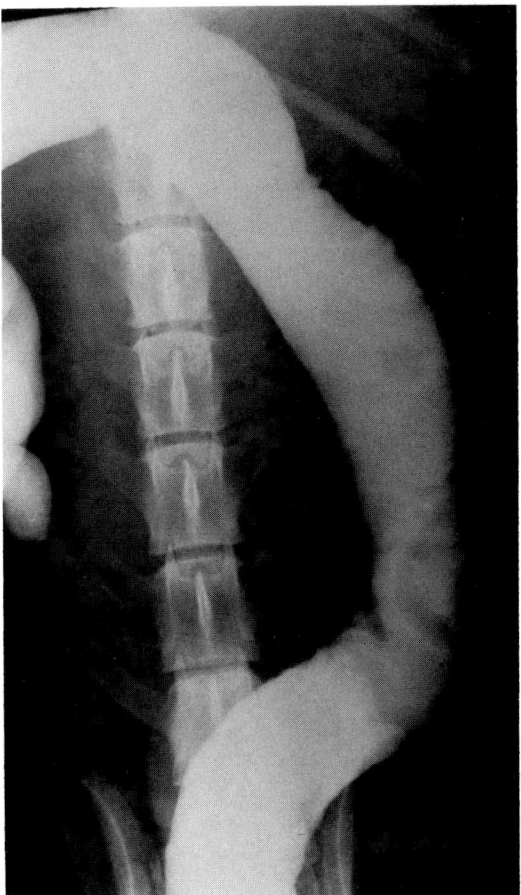

Figure 59–3. A ventrodorsal radiograph (following barium enema) of a seven-year-old male hound with idiopathic ulcerative colitis. The descending colonic wall is irregular in outline with some projections that represent ulcers and masses. Proctoscopy and biopsy findings confirmed the diagnosis of ulcerative colitis. (Courtesy of Dr. Robert Lewis, UGA.)

of possible etiologies and diagnosis. Treatment is discussed in the section dealing with therapy of chronic ulcerative colitis.

EOSINOPHILIC ULCERATIVE COLITIS

Etiology. Eosinophilic ulcerative colitis may occur as a primary disease entity of the colon and rectum or may occur as the colonic component of a broader syndrome, eosinophilic gastroenteritis. The cause of the disease in both men and dogs is unknown. Possible causes include an allergic or hypersensitivity phenomenon, parasitic infections, or foreign body reactions (Kumar, 1972).

In man, elimination of certain foods such as meat, cereals, and milk may be beneficial in resolving milder forms of eosinophilic gastroenteritis. Hypoallergenic diets and other forms of dietary management have not benefited the patients with eosinophilic ulcerative colitis treated by the author. Controlled studies to determine the role of food antigens in the etiology of this disease in dogs are lacking. However, clinical evidence accumulated to date does not support food allergy as the cause of this disease. Food allergy colitis has been described by Povar (1947) and Van Kruiningen (1972). Diagnosis apparently was based solely upon improvement of signs following the omission of horse meat from the diet of affected dogs. Biopsy studies were not reported, and thus a comparison with eosinophilic ulcerative colitis cannot be made.

Recently, visceral larva migrans has been associated with a canine syndrome similar to eosinophilic gastroenteritis (Hayden and Van Kruiningen, 1973). However, the dogs reported in this study had lesions confined to the stomach, small intestine, regional lymph nodes, and lungs. Lesions in the colon were not reported. The role of visceral larva migrans in the pathogenesis of eosinophilic infiltration of the canine colon cannot be assessed from this study.

Pathology. Characteristically, the lamina propria and submucosa of the colon are infiltrated by eosinophils. In some cases, the eosinophilic aggregates have the appearance of granulomas. Some neutrophils, macrophages, and fibroblasts may also be present (Hall, 1967). The luminal epithelium may be ulcerated, but the severity of ulceration is usually less than that noted with histiocytic ulcerative colitis. The pathogenesis of the mucosal ulceration and the function of histamine in the pathogenesis of this lesion are not known.

Clinical Signs. Early reports of this disease indicate a predisposition for the cocker spaniel and German shepherd dog (Theran, 1968). However, dogs of many different breeds can be affected. Younger dogs may be more frequently affected, but the author has documented eosinophilic ulcerative colitis in middle-aged and older dogs.

The outstanding clinical sign of eosinophilic ulcerative colitis is chronic, intermittent, or constant hemorrhagic diarrhea. Affected dogs are presented with signs similar to those of other ulcerative diseases of the colon and rectum.

Diagnosis. Hematologic examinations reveal a marked circulating eosinophilia frequently exceeding 3000 eosinophils/cm. The presence of a circulating eosinophilia in the absence of other diseases that could explain the elevated blood eosinophil count is highly suggestive of eosinophilic ulcerative colitis. The patient should always be evaluated for other causes of eosinophilia, including concomitant parasitism (internal and external), respiratory or dermatologic allergy, and adrenal cortical insufficiency. If colonic hemorrhage is severe, moderate anemia may also be present.

Microscopic examination of the hemorrhagic feces may reveal a high concentration of eosinophils (Legendre and Krehbiel, 1973). Numerous fecal examinations are also necessary to rule out parasitism of the colon.

The best documentation of eosinophilic ulcerative colitis is made by proctoscopy, followed by biopsy of the affected colonic wall. The mucosa appears granular and friable upon proctoscopic examination. The mucosal folds may have a corrugated or pebble-like appearance. Small erosions and ulcers are commonly found. Strictures are usually absent. Biopsy reveals infiltration of the lamina propria and submucosa by eosinophils.

Treatment. Therapy of eosinophilic ulcerative colitis is presented in the following section, which deals with management of chronic ulcerative colitis.

TREATMENT OF CHRONIC ULCERATIVE COLITIS

Although the histopathological lesions of histiocytic and idiopathic ulcerative colitis are different, both conditions may be treated with similar methods. The etiology of both conditions is unknown and treatment regimens have been based primarily upon those used for the management of human ulcerative and granulomatous (Crohn's) colitis. The prognosis for total remission of signs is guarded, and the owner should be warned to expect several relapses during therapy. Remissions can be achieved in less advanced cases, but once the disease becomes severe and scar tissue is present, the chances for successful therapy are poor. Eosinophilic ulcerative colitis responds well to corticosteroid therapy. Although relapses may occur, the prognosis is usually good.

Immediate Management. The immediate objectives of medical therapy for severe ulcerative colitis or acute fulminating exacerbations include colonic rest with attempts to restore normal intestinal function, maintenance of nutrition, correction of electrolyte and fluid imbalances, and correction of anemia that may accompany prolonged colonic hemorrhage.

Affected dogs should be placed in a quiet environment where they are not likely to be disturbed by daily hospital activities. If at all possible, therapy should be carried out at home. Various sedatives such as phenobarbital or tranquilizers such as chlorpromazine (Thorazine) allow the patient to rest. Chlorpromazine and prochlorperazine (Compazine) help to control signs of anxiety and vomiting that may occur in highly nervous dogs. Anticholinergic antispasmodics have variable, oftentimes disappointing effects in controlling the diarrhea or tenesmus. These agents may be most effective if administered 30 minutes to one hour prior to feeding, because they tend to abolish the gastrocolic reflex. Propantheline bromide (Pro-Banthine L.A.), 15 to 30 mg every 12 hours, may be quite helpful. Excessive use of potent antispasmodics should be avoided because they may totally suppress intestinal motility and produce ileus. The author prefers to administer propantheline bromide tablets before each meal and to use the long-acting tablets at night to prolong nocturnal effects. Diphenoxylate (Lomotil) therapy may also be beneficial; however, it should be used for brief periods of time or discontinued if colonic perforation appears likely. Hydrophilic agents such as Metamucil or binding agents such as aluminum hydroxide gel may thicken the consistency of stools and reduce the frequency of diarrheal movements. These agents should be given four times a day, usually after meals and at night.

In fulminant ulcerative colitis or in prolonged cases with profuse diarrhea, parenteral fluid and electrolyte replacement therapy may be necessary to correct dehydration and electrolyte imbalances. To fully evaluate the patient, a complete blood count and biochemical profile should be performed. If bleeding has been prolonged or severe, whole blood transfusions may be indicated. In most cases, the patient is rehydrated over three to four days with lactated Ringer's solution supplemented with potassium chloride, if needed. For the first 48 hours, it may be desirable to permit nothing by mouth to avoid gastrocolic stimulation, which may reduce tenesmus. In the dog, it is usually not possible to achieve total parenteral hyperalimentation for several weeks, as is commonly done for human patients (Driscoll and Rosenburg, 1978). Therefore, to assure adequate caloric intake, affected dogs are placed on bland, low residue diets on the third day of treatment. Dietary substances that are allowed include corn oil, cooked refined corn or rice, rice and wheat cereals, oatmeal, white bread, lean meat, poultry, potatoes, macaroni, and spaghetti. Commercial low residue diets (I/D) may be substituted for part or all of the diet. The total ration should be divided into three equal meals. B complex and fat-soluble vitamins should be given by intramuscular injection for three days, followed by oral vitamin supplementation with each meal. Evidence of iron deficiency anemia secondary to chronic blood loss is an indication for daily hematinic therapy.

Antibiotic Therapy. Dogs severely affected with histiocytic or idiopathic ulcerative colitis should be immediately started on salicylazosulfapyridine (Azulfidine) therapy. This drug is seldom necessary in cases of eosinophilic ulcerative colitis. The value of this drug in the management of ulcerative colitis is debatable, since no controlled studies in the dog are available. Yet, on a clinical basis, this drug appears to benefit many dogs (Ewing and Gomez, 1973), particularly where client cooperation allows a long-term trial. Studies indicate that intestinal bacteria split the compound into 5-aminosalicylate and sulfapyridine (Goldman, 1973). The anti-inflammatory action of 5-aminosalicylate may be responsible for the beneficial effects, in that this compound apparently is concentrated in the colonic wall. If the proposed mechanism of Azulfidine is correct, one should avoid concomitant antibiotic therapy. The dose of Azulfidine is 60 mg/kg every eight hours; however, in most cases a maximum dose of one gm every eight hours is effective. A total daily dose of four to five gm should not be exceeded. Complications in the dog are not common. Vomiting, depression, hemolytic anemia, dermatitis, keratitis sicca, and cholestatic jaundice have been reported. Response to this drug may be delayed, so therapy should be continued several weeks before it is decided that the treatment is not effective.

In early cases, chloramphenicol or tetracycline may be beneficial and should be given for three to four weeks. During this time, the patient must be closely monitored for improvement. Worsening of signs during this time is an indication to stop the antibiotics and begin treatment with Azulfidine as recommended above. Dogs with eosinophilic ulcerative colitis are given tetracycline orally for ten days. In a cat with chronic histiocytic colitis, clinical recovery was completed with seven months of chloramphenicol therapy (Van Kruiningen and Dobbins, 1979).

Corticosteroid Therapy. Systemic corticosteroid therapy produces rapid and dramatic improvement in dogs with eosinophilic ulcerative colitis (Fig. 59–4). In the other forms of ulcerative colitis, however, systematic corticosteroids should be given with great caution and probably not until all other measures have been given a fair trial. For eosinophilic ulcerative colitis, prednisolone, 2 mg/kg in divided doses twice daily is given for five to seven days or until signs of tenesmus, diarrhea, and colonic hemorrhage have greatly improved. Thereafter,

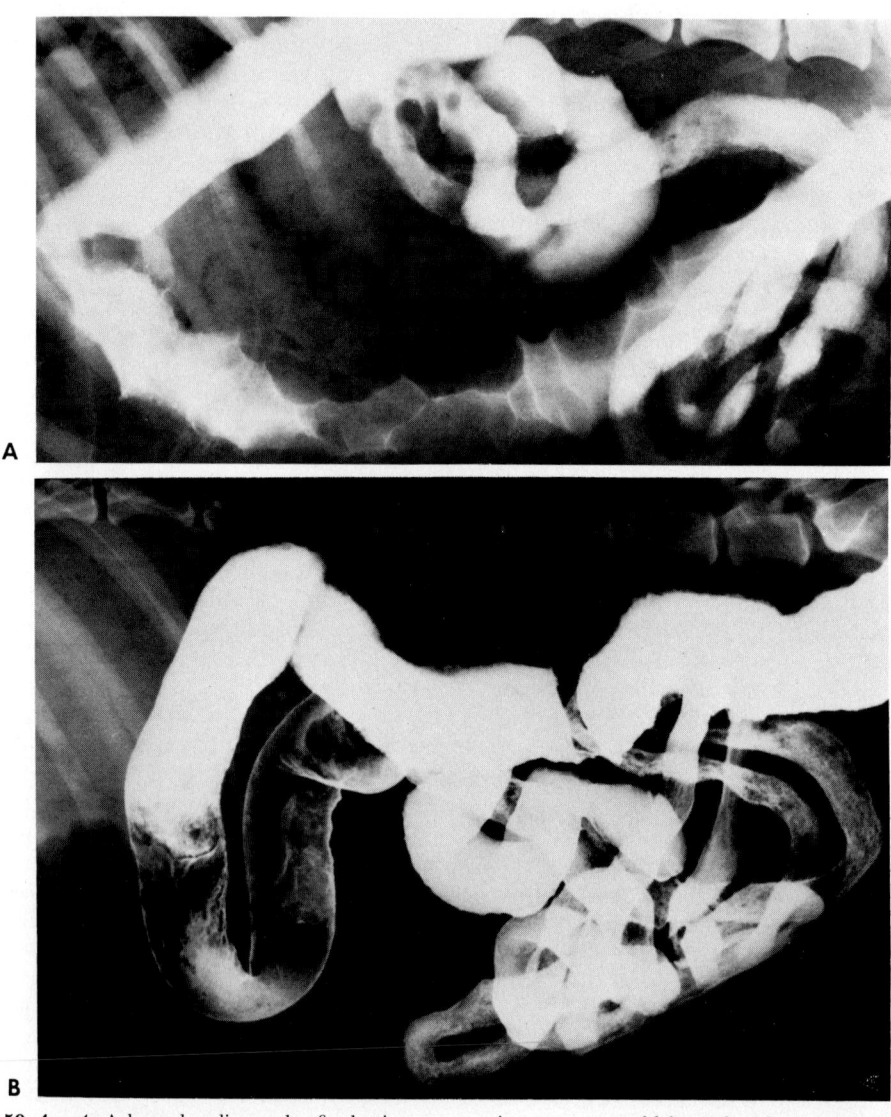

Figure 59–4. *A,* A lateral radiograph of a barium enema in a two-year-old hound with eosinophilic ulcerative colitis. The colon is irregular in outline with multiple large defects throughout the colonic wall. (Courtesy of Dr. Robert Lewis, UGA.) *B,* Subsequent barium enema radiograph taken two and one half weeks after therapy with daily oral prednisolone. The contour of the colonic wall is nearly normal, and the filling defects are reduced in size. (Courtesy of Dr. Robert Lewis, UGA.)

the dose is gradually reduced every three days until the medication is discontinued. Many cases do not require constant therapy; however, periodic therapy may be necessary, because relapses are occasionally encountered. During initial steroid therapy when the colon is severely ulcerated, broad spectrum antibiotics such as tetracycline or chloramphenicol are administered.

Systemic corticosteroids should not be routinely given to dogs with idiopathic or histiocytic ulcerative colitis until Azulfidine therapy has been thoroughly evaluated. Azulfidine therapy should be continued during corticosteroid administration. Prednisolone, 1.0 to 2.0 mg/kg, should be given in divided doses for two weeks. Failure to achieve improvement with corticosteroids during this period of time is an indication to stop these agents. If improvement occurs, alternate day steroid therapy for several months is maintained. Any indication that the dog's condition is worsening necessitates withdrawal of steroid therapy. Some dogs may respond to corticotropin (ACTH) gel, 1.0 unit/kg, given daily by intramuscular injection. Critical evaluations of ACTH therapy in the dog have not been reported, although this therapy is known to be beneficial in many human patients.

Corticosteroid retention enemas may be quite beneficial (although somewhat expensive) in the initial therapy of chronic ulcerative colitis. Hydrocortisone retention enemas (Cortifoam, Cortenema) should be given three times a day for three to five days and then decreased to once a day, usually at night. Hydrocortisone suppositories (Cort-Dome suppositories) inserted intrarectally three times a day may be beneficial in those cases with severe rectal involvement. Variable systemic absorption may occur following local therapy, and the dosage of systemic corticosteroids should be lowered if steroid side effects become severe.

Immunosuppressive Therapy. In dogs that do not respond to Azulfidine or corticosteroid therapy, immunosuppressive therapy should be considered. Although numerous studies have been reported in humans, studies related to the effects of immunosuppressive agents in the treatment of canine ulcerative colitis are lacking. Recently, immunotherapy in human inflammatory bowel disease has been thoroughly reviewed (Sachar and Present, 1978). These authors conclude that immunosuppressive drugs are potentially dangerous and that

their routine use in ulcerative colitis is not advisable, except as a short-term measure in patients unresponsive to or intolerant of Azulfidine or corticosteroid therapy. In the treatment of Crohn's colitis (granulomatous colitis), these agents appear to have a steroid-sparing effect and are as beneficial as Azulfidine. The interested reader should consult this article for the various regimens that are reviewed (Sachar and Present, 1978).

Metronidazole (Flagyl) may have immunosuppressive and granuloma-inhibiting properties (Grove et al., 1976). Some human patients have experienced marked clinical improvement (Ursing and Kamme, 1975). Long-term follow-up studies were not reported. One must wonder whether this drug has any role in the treatment of canine ulcerative colitis, in that it is apparently safe for chronic administration in this species.

Other Potentially Beneficial Treatments. Various clinicians have reported favorable results when oral tylosin therapy has been given for several months. This drug can be given as tablets or as a powder placed in the dog's drinking water. This author has no experience with this therapy, and controlled studies have not been reported.

Hypoallergenic diets are thought to benefit some dogs with ulcerative colitis, and food allergy has been suggested as a cause of this disease. These diets have not benefited cases treated by the author. In the long-term management of ulcerative colitis, bulky diets may help some patients (used only after the colon has healed). The addition of wheat bran or hydrophilic agents such as Metamucil to the diet may be of benefit.

PROTOTHECOSIS OF THE COLON

Etiology. The cause of canine protothecosis is a colorless algae of the family Chlorellaceae. The algal genus *Prototheca* has been infrequently reported to cause disease of the canine colon associated with other systemic manifestations (Van Kruiningen et al, 1969; Povey et al., 1969; Van Kruiningen, 1970). Cases of feline protothecosis have not been reported. As a primary pathogen, the *Prototheca* have little virulence and slowly involve the host. The algae cause little destruction of tissue and do not provoke a febrile response.

The source of protothecal infection is

usually undetermined, since the organism is ubiquitous in the environment. It would appear that the potential for exposure is high but infection is rare. Infection, resulting in lesions, may depend on failure of the host's immune competence. The disease may result in disseminated CNS disease without evidence of GI involvement (Tyler et al., 1978).

Pathology. The algae colonize the lamina propria and submucosa of the small intestine and colon. The rectum is most severely involved, and patchy ulceration of the mucosa is found, although inflammatory cellular response is minimal. The mucosa and submucosa become corrugated, owing to the presence of large numbers of algae. The algae enter other tissues, such as the liver, kidney, heart, brain, and eye, via the lower digestive tract.

Clinical Signs. Affected dogs usually have signs referable to lower colonic disease. In addition, signs of associated diseases may be present, including blindness, renal failure, and arthritis (Van Kruiningen et al, 1969). Povey et al. (1969) report vague neurologic signs referable to the rear legs, and their canine patient experienced shock and hypothermia. Fever is apparently uncommon.

Diagnosis. Proctoscopic examination may reveal thickened, friable mucosal folds. Ulceration is variable and patchy in distribution. Biopsy of affected tissue is diagnostic. The *Prototheca* range in size from 5 by 5 to 10 by 16 μ. They are characterized by endosporulation, and each organism may contain two to eight endospores.

Microscopic examination of the feces may reveal clusters of the organisms. *Prototheca* can also be grown on Sabouraud's media.

Therapy. Successful therapy in the dog has not been reported.

BALANTIDIASIS

Etiology. *Balantidium coli* is a large protozoan parasite capable of infecting both the canine and human colon. The organism measures 50 to 70 μ in length by 30 to 60 μ in width. The trophozoite of *B. coli* is identified by its spiral longitudinal rows of cilia and its large oral macronucleus (Fig. 59–5). Both the trophozoite form and the infective resistant cyst form are passed in the feces. *B. coli* is commonly found in swine, which are considered the primary host. Dogs are probably infected after ingesting pig feces containing the infective cysts (Hayes and Jordan, 1956).

In the dog, balantidiasis may be associated with concomitant *Trichuris* infections (Hayes and Jordan, 1956; Ewing and Bull, 1966). The inflammation and colonic mucosal ulceration produced by the whipworms may allow *B. coli* to penetrate the mucosal surface. Once penetration has occurred, the proteolytic secretions of *B. coli* produce extensive necrosis and further ulceration of the colonic mucosa. Once the organism be-

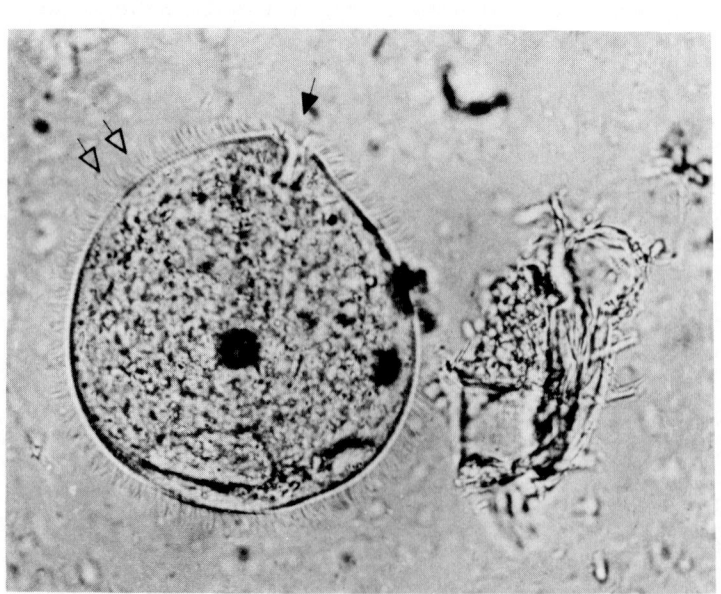

Figure 59–5. Trophozoite of *B. coli* as it may appear in dog feces. Note the large mouth pore (solid arrow) and ciliated outer membrane (clear arrows). A large nucleus can be observed in the center of the organism. (Courtesy of Dr. Ed Roberson, UGA.)

comes firmly established in the submucosa, extensive indurated ulcers are produced in the mucosa. The pathology and diagnosis of *B. coli* are similar to those previously presented for amebiasis.

Treatment. Therapy for the *Trichuris vulpis* is reported to be effective in resolving canine balantidiasis (Hayes and Jordan, 1956).

DISEASES OF ALTERED COLONIC MOTILITY

IRRITABLE COLON SYNDROME

Etiology. The irritable colon syndrome encompasses a variety of disturbances of colonic function that accompany emotional stress or other psychological problems. This syndrome is also known as mucous colitis, spastic colon, and psychologically induced colitis. Specific studies of this syndrome in the dog and cat have not been published, and its existence has been based entirely on clinical observations. Disorders of colonic motility (characterized by soft mucoid feces and frequent defecation) that are unrelated to other known colonic diseases occur in dogs. The absence of clinical and laboratory evidence incriminating other colonic diseases supports the hypothesis that these cases represent the irritable colon syndrome.

The cause of the irritable colon syndrome is unknown. In man, the onset or recurrence of this syndrome may coincide with stressful or emotional conflict. The signs may subside once the stressful period has passed. In humans, reactions to pain, fear, and anxiety can produce pallor of the colonic mucosa, reduced secretion of mucus, and inhibition of motility. Constipation may result. Anger, resentment, and hostility are associated with hyperemia, engorgement of the mucosa, and increased motility. Mucoid diarrhea may occur as a sequela to these events. These reactions are probably mediated through the central and peripheral portions of the autonomic nervous system. Comparable disturbances of colonic function have been produced by the administration of methacholine or neostigmine.

Clinical Signs. In dogs suspected of having the irritable colon syndrome, the primary clinical sign is soft mucoid feces accompanied by frequent attempts to defecate. At times, only mucus is passed. Blood in the feces is not common unless the clinical signs are of long duration. Even in these cases, blood in the feces is sporadic and may be lightly intermingled with the fecal column.

Signs are generally episodic. Affected dogs may be timid and may whine, pace, or bark excessively. The dog is usually psychologically dependent on one person and is disturbed when its master leaves. The colonic disturbance frequently follows several hours' separation from the owner. Certain dogs that are worked in obedience trials or as Seeing-Eye dogs may experience mucoid diarrhea during times of stressful duty. In a few cases, the birth of a child in the family has been associated with suspected irritable colon syndrome in the family pet. A definite cause-and-effect relationship between a psychological disorder and diarrhea is extremely difficult to document in pets.

Diagnosis. The diagnosis of irritable colon syndrome is justified only after the clinician has systematically eliminated all other causes of colonic disease. Frequent fecal examinations are indicated. Proctoscopic examination is usually normal. Occasionally, hyperemia of the colon is noted; rarely, punctate ulcers are found. Barium enema is normal and of value only as a means of ruling out disease of the cecum and proximal colonic segments.

Therapy. Some cases respond to anticholinergic therapy. Propantheline bromide, 15 mg three times per day, provides good control in these cases. Diphenoxylate, 1.0 to 2.5 mg every six hours, is the antidiarrheal agent of choice for the relief of intractable diarrhea. Excessively nervous dogs may require mild sedation or tranquilization during periods of anticipated stress. Chlorpromazine is a reliable tranquilizer for this purpose. Phenobarbital, 1 to 3 mg/lb once or twice a day, is also effective for mild sedation. Anti-anxiety drugs such as hydroxyzine hydrochloride (Atarax) 10 to 25 mg three times per day, or diazepam sodium (Valium) 10 to 30 mg three times per day, may be beneficial.

Dietary management of the irritable bowel syndrome may help to improve the condition in a few cases. Low bulk diets help to decrease the frequency of defecation. If constipation accompanies the syndrome, low bulk diets are not indicated, and the addition of bran to the diet may be beneficial.

MEGACOLON

Etiology. The term megacolon is often used to describe any unusually dilated or elongated colon recognized by radiography or at laparotomy. Congenital megacolon, or Hirschsprung's disease, is a specific disorder of colonic motility that results in severe constipation. The basic lesion is a congenital absence of myenteric ganglion cells in a distal colonic segment. Although ganglion cells of the myenteric plexus are absent, there are abundant nerve fibers that represent the terminal branches of preganglionic cholinergic parasympathetic fibers. The muscle of the affected segment is persistently contracted and creates a functional obstruction to the passage of feces. The normal colon proximal to the aganglionic segment is dilated, and the muscle layers become hypertrophied. Upon injection of methacholine, the affected narrow segment fails to relax because of its disturbed innervation.

Megacolon has been reported in dogs and cats (Wolf and Schlotthaver, 1936; McClure, 1956; Duncan, 1957; Yoder et al., 1968). Dogs and cats may be adults before the disorder is discovered. In fact, true congenital megacolon is not usually the underlying cause of colonic dilatation in older animals. Chronic constipation due to other causes may produce a clinical syndrome termed acquired megacolon. A narrowed aganglionic segment of colon is usually not present in this disease. Acquired megacolon may be caused by obstructive rectal or colonic neoplasia, strictures, or foreign bodies such as bone chips. Healed pelvic fractures may mechanically obstruct the pelvic canal of cats and small dogs and thus predispose these patients to megacolon. Injury to the terminal spinal cord may also predispose an animal to develop megacolon. Severe chronic prostatic enlargement is an uncommon cause in male dogs.

Clinical Signs. Animals with congenital megacolon may develop clinical signs at any age, although the signs usually occur during the first few weeks of life. The severity of the signs depends largely upon the degree of obstruction produced by the narrowed aganglionic colonic segment. Many cases are not presented for medical attention until the patient has had recurrent episodes of constipation for months or years. In cases of acquired megacolon, the history may reveal that the patient is fed bones on a regular basis. Stools are not passed for days to weeks. The frequency of defecation may be normal or excessive. Blood-streaked mucus containing little or no fecal material may be passed. Rarely, a brownish watery diarrhea may be observed, even though hardened feces are in the colon. Systemic signs of depression, weakness, dehydration, and unthrifty condition may accompany very chronic cases. Most cases are in relatively good physical condition even though the disease has been present for many weeks. Vomiting occurs in a few cases.

Diagnosis. The dilated colonic segment packed with feces can be easily palpated through the abdomen. In congenital megacolon, the rectum distal to the affected segment is usually empty. Digital examination of the rectum may confirm this finding. In simple constipation or acquired megacolon, feces may be easily palpated in the rectum.

Survey radiographs will confirm the presence of colonic dilatation and impaction. Barium enema studies, following complete removal of the fecal mass, will help establish the presence of a narrow segment of colon characteristic if congenital megacolon is present. Every effort should be made to establish the cause of acquired megacolon. Proctoscopy and barium enema are often necessary to identify obstructive tumors, strictures, or other masses. Abdominal and rectal palpation of the prostate gland is indicated in all affected male dogs.

Treatment. The patient with megacolon should be thoroughly evaluated for fluid and electrolyte balance and nutritional status. Improvement of the patient's physical condition and alleviation of the impacted colon should be the clinician's initial concern. Fluid, electrolyte, and acid-base therapy is based upon clinical and laboratory evaluation of the patient. Fluid therapy is indicated in debilitated patients prior to treatment for removal of the impacted fecal mass. Repeated large-volume soapy-water and mineral oil enemas are helpful in removal of the fecal mass. In severe cases, gentle manipulations with a "clamshell"-type forceps inserted through the anus may be necessary to break down and remove the fecal mass. Light sedation may be necessary for restraint. General anesthesia is usually not indicated except in the most severe cases or in animals difficult to restrain (such as some cats). The fecal impaction is best removed over a period of two to three days, during which time the physical condition of the patient can be improved with fluid therapy.

Once the impaction is removed and the physical condition of the patient is improved, definitive therapy for the underlying cause of the dilated colon should be undertaken. Congenital megacolon can be surgically corrected by removal of the narrowed aganglionic segment of colon or rectum. The "Swenson pull-through technique" has been a satisfactory procedure for treating megacolon when the narrow segment involves the rectum (Swenson and Bill, 1948; Archibald and Horney, 1965). This procedure may be satisfactory for dogs and larger cats. Partial distal colectomy with anastomosis of the proximal colon to the rectum has been reported as successful therapy for megacolon in the adult cat (Yoder et al., 1968). Obstructive tumors, strictures, or other masses are best managed by surgical intervention.

In cases of acquired megacolon, or obstipation, medical therapy should be tried prior to surgical intervention. The primary goal is to produce a soft stool and to encourage the patient to regularly evacuate the colon. A laxative diet such as dog meal mixed with bran or Metamucil may be beneficial in mild cases. Periodic soapy-water enemas or glycerine suppositories are used to relieve mild constipation. Bones in the diet are forbidden. Numerous laxative preparations containing molasses, mineral oil, and fish oil are available for use in cats. These preparations are most beneficial in feline cases of megacolon resulting from the ingestion of hair during the cat's normal grooming process. Dioctyl sodium sulfosuccinate in the diet is also effective as a fecal softener. To encourage regular defecation, the cat should have constant access to a litter pan, and canine patients should be exercised frequently. Severe cases are only temporarily benefited by medical therapy, and repeated episodes of colonic impaction are common. These cases should be managed by surgical correction of the primary defect.

COLONIC AND CECAL NEOPLASIA

Neoplasms of the canine intestinal tract are uncommon compared with tumors of the skin, mammary gland, or testicles. Cotchin (1959) reported 130 intestinal tumors in a survey of 4187 canine tumors at the Royal Veterinary College, London. Five hundred and eighty-eight alimentary tumors were studied. Brodey and Cohen (1964) found 70 intestinal tumors in the 99 gastrointestinal tumors studied at the University of Pennsylvania. Other sources report the incidence of alimentary neoplasia at two per cent (Smith and Jones, 1966) and 4.2 per cent (Ontario Veterinary College, 1968). Hayden and Nielsen (1973) studied 30 canine cases of alimentary neoplasia and found 18 benign and 8 malignant intestinal tumors. In all studies, dogs more than five years old are most commonly affected.

Benign Tumors. Benign colonic and rectal tumors include adenomatous polyps, leiomyomas, and papillary adenomas. In one study (Hayden and Nielsen, 1973), adenomatous polyps were the most common benign neoplasms of the rectum and colon, with most of the polyps occurring in the rectum. Colorectal polyps may undergo carcinomatous change. Carcinoma in situ has been reported in an adenomatous polyp of the rectum in a dog (Silverburg, 1971). Seiler (1979) has classified colorectal polyps in the dog into five histopathological categories: hyperplastic polyp, papillary adenoma, tubular adenoma, papillulotubular adenoma, and unclassified. The majority of polyps encountered were papillulotubular adenomas. Severe epithelial atypia, suggestive of carcinoma in situ, was present in five papillulotubular adenomas. Large polyps more frequently had these malignant changes (Seiler, 1979). Leiomyomas also occur most frequently in the canine rectum. Benign tumors found in the cecum include a neurilemoma (Singleton, 1956) and a leiomyoma (Hayden and Nielsen, 1973).

Malignant Tumors. Carcinoma, adenocarcinoma, and lymphosarcoma are the most common tumors of the canine colon and rectum. Carcinoma or adenocarcinoma may be mucoid or scirrhoid in type (Fig. 59–6). Malignant neoplasms of the large bowel account for 45.6 per cent of the alimentary tumors in the dog (Hayden and Neilsen, 1973). Hayden and Neilsen (1973) report an equal distribution of these tumors between colon and rectum. Other studies indicate that carcinomas occur most frequently in the rectum (Brodey and Cohen, 1964). Metastasis to the regional lymph nodes, peritoneal cavity, and liver is common. Lymphosarcoma arising in the large

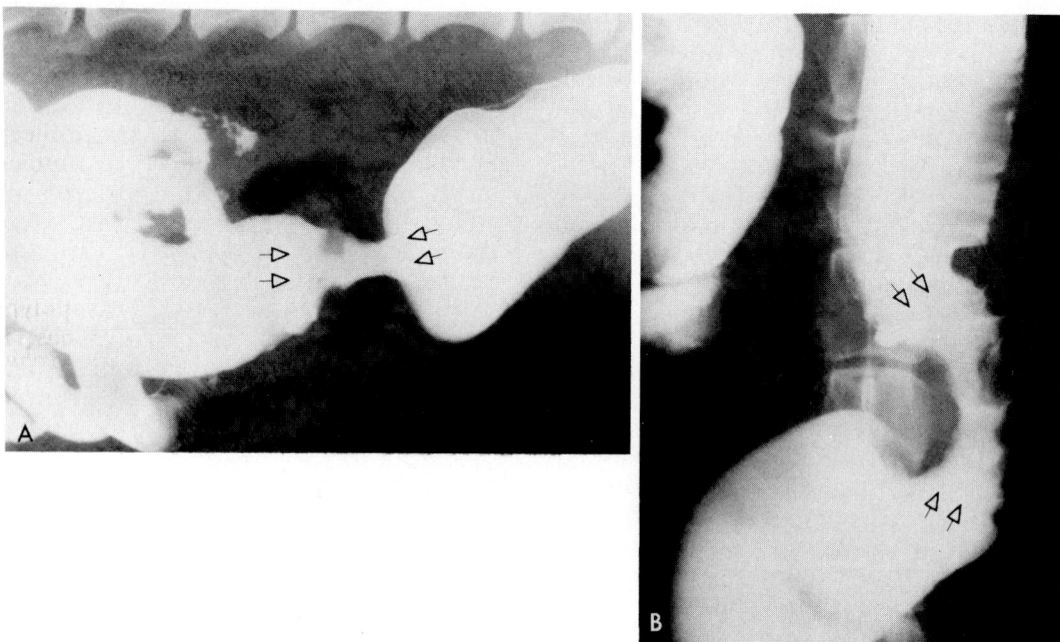

Figure 59–6. Lateral (*A*) and ventrodorsal (*B*) abdominal radiographs of an eight-year-old Bassett hound examined because of lethargy and weight loss. The barium enema demonstrates a rough annular lesion of the descending colon (between sets of arrows). The lesion was caused by a colonic adenocarcinoma which metastasized to the regional lymph nodes, liver, and lungs. (Courtesy of Dr. Donald Barber, UGA.)

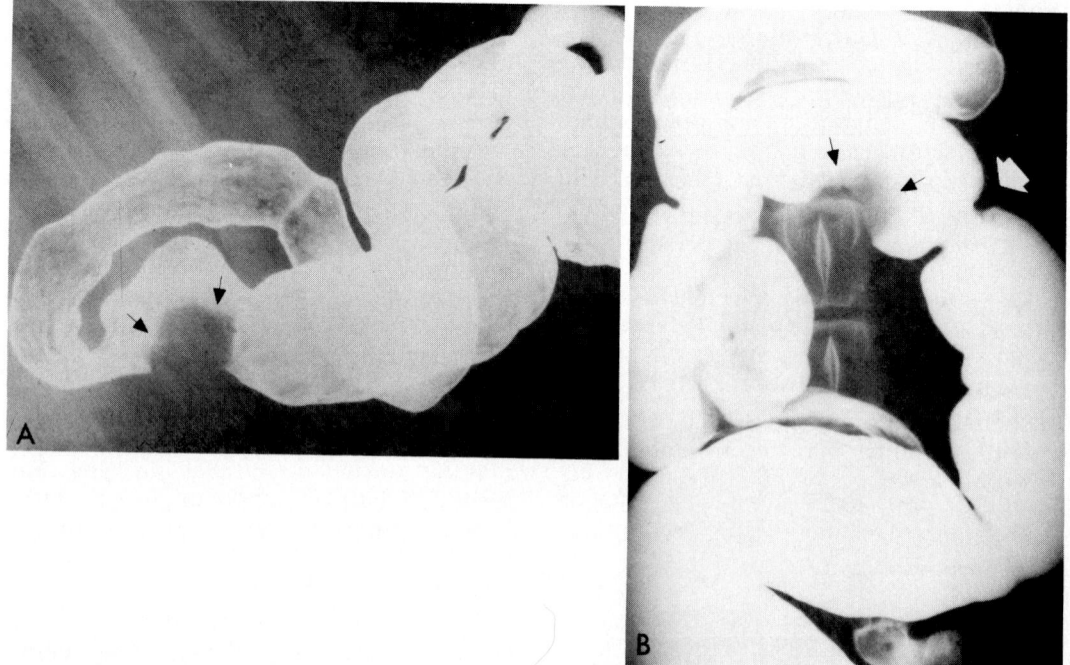

Figure 59–7. Lateral (*A*) and ventrodorsal (*B*) abdominal radiographs of a three-year-old English pointer with chronic mucoid bloody diarrhea. Palpation suggested an abdominal mass. The barium enema demonstrates a murial lesion (between arrows) three to four cm in diameter near the splenic flexure of the colon. The annural ring, apparent in *B* (large white arrow), did not persist and was thought to represent a peristaltic contraction.

bowel may be localized to one area of the colonic wall (Fig. 59–7) or may diffusely infiltrate the mucosa of the rectum or colon. Regional lymph node involvement is more common in the diffuse form of the disease. Diffuse rectal involvement may result in partial rectal prolapse. A malignant anaplastic sarcoma has been reported in the cecum of a dog (Hayden and Nielsen, 1973). Apparently, malignant tumors of the cecum are rare.

Neoplasia of the feline large intestine is uncommon. In a study of 46 feline alimentary tract neoplasms by Brodey (1966), 17 gastrointestinal neoplasms were identified. Of these 17 neoplasms, five were involved in the large intestine or cecum. Three adenocarcinomas and two lymphosarcomas were described. In contrast to the finding of benign colonic neoplasms in the dog, none were reported in the cat by Brodey (1966). Lymphosarcoma is a common neoplasm of the feline small intestine but apparently occurs less frequently in the feline colon.

Clinical Signs. Tenesmus and bloody mucoid diarrhea are the outstanding signs of colonic and rectal polyps. Occasionally, rectal prolapse may occur secondary to tenesmus caused by colonic or rectal polyps. Other benign tumors may produce signs similar to those associated with intestinal polyps.

The clinical signs associated with colonic carcinoma depend largely upon the type of tumor. Tenesmus is common to all types if the rectum is diseased. Blood in the stool is a sign of the ulcerative form of colonic carcinoma. Colonic carcinoma more commonly tends to be infiltrative and obstructive. Stenosis of the large bowel results in the clinical signs of constipation with intermittent mucoid bloody diarrhea. Carcinoma may form a ringlike stricture in the colon and may functionally obstruct the colonic lumen (Fig. 59–6). Carcinoma may be an underlying cause of acquired megacolon in older dogs. Dogs with diffuse rectal lymphosarcoma have tenesmus and pass mucoid stools that are occasionally streaked with fresh blood. Partial rectal prolapse may occur. The rectal mucosa is thickened and edematous. Localized lymphosarcoma presents no unique clinical signs except those of large bowel diarrhea. Bloody mucoid stools may be passed; however, this neoplasia may not result in mucosal ulceration in all cases.

Therefore, bloody stools may not be passed even though the colon is seriously diseased.

Diagnosis. Digital examination of the rectum may reveal a polypoid mass or a stenotic area. Definitive diagnosis can be made by proctoscopy and biopsy. Polyps have the gross appearance of grapelike clusters with a pedunculated base. They are reddish-purple in color, and the surface bleeds easily. The surrounding colonic mucosa is usually normal. Carcinomas may appear as a grossly ulcerated area in the colonic wall. The affected tissue may bleed easily if manipulated with the proctoscope. In other cases, the lumen may be stenotic, and the clinician may have difficulty passing the proctoscope through the diseased segment. The mucosa overlying the stenotic lesion is usually intact. Any abnormal tissue should be biopsied at the time of proctoscopy.

Barium enema studies are indicated to delineate lesions in the transverse and ascending colon. Insufflation of air into the colon after evacuation of the barium is especially beneficial in outlining colonic polyps.

Treatment. Surgical removal of rectal and colonic polyps is indicated and is described in Chapter 64. Because frequent metastasis is associated with carcinoma, it warrants a poor prognosis. Surgical intervention is indicated in early cases in which metastasis may not yet have occurred. (The medical management of acquired megacolon as the result of obstructive tumors has been previously described in this chapter.) Lymphosarcoma occurring as a solitary lesion should be surgically excised. Surgery can be followed with chemotherapy. Diffuse lymphosarcoma lesions are best treated with chemotherapy alone. Solitary lesions usually respond well to surgical therapy and the prognosis is favorable. Diffuse lesions have a guarded prognosis.

MISCELLANEOUS DISEASES OF THE CECUM AND COLON

CECAL INVERSION

Inversion of the cecum into the colon is not a common canine disorder. Apparently, the ileocecal colic ligament is responsible for preventing cecal inversion except upon rare occasions. Canine cecal inversion has been reported to mimic ileocolic intussusception

(Guffy et al., 1970). Other cases may be presented with signs of chronic diarrhea of colonic origin with no signs of obstruction.

Clinical Signs. Chronic blood-stained feces are associated with cecal inversion. Tenesmus is not common because the rectum is clinically normal. Weight loss is minimal unless obstruction of the ileocolic sphincter results in chronic vomiting. Weight loss and dehydration may be severe in long-standing obstructed cases. The clinical course of cecal inversion is usually more chronic than that of ileocolic intussusception.

Diagnosis. The inverted cecal mass may be palpated as a firm mass in the midventral abdomen. Definitive diagnosis of cecal inversion is made by barium enema studies. The inverted cecum may appear as "accordion pleating" of the first four to six centimeters of the colon (Guffy et al., 1970) (Fig. 59–8). Insufflation of air into the colon after evacuation of the barium helps to outline the inverted cecal mass. Gaseous distention of the small intestine may be present in the abdominal radiographs of obstructed cases.

Therapy. Surgical removal of the inverted cecum is curative in most cases. The inverted cecum is usually removed via laparotomy through an incision in the colon just distal to the ileocecocolic junction (Fig. 59–8). The cecal vessels are ligated, and the inverted cecal mass is amputated at its base through the colonic incision. The base is then everted and sutured. The colonic incision is then routinely closed. The patient is managed postoperatively in a fashion similar to other cases requiring intestinal surgery.

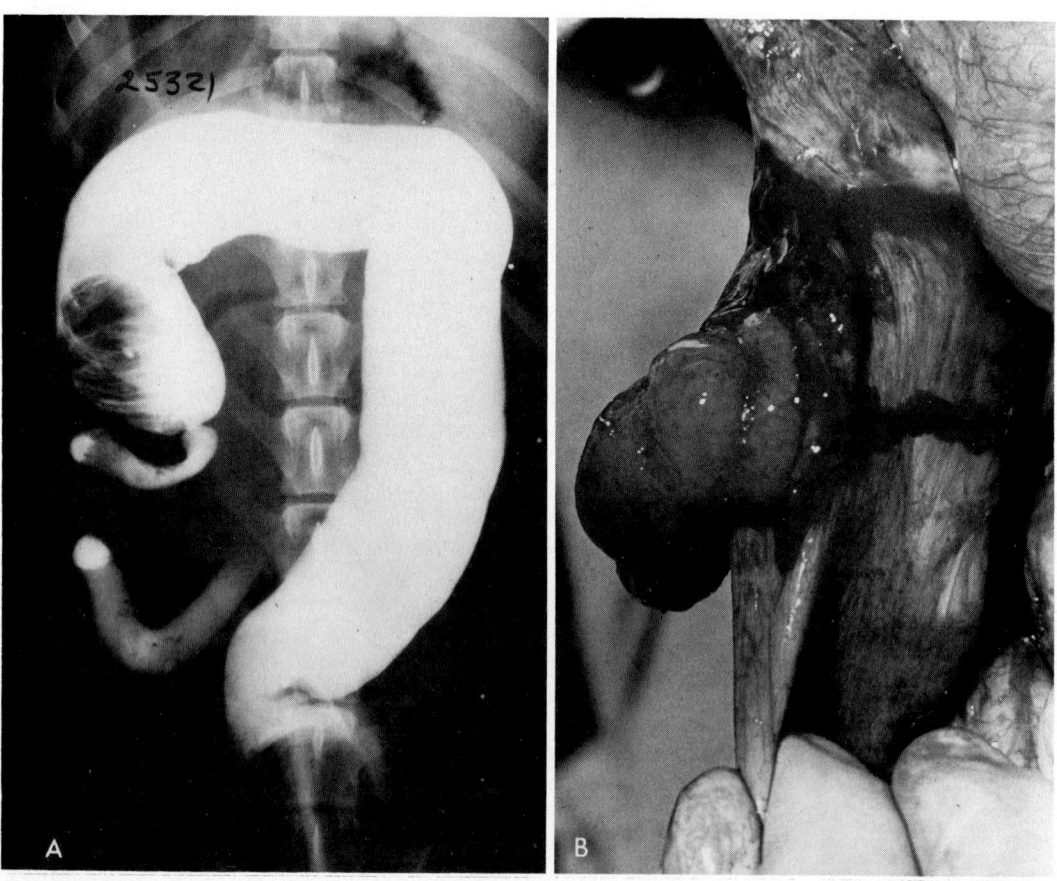

Figure 59–8. *A,* A ventrodorsal radiograph following a barium enema in a two-and-one-half-year-old male mixed breed dog with cecal inversion (cecocolic intussusception). The colon is evenly filled with barium except for a filling defect in the ascending colon (see arrows). The primary air-dense filling defect in the colon has a coiled spring appearance and represents the inverted cecal mass. (Courtesy of Dr. Robert Lewis, UGA.) *B,* The inverted cecum in the previous case is surgically exposed through an incision in the colon. Typhlectomy is performed through the colonic incision.

COLONIC PERFORATION

Perforation of the colon may be caused by trauma, biopsy procedures, erosion by neoplasia, or perforating ulcers from chronic inflammation. Recently, colonic perforation has been observed in dogs following neurosurgical procedures and the parenteral use of dexamethasone (Toombs et al., 1980). The four dogs studied developed clinical signs four to eight days after surgery. The signs were those of nonspecific gastrointestinal disease (vomiting, anorexia, depression, fever, and occasionally abdominal pain). All dogs died within 48 hours after signs developed. Perforations occurred in the proximal descending colonic wall, and fecal contents were present in the abdominal cavity. Cause of death was peritonitis and possible endotoxic shock. The cause of the perforations was not identified; however, corticosteroids and neurologic factors may play a role.

REFERENCES

Archibald, J., and Horney, F.: Colon, Rectum, and Anus. *In* Archibald, J. (ed.): Canine Surgery. American Veterinary Publications, Inc., Santa Barbara, Calif., 1965.

Brodey, R. S.: Alimentary tract neoplasms in the cat: A clinicopathologic survey of 46 cases. Am. J. Vet. Res. *27*:74–80, 1966.

Brodey, R. S., and Cohen, C.: An epizootiologic and clinicopathologic study of 95 cases of gastrointestinal neoplasms in the dog. Proc. 101st Ann. Meeting A.V.M.A., 1964, pp. 167–179.

Brown, J., and Lorenz, M.: Unpublished data. University of Georgia, 1973.

Buckner, T. G., and Ewing, S. A.: Trichomoniasis. *In* Kirk, R. W. (ed.): Current Veterinary Therapy IV. W. B. Saunders, Co., Philadelphia, 1971.

Burrows, R. B., and Hillis, W. G.: Intestinal protozoan infections in dogs. J.A.V.M.A., *150*:880–883, 1967.

Cockrell, B. Y., and Krehbiel, J. D.: Ultrastructural changes in histiocytic ulcerative colitis in a boxer. Am. J. Vet. Res. *33*:453–459, 1972.

Cotchin, E.: Some tumors of dogs and cats of comparative veterinary and human interest. Vet. Rec. *71*:1040–1050, 1959.

Driscoll, R. H., and Rosenberg, I. H.: Total parenteral nutrition in inflammatory bowel disease. Med. Clin. North Am. *62*:185–201, 1978.

Duncan, J. R.: Megacolon in the canine. Southeast. Vet. *9*:178–179, 1957–58.

Ewing, G. O., and Gomez, J. A.: Canine ulcerative colitis. J.A.A.H.A. *9*:395–406, 1973.

Ewing, S. A., and Bull, R. W.: Severe chronic canine diarrhea associated with *Balantidium trichuris* infections. J.A.V.M.A. *149*:519–520, 1966.

Eyles, D. E., Jones, F. E., Jumper, J. R., and Drinnon, V. P.: Amebic infections in dogs. J. Parasitol. *40*:163–166, 1954.

Faust, E. C., and Kagy, E. S.: Studies on the pathology of amebic enteritis in dogs. Am. J. Trop. Med. *14*:221, 1934.

Gaefer, S. M.: Protozoal Infection. *In* Catcott, E. J. (ed.): Canine Medicine. American Veterinary Publications, Inc., Santa Barbara, California, 1968.

George, W. L., Rolfe, R. D., Sutter, V. L., and Finegold, S. M.: Diarrhea and colitis associated with antimicrobial therapy in man and animals. Am. J. Clin. Nutr. *32*:251–257, 1979.

Goldman, P.: Therapeutic implications of the intestinal microflora. N. Engl. J. Med. *289*:623–628, 1973.

Gomez, J. A., Russell, S. W., Trowbridge, J. O., and Lee, J.: Canine histiocytic ulcerative colitis. An ultrastructural study of the early mucosal lesion. Am. J. Dig. Dis. *22*:485–496, 1977.

Grove, D. I., Mahumoud, A. A. F., and Warren, K. S.: Suppression of cell mediated immunity by metronidazole (Abstract). Clin. Res. *24*:286A, 1976.

Guffy, M. M.: Radiology of the gastrointestinal tract. Vet. Clin. North Am. *2*:105–129, 1972.

Guffy, M. M., Wallace, L., and Anderson, Neil, V.: Inversion of the cecum into the colon of a dog. J.A.V.M.A. *156*:183–186, 1970.

Hall, C. L.: Three clinical cases of eosinophilic enteritis. Southwest. Vet. Fall, 1967, pp. 41–42.

Haubrich, W. S., Watson, J. H. L., and Siaracki, J. C.: Unique morphologic features of Whipple's. A study of light and electron microscopy. Gastroenterology *39*:45, 1960.

Hayden, D. W., and Neilsen, S. W.: Canine alimentary neoplasia. Zentralbl. Veterinaermed. *20*:1–22, 1973.

Hayden, D. W., and Van Kruiningen, H. J.: Eosinophilic gastroenteritis in German shepherd dogs and its relationship to visceral larva migrans. J.A.V.M.A. *162*:379–384, 1973.

Hayes, F. A., and Jordan, H. E.: Canine helminthiasis complicated with Balantidium species. J.A.V.M.A. *129*:161, 1956.

Jordan, H. E.: Amebiasis in the dog. Vet. Med. Small Anim. Clin. *62*:61–64, 1967.

Koch, S. A., and Skelley, J. F.: Colitis in a dog resembling Whipple's disease in man. J.A.V.M.A. *150*:22–26, 1967.

Kumar, P.: Eosinophilic infiltration of the gastrointestinal tract. Proc. R. Soc. Med. *65*:287, 1972.

Lawson, T. L., Gomez, J. A., Stewart, E. T., Rambo, O. N., and Margulis, A. R.: Roentgenographic appearance of canine histiocytic ulcerative colitis. Am. J. Roentgenol. Radium Ther. Nucl. Med. *110*:337–384, 1970.

Legendre, A. M., and Krehbiel, J. D.: Eosinophilic enteritis in a Chesapeake Bay retriever, J.A.V.M.A. *163*:258–259, 1973.

Marsaen, P. D.: Amebiasis. *In* Beeson, R. B., and McDermott, W. (eds.): Textbook of Medicine. 13th ed. W. B. Saunders Co., Philadelphia, 1971.

McClure, J. H.: Congenital aganglionic megacolon. J.A.V.M.A. *128*:80–81, 1956.

Ontario Veterinary College Graduate Symposium, June, 1968.

Pavar, R.: Food allergy in dogs. J.A.V.M.A. *111*:61–63, 1947.

Povey, R. C., Austwick, P. K. C., Pearson, H., and

Smith, K. C.: A case of protothecosis in a dog. Pathol. Vet. 6:396–402, 1969.

Russell, S. W., Gomez, J. A., and Trowbridge, J. O.: Canine histiocytic ulcerative colitis. The early lesion and its progression to ulceration. Lab. Invest. 25:509–515, 1971.

Sachar, D. B., and Present, D. H.: Immunotherapy in inflammatory bowel disease. Med. Clin. North Am. 62:173–183, 1978.

Sanders, C. H., and Langham, R. F.: Canine histiocytic ulcerative colitis. A condition resembling Whipple's disease, colonic histiocytosis, and malakoplakia in man. Arch. Pathol. 85:94–100, 1968.

Seiler, R. J.: Colorectal polyps of the dog: A clinicopathologic study of 17 cases. J.A.V.M.A. 174:72–75, 1979.

Silverburg, S. G.: Carcinoma arising in adenomatous polyps of the rectum in a dog. Dis. Col. Rect. 14:191–194, 1971.

Singleton, W. B.: An unusual neoplasm in a dog (a probable neurilemmoma of the cecum). Vet. Res. 68:1046, 1956.

Smith, H. A., and Jones, T. C.: Veterinary Pathology. 3rd ed. Lea and Febiger, Philadelphia, 1966.

Starnes, D. D.: Granulomatous colitis in a dog. Southwest. Vet., 1969, pp. 234–235.

Swartzwelder, J. C., and Avant, W. H.: Immunity to amebic infections in dogs. Am. J. Trop. Med. Hyg. 1:567, 1952.

Swenson, O., and Bill, A. H.: Resection of rectum and rectosigmoid with preservation of the sphincter for benign spastic lesions producing megacolon. Surgery 24:212–220, 1948.

Theran, Peter: Eosinophilic Gastroenteritis. In Kirk, R. W. (ed.): Current Veterinary Therapy III. W. B. Saunders Co., Philadelphia, 1968.

Thomas, P. J.: Identification of some enteric bacteria which convert obic acid to hydroxystearic acid in vitro. Gastroenterology 62:430–435, 1972.

Thompson, H., and Wright, N. G.: Canine salmonellosis. J. Small Anim. Pract. 10:579–582, 1969.

Thorson, R. E., Seibold, H. R., and Bailey, W. S.: Systemic amebiasis with distemper in a dog. J.A.V.M.A. 129:335, 1956.

Toombs, J. P., Caywood, D. D., Lipowitz, A. J., and Stevens, J. B.: Colonic perforation following neurosurgical procedures and corticosteroid therapy in four dogs. J.A.V.M.A. 177:68–72, 1980.

Tyler, D. E., Lorenz, M. D., Blue, J. L., Munnell, J. F., and Chandler, F. W.: Disseminated protothecosis with central nervous system involvement in a dog. J.A.V.M.A. 176:987–993, 1980.

Ursing, B., and Kamme, C.: Metronidazole for Crohn's disease. Lancet 1:775–777, 1975.

Van Kruiningen, H. J.: The ultrastructure of macrophages in granulomatous colitis of boxer dogs. Vet. Pathol. 12:446–459, 1975.

Van Kruiningen, H. J.: Canine colitis comparable to regional enteritis and mucosal colitis of man. Gastroenterology 62:1128–1142, 1972.

Van Kruiningen, H. J.: Interpreting problem diarrheas of dogs. Vet. Clin. North Am. 12:29–47, 1972.

Van Kruiningen, H. J.: Prothecal enterocolitis in a dog. J.A.V.M.A. 157:56–63, 1970.

Van Kruiningen, H. J., and Dobbins. W. O.: Feline histiocytic colitis. Vet. Pathol. 16:215–222, 1979.

Van Kruiningen, H. J., Garner, F. M., and Schiefer, B.: Protothecosis in a dog. Pathol. Vet. 6:348–354, 1969.

Van Kruiningen, H. J., Montali, R. J., Strandberg, J. D., and Kirk, R. W.: A granulomatous colitis in dogs with histologic resemblance to Whipple's disease. Pathol. Vet. 2:521–544, 1965.

Wolf, L. H., and Schlotthaver, C. F.: Megacolon in a dog. J.A.V.M.A. 88:451–459, 1936.

Yoder, J. T., Dragstedt, L. R., and Starch, C. J.: Partial colectomy for correction of megacolon in a cat. VM SAC, 63:1049–1052, 1968.

Zetzel, L.: Inflammatory Diseases of Intestine. In Beeson, P. B., and McDermott, W. (eds.): Textbook of Medicine. 13th ed. W. B. Saunders Co., Philadelphia, 1971.

CHAPTER **60**

Diseases of the Liver

ROBERT M. HARDY

INTRODUCTION

The liver is essential to the maintenance of life and is the largest and one of the most important secreting/excreting organs in the body. It functions in hundreds of diverse metabolic activities that maintain the body's normal homeostatic mechanisms. The most prominent of these functions are the synthesis of most plasma proteins; catabolism and storage of carbohydrates; synthesis, degradation, and mobilization of lipids; detoxification and excretion of many toxic agents and drugs; and the formation and elimination of bile. Because of its key role in many metabolic processes, the liver is subject to injury by a wide variety of infectious, metabolic, and toxic diseases. It has been estimated that hepatic diseases account for three per cent of all diseases seen by the veterinarian (Candlin, 1968). With the recent heightened interest in hepatic diseases and availability of diagnostic aids, this figure is probably low.

Our knowledge of hepatic diseases in dogs and cats has increased significantly in the last several years. Reports of several previously undescribed clinical entities have appeared, and great advances in hepatic therapy have been made.

PATHOPHYSIOLOGY OF HEPATIC DISEASE

Signs of hepatic disease or failure are often clinically silent until the disease process is quite advanced. This results from both the amazing regenerative capability of the liver and its large functional reserve. As much as 70 to 80 per cent of the liver's mass must be impaired before signs of functional impairment are noted. Under optimal conditions, the liver is capable of regenerating up to three fourths of its functional mass within a few weeks. This combination of large functional reserve and "embryonic" regenerative ability makes the diagnosis and treatment of hepatic disease a challenging and exacting task for the veterinarian.

BILE METABOLISM

One of the most prominent hepatic functions is formation and elimination of bile. Abnormalities in this process produce one of the classic signs of hepatic disease, jaundice.

Bile is a complex aqueous solution of organic and inorganic compounds. Primary bile components include bile pigments (mainly conjugated bilirubin), bile acids and their salts, cholesterol, phospholipids (primarily lecithin), and alkaline phosphatase (Ingelfinger, 1967). Bile alkalinizes intestinal juice, aids in the emulsification and absorption of dietary fat, and prevents intestinal putrifaction.

Bilirubin is derived primarily from the metabolism of hemoglobin from red blood cells (RBCs). Senescent RBCs are removed from circulation by cells of the reticuloendothelial (RE) system in the spleen, liver, and bone marrow. Within RE cells the heme molecule is converted to a green pigment, biliverdin, and then to the lipid soluble, water insoluble compound known as free, unconjugated, or indirect-reacting bilirubin. Unconjugated bilirubin, once released from the RE cell, is bound to albumin for transport to the liver. Under unusual circumstances unconjugated bilirubin may escape albumin binding and is extremely toxic to host cells. The central nervous system of neonates is particularly susceptible to injury by unconjugated bilirubin, and such damage is termed kernicterus (Cornelius and Himes, 1973). An increase in nonprotein bound unconjugated bilirubin occurs whenever serum albumin concentrations are depressed or when increases in other organic ions that compete for bilirubin binding — i.e., thyroxine, sulfonamides, fatty acids, salicylates, hydrocortisone, digoxin, and valium — are elevated (Schmid, 1972). Significant increases in unconjugated bilirubin (over 20 mg/dl) must occur in order to exceed normal plasma albumin binding capacity for bilirubin. Nonerythroid sources of bilirubin account for 15 to 20 per cent of the bilirubin excreted in bile. Unconjugated bilirubin is removed from the circulation by the liver and conjugated primarily with glucuronic acid to produce water soluble, conjugated, direct-reacting bilirubin. Bilirubin conjugation serves two important functions: it increases the water solubility of bilirubin and reduces its access to host cells. Both of these characteristics facilitate its excretion in bile. Once conjugated, bilirubin is transported across the hepatocyte and eventually is excreted into bile canaliculi. Bile canaliculi join main hepatic bile ducts and then the gallbladder and the common bile duct, with bilirubin ultimately entering the upper duodenum. Upon entering the intestinal tract conjugated bilirubin is reduced by intestinal bacteria to a poorly characterized group of colorless compounds known collectively as urobilinogens or stercobilinogens. Most of the urobilinogens are eliminated in the feces after further bacterial degradation to pigmented compounds, of which urobilin (stercobilin) predominates (Cornelius, 1970). Urobilins impart the normal color to stool, and a visual stool exam usually indicates if bile is entering the intestines. Acholic stools are usually a pale gray color and indicate that a total absence of bile flow has occurred.

A small percentage (10 to 15 per cent) of intestinal urobilinogen is reabsorbed by the portal circulation of the ileum and colon; most is then rapidly reexcreted into bile, producing an enterohepatic circulation of bilirubin. Approximately 20 per cent of this reabsorbed urobilinogen escapes hepatic portal clearance, enters the systemic circulation, and is excreted in urine as urine urobilinogen (Fig. 60–1). Thus, the presence of urine urobilinogen indicates that bilirubin entered the intestine, was reabsorbed as urobilinogen, and was ultimately excreted in urine.

JAUNDICE

Jaundice, or icterus, is the yellow discoloration of the skin, mucous membranes, and plasma caused by an abnormal accumulation of conjugated and/or unconjugated bilirubin. Jaundice occurs whenever the rate of production of bilirubin exceeds its rate of elimination. The subjective depth of jaundice depends on many factors, including the serum concentration of bilirubin, capillary permeability, diffusion from plasma to lymph, and tissue binding of bilirubin (Jeffries, 1971).

The conjugated product stains superficial tissues more readily than the free or unconjugated product and is usually detectable

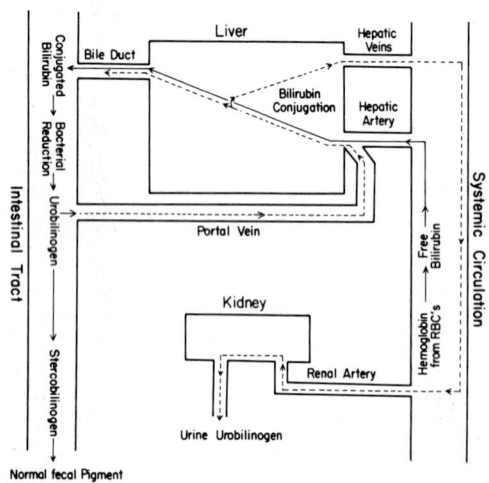

Figure I

Figure 60–1. Enterohepatic circulation of bilirubin. Solid lines (→) indicate metabolic pathways for bilirubin. Broken lines (————→) indicate metabolic pathways for urobilinogen.

clinically when serum concentrations reach 2 to 3 mg/dl. Conjugated bilirubin has an affinity for areas high in elastic fibers such as the sclera and skin. Free bilirubin, being lipid soluble, preferentially enters fat depots and requires higher levels in the peripheral blood to be clinically apparent (Weisberg, 1949; Jeffries, 1971). Areas of high capillary density do not become jaundiced until serum bilirubin levels are quite high, as the intensity of the hemoglobin pigment overrides that of bilirubin. Therefore, the degree of tissue staining is as important as the actual serum bilirubin levels in determining the severity of clinical jaundice.

Whenever increased production or decreased uptake, conjugation, and excretion of bilirubin occurs, jaundice may develop. It is most often classified as to its source of origin, i.e., prehepatic or hemolytic, hepatic, or posthepatic (obstructive). Increased production of free bilirubin (unconjugated hyperbilirubinemia) is most commonly seen with hemolytic states, when the rate of RBC breakdown and unconjugated bilirubin production exceed the ability of the liver to conjugate and excrete it. The presence of clinically evident anemia and jaundice suggests an uncomplicated diagnosis of the prehepatic form.

Hepatocellular jaundice is the most frequent type observed in the dog and cat and is produced by a variety of etiologic agents that cause cholestasis. Cholestasis refers to the stagnation of bile formed by hepatocytes within the intra- or extrahepatic biliary passages and the subsequent retention and regurgitation of all biliary substances into the blood (Popper, 1968). Over 30 clinical entities leading to varying types of cholestasis have been documented in man (Zimmerman, 1979d). Many of the intrahepatic cholestatic syndromes are due to biochemical interruption of bilirubin secretory mechanisms and are not detectable by light microscopy (Cornelius, 1979).

Although jaundice is a common finding in animals with severe liver disease, many patients have no detectable jaundice in spite of severe hepatic failure. The failure to develop jaundice has been explained in such patients by the location of the lesion within the hepatic lobule (Gopinath and Ford, 1972). Periportal lesions (peripheral-lobular), even of a mild degree, cause severe hyperbilirubinemia. Lesions primarily of a centrolobular nature, however, rarely have an effect on the circulating bilirubin levels until the periportal cells become involved, because centrolobular lesions cause minimal interruption of bile flow.

The pathways by which conjugated bilirubin reaches the circulation are through hepatic lymphatics following increased permeability of the biliary tract. Metabolic parenchymal functions, other than bilirubin formation and excretion, are not initially affected by cholestasis. Eventually, prolonged cholestasis results in secondary parenchymal injury, which may ultimately lead to hepatic failure. Intrahepatic cholestasis and conjugated hyperbilirubinemia are caused by many therapeutic agents in man, such as anabolic steroids, phenothiazines, thiazides, oral hypoglycemic agents, erythromycin, and organic arsenicals (Popper, 1968; Zimmerman, 1978). Although similar situations may exist in the dog and cat, they have not been reported.

Extrahepatic cholestasis (posthepatic jaundice) may result from conditions partially or completely obstructing main bile ducts. This condition is infrequent in the dog and cat, but has been reported secondary to tumors compressing the common bile duct, cholelithiasis, and inflammation or strictures involving the common bile duct or duodenum. Complete biliary obstruction eventually progresses to total parenchymal failure. In cases of partial obstruction, sufficient numbers of parenchymal cells survive, so that metabolic functions are only moderately depressed (Ingelfinger, 1967).

The gallbladder functions to store and concentrate bile. In cases of obstruction to the common bile duct, the gallbladder cushions the effects of biliary back pressure upon hepatic parenchymal cells until cholestasis is so advanced that secretory pressure is arrested. If the obstruction involves the hepatic bile ducts proximal to the gallbladder, a significant degree of hepatomegaly develops. Occasionally, "white bile" is formed following prolonged, total biliary obstruction. In such cases, bile pigments are reabsorbed from the bile ducts and a whitish mucus is secreted into the bile ducts and biliary tree from biliary epithelial cells.

BILE ACID METABOLISM

Bile acids are the major solute in bile. They are synthesized by the liver and secreted into the bile ducts and then into the intestine, where they undergo a highly efficient enterohepatic circulation, small amounts eventually being lost in the feces (Fig. 60–2). Absorbed bile acids are efficiently removed from the portal blood by the liver and are then available for biliary reexcretion. Very little of the absorbed bile acids reaches the systemic circulation because of this highly efficient hepatic extraction in normal animals. Peripheral blood bile acid concentrations remain quite stable and low in nondiseased states (Matern and Gerok, 1979a). Small, transient increases occur postprandially. Bile acid synthesis is stimulated by decreased concentrations and altered composition of bile acids returning from the intestinal tract. Hepatic synthesis of bile acids is of limited capacity. The liver primarily synthesizes sufficient new bile acids to match fecal losses. This efficient recycling of bile acids (20 to 30 gm/day) enables the total bile acid pool (three to five gm) to be maintained. During a single meal, the total bile acid pool may be recycled two to three times through the enterohepatic circulatory pathway, and in a given day bile acid turnover equals six to ten times the available pool size.

Bile acids serve as the major route for cholesterol elimination from the body. Cholesterol is metabolized to two primary bile acids, cholic and chenodeoxycholic acid. The liver conjugates these bile acids with taurine and glycine prior to their excretion into the bowel. Ninety-five per cent of intestinal bile acids are actively absorbed in the ileum. The remaining five per cent enter the colon and are deconjugated by anaerobic bacteria. Cholic acid is converted to deoxycholic acid, and chenodeoxycholic acid to lithocholic acid. Most deoxycholate is reabsorbed, while most lithocholate is excreted in the feces. When the unconjugated bile acids reenter the liver they are reconjugated to their parent compounds prior to reexcretion into the duodenum. In the intestines, bile acids disperse complex ingested lipids into micellular solutions so that absorption can occur. Bile acids also enhance the activity of pancreatic lipase (Matern and Gerok, 1979a) and stimulate pancreatic enzyme release. Within the biliary system, bile acids are important for maintaining cholesterol solubility (Campbell, 1977; Cowan, 1977) and have been used therapeutically to dissolve choleliths in man. Conjugated bile acids are inefficiently ab-

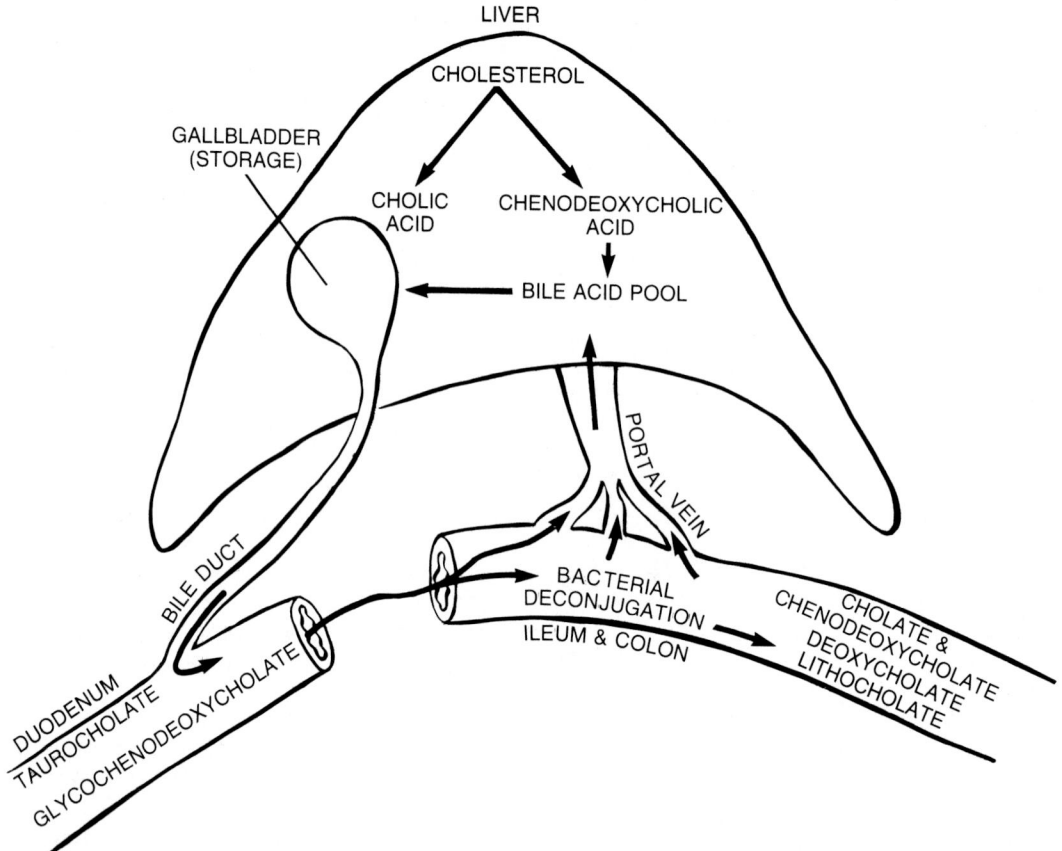

Figure 60-2. Enterohepatic circulation of bile acids. Adapted from, Strombeck, D. R.: Small Animal Gastro-enterology, Davis, California: Stonegate Publishing Co., 1979.

sorbed in the upper small intestine, which allows them to perform these lipid digesting functions. Deconjugated bile acids, however, are efficiently absorbed proximally in the intestine, which reduces lipid absorption significantly.

Because of the importance of the liver, portal blood supply, and small intestine in bile acid metabolism, abnormalities of any of these areas result in changes in circulating bile acids with resulting systemic alterations. Increases in circulating bile acid concentrations occur with most hepatic parenchymal or biliary tract diseases. The liver is less able to extract bile acids from the circulation, and bile acids may back diffuse into the circulation during cholestasis. Extensive portal-systemic shunting, as occurs in chronic fibrotic livers or congenital portal vascular anomalies, bypasses hepatic parenchyma, allowing absorbed bile acids direct access to the systemic circulation. Increased serum bile acids have been used recently in human medicine as a sensitive indicator of

hepatobiliary disease. The diagnostic use of these compounds will be discussed further in the section on diagnosis of liver disease.

The pathophysiologic effects of bile acids are related to a direct hepatotoxic action, induction of gastric ulcers and diarrhea (Campbell and Cowen, 1977; Goldman et al., 1979; Matern and Gerok, 1979a). Lithocholic acid is known to have a direct hepatotoxic effect. Cholestasis and other pathologic alterations in the liver may lead to abnormal bile salt metabolism, retention, and reduced lithocholate conjugation and subsequent hepatic injury. Bile salts also stimulate gastrin release and have been associated with gastric ulcer formation in chronic liver disease patients. In terms of small bowel function, bacterial overgrowth into the small bowel leads to increased deconjugation of bile acids, which induces both functional and morphologic alterations in the mucosa. Decreased availability of conjugated bile salts impairs fatty acid absorption, thus promoting steatorrhea. Augmented ileal deconjugation also increases lithocholate formation and absorption, which could be potentially hepatotoxic. With ileal dysfunction (regional ileitis, abnormal motility) or pancreatic insufficiency, increased concentrations of bile acids enter the colon. Deoxycholic acid inhibits colonic water and electrolyte absorption, producing diarrhea. Therapy to control intestinal bacterial overgrowth (antibiotics) or cation exchange resins that bind bile salts in the intestine (cholestyramine) help eliminate these adverse effects of bile acids.

URINARY BILE PIGMENTS

Urinary bile pigments, conjugated bilirubin, urobilinogen, and urobilin are valuable aids to the differential diagnosis of jaundice, and in nonjaundiced animals may be one of the earliest indications that hepatic disease is present.

Bilirubin. Urine bilirubin is always in the conjugated form. Unconjugated bilirubin, owing to its albumin binding, is too large to pass through the glomerular capillary membrane and is not detected in the urine of dogs and cats. The renal threshold for bilirubin is very low in the dog, and even slight serum elevations result in detectable amounts appearing in the urine. Between 20 per cent (Hoe and Harvey, 1961) and 60 per cent (Cornelius, 1970) of normal dogs excrete detectable amounts of bilirubin in their urine. It is common to detect a positive (1+) Ictotest reaction during any febrile state or during periods of starvation in dogs. Bilirubinuria is not a normal finding in the feline, however, and when detected is always associated with significant hepatic disease.

The highest levels of bilirubinuria occur in hepatocellular diseases or in association with extrahepatic bile duct obstructions. In both these conditions, conjugated bile is regurgitated into the blood and eliminated in urine. Urinary levels of conjugated bilirubin are dependent upon the degree of intra- or extrahepatic obstruction and the level of serum bilirubin.

Animals with hemolytic anemias often have mild elevations of urine bilirubin, presumed to be secondary to anoxic hepatocellular damage and regurgitation. Elevated urine bilirubin will be detected in the rare event that circulating hemoglobin levels exceed the plasma haptoglobin-binding capacity (> 50 mg/dl) in severe hemolytic anemias (DeSchepper, 1974). It has been suggested by Cornelius and Himes (1973) that this is due to the conversion of free hemoglobin to bilirubin by the renal tubular epithelial cells and not to hepatocellular or obstructive liver disease.

Male dogs excrete greater quantities of bilirubin in their urine than do female dogs. A sex-linked difference in renal handling and excretion of bilirubin has been hypothesized as the explanation (DeSchepper, 1974).

Urobilinogen. Urobilinogen is the second bilirubin pigment detected in the urine. Urobilinogen is formed by the bacterial reduction of conjugated bilirubin in the intestine. Subsequent absorption of urobilinogen by the portal circulation is necessary if later urinary excretion is to occur. Ten to 20 per cent of the total intestinal urobilinogen is absorbed from the intestine and filters through the liver. A small percentage escapes biliary reexcretion and enters the systemic circulation to be excreted by the kidneys.

The primary significance of urine urobilinogen is as an indicator of the patency of the common bile duct and the integrity of the enterohepatic circulation. Urine urobilinogen is a colorless compound that, upon exposure to sunlight, is oxidized to urobilin, a highly pigmented product that imparts some of the normal color to urine left standing.

Ingelfinger (1967) lists the following factors that affect the quantity of urobilinogen excreted in the urine: the amount of bile reaching the intestine, the efficiency of bacterial reduction of bilirubin to urobilinogen, the proportion of urobilinogen absorbed by the intestine, and the amount of urobilinogen reexcreted by the liver. Urine urobilinogen is decreased in obstructive hepatic disease, in states of impaired intestinal absorption, in polyuric states (dilution), and following the use of intestinal antibiotics that sterilize the gut and prevent bacterial reduction of bilirubin to urobilinogen. Increased urobilinogen is found in a number of conditions (Benjamin, 1961; Cornelius, 1970). In hepatocellular diseases, because of the deficient hepatic reexcretion of urobilinogen into bile, excess quantities are eliminated in the urine. Normally, 80 per cent of the urobilinogen absorbed by the portal vein is reexcreted by the liver. Following hepatocellular damage, equal quantities of urobilinogen reach the general circulation and bile ducts, so that quantitatively more is available for renal excretion (Cornelius, 1970). Following a hemolytic crisis, the total volume of bile pigment excreted by the liver is increased, so that an absolute increase in all types of bile pigments and their breakdown products occurs.

ASCITES

Ascites is the localized collection of extracellular fluid in the peritoneal cavity and is one of the more dramatic signs associated with hepatic failure. Controversy exists over the exact pathophysiologic mechanisms responsible for ascites formation in hepatic diseases. A more detailed discussion of ascites and abdominal enlargement can be found in Chapter 17.

Ascites results initially from alterations in Starling forces (within the liver and portal vascular bed) that operate across peritoneal capillaries and determine the rate and direction of transperitoneal fluid movement (Shear, 1973). The forces that tend to increase ascites formation are intraperitoneal oncotic pressure and elevated intravascular (portal) hydrostatic pressure. Conversely, forces tending to limit ascites formation are the intraperitoneal hydrostatic pressure and the intravascular oncotic pressure. Three mechanisms responsible for the altered Starling forces in hepatic failure are (1) pre- and postsinusoidal hepatic venous outflow block, which produces portal hypertension and increased hepatic lymph flow; (2) decreased plasma oncotic pressure due to hypoalbuminemia; and (3) abnormal renal salt and water retention (Shear, 1973; Sherlock, 1970).

Portal hypertension plays a significant role in the pathophysiology of hepatic disease and is associated with the formation of ascites, the development of collateral venous drainage for abdominal organs, and occasionally, splenomegaly. Portal hypertension results from lesions that increase portal blood flow (arteriovenous [A-V] fistulas) or, more commonly, lesions that impair portal venous drainage. Normal portal vein pressure has been reported to be from 8 to 26 cm H_2O, but 8 to 13 cm H_2O is a more likely range (Strombeck, 1979).

Portal hypertension is frequently classi-fied on the basis of the location of the lesion in the portal venous system, i.e., prehepatic portal hypertension causing impaired blood flow proximal to the hepatic sinusoids, in this case involving the portal vein only; hepatic portal hypertension involving intrahepatic lesions, which compress sinusoids; and posthepatic portal hypertension associated with lesions affecting the hepatic veins, thoracic post cava, or heart (Schmidt and Suter, 1981). Prehepatic portal hypertension can be caused by compression, invasion, or thrombosis of the portal vein and arteriovenous malformations (Hoskins et al., 1979; Legendre et al., 1976; Schmidt and Suter, 1981). Intrahepatic portal hypertension has been associated with lipidosis, chronic active hepatitis, biliary obstruction, diffuse hepatic fibrosis, metastatic neoplasia, hepatic vein thrombosis and intrahepatic A-V fistulas (Rogers et al., 1977; Schmidt and Suter, 1981). Posthepatic portal hypertension has been reported secondary to congestive heart failure, constrictive pericarditis, cardiac tamponade, obstruction of the caudal vena cava by tumor or thrombi, and hepatic vein thrombosis (Edwards et al., 1978; Schmidt and Suter, 1981).

The most common cause of portal hypertension when associated with hepatic disease is cirrhosis. Anastomoses develop between hepatic arterioles and the portal venous system early in cirrhosis and contribute to hypertension. Cirrhotic nodules and fibrosis that develop produce a postsinusoidal outflow block to hepatic venous blood flow (Popper et al., 1970). Postsinusoidal outflow block causes sinusoidal hypertension, a near prerequisite for the development of ascites. Animals with portal vein ligation and portal hypertension, without sinusoidal hypertension, rarely develop ascites (Jeffries, 1971). Hepatic sinusoids are lined by discontinuous endothelium. Large gaps exist and permit nearly free passage of plasma proteins in the hepatic interstitium. Fluid transudation out of hepatic sinusoids is minimal in the normal state, owing to the extremely low venous pressure in the portal vein, i.e., ~ 8 to 13 cm H_2O (Witte et al., 1980). Even slight increases in portal pressure, however, produce massive increases in hepatic lymph formation. When the carrying capacity of peritoneal lymphatics is exceeded, the liver weeps a high protein fluid into the abdomen. Large amounts of hepatic lymph, which has nearly five-sixths the protein content of plasma, drains from the congested liver sinusoids into hilar lymphatics and the thoracic duct (Smith and Hamlin, 1965).

The development of portal hypertension forces blood draining from the abdominal viscera to use alternative channels to the heart. These naturally occurring portal-systemic communications have been well studied by Vitums (1961) and Khan and Vitums (1971) in experimental portal hypertension in the dog and cat.

Two major groups of collateral vessels develop, the portoprecaval and the portopostcaval systems. Normally, these anastomoses between the portal and systemic veins are quite small and carry minimal amounts of blood. Only after portal hypertension develops do they become important physiologically.

Splenomegaly does not occur with any frequency in the dog and cat, as collateral velar omental anastomoses aid splenic venous outflow (Vitums, 1961).

Since the liver is the sole source of albumin production, serum albumin synthesis is depressed and levels begin to fall following prolonged hepatocellular damage. Because of its relatively low molecular weight, albumin is quantitatively and qualitatively the most important substance contributing to the oncotic pressure of plasma. Once serum albumin concentrations fall, the ability to retain fluids within the capillary tree is diminished and fluid leaks into interstitial spaces or into the peritoneal cavity. Neither hypoalbuminemia nor portal hypertension alone regularly causes ascites to form, but in combination, these two factors appear to be the most important causes of the initiation of ascites formation (Sherlock, 1970). Hypoalbuminemia increases fluid transudation from hepatic sinusoids and augments lymph flow from congested vascular beds. With normal colloidal osmotic pressure, portal pressures must reach 37 cm H_2O for ascites to develop. Even when serum albumin concentrations decrease to 2.0 gm/dl, ascites does not form until portal pressures exceed 20 cm H_2O (Suter, 1975).

The protein content of ascites associated with alterations in portal pressure is useful diagnostically (Greene, 1979). High protein ascitic fluid, i.e., > 2.5 gm/dl, is usually associated with postsinusoidal causes of hypertension such as early cirrhosis, congestive heart failure, heartworms, or hepatic vein or postcaval thrombosis or compres-

sion. Low protein ascites, however, is most often associated with diseases causing presinusoidal portal hypertension, i.e., portal vein thrombosis, compression or atresia of the portal vein, and A-V fistulas. The ascites develops secondary to increased outflow of intestinal lymph, which is of lower protein content than hepatic lymph.

The greatest amount of new and controversial information regarding the pathophysiology of ascites relates to renal salt and water retention. The traditional theory suggests that hypoalbuminemia and portal hypertension initiate ascites formation, while altered renal salt and water metabolism serve to perpetuate the problem. The production of ascites has been thought to lead to a decrease in "effective" blood volume perfusing the kidneys. Such a drop in vascular volume stimulates the renin-angiotensin-aldosterone mechanism to reabsorb salt and water (Ingelfinger, 1967; Sherlock, 1970). The restoration of plasma volume further augments splanchnic lymph flow and perpetuates a vicious circle leading to increased ascites formation (Witte et al., 1971). In addition to the increased production of aldosterone in severe hepatic failure, hepatic inactivation of aldosterone is impaired, leading to prolongation of its action.

Recent findings in both man and dog tend to contradict this "traditional" theory of ascites formation in hepatic failure (Levy, 1977a; 1977b; Wilkinsen et al., 1978; Witte et al., 1980). This alternative "overflow theory" proposes that abnormal renal salt and water retention is the primary initiating event in the formation of ascites in cirrhosis. In the early stages of cirrhosis, prior to the development of ascites, the kidney begins reabsorbing sodium and water. The vascular volume is expanded, not contracted, leading to portal hypertension. Eventually, as hypoalbuminemia develops and portal hypertension reaches a critical level, ascites begins to form. The alterations in Starling forces within the abdomen favor fluid accumulation there rather than in other regions of the body. Experimental work in dogs using a chemical-induced cirrhosis model lends strong support to the "overflow" theory. Renal sodium retention and an expansion of extracellular fluid (ECF) volume occurred several days prior to the development of ascites. These dogs had no decrease in glomerular filtration rates or renal blood flow. The serum concentrations of albumin, renin, aldosterone, estrogen, and progesterone were all normal in the salt-retaining phase of their disease. Once ascites developed and cirrhosis reached advanced stages, aldosterone concentrations increased and hypoalbuminemia was present. Nonascitic, salt-retaining dogs developed ascites very rapidly when given high salt diets (150 mEq/day). When the ascites was removed by paracentesis, it did not re-form as long as salt was restricted from the diet (Levy, 1978). The relative importance of aldosterone in hepatic ascites is underscored by data indicating that adrenalectomized dogs still have significant salt and water retention (Epstein, 1977).

The factor(s) that initiate renal salt and water retention in cirrhosis have not been identified, but several possibilities have been proposed (Epstein, 1978; Wylie et al., 1980). An increased sensitivity to aldosterone or the release or failure to inactivate other salt-retaining factors is being considered. In addition, a failure to release natriuretic hormone in response to an expanded ECF may occur. Natriuretic hormone induces renal salt and water loss (natriuresis) in response to an expansion in ECF. A deficiency of this hormone or inhibition of its release in cirrhosis could explain the augmented renal salt and water retention. Regardless of the mechanism leading to increased renal salt retention, salt restriction of patients with hepatic induced ascites is critical for its management.

HEPATIC ENCEPHALOPATHY

Hepatic encephalopathy or coma has received a great deal of attention in recent veterinary literature (Sherding, 1979; Srombeck et al., 1975b). This reflects both increased awareness by veterinarians of its signs and also improvement in and increased availability of diagnostic tests. Hepatic encephalopathy is recognized more frequently in association with congenital hepatic disorders than with acquired, acute, or chronic progressive liver disease. On a percentage basis, congenital portal-systemic shunts are the most commonly diagnosed cause for signs of hepatic encephalopathy, while acute or chronic hepatic failure is only occasionally associated with such signs, and very rare cases of congenital urea cycle enzyme deficiencies have histories of encephalopathy.

Hepatic encephalopathy is defined as a neuropsychiatric syndrome consisting of intellectual deterioration, an altered state of consciousness, and abnormal neurologic function in a patient with advanced liver disease and/or portal-systemic shunting (Maddrey and Weber, 1975).

Encephalopathy ultimately results from a failure of the diseased liver to remove toxic products of gut metabolism from the portal circulation. This inability to effectively clear portal blood is caused by a decrease in the functional mass of the liver following parenchymal injury and/or by portal-systemic shunts that bypass hepatic parenchyma. The signs associated with hepatic encephalopathy in dogs can be grouped into two general categories, (1) signs of a nonspecific nature, often seen with non-neurological and nonhepatic associated diseases; and (2) signs most often associated with cerebral disease. Nonspecific signs include anorexia, depression, weight loss, lethargy, polydipsia, polyuria, vomiting, and diarrhea (Strombeck et al., 1975b). Since such signs are characteristic of hundreds of disorders and have little localizing value, the author considers them to have little clinical usefulness in the diagnosis of hepatic encephalopathy. The second group of signs, however, can be very helpful to clinicians in leading them to consider hepatic encephalopathy in a list of diagnostic rule-outs. The most useful signs include incessant pacing or circling; head pressing; transient amaurotic blindness; seizures; generalized dementia; hysteria; and episodic, nonpurposeful aggression. These types of signs often are intermittent and may be associated with ingestion of high protein meals.

There is increasing evidence that hepatic encephalopathy is not a homogenous entity. A very often fatal syndrome is seen following viral or toxic hepatitis. A more insidious, relapsing form is seen in association with progressive hepatic diseases (cirrhosis) and with extensive portal vein shunting (acquired or congenital) (Fischer and Baldessarini, 1976). In most cases of fulminant hepatic coma, no morphologic abnormalities are noted in the brain, although recent evidence for cerebral edema has been documented in a few cases. In dogs with encephalopathy following chronic liver injury, increases in number and size of protoplasmic astrocytes may be seen. The functional significance of such anatomic changes is not completely understood. Since the coma associated with acute fulminant hepatic failure is not associated with structural changes in the brain and since the coma of both acute and chronic hepatic failure are rapidly and completely reversible, it is assumed that neither clinical syndrome results from permanent morphologic abnormalities of the brain. Based on the above observations, hepatic encephalopathy is considered a metabolic abnormality induced by biochemical alterations in cerebral metabolism.

Proposed Factors Inducing Hepatic Encephalopathy

Three interrelated factors have been implicated as the cause of the cerebral dysfunction of hepatic coma. These are increased cerebral sensitivity, cerebral toxins, and metabolic abnormalities (Breen and Schenker, 1972).

Increased Cerebral Sensitivity. A number of clinical observations form the basis for the concept that the brain has an increased sensitivity to exogenous and endogenous substances (Breen and Schenker, 1972). Coma is often precipitated in alert individuals with hepatic disease by a variety of factors that are well tolerated in normal individuals (infection, sedatives, electrolyte imbalances, hypoxia). Experimental evidence has indicated that the liver synthesizes compounds necessary for normal brain activity and in their absence, electrical and metabolic activity of the brain is impaired. Ammonia, a primary cerebral toxin, is known to depress brain oxygen consumption and thus impair cerebral function. The concept of increased cerebral sensitivity is most appropriate for patients with long-standing, stable liver disease who lapse into coma following an exogenous insult (sedatives, diuretics, analgesics). Cerebral sensitivity suggests a gradual accumulative effect of a single toxin over time or the combined effect of a number of metabolic toxins that have a synergistic action. Sensitivity is due in some cases to the inability of the diseased liver to remove a number of potentially toxic substances from the circulation (ammonia, false neurotransmitters, short-chain fatty acids). The liver may elaborate toxic products itself because of altered metabolic capabilities in diseased states.

Cerebral Toxins. A number of substances have been incriminated in the induction of hepatic coma. The most important include ammonia; circulating amino acids, in particular, methionine and its metabolic by-products; short-chain fatty acids (SCFA); and beta hydroxylated biogenic amines, which act as false neurotransmitters.

For years, ammonia has been implicated as a key cerebral toxin in hepatic failure. It was first associated with encephalopathy in Eck fistula dogs that developed what was then known as "meat intoxication" (Fischer and Baldessarini, 1976). Ammonia is increased in blood and CSF fluid of most patients with hepatic coma, and its concentration generally parallels the severity of coma. Blood ammonia concentrations remain the primary diagnostic test for hepatic encephalopathy. The administration of ammonium salts or other substances that lead to ammonia production (meat, blood, urea) will induce coma in susceptible individuals. Therapy to decrease blood ammonia is often associated with clinical improvement (Breen and Schenker, 1972; Fischer and Baldessarini, 1976; Madrey and Weber, 1975). Arguments against ammonia involvement cite its being normal in ten per cent of patients with hepatic coma and poor correlations with blood ammonia concentrations and the severity of clinical signs in other patients.

The primary sources of blood ammonia are the colon and endogenous renal tubular synthesis from glutamine. Colonic ammonia production arises primarily from conversion of urea to ammonia by urease-containing bacteria. Secondary colonic ammonia arises from dietary amines (Strombeck et al., 1975b). Ammonia diffuses readily out of the colon, entering the portal vein. The liver extracts from 81 to 87 per cent of the portal vein ammonia, converting it to urea in the Krebs-Henseleit urea cycle. Approximately 16 per cent of the absorbed ammonia is thus left to enter the systemic circulation (Aldrete, 1975). Resting venous blood ammonia in the dog is from 60 to 120 μg/dl, while mesenteric venous ammonia concentrations of 365 μg/dl are common (Strombeck et al., 1975b). Approximately 25 per cent of the circulating urea pool escapes renal excretion and diffuses into the colon, where it is hydrolized to ammonia and reabsorbed, only to be reconverted to urea again. The liver is the only site of urea synthesis in the body and the major route for NH_3 detoxification.

Hyperammonemia associated with liver disease occurs secondary to several factors. With severe parenchymal failure, insufficient numbers of functional hepatocytes remain to convert the normal daily load of NH_3 to urea. In other cases, acquired or congenital portal vein shunting leads to NH_3 bypassing hepatic parenchyma and entering the systemic circulation. Finally, increased NH_3 production by the kidney and colonic urease-containing bacteria, or augmented intake of substances producing NH_3 may occur. The exact mechanism by which ammonia induces cerebral injury is unknown. It has been proposed that NH_3 interferes with brain energy metabolism, causes an increased cerebral concentration of inhibitory neurotransmitters and a decreased synthesis of acetylcholine, or has a direct inhibitory effect on neuronal cell membranes (Stombeck et al., 1975a).

Oral methionine and its metabolic by-products are important inducers of hepatic coma in dogs (Merino et al., 1975). Methionine is degraded by gut flora to a group of by-products collectively termed mercaptans (methanethiol, ethanethiol, dimethylsulfide). Dimethylsulfide has been measured in the breath of cirrhotics and is considered responsible for the typical breath odor of patients with hepatic failure called fetor hepaticus. The formation of dimethylsulfide may serve as one excretory route for methionine. The toxicity of methionine relates to its metabolism by gut flora to NH_3 and other metabolites in the bowel, since only orally administered methionine produces encephalopathy, whereas the intravenous route of administration produces no signs. Signs of methionine toxicity can also be reversed by prior oral antibiotic therapy (Breen and Schenker, 1972). Methanethiol appears to be the most toxic metabolite of methionine. It may induce coma alone, or in subcoma doses may act synergistically with NH_3 and SCFA to induce encephalopathy (Zieve et al., 1974). When dogs with experimentally created porta caval shunts were given oral 25 gm doses of methionine every four hours, all dogs became comatose after one to four doses. All dogs were hyperammonemic prior to the oral methionine, and the higher their resting blood ammonia concentration, the lower the dose needed to induce coma (Merino et al., 1975). In normal dogs even 150 gm methionine/day did not induce coma or hyperammonemia. The longer hepatic disease has been present, the lower the quantity of methionine, methanethiol, or NH_3 required to induce coma.

The metabolism of other amino acids also plays an important role in the production of hepatic coma. Significantly deranged amino acid metabolism occurs in hepatic failure. In normal dogs, the ratio of branched chain amino acids (valine, leucine, and isoleucine) to aromatic amino acids (phenylalanine, tyrosine, tryptophan) is 3.03:1 (Fischer and Baldessarini, 1976). The branched chain amino acids are primarily metabolized by muscle tissue, while the aromatic amino acids are metabolized by the liver (Striebel et al., 1979). In hepatic failure there is decreased clearance of the aromatic compounds, owing to cellular damage and/or vascular shunting and increased utilization of the branched chain amino acids. This leads to a shift in the branched chain:aromatic amino acid ratio from 3.03:1 to 1 to 1.5:1 or less. Since both groups of amino acids compete for entry into the brain by a similar mechanism, the great increase in aromatic amino acids serves to augment their entry into the central nervous system. Normal synthesis of the physiologic neurotransmitters norepinephrine and dopamine depends on adequate brain uptake of the branched chain amino acids. When branched chain amino acid uptake is impaired and aromatic amino acid uptake enhanced, the synthesis of false neurotransmitters exceeds that of normal neurotransmitters. Both tyrosine and phenylalanine serve as precursors of two such false neurotransmitters, octopamine and β-phenylethanolamine. Large quantities of these false neurotransmitters also arise from the bowel following bacterial degradation of the aromatic amino acids. Failure of the liver to remove these products allows them access to the brain, where they "flood" presynaptic nerve endings and displace the normal neurotransmitters, preventing the brain and peripheral nerve endings from responding normally to stimuli. Tryptophan also increases in the brains of patients with hepatic coma. Tryptophan is a precursor to serotonin, a potent inhibitory neurotransmitter. Thus, the increased production of both weak neurotransmitters and inhibitory neurotransmitters serves to severely depress brain function in hepatic encephalopathy.

Short-chain fatty acids (SCFA) (5-6-8 carbon; butyric, valeric, and octanoic acids) have also been implicated in the pathogenesis of hepatic coma (Breen and Schenker, 1972; Fischer and Baldessarini, 1976;

Schenker et al., 1974). Short-chain fatty acids are routinely increased in both CSF and blood in patients with encephalopathy. In experimental animals, short-chain fatty acids, particularly octanoic acid, have been shown to act synergistically with either ammonia or methionine to induce coma. SCFA are derived primarily from ingested medium-chain triglycerides, although some are synthesized by intestinal bacteria from carbohydrates and amino acids.

Metabolic Abnormalities. A number of precipitating causes for hepatic coma have been identified in man and are probably important in the induction of encephalopathy in animals as well (Breen and Schenker, 1972; Fischer and Baldessarini, 1976; Maddrey and Weber, 1975) (Table 60–1). Clinicians must search for such underlying causes for encephalopathy if therapy is to be successful. In 100 human cases of hepatic coma, the leading precipitating factors, in order of occurrence, were azotemia, sedative or tranquilizer use, analgesics, gastrointestinal hemorrhage, hypokalemia, alkalosis, and protein intoxication (Fischer and Baldesserini, 1976). Prerenal, renal, or postrenal causes for azotemia may all precipitate hepatic encephalopathy. Urea nitrogen retention increases its enterohepatic circulation, promoting increased intestinal ammonia production. The depressive effects of uremia on cerebral function may also contribute to some of the CNS signs. Because of the impaired hepatic conversion of NH_3 to urea in these patients, the magnitude of rise in blood urea nitrogen will be less than expected for the degree of renal damage. Creatinine concentrations are more reliable and consistent in patients with combined hepatic and renal failure, because they are not affected by hepatic disease per se. In patients with normal renal function and hepatic failure, the BUN may be subnormal as a result of failure of the liver to synthesize sufficient urea to attain even low normal blood concentrations (Sherlock, 1970).

Acute upper gastrointestinal hemorrhage

Table 60–1. Common Precipitating Causes of Hepatic Coma

Cause	Proposed Mechanism Producing Coma
Increased dietary protein	Source for NH_3, false neurotransmitters, SCFA
Gastrointestinal hemorrhage	Provides substrate for increased ammonia (100 ml blood yields 15 to 20 gm of protein).
	Hypovolemia may compromise hepatic, cerebral, and renal function. Decreased renal perfusion leads to urea retention and increased ammonia production.
	Transfusions: Storage of blood for 1 day = 170 μg/100 ml, 4 days = 330 μg/100 ml, 21 days = 900 μg/100 ml.
	Role of shock and/or hypoxia.
Diuretics	Induced hypokalemic alkalosis, increased renal vein ammonia, enhanced ammonia transfer across blood brain barrier.
	Overzealous diuresis (+ paracentesis) may lead to hypovolemia and prerenal uremia.
	Separate role of acetazolamide and hypokalemia on cerebral function.
Sedatives and anesthetics	Direct depressive effect on brain.
	Hypoxia
Uremia	Increased enterohepatic circulation of urea nitrogen and thus ammonia production.
	Direct cerebral effect of uremia.
Infection	Increased tissue catabolism, leading to increased endogenous urea nitrogen load and increased ammonia.
	Dehydration and diminished renal function.
	Hypoxia and hyperthermia may potentiate ammonia toxicity.
Constipation	Increased production and absorption of ammonia and other nitrogenous derivatives.

is a serious precipitating cause of hepatic coma in man. The frequency of such an event in animals is unknown, although terminal hemorrhage from coagulation abnormalities in end-stage hepatic failure is seen fairly often and undoubtedly plays a significant role in the death of these animals. Blood provides a significant quantity of protein to the GI tract (100 ml yields 15 to 20 gm protein), which is a major source of intestinal NH_3 production. Hypovolemia may further compromise hepatic, cerebral, and renal function. Transfusions of stored blood are particularly dangerous. Blood stored for one day contains 170 μg/dl of NH_3; by four days the NH_3 content is 330 μg/dl, and by 21 days it is 900 μg/dl. If blood transfusions are indicated, only fresh, whole blood should be used or more severe encephalopathy may develop.

The use of diuretics may induce hepatic coma by several mechanisms. Potassium-losing diuretics such as the thiazides, the mercurials, and furosemide or ethacrynic acid can induce hypokalemic alkalosis. In hypokalemic states, renal NH_3 production is increased, augmenting blood NH_3 concentrations. Alkalosis also plays a major role in the tissue availability of NH_3. At a normal blood pH of 7.4, most NH_3 is ionized to NH_4^+ (ammonium). Ammonium is relatively nondiffusible and has limited access to the brain. Any conditions that increase blood pH shift the equilibrium of NH_4^+ towards NH_3. Since NH_3 is highly diffusible, it readily enters the brain cells. Once NH_3 is inside the cell, the low cellular pH (7.0) shifts NH_3 back to NH_4^+, trapping it in the cell and increasing its toxic cerebral effect (Breen and Schenker, 1972; Gabuzda, 1962). In addition to the metabolic alkalosis induced by potassium-losing diuretics, a respiratory alkalosis develops in many humans in coma. Although the reason why these people hyperventilate is in dispute, alkalosis favors the entry of NH_3 into the brain, enhancing its toxicity. Blood gas analysis of a limited number of dogs in hepatic coma has indicated that respiratory alkalosis also occurs in this species but is inconsistent (Riveron et al., 1967).

Protein overload is a particularly important cause of encephalopathy in dogs. Many dogs presented in hepatic coma have histories of ingesting high protein diets, or the onset of their CNS signs frequently is associated with meals. Young dogs with portal vascular anomalies are uniquely predisposed to this problem, as they are often purposefully given high protein diets during their rapid growth period. Protein serves as a source of NH_3, false neurotransmitters, and short-chain fatty acids, all of which can induce coma in susceptible animals.

Other, less important precipating factors in coma are sedatives and anesthetics, infections, and constipation. Sedatives and anesthetics have a depressive effect on cerebral function and, with the increased cerebral sensitivity seen in patients with hepatic failure, may induce coma easily at usual therapeutic dosages. These agents may also induce hypovolemia, which can impair brain oxygenation and produce prerenal uremia. Serious infections increase tissue catabolism, thus increasing the endogenous ammonia load on the liver. They may also lead to dehydration, which can compromise renal perfusion and lead to urea retention. Hyperthermia may also potentiate ammonia toxicity in the brain. Constipation leads to increased production and absorption of ammonia and other cerebrotoxic compounds from the colon.

ENDOTOXINS

The reticuloendothelial system of the liver plays a major role in removing bacteria and endotoxins from the portal circulation, preventing systemic effects. The liver serves as a filtration barrier for bacterial by-products that escape intestinal defense mechanisms and gain entry to portal blood (Nolan, 1975; Liehr et al., 1976). Endotoxins may induce both severe hepatocellular injury and extrahepatic systemic signs of disease. Although endotoxins may induce or contribute to massive cellular necrosis, most often they are associated with inducing mild degrees of hepatic lipidosis. The impaired RE function occurs secondary to hepatic injury by other toxins, pharmacologic dosages of glucocorticoids, portal-systemic shunting, or infection itself (Liehr et al., 1976). Extrahepatic manifestations of endotoxemia include a nonspecific hypergammaglobulinemia, renal vasoconstriction with occasional cases of acute tubular necrosis, disseminated intravascular coagulation, fever, and depressed myocardial function. Therapy directed at controlling endotoxin production with oral antibiotics or oral toxin absorbing agents such as cholestyramine has reduced the incidence of endotoxin-related complications.

NUTRITIONAL AND METABOLIC ABNORMALITIES

Multiple abnormalities of a nutritional or metabolic nature are present in hepatic failure. Signs of such abnormalities are most often observed in animals with long-standing, advanced disease.

Endocrine Abnormalities

Chronic hepatic disease has been incriminated as the cause of many endocrine-related abnormalities in man (Ingelfinger, 1967). Whether or not a similar situation exists in the dog and cat with chronic hepatic disease is unresolved. Multiple factors may be responsible for the observed endocrine abnormalities. Malnutrition, chronic illnesses, or primary endocrinopathies may coexist with hepatic disease, or actual altered hepatic metabolism of the hormones may be responsible for observed signs.

The liver plays a major role in the metabolism of estrogen, progesterone, androgens, thyroxine, corticosteroids, and the pituitary hormones. These functions may be altered in hepatic disease. The three primary means of inactivation of hormones by the liver are (1) reduction, hydroxylation, or oxidation; (2) conjugation; and (3) biliary excretion or reexcretion. The liver also may be necessary for activating hormones for forming hormonal precursors, or for changing one active agent to another (Ingelfinger, 1967). Several plasma alpha globulin–binding proteins are synthesized in the liver, and their altered production may affect hormone activity. Because of the feedback controls over most trophic hormones, depressed hepatic inactivation will not necessarily result in hypersecretion or clinical signs.

The male feminizing syndrome is a common sequela to cirrhosis in man. Gynecomastia, testicular atrophy, thinning of the skin, and hair loss are noted. Interruption of the enterohepatic circulation of estrogens, changes in hepatic blood flow, and decreased uptake of estrogens by hepatocytes appear to be responsible for the observed physical changes (Fischer and Eisenfeld, 1971).

Occasionally, signs suggestive of hyperadrenocorticism are seen in human cirrhotic patients. Measurement of plasma cortisol and corticosterone are normal, however. Furthermore, it has been found experimentally that although there is depressed hepatic metabolism of cortisol in cirrhosis, adrenal synthesis is also depressed, so that plasma levels remain normal (Peterson, 1960). Urine corticoids and 17-ketosteroids are often depressed.

Hyperaldosteronism occurs in cirrhosis and was briefly discussed in the section on ascites. The elevations seen in cirrhosis appear to be secondary to increased secretion, although the biologic half-life of aldosterone is also increased because of decreased hepatic inactivation (Ayers et al., 1962; Barnardo et al., 1969).

Malnutrition

Malnutrition accompanies hepatic cirrhosis in many cases and aggravates the disease. Malabsorption in hepatic cirrhosis is responsible for potentiation of a malnutritive state and is usually associated with either quantitative (bile duct obstruction) or qualitative (hepatocellular damage) alterations of bile salts that reach the intestine. The malabsorption syndrome primarily concerns the absorption of fats, fat-soluble vitamins, and calcium, although other nutrients may be involved.

The presence of increased amounts of unconjugated bile salts in the intestine of cirrhotics may cause diarrhea and may inhibit certain activities of the conjugated product necessary for fat digestion (Linscheer, 1970). The fat-soluble vitamins A, D, E, and K are almost completely dependent upon the action of bile for absorption. Calcium is also often unavailable for absorption because of the formation of insoluble calcium soaps with undigested fatty acids.

Osteomalacia and osteoporosis may occur singly or in combination in advanced cirrhosis. Vitamin D absorption, as with calcium, is dependent upon proper micelle formation within the intestine. Vitamin D storage is also somewhat impaired in cirrhosis.

The clinical signs related to malabsorption in cirrhosis are steatorrhea, weight loss, night blindness (man, animals?), osteomalacia, osteoporosis, and hemorrhagic diatheses.

Hepatic failure is often accompanied by

hypovitaminosis. Primary deficiencies of folic acid, B_6, thiamine, and vitamins A and E are most often reported in man. The reasons for this have been discussed by Leevey et al. (1970) and Russell (1979). Primary causes are anorexia and decreased intake; less impotant but still significant are increased metabolic demand for repair and regeneration of cells, intestinal malabsorption, reduced hepatic uptake, failure of hepatic conversion of vitamins to their metabolically active forms, reduced storage capacity, and a decrease in circulating carrier protein (alpha and beta globulins), all of which combine to cause hypovitaminemia. The B-complex vitamins are often depleted secondary to release from damaged hepatic cells, inadequate replacement, and an increased demand for nucleic acid synthesis during liver regeneration (Leevy et al., 1970; Rosenthal and Glass, 1970). Even though patients receive a nutritious diet and vitamin supplementation, malutilization of vitamins will occur as long as the disease is progressing. Presumably, this is due to a lack of conversion of the vitamin to a metabolically active form or to intestinal malabsorption.

The liver is the primary source of 90 to 95 per cent of the serum proteins. It synthesizes all the serum albumin as well as 80 per cent of the serum globulins, (i.e., not the gamma fraction) (Hoe and Wilkinson, 1973). Other important proteins dependent upon the liver for formation are fibrinogen and most of the blood clotting factors. Amino acids derived from the diet are almost completely cleared from the blood by the liver and either catabolized for energy or used for protein synthesis. Serum proteins are important in maintaining serum colloidal osmotic pressure and normal blood hemostatic mechanisms, and in transporting such substances as iron, vitamin B_{12}, many hormones, hemoglobin, bilirubin, and many drugs.

Serum albumin concentrations are maintained within fairly narrow limits in normal animals. The half-life for canine albumin is reported to be seven to ten days (Schall, 1976). The exact stimulus for albumin synthesis is unresolved, but hypotheses suggest that plasma oncotic pressure or hepatic interstitial oncotic pressure may be responsible (Taville, 1972). The liver has a fairly limited ability to increase synthesis of albumin in response to hypoalbuminemia.

Data in the rat indicate that a fivefold increase in basal synthetic levels is maximal (Peters, 1977). Synthesis is critically dependent on appropriate supplies of dietary amino acids. Overgrowth of small intestinal bacteria decreases amino acid uptake significantly and grossly alters albumin synthesis. Approximately 25 per cent of the total daily hepatic protein synthesis is directed towards albumin. Interestingly, glucocorticoids augment hepatic albumin synthesis markedly even though they result in significant catabolism of muscle protein. Even more important than synthesis augmentation for maintaining serum albumin concentration is the ability of the liver to decrease its rate of catabolism (Taville, 1972). Albumin catabolism occurs to a limited extent in the liver (ten per cent) and another ten per cent of albumin is lost through the GI tract. The remaining 80 per cent is catabolized in other poorly identified areas of the body. In response to declining albumin concentrations, the rate at which albumin is degraded is significantly decreased, thus prolonging its functional half-life without having to increase synthesis. Because of these compensatory mechanisms, hypoalbuminemia is not seen until significant hepatic parenchymal injury has existed for several days to weeks. An 80 per cent decrease in hepatic mass is necessary in order for significant hypoalbuminemia to be detected. Diseases often associated with hypoalbuminemia are hepatic fibrosis (cirrhosis), subacute hepatitis, and congenital hepatic atrophy.

Globulin changes in hepatic diseases are fairly nonspecific. The alpha and beta globulins may be depressed by hepatocellular damage, as 75 per cent to 90 per cent of the alpha globulins and 50 per cent of the beta globulins are synthesized by the canine liver (Kukral et al., 1963). The gamma globulins, conversely, often show a wide electrophoretic peak in hepatopathies (Cornelius, 1970). The serum globulins usually increase in hepatitis and diffuse fibrosis, although the exact mechanisms responsible for this rise are still uncertain. It is possible that the increase is a response to foreign antigens (bacterial or viral) that escape hepatic clearance in inflammatory diseases, or it may occur secondary to the formation of homologous tissue antibodies after hepatic parenchymal damage. The elevation in gamma globulins has been demonstrated to be a result of increased production rather than of decreased removal from the blood (Havens et al., 1954).

The liver is the sole site of urea production from deamination of amino acids (Bollman et al., 1924). It is possible for blood urea nitrogen levels to occasionally decrease below normal with severe hepatic failure in animals, but it is seen only with very advanced hepatic disease in man. In advanced human cirrhosis, maximal urea production may be as low as five per cent of normal, yet serum levels are still within normal limits (Rudman et al., 1969). Two canine hepatic diseases often associated with decreases in BUN are end stage cirrhosis and portal vascular anomalies with severe hepatic atrophy.

The liver plays a central role in carbohydrate metabolism of the body. The liver extracts monosaccharides from the portal blood and converts them to energy or forms glycogen as a storage product for later utilization. Although experimentally hepatectomized animals will die within a few hours from hypoglycemia, clinical, symptomatic hypoglycemia from hepatic disease is infrequent and often represents a preterminal event. Peripheral gluconeogenesis and hepatic reserve function apparently maintain blood glucose levels within physiologically acceptable limits even though severe liver disease is present.

The liver plays a major role in the metabolic pathways involved with the utilization and storage of fat. Large amounts of fat may accumulate in the liver, a condition variously referred to as hepatic lipidosis, steatosis, fatty metamorphosis, fatty degeneration, and fatty hepatosis. The exact cause(s) in many cases remains unknown.

Normal and abnormal lipid metabolism is a complex process that has recently been well reviewed by Hoyumpa et al. (1975). Normal hepatic lipid arises from three primary sources, the diet, mobilization of peripheral fat depots, and endogenous hepatic fatty acid synthesis. Fatty acids entering the liver are either converted to a triglyceride-phospholipid-cholesterol lipoprotein complex or directly oxidized for energy. The balance between triglyceride esterification and oxidation is determined by the body's hormonal state and the availability of biochemical intermediates necessary for fatty acid esterification or oxidation. Triglyceride buildup (lipidosis) develops when the rate of

formation exceeds the liver's capacity to mobilize triglycerides from the liver. The influx of hepatic fatty acids depends upon their rate of entry (dietary or fat depot sources) or upon de novo synthesis of fatty acids by hepatocytes and their subsequent esterification. Efflux of hepatic lipids depends on the formation of very low density lipoproteins from triglycerides or the oxidation of fatty acids to CO_2, water, or ketones. In removing stored hepatic triglycerides, a large proportion must be converted to phospholipids. Phospholipid synthesis requires choline or one of its precursors, methionine. Thus, fatty livers that respond to lipotropic agents such as choline, methionine, betaine, casein, or raw pancreas are physiologic fatty livers and are due to deficiencies of lipotropic compounds. In most diseases associated with lipidosis, supplementation with lipotropic drugs does no good and may be harmful (see therapy section). Either the liver is unable to synthesize adequate amounts of phospholipids or the rate of delivery of fatty acids to the liver exceeds its maximal physiologic ability to utilize them; thus they accumulate within hepatocytes.

The most important clinical disorders associated with hepatic lipidosis are starvation, obesity, diabetes mellitus, drug-induced disorders, and toxic disorders. The lipidosis associated with starvation is usually mild. Lipidosis develops secondary to a decreased availability of glucose and increased release of growth hormone and catecholamines, all of which augment fatty acid synthesis within the liver and their release from peripheral fat stores. Severe protein-calorie malnutrition impairs hepatic lipoprotein synthesis and subsequent hepatic triglyceride release. Obesity frequently leads to lipidosis. The causes are many but primary abnormalities revolve around an increased intake of dietary fatty acids and imbalances of protein and calories (high carbohydrate, low protein diets). The liver serves as one of many lipid storage organs. Dieting uniformly results in decreases in stored hepatic lipids. Diabetes mellitus is an important cause of lipidosis in dogs and cats. Lipidosis in this disease is often severe. Although it has generally been considered that the severity of lipidosis correlates with inadequacy of insulin therapy, newer information indicates that adequacy of control and duration of illness do not correlate with lipidosis severity. The presence or absence of antecedent obesity appears to be the primary determinant of the severity of diabetic fatty liver in man. Certainly, it is known that in the unregulated diabetic a tremendous increase in circulating fatty acids occurs. Insulin inhibits peripheral lipolysis and thus decreases the availability of fatty acids flooding the liver for incorporation into triglycerides. Two important drug-related causes for lipidosis are tetracycline and glucocorticoid administration. Oral tetracyclines are associated with mild lipidosis in dogs, which is reversible upon withdrawal of the drug. A much more important disease entity is that seen one to two weeks following parenteral (IV) administration of large doses of tetracycline in man. The milder forms of tetracycline-induced lipidosis are thought to result from impaired hepatic protein synthesis and decreased lipoprotein formation. Glucocorticoids induce significant hepatic morphologic lesions. Such abnormalities were once interpreted as lipidosis, although newer information indicates that most of the vacuolar changes are not lipid associated. Lipidosis does exist in steroid hepatopathy, but it is mild. The exact mechanism responsible for increases in hepatic lipid in dogs given steroids is unknown. Steroids are known to increase peripheral fatty acid mobilization and inhibit hepatic triglyceride reesterification, both of which could lead to abnormal accumulation of lipid. Toxic injury is another important cause for fatty liver. Many toxins can induce fatty metamorphosis of the liver. Bacterial toxins (endotoxins) absorbed from the gut are well established as causes of lipidosis. Such toxins are thought to inhibit hepatic lipoprotein synthesis. Treatment with oral antibiotics significantly reduces the severity of these lesions by suppressing colonic bacterial toxin formation.

HEMATOLOGIC ABNORMALITIES

Numerous alterations in normal hemostatic mechanisms may exist in patients with hepatic disease. These include multiple aberrations in normal blood clotting mechanisms, as well as anemias unrelated to blood losses. The clinical significance of clotting abnormalities from spontaneous hepatic diseases in veterinary medicine has received little attention. The importance of the liver in normal blood clotting homeostasis is indicated by the fact that hepatectomized dogs supported with glucose invariably die from overwhelming hemorrhage (Schenk et al., 1957).

In clinical hepatic disorders, abnormalities in coagulation tests are usually multiple (Feldman, 1980). Often, the activated clotting time, prothrombin time, and partial thromboplastin time are all prolonged. Significant clotting abnormalities are most often of clinical importance in acute, severe hepatic failure, rather than in chronic hepatic diseases (Aledort, 1976). The liver is the site of production of most of the plasma procoagulants, including factors, I, II, V, VII, IX, and X. The liver also synthesizes both activators and inhibitors of the fibrinolytic system and is involved with the catabolism of many coagulants and procoagulants. Factors II, VII, IX, X, and prothrombin are vitamin K-dependent factors; i.e., they require this vitamin for normal hepatic synthesis (Corn, 1968). Abnormally prolonged prothrombin time is a common event in human hepatic diseases and occurs following administration of experimental hepatotoxic agents in dogs (Brinkhous and Warner, 1940; Osbaldiston and Hoffman, 1971). Two mechanisms exist by which prothrombin time is prolonged in hepatic disease. With severe hepatocellular damage, the ability of the liver to synthesize prothrombin and the prothrombin-dependent clotting factors is impaired. Such cases will not respond to parenteral vitamin K administration until the hepatocellular damage is corrected. The second cause is related to impaired bile release into the intestines. Vitamin K is a fat-soluble vitamin and requires the presence of adequate amounts of bile salts for absorption from the intestine. In obstructive biliary tract disease, prolonged prothrombin times will occur fairly readily, because vitamin K is stored in minimal amounts in the dog. Parenteral administration of vitamin K will return prothrombin levels to normal within 48 hours in cases of obstructive biliary disease (Ingelfinger, 1967). Other factors related to absorption and production of vitamin K are the use of long-term intestinal antibiotics that suppress bacterial synthesis of this vitamin and result in a deficiency state even in the presence of adequate bile flow. Malabsorption of fat-soluble vitamins may also result in prolonged prothrombin times.

Abnormalities in circulating platelets may exist in hepatic disease and produce hemorrhagic diatheses. Thrombocytopenia in man has been related to hypersplenism and platelet sequestration associated with portal hypertension, slightly decreased platelet life-span, and a mild decrease in production (Corn, 1968; Roberts and Cederbaum, 1972).

A last factor that is theorized to be responsible for hemorrhage in hepatic failure is the development of disseminated intra-vascular coagulation. The release of thromboplastin-like substances from dam-aged hepatocytes and a decreased ability of the diseased liver to clear clot-promoting factors are potential causes for this phenom-enon (Roberts and Cederbaum, 1972; Ale-dort, 1976). The development of severe DIC has been reported in a dog with severe hepatic necrosis (Strombeck et al., 1976a). Evidence for accelerated fibrinolysis asso-ciated with a diaphragmatic hernia in a dog was reported (Engen et al., 1974). It was hypothesized that a reduction in fibrinolytic inhibitors, an increased release of fibrinoly-tic activators, and impaired hepatic clear-ance of plasminogen activators led to accel-erated clot lysis in this dog. No evidence for DIC was present. Therapy with an inhibitor of plasminogen, ϵ-aminocaproic acid, was associated with partial correction of the fi-brinolytic state.

Mild anemia is a frequent finding in do-mestic animals with chronic liver disease. Potential causes for the anemia are blood loss, prolonged prothrombin time, throm-bocytopenia, macrocytic anemias from folic acid and vitamin B_{12} deficiencies, and occa-sionally hemolytic disorders related to al-tered serum lipids and proteins leading to an imbalance of prohemolytic and antihe-molytic substances in the blood (Norcross, 1966; Zieve, 1966; Ingelfinger, 1967). Dhar et al. (1968) report finding no detectable levels of erythropoietin in 75 per cent of a series of cases of human cirrhotics with anemia. Spur cell anemia has been de-scribed in a 2.5-year-old cat with severe inflammatory liver disease (Shull et al., 1978). The spleen and RE system remove such cells from the circulation because they are noncompliant compared with normal RBCs.

RENAL ABNORMALITIES

An occasional complication of severe he-patic failure in man is the development of acute oliguric renal failure. This is a major

concern, not only because of the uremia that ensues but also because of the deleterious effect that retained urea has in inducing hepatic coma. When the kidneys from pa-tients with hepatorenal syndrome are exam-ined, no significant lesions are found. In fact, when kidneys from patients dying of this syndrome have been transplanted into other patients without liver disease, the pre-viously failing kidneys function normally. This has led to the proposal that the hepa-torenal syndrome is a neurovascular compli-cation of hepatic failure, although the exact pathogenesis of this serious complication has not been elucidated. No data are cur-rently available on spontaneous canine or feline hepatic failure to support the concept that a hepatorenal syndrome similar to that of man occurs in these species.

The mechanism(s) responsible for poly-dipsia and polyuria in canine hepatic dis-orders have perplexed veterinarians for years. It is a widely accepted clinical fact that a significant number of dogs with hepatic diseases due to multiple etiologies have polydipsia and polyuria as a historical com-plaint. Low (1972) reported the urine spe-cific gravity of cirrhotic dogs to be consistently below that of dogs with hepa-toma, and a reversible defect in urine con-centrating ability is known to occur in many patients (human) with cirrhosis (Jick et al., 1964; Vaamonde et al., 1967). Although the exact mechanisms for this are subject to debate, several plausible mechanisms have been experimentally investigated. These in-clude psychogenic polydipsia, decreased medullary urea concentration, medullary washout, hypokalemia, and alterations in portal vein osmoreceptor response. The au-thor has investigated several dogs with pro-found polydipsia and polyuria as primary complaints that had hepatic failure as the only identified cause for the signs. Follow-ing water deprivation, these dogs concen-trated well (i.e., 1.035), but not maximally. When free access to water was allowed, they rapidly returned to hyposthenuric levels (1.001 to 1.004). The author has concluded that the dogs had mildly impaired concen-trating abilities but were able to significantly conserve water following dehydration. They had no physiologic need for the volumes they drank. The polydipsia was considered primary, with the polyuria being compensa-tory to eliminate the excess water load. When these dogs were treated for their hepatic disease, the clinical signs disappeared. Presumably, the polydipsia had a psychogenic component and is but one of many manifestations of hepatic encephalopathy.

A significant decrease in the renal medullary solute concentration occurs in cirrhotic dogs and dogs whose bile ducts have been ligated (Massry and Klein, 1978; Vaamonde, 1978; Whang and Popper, 1974). Several factors lead to this reduction in medullary solute concentration. A shift in blood flow occurs from the outer cortical nephrons to the juxtamedullary nephrons. The resulting high blood flow to juxtamedullary nephrons impairs the renal countercurrent mechanism and leads to a "washout" of interstitial solutes necessary for normal concentrating ability. In addition, owing to reduced protein intake associated with anorexia and the liver's inability to effectively convert ammonia to urea, the renal medullary urea concentration can be severely depleted in cirrhosis. Urea accounts for 50 per cent of the total medullary solute concentration in the dog (Levinsky et al., 1959). Thus, even if other factors are kept constant, a reduction in renal urea concentration would reduce a dog's maximal renal concentrating ability by 50 per cent, i.e., from 1.060 to 1.030. A third mechanism favoring the production of dilute urine is the augmented renal sodium reabsorption that occurs in hepatic failure, as discussed in the section on ascites. With decreased delivery of sodium to the distal tubules and collecting ducts, sodium excretion is minimal and a reduction in urine osmolality is seen. In dogs whose bile ducts have been ligated, renal medullary osmolality decreased from 1528 mOsm/kg to 900 mOsm/kg in four to seven days following ligation (Vaamonde, 1978).

Hypokalemia has been proposed for a number of years as a cause for the polydipsia and polyuria of hepatic failure. Total body exchangeable potassium is often severely depleted in cirrhosis, even though serum potassium concentrations usually remain normal (Casey et al., 1965). The reduction in total body potassium is most likely due to renal wasting secondary to chronically increased aldosterone concentrations in long-standing cirrhosis and/or prolonged diuretic use. Hypokalemia is known to induce a severe defect in renal concentrating ability; however, since serum potassium concentrations are usually normal and no morphologic tubular lesions characteristic of hypokalemia have been documented in patients with impaired concentrating ability, it is an unlikely cause for the disorder (Whang and Popper, 1974). Lastly, recent evidence indicates that osmoreceptors that are highly sensitive to increases in portal vein osmolality are present within the canine portal circulation (Kozlowski and Orzewrecki, 1973). Input regarding portal venous osmolality is mediated through the vagus nerve to the brain. Infusions of mildly hypertonic solutions into the portal vein induced dramatic water drinking in dogs. It is conceivable that portal vein osmoreceptors are altered in hepatic disease so that they respond abnormally and induce a thirst response in the absence of portal vein osmolality changes.

DIAGNOSIS OF HEPATIC DISEASE

ANAMNESIS AND PHYSICAL FINDINGS IN HEPATIC DISEASES

The history and physical examination obtained on an animal with hepatic disease are often vague and nonspecific. Because of the wide diversity of metabolic functions the liver performs and its great reserve capacity and regenerative ability, clinical signs rarely are evident until the disease is far advanced. Even when signs do exist, the clinician must maintain a high index of suspicion for hepatic disease because of the tendency for similar signs to be initially associated with many other diseases. The history is often one of intermittent abdominal disorders, anorexia, vomiting, and diarrhea or constipation. The owners may notice progressive depression and lethargy or the tendency for the abdomen to enlarge (ascites). Observant owners may note the presence of acholic feces associated with complete bile duct obstruction or the "orange" urine associated with hyperbilirubinuria. The development of jaundice in the sclera and oral mucous membranes is rarely observed by the client but may be the sole complaint on admission. The development of petechiation, hemorrhagic enteritis, or hematuria associated with hemorrhagic diatheses is an infrequent occurrence in hepatic diseases. Signs of hepatic encephalopathy such as dementia, circling, head pressing, aggression, and transient blindness can also be misinterpreted as signs of primary CNS disease. Polydipsia and polyuria are commonly present in dogs with hepatic failure and may be the only historical complaint of significance.

The physical examination of patients with hepatic disease is often no more rewarding than the history. The presence of jaundice, a palpably enlarged liver, and ascites makes the diagnosis uncomplicated, but rarely are all these findings present. Acholic feces and hepatomegaly are the only two definitive signs of hepatic abnormalities, since jaundice may be prehepatic in origin. The presence of normally pigmented stools in a constipated animal does not indicate the current status of bile flow. A fresh fecal sample should always be evaluated for the presence of normal bile pigmentation. Acholic feces tend to be fatty and clay- or slate-colored from a lack of stercobilin. Jaundice, in the absence of anemia, is good evidence for hepatocellular or posthepatic biliary disease. Pain on palpation of the liver results from tension on Glisson's capsule and is indicative of acute disease processes (congestion or inflammation), as chronic hepatic disorders are rarely painful. The liver should be palpated, if possible, for size, shape, and location. The normal liver is difficult to palpate in the dog and cat. The borders are sharp and the liver substance is firm.

The most common causes or processes associated with hepatomegaly are severe congestion and edema, bile engorgement, diffuse inflammation, nodular hyperplasia, infiltrative diseases (lipidosis or amyloidosis), and primary or secondary neoplasias. A decrease in hepatic size may exist in acute or subacute necrosis, hepatic atrophy, and cirrhosis. Ascites, although not a specific sign of hepatic disease, should make one suspicious of its existence. Abdominal palpation in the presence of ascites is often difficult, or even impossible, until the fluid is removed.

LABORATORY EVALUATION OF LIVER DISEASE

Well over a hundred tests are currently available for the evaluation of hepatic disease. Most of these tests are more useful for evaluating the large number of metabolic activities of the liver than they are as diagnostic aids. It is important that the clinician select a few specific tests that fully evaluate the major anatomicophysiologic divisions of the liver and understand their significance, rather than run a barrage of randomly selected evaluations. Cornelius (1970) stresses the importance of recognizing the quantitative association of various liver function tests as they relate to the liver as a whole, rather than emphasizing the qualitative dissociation of partial function.

Whether the liver performs its functions well is determined largely by the integrity and vitality of its enzyme systems. Alterations in diagnostic tests are usually associated with cell damage, resulting either in an inability of the liver to perform a function, or in the release of intracellular components that are measured in the blood.

Indications and Limitations of Diagnostic Tests

The primary clinical reasons for carrying out liver function tests are (1) to establish the diagnosis of primary and secondary hepatic diseases in jaundiced and nonjaundiced animals, (2) to differentiate between the various causes of jaundice, (3) to provide information necessary to establish a valid prognosis, and (4) to evaluate the effects of therapy in hepatic disease.

The limitations of liver function tests must be taken into consideration when laboratory results are interpreted. No single test has been developed that will assess the total functional status of the liver. Biochemical functions of the liver do not become impaired equally in every disease, as varying degrees of reserve function exist for each. Often, some functions are severely impaired (bile secretion), while others are totally unaffected, e.g., albumin synthesis. The sequence of loss and return of biochemical functions will vary from one disease to another. The lack of specificity of many tests makes interpretation of their significance difficult. Lastly, many extrahepatic factors affect specific hepatic function tests or studies (Benjamin, 1961; Cornelius, 1970).

Because of the many limitations indicated for liver function tests, the concept of battery testing has gained favor in the evaluation of hepatic diseases. A relatively small group of tests is selected for evaluating each of the four major hepatic cell types. This provides an indication of the status of the whole organ.

Even though the presence of hepatic disease may be established, it is often impossible to determine a morphologic or etiologic diagnosis from function tests alone. This is because many different diseases with widely varied histologic pictures produce similar biochemical results. Because of the potentially rapid changes in the status of liver functions, diagnosis and prognosis must be made on serial evaluations of specific functions rather than on single, isolated diagnostic panels.

The proper interpretation of laboratory data is one of the greatest challenges in internal medicine. The decision of what is "normal" for a given species in a given lab is critical. The normals discussed in this section are those the author is familiar with and may be quite different in other laboratories. Accurate normal ranges for the species in question should always be established by each particular laboratory used by the clinician.

Tests of Hepatic Excretory and Secretory Function

A number of valuable and relatively simple laboratory determinations are available for the assessment of the excretory or secretory capabilities of the liver. The estimation of serum concentrations of free and conjugated bilirubin and urinary and fecal bile pigments is used primarily in the differential diagnosis of jaundice. The history and physical examination of the patient, including examination of urine and fecal color, will usually serve to establish whether jaundice is prehepatic, hepatic, or posthepatic in origin. The use of laboratory evaluations confirms the clinical findings and establishes baseline data for future use in evaluating therapy or prognosis.

Total and Conjugated Bilirubin. The Van den Bergh test evaluates the amount of conjugated and total bilirubin in the serum and is used primarily to separate cases of hyperbilirubinemia into conjugated or unconjugated forms. The Van den Bergh reaction is of little or no value in differentiating hepatocellular from posthepatic jaundice. Increased levels of the unconjugated product are seen in hemolytic states. Normal total serum bilirubin is less than 0.6 mg/dl in the dog and 0.2 mg/dl in the cat, most of it being unconjugated. In hepatocellular diseases total serum bilirubin levels are increased, with more than 50 per cent being the conjugated product. The diseased liver cells still maintain some conjugating ability, but intrahepatic cholestasis causes

regurgitation of the conjugated bilirubin into the blood. With extrahepatic obstruction, total serum bilirubin levels are even higher, with 60 to 90 per cent of the bilirubin being in the conjugated form (Van Fleet and Alberts, 1968).

Most hepatocellular diseases have total serum bilirubin levels below 4 mg/dl, while prolonged posthepatic biliary obstruction may cause levels to reach 20 mg/dl. It is important to determine the levels of serum bilirubin early in the disease, as the ratio of the conjugated to unconjugated product changes with time, making valid interpretations later in the disease more difficult (Medway, 1968).

Bile Pigments. The two urine bile pigments of greatest clinical significance are urine bilirubin and urobilinogen. Owing to the low renal threshold, bilirubin is seen in the urine of 20 to 60 per cent of all dogs and is present in any febrile condition. The test most commonly used to detect bilirubinuria is the tablet diazo reaction (Ictotest). Pathological bilirubinemia is indicated by a 2^+ to 3^+ Ictotest reaction if the urine specific gravity is 1.035 or less. Any hepatocellular or posthepatic liver disease will produce elevated levels of urine bilirubin, and bilirubinuria may be the first indication of disease. In animals with hemolytic anemia, bilirubinuria is occasionally found and is a result of secondary hepatic damage from anoxia and/or renal conjugation of hemoglobin and its urinary excretion (Cornelius and Himes, 1973).

Urine urobilinogen results from the enterohepatic circulation of reduced bilirubin and its subsequent renal clearance. The presence of urine urobilinogen is evidence that the bile duct is at least partially patent, while its absence (unless absent on repeated urinalyses) carries little significance. If repeated negative urine urobilinogen determinations are recorded, an obstructed biliary system is most likely present.

Factors that may alter urine urobilinogen have been discussed (see Urobilinogen, this chapter).

Urine urobilinogen, if exposed to sunlight, is oxidized to a colored pigment, urobilin. It will not be detected in normal reactions for urobilinogen and must be tested for separately. Urine samples to be tested for urobilinogen should be kept in opaque containers or protected from sunlight if analysis is delayed for several hours.

Stercobilinogen. Fecal stercobilinogen

concentration and its oxidation product, stercobilin, can be determined but are usually impractical clinically. Stool color is a good indication of the presence or absence of bile pigments, as acholic feces are pale and slate gray in color, indicating bile duct obstruction or progressive hepatic fibrosis, while cholic stools appear normally pigmented. Feces from animals with chronic pancreatitis or pancreatic atrophy may also be pale but usually are fawn colored, while those associated with hemolytic diseases are very dark from excessive bilirubin production and excretion. Fecal stercobilin levels reflect the quantity of bile reaching the intestinal tract, the amount of bacterial conversion of bilirubin to urobilinogen, and the capacity of the liver to secrete reabsorbed urobilinogen (Jeffries, 1971). Decreased fecal stercobilin is seen in hepatobiliary diseases impairing bile excretion or after inefficient bacterial conversion of stercobilinogen to stercobilin following the use of intestinal antibiotics.

Clearance Tests. Uptake and excretion of a number of organic dyes have been used as a sensitive index of hepatic function for many years. The purpose of using such clearance tests is to evaluate the functional mass of the liver. They assess the ability of the liver to remove a given volume of a substance per unit of time. Some of these tests are the most reliable and sensitive indicators of hepatic function available (Brody and Leichter, 1979). Such tests are useful for assessing liver function when hepatic enzyme tests are normal but hepatic disease is still suspected. Of these dyes, sulfobromophthalein (BSP) and indocyanine green (ICG) have the greatest clinical application. Both are primarily excreted from the body via the bile after uptake and conjugation by the liver. Because of hepatic metabolic pathways involved in their excretion, they are sensitive indicators of hepatic disease. In addition to normal hepatic biochemical integrity, the excretion of these dyes requires a normal hepatic blood flow for proper elimination. Thus, elevated BSP and ICG retention will occur in conditions altering hepatic blood flow, such as congestive heart failure or other diseases that induce chronic passive congestion. Unfortunately, owing to rare anaphylactic reactions to BSP in man, this test is no longer used in human medicine, which has made the dye difficult to obtain for veterinarians. It can still be purchased through chemical supply houses, but its availability is limited.

Measurement of BSP is the simpler and more economical of the two tests. A standard dose of 5 mg/kg body weight is injected intravenously after a heparinized blood sample is taken. Thirty minutes later, a second blood sample is taken from an alternate vein. Normal dogs have less than five per cent retention of the dye after 30 minutes, although values up to ten per cent retention have been found in dogs with no histologic evidence of hepatic disease (Coles, 1967). Delayed BSP excretion is seen in such diseases as infectious canine hepatitis, fibrosis, lipidosis, diabetes mellitus, leptospirosis, portal vascular anomalies, and carbon tetrachloride toxicosis. Normals should be determined for each clinical situation, as different laboratories have variable techniques for interpreting the percentage dye retention. Determinations of BSP retention in jaundiced animals is not recommended, as bilirubin competes with BSP for uptake, and delays in excretion will be difficult to interpret accurately. It has been reported that total bilirubin concentrations of less than 5 mg/dl will not interfere with BSP uptake by the liver (Feldman, 1980). The results of BSP testing may be significantly altered in hypoalbuminemic patients. BSP is bound to a great degree to albumin in the blood. Only the small fraction of unbound or free BSP is actively cleared by the liver. In hypoalbuminemic states, more of the injected BSP is unbound and available for excretion in any given time period. Therefore, it has been proposed that BSP retention may be falsely lowered in hypoalbuminemic patients with hepatic disease (Grausz and Schmidt, 1971). This has not been substantiated in clinical patients, however. Phenobarbital has also been reported to significantly increase the rate of removal of BSP from the circulation (Yeary and Wise, 1975).

Indocyanine green is also a sensitive clearance test for canine liver function, although it requires more sophisticated equipment and is somewhat more expensive to use. After intravenous administration, ICG has an exponential disappearance from the blood during the first 15 minutes. By taking three timed blood samples during that interval, the half-time for ICG clearance can be determined. The advantages of ICG over BSP are that in addition to measuring dye clearance, it can be used to estimate hepatic blood flow and plasma volume. Cornelius (1970) lists the range for the fractional clearance of ICG as 5.5 to 9.8 per cent per minute. For most clinical situations, the BSP retention test is as satisfactory as ICG determinations.

Bile Acid Concentrations. Another hepatic function test that has been receiving increased usage in the human field and preliminary investigations in veterinary medicine is quantitation of serum bile acid concentration. Four types of bile acid measurements can be used diagnostically: (1) fasting, (2) two-hour postprandial, (3) serum concentration following oral bile salt loading, and (4) rate of removal of intravenously administered radiolabeled bile salts (Matern and Gerok, 1979b). Most hepatobiliary diseases result in increased concentrations of serum bile acids. With hepatocellular failure, extraction from portal blood is reduced. In cholestatic diseases, bile acids are regurgitated into the peripheral blood in increased quantities. Lastly, in diseases associated with the formation of portal systemic shunts, much of the intestinally absorbed bile acid pool is diverted around the liver, reaching the general circulation. Either fasting or two-hour postprandial levels are considered sensitive indices of hepatic functional disease and are used as screening tests in man. Combinations of SGOT and bile salt concentrations are considered very sensitive indicators of hepatic injury.

Unfortunately, insufficient data are available on bile acid alterations in spontaneous hepatic disorders of dogs and cats for conclusions regarding their diagnostic usefulness to be made at this time. It is possible that bile acid concentrations will serve as a replacement for BSP clearance, since the latter is becoming difficult to obtain. The author has evaluated serum bile salt concentrations in a limited number of dogs with hepatic disease and found them to parallel abnormalities detected by other, more commonly used tests of hepatic function.

Serum Enzymes

Numerous serum enzyme determinations are available for evaluation of hepatocellular and biliary tract integrity. Unfortunately, the great majority of these enzymes are not liver-specific; that is, they are also found in many other tissues, and if elevated, all nonhepatic sources of the enzyme must be eliminated before a diagnosis of hepatic disease can be made. Serum enzymes are elevated in hepatic disease for several reasons. Necrosis of cells or increased membrane permeability is responsible for elevations of serum alanine aminotransferase (ALT), serum aspartate aminotransferase (AST), serum isocitric dehydrogenase (ICD), arginase, sorbitol dehydrogenase (SD), ornithine carbamyl transferase (OCT), and lactic dehydrogenase (LDH). Retention and increased production cause increased levels of serum alkaline phosphatase (AP) in association with biliary tract disease, and decreased synthesis causes depression of cholinesterase levels in the blood.

Serum Alanine Aminotransferase. The serum alanine aminotransferase enzyme is liver-specific in the dog and cat and should be the enzyme used for the detection of hepatocellular necrosis and inflammation. Serum ALT enzymes are localized to the cytoplasm of hepatocytes and are easily lost to the interstitial spaces and venous system with minor cellular injury. The intracellular concentrations of S-ALT and Serum-AST are 10,000 times those of extracellular fluid (Cornelius, 1979). In addition to leakage from cells associated with injury, Serum ALT concentrations may increase secondary to enzyme induction by drugs. Certain chemical agents are known to dramatically increase the basal intracellular concentration of this enzyme. This can result in mild increases in the "normal" serum concentration, and with hepatic injury, very high serum concentrations will be produced by mild lesions. The half-life of both Serum ALT and Serum AST is two to five hours (Feldman, 1980); thus, if injury to the liver is transient, serum concentrations should return to normal fairly rapidly. Since Serum ALT concentrations may remain elevated for up to three weeks following acute experimental toxic hepatitis in dogs, it has been proposed that the continued serum activity may reflect the involvement of this enzyme system in protein synthesis associated with hepatic regeneration and not with progressive injury (Cornelius, 1979). Elevations occur after leakage either from necrotic cells or from cells surrounding the necrotic area that are stimulated to produce abnormal amounts of this enzyme (Hoe, 1969). Small quantities of Serum ALT do exist in the kidney and myocardium. With severe renal or cardiac disease (necrosis), mild elevations in Serum ALT, unrelated to the liver, could occur (Cornelius et al., 1959). Elevations in Serum ALT in dogs are seen with infectious canine hepatitis, cholestasis, neoplasia, lipidosis, suppurative necrosis, anemias, and any other conditions resulting in active hepatocellular necrosis or inflammation. Normal values for Serum ALT in the dog and cat are 10 to 50 Sigma Frankel units (SFU) or 80 IU. Levels between 50 and 400 SFU are considered indicative of moderate necrosis, while those over 400 SFU indicate severe hepatocellular damage.

Only a brief discussion of other available hepatic enzyme tests of hepatic inflammation will be made, since they are usually of less value than serum ALT and are more rigorous and expensive. LDH, serum ICD, and serum AST are all present in multiple body tissues and are of no more value and less specificity than serum ALT. Serum OCT and SD are quite liver-specific for the dog and are of diagnostic value equal to serum ALT determination.

Plasma Arginase. Plasma arginase determinations may be of prognostic value when used in conjunction with serum ALT levels. Arginase is a mitochondrial-bound enzyme and thus is less sensitive to release from mild hepatic injury. Arginase elevations in serum are associated with overt cell necrosis rather than with membrane injury alone. Normal serum values are 0 to 14 IU/L. In carbon tetrachloride toxicosis, values of 44 to 1815 IU/L were observed (Mia and Koger, 1979). In severe hepatic necrosis both enzymes are elevated, but when regeneration begins, arginase levels return to normal more rapidly. If necrosis is continuing, both levels remain elevated (Cornelius et al., 1962, Mia and Koger, 1979). The author has not found serum arginase values to be particularly useful in clinical practice. In many spontaneous liver diseases in dogs associated with mild to moderate degrees of serum ALT elevation, arginase concentrations remain normal. Only in severe cases of hepatic necrosis has arginase been pathologically elevated and other enzymes reflected the severity of the diseases as well.

Serum Alkaline Phosphatase. Serum alkaline phosphatase determinations are a very important part of any liver disease workup. A great deal of useful information regarding serum AP in both dogs and cats has recently appeared in the veterinary literature. Since there are dramatic differences between the cat and dog in terms of serum AP interpretation and metabolism, they will be considered separately.

The serum concentration of alkaline phosphatase in the dog reflects the total activity of several isoenzymes derived from a number of different tissues. To date, four serum isoenzymes have been identified by cellulose acetate electrophoresis (Hoffman, 1977; Hoffman and Dorner, 1975). These include enzymes derived from liver and bone, a glucocorticoid-induced isoenzyme, and an isoenzyme from an as yet unidentified source. Although other isoenzymes of alkaline phosphatase exist within placental, renal, and intestinal tissue, their half-lives are so short in the circulation (less than six minutes) that significant serum concentrations do not develop (Hoffman, 1976; Hoffman and Dorner, 1977). The half-lives of both the hepatic and steroid isoenzymes is similar, i.e., 66 hours for the former and 70 hours for the latter (Hoffman and Dorner, 1977). Normal serum AP is primarily of hepatic origin, with the bone isoenzyme of minor importance (Saini and Saini, 1978). Once within the circulation, alkaline phosphatase is not cleared by the liver but is catabolized like other serum proteins (Young, 1974).

Many theories concerning the mechanism of serum AP increases in hepatic disease have been proposed, but present evidence favors a modification of the regurgitation concept. Experimental work has confirmed that the rise in serum AP associated with liver disease is secondary to varying degrees of intra- or extrahepatic cholestasis. Cholestasis induces massive increases in the synthesis of alkaline phosphatase by both bile duct epithelial cells and hepatocytes. This massive increase in production in a dog who is unable to excrete the enzyme through blocked bile canaliculi or ducts leads to regurgitation of alkaline phosphatase into the circulation.

Pathologic increases in serum AP occur primarily in association with a variety of hepatic disorders, in association with increased endogenous or exogenous glucocorticoids, in certain diseases of bone, occasionally with nonhepatic or osseous neoplasms, and following enzyme induction by a number of therapeutic agents. Hepatic disorders are the most frequent cause of serum AP elevations in the dog. Any hepatic disease that has a degree of cholestasis will be associated with variable increases in serum AP concentration. Extrahepatic obstructive biliary tract diseases tend to produce the greatest rise, often seven to ten times normal (Young, 1974). Severe intrahepatic cholestasis will also result in massive increases in serum AP. Diseases that are primarily centrolobular in location cause very mild increases in serum AP, while those at the periphery of the lobule, since they cause much more severe impairment to bile flow, often have very elevated concentrations. With early extrahepatic obstruction the serum AP and bilirubin are markedly increased, while serum ALT is mildly elevated. With time, however, obstructive jaundice induces cholangitis and pericholangitis, which result in significant alterations in serum ALT concentrations.

The identification of a steroid-induced isoenzyme of serum AP has been of great diagnostic help to veterinarians. The dog is uniquely sensitive to the effects of glucocorticoids, which induce hepatic synthesis of a steroid specific isoenzyme. Most dogs, but not all, will have increases in serum AP following the administration of glucocorticoids or ACTH. In addition, dogs with spontaneous hyperadrenocorticism or functional adrenal cortical tumors, frequently develop massive increases in serum AP. The magnitude of rise in serum AP associated with steroids may be 100 times normal, which is generally higher than that seen in hepatobiliary disorders (Hoffman, 1977). The initial rise in serum AP following steroid administration is quite rapid, often within a few days (Dorner et al., 1974). The magnitude of the rise appears to be dependent on the dose, type of steroid, duration of administration, and individual patient response (Hoffman, 1977). Since hepatomegaly and increased serum AP may be identified in many early cushingoid dogs without other evidence for this disease, clinicians must elect to obtain serum AP isoenzyme analyses, hepatic biopsy, or ACTH stimulation data to identify the cause of hepatic pathology. Steroid hepatopathy will be considered in more detail later in this chapter.

Abnormalities involving bone synthesis of serum AP are uncommon, but situations reported to produce mild increases in serum AP of osseous origin include primary and secondary hyperparathyroidism, bone neoplasia, rickets, osteomalacia, and osteoporosis (Harvey, 1967). Young, growing puppies will also have mildly increased levels. Although increases in serum AP may occur in these conditions, it usually remains normal. When a rise is detected, its magnitude is less than five times normal (Hoffman and Dorner, 1975; Hoffman, 1977). Bone neoplasia may be associated with two- to threefold increases in SAP.

Several commonly used therapeutic agents have been shown to result in enzyme induction of the hepatic serum AP isoenzyme (Sturtevant et al., 1977). The most important include primidone, phenobarbital, and phenytoin, all commonly used anticonvulsants. The magnitude of rise for phenobarbital was 30-fold, that for primidone fivefold, and that for phenytoin threefold. The latter drug also caused a parallel increase in serum ALT concentrations. Clinicians must be aware that drugs used to treat nonhepatic diseases may induce biochemical and/or morphologic changes in the liver.

Recent experimental work in the cat following bile duct ligation or carbon tetrachloride–induced hepatitis has clarified the value of serum AP as a diagnostic aid in this species. Older experimental data indicated that serum AP was not useful in cats, since it was excreted in the urine following bile duct ligation, preventing significant serum increases (Flood et al., 1937). Newer information negates these earlier conclusions. In general, although serum AP does increase in serum of cats with hepatobiliary disorders, the frequency and magnitude of such pathological increases is low in spontaneous feline hepatic diseases. The reasons for this are several (Hoffman et al., 1977). Feline hepatic tissue contains only one-third the concentration of serum AP per gram present in the dog. The serum half-life of feline serum AP is considerably shorter than dogs, six hours versus 66 hours; thus, it is catabolized so rapidly that only in major cholestatic disease does its serum activity rise to a diagnostically useful concentration. The half-lives of other tissue AP isoenzymes (intestines and placenta) are so short (two minutes) that the only serum isoenzyme identified is that of the liver. Normal serum AP values for the cat are less than those for the dog (less than 30 μU/L or 10 to 80 IU versus 90 μU/L or 10 to 120 IU for the dog). Total bile duct ligation in cats produces a seven- to tenfold increase in serum AP (Hoffman et al., 1977; Mehain et al., 1978), while ligating one hepatic lobe caused a fourfold rise in activity. Carbon tetrachloride toxicosis caused a fivefold increase in serum AP activity and a 100-fold rise in serum ALT (Everell et al., 1977). In conclusion, although serum AP will rise in feline hepatobiliary disorders, only those with the most severe cholestatic diseases have diagnostically useful increases in this enzyme. Diseases the author has associated with increased serum AP include lymphosarcoma, chronic pancreatitis, cholangiohepatitis, and severe lipidosis. Most feline hepatic disorders that have been evaluated in the author's hospital have not shown significant increases in serum AP.

The use of another hepatobiliary-associated enzyme in man, gamma glutamyltransferase (γ-GGT), has helped to eliminate the need for serum AP isoenzyme determinations. γ-GGT exists in high concentrations within the biliary tract and increases are common in obstructive biliary tract disease in man. This enzyme has been evaluated in the dog for diagnostic usefulness (Shull and Hornbuckle, 1979). The conclusions reached are that γ-GGT has diagnostic implications similar to serum AP but no increased usefulness. This may be because canine liver contains less of this enzyme per gram of tissue than do other species. The magnitude of γ-GGT rise in dogs with ligated bile duct was less than serum AP increases in the same animals.

Selecting several laboratory tests in the initial evaluation of patients suspected to have liver disease is more likely to lead to a correct diagnosis. The two most widely available and used tests are serum ALT and serum AP. Hoe and O'Shea (1962) combined serum ALT and serum AP as a screening test for diverse hepatic disorders and detected 80 to 100 per cent of all diagnosed cases of lipidosis, malignant neoplasia, hepatoma, cirrhosis, and hepatitis. Two more recent articles assessed the relative value of serum ALT and serum AP for detecting occult or known hepatic disease (Brunson et al., 1980; Schull et al., 1978b). Although there were some differences in the relative value of serum ALT versus serum AP between the two studies, it can be concluded that both tests together yield significantly greater diagnostic accuracy than either test alone.

Biochemical Function Tests

Tests to evaluate the integrity of hepatic protein synthetic capabilities are useful in diagnosing hepatic diseases. All the plasma albumin, fibrinogen, and prothrombin synthesis occurs in the liver. With impairment of hepatocellular function, synthesis of plasma proteins is depressed and levels fall. Since many other conditions will depress plasma protein levels, hypoalbuminemia is not specific for hepatic damage and must be interpreted in conjunction with other hepatic function tests.

Normal total plasma protein levels in the dog and cat are between 6.0 and 7.5 gm/dl. The normal half-life of plasma albumin is seven to 12 days; thus, levels decrease slowly even if synthesis is totally interrupted. A separation of serum protein into albumin and globulin fractions is necessary if proper interpretation of total serum protein values is to be made. Serum albumin levels can become quite depressed with longstanding hepatic diseases ($<$1 to 2 gm/dl), but because gammaglobulin levels are often elevated, total serum protein determinations may be near normal.

Serum gamma globulins are often elevated in hepatic disorders (hepatitis, diffuse fibrosis), although the mechanisms for this elevation are poorly understood. Hoe (1961) and Hoe and Harvey (1961) have studied the electrophoretic patterns of serum proteins for a wide variety of hepatic disorders and concluded that albumin levels are depressed in most cases, alpha-2 globulin changes are nonspecific, beta-1 peaks are associated with neoplastic conditions but are decreased in all other diseases, beta-2 globulins are increased in all jaundiced animals, and the gamma globulin fraction is increased in jaundice and cirrhosis, with all cirrhotic dogs having a characteristically poor resolution of the beta and gamma bands. The practice of using albumin-globulin ratios alone should be discontinued in deference to careful electrophoretic study of the albumin and globulin protein fractions.

Measurement of serum cholesterol and cholesterol esters has been used as supportive evidence for the presence of hepatic disease and may be of limited value in prognosis. The liver is the main source of serum cholesterol. Large amounts are excreted in the bile and partially converted to bile acids and their salts. The liver is also responsible for the normal esterification of cholesterol, esterified cholesterol comprising 60 to 80 per cent of the total serum levels. Total serum cholesterol levels are often elevated in obstructive biliary disease. The elevations are due, in part, to regurgitation but are also a result of increased bile salt release to plasma, which holds cholesterol and other lipids in solution, preventing their tissue uptake (Ingelfinger, 1967).

With hepatocellular disease, both total and esterified fractions tend to fall as the disease progresses. Progressively decreasing total and esterified cholesterol values are considered a poor prognostic sign in man. Normal total cholesterol values range from 125 to 250 mg/dl and are affected by such variables as diet, exercise, and metabolic diseases (diabetes mellitus, Cushing's syndrome, hypothyroidism, and nephrotic syndrome). Hoe and Harvey (1961) have concluded that although animals with normal total cholesterol and cholesterol ester values are unlikely to have hepatic disease, the presence of abnormal cholesterol values is not necessarily indicative of hepatic disease.

Uric acid levels in serum were used at one time as an indication of hepatocellular damage since, in the dog, uric acid is converted in the liver to allantoin for excretion. With liver cell damage, uric acid will increase (> 1.5 mg/dl). Since the advent of newer and more sensitive tests (BSP, serum AP, serum ALT), the use of uric acid as a diagnostic test has little value.

Ammonia tolerance tests have been well evaluated in clinical and experimental hepatic disorders in dogs and cats in recent years (Meyer et al., 1978; Strombeck et al., 1975b). The test involves the oral administration of an ammonia salt (ammonium chloride) and measuring of the blood NH_3 concentration 30 minutes later. The test is particularly useful for assessing the integrity of the hepatic portal system. The orally administered drug enters the small bowel, and the ammonium is converted to ammonia by the alkaline intestinal contents and absorbed. If significant portal vascular shunting, hepatocellular failure, or deficiencies of urea cycle enzymes exist, blood ammonia concentrations will be significantly elevated. The procedure involves oral administration of NH_4Cl at a dosage of 100 mg/kg body weight up to a maximum of 3 gm. The animal should be fasted for 12 hours and the ammonium salt diluted in 20 to 50 ml of water before administration to prevent vomiting. It may be given by syringe or stomach tube. This procedure has been well tolerated by many dogs with severe hepatic failure, except for occasional vomiting or nausea. Samples of heparinized blood are drawn at zero time and 30 minutes after administering the drug. Normal values for the dog are between 60 and 120 μg/dl on fasting samples and less than 200 μg/dl at 30 minutes. Although many animals with signs of hepatic encephalopathy have raised fasting blood ammonia concentrations, a significant number of dogs with severe hepatic failure will be normal, so that resting concentrations alone may not be diagnostic. The author, therefore, routinely performs ammonia challenge tests unless the animal shows obvious signs of encephalopathy. Significant increases are most often seen in portal vascular anomalies or chronic cirrhotics. The author has found blood NH_3 concentrations to be particularly useful in dogs with congenital vascular anomalies, while the BSP test has had greater reliability than NH_3 in a limited number of chronic fibrotic liver diseases. More clinical data are needed on cases in which both tests have been run simultaneously in order to determine whether or not one has greater diagnostic accuracy than the other in selected hepatic disorders.

BIOPSY

Liver biopsy is one of the most important diagnostic aids available for clinical evaluation of patients with hepatic disease. In many cases, even after a careful clinical and laboratory evaluation, a specific etiologic or morphologic diagnosis is lacking and biopsy is the only method of obtaining such information. Liver biopsy is not an innocuous procedure and should only be considered when the potential benefit to the patient outweighs the inherent risks of the technique (Osborne et al., 1969). Biopsy of the liver is indicated primarily when a specific diagnosis cannot be reached, as an aid to determine or evaluate therapy, and to establish a prognosis. Successful results of liver biopsy are most often obtained when diffuse hepatic diseases are involved (lipidosis, amyloidosis, glycogen storage diseases), or when diffuse necrosis and fibrosis exist, rather than with focal lesions, since the sample is small and is usually obtained by a blind technique.

Prior to performing liver biopsy, the clinician must be thoroughly familiar with the techniques available and be prepared to control any of the potential complications following biopsy (discussed below). As prebiopsy considerations, a complete clinical and laboratory evaluation must be performed and an activated clotting time determined. Impression smears and cultures of the biopsy material should be taken prior to fixation in formalin and may yield useful diagnostic information. Special stains for determining if fat or glycogen is present should be available.

Potential postbiopsy complications are bile peritonitis (following inadvertent penetration of the gallbladder or an engorged bile duct under pressure), hemorrhage, injury to other organs, and pneumothorax (Osborne et al., 1969). Patients should be kept quiet for 24 to 48 hours after biopsy, and the clinician should avoid any deep or excessive palpation. Any postbiopsy hemorrhage can usually be controlled by fresh, whole blood transfusions.

Needle biopsy is the most efficient in terms of time and is less expensive than other procedures available for obtaining hepatic tissue. The needles used most often are the Tru-Cut, Menghini, or modified Vim-Silverman (Osborne et al., 1974). The choice of needle or surgical approach depends largely on a clinician's preference rather than on scientific evidence. Aspiration needles like the Menghini have been considered to be less reliable for obtaining tissue from fibrotic livers and also generally obtain smaller samples. A recent study comparing the Menghini needle with the Tru-Cut indicates that except for greater fragmentation of samples, both needles obtained similar volumes of hepatic tissue and neither had better success in fibrotic livers.

Two recent reports summarized the results of a large number of liver biopsies obtained either by the transthoracic approach (Feldman and Ettinger, 1976; Feldman and Ettinger, 1977) or by a blind percutaneous transabdominal approach using a Menghini needle (Edwards, 1977). Of these 182 total cases only one mortality associated with the procedure was recorded. Significant complications were observed in six per cent, including six gallbladder punctures, of which two required surgery to

correct and four sealed spontaneously; biopsy of adjacent organs (three cases, no complications); one case of hemoperitoneum, which resolved with cage rest; and one case of transfer of ascites into the thorax through a diaphragmatic puncture, which was controlled using thoracentesis and diuretics. The histopathological results from these two studies are difficult to compare because of the variability between pathologists who read hepatic biopsies. The ten most frequent diagnoses were (1) steroid hepatopathy, which was reported by only one group (18.1 per cent) and which included both Cushing's disease and exogenous steroid administration; (2) normal liver tissue (15.9 per cent); (3) neoplasia (14.8 per cent); (4) inflammatory hepatitis, including chronic active hepatitis, which was diagnosed by only one group (14.8 per cent); (5) acute necrosis (11.5 per cent); (6) lipidosis (9.3 per cent); (7) no tissue obtained (6.0 per cent); (8) cholestasis (4.3 per cent); (9) cholangitis (2.2 per cent); and (10) cirrhosis (1.1 per cent). Twenty five of these 182 cases eventually had necropsies, and necropsy diagnoses correlated with the previous needle biopsies in 80 per cent of the cases. It is obvious that the biopsy information obtained in these cases significantly affected the prognosis and therapy of many of these animals, and this type of information was available by no other diagnostic means. Because proficiency at needle biopsy is easy to learn, veterinarians should strive to master this technique so that it can become a routine part of hepatic disease workups.

RADIOGRAPHY

Plain and contrast radiographs can be used to evaluate the liver in suspected cases of hepatic disease. If ascites is present, it must be removed prior to radiographic evaluation for consistently reliable results to be obtained. Survey films enable the size, shape, and position of the liver to be ascertained. Normal radiographic liver size has not been precisely determined, partly because of the great variability between dogs and partly because the liver changes position with respirations, positioning, obesity, and disease in adjacent organs (Ackerman and Silverman, 1977). Liver size is best evaluated in the lateral projection, because the liver shadow on the ventrodorsal view is often obscured by adjacent organs. In later-

moves caudally and, on expiration, cranially. The normal caudal liver margin on the lateral projection thus may shift approxial recumbency the diaphragmatic crura are very mobile. The dependent crus sags forward more than the upper crus, causing the liver to look larger in right lateral recumbency (Grandage, 1974). Respiratory movements also cause the liver to shift its position significantly. Upon inspiration the liver mately one centimeter cranially or caudally to the costal arch. Root (1974) has described in detail the radiographic changes that occur in association with liver enlargement. Hepatomegaly is not difficult to interpret. Reduced hepatic size, however, is often not fully appreciated radiographically. Microhepatia most often is seen with congenital vascular anomalies and the associated hepatic atrophy, or in chronic, fibrotic liver disease with scar tissue contracture and cellular collapse. Small livers can only be assessed by the position of adjacent organs or by pneumoperitoneography. When the liver is reduced in size, adjacent abdominal viscera—i.e., the stomach, pylorus, spleen, and duodenum — shift cranially. The stomach angle, rather than being vertical or angled slightly cranial to caudal, consists of the pylorus shifted cranially while the cardia remains fixed in its normal position. Putting a small quantity of gas (air) into the stomach with a stomach tube is an easy method of assessing the position of the caudal liver margin relative to the stomach.

Contrast angiography of the liver has received intense investigation as clinicians have become increasingly aware of the importance of congenital vascular anomalies as a clinical entity. Contrast angiography is at present the only dependable method of determining whether a vascular shunt exists and whether or not it is surgically correctable (Suter, 1975). In addition to identifying congenital vascular anomalies, angiography can determine if portal hypertension is due to intra- or extrahepatic portal vein obstruction and can aid in the diagnosis of hepatic and pancreatic neoplasia. Four radiographic techniques have been used to evaluate hepatic blood supply, cranial mesenteric arteriography, transabdominal splenoportography, operative mesenteric portography, and celiac arteriography. Of these techniques, splenoportography and cranial mesenteric angiography have provided the most information (Ewing et al., 1974). Splenoportography and cranial mesenteric portogra-

phy are the easiest techniques to use and do not require sophisticated radiographic equipment to perform. These will be discussed further in the section on portal vascular anomalies. Although the techniques for both oral and intravenous cholangiography have been well worked out in dogs and cats, they have very limited clinical usefulness because of the infrequency of obstructive biliary tract disease.

HEPATIC DISEASES

Because the liver is intimately involved with so many diverse metabolic functions within the body, any factors that significantly alter normal physiology will often produce hepatic damage. Such damage may result from multiple infectious, toxic, metabolic, degenerative, and neoplastic diseases. Hepatic disease may be primary, as with infectious canine hepatitis and leptospirosis, or secondary to such diseases as diabetes mellitus, hypothyroidism, and hyperadrenocorticism. Owing to the close association of the four functional units of the liver, preferential attack by specific agents on any one of them results, in time, with unavoidable damage to the others. Thus, the clinical and histologic picture is similar for many generalized hepatic disorders.

Unfortunately, much of the recent increase in knowledge of the diagnosis, etiology, and therapy of spontaneous hepatic diseases in dogs and cats is rather speculative, and a great deal still remains to be learned. The hepatic disease classification that follows is in certain respects arbitrary, as is generally true of manmade schemes for nature's diseases; nevertheless, it should enable the reader to organize his/her thoughts in a logical approach to patients with hepatic disease, with the ultimate goal of better patient care.

From a diagnostic and pathologic point of view, hepatic diseases tend to fall into one of three major categories: (1) diseases primarily characterized by hepatocellular necrosis or inflammation, (2) diseases characterized by cholestasis, and (3) diseases associated with hepatic atrophy or fibrosis (Cornelius, 1979).

INFLAMMATORY DISEASES

Inflammation or necrosis characterizes the majority of hepatic disorders diagnosed in clinical practice. Inflammation is defined as significant elevation in the enzymes associated with hepatocyte injury, serum ALT, serum AST, arginase, and others. Serum ALT is a very sensitive index of hepatic parenchymal injury, and most hepatic diseases that cause functional impairment show an increase in serum ALT. Inflammatory hepatopathies may be either infectious or noninfectious and acute or chronic in nature. Noninfectious inflammatory diseases predominate. Unfortunately, diagnosing a patient as having "hepatitis" does little towards establishing an etiologic diagnosis, nor does it help in terms of prognosis or therapy. Nearly all cases of significant inflammatory hepatic disease require biopsy for diagnostic specificity. Hematologic, biochemical, radiographic, and urinalysis data are not definitive enough in most inflammatory diseases.

Infectious Inflammatory Hepatic Diseases

The liver is prone to infection by a number of primary or secondary infectious agents. The adenovirus of infectious canine hepatitis and canine herpesvirus are the only known viral hepatic diseases in the dog; none are known to exist in the cat. These diseases are discussed in Chapter 27. In addition to viruses, the liver may be invaded by pyogenic and granulomatous bacteria, systemic fungi (blastomycosis, histoplasmosis, and coccidioidomycosis), protozoans (toxoplasmosis), spirochetes (leptospirosis), and parasites.

The canine liver harbors a normal resident bacterial population; however, only under exceptional circumstances is bacterial hepatitis a significant problem (Speaman et al., 1979). Infection may progress through the hematogenous and lymphatic routes, through the biliary system, and by direct extension from adjacent organs. Most adult dogs have one to several species of bacteria within their liver by 10 to 12 months of age, with *Clostridia spp* predominating (Cobb and McKay, 1962; Lykkegaard et al., 1974). Hepatic anaerobes develop pathological potential only if hepatic arterial blood supply is compromised, leading to hypoxic conditions within the liver. Death following hepatic artery ligation in the dog is prevented by administering broad spectrum antibiotics. Bacterial abscesses of the liver are rare, and diagnosis is extremely difficult, except by laparotomy or radiographic evidence of gas pockets within the liver caused by gas-forming organisms (Fig. 60–3).

Parasitic infestations of the liver do occur but are infrequently reported. Heavy infestations by trematodes have produced cirrhosis in the dog and cat. Reported species include *Opisthorchis felineus, Amphimerus pseudofelineus, Metorchis conjunctis, M. albidis*, and *Clonorchis sinensis* (Rothenbacher and Lindquist, 1963; Levine et al., 1958). Flukes invade the bile ducts and gallbladder, producing chronic cholangitis and eventually biliary cirrhosis. Cats are the most frequently affected species, probably owing to their ingestion of the suspected intermediate hosts (fish and snails). Most of the life cycles of these trematodes are unknown, and no proven therapeutic measures exist at present. Diagnosis is based on finding eggs in the stool or hepatic biopsy.

Dirofilariasis in dogs is infrequently associated with acute hepatic failure and death, a condition referred to as the vena cava syndrome. It is characterized by sudden weakness, bilirubinuria, hemoglobinuria, azotemia, marked elevation of BSP and serum ALT, and death. Large numbers of adult heartworms are found in both the pre- and postcava, and severe passive congestion of the liver is seen pathologically.

Systemic mycoses, particularly histoplasmosis, may cause significant hepatic pathology. Because these organisms are polysystemic in nature, the liver is usually but one of several organ systems invaded (pulmonary, skin, gastrointestinal, RE). From a diagnostic standpoint, the liver may assume prominence, since confirming the diagnosis of deep mycoses requires identification of the organism in tissue specimens. Hepatic biopsy is much less complicated and generally carries less risk than do intestinal biopsies. As such, the easiest access to RE cell–containing tissues may involve hepatic biopsy to establish an etiologic diagnosis.

Noninfectious Inflammatory Diseases

Noninfectious inflammatory hepatic diseases account for the majority of liver disease in clinical practice. They include injuries to the liver that are secondary to disease in other organs, i.e., acute pancreatitis or chronic inflammatory colitis, or that following severe trauma. They may also be related to primary liver disorders, such as chronic hepatitis/chronic active hepatitis,

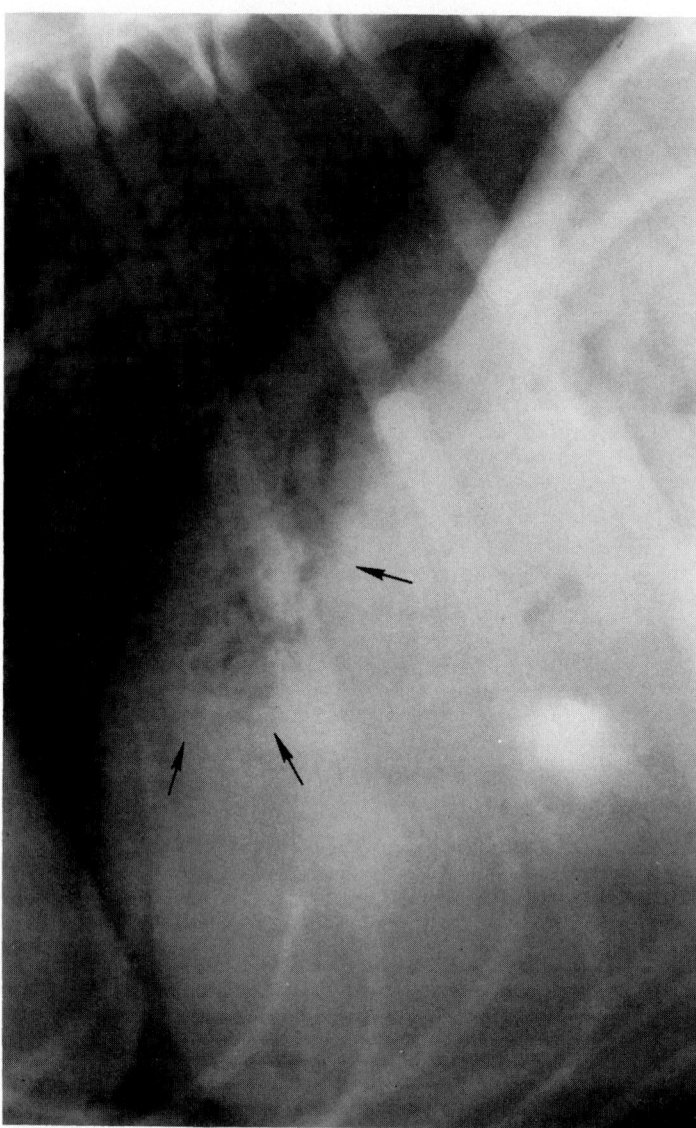

Figure 60–3. Abscess is visible within the liver because of gas produced by *Clostridia* organisms (arrows).

toxic and drug-induced hepatic disease, chronic copper toxicity of Bedlington terriers, and cirrhosis. Acute pancreatitis in the dog is commonly associated with hepatic injury. Typical lesions in experimental pancreatitis are hemorrhage, necrosis, and fatty infiltration (Tuzhilin et al., 1975). The severity of hepatic injury correlates with the duration of the pancreatitis. Lymphatic introduction of toxic products from the pancreas to the liver is considered responsible for most of the damage. The hepatic lesions are reversible once the pancreatitis is brought under control.

Chronic inflammatory bowel disease in man has a fairly high incidence of associated hepatic inflammatory disease (Dew et al.,

1979). The bowel disease most often associated with hepatic pathology is ulcerative colitis. Increases in serum AP are observed most often, and a pericholangitis is usually found pathologically. Therapy for colitis or colectomy has been associated with significant improvement in the hepatic abnormalities. Abdominal trauma may result in significant injury to the liver or biliary tract. In most cases in which only hepatic contusions have occurred without lacerations of parenchyma or biliary system, enzyme activity will be increased for several days, but repair should be complete. Lacerations of the liver can produce significant hemoperitoneum, which will require exploratory surgery to control. Rarely, the gallbladder or bile ducts may be torn, leading to bile peritonitis. If the bile remains sterile (as is often the case), the dog will tolerate the peritonitis well and the first abnormality noted may be abdominal distension. Septic bile peritonitis is a particularly aggressive disease, and it needs to be diagnosed and treated rapidly.

Chronic Hepatitis, Chronic Active Hepatitis

The spectrum of chronic inflammatory liver diseases in the dog is only just beginning to be clarified. A number of articles have recently appeared in the veterinary literature describing an entity called "chronic active hepatitis" (Bishop et al., 1979; Strombeck and Gribble, 1978; Meyer et al., 1980; Strombeck et al., 1976b). Attempts have been made to compare chronic active hepatitis (CAH) of man with a syndrome observed in the dog. Whether the etiology, pathogenesis, and therapy of these diseases are similar in the two species is still subject to debate.

The human disease known as CAH has been much refined in terms of diagnostic specificity in recent years. Originally, this disease was considered to occur primarily in females and to be of unknown etiology, progressive, and usually fatal. Affected individuals were often LE cell–positive and had increased concentrations of circulating antinuclear antibody (ANA) and antibodies to smooth muscle. Terms other than CAH used to describe the syndrome were lupoid hepatitis, autoimmune hepatitis, chronic aggressive hepatitis, and chronic persistent hepatitis (Redeker, 1981). Fortunately, this confusing game of semantics is improving. Chronic active liver disease is now considered to be composed of two major categories, CAH and chronic persistent hepatitis (Whitcomb, 1979). CAH is a potentially serious disorder that often progresses to macronodular cirrhosis, hepatic failure, and death. Chronic persistent hepatitis, in contrast, is a relatively benign disorder reflecting residual viral or drug-induced hepatic injury. Patients remain asymptomatic and are characterized by mild increases in transaminases, inflammation is confined to portal triads, necrosis is minimal, and the disease does not progress to cirrhosis.

CAH of man is characterized by a fairly distinct histologic picture and by dramatic increases in serum ALT for at least 12 weeks, with serum ALT concentrations remaining at five to ten times normal during this period. In addition, a number of immunologic abnormalities are often associated with CAH. Increased concentrations of IgG are almost always present; antibodies to smooth muscle, mitochondria, and nucleoproteins are present; LE cells are found in 30 per cent of patients; and antibody to hepatitis B surface antigens exist in 25 per cent of affected individuals. Although the exact cause of CAH in most human cases is unknown, viruses probably initiate ten to 30 per cent of cases and drugs may induce a significant number of others. Three therapeutic agents known to induce CAH are α-methyldopa, oxyphenisatin (found in some laxatives), and isoniazid (Eddleston and Williams, 1976; Zimmerman, 1979a). Withdrawal of these drugs leads to clinical improvement, while readministration initiates a rapid return of signs.

The pathogenesis of CAH in man, whether in the idiopathic, viral, or drug-induced cases, involves autoimmune reactions against hepatocytes and probably a genetic predisposition as well. Patients with CAH have a high incidence of a certain pattern of histocompatibility antigens. Until recently, only nonspecific autoantibodies had been detected in sera of patients with CAH. These included ANA, anti–smooth muscle, and anti-mitochondrial antibodies. Although nonspecific as to the tissue of origin, they are identified only rarely in inflammatory liver diseases other than CAH. They are thought to reflect a generalized immunologic abnormality rather than being responsible for the disease. However, the identification of antibodies to two liver-specific antigens in patients with CAH solidified the importance of autoimmunity to the pathogenesis of the disease. Antibodies against liver-specific cell surface lipoprotein antigens and a cytoplasmic "F" antigen have been consistently identified in patients with CAH but are rarely found in other forms of chronic inflammatory liver disease (Chen et al., 1979; Kakumu et al., 1979). Chronic immunization of rabbits with these two antigens in Freund's adjuvant leads to hepatic lesions typical of CAH (Glynn, 1976). *In vitro* culturing of hepatocytes from normal humans or laboratory animals with lymphocytes of patients with CAH results in lysis of the autologous or heterologous hepatocytes. Isolated hepatocytes from patients with

CAH have been shown to have membrane-fixed IgG on their surface, and an antibody dependent and immune complex-mediated cytotoxicity has been demonstrated against hepatocytes from CAH patients (Chen et al., 1979). EM studies of hepatocytes from these patients show lymphocytes closely attached to the liver cell surface, and fatal degenerative changes in the liver cell walls occur adajcent to these "killer" lymphocytes (Kawanishi, 1977).

The overall sequence of events leading to CAH is as follows. Some initiating event occurs that leads to injury to hepatocytes (viruses, drugs, others). Binding of drugs or their metabolites or viruses to the cell surface results in antibodies and sensitized lymphocytes being directed against these altered hepatocyte membranes, and eventually cellular death occurs. Once hepatocyte-specific antigens are released, additional immunologic reactions are initiated, leading to complement-mediated cytotoxic reactions, which may then be self-perpetuating. Such immunologic injury is critical in the early phases of the disease but may be of less importance in chronic phases. It is probable that vascular factors or changes in collagen formation are dominant factors late in the disease course (Eddleston and Williams, 1976).

Hepatic histopathology is essential to the diagnosis of CAH in man, but the lesions observed are not pathognomonic for this disease. Biopsy lesions must have been present for three months, although this time designation is somewhat arbitrary (Whitcomb, 1979). The lesions of CAH are characterized by bridging necrosis, piecemeal necrosis, and active cirrhosis. Inflammatory infiltrates are localized primarily to portal and periportal areas, with the primary cell types being lymphocytes, plasma cells, and eosinophils. Piecemeal necrosis involves the spread of inflammation, necrosis, and fibrosis from the portal triad area into the liver lobule, obscuring or destroying the limiting plate. Bridging necrosis involves an extension of the inflammatory process from portal triad to adjacent portal triads or central veins (Whitcomb, 1979). The diagnosis of CAH in man is based on fulfilling a number of criteria: (1) clinical data supporting active hepatic disease for 12 weeks or longer, (2) the presence of multiple immunologic abnormalities as described earlier, and (3) biopsy confirmation of typical histopatho-logical changes. Not all of these criteria have been confirmed to exist in dogs with so-called CAH.

Reports describing a canine disease resembling human CAH have appeared in the veterinary literature. A study of 11 cases by Strombeck and Gribble (1978) probably is the best documented report on a canine disease resembling CAH in humans. The clinical signs were typical of most liver diseases with primary complaints of depression, weakness, and anorexia in all dogs. Polydipsia and polyuria were observed in 8 of 11, jaundice in 6 of 11, vomiting in 5 of 11, ascites and/or weight loss in 4 of 11, hepatomegaly in 2 of 11, and encephalopathy in one animal. In general, transaminases were significantly increased (mean = 15 times normal), serum AP concentrations averaged five times normal and the total bilirubin was increased in 9 of 11 (mean = 2.6 mg/dl). BSP retention ranged from 6 to 48 per cent (mean = 33 per cent). Hypoalbuminemia and hypergammaglobulinemia were observed in only 3 of 11 animals. Again, hepatic biopsy alterations were used as the single confirmatory test to suggest a diagnosis of CAH in these dogs and also dictated whether glucocorticoid therapy was used to augment other supportive measures. Unfortunately, the typical lesions of CAH as it occurs in man do not represent unique morphologic changes in the dog. Piecemeal necrosis, bridging necrosis, and mononuclear cell infiltrates may be seen in canine liver disease that are not necessarily associated with immunologic injury and do not need steroid therapy for treatment. Because we are hampered diagnostically in terms of definite immunologic criteria similar to those of the human disease, it is very difficult to be certain that CAH actually exists in the dog at all, at least as it has been defined in man. This is particularly important in terms of therapy, because steroids and even immunosuppressive therapy are becoming more widely employed as part of a treatment schedule for canine inflammatory liver diseases with biopsy evidence of lymphocytes and plasma cells in areas of inflammation. Recent data in man suggest that steroids are harmful in hepatitis-B surface antigen positive patients with CAH (Lam et al., 1981; Redeker, 1981). It would seem wise for veterinarians to be prudent in their use of glucocorticoids in dogs suggested to have CAH until more data from controlled clinical trials are available. It is just as likely that steroids will be found to be harmful in many cases rather than clinically beneficial, as has been claimed.

The therapy of confirmed CAH is well defined in human medicine, but it has taken 20 years of controlled clinical trials to establish a rational treatment protocol. General supportive measures for the treatment of liver failure will be discussed in the section on therapy at the end of this chapter. Only those drugs that are unique to the therapy of CAH will be considered here. These drugs include steroids (glucocorticoids), immunosuppressants (azathioprine), and penicillamine. Steroids are used alone or in combination with azathioprine (Imuran). Dosages used in adults are 60 mg prednisone daily for one to two weeks, then 10 to 20 mg daily is administered until clinical, biochemical, and histologic evidence for remission has been obtained (Popper and Schaffner, 1976; Summerskill et al., 1975; Whitcomb, 1979). Clinical signs often require six months for remission, biochemical and immunologic abnormalities require 12 months, and histologic improvement often requires 12 to 24 months to resolve. Biopsies are performed at six-month intervals until morphologic resolution is complete. Steroid administration is often necessary on a daily basis for two years or more. In order to reduce steroid side effects in man, a combination of 10 mg prednisone and 50 mg azathioprine once daily has been evaluated. This combination had therapeutic effectiveness identical to that of large steroid dosages. Azathioprine alone had no better response than the placebo. Once complete remission has occurred, drugs are slowly withdrawn for six weeks. If relapses are noted, patients are started back on maintenance therapy. Relapses are particularly prominent if cirrhosis or bridging necrosis is present on initial biopsy. Cyclophosphamide was also evaluated for potential use in CAH. It had no benefit over placebo. It is interesting to note that four of ten human patients receiving placebo alone underwent complete clinical remissions (Gilmore et al., 1979). Of particular importance is the recent observation that when steroids are administered to humans with hepatitis B–associated CAH, they have increased incidences of biochemical relapses, more complications, and higher death rates than if given placebo alone (Lam et al., 1981).

This further stresses the importance of critically defining the criteria for instituting steroid therapy in dogs suspected of having CAH. In addition to steroids, penicillamine has had limited clinical trials as an antifibrosis drug in CAH (Chen. et al., 1979; Popper and Schaffner, 1976). Penicillamine inhibits collagen synthesis, causes reductions in IgM and circulating immune complexes, and may inhibit cell-mediated immunity. Steroids have not been effective in reversing or delaying hepatic fibrosis in human CAH, while penicillamine has been shown to have a beneficial effect.

Only one report of clinical usage of steroids in canine CAH has appeared (Strombeck and Gribble, 1978). Five of nine dogs treated were considered to have improved. However, since multiple approaches to therapy were used on this group of dogs, and since no control group in which steroids were withheld was evaluated, conclusions regarding the efficacy of steroids in CAH in dogs remain speculative, at best. Recommended dosages were 1 to 2 mg/kg body weight per day of prednisone until clinical remission occurred, and then reduced dosages of 0.4 mg/kg body weight or less were given.

TOXIC AND DRUG-INDUCED LIVER DISEASE

Toxic Liver Disease

The liver is subject to damage by a wide variety of chemical products by virtue of its central role in metabolism and detoxification of the body. Hepatotoxins are agents that cause a predictable pattern of hepatic damage in animals, usually associated with a short latent period (Jeffries, 1971). Some of the more common toxins are chemicals and heavy metals, e.g., copper, iron, selenium, arsenic, phosphorus, mercury, chloroform, chlordane, dieldrin, tannic acid, tetrachlorethylene, trinitrotoluene, cinchophen, tetrachlorethane, dimethylnitrosamine, carbon tetrachloride, coal tar pitch, and gossypol. Certain plants, especially those associated with fungal growth and aflatoxin production (moldy corn poisoning), and metabolic or nutritional deficiencies (i.e., methionine, and choline) also produce toxic hepatitis (Smith et al., 1972). In cases of severe, acute, diffuse toxic reactions, the animal only survives a few days, as most of the hepatocytes are injured.

In others, complete recovery may be possible. Certain toxins associated with nutritional deficiencies may develop so slowly that no acute signs are seen, and chronic fibrotic liver disease is the first indication that a toxic process is present. Hepatotoxins may cause necrosis of parenchymal cells and its sequelae, biochemical evidence of disease, or morphologic alterations in the liver, e.g., lipidosis or fibrosis.

Multiple factors appear to predispose an animal to toxic liver injury. Individual host susceptibility is related to the animal's sex and nutritional status. Females appear to be more susceptible to hepatotoxins than males, while diets high in fat increase the toxic effect of many poisons, especially lipid-soluble ones (Jubb and Kennedy, 1970). Diets deficient in carbohydrate and protein also increase the animal's susceptibility to toxic damage. Diets adequate in quantity and quality of protein, specifically the lipotrophic substances methionine and choline, protect against carbon tetrachloride and chloroform injury. Other factors that determine host response to toxic agents are dose, duration of exposure, and type of agent. The duration of exposure is critical with toxins that have a cumulative effect, and exposure may require weeks for effects to be seen. Once hepatocellular necrosis begins, it is resolved with fibrosis, a process that may be self-perpetuating even if the agent is no longer present.

Drug-Induced Liver Disease

Drug-induced liver injury is merely one spectrum of toxic hepatitis. While we commonly do not associate hepatic injury with the use of therapeutic agents, drug-induced liver disease accounts for five per cent of all jaundice cases in man (Zimmerman, 1978). Drugs are an even more important cause of severe acute hepatic failure in man, as 25 per cent of all cases of acute hepatic failure are associated with drug reactions. In fact, Mitchell and Potter (1975) indicate that hepatic drug reactions are expected from all new drugs introduced into medicine. Acute drug-related hepatic injury typically manifests itself as cytoxic, cholestatic, or mixed. Cytoxic reactions induce either necrosis or steatosis. In general, cytotoxic injury carries a much more grave prognosis than do cholestatic types of injury, although cholestasis may be very chronic (Zimmerman, 1975).

Following chronic drug administration, neoplasias may develop. Histopathologic entities caused by drugs include CAH, steatosis, cirrhosis, fibrosis, hepatoportal sclerosis, hepatic vein thrombosis, adenomas, carcinomas, and angiosarcomas (Zimmerman, 1978). Two major factors appear to determine why the liver is so often involved in adverse drug reactions. The first relates to the central role of the liver in drug metabolism. Hepatocytes metabolically alter stable chemical compounds to potent alkylating, arylating, or acetylating agents that are toxic to the liver. Second, because the liver is anatomically situated between the venous effluent of the intestinal tract and the systemic circulation, noxious compounds gain access to the liver prior to the rest of the body being exposed (Mitchell and Potter, 1975). Preexisting hepatic disease was once considered to be important in determining whether a drug toxicity developed. Clinical observations in man tend to suggest that this is not the case. The recognition that drug-induced hepatic injury is taking place in nonjaundiced patients is difficult. For such injury to be documented, all patients receiving drugs must be biochemically monitored. Even if slight damage is detected, unless it is likely to progress to more severe injury, such monitoring is questionable (Zimmerman, 1978). This is the dilemma faced by practitioners. It is highly probable that adverse drug reactions involving the liver are occurring frequently in clinical practice, but unless one is aware of the probability of such occurrences and attempts to document them, veterinary medicine will be no better off in 20 years than it is today, in terms of recognizing and correcting drug-induced liver disease.

Drugs may be classified as either intrinsic (predictable) hepatotoxins or idiosyncratic (unpredictable) hepatoxins (Schaffner and Popper, 1977; Zimmerman, 1975). Intrinsic hepatotoxins are further classified as direct or indirect, according to the way they induce hepatic injury. Intrinsic direct hepatotoxins induce injury primarily by damaging the structural integrity of the hepatocyte, which then leads to functional and metabolic changes. Such drugs were essentially eliminated from clinical use, once their toxicity was identified, for example, carbon tetrachloride, chloroform, and tannic acid. Intrinsic indirect hepatotoxins selectively block essential metabolic pathways and, by inducing specific biochemical injuries, lead secondarily to structural changes. Indirect hepatotoxins may be either cytoxic or cholestatic. Important indirect hepatotoxins in man include methotrexate, ethanol, tetracycline, paromycin, L-asparaginase, azaserine, azacytidine, azauridine, acetaminophen, urethane, 6-mercaptopurine, mithramycin, contraceptive steroids, C-17 alkylated steroids, lithocholic acid, flavaspidic acid, cholecystographic dyes, rifampicin, and novobiocin (Zimmerman, 1978). Characteristics of intrinsic hepatotoxins, whether direct or indirect, include (1) a high incidence of injury in an exposed population, (2) a dose-dependent toxic effect, and (3) injury is usually produced in experimental animals.

Idiosyncratic (unpredictable) hepatotoxins differ from intrinsic hepatotoxins in several ways (Schaffner and Popper, 1977; Zimmerman, 1978). Detectable hepatic injury occurs in very few individuals given the drug (< one per cent); little, if any, dose dependency for toxicity is present; and toxic injury is rarely reproduced in experimental animals. This particular group of hepatotoxins is very difficult to identify and to substantiate that they are actually responsible for disease because they require widespread usage before sufficient numbers of toxic events are recognized. The proposed mechanism of injury with these drugs is both immunologic and metabolic in nature. Hypersensitivity-type reactions occur following the administration of some drugs. Polysystemic allergic reactions such as fever, rash, and eosinophilia accompany the hepatic disease. Hepatic lesions often have a heavy eosinophilic infiltrate or granulomas present. "Allergic"-type drug reactions typically have a relatively short sensitization period of one to four weeks, and prompt recurrence of jaundice or hepatocellular injury follows readministration of small doses of the drug. In some cases hepatic pathology appears only after months of therapy. Such a situation occurs following isoniazide, oxyphenisatin, or α-methyldopa administration (Schaffner and Popper, 1977). The latter three drugs have already been mentioned as causes of CAH. Provided these drugs are withdrawn immediately upon the detection of hepatic injury, the CAH lesions are totally resolvable with drug withdrawal alone and steroids are not required. Metabolic aberrations also are responsible for hepatic injury with some idiosyncratic hepatotoxins. Some drugs are metabolized to toxic products in susceptible individuals. Such metabolites are proposed to exist in higher concentrations or to persist for prolonged periods in genetically or environmentally predisposed individuals. The sensitization period for idiosyncratic hepatotoxins that cause metabolic abnormalities may be weeks to 12 months or more, and the response to challenge doses of the drug may not be evident for many days or weeks (Zimmerman, 1978). Acetaminophen (Tylenol) and furosemide in massive doses may lead to increases in toxic intermediates that induce hepatic injury (Mitchell and Potter, 1975).

Drug toxicity should be suspected in all cases of unexplained jaundice or inflammatory liver disease. A history of exposure, a characteristic clinical picture, and documentation of other supportive evidence of a toxic injury is necessary. Recurrence of hyperbilirubinemia following a test dose of the drug is highly suggestive of its role in cholestatic diseases; however, only 40 to 60 per cent of patients with drug induced cholestasis develop jaundice following a single test dose of the suspected drug (Zimmerman, 1975). Challenge testing should be restricted to drugs whose primary pathology is cholestasis, in which only one dose is administered and the patient is likely to require the drug again. Drug testing of agents known to induce cytotoxic reactions could produce serious hepatocellular injury and is not warranted unless the patient is likely to need the drug again (phenytoin, isoniazid).

Reports of confirmed or suspected hepatotoxic drug reactions in companion animals are extremely uncommon. Compounds reported to induce hepatic injury in dogs and cats include arsenicals, phenytoin, primidone, glucocorticoids, metophane, mebendazole, tolbutamide, phenazopyridine, and acetaminophen. All these drugs produce a cytotoxic injury or combined cytotoxic and cholestatic injury. No references have been found regarding a purely cholestatic jaundice induced by drugs in dogs and cats. Inhalant anesthetics have been associated with fulminant hepatic failure in man following repeated exposures. Similar reports in the veterinary literature are meager and circumstantial. Ndiritu and Weigel (1977) reported a dog with fulminant hepatic necrosis following multiple anesthesias with methoxyflurane. Lesions seen at necropsy were suggestive of those observed in humans with idiosyncratic halothane or methoxyflurane-associated hepatic toxicity. Anticonvulsants, particularly phenytoin and primidone, are known to induce hepatic enzyme changes in many dogs (Meyer and Noonan, 1981). Whether such biochemical alterations result in significant functional impairment is open to question. Acute hepatic failure has been reported in a dog on long-term primidone therapy that had a five-day course of phenytoin added to the other drug. Acute toxicity was proposed as the cause of the hepatic failure (Nash, 1977). Of particular importance is the report of acute hepatic failure associated with the use of mebendazole in dogs (Polzin et al., 1981). Of nine dogs administered the drug in a kennel, two died and four had biochemical and clinical evidence of mild to severe hepatic disease. Signs of vomiting, depression, anorexia, and jaundice appear following single or repeat administrations of the drug. Forty-five additional cases of possible adverse drug reactions to mebendazole have been reported to the Food and Drug Administration. Biochemical evaluations were done on 34 of the 45 dogs, and all had increased serum ALT concentrations. This drug is most likely an indirect, intrinsic hepatotoxin with a low order of toxicity. Other infrequently used therapeutic agents can induce hepatic failure in dogs and cats. Tolbutamide, an oral hypoglycemic agent used to control mild diabetes in man, is hepatotoxic to dogs at doses over 65 mg/kg body weight and should not be used except for diagnostic purposes (Wilson and Wilson, 1970). Lastly, two drugs have been reported to induce hepatotoxicity in cats, acetaminophen (Tylenol) and phenazopyridine. Acetaminophen induces methemoglobinemia and increases serum ALT in cats, and should not be used as an anti-inflammatory drug in cats (St. Omar and McKnight, 1980). Phenazopyridine, a human urinary tract analgesic, was administered to a cat with feline urologic syndrome. The cat developed a Heinz body hemolytic anemia and hepatic injuries and died. The hepatic injuries were mild but probably contributed to the cat's death (Harvey and Kornick, 1976).

Therapy of drug-induced hepatic disease is primarily supportive. Major goals involve removing the offending drug, providing supportive care, and waiting for the resolution of a self-limited bout of necrosis (Black, 1979). General principles of supportive care will be covered in the section on hepatic therapy.

Copper-Associated Hepatitis in Bedlington Terriers

Bedlington terriers have a unique, genetically predisposed liver disease that is caused by marked accumulation of copper within hepatocytes. This disorder was first described by Hardy et al., in 1975. Although the disease is inherited as an autosomal recessive trait (Johnson et al., 1980), its prevalence within this breed appears to be quite high. Of 144 Bedlingtons screened, 66 per cent had biochemical and /or histologic evidence of hepatic pathology.

Clinical signs and physical findings associated with Bedlington liver disease are highly variable. Affected dogs generally can be divided into one of three groups. The first group includes young adults of either sex. They have a relatively short, often fulminant clinical course, in which the onset of signs frequently follows some stressful event (whelping, showing). The second group has a more chronic course, typical of slowly progressive, hepatic disease. The third group is clinically asymptomatic, and suspicion of hepatic disease is based on biochemical evidence of active hepatocellular damage or necrosis, i.e., elevated serum ALT or biopsy abnormalities.

Animals in the first group tend to be young (two to six years of age) and usually have had no apparent illnesses prior to the onset of hepatic failure. The association of stress preceding the illness, as observed by breeders, appears to be a valid one. Female Bedlington terriers are particularly prone to acute hepatic failure within a few weeks of whelping.

Signs exhibited by the dogs are relatively nonspecific. They include depression, lethargy, anorexia, and vomiting, all of acute onset. Jaundice tends to be prominent in the more severely affected dogs, appearing one to two days following the onset of signs. Another physical finding of localizing value is hepatomegaly. Generally, biochemical profiles are necessary to confirm the existence of hepatic failure. A less common but more dramatic physical finding is severe hemolytic anemia. It is characterized by a rapid fall in packed cell volume, severe jaundice, hemoglobinemia, and hemoglobinuria. Serum copper concentrations have been noted to elevate dramatically during the hemolytic crisis.

The acute hepatic failure group is characterized by high mortality in spite of massive supportive care. Death may occur within 48 to 72 hours following the onset of signs. Animals surviving an acute attack may remain clinically asymptomatic for years or suffer recurrent attacks of a similar but less severe nature later in life.

The second group of animals is composed of middle-aged to older dogs. Their clinical signs are similar to, although less severe than, those of the first group. Appropriately, chronic weight loss and ascites may be evident. Previous attacks of acute hepatitis have generally not been observed or recognized. The liver is nonpalpable and will appear reduced in size radiographically.

The third group is an arbitrary one, composed of clinically normal but affected dogs. This group is only detected via abnormal biochemical tests (serum ALT) and/or biopsy evidence characteristic of the disease. This segment of the Bedlington terrier population probably represents younger dogs that have not experienced an acute crisis or the preclinical stages of the chronic progressive group. Until large numbers of Bedlington terriers were screened for evidence of hepatic disease, this group went undetected.

The pathogenesis of this disease is not completely understood, but of primary importance is the progressive accumulation of dietary copper within hepatocytes. Copper is known to be hepatotoxic once significant intracellular concentrations develop. In affected Bedlingtons, hepatic copper concentrations may be increased by 8 to 12 weeks of age or require as long as one year for pathologic increases to be detected. Generally, hepatic copper concentrations continue to increase until the dogs reach five to six years of age; after that time, assuming the dog does not die of acute failure, hepatic copper levels slowly decline but never return to normal (Ludwig et al., 1980; Twedt et al., 1979). Normal hepatic copper concentrations range from 91 to 377 μg/gm on a dry weight basis. From a diagnostic standpoint, dogs are considered to be affected if hepatic copper concentrations exceed 350 μg/gm on a dry weight basis. Most affected Bedlingtons have hepatic copper concentrations 5 to 50 times normal. The copper accumulates within lysosomes of hepatocytes and gives them a somewhat characteristic histologic picture (Fig. 60–4). Hepatic copper concentrations above 2000 μg/gm dry weight have been consistently associated with signs of progressive disease both morphologically and functionally (Twedt et al., 1979).

The mechanism by which copper continues to accumulate in these dogs is unknown. It is theorized that dogs remain relatively asymptomatic until the ability of hepatic lysosomes to store copper is exhausted. Once the lysosomal storage capacity is exceeded, copper is released to the cytoplasm of the hepatocytes, where it becomes toxic. When massive numbers of hepatocytes undergo rapid lysis, large quantities of copper

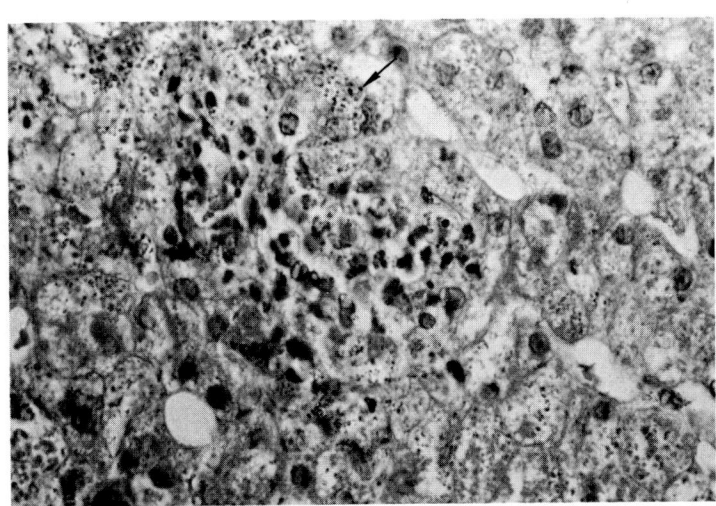

Figure 60–4. Foci of neutrophils associated with necrotic hepatocytes in a liver biopsy from a Bedlington terrier with a copper storage disease. Large copper-containing lysosomal granules are prominent throughout the specimen (arrow). ×320.

are released to the circulation. This phenomenon has occasionally been associated with acute hemolytic crises.

Initial clinical, biochemical, and histologic findings in the disease strongly resemble an inherited human disorder, Wilson's disease (hepatolenticular degeneration). Although many features of these two disorders are similar, enough differences exist such that they are no longer considered identical genetic disorders. Nonetheless, the canine disease has served as a valuable biomedical model for copper storage disorders of man.

A definitive diagnosis of this disease requires liver biopsy. Occasionally, biopsy and quantitative hepatic copper assays are necessary. Biochemical evidence of hepatocellular inflammation, i.e., a rise in serum ALT, is only suggestive of the disease. Conversely, a normal serum ALT does not rule out Bedlington liver disease, since significant numbers of affected dogs confirmed by biopsy have normal serum ALT concentrations. Histologically, these livers vary greatly in terms of lesions observed. Some dogs have no structural injury present, the only pathology being increased copper concentrations as determined histochemically. More severe pathology is indicated by focal hepatitis, which progresses to lesions identical to those described for chronic active hepatitis and ultimately leads to micro- or macronodular cirrhosis. Hepatocyte cytoplasm contains numerous brownish eosinophilic granules that react strongly to three stains used to detect copper (rubeanic, Timm's, and rhodanine). In cases in which histochemical determination of hepatic copper content is equivocal, quantitative copper assay is the only way to confirm a diagnosis.

Therapy of this disorder is both specific and symptomatic. This is one of only a few hepatic diseases wherein a specific mode of therapy exists. Drugs thought to have a beneficial effect in this disease include D-penicillamine, glucocorticoids, and ascorbic acid. D-Penicillamine is the only one of this group for which objective data are available to substantiate its efficacy. This drug has been used for years to treat Wilson's disease, and its beneficial effects are thought due to its ability to chelate copper within the circulation; the copper is ultimately eliminated in urine. Quantitative hepatic copper concentrations from an affected dog treated 26 months with D-penicillamine were reduced from 5298 μg/gm to 228 μg/gm dry weight (Ludwig et al., 1980). Recommended dosages are 125 to 250 mg per day in adult dogs, given 30 minutes prior to feeding. No toxic side effect except vomiting has been observed in dogs treated for over three years. Dividing the total daily dose into two to three doses will usually stop any vomiting problems. Corticosteroids, because of their lysosomal stabilizing effect, may be useful in this disease, particularly in acute crisis states; administration of 0.5 to 1.0 mg/kg body weight per day may be useful in acute therapy. Ascorbic acid is known to augment copper excretion in urine. Dosages have been empirical, 500 to 1000 mg/day being administered. Other therapy used for these patients is supportive and symptomatic. Objective evidence of therapeutic efficacy — reduction in serum ALT or hepatic copper content — often requires weeks or months of continuous therapy. Clinical improvement, however, is frequently seen much more quickly. Patients often gain weight, improve in activity, condition, and alertness in a few weeks. No objective criteria have as yet been established for determining which affected Bedlingtons should receive therapy with D-penicillamine. The author routinely initiates therapy in any dogs that have had one attack of liver disease and are not exhibiting gastrointestinal signs. Therapy is also indicated in asymptomatic dogs with persistently increased serum ALT concentrations of 300 to 400 IU or higher, as an attempt to prevent an acute crisis. At this time, the author recommends treating such dogs for life on the premise that hepatic injury will continue unless therapy is maintained.

Cirrhosis

Cirrhosis should be considered the end stage of many inflammatory hepatic diseases. It is the end result of multiple pathologic processes affecting the liver. No universally accepted definition for cirrhosis exists. Jubb and Kennedy (1970) and Smith et al. (1972) characterize cirrhosis by the presence of widespread hepatic fibrosis or scarring. Cirrhotic livers typically have diffuse increases in connective tissue associated with varying degrees of necrosis and attempts at parenchymal cell regeneration. The result is loss of normal hepatic lobular architecture and development of multiple fine to coarse regenerative nodules separated by connective tissue septae. Often, the pathological appearance of an end-stage liver gives little clue to the initiating factors responsible for its failure. Many different agents or processes can produce a similar gross and histologic picture. Cirrhosis tends to be an active, chronic, and progressive disease that ultimately leads to hepatic failure and death.

Because of the factors mentioned previously, the etiology of cirrhosis is undetermined in the majority of cases. Known causes may originally be of acute toxic origin, or secondary to chronic drug administration when inflammation progresses to cirrhosis. Regenerative nodules expand and compress sinusoids and bile ducts at their periphery, producing further anoxia and cholestasis. As fibrous scar tissue contraction occurs, anoxic conditions result, producing new areas of necrosis, which stimulate further fibrosis, thus perpetuating the process. It is interesting to speculate on the role of viral infections in this process. Gocke et al. (1970) have described the experimental production of cirrhosis by ICH virus in partially immune dogs. A form of chronic active hepatitis was produced in several dogs that eventually developed cirrhosis. Chronic biliary tract disease also will eventually result in parenchymal cell death, scarring, and cirrhosis if unresolved.

Animals with congestive heart failure and chronic passive congestion develop a mild degree of "cardiac cirrhosis." Anoxia and centrolobular necrosis are thought to be responsible for the changes observed. Other causes of chronic passive congestion are dirofilariasis and heart base tumors. Ascites will develop in advanced cases, but jaundice is rare. Rarely will hepatic failure result from chronic passive congestion. The animal usually succumbs to the primary disease prior to liver failure. Laboratory evaluations usually indicate a mild hyperbilirubinemia, slightly increased serum ALT (240 SFU) and serum AP concentrations, and mild BSP retention (Ettinger and Suter, 1970).

Autoimmune reactions are increasingly incriminated as causative factors in chronic active hepatitis in man, in which the term "lupoid hepatitis" has developed. The possibility of autoimmune disease being responsible for initiating or perpetuating some cases of active hepatitis and cirrhosis in

animals needs continued investigation. Recent reports of a CAH-like condition in dogs suggests that such diseases may progress to cirrhosis.

Nutritional factors are known to be important in the development of cirrhosis (see discussion, pp. 1385–1388).

There is a frequent association of cirrhosis with diabetes mellitus in man. Hepatic disease is also a common complication of diabetes in animals. Statistical studies in man have indicated that the cirrhosis most likely precedes the development of diabetes mellitus in the majority of the cases studied (Conn et al., 1969). The changes seen in hepatic cirrhosis predispose to persistent mild hyperglycemia and to the subsequent development of diabetes mellitus.

The clinical manifestations of cirrhosis are impaired liver function, jaundice, portal hypertension, and ascites. There is little unique to the clinical presentation of cirrhotic dogs, except their signs are more typical of chronic than acute hepatic failure. The onset of signs is generally gradual, taking weeks or months for owners to appreciate that serious disease is present. Evidence of marked weight loss and ascites is often noted. Signs of CNS derangement other than depression, anorexia, lethargy, polydipsia, and polyuria are very uncommon. Rare animals will have encephalopathy characterized by dementia, circling, pacing, amaurotic blindness, and ultimately, coma.

Diagnostic information in cirrhotic dogs is fairly typical, although great individual variation from this characteristic pattern may be noted. Biochemical evidence of inflammation is nearly always present but may be mild. In very advanced cases, serum ALT concentrations may be normal, presumably because few residual hepatocytes remain. Alkaline phosphatase concentrations are also increased, often in the moderate to severe range. Hyperbilirubinemia is inconsistent and depends on the location of lesions within the liver. Biochemical evidence of functional derangements typify end-stage livers. Serum albumin concentrations become depressed, often less than 2 gm/dl. BSP retention, ten to 30 per cent in 30 minutes is common, probably reflecting altered hepatic blood flow that typifies these disorders. Ammonia tolerance test results have been too few for generalities to be made. The author has found them generally to be normal in dogs with severe failure without signs of coma but abnormal in those few cirrhotics that have signs of cerebral dysfunction. Radiographs are helpful, as they often demonstrate a small liver. In acquired hepatic disorders, microhepatica generally reflects progressive fibrosis and scar tissue contraction, along with loss of parenchymal tissue. Small livers generally warrant a poor prognosis.

Therapy for cirrhosis generally involves supportive and symptomatic care, as the lack of an etiology and advanced stage of the disease usually precludes specific therapy from being beneficial. These will be discussed later.

NONINFLAMMATORY HEPATIC DISEASES

Noninflammatory hepatic diseases, although less frequent than inflammatory ones, form an important group of clinical disorders. They often differ dramatically from inflammatory hepatic diseases in terms of diagnosis, prognosis, and therapy. Disorders to be considered include (1) portal vascular anomalies, (2) congenital urea cycle enzyme deficiencies, (3) steroid hepatopathy, (4) lipidosis, (5) amyloidosis, and (6) glycogenosis.

Portal Vascular Anomalies

Numerous reports of congenital portal vascular anomalies in both dogs and cats

have appeared since 1974 (Audell et al., 1974; Barrett et al., 1976; Cornelius et al., 1975; Ewing et al., 1974; Lohse et al., 1976; Maretta et al., 1981; Simpson and Hribernik, 1976; Valgamott et al., 1981). The spectrum of disease induced by these anomalies is very diverse, and clinicians must be constantly alert to avoid missing portal systemic shunts (PSS) in clinical practice. Congenital portal systemic shunts develop between the portal vein and major systemic veins, so that blood from the intestinal tract bypasses hepatic parenchyma and enters the systemic circulation. To date, five major types of shunt have been recognized: (1) patent ductus venosus, (2) portal vein atresia with development of multiple collateral portal systemic communications, (3) drainage of the portal vein into the caudal vena cava (portal-caval shunt), (4) drainage of the portal vein into the azygous vein, and (5) drainage of the portal vein and caudal vena cava into the azygous vein with discontinuation of the prerenal post cava (Fig. 60–5). Diversion of portal blood around or through (patent ductus venosus) the liver leads to hepatic atrophy. The severity of clinical signs depends on the volume of blood shunted and the location of the shunting vessels. Blood draining the gastric, pancreatic, duodenal, and splenic areas is most critical for normal hepatic growth. Insulin plays a particularly important hepatotropic role, although other nonpancreatic factors are also necessary (Starzl et al., 1975; Starzl

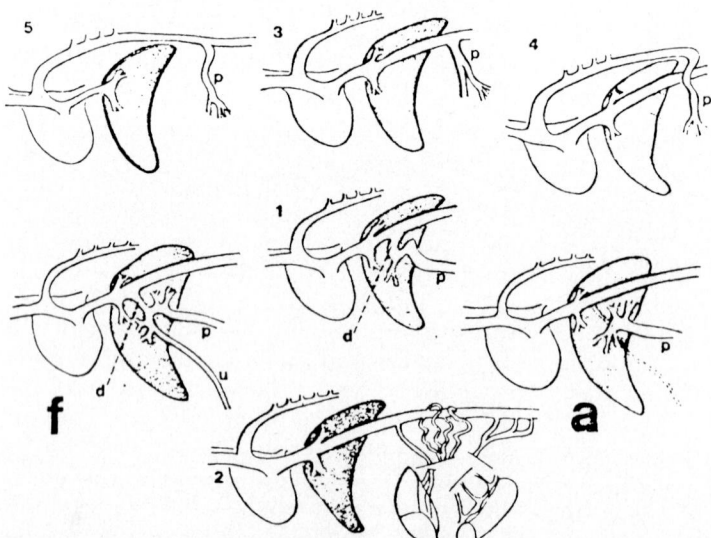

Figure 60–5. The five types of congenital portal vein anomalies found in dogs. In addition, the normal fetal (*f*) and adult (*a*) portal systems are illustrated. In the fetus, the umbilical vein (u) perfuses the liver, but most of its volume is diverted through the ductus venosus (d) to the fetal heart. Soon after birth, the umbilical vein and ductus venosus atrophy. Portal vein blood (p) then perfuses hepatic sinusoids completely, being collected by the hepatic veins. The abnormal portal systemic shunts are (1) patent ductus venosus (d) with or without a hypoplastic portal system; (2) portal vein atresia, associated with the development of multiple portopostcaval anastomoses; (3) major solitary portopostcaval anastomosis; (4) isolated, major portal azygous shunt; (5) Portal azygous shunt with discontinuation of the prerenal segment of the caudal vena cava. (Reprinted with permission, Suter, P. F., Portal vein anomalies in the dog: their angiographic diagnosis. J. Amer. Vet. Radiol. Soc., *16*:84–97, 1975.)

and Terblanche, 1976). Thus, clinical signs and hepatic atrophy are most severe in animals with gastroduodenal-pancreatic venous shunting.

Clinical signs in dogs with PSS are highly variable, but all result from hepatic encephalopathy or progressive functional impairment. In many cases the clinical signs have an episodic nature, being present for a few hours or a day or two, with the animal then "recovering" for a variable period of time. The association of clinical signs with eating, particularly high protein meals, is helpful diagnostically. Such an association is inconsistent, at best, however. The majority of animals have been diagnosed under one year of age, but dogs over eight years old have also been reported with congenital anomalies of the portal vascular system. No breed or sex predisposition has been identified. Many dogs are reported to be stunted, and many have difficulty gaining weight, are depressed or weak, and generally are in poor physical condition. One term that summarizes many of these animals is that they are "chronic poor doers." Gastrointestinal signs are often noted but usually are mild; these include vomiting, diarrhea, and anorexia. Central nervous system signs may be the best diagnostic clue for the clinician. When present, such signs become almost pathognomonic for these anomalies. Particularly bizarre behavioral changes or dementia characterized by hysteria, unpredictable bouts of aggression, staggering, head pressing, circling or pacing, amaurotic (cortical) blindness, or coma should put PSS high on a rule-out list. Grand mal seizures and intermittent ataxia or incoordination have also been reported. Signs of less localizing value include polydipsia and polyuria, ascites, and anesthetic/tranquilizer intolerance. Recently, a report stressing the importance of recurrent urinary calculi as one additional type of symptomatology has appeared (Maretta et al., 1981). In one of the six cases reported, the primary complaint was that of recurrent bladder calculi unassociated with other significant signs. Physical examination of these animals is usually unrewarding. The most severely affected dogs are stunted and thin to the point of cachexia, and may have ascites, but there is little of localizing value in such findings. If a patient exhibits signs of dementia as described, however, PSS becomes a very real probability.

The diagnosis of portal vascular anomalies may require a combination of hematologic, biochemical, urinalysis, and radiographic evaluations. Hematologic data are generally nonspecific. Mild anemia is present in approximately 25 per cent of the dogs, and it may be microcytic and hypochromic. Impaired iron uptake and utilization and deficient hemoglobin synthesis have been noted in experimental dogs with portal-caval shunts (Ewing et al., 1974). The author has observed marked increases in target cells in dogs with PSS (Fig. 60–6). This finding is uncommon in other clinical diseases. One of the most consistent abnormalities is a reduction in total plasma proteins as estimated with a refractometer, often in the range of 4 to 5 gm/dl.

Biochemical data, although not providing a definitive diagnosis, does provide significant evidence that hepatic failure is present. This disease is fairly unique in that routine screening tests of hepatic disease — i.e., serum ALT and serum AP — are either normal or only slightly increased. This reflects the type of pathology in the liver, primarily atrophy, secondary to reduced hepatic portal perfusion, rather than any inflammatory process. Total serum bilirubin and urine bilirubin are within normal limits. No significant cholestasis develops in this disorder. Biochemical tests that have the greatest diagnostic value are those that assess the functional capacity of the liver, such as BSP, ammonia tolerance, serum albumin, uric acid, total cholesterol, BUN, and glucose. BSP retention and ammonia tolerance are the two most useful biochemical tests for supporting a diagnosis. Nearly all dogs with PSS have mild to severely increased BSP retention. Some may be between five and ten per cent, however, which is in the equivocal diagnostic range. The ammonia tolerance test has been consistently abnormal in all dogs with PSS in the author's clinic, and no false negatives have been reported in the literature. If dogs are symptomatic, only a resting blood ammonia is necessary, and a challenge test could precipitate more severe encephalopathy. In the absence of signs of encephalopathy, however, an exogenous ammonia load is administered because some dogs with PSS have normal fasting blood ammonia concentrations, and inability to efficiently clear portal blood ammonia is only detected upon oral challenge.

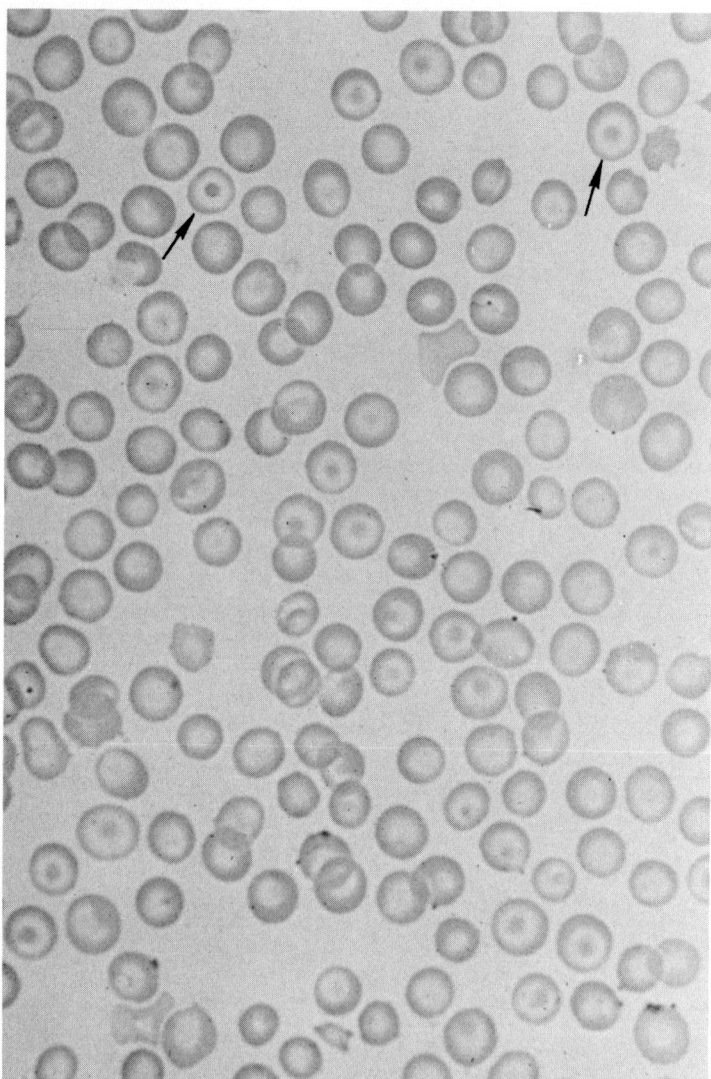

Figure 60–6. Multiple target cells (arrows) as seen in a blood smear from a dog with a congenital portal systemic shunt. ×450.

Serum albumin concentrations are usually depressed, reflecting the liver's inability to synthesize sufficient albumin to maintain normal serum concentrations. The BUN concentration is often subnormal in dogs with PSS. This probably represents the inability of the atrophic liver to effectively convert absorbed ammonia to urea. Fasting blood glucose concentrations have been reported to be reduced in 25 per cent of dogs with PSS (Ewing et al., 1974). However, most of these dogs had no clinical signs of hypoglycemia at the time they were sampled. Uric acid concentrations are often increased in serum in these patients. A major hepatic function is the conversion of uric acid to allantoin. With decreased conversion of uric acid more is able to be eliminated in the urine and may be the reason for the occurrence of uric acid or ammonium urate calculi in dogs with PSS (Maretta et al., 1981). Studies documenting that renal uric acid excretion is increased in this disease have not been reported. Hypocholesterolemia is a common biochemical finding. Since endogenous cholesterol synthesis is a function of the liver and is dependent on normal hepatic blood flow, cholesterol synthesis is often reduced, as evidenced by reductions in the serum concentration. The biochemical abnormalities associated with PSS reflect the severity of portal shunting and the degree of hepatic functional insufficiency. They are not unique to PSS and would be expected to occur in any advanced, generalized hepatic disease. Definitive diagnosis requires radiographic or pathologic confirmation.

The finding of ammonium urate crystals in urine sediment occurs in about one third of dogs with PSS (Fig. 60–7). These crystals are infrequently observed in other types of hepatic disease but are common in Dalmatians in which enzyme defects prevent conversion of uric acid to allantoin. Although finding ammonium urate crystals is helpful in establishing a diagnosis, they appear unpredictably in any given dog. Urine-specific gravities are often low in dogs with PSS. Most respond reasonably well to water deprivation but cannot concentrate maximally for reasons already discussed. The recent observation that recurrent renal or cystic calculi may occur in association with PSS expands further the clinical symptomatology one must consider in this syndrome. Nine cases have been described in the literature, and the author has had clinical evidence of six additional cases at the University of Minnesota. The majority of the calculi have been uric acid or ammonium urate. Occasional mixed calculi containing uric acid and ammonium magnesium phosphate also occur. Any non-Dalmatian in which a uric acid calculus is identified should be evaluated as a possible PSS dog.

Radiography is one of the most important diagnostic procedures in dogs with PSS. Survey abdominal radiographs are valuable initial screening procedure for dogs with suspected PSS. Nearly all animals evaluated will have reductions in liver size. This is particularly evident on lateral projections. Because abdominal contrast is generally poor in these dogs, owing to a lack of fat, administering a small quantity of positive or negative contrast material into the stomach will allow a better appreciation of hepatic size. Pneumoperitoneography may also be used if preliminary studies are equivocal. The author has used reduction in liver size as a valuable initial diagnostic procedure in dogs with PSS. Renomegaly has also been noted to occur in many dogs with this disease.

Radiography provides the only method of confirming the diagnosis short of major surgery and determines whether medical or surgical therapy should be considered. Several contrast radiographic procedures have been evaluated for use in dogs with PSS. Four that provide useful information include cranial mesenteric arteriography, transabdominal splenoportography, operative mesenteric portography, and celiac arteriography (Suter, 1975). Cranial mesenteric arteriography or splenoportography provide the most diagnostic information (Ewing et al., 1974). The author has used operative splenoportography in most cases and feels it is highly adaptable to clinical practice. It does not require special injection equipment or rapid speed cassette changers for diagnostic films to be made. Approximately 0.25 ml/kg body weight of intravenous contrast agent is injected into a cannulated splenic vein or directly into the splenic pulp. Films may be exposed as soon as the injection is completed or delayed for four to eight seconds. We have found that films taken immediately upon completion of the injection are usually sufficient. Lateral

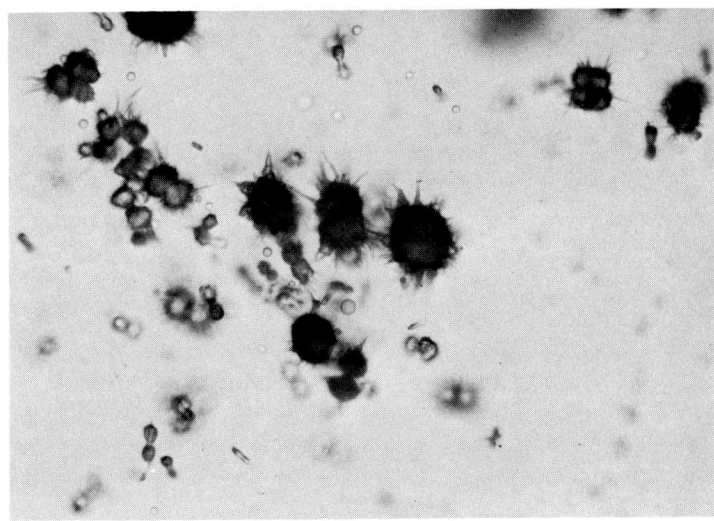

Figure 60–7. Ammonium urate (biurate) crystals from the urine sediment of a dog with a portal vascular anomaly. ×450.

views are most diagnostic; however, ventrodorsal views following a second dye injection may occasionally add useful information. If radiographs indicate that a surgically correctable shunt exists, the author normally proceeds at that time with surgery.

Therapy for dogs with PSS may be surgical, medical, or a combination of the two. Various reports of surgical correction of portal vein anomalies have appeared (Breznock, 1979; Gofton, 1978; Simpson and Hribernik, 1976; Strombeck et al., 1977). Several presurgical considerations are critical for any degree of success. The type of anomaly determines if surgery should be considered. Patients with either a patent ductus venosus or portal vein atresia are poor surgical candidates. Patent ductes are surgically very difficult to approach. Patients with portal vein atresia have severely hypoplastic intrahepatic portal venous systems, usually already have portal hypertension, and die of vascular collapse if shunting collaterals are ligated. On the other hand, portal-caval and portal azygous shunts are usually surgical approachable.

Although angiography usually clearly delineates the type of shunt present, it rarely indicates whether any rudimentary hepatic portal perfusion exists. At surgery, remnants of the portal circulation can be visualized entering at the hilus of the liver. It is this residual portal blood flow that will expand as the shunt is partially ligated, diverting shunting blood back into hepatic parenchyma. It has been suggested that portal venous pressures should be measured prior to attempting any attenuation of the shunting vessel(s) (Schmidt and Suter, 1981). Increases in portal vein pressure above 20 to 30 cm H_2O indicate portal hypertension already exists, and ligating the shunt is likely to lead to venous stagnation of the bowel, shock, and death. Surgical correction involves partial ligation of the shunting vessels (75 per cent reduction in luminal diameter) rather than complete occlusion. This allows a safety valve to reduce the chance of a shock bowel and usually results in complete amelioration of clinical and biochemical evidence of disease. The most significant postoperative complication is ascites, if shock is avoided. This can usually be controlled with diuretics and salt restriction in a few days. Biochemical functions return to normal remarkably fast. Albumin concentrations, BSP retention, and ammonia tolerance are often normal within a few days to a few weeks. Although long-term followups of postsurgical cases have been limited, these dogs have been reported to be doing well up to two years after ligation.

Medical therapy involves measures used to control the signs of hepatic encephalopathy and maximize remaining hepatic function. These measures are covered in detail in the section on hepatic therapy. Although medical therapy may provide dramatic short-term improvement, hepatic atrophy will progress in spite of adequate medical therapy. Thus, the author would expect most animals with PSS to eventually succumb to their disease; however, a number of dogs have been treated medically for over three years with no signs that their disease is progressing. It appears that some animals will plateau and that medical therapy can maintain them at a constant level of function.

Only two cats have been reported with PSS (Vulgamott et al., 1981). Signs include CNS derangement and stunting. Diagnosis was based on abnormal BSP retention and ammonia tolerance tests. Normal blood ammonia in cats was reported to range from 100 to 350 μg/dl after ammonium chloride therapy. Both resting and post-administration blood ammonia concentrations were increased in the two cats. Splenic pulp injections confirmed that both cats had large porto-postcaval shunts. The cats were euthanatized.

It is only since an understanding of the many manifestations of hepatic encephalopathy has developed that PSS patients are being correctly diagnosed and treated. Clinicians must not ignore this disease as some rarity seen only in academic institutions. Portal vascular anomalies are one of the most common causes of CNS signs in young dogs in the author's practice.

Urea Cycle Enzyme Deficiencies

Two dogs have been described with signs of hepatic encephalopathy that were determined to have deficiencies of hepatic urea cycle enzymes (Strombeck et al., 1975a). One dog was a four-month-old golden retriever with neurologic signs of hepatic coma, including stunting. The other animal was a stunted four-year-old beagle with a history of seizures since nine months of age.

The only abnormalities detected during a medical workup were hypoalbuminemia and increased blood ammonia concentrations. Hepatic biopsy material was quantitatively analyzed for enzymes important in the conversion of ammonia to urea. Both dogs had significant reductions in the urea cycle enzyme, arginosuccinate synthetase, which would lead to inability to handle endogenous ammonia and signs of encephalopathy. Portal angiographic studies were normal. Dietary and antibiotic therapy designed to reduce intestinal ammonia production resulted in significant amelioration of clinical signs in both dogs. These cases might not be as rare as first supposed. Since blood ammonia determinations are not routinely available, it is entirely possible that many other dogs with seizures or behavior changes could be manifesting signs of hepatic encephalopathy and not be diagnosed because of the selective nature of the defect. Obviously, a definitive diagnosis requires very sophisticated techniques to assay for intracellular enzymes.

Steroid Hepatopathy

The canine liver appears to be uniquely sensitive to the development of microscopic lesions and biochemical abnormalities following exogenous administration or endogenous production of excess glucocorticoids. This condition has been termed steroid hepatopathy (Rogers and Ruebner, 1977). Of 22 biopsy confirmed cases, 18 were deemed secondary to iatrogenic administration of steroids and four secondary to hyperadrenocorticism. Little data are available regarding the effects of dose, type, or duration of steroid administration necessary to induce pathologic changes. It appears that all types of steroids are capable of inducing changes in some dogs. In one experimental study, prednisolone acetate was administered intramuscularly at 2 mg/kg body weight twice daily to normal dogs for 3, 7, 14, and 28 days (Dillon et al., 1980). Microscopic lesions compatible with steroid hepatopathy occurred in all dogs. However, only dogs treated for 14 and 28 days had induction of the steroid specific isoenzyme. There were also no correlations between alterations in serum AP or serum ALT concentrations and hepatic lesions.

Steroids are known to produce significant increases in serum ALT and serum AP concentrations and in BSP retention. Serum ALT levels are increased in 75 per cent of dogs on glucocorticoids, the mean rise is mild, about two to three times normal. Induction of a steroid isoenzyme of alkaline phosphatase is the most dramatic biochemical abnormality. Serum AP values increase rapidly and massively once glucocorticoids are administered. Mean increases are ten fold above normal and may rise much higher. BSP retention averages 11 per cent in 30 minutes and ranges from 6 to 43 per cent (Rogers and Ruebner, 1977). In addition to these biochemical changes, polydipsia, polyuria, and hepatomegaly will be noted in approximately 50 per cent of dogs with steroid hepatopathy.

In the absence of obvious clinical signs of hyperadrenocorticism or knowledge of iatrogenic steroid administration, the presence of hepatomegaly and hepatic enzyme abnormalities would warrant biopsy. Typical steroid lesions are obvious microscopically and probably represent hydropic degeneration (Fig. 60–8). Attempts to define the nature of the prominent vacuoles in the hepatic cytoplasm indicate they are not lipid, glycogen, polysaccharides, protein, acid or alkaline phosphatase (Thompson et al., 1977). The diffuse swelling and vacuolation probably represent imbibition of water or dilute protein solutions. Such lesions, although typical for steroid-induced pathology, are also seen in other types of toxic hepatosis.

Lesions induced by glucocorticoids are apparently reversible upon withdrawal of the drug or treatment for hyperadrenocorticism. The time necessary for return of hepatic size and enzymes to normal has not been precisely defined, but data on clinical cases indicate that resolutions may require several weeks or months.

The importance of this disease as a cause of overt signs of hepatic failure is unknown. Other than signs of polydipsia, polyuria, and hepatomegaly, dogs appear to remain asymptomatic. It is more important for clinicians to recognize the typical pattern of steroid hepatopathy in dogs receiving steroids and not assume major hepatic disease exists. In addition, once dogs are given steroids, the clinician should expect typical biochemical changes to occur. In dogs with hyperadrenocorticism without skin changes, liver biopsy may prove an efficient means of establishing a tentative diagnosis.

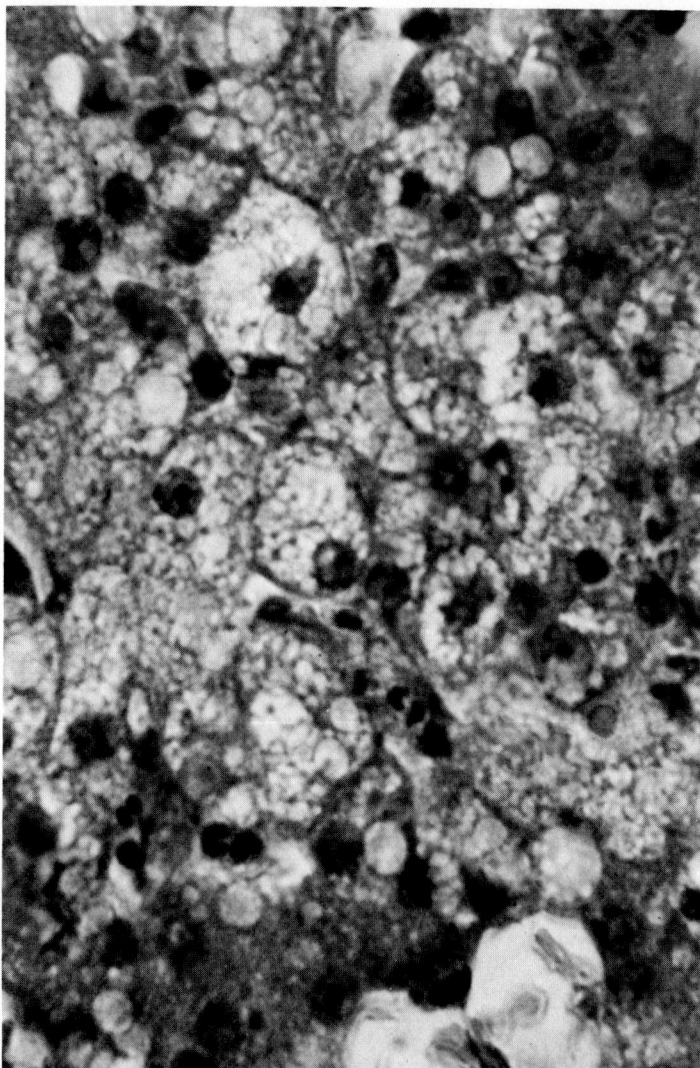

Figure 60–8. Diffuse vacuolation of hepatocytes typical for dogs with glucocorticoid-induced hepatopathy. ×100.

Lipidosis

Major diseases associated with lipidosis and mechanisms for lipid accumulation were previously considered under pathophysiology of hepatic failure. Since lipidosis is caused by a number of disease entities, the clinical significance of lipidosis depends on the identification of the underlying disease responsible for its buildup. Lipidosis caused by starvation or obesity is infrequently of great clinical importance. However. lipid buildup secondary to diabetes, toxins, or drugs may be significant, and efforts to identify the precipitating factors are warranted. Hepatomegaly may be the only obvious clinical abnormality. Signs of hepatic failure are not often present until late in the disease course. Laboratory findings are nonspecific but localize disease to the liver.

Serum ALT concentrations increased in 50 per cent of the dogs with lipidosis, but such increases are generally mild. In contrast, serum AP concentrations are nearly always increased. The magnitude of the rise is variable, but three- to five-fold increases are common. BSP retention ranges from 6 to 12 per cent, particularly in diabetic lipidosis (Ling et al., 1977). Hyperbilirubinemia is uncommon and, when present, is mild.

Therapy for hepatic lipidosis should be successful if its cause is related to over- or under-nutrition, dietary imbalances, or toxicities that can be corrected. Diabetic lipidosis is difficult to reverse clinically. Successful regulation does not reverse human diabetic fatty liver, and this may be the case in dogs. Dietary control is more successful than strict insulin regulation in reversing the lipidosis.

Lipotropic drugs such as methionine and choline have not been shown to have any beneficial therapeutic effects in diabetic lipidosis. Oral antibiotics may be useful in correcting some forms of toxic lipidosis. Endotoxins absorbed from the intestine are known to cause hepatic lipidosis. A reduction in bacterial numbers or a change in flora types has been shown to reduce the severity of endotoxin-induced lipidosis. Reductions in intestinal bacterial numbers also occur if highly digestible, low-residue diets are fed. Such diets are almost completely absorbed in the small intestine, leaving little substrate for colonic bacteria to feed on. Thus, bacterial numbers decline and harmful byproducts of bacterial metabolism are reduced.

Lipidosis in the cat has a much more serious prognosis (Barsanti et al., 1977). The majority of cats presented to the author's clinic in hepatic failure secondary to severe lipidosis have died of their disease. Most of these cats were very overweight at the start of their illness, have lost over 50 per cent of their body weight, and have a course of anorexia lasting four to six weeks. Clinical signs are usually unremarkable, except that mild to severe jaundice is often present and hepatomegaly is frequent. Biochemical parameters indicate elevations in serum ALT, AP, and bilirubin. Bilirubinuria is also frequent in these cats, reflecting the severity of cholestasis. Hepatic biopsy indicates whether massive lipidosis is present. These cats probably suffer from a severe starvation-induced lipidosis. It is probable that the initial cause of their anorexia is not liver disease, but fasting induces marked lipidosis and, later, signs of encephalopathy (depression, anorexia), which further aggravates the disease. If the diagnosis can be established early enough in the clinical course, it should be reversible with force feeding of a high protein, high carbohydrate diet. The author has had success in a few cats by inserting pharyngostomy tubes into the cats and maintaining them for several weeks. Suggestions have been made that this severe form of lipidosis represents a prediabetic state in the cat and that low dose insulin therapy should be used. The author has no data to substantiate such claims, and insulin therapy in cats carries too high a risk of complications for it to be used indiscriminately.

Amyloidosis

Amyloidosis refers to the accumulation of abnormal types of hyaline-like deposits primarily within the liver, spleen, kidneys, and adrenal glands. Primary amyloidosis is very uncommon and occurs principally in the islet cells of the feline pancreas. Secondary amyloidosis occurs most often in the dog, and its presence is associated with various chronic antigen-antibody diseases that stimulate the production of amyloid. Amyloidosis is most often seen in association with chronic infections, such as osteomyelitis, tuberculosis, or neoplastic conditions. Amyloid fibrils have an amino acid sequence identical to that of light chain immunoglobulins. On this basis, amyloid is thought to be an abnormal degradation product of the antibody molecule, which remains as an extracellular accumulation in various organs.

Liver amyloid accumulates within the space of Disse adjacent to the cords of hepatocytes lining the liver sinusoids. As this material accumulates, sinusoidal blood supply is reduced and anoxia and necrosis develop. The liver becomes quite enlarged with palpably rounded edges. Liver failure may be the cause of death from amyloidosis. Only one case of hepatic failure secondary to amyloidosis has been reported (Thornburg and Moody, 1981). The amyloidosis was secondary to coccidioidomycosis.

Liver function tests indicate gradual deterioration of parenchymal cell activities. BSP retention is increased initially because of impaired hepatic blood flow. As the disease progresses, parenchymal cell necrosis and bile duct obstruction occur, causing serum AP and ALT levels to become elevated. A definitive diagnosis requires biopsy and special staining techniques to detect the presence of amyloid. Amyloidosis is a progressively fatal disorder; there is no specific therapy. Therapeutic efforts are aimed at the primary stimulus for antigen-antibody production, although success has not been documented in domestic animals.

Glycogen Storage Diseases

A number of hereditary deficiencies of enzymes necessary for the breakdown of hepatic glycogen have been documented in human literature. A similar condition may exist in the dog and has been reported by

Bardens (1961; 1966). Hepatic glycogen is necessary for the maintenance of normal fasting blood glucose levels, and an inability to mobilize hepatic glycogen results in hypoglycemic attacks. Additionally, because no defect in hepatic synthesis of glycogen exists in this condition, the continued accumulation of glycogen without degradation leads to hepatomegaly. The disease occurs in puppies, usually miniature breeds six to 12 weeks of age. It begins in association with some form of stressful situation such as excessive handling, shipment, new owners, or illnesses (diarrhea, vomiting). The animals become incoordinated, weak, and depressed. Eventually the depression progresses to coma, and seizures are common. Blood glucose determinations are usually in the hypoglyconic range.

Bardens (1966) describes three separate types of glycogen storage diseases that are clinically identical. One is a generalized glycogen storage deficiency that responds to glucagon and is age-limited to puppies. Usually they outgrow the disease, if treated. Strombeck et al. (1978) reported on a similar syndrome in a young Pomeranian puppy. They were unable to confirm that any form of glycogenosis was present. Rather, the persistent hypoglycemia was attributed to a normal inability of immature dogs to tolerate fasting. Frequent feedings completely reversed the dog's disease, which was self-correcting with age. Another form is a Von Gierke's-like syndrome, associated with a glucose-6-phosphatase deficiency in man. These animals do not respond to glucagon, either after starvation or when given exogenous glucagon, but will respond to five per cent dextrose. Many of this group are prone to relapse and may die. The third group resembles the human Cori's disease, in which a deficiency of a debranching amyloclastic enzyme, amylo-1-6-glucosidase, exists. In non-fasted animals, a normal glucagon response is seen, but in the fasted state, no elevation in blood glucose occurs following glucagon injections. This may be responsible for the intermittent hypoglycemia observed with some hunting breeds after exercise. Frequent feedings and glucocorticoids control this type. Two reports of a well-documented Type III glycogenosis (Cori's disease) have appeared (Ceh, et al., 1976; Rafiquazzaman et al., 1976). The disease was diagnosed in four female German shepherds of similar genetic background.

The most obvious clinical sign was massive hepatomegaly. Other signs included poor weight gains and muscle weakness. Signs began as early as two months of age and progressed slowly. Significant pathological findings included massive increases in the glycogen content of the liver, cardiac and skeletal muscle, and brain. A reduction in the hepatic concentration of the glycogen debranching enzyme amylo-1-6-glucosidase was confirmed. Hepatic concentrations were zero to seven per cent of normal in these German shepherd dogs.

Hepatic Neoplasia

The liver is a frequent site for both primary and metastatic neoplasms. The most common primary tumors in order of frequency are hepatocellular carcinoma, hepatomas, cholangiocarcinoma, fibroma/fibrosarcoma, hemangioma/hemangiosarcoma, and hamartomas. Strombeck (1978) lists the frequency of primary hepatic tumors as 1 per 2000 admissions, while that of metastatic hepatic tumors is 1 per 1000 admissions. Metastatic tumors arise from multiple sites, but the most important are the mammary gland, the spleen, the lymph nodes, the adrenal glands, the pancreas, bone, and the lung.

The clinical signs induced by primary hepatic tumors are similar to those observed in inflammatory liver disease. They include anorexia, depression, vomiting, polyuria, and polydipsia. Hepatomegaly is an important differential feature, as it is usually marked with primary tumors. Hepatocellular carcinomas have dramatic biochemical alterations. Serum ALT concentrations are increased ten fold, serum AP activity is often 20 times normal, albumin concentrations are often depressed (<2.0 gm/dl), hypergammaglobulinemia (4.9 gm, mean) is noted in most, hypoglycemia was observed in one third of the cases, hyperbilirubinemia was mild and present in only one quarter of the dogs, and slight increases in BSP retention were measured, six to 11 per cent in 33 per cent of the cases (Strombeck, 1978). Diagnosis of primary hepatic tumors is most often established via biopsy during exploratory surgery. Hepatomas and hepatocellular carcinomas grow very slowly and are often localized to single hepatic lobes such that surgical resection is feasible. Cholangiocarcinomas are usually associated with weight loss and jaundice. Patients usually have multicentric infiltrates with this tumor and are inoperable. Death usually results within a few months following diagnosis.

The majority of tumors metastatic to the liver are diagnosed by identifying the primary tumor first. In occasional cases, however, the liver may prove the most accessible site for a tissue diagnosis (gastrointestinal lymphosarcoma). Clinical signs referrable to metastatic hepatic tumors are highly variable owing to the numerous primary sites that may be involved. Biochemical and radiographic evaluation of the liver is most often normal, even in cases of widespread metastases. Mild increases (one-fold) in serum ALT occur in 46 per cent of cases, serum AP activity is increased in 50 per cent of patients approximately three times normal, and a doubling of serum bilirubin concentration may occur in 46 per cent of the metastatic neoplasms. Diagnosis of metastatic hepatic tumors is often made at necropsy or on exploratory coeliotomy. Signs of liver disease are usually subtle or absent, and a search for the primary tumor should be the clinician's main concern. Therapy is directed at the primary tumor, and chemotherapy is the only available mode of treating such cases.

THERAPY

General objectives for therapy of hepatic failure revolve around attempts to eliminate causative agents, if known; to suppress or eliminate mechanisms that potentiate the illness; to provide optimum conditions for liver regeneration; and to control manifestations of any complications that may occur (Hoenig, 1970; Schaffner, 1969). Clinical manifestations of hepatic failure are often similar in acute or chronic diseases, differing primarily in the severity and number of complications that develop. Unfortunately, little controlled work has been done on therapy of spontaneous hepatic diseases in the dog and cat. Most therapeutic recommendations are based on conclusions obtained from trials in experimental animals or man.

SPECIFIC THERAPY FOR HEPATIC FAILURE

Therapy for hepatic diseases may be either specific (directed at a causative agent) or supportive and symptomatic (directed at the signs of failure regardless of the etiology). Unfortunately, little in the way of specific therapy for hepatic diseases exists at present, most often because specific etiologic agents are never defined. Even when causative agents are known, they may not be susceptible to current modes of treatment (viruses), or they are no longer present when the disease is diagnosed (cirrhosis). Clinicians are compelled to treat the manifestations of hepatic failure symptomatically in an attempt to prolong the patient's life so that an etiologic diagnosis can be made and specific therapy instituted, if possible.

Acute hepatic failure is most often the result of trauma, viruses, drugs, or toxins. Viral hepatitis has no specific therapy once the disease process has been initiated. With drug-induced hepatitis, the only specific therapy involves recognizing that drugs may be responsible and withdrawing them. Since the liver is the main organ for the metabolism of endogenous and exogenous noxious substances, it is often damaged by toxic products. Because of the great reserve capacity of the liver and the fact that many toxins (lead, arsenic, mercury) damage multiple organs with less compensatory reserve (brain, kidney), animals often die from damage to these organs prior to the time that signs of fulminant hepatic failure develop. In other cases, although the toxin is liver-specific (carbon tetrachloride), therapy is nonspecific, and, of necessity, is supportive and symptomatic. In the great majority of cases, toxicity may be suspected from laboratory data and biopsy material but a specific agent is never discovered. Obviously, when a known toxin is incriminated, specific antidotes are used in addition to supportive measures.

Of the chronic hepatic diseases for which an etiology is known — i.e., neoplasms, amyloidosis, lipidosis — little in the way of specific therapy is available. Hepatic neoplasms advanced enough to cause signs of liver failure, except for extrahepatic jaundice, usually warrant a poor prognosis. No specific therapy exists for amyloidosis. Severe hepatic lipidosis occurs secondary to a number of metabolic diseases. Advanced lipidosis may result in varying degrees of hepatic failure. Specific therapy is directed at correcting the underlying metabolic abnormality. Lipidosis is potentially reversible in hypothyroidism, hyperadrenocorticism, lipoprotein abnormalities, and malnutritive states. Lipidosis secondary to diabetes in the dog appears to be progressive, irrespective of the adequacy of insulin regulation or supplementation with lipotropic agents, as is often recommended.

SUPPORTIVE AND SYMPTOMATIC THERAPY

The animal with hepatic failure from carbon tetrachloride toxicity may present a clinical picture similar to that of one dying from advanced cirrhosis. The therapy is, in general, the same for both, in the hope that liver regeneration is still possible, that the individual crisis may be overcome, and that efforts toward prevention and control of the complications of hepatic failure are successful. The primary means of supporting hepatic function continue to be confinement and dietary modifications. In addition, a number of drugs may be indicated for patients in hepatic failure, while others are contraindicated. Lastly, therapy may be directed specifically at the major complications of hepatic failure, coma, ascites and edema, infection, malabsorption, hemorrhage or anemia, and fulminant hepatic failure.

Rest and Confinement. Rest and confinement of animals with hepatic failure is important for several reasons. Rest facilitates liver regeneration by increasing its blood flow and reducing the workload presented to it. Decreased activity will reduce pain and tenderness associated with stretching of the liver capsule. Lastly, the subjective signs of illness reported by human patients (malaise, nausea, and anorexia) are reduced if activity is curtailed, and presumably the same is true for animals. Once biochemical evidence of improvement in hepatic function occurs, exercise restriction is unnecessary. Fortunately, most dogs and cats with symptomatic liver disease are depressed enough that excessive physical activity is not a problem until their disease begins to improve.

Dietary Modifications. Dietary therapy is probably the single most important method of modifying the course of most spontaneous liver diseases. Dietary modifications are particularly effective in chronic liver diseases because these patients will usually consume adequate quantities of nutrients and calories if proper dietary adjustments are made. Dogs and cats with more severe acute hepatopathies are usually totally anorectic, as voluntary intake is impaired and forced feeding is poorly tolerated. The goals of dietary modifications are to reduce the symptoms of hepatic failure and at the same time to provide optimal conditions for hepatocellular repair and regeneration.

Dietary therapy involves adjusting the diet so that optimal quantities and types of protein, carbohydrate, fat, vitamins, and minerals are provided to the animal. The attempt is to balance the intake of the patient with its ability to metabolize these foodstuffs in a failing liver. Protein restriction and modification is of primary importance. The goal is to minimize the alterations in nitrogen metabolism induced by hepatic failure, that is, to reduce blood ammonia concentrations and return circulating plasma amino acid concentrations toward normal. The type and quantity of protein, as well as the frequency of feeding are all important in reducing signs of hepatic failure (Strombeck and Gribble, 1978).

Cottage cheese has recently been recommended as an excellent protein source for animals in hepatic failure (Strombeck, 1980; Strombeck and Gribble, 1978). Cottage cheese is a high biologic value protein source, contains no additives, is easily and completely digested and has a good ratio of branched chain to aromatic amino acids. Cottage cheese was much better tolerated than when either red meat or a mixed protein diet was used as a protein source in humans with hepatic failure, even though the amino acid ratios of these protein sources are very similar. It was hypothesized that the beneficial effects of cottage cheese over the other proteins were related to three factors: (1) reduced putrefaction and ammonia production by intestinal bacteria prior to absorption, (2) a reduction in urease positive bacteria within the colon, and (3) the high bacterial content of cottage cheese, which may have repopulated the intestine with a more favorable flora (Fenton et al., 1966). Cottage cheese has also been shown to be superior to intravenous casein hydrolysates in terms of both nitrogen retention and stabilization of plasma amino acid ratios (Patel et al., 1973). The lack of food additives in these formulated diets is important, as commercial pet foods contain certain additives that are metabolized by intestinal bacteria to potent hepatotoxins (Strombeck, 1980). The efficient digestion of cottage cheese within the small bowel leaves little residue for colonic bacteria to metabolize; this reduces both the numbers of bacteria and the toxic nitrogenous byproducts of bacterial metabolism. In order for this efficient assimilation to occur, the animal should be fed frequently, three to four times a day, and quantities kept small.

Low residue diets further decrease intestinal ammonia production and absorption by reducing desquamation of intestinal epithelium. Reduced cell turnover results in smaller intestinal protein loss from lymphatics. The minimum protein intake for dogs has been reported to be one gm of protein for each 20 calories required per day (Strombeck and Gribble, 1978). In estimating protein requirements for patients, it is important to know the serum albumin concentration. Severe protein restriction in hypoalbuminemic patients will likely serve to further deplete serum albumin concentrations. Protein intake can and should be adjusted upwards from the minimal figure unless signs of encephalopathy intervene.

An easily digested carbohydrate source should form the basis for the bulk of required daily calories. The carbohydrate selected should be easily digested, with few colonic residues to reduce colonic bacterial production of volatile fatty acids. Boiled white rice serves this purpose well. A high carbohydrate diet provides an easily assimilated source of nonprotein calories, which spares body tissues from catabolizing muscle protein for energy and reduces the catabolism of dietary protein for energy.

Fats should not comprise a major part of the diet in animals with hepatic failure. Minimal amounts, four to six per cent on a dry weight basis, should supply sufficient essential fatty acids and fat soluble vitamins to meet nutritional requirements. Fat also significantly improves palatability. Excessive dietary fat intake may aggravate signs of encephalopathy, as certain fatty acids have been shown to induce hepatic encephalopathy. Cholestatic liver disease may be associated with reduced bile salt excretion and steatorrhea.

Vitamin and mineral supplementation can be important, especially when diets are being formulated at home. Hypovitaminosis is common in liver disease and is secondary to multiple factors. Decreased intake and anorexia in patients play important roles. In addition, increased physiologic demands,

accelerated intestinal loss, malutilization, and impaired storage capacity contribute to hypovitaminosis (Russell, 1979; Twedt, 1981). Certain drugs used to treat hepatic failure may impair both fat and fat soluble vitamin absorption, i.e., neomycin and cholestyramine (Russell, 1979). Clinical signs of hypovitaminosis occur in 70 per cent of humans with hepatic disease and include glossitis, peripheral neuropathies, hyperkeratosis, night blindness and macrocytic anemias. Vitamins most often deficient in humans with hepatic failure include folic acid, B_6, B_{12}, thiamine, A, E, riboflavin, nicotinic acid, pantothenic acid and the minerals zinc and cobalt. Vitamin B_6 and B_{12} are particularly important for cell regeneration. It is recommended that daily B-complex vitamin requirements be doubled. Of the fat soluble vitamins, K and D are most important. Vitamin K may require parenteral administration if biliary obstruction is severe.

The routine use of lipotropic agents (methionine and choline) in dogs with hepatic disease should be avoided. Recent experimental work on dogs indicates that oral methionine can induce hepatic encephalopathy quite easily and that it acts synergistically with short chain fatty acids and ammonia to induce coma. Lipotropic drugs are of proven value only in cases in which true deficiencies of these substances exist. Animals receiving a nutritious diet with adequate quantities of protein have no need for such drugs and they may prove harmful.

Drugs in Hepatic Failure

The liver is quantitatively the most important organ involved with drug metabolism, although the kidney, brain and other organs make significant contributions. The duration and intensity of action may be increased for many drugs metabolized in the liver. Not all enzyme systems are equally affected by hepatic failure, however, and many agents produce nonspecific enzyme induction, even in the failing liver, resulting in increased metabolism of many drugs. Most commonly used drugs can be used in patients with hepatic failure, but a balance must be maintained between what is given to the patient and the patient's ability to tolerate the prescribed amount.

Antibiotics. Adequate hepatic function does not seem to be a critical factor in the handling of most antibiotics by patients with hepatic disease. In general, they may be given at the standard recommended levels (Rosenoer and Gualberto, 1972). Antibiotics are of value in the treatment of primary bacterial hepatitis or cholangitis and in the suppression of the proliferation of the normal population of anerobic bacteria within the liver. Oral antibiotics are particularly of value in treating hepatic coma (see Complications of Hepatic Failure).

The selection of antibiotics to be used for the treatment of nonhepatic infections should be made with caution. Avoid drugs requiring hepatic inactivation or excretion, and any nonantibiotic hepatotoxic agents. Conversely, antibiotics metabolized and/or excreted by the liver are theoretically ideal for treating acute infections of the liver and biliary tract (Jacobs, 1969).

All tetracyclines are concentrated in the liver and excreted in bile. Biliary concentration may reach 5 to 32 times the serum concentration. Parenteral preparations are known to be toxic in high dosages in man, and in one half to two thirds of the human patients, a reversible lipidosis occurs. Chlortetracycline is the most hepatotoxic of this group of antibiotics and should be avoided. The prolonged use of tetracycline may suppress vitamin K and urobilinogen production by intestinal bacteria, resulting in a decrease in urine urobilinogen. Tetracyclines generally are useful in hepatic failure, especially with biliary tract diseases.

Penicillin and streptomycin are only minimally eliminated by the liver, but appreciable hepatic tissue levels are developed and they may be used safely in hepatic disease.

Chloramphenicol is conjugated by the liver and then excreted renally. Concentrated hepatic tissue levels develop. The plasma half-life is increased in cirrhosis and the potential for toxicities exists, although they have not been reported. A potential contraindication in the use of chloramphenicol is its depressing effect on hepatic microsomal enzyme systems. Because it is a profound enzyme repressor it impairs the liver's ability to metabolize many substances and should be avoided in patients with known hepatic failure.

Lincomycin is primarily metabolized and excreted by the liver. The serum half-life may double in hepatic failure and toxicities may develop. The dosage should be reduced or the medication stopped, if possible.

Sedatives. Sedatives should be avoided in hepatic failure, since their use is commonly associated with the development of hepatic coma. Phenobarbital, being primarily excreted by the kidneys, is the safest hypnotic. Convulsive states are best controlled using diazepam (Valium) and chlordiazepoxide (Librium) at reduced dosages (Schaffner and Raisfeld, 1969). The potential toxicities of phenytoin and primidone (Mylepsin) have already been discussed.

Avoid analgesics, anesthetics, and barbiturates in patients with hepatic failure. If analgesia is required, meperidine, codeine, and acetaminophen in subnormal dosages appear better tolerated than morphine. Of the inhalant anesthetic agents, halothane has been frequently incriminated in cases of fulminant hepatic failure in man following repeated exposures. Similar evidence is lacking for domestic species of animals, but halothane in combination with hypoxia and metabolic acidosis has been shown to be hepatotoxic (Hoenig, 1970). In spite of the potential for halothane-induced hepatitis, no documented halothane-associated hepatic disease has been observed at the author's hospital; however, the author rarely, if ever, subjects animals with severe hepatic disease to multiple anesthesias with inhalant anesthetics.

Anabolic Agents. A number of recent reports have attributed beneficial effects to the use of anabolic steroids in the therapy of chronic liver disease in man (Figueroa, 1973; Islam and Islam, 1973; Puliyel et al., 1977). Mesterolone, a synthetic androgen, was evaluated in alcoholic cirrhosis and other forms of chronic active liver disease that had progressed to cirrhotic stages. Patients were given 75 mg/day divided three times daily for several weeks. Significantly greater clinical and biochemical improvement occurred in the treated group over nonandrogen treated individuals (Figueroa, 1973). Two clinical trials in man, one controlled and the other uncontrolled, using testosterone proprionate, gave similar results in the treated groups. Significant reductions in ascites and mortality and increases in serum albumin and body weight occurred in androgen-treated patients (Islam and Islam, 1973; Puliyel, 1977). No information is available on the therapeutic benefit of anabolic steroids in spontaneous hepatic diseases of dogs and cats. Whenever such agents are utilized, however, their anabolic effects develop only if sufficient non-protein calories are ingested along with a high biologic value protein source to meet caloric requirements. Methyltestosterone has been shown to have a low order of toxicity in dogs and should be avoided in hepatic failure of dogs and cats (Heywood et al., 1977).

Glucocorticoids. The use of glucocorticoids in hepatic failure remains a controversial subject. The only hepatic disease in which glucocorticoids have proven efficacy in man is chronic active hepatitis. Recent reports in the veterinary literature have also advocated glucocorticoids in a syndrome resembling chronic active hepatitis (Strombeck and Gribble, 1978). This was an uncontrolled clinical trial, and proven efficacy in this canine syndrome remains to be demonstrated. Although they may be used widely in other forms of hepatic failure, their value is questionable. Beneficial effects of steroids include increased appetite, reductions in serum bilirubin concentrations, reductions in serum transaminases, reduced BSP retention, and increased serum albumin concentration (Schiff, 1966). In spite of these beneficial effects, a number of disadvantages are also known. They fail to prevent the progression of acute to chronic liver diseases, may increase the possibility of intercurrent infections, usually do not increase life expectancy, fail to change the histologic picture of most diseases, and can aggravate the management of ascites (Rogers, 1971; Schiff, 1966). In general, patients in which steroids may have a positive effect are those with prolonged anorexia and weight loss when increased food intake would be beneficial and patients with immunologically mediated hepatic disease, as indicated by biopsy information.

The dosage and type of glucocorticoid used may be more critical in patients with hepatic failure than other steroid responsive disorders. Prednisone and prednisolone are the two most commonly used steroids in hepatic disease. Prednisone must be converted to prednisolone in the liver in order to be biologically active. Thus, prednisolone has the theoretic advantage of not requiring hepatic biotransformation for activity. Experimental evidence in man on patients with cirrhosis or chronic active liver disease receiving either prednisone or prednisolone indicate that blood levels of the biologically active drug are significantly lower in

prednisone-treated patients (Madsbad et al., 1980; Powell and Axelson, 1972; Tanner and Powell, 1979). However, this problem is likely to have clinical importance only in patients with the most severe degrees of hepatic failure. One additional complication of glucocorticoid therapy involves a decreased hepatic catabolism of the active compound, thus prolonging its duration of activity. Exact dosage recommendations for treating hepatic failure patients have not been established for animals. In man, the lowest dosage that results in sustained clinical or biochemical improvement is used. Recommended dosages for dogs with suspected CAH are 1 to 2 mg/kg body weight per day in divided dosages.

Drugs to Control Hepatic Fibrosis. One of the most significant pathologic changes occurring in chronic liver diseases is the development of fibrosis. Hepatic fibrosis refers to an absolute increase in hepatic collagen content and is due primarily to increased synthesis. In cirrhosis, normal collagen synthesis in the liver is greatly accelerated (Rojkind and Kershenobich, 1976). Experimental hepatic fibrosis in rats can be completely reversed if the etiologic agent is removed early in the disease. However, there appears to be a point of no return, after which the fibrosis becomes self-perpetuating even if the inciting agent is removed. Immunologic factors probably play an important role in the development and progression of hepatic fibrosis in many liver diseases. Lymphocytes from cirrhotic patients stimulate increased collagen synthesis by normal fibroblasts. Fibroblasts and lymphocytes from cirrhotic humans have been shown to release increased quantities of migration inhibitory factors, which may help to perpetuate the inflammatory process in the absence of an identifiable etiologic agent (Chen et al., 1979).

A number of drugs have been used experimentally to reduce hepatic fibrosis with encouraging success. Colchicine has been used in human cirrhotics in a controlled clinical trial (Kershenobich et al., 1979), and resulted in significant reductions in liver fibrosis, reductions in transaminases, bilirubin and globulin concentrations, and increased serum albumin and alkaline phosphatase concentrations (Rojkind and Kershenobich, 1973). Unfortunately, although clinical, histologic, and biochemical improvement was noted, no significant increases in survival between colchicine treated and nontreated controls were noted. Colchicine acts by inhibiting microtubular assembly of collagen, interrupting intracellular collagen transport, and accelerating collagen degradation by increasing collagenase activity. Penicillamine is another agent used to modify hepatic fibrosis. When used in high doses (300 mg/kg/day) in rats with experimental cirrhosis, significant decreases in hepatic fibrous tissue were observed (Brunner et al., 1973). This dose would be highly toxic to dogs. Two other experimental antifibrotic agents have also had encouraging reports, TECA-Medecassol, an extract of the plant *Centella asiatica*, and L-azetidine-carboxylic acid (AZC). TECA-Medecassol suppresses fibroblast proliferation and when used in schistosomiasis-induced human cirrhosis at 20 mg SID for two months, significantly decreased hepatic fibrosis in biopsy samples (El-Zawabry et al., 1975). AZC, a proline analog, when given to rats with CCl_4-induced cirrhosis, reduced fibrosis dramatically. AZC inhibits collagen synthesis (Rojkind and Kershenobich, 1976).

THERAPY FOR COMPLICATIONS OF HEPATIC FAILURE

A number of potentially serious complications of hepatic failure may develop in any given patient. Often, one or more of these complicating factors results in death of the patient; thus, they must be managed vigorously if any degree of therapeutic success is to be obtained.

Hepatic Coma. Hepatic coma is a serious complication of hepatic failure. It is most often seen in young dogs with congenital portal vascular anomalies but may occasionally develop in dogs with acquired hepatic disease. The goal of therapy is to control the pathophysiologic mechanisms responsible for inducing the encephalopathy. This is accomplished by reducing the entry, production, and absorption of gastrointestinal toxins and by administering systemic therapy to counteract the effects of absorbed toxins.

The mainstays of therapy for encephalopathy involve reduction of protein intake, gut "sterilization," and catharsis. For dogs with encephalopathy, all oral intake, but especially protein intake, should cease until CNS signs abate. Cessation of protein intake eliminates exogenous sources of ammonia, toxic amines, aromatic amino acids, and short chain fatty acids that may aggravate the encephalopathy. The next step involves complete catharsis of the colon to reduce the numbers of colonic bacteria and empty the colon of potentially toxic by-products of microbial metabolism. Although warm water enemas are most often used, mildly acidic enema solutions of vinegar and water (1:10 ratio) or povidone iodine in a ten per cent solution may have a better initial effect. Reducing the colonic pH traps NH_3 within the colon as NH_4^+ and prevents its absorption. Magnesium citrate used for several days maintains a mild catharsis and prevents prolonged retention of colonic contents. Gut "sterilization" is the next important step. Nonabsorbable intestinal antibiotics are used for this purpose. The most commonly used antibiotic in man is neomycin, although kanamycin, vancomycin, and paromomycin may be used interchangeably. Neomycin is normally administered in man at dosages of 6 to 8 gm/day, with maintenance dosages of 2 to 4 gm/day. No controlled studies have been designed to determine the minimally effective dose of nonabsorbable antibiotics to use in hepatic coma. Intestinal antibiotics significantly reduce numbers of urease-containing bacteria, decrease bacterial deamination of amino acids, and reduce aromatic amino acid absorption, as well as circulating false neurotransmitters and short chain fatty acids (Breen and Schenker, 1972; Fischer et al., 1974; Schenker et al., 1974). Neomycin is also known to induce a degree of intestinal malabsorption, which may be the most important reason for its therapeutic success (Fischer and Baldessarini, 1976). Neomycin may be given orally or per rectum using retention enemas. No data are available to substantiate increased value of one route over another. Rare, but important, complications of prolonged neomycin therapy include oto- and nephrotoxicity, severe diarrhea, and intestinal malabsorption (Madrey and Weber, 1975).

Lactulose is a nonabsorbable synthetic disaccharide (B-1,4-galactoside fructose). The drug is neither absorbed nor metabolized in the small intestine. Colonic bacteria contain lactulases that convert it into acetic and lactic acid. The fermentation of lactulose results in an increase in colon gas formation and a reduction in colon pH. The nonabsorbable organic acids serve as an osmotic cathartic, and lactulose in large doses induces profound diarrhea. Several controlled clinical trials using neomycin or lactulose for human hepatic coma indicate they have nearly equal efficacy (80 per cent) in reversing signs of coma (Atterbury et al., 1978; Conn et al., 1977). Recent evidence suggests that a combination of lactulose and neomycin is better than either drug alone (Pirotte et al., 1974). In dogs 5 to 15 mls TID will usually produce two to three soft bowel movements per day. The dose is titrated to each dog so that several soft but not diarrheic stools are produced each day. Other means of controlling colonic ammonia production that are less effective than neomycin or lactulose may be tried; these include lactobacillus colonization and acetohydroxamic acid (Fischer and Baldessarini, 1976). Attempting to repopulate the colon with lactose fermenting, nonurease-containing bacteria is a logical goal. Unfortunately, using lactobacillus-containing drugs or yogurt in quantities sufficient to maintain desirable flora in adequate numbers has not had much clinical success. The absorption of endotoxins from the colon may play a significant role as a complicating factor in hepatic encephalopathy. Methods to control endotoxin absorption include the use of oral intestinal antibiotics and cholestyramine. Cholestyramine, a cation exchange resin used primarily to bind bile salts within the colon in cholestatic diseases, is also known to bind E. coli endotoxin (Nolan, 1975).

In addition to the methods discussed that reduce or eliminate the production and absorption of toxic products from the intestinal tract, other supportive measures may be employed to improve the recovery from hepatic coma. The use of five per cent glucose intravenously prevents hepatic induced hypoglycemia, adds a moderate number of calories, and aids in the reversal of coma by stimulating the combining of NH_3 with glutamic acid to form glutamine (Schenker et al., 1974). The type of fluid used in hepatic coma is controversial. Most patients in severe coma have a respiratory alkalosis, and commonly used rehydrating fluids, such as lactated Ringer's solution, would seem to be contraindicated. However, when humans in coma with respiratory alkalosis were given alkalinizing therapy they had dramatic improvement in their electroencephalograms and clinical signs, rather than deteriorating, as might have been expected (James et al., 1969). It has been suggested that the respiratory alkalosis was compensatory for intracellular (cerebral) acidosis.

The use in dogs of specially formulated amino acid solutions (F080) high in branched-chain and low in aromatic amino acids has resulted in marked improvement in encephalopathy (Freund et al., 1979; Smith et al., 1979). These solutions are designed to normalize the plasma amino acid patterns by reducing brain uptake of aromatic amino acids and decreasing endogenous muscle catabolism, which would result in the production of large quantities of aromatic amino acids. In addition, dogs with experimental portal-caval shunts fed an oral diet of 35 per cent branched chain amino acids that was low in aromatic amino acids did as well as those on the IV solution. Clinicians must be extremely cautious when using commercial protein hydrolysates parenterally in patients in hepatic failure. Such solutions have extremely high ammonia concentrations, 1500 to 1900 $\mu g/dl$ (Strombeck et al., 1975). Stored blood is also dangerous in this regard.

Ascites and Edema. Ascites is a fairly common complication of chronic hepatic failure, while peripheral edema is seen infrequently. Ascites, although varying in severity, is not necessarily harmful. Moderate amounts have minimal physiologic importance. Therapy should be directed not only at reducing the severity of ascites pharmacologically or mechanically, but also towards measures that will improve hepatic function. Patients with severe hepatic failure and ascites may not have significant diuresis until improvement in hepatic function has occurred.

The most commonly used means of controlling ascites formation and augmenting its elimination are low sodium diets, diuretics, paracentesis, and peritoneovenous or portacaval shunts. Low sodium diets and diuretics form the backbone of therapy for ascites. Bed rest and sodium restriction alone result in a spontaneous diuresis in 5 to 15 per cent of ascitic humans. Sodium restriction must be severe. In man, salt restriction for patients with hepatic failure and ascites is four times more severe than in those with congestive heart failure, i.e., 250 mg/day vs. 1200 to 1500 mg/day (Arroyo and Rodes, 1975). Commercially available low sodium diets may be tried initially, but if a poor response is noted, home formulated diets should be tried.

Since sodium retention in hepatic-induced ascites occurs at both proximal and distal sites along the nephron, potent "loop" diuretics are the most successful at counteracting this sodium reabsorbing tendency. Either furosemide or ethacrynic acid are good choices for inducing a diuresis. Distal tubular diuretics, i.e., those that interfere with aldosterone activity, such as spironolactone (Aldactone or Aldactone-A) or triamterene should also be used. These latter diuretics may also help reduce the potassium wasting caused by "loop" diuretics. Procedures followed in man that appear as though they could apply to the dog begin with marked sodium restriction and the addition of spironolactone. Spironolactone is dosed at 1 to 2 mg/kg body weight twice daily. Response to aldosterone antagonists often requires three to four days for an obvious diuresis to develop. If no response is noted, the spironolactone dosage should be doubled for an additional three to four days. This regimen results in a significant diuresis in 40 to 60 per cent of humans. If these initial two methods are ineffective, furosemide or ethacrynic acid are added to the foregoing regime. The furosemide dosage (0.25 to 0.5 mg/kg body weight divided twice daily) may also be doubled if no response is noted in four to seven days. Patients should not be allowed to become dehydrated by overvigorous use of diuretics. Ascitic fluid has a maximal rate of mobilization of 700 to 900 ml/day in man. Any net body fluid losses beyond this are at the expense of plasma water. Patients are normally not allowed more than 200 to 300 ml net water loss per day. Animals should be weighed daily and the owners instructed in methods to detect severe dehydration. Periodic serum electrolyte determinations should be made on any animal given potent diuretics over sustained periods. Although clinically significant electrolyte abnormalities would appear to occur infrequently, monitoring is essential for their detection. If salt restriction and diuretics do not result in significant mobilization of ascites in two weeks, more heroic measures should be considered.

Paracentesis for removal of ascites should be avoided unless dyspnea or patient discomfort are noted and the ascites has not responded to medical therapy, or as a temporary expedient to provide abrupt relief. Small quantities may be removed for diagnostic purposes. Many complications of paracentesis can occur in patients in hepatic failure, including albumin depletion, peritonitis, hypovolemia, hepatic coma, and oliguria (Zeegen et al., 1968) Two surgical procedures have been used clinically in man and experimentally in dogs to control chronic, diuretic refractory ascites. The first is the LaVeen shunt, initially developed in 1972. The LaVeen shunt is a one-way pressure-actuated valve. The valve is inserted into the peritoneal cavity and connected by subcutaneous tubing to the jugular vein. Ascitic fluid is propelled into the venous system by the pumping action of the diaphragm (Wyllie et al., 1980). Such surgical drainage systems have been well tolerated by experimental cirrhotic dogs (Levy et al., 1979). An alternative surgical procedure for ascites control in cases of acquired or congenital portal hypertension is the creation of a portal-systemic venous shunt. Creating a large communication between the portal vein and a major systemic vein decompresses the hypertensive portal system. The major drawbacks to this procedure lie in the high surgical risk to patients in hepatic failure and the increased tendency for operated animals to develop hepatic coma. The trade-off lies in whether the ascites is worse than managing encephalopathy.

Intercurrent Infection. Intercurrent infections are one of the most frequent complications of hepatic cirrhosis. Gram-negative septicemias are a frequent occurrence, the bowel being the presumed source of infection (in man). Since many cases of chronic active liver disease are associated with a nonseptic fever, an infection tends to be overlooked and must be guarded against. The normal dog liver harbors anerobic gram-positive organisms that may proliferate in hepatic failure. The addition of prophylactic antibiotics to the therapeutic regime is justified in such cases.

Malabsorption. Clinically significant malabsorption associated with chronic hepatic and biliary tract diseases is uncommon in animals. When it occurs, a number of therapeutic agents may be used to alleviate or reduce the severity of the problem. Oral bile salts may increase the emulsification, digestion, and absorption of intestinal fats but often contain unconjugated fractions that are irritating to the bowel and may cause diarrhea. The addition of neutral fats in the form of H_2O-soluble medium chain triglycerides (Portagen) that do not require the action of lipase or bile salts for absorption may increase caloric intake and promote weight gains; however, they may aggravate patients in coma. Lastly, occasional cases of biliary tract disease with steatorrhea may benefit from the addition of pancreatic enzymes to the diet.

Hemorrhage and Anemia. Therapy for hemmorhage and anemia associated with hepatic failure is often difficult until the hepatic disease starts to repair itself. Hypovitaminosis K associated with prolonged prothrombin time secondary to impaired bile drainage can be alleviated by parenteral injections of aqueous vitamin K. If associated with depressed synthesis of prothrombin due to severe hepatocellular damage, vitamin K will have no effect on alleviating the bleeding problem. Anemia associated with hypersplenism and portal hypertension may be corrected by splenectomy or portacaval shunting, but the patient's condition often precludes such procedures. The nutritional anemias are managed by a balanced diet and parenteral vitamin therapy, if necessary. In general, bleeding tendencies are uncommon except in terminal stages of hepatic failure or in those situations in which DIC becomes a problem (diaphragmatic hernias, massive liver necrosis). Bleeding into the gastrointestinal tract is particularly catastrophic, as blood is a highly effective protein source for inducing severe hepatic coma.

Fulminant Hepatic Failure. Acute hepatic failure is often of a fulminant nature, the clinical syndrome being associated with massive necrosis of parenchymal cells and sudden severe impairment of hepatic function. Fulminant hepatic failure most commonly follows viral hepatitis or exposure to hepatotoxins or drugs. Primary goals of therapy are to preserve life until sufficient hepatic regeneration occurs to allow recovery and to manage any complications that develop during the early recovery period. Such therapy is primarily supportive in nature but also may involve a number of heroic measures that, as yet, have not been documented as to efficacy. Supportive care involves frequent monitoring of the animal's vital signs; repeated physical exams, particularly noting changing mental status or the development of neurologic signs, discontinuing all drugs not absolutely indicated; preventing hypoglycemia; monitoring acid base, electrolyte, and volume status; instituting measures to control blood ammonia; and promptly detecting and treating any infections, bleeding, or respiratory complications (Scharschmidt, 1975). Glucocorticoids have been used for years in the therapy of fulminant hepatic failure. Recent results of controlled clinical trials indicate they have no beneficial effects and may be detrimental (Tanner and Powell, 1979).

REFERENCES

Ackerman, N., and Silverman, S.: Radiographic interpretation: liver enlargement. Mod. Vet. Pract. *58*:949–954, 1977.

Aldrete, J. S.: Quantification of the capacity of the liver to remove ammonia from the circulation of dogs with portacaval transposition. Surg. Gynecol. and Obstet. *141*:399–404, 1975.

Aledort, L. M.: Blood Clotting Abnormalities in Liver Disease. *In* Popper, H., and Schaffner, F. (eds.): Progress in Liver Diseases. Vol. 5. Grune and Stratton, New York, 1976.

Arhelger, R. B.: Experimental cholemia in dogs. Electron microscopy of glomerular lesions. Arch. Pathol. *89*:355, 1970.

Arroyo, V., and Rodes, J.: Treatment of ascites — a rational approach to the treatment of ascites. Post. Grad. Med. J. *51*:558–562, 1975.

Atterbury, C. E., Maddrey, W. C., and Conn, H. O.: Neomycin-sorbitol and lactulose in the treatment of acute portal systemic encephalopathy. Dig. Dis. Sci. *23*:398–406, 1978.

Audell, L., Jonsson, L., and Lannek, B.: Congenital portal caval shunts in the dog. A description of three cases. Zentralbl. Veterinaermed. *21*:797–805, 1974.

Ayers, C. R., Davis, J. O., Lieberman, F., Carpenter, C. J., and Berman, M.: Effects of chronic hepatic venous congestion in metabolism of d,1-aldosterone and d-aldosterone. J. Clin. Invest. *41*:884, 1962.

Barnardo, D. E., Strong, C. G., and Baldus, W. P.: Failure of the cirrhotic liver to inactivate renin: Evidence for a splachnic source of renin-like activity. J. Lab. Clin. Med. *74*:495, 1969.

Barrett, R. E., DeLahunta, A., Roenick, W. J., Hoffer, R. E., and Coons, F. H.: Four cases of congenital portalcaval shunt in the dog. J. Small Anim. Pract. *17*:71–85, 1976.

Barsanti, J. A., Jones, B. D., Spano, J. S., and Taylor, H. W.: Prolonged anorexia associated with hepatic lipidosis in three cats. Feline Pract. 7:52–57. 1977.

Benjamin, M. J.: Outline of Veterinary Clinical Pathology. Iowa State University Press, Ames, 1961.

Bishop, L., Strandberg, J. D., Adams, R. J., Brown-stein, D. B., and Patterson, R.: Chronic active hepatitis associated with leptospires. Am. J. Vet. Res. 40:839–844, 1979.

Black, M.: Hepatotoxicity: Pathogenesis and therapeutic intervention Clin. Gastroenterol. 8:89–104, 1979.

Bollman, J. L., Mann, F. C., and Magath, T. B.: Effect of total removal of liver on formation of urea. Am. J. Physiol. 69:371, 1924.

Breen, K. J., and Schenker, S.: Hepatic Coma: Present Concepts of Pathogenesis and Therapy. In Popper, H., and Schaffner, F. (eds.): Progress in Liver Diseases. Vol. 4. Grune and Stratton, New York, 1972.

Breznock, E. M.: Surgical manipulations of portosystemic shunts in dogs. J.A.M.A. 174:819–826, 1979.

Brinkhous, K. M., and Warner, E. D.: Effect of vitamin K on hypoprothrombininemia of experimental liver injury. Soc. Exp. Biol. & Med. 44:609, 1940.

Brody, D. H., and Leichter, L.: Clearance tests of liver function. Med. Clin. North Am. 63:621–630, 1979.

Brunson, D. B., Stevens, J. B., and McGrath, C. J.: Preoperative liver screen selection: a comparison of serum glutamic-pyruvic transaminase and serum alkaline phosphatase. J.A.A.H.A. 16:209–214, 1980.

Campbell, C. B., and Cowen, A. E.: Bile salt metabolism II-bile salts and disease. Aust. N.Z. J. Med. 7:587–595, 1977.

Candlin, F. T.: Diseases of the liver, pancreas and peritoneum. In Catcott, E. J. (ed.): Canine Medicine. 1st Catcott ed. American Veterinary Publications, Inc., Wheaton, 1968.

Casey, T. H., Summerskill, W. H. J., and Orvis, A. L.: Body and serum potassium in liver disease. Gastroenterol., 48:198–207, 1965.

Ceh, L., Hauge, J. G., Svenkerud, R., and Strande, A.: Glycogenosis type III in the dog. Acta. Vet. Scand. 17:210–222, 1976.

Chen, T. S., Zaki, G. F., and Leevy, C. M.: Studies of nucleic acid and collagen synthesis: current status in assessing liver repair. Med. Clin. North AM. 63:583–592, 1979.

Cobb, L. M., and McKay, K. A.: A bacteriological study of the liver of the normal dog. J. Comp. Pathol. 72:92, 1962.

Coles, E. H.: Veterinary Clinical Pathology. W. B. Saunders Co., Philadelphia, 1967.

Conn, H. O., Leevy, C. M., Vlahcevic, Z. R., Rogers, J. B., and Maddrey, W. C.: Comparison of lactulose and neomycin in the treatment of chronic portal systemic encephalopathy. Gastroenterology 72:573–583, 1977.

Corn, M.: Hemostasis and hemorrhage in patients with liver disease. Med. Times 96:76, 1968.

Cornelius, C. E.: Liver Function. In Kaneko, J. J., and Cornelius, C. E. (eds.): Clinical Biochemistry of Domestic Animals. Academic Press, New York, 1970.

Cornelius, C. E.: Biochemical evaluations of hepatic function in dogs. J.A.A.H.A. 15:259–269, 1979.

Cornelius, C. E., and Himes, J. A.: New concepts in canine hepatic function. J.A.H.A. 9:147, 1973.

Cornelius, C. E., Bishop, J. A., Switzer, J., and Rhode, E. S.: Serum and tissue transaminase activities in domestic animals. Cornell Vet. 49:116, 1959.

Cornelius, L. M., Thrall, D. E., Halliwell, W. H., Frank, G. M., Kern, A. J., and Woods, C. B.: Anomalous portosystemic anastomoses associated with chronic hepatic insufficiency in six young dogs. J.A.V.M.A. 167:220–228, 1975.

Cowen, A. E., and Campbell, C. B.: Bile salt metabolism — the physiology of bile salts. Aust. N.Z. J. Med. 7:579–586, 1977.

DeSchepper, J.: Degradation of haemoglobin to bilirubin in the kidney of the dog. Tijdschr. Diergeneeskd. 99:699–707, 1974.

Dew, M. J., Thompson, H., and Allan, R. N.: The spectrum of hepatic dysfunction in inflammatory bowel disease. Quart. J. Med. 48:113–135, 1979.

Dhar, P., Gupta, N. N., and Mehrotra, R. M. L.: Plasma erythropoietin as a parameter in the evaluation of anemias associated with hepatic and renal disorders. Indian J. Med. Sic. 22:91, 1968.

Dillon, A. R., Spano, J. S., and Powers, R. D.: Prednisolone-induced hematologic biochemical and histologic changes in the dog. J.A.A.H.A. 16:831–837, 1980.

Dorner, J. L., Hoffman, W. E., and Long, G. E.: Corticosteroid induction of an isoenzyme of alkaline phosphatase in the dog. A.J.V.R. 35:1457–1458, 1974.

Eddleston, A. L., and Williams, R.: The role of immunological mechanisms in chronic hepatitis. Ann. Clin. Res. 8:162–173, 1976.

Edwards, D. F.: Blind percutaneous liver biopsy: A safe diagnostic procedure. Calif. Vet. 4:9–15, 1977.

EL-Zawahry, M. D., Kahlil, A. M., and EL-Banna, M. H.: Medeccasol. A new therapy for hepatic fibrosis. Bull. Soc. Int. Chir., 6:573–577, 1975.

Engen, M. H., Weirsch, W. E., and Lund, Y. E.: Fibrinölysis in a dog with diaphragmatic hernia. J.A.V.M.A. 164:152–153, 1974.

Epstein, M.: Renal Sodium Handling in Cirrhosis. In Epstein, M. (ed.): The Kidney In Liver Disease. Elsevier-North Holland, Inc. New York, 1978.

Epstein, M.: Deranged renal function in liver disease. Contrib. Nephrol. 7:250–271, 1977.

Ettinger, S. E., and Suter, P. F.: Canine Cardiology. W. B. Saunders Co., Philadelphia, 1970.

Everell, R. M. Duncan, J. R., and Prasse, K. W.: Alkaline phosphatase, leucine aminopeptidase, and alanine aminotransferase activities with obstructive and toxic hepatic disease in cats. A.J.V.R. 38:963–966, 1977.

Ewing, G. O., Suter, P. F., and Bailey, C. S.: Hepatic insufficiency associated with congenital anomalies of the portal vein in dogs. J.A.A.H.A. 10:463–476, 1974.

Feldman, B. F.: Clinical Pathology of the Liver. In Kirk, R. W. (ed.): Current Veterinary Therapy. Vol. 7. W. B. Saunders Co., Philadelphia, 1980.

Feldman, E. C., and Ettinger, S. J.: Percutaneous transthoracic liver biopsy in the dog: A review of 75 cases. Calif. Vet. 13:17–22, 1977.

Feldman, E. C., and Ettinger, S. J.: Percutaneous transthoracic liver biopsy in the dog. J.A.V.M.A. 169:805–810, 1976.

Fenton, J. C. B., Knight, E. J., and Humpherson, P. L.: Milk and cheese diet in portal systemic encephalopathy. Lancet 1:164–166, 1966.

Figueroa, R. B.: Mesterolone in steatosis and cirrhosis of the liver. Acta Hepato-Gastroenterol. 20:282–290, 1973.

Fischer, J. E., and Baldessarini, R. J.: Pathogenesis and Therapy of Hepatic Coma. In Popper, H., and Schaffner, F., (eds.): Progress in liver diseases. Vol. 5. Grune and Stratton, New York, 1976.

Fischer, J. E., and Eisenfeld, A.: Alterations in H-estradiol distribution following portal caval shunt. Surgery, 69:655, 1971.

Fischer, J. E., Keane, J., Dodsworth, J., and Funories, J. M.: An alternative mechanism for beneficial effects of intestinal sterilization in hepatic encephalopathy. Surg. Forum 25:369–372, 1974.

Flood, C. A., Gutman, E. B., and Gutman, A. B.: Serum and urine phosphatase activity in the cat after ligation of the common bile duct. Am. J. Physiol. *120*:120–696, 1937.

Freund, H., Yoshimura, N.,and Fischer, J.: Chronic hepatic encephalopathy. Long-term therapy with a branched-chain amino acid enriched diet. J.A.M.A. *24*:347–349, 1979.

Gabuzda, G. J.: Symposium on liver disease II: Treatment of ascites and hepatic insufficiency. A. J. Gastroenterol. *38*:15, 1962.

Gocke, D. J., Morris, T. Q., and Bradley, S. E.: Chronic hepatitis in the dog: The role of immune factors. J.A.V.M.A. *156*:1700, 1970.

Gilmore, I. T., Cowan, R. E., Axon, A. T. R., and Thompson, R. H.: Controlled trial of cyclophosphamide in active chronic hepatitis. Br. Med. J. *1*:1120–1121, 1979.

Glynn, L. E.: Immunopathology of the Liver. *In* Popper, H., and Schaffner, F. (eds.): Progress in Liver Diseases. Vol. 5. Grune and Stratton, New York, 1976.

Gofton, N.: Surgical ligation of congenital portosystemic shunts in the dog: A report of three cases. J.A.A.H.A. *14*:728–733, 1978.

Goldman, M. A., Schwartz, C. C., Swell, L., and Vlachevic, Z. R.: Bile Acid Metabolism in Health and Disease. *In* Popper, H., and Schaffner, F. (eds.): Progress in Liver Diseases. Vol. 6. Grune and Stratton, New York; 1979.

Grandage, J.: The radiology of the dog's diaphragm. J. Small Anim. Pract. *15*:1–17, 1974.

Grausz, H., and Schmidt, R.: Reciprocal relationship between plasma albumin level and hepatic suffobromophthalein removal. N. Engl. J. Med. *284*:1043–1405, 1971.

Greene, C. E.: Ascites: diagnostic and therapeutic considerations. Comp. Cont. Ed. *1*:712–719, 1979.

Hardy, R. M., Stevens, J. B., and Stowe, L.: Chronic progressive hepatitis in bedlington terriers associated with elevated liver copper concentrations. Minn. Vet. *15*:13–24, 1975.

Harvey, D. G.: The estimation of serum alkaline phosphatase in the dog. J. Small Anim. Pract. *8*:557, 1967.

Harvey, J. W., and Kornick, H. P.: Phenazopyridine toxicosis in the cat. J.A.V.M.A. *169*:327–331, 1976.

Havens, W. P., Jr., Dickensheets, J., Bierly, J. N., and Eberhard, T. P.: the Half-life of I[131]-labeled normal human gamma globulin in patients with hepatic cirrhosis. J. Immunol. *73*:256, 1954.

Heywood, R., Chesterman, H., Ball, S. A., and Wadsworth, P. F.: Toxicity of methyl testosterone in the beagle dog. Toxicology *7*:357–365, 1977.

Hoe, C. M.: Liver Function Tests. *In* Medway, W., Prier, J. E., and Wilkinson, J. S. (eds.): Textbook of Veterinary Clinic Pathology. Williams & Wilkins Co., Baltimore, 1969.

Hoe, C. M.: Tests for liver dysfunction in dogs. Nature (London) *192*:1045, 1961.

Hoe, C. M., and Harvey, D. G.: An investigation into liver tests in dogs. Part 2. Tests other than transaminase estimations. J. Small. Anim. Pract. *2*:109, 1961.

Hoe, C. M., and O'Shea, J. D.: The correlation of biochemistry and histopathology in liver disease in the dog. Vet. Rec. *77*:1164, 1965.

Hoenig, V.: Management of Acute Liver Damage in Man. *In* Popper, H., and Schaffner, F. (eds.): Progress in Liver Diseases. Vol. 3. Grune and Stratton, New York, 1970.

Hoffman, W. E.: The diagnostic value of canine serum alkaline phosphatase and alkaline phosphatase isoenzymes. 26th Gaines Veterinary Symposium, Oct. 1976, pp. 2–6.

Hoffman, W. E.: Diagnostic value of canine serum alkaline phosphatase and alkaline phosphatase isoenzymes. J.A.A.H.A. *13*:237–241, 1977.

Hoffman, W. E., and Dorner, J. L.: Disappearance rates of intravenously injected canine serum alkaline phosphatase isoenzymes. Am. J. Vet Res. *38*:1553–1556, 1977.

Hoffman, W. E., and Dorner, J. L.: Separation of isoenzymes of canine alkaline phosphatase by cellulose acetate electrophoresis. J.A.A.H.A. *11*:283–285, 1975.

Hoffman, W. E., Reneger, W. E., and Dorner, J. L.: Serum half-life of intravenously injected intestinal and hepatic alkaline phosphatase isoenzymes in the cat. Am. J. Vet. Res. *38*:637–639, 1977.

Hoskins, J. D., Ochoa, R., and Hawkins, B. J.: Portal vein thrombosis in a dog: A case report. J.A.A.H.A. *15*:497–500, 1979.

Inglefinger, F. J.: The Liver. *In* Sodeman, W. A., and Sodeman, W. A., Jr. (eds.): Pathologic Physiology. W. B. Saunders Co., Philadelphia, 1967.

Islam, N., and Islam, A.: Testosterone propionate in cirrhosis of the liver. Br. J. Clin. Pract. *27*:125–128, 1973.

Jacobs, I.: Antibiotics and liver disease. Calif. Med. *111*:382, 1969.

James, I. M., Sashat, S., Sampson, D., Williams, H. S., and Garassini, M.: Effect of induced metabolic alkalosis on hepatic encephalopathy. Lancet *2*:1106–1107, 1969.

Jeffries, G. H.: Diseases of the Liver. *In* Beeson, P. B., and McDermott, W. (eds.): Cecil and Loeb Textbook of Medicine. 13 ed. W. B. Saunders Co., Philadelphia, 1971.

Jick, H., Kamm, D. E., Synder, J. G., Morrison, R. S., and Chalmers, T. C.: On the concentrating defect in cirrhosis of the liver. J. Clin. Invest. *43*:258, 1964.

Johnson, G. F., Sternlieb, I., Twedt, D. C., Grushoff, P. S., and Scheinberg, I.: Inheritance of copper toxicosis in Bedlington terriers. Am. J. Vet. Res. *41*:1865–1866, 1980.

Jubb, K. V. F., and Kennedy, P. C.: The Liver and Biliary Systems, Vol. 2. *In* Jubb, K. V. F., and Kennedy, P. C. (eds.): Pathology of Domestic Animals. 2nd ed. Academic Press, New York, 1970.

Kakumu, S., Arakawa, Y., Goj, H., Kashio, T., and Yata, K.: Occurrence and significance of antibody to liver specific membrane lipoprotein by double antibody immune precipitation method in sera of patients with acute and chronic liver disease. Gastroenterology *76*:665–672, 1979.

Kawanishi, H.: Morphologic association of lymphocytes with hepatocytes in chronic liver disease. Arch. Pathol. Lab Med. *101*:286–290, 1977.

Kershenobich, D., Uribe, M., Suares, G. I., Mata, J. M., Peres-Tamayo, R., and Rojkind, M.: Treatment of cirrhosis with cholchicine: A double-blind, randomized trial. Gastroenterology *77*:532–536, 1979.

Khan, I. R., and Vitums, A.: Portosystemic communications in the cat. Res. Vet. Sci. *12*:215, 1971.

Kozlowski, S., and Drzewiecki, K.: The role of osmoreception in portal circulation in control of water intake in dogs. Acta Physiol. Polonica *24*:325–330, 1973.

Kukral, J. C., Spom, J., Louch, J., and Winzler, R. J.: Synthesis of alpha and beta globulins in normal and liverless dogs. Am. J. Physiol. *204*:262, 1963.

Lam, K. C., Lai, C. L., Mg, R. P., Trepo, C., and Wu, P. C.: Deleterious effect of prednisolone in HBsAg-positive chronic active hepatitis. New Engl. J. Med. *304*:380–386, 1981.

Leevy, C. M., Thompson, A., and Baker, H.: Vitamins and liver injury. Am. J. Clin. Nutr. *23*:493, 1970.

Legendre, A. M., Krahwinkel, D. J., Carrig, C. B., and Michel, R. L.: Ascites associated with intrahepatic arteriovenous fistula in a cat. J.A.V.M.A. *168*:589–592, 1976.

Levine, N. D., Beamer, P. D., and Maksic, D.: Hepatitis due to *Amphimerus pseudofelineus* in a cat. Ill. Vet. *1*:47, 1958.

Levinsky, N. G., Davidson, D. G., and Berliner, R. W.: Change in urine concentration during prolonged administration of vasopressin and water. Am. J. Physiol. *196*:451, 1959.

Levy, M., Wexler, M. J., and McCaffrey, C.: Sodium retention in dogs with experimental cirrhosis following removal of ascites by continuous peritoneovenous shunting. J. Lab. Clin. Med. *94*:933–946, 1979.

Liehr, H., Grun, M., and Brunswig, D.: Endotoxemia in acute hepatic failure. Acta. Hepato-Gastroenterol. *23*:235–240, 1976.

Ling, G. V., Lowenstine, L. G., Pulley, L. T., and Kaneko, J. J.: Diabetes mellitus in dogs: A review of initial evaluation, immediate and long-term management and outcome. J.A.V.M.A. *170*:521–530, 1977.

Linscheer, W. G.: Malabsorption in cirrhosis. Am. J. Clin. Nutr. *23*:488, 1970.

Lohse, C. L., Selcer, R. R., and Suter, P. F.: Hepatoencephalopathy associated with situs inversus of abdominal organs and vascular anomalies in a dog. J.A.V.M.A. *168*:687–688, 1976.

Low, D. G.: Diseases of the Liver. *In* Scientific Presentations and Seminar Synopses of the 39th Annual Meeting of the A.A.H.A. 1972, p. 348.

Ludwing, J., Owen, C. A., Barham, S. S., McCall, J. T., and Hardy, R. M.: The liver in the inherited copper disease of Bedlington terriers. Lab. Invest. *43*:82–87, 1980.

Lykkegaard, N. M., Justeses, T., and Asnaes, S.: Anaerobic bacteriological study of the human liver, with a critical review of the literature. Scand. J. Gastroenterol. *9*:671–677, 1974.

Maddrey, W. C., and Weber, F. L.: Chronic hepatic encephalopathy. Med. Clin. North Am. *59*:937–944, 1975.

Madsbad, S., Bjerregaard, J. B., Henrickson, J. H., and Julin, E.: Impaired conversion of prednisone to prednisolone in patients with liver cirrhosis. Gut *21*:52–56, 1980.

Maretta, S. M., Pask, A. J., Greene, R. W., and Liu, S. K.: Urinary calculi associated with portosystemic shunts in six dogs. J.A.V.M.A. *178*:133–137, 1981.

Massry, S. G., and Klein, K. L.: Effects of Bile Duct Ligation on Renal Function. *In* Epstein, M. (ed.): The Kidney in Liver Disease. Elsevier, North Holland, Inc., New York, 1978.

Matern, S., and Gerok, W.: Pathphysiology of the enterohepatic circulation of bile acids. Rev. Physiol. Biochem. Pharmacol. *85*:125–204, 1979a.

Matern, S., and Gerok, W.: Diagnostic value of serum bile acids. Acta Hepatogastroenterol. (Stutt) *26*:185–189, 1979b.

Medway, W.: Assessment of liver function. Norden News, *43*:30, 1968.

Mehain, D. L., Nagode, L. A., Wilson, G. P., and Kociba, G. L.: Alkaline phosphatase and its isoenzymes in normal cats and in cats with biliary obstruction. J.A.A.H.A. *14*:94–99, 1978.

Merino, G. E., Jetzer, T., Dorzaki, W. M. D., and Najarian, J. S.: Methionine induced hepatic coma in dogs. Am. J. Surg. *130*:41–46, 1975.

Meyer, D. J., and Noonan, N. E.: Liver tests in dogs receiving anticonvulsant drugs (diphenylhydantoin and primidone). J.A.A.H.A. *17*:261–264, 1981.

Meyer, D. J., Iverson, W. D., and Terrell, T. G.: Obstructive jaundice associated with chronic active hepatitis. J.A.V.M.A. *176*:41–44, 1980.

Meyer, D. J., Strombeck, D. R., Stone, E. A., Zenoble, R. D., and Buss, D. D.: Ammonia tolerance test in clinically normal dogs and in dogs with portosystemic shunts. J.A.V.M.A. *173*:377–379, 1978.

Mia, A. S., and Koger, H. D.: Comparative studies on serum arginase and transaminases in hepatic necrosis in various species of domestic animals. Vet. Clin. Pathol. *8*:9–15, 1979.

Mitchell, J. R., and Potter, W. Z.: Drug metabolism in the production of liver disease. Med. Clin. North Am. *59*:877–885, 1975.

Morgan, M. Y., Jakovovits, A., Elithorn, A., Jamer, I. M., and Sherlock, S.: Successful use of bromocriptine in the treatment of a patient with chronic portosystemic encephalopathy. New Engl. J. Med. *296*:793–794, 1977.

Nash, A. J.: Phenytoin toxicity: A fatal case in the dog with hepatitis and jaundice. Vet. Rec. *1*:280–281, 1977.

Ndiritu, C. G., and Weigel, J.: Hepatorenal injury in a dog associated with methoxyflurane (a case report). VM SAC *72*:545–550, 1977.

Nolan, J. P.: The role of endotoxin in liver injury. Gastroenterology *69*:1346–1356, 1975.

Norcross, J. W.: The anemia of liver disease. Med. Clin. North Am. *50*:543, 1966.

Osbaldiston, G. W., and Hoffman, M. W.: Coagulation defects in experimental hepatic injury in the dog. Can. J. Comp. Med. *35*:129, 1971.

Osborne, C. A., Hardy, R. M., Stevens, J. B., and Perman, V. P.: Liver biopsy. Vet. Clin. North Am. *4*:333–350, 1972.

Osborne, C. A., Stevens, J. B., and Perman, V.: Needle biopsy of the liver. J.A.V.M.A. *155*:1605, 1969.

Patel, D., Anderson, G. H., and Jeyeebhoy, K. N.: Amino acid adequacy of parenteral casein hydrolysate and oral cottage cheese in patients with gastrointestinal disease as measured by nitrogen balance and blood aminogram. Gastroenterology *65*:427–437, 1973.

Peters, T.: Serum albumin: recent progress in the understanding of its structure and biosynthesis. Clin. Chem. *23*:5–12, 1977.

Pirotte, J., Guffens, J. M., and Devos, J.: Comparative study of basal arterial ammonia and of orally induced hyperammonemia in chronic portal-systemic encephalopathy treated with neomycin, lactulose and an association of neomycin and lactulose. Digestion *10*:435–444, 1974.

Polzin, D. J., Stowe, C. J., O'Leary, T. P., Stevens, J. B., and Hardy, R. M.: Acute hepatic necrosis associated with the administration of mebendazole. J.A.V.M.A. *179*:1013–1016, 1981.

Popper, H., and Schaffner, F.: Chronic Hepatitis: Toxonomic, Etiology and Therapeutic Problems. *In* Popper, H., and Schaffner, F. (eds.): Progress in Liver Diseases. Vol. 5. Grune and Stratton, New York, 1976.

Powell, L. W., and Axelsen, E.: Corticosteroids in liver disease: studies on the biological conversion of prednisone to prednisolone and plasma protein binding. Gut *13*:690–696, 1972.

Pulliyel, M. M., Vyas, G. P., and Mehta, G. S.: Testosterone in the management of cirrhosis of the liver — a controlled study. Aust. N.Z. J. Med. 7:596–599, 1977.

Rafiquazzaman, M., Svenkernd, R., Strande, A., and Hauge, J. G.: Glycogenosis in the dog. Acta Vet. Scand. 17:196–209, 1976.

Redeker, A. G.: Treatment of chronic active hepatitis, good news and bad news. New Engl. J. Med. 304:420–421, 1980.

Riveron, E., Abtahi, H., Kukral, J. C., Zeineh, R. A., and Henegar, G. C.: Syndrome of metabolic alkalosis, hypokalemia and hyperammonemia in patients with cirrhosis. Surg. Forum 18:341, 1967.

Roberts, H. S., and Cederbaum, A. I.: The liver and blood coagulation — physiology and pathology. Gastroenterology 63:297, 1972.

Rogers, A. E.: Therapeutic considerations in selected forms of acute and chronic liver disease. Med. Clin. North Am. 55:373, 1971.

Rogers, W. A., and Ruebner, B. H.: A retrospective study of probable glucocorticoid induced hepatopathy in dogs. J.A.V.M.A. 170:603–606, 1977.

Rojkind, M., and Kershenobich, D.: Regulation of Collagen Synthesis in Liver Cirrhosis. In Popper, H., and Becker, K. (eds.): Collagen Metabolism in the Liver. Stratton Intercontinental Medical Book Corp., New York, 1973.

Rojkind, M., and Kershenobich, D.: Hepatic Fibrosis. In Popper, H., and Schaffner, F. (eds.): Progress in Liver Diseases. Vol. 5. Grune and Stratton, New York, 1976.

Root, C. R.: Interpretation of abdominal survey radiographs. Vet. Clin. North Am. 4:763–804, 1974.

Rosenoer, V. M., and Gualberto, G., Jr.: Management of patients with chronic obstructive jaundice. Med. Clin. North Am. 56:759, 1972.

Rosenthal, W. S., and Glass, G. B. J.: Vitamin B_{12} and the Liver. In Popper, H., and Schaffner, F. (eds.): Progress in Liver Diseases. 3rd ed. Grune and Stratton, New York, 1970.

Rothenbacker, H., and Lindquist, W. D.: Liver cirrhosis and pancreatitis in a cat infected with Amphimerus pseudofelineus. J.A.V.M.A. 143:1099, 1963.

Rudman, D., Akgun, S., Galambos, J., Cullen, A., and Gerron, G.: Defective urea synthesis in cirrhotics. Clin. Res. 17:461, 1969.

Russell, R. M.: Vitamin and mineral supplements in the management of liver disease. Med. Clin. North Am. 63:537–544, 1979.

Saini, P. K., and Saini, S. K.: Origin of serum alkaline phosphatase in the dog. Am. J. Vet. Res. 39:1510–1513, 1978.

Schaffner, F.: Treatment of liver disease. Modern Treatment 6:121, 1969.

Schaffner, F., and Popper, H.: Adverse drug reactions involving the liver: probable mechanisms. Mt. Sinai J. Med. 44:813–819, 1977.

Schall, W. D.: Laboratory diagnosis of hepatic disease. Vet. Clin. North Am. 6679–686, 1976.

Scharschmidt, B. F.: Approaches to the management of fulminant hepatic failure. Med. Clin. North Am. 59:927–935, 1975.

Schenk, W. G., Jr., Fopeano, J., Cosgriff, J. H., Jr., and Gray, J. G.: The coagulation defect after hepatectomy. Surgery 42:822, 1957.

Schenker, S., Breen, K. J., and Hoyumpa, A. M.: Hepatic encephalopathy: current status. Gastroenterology 66:121–151, 1974.

Schiff, L.: The use of steroids in liver disease. Medicine 45:565, 1966.

Schmid, R.: Bilirubin metabolism in man. N. Engl. J. Med. 287:703. 1972.

Schmidt, S., and Suter, P. F.: Indirect and direct determination of the portal vein pressure in normal and abnormal dogs and normal cats. Am. J. Vet. Rad. Soc. 21:246–259, 1980.

Sherding, R. G.: Hepatic encephalopathy in the dog. Comp. Cont. Ed. 1:55–63, 1979.

Sherlock, S.: Advances in the treatment of disease of the liver. Practitioner 205:494, 1970.

Shull, R. M., and Hornbuckle, W.: Diagnostic use of serum gamma glutamyltransferase in canine liver disease. Am. J. Vet. Res. 40:1321–1324, 1979.

Shull, R. M., Tasker, J. B., and Hiltz, F. L.: A computerized retrospective study of liver enzyme concentrations in dogs. Vet. Clin. Pathol. 7:13, 1978.

Simpson, S. T., and Hribernik, T. N.: Portosystemic shunts in the dog. Two case reports. J. Small Anim. Pract. 17:163–170, 1976.

Smith, H. A., Jones, T. C., and Hunt, R. D.: Veterinary Pathology. Lea & Febiger, Philadelphia, 1972.

Smith, A. R., Rossi-Fanelli, F., Freund, H., and Fischer, J. E.: Sulfur-containing amino acids in experimental hepatic coma in the dog and monkey. Surgery 85:677–683, 1979.

Speaman, J. G., Hunt, P., and Nayar, P. S. G.: Yersinia (Pasturella) pseudotuberculosis infection in a cat. Can. Vet. J. 20:361, 1979.

Starzl, T., and Teiblanche, J.: Hepatotrophic Substances. In Popper, H., and Schaffner, F. (eds.): Progress in Liver Diseases. Vol. 6. Grune and Stratton, New York, 1979.

Starzl, T. E., Porter, K. A., and Putnam, C. W.: Intraportal insulin protects from the liver injury of portacaval shunt in dogs. Lancet 2:1741–1742, 1975.

St. Omar, V. D., and McKnight, E. D.: Acetylcysteine for treatment of acetaminophen toxicosis in the cat. J.A.V.M.A. 176:911–913, 1980.

Striebel, J. P., Holm, E., Lutz, H., and Storz, L. W.: Parenteral nutrition and coma therapy with amino acids in hepatic failure. J. Parent. Ent. Nutr. 4:240–246, 1979.

Strombeck, D. R.: Management of Chronic Active Hepatitis. In Kirk, R. W. (ed.): Current Veterinary Therapy. Vol. 7. W. B. Saunders Co., Philadelphia, 1980.

Strombeck, D. R.: Small Animal Gastroenterology. Stonegate Publishing Co., Davis, Calif., 1979.

Strombeck, D. R.: Clinicopathologic features of primary and metastatic neoplastic diseases of the liver in dogs. J.A.V.M.A. 173:267–269, 1978.

Strombeck, D. R., and Gribble, D.: Chronic active hepatitis in the dog. J.A.V.M.A. 173:380–386, 1978.

Strombeck, D. R., Breznock, E. M., and McNeel, S.: Surgical treatment for portosystemic shunts in two dogs. J.A.V.M.A. 170:1317–1319, 1977.

Strombeck, D. R., Krum, S., and Rogers, D.: Coagulopathy and encephalopathy in a dog with acute hepatic necrosis. J.A.V.M.A. 169:813–816, 1976a.

Strombeck, D. R., Meyer, D. J., and Freedland, R. A.: Hyperammonemia due to a urea cycle enzyme deficiency in two dogs. J.A.V.M.A. 166:1109–1111, 1975a.

Strombeck, D. R., Rogers, W., and Gribble, D.: Chronic active hepatic disease in a dog. J.A.V.M.A. 169:802–804, 1976b.

Strombeck, D. R., Rogers, Q. R., Freedland, R., and McVan, L. C.: Fasting hypoglycemia in a pup. J.A.V.M.A. 173:299–300, 1978.

Strombeck, D. R., Weiser, M. G., and Kaneko, J. J.: Hyperammonemia and hepatic encephalopathy in the dog. J.A.V.M.A. *166*:1105–1108, 1975b.

Sturtevant, F., Hoffman, W. E., and Dorner, J. C.: The effect of three anticonvulsant drugs and ACTH on canine serum alkaline phosphatase. J.A.A.H.A. *13*:754–757, 1977.

Summerskill, W. H. J., Korman, M. G., Ammon, H. V., and Baggenstross, A. H.: Prednisone for chronic active liver disease: dose titration, standardized dose and combination with azathioprine compared. Gut *16*:876–883, 1975.

Suter, P. F.: Portal vein anomalies in the dog: Their angiographic diagnosis. J. Am. Vet. Radiol. Soc. *16*:84–97, 1975.

Tanner, A. R., and Powell, L. W.: Corticosteroids in liver disease: Possible mechanisms of action, pharmacology and rational use. Gut *20*:1109–1124, 1979.

Taville, A. S.: The synthesis and degradation of liver produced proteins. Gut *13*:225–241, 1972.

Thompson, S. W., Sparano, B. M., and Diener, K. M.: Vacuoles in the hepatocytes of cortisone treated dogs. Am. J. Pathol. *63*:135–145, 1971.

Thornburg, L. P., and Moody, G. M.: Hepatic amyloidosis in a dog. J.A.A.H.A. *17*:721–723, 1981.

Tuzhilin, S. A., Podolsky, A. E., and Dreilling, D. A.: Hepatic lesions in pancreatitis: clinicoexperimental data. Am. J. Gastroenterol. *64*:108–114, 1975.

Twedt, D. C.: Jaundice hepatic trauma and hepatic encephalopathy. Vet. Clin. North Am. *11*:121–146, 1981.

Twedt, D. C., Sternlieb, I., and Gilbertson, S. R.: Clinical, morphologic and chemical studies in copper toxicosis of Bedlington terriers. J.A.V.M.A. *175*: 269–275, 1979.

Uribe, M., Farca, A., Marquez, M. A., Garcia-Ramos, G., and Guevara, L.: Treatment of chronic portalsystemic encephalopathy with bromocriptine: A double-blind controlled trial. Gastroenterology *76*:1347–1351, 1979.

Vaamonde, C. A.: Renal Water Handling in Liver Disease. *In* Epstein, M. (ed.): The Kidney in Liver Disease. Elsevier-North Holland, Inc., New York, 1978.

Vaamonde, C. A., Vaamonde, L. S., Morosi, H. J., Klingler, E. L., and Papper, S.: Renal concentrating ability in cirrhosis: I. Changes associated with the clinical status and course of the disease. J. Lab. Clin. Med. *70*:179, 1967.

Vitums, A.: Portosystemic communications in animals with hepatic cirrhosis and malignant lymphoma. J.A.V.M.A. *138*:31, 1961.

Vulgamott, J. C., Tumwald, G. H., King, G. K., Herring, D. S., Hansen, J. F., and Booth, H. W.: Congen-ital portalcaval anomalies in the cat: Two case reports. J.A.A.H.A. *16*:915–919, 1981.

Weber, F. L.: The effect of lactulose on urea metabolism and nitrogen excretion in cirrhotic patients. Gastroenterology *77*:518–523, 1979.

Weisburg, H. F., Friedman, A., and Levine, R.: Inactivation or removal of insulin by the liver. Am. J. Physiol. *158*:332, 1949.

Whang, R., and Popper, S.: The possible relationship of renal cortical hypoperfusion and diminished renal concentrating ability in Laennec's cirrhosis. J. Chronic dis. *27*:263–265, 1974.

Whitcomb, F. F.: Chronic active liver disease: definition, diagnosis and management. Med. Clin. North Am. *63*:413–421, 1979.

Wilson, R. B., and Wilson, W. D.: Hepatotoxicity of tolbutamide in dogs. J.A.V.M.A. *156*:1557–1566, 1970.

Witte, C. L., Witte, M. H., and Dumont, A. E.: Lymph imbalance in the genesis and perpetuation of the ascites syndrome in hepatic cirrhosis. Gastroenterology *78*:1059–1068, 1980.

Witte, M. H., Witte, C. L., and Dumont, A. E.: Progress in liver disease: physiological factors in the causation of cirrhotic ascites. Gastroenterology *61*:742, 1971.

Wyllie, R., Arasu, T. S., and Fitzgerald, J. F.: Ascites: pathophysiology and management. J. Pediatr. *97*:167–176, 1980.

Yeary, R. A., and Wise, K. J.: Plasma disappearance of sulfobromophthalein or indocyanine green in unconjugated hyperbilirubinemia. Res. Commun. Chem. Pathol. Pharmacol. *12*:125–136, 1975.

Young, J. T.: Source, fate and possible significance of elevated serum alkaline phosphatase in nonicteric animals with partial biliary obstruction. J.A.A.H.A. *10*:415–419, 1974.

Zeegen, R., and Dawson, A. M.: The Neuro-psychiatric disturbances of liver disease. Br. J. Clin. Pract. *22*:170, 1968.

Zieve, L.: Hemolytic anemia in liver disease. Medicine (Balt.) *45*:497, 1966.

Zieve, L., Doizaki, W. M., and Zieve, F. J.: Synergism between mercaptans and ammonia or fatty acids in the production of coma: A possible role for mercaptans in the pathogenesis of hepatic coma. J. Lab. Clin. Med. *83*:16–28, 1974.

Zimmerman, H. J.: Drug-induced chronic hepatic disease. Med. Clin. North Am. *63*:567–582, 1979a.

Zimmerman, H. J.: Intrahepatic Cholestasis. Arch. Int. Med. *139*:1038–1045, 1979b.

Zimmerman, H. J.: Drug-induced liver disease. Drugs *16*:25–45, 1978.

Zimmerman, H. J.: Liver disease caused by medicinal agents. Med. Clin. North Am. *59*:897–907, 1975.

CHAPTER 61

WILLIAM A. ROGERS

Diseases of the Exocrine Pancreas

INTRODUCTION

Pancreatic disorders occur frequently in the dog and cat. Response to injury by the pancreatic acinar tissue is somewhat unique inasmuch as the acinar cells contain packets of digestive enzymes, known as zymogen granules. If digestive enzymes become activated within the pancreas, autodigestion occurs, causing severe inflammation of the gland. In other cases, failure of the acinar cells to secrete digestive enzymes into the small intestine results in maldigestion of food and subsequent malnutrition.

To understand acute pancreatitis and exocrine pancreatic insufficiency, one must study normal pancreatic function. Then, dysfunction of the pancreas and the clinical manifestations of pancreatic disease will be appreciated. With this knowledge in hand, successful clinical management of pancreatic disease in the dog and cat can often be achieved.

FUNCTIONAL AND ANATOMIC CONSIDERATIONS

The pancreas is a compound, tubuloacinar gland lying adjacent to the greater curvature of the stomach and the duodenum (DeHoff and Archibald, 1974; Miller, et al., 1964). It is a soft, lobular, pinkish-gray gland whose long narrow "boomerang" shape gives one the impression that it is small, although it is, in fact, a rather substantial gland. Because portions of the pancreas lie adjacent to or in close proximity to other organs (liver, pylorus, duodenum, jejunum, cecum, ascending and transverse colon, spleen, and kidneys), pancreatitis can cause inflammation of these organs as well.

The exocrine function of the pancreas is to secrete fluid containing digestive enzymes and sodium bicarbonate into the intestinal lumen. These secretions accomplish diges-tion of food and neutralize hydrochloric acid of gastric origin. Important digestive enzymes include proteases (trypsin, chymotrypsin, carboxypeptidases, elastase), amylases, and lipases. There are more than 25 enzymes that occur in the zymogen granules of acinar cells. Many enzymes occur in an inactive form (proenzyme) and are activated after secretion, for example,

$$\text{trypsinogen} \xrightarrow{\text{enterokinase}} \text{trypsin.}$$

Enzyme inhibitors (α_1-antitrypsin, α_2-macroglobulin) are located within the pancreas, probably to prevent autodigestion of the small amounts of enzyme that become activated within the pancreatic parenchyma (Ohlsson and Eddeland, 1975).

Adequate exocrine pancreatic function is vital to the health of the animal, since without enzyme secretion absorbable nutrients become unavailable to the body, resulting in starvation. Also, acidification of the small intestinal lumen caused by lack of pancreatic bicarbonate may lead to serious impairment of small bowel function.

The duct systems that deliver the pancreatic secretions to the duodenum differ significantly in the dog and cat (Nielsen and Bishop, 1954; Miller et al., 1964). Most dogs have two ducts that enter the duodenum, although many variations in duct anatomy occur (Nielsen and Bishop, 1954; DeHoff and Archibald, 1974; Miller et al., 1964). Usually, the lesser (accessory) duct of the dog (Wirsung's duct) enters the duodenum adjacent to the common bile duct at the major duodenal papilla. In the cat this same duct (entering at the major papilla) is the major pancreatic duct and frequently joins the common bile duct to form the ampulla of Vater (Nielsen and Bishop, 1954). In the dog, a second pancreatic duct enters the duodenum at the minor duodenal papilla about three cm downstream from the major duodenal papilla. This second duct is the major duct of the dog (Santorini's duct). Thus, a much larger lesion would be required to cause obstruction of both common bile duct and pancreatic ducts in the dog than in the cat.

The major arterial blood supply to the pancreas is via the cranial pancreaticoduodenal artery, caudal pancreaticoduodenal artery, gastroduodenal artery, and branches of the splenic artery (DeHoff and Archibald, 1974). Familiarity with this blood supply is important to the surgeon in order to prevent ischemic damage to the pancreas by inadvertent disruption of its blood supply. The venous drainage of the pancreas is via the pancreaticoduodenal veins, which empty into the anterior-mesenteric vein and then into the portal vein. The passage of pancreatic venous blood through the liver prior to entering the systemic circulation may be important in the pathogenesis of the extrapancreatic manifestation of acute pancreatitis (such as hepatitis).

Blood flow to the pancreas (about .6 ml/min-gm) is important in pancreatic disease, especially acute pancreatitis (Delaney and Grim, 1966). Administration of secretin or norepinephrine increases pancreatic blood flow, whereas epinephrine and vasopressin decrease the rate of blood flow. Agents that alter the pancreatic circulation have been proposed as therapy in pancreatic disease.

The exocrine secretions of the pancreas are under complex neural and hormonal control (Singh and Webster, 1978). Hormonal regulation appears to be of much greater physiologic importance than neural control, although neural and hormonal control mechanisms can take over for each other when one or the other is lost.

Intestinal hormones known to play major physiologic roles in the regulation of pancreatic secretion include cholecystokinin-pancreozymin (CCK-PZ) and secretin. These hormones are released from intestinal endocrine cells in response to chemical stimulation by food or by gastrointestinal secretions. CCK-PZ is a potent secretagogue of enzyme-rich pancreatic juice and a weak stimulant of watery, bicarbonate-rich pancreatic fluid. CCK-PZ acts at the cellular level by attaching to a basolateral cell membrane receptor that sets off a series of intracellular events, including increased availability of calcium and exocytosis of zymogen granules (Williams, 1980). The hormone secretin is a weak secretagogue of enzyme-rich fluid but a potent stimulator of watery bicarbonate-rich secretion. Secretin-induced secretion is mediated via cyclic-AMP.

An important interaction occurs between CCK-PZ and secretin. The effect of secretin is markedly enhanced by the presence of CCK-PZ and the converse is also true. Inasmuch as these two hormones have different acinar cell membrane receptors, their synergism is probably a result of mutually enhancing intracellular events, possibly increased calcium availability (Williams, 1980).

Other hormones may also play important roles in controlling pancreatic secretion. Gastrin is trophic to the exocrine pancreas and causes release of enzyme-rich fluid in a manner similar to CCK-PZ. Insulin released from pancreatic β-cells also has a trophic effect on acinar cells. In fact, blood flows through the pancreatic islets into the acinar pancreas carrying islet hormones with it, including insulin. Thus, pancreatic exocrine and endocrine function are not unrelated (Henderson et al., 1981). Other hormones such as glucagon, pancreatic polypeptide, somatostatin, bombesin, motilin, and chymodenin may have important roles in health and disease, but these hormones need further evaluation to determine their significance (Susim et al., 1978).

Neural control of the exocrine pancreas is primarily mediated by cholinergic vagal nerves. Cholinergic vagal nerve stimulation results in secretion of enzyme-rich pancreatic juice. This secretion may be a direct effect of acetylcholine on acinar cells or it may be mediated via CCK-PZ and secretin, both of which may be released by vagal stimulation. Sympathetic innervation has little apparent physiologic importance in controlling pancreatic secretion. Sympathetic nerve endings are located in the pancreatic blood vessels and alter pancreatic blood flow. Their effects on pancreatic secretion are variable.

Complex interactions between hormones and between neural and hormonal factors occur in the regulation of exocrine pancreatic function. The role of gut hormones and neural inputs in pancreatic disease will receive greater emphasis in the future as more data become available.

FREQUENCY AND IMPORTANCE OF EXOCRINE PANCREATIC DISEASE

The clinical importance of exocrine pancreatic disease is difficult to determine from examination of the veterinary literature (Kleine and Hornbuckle, 1978; Duffell, 1975; Anderson and Low, 1965; Small, 1964; Anderson and Strafuss, 1971; Owens, 1975; Coffin, 1953; Ruwitch, 1964). In many discussions, the criteria for diagnosis are not given, a critical factor, inasmuch as definitive diagnosis of pancreatic disease may be difficult. Necropsy studies, in which histologic evidence of pancreatic disease is the main criterion for diagnosis, indicate that parenchymal pancreatic disorders are common in the dog and important in the cat (Duffell, 1975). Retrospective necropsy data also indicate that pancreatic adenocarcinomata are important neoplasms of the gastroenteric system (Anderson and Johnson, 1967; Ruwitch, 1964).

CLASSIFICATION OF EXOCRINE PANCREATIC DISEASE

Various classification schemes have been used (Perman and Stevens, 1969; Coffin, 1953). The author finds that shown in Table 61–1 to be the most useful on a clinical basis. This scheme will be described and then each entity will be discussed.

Acute pancreatitis can be of two types. A mild edematous or interstitial form is the more common form in the dog and has a good prognosis. A very severe form, acute hemorrhagic or necrotic pancreatitis, is un-common in the dog but is often fatal (Coffin, 1953).

When acute pancreatitis occurs repeatedly, it is called chronic relapsing pancreatitis. Each relapse is usually of the edematous type, probably because dogs do not usually survive multiple episodes of relapsing hemorrhagic pancreatitis. Chronic interstitial pancreatitis is characterized by constant low-grade inflammation of the pancreas and is most common in the cat. The clinical differentiation between chronic relapsing pancreatitis and chronic interstitial pancreatitis is often indistinct.

Exocrine pancreatic insufficiency occurs when deficient acinar function results in maldigestion. In the dog, an idiopathic atrophy of the acinar cell mass (pancreatic acinar atrophy) causes severe maldigestion. A secondary exocrine pancreatic insufficiency can result from destruction of the acinar cells by chronic relapsing pancreatitis or by an episode of severe acute pancreatitis. These patients may also develop diabetes mellitus if the islets of Langerhans are damaged (Coffin, 1953). Functional secondary pancreatic insufficiency may also occur during states of marked protein-calorie malnutrition, such as in patients with severe small bowel disease. In this form, negative protein or calorie balance causes decreased secretion of protein-rich pancreatic juice (Barbezat and Hansen, 1968).

Primary neoplasms of the exocrine pancreas originate from the duct system (ductular adenocarcinoma) or acinar cells (acinar cell carcinoma).

Table 61–1. Classification Scheme for Exocrine Pancreatic Disorders in the Dog and Cat

I. Acute pancreatitis
   A. Acute interstitial (edematous) pancreatitis
   B. Acute hemorrhagic (necrotic) pancreatitis
II. Chronic Pancreatitis
   A. Chronic relapsing pancreatitis
   B. Chronic interstitial (persistent) pancreatitis
III. Exocrine Pancreatic Insufficiency
   A. Pancreatic acinar atrophy
   B. Secondary pancreatic insufficiency
      1. Relapsing pancreatitis (II a)
      2. Sequel to severe acute pancreatitis (I b)
      3. Protein-calorie malnutrition
IV. Neoplasms of the pancreas
   A. Ductular carcinoma
   B. Acinar cell carcinoma

ACUTE PANCREATITIS

Dogs afflicted with acute edematous pancreatitis exhibit varying degrees of lethargy, anorexia, and vomiting (Kleine and Hornbuckle, 1978; Small, 1964). Diarrhea may be present and is sometimes bloody (Coffin, 1953). Some dogs assume a prayer-like stance (the position of relief) and some may seek a cool surface upon which to lie. The latter signs indicate abdominal distress. The onset of signs often follows ingestion of a fatty meal or garbage containing rancid food.

Surveys conflict as to whether acute pancreatitis is more common in the female or in the male dog, but many clinicians believe that it is more common in the female. Pancreatitis

appears to be more common in middle-aged
dogs, although all ages may be affected
(Kleine and Hornbuckle, 1978).

During physical examination, a pain reaction can be elicited by palpation of the
anterior abdomen (Coffin, 1953). However,
absence of abdominal pain does not rule out
acute pancreatitis, inasmuch as it is an inconsistent sign in both naturally occurring
cases and in experimental pancreatitis.
Fever — 39.44° to 40° C (103° to 104° F) —
is often present.

Clinical signs in dogs with acute hemorrhagic pancreatitis are similar to those in
dogs with acute edematous pancreatitis except they are much more severe. Abdominal
pain is a more consistent feature and it may
be diffuse rather than localized to the anterior abdomen. Bloating or abdominal distention may be noted. The diarrhea and
vomiting are more severe than in acute
edematous pancreatitis and are likely to be
bloody. Dogs with acute hemorrhagic pancreatitis may be presented in shock, and all
cases are in danger of developing shock.

ETIOLOGY

Almost every review of acute pancreatitis
contains a detailed discussion concerning
the etiology of pancreatitis. Many of the
same theories that were entertained in the
late nineteenth century are still viable
theories today (Schiller et al., 1974). General
agreement by experts concerning the validity of any single event as an essential pathogenetic mechanism in acute pancreatitis is
lacking. Acute pancreatitis probably has
many causes, and injury may be manifested
in more than one way, so that no single
theory of the etiology or pathogenesis will
prevail. Clinical studies are needed to detect
the most common causes of acute pancreatitis in the dog and cat. At present, very few
data are available.

One must be cautious in drawing conclusions from data derived from experimental
acute pancreatitis, because most experimental canine models have hemorrhagic pancreatitis, whereas the milder edematous
pancreatitis is the more common naturally
occurring form in the dog.

Obesity. Many dogs with acute pancreatitis are obese (Coffin, 1953). Conversely,
thin dogs rarely develop acute pancreatitis.
Acute pancreatitis can be induced in dogs by
feeding a diet high in fat content, and

experimental pancreatitis in obese dogs is
more severe than in thin dogs, suggesting a
permeability defect of the acinar cell membrane of obese dogs (Haig, 1969). Increased
dietary fat may also alter the enzyme content of pancreatic acinar cells, making them
more subject to autodigestion (Haig, 1970).
Thus, one must conclude that the dietary fat
content and nutritional status of the animal
are important factors in acute pancreatitis
(Goodhead, 1971). Whether they actually
cause or simply predispose the pancreas to
injury is not understood.

Hyperlipemia. Hyperlipemia (lactescent
serum) is not unusual in dogs with acute
pancreatitis. Hyperlipemia can cause pancreatitis, and conversely, acute pancreatitis
can cause lipemia and altered plasma lipoproteins. Thus, the relationship of lipemia
to pancreatitis in the individual patient is
usually obscure. That lipemia can cause
pancreatitis may help explain the relationship between ingestion of a fatty meal and
subsequent acute pancreatitis. The fatty
meal could cause marked dietary lipemia
(chylomicronemia) and subsequent pancreatitis, especially if the mechanism for
clearing chylomicrons from the blood is
impaired (as in dogs with hypothyroidism or
diabetes mellitus).

Exactly how lipemia results in pancreatitis
is not known. One theory is that lipase
located in the pancreatic capillary bed hydrolyzes fat in the blood stream, releasing
fatty acids. These fatty acids cause localized
acidosis and vasoconstriction within the
pancreas. The resultant ischemia and inflammation release even more lipase into
the circulation, setting up a process that
perpetuates the pancreatitis (Fig. 61–1).

Biliary Tract Disease. A relationship between biliary tract disease and pancreatitis
has been observed in dogs, cats, and human
beings (Banks, 1971; Jubb and Kennedy,
1970; Kelly et al., 1975). How this may
occur is unknown. One theory is based on
the finding of intercommunicating lymphatic channels between the biliary tree and the
pancreatic interstitium (Weiner et al., 1970).
Thus, disease in one organ system could
spread to the other via lymphatic ducts.

Drug Factors. Several drugs have been
implicated as causes of acute pancreatitis
(Banks, 1971). None have been proved in
the dog or cat, but there is little reason to
believe that drug-induced pancreatitis does
not affect dogs and cats. Many veterinary

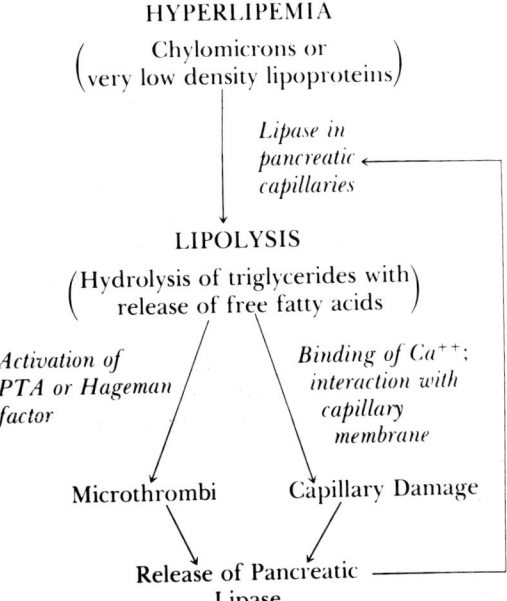

HYPERLIPEMIA

$\left(\begin{array}{c}\text{Chylomicrons or}\\ \text{very low density lipoproteins}\end{array}\right)$

Lipase in
pancreatic
capillaries

LIPOLYSIS

$\left(\begin{array}{c}\text{Hydrolysis of triglycerides with}\\ \text{release of free fatty acids}\end{array}\right)$

Activation of
PTA or Hageman
factor

Binding of Ca^{++};
interaction with
capillary
membrane

Microthrombi   Capillary Damage

Release of Pancreatic
Lipase

Figure 61–1. A proposed mechanism for lipemia-induced pancreatitis. (From Havel, R. J.: Adv. Intern. Med. *15*:117–150, 1969, with permission.)

clinicians believe that corticosteroids can cause pancreatitis in dogs. Indeed, experimental studies indicate that pancreatic secretions are altered by glucocorticoid administration and that ductular hyperplasia may occur (Riemenschneider et al., 1968).

Infectious Disease. Pancreatitis is a feature of several infectious diseases in the dog and cat. Toxoplasmosis and feline infectious peritonitis (FIP) in the cat are infectious diseases that involve the pancreas (Sherding, 1979). Since cholangiohepatitis or pancreatitis can also be caused by *Toxoplasma gondii* or the FIP virus, it is important to consider these diseases in cats with signs of hepatic and/or pancreatic disease. Other viral infections may be possible and also warrant future study (Ross et al., 1974).

Duodenal Reflux. Reflux of duodenal contents or bile into the pancreatic duct and then into the pancreatic interstitium has been entertained as a cause of acute pancreatitis for many years (Banks, 1971). Small amounts of duodenal contents may reflux into the main pancreatic duct of dogs in the postprandial period (Hendricks, 1980; Owyand et al., 1977). Bacteria in refluxed duodenal contents are probably not important, since closed duodenal loops cause equally severe pancreatitis in both conventional and germ-free dogs (Nance and Cain, 1968). Studies on experimental models using closed duodenal loops to cause pancreatitis have not provided convincing evidence that reflux of duodenal contents into the pancreatic ducts is an important cause of naturally occurring acute pancreatitis in the dog or cat.

This theory is still controversial, however. Inasmuch as the bile duct and pancreatic duct have separate duodenal openings and do not form an ampulla of Vater in the dog, it is unlikely that bile could reflux into the pancreatic duct system. The anatomy of the cat's duct system is such that reflux of bile into the pancreatic duct is feasible. Two components of bile, lysolecithin and unconjugated bile salts, are very toxic to the pancreas (Banks, 1971).

Duct Obstruction. Obstruction of the pancreatic ducts does not appear to be a likely cause of acute hemorrhagic pancreatitis (Hiatt and Warner, 1969). Edematous pancreatitis can be caused by duct ligation, however, especially when the pancreas is simultaneously stimulated to secrete (Bockman et al., 1973). Nevertheless, there is no evidence that duct obstruction causes naturally occurring acute pancreatitis in the dog. In the cat, pancreatic duct obstruction may be caused by the flukes *Amphimerus pseudofilineus* or *Eurytrema procyonis* (Rothenbacker and Lindquist, 1963; Sheldon, 1966). Usually parenchymal inflammation of the pancreas is minimal in these cases, although atrophy and fibrosis may occur.

Hyperparathyroidism or Hypercalcemia. Unlike human cases, acute pancreatitis is not a recognized feature of primary hyperparathyroidism in the dog or cat, but further evaluations are needed in this regard (Dubost et al., 1979). Hypercalcemia has also been incriminated as a cause of pancreatitis. However, dogs with hypercalcemia associated with lymphosarcoma do not appear to have a predisposition to acute pancreatitis. One case of pancreatitis induced by calcium infusion has been reported, but it was not determined whether or not the dog had pancreatitis prior to calcium infusion (Neuman, 1975).

Uremia. Acute pancreatitis has been observed in human patients with uremia. A recent retrospective survey indicates that pancreatic disease is an important complication in human patients with kidney failure (Avram, 1977). The importance of pancreatic disease in dogs with kidney failure warrants study, especially since increased serum amylase values often occur in uremic dogs. The increased amylase values are usually attributed to decreased renal clearance of amylase (Hudson and Strombeck, 1978). However, one should also consider the diagnosis of pancreatitis.

Immune Mechanisms. The role of immune mechanisms in acute pancreatitis is unknown. Experimental production of immune-mediated pancreatitis has been accomplished. The pancreas contains tissue-specific antigens, and circulating isoantibodies have been identified in human beings after development of pancreatitis (Shutt et al., 1975). Thus, immune factors may perpetuate pancreatitis after the initial injury has resulted in autoantibody formation.

Trauma. Trauma is probably not a common cause of pancreatitis in the dog or cat. It should be considered in cats that have fallen from high buildings (high-rise syndrome), and it is seen occasionally after traumatic surgery (Owens et al., 1975).

PATHOGENESIS

Regardless of the cause of acute pancreatitis, most experts agree that enzymatic autodigestion of the gland is an important common denominator, at least in patients with acute hemorrhagic pancreatitis. Two enzymes, elastase and phospholipase A, are especially potent destructive factors in acute hemorrhagic pancreatitis. What initiates autodigestion probably varies, depending on the etiology. Enzyme inhibitors produced by the pancreas protect it to some degree from autodigestion. These inhibitors must be overcome before autodigestion occurs (Ohlsson and Eddeland, 1975). The true importance of these enzyme inhibitors (α_1-antitrypsin, α_2-macroglobulin) in preventing pancreatitis is not known, but it is possible that saturation of the inhibitors is a factor that determines whether or not acute edematous pancreatitis will progress to acute hemorrhagic pancreatitis.

Extrapancreatic manifestations of pancreatic disease contribute to the pathology caused by acute pancreatitis. In general the extrapancreatic features have been attributed to release of pancreatic factors, including enzymes, kallikrein, bradykinin, and myocardial depressant factors (Bockman et al., 1973). Hepatic lesions seen in dogs with acute pancreatitis include hemorrhage and focal hepatic necrosis. Perfusion of the liver by the portal blood, which contains a high content of pancreatic enzymes, may be the cause of this hepatitis (Bockman, 1973; Tuzhilin et al., 1975). Cholecystitis also accompanies experimental acute pancreatitis in the dog, possibly because of interconnecting lymphatic channels between the pancreas and biliary tree (Weiner et al., 1970). Nephrosis has also been attributed to the effect of toxins released from the pancreas (Goldstein et al., 1976).

Notable biochemical effects of pancreatitis include hypocalcemia and hyperglycemia. Several theories have been advanced to explain hypocalcemia, including (1) precipitation of calcium in the soaps that form in necrotic fat, (2) low plasma protein with decreased calcium carrying capacity, and (3) blunted parathormone response (Robertson, 1976; Shieber, 1970; Weir et al., 1975). Hyperglucagonemia and hypercalcitonism have been considered as possible causes but are not favored theories as causes of hypercalcemia.

Hyperglycemia in acute pancreatitis can be caused by either insulinopenia or hyperglucagonemia, both of which are known to occur in pancreatitis. Diabetes mellitus during acute pancreatitis may be transient, complete resolution occurring upon abatement of the pancreatitis (Donowitz et al., 1975).

Less well documented extrapancreatic effects of acute pancreatitis include cardiomyopathy, pulmonary edema, and clotting disorders (Bockman, 1973; Lees et al., 1978; Kwaan et al., 1971). Disseminated intravascular coagulopathy can be produced consistently in experimental acute necrotizing pancreatitis (Feldman et al., 1981).

DIAGNOSIS

Definitive diagnosis of acute pancreatitis is extremely difficult in many cases, because there are no pathognomonic signs or laboratory tests. Therefore, one often elects to treat dogs for acute pancreatitis based on a presumptive diagnosis. The difficulty in making a diagnosis also confuses the data in the veterinary literature, because many studies are based on presumptive unproven cases.

Clinical Signs. The clinical signs of acute pancreatitis (as already described) are of diagnostic importance, although they are not pathognomonic. The diagnostic value of abdominal pain is controversial. Whereas this author agrees that acute pancreatitis may not be accompanied by abdominal pain, it is his opinion that dogs with severe acute hemorrhagic pancreatitis invariably demonstrate signs of abdominal pain or distress on palpation. In less severe cases, abdominal pain reactions are quite variable.

Radiology. Plain abdominal radiographs are indicated in suspected cases of acute pancreatitis (Kleine and Hornbuckle, 1978; O'Brien, 1978; Suter and Lowe, 1972). Radiographic signs include "ground glass appearance" and increased radiographic density in the cranial right quadrant of the abdomen (Fig. 61–2). Displacement of the duodenum to the right and displacement of the pyloric antrum to the left are often seen. Less commonly, a static duodenal gas pattern, a thickening of the wall of the descending duodenum, a static gas pattern of the transverse colon, or a caudal displacement of the transverse colon are observed in abdominal radiographs. The absence of abnormal radiographic findings does not rule out acute pancreatitis.

Laboratory Studies. Laboratory evaluation of suspected cases of acute pancreatitis is helpful but not usually confirmatory. Results of a complete blood count usually indicate an inflammatory process or stress (Perman and Stevens, 1969; Coffin, 1953; Gage and Anderson, 1967). That is, leukocytosis, neutrophilia, lymphopenia, and sometimes a monocytosis are detected. In cases of severe acute hemorrhagic pancreatitis or those with infection, a very high white blood cell count may develop.

The value of plasma amylase in detecting acute pancreatitis is confusing and controversial (Challis et al., 1957). The dog and cat normally have relatively high serum amylase activity (for example ≤1200 IU/dl) and have low or absent urine amylase activity, compared to some other species, such as man. Saccharogenic methods should be avoided in measuring amylase in dogs because they have a serum maltase, which may cause falsely high values (Rapp, 1962).

The source of normal serum amylase in the dog and cat is uncertain, but it is thought to originate from many organs, including the pancreas (Jacobs and Hall, 1981; Stickle et al., 1980). In pancreatitis, therefore, interpretation of increased amylase values may be confused by a baseline amylase value that is predominantly nonpancreatic amylase. Serum amylase is composed of isoamylase from many tissues (Fig. 61–3). Earlier suspicion that dog serum amylase was primarily of liver origin has been refuted by recent studies that fail to demonstrate the presence of an hepatic amylase isoenzyme (Notheman and Callow, 1971; Stickle et al., 1980; Jacobs and Hall, 1981).

The issue is clouded by the observation that increased serum amylase values have been detected in nonpancreatic disease (Wanke, 1970). Conversely, pancreatitis has been diagnosed without increased serum amylase activity (Gage and Anderson, 1967), although experimental pancreatitis causes hyperamylasemia with fair consistency (Wanke, 1970). Thus, the amylase value can serve only as a clue that pancreatitis may be present.

Nonpancreatic diseases that could increase serum amylase activity include those affecting the intestine and kidney. Since the kidney and intestine are potential sources of amylase, many clinicians believe that gastroenteritis is a common cause of an increased amylase value, although this has been refuted (Finco and Stevens, 1969). The empirical judgment that intestinal disease can increase serum amylase activity should not be trusted, since clinical signs of intestinal disease and pancreatitis overlap.

Uremic dogs often have increased amylase values (Finco and Stevens, 1969). Ligation of the renal artery appeared to decrease the clearance rate of infused amylase in the dog (Hudson and Strombeck, 1978). However, the potential contribution of endogenous pancreatic amylase or renal amylase (to the clearance in response to renal ischemia) values was not controlled. Bilateral renal artery ligation alone also caused the serum amylase to increase until high serum urea nitrogen was reached, at which point the amylase value failed to go up as expected (Hudson and Strombeck, 1978). Thus, it is difficult to blame the increased amylase values in dogs with kidney failure on decreased renal clearance of amylase alone. Furthermore, many dogs with severe kidney failure have normal amylase values. Therefore, one should consider concomitant pancreatitis a possible cause of high amylase values in uremic dogs. A high incidence of pancreatic disease has been detected in human patients with kidney failure, and the presence of kidney disease does not preclude the presence of acute pancreatitis (Avram, 1977).

Thus, it can be seen that increased amylase values suggest the presence of pancreatitis, but a definitive diagnosis of acute pancreatitis cannot be made based on hyperamylasemia alone.

Plasma lipase has been purported to be a better test than the serum amylase for the diagnosis of acute pancreatitis in the dog, although there are no studies to support this contention. The lipase test is technically more difficult to perform than the amylase test, and there is marked variation in lipase values in dogs with experimental pancreatitis (Brobst and Brester, 1967; Wanke, 1970). It appears that the lipase test is not a more effective diagnostic aid than the amylase test but that simultaneous measurement of both amylase and lipase activities will detect more cases of pancreatitis than either test performed alone (Mia et al., 1978a). In experimental canine pancreatitis the amylase and lipase values tend to fluctuate in concert (Mia et al., 1978b). Many of the same questions concerning amylase apply to lipase, except that basal levels appear to be of pancreatic origin in the dog.

The diagnostic value of amylase and lipase tests will not be appreciated until a clinical study is performed in which the enzyme values are correlated with the presence or absence of pancreatic and nonpancreatic disease and in which the diagnoses of pancreatitis are confirmed histologically. Amylase isozyme determinations also await studies to determine their diagnostic efficiency and practical value.

Severe cases of pancreatitis may have ascites caused by effusion of fluid from the inflamed pancreas and adjacent organs. In these cases, amylase content of the ascitic fluid is of diagnostic value. A higher amylase value in ascitic fluid than in serum is indicative of effusive pancreatitis. Perforation of the small bowel may also cause high amylase values in ascitic fluid, but cytology of the fluid usually differentiates it from pancreatic ascitic fluid.

Other laboratory tests that are helpful in detecting pancreatitis include the serum calcium, blood glucose, liver enzymes, methemalbumin, and examination of serum for lipemia (Perman and Stevens, 1969). Hypocalcemia occurs in some cases of acute pancreatitis; thus, acute pancreatitis should receive diagnostic consideration in hypo-

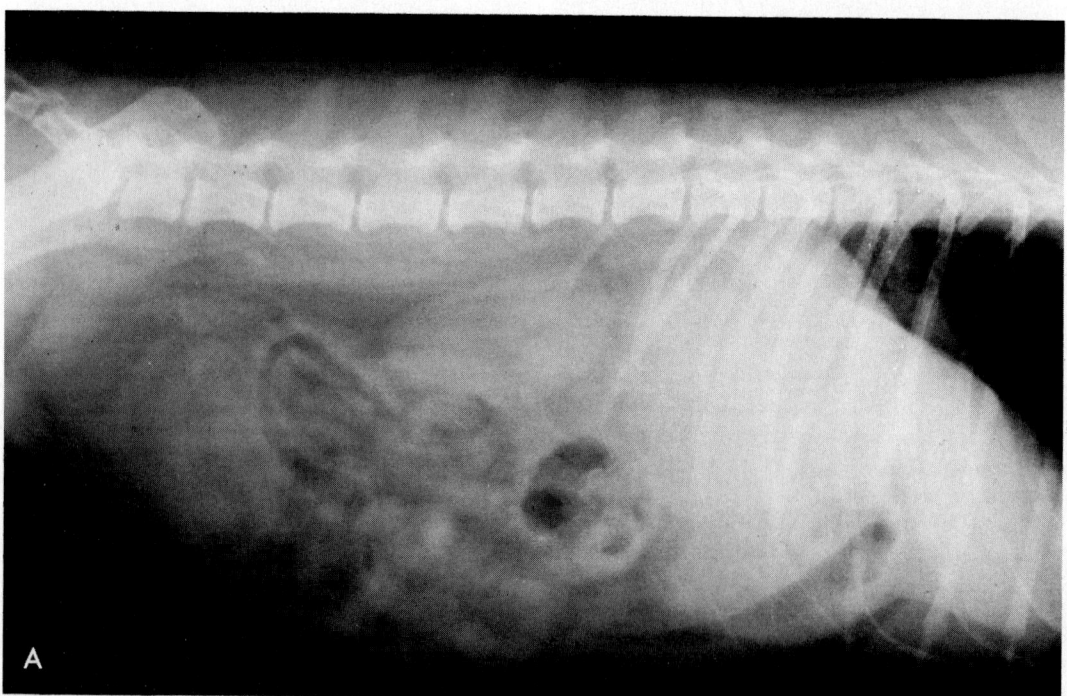

A

Figure 61–2. Plain abdominal radiographs (A = lateral view; B = ventrodorsal view) from a dog with acute pancreatitis demonstrate localized peritonitis in the region of the pancreas and displacement of the duodenum to the right. (Courtesy of Dr. C. W. Myer, Radiology Section, College of Veterinary Medicine, Ohio State University.)

Illustration continued on opposite page.

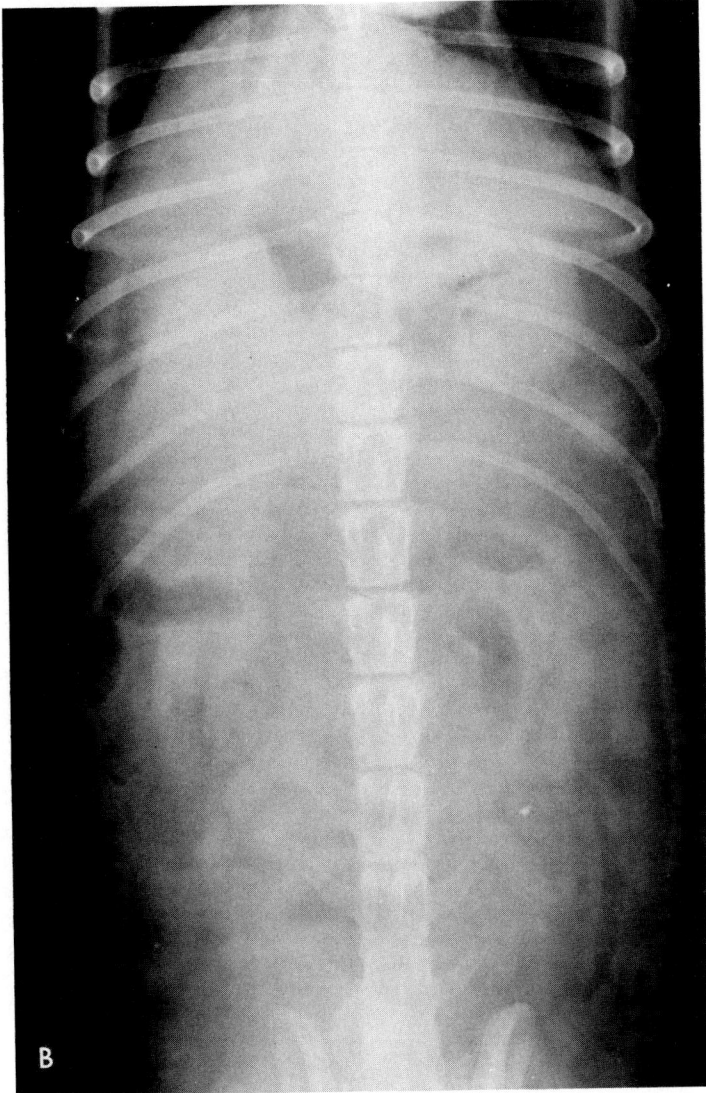

Figure 61–2 *Continued.*

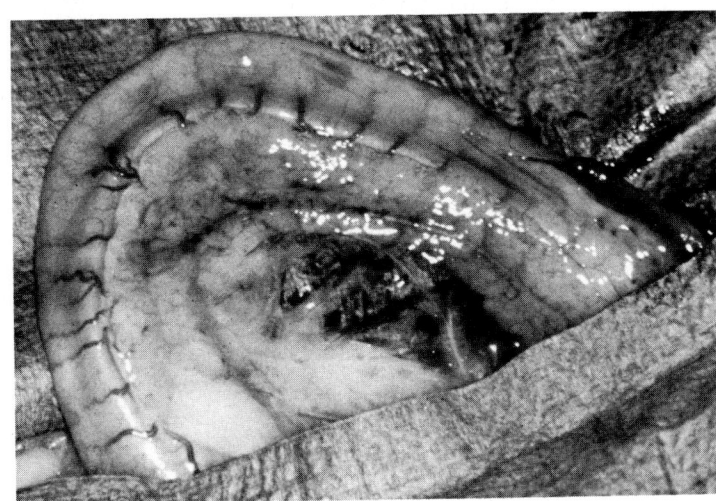

Figure 61–3. A case of acute hemorrhagic pancreatitis as observed at laparotomy. The pancreas is swollen and hyperemic, and has many petechial hemorrhages. The severity of pancreatitis is often difficult to assess by visual inspection, since histopathology often reveals a much more severe process than is evident grossly.

calcemic dogs. Hyperglycemia may also be observed and is usually transient, although persistent diabetes may be a sequel of acute pancreatitis. Increased activity of hepatic enzymes (such as SGPT, SAP) may signal pancreatitis-associated hepatitis (Perman and Stevens, 1969). Methemalbuminemia is considered to be diagnostic of acute hemorrhagic pancreatitis (uncommon in the dog), since it is indicative of hemorrhage that has taken place within the pancreas (Geokas et al., 1974); Anderson and Strafuss, 1971). One may wish to perform a methemalbumin test in cases of suspected acute hemorrhagic pancreatitis when other diagnostic aids are inadequate.

Lipemia may herald acute pancreatitis, and the lipoprotein electrophoresis may be characteristically abnormal (Bass et al., 1976; Rogers, 1977). The diagnosis of acute pancreatitis should be considered in dogs with fasting hyperlipemia, and dogs with lipemia should be considered to be at risk for development of acute pancreatitis.

In rare cases a definitive diagnosis is imperative. In this event, an exploratory laparotomy or laparoscopic examination of the abdomen is indicated (Fig. 61–4).

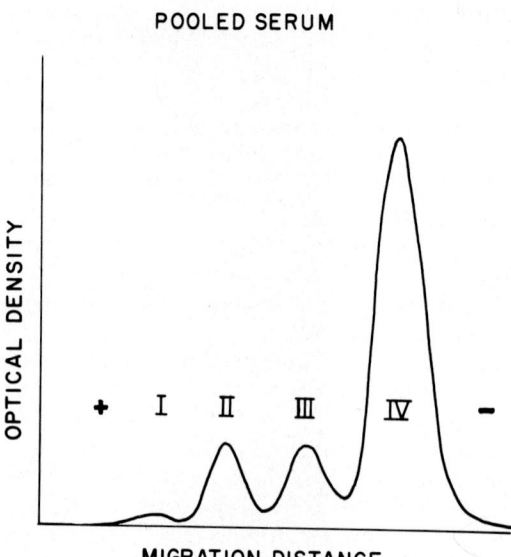

POOLED SERUM

Figure 61–4. An electrophoretic separation of amylases from the serum of dogs. Four peaks (bands) are observed. Pancreas isoenzymes are found in peaks 3 and 4. (Courtesy of Dr. R. M. Jacobs, Clinical Pathology Section, College of Veterinary Medicine, Ohio State University.)

TREATMENT

Clinical trials of therapy in canine acute pancreatitis are not available. Therefore, current therapeutics are empirical or are derived from experimental data. Nevertheless, certain therapeutic measures appear to be warranted in dogs with acute pancreatitis.

Probably the most important measure is to withhold administration of all oral substances (food, water, and medications), in order to avoid stimulation of pancreatic secretion. Dehydration must then be corrected or avoided by appropriate intravenous or subcutaneous fluid therapy. Usually a balanced electrolyte solution such as lactated Ringer's solution is selected, although the solution may require tailoring to correct electrolyte imbalance (most commonly potassium depletion). During recovery, oral alimentation should be reinstituted gradually by feeding small meals of low fat content. These feedings can be increased in quantity and mixed with the dog's usual foodstuff until a return to normal dietary habits has been achieved. Chronic dietary manage-

ment includes avoidance of fatty meals such as meat trimmings or fat supplements. Obese dogs are placed on a weight reduction program. Inability to lose weight in the face of a low-calorie diet should prompt one to evaluate for hypothyroidism (and hyperlipemia). If the dog has relapsing acute pancreatitis while consuming standard foods, an evaluation of plasma lipids should be made and the dog should be placed on a low-fat diet (e.g., R/d).

The lipid profile is used to detect fasting hyperlipemia and to evaluate whether or not diseases that may cause hyperlipemia (e.g., diabetes mellitus, hypothyroidism) should be considered. Since lipemia itself may cause pancreatitis, it should probably be treated. Treatment of lipemia secondary to other disease is accomplished by specific therapy of the primary disease, such as thyroid hormone replacement in hypothyroidism. Primary lipemia as seen in idiopathic lipemia of the miniature schnauzer is usually of dietary origin and can usually be resolved by feeding low fat diet (e.g., R/d). Low fat diet fits in well with weight reduction programs and may decrease the susceptibility of the pancreas to injury.

Measures to decrease pancreatic secretion have also been used to treat canine acute pancreatitis. Anticholinergics may be useful in this regard, although their effect on pancreatic secretion is not marked and their usage is controversial. Examples include atropine (0.04 to 0.08 mg/kg), isopropamide (0.06 mg/kg), propantheline (15.0 to 30 mg), and glycopyrrolate (0.01 mg/kg) given three to four times per day. Propantheline hydrobromide was effective in reducing the severity of experimental acute edematous pancreatitis (duct-ligated dogs) and experimental acute hemorrhagic pancreatitis (Shingleton et al., 1952). A controlled clinical evaluation of anticholinergics in canine acute pancreatitis has not been reported.

Cimetidine has been suggested as a drug for use in acute pancreatitis, according to the rationale that decreased gastric acid secretion induced by cimetidine would decrease the stimulus for pancreatic secretion (less duodenal acidity). However, cimetidine was ineffective in the treatment of human beings with alcoholic pancreatitis (Meshkinpour et al., 1979).

Antibiotics may be indicated in dogs with acute pancreatitis to prevent pancreatic infection and abscess formation. Whether antibiotics would effectively prevent abscess formation is unknown; broad spectrum antibiotics such as ampicillin or chloramphenicol are often administered parenterally. Evidence is lacking that antibiotics alter the clinical course of naturally occurring pancreatitis, and studies in this regard are needed.

Severe acute hemorrhagic pancreatitis is characterized by peritonitis and remarkable abdominal pain. Pain not only causes severe distress but also may cause or contribute to shock. Hence, analgesics have been recommended for use in acute pancreatitis to control pain. Meperidine hydrochloride (Demerol) has been used most often, but because it has a very short plasma half-life in the dog, it may not be a good analgesic choice. Morphine sulfate, on the other hand, appears to be a potent analgesic. Use of morphine sulfate in acute pancreatitis has been avoided in the past because it reportedly increases tone of the pancreatic duct sphincters, thus potentially impeding the flow of pancreatic secretions. This fear may be exaggerated inasmuch as morphine also reduces pancreatic secretion (Konturek et al., 1978). Reduced secretion and control of pain may outweigh potential disadvantages of increased sphincter tone. The initial emetic action of morphine may also be a disadvantage, although this effect is transient and its antiemetic effect rapidly ensues. Morphine sulfate administration apparently does not cause hyperamylasemia in the dog (Konturek et al., 1978). Analgesics are not indicated in the vast majority of dogs with acute pancreatitis and should be reserved for cautious use in those with severe pain.

Other treatments for acute pancreatitis in the dog are even less understood than those already mentioned. Glucocorticoids have been used for their anti-inflammatory effect but are considered by some to be contraindicated because they may in fact cause pancreatitis and have been shown to cause ductular hyperplasia and increase viscosity of pancreatic juice (Riemenschneider et al., 1968). However, other studies do not demonstrate any effect of cortisol on pancreatic secretion (Gullo et al., 1980). Thus, their use will remain controversial until futher studies are performed to clarify this issue. Glucocorticoids should be used when needed to treat shock.

Heparin decreases the severity of experimental acute pancreatitis, possibly by preventing clot formation within the pancreatic microcirculation and thus improving pancreatic blood flow and preventing ischemia (Wright and Goodhead, 1970). Heparin also activates lipoprotein lipase in the capillary bed. Lipoprotein lipase is an enzyme that clears the blood of triglyceride-rich lipoproteins (chylomicrons and very low density lipoproteins). The lipemia often seen in acute pancreatitis may therefore be cleared by an intravenous dose of heparin sulfate (150 IU/kg body weight). If the lipemia is a cause or contributing factor in the pancreatitis, clearing of the lipemic serum should be beneficial.

Vasopressin has been shown to decrease severity of experimental pancreatitis, possibly by stabilizing pancreatic blood flow and thus preventing ischemic damage to the pancreas (Schapiro et al., 1976). Vasopressin has not been evaluated in naturally occurring canine acute pancreatitis.

Glucagon is a suppressor of exocrine pancreatic secretion. Efficacy of glucagon administration in the treatment of experimental acute pancreatitis or pancreatitis in human beings is variable and has not found a place in the standard regimen of therapy (Papp et al., 1975; Gilsanz et al., 1978; Olazabal and Fuller, 1978). Glucagon levels are increased in experimental pancreatitis in the dog, making it doubtful if additional glucagon would be of value (Donowitz et al., 1975; Rosi et al., 1974; Paloyan et al., 1966).

Pancreatic enzyme inhibitors such as aprotinin have not yet found a place in treatment of canine acute pancreatitis.

Peritoneal lavage has been recommended for dogs with severe acute pancreatitis, but its efficacy is unknown (Parks et al., 1973). Removal of enzyme-rich peritoneal fluids may be of value to lessen the severity of chemical peritonitis, and if septic peritonitis is present, drainage may be beneficial (Rodgers and Carey, 1966). The risks of bacterial contamination of an insulted peritoneum by the lavage solution require caution. Furthermore, the percentage of dogs with acute pancreatitis that might benefit from lavage is small, and it should only be considered in cases with severe refractory peritonitis.

CHRONIC PANCREATITIS

Dogs with chronic pancreatitis usually have a relapsing form characterized by frequent recrudescence of acute pancreatitis. These dogs often have a history of episodic abdominal distress, gastrointestinal upsets, and other signs compatible with acute pancreatitis. Laboratory parameters are altered in the same manner as in a single episode of pancreatitis. Between episodes, the dogs are clinically normal, but each episode of acute pancreatitis causes some destruction of the gland. Eventually, some dogs develop exocrine pancreatic insufficiency and/or diabetes mellitus. Exocrine pancreatic insufficiency will be dealt with later in this chapter.

In contrast to the disease in dogs, chronic pancreatitis in cats usually is persistent, producing smoldering inflammation and vague signs of illness (Duffell, 1975). In fact, cats with chronic persistent pancreatitis are seldom diagnosed ante mortem. Chronic persistent pancreatitis is more common in the male than in the female cat. Abdominal pain is not a feature of the disease. Most of the cats have anorexia, weight loss, and variable degrees of depression. Many of them also have polydipsia. Laboratory data in cats with chronic pancreatitis are often unremarkable. Amylase values may be increased but are just as often within the normal range. Serum lipase values are not of diag-

nostic value in these cats. The blood glucose may be increased. Hyperglycemia may indicate diabetes mellitus caused by destruction of the islets of Langerhans or may be a result of stress.

There is an increased incidence of azotemia in cats with pancreatitis (Duffell, 1975). The azotemia is caused by a chronic interstitial nephritis. The cause and effect relationships that are operative in cats with concomitant nephritis and pancreatitis are not understood.

As previously mentioned, feline pancreatitis may also be associated with cholangitis (Duffell, 1975; Jubb and Kennedy, 1970). The cholangitis may cause increased serum activity of liver enzymes such as alanine aminotransferase and alkaline phosphatase. Cats may develop exocrine pancreatic insufficiency when acinar damage by chronic persistent pancreatitis becomes extensive (Jubb and Kennedy, 1970).

Treatment of chronic relapsing pancreatitis in the dog is essentially the same as for each episode of acute pancreatitis. In addition, careful attention should be paid to diet and obesity should be controlled. Underlying conditions that may cause chronic hyperlipemia and lipemia-associated pancreatitis, such as hypothyroidism or diabetes mellitus, should be ruled out.

Treatment of cats with chronic pancreatitis is undefined.

EXOCRINE PANCREATIC INSUFFICIENCY

When acinar cell function is severely impaired, a syndrome of nutrient maldigestion and malnutrition ensues (Sherding, 1980; Small et al., 1964; Sateri, 1975; Johnson, 1980). Exocrine insufficiency is seen in chronic pancreatitis, less commonly as a sequel of severe acute hemorrhagic pancreatitis, as an idiopathic atrophy in young dogs, and as a functional defect in protein-calorie malnutrition (Gyr et al., 1978; Tandon et al., 1970; Hashimoto et al., 1979; Prentice et al., 1980; Szabo et al., 1978). These disorders will be considered separately after the syndrome of exocrine pancreatic insufficiency itself is discussed.

PATHOGENESIS

Insufficient secretion of digestive enzymes precipitates a series of negative self-perpetuating events (Fig. 61–5). The initial event is failure to secrete adequate amounts of pancreatic juice. Significant pancreatic insufficiency does not become clinically evident until most (> 90 per cent) of the pancreatic acinar mass is destroyed or nonfunctional. Lack of digestive enzymes results in maldigestion of food. Inadequate bicarbonate secretion results in acidification of the small bowel by gastric acid (Regan et al., 1979; Dutta et al., 1979a; 1979b). End-products of digestion are not available for absorption, leading to malnutrition with weight loss. Partial digestion of food produces nonabsorbable, osmotically-active particles that retain water within the intestinal lumen. Increased stool water combined with increased fecal fat (steatorrhea) results in

production of voluminous stools. Chronic steatorrhea may lead to fecal loss of fat-soluble vitamins. Other vitamins such as folic acid may also be lost. These vitamin deficiencies may contribute to the animal's debility.

Acidification of the small intestine has a detrimental effect on mucosal function. Altered pH, combined with increased availability of unabsorbed nutrients, favors intestinal bacterial overgrowth, which may further impair intestinal function. In fact, mucosal lesions, including blunting of intestinal villi, can occur in patients with chronic exocrine pancreatic insufficiency. Mucosal enzyme function may also be depressed by this abnormal intestinal milieu.

Bile salt malabsorption and precipitation of bile acids in the acid environment of the

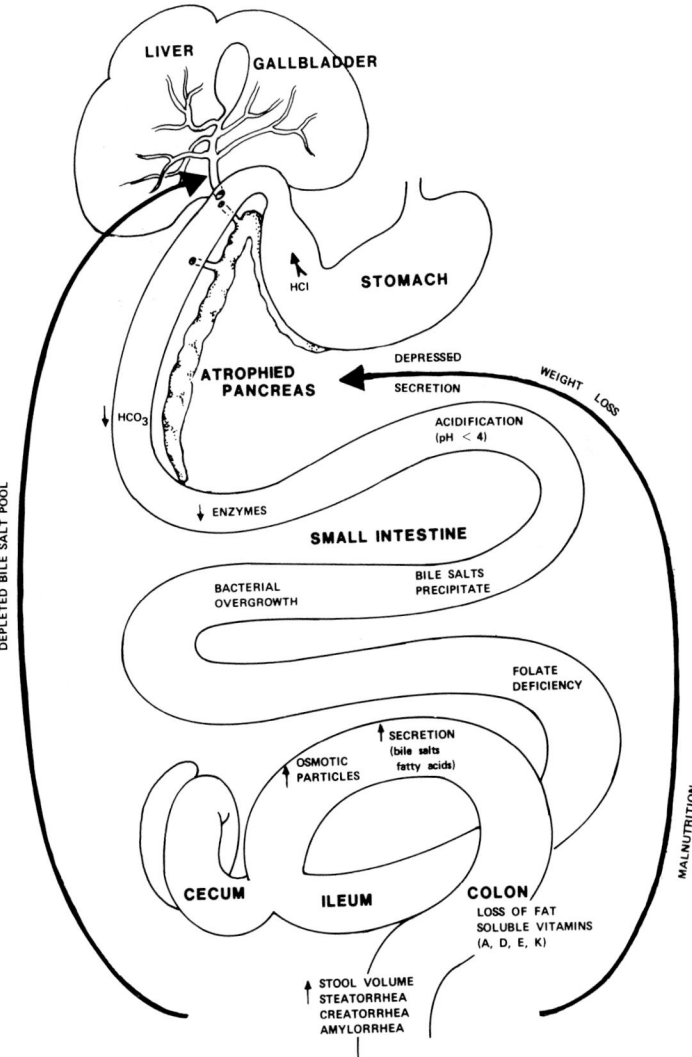

Figure 61–5. A scheme illustrating the self-perpetuating events responsible for the malabsorption and malnutrition in dogs or cats with decompensated exocrine pancreatic insufficiency.

small bowel can occur in cases of pancreatic insufficiency. This malabsorption leads to depletion of the bile salt pool, further impairing fat digestion and worsening steatorrhea.

Imbalances in the intraluminal environment of the intestine and deterioration of intestinal function may lead to further impairment of pancreatic function by virtue of protein-calorie malnutrition and/or impaired release of intestinal hormones that regulate the pancreas. Thus, a state of decompensation and self-perpetuating malfunction may develop in animals with exocrine pancreatic insufficiency.

DIAGNOSIS

Laboratory Procedures

Diagnosis of exocrine pancreatic insufficiency is usually not difficult, since the clinical signs are rather characteristic. Furthermore, several simple tests that can be performed in the clinician's practice are very helpful in making the diagnosis.

Microscopic examination of a fecal smear stained with Sudan III or Sudan IV dye usually reveals numerous fat globules (Table 61–2; Fig. 61–6) (Drummey et al., 1961; Luk and Hendrix, 1978). Since direct Sudan III dye will only stain undigested fat, maldigestion must be present if these fat globules are detected (normal dogs absorb nearly all of their dietary fat, and only an occasional fat globule can be found on a direct Sudan III stain of a fecal smear). Inasmuch as pancreatic insufficiency is by far the most common cause of maldigestion in the dog, the combination of appropriate clinical signs and a strongly positive direct Sudan III test is highly suggestive of pancreatic insufficiency, and the clinician may elect to treat the dog based on these findings alone.

Occasionally, a dog or cat with pancreatic insufficiency has steatorrhea consisting of digested fat rather than of undigested fat. This type of steatorrhea may be a result of bacterial degradation of unabsorbed neutral fat. In such case, the direct Sudan III smear is negative. Steatorrhea characterized by digested fat can be detected by examining a fecal smear prepared by the indirect method (Table 61–2) (Drummey et al., 1961). Thus, steatorrhea characterized by undigested fat (direct Sudan III positive) indicates

Table 61–2. Instructions for Performing Simple Screening Tests in Dogs and Cats With Diarrhea and Suspected Exocrine Pancreatic Disease

Direct Sudan Stain (unsplit fat)
1. Smear small amount of fresh feces onto a glass slide.
2. Mix thoroughly with 2 to 3 drops of Sudan III.
3. Add cover slip.
4. Examine microscopically for fat droplets. Positive test results (many fat droplets) indicate steatorrhea with maldigestion of fat.

Indirect Sudan Stain (split fat)
1. Smear small amount of fresh feces onto a glass slide.
2. Mix thoroughly with 2 drops of 36 per cent acetic acid.
3. Mix thoroughly with 2 drops of Sudan III; add cover slip.
4. Heat gently on a hot plate or over a flame until it begins to bubble (boil).
5. Examine microscopically while warm. Fat droplets (positive results) indicate steatorrhea. Either malabsorption or maldigestion may be the cause.

X-ray Film Digestion Test
1. Mix 1 part fresh feces with 9 parts (9 ml) of 5 per cent sodium bicarbonate in a vial or test tube. A control (normal) feces and the patient feces should be tested concomitantly.
2. Cut a long strip of x-ray film that will fit into the test tube.
3. Insert the film strip into the test tube and incubate for 2.5 hours at room temperature.
4. Lift up the film strip every 30 minutes and examine the submerged part for digestion (clearing) of the gel from the film strip. Clearing indicates the presence of proteolytic enzyme

maldigestion and suggests a diagnosis of pancreatic insufficiency, whereas steatorrhea characterized by digested fat (indirect Sudan III positive) indicates steatorrhea caused by either pancreatic insufficiency or other gastroenteric disease.

Fecal smears may also be stained with a two per cent tincture of iodine solution and examined both grossly and microscopically for blue starch particles. Amylorrhea (starch in the feces) may indicate maldigestion of dietary starches, but test results may be false positive in normal dogs or cats if they have consumed poorly digestible carbohydrates, such as cardboard or paper.

Creatorrhea (undigested muscle fibers in the feces) may be detected by observing striated muscle fibers on the fecal smear.

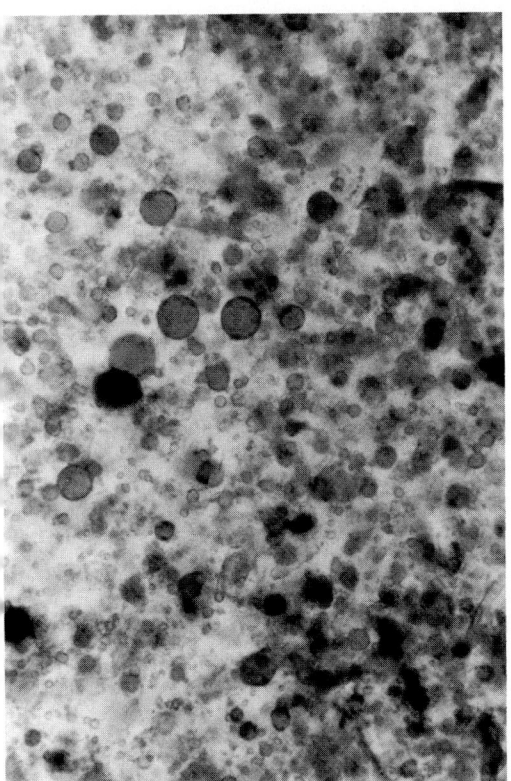

Figure 61–6. Microscopic fat droplets in a fecal smear prepared with Sudan III indicating steatorrhea.

Staining the slide with new methylene blue will facilitate detection of these muscle fibers.

Another simple laboratory test is the x-ray film gel digestion test. In this test, an alkaline solution of feces is incubated with strips of x-ray film. Clearing of the x-ray film indicates that the film's proteinaceous gel has been digested, presumably by pancreatic proteolytic enzymes. Thus, digestion of the gel would indicate that pancreatic insufficiency is not present. Unfortunately, false positives (possibly because of bacterial degradation of the x-ray film gel) and false negatives occur. A test tube gel-digestion test may also be performed according to the same rationale.

Another easy test to perform in a practice situation is the plasma turbidity test, although results must be interpreted with caution. This test is performed by feeding a bolus of corn oil (3 ml/kg body weight) and examining plasma samples (two, three, and four hours post-feeding) for subsequent lactescence (lipemia). If lipemia occurs, ability to assimilate fat is intact and the presence of significant exocrine pancreatic insufficiency

is unlikely. If lipemia does not result from the fatty meal, malabsorption or maldigestion of fat may be present and further diagnostics are indicated (see Chapter 58). If the test is repeated with the addition of pancreatic enzymes to the corn oil, and lipemia is produced, pancreatic insufficiency is the likely diagnosis. A problem with the plasma turbidity test is that marked delay of gastric emptying (fat is a potent inhibitor of gastric emptying) may prevent the formation of lipemia. Therefore, the plasma turbidity test is a more useful procedure for ruling out pancreatic insufficiency or malabsorption syndromes (when the results are positive, lipemia occurs) than for confirming the diagnosis of pancreatic insufficiency.

In most cases, these simple tests provide adequate information for the presumptive diagnosis of exocrine pancreatic insufficiency and treatment is instituted. Response to treatment is also a useful diagnostic aid. One must be careful, however, not to cause delay in the definite diagnosis of the cause of chronic diarrhea by attempting various treatments, because a point may be reached when the patient is so debilitated that the stress of further diagnostic tests precludes performing them.

When the diagnosis is still in question, more sophisticated tests are indicated to detect pancreatic insufficiency. Tests of value include the peptide — para-aminobenzoic acid (BT-PABA) test (Fig. 61–7), the 72-hour fecal fat measurement, and the D-xylose absorption test (see Chapter 58). The BT-PABA test involves feeding a solution of BT-PABA and measuring plasma or urinary PABA content (Imondi, 1972; Strombeck, 1978; Freudiger, 1977). BT-PABA is not absorbed from the intestine. However, if chymotrypsin cleaves the molecule, free PABA is liberated and is subsequently absorbed from the intestine. The plasma PABA values then increase and PABA appears in the urine. If chymotrypsin is absent (as in pancreatic insufficiency), BT-PABA is not digested and plasma or urinary PABA content does not increase as expected. Furthermore, since free PABA is well-absorbed even in malabsorption states, PABA malabsorption is not likely to interfere with the test. The ease of performance of the BT-PABA test makes it a very convenient pancreatic function test, and it should be commercially available in the near fu-

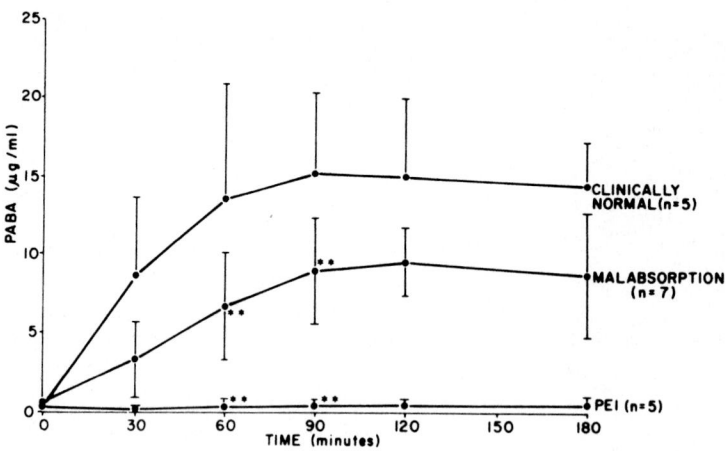

Figure 61–7. Plasma PABA curves obtained from clinically normal dogs, dogs with intestinal malabsorption, and dogs with pancreatic exocrine insufficiency. Brackets indicate standard deviation. ** = different from other groups (P < 0.05). Note that the 60 minute and 90 minute values can be used to differentiate these diagnoses. (From Rogers, W. A., et al., J.A.V.M.A. *177*:1130, 1980, with permission.)

ture. The BT-PABA test and D-xylose absorption test can be performed simultaneously, allowing one to evaluate intestinal function and pancreatic function at the same time (Stradley et al., 1979; Rogers et al., 1980). Malabsorption states usually depress the D-xylose curve (see Chapter 58).

The 72-hour fecal fat assay is easy to perform, collection of feces being the most difficult step, especially when the feces are watery. Dogs with complete pancreatic acinar atrophy have marked steatorrhea (average 3.38 gm/kg body weight/day; normal 0.17 ± 0.08 gm/day), usually greater than that occurring in malabsorption states (Burrows et al., 1979; Rogers et al., 1980). In the author's experience, cats with exocrine pancreatic insufficiency also have marked increase in 72 hour fecal fat excretion (>3.5 gm/day, Lewis and Boulay, 1979).

Although less readily available, quantitative fecal trypsin analysis has been used in the dog and is considerably more reliable than the qualitative test for diagnosing EPI (Burrows, 1979). Dogs with EPI in one study excreted 0.49 ± 0.22 gm/kg/day of fecal trypsin as compared with normal dogs which excreted 4.96 ± 1.66 gm/kg/day (Burrows, 1979). Fecal trypsin output appeared to be higher than normal (15.2 ± 1.94 gm/kg/day) in dogs with intestinal mucosal disease and malabsorption.

The combination of oral starch digestion test and glucose tolerance test can be used (Hill, 1972). If a starch meal is not followed by an expected increase in blood glucose, maldigestion of starch or malassimilation of glucose is present. If results of subsequent oral glucose tolerance tests are normal, amy-

lase deficiency (exocrine pancreatic insufficiency) may be presumed to be present, since glucose malassimilation is ruled out as the cause of the flat starch digestion test results. A major difficulty with this procedure is that the differences between the glucose curve produced by the starch digestion test and glucose tolerance test are small, even in normal dogs, making detection of abnormal curves in individual cases difficult. Furthermore, the metabolism of glucose may have a marked effect on the glucose curve. An advantage of these tests is that glucose determinations are readily available to the general practitioner.

Sophisticated tests of pancreatic function such as the Lundh test and the triolein-olein absorption test have little clinical value because of technical difficulties.

Pancreatic Acinar Atrophy

Pancreatic acinar atrophy is a disorder of young dogs characterized by idiopathic atrophy of the pancreatic acinar cells, but the islets of Langerhans remain intact (Coffin, 1953; Hashimoto, 1979; Prentice, 1980; Sateri, 1975). It has been called a disease of exocrine-endocrine dissociation (Szabo et al., 1978). It is more common in large breeds of dogs, particularly German shepherds (Anderson and Low, 1965), and there may be a sex predilection favoring females.

Dogs afflicted with pancreatic acinar atrophy are apparently born with adequate pancreatic function, for they usually grow to a normal size without evidence of pancreatic insufficiency. Usually the pancreas atrophies sometime during their first year of life and the dog develops signs of pancreatic insufficiency, including polyphagia, weight loss, and voluminous stools. The polyphagia is a remarkable feature of this disease and is of some differential value inasmuch as dogs with malnutrition secondary to primary small bowel disease are usually anorexic. In some cases, the polyphagia is so severe that the dog exhibits pica and becomes so obnoxious that the owner cannot tolerate the dog. A recent example was a dog that robbed all of the zucchini squash from the owner's garden. Coprophagia is common. Polyphagia combined with maldigestion of food may result in palpably distended intestines and abdominal distention (Coffin, 1953; Jubb and Kennedy, 1970).

Diagnosis of pancreatic acinar atrophy is usually not difficult, because the clinical signs are rather characteristic and the simple tests already described are very helpful diagnostic aids. As a group, serum amylase activity in such dogs is less than that in normal dogs, but the difference is not great enough to be helpful on an individual basis. Dogs with pancreatic acinar atrophy also have mildly elevated SGPT values (Sateri, 1975).

Exocrine Pancreatic Insufficiency Secondary to Pancreatitis

History and clinical signs in dogs with exocrine pancreatic insufficiency secondary to pancreatitis differ from those in pancreatic acinar atrophy. Usually parenchymal destruction resulting in exocrine pancreatic insufficiency is caused by chronic relapsing pancreatitis. Thus, a history of episodic gastrointestinal distress may be obtained from the owner. Since this is the result of chronic disease, the dogs are usually older than those with pancreatic acinar atrophy. Many of these dogs have concomitant diabetes mellitus, because the endocrine cells are also affected by the inflammatory process. Thus, the signs of diabetes mellitus may also be observed. Since the signs of diabetes mellitus and exocrine pancreatic insufficiency overlap (weight loss, polyphagia), one must be on the lookout for both diseases when one or the other is diagnosed. The onset of exocrine pancreatic insufficiency in dogs may precede or follow the onset of diabetes mellitus when they are caused by pancreatitis.

The same techniques used to detect maldigestion in pancreatic acinar atrophy can be applied to diagnose exocrine pancreatic insufficiency caused by chronic pancreatitis.

Functional Pancreatic Insufficiency

The fact that decreased exocrine pancreatic function occurs in states of protein-calorie malnutrition has recently been appreciated (Gyr et al., 1978; Barbezat and Hansen, 1968; Tandon et al., 1970). This type is usually a partial pancreatic insufficiency, compared with the complete lack of function characteristic of pancreatic acinar atrophy or exocrine pancreatic insufficiency secondary to pancreatitis. When an animal suffers from inadequate intake of calories or from protein depletion, the ability to secrete its protein-rich digestive juices is severely impaired. Exocrine function returns to normal upon repletion of adequate nutrient intake (Barbezat and Hansen, 1968; Tandon et al., 1970). Thus, decreased pancreatic function with some degree of malnutrition may be detected in patients with chronic diarrhea and weight loss or in energy-deficient states such as diabetes mellitus (Rogers et al., 1980; Strombeck, 1978).

Pancreatic function may also be depressed when gut endocrine secretion is impaired by primary bowel disease, e.g., malabsorption syndromes. In these cases, both lack of endocrine stimulation and protein calorie malnutrition probably contribute to depressed exocrine pancreatic function (Rhodes et al., 1978).

Deficient pancreatic function has been detected in these catabolic disease states by the BT-PABA test. This concept of functional pancreatic deficiency is clinically important for accurate interpretation of pancreatic function test results; moreover, therapy may be indicated even though primary pancreatic disease is not present (Gyr et al., 1978).

TREATMENT OF EXOCRINE PANCREATIC INSUFFICIENCY

Pancreatic insufficiency should be treated regardless of its etiology. Efforts to treat dogs with pancreatic insufficiency are usually rewarded with a favorable response. The expense of treatment, rather than ineffectiveness of the treatment regimen itself, is most often the reason that successful treatment is not accomplished.

The basis of therapy is dietary replacement of pancreatic digestive enzymes. Pancreatic enzymes are administered orally with each meal (Graham, 1977). Various enzyme preparations are on the market (Graham, 1979). Enteric-coated tablets should be avoided. They are relatively ineffective, because the enteric coating cannot be effectively removed from the tablets in patients with pancreatic insufficiency. The preparations containing enteric-coated microspheres are an exception to this rule (Graham, 1979). When pancreatic enzymes are given orally, a high percentage of them are inactivated by gastric acid. They are also rendered ineffective when the duodenal intraluminal pH is less than 4, an acidity that is reached in pancreatic insufficiency. Even though only a fraction of the enzymes administered reach the small intestine intact (active), they are still effective, because only a slight increase in duodenal digestive enzyme activity is needed to achieve a marked clinical improvement.

Various measures have been devised to spare the pancreatic enzymes from gastric inactivation (Strombeck, 1979). Sodium bicarbonate (20 to 40 mg/kg body weight) may be administered, along with pancreatic enzyme preparations. Beneficial effects of bicarbonate include increased intraduodenal pH, thus correcting the acidification of the small intestine caused by lack of pancreatic bicarbonate secretion.

Cimetidine (10 mg/kg body weight) has also been given, along with replacement digestive enzymes to protect them from gastric acid inactivation (Regan et al., 1977; Durie et al., 1980). Cimetidine antagonizes histamine-mediated gastric acid secretion. It also acts directly on parietal cells to decrease hydrochloric acid secretion (Regan et al., 1978). Cimetidine effectively spares pancreatic enzymes from gastric inactivation and improves intraduodenal pH. Bile acid deficiency caused by bile acid precipitation at low duodenal pH may be reversed by cimetidine, making the enzymes once more available for fat emulsification and micelle formation. Because of its expense, cimetidine therapy will probably be reserved for those cases that do not respond satisfactorily to pancreatic enzymes and bicarbonate. The effectiveness of enzyme replacement therapy can also be improved by incubating the food and pancreatic enzymes for several hours before feeding.

Ancillary treatment of pancreatic insufficiency is important in severe cases. Vitamins that may be indicated include the fat-soluble vitamins A, D, E, and K. Vitamin B_{12}, folic acid, and other suspected vitamin deficiencies should be treated. As previously stated, bile salt malabsorption can occur in exocrine pancreatic insufficiency, and short-term therapy with bile salts may be needed to replenish the bile salt pool.

Body weight and stool character should be monitored during treatment. Stool volume should decrease precipitously, and gains in body weight should begin soon after therapy is started. Chronic therapy should consist of pancreatic enzymes given with the food, and in some cases, bicarbonate therapy will also have to be continued.

NEOPLASMS OF THE EXOCRINE PANCREAS

Primary neoplasms of the exocrine pancreas include ductular adenocarcinoma and acinar cell adenocarcinoma. These tumors are more common in older dogs. They are rare in cats (Prieter, 1974; Theilen and Madewell, 1979; Anderson and Johnson, 1967).

Dogs with adenocarcinoma of the pancreas are not usually presented to the hospital with clinical signs of pancreatic disease. More commonly, they exhibit signs of liver disease such as jaundice, ascites, vomiting, and weight loss. These signs of liver disease are caused by hepatic metastasis of the pancreatic tumor. Metastasis has usually occurred by the time that the dog is presented to the hospital (Anderson and Johnson, 1967). Subsequent metastasis to the lungs is frequent and can cause signs of respiratory disease such as dyspnea and cough. Only rarely are signs of acute or chronic pancreatitis exhibited. Palpation of a nodular mass in the area of the pancreas is a very helpful clue leading to suspicion of a pancreatic carcinoma.

Plain radiographs often reveal hepatomegaly and nodular pulmonary densities compatible with tumor metastasis. Increased soft tissue density in the area of the pancreas may suggest a mass lesion. Occasionally the radiographic features of pancreatitis are present.

Laboratory test results are variable in

dogs and cats with pancreatic tumors. Serum amylase and lipase values may be moderately increased but are often within normal limits. Abnormal liver function tests, hyperbilirubinemia, and liver enzyme elevations are common. These results may indicate diffuse hepatic parenchymal infiltration of tumor or extrahepatic ductular obstruction by tumor mass. Occasionally, a laboratory diagnosis of diabetes mellitus is made and indicates destruction of islet tissues by tumor mass and by tumor-associated inflammation. Steatorrhea caused by exocrine insufficiency can occur (Cornelius, 1976).

Antemortem diagnosis of pancreatic adenocarcinoma is usually made by exploratory laparotomy or by liver biopsy upon detection of metastatic lesions.

Pancreatic adenocarcinomata are not successfully treatable at present and they carry a grave prognosis.

REFERENCES

Anderson, N. V., and Johnson, K. H.: Pancreatic carcinoma in the dog. J.A.V.M.A. *150*:286–295, 1967.

Anderson, N. V., and Low, D. G.: Diseases of the canine pancreas: a comparative summary of 103 cases. Anim. Hosp. *1*:189–194, 1965.

Avram, M. M.: High prevalence of pancreatic disease in chronic renal failure. Nephron *18*:68–71, 1977.

Banks, P. A.: Progress in gastroenterology, acute pancreatitis. Gastroenterology *61*:382–397, 1971.

Barbezat, G. O., and Hansen, J. D. L.: The exocrine pancreas and protein-calorie malnutrition. Pediatrics *42*:77–92, 1968.

Bass, V. D., Hoffmann, W. E., and Dorner, J. L.: Normal canine lipid profiles and effects of experimentally induced pancreatitis and hepatic necrosis on lipids. Am. J. Vet. Res. *37*:1355–1357, 1976.

Batt, R. M., and Mann, L. C.: Specificity of BT-PABA for diagnosis of exocrine pancreatic insufficiency in the dog. Vet. Rec. *108*:303–307, 1981.

Bockman, D. E., Schiller, W. R., Suriyapa, C., Mutchler, J. H. W., and Anderson, M. C.: Fine structure of early experimental acute pancreatitis in dogs. Lab. Invest. *18*:584–592, 1973.

Brobst, D., and Brester, J. E.: Serum lipase determination in the dog using a one hour test. J.A.V.M.A. *150*:767–771, 1967.

Burrows, C. R., Merritt, A. M., Chiapella, A. M.: Determination of fecal fat and trypsin output in the evaluation of chronic canine diarrhea. J.A.V.M.A. *174*:62–66, 1979.

Challis, T. W., Reid, L. C., and Hinton, J. W.: Study of some factors which influence the level of serum amylase in dogs and humans. Gastroenterology *33*:818–822, 1957.

Coffin, D. L., and Thordal-Christensen, A.: The clinical and some pathological aspects of pancreatic disease in dogs. Vet. Med. *48*:193–198, 1953.

Cornelius, L. M.: Laboratory diagnosis of acute pancreatitis and pancreatic adenocarcinoma. Vet. Clin. North Am. *6*:671–678, 1976.

DeHoff, W., and Archibald, J.: Pancreas. In Archibald, J. (ed.): Canine Surgery. American Veterinary Publications, Santa Barbara, CA. 1974, pp. 827–843.

Delaney, J. P., and Grim, E.: Influence of hormones and drugs on canine pancreatic flow. Am. J. Physiol. *211*:1398–1402, 1966.

Donowitz, M., Hendler, R., Spiro, H. M., Binder, H. F., and Felig, P.: Glucagon secretion in acute and chronic pancreatitis. Ann. Intern. Med. *83*:778–781, 1975.

Drummey, G. D., Benson, J. A., and Jones, C. M.: Medical intelligence. Microscopic examination of the stool for steatorrhea. N. Engl. J. Med. *264*:83–87, 1961.

Dubost, C., Testart, J., Choguart, P., and Kaswin, R.: Les pancreatitis de l'hyperparathroidie. Gastroenterol. Clin. Biol. *3*:621–630, 1979.

Duffell, S. J.: Some aspects of pancreatic disease in the cat. J. Small Anim. Pract. *16*:365–374, 1975.

Durie, P. R., Bell, L., Linton, W., Corey, M. L., and Forstner, G. G.: Effect of cimetidine and sodium bicarbonate on pancreatic replacement therapy in cystic fibrosis. Gut *21*:778–786, 1980.

Dutta, S. K., Russel, R. M., and Iber, F. L.: Impaired acid neutralization in the duodenum in pancreatic insufficiency. Dig. Dis. Sci. *24*:775–780, 1979a.

Dutta, S. K., Russel, R. M., and Iber, F. L.: Influence of exocrine pancreatic insufficiency on the intraluminal pH of the proximal small intestine. Dig. Dis. Sci. *24*:529–534, 1979b.

Feldman, B. F., Attix, E. A., Strombeck, D. R., and O'Neill, S.: Biochemical and coagulation changes in a canine model of acute necrotizing pancreatitis. Am. J. Vet. Res. *42*:805–809, 1981.

Finco, D. R., and Stevens, J. B.: Clinical significance of serum amylase activity in the dog. J.A.V.M.A. *155*:1686–1691, 1969.

Freudiger, M., and Bigler, B.: The diagnosis of chronic exocrine pancreatic insufficiency by the PABA test. Keintier-Praxis (Bern) *22*:73–79, 1977.

Gage, E. D. G., and Anderson, N. V.: Acute pancreatitis in a dog. Anim. Hosp. *3*:151–159, 1967.

Geokas, M. C., Rinderknecht, H., Walberg, C. B., and Weissman, R.: Methemalbumin in the diagnosis of acute hemorrhagic pancreatitis. Ann. Intern. Med. *81*:483–486, 1974.

Gilsanz, V., Oteyza, C. P., and Rebollar, J. L.: Glucagon vs. anticholinergics in the treatment of acute pancreatitis. Arch. Intern. Med. *138*:535–538. 1978.

Goldstein, D. A., Llach, F., and Massry, S. G.: Acute renal failure in patients with acute pancreatitis. Arch. Intern. Med. *136*:1363–1365, 1976.

Goodhead, B.: Importance of nutrition in the pathogenesis of experimental pancreatitis in the dog. Arch. Surg. *103*:724–727, 1971.

Graham, D. Y.: An enteric-coated pancreatic enzyme preparation that works. Dig. Dis. Sci. *24*:906–909, 1979.

Graham, D. Y.: Enzyme replacement therapy of exocrine pancreatic insufficiency in man. N. Engl. J. Med. *296*:1314–1317, 1977.

Gullo, L., Costa, P. L., Fontana, G., Tessari, R., Serra,

D., and Labo, G.: Cortisol and pancreatic secretion. Observations on pure pancreatic juice. Scand. J. Gastroenterol. 15:45–47, 1980.

Gyr, K., Felsenfeld, O., and Zimmerli-Ning, M.: Effect of oral pancreatic enzymes on the course of cholera in protein-deficient vervet monkeys. Gastroenterology 74:511–513, 1978.

Haig, T. H. B.: Pancreatic digestive enzymes: influence of a diet that augments pancreatitis. J. Surg. Res. 10:601–607, 1970.

Haig, T. H. B.: Cellular membranes in the etiology of acute pancreatitis. Surg. Forum 20:380–382, 1969.

Hardy, R. M., and Stevens, J. B.: Canine Exocrine Pancreatic Diseases. In Ettinger, S. J. (ed.): Textbook of Veterinary Internal Medicine, W. B.Saunders Co., Philadelphia, 1975, pp. 1247–1269.

Hashimoto, A., Kita, I., Okada, K., and Fujimoto, Y.: Juvenile acinar atrophy of the pancreas of a dog. Vet. Pathol. 16:74–80, 1979.

Henderson, J. R., Daniel, P. M., and Fraser, P. A.: Progress Report. The pancreas as a single organ: the influence of the endocrine upon the exocrine part of the gland. Gut 22:158–167, 1981.

Hendricks, J. C., DiMagno, E. P., and Go, V. L. W.: Reflux of duodenal contents into the pancreatic duct of dogs. J. Lab. Clin. Invest. 96:912–921, 1980.

Hiatt, N., and Warner, N. E.: Serum amylase and changes in pancreatic function and structure after ligation of pancreatic ducts. Am. Surg. 35:30–33, 1969.

Hill, F. W. G., and Kidder, D. E.: The oral glucose tolerance test in canine pancreatic malabsorption. Br. Vet. J. 128:207, 1972.

Hill, F. W. G., and Kidder, D. E.: The estimation of daily fecal trypsin levels in dogs as an indication of gross pancreatic exocrine insufficiency. J. Small Anim. Pract. 11:191–195, 1970.

Hudson, E. B., and Strombeck, D. R.: Effects of functional nephrectomy on the disappearance rates of canine serum amylase and lipase. Am. J. Vet. Res. 39:1316–1321, 1978.

Imondi, A. R., Stradley, R. P., and Wolgemuth, R.: Synthetic peptides in the diagnosis of exocrine pancreatic insufficiency in animals. Gut 13:726–731, 1972.

Jacobs, R. M., and Hall, R. L.: Isoamylases in clinically normal dogs. 1981, (in press).

Johnson, G. F.: Exocrine Pancreatic Insufficiency. In Anderson, N. V. (ed.) Veterinary Gastroenterology. Lea and Febiger, London, 1980, pp. 637–643.

Jubb, K. V. F., and Kennedy, P. C.: The Pancreas. In Pathology of Domestic Animals. Academic Press, New York, 1970, pp. 263–276.

Kelly, D. F., Baggot, D. G., and Gaskell, C. J.: Jaundice in the cat associated with inflammation of the biliary tract and pancreas. J. Small Anim. Pract. 16:163–172, 1975.

Kleine, L. J., and Hornbuckle, W. E.: Acute pancreatitis: the radiographic findings in 182 dogs. J. Am. Vet. Rad. Soc. 19:102–106, 1978.

Konturek, S. J., Tasler, J., Cieszkowski, M., Jaworek, J., Coy, D. H., and Schally, A. V.: Inhibition of pancreatic secretion of enkephalin and morphine in dogs. Gastroenterology 74:851–855, 1978.

Kwaan, H. C., Anderson, M. C., and Aramatica, L.: A study of pancreatic enzymes as a factor in the pathogenesis of disseminated intravascular coagulation during acute pancreatitis. Surgery 69:663–672, 1971.

Lees, G. E., Suter, P. F., and Johnson, G. C.: Pulmona-

ry edema in a dog with acute pancreatitis and cardiac disease. J.A.V.M.A. 172:690–696, 1978.

Lewis, L. D., and Boulay, J. P.: Fat excretion and assimilation by the cat. Feline Practice 9:46–49, 1979.

Loeb, W. F., and Edge, L. I.: A method for the determination of serum amylase in the dog. Am. J. Vet. Res. 23:1117–1119, 1972.

Luk, G. D., and Hendrix, T. R.: Microscopic examination of stool as a screening test for steatorrhea. Abstract Gastroenterology 74:1134, 1978.

Meshkinpour, H., Molinari, M. D., Gardner, L., Berk, J. E., and Hoehler, F. K.: Cimetidine in the treatment of acute alcoholic pancreatitis. Gastroenterology 77:687–690, 1979.

Mia, A. S., Koger, H. D., and Tierney, M. M.: Rapid turbidimetric determination of serum pancreatic lipase in the dog. Am. J. Vet. Res. 39:317–318, 1978a.

Mia, A. S., Koger, H. D., and Tierney, M. M.: Serum values of amylase and pancreatic lipase in healthy mature dogs and dogs with experimental pancreatitis. Am. J. Vet. Res. 39:965–969, 1978b.

Miller, M. E., Christenson, G. C., and Evans, H. E.: Anatomy of the Dog. W. B. Saunders Co., Philadelphia, 1964.

Neuman, N. B.: Acute hemorrhagic pancreatitis associated with iatrogenic hypercalcemia in a dog. J.A.V.M.A. 166:381–382, 1975.

Nielsen, S. W., and Bishop, E. J.: The duct system of the canine, pancreas. Am. J. Vet. Res. 15:266–271. 1954.

Notheman, M. M., and Callow, A. D.: Investigations on the origin of amylase in serum and urine. Gastroenterology 60:82–89, 1971.

O'Brien, T.: Pancreas. In Radiographic Diagnosis of Abdominal Disorders in the Dog and Cat. W. B. Saunders Co., Philadelphia, 1978.

Ohlsson, K., and Eddeland, A.: Release of proteolytic enzymes in bile-induced pancreatitis in dogs. Gastroenterology 69:668–675, 1975.

Olazabal, A., and Fuller, R.: Failure of glucagon in the treatment of alcoholic pancreatitis. Gastroenterology 74:489–491, 1978.

Owens, J. M., Drazner, F. H., and Gilbertson, S. R.: Pancreatic diseases in the cat. J.A.A.H.A. 11:83–90, 1975.

Owyand, C., Dozois, R. R., Dimagno, E. P., and Go, V. L. W.: Relationships between fasting and postprandial pancreaticoduodenal pressures, pancreatic secretion, and duodenal volume flow in the dog. Gastroenterology 3:1046–1049, 1977.

Paloyan, D., Payoyan, E., Worobec, R., Ernst, K., Deininger, E., and Harper, P. V.: Serum glucagon levels in experimental acute pancreatitis in the dog. Surg. Forum 17:348–349, 1966.

Papp, M., Ribet, A., Fodor, I., Nemeth, P. E., Feher, S., Horvath, J. E., and Folly, F.: Glucagon treatment in experimental acute pancreatitis. Acta Med. Acad. Sci. Hung. 32:105–116, 1975.

Parks, J. L., Gahring, D., and Greene, R. W.: Peritoneal lavage for peritonitis and pancreatitis in seventy-two dogs. J.A.A.H.A. 9:442–446, 1973.

Perman, V., and Stevens, J. B.: Clinical evaluation of the acinar pancreas in the dog. J.A.V.M.A. 155:2053–2058, 1969.

Prentice, D. E., James, R. W., and Wadsworth, P. F.: Pancreatic atrophy in young beagle dogs. Vet. Pathol. 17:575–580, 1980.

Prieter, W. A.: Data from eleven United States and

Canadian colleges of veterinary medicine on pancreatic carcinoma in domestic animals. Cancer Res. 34:1372, 1974.

Rapp, J. P.: Normal values for serum amylase and maltase in dogs, and the effect of maltase on the saccharogenic method of determining amylase in serum. Am. J. Vet. Res. 23:343–350, 1962.

Regan, P. T., Malogelada, J., DiMagno, E. P., and Go, V. L. W.: Postprandial gastric function in pancreatic insufficiency. Gut 20:249–254, 1979.

Regan, P. T., Malogelada, J., DiMagno, E. P., and Go, V. L. W.: Rationale for the use of cimetidine in pancreatic insufficiency. Mayo Clin. Proc. 53:79–83, 1978.

Regan, P. T., Malogelada, J., DiMagno, E. P., Glanzman, S. L., and Go, V. L. W.: Comparative effects of antacids, cimetidine and enteric coating on the therapeutic response to oral enzymes in severe pancreatic insufficiency. N. Engl. J. Med. 297:854–858, 1977.

Rhodes, R. A., Hsin-Hsiung, T., and Chey, W. Y.: Impairment of secretin release in celiac sprue. Dig. Dis. 23:833–839, 1978.

Riemenschneider, T. A., Wilson, J. F., and Vierner, R. L.: Glucocorticoid induced pancreatitis in children. Pediatrics 41:428–437, 1968.

Robertson, G. M., Moore, E. W., Switz, D. M., Sizemore, G. W., and Estep, H. L.: Inadequate parathyroid response in acute pancreatitis. N. Engl. J. Med. 294:512–516, 1976.

Rodgers, R. E., and Carey, L. C.: Peritoneal lavage in experimental pancreatitis in dogs. Am. J. Surg. 111:792–794, 1966.

Rogers, W. A.: Lipemia in the dog. Vet. Clin. North Am. 7:637–647, 1977.

Rogers, W. A., Stradley, R. P., Sherding, R. G., Powers, J., and Cole, C. R.: Simultaneous evaluation of pancreatic exocrine function and intestinal absorptive function in dogs with chronic diarrhea. J.A.V.M.A. 177:1128–1131, 1980.

Rosi, T. C., Pissiotis, C. A., Taube, R. R., and Condon, R. E.: Hemodynamic and metabolic effects of glucagon in acute hemorrhagic pancreatitis. Eur. Surg. Res. 6:209–218, 1974.

Ross, M. E., Hayashi, K., and Notkins, A. L.: Virus-induced pancreatic disease: alterations in concentration of glucose and amylase in blood. J. Infect. Dis. 129:669–676, 1974.

Rothenbacker, H., and Lindquist, W. D.: Liver cirrhosis and pancreatitis in a cat infected with Amphimerus pseudofelineus. J.A.V.M.A. 143:1099–1102, 1963.

Ruwitch, J., Bonertz, H. E., and Carlson, R. E.: Clinical aspects of pancreatic diseases of dogs and cats. J.A.V.M.A. 145:21–24, 1964.

Sateri, H.: Investigations on the exocrine pancreatic function of dogs suffering from chronic pancreatic insufficiency. Acta Vet. Scand. Suppl. 53:1–86, 1975.

Schapiro, H., McDougal, H. D., Morrison, E. J., and Wan, A. T.: Acute hemorrhagic pancreatitis in the dog, IV. Intravenous treatment with vasopressin. Dig. Dis. 21:286–290, 1976.

Schiller, W. R., Suriyapa, C., and Anderson, M. D.: Current Research Review, a review of experimental pancreatitis. J. Surg. Res. 16:69–90, 1974.

Sheldon, W. G.: Pancreatic flukes (Eurytrema procyonis) in domestic cats. J.A.V.M.A. 148:251–253, 1966.

Sherding R. G.: Canine exocrine pancreatic insufficiency. Comp. Cont. Ed. 1:816–820, 1979.

Sherding, R. G.: Feline infectious peritonitis. Comp. Cont. Ed. 1:95–101, 1979.

Shieber, W.: Why hypocalcemia in pancreatitis? Am. J. Surg. 120:685–686, 1970.

Shingleton, W. W., Anlyan, W. G., and David, A. K.: Treatment of experimental acute pancreatitis with banthene. Surgery 31:490–494, 1952.

Shutt, C., Friemel, H., Schulze, H. A., and Zubaidi, G.: Specific lymphocyte sensitization in chronic pancreatitis. Digestion 13:308–311, 1975.

Singh, M., and Webster, P. D.: Progress in gastroenterology. Neurohormonal control of pancreatic secretion, a review. Gastroenterology 74:294–309, 1978.

Small, E., Olsen, R., and Fritz, T.: The canine pancreas. VM SAC 59:627–642, 1964.

Stickle, J. E., Carlton, W. W., and Boon, G. D.: Isoamylases in clinically normal dogs. Am. J. Vet. Res. 41:506–509, 1980.

Stradley, R. P., Stern, R. J., Heinhold, N. B.: A method for the simultaneous evaluation of exocrine pancreatic function and intestinal absorptive function in dogs. Am. J. Vet. Res. 40:1201–1205, 1979.

Strombeck, D. R.: Small Animal Gastroenterology. Stonegate Publishing, Davis, California, 1979.

Strombeck, D. R.: New method for evaluation of chymotrypsin deficiency in dogs. J.A.V.M.A. 173:1319–1323, 1978.

Susni, C., Esteve, J. P., Bommelaer, G., Vayasse, N., and Ribet, A.: Inhibition of exocrine pancreatic secretion by somatostatin in dogs. Digestion 18:384–393, 1978.

Suter, P. F., and Lowe, R. Acute pancreatitis in the dog: a clinical study with emphasis on radiographic diagnosis. Acta Radiol. Suppl. 319:195, 1972.

Szabo, T., Greenstein, A. J., Geller, S. A., and Dreiling, D. A.: Pancreatic atrophy in the canine: an entity of exocrine-endocrine dissociation. M. Sinai J. Med. 45:503–508, 1978.

Tandon, B. N., Banks, P. A., George, P. K., Sama, S. K., Ramachandran, K., and Gandhi, P. C.: Recovery of exocrine pancreatic function in adult protein-calorie malnutrition. Gastroenterology 58:358–362, 1970.

Theilen, G. H., and Madewell, B. R.: Tumors of the Digestive Tract. In Theilen, G. H., and Madewell, B. R. (eds.): Veterinary Cancer Medicine. Lea and Febiger, Philadelphia, 1979.

Tuzhilin, S. A., Podolosky, A. E., and Dreiling, D. A.: Hepatic lesions in pancreatitis. Am. J. Gastroenterol. 4:108–114, 1975.

Wanke, M.: Experimental acute pancreatitis. Curr. Top. Pathol. 52:64–142, 1970.

Weiner, S., Gramatica, L., Voegle, L. D., Hauman, R. L., and Anderson, M. C.: Role of the lymphatic system in the pathogenesis of inflammatory disease in the biliary tract and pancreas. Am. J. Surg. 119:55–62, 1970.

Weir, G. C., Lesser, P. B., Drop. L. J., Fischer, J. E., and Warshaw, A. L.: The hypocalcemia of acute pancreatitis. Ann. Int. Med. 83:185–189, 1975.

Williams, J. A.: Regulation of pancreatic acinar function by intracellular calcium. Am. J. Physiol. 238:269–279, 1980.

CHAPTER 62

Diseases of the Gallbladder

WILLIAM D. SCHALL
and THOMAS P. GREINER

ANATOMY

The gallbladder in the dog is located in the depression on the visceral surface of the liver between the quadrate and right medial lobes. The feline gallbladder lies on the fissure of the right medial lobe. Blood supply to the gallbladders of both species is via the cystic artery which arises from the left branch of the proper hepatic artery and ramifies on the surface of the gallbladder. Proximal to the junction of the common and cystic ducts, the extrahepatic bile ducts of the dog and cat vary greatly (Mann et al., 1920). Sleight and Thomford (1970) have described variations in the canine duct system in detail. The intrahepatic bile-duct system in dogs is characterized by small collateral channels that connect the intrahepatic bile ducts of adjacent lobes. These channels allow drainage of bile from lobes in which primary pathways are obstructed (Sleight and Thomford, 1970). It is not known whether similar channels exist in the cat.

DISEASES OF THE GALLBLADDER

The incidence of gallbladder disease in the cat and dog is extremely low. Associated signs are often nonexistent, but can be dramatic and life threatening. The ante mortem diagnosis of gallbladder disease is often difficult because of the lack of specific physical, laboratory, and radiographic findings.

CHOLELITHIASIS AND CHOLEDOCHOLITHIASIS

Choleliths are rare in cats and dogs. Their occurrence in dogs has been reviewed (Schall et al., 1973) and three cases have been reported in cats (Gibson, 1952; Wigderson, 1955; O'Brien and Mitchum, 1970). There is no known breed or sex predilection, but most animals are over two years of age at the time of diagnosis.

The cause of gallstones remains debatable. The major theories implicate bile stasis, infection, and changes in bile composition. The small number of canine and feline choleliths subjected to quantitative analysis precludes generalization regarding their composition. Cholesterol, bilirubin, calcium, magnesium, and oxalates have been identified as constituents of canine and feline choleliths. Normal canine bile has been found to be less saturated with cholesterol than human bile (Nakayama, 1969). It is unlikely, therefore, that canine gallstones are composed predominately of cholesterol.

Cholelithiasis does not usually cause overt disease. Emesis and abdominal pain are occasionally associated. Bile peritonitis can result if the choleliths erode the gallbladder wall. Rarely, the mineral content of canine and feline gallstones is sufficient to make them radiopaque, and they may be detected when abdominal radiographs are obtained for other purposes. In most instances, however, the gallstones are discovered at necropsy and are not associated with clinical signs.

Choleliths, formed either in the bile ducts or, more likely, in the gallbladder, may pass into the common bile duct and cause permanent or temporary obstruction. Permanent obstruction of the common bile duct demands surgical intervention. Recurrent temporary obstruction is associated with recurrent icterus and occurs as commonly as permanent obstruction.

Choledocholithiasis is reliably associated with icterus. As is the case with any cause of either intra- or extrahepatic biliary obstruction, the icterus is usually characterized by conjugated bilirubin levels in excess of 50 per cent of the total. Depending on

1456

the duration of the obstruction, serum-transaminase activity may be increased because of secondary hepatic necrosis. Serum-alkaline-phosphatase activity is more likely to be increased because of induced increase in production (Kaplan, 1972), hepatic necrosis, and lack of biliary excretion.

RUPTURE OF THE GALLBLADDER AND BILE DUCTS

Rupture of the gallbladder or bile ducts in the dog and cat is uncommon. It results from a variety of causes, which, in decreasing order of frequency, are (1) blunt trauma, such as an automobile accident; (2) sharp trauma, such as knife or gunshot wounds; (3) iatrogenesis, as a result of percutaneous liver biopsy or manipulation at laparotomy; and (4) pathologic rupture, as a sequela of calculi, inflammation, or neoplasia. There is no breed, age, or sex predilection.

Traumatic gallbladder or bile-duct rupture in the cat and dog is usually accompanied by other disorders, such as shock, hemorrhage, liver fracture, bone fracture, muscle injury, and pneumothorax (Suter and Olsson, 1970). As a consequence, signs strictly referable to gallbladder or bile-duct rupture are often obscured. Clinical signs associated with relatively uncomplicated rupture are dependent upon the extent and duration of the resultant bile peritonitis. Mild to moderate abdominal pain, which often subsides within 48 hours, is the only consistent sign after rupture of the gallbladder or bile duct. As a result, the average delay in diagnosis after traumatic rupture is about five days, by which time abdominal distention due to the accumulation of bile-tinged peritoneal effusion is usually present. Other clinical signs that may be present five to seven days after bile-duct or gallbladder rupture are anorexia, depression, dehydration, fever, and icterus.

Hematologic and serum-chemistry findings are not specific. If dehydration is present, blood urea nitrogen (BUN), packed-cell volume (PCV), and plasma-protein determinations will be increased. If icterus is associated, it is usually characterized by increased amounts of conjugated bilirubin. Confirmation of bile peritonitis is possible if fluid obtained by abdominocentesis is bilirubin positive. Failure to obtain such fluid does not, however, rule out bile-duct or gallbladder rupture. It may be possible to obtain bilirubin-positive aspirates after irrigation of the peritoneal cavity with saline when bile peritonitis has not resulted in sufficient fluid production for aspiration. If bile peritonitis is determined to be present on the basis of abdominocentesis, it is not possible to distinguish between a leak in the biliary tree and perforation of the upper small intestine with leakage of bile-rich intestinal juice. Plain abdominal radiographs either are noncontributory or simply confirm the presence of fluid in the peritoneal cavity. Oral cholecystography (if the patient is not vomiting) or intravenous cholangiography may confirm the presence of bile leakage and may aid in localizing the site. Laparotomy is usually required for definitive location.

CYSTIC MUCINOUS HYPERTROPHY

Cystic mucinous hypertrophy of the gallbladder has been observed at necropsy in dogs without associated clinical signs (Kovatch et al., 1965). No breed or sex predilection has been identified, but all affected dogs have been over six years of age. The gallbladder mucosa contains epithelium-lined cysts that are filled with mucin. Inflammatory infiltrate is minimal. In some instances, the cysts are grossly visible. Although the cause is unknown, similar changes have been observed in dogs to which carbomycin and progestational compounds have been administered. At present, the clinical significance of these observations is unknown.

NEOPLASIA

Tumors of the feline and canine gallbladder are very rare. Adenomas and adenocarcinomas have been reported, but the scant number precludes generalization regarding associated signs and biological behavior. Bile-duct carcinomas may cause obstructive icterus but are virtually always intrahepatic in location.

CHOLECYSTITIS

Acute and chronic inflammation of the gallbladder has been reported rarely (Endres et al., 1971). Cholecystitis may be present with or without choleliths, and associated signs are not specific.

THERAPEUTIC CONSIDERATIONS

Medical therapy for gallbladder disease is restricted to efforts directed against the secondary effects of the disease. Specific therapy for cholelithiasis and choledocholithiasis, rupture of the gallbladder or bile ducts, and neoplasia is surgical.

A number of surgical procedures have been described to treat various conditions of the gallbladder, including cholecysto-duodenostomy, cholecystectomy, cholecystotomy, and anastomosis of the gallbladder to the common bile duct utilizing a T tube (Pennock et al., 1969; Hoffer et al., 1971; Schall et al., 1973). However, the indications for these procedures are limited, and all may induce postoperative complications. The most commonly performed procedure in the dog and cat is cholecystectomy.

SURGICAL PROCEDURE (CHOLECYSTECTOMY)

There are two basic approaches to the canine gallbladder, the thoracic approach through the eighth intercostal space and diaphragm and the abdominal approach. The abdominal approach is simpler, but exposure may be poor and mobility is difficult, especially in the deep-chested dog. It may be combined with a paracostal incision for greater exposure. The right thoracic approach has the advantage of offering greater exposure and visualization of the gallbladder and surrounding structures, but has an added disadvantage of requiring respiratory assistance and postoperative thoracotomy management.

The thoracic approach is through the eighth intercostal space on the right side. The diaphragm is incised, and the right medial lobe of the liver is retracted to expose the gallbladder. The abdominal approach is made from the xiphoid posteriorly to allow sufficient exposure of the liver and gallbladder. The surrounding viscera are then packed away utilizing laparotomy pads, and the gallbladder is identified. Next, the apex is grasped with an Allis clamp or a stay suture is placed in the wall for retraction, and the gallbladder is gently dissected from its fossa. The cystic artery is identified and ligated close to the surface of the gallbladder. The cystic duct is dissected to its point of junction with the common bile duct and ligated. The ligature is placed between two clamps one-fourth inch from the junction to prevent the ligature from causing a narrowing of the common duct. Penrose drains are placed in the fossa and brought out through the abdominal wall via separate incisions.

Dilatation of the common duct after canine cholecystectomy has been documented (Mahour et al., 1969). This dilatation has no known clinical significance. The use of the T tube to facilitate bile drainage and minimize bile seepage from the raw surface of the liver after canine cholecystectomy has been advocated (Hoffer et al., 1971); however, recently it has been criticized because of complications in man (Lucas, 1970). Another disadvantage of this procedure in the dog and cat is the small size of the bile ducts, which makes them extremely difficult to cannulate for drainage. Moreover, the T tube itself may cause obstruction.

After removal of the gallbladder, some form of drainage may be provided to remove seepage of bile from the gallbladder fossa, as total reperitonealization after removal is impossible in the dog and cat. Drainage can be accomplished by instilling Penrose drains into the area from which the gallbladder was removed and leaving them there for a minimum of three to five days (DeHoff et al., 1972). If a great deal of bile is present, sump-suction catheters should be placed in the area and lavage provided for 48 to 72 hours. An effective sump drain can be made by placing No. 14 or 16 Foley catheters, in which additional holes have been cut, through the Penrose drains. Suction may then be applied to the drains. Lavage is provided by introducing a Foley catheter through the skin on the posterior dorsal aspect of the last rib with the tip placed in the gallbladder area. A sterile solution of saline and antibiotics may then be flushed into the area, and it will drain through the sump drain.

The generalized peritonitis that is present must also be treated. This may be accomplished by a thorough irrigation of the peritoneal cavity at the time of surgery, followed by peritoneal lavage and drainage with sump drains for a minimum of two to four days postoperatively. Massive doses of antibiotics should be given for seven to ten days postoperatively to combat gram-negative organisms. Adequate fluid therapy should also be provided, as large quantities of fluid may be lost through the irritated peritoneal surfaces.

REFERENCES

DeHoff, W. D., Greene, R. W., and Greiner, T. P.: Surgical management of abdominal emergencies. Vet. Clin. N. Am. *2*:301, 1972.

Endres, W., Johnson, M. E., and Graber, E. R.: Acute cholecystitis in a canine: A case report. Anim. Hosp. *7*:107, 1971.

Gibson, K. S.: Cholelithiasis and choledocholithiasis in a cat. J.A.V.M.A. *121*:288, 1952.

Hoffer, R. E., Niemeyer, K. H., and Patton, M.: Common bile duct repair utilizing the gallbladder and T-tube. Vet. Med. Small Anim. Clin. *66*:889, 1971.

Kaplan, M. M.: Alkaline phosphatase. N. Engl. J. Med. *286*:200, 1972.

Kovatch, R. M., Hildebrandt, P. K., and Marcus, L. C.: Cystic mucinous hypertrophy of the mucosa of the gallbladder in the dog. Path. Vet. *2*:574, 1965.

Lucas, C. E.: What is the role of biliary drainage in liver trauma? Am. J. Surg. *120*:509, 1970.

Mahour, G. H., Wakim, K. G., Ferris, D. O., and Soule, E. H.: Canine common bile duct: Chronologic changes in caliber after cholecystectomy. Arch. Surg. *98*:239, 1969.

Mann, F. C., Brimhall, S. D., and Foster, J. P.: The extrahepatic biliary tract in common domestic and laboratory animals. Anat. Rec. *18*:47, 1920.

Nakayama, F.: Composition of gallstone and bile: Species difference. J. Lab. Clin. Med. *73*:623, 1969.

O'Brien, T. R., and Mitchum, G. D.: Cholelithiasis in a cat. J.A.M.A. *156*:1015, 1970.

Pennock, P. W., Archibald, J., and Putnam, R. W.: Emergency surgery of the abdomen. Mod. Vet. Pract. *50*:47, 1969.

Schall, W. D., Chapman, W. L., Jr., Finco, D. R., Greiner, T. P., Mather, G. W., Rosin, E., and Welser, J. R.: Cholelithiasis in dogs. J.A.V.M.A. *163*:469, 1973.

Sleight, D. R., and Thomford, N. R.: Gross anatomy of the blood supply and biliary drainage of the canine liver. Anat. Rec. *166*:153, 1970.

Suter, P. F., and Olsson, S. E.: The diagnosis of injuries to the intestines, gallbladder and bile ducts in the dog. J. Small Anim. Pract. *11*:575, 1970.

Wigderson, F. J.: Cholelithiasis in a cat. J.A.V.M.A. *126*:287, 1955.

CHAPTER **63**

THOMAS P. GREINER
and RICHARD G. JOHNSON

Diseases of the Prostate Gland

THE PROSTATE GLAND

Much new information regarding the treatment of diseases of the prostate gland has appeared in the literature in the last five years. New techniques for the surgical correction of prostatic abscesses have been developed; new antibiotics are available that cross the prostatic barrier and can be used as a conservative mode of therapy.

Enlargement of the gland is common in both the dog and man (with incidence of 60 per cent in all male dogs over five years of age) (Matera and Archibald, 1965). The gross appearance of the organ and clinical signs of disease are also similar in the two species. Because of the similarities, the canine prostate continues to be used as a model for the study of prostatic disease conditions in man. As a result, much continues to be learned about canine prostatic disease, and better methods of therapy are being developed from this increased knowledge.

ANATOMY

The prostate gland is a retroperitoneal, bilobate, musculoglandular structure that completely encircles the proximal end of the urethra and the neck of the bladder. It is classified as an accessory sex gland and is the only one present in the dog. Embryologically, it develops as multiple outgrowths of the entodermal epithelium of the urethra, both anterior and posterior to the entrance of the male ducts or future ductus deferens. These outgrowths begin to bud early in fetal life and develop as two groups, each constituting a future lobe of the gland. As the buds develop, the surrounding mesenchymal tissue differentiates into connective tissue and smooth muscle fibers. The buds grow into differentiating mesenchymal tissue, eventually forming glandular tissue interspersed with the stromal tissue (Arey, 1965).

In the developed embryo, the gland consists of numerous, compound tubuloalveolar glands, which are enclosed in interstitial connective tissue and smooth muscle and form tubules and excretory ducts that enter the urethra. The gland is surrounded by a relatively thick fibromuscular capsule and is divided into two lobes by a medium septum on the dorsal surface. It is ovoid in shape.

O'Shea (1962) reported that the prostate of the adult dog passes through three phases of growth in relation to age: normal growth in the young adult, hyperplasia during middle age, and involution in old age. This is important in differentiating abnormal growth (hyperplasia) from normal enlargement of the gland during mature adult life. The average gland in a mature 25-pound dog weighs 6.5 gm and measures two cm in length and transverse diameter. The normal size and weight of the prostate vary, depending on age, breed, and body weight (Miller et al., 1964).

In the normal adult, it is situated in the pelvic canal at the pelvic brim and lies on the pelvic symphysis. Dorsally, it lies near the ventral surface of the rectum and is attached to it by a fibrous band (Gordon, 1960). The location of the prostate at the pelvic brim varies according to the cranial displacement of the full urinary bladder. Ventrally, a large accumulation of adipose tissue covers the gland and vessels; this must be separated at the midventral portion of the prostate and reflected laterally to view the gland. The prostate gland is usually considered to be retroperitoneal (Gordon, 1960) and is covered by the peritoneum only on its craniodorsal side.

Knowledge of the extensive blood and nerve supply to the prostate is important for avoiding unnecessary surgical complications (Fig. 63–1). The main arterial supply comes from the urogenital artery, which is a branch of the visceral branch of the internal iliac artery. This vessel can be seen readily when the adipose tissue overlying the prostate gland has been reflected and the gland has been rotated slightly. At the mid-dorsolateral surface of each lobe, the urogenital artery gives rise to two or, occasionally, three branches to the prostate gland, the prostaticovesical artery, and the prostaticourethral artery. The vessels are quite short in the normal animal but may be two to three cm in length in an abnormal gland. These arteries ramify on the surface of the gland and send small branches to the prostatic urethra and a few minor branches to

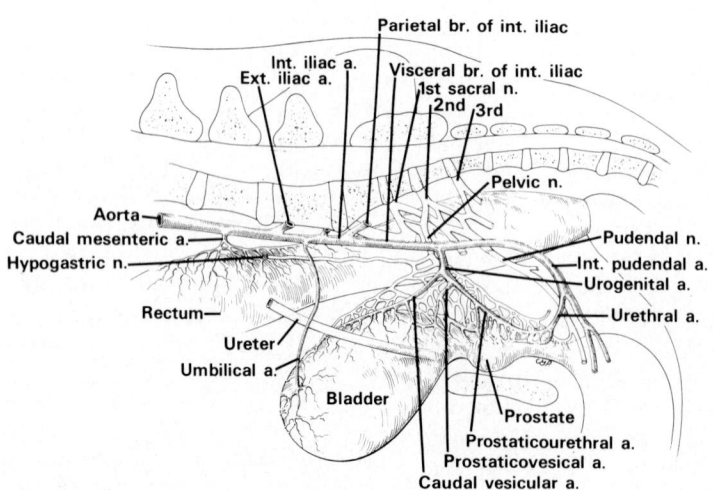

Figure 63–1. Diagrammatic illustration of the normal anatomic relationship between canine prostate and bladder. (Adapted from Miller, M. E., et al.: Anatomy of the Dog. W. B. Saunders Co., Philadelphia, 1964.)

the neck of the bladder. The urogenital artery continues as the vesicular artery and ramifies on the surface of the bladder.

As it courses to the bladder, the vesicular artery lies close to the dorsolateral surface of the prostate gland. Special care must be taken to avoid cutting this artery when identifying the prostatic arteries, as it is the major blood supply to the urinary bladder. The nerve supply of this area closely parallels the blood supply. The hypogastric nerve from the caudal mesenteric ganglion provides sympathetic innervation and is accompanied by a small branch of the prostaticovesical artery. The parasympathetic innervation is via the pelvic nerve, which arises from the second sacral nerve. The pelvic nerve runs parallel to the urogenital artery and vein for a distance, then it divides into numerous branches, which unite with branches from the hypogastric nerve to form the pelvic plexus.

The pelvic plexus consists of three parts — the cranial vesical plexus, the middle genital plexus, and the caudal hemorrhoidal plexus — and is located on the ventrolateral surface of the rectum overlying the prostate. The vesical plexus is formed mainly by a large branch from the hypogastric nerve and a large branch from the pelvic nerve. It sends nerves to the bladder and closely parallels the prostaticovesicular artery. The genital plexus sends branches to the prostate, the ductus deferens, and the cranial portion of the urethra. The somatic innervation to the bladder and urethra is from the pudendal nerve, derived from sacral nerves one to three. Branches from the pudendal nerve are distributed throughout the striated muscles of the urethra and external sphincter of the bladder as the nerve courses along the ventral surface of the urethra (Gordon, 1960; Miller et al., 1964).

The anatomy of the trigone and bladder-neck area is also of surgical importance. In recent years, anatomic studies by Hutch (1966) and Tanagho and Smith (1966) have established that there are no true sphincter or circular muscle fibers in the bladder-neck area, but rather an intertwining extension of the detrusor and trigonal muscle layers. Normal micturition involves a coordination of the autonomic systems under sympathetic and parasympathetic control. Sympathetic-induced contractions open the bladder-neck area, while the detrusor muscle contracts owing to parasympathetic stimulation (Rohner et al., 1971). To prevent urinary incontinence following a total prostatectomy, one must preserve the reflex arc that controls micturition. Thus, protection of the innervation described above takes on great significance. Preservation of the caudal vesicular artery is also important to prevent necrosis of the posterior portion of the bladder. When performing a prostate resection, the surgeon must isolate and gently retract the vessels and nerves described, especially on the ventrolateral surface of the gland.

PHYSIOLOGY

The prostate gland is the only accessory sex gland in the male dog and, like all accessory sex glands, is remarkably dependent upon androgen. Its only known function is the secretion of seminal plasma, a milky fluid that thins and increases the volume of the ejaculate, to aid in the transport and support of sperm.

Under parasympathetic stimulation, during erection, the prostate increases the rate of fluid production and under sympathetic stimulation ejects the fluid during ejaculation. Several authors have reported the alkaline character of prostatic secretion, and its importance in successful sperm mobility and fertilization (Matera and Archibald, 1965; Swenson, 1970; Guyton, 1971). Experimental studies, however, have shown a pH range of 6.0 to 7.4 (Stamey et al., 1968). Prostatic fluid pH is important in determining antibiotic efficacy, as will be discussed.

Prostatic secretions are produced by the epithelial cells of the gland but are dependent on androgens produced in the testis and other parts of the body. Castration will cause cytologic changes in the gland epithelial cells, characterized by a low cuboidal epithelium reduction in cell height, prominent basal cells, loss of basement membrane, diminished cytoplasm, and a pyknotic nucleus (Leav and Cavazos, 1974). Castration almost abolishes the secretion of prostatic fluid; injections of testosterone completely reverse this effect.

Estrogens also have a marked effect on both the size and the amount of secretion of the prostate gland. When administered to the male, estrogen depresses the secretion of gonadotropin by the pituitary gland

(Huggins and Clark, 1940), which reduces the level of androgen secretion by the testes and results in prostatic atrophy (O'Shea, 1962). Markowitz et al. (1964) demonstrate that as little as 0.1 mg of diethylstilbestrol injected daily into normal dogs abolishes prostatic secretions and causes squamous cells to appear in the prostatic secretions after about a week. They further demonstrated that the estrogen injections neutralize the effects of androgens before decreasing prostatic secretions. All dogs showed spermatogenesis and an apparent decrease of Leydig cells in the testes. These facts are of clinical significance when one considers the widespread use of estrogens in treating hyperplasia of the prostate, as well as disorders such as perineal adenomas. Squamous metaplasia can result from the indiscriminate use of estrogens, which cause enlargement and predispose the gland to inflammatory changes (O'Shea, 1963).

The prostate gland also secretes acid phosphatase and alkaline phosphatase, depending on the activity of the gland. This is clinically important in human medicine because acid phosphatase levels are used as an aid in the diagnosis of prostatic adenocarcinoma. Acid phosphatase does not normally enter the bloodstream, but when prostatic tissue becomes disseminated, as in cancer, there is a great secretion of this enzyme into the bloodstream. No pertinent data concerning the diagnostic value of this test for the dog now exist (Leav and Ling, 1968).

Recent studies on the immunologic properties of the canine prostate have shown that it contains three prostatic-specific antigens (Albin and Soanes, 1971). Dogs inoculated with rabbit antisera developed severe progressive histodegenerative changes in the prostate gland. This may be of clinical significance as a future method of treating benign hypertrophy.

DISEASES OF THE PROSTATE GLAND

PROSTATITIS (INFECTIOUS DISEASE)

Prostatitis, or infectious conditions of the prostate, can be divided into four groups for the purpose of description: (1) specific infections, (2) acute prostatitis, (3) chronic prostatitis, and (4) prostatic abscess or suppurative prostatitis. Each form is based on clinical and pathological evidence that the lesion is inflammatory. Each will be dis-

cussed individually, but one form may progress to the next if not properly treated, or more than one form may coexist with another.

Specific Infections

Specific infections of the prostate gland, such as blastomycosis and tuberculosis, have been reported by Matera and Archibald (1965) but are seldom encountered. *Brucella canis* can also cause prostatitis and because of the public health significance should be considered as a differential.

Acute Prostatitis

Acute prostatitis is an acute inflammatory condition of the prostate gland that may occur with or without hyperplasia of the gland. O'Shea (1963) reported that inflammatory changes are common in benign prostatic hyperplasia exhibiting squamous metaplasia, because multiplication of bacteria is likely when secretory stasis has occurred, such as with squamous metaplasia. The bacterial organisms most frequently isolated are the gram-negative bacteria, *Escherichia coli*, *Proteus* spp., and *Pseudomonas* spp., as well as gram-positive organisms such as *Staphylococcus* spp. and *Streptococcus* spp. The most common route of bacterial entry is via an ascending infection from the urinary tract; however, the infection may be bloodborne.

Diagnosis. The diagnosis of acute prostatitis is based on clinical and laboratory findings. The outstanding clinical signs seen with acute prostatitis are those of an acute infection with systemic signs of illness, fever, anorexia, depression, listlessness, and, occasionally, emesis (Hornbuckle et al., 1978). In addition, pain is usually a consistent finding. The animal may stand with an arched back and resist posterior abdominal palpation. Palpation per rectum will cause pain. The prostate gland will be swollen and warm to the touch; it may be spongy in some cases but is usually uniformly enlarged and firm. The characteristic signs of prostatic disease (dysuria, urinary incontinence, hematuria, pyuria, and tenesmus) may or may not be present, depending on the duration of the disease. Initially, urinary symptoms may be absent. However, as the disease progresses, stranguria, hematuria, and pyuria usually develop, as do cystitis and urethritis (Hornbuckle et al., 1978). Rectal tenesmus may occur when the acute process is accompanied by benign hypertrophy.

Laboratory examination of the blood and urine will be helpful in arriving at a diagnosis. A marked leukocytosis with many immature neutrophils is common. Urinalysis will reveal evidence of hematuria, pyuria, and bacteria. Urine culture will usually reveal the causative organisms.

Radiographic examination of the pelvic region is usually unrevealing in acute prostatitis. Abnormal enlargement and malposition of the prostate gland are not usually evident unless the condition is accompanied by benign hypertrophy (Borthwick and MacKenzie, 1971).

Treatment. Medical treatment is aimed at eliminating the causative bacterial organism. Animals that are acutely ill should be given supportive therapy. Fluids and electrolytes should be given to correct deficits that may have resulted from vomiting. If stranguria and hematuria are severe, catheterization and irrigation of the bladder and urethra with cold, sterile saline solution and an appropriate antibiotic may be helpful. Smooth muscle relaxants may be beneficial in relieving urethral spasms associated with the cystitis and urethritis that often accompany the disease.

The selection of an effective antibiotic is important in treating the disease. Urine culture will frequently isolate the infective organism; however, the organism may be present only in the prostatic secretions and not in the urine. Bacteriologic cultures of ejaculates from normal dogs have not been evaluated. It has been shown that a high number of contaminants exist at the distal urethra. It is therefore optimal for both urine cultures and prostatic samples to be cultured quantitatively and compared.

To isolate bacteria from the prostate, the bladder is catheterized and emptied, using aseptic technique. The bladder is then flushed using five ml of sterile saline and this sample is saved. The catheter is now retracted so the tip is distal to the prostate and the prostate is massaged per rectum. Five to ten ml of sterile saline are injected slowly by the prostate and into the bladder. This sample is now collected by advancement of the catheter into the bladder. Both samples are evaluated for culture and antibiotic sensitivity.

Efficacy of an antibiotic is in part due to its ability to cross the blood-prostatic fluid barrier into the prostatic fluid. Stamey et al. (1970), Wolf et al. (1967), and Madsen et al. (1968) showed most antibiotics unable to cross the prostatic epithelium in normal dogs. It is thought that with acute bacterial prostatitis, an alteration occurs in the blood-prostatic fluid barrier that enables most antibiotics to enter the prostatic fluid. This may explain why antibiotics commonly used against gram-negative enteric pathogens in urinary tract infections such as ampicillin, penicillin G and K, cephalothin, kanamycin, polymyxin, oxytetracycline, nitrofurantoin, sulfisoxazole, and sulfamethazone have been reported to be successful in the treatment of acute prostatitis. With chronic prostatitis, however, the barrier remains intact and limits the choice of antibiotics (Barsanti and Finco, 1979). Of the commonly used antibiotics, only erythromycin, oleandomycin, and trimethoprim sulfonamide (Tribrissen) have been shown to be present in sufficient concentrations in the prostatic fluid to be valuable in treating the disease. However, there are insufficient clinical data to substantiate their use. Information on chloromycetin and streptomycin is not available in the veterinary literature. Regardless of the type of prostatitis, i.e., chronic or acute, antibiotics should be chosen based on culture and sensitivity testing of prostatic fluid. In addition, it is important to administer high levels for long periods of time (four to six weeks), as too short a course may predispose the animal to chronic prostatic abscesses.

It is wise to perform culture and sensitivity tests at regular intervals after antibacterial therapy to ensure that the infection has been cured. Along with prolonged, vigorous antibacterial therapy, castration should be considered in order to decrease the size and secretions of the prostate. Estrogen therapy has been proposed by some (Matera and Archibald, 1965; Betts and Finco, 1974); however, since prolonged estrogen therapy, even in small dosages, produces squamous metaplasia with resultant secretory stasis (O'Shea, 1963), castration should be considered after recurrent attacks.

Chronic Prostatitis

Chronic prostatitis in the dog reportedly occurs less frequently than acute prostatitis (McEntee et al., 1970); however, owing to the relative lack of clinical signs, it may be more common but not diagnosed. It is thought to be an extension of, or a sequela to, acute prostatitis.

Diagnosis. The diagnosis of chronic prostatitis is difficult to make based on clinical signs alone. The disease should be suspected in dogs with a history of recurrent intermittent attacks of cystitis and acute prostatitis. Characteristic clinical signs of the disease are few. In man, chronic prostatitis is the most common cause of recurrent bladder and kidney infections (Stamey et al., 1970); it should also be considered a cause of these infections in the dog. In one study, 85 per cent of dogs with chronic prostatitis presented with problems referable to the urinary tract (Hornbuckle et al., 1978). Because most antimicrobial drugs cannot cross the prostatic epithelium, small numbers of bacteria may remain in the prostatic fluid during therapy and act as a chronic source of infection.

On rectal palpation, the gland is usually small, hard, and not painful. The gland may shrink in size, creating a stricture of the urethra (Borthwick and MacKenzie, 1971). Histopathologically, chronic prostatitis is distinguished by increased amounts of connective tissue in which there are inflammatory cells. The condition should be differentiated from the aggregations of lymphocytes seen in the fibromuscular stroma of the older dog.

Treatment. Vigorous antibiotic therapy should be instituted to eliminate the causative bacteria, and the prostatic secretions and urine should be cultured intermittently. This should be continued until the organism is eliminated. An alternative is continuous low-dosage antimicrobial therapy, which produces a bactericidal bladder urine. Castration should be performed to reduce or eliminate prostatic secretions.

Prostatic Abscesses (Suppurative Prostatitis)

Prostatic abscesses are defined as localized collections of pus within the parenchyma of the prostate gland. Other terms used to describe this condition are *suppurative prostatitis* (Matera and Archibald, 1965), *infected prostatic cysts,* and *benign hyperplasia* with abscess formation (Borthwick and MacKenzie, 1971). Prostatic abscesses may be minute or large, diffuse or focal (Fig. 63–2). Usually,

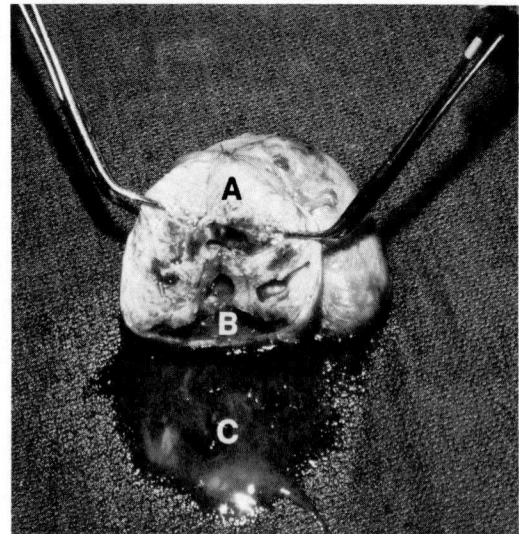

Figure 63–2. Prostate gland removed from a dog with suppurative prostatitis and abscessation. One lobe has been incised to show abscess cavities. A, Prostate gland parenchyma showing benign hyperplasia. B, Large abscess cavity surrounded by many small abscesses. C, Purulent material that was in the gland.

the smaller abscesses coalesce to form one or more larger abscesses (Lord et al., 1956), and it is not uncommon to find one large abscess in each lobe, which may extend into the urethra. The disease has been reported to be rare (Hogg, 1947; Schlotthauer, 1955); however, it may occur more commonly than is actually diagnosed (Borthwick and MacKenzie, 1971; Pollock, 1956). Hornbuckle et al. (1978) reported 23 cases of prostatic abscesses in a retrospective study of 140 cases of prostatic disease. Because it frequently occurs with benign hyperplasia (Borthwick and MacKenzie, 1971), it may often be overlooked.

The exact pathogenesis of the disease is not clearly understood, but it is thought to be an extension of acute prostatitis (McEntee et al., 1970). O'Shea (1963) has suggested that benign hyperplasia and associated squamous metaplasia due to prolonged estrogen therapy may be predisposing causes. Squamous metaplasia may lead to secretory stasis within the gland, creating an environment favorable for bacterial multiplication that may, in turn, lead to abscess formation. The occurrence of prostatic abscesses in conjunction with benign hyperplasia partially explains why approximately one third of the cases of prostatic enlargement do not respond to castration therapy. The infecting agents are those common in urinary tract infections, *Proteus* spp., *Pseudomonas* spp., and *E. coli*. Frequently, pure cultures of staphylococcus and streptococcus are also obtained from the abscess.

It has been reported the disease occurs most frequently in dogs greater than five years of age, 91.3 per cent (Hornbuckle et al., 1978). Though no breed predilection has been reported, in the authors' experience it occurs more frequently in large breed dogs, especially the German shepherd dog.

A good history is a valuable aid in differentiating prostatic abscesses from other diseases of the prostate. Typically, the animal has been treated with synthetic estrogens and antibiotics for a prostatic condition, such as acute prostatitis or benign hyperplasia, for six months to one year prior to presentation. Response to therapy was initially satisfactory but was followed by intermittent relapses with stranguria and blood at the end of every urination.

Clinical Signs. The clinical signs associated with prostatic abscesses are similar to those seen with other prostatic diseases, especially chronic prostatitis. In the authors' experience, pain and fever are not usually observed unless the disease is associated with an episode of acute prostatitis with systemic signs. Hornbuckle et al. (1978) found 82 per cent of dogs with prostatic abscesses had systemic signs of illness characterized primarily by weight loss, cachexia, degrees of pain, lethargy, loss of appetite, and vomiting. The animal is usually alert and in fair to good health, although somewhat underweight. Moderate dehydration may be present. Rectal tenesmus and constipation are usually observed in varying degrees of severity, depending on the size of the prostate gland. The most consistent clinical signs are those associated with urinary tract abnormalities. Dysuria and stranguria without urinary retention are commonly seen. Blood at the end of urination is a consistent finding, with the amount varying from a few drops to several milliliters. After urination, the animal may remain postured and strain for several seconds before the appearance of blood. Blood may also be mixed with the urine, since cystitis almost always accompanies the disease.

Between urinations, there may be an intermittent sanguinopurulent discharge from the penis. On rectal palpation, the gland is enlarged and usually displaced into the abdominal cavity, except for its posteri-

or part. Some discomfort may be evidenced on palpation, but the extreme discomfort associated with acute prostatitis is usually not seen. At times, the entire gland may be difficult to palpate because of its abdominal location; however, when palpable, it appears firm and somewhat asymmetric. The area over the abscess may feel smooth and fluctuant. Abdominal palpation reveals that the prostate is in the location that the bladder normally occupies. Manipulating the gland into the pelvic canal by abdominal palpation while simultaneously palpating per rectum will allow a better examination of the gland.

Laboratory Findings. Laboratory examination of the urine reveals varying degrees of hematuria and pyuria. The marked elevation of the white blood cell count reported by some (Pollock, 1956; Matera and Archibald, 1965; Hornbuckle et al., 1978) differs from the authors' findings. In 40 cases confirmed by surgical exploration, the majority exhibited white blood cell counts of 9000 to 17,000. The higher elevations occured infrequently and were associated with rupture of the abscess, with evidence of peritonitis.

Pathological Findings. The gross pathological changes seen with prostatic abscesses are similar to those seen in other abscessed organs. The gland may be diffusely involved with many small abscesses, giving it an asymmetric appearance and a spongy consistency, while pressure causes escape of pus on its cut surface; or the small abscesses may coalesce to form one or more large abscesses (Fig. 63–3) in one or both lobes. The abscess may develop tracts that communicate directly with the urethra. If the ab-

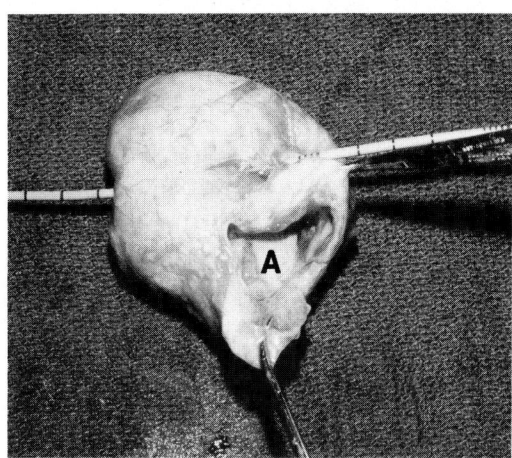

Figure 63–3. Prostate gland with abscessation showing one large abscess cavity (A).

scess is quite large, it may project above the surface, making the gland appear asymmetric, soft, and fluctuant when palpated directly (Fig. 63–4).

Radiographic Findings. Radiographic examination of the prostate gland should include both plain and contrast radiography. The contrast radiography technique preferred by the authors is cystourethrography, which consists of injecting radiopaque dye through the urethra into the bladder. Plain films will reveal an enlarged prostate that is located either at the anterior pelvic brim or in the abdominal cavity, with dorsal displacement of the colon or rectum (Fig. 63–5) (Archibald and Bishop, 1956). Contrast studies may show reflux of dye into the prostatic parenchyma during retrograde cystourethrography. This finding must be evaluated cautiously, as it has been shown that reflux occurs in all categories of prostatic disease (Stone et al., 1978). In the authors' experience, large quantities of dye reflux have been shown to be associated with prostatic abscesses (Fig. 63–6). Radiographic changes characteristic of cystitis are frequently seen, since the disease often is accompanied by cystitis.

Diagnosis. Diagnosis of prostatic abscesses or suppurative prostatitis may be based on clinical and radiographic findings. The typical history and clinical findings of dysuria, blood at the end of urination, and an enlarged gland should be suggestive. The radiographic changes will frequently afford a diagnosis. If clinical signs and radiographs are not diagnostic and the disease cannot be ruled out, an exploratory laparotomy is recommended. Percutaneous biopsy of the gland or needle aspirations are not recommended by the authors because of the danger of rupturing the large abscess, which may lead to a fatal peritonitis.

Treatment. Conservative treatment of prostatic abscesses is frequently unrewarding, and more drastic measures may be required to effect a cure. Castration is recommended in all cases to reduce the size of the gland and stop secretion. Synthetic estrogen therapy should not be used because it may exacerbate rather than cure the disease (O'Shea, 1963). The prostatic secretions should be cultured by methods described earlier and sensitivity tests performed to determine the appropriate antibiotic to use. Antibiotic therapy should be continued for long periods of time, with intermittent culturing of the secretions to determine whether the bacteria are still present.

That many of the commonly used antibacterials do not cross the prostatic epithelium may account for the large number of cases that do not respond to therapy. In these cases, usually one or two large abscesses occupy the gland, and surgical drainage or removal is necessary to effect a cure. Several techniques have been described to drain the abscess (Pollock, 1956; Gourley and Osborne, 1966); however, the authors do not recommend aspiration through the abdominal wall because fatal peritonitis may

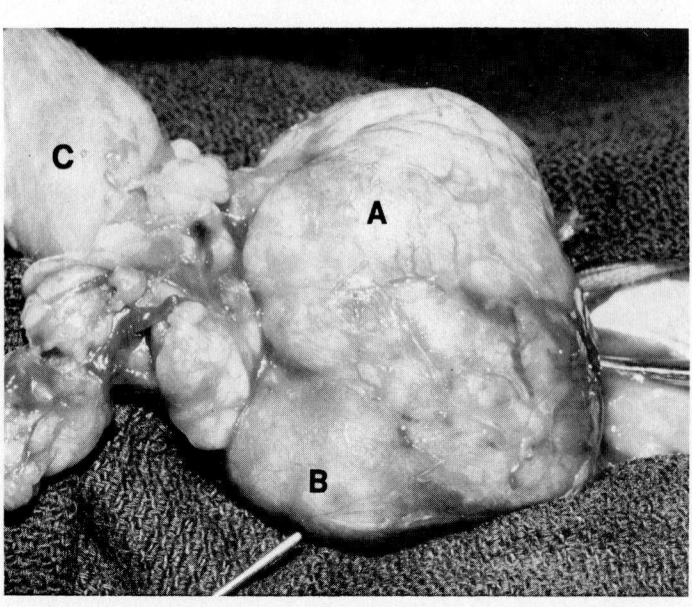

Figure 63–4. Prostate gland with prostatic abscess exposed through a posterior abdominal laparotomy incision. A, Prostate gland showing abnormal enlargement. B, Abscess cavity located on anterior dorsal pole of the prostate gland producing an asymmetric appearance of the gland. C, Bladder.

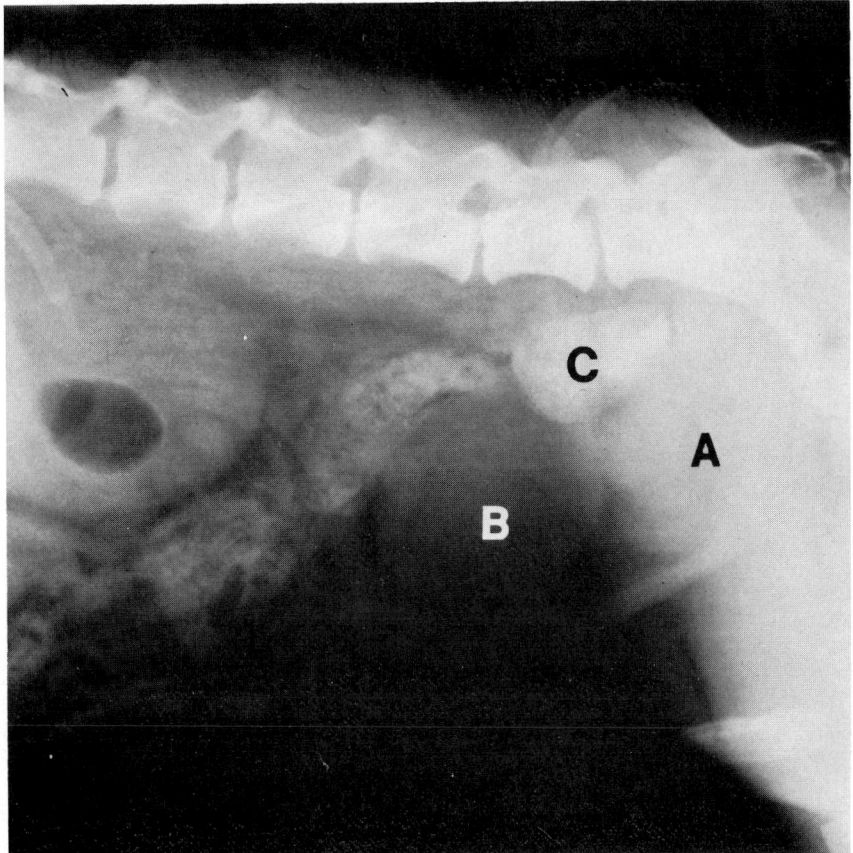

Figure 63–5. Lateral radiograph of posterior abdomen showing that the prostate gland is enlarged and contained in the posterior abdominal cavity. A, Enlarged prostate gland extending over pelvic brim. B, Bladder. C, Fecal accumulation in colon and rectum.

result from leakage of the contents into the abdominal cavity. Drainage through the rectum or perirectal area is less dangerous, but thorough drainage is usually not possible owing to the location of the gland (McKee, 1954) and recurrence of the abscess is frequent. Marsupialization of the abscess has been advocated (Gourley and Osborne, 1966), but the aftercare and results may be undesirable.

The currently recommended technique for treatment of prostatic abscesses is ventral abdominal drainage via insertion of Penrose drains into the prostatic parenchyma (Zolton and Greiner, 1978; Zolton, 1979) (see Operative Procedures). Total prostatectomy is advised only as a last resort.

PROSTATIC TRAUMA

Traumatic injuries to the prostate gland are either rare or infrequently diagnosed.

The most common apparent cause is blunt trauma, such as that sustained in an automobile accident, resulting in a fractured pelvis. Capsular rupture and subcapsular hematomas have been seen as results of pelvic fractures. Lacerations of the prostatic urethra will require treatment.

Diagnosis. Clinical signs associated with traumatic injuries are usually absent or are masked by symptoms of shock and pain associated with other injuries, such as the pelvic fracture. Extravasation of urine into the perineum and abdominal cavity occurs in rupture of the prostatic urethra. Extravasation of urine into the perineum is evidenced by a purplish swelling in the perineal area, as well as by edema and the appearance of bruising in the posterior penile area. Prostatic trauma without urethral rupture is usually discovered incidentally on exploratory laparotomy. The diagnosis of rupture of the prostatic urethra can be confirmed by contrast radiography.

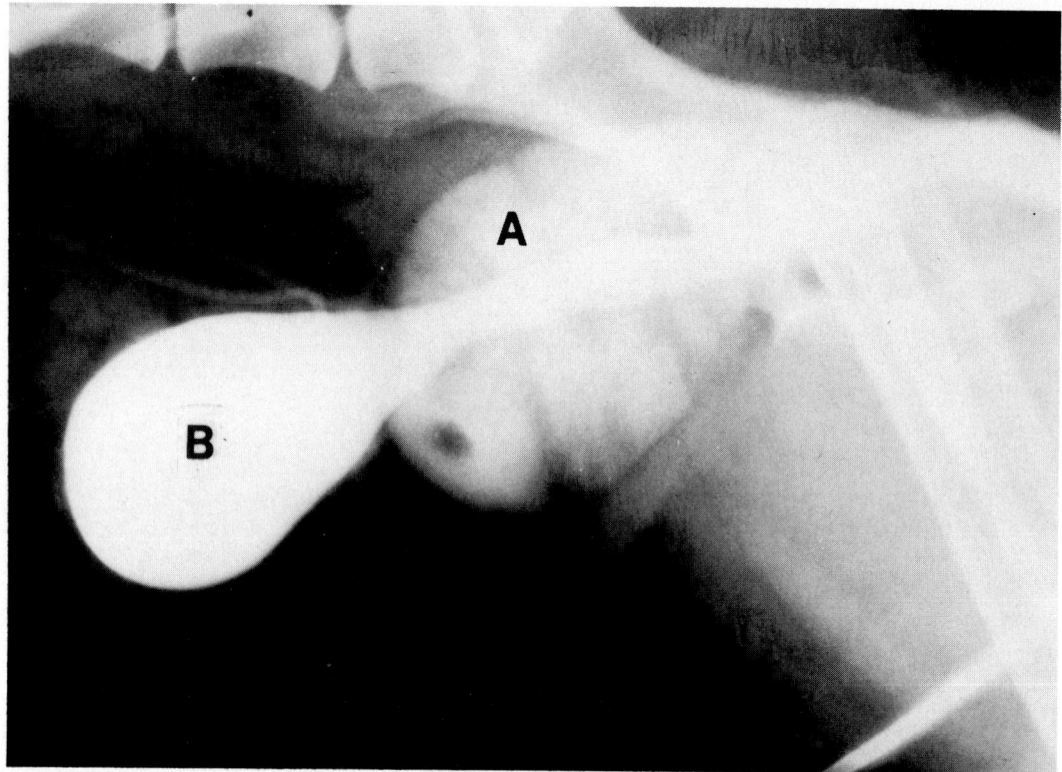

Figure 63–6. Lateral radiograph of a prostate gland with a prostatic abscess showing dye reflux into parenchyma of gland. A, Prostate gland with reflux into parenchyma of gland. B, Bladder containing contrast material. Note also reflux of contrast material into ureters indicating the presence of cystitis.

Treatment. Minor traumatic injuries will not require treatment. Extensive tearing of the capsule should be treated by providing ventral abdominal drainage and irrigation. Hematomas should be aspirated and the bleeding vessel ligated. Rupture of the prostatic urethra may require removal of the prostate gland. Small lacerations may be treated by traction with a Foley catheter, allowing the injury to heal over the catheter. Good ventral drainage should be provided. More extensive injuries, in which there is severe trauma to the surrounding tissue, should be treated initially with a traction catheter such as a Foley catheter. Later, when excessive inflammation and infection subside, the urethra can be sutured or the prostate removed. Suturing an acutely traumatized prostatic urethra is usually unrewarding, but sutures may be used to appose the edges of the urethra over the catheter.

Antibiotics effective against the common urinary tract bacteria should be given. Ventral abdominal drainage using sump or Penrose drains should be provided, and drains should be placed in the perineal area when the perineum is edematous and discolored.

BENIGN PROSTATIC HYPERPLASIA

Benign prostatic hyperplasia (BPH) (Matera and Archibald, 1965), benign hypertrophy or adenomatous hypertrophy (Schlotthauer, 1955), and parenchymatous hypertrophy (Berg, 1958a) are benign enlargements of the prostate gland that are thought to result from hormonal imbalance. Clinically, the disease occurs almost exclusively in man and dog and is generally considered a geriatric condition in both species. Hornbuckle et al. (1978) reported it in 87 per cent of the dogs over five years of age, although it has been observed in younger animals one to three years of age (Berg, 1958; Hornbuckle et al., 1978). BPH occurs commonly; the prevalence has been reported to be as high as 50 per cent of all adult dogs (Schlotthauer, 1932). This estimate was based on histologic changes within the gland, but not all the changes are accompanied by prostatic enlargement or clinical signs of prostatic disease, and the disease cannot be substantiated clinically (Berg, 1958a; Borthwick and MacKenzie, 1971; Campbell and Lawson, 1963). Borthwick and MacKenzie (1971) report an occurrence of 61 per cent of benign hyperplasia alone and an 85 per cent prevalence when the condition is accompanied by some other form of prostatic disease.

The etiology of benign hyperplasia is not known, but it has been postulated that it is caused by a testicular hormonal imbalance that develops when testicular function decreases in the aging animal. The testicles normally produce estrogenic hormone in the Sertoli cells and androgenic hormones in the interstitial cells of Leydig. The imbalance of these hormones within the testicles may explain the hypertrophy of the gland, although an exact imbalance has never been demonstrated. Some investigators (Zuckerman and Groome, 1937; Huggins, 1948) hypothesize that estrogen production is decreased, while the androgen production is unaffected. Hypertrophy would then be a result of excess androgen. Another theory is that hypertrophy results from a relative increase in estrogens owing to decrease in production of androgens (Thorberg, 1948).

A third theory is that stimulation by either hormone may cause hypertrophy, but in different ways. Androgen stimulation results in hyperplasia of the glandular structures, while estrogen stimulation results in squamous metaplasia and proliferation of the fibromuscular stroma, and both result in enlargement of the prostate gland (Zuckerman and McKeown, 1938). This theory most adequately explains the pathologic process. Enlargement due to glandular hyperplasia is more common and occurs as an isolated condition. The metaplastic type is usually associated with pathological conditions, such a Sertoli-cell tumor. Therefore, regardless of which hormone predominates, enlargement of the prostate gland will occur. The parenchymatous form of hypertrophy is more common than the adenomatous form and is due to excess androgen stimulation (Logan, 1947).

There appears to be no definite breed predisposition, although one has been suggested by Hogg (1947). The authors' experience indicates that benign hyperplasia affects all breeds, although it is more common in large and medium-sized breeds. Of interest, however, is the Scottish terrier, whose prostate is four times as large (on a weight basis) as the normal prostate of any other adult dog (O'Shea, 1962).

Clinical Signs. The most consistent clinical signs associated with benign hyperplasia are constipation and tenesmus. As the disease develops progressively over many months, these signs may not be noticed until the gland is extremely enlarged, at which time the enlargement partially occludes the lumen of the large bowel. This partial occlusion may lead to tenesmus, which forces the prostate into the pelvic cavity, further occluding the lumen of the bowel.

Hornbuckle et al. (1978) reported 56 per cent of cases with BPH have signs referable to the urinary tract. In the authors' experience, however, urinary tract signs are infrequently seen. Stranguria and dysuria associated with overdistention of the bladder and incontinence, as well as urinary obstruction, have been reported. Stranguria and dysuria are less common than constipation but frequently occur in concert (Borthwick and MacKenzie, 1971). Hematuria may be seen, but it seldom occurs with uncomplicated benign hyperplasia. It is usually associated with a coexisting cystitis or posterior urethritis (due to stagnation of the urine), which may be a sequela to benign hyperplasia. Pyuria is rare, but is usually associated with disease of the kidneys (which may coexist with benign hyperplasia, since both are frequently seen in older dogs). Uremia will occur with total obstruction or overdistention of the bladder. In uncomplicated cases, the animal is usually in good general health, although gradual weight loss usually occurs; weakness in the hindquarters may develop as the disease progresses. A perineal hernia frequently occurs with the disease, but the exact pathophysiology is unknown. The type of enlargement of the gland seen with a perineal hernia is a proliferation of the fibromuscular elements and cyst formation. This type is more characteristic of excess estrogen stimulation and occasionally exists with Sertoli-cell tumors of the testes.

The abdomen may appear pendulous in some cases, probably owing to the gradual decline of the animal, rather than to the presence of an enlarged prostate. Often the prostate can be palpated abdominally. A thorough digital examination of the prostate per rectum may be difficult because the enlarged gland will be at the pelvic brim (hanging over it) or located in the abdominal cavity. Pain, frequently a symptom of other conditions of the prostate, is usually absent. The gland is usually firm and symmetric on palpation, although in some instances it may be soft and spongy. Abdominal palpation and manipulation of the gland to the pelvic canal and simultaneous palpation per rectum will facilitate examination. Berg (1958a) states that there is considerable variation in the size of the gland, but any gland that measures more than 3 to 3.5 cm in length, width, and height is probably diseased.

Laboratory Findings. Laboratory tests of the blood and urine are usually unremarkable. The absence of blood and pus in the urine in uncomplicated cases is significant in differentiating the condition from other diseases of the prostate. Uremia and hematuria, however, may occur with urethral obstruction or overdistention of the bladder.

Radiographic Findings. Radiographically, the hypertrophied prostate gland will appear enlarged, particularly in the lateral view. Plain radiographs without the use of contrast media frequently demonstrate the enlargement, but for a detailed outline of the gland and urethra, cystourethrography must be used.

On plain films, the enlarged prostate will appear as a round mass of increased density located at the pelvic brim or in the abdominal cavity. Normally, only the neck of the bladder can be visualized.

Cystourethrography will clearly outline the bladder and urethra, and the prostate will then be more readily visible. Frequently, the prostatic urethra may appear narrowed owing to the benign hyperplasia. In the authors' experience, this finding has been of value in differentiating benign hyperplasia from prostatic abscess with hyperplasia, which frequently exhibits a marked dilatation of the prostatic urethra. Dorsal displacement of the rectum and varying degrees of constipation will also be seen on the radiograph. In marked enlargement, the bladder will be displaced cranially in the abdominal cavity (Fig. 63–7).

Diagnosis. The diagnosis of benign hyperplasia is based on a clinical history of intermittent constipation, urinary abnormality, and a gradual decline in the animal's condition. The demonstration of an enlarged prostate unaccompanied by hema-

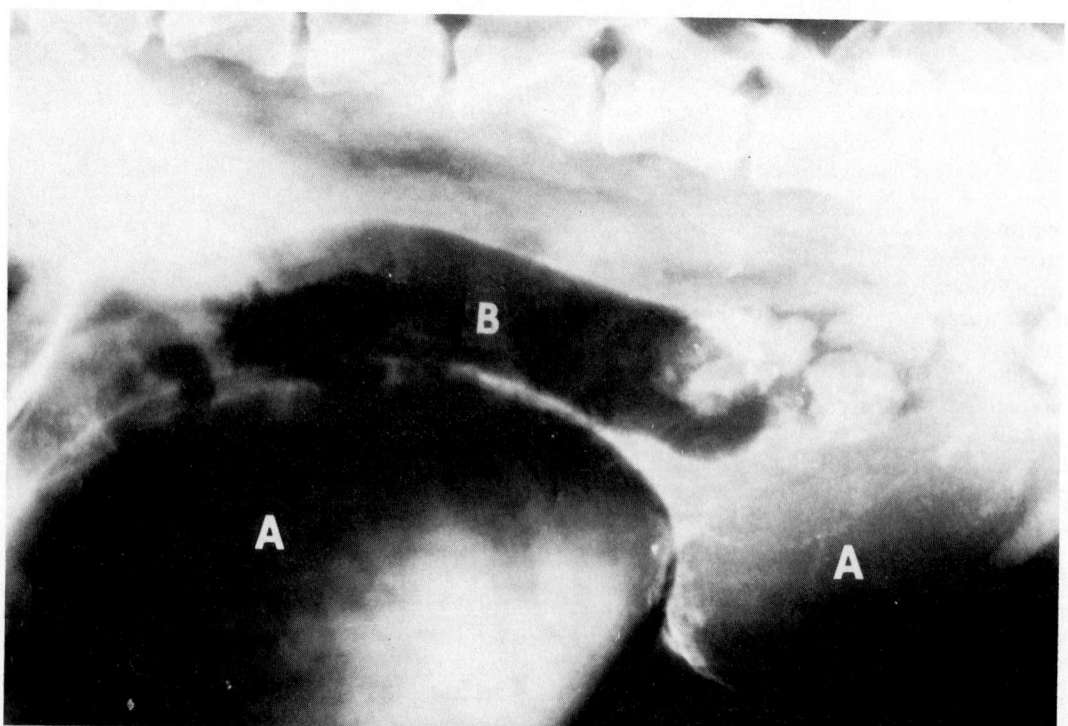

Figure 63–7. Lateral radiograph of a dog with benign hyperplasia. A, Cranial displacement of bladder and prostate gland. B, Deviation of the colon and rectum in a dorsal direction.

turia, pyuria, and pain on palpation is characteristic of this disease. Radiographic demonstration of an enlarged gland is suggestive of disease. The definitive diagnosis can be made only by percutaneous biopsy or on surgical exploration or necropsy; however, a biopsy of the gland as reported by Leeds and Leav (1969) may be definitive. Since a large, obscure abscess may rupture when a biopsy is taken, this procedure is not performed without risk. In addition, abscessation frequently occurs with benign hyperplasia, and diagnosis of benign hyperplasia may be misleading.

Treatment. The treatment of benign hyperplasia should be aimed at reducing the size of the gland and eliminating the abnormal effects of the hypertrophy. Supportive therapy and good nursing care should be provided, as well as dietary adjustments. Gentle, cleansing enemas and laxatives should be provided until constipation is alleviated, and then the diet should be adjusted to further reduce constipation. Urinary abnormalities should be treated symptomatically. When the bladder is overdistended and incontinent, parasympathomimetics such as bethanechol chloride may be used to stimulate the bladder, provided the urethra is patent.

Along with nursing care, a medical or surgical method must be used to reduce the size of the enlarged gland. To date, castration is the most effective procedure. Synthetic estrogens have been used for many years but not without unwanted effects. Used in small doses and over short periods of time (not more than one mg every third day), synthetic estrogens will cause atrophy of the gland; however, improper use may cause squamous metaplasia and enlargement of the gland. O'Shea (1963) reports that squamous metaplasia results in secretory stasis, which favors bacterial multiplication and may lead to abscess formation, a more serious condition than benign hyperplasia. Castration, on the other hand, leads to a longer period of regression with fewer complications.

Various other drugs are currently being investigated for the treatment of benign hyperplasia. Nonsteroidal antiandrogen compounds have been beneficial in reducing the secretions and the size of the gland (Neri et al., 1972). With discontinued use, however, the gland reverted to a hypertrophied form. Some antimycotics also have a pronounced effect on reducing the size of the prostate. The experimental administration of candicidin and amphotericin B have produced marked reductions in size and histologic appearance of the gland in the dog (Aalkjaer, 1970; Gordon and Schaffner, 1968), but not in man.

Chelating agents (such as sodium diethyldithiocarbamate, which combines with zinc) have been reported to be beneficial (Kirk et al., 1968). The recent discovery of prostatic-specific antigens may be of value in the future treatment of prostatic hyperplasia (Peel, 1967; Albin and Soanes, 1971).

Cases that do not respond to castration or medical therapy may require other surgical procedures to remove or cause regression in the size of the gland. Capsulotomy, partial prostatectomy, total prostatectomy, and ligation of the prostatic blood supply have been advocated (Matera and Archibald, 1965). The partial prostatectomy and capsulotomy procedures may be of value, but they cause a temporary regression only. Ligation of the prostatic blood vessel has been reported effective in reducing the size of the gland in one case (Kopp and Stockton, 1960); however, Hodson (1968) reported that in 37 cases it was impossible to achieve atrophy of the prostate, in normal glands as well as those with benign hyperplasia. In such cases, total prostatectomy should be considered.

Pathological Findings. Grossly, the hyperplastic prostate gland appears uniformly enlarged (Fig. 63–8), and the bilobate structure characteristic of the normal gland may have almost disappeared. The surface of the gland is usually irregularly nodular when palpated, and fluctuating cysts may be felt beneath the capsule. On firm palpation, the gland may appear tense and elastic, or spongy, depending on the number and size of cysts present. On cut surface, the outer portion appears swollen, and a milky substance may exude from the parenchyma of the gland. Lobules may be distinguishable and will vary in size. In the metaplastic type of hyperplasia, there may be an abundance of fibromuscular tissue. The prostatic urethra may be distorted, but because of its structure, such distortion would not obstruct urine outflow. Stricture of the urethra does occur in man, but it is the result of obstruction by the middle lobe of the prostate gland, which is absent or poorly developed in the dog.

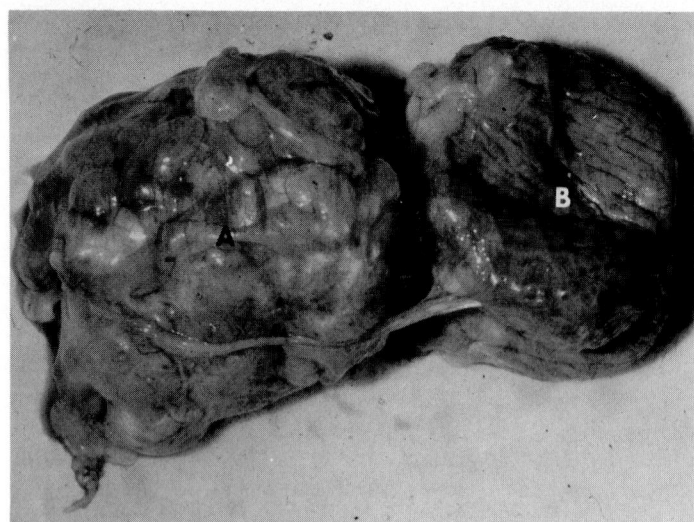

Figure 63–8. Necropsy specimen of prostate (A) and bladder (B) showing the uniformly enlarged appearance of benign prostatic hyperplasia. Note the irregular nodules and cysts on surface of gland.

The clinical sign of an overdistended bladder with stranguria and urinary dribbling (frequently seen in the markedly hyperplastic glands) has been attributed to nodules of hyperplastic tissue projecting into the lumen beneath the urethral mucosa (Smith et al., 1972). Others (Lord et al., 1956) believe this symptom is due to the pinching effect created by stretching the urethra over the pelvic brim when the gland is located in the abdomen. However, neither structural abnormality demonstrates compression in the post-mortem specimen. As urine will readily flow through the urethra with moderate pressure on the bladder, the symptom probably results from pressure of the enlarged gland on the sacral parasympathetic outflow, causing paresis of the bladder (McEntee et al., 1970).

Microscopically, the enlarged gland exhibits a marked glandular hyperplasia, varying degrees of interstitial tissue response, and cystic formations variously interspersed. The glandular hyperplasia consists of epithelial hyperplasia without hypertrophy. The epithelial proliferation may be seen as an ingrowth of papilliform processes or as a stacking of lining cells. Owing to retained secretion, some of the glands and ducts are distended into cysts of various sizes, lined by only one layer of flattened or cuboid cells. The interlobular fibromuscular tissue is frequently increased along with the glandular elements.

Another type of prostatic enlargement, described by Zuckerman and Groome (1937), is associated with Sertoli-cell neoplasms and corresponds to the changes seen with experimental estrogen stimulation (Fig. 63–9). These glands contain many cysts, some very large, and normal glandular tissue is absent. The most consistent change is squamous epithelial metaplasia. The ducts become cystic and are lined by irregular squamous epithelium, and their lumens contain desquamated cells.

PROSTATIC NEOPLASMS

Although carcinoma of the prostate is the second most common cause of death from cancer in man, adenocarcinomas of the canine prostate are rare. The incidence in dogs has been reported as less than one per cent by some investigators (Leav and Ling, 1968). Another study reported 22 cases of adenocarcinoma out of 140 randomly selected case studies of prostatic disease in the canine (Hornbuckle et al., 1978). Explanations for the low frequency have been suggested by Leeds and Leav (1969). The neoplasm may be more common than is reported, owing to difficulties encountered in the diagnosis. In addition, the dog may possess some unknown mechanisms that protect it from the neoplasm, or the etiology of the neoplasm may not the same in the dog as it is in man. In both man and dog, however, prostatic neoplasm appears to be a disease of the geriatric patient. In experimental studies, the majority of animals were over ten years of age (O'Shea, 1963; Leav and Ling, 1968; Hornbuckle et al., 1978). There appears to be no breed predilection. The etiology of the disease is not known; however, the aging process and its relation-

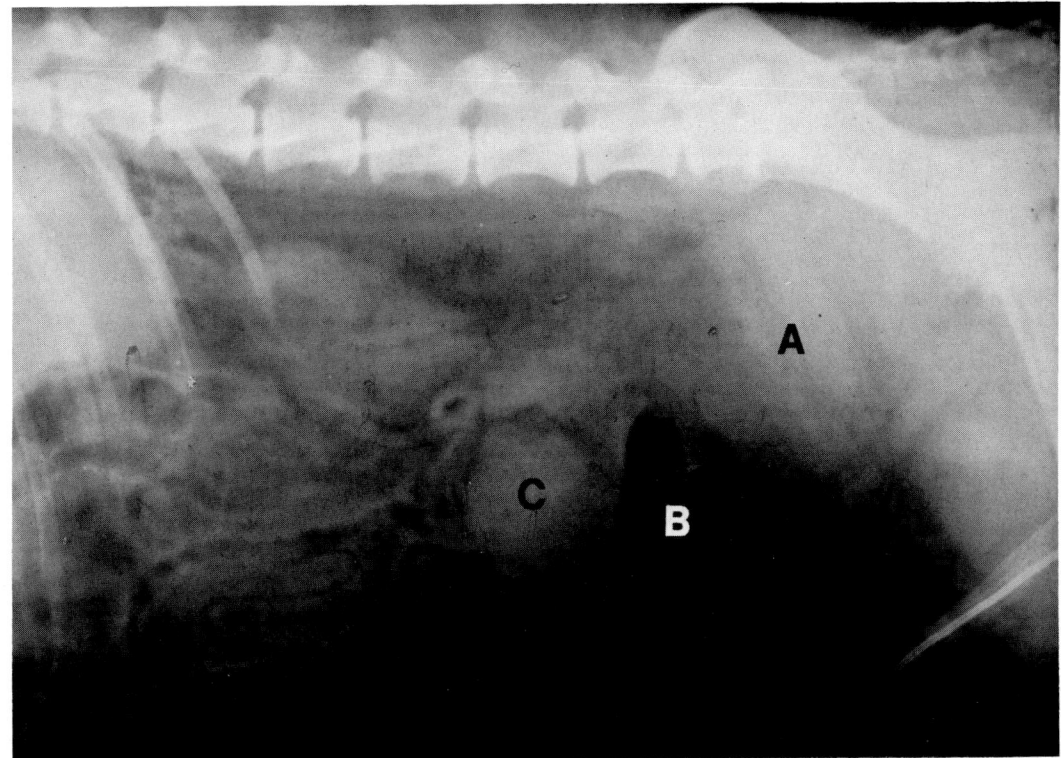

Figure 63–9. Lateral radiograph of a dog with an adenocarcinoma of the prostate gland associated with a Sertoli-cell tumor of an abdominally retained testicle. Note the irregular surface and loss of detail at the anterior dorsal surface of the prostate. A, Enlarged prostate with irregular anterior dorsal surface. B, Bladder with air contrast. C, Abdominally retained testicle with a Sertoli-cell tumor.

ship to hormones appear to be of prime importance in prostatic carcinogenesis (Leav and Ling, 1968). Although some neoplasms seem to develop at sites of metaplastic tissue, squamous metaplasia has not been shown to be a preneoplastic change (O'Shea, 1963; Smith et al., 1972).

Clinical Signs. The clinical signs of prostatic adenocarcinoma are often difficult to differentiate clinically from those of prostatic hyperplasia occurring with prostatitis. Frequently, the glands affected with adenocarcinoma also exhibit benign hyperplasia, and in both cases, the gland is usually enlarged and impinges on the colon and rectum.

As in many neoplastic conditions, the clinical signs may not be noticed until the condition is terminal. The most common signs are rectal tenesmus, stranguria, and weakness in the hindquarters or hindleg lameness. Emaciation is usually marked, and the animal exhibits posterior abdominal and lumbar pain. Various other urinary abnormalities, such as pyuria and hematuria, may be present, as well as infection and necrosis, depending on the duration of the condition.

Many of the clinical signs may be related to metastasis. Respiratory complications may occur secondary to lung metastasis. Direct extension of the neoplasm to the trigone area of the bladder and partial occlusion of one or both ureters occur frequently. Partial to total hydronephrosis of one or both kidneys can result. Rectal palpation will usually reveal that the gland is enlarged, firm, and irregularly nodular with loss of the bilobate appearance. Pain in varying degrees is usually a constant symptom. Frequently, the gland will appear to be attached to the pelvic floor and shafts of the ileum. Terminally, the growth of the neoplasm may occlude the entire pelvic canal, so that digital examination is initially impossible. The sublumbar lymph nodes may be involved by metastasis and can be palpated.

Laboratory Findings. Results of laboratory examinations of the blood and urine are usually nonspecific. A neutrophilia with a left shift occurs in most cases. The blood urea nitrogen may be elevated when the lower urinary tract has been occluded. Hematuria and pyuria are usually evident in the terminal stages; proteinuria has also been reported as a constant finding.

Elevated serum acid phosphatase levels are a valuable aid in the diagnosis of prostatic adenocarcinoma in man, but no satisfactory data concerning their use in dogs have been reported. They have been used, however, to evaluate antiandrogen therapy for benign hyperplasia, and show a decrease or loss from the cells when the drug is effective (Neri et al., 1968).

Radiographic Findings. Radiographically, metastatic lesions and those invading the prostate are seen. Early prostatic adenocarcinoma will be difficult to differentiate from benign hyperplasia. If the gland appears enlarged and the surfaces irregular, adenocarcinoma should be suspected. As the disease becomes more advanced, complete occlusion of the pelvic canal by a mass with an irregular outline may be seen. Contrast cystourethrography may reveal an elongated neck of the bladder with an irregular outline in the area of the trigone, and the prostatic urethra may appear narrowed. If prostatic adenocarcinoma is suspected, radiographs of the common sites of metastasis (Leav and Ling, 1968) should be taken. These include the iliac lymph nodes, the lung, the urinary bladder, and the long bones and pelvis. Metastatic bony lesions may appear as destructive or proliferative, or a combination of both. Bony lesions of the shaft of the ileum and vertebral bodies due to direct extension have been seen (Figs. 63–10 and 63–11). Hydronephrosis

and hydroureter, involving one or both kidneys as a result of encroachment of the neoplasm on the ureteral orifice, are not uncommonly seen.

Diagnosis. Early diagnosis of prostatic adenocarcinoma is difficult; however, as the disease progresses, the clinical signs of prostatic enlargement with an irregular outline and pain should be strongly suggestive. Radiographs can be diagnostic when the disease has advanced so that the gland occupies most of the pelvic canal and has an irregular outline, and urinary symptoms and metastatic lesions have developed. An early definitive diagnosis will require a biopsy; however, results may be misleading, as the neoplasm may be missed in the biopsy sample if the gland is not diffusely involved. Therefore, it is advisable to biopsy one of the iliac lymph nodes simultaneously, since these tissues frequently contain neoplastic cells.

Pathological Findings. The pathological appearance of adenocarcinomas of the prostate varies, both grossly and microscopically. Grossly, the neoplastic gland is usually enlarged, is irregular in shape, and has a nodular surface. The cut surface of the neoplastic prostate is dominated by dense firm white tissue (Leav and Cavazos, 1973). Prostatic hyperplasia frequently accompanies the disease. The gland may give the appearance of benign hyperplasia, and there may be neoplastic foci within it. The neoplasms originate in one lobe and spread to the other by direct extension; in the early stages of the disease, this may account for a unilateral enlargement. As the disease progresses, the gland loses its well-defined ap-

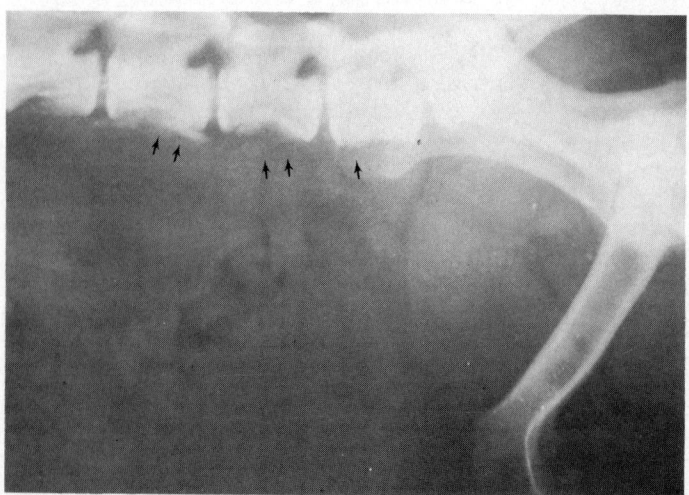

Figure 63–10. Early radiographic changes due to prostatic adenocarcinoma. Proliferative changes (arrows) indicative of early metastasis (L5–L7).

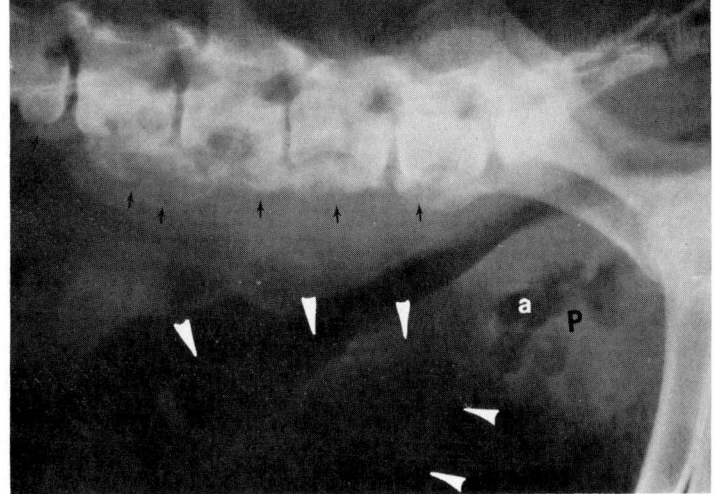

Figure 63–11.   Same case as presented in Figure 63–10, one month later. Note the marked lytic and proliferative changes along the vertebral bodies (small arrows) (L3–L7, S1) due to metastasis of prostatic adenocarcinoma. Air reflux (a) in prostate (P) due to concomitant cystic formation. Bladder outlined by white arrows.

pearance. Direct invasion and adherence of the gland to the pelvis, pelvic musculature, colon, and rectum is common, as is extension onto the neck and trigone area of the bladder causing occlusion of the ureteral opening (Fig. 63–12). Fluid-filled cysts, abscesses, and areas of hemorrhage are seen within the neoplasm. Erosion of the prostatic urethra and breakthrough of the neoplastic tissue to form papillomatous projections into the lumen have been reported (Clark and English, 1966).

Microscopically, extensive pleomorphism exists between and within the neoplasms. Leav and Ling (1968) have divided these various forms of the neoplasm into four types on the basis of predominant histologic pattern: type 1 — intraalveolar proliferative type; type 2 — small acinar type; type 3 — syncytial type; and type 4 — discrete epithelial type. The first two types are the most common and form definite adenocarcinomatous structures, whereas the latter two types are much less common and the cells bear little resemblance to prostatic epithelium. Adenocarcinoma is the most common

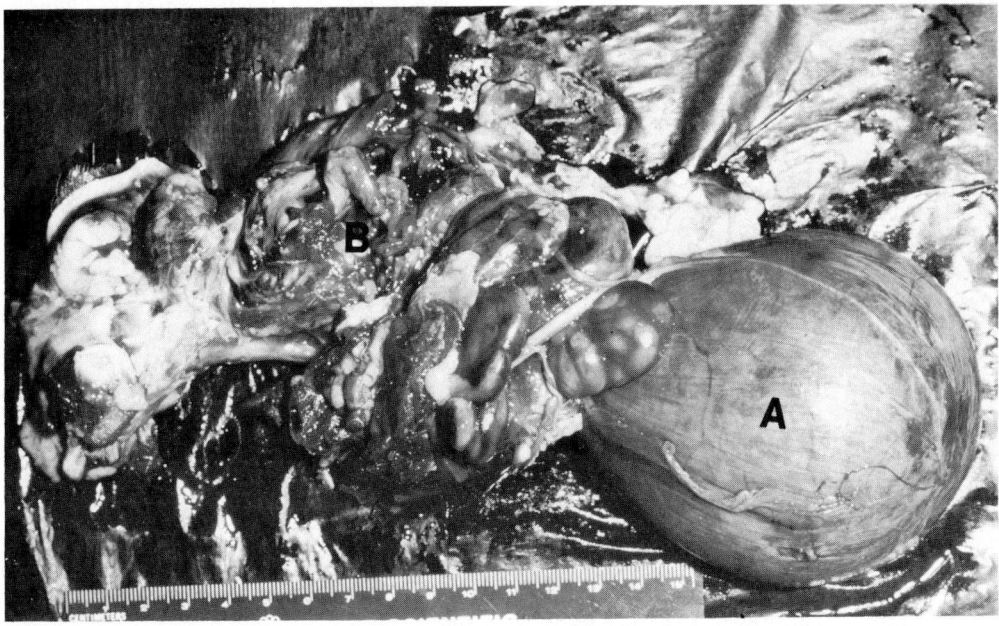

Figure 63–12.   Necropsy specimen of an adenocarcinoma of the prostate gland. Note loss of well-defined appearance of gland and invasion into neck of bladder. Cystlike structures are also visible on surface of the gland. A, Bladder. B, Prostate gland.

histologic type, though leiomyosarcomas have been reported (Leav and Cavazos, 1973). The well-differentiated carcinomas are difficult to diagnose until they have penetrated the capsule. Invasion of the capsule, blood vessels, and perineural spaces is common. An interesting feature of the neoplasm is the production of a mucosal secretion that differs from the normal prostatic secretion (O'Shea, 1963).

Widespread metastasis is common with this neoplasm and occurs regionally via the rich lymphatic supply. The vertebral venous plexus and the venous canal system are the suspected routes of dissemination to other bodily organs. The external and internal iliac lymph nodes are the most frequent sites of metastasis. The lungs, omentum, and mesentery are also often involved. O'Shea (1963), McEntee et al. (1970), Bloom (1954), and Leav and Ling (1968) found metastasis to bones to be common. Bony invasion characterized by dense fields of fibrosis, bone destruction, and new bone formation has been seen in the pelvis, the lumbar vertebrae, and the long bones of the hindlegs. Local invasion of the capsule, urethra, bladder, rectum, periprostatic fat, and soft tissue of the pelvis occurs as a result of direct extension. Occasionally, clinical signs of the metastatic lesion will be more evident than those relating to the primary neoplasm.

Treatment. The only effective therapy for prostatic adenocarcinoma is surgical removal of the gland before metastasis has occurred. Owing to the diagnostic difficulties and the lack of clinical signs, the disease is only rarely recognized before extensive invasion and metastasis have occurred. Therefore, surgical removal is unrewarding in most cases. At the present time, estrogen therapy and castration are the most effective temporary methods of controlling the growth of the neoplasms. There are no extensive studies available on the effects of castration or estrogen therapy on prostatic adenocarcinoma in the dog. Howver, clinical reports suggest that these methods are beneficial (Leav and Ling, 1968). The recent discovery of prostate-specific antigens may permit the treatment of adenocarcinoma of the prostate with immunotherapy, but at the present time, the techniques are not perfected for clinical application. Cryosurgery has also been suggested as a treatment for prostatic cancer, but in the authors' experience this mode of therapy has not yielded successful results.

PROSTATIC CYSTS

Prostatic cysts that develop independently of the cysts commonly associated with benign hyperplasia are a specific disease entity. The two conditions also frequently occur together. These cysts are characterized by their large size. In most cases, the animals affected remain asymptomatic until the cysts grow large enough to impinge on the bladder or rectum.

Although the exact etiology is not known, prostatic cysts are thought to develop from vestiges of the müllerian ducts, the utriculus prostaticus. It has been suggested, but not proved, that the cysts develop when blocked ducts accumulate the prostatic secretion. They may be the end stage of a long-standing prostatic hematoma with calcification of the fibrous wall (Brody, 1962).

Clinical Signs. Clinical signs of prostatic cysts are usually absent until the cyst becomes large enough to impinge on the bladder and rectum, resulting in constipation and dysuria. Frequently, the cysts become large enough to occupy the entire posterior abdominal cavity, giving a pear-shaped appearance to the abdomen. When they are large, they are easily palpated as a firm cystic mass in the posterior abdomen. Occasionally, they may extend along the rectum, creating a bulge in the perineal area that may be confused with a perineal hernia. Palpation per rectum is difficult. The cysts are frequently located at the anterior pole of the prostate gland and are usually located entirely within the abdominal cavity (Fig. 63–13). Those that extend along the rectum may be palpated as tubular cystic masses. Rectal tenesmus, constipation, and frequent urination are the most characteristic signs. Hematuria, pyuria, and stranguria may develop when the cysts become infected or when prostatitis accompanies the disease.

When prostatitis is a complicating feature, the animal will exhibit both local and systemic signs. It is important not to overlook the prostatic cyst because of the other signs. Infrequently, the cysts become infected and rupture, creating a syndrome of acute peritonitis and shock.

Laboratory Findings. In the uncomplicated case, results of laboratory examination of the blood and urine will be unremarkable. Hematuria and pyuria may be present when the cyst is infected or when prostatitis accompanies the disease. Paracentesis of the fluid-filled cyst is of value in the diagnosis.

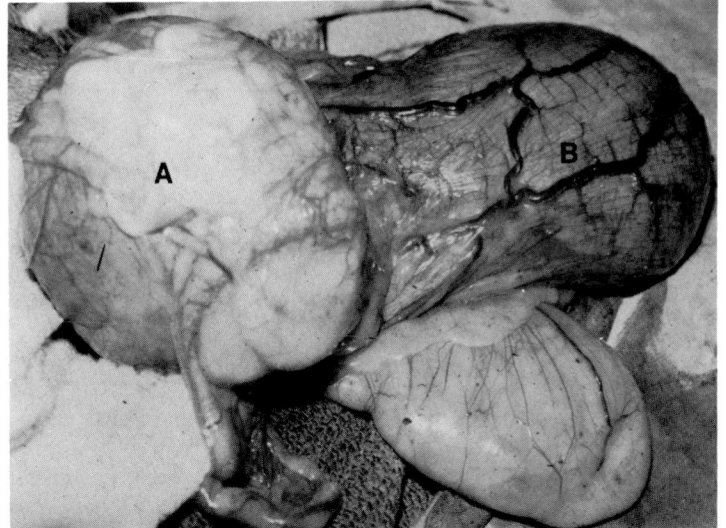

Figure 63–13. Prostatic cyst (A) extending from anterior pole of prostate gland. Bladder (B) has been exteriorized and reflected posteriorly so that the dorsal surface of bladder is exposed to better visualize the prostatic cyst. Cysts are occasionally large enough to occupy posterior abdominal cavity.

The fluid will vary in color, but usually it is pale yellow with varying degrees of cloudiness. Occasionally, it will be serosanguineous. The fluid must be differentiated from urine; it lacks the characteristic urine odor, and the microscopic appearance is different. Erythrocytes and degenerated neutrophils may be present. Infected cysts contain a more flocculent fluid that gives the appearance of a purulent exudate.

Radiographic Findings. Radiographically, the cyst is best visualized in the lateral view. There may appear to be two bladders or two masses in the prostate-bladder region. To demonstrate which is the bladder, contrast cystourethrography will be helpful, because the dye will outline the contour of the bladder (Fig. 63–14). Frequently, the cysts will be large enough to occupy most of the abdominal cavity, compressing the blad-

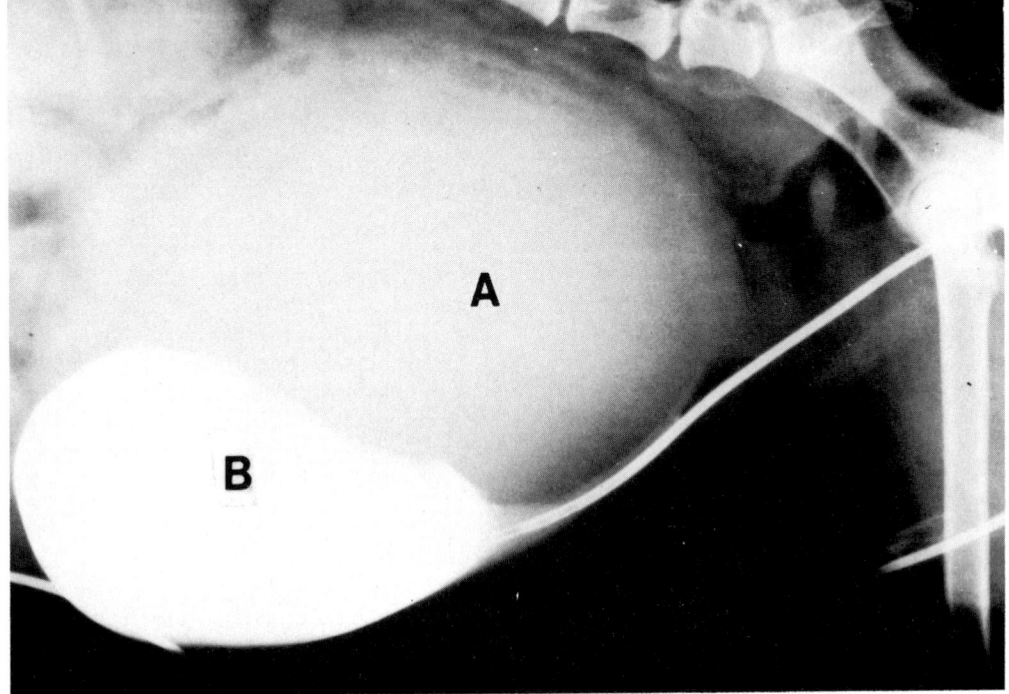

Figure 63–14. Large prostatic cyst (A) demonstrated with use of contrast material to outline the bladder. Cyst occupies most of posterior abdominal cavity (B).

der so that it is not visible with plain radiography, and the cyst appears to be the bladder. Occasionally, reflux of contrast material into the cyst will be seen; however, this only occurs when the cyst communicates with the prostate gland and urethra. Radiographic differentiation of prostatic cysts (especially the smaller cysts) from prostatic abscesses is difficult.

Diagnosis. The diagnosis of prostatic cysts can frequently be based on the clinical signs and radiographic findings. However, the smaller cysts must be differentiated from prostatic abscesses. Uncomplicated prostatic cysts lack the systemic signs and urinary abnormalities seen with abscessation. The demonstration of two bladder-like structures in the prostate-bladder region, coupled with aspiration of a straw-colored or serosanguineous fluid, should be highly suggestive of a prostatic cyst. Cysts with perineal extensions must be differentiated from perineal hernias with retroflexion of the bladder. Paracentesis of the fluid will usually provide the differential diagnosis. In many cases, an exploratory laparotomy will be necessary for a definitive diagnosis.

Pathological Findings. Only a few isolated case reports concerning the gross and microscopic pathology of prostatic cysts are found in the veterinary literature (Brody, 1962; Matera and Archibald, 1965). Some reports and the authors' experience indicate that there are two types of prostatic cysts, although one may be an extension or a long-standing form of the other. The type most frequently encountered is small (up to three inches in diameter) and thin walled (ranging from two to five mm in thickness), whereas the other type is larger, thick walled, and characterized by osteocollagenous tissue in the cyst wall. The majority of cysts appear to originate from the anterior pole of the gland and extend over the dorsal part of the bladder into the abdominal cavity. Direct communication with the prostate gland and prostatic urethra has been seen in a few cases, but most cysts appear to be attached to the gland at a small localized area without a definite stalk. Extensions posteriorly along the rectum and into the perineum are occasionally encountered.

Histologically, the walls of the osteo-collagenous-type cysts are composed of a dense, collagenous outer portion infiltrated with foci of inflammatory cells and an inner portion consisting of a zone of granulation tissue in which spicules and masses of osteoid are embedded. An accumulation of a layer of fibrin on the inner aspect of the cyst, as well as cauliflower-like bony lesions extending into the lumen, is common. The thin-walled cysts lack the osteoid that is seen in the larger cysts. Both types appear to be secretory, as they are lined with a layer of epithelial tissue. Biopsies of the cyst wall should be taken when treating the cyst, because adenocarcinomatous tissue may be present. One case reported in the literature (Brody, 1962) and a number of cases treated by the authors have been diagnosed as adenocarcinoma on histopathological examination.

Treatment. Conservative medical treatment of prostatic cysts is unrewarding. Estrogen therapy will frequently cause the cysts to enlarge. Castration alone will not be beneficial; aspiration of the cyst in conjunction with irrigation is only a temporary measure. The treatment of choice initially is surgical excision of the cyst. Many prostatic cysts will come to a stalk at their base and by careful dissection may be removed from the anterior pole of the prostate gland. It is imperative that the surgeon identify all major anatomic structures, including vascular supply, nervous innervation, urethra and both ureters. Not all cysts are amenable to total excision. In these cases treatment of choice is marsupialization of the cyst (Hoffer and Greiner, 1977) (see Operative Procedures). The marsupialization opening should be kept patent for seven to ten days, using a Penrose drain and daily irrigation with an antiseptic solution. Drainage from the marsupialization site for up to three weeks can be expected. It is important to clean the area daily and apply a petrolatum-base ointment to prevent excessive skin irritation. Systemic antibiotics should be given for ten days to two weeks. Healing takes place over several weeks; the cyst eventually forms a fibrous band between the prostate gland and the abdominal wall. Whichever mode of therapy is used, castration is always included in conjunction with the operative procedure.

PROSTATIC CALCULI

Prostatic calculi in the dog have been described (Lumb, 1952); however, they are not of major clinical importance. They are seen infrequently as an incidental finding on routine abdominal radiography and may be classified as exogenous or endogenous. The exogenous calculi originate in the urinary tract, lodge in the prostatic urethra, and burrow into the prostatic parenchyma. The endogenous calculi originate in the prostatic gland, usually within a cyst. If they are numerous, they may create a clinical prostatic disease, in which case surgical excision (prostatotomy) may be necessary.

OPERATIVE PROCEDURES

MARSUPIALIZATION

Marsupialization is defined as "the creation of a pouch . . . by resection of the anterior wall and suture of the cut edges of the remaining cyst to the adjacent edges of the skin . . ." (Dorland, 1981). Prostatic marsupialization is indicated only for diseases that require constant drainage. The surgical procedure has been described for drainage of prostatic abscesses (Gourley and Osborne, 1966). Extreme care must be exercised when using this procedure because fatal peritonitis may follow if the cystic contents are allowed to leak into the abdominal cavity. It is, however, the recommended procedure for the treatment of prostatic cysts that cannot be totally excised. The stoma of the marsupialization may be made in a number of areas, but it is important that the opening be made at the most ventral portion of the cyst or abscess to ensure maximal drainage.

General anesthesia (preferably the inhalation type) is used, and the animal is prepared for major abdominal surgery, with supportive electrolyte and fluid therapy provided. A ventral midline incision is the preferred approach. The skin incision is made from approximately three cm posterior to the umbilicus, around the prepuce, to the pubic bone; the prepuce is reflected laterally. The abdominal cavity is entered through the linea alba on the midline. Exploration of the prostate gland and its accompanying cysts or abscess should be performed. The cyst is then visualized to determine where it touches the inner aspect of the abdominal wall on the ventral surface, approximately three cm from the midline (Fig. 63–15). A stab incision into the cyst is made at this point and the contents aspirated (Fig. 63–16). Antibiotic culture and sensitivity samples as well as biopsy specimens are then taken. The opening is then enlarged to three to four cm in length, and the inner aspect of the cyst is explored to break down any cavitations or pockets and remove any growths that may be present.

The cyst is irrigated with an antiseptic solution, and prior to exteriorizing, the lining is cauterized with tincture of iodine. Next, the cyst is exteriorized through a separate abdominal and skin incision two to three cm lateral but parallel to the abdominal incision. The incision should be three to four cm in length to allow good drainage and prevent it from healing too rapidly (Fig. 63–17). As the cyst is brought through the abdominal musculature, it is sutured to the

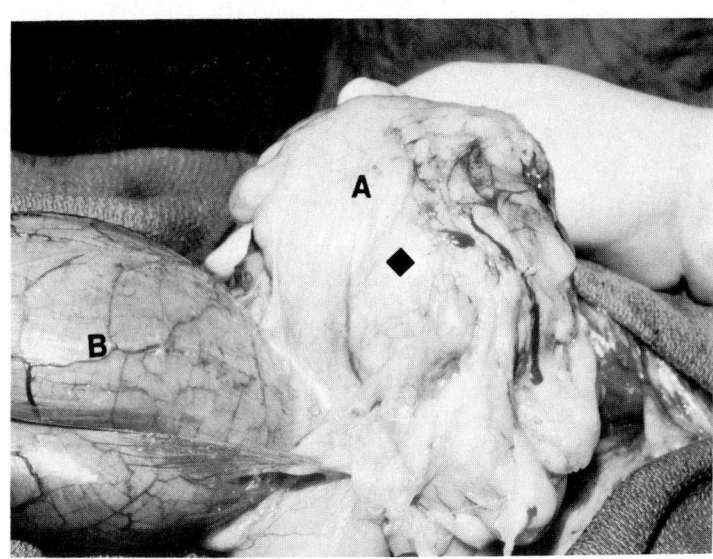

Figure 63–15. Prostatic cyst (A) exposed and area where it comes in contact with ventrolateral abdominal wall identified (diamond). Stab incision is made here for marsupialization. B, Bladder.

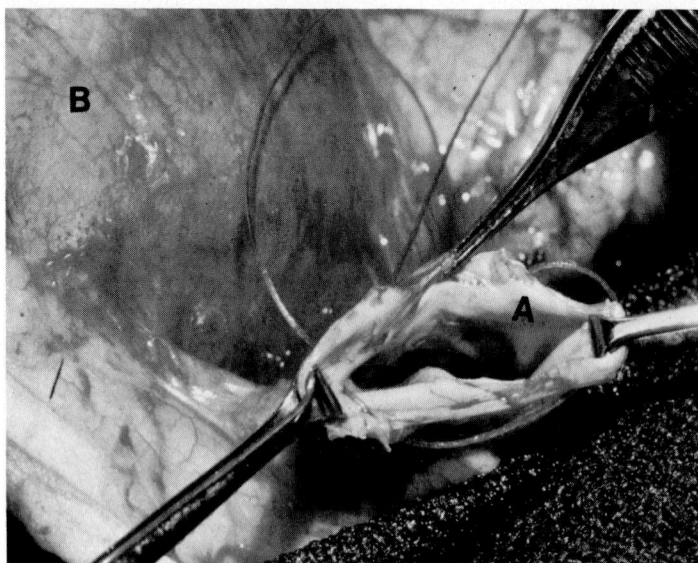

Figure 63–16. Incision made at predetermined area on cyst and contents aspirated. A, Note thick wall of the cyst. B, Bladder.

musculature with 0 or 2–0 chromic catgut, incorporating the peritoneum in the sutures (Fig. 63–18). The cyst wall is then sutured to the skin with monofilament nonabsorbable material. The abdominal cavity is irrigated with an antiseptic solution and closed in a routine fashion. The authors prefer stainless steel wire or other nonabsorbable monofilament to close the abdominal muscula-

ture to prevent dehiscence (Fig. 63–19). The stoma created should be approximately three to four cm in length after it has been sutured and the abdomen closed. A one-half inch Penrose drain is inserted through the stoma into the cyst cavity, sutured in place, and left for seven to eight days (Fig. 63–20).

Aftercare consists of daily irrigation of

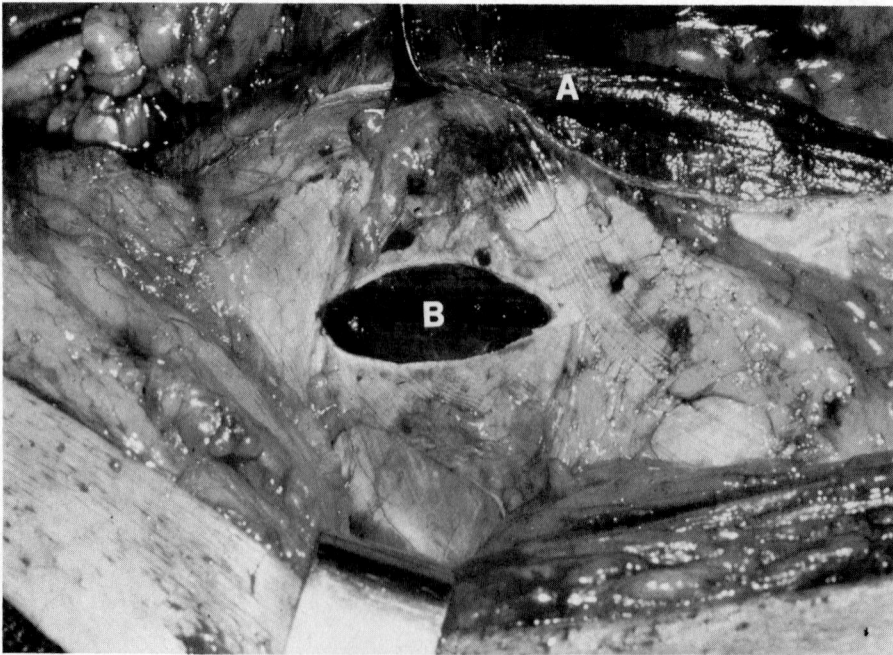

Figure 63–17. Location of incision in abdominal musculature through which cyst is to be marsupialized. A, Edge of laparotomy incision. B, Incision should be three to four cm in length to prevent premature closure of marsupialization site.

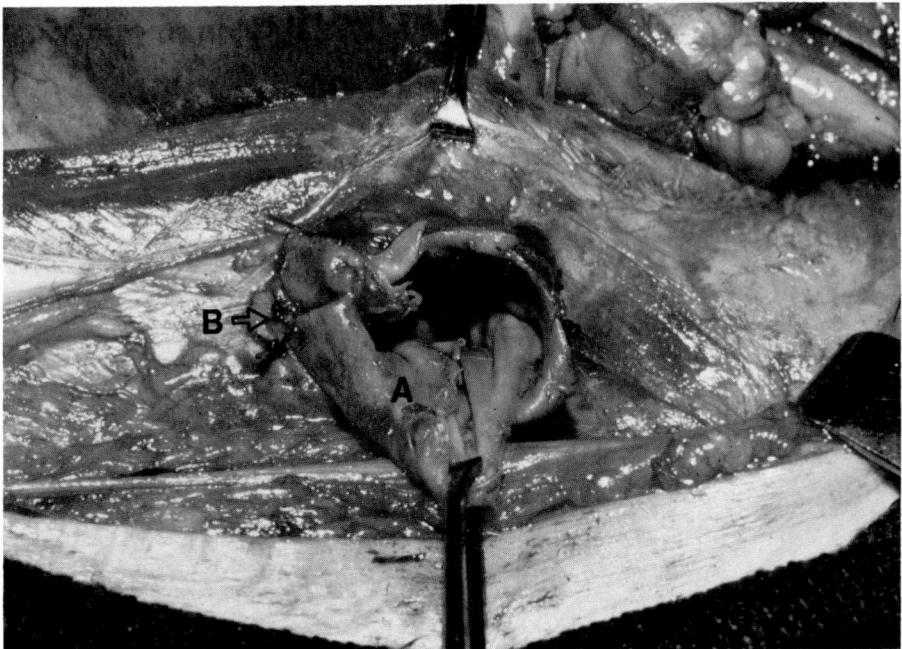

Figure 63–18. Cyst wall (A) is brought through previously incised abdominal opening and sutured to peritoneum and abdominal musculature (B) with 2–0 chromic catgut in a simple interrupted pattern.

the cyst with an antiseptic solution such as 20 per cent providone-iodine for one week. A petrolatum-base ointment should be applied around the marsupialization opening to prevent excessive skin irritation. After the first week, drainage will gradually subside over a seven- to ten-day period, then the condition may be considered healed.

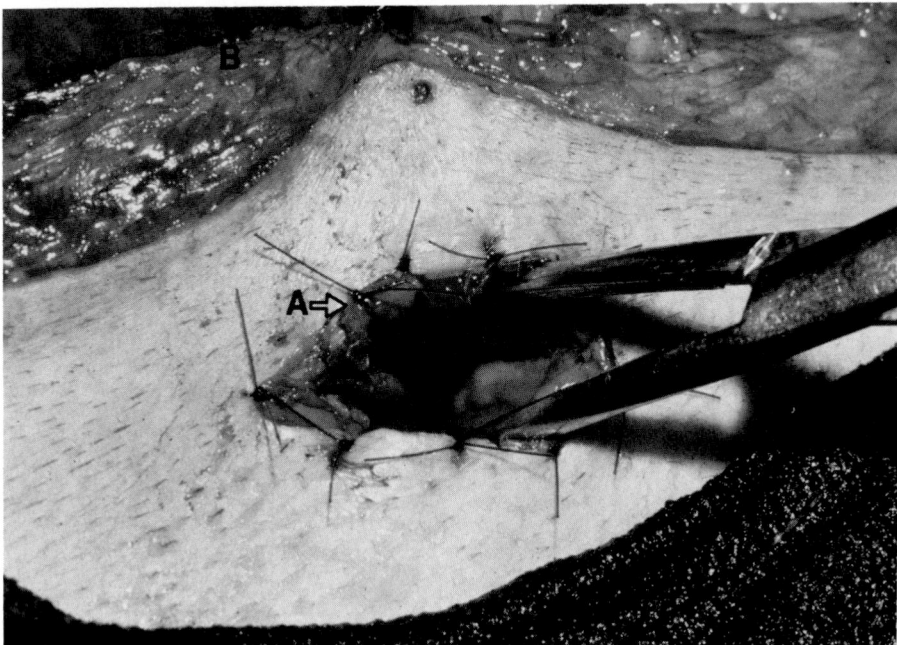

Figure 63–19. Cyst wall (A) sutured to skin and abdominal incision (B) closed with simple interrupted sutures of monofilament nonabsorbable suture material such as nylon.

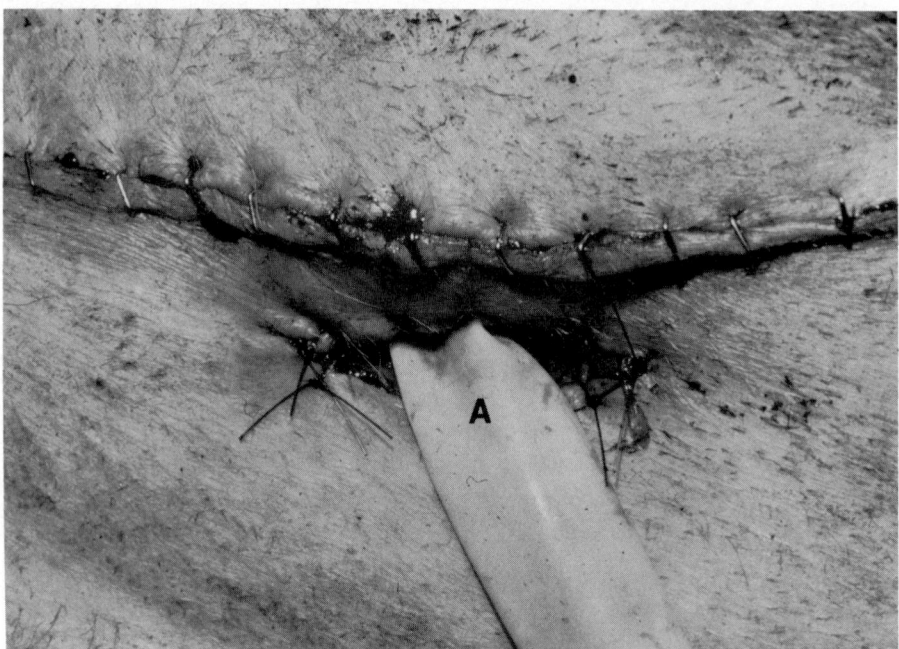

Figure 63–20. Abdominal closure complete and Penrose drain (A) placed in cyst and sutured to marsupialization opening. Drain is left in place for seven to eight days.

Occasionally, drainage may occur for four to six weeks. Healing of the prostatic cysts occurs by the formation of a large fibrous band from the prostate gland to the abdominal wall (Fig. 63–21).

PROSTATIC BIOPSY

Prostatic biopsies may be obtained via an open or closed approach. In the open approach, done in conjunction with exploratory abdominal surgery, a wedge-shaped

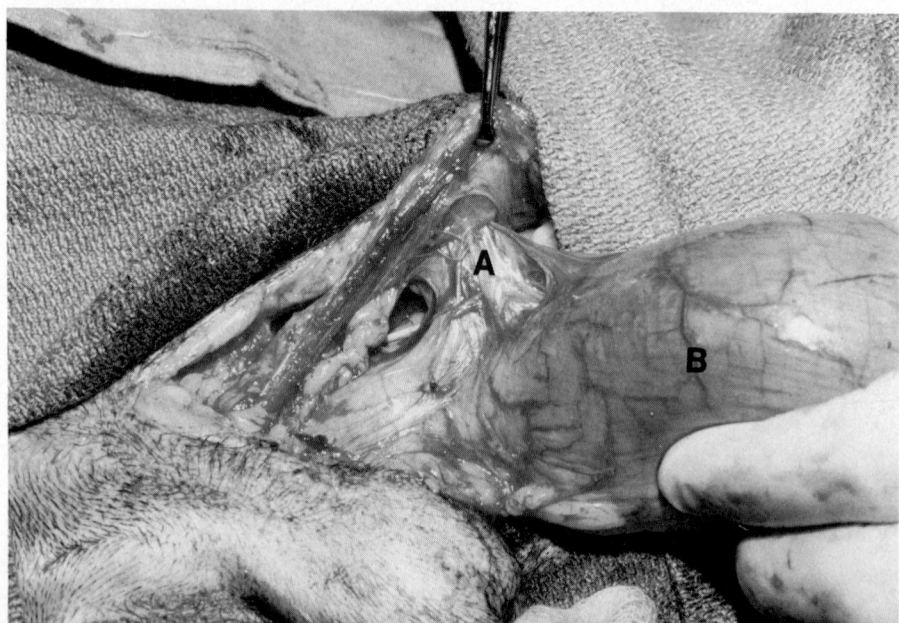

Figure 63–21. Healed prostatic cyst. A, Fibrous band that is remnant of a cyst two years after marsupialization. B, Bladder.

piece of prostatic tissue may be removed by cutting between mattress sutures placed deep in the parenchyma of the gland. Upon removal of the tissue, the mattress sutures are tied, apposing the cut edges of the prostate. Hemorrhage can be controlled by applying pressure with a gauze sponge.

A closed technique has been described for obtaining prostatic tissue through a perineal approach, using a biopsy needle (Leeds and Leav, 1969). In this procedure, a Franklin-Silverman biopsy needle is inserted through a previously made skin incision ventrolateral to the anus. The needle is guided to the site of biopsy by a finger inserted into the rectum, which also helps to stabilize the prostate gland when the biopsy is taken. Unfortunately, in this procedure, the gland is not visualized and a biopsy of the diseased area may be missed.

ASPIRATION

It is the authors' belief that the indications for aspiration of prostatic cysts and abscesses are few. Blind aspiration of prostatic abscesses is dangerous and frequently can cause the death of the animal because of peritoneal contamination and subsequent peritonitis. Aspiration of prostatic cysts is only a palliative measure, and the cysts must eventually be surgically drained or removed. Aspiration may be of value when the animal is severely debilitated and cannot undergo a major surgical procedure.

TOTAL PROSTATECTOMY

Certain disease conditions of the prostate gland will require removal of the gland to effect a cure. Although it is not an easy procedure, it should not be viewed as a last resort, nor should it be delayed until the animal is severely debilitated. Success depends on recognizing the disease and operating when the animal is in reasonably good physical condition.

The most common indication for total removal of the gland is prostatic adenocarcinoma that has not metastasized. Chronic recurrent cystitis caused by a deep-seated infection in the prostate gland that does not respond to therapy is also an indication. Benign prostatic neoplasms, and recurrent prostatic cysts will require total removal, as well as the infrequent cases of benign hyper-

plasia that fail to respond to the conventional method of treatment.

Several procedures have been described for total removal of the prostate (Archibald and Cawley, 1956; Archibald, 1957; Pettit, 1960; Matera and Archibald, 1965; Knecht and Schiller, 1966; Howard, 1975). The prepubic approach is preferred because total visualization of the gland and associated structures is possible. Techniques that use splitting of the pubic symphysis (Knecht and Schiller, 1966), partial reflection, and subsequent replacement of the pubic bones have been described as offering better exposure (Howard, 1969); however, it is the authors' opinion that few cases require these additional techniques. Most dogs with prostatic disease that requires prostate removal will have an enlarged gland located intraabdominally, and adequate exposure will be afforded through the usual prepubic approach. Additional, time-consuming steps should be avoided when possible with this procedure.

The perineal approach is useful when the gland is small and can be drawn through the pelvic canal, or when the gland is contained in the contents of a perineal hernia and cannot be replaced in its anatomic position for the correction of the hernia.

Preoperative Considerations. Renal function should be thoroughly evaluated prior to surgery, since the procedure is most frequently performed in the geriatric patient in which coexisting renal disease may be present. Therapy to reduce blood-urea-nitrogen or creatinine values, as well as therapy for coexisting infection of the urinary tract and dehydration, should also be started prior to surgery. It is wise to obtain a culture and sensitivity test of the urine to specifically treat the infecting organism. Intravenous fluid administration in the form of buffered lactated Ringer's solution is essential during surgery to help prevent shock and acute renal shutdown. The administration of intravenous steroids (hydrocortisone, succinate, 20 to 40 mg/kg, or dexamethasone, 4 to 8 mg/kg) is also helpful in preventing shock. Urine production during surgery is a valuable parameter that can be monitored by the surgeon. When anuria or poor urine production is observed, intravenous mannitol or furosemide should be given to establish urine flow.

Anesthesia. The choice of anesthesia

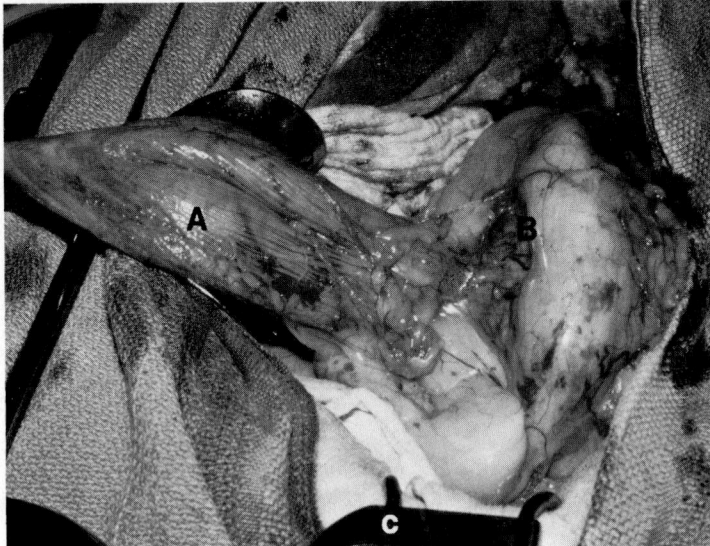

Figure 63–22. Bladder (A) and prostate gland (B) covered with fold of peritoneum containing fat have been exposed and prepared for dissection from surrounding tissue. Balfour abdominal retractors (c) assist in exposing the prostate gland to be removed.

rests with the surgeon. The authors prefer premedication with atropine and acepromazine, followed by induction with a short-acting barbiturate and maintenance on halothane (Fluothane) in combination with nitrous oxide and oxygen.

Surgical Technique. The surgical procedure is the technique described by Archibald and Cawley (1956), with minor modifications. The animal is positioned in dorsal recumbency with the hindlegs drawn posteriorly and secured. A suitably sized Foley catheter is inserted in the bladder. After routine abdominal preparation, a skin incision is made from the umbilicus posteriorly, curving around the prepuce, to a point two inches posterior to the anterior brim of the pubic bone. The prepuce is reflected laterally and packed away from the operating site. The linea alba is then incised from the umbilicus to the brim of the pubic bone. The incision is carried laterally approximately one-half inch on each side of the anterior brim of the pubic bone at the insertion of the rectus abdominis muscle. The lateral incision allows better exposure of the posterior abdominal cavity.

A Balfour self-retaining abdominal re-

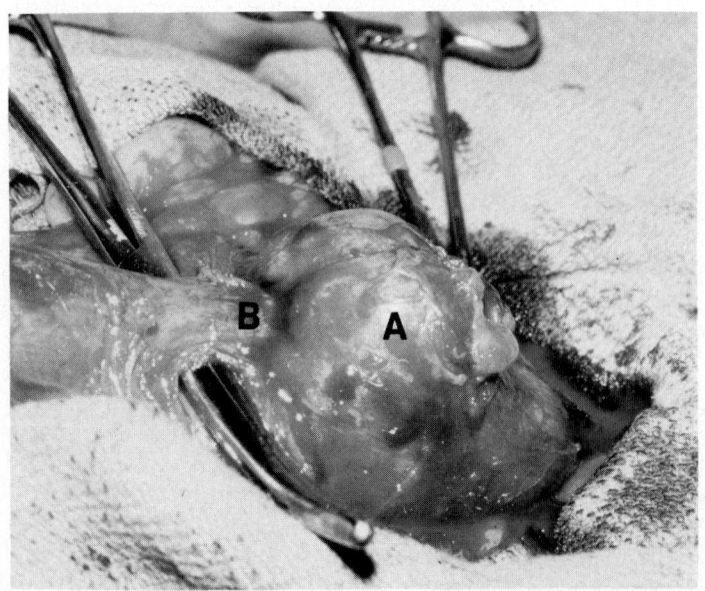

Figure 63–23. Peritoneal fold containing fat has been gently reflected from the ventral and lateral surfaces of the prostate gland (A). The neck of the bladder (B) is also freed from surrounding tissue. Care must be taken to stay close to the surface of the prostate gland when dissecting it from surrounding tissue.

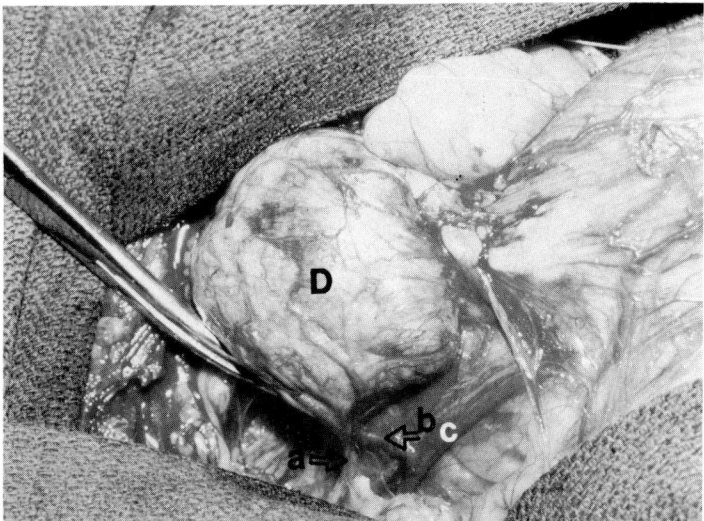

Figure 63–24. The prostatic vessels (a and b), which are branches of the urogenital vessels (c), are isolated and ligated on each side. Note the proximity of the urogenital vessels to the prostate gland (D).

tractor is then used to spread the edges of the abdominal wall apart (Fig. 63–22). The contents of the abdominal cavity should be explored for evidence of other disease. The small intestines should be packed into the anterior abdominal cavity using saline-moistened laparotomy pads. The bladder is grasped, pulled anteriorly, and held by stay sutures placed in the muscularis of the bladder wall. Overlying the ventral surface of the neck of the bladder, the prostate, and the urethra is a fold of peritoneum containing variable amounts of fat. This fold of peritoneum should be incised over the ventral surface of the prostate, leaving it attached at the neck of the bladder and re-

flected laterally. Reflection of the peritoneal fold will expose the ventral surface of the prostate, the neck of the bladder, and the pelvic urethra (Fig. 63–23). Careful dissection should then be done to identify the prostatic vessels as they join the prostate gland on the dorsolateral surface. This is best accomplished by blunt dissection, working from the ventral surface around the gland and staying close to it until the two prostatic vessels on each side are isolated and ligated (Fig. 63–24). Extreme care should be taken to avoid injury to the urogenital artery and nerves, as they lie close to the prostate gland at this point.

After ligation of the prostatic vessels, the

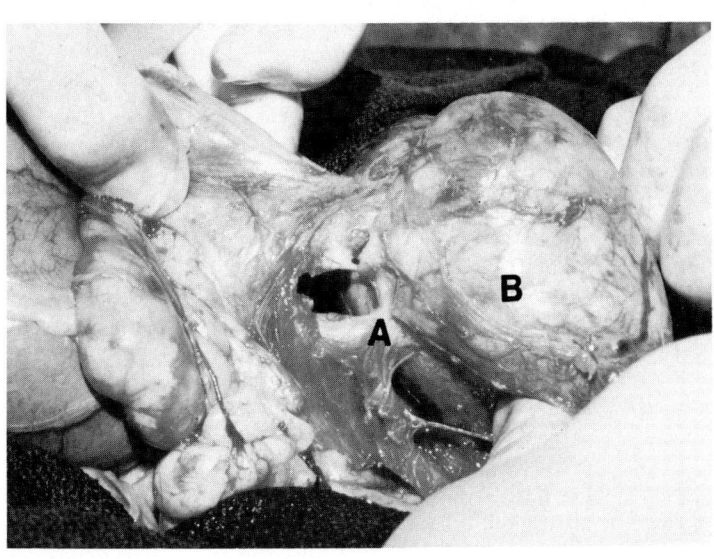

Figure 63–25. After isolation and ligation of the prostatic vessels, the remaining surface of the prostate gland is freed from surrounding tissue and the entrance of the ductus deferens into the urethra (A) is ligated and separated from the prostate and urethra (B).

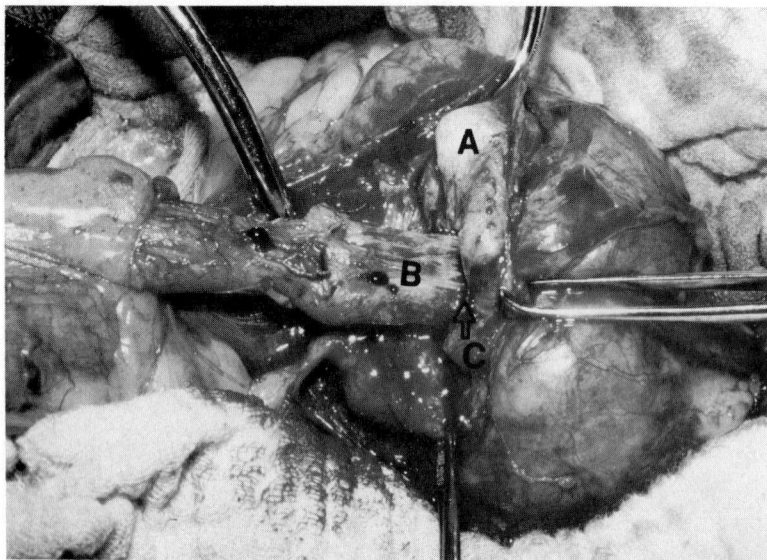

Figure 63–26. Starting at the anterior margin of the prostate gland, prostatic tissue (A) is dissected from the prostatic urethra (B) posteriorly to the area where the ductus deferens enters the urethra (C). At this point, the urethra is incised transversely from the prostate gland. The urethra is also incised one cm posterior to the prostate gland, thus freeing the gland for removal.

prostate should be separated from the surrounding tissue by blunt dissection. On the dorsal surface of the gland, a fibrous band attaching the prostate to the rectum will be encountered and should be incised. The ductus deferens and its blood supply should be isolated and ligated where it enters the dorsal surface of the gland (Fig. 63–25). Starting at the anterior part of the gland, it should be dissected from the neck of the bladder and urethra posterior to the point where the ductus deferens enters the urethra (Fig. 63–26). Dissection from the urethra to this point ensures that the muscles concerned with urinary control will not be resected. The pelvic urethra posterior to the prostate gland should be freed from the surrounding tissue and its blood supply maintained. By blunt dissection with a finger, the urethra can be mobilized anteriorly to gain better exposure. Umbilical tape placed around the urethra and secured with a hemostat posterior to the prostate will hold the urethra and prevent it from slipping into the pelvic cavity once the gland is resected. Umbilical tape also can be used to hold the bladder portion of the urethra and prevent urine leakage into the abdominal cavity.

The prostatic urethra is incised over the catheter where the ductus deferens enters and at the posterior end of the gland. The gland is slipped over the anterior end of the catheter, and the catheter is reintroduced into the bladder (Fig. 63–27). The cut ends of the urethra are apposed and sutured. Suturing is facilitated by preplacing three or four sutures on the dorsal surface of the urethra before tying (Fig. 63–28). The anastomosis is continued, using 2–0 nylon or a synthetic absorbable in a simple interrupted pattern (Fig. 63–29). It is important that the

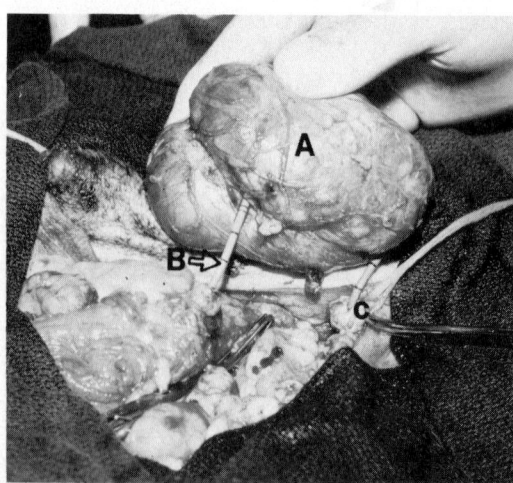

Figure 63–27. Prostate gland (A) being removed by removing urinary catheter (B) from the bladder, sliding gland over catheter, and then reintroducing catheter into the bladder. The posterior urethra (c) is secured with umbilical tape to prevent it from retracting into the pelvic canal.

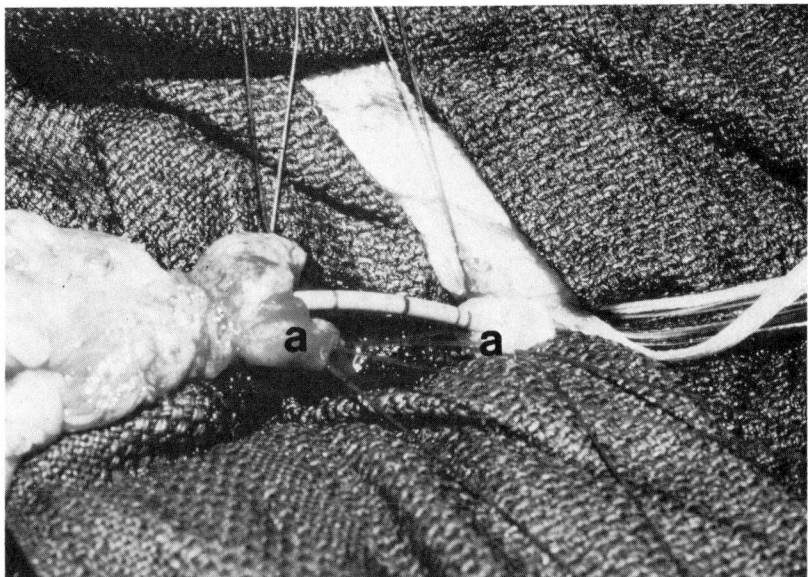

Figure 63–28. Three simple interrupted through-and-through sutures of monofilament nonabsorbable nylon are preplaced in the incised edges (a) on the dorsal surface of the urethra to facilitate the anastomosis.

urethral mucosa be incorporated in the suture to help prevent breakdown and postoperative stricturing of the urethra. After the anastomosis is completed, it is wise to attempt to place the omentum around the suture line (Fig. 63–30). This will help seal leaks that may be present in the anastomosis. When the gland has been removed because of abscessation, the abdominal cavity should be irrigated with an antibiotic solution, and Penrose drains should be placed in the posterior abdominal wall. The linea alba is sutured with 2–0 stainless steel wire to the remaining layers in a routine fashion.

Postoperative Care. The Foley catheter should be left in place for 48 to 72 hours, or longer when the urethra appears devitalized. It can be held in position by placing a

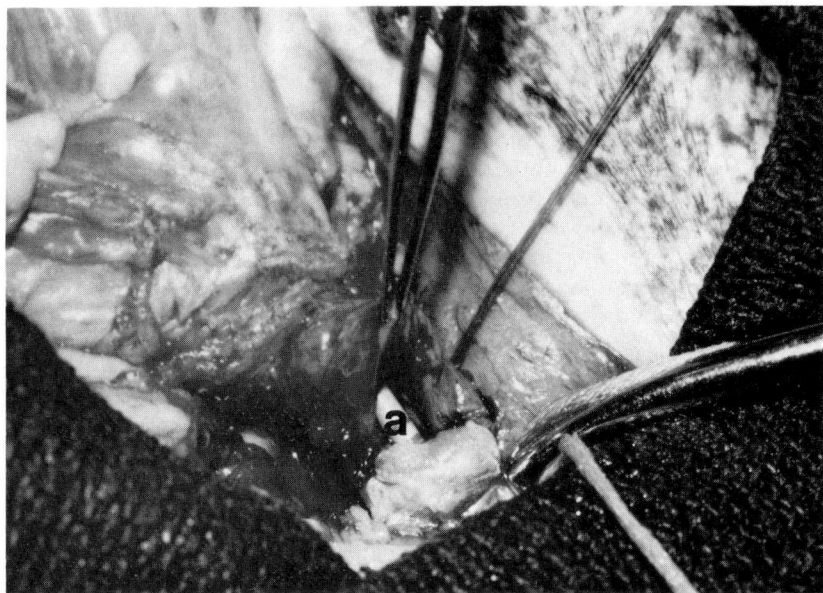

Figure 63–29. The anastomosis is completed using simple interrupted sutures of monofilament material. A urinary catheter (a) is visualized in the lumen of the urethra.

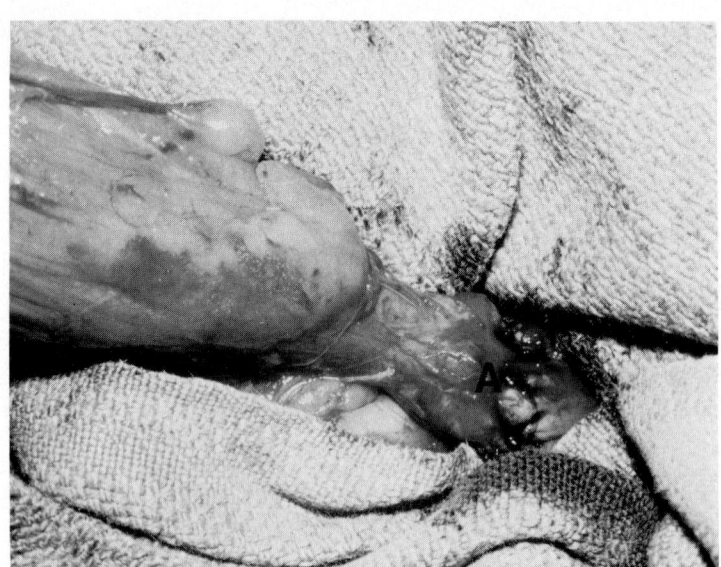

Figure 63–30. Urethral anastomosis (A) completed. An attempt should be made to mobilize omentum over the anastomosis site to help prevent any extravasation of urine. Abdominal cavity is irrigated and closed in the manner described in the text.

piece of tape in a butterfly fashion around the end as it emerges from the prepuce, and suturing the tape to the prepuce. Inflation of the balloon on the tip of the Foley catheter also will help maintain it in the bladder. The catheter should be intermittently flushed with a bladder irrigant to prevent formation of clots in the catheter. A continuous infusion of lactated Ringer's solution is given for 24 hours after surgery. Six mg/kg of prednisolone sodium succinate or dexamethasone is given every four hours for three doses to prevent shock. The animal's urine output is monitored. If urine production falls below one ml per lb body weight per hour, an osmotic diuretic is given. Fluid therapy is diminished gradually during the second postoperative day when the animal begins eating and drinking. The serum electrolyte, sodium, and potassium should be monitored and corrections made when abnormalities are noted. Diuresis may lower the serum potassium. A complete blood count should be taken, and blood urea nitrogen should be monitored daily for three to four days. An elevation in the blood-urea-nitrogen level may signal a breakdown of the anastomosis. Systemic antibiotics, effective against the common urinary tract bacteria, should be given for ten days to two weeks.

Postoperative Complications. The most common complication encountered postsurgically, other than the shock created by the surgery, is breakdown of the anastomosis. This occurs most frequently on the second or third postoperative day and probably results from improper suturing or interference with the blood supply to the pelvic urethra. The use of an indwelling Foley catheter will greatly reduce the number of breakdowns. Postsurgical urinary incontinence has also been described as a frequent complication (Gordon, 1960; Matera and Archibald, 1965). However, when care has been taken to avoid undue trauma to the urogenital artery and its satellite nerve supply, and the prostate has been dissected from the urethra to the vas deferens, incontinence has not been a major problem. If it is encountered, satisfactory correction has been obtained by attaching a prosthesis, such as a rib graft, to the ischiatic tuberosities to compress and elevate the bulbocavernous muscle and urethra (Schmaelzle et al., 1968). Other complications, such as urethral stricturing and formation of urinary fistulas, are encountered infrequently.

PROSTATIC ABSCESS DRAINAGE

Surgical Technique. The previously described ventral abdominal approach is used. Techniques of pelvic splitting have been described (Knecht, 1979) but are seldom necessary, owing to the cranial displacement of the prostate. Blunt dissection laterally through the periprostatic fat will expose the parenchyma of the prostate. The prostate is packed off, using saline-moistened laparotomy pads. Prior placement of a male urinary catheter will aid in the identification of

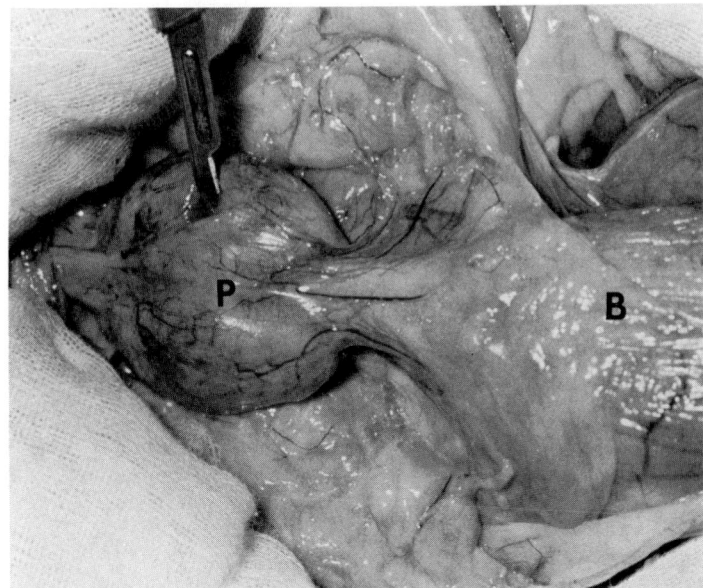

Figure 63–31. Stab incision is made into the ventral aspect of the prostatic parenchyma (P). B, Bladder. Biopsy, culture, and antibiotic sensitivity specimens are taken at this time.

the urethra. A stab incision is made into the ventral aspect of the prostatic parenchyma and into the abscess cavity, which facilitates drainage of the abscess via suction (Fig. 63–31). The numerous, pus-filled cystic cavities can now be broken down by digital palpation, creating one large cavity. The prostatic cavity is copiously irrigated with a sterile saline-antibiotic solution (saline-kanamycin or saline-ten per cent povidone-iodine solution). At this time a second stab incision, dorsal to the initial incision (on the dorsal surface of the prostatic lobe) is made to allow passage of two ¼- or ½-inch Penrose drains through the pa-

renchyma of the gland (Figs. 63–32 and 63–33). With diffuse bilateral involvement, drains are placed to the opposite lobe of the prostate in a similar fashion. The Penrose drains are now sutured to the prostatic capsule with one 4–0 chromic catgut suture. The opposite ends of the drains are exteriorized via stab incisions penetrating the abdominal wall and sutured to the skin using monofilament nonabsorbable suture (Fig. 63–34). Four additional drains are placed on each side lateral to the prostate and exteriorized in a similar fashion to allow drainage of the periprostatic and caudal abdominal regions (Fig. 63–35). The pro-

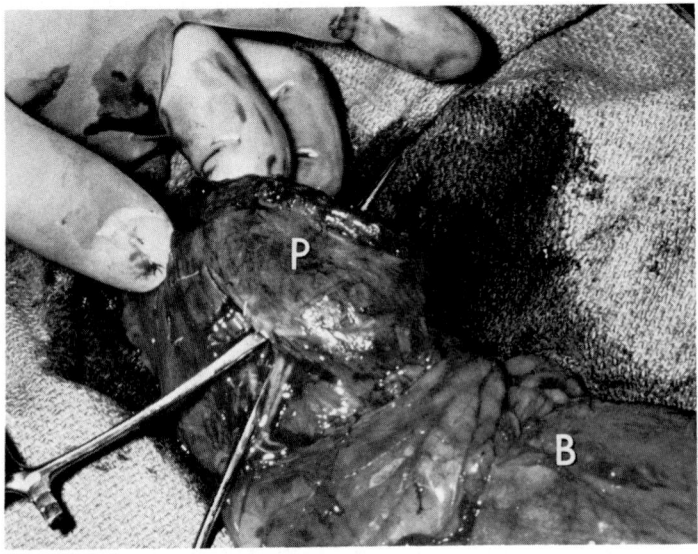

Figure 63–32. The pus-filled cystic cavities are broken down and a second stab incision is made through the dorsal surface of the prostatic lobe (P). B, Bladder.

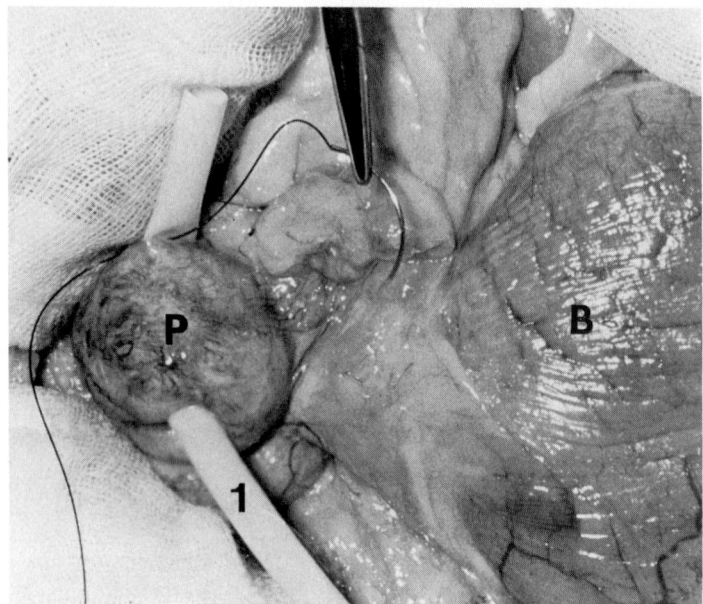

Figure 63-33. Penrose drains (1) are passed through the prostatic parenchyma (P) and secured with a single 4–0 chromic catgut suture. B, Bladder.

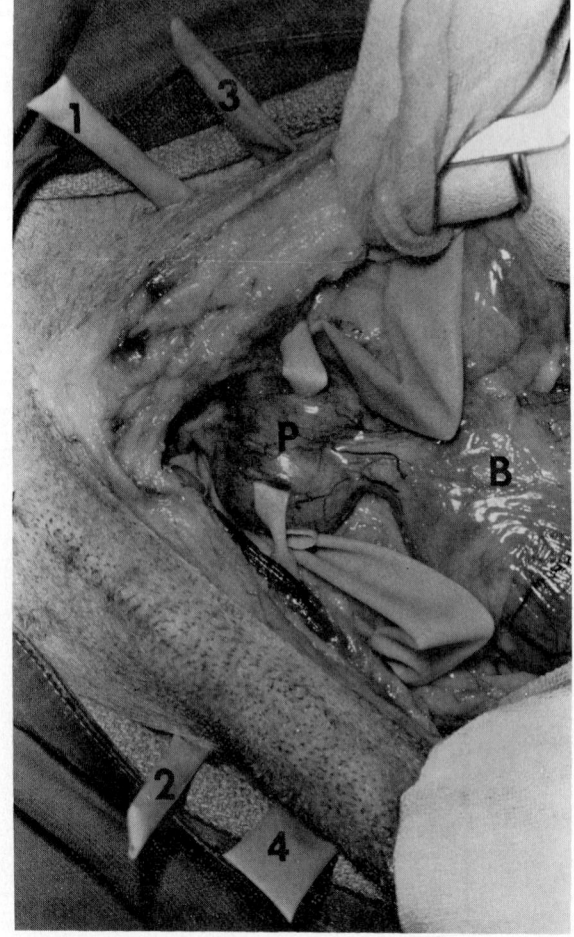

Figure 63-34. Diffuse involvement requires bilateral drain placement to the prostatic parenchyma. The prostatic drains (1 and 2) are exteriorized and the periprostatic drains (3 and 4) are placed. Exteriorized drains are secured with monofilament nonabsorbable suture materials prior to routine abdominal closure. P, Prostate. B, Bladder.

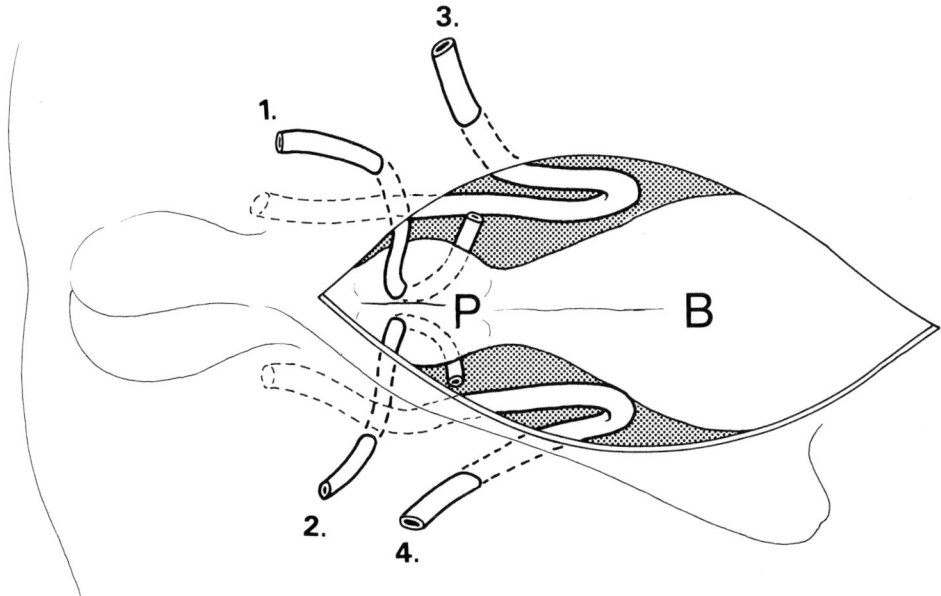

Figure 63–35. Schematic representation of prostatic drainage system for prostatic abscesses. Prostatic drains are placed in the parenchyma and secured with 4–0 chromic catgut, then exteriorized through the abdominal wall drains 1 and 2. Periprostatic drains placed laterally to the prostate and exteriorized through the abdominal wall drains 3 and 4.

static drains are exteriorized caudal to the periprostatic drains for easy identification and sequential removal postoperatively.

The prostatic abscess and surrounding areas are again thoroughly irrigated prior to routine abdominal closure. If not previously done, castration is now performed.

Postoperative Care. Postoperatively, the dog is fitted for an Elizabethan collar or plastic bucket. Antibiotics, as previously discussed, are continued until culture and sensitivity results are available. The prostatic abscess drains are pulled four to seven days after surgery, depending upon quantity of fluid drainage. The periprostatic drains are pulled one to two days after the abscess drains.

Postoperative Complications. Occasionally, there will be postoperative urine leakage through the drains as a result of a communication of the urethra and prostatic abscess. Placement of a Foley traction catheter for four to five days will usually resolve this problem; if it persists, however, it may be necessary to close this communication.

REFERENCES

Aalkjaer, V.: Antimycotics in hypertrophy of the prostate. Urol. Int. 25:196, 1970.

Albin, R. J., and Soanes, W. A.: Antigens of canine prostatic tissue. Indian J. Exp. Biol. 9:439, 1971.

Archibald, J.: The canine prostate. North Am. Vet. 38:253, 1957.

Archibald, J., and Bishop, E. J.: Radiographic visualization of the canine prostate gland. J.A.V.M.A. 128:337, 1956.

Archibald, J., and Cawley, A. J.: Canine prostatectomy. J.A.V.M.A. 128:173, 1956.

Arey, L. B.: Developmental Anatomy. 7th ed. W. B. Saunders Co., Philadelphia, 1965.

Barrett, R. E., and Theilen, G. H.: Neoplasms of the Canine and Feline Reproductive Tract. In Kirk, R. W. (ed.): Current Veterinary Therapy VI. W. B. Saunders Co., Philadelphia, 1977, pp. 1263–1267.

Barsanti, J. A., and Finco, D. R.: Canine Bacterial Prostatitis. Vet. Clin. North Am. 9:679–699, 1979.

Berg, O. A.: Parenchymatous hypertrophy of the canine prostate gland. Acta Endocrinol. 27:140, 1958a.

Berg, O. A.: Effects of stilbestrol on the prostate gland in normal puppies and adult dogs. Acta Endocrinol. 27:155, 1958b.

Betts, C. W., and Finco, D. R.: Diseases of the Canine Prostate Gland. In Kirk, R. W. (ed.): Current Veterinary Therapy V. W. B. Saunders Co., 1974.

Bloom, F.: Pathology of the Dog and Cat. American Veterinary Publications, Inc., Santa Barbara, Calif., 1954.

Borthwick, R., and MacKenzie, C. P.: The signs and results of treatment of prostatic disease in dog. Vet. Rec. 89:374, 1971.

Brody, R. S.: Clinico pathologic conference. J.A.V.M.A. *140*:1339, 1962.

Campbell, J. R., and Lawson, D. D.: The signs of prostatic disease in the dog. Vet. Rec. *75*:4, 1963.

Clark, L., and English, P. B.: Carcinoma of the prostate gland in a dog. Aust. Vet. J. *42*:214, 1966.

Dorland's Illustrated Medical Dictionary. 26th ed. W. B. Saunders Co., Philadelphia, 1981.

Gordon, H. W., and Schaffner, C. P.: The effect of polyene macrolides on the prostate gland and canine prostatic hyperplasia. Appl. Biol. *60*:1201, 1968.

Gordon, N.: Surgical anatomy of the bladder, prostate and urethra in the male dog. J.A.V.M.A. *136*:215, 1960.

Gourley, I. M. G., and Osborne, C. A.: Marsupialization. A treatment for prostatic abscess in the dog. Anim. Hosp. *2*:100, 1966.

Guyton, A. C.: Textbook of Medical Physiology. 4th ed. W. B. Saunders Co., Philadelphia, 1971.

Hodson, N.: On the intrinsic blood supply to the prostate and pelvic urethra in the dog. Res. Vet. Sci. *9*:274, 1968.

Hoffer, R. E., Dykes, N. L., and Greiner, T. P.: Marsupialization as a treatment for prostatic diseases. J.A.A.H.A. *13*:98–104, 1977.

Hogg, A. H.: Prostatic disease in the dog. Clinical manifestations. Vet. Rec. *59*:47, 1947.

Hornbuckle, W. E., et al.: Prostatic disease in the dog. Cornell Vet. *68*(7):284–305, 1978.

Howard, D. R.: The Prostate Gland. *In* Bojrab, M. J. (ed.): Current Techniques in Small Animal Surgery I. Lea and Febiger, Philadelphia, 1975.

Howard, D. R.: Surgical approach to the canine prostate. J.A.V.M.A. *155*:2026, 1969.

Huggins, C.: The physiology of the prostate gland. Physiol. Rev. *25*:287, 1948.

Huggins, C., and Clark, P. J.: Quantitative studies of prostatic secretion. II. The effect of castration and estrogen injection on the normal and on hyperplastic prostate glands of dogs. J. Exp. Med. *72*:747, 1940.

Hutch, J. A.: A new theory of the anatomy of the internal urinary sphincter and the physiology of micturition. II. The base plate. J. Urol. *96*:182, 1966.

Julian, L. M.: The pathology of the prostate gland in man and the dog. A review. Cornell Vet. *37*:241, 1947.

Kirk, R. W., McEntee, K., and Bentick-Smith, J.: Diseases of the Urogenital System. *In* Catcott, E. J. (ed.): Canine Medicine. American Veterinary Publications, Inc., Santa Barbara, Calif., 1968.

Knecht, C. D.: Diseases of the canine prostate gland (Part I). Comp. Cont. Ed. *1*:385–391, 1979.

Knecht, C. D.: Diseases of the canine prostate gland (Part II). Surgical Techniques. Comp. Cont. Ed. *1*:426–433, 1979.

Knecht, C. D., and Schiller, A. G.: Prostatectomy in the dog by incision of the pelvic symphysis. J.A.V.M.A. *149*:1186, 1966.

Kopp, H., and Stockton, N.: Ligation of blood supply in the treatment of canine prostatic hyperplasis. J.A.V.M.A. *136*:327, 1960.

Leav, I., and Cavazos, L. F.: Some Morphologic Features of Normal and Pathologic Canine Prostate. *In* Goland, M. (ed.): Normal and Abnormal Growth of the Prostate. Charles C Thomas, Springfield, 1973.

Leav, I., and Ling, G. V.: Adenocarcinoma of the canine prostate gland. Cancer *22*:1329, 1968.

Leeds, E. B., and Leav, I.: Perineal punch biopsy of the canine prostate gland. J.A.V.M.A. *154*:925, 1969.

Logan, J. M.: The pathology of the prostatic gland of man and the dog: A review. Cornell Vet. *37*:241, 1947.

Lord, L. H., Rowsell, H. C., Cawley, A. J., and Archibald, J.: Suppurative prostatitis corrected by prostatectomy. North Am. Vet. *37*:963, 1956.

Lumb, W. V.: Prostatic calculi in a dog. J.A.V.M.A. *121*:14, 1952.

Madsen, P. O., Wolf, H., Barquin, O., and Rhodes, P.: The nitrofurantoin concentration in prostatic fluid of humans and dogs. J. Urol. *100*:54, 1968.

Markowitz, J., Archibald, J., and Downie, H. G.: Experimental Surgery. 5th ed. The Williams and Wilkins Co., Baltimore, 1964.

Matera, E. A., and Archibald, J.: Prostate gland. *In* Archibald, J. (ed.): Canine Surgery. American Veterinary Publications, Inc., Santa Barbara, Calif., 1965.

McEntee, K., Jubb, K. V. F., and Kennedy, P. C.: Prostate. *In* Jubb, K. V. F., and Kennedy, P. C. (eds.): Pathology of Domestic Animals. Academic Press, Inc., New York, 1970.

McKee, G. S.: A simplified method of surgical correction of prostatitis of the dog. J.A.V.M.A. *124*:442, 1954.

Miller, M. E., Christensen, G. C., and Evans, H. E.: Anatomy of the Dog. W. B. Saunders Co., Philadelphia, 1964.

Neri, R. O., and Monahan, M.: Effects of a novel nonsteroidal antiandrogen on canine prostatic hyperplasia. Invest. Urol. *10*:123–130, 1972.

O'Shea, J. D.: Squamous metaplasia of the canine prostate gland. Res. Vet. Sci. *4*:431, 1963.

O'Shea, J. D.: Studies on the canine prostate gland. J. Comp. Pathol. *73*:244, 1962.

Peel, S.: An immunologic study of dog prostate and the effects of injecting anti-dog prostate serum. Invest. Urol. *5*:427, 1967.

Pettit, G. D.: Prostatectomy in the dog. J.A.V.M.A. *136*:486, 1960.

Pollock, S.: Prostatic abscess in the dog. J.A.V.M.A. *128*:274, 1956.

Proceedings of a Symposium on Trimethoprim-Sulfadiazine. Burroughs Wellcome Co., North Carolina, Jan. 1978.

Rohner, T. J., Raezer, D. M., Wein, A. J., and Schoenberg, H. W.: Contractile responses of the dog bladder neck muscles to adrenergic drugs. J. Urol. *105*:657, 1971.

Schlotthauer, C. F.: Observations on the prostate gland of the dog. J.A.V.M.A. *81*:645, 1932.

Schlotthauer, C. F.: Diseases of the prostate gland in the dog. J.A.V.M.A. *90*:176, 1955.

Schmaelzle, J. F., Cass, A. S., and Hinman, F., Jr.: Autogenous bone graft for post prostatectomy incontinence, I. Animal experiments. J. Urol. *99*:656, 1968.

Smith, H. A., and Jones, T. C.: Veterinary Pathology. Lea and Febiger, Philadelphia, 1972.

Stamey, T. A., Meares, E. M., and Winningham, D. G.: Chronic bacterial prostatitis and the diffusion of drugs into prostatic fluid. J. Urol. *103*:187, 1970.

Swenson, M. J.: Duke's Physiology of Domestic Animals. 8th ed. Comstock Publishing Associates, Ithaca, N.Y., 1970.

Tanagho, E. A., and Smith, O. R.: The anatomy and function of the bladder neck. Brit. J. Urol. *38*:54, 1966.

Thorberg, J. U.: Acta Endocrinol. *I*(Suppl. 2):155, 1948.

Winningham, D. G., and Stamey, T. A.: Diffusion of sulfonamides from plasma into prostatic fluids. J, Urol. *104*:559, 1970.

Wolf, H., Madsen, P. O., and Rhodes, P.: The ampicillin concentration in prostatic tissue and prostatic fluid. Urol. Int. *22*:453, 1967.

Zolton, G. M.: Surgical techniques for the prostate. Vet. Clin. North Am. *9*:349–356, 1979.

Zolton, G. M., and Greiner, T. P.: Prostatic abscesses. A surgical approach. J.A.A.H.A. *14*:698–702, 1978.

Zuckerman, S., and Groome, J. R.: The etiology of benign enlargement of the prostate in the dog. J. Pathol. Bact. *44*:113, 1937.

Zuckerman, S., and McKeown, T.: Canine prostate in relation to normal and abnormal testicular changes. J. Pathol. Bact. *46*:7, 1938.

CHAPTER 64

THOMAS P. GREINER,
RICHARD G. JOHNSON,
and C. WILLIAM BETTS

Diseases of the Rectum and Anus

Anorectal problems are encountered frequently in veterinary medicine. They are variable in nature, and are common in dogs and less common in cats. Lesions generally respond well to conservative therapy if diagnosed and treated early in their course. The majority of problems are due to dietary imbalances, anal sac disorders, proctitis, and the rectal effects of prostatic hypertrophy (Levene, 1968). These disorders are characterized by a relatively restricted group of symptoms: pruritus, pain, bleeding, passage of excess mucus or flatus, tenesmus, diarrhea, and constipation. Any one of these signs indicates the need for a complete examination of the anorectal area (Rodkey, 1973). Of special significance because of its devastating consequences are problems related to fecal incontinence.

When presented with problems of the anorectal region, as with all problems, it is imperative that the veterinarian begin with a thorough history and physical examination. Owner education and awareness are important as aids in the early recognition and management of anorectal problems as well.

HISTORY AND PHYSICAL EXAMINATION

The most common presenting complaints referable to anorectal problems are usually associated with prolonged treatment for unresponsive diarrhea, tenesmus (straining to defecate), or dyschezia (painful defecation) (Greiner, 1972). Items of primary concern include

1. *Diet:* Type, frequency of feeding, and recent changes.

2. *General health:* Alertness, activity, vomiting, diarrhea, water consumption, micturition, appetite (normal, depressed, or pica).

3. *Defecation:* Feces color and consistency (bloody, mucous, hard, soft, or with foreign debris) (Palminteri, 1968); frequency and nature of elimination (normal, scant, voluminous, foul, or with excessive flatulence); and straining (moderate or severe, constant or intermittent, productive or unproductive, of long or short duration, before, during, or after act of defecation) (Palminteri, 1968).

4. *Vaccination history and intestinal parasite control.*

5. *Previous trauma, surgery, harsh laxatives, vermifuges, or diseases.*

Propensities for certain types of anorectal problems are determined by age, sex, and breed. Puppies and kittens are more prone to digestive disturbance from dietary changes, intestinal parasites, ingestion of foreign bodies, infectious diseases, rectal prolapse, prolapsed intussusception, and congenital abnormalities. Mature animals tend to have dietary imbalance, anal sac impaction, constipation, and perianal fistulas; cats are prone to obstipation. Middle-aged and older animals are prone to perineal hernia, perianal adenoma, neoplasms, and anal sac abscess.

Rectovaginal fistulas are found in the female, and perineal hernia and perianal adenoma in the male (Levene, 1968).

Pseudocoprostasis (matting of escutcheon with feces) occurs in young poodles and schnauzers; the German shepherd and the Irish setter are prone to perianal fistulas (Palminteri, 1968; Greiner, 1972).

Other diseases with symptoms similar to those of anorectal disorders must be considered prior to initiating definitive therapy. It is not unusual for owners to complain of constipation in their cat, which is obstructed by urolithiasis. The authors have seen animals with an open, draining pyometra presented for diarrhea. Cystitis, cystic calculi, carcinoma of the bladder, and dystocia can be confused with or misdiagnosed as the straining associated with an anorectal disorder. Dyschezia may be secondary to prostatitis, advanced benign prostatic hypertrophy, proctitis, anusitis, or long-standing diarrhea (Palminteri, 1968).

Clinical history and symptomatology should not be given precedence over a thorough physical examination. Many German shepherds have been treated symptomatically for weeks, and occasionally for months, for tenesmus or dyschezia or both in order to alleviate what appeared to be a chronic, intractable diarrhea or a constipation problem, because no one happened to observe the fistulous tracts hidden by the dog's apprehensively clamped-down tail. Occasionally, more than one anorectal problem will be present.

Once the general bodily systems have been checked, the clinician should closely examine the perineum and anorectal areas. Visual examination of the external anal area may reveal the following disorders: anal sacculitis, neoplasms, abnormal swellings, perineal hernia, imperforate anus, perineal fistulas, eversion of anal mucosa, rectal prolapse, and, rarely, prolapsed intussusception (Palminteri, 1968; Greiner, 1972).

Digital examination should always be performed. If the procedure is extremely painful for the animal, it should be sedated or anesthetized. Disposable rectal examination gloves enable the finger to advance easily into the pelvis. Generous use of lubrication

and slow, gentle introduction of the finger into the anal orifice, while slightly elevating the tail, will be well tolerated by most patients. A painful response to internal examination may indicate anal sac infection, perianal abscess, rectoanal fistulas, severe anusitis, rectal foreign body, acute prostatitis, or carcinoma (Palminteri, 1968). In addition to noting the presence or absence of pain, the veterinarian should evaluate anal sphincter tone and check for rectal deviation associated with sacculation or diverticulum and perineal hernia, perirectal masses or abscesses, interference by constriction, and the presence of a rectal foreign body. The anal sacs should be discrete structures that are easily palpated and expressed. The rectal mucosa should be smooth to the touch, with normal corrugations. No bleeding should result from the digital palpation. During this examination, a fecal sample can be easily obtained and should be evaluated for abnormal color or consistency, foreign debris, excessive mucus, or streaking with blood. A wet mount can be quickly examined for protozoa, intestinal parasites, and occult blood. A routine fecal flotation should also be done.

Internal visualization should follow the digital examination. Anoscopy can be performed with minimal discomfort to the animal and enables visualization of the rectum and distal colon. Proctoscopy is best performed under tranquilization and, preferably, under anesthesia. A healthy, pink-looking mucosa with normal corrugations should be present. Neoplasms, ulcers, foreign bodies, polyps, or trauma may be noted. Numerous, small, punctate grayish areas will frequently be seen; these are normal lymphoid aggregates of the rectal mucosa (Miller et al., 1964; Palminteri, 1968; Greiner, 1972).

ANATOMY

The pelvic brim is the cranial boundary of the rectum, which is continuous with and indistinguishable from the descending colon. The rectum courses caudally through the pelvic canal as a tubular structure that is flattened from side to side at rest. Caudally, the rectum is delimited by the anal canal at the anal sphincters. Together, the rectum and anal canal compose an epithelial tube that is continuous with the perineal skin forming the mucocutaneous junction at the anus. The anus is the terminal opening of the alimentary canal (Miller et al., 1964; Ashdown, 1968).

The medial coccygeus (levator ani) and the lateral coccygeus (coccygeus) muscles form a funnel-shaped diaphragm through which the rectum courses. The rectum is bounded dorsally by the right and left sacro-coccygeus muscles, and ventrally by the vagina in the female and the urethra in the male. The rectum is supported dorsally by a thin band of tissue, the mesorectum; this contributes the parietal peritoneum of the rectum, which blends with visceral peritoneum as it reflects forward at the terminal portion of the rectum. This conjoined reflection forms the pararectal fossa. Caudal to this fossa, the rectum and anus are supported by superficial and deep fascia (Miller et al., 1964; Ashdown, 1968).

Blood is supplied to the rectum and anus by the caudal mesenteric artery and the visceral branch of the internal iliac artery (Fig. 64–1). The caudal mesenteric artery runs posteriorly on the dorsal wall of the rectum and becomes the cranial rectal artery, which terminates at the anal canal. The visceral branch of the internal iliac artery continues as the internal pudendal artery

and branches into the perineal artery and the caudal rectal artery (hemorrhoidal artery), which passes under the external anal sphincter and supplies the perianal structures, including the perianal glands. The internal pudendal artery branches and supplies the cutaneous and subcutaneous tissues of the pararectal fossa.

Innervation to the anorectal area is derived from the pudendal nerve, which is formed from the first three sacral nerves and provides voluntary motor control to the external anal sphincter. The pudendal nerve also branches and supplies the skin of the anus and perianal region. The sole motor supply to the external anal sphincter is the rectal branch of the pudendal nerve. The internal anal sphincter and rectum receive nerve branches from the pelvic plexus (Miller et al., 1964).

Draining the anorectal region is a plexus of lymphatics located on the dorsal wall of the rectum and anal canal; these empty into the left colic, internal iliac, and the external iliac nodes. There are also small pelvic lymph nodes in the areolar tissue of the ventrolateral rectal wall (Ashdown, 1968).

The smooth muscle of the rectum consists of an inner circular and an outer longitudinal layer. The longitudinal muscle layer

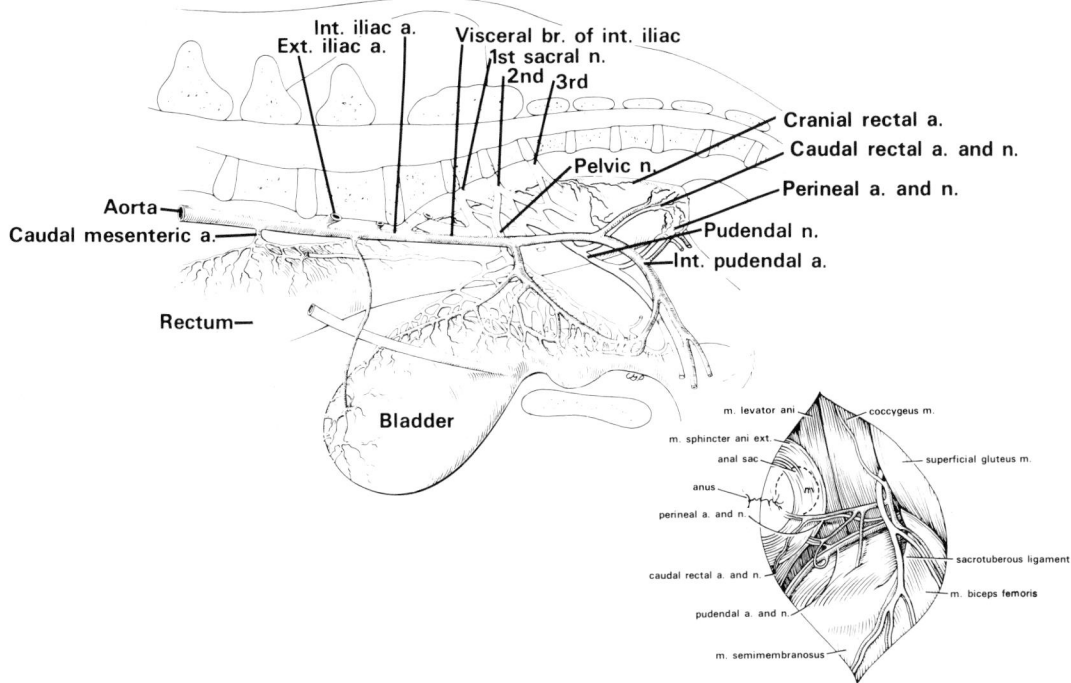

Figure 64–1. Diagrammatic representation of blood supply and innervation to the anorectal area.

ends in the region of the perianal glands, except for a part of the longitudinal muscle that passes from the rectum bilaterally and attaches to coccygeal vertebrae five and six as the rectococcygeus muscle. The circular layer ends at the perianal glands and is thickened to form the internal anal sphincter (Ashdown, 1968), which functions involuntarily (Miller et al., 1964). In contrast, the external anal sphincter is largely a circular band of striated muscle that invests the anal canal and the anal sacs and functions voluntarily (Miller et al., 1964).

The rectal wall is essentially the same in structure as the colon. The rectal mucosa contains glands of Lieberkühn, with more mucous cells than the colon (Strombeck, 1980). The rectal mucosa merges with the external skin to form four zones: a columnar zone composed of the longitudinal columns of mucosal tissue; a thin intermediate zone; the inner cutaneous, hairless zone in which the anus is located; and an ill-defined outer cutaneous, hair-bearing zone (Miller et al., 1964; Ashdown, 1968). Located in the first zone are the mucosal pouches analogous to the crypts and pillars of Morgagni in man (Shaffer and Block, 1961; Archibald and Horney, 1975). There are also three special glandular zones: the glands of the perianal skin, which will eventually form a circular mound of tissue; the anal glands in the columnar zone; and the anal sacs, which are diverticula of the inner cutaneous zone (Miller et al., 1964; Ashdown, 1968) (Fig. 64–2).

PHYSIOLOGY

The basic function of the rectum is to serve as a passageway for the expulsion of feces (Palminteri, 1968; Greiner, 1972). This seemingly simple function is actually a complex, integrated process that is influenced by several voluntary and involuntary factors. Disease processes can alter the normal excretory process and directly affect the animal's ability to defecate.

Some consideration must be given to the manner in which fecal material is moved through the colon in order to appreciate the role of the rectum and anus. In the colon, segmental contraction signifies compression of a haustral segment between two constricting folds. This results in random movement of a fecal bolus to the adjacent proximal or distal segment. Forward propulsion need

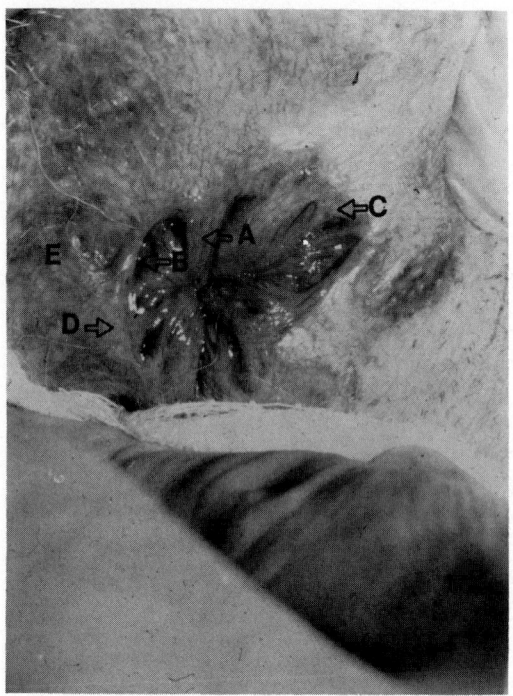

Figure 64–2. Anatomy of anus. A, Longitudinal columns of rectal mucosa, which reflect at beginning of anus to form anal crypts (B). C, Thin intermediate zone of anal canal; D, inner cutaneous, hairless zone of anus; and E, outer hair-bearing zone of anus.

not occur, but if sequential movement for a few short segments occurs in an aboral direction, the net progress is distal and is termed *haustral propulsion*. If the net progress is proximal, it is termed *haustral retropulsion*. This oscillatory action facilitates absorption of water from the fecal mass. Often, several segments will contract in unison, which is termed *multihaustral propulsion*. This contraction is common in the ascending colon and is more effective on semisolid stool.

These segmental contractions are caused by the peristaltic action inherent in the bowel. There is progression of a narrow contracting ring of circular smooth muscle, preceded by a variable distance of distal relaxation or inhibition of circular muscle and contraction of longitudinal muscle. This progression is usually followed by tonic contraction from behind, which propels the fecal bolus distally for some distance. This tonic action occurs more frequently in the descending colon, but it may start and end anywhere. Antiperistalsis is rare in man but is commonly seen postprandially on the right side in animals.

Multihaustral contractions of the ascending colon often precede mass propulsion or action in the transverse colon. The net effect is to propel the fecal bolus into the descending colon or rectum. The mass peristaltic action of the colon results in evacuation of unneeded material from the colon (Hagihara and Griffen, 1972).

These mass movements have been associated with distention of the stomach, which stimulates the gastrocolic reflex, resulting in rectal contractions and a desire to defecate. This reflex seems to be an established pattern in children and animals (Ganong, 1967; Palminteri, 1969). Recently, a humoral factor has been demonstrated in cross-circulation experiments, which suggests that the term *gastrocolic reflex* is probably a misnomer (Hagihara and Griffen, 1972).

The rectal mucosa is lined by numerous simple tubular glands containing goblet cells. The goblet-cell secretion rate is determined by direct, tactile stimulation. Local nervous reflexes may stimulate the goblet cells in the crypts of Lieberkühn. In addition, parasympathetic stimulation results in a marked increase in mucus production. Goblet cells secrete mucus to protect the rectal mucosa against excoriation, to lubricate the feces, and to bind the fecal particles. The mucus also protects the rectal wall from the great amount of bacterial activity occurring inside the fecal mass. The mucus and the alkalinity of the secretion (pH 8.0) prevent the acids formed by bacteria deep in the feces from irritating the rectal wall. The mucus contains important protein radicals, with a total nitrogen content of seven to 12 per cent. Any loss of large amounts of mucus and nitrogen can contribute to malnutrition and inanition. In addition, the rectum has almost no resorptive capacity (Guyton, 1966; Palminteri, 1969).

In order to defecate, an animal assumes a squatting position that is facilitated by a reflex contraction of the hamstring muscles. By closure of the glottis and application of an abnormal press (Valsalva maneuver), the intra-abdominal pressure increases. When the external anal sphincter relaxes, the fecal mass is expelled by development of pressures of 100 to 200 mm Hg within the rectum, which shortens and descends. Subsequent contractions of the levator ani and other pelvic floor muscles enhance the increased abdominal pressure. This pressure contracts the rectum over the last part of the fecal bolus and prevents the anus from being forced too far downward. The entire descending colon may be evacuated if mass peristalsis accompanies defecation.

Sensory activity of the rectum is extremely important during defecation. Stretch receptors stimulated by the fecal mass entering the rectum initiate the defecation reflex. Impulses pass via visceral afferent nerves, through a dorsal root ganglion, to the respective spinal segment. Impulse distribution occurs (1) cephalad to the cerebral cortex to elicit all the necessary voluntary actions, i.e., closure of the glottis and fixation of the diaphragm; (2) to ventral horn cells to mediate relaxation of the external anal sphincter and perineal muscles and contraction of the abdominal muscles; and (3) via neuronal connections to the pelvic autonomic nervous system to stimulate the rectal circular and longitudinal muscles to expel the fecal mass. In addition to these three major impulses, the internal anal sphincter is also instructed by local intrinsic ganglia to dilate. This intensifies the peristaltic waves sufficiently to empty the large bowel (Guyton, 1966; Scharli and Kiesewitter, 1970; Rawlings and Capps, 1971; Hagihara and Griffen, 1972; Rodkey, 1973).

FECAL CONTINENCE

Fecal continence is defined as the ability to retain feces until their delivery is convenient (Gaston, 1951). Since correction of most disease conditions of the anorectal area will require some form of surgical intervention, familiarity with the physiology of the act of defecation is necessary in order to prevent accidental destruction of structures that ultimately control elimination. Although the exact mechanism is controversial, it is generally agreed that fecal continence has two components, sphincter continence and reservoir continence, which act together in a complicated, highly integrated manner. Sphincter continence results from contraction of the external anal sphincter in resisting propulsive forces created by peristaltic waves in the colon and rectum, whereas reservoir or colonic continence results from the plastic adaption of the smooth muscle of the colon, due to an enlarging fecal mass. Functional sphincter continence depends on various intact components, such as the afferent nerve fibers (with endings located in the wall of the rectum) and the efferent nerve fibers (terminating in the external anal sphincter), which connect at the cerebral level to form a nervous reflex arc. Reservoir continence depends on the ability of the descending colon to distend, which reduces fecal volume by resorption and decreases the frequency of defecatory impulses.

Normal fecal continence in man, which is thought to be similar to that in the dog, is accomplished by an interplay of anorectal reflexes. The rectum and lower colon are normally empty of fecal content and maintain a normal, resting intrarectal pressure by reflex activity of the internal anal sphincter, the external anal sphincter, and the puborectalis muscle. In the dog, the puborectalis muscle is probably represented by the caudal part of the medial coccygeus (Ashdown, 1968). Slight distention of the rectal luminal fibers by peristaltic waves from the upper colon initiates brief involuntary contraction of the puborectalis muscle, after which the muscle returns to a normal state, thus preventing fecal movement into the rectum. The patient is not aware of slight or minor rises in intrarectal pressure but is aware of increases of high amplitude and reacts with a conscious, active contraction of the external anal sphincter. There is controversy about which of the three muscles is responsible for maintaining the resting resistance of the rectum. Scharli and Kiesewitter (1970) report that although the three reflexes are diverse in nature, they probably work synergistically in maintaining the resting resistance.

The act of defecation proceeds when fecal material passes into the rectum. Sensitive nerve endings on the rectum are stimulated, creating the desire to defecate. The internal anal sphincter dilates and readies the anal canal for evacuation. When the desire to defecate is initiated, the patient can either voluntarily contract the external anal sphincter until the desire to defecate disappears and the rectum adjusts to the new volume, or allow the stool to pass out the anal canal with the assistance of intra-abdominal pressure. When the external anal sphincter is contracted, delaying the elimination, the desire to defecate subsides until more fecal mass is moved into the rectum, which initiates a new reflex more powerful than the previous one. Eventually, when the rectal reservoir is filled, the anal sphincter can no longer repel the mass, and elimination must occur.

From a surgical standpoint, it is desirable to know which anorectal structures should not be removed or traumatized if complete continence is to be maintained. The rectum itself, especially the posterior part, should be preserved. Karland et al. (1959) report that the reflexes invoked in voluntary sphincter function are maintained or only minimally disturbed by preservation of a short length of distal rectum denuded of mucosa, whereas removal of the rectum and anastomosis of the ileum to the dentate line of the anal canal result in complete loss of continence. Swenson and Bill (1948) show similar results with the pull-through procedure. Removal of the anterior portion of the rectum and some of the distal colon does not disturb fecal continence or interfere with sphincter function. Extensive removal of the colon and rectum, however, reduces normal alimentary transit time by one third (Glotzer and Scharmer, 1964).

Sphincter continence is lost in dogs when there is complete division of the external anal sphincter (Gaston, 1951). Another way of destroying sphincter continence is destruction of the efferent fibers of the external anal sphincter. In the dog, these fibers compose the rectal or hemorrhoidal nerve (a branch of the pudendal nerve), and appear to be the sole motor innervation to the sphincter. Removal of the afferent fibers of the rectoanal reflex, by removal of the rectum or destruction of the nerves or component of the pelvic plexus, also destroys sphincter action. Transection of the spinal cord also results in complete loss of continence and may be confusing in traumatic injuries in which extensive trauma has occurred to the anorectal area.

Loss of continence can occur in varying degrees. Total loss, by the causes mentioned, can create a nonfunctional pet, but partial loss of continence, such as that encountered in surgical removal of perianal fistulas, can be managed. This partial loss is manifested by the inability to control flatulence; by soiling or accumulation of fecal material at the anal opening between defecations; and by the forceful, unconscious elimination of feces when the animal is excited, caused by increased intraabdominal pressure due to the Valsalva reflex. Partial loss of continence usually results from partial removal of the external anal sphincter. Patients with this loss can be managed by being fed twice daily with low bulk (lean meat) diets and by being taken to eliminate shortly after feeding, in addition to being walked frequently during the day.

CONGENITAL DISEASES OF THE ANUS

Imperforate anus (atresia ani), segmental aplasia, and rectovaginal fistula are the three most common congenital diseases involving the rectum and anus (Fig. 64–3). Congenital abnormalities of this region are rare but significant when they occur (Palminteri, 1969; Greiner, 1972), and have been reported to occur concomitantly (Rawlings, 1971).

IMPERFORATE ANUS

In uncomplicated imperforate anus, the rectal portion of the cloacal membrane per-

sists. There will be a depression at the anal dimple, and the sphincters will be normal (Archibald and Horney, 1975; Ashdown, 1968). Normally, the cloacal membrane is resorbed or ruptures by the seventh to eighth week of embryonal development, establishing continuity between the rectum and anus (Arey, 1965).

There does not seem to be a breed or sex predilection. The diagnosis is usually made within the first few weeks of life, and the condition is often noted by the owner. The clinical signs are tenesmus, no visible anal opening, bulging of the perineum, and manifestations of abdominal discomfort. If abdominal discomfort is extreme, the patient may whine constantly, and the abdomen may be distended (Archibald and Horney, 1975; Greiner, 1972) (Fig. 64–4).

A horizontal beam radiograph, with the patient held upside down by its hindfeet,

Congenital Diseases of the Anus

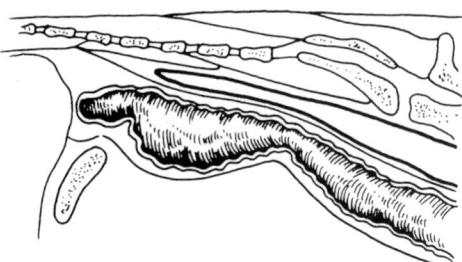

Type 1. Thin membrane over anus

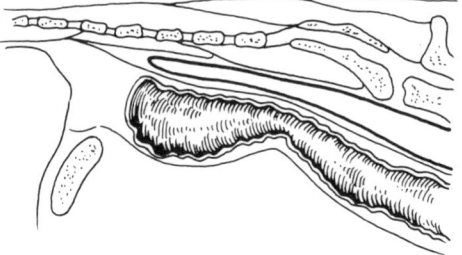

Type 2. Blind pouch receded from anal dimple

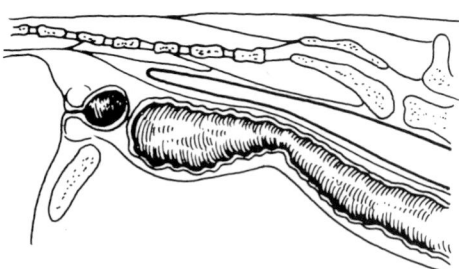

Type 3. Atresia of rectum with normal anus

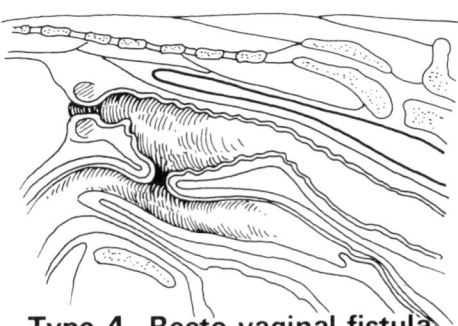

Type 4. Recto-vaginal fistula

Figure 64–3. Diagrammatic representation of congenital diseases of the anorectal region. Adapted from The Ciba Collection of Medical Illustrations.

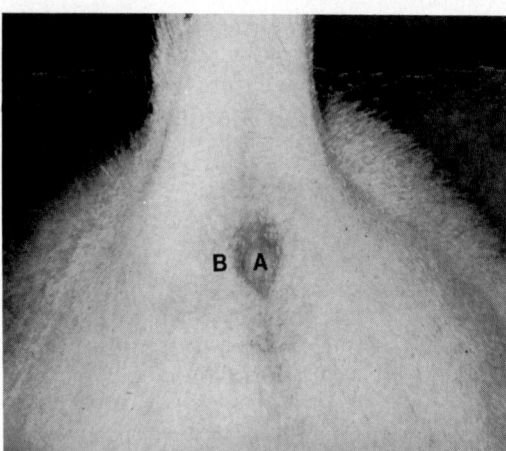

Figure 64–4. Imperforate anus in a four-week-old mixed breed pup. A, persistent cloacal membrane; B, bulging perineum.

will aid in distinguishing imperforate anus from segmental aplasia. Colonic gas will migrate to the distal colon and rectum in this position (Fig. 64–5).

Correction of atresia ani is surgical. A stab incision into the anal dimple is made under local anesthesia. Resection of the membrane is usually sufficient for correction. If necessary, mucocutaneous sutures can be placed. In some instances, a cruciate incision may facilitate dissection. The prognosis is good unless bowel stasis has resulted in malaise,

inanition, and deterioration of general health.

SEGMENTAL APLASIA

In segmental aplasia, the rectal tube ends blindly in the pelvic canal. Rarely, there is compartmentalization. Radiographic examination will reveal the extent of the lesion if surgical correction is contemplated.

Segmental aplasia is more difficult to correct than imperforate anus and requires a guarded prognosis. After a general anesthetic is administered, a midline incision extending a short distance above and below the anal sphincter is made over the anal dimple. The anal sphincter is identified by careful dissection. Dissection is continued bluntly through the pelvic area to the rectal pouch. At this point an Allis tissue forceps or stay sutures are used to secure the pouch while adjacent tissue is carefully dissected to free the rectum. When the rectum has been mobilized sufficiently to be exteriorized, the blind pouch is incised and the rectal edges sutured to the edges of the skin around the anal orifice, using 5–0 or 6–0 chromic catgut in a simple interrupted pattern (Greiner, 1972). In man, every effort is made to maintain the rectum within the puborectalis sling and the external anal sphincter (Scharli and Kiesewitter, 1970).

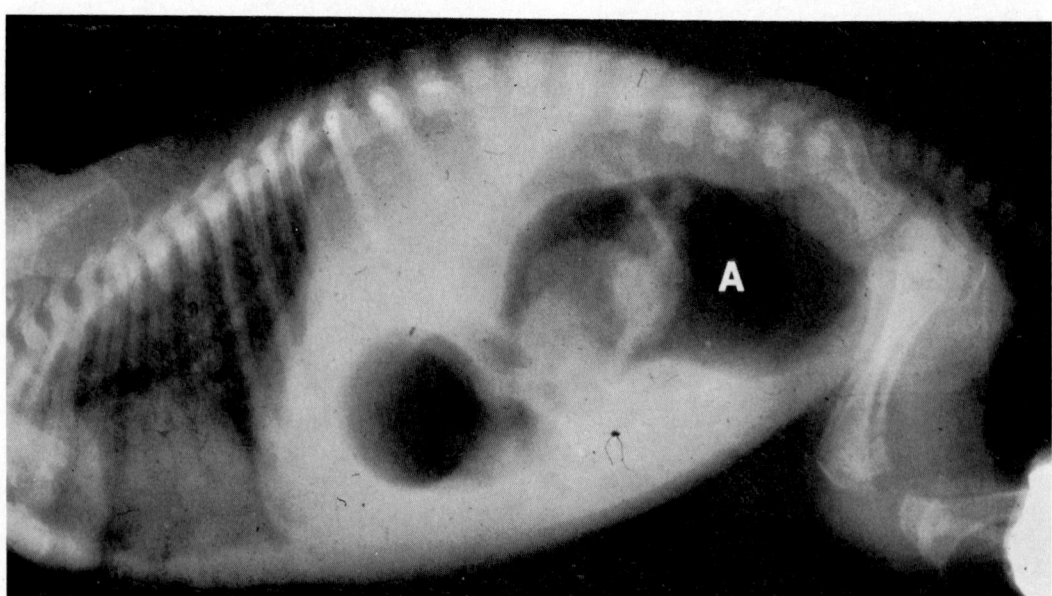

Figure 64–5. Lateral radiographic view of puppy with imperforate anus. A, Gaseous distention of colon. A horizontal beam radiograph with the puppy held upside down should also be taken to differentiate imperforate anus from segmental aplasia.

RECTOVAGINAL FISTULA

Of the three congenital anal diseases listed, rectovaginal fistula is the most difficult for the owner to determine. The presenting complaint may be that the pet exhibits tenesmus and passes a scant amount of thin, watery feces. This lesion occurs more rarely than imperforate anus and segmental aplasia (Palminteri, 1969), and the animals are seldom sick. There may be an associated vaginitis and cystitis. Visual inspection will demonstrate either the presence or the absence of an anus, feces coming from the vulva, and perivulvar irritation (Fig. 64–6). If there is an anus, a barium enema will confirm the diagnosis by outlining the communication with the vulva (Fig. 64–7). Surgical correction consists of eliminating the fistulous tract by closure of the rectal and vaginal defects. This restores the separate lumens of the rectum and vagina (Rawlings and Capps, 1971; Greiner, 1972).

DISEASES OF THE ANAL SACS

The archaic anal sacs of the dog and cat have no known function. Scent marking and anointing of territory is a well-accepted behavioral pattern in many mammalian species (Donovan, 1969); some dogs and cats manifest this instinct by expressing their anal sacs. The normal secretion of these sacs is a serous to somewhat viscid, slightly granular, brownish liquid with a distinct, disagreeable odor (Archibald and Horney, 1975).

Anatomy. In the cat, the anal sacs are paired, glandular organs about one cm in length. The anal sacs are situated on each side of the anus, into which they open by narrow, paired ducts about 3.5 mm long. The walls of the sacs consist of white, fibrous connective tissue and contain sebaceous gland complexes and tubular apocrine glands. The sacs and ducts are lined with keratinized stratified squamous epithelium. The blood supply is derived from branches of the middle hemorrhoidal artery. The excretory product is a mixture of fatty and serous material plus cellular debris (Greer and Calhoun, 1966).

The anatomy of the dog is similar. The sacs are located at approximately a five and seven o'clock position with respect to the anus. The squirting of the fluid (0.25 to 0.5 ml) from the sacs may precede or follow elimination of feces. Expression occurs as the overlying anal sphincter squeezes the sacs against stool present in the anal canal (Ashdown, 1968). Halnan (1978) suggested that an earlier predisposing factor to disease was a mild attack of diarrhea, reasoning that the normal mechanism of emptying the sac was a passive squeezing of the sacs by the passage of a well-formed firm fecal bolus. It is doubtful that anal sac fluid functions as a lubricant.

ANAL SAC IMPACTION

Anal sacs are highly prone to problems. The classic complaint of the owner is that the animal frequently "scoots," "drags," or "rubs" its rump on the floor. In a puppy, this may be associated with intestinal parasites, but usually it is an effort to relieve the discomfort associated with impacted anal sacs. In the adult animal, anal sac impaction is common and influenced in some cases by the social restrictions of the environment. An animal with impacted anal sacs may rub the perineum on the ground, bite or chew at its rump, and occasionally excoriate the skin by constant aggravation of the anal area (Hansen, 1972).

The incidence and distribution of anal sac impaction was described by Harvey (1974), who found an overall incidence of 61 of 3027 cases (2.0 per cent). The median age was three years (range — three months to

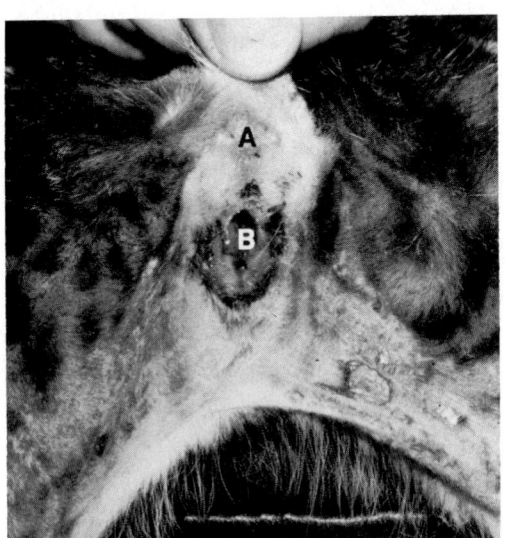

Figure 64–6. Rectovaginal fistula in a four-week-old female kitten. A, Anal dimple without anal orifice; B, vulvar orifice enlarged as a result of the rectal fistulas. Note fecal soilage around the perivulvar area.

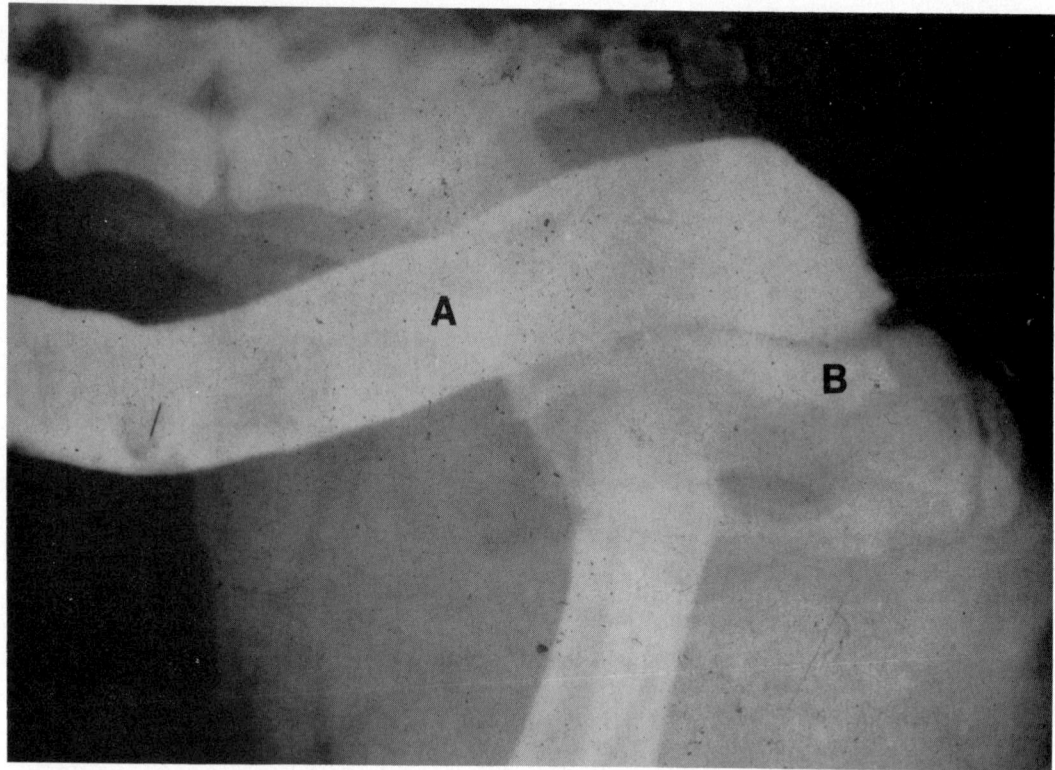

Figure 64–7. Lateral radiographic view of a dog given a barium enema. A, Contrast material in distal colon and rectum; B, contrast material in vagina that has passed through rectovaginal fistula. Fistula is not demonstrated on radiograph.

15 years), with poodles and Chihuahua breeds significantly overrepresented. Fortunately, the incidence of anal sac disorders in the feline population is quite low (Myrilos, 1967).

Proper early treatment of anal sac impaction will prevent development of a more serious condition. The anal sacs should be routinely checked at every physical examination. Often the owner is not aware of anal sac problems, or even of the fact that his pet has these glands and that they may need attention. As with many routine problems that can affect a pet's health, owner education regarding the premonitory signs associated with anal sac disorders can eliminate many unnecessary telephone calls and office visits. Willing clients should be shown how to express anal sacs at home. They must also be taught the difference between a mild impaction and an infection or abscess that needs professional attention.

Impaction characterized by the accumulation of a thick, pasty secretion can result from abnormal bowel elimination that fails to empty the sacs. Hypersecretion may occur in obese dogs with generalized seborrhea and poor muscle tone. If the secretion is inspissated, a thin ribbon-like material can be expressed with difficulty and discomfort to the dog.

Taenia proglottides have also been responsible for anal sac impaction. Diagnosis is based on visualization of the proglottids after the sacs have been expressed manually, and good response to therapy with Yomesan (Niclosamide). *Dipylidium* spp have also been implicated, but no cases were seen over a 15-month period in a high-incidence area (Myrilos, 1967).

When expressing anal sacs internally, well lubricated rectal examination gloves should be worn. External expression of the sacs is often adequate for the normal dog (particularly small breeds), but the rectal procedure enables one to palpate the size, configuration, and consistency of the sacs and to evaluate the degree of discomfort induced during expression. The internal procedure is well tolerated by most animals and enables the clinician to palpate the rectum, pelvic canal, and prostate gland for signs of possible abnormalities. A softening agent such as sulfaurea solution, mineral oil, furacin solution, or mastitis ointment should be instilled in the sacs if the secretion is dry and difficult to express (Severin, 1968). If the anal sac area seems painful and the animal has been exhibiting prior symptoms of discomfort, anal sac infection is probable. The secretion of infected sacs is often thin and watery and of a yellow or greenish color. Antibiotic ointment should be instilled in the sacs through the ducts, which run slightly cranially in a ventrolateral direction. The condition may be unilateral. The use of systemic antibiotics is a matter of judgment, but hemolytic streptococcus and staphylococcus organisms are often cultured from the sacs (Severin, 1968). The animal should be made comfortable by such means as cleansing enemas to relieve straining associated with constipation, a mildly laxative diet, and treatment of coexisting problems, such as self-induced dermatitis. If impaction becomes a chronic, recurring condition, the anal sacs will become firm and fibrotic, and should be removed (Severin, 1968; Panel Report, 1969).

ANAL SAC ABSCESSES

Anal sac abscesses are characterized by an increased degree of pain associated with rectal palpation of the involved sac and by

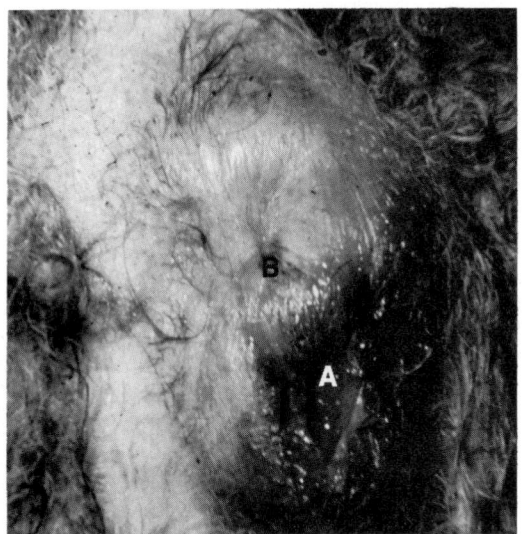

Figure 64–8. Ruptured anal sac abscess (A) in a dog. The location, ventrolateral to the anus (B), is characteristic in the dog. A firm, erythematous, painful swelling is usually present two to three days prior to rupture.

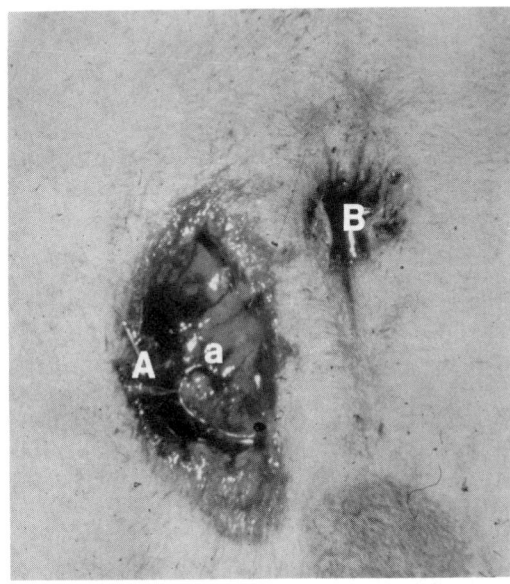

Figure 64–9. Ruptured anal sac abscess (A) in a cat; a, glistening membranous structure is inner lining of anal sac; B, anus. In the authors' experience, excision is preferred to cauterization in the acute ruptured state in the cat.

visualization of a raised, inflamed, and often hairless area covered by thin, tenuous skin. Many cases are presented after the abscess has spontaneously ruptured and drained, but pain is usually a constant feature (Figs. 64–8 and 64–9).

The area should not be lanced if cellulitis is present and the abscess has not pointed. If the abscess is not ready to be lanced, hot packs should be instituted. When the abscess is ready to be lanced, a No. 11 BP blade is effective. Highly intractable animals should be tranquilized or anaesthetized. Manual restraint is sufficient for most patients and, in the authors' experience, anesthesia is rarely necessary. There is very little pain associated with the lancing, but irrigation of the cavity with an antiseptic solution and mild cauterization of the sac elicit considerable pain and squirming for a short period of time. After the abscess is lanced, the sac should be expressed by rectal and external pressure, followed by debridement and drainage. Evaluation of the anal sac duct should be done to insure patency.

After expression and irrigation, many clinicians routinely cauterize the anal sac with tincture of iodine or ten per cent silver nitrate solution (Archibald and Horney, 1975; Severin, 1968; Panel Report, 1969). This should be done with care, or a less caustic agent such as Betadine solution should be used. Excessive cauterization can result in extensive cellular necrosis, pseudomembrane formation, and the trapping of infective organisms beneath the pseudomembrane. Recurrent abscesses may be due in part to overly vigorous cauterization or inadequate debridement.

Systematic antibiotics are indicated, and the owner should continue to apply hot packs and an antiseptic to the wounds. Cotton-tipped applicator sticks can be used to probe, clean, and apply antiseptic to the wound daily. Daily probing ensures that the wound will stay open to heal from the inside out. This procedure is well tolerated after a few days by most animals, but the owner should be cautioned to be gentle as well as thorough.

Recurrent anal sac abscesses are an indication for anal sac excision. In the dog, when the area is infected, excision of the anal sacs should not be performed. In the authors' experience with the cat, however, excision in the acute ruptured state will reduce the healing period postoperatively and is preferred to cauterization. Preoperative management should include control of any preexisting infection, fasting, an enema, and evacuation of the anal sacs (Archibald and Horney, 1975). Open and closed procedures have been advocated, both with good results (Spira et al., 1971). The authors prefer a closed procedure, although an open procedure takes less time.

Anal Sac Excision. In the closed operating procedure, scissors can be inserted into the duct and the duct and overlying skin incised; the anal sac is then excised intact (Bloom, 1971). Dissection is facilitated by infusing the sac with melted paraffin or commercial gels, or by packing the sac with string, yarn, or similar materials (Frye et al., 1970; Spira et al., 1971). The sacs are easily palpated when filled with a suitable preparation, though the authors seldom find this necessary.

An alternate approach uses a perirectal incision over the involved anal sac and dissection to the sac through the overlying subcutaneous tissue. Closure in both cases is routine.

The open method is accomplished by incising with scissors, or over a groove director, inserted into the lumen of the anal sac. Dissection of the duct and anal sac exposes the contents of the sac to the surrounding tissue but does not seem to be deleterious. Using a local excision and allowing the wound to heal by granulation are reported to be successful (Spira et al., 1971). The inherent resistance of this area to infection favors granulation, but the minimal time necessary for surgical closure of the wound assures healing and satisfies a sense of surgical aesthetics.

Cryosurgery has been advocated by some but seems to have met with little success.

DISEASES OF THE ANORECTUM

ANAL ULCERS (PERIANAL IRRITATION)

Infrequently, a disease of the anal and surrounding perianal area is encountered that is characterized by excessive irritation and inflammation that, if left untreated, may progress to ulceration of the skin surrounding the anal orifice (Fig. 64–10).

Perianal irritation appears to be most common in large breed dogs; the German shepherd and mixed breeds are most commonly affected. The etiology of the disease is unknown; however, chronic anal sacculitis or infection in the anal crypts may produce an irritation that results in severe pruritus

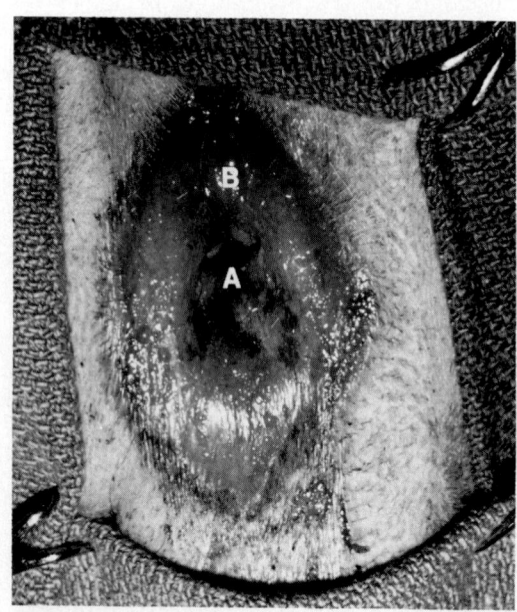

Figure 64–10. Perianal ulceration in a dog. Ulceration is characterized by severe pruritus with superficial ulceration of the skin. The area is usually markedly inflamed and quite painful. A, Anal orifice; B, ulcerated skin surrounding anal orifice.

of the anal areas, with trauma caused by resultant licking and rubbing of the area.

Treatment with antibiotic steroid ointments usually affords only temporary relief, and the irritated condition persists. Elevating the tail to prevent contact with the anal area and cauterizing with chemicals such as silver nitrate or electrocautery give the best results. Recurrence of this disease after treatment is not uncommon.

PERIANAL FISTULAS

Perianal fistulas (also called perianal sinus, perianal fissures, anal furunculosis, anusitis, and anorectal abscesses) are a specific disease of the canine, characterized by chronic, ulcerating fistulous tracts, together with a malodorous, purulent discharge around the anal orifice. The disease appears in the following breeds, listed in order of frequency of reported infection: the German shepherd, the Irish setter and English setter, and rarely, the Labrador and collie cross (Levene, 1968; Bloomberg, 1980). Perinanal fistulas may occur in the aged dog but appear most commonly in the middle-aged animal (Harvey, 1972). Although Lacroix and Lacroix (1945), Lewis (1968), and Palminteri (1968, 1969) report the disease to be more common in the male, recent reports indicate that it occurs in both sexes with approximately equal frequency (Borthwick, 1971; Harvey, 1972; Palminteri, 1974).

Etiology. Although the etiology of the disease is not clear, possible causes have been suggested. Minute fecoliths lodging in the anal crypts may cause necrosis and focal abscessation in the surrounding tissue, with inflammation and infection proceeding along the ducts of the circumanal glands, resulting in eventual exterior fistulation. Anal crypts are normal anatomic structures that are thought to be similar to the crypts of Morgagni in man, in whom they are thought to function as a valve of the anal canal (Netter, 1962). Lewis (1968) and Palminteri (1974) have suggested that the conformation of the German shepherd dog is a predisposing factor in the development of the disease, since the close proximity of the tail to the anus does not allow for proper ventilation of the anal area. Harvey (1972) postulates that the broad-based tail of the German shepherd and other affected breeds might result in a film of fecal materi-

al being spread over the perianal area, with abscesses and fistulas proceeding from infection of the sebaceous and tubular glands or hair follicles scattered throughout the cutaneous zone of the anus. The possibility of the disease being caused by infection spreading from abscessed anal glands has been reported by Lacroix and Lacroix (1945), Archibald and Horney (1975), and Lewis (1968). Harvey (1974), however, suggests that because of the low incidence of anal sac disease in the German shepherd there is probably no relationship.

Until detailed anatomic and pathologic studies of the anus and perianal area of the dogs affected with perianal fistulas and of clinically normal German shepherds are performed, the etiology of this condition will be speculative. The uncertainty of the etiology probably accounts for the number of treatments recommended for the disease, none of which seem to achieve a 100 per cent cure.

Clinical Signs. The outstanding clinical signs of perianal fistulas are tenesmus, constipation, and dyschezia, with frequent attempts to lick and bite the anal area. Occasionally, rectoanal hemorrhage will occur. The early signs will be mild. As the disease progresses, intermittent diarrhea, anorexia, and weight loss may occur. In severe cases, there will be a copious, offensive-smelling, mucopurulent discharge that may create considerable soiling around the tail and perianal area. A mild fecal incontinence may occur if the disease is advanced.

Direct observation of the perianal area will reveal the fistulous lesions, which vary according to the chronicity of the disease. Early in the disease only one or two fistulous openings located in the cutaneous hairless zone around the periphery of the anus may be seen, but as the disease progresses, the entire perianal area may become involved (Figs. 64–11 and 64–12).

Ulceration and necrosis of the skin surrounding the entire anus are common. The lesions usually extend two to five cm radially and further in severe cases. The fistulous tract may be seen extending deep into the tissue of the ischiorectal fossa and may contain hair and fecal material. Fibrous bands and necrotic tags of skin may connect the edges of the skin. Considerable amounts of granulation tissue are seen between the fibrous tracts. Often, a foul-smelling, mucopurulent discharge may be seen in the

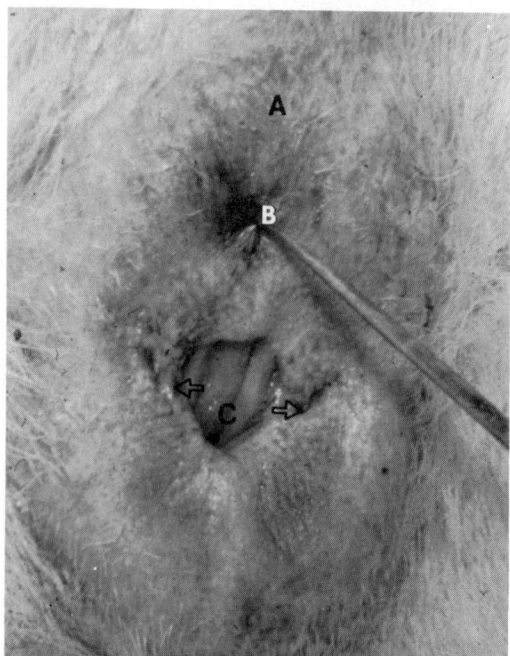

Figure 64–11. Perianal fistula early in the course of the disease. Only one fistulous opening is present. If untreated, the disease can progress to multiple fistulous openings that coalesce to form a large ulceration around the periphery of the anus. A, Base of tail; B, opening of fistulous tract; and C, anal orifice. Anal sac orifices are indicated by arrows.

deeper sinuses. Fibrous tissue around the anus will prevent easy dilatation of the anal orifice, and in some cases the opening will be strictured owing to excessive fibrosis. Fecal impaction may occur in the rectum as a result of the stenosis of the anal orifice. Rectal palpation will create considerable discomfort for the animal (Fig. 64–13).

Diagnosis. Although the diagnosis of perianal fistulas can usually be based on breed association, clinical signs, and the nature of the lesions, there are other disease conditions from which it must be differentiated. Chronic anal sac abscesses with resulting fistulous tracts may be confused with perianal fistulas, but these two disorders can usually be differentiated by following the sinus or tracts to the anal sacs and locating the sinus over the anal sac area. The massive ulceration that develops in perianal fistulas is absent in anal sac abscesses. Perianal adenocarcinomas will present lesions of fistulization and ulceration very similar to perianal fistulas; on palpation, however, the perianal gland tissue around the anus will be considerably thickened. In most cases, a biopsy is necessary to differentiate the two

diseases. Other anal neoplasms, perianal irritation, and ulcers will be less frequently confused with perianal fistulas. Biopsy specimens of the fistulas should be taken when the disease is treated surgically, because infrequently, the removed perianal fistulous tissue will show anaplastic changes.

Pathology. Grossly, the tissue immediately surrounding the anal area is composed of fistulous tracts and sinuses, with granulation tissue interspersed. The tracts radiate for some distance into the surrounding subcutaneous and muscular tissue and frequently into the external anal sphincter. Ulceration around the entire anus and rectum is common. Within the rectal lumen, tags of rectal mucosa are frequently seen one to three cm anterior to the anal orifice. The anal crypts are exaggerated, and frequently two or three cysts coalesce to form one large crypt.

Microscopically, the fistulous tracts are lined by chronic granulation tissue or stratified squamous epithelium. Within the tracts, there may be a purulent exudate containing hair and keratin. The perianal skin surrounding the area shows necrosis, and the tubuloalveolar glands and sebaceous glands in the perianal skin may show dilatation of the ducts, with the glands themselves surrounded by chronic inflammation (Harvey, 1972).

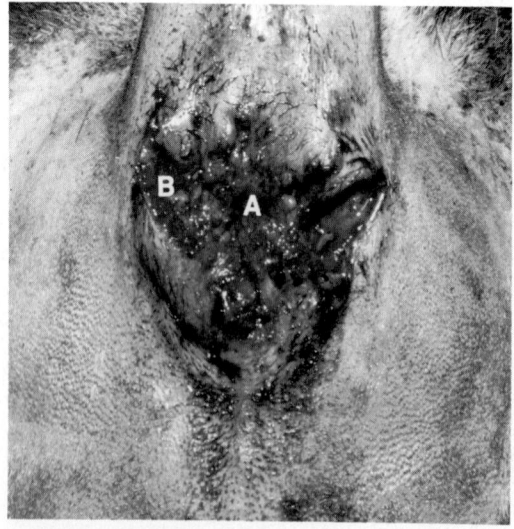

Figure 64–12. Perianal fistula in moderately advanced state. Fistulas have coalesced to form deep ulcerations with fibrous tissue formation. Disease frequently progresses to this stage before the animal is presented to the veterinarian. A, Anal orifice; B, ulcerated, fistulous perianal area.

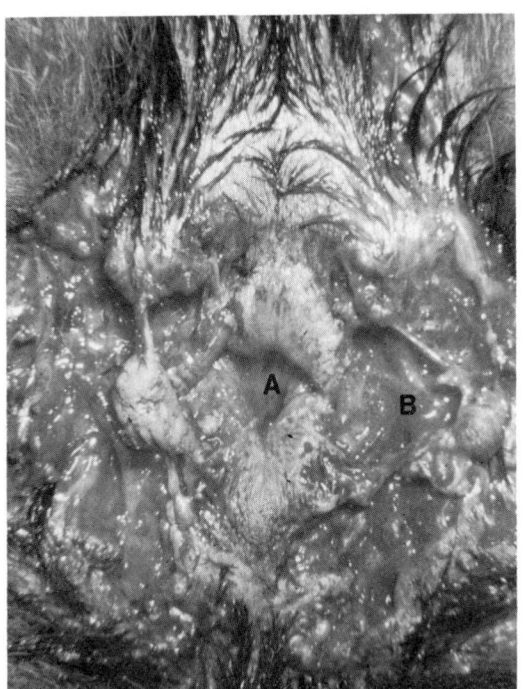

Figure 64–13. Perianal fistulas in severely advanced stage. Fistulous tracts extend well beyond anal orifice and deep into perianal tissues. At this stage, the external anal sphincter is frequently involved in the disease process. A, Anal orifice; B, coalesced fistulous tracts with severe fibrous tissue formation.

Treatment. Conservative treatment involving the application of topical ointments and systemic antibiotics is unrewarding. Successful treatment requires destruction or removal of the fistulous tracts and sinuses.

Surgical removal of the fistulas early in the course of the disease will avoid the complications associated with the more radical excisions that are necessary when the disease is at an advanced stage. If a major surgical procedure is contraindicated because of age or because of some coexisting problem that may subject the dog to unnecessary risk, the disease process may be controlled to ease the discomfort of the patient. Palminteri (1974) reports successful control, but not a cure, with the use of systemic antibiotics, laxatives, topical enzyme preparations, and opposite sex hormone therapy. These methods, along with regular nursing care and radiation therapy for the fistulas, will bring a temporary regression of the disease (Severin, 1968).

Shaffer and Block (1961) report success by lancing the anal crypts and the fistulous tracts to provide drainage. A speculum is inserted into the anus to facilitate location of the crypts. A bent probe is inserted into the crypt, and traction is applied to outline the crypt. The crypt is incised over the probe, and the incision is carried down to lance the fistulous tract. The two mucosal flaps of tissue created by the incision are excised, and the area is left to granulate. Failure of this surgical procedure results from incomplete lancing of the fistulous tracts. In the authors' experience, this lancing procedure is not successful in the more severe cases, in which fistulous tracts coalesce to form ulcerated areas around the anal area.

Cryosurgery has been successful in the treatment of fistulas but is not in widespread use at this time (Borthwick, 1971; Lane, 1975).

Complete excision of the fistulous tracts and all diseased tissue around the perianal area is the most successful treatment of perianal fistulas. The patient is fasted for 24 hours and given cleansing enemas at least three hours prior to surgery. Preoperative antibiotic therapy may be given but is not essential. Local excision of fistulous tracts is performed when possible, but when extensive involvement is present, a 360-degree excision of the perianal glands is necessary.

For the surgical procedure, the dog is placed on a well-padded stand in the perineal position. The surgical site is clipped, scrubbed, and draped. The initial incision is made at the periphery of the diseased skin and curved around the entire anal orifice as close to the anal opening as possible without entering necrotic skin. Sharp dissection with dissecting scissors directed radially to encompass all the fistulous tracts and granulation tissue is performed. When the depth of the fistulous tracts and abnormal tissue is reached, dissection is directed posteriorly toward the anal orifice. At this point, the external anal sphincter becomes visible. This structure should be preserved unless major fistulous tracts extend into it, in which case only the fistulous tracts are removed, preserving as much of the sphincter as possible. Anal sacs routinely should be removed at this stage of the procedure. Dissection then is carried posteriorly to the anal orifice and the diseased tissue excised. The diseased portion of the rectum is usually amputated to the normal tissue. A modification of this part of the procedure involves removing only the mucosa of the diseased rectum. Maintenance of fecal continence is enhanced by preserving the posterior quarter of the rectal wall.

The only major vessels and nerves encountered during the surgical procedure are the cranial and caudal rectal arteries and the caudal rectal nerve. The caudal and cranial rectal arteries are located close to the rectum on its dorsal and ventral surfaces. The caudal rectal nerve, which is the sole motor nerve supply to the external anal sphincter, is located at the anterior surface of the external anal sphincter, lying close to the rectum on the ventrolateral aspect. This structure is hard to identify, but the surgeon should be aware of its presence.

After removal of all of the diseased tissue, the anorectal area is irrigated with an antiseptic solution, and subcutaneous sutures are placed through the subcutis of the skin and into, but not through, the posterior rectal wall, excluding the anal sphincter. Through-and-through sutures are placed in the skin and rectum to achieve rectocutaneous anastomosis.

It is essential to remove at least the major portion of the fistulous tracts or the disease will recur. If the fistulous tracts extend so far that sharp excision is impossible without severe disruption of the normal anatomy, the fistulas may be cauterized with electrocautery to sear the fistulous tissue. Recent experimentation with an argon laser to remove the fistulous tracts has shown excellent results. With the laser, the diseased tissue is desiccated, and a rectocutaneous anastomosis is performed.

Postoperatively, systemic antibiotics should be administered for one week. Tetracycline or penicillin-streptomycin combination is preferred by the authors. If necessary, an Elizabethan collar is placed on the animal for seven to ten days to prevent self-mutilation. Food is withheld for 24 hours, and the animal is maintained on fluid therapy. A highly digestible, low-carbohydrate, and low-residue diet is given on the second postoperative day to reduce bulk and flatulence postsurgically. If the animal exhibits considerable discomfort upon handling or is extremely apprehensive, no attempt is made to raise the tail to observe the incision until the third postoperative day. Tension on the incision line should be avoided. Diarrhea frequently occurs immediately after surgery and is controlled with antispasmodics. Although it is not essential, the authors prefer hospitalization of the patient for four to seven days. If perianal fistulas recur, it is necessary to excise the involved tissue.

Complications. The major immediate postoperative complication is wound dehiscence. This usually occurs on approximately the third postoperative day and may then be resutured with only minimal debridement. Fecal incontinence, ranging from an occasional accident to severe constant dribbling of stool, is the primary postoperative complaint. The main cause of incontinence is removal or destruction of the external anal sphincter during the surgical excision of the fistulous tissue. Removal of too much of the posterior rectum will also create incontinence, but this may be partially avoided by resection of the diseased mucosa, leaving only the rectal wall.

Anal strictures forming a fibrous ring around the rectocutaneous anastomosis may occur as healing progresses. This is treated by making four to six small incisions equidistant around the circumference of the fibrous ring, and then dilating the ring by inserting two or three fingers into the rectum or by using a vaginal speculum or one of the various bougienages. The torn rectal mucosa is sutured to the skin at right angles to where it was torn, using 2–0 chromic catgut.

RECTAL DEVIATION AND RECTAL DIVERTICULUM

Deviation or sacculation of the rectum is usually seen in male animals over six years of age. It is often associated with relaxation of the pelvic diaphragm and formation of a perineal hernia. The rectum deviates laterally, forming a flexure and causing subsequent impaction of feces (Archibald and Horney, 1975). (Perineal hernia will not be dealt with specifically in this chapter, except as it relates to the rectum.) The degree of rectal deviation can vary from slight distortion to obvious convolution or gross sacculation. The deviation is thought to result from unproductive straining that forces the lower bowel into an enlarged pelvic space (Lewis, 1968). The disorder has been noted in German shepherd, Doberman pinschers, Boston terriers, bulldogs, and Pekingese (Palminteri, 1969; Greiner, 1972).

Rectal diverticulum is usually related to some form of trauma that causes a rupture in the smooth muscle of the rectal wall. This rupture may be a subtle change that is difficult to palpate, but it usually can be demonstrated histologically. The disorder may be related to conformation or a hereditary, primary weakening in the external anal sphincter and levator ani muscle (Lewis, 1968).

The symptoms of both rectal deviation and rectal diverticulum are tenesmus and a noticeable bulge lateral to the rectum, caused by the accumulation of feces (Archibald and Horney, 1975; Lewis, 1968; Palminteri, 1969). If the rectal examination reveals a flaw in the muscular coat, the diagnosis is rectal diverticulum. If the muscle wall is intact, the condition is more likely to be a rectal deviation (sacculation) in association with a perineal hernia (Lewis, 1968).

These conditions are the manifestations of tenesmus, which is secondary to the primary cause of the disorder. The differential diagnosis must include other possible causes of tenesmus, such as perineal hernia, tumors obstructing the pelvic canal, previous trauma, benign prostatic hypertrophy, and chronic constipation. If a rectal deviation or diverticulum is not present, the contents of a perineal hernia may include the bladder, uterus, periprostatic fat, or the small intestine (Barchfeld, 1970).

Correction of both lesions is usually surgical. Castration was thought to favorably influence a gradual recovery of normal tonus of the pelvic diaphragm and is indicated if benign prostatic hypertrophy is present. Although some reports do not advocate castration, the authors recommend it when the condition occurs in conjunction with a perianal hernia (Burrows and Harvey, 1973). A low-residue diet and stool softener will be beneficial, particularly in an older, debilitated animal that is not a good candidate for surgery (Archibald and Horney, 1975; Palminteri, 1969). If a perineal hernia is present, repair will resolve the deviation. If the defect is due to a diverticulum, it may be possible to use imbricating sutures to close the defect. However, it is often necessary to excise the weakened area and perform an inverting closure to maintain the rectal wall (Palminteri, 1969).

RECTAL STRICTURE

Rectal strictures have been noted in German shepherds, beagles, and poodles. Anorectal abscesses, perianal fistulas, trauma, and chronic anal sac disease predispose an animal to rectal strictures. This condition is also a complication of rectal surgery, particularly perianal fistula excision. The clinical signs are tenesmus, dyschezia, thin stools, and hematochezia (Palminteri, 1969).

Diagnosis of rectal strictures is based on palpation of a firm constricting bowel during rectal examination. When the stricture is cranial, contrast radiography can be used to determine the extent of the lesion (Greiner, 1972). The lesions may be anular and may vary in length from short to several inches long (Lewis, 1968). This lesion should not be confused with spastic colon. Palpation will reveal a consistently firm, inelastic, fibrous area of tissue that does not relax when the patient is anesthetized.

Mild cases may respond to bougienage and dilatation (Archibald and Horney, 1975; Lewis, 1968; Palminteri, 1969; Greiner, 1972; Rodkey, 1973). If these methods are not satisfactory, surgery is required. A myotomy can be done (Archibald and Horney, 1975; Greiner, 1972). Fibrotic rings of tissue near the anal orifice should be resected. The lesions are seldom extensive enough to require a pull-through procedure for correction (Swenson and Bill, 1948).

NEOPLASMS OF THE ANORECTUM

POLYPS

Rectal polyps are infrequent in the dog. One study showed similar incidence in males (7/17) and females (9/17), with a mean age of 6.9 years (range 1.5 to 12 years) and a higher prevalence in the collie breed (Seiler, 1979). A typical history includes tenesmus preceding defecation and a chronic diarrhea unresponsive to treatment (Palminteri, 1966, Greiner, 1972). Stools are bloody or mucoid. Clinical signs demonstrated during the general physical examination are generally normal, but palpation per rectum is usually diagnostic. The polypoid masses are friable, with surface ulceration, bleed easily, and often are visible with slight digital eversion of the rectum (Fig. 64–14). If no masses are palpated, anoscopic or proctoscopic examination should be done. Air-insufflation or double-contrast radiography often outlines these lesions clearly (Fig. 64–15).

Grossly, the masses appear as lobulated, grape-like clusters with a pedunculated or

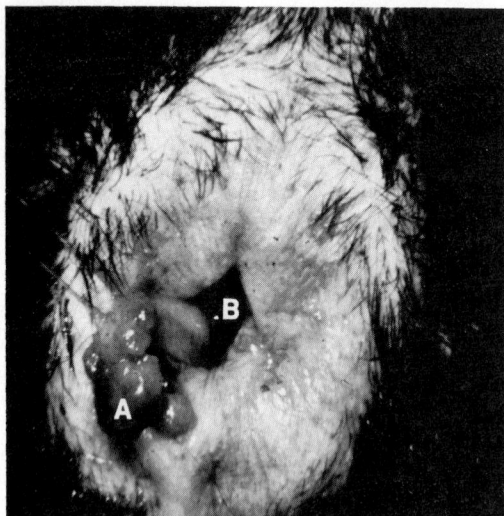

Figure 64–14. Rectal polyp (A) everted through anal orifice (B). Polyps can occur throughout entire colorectal area. Polypoid masses located near anal orifice can be removed from exterior by ligation at peduncle.

sessile base. They are deep red to purplish in color and vary from one to many in number and from a few millimeters to several centimeters in diameter (Fig. 64–16).

Histologically, the outer epithelial layer is continuous with the epithelium of the bowel, and the inner portion of the polypoid stalk continues into the fibrous tissue of the submucosa (Greiner, 1972). There may be foci of epithelial atypia, and carcinomatous colorectal polyps have been observed (Silverberg, 1971; Greiner, 1972; Seiler, 1979). One case of malignant lymphoma has been reported in the dog (Palminteri, 1969).

Surgical excision of rectal polyps is the recommended treatment. A rectal approach is satisfactory for pedunculated masses near the anal orifice. Pedicle ligation is sufficient for small polyps, but if the stalk is large, the clamp should be oversewn. Anoscopy is used to define polyps that are further than two cm into the rectum, before they are excised with pedicle ligation, electrocautery, or a tonsil snare (Palminteri, 1966, 1969; Greiner, 1972). A laparotomy and colotomy are necessary for the removal of polyps in the anterior rectum, and proper precaution must be taken to prepare the bowel for surgery and to prevent contamination.

In most cases, polypectomy is followed by

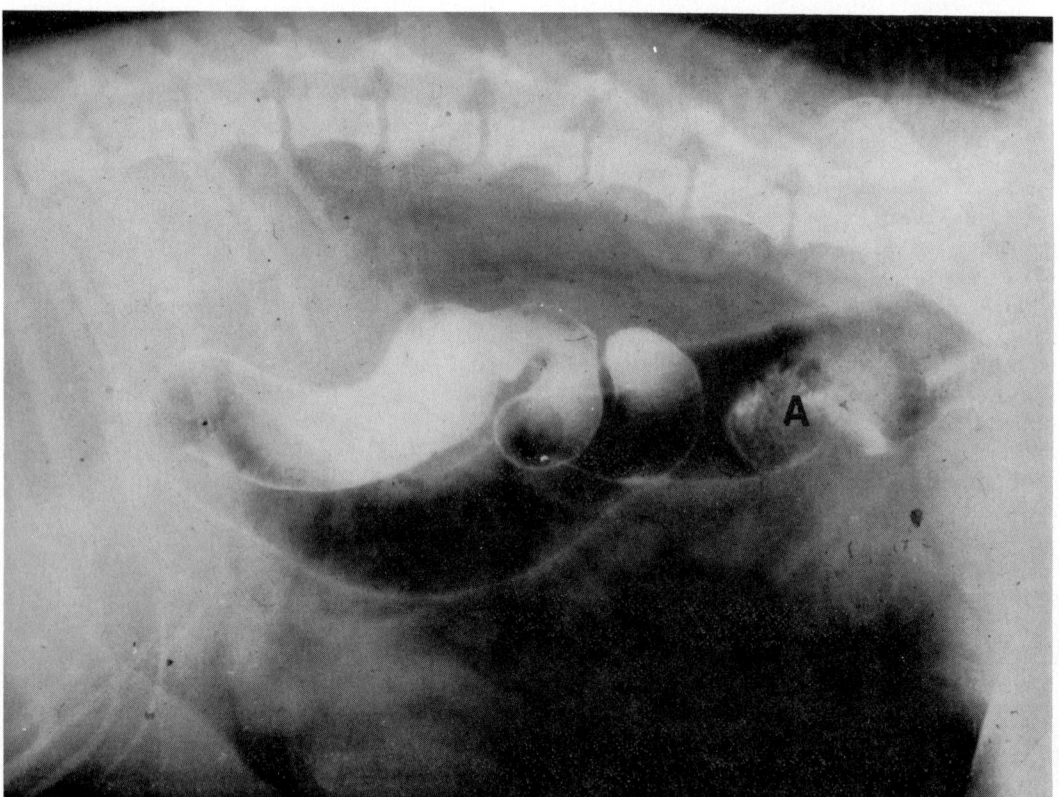

Figure 64–15. Lateral radiograph using double contrast technique to outline mass at anterior rectum. A, Polyp located at anterior rectum. Lesion located in this region is best removed by colotomy.

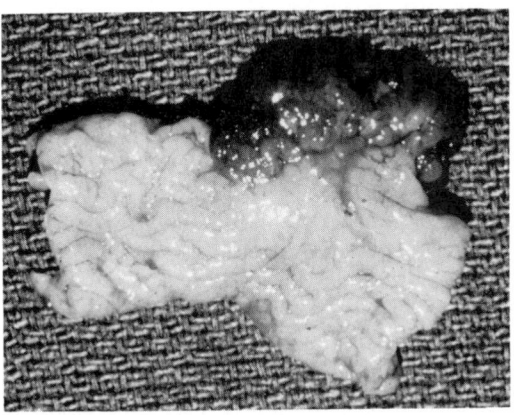

Figure 64–16. Colorectal polyp excised from anterior part of rectum. Note grape-like cluster growth that is characteristic of the lesion. Mass is friable and hemorrhages easily.

clinical recovery and lengthy survival times; the possibility of recurrence or of neoplastic invasion should be considered, however, and care should be taken to provide biopsy material to rule out carcinomatous lesions of the rectal region (Seiler, 1979). Polyp size is currently regarded as an indication of malignant potential in human rectal and colonic polyps, and polyps greater than one cm in

diameter have a higher potential for malignancy. Intraepithelial carcinomatous change or malignant transformation has been reported in rectal polyps of dogs (Lungeman, 1972; Shaffer and Schieffer, Silverberg, 1971), and in one study carcinoma in situ was diagnosed in 5 of 17 dogs with rectal polyps (Seiler, 1979).

RECTAL AND ANAL CARCINOMA

Intestinal carcinomas are uncommon; when they do occur, however, colorectal and anal involvement is most frequently seen (Moulton, 1961; Jubb and Kennedy, 1963; Archibald and Horney, 1975; Patnaik, 1977). The anal canal is an area prone to metaplasia, which can ultimately become some form of epidermoid carcinoma (Brennan and Stewart, 1972). In dogs, these neoplasms generally are epithelial in origin (Archibald and Horney, 1975).

Rectal neoplasms are adenocarcinomas of an infiltrative, ulcerative, or proliferative nature (Levene, 1968; Severin, 1968). The infiltrative lesions spread within the wall of the rectum, and an associated fibrosis with resultant stricture is often seen (Fig. 64–17).

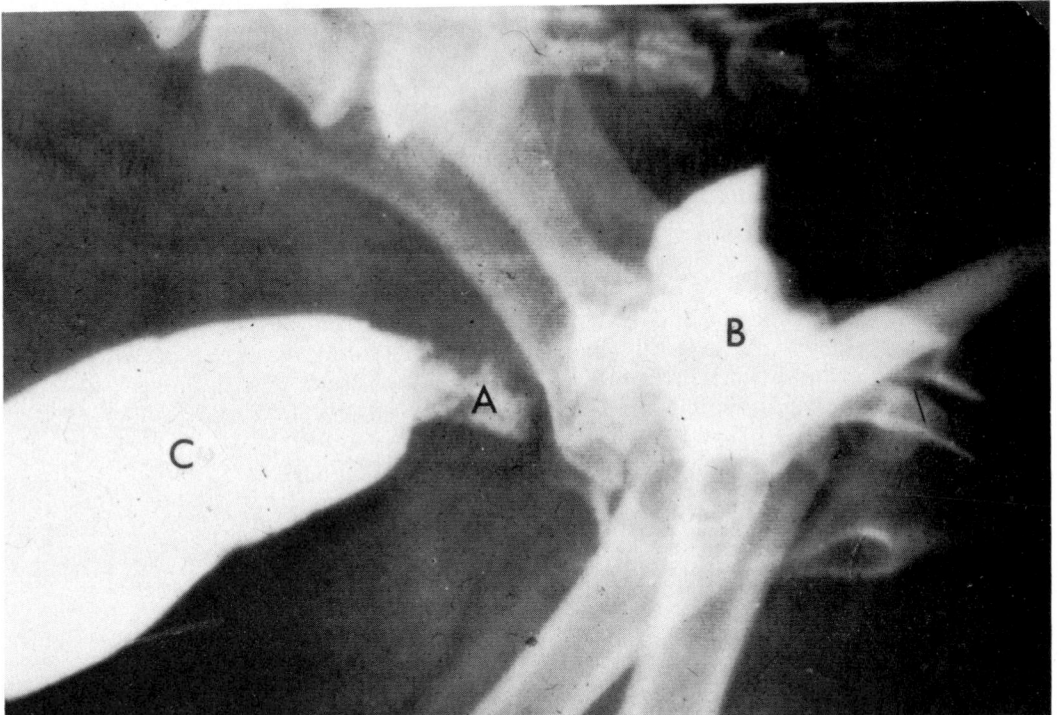

Figure 64–17. Lateral radiograph of colon and rectum, using barium as a contrast medium to demonstrate grossly infiltrative-type adenocarcinoma of rectum and posterior colon. A, Stricture created by infiltration of neoplasm into wall of rectum with resultant fibrosis and narrowing of rectocolonic lumen; B, rectum; and C, colon.

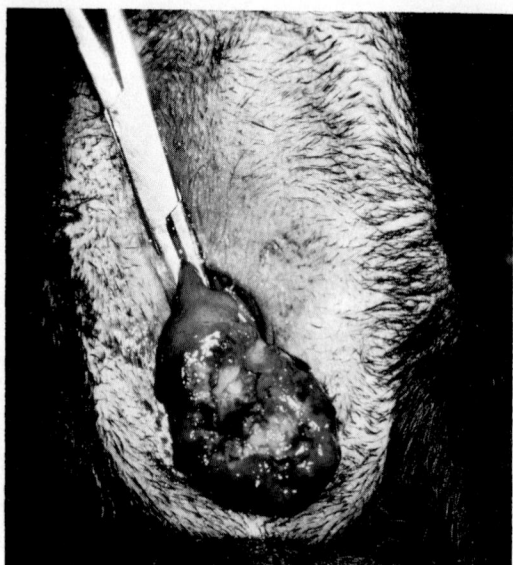

Figure 64–18. Malignant ulcerative adenocarcinoma of rectum exposed through anal orifice. This type of adenocarcinoma is characterized grossly by having raised edges with a denuded, ulcerative surface.

Malignant ulcerative lesions are characterized by a hard, raised edge and a raw or denuded surface (Fig. 64–18). In contrast, proliferative lesions often appear warty (Levene, 1968) (Fig. 64–19). To some degree, all three conditions may be present simultaneously. These tumors are usually slow growing and may be present for months or even years before causing problems. Unfortunately, local or systemic metastasis may have become extensive by the time the animal is presented.

In a 12-year period, 14 rectal carcinomas were confirmed histologically out of 12,456 necropsies and surgical specimens. In addition, one polypous adenoma and six mesenchymal tumors were diagnosed. There was lymphatic or venous metastasis in 9 of the 14 cases (Shaffer and Schieffer, 1968).

Adenocarcinomas with mucin production (Lassoie and Hennan, 1971; Greiner, 1972; Josen et al., 1972) are usually more prevalent than scirrhous carcinomas and undifferentiated carcinomas. Clinical evaluation of malignancy is based on the actual extent of the spread of the tumor by metastasis or local invasion, and histologic evaluation is based on whether the tumor is well differentiated, anaplastic, or poorly differentiated (Levene, 1968).

Squamous cell carcinoma seldom occurs in a mucous membrane; if it does occur, it usually originates within the anal region (Shaffer and Schieffer, 1968) (Fig. 64–20). Usually, these tumors have a typical ulcerated appearance and irregular edges. They metastasize to the regional lymph nodes and may be effectively removed by early, radical excision (Levene, 1968; Greiner, 1972). Occasionally, this lesion is confused with perianal fistulas.

Malignant melanoma occasionally involves the anus, especially in the breeds with heavily pigmented skin. Clinically, any ulcerated, black lesion in the anal area should be considered a malignant melanoma until disproved by biopsy. The gross apperance of the lesion can be misleading, since the color of the lesion can vary from black to gray to white, depending on the amount of melanin present (Levene, 1968). Amelanotic melanomas are frequently difficult to diagnose on routine histopathologic examination, but electron microscopy may provide a definitive diagnosis. These lesions are highly malignant, and the tumor tends to metastasize early (Greiner, 1972). Only a radical excision justifies surgery, since surgical prognosis is very poor. In most cases, surgical or medical therapy is futile.

Perianal adenomas are some of the most common tumors encountered in dogs. Perianal adenocarcinoma is far less com-

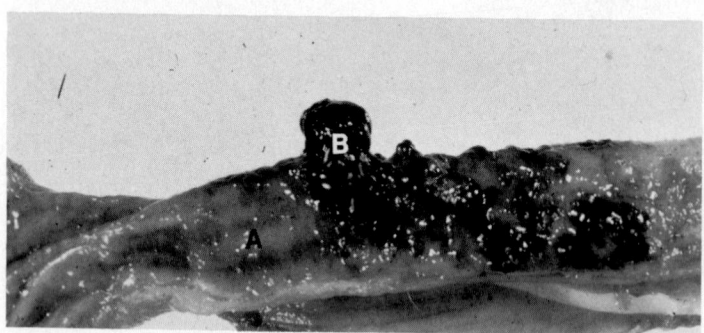

Figure 64–19. Necropsy specimen of rectal muscle longitudinally illustrating gross appearance of proliferative-type adenocarcinoma of rectum and colon. A, Normal rectal mucosa; B, neoplastic growths giving mucosa a warty appearance.

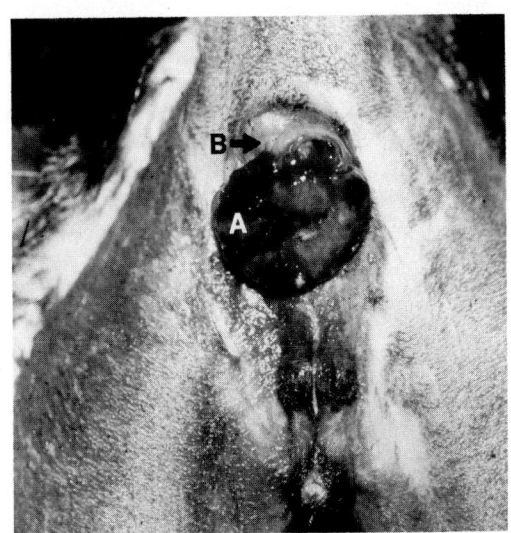

Figure 64–20. Squamous cell carcinoma of anus in a cat. The exposed surface of this type of tumor has a typically ulcerated appearance. Neoplasm (A) partially overlies anal orifice (B).

mon, and metastasis is rare (Wilson and Brown, 1964; Greiner, 1972). Ulceration and fistulization with suppuration are commonly associated with perianal adenocarcinoma, and the condition should be differentiated from circumanal fistulas (Greiner, 1972) (Fig. 64–21). Rectal palpation may reveal a thickened anal ring. Early resection of the anal ring may be successful in preventing spread of the tumor to regional lymph nodes. The prognosis is fair if the tumors are small and are excised early.

Anal gland adenocarcinomas seldom occur and are without breed predilection. Clinical symptoms reflect obstruction of the anal canal. Early radical resection may effect a cure, but metastasis usually occurs prior to the diagnosis, making the surgical prognosis guarded to poor (Greiner, 1972).

Prior to surgical excision, any suspicious lesions should be biopsied as part of a complete work-up. The gross appearance of anorectal neoplasms may be misleading, but histopathologic evaluation can often aid in deciding the best mode of treatment, as well as in providing an accurate prognosis. All excisional biopsies should also be examined. Local tissue invasion can be evaluated, as can the success of the surgery with respect to the primary site.

Orifices that provide a portal of entry into the body seem to possess an inherent capacity to resist infection that is superior to that of other areas of the body. Occasionally, this

strong resistance to infection will be reflected in a tumor specimen. If, on histologic examination, the surrounding tissue seems to be walling off the offending neoplasm (as indicated by the presence of large numbers of plasma cells), the surgical prognosis is better. This form of resistance to infection may reflect an immune-mediated phenomenon, and small islands of tumor tissue not removed will probably remain (Levene, 1968).

Treatment of anorectal neoplasms in animals and human beings is difficult and unrewarding. In man, epidermoid or cloacogenic carcinoma is a common lesion. Abdominoperineal resection is the treatment of choice, and a 37 per cent, five-year survival rate can be expected. Whether or not a local excision will be sufficient is determined by the location, size, depth, and aggressiveness of the tumor (Brennan and Stewart, 1972).

Some anorectal tumors are radioresponsive. A two-year cure rate of 69 per cent for perianal tumors, 74 per cent for squamous cell carcinomas, 56 per cent for fibrosarcomas, and 54 per cent for mast-cell tumors has been reported. Perianal tumors had an ultimate rate of recurrence of 32 per cent. Combination chemotherapy, radiotherapy, and surgery has been suggested as a mode of therapy, with good response in the human literature (Sischy et al., 1980).

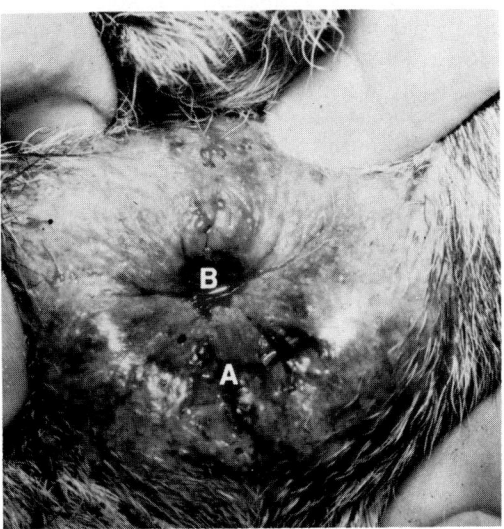

Figure 64–21. Perianal gland adenocarcinoma involving the hairless portion of the anus. Ulceration and fistulization are typical of this neoplasm, which must be differentiated from perianal fistulas. Fistulous openings (A) around anal orifice (B).

The size and location of a tumor are important factors in determining radiocurability. The possibility of successful treatment lessens as tumor size increases. Ionizing radiation effectively kills rapidly dividing cells, but occasionally cancer cells may divide more slowly than proliferating cells of normal tissue (Gillette, 1970).

Surgical excision of the tumor may be successful if it is done early and if metastasis has not occurred. When possible, a wide excision should be made. Although the vascular system of the pelvic organs has a high plasticity and adaptability to disturbance of blood supply (Minin, 1968), one should attempt to preserve the normal anatomy as much as possible.

In order to satisfactorily remove sufficient tissue in rectal tumor resection, the involved segment of bowel may have to be removed and an anastomosis performed. If the lesion is caudal, it may be possible to evert the mass through the anus for excision. If a resection is preferred, one should mobilize the anorectum, amputate the involved rectum and anus, and anastomose the remaining rectum to the skin.

A pull-through procedure can be used to remove more cranial lesions. This requires a coordinated effort, preferably by at least two surgeons, and involves a laparotomy as well as the exteriorized anastomosis. In man, this procedure is also successful in treating congenital megacolon (Hirschsprung's disease). The authors have successfully used this procedure in selected cases, and the surgical technique is well described in the literature (Swenson and Bill, 1948; Archibald and Horney, 1975). Successful ileorectal anastomoses were performed on 42 dogs. Twelve to 15 months following total colectomy, the mucosa of the ileum was similar morphologically to the large intestine and performed colonic functions (Bokeria and Ekhiskelashvili, 1969).

The success of bowel surgery depends on many factors. Absolute asepsis is essential. Secondary bacterial invasion from direct contamination or leakage of the surgical incision can be devastating (Dencker et al., 1969). Absolute requirements for successful anastomosis include healthy bowel margins, good blood supply, absence of tension, and accurate placement of sutures to ensure a watertight seal. Anastomotic leakage during surgery is increased in older patients and in anemic patients. Preexisting infection, intraoperative transfusions, extraperitoneal anastomoses, and the lengthy duration of the operation all adversely affect the anastomotic success rate. The use of glucocorticoids does impair synthesis of collagen in cutaneous wounds and, by inference, in gastrointestinal wounds. In man, anastomosis to the rectum has a reputation for frequent breakdown of poor blood supply and exclusion from the peritoneal cavity (Shrock et al., 1973).

PERIANAL GLAND ADENOMA

Perianal gland adenomas are unique to the dog and are commonly encountered; in the male they are the third most frequently diagnosed tumor. They are usually seen in male dogs over seven years of age and occur less often in younger animals and females (Levene, 1968; Greiner, 1972). Oophorectomized females have a higher incidence of such tumors (three times the risk) than do intact females (Baker, 1967; Ellis, 1968; Levene, 1968; Wilson, 1979), and the intact male dog has 12 times the risk of the intact female. An excessive risk has been noted in both sexes of the cocker spaniel breed and male dogs of the English bulldog, Samoyed, and beagle breeds (Hayes and Wilson, 1977).

Perianal adenomas can be found at almost any site near the perineum or genitalia but usually grow in the skin surrounding the anus (Fig. 64–22). These glands continue to grow throughout the life of an unaltered male until senility. Prior to cessation of growth, cystic degeneration (but no atrophy) may be seen in the glands. Perianal glands should not be confused with the anal sacs or small clusters of glands immediately around the anus. The perianal glands surround the anus in an irregular circle at the mucocutaneous junction. They consist of a major hepatoid glandular element, plus a minor sebaceous element. They develop as buds from compound hair follicles and enlarge rapidly after birth (Baker, 1967; Severin, 1968; Isitor, 1979).

The glandular cells contain nonproteinaceous, nonlipid granules. It is suggested that the perianal glands are endocrine in nature and that the secretory granules are passed into surrounding vessels. Initially, these glands are under the control of the *pars distalis* of the pituitary gland. After puberty, the gonads exert a controlling influence on the perianal glands in the male, and androgen secretion from the adrenal cortex is

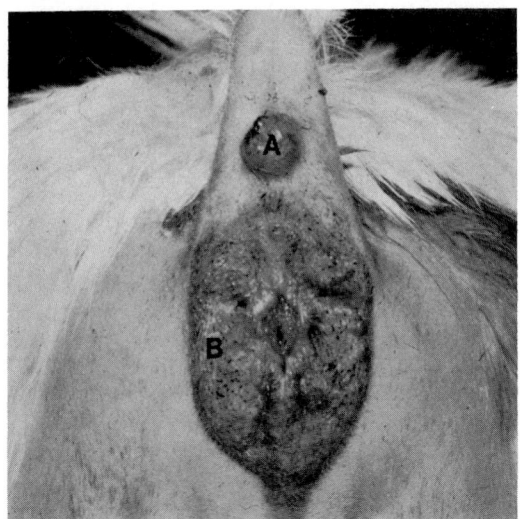

Figure 64–22. Typical appearance of perianal adenoma (A) located on base of tail. Hypertrophy of circumanal glands (B) surrounding anal orifice. These neoplasms are most frequently seen in the area immediately surrounding the anal orifice but may occur on the tail and in the prepuce in the male.

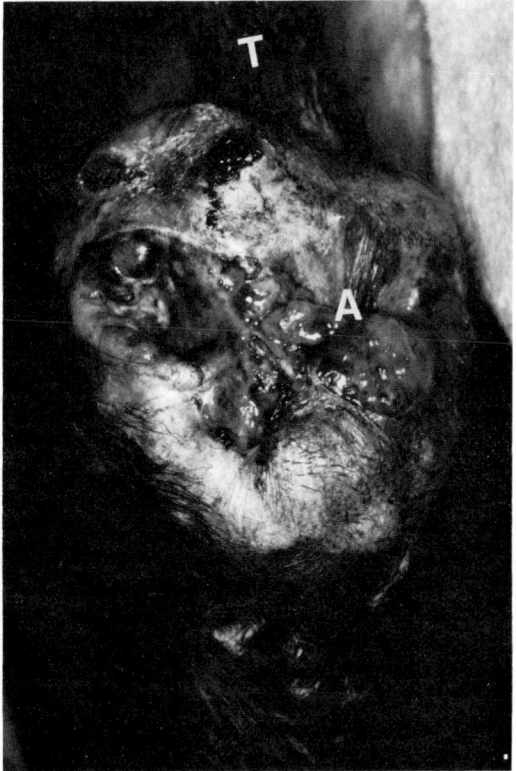

Figure 64–23. Appearance of extensive perianal gland adenoma treated only by castration (also see Fig. 64–24). Note the extensive ulceration lateral to anal orifice (A) and ventral to the tail (T). (Photo courtesy of Dr. Lloyd Prashum, Lake Shore Animal Hospital, Chicago, IL.)

the controlling factor in the female. There may be an associated glandular protective function involving sebum production to prevent soiling of the hairless area immediately around the anus (Baker, 1967). Histologically, the cell clusters resemble liver lobules with a hematoxylin and eosin stain, hence the term *hepatoid circumanal glands* (Baker, 1967; Levene, 1968).

Perianal gland tumors begin as small, firm nodules but can become quite large, maintaining an intact skin covering. They frequently ulcerate and necrose, and may hemorrhage enough when abraded to cause owner concern (Severin, 1968). Preoperative diagnosis is easily confirmed by aspiration biopsy and histopathologic evaluation. Malignancy is rare and metastasis infrequent (Wilson and Brown, 1964; Baker, 1967).

Perianal gland tumors are hormone dependent and estrogen sensitive (Levene, 1968; Evans, 1975). Early suppression of tumor growth, and in some cases regression in tumor size, can be achieved through estrogen therapy. There is some preliminary laboratory evidence indicating that the addition of some estrogens to tissue cultures of cancer cells has an inhibiting effect on cell growth (Burch and Vaughn, 1973). The authors feel that this should be an interim therapy only. The results of estrogen treatment are not completely reliable, and therapy is not without side effects, including bone marrow suppressing effects, anemia, vascular pancytopenia, and thrombocytopenia (Lowenstine, 1972).

Perianal adenomas are also radioresponsive. A cure rate of 69 per cent was reported in one study (Gillette, 1970). Some authors have advocated cryosurgery as a means of treatment. Liska and Withrow (1978) reported good success in the cryosurgical removal in 42 dogs. Postoperative complications were minimal and occurred in only two dogs.

Many small and some large tumors may regress completely with castration alone (see Figs. 64–23 and 64–24). Castration decreases the probability that new tumors will develop and can be performed at the time of radiation therapy or surgical excision (Severin, 1968). Wilson found that out of 123 dogs treated by castration, only five developed another adenoma and only one

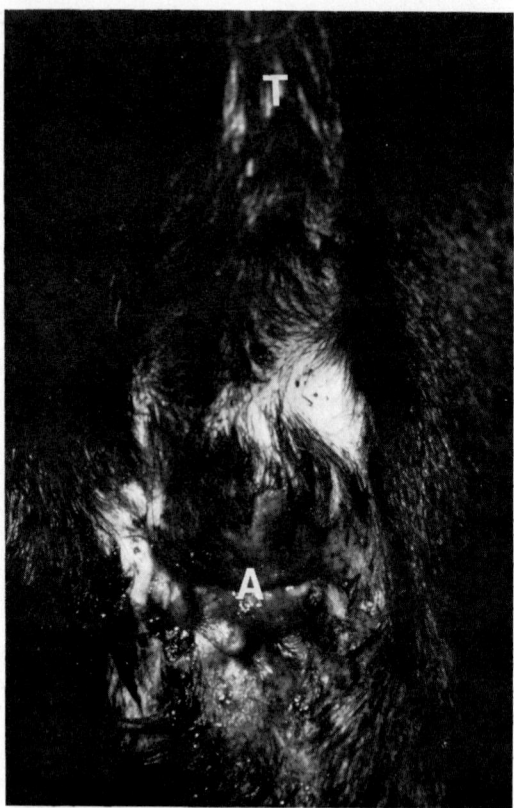

Figure 64–24. Same tumor pictured in Fig. 64–23, six months after castration. Tumor regressed and anal region was normal in appearance. Orientation, tail (T) and anal orifice (A).

developed a carcinoma. If castration of the pet is aesthetically displeasing to the owner, estrogen therapy can be used instead. The authors prefer surgical excision with castration, if feasible, and the prognosis is generally good (Baker, 1967; Ellis, 1968; Levene, 1968; Severin, 1968; Greiner, 1972). Between 10 per cent and 20 per cent of the tumors are malignant (Wilson, 1979), however; therefore biopsy specimens should always be submitted for histopathology.

ANORECTAL TRAUMA

Injuries of the anorectum resulting from bite wounds and automobile accidents are occasionally encountered. These may vary from mild puncture wounds to severe disruption of the anatomy of the anorectal area, including perforation of the rectum and severance of the external anal sphincter. A thorough examination of the area, as well as the animal, should be performed. The injured area may appear to have lost its innervation, with the anus dilated and flaccid and with loss of sensation to the skin immediately surrounding the area. Care should be taken not to overlook a fractured spine, as it may create similar symptoms.

The traumatized area should be cleaned and irrigated with an antiseptic solution, and debridement of the devitalized tissue should be performed. After debridement of the wound edges, lacerations in the rectum can be sutured with chromic catgut in a simple interrupted pattern. If the external anal sphincter is severed, an attempt should be made to suture it. Healing of the structure usually results. The skin and subcutaneous tissue should be debrided and sutured, and good drainage should be provided. Systemic antibiotics should be given postoperatively. Normal tone and sensation usually returns to the anal area in two to three days, provided severe nerve destruction has not occurred.

CONSTIPATION

Some of the possible causes of constipation are an improper diet, pica, benign prostatic hypertrophy, and an inadequate pelvic canal. Obstipation results when evacuation of feces is no longer possible. The primary clinical sign of constipation is tenesmus.

Mild cases of constipation can be treated sucessfully with warm water enemas. A stool softener added to the water will facilitate elimination. More severe cases will require anesthesia or heavy sedation to permit manual extraction of the fecal mass. Sponge forceps enable the doctor to selectively break down and remove the fecal material. Insertion of water into the rectum through a hose should be done very cautiously, especially in cats, since it is not difficult to penetrate the rectal wall.

An unusual cause of constipation is seen occasionally in Boston terriers and English bulldogs, when the screwtail grows into or presses on the anal region. The associated discomfort and mechanical impairment of defecation can result in fecal retention. Surgical amputation of the impeding part solves the problem.

DISEASES OF THE RECTUM

PROCTITIS

Proctitis is characterized by inflammation of the rectum and may be caused by a variety of conditions, the most common of which is rectal foreign bodies. A number of types of foreign bodies, such as needles, bones, and various other sharp objects, can traverse the entire alimentary canal and lodge in the rectum.

Certain infectious diseases of the alimentary tract may produce inflammation in the rectum, but the lesions of these diseases are usually more evident in other parts of the gastrointestinal tract, and the clinical signs are referable to these other regions.

The clinical signs of proctitis are characterized by an unproductive tenesmus. Digital rectal examination will reveal the lesions. The mucosa often will be quite hyperemic and thickened.

Treatment of proctitis is aimed at eliminating the cause while providing symptomatic relief through soothing enemas with coating agents and other anti-inflammatory products.

RECTAL PROLAPSE

Rectal prolapse is a condition in which one or more layers of the rectum protrude from the anal orifice. The severity of the prolapse depends upon the part or parts of the rectum that are prolapsed. Prolapses are classified as incomplete and complete. In incomplete prolapse, only the rectal mucosa

protrudes (Fig. 64–25), whereas in complete prolapse (also called procidentia), all layers of the rectum are involved (Fig. 64–26). Occasionally, a portion of the lining of the anal canal also prolapses. Rectal prolapse results from a variety of causes, and there are certain predisposing factors. Defects in the supporting structures of the anorectum could conceivably be produced by tenesmus or strangury associated with chronic constipation and urinary tract infections. Any mechanical interference with the external anal sphincter, such as disruption of its nerve supply (which might occur during repair of a perineal hernia), will predispose to rectal prolapse.

In incomplete prolapse, only the mucosa protrudes. It is most often associated with severe diarrhea in the young animal. Soiling of the perianal area and severe enteritis create considerable tenesmus and resultant prolapse of the mucosa. Foreign bodies — such as needles or bones — lodged in the rectum may also be associated with marked

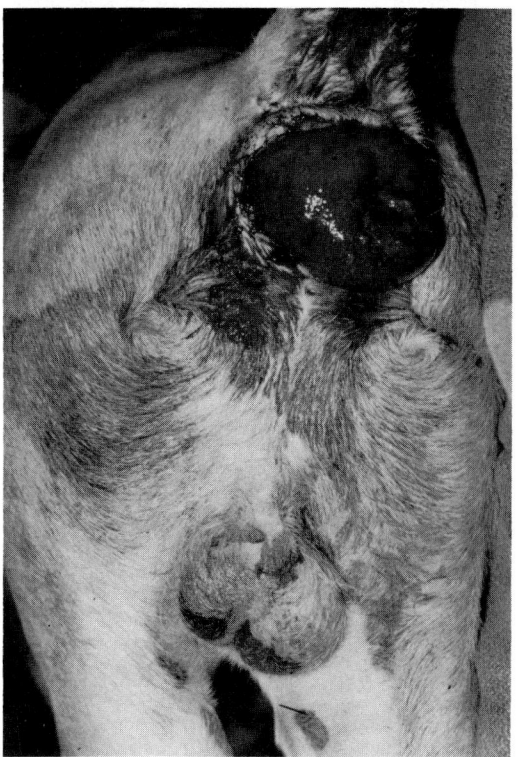

Figure 64–26. Complete rectal prolapse (procidentia). All layers of rectum are prolapsed through anal orifice. This condition must be differentiated from an incomplete rectal prolapse and an ileocolic intussusception in which the ileum has prolapsed through the anal orifice.

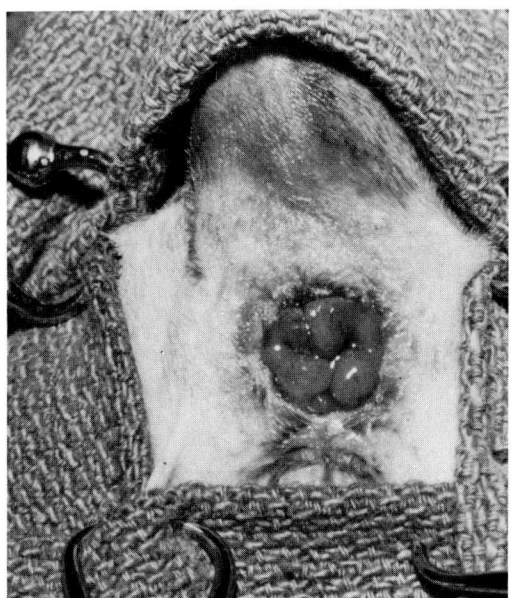

Figure 64–25. Incomplete rectal prolapse. This is differentiated from complete prolapse in which all the layers of the rectum are prolapsed through the anal orifice.

tenesmus, leading to an incomplete prolapse. Diseases of the genitourinary tract that lead to severe tenesmus, such as urethral obstruction, prostatic disease, and dystocia, are more often responsible for a complete prolapse.

There appears to be no age or sex predilection, although some breeds may be predisposed by a congenital weakness of the anal sphincter (Archibald and Horney, 1975).

Clinical Signs. The clinical signs associated with prolapse of the rectum are usually quite evident. The presence of an elongated, cylindric mass protruding from the anal orifice is usually diagnostic. However, this protrusion must be carefully differentiated from the protrusion of a portion of the ileum that can occur as a result of an ileocolic intussusception. Differentiation can be made by passing a blunt instrument or a finger between the prolapsed mass and the inner rectal wall. In rectal prolapse, a fornix can be felt between the prolapsed mass and the anal orifice. The intussusception can be demonstrated also by contrast radiography. The intussuscepted portion of the ileum will be visible in the colon on lateral radiographs.

Treatment. In addition to searching for and eliminating the cause of rectal prolapse, the treatment of the disease should be aimed at replacing the prolapsed rectum in its anatomic position or amputating the prolapsed portion if it is necrotic.

Incomplete prolapse, in which only the mucosa protrudes, will usually respond to conservative therapy. The mucosa should be replaced inside the anal orifice, and antibiotic steroid ointments should be applied topically to the irritated perianal area for at least a week. Since this type of prolapse is usually associated with a severe enteritis and perianal soiling, effective medication should be given to treat the enteritis and subsequent diarrhea. Along with the antibiotics and anticholinergics (antispasmodics) used to treat enteritis, an enema consisting of from 10 to 20 ml Kaopectate is beneficial in bringing prompt relief.

If the mucosa continues to prolapse after repeated replacements and elimination of the cause, resection may be indicated. This is accomplished under general anesthesia. The prolapsed mucosa is grasped and pulled beyond the anal orifice so that the prolapsed portion can be easily excised (see Surgical Technique). After excision of the prolapsed portion, stay sutures are placed to hold the edges of mucosa in apposition until suturing can be performed, using 3–0 to 4–0 chromic catgut in a simple interrupted pattern. After suturing, the anastomosis of the rectal mucosa should shrink back into the anal canal. Postoperatively, enteric antibiotics should be given for five to seven days, along with medication to control any diarrhea that may be present.

The treatment of total rectal prolapse varies with the etiology and duration of the prolapse. The cause should always be corrected. In the less severe cases of short duration, when the cause is evident, the rectum is replaced in its anatomic position. Before attempting replacement, the area should be thoroughly irrigated and cleaned with sterile saline solution. Placement of a purse-string suture around the anal orifice prevents recurrence. The purse-string suture can be loosened on consecutive days for five to seven days until it is removed. This allows the animal to pass some stool while avoiding a reprolapse.

If the prolapsed mass is edematous and engorged, the application of ice-cold saline or a hyperosmotic solution of glucose will be beneficial in reducing the size, thus facilitating replacement. Replacement is best accomplished by holding the animal in a head-down position and by milking the prolapse back through the anal orifice. The rectum must be replaced in its anatomic position; otherwise, strangulation of the intussuscepted portion at the anal orifice may occur. To ensure total replacement, a smooth, rounded probe, such as the probang of a proctoscope, should be gently passed through the rectum. Occasionally, a viable-looking prolapse will not respond to external reduction. A laparotomy may be performed and the prolapse reduced by applying gentle traction on the descending colon. A colopexy should be done to maintain the reduction. Epidural anesthesia will be beneficial in some cases to control straining after replacement.

SURGICAL TECHNIQUE

Colopexy. Although this technique has not gained widespread acceptance, when performed properly it is beneficial in preventing reprolapse of the rectum. The procedure is performed under general anesthesia through a ventral midline incision

Figure 64–27. Photograph demonstrates surgical procedure for colopexy. A, Incised edge of abdominal wall; B, ventrolateral peritoneal surface of abdominal wall; C, rectum; D, deep mattress sutures placed into submucosa of rectum securing it to ventrolateral abdominal wall; and E, anterior margin of rectum and beginning of colon. It is wise to place two rows of mattress sutures to secure the bowel in place.

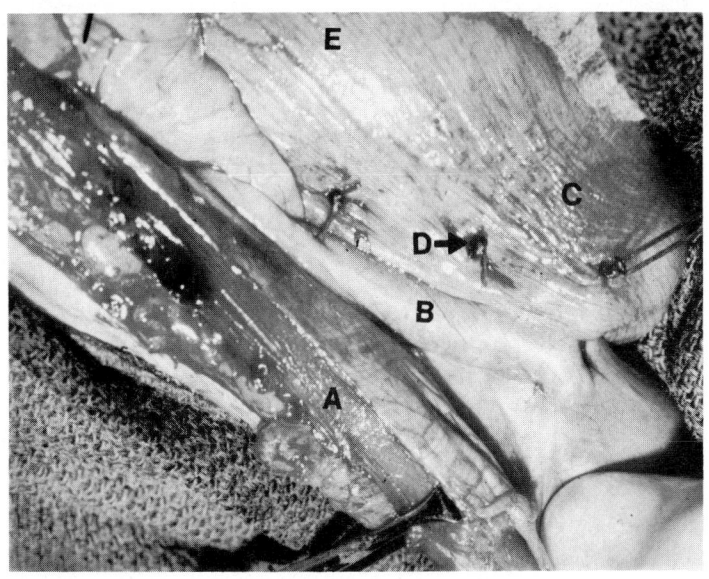

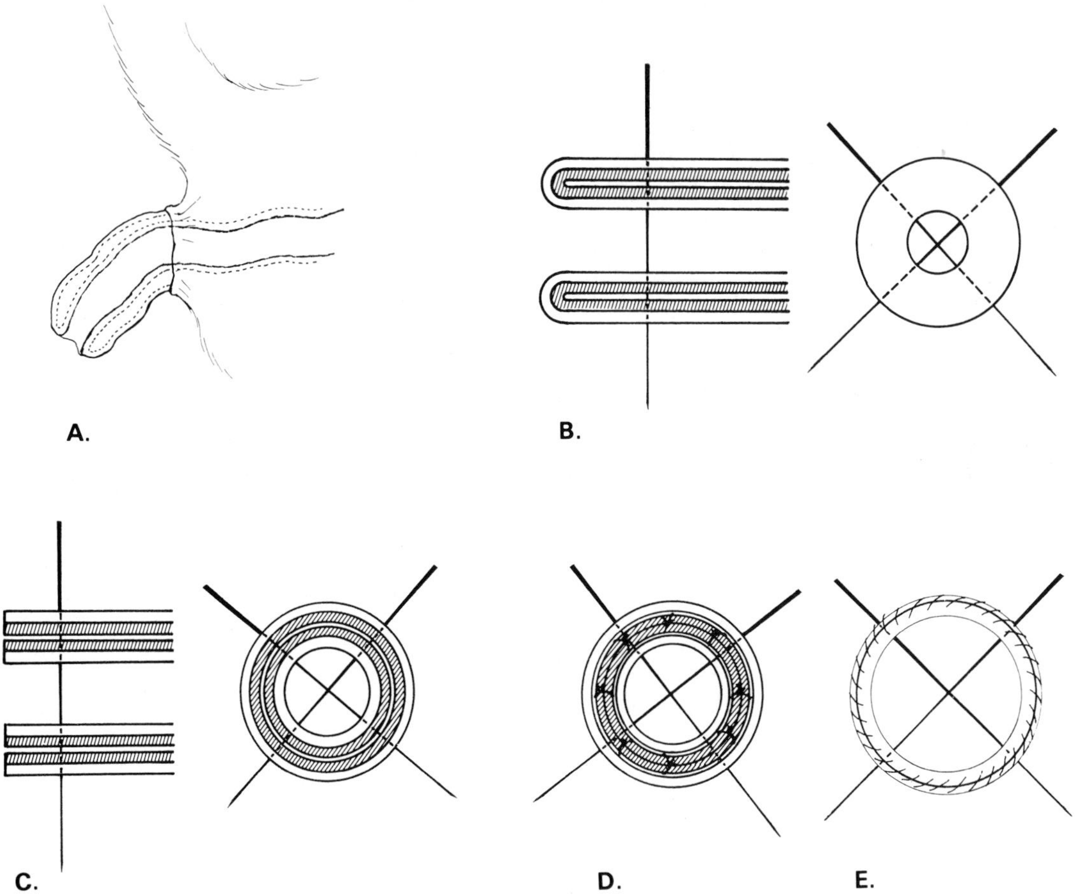

A.

B.

C.

D.

E.

Figure 64–28. Diagrammatic representation of rectal amputation using straight needles to prevent retraction of the layers during suturing. A, Rectal prolapse with mucosal surface (solid line) and muscularis surface (dotted line) inverted and exposed. B, Straight needles are placed perpendicular and through all layers of the prolapsed rectum (mucosa-submucosa solid line, muscularis hashed line). C, Prolapsed portion is excised approximately 0.5 cm posterior to the needles, exposing the tissue layers to be apposed. D, Muscularis is apposed (hashed lines) using 2.0 chromic catgut or monofilament nonabsorbable such as nylon in a simple interrupted pattern. The mucosa and submucosa (solid line) are then oversewn using a simple continuous pattern. The needles are now removed, allowing the bowel to retract through the anal orifice.

extending six to eight inches anterior to the anterior brim of the pelvis. The descending colon is grasped, and slight tension is placed in an anterior direction. The colon is sutured to the ventrolateral abdominal wall on the left side, using six to eight mattress sutures of 0 or 00 chromic catgut (Fig. 64–27). The sutures are placed through the serosa extending into the submucosa of the colon, which is sutured to the muscle and peritoneum of the abdominal wall. Care should be taken not to suture the colon too close to the midline, in order to prevent it from being incorporated in the abdominal incision. Postoperatively, a low-residue diet should be fed for five to seven days.

Rectal Amputation. In those cases in which a large portion of the rectum is protruding and the etiology is not immediately known, more radical methods of treatment may be necessary. If there is a question regarding viability of the tissue, the affected rectal portion should be amputated (Fig. 64–28). This excision is best performed under general anesthesia, with the animal in sternal recumbency and the hindquarters elevated. The necrotic portion is cleaned and irrigated with an antiseptic solution, and the area is sterilely draped. Straight needles are placed perpendicular through the prolapsed rectum approximately 0.5 cm from the anal orifice. These needles should penetrate all layers of the prolapsed bowel. After placement of the needles, the rectum is excised just 0.5 cm posterior to the needles. Anastomosis of the rectum should then be performed using 2–0 chromic catgut or monofilament nonabsorbable suture material. The first layer to be opposed is the muscularis, using a simple interrupted pattern. Next, the mucosal and submucosal layers are closed using a simple continuous pattern. The needles are now removed and the bowel is left to retract through the anal orifice. The anastomosis will be inverted, with the muscularis, submucosa, and mucosal surfaces apposed. Postoperative care consists of the administration of enteric antibiotics for five to seven days, along with feeding of a low-residue diet for the same period.

REFERENCES

Archibald, J., and Horney, F. S.: Colon, Rectum, and Anal Canal. *In* Archibald, J. (ed.): Canine Surgery. 2nd ed. American Veterinary Publications, Inc., Wheaton, Ill., 1975.

Arey, L. B.: Developmental Anatomy. 7th ed. W. B. Saunders Co., Philadelphia, 1965.

Ashdown, R. R.: Symposium on canine recto-anal disorders — I: Clinical anatomy. J. Small Anim. Pract. *9*:315, 1968.

Baker, K. P.: The histology and histochemistry of the circumanal hepatoid glands of the dog. J. Small Anim. Pract. *8*:639, 1967.

Barchfeld, W. P.: Perineal hernia in a bitch: Clinical briefs. Mod. Vet. Pract. *51*:61, 1970.

Bloom, H. F.: Synopsis of a technic for resection of the canine anal sacs. VM SAC *66*:782, 1971.

Bloomberg, M. S.: The clinical management of perianal fistulas in the dog. Comp. Cont. Ed. *2*:615–623, 1980.

Bokeria, R. I., and Ekhiskelashvili, D. M.: On ileorectal anastomosis. Akad. Nauk. Gruz. SSR. Tiflis Seob. *53*:477, 1969.

Borthwick, R.: The treatment of multiple peri-anal sinuses in the dog by cryosurgery. Am. Col. Vet. Tox. News 7:45, 1971.

Brennan, J. T., and Stewart, C. F.: Epidermoid carcinoma of the anus. Ann. Surg. *176*:787, 1972.

Burch, J. C., and Vaughn, W. K.: Significance of postoperative estrogen therapy on the occurrence and clinical course of cancer. Ann. Surg. *177*:626, 1973.

Burrows, C. F.: Diseases of the Colon, Rectum and Anus in the Dog and Cat. *In* Anderson N. V. (ed.): Veterinary Gastroenterology. Lea and Febiger, Philadelphia, 1980.

Burrows, C. F., and Harvey, C. E.: Perineal hernia in the dog. J. Small Anim. Pract. *14*:315, 1973.

Dencker, H., Lingardh, G., Muth, T., et al.: Massive gangrene of the colon secondary to carcinoma of the rectum. Acta Chir. Scand. *135*:357, 1969.

Donovan, C. A.: Canine anal glands and chemical signals (pheromons). J.A.V.M.A. *155*:1995, 1969.

Donovan, C. A.: *Taenia proglottides* in canine anal sacs. J.A.V.M.A. *154*:803, 1969.

Ellis, T. H.: Opening address on the discussion at the symposium on canine recto-anal disorders. J. Small Anim. Pract. *9*:339, 1968.

Evans, E. R., and Pierrepoint, C. G.: Tissue-steroid interactions in canine hormone-dependent tumors. Vet. Rec. *97*:1975.

Frye, F. L., Hoeft, D. J., Cucuel, J. P., and Hardy, R. J.: Silicone sealant for preoperative packing of canine anal sacs. J.A.V.M.A. *156*:1030, 1970.

Ganong, W. F.: Review of Medical Physiology. 3rd ed. Lange Medical Publications, Los Altos, Cal., 1967.

Gaston, E. A.: Physiologic basis for preservation of fecal continence after resection of rectum. J.A.M.A. *146*:1486, 1951.

Gillette, E. L.: Veterinary radiotherapy. J.A.V.M.A. *157*:1707, 1970.

Glotzer, D. J., and Scharmer, A. N.: Experimental total abdominoperineal colectomy with preservation of sphincters. Surg. Gynecol. Obstet. *119*:338, 1964.

Greer, M. B., and Calhoun, M. L.: Anal sacs of the cat *(Felis domesticus)*. Am. J. Vet. Res. *27*:773, 1966.

Greiner, T. P.: Surgery of the rectum and anus. Vet. Clin. North Am. *2*:167, 1972.

Guyton, A. C.: The Alimentary Tract: Textbook of Medical Physiology. 3rd ed. W. B. Saunders Co., Philadelphia, 1966.

Hagihara, P. F., and Griffen, W. O., Jr.: Physiology of the colon and rectum. Surg. Clin. North Am. *52*:4, 1972.

Halvan, C. R. E.: Canine Anal Sac Disease. Veterinary Annual No. 18. Grunsell, C. S., and Hill, F. W. G., (eds.) Bristol, England, Scientechnica, p. 225, 1978.

Hansen, J. H.: A visual aid for clients: the problems of anal sacs in dogs. VM SAC *67*:143, 1972.

Harvey, C. E.: Incidence and distribution of anal sac disease in the dog. J. A.A.H.A. *10*:573, 1974.

Harvey, C. E.: Perianal fistula in the dog. Vet. Rec. *91*:25, 1972.

Hayes, H. M., and Wilson, G. P.: Hormone-dependent neoplasms of the canine perianal gland. Cancer Research *37*(7 Pt 1):2068–2071.

Isitor, G. N., and Weinman, D. E.: Origin and early development of canine circumanal glands. Am. J. Vet. Res. *40*:4, 487–492, 1979.

Josen, A. S., Ferrer, J. M., Jr., Forde, K. A., and Bashir, A. Z.: Primary clsoure of civilian colorectal wounds. Ann. Surg. *176*:782, 1972.

Jubb, K. V., and Kennedy, P. C.: Pathology of Domestic Animals. Vol. II. Academic Press, Inc., New York, 1963.

Karland, M., McPherson, R. C., and Watman, R. N.: An experimental evaluation of fecal continence — sphincter and reservoir — in the dog. Surg. Gynecol. Obstet. *108*:469, 1959.

Lacroix, J. V., and Lacroix, L. J.: Pararectal fistula. North Am. Vet. *26*:39, 1945.

Lane, J. G., and Bench, D. S.: The cryosurgical treatment of canine anal furunculosis. J. Small Anim. Pract. *16*:387–392, 1975.

Lassoie, L., and Hennan, A.: Anesthésie de la région anale et périneale du chien par infiltration des nerfs sacrés. Ann. Med. Vet. *115*:87, 1971.

Levene, A.: Symposium on canine recto-anal disorders — II: The surgical pathology of ano-rectal disease in the dog. J. Small Anim. Pract. *9*:323, 1968.

Lewis, D. G.: Symposium on canine recto-anal disorders — III: Clinical management. J. Small Anim. Pract. *9*:329, 1968.

Liska, W. D., and Withrow, S. J.: Cryosurgical treatment of perianal gland adenomas in the dog. J.A.A.H.A. *14*:457–463, 1978.

Lowenstine, L. H., et al.: Exogenous estrogen toxicity in the dog. Calif. Vet. *26*:37–39, 1972.

Lungeman, C. H., and Garner, F. M.: Comparative study of intestinal adenocarcinoma of animals and man. J. Natl. Cancer Inst. *48*:1972.

Miller, M. E., Christensen, G. C., and Evans, H. E.: Anatomy of the Dog. W. B. Saunders Co., Philadelphia, 1964.

Minin, N. P.: Arteries of rectum and bladder in elimination of branches of caudal end of aorta. Arkh. Anat. Gistol. Embriol. *55*:104, 1968.

Moulton, J. E.: Tumors of Domestic Animals. Universi-ty of California Press, Berkely and Los Angeles, 1961.

Myrilos, P. M.: Anal sac impaction in the dog. Vet. Rec. *80*:211, 1967.

Netter, F. H.: Digestive System, Part 2. The Ciba collection of Medical Illustrations, Vol. 3. Ciba Pharmaceutical Company, New York, 1962.

Palminteri, A.: Anorectal Disease. *In* Kirk, R. W. (ed.): Current Veterinary Therapy V. W. B. Saunders Co., Philadelphia, 1974.

Palminteri, A.: Rectal disease and surgery of dogs. Scientific Presentations and Seminar Synopses, 36th Annual Meeting of Am. Anim. Hosp. Assoc., 1969.

Palminteri, A.: The implications of rectal tenesmus in the dog. J.A.A.H.A. *4*:171, 1968.

Palminteri, A.: The surgical management of polyps of the rectum and colon of the dog. J.A.V.M.A. *148*:771, 1966.

Panel Report: Clinical report. Treatment of anal gland infection in the dog. Aust. Vet. J. *45*:257, 1969.

Patnaik, A. K., et al.: Canine gastrointestinal neoplasms. Vet. Pathol. *14*:547–555, 1977.

Rawlings, C. A., and Capps, W. F.: Rectovaginal fistula and imperforate anus in a dog. J.A.V.M.A. *159*:320, 1971.

Rodkey, G. V.: Office treatment of rectal and anal diseases. J.A.M.A. *223*:676, 1973.

Scharli, A. F., and Kiesewitter, W. B.: Defecation and continence: Some new concepts. Dis. Colon Rectum *13*:81, 1970.

Schrock, T. R., Deveney, C. W., and Dunphy, J. E.: Factors contributing to leakage of colonic anastomoses. Ann. Surg. *177*:513, 1973.

Seiler, R. J.: Colorectal polyps of the dog: a clinicopathologic study of 17 cases. J.A.V.M.A. *1074*(1):72–75, 1979.

Severin, G. A.: Digestive System Disorders. *In* Catcott, E. J. (ed.): Canine Medicine. American Veterinary Publications, Inc., Wheaton, Ill., 1968.

Shaffer, A., and Block, I. R.: Pathology and surgical correction of perianal fistulous tracts in a dog. J.A.V.M.A. *138*:22, 1961.

Shaffer, A., and Schieffer, B.: Incidence and types of canine rectal carcinomas. J. Small Anim. Pract. *9*:491, 1968.

Silverberg, S. G.: Carcinoma arising in adenomatous polyps of the rectum in a dog. Dis. Colon Rectum *14*:191, 1971.

Sischy, B., et al.: Treatment of carcinoma of the rectum and squamous carcinoma of the anus by combination chemotherapy, radiotherapy and operation. Surg. Gynecol. Obstet. *151*:369–371, 1980.

Spira, E., Spira, A., and Porteus, D.: A new gel medium for use in the surgical removal of canine anal sacs. VM SAC *66*:688, 1971.

Strombeck, D. R.: Rectum and Anal-Canal Intestinal Neoplasms. *In* Strombeck, D. R. (ed.): Small Animal Gastroenterology. Stonegate Publishing Co., Davis, Calif., 1979.

Swenson, O., and Bill, A. H., Jr.: Resection of the rectum and rectosigmoid with preservation of the sphincter for benign spastic lesions producing megacolon. An experimental study. Surgery *24*:212, 1948.

Wilson, G. P., and Hayes, H. M., Jr.: Castration for treatment of perianal gland neoplasms in the dog. J.A.V.M.A. *174*:1301–1303, 1979.

Wilson, J. E., and Brown, D. E.: Malignant perianal gland tumor with metastasis in a dog. J.A.V.M.A. *144*:389, 1964.

SECTION XI

The Endocrine System

CHAPTER 65

CHARLES C. CAPEN
and SHARRON L. MARTIN

Diseases of the Pituitary Gland

INTRODUCTION

Endocrine glands such as the pituitary are concerned exclusively with endocrine function. They are small in comparison with other body organs, widely distributed in the body, and connected with one another only by the bloodstream. They are richly supplied with blood, and there is a close anatomic relationship between endocrine cells and the capillary network. The peripheral cytoplasmic extensions of capillary endothelial cells have fenestrae covered by a single membrane in order to facilitate rapid transport of raw materials and secretory products between the bloodstream and endocrine cells.

Endocrine glands are collections of specialized cells that synthesize, store, and release their secretions directly into the bloodstream. Since they lack a duct system, they are often referred to as ductless glands of internal secretion. They are interposed as sensing or signalling organs to detect changes in constituents of the extracellular fluid compartment (Fig. 65–1). The secretory products of specialized endocrine cells are hormones, which are released into the extracellular fluids and transported via the blood to influence the rates of existing chemical reactions in populations of target cells in other tissues of the body. Other populations of cells in the body are concerned with the degradation of hormones by proteases on the cell surface or lysosomal enzymes within the cell, or by conjugation with glucuronic acid or sulfate and excretion in the bile or urine (Fig. 65–1). Endocrine glands working in concert with the nervous system integrate and coordinate a wide variety of physiologic activities concerned with maintaining a constant internal environment.

Polypeptide hormones, such as those secreted by the adenohypophysis, (1) have their primary site of action at the plasma membrane of target cells (Fig. 65–2), (2) have receptor proteins for the hormone bound on the outer surface of the plasma membrane, (3) are water soluble, (4) have a short half-life in blood (usually measured in minutes), and (5) lack specific plasma-binding proteins.

The receptors for a particular polypeptide hormone on the plasma membrane of target cells perform two key functions. The first is the recognition of the active hormone from among all other proteins (10^{-3} to 10^{-4}M) to which the cell is exposed, since the concentration of hormone in extracellular fluids is low (10^{-10}M). It provides this recognition by binding the hormone to the receptor site and forming a reversible hormone-receptor complex. The second important function of the receptor is to convey the "message" of the hormone bound to the plasma membrane from the outside to the inside of the target cell (Fig. 65–2). The magnitude of this transmembrane signal depends upon the concentration of hormone to which the target cell is being exposed, the affinity of the receptor for the hormone, and the concentration of receptors per unit of target cell.

There appears to be a single common intracellular pathway for many different polypeptide hormones. It begins with the activation of the enzyme adenylate cyclase in the plasma membrane of target cells, followed by the intracellular formation of cyclic adenosine monophosphate (cAMP) from ATP, and the activation of cAMP-dependent protein kinases (Fig. 65–2). These protein kinases activate and inactivate a variety of enzymes by phosphorylating them, using ATP as a source of phosphate. At this point the intracellular pathway for each polypeptide hormone appears to branch, resulting in a multiplicity of

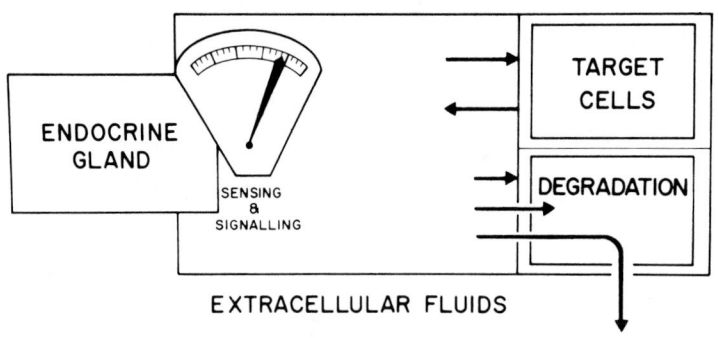

Figure 65–1. Schematic representation of the endocrine system. Endocrine glands are interposed as sensing and signaling devices to detect changes in constituents of the extracellular fluid compartment. Hormones interact with specific target cells in the body to elicit a biologic response. In addition, hormones are degraded by cell surface enzymes or lysosomal enzymes within the cells, or are conjugated with glucuronic acid and sulfate for excretion in the urine or bile. (From Roth, J.: *In* Beers, R. F., and Bassett, E. G. (eds.): Cell Membrane Receptors for Viruses, Antigens and Antibiotics, Polypeptide Hormones, and Small Molecules, Raven Press, New York, 1976.)

different pathways being activated and leading to a variety of effects on any given target cell.

Cells concerned with the reproduction of polypeptide hormones, such as the adenohypophysis, have a well-developed endoplasmic reticulum, with many attached ribosomes for assembly of hormone and a prominent Golgi apparatus for packaging of hormone into granules for intracellular storage and transport (Fig. 65–3). Secretory granules are unique to polypeptide hormone–secreting endocrine cells and provide a mechanism for intracellular storage of substantial amounts of preformed hormone. These membrane-limited granules represent macromolecular aggregations of active hormone, often in association with specific binding proteins. Upon receipt of an appropriate signal for hormone secretion, secretory granules are directed to the periphery of the endocrine cell, probably by the contraction of microfilaments, and the limiting membrane of the granule fuses

with the plasma membrane of the cell. The hormone-containing granule core is extruded into the extracellular perivascular space by either emiocytosis or exocytosis. Subsequently, the granule core is fragmented and rapidly transported through capillary fenestrae into the circulation. Hormone synthesized in excess of the body's requirement is degraded by fusion of the hormone-containing granules with lysosomes, a process termed crinophagy.

STRUCTURE AND FUNCTION OF THE PITUITARY GLAND

The pituitary gland in the adult is completely separated from the oral cavity. It is situated in the sella turcica, a concavity of the sphenoid bone, and enveloped by an extension of dura mater. The pituitary gland (hypophysis) is subdivided anatomically into the adenohypophysis (anterior lobe) and neurohypophysis (posterior lobe).

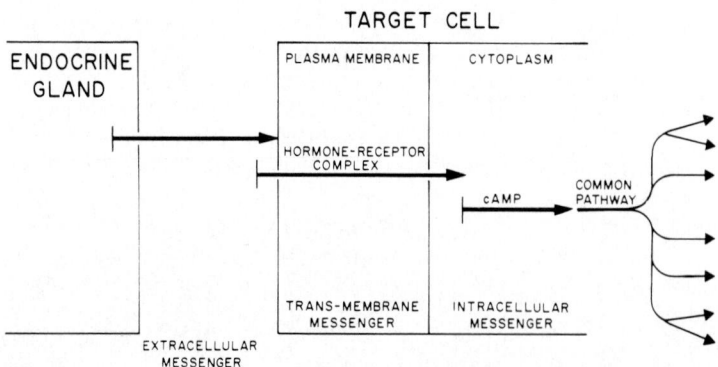

Figure 65–2. Mechanism of action of polypeptide hormones at target cells. Many polypeptide hormones act on target cells by binding to specific receptors on the cell surface and activating the membrane-limited enzyme, adenylate cyclase, resulting in the intracellular formation of cyclic adenosine monophosphate (cAMP). This second messenger conveys the hormonal information within the target cell, and by either common pathways (e.g., activation of protein kinases) or branch pathways, which are unique for a particular hormone, elicits the biologic response of the hormone. (From Roth, J.: Receptors for peptide hormones. *In* DeGroot, L., and Cahill, G., Jr. (eds.): Endocrinology. Vol. III. Grune and Stratton, New York, 1979.)

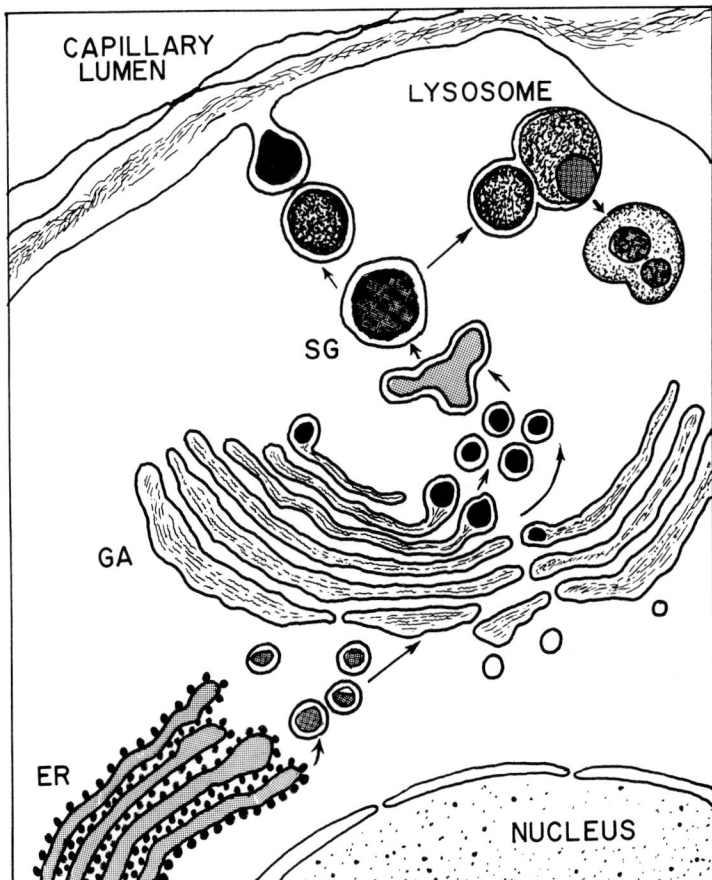

Figure 65–3. Synthesis of polypeptide hormones from endocrine glands, such as the adenohypophysis, begins on ribosomes attached to membranes of the rough endoplasmic reticulum (ER). Precursor hormone molecules accumulate within the cisternae of the ER and are transported to the Golgi apparatus (GA), where they are concentrated and packaged into membrane-limited secretory granules. Secretory granules (SG) are macromolecular aggregations of pre-formed hormone that are moved to the periphery of the cell by contraction of microfilaments and released into the perivascular spaces either by exocytosis or emiocytosis. Hormone synthesized in excess of the body's requirement is degraded by fusion of secretory granules with lysosomes, a process termed "crinophagy."

ADENOHYPOPHYSIS

In the dog and cat the adenohypophysis completely surrounds the pars nervosa of the neurohypophyseal system (Fig. 65–4). The adenohypophysis consists of three portions, the pars distalis, the pars tuberalis, and the pars intermedia. The pars distalis is the largest of the three portions and contains the multiple populations of endocrine cells that secrete the pituitary tropic hormones. The secretory cells are supplied with abundant capillaries that have fenestrae in the cytoplasm and are supported by the cytoplasmic processes of stellate follicular (substentacular) cells. The pars tuberalis consists of dorsal projections of cells along

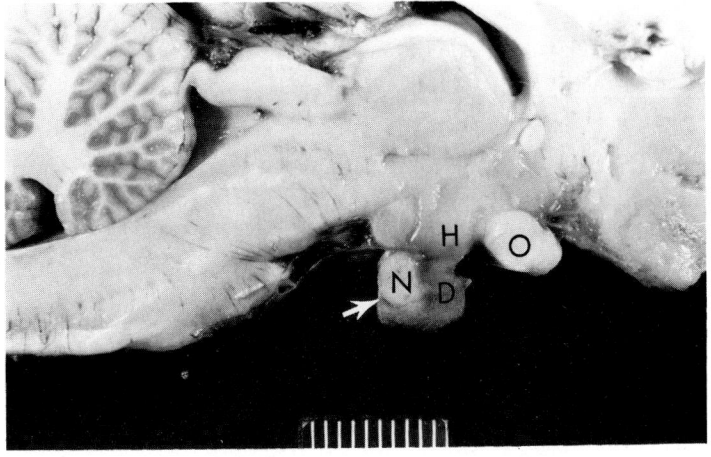

Figure 65–4. The pituitary region from a dog illustrating the close relationship to the optic chiasm (O), hypothalamus (H), and overlying brain. The pars distalis (D) forms a major part of the adenohypophysis and completely surrounds the pars nervosa (N). The residual lumen of Rathke's pouch (white arrow) separates the pars distalis and pars nervosa, and is lined by the pars intermedia. The scale at the bottom represents 1 cm.

the infundibular stalk. It functions primarily as a scaffold for the capillary network of the hypophyseal portal system during its course from the median eminence to the pars distalis. The pars intermedia forms the junction between the pars distalis and pars nervosa (Howe, 1973). It lines the residual lumen of Rathke's pouch and contains two populations of cells in the dog, one of which synthesizes adrenocorticotropic hormone (ACTH) (El Etreby and Dubois, 1980; Halmi et al., 1981).

A specific population of endocrine cells is present in the pars distalis (and in the pars intermedia for ACTH in the dog) that synthesize and secrete each of the pituitary tropic hormones (Ricci and Russolo, 1973). Secretory cells in the adenohypophysis are subdivided into acidophils, basophils, and chromophobes based on interaction of their secretory granules with pH-dependent histochemical stains. Pituitary cells have a secretory cycle and enter an actively synthesizing phase in response to increased demand for a particular tropic hormone (Fig. 65–5). During this phase the cytoplasm is chromophobic, because it contains predominately rough endoplasmic reticulum and Golgi apparatus but few secretory granules. As the batch of recently synthesized hormone is packaged into secretory granules by the Golgi apparatus, the cell enters the storage phase and can be selectively stained by histochemical procedures as either acidophils, basophils, or chromophobes.

Acidophils are further subdivided into somatotrophs and luteotrophs that secrete growth hormone (GH, somatotropin) (Wil-

helmi, 1968) and luteotropic hormone (LTH, prolactin) (Papkoff, 1976), respectively. Basophils include both gonadotrophs that secrete luteinizing hormone (LH) and follicle-stimulating hormone (FSH) (El Etreby and Fath El Bab, 1978) and thyrotrophs that secrete thyrotropic hormone (TTH) (El Etreby and Fath El Bab, 1978b). Chromophobes are pituitary cells that do not have obvious cytoplasmic secretory granules by light microscopy. They include the endocrine cells concerned with the synthesis of ACTH and melanocyte-stimulating hormone (MSH), nonsecretory follicular cells, and undifferentiated stem cells.

The recent development of radioimmunoassays for plasma ACTH in the dog has demonstrated a mean concentration of 45.8 pg/ml (range 17 to 98 pg/ml) (Feldman et al., 1977). Assays for plasma ACTH should be useful in differentiating between pituitary-dependent and other causes of adrenal cortical hyperplasia and the syndrome of cortisol excess. Dogs with functional adrenal cortical neoplasms have plasma ACTH concentrations two standard deviations or more below the mean value for normal dogs (Feldman, 1981). In addition, the development of a homologous radioimmunoassay for canine thyrotropin will facilitate the evaluation of the pituitary-thyroid axis and the diagnosis of certain thyroid diseases. Quinlan and Michaelson (1981) reported mean serum thyrotropin levels of 7.0 ± 0.9 ng/ml in euthyroid dogs (9 to 10 years of age, 7 to 14 kg body weight), which increased in response to propylthiouracil administration (334 mg/day intramuscularly)

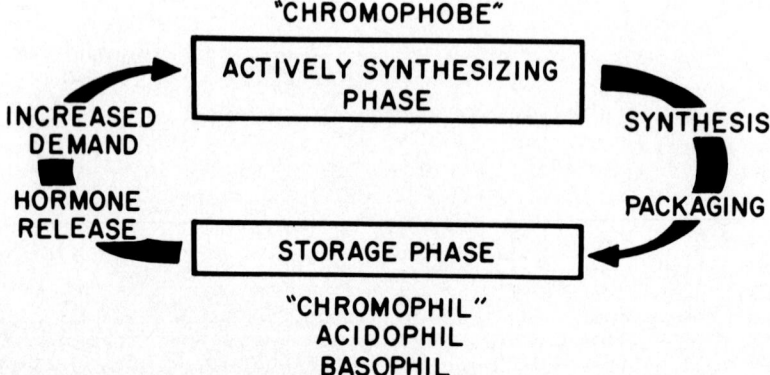

Figure 65–5. Secretory cycle of cells in the adenohypophysis. During the actively synthesizing phase all pituitary cells are "chromophobic," since their cytoplasm contains abundant endoplasmic reticulum and Golgi apparatus but few secretory granules. When the cell enters the storage phase, the accumulation of hormone-containing secretory granules permits the cells to be subdivided into acidophils, basophils, or chromophobes, based upon their reaction with specific pH-dependent stains.

for one week. This response was abolished by moderately high doses (1000 Rad) of x-radiation to the head.

Immunocytochemical staining demonstrated that ACTH- and MSH-staining cells (antisera to porcine ACTH, synthetic $ACTH^{\beta(1-24)}$ and $ACTH^{\beta(17-39)}$, and bovine β-MSH) were polyhedral to round, sparsely granulated, and most numerous in the ventrocentral and cranial portions of the pars distalis in dogs, where they occurred in large groups (El Etreby and Dubois, 1980). They were less numerous in the dorsal and caudal regions of the pars distalis and throughout the pars tuberalis. In the pars intermedia of dogs most cells demonstrated immunoreactivity to either pACTH, α-MSH, or β-MSH. Thyrotrophs in the dog were large polyhedral cells situated singly or in small groups ventrocentrally in the paramedian plane of the pars distalis (El Etreby and Fath El Bab, 1978a). Gonadotrophs (cells reacting with antisera to human FSH^{β} and/or bovine LH^{β}) were oval to polyhedral and distributed singly in the pars distalis, particularly in the dorsal-cranial region and in caudal extensions along the pars intermedia (El Etreby and Fath El Bab, 1978). Immunoreactive prolactin cells occurred in small groups of large polygonal cells with prominent granules in the ventrocentral and cranial portion of the canine pars distalis (El Etreby and Fath El Bab, 1977). A diffuse increase in this population of cells occurs in female dogs near parturition (El Etreby et al., 1980). Growth hormone–secreting cells were present singly along capillaries in the dorsal region of the pars distalis near the pars intermedia (El Etreby and Fath El Bab, 1977). They were small, round to oval, and had fine cytoplasmic granules. Somatotrophs frequently undergo diffuse hyperplasia and hypertrophy in old dogs, especially females with mammary dysplasia or neoplasia (El Etreby et al., 1980).

Each population of endocrine cells in the adenohypophysis is under the control of a corresponding releasing hormone (factor) from the hypothalamus (Fig. 65–6). These releasing hormones are small peptides synthesized by neurosecretion by neurons in the hypothalamus (Schally, 1978). They are transported by axonal processes to the median eminence, where they are released into capillaries and conveyed by the hypophyseal portal system to specific endocrine cells in the adenohypophysis; there they stimulate

the rapid release of preformed tropic hormones (Fig. 65–7).

There appear to be seven different hypothalamic releasing hormones that regulate the rate of secretion of each tropic hormone secreted by the adenohypophysis. For most pituitary tropic hormones, negative feedback control is accomplished by the blood concentration of the hormone produced by the target endocrine gland (e.g., thyroid gland, adrenal cortex, ovary, and testis). The hormone produced by the endocrine glands exerts negative feedback control on the neurosecretory neurons in the hypothalamus that synthesize the corresponding releasing hormone. Growth hormone, prolactin, and MSH do not act on target endocrine organs to stimulate secretion of a hormone, however. Negative feedback control of these three pituitary hormones is effected by production of a corresponding release-inhibiting hormone (factor) by neurons in the hypothalamus. The relative local concentrations of the specific releasing hormone and release-inhibiting hormone appear to govern the rate of release of GH, LTH, and MSH from the adenohypophysis. The feedback mechanism of homeostatic control of adrenal cortical secretion is functional in the dog at birth. The newborn dog responds to the administration of ACTH (two units) or dexamethasone (0.01 to 0.02 mg/kg body weight) with the expected increase or decrease in plasma cortisol concentrations (Muelheims et al., 1973).

NEUROHYPOPHYSIS

The neurohypophysis consists of three anatomic subdivisions. The pars nervosa (posterior lobe) represents the distal component of the neurohypophyseal system. It is composed of numerous capillaries that are supported by modified glial cells (pituicytes). The capillaries in the pars nervosa are termination sites for the nonmyelinated axonal processes of neurosecretory neurons in the hypothalamus. Secretion granules that contain the neurohypophyseal hormones, i.e., oxytocin and antidiuretic hormone, are synthesized in hypothalamic neurons but are released into the bloodstream in the pars nervosa. The infundibular stalk joins the pars nervosa to the overlying hypothalamus and is composed of axonal processes from neurosecretory neurons. Neurosecretory neurons in the hy-

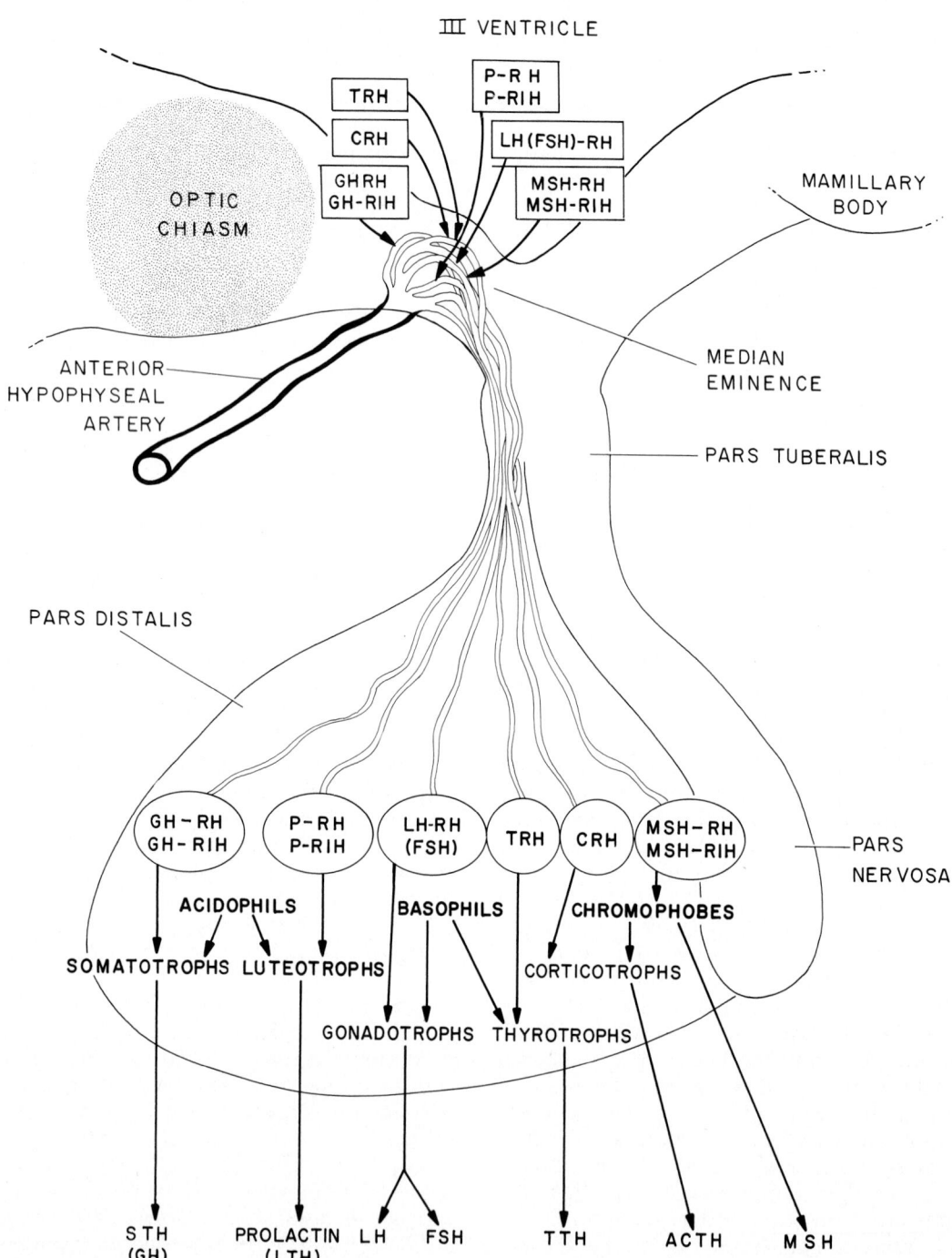

Figure 65–6. Control of tropic hormone secretion from the adenohypophysis by hypothalamic releasing hormones (RH) and release-inhibiting hormones (R-IH). The releasing and release-inhibiting hormones are synthesized by neurones in the hypothalamus, transported by axonal processes, and released into capillary plexus in the median eminence. They are transported to the adenohypophysis by the hypothalamic-hypophyseal portal system where they interact with specific populations of tropic hormone–secreting cells to govern the rate of release of preformed hormones, such as somatotropin (GH, STH), prolactin (LTH), lutenizing hormone (LH), follicle-stimulating hormone (FSH), thyrotropin hormone (TTH), adrenocorticotropic hormone (ACTH), and melanocyte-stimulating hormone (MSH).

Figure 65–7. Highest order of endocrine control involving interrelationship with the central nervous system. Receptors in the nervous system detect changes in the internal or external environment and convey this information through neural impulses to neurosecretory neurons in the hypothalamus. Releasing hormones (H_1) produced in response to the neural input stimulate the rapid release of corresponding tropic hormone (H_2) from the adenohypophysis. Tropic hormones influence the rates of

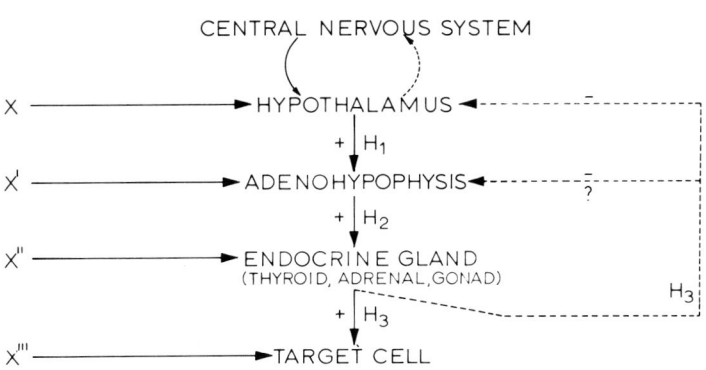

existing reactions in the corresponding endocrine gland (thyroid, adrenal cortex, gonad) and increase the secretion of their hormone (H_3), which is carried by the bloodstream to specific target cells to elicit a biologic response. Negative feedback control is affected primarily by the blood concentration of the final endocrine product (H_3), primarily on cells in the hypothalamus. Local autoregulatory mechanisms (X) influence the functional activity of each component of the endocrine control system.

pothalamus receive neural input from higher centers and translate this into endocrine output in the form of hormonal secretion. In addition to the usual structural features of neurons they contain prominent arrays of rough endoplasmic reticulum, large Golgi apparatuses, and numerous membrane-limited secretory granules in the cell body and axonal process (Fig. 65–8). The neurosecretory neurons concerned with hormone synthesis are segregated into anatomically defined regions called nuclei in the hypothalamus. The supraoptic nucleus is concerned primarily with the synthesis of antidiuretic hormone, whereas oxytocin is produced predominately by neurons in the paraventricular nucleus.

The neurohypophysis in most animals is supplied directly by the posterior (inferior) hypophyseal arteries that branch from the internal carotid arteries (Fig. 65–9). Branches of the anterior (superior) hypophyseal arteries originate from the internal carotid arteries and from the posterior communicating arteries of the circle of Willis. Arteriolar branches penetrate the pars tuberalis (infundibularis), lose their muscular coat, and form a capillary plexus near the median eminence. These vessels subsequently drain into hypophyseal portal veins that supply the pars distalis. There also may be a small direct arterial supply to the adenohypophysis of minor physiologic importance that arises from the posterior hypophyseal arteries (Fig. 65–9).

Antidiuretic hormone (ADH; vasopressin) is an octapeptide synthesized by neurons situated primarily in the supraoptic nucleus

of the hypothalamus. The hormone is packaged into membrane-limited granules with a corresponding binding protein (neurophysin) and transported to the pituitary gland by axonal processes of the neurosecretory neurons (Fig. 65–8). These axons terminate on fenestrated capillaries in the pars nervosa and release ADH into the circulation.

ADH is transported by the bloodstream to the kidney, where it binds to specific isoreceptors in the distal part of the nephron and collecting ducts. The overall effect of ADH on the kidney is to increase the active renal tubular reabsorption of water from the glomerular filtrate. The hormone(ADH)-receptor complex activates the membrane-bound enzyme, adenylate cyclase, resulting in the intracellular formation of cyclic adenosine monophosphate (cAMP) from ATP (Dousa, 1974) (Fig. 65–10). The accumulation of cAMP appears to activate protein kinases involved in the phosphorylation of proteins in the luminal membrane that increase the permeability of the cell to water.

Pathophysiology of Neurohypophysis

Diabetes insipidus is a disorder in which inadequate ADH is produced or target cells in the kidney lack the biochemical machinery necessary to respond to the secretion of normal or elevated circulating levels of hormone. The hypophyseal form of diabetes insipidus develops as a result of compression and destruction of the pars nervosa, infundibular stalk, or supraoptic nucleus in the hypothalamus. The lesions responsible for this disruption of ADH synthesis or

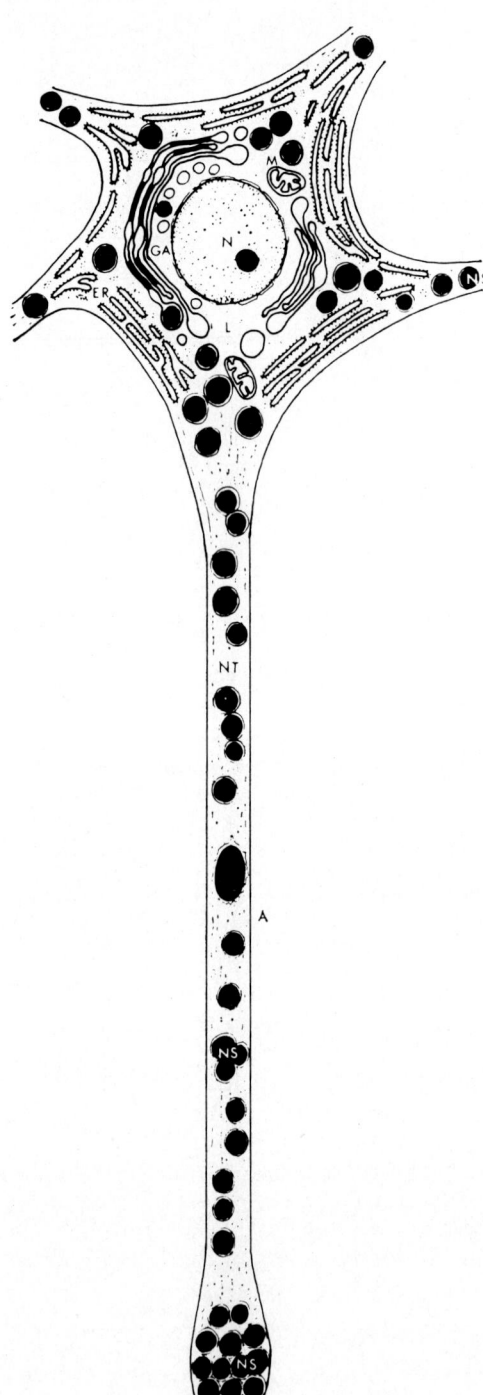

Figure 65–8. Structural characteristics of a neurosecretory neurone in the hypothalamus. The nerve cell body (N, nucleus) has dendritic and axonal (A) processes with arrays of rough endoplasmic reticulum, a prominent Golgi apparatus, and neurotubules (NT). Hormone-containing, membrane-limited neurosecretory granules (NS) are formed in the Golgi apparatus and transported along the axon to the site of release at the termination on capillaries. Neurosecretory neurones synthesize the releasing and release-inhibiting hormones of the adenohypophysis and the hormones of the neurohypophysis (oxytocin, antidiuretic hormone).

secretion in dogs and cats include large pituitary neoplasms (Koestner and Capen, 1967), a dorsally expanding cyst or inflammatory granuloma, and traumatic injury to the skull with hemorrhage and glial proliferation in the neurohypophyseal system (Rogers et al., 1977). Axons in the compressed pars nervosa of dogs with hypophyseal diabetes insipidus associated with pituitary neoplasms are depleted of ADH-containing dense secretory granules (Fig. 65–11), compared with normal dogs (Fig. 65–12).

Sporadic cases of hypophyseal diabetes insipidus may be the result of an inherited biochemical defect in the synthesis of ADH

Figure 65–9. Diagrammatic representation of the pituitary gland and its vascular supply. 1, superior hypophyseal artery; 2, inferior hypophyseal artery; 3, primary plexus of the infundibular stem; 4, primary plexus of the infundibular process; 5, long portal vessels; 6, short portal vessels; 7, secondary plexus in the adenohypophysis; 8, collecting vein; 9, pars tuberalis (infundibularis) of the adenohypophysis; 10, pituitary stalk; 11, pars distalis; 12, residual hypophyseal lumen (intraglandular cleft); 13, pars intermedia; 14, infundibular process of the neurohypophysis; III, infundibular recess of the third ventricle. From Meijer, J. C.: An investigation of the pathogenesis of pituitary-dependent hyperadrenocorticism in the dog. Utrecht, The Netherlands, 1980.

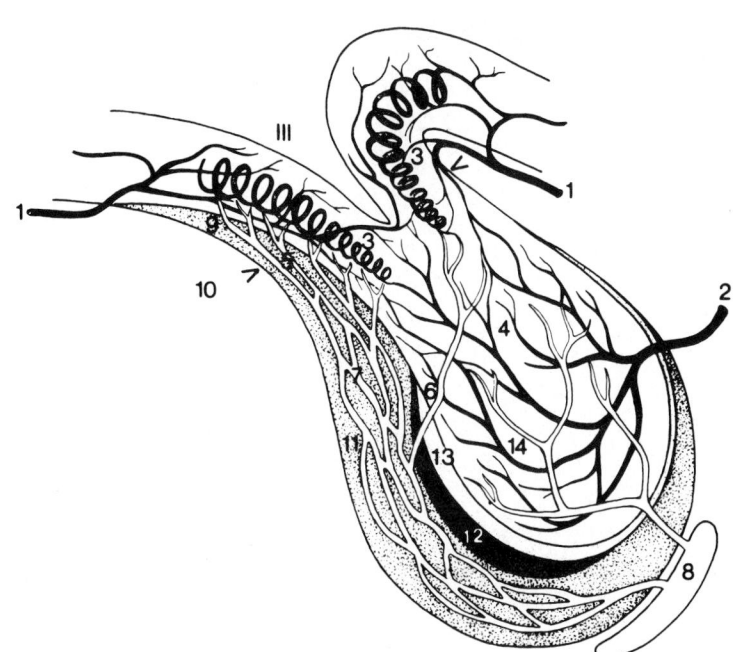

and its corresponding neurophysin I, as has been well characterized in the Brattleboro strain of rats (Sokol and Vatlin, 1965; Kalimo and Rinne, 1972). In the nephrogenic form of diabetes insipidus blood levels of ADH are normal or elevated, but target cells in the distal nephron and collecting ducts are unable to respond owing to a lack of adenylate cyclase in the plasma membrane.

Dogs and cats with diabetes insipidus excrete large volumes of hypotonic urine, which in turn obligates the intake of equally large amounts of water to prevent hyperos-

molality of body fluids and dehydration (Koestner and Capen, 1967; Green and Farrow, 1974) (refer to Chapter 19 on polyuria and polydipsia for details). Urine osmolality is decreased below normal plasma osmolality (approximately 300 mOsM/kg) in both hypophyseal and nephrogenic forms of diabetes insipidus (Figs. 65–13 and 65–14). In response to water deprivation, urine osmolality remains below that of plasma in both forms of diabetes insipidus in contrast to that observed in normal animals. The elevation of urine osmolality above that of

Figure 65–10. Subcellular mechanism of action of antidiuretic hormone (vasopressin) in the kidney. The hormone (VP) binds to isoreceptors on target cells of collecting ducts and activates adenylate cyclase (AC) in the plasma membrane on the basilar aspect of the cell. The intracellular accumulation of cyclic adenosine monophosphate (cAMP) may activate certain protein kinases that phosphorylate proteins in the luminal plasma membrane that increase the permeability to water. From Dousa, T. P.: Cellular action of antidiuretic hormone in nephrogenic diabetes insipidus. Mayo Clin. Proc. *49*:188, 1974.

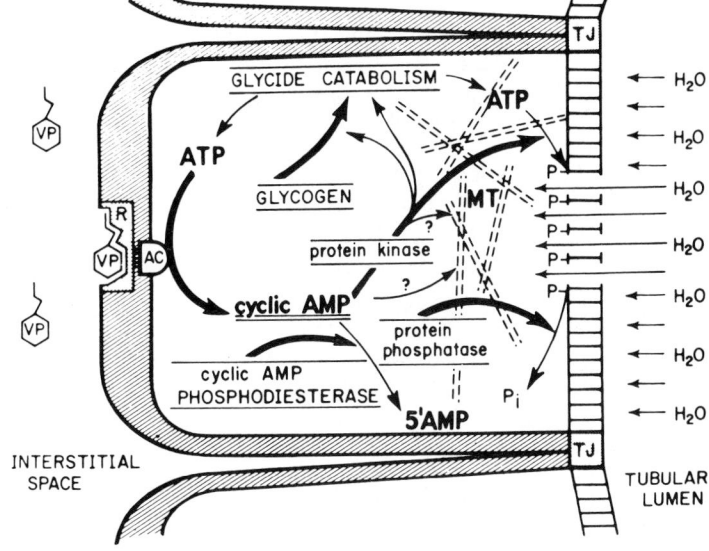

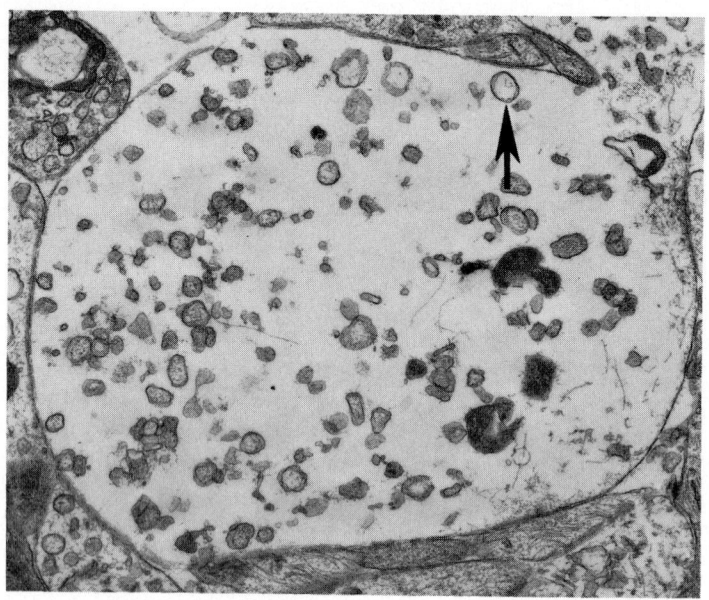

Figure 65–11. Axonal process in pars nervosa from a dog with hypophyseal diabetes insipidus associated with a large pituitary adenoma. The axonal swelling contains few secretory granules with dense cores but occasional irregularly shaped, empty vesicles. × 19,800.

plasma in response to exogenous ADH in the hypophyseal form (Fig. 65–13), but not in nephrogenic diabetes insipidus (Fig. 65–14), is useful in the clinical separation of these two forms of the disease (Richards, 1970; Lage, 1973).

NEOPLASTIC DISEASE OF THE PITUITARY GLAND

Endocrinologically Inactive Chromophobe Adenoma Arising in the Pars Distalis

Nonfunctional pituitary tumors occur frequently in dogs, cats, and horses but are uncommon in other species (Capen, 1978). There does not appear to be any breed or sex predisposition. Although chromophobe adenomas appear to be endocrinologically inactive, they may result in significant functional disturbances and clinical signs by virtue of compression atrophy of adjacent portions of the pituitary gland and dorsal extension into the overlying brain.

Dogs and cats with nonfunctional pituitary adenomas are presented with clinical disturbances related to lack of secretion of pituitary tropic hormones and diminished target organ function or dysfunction of the

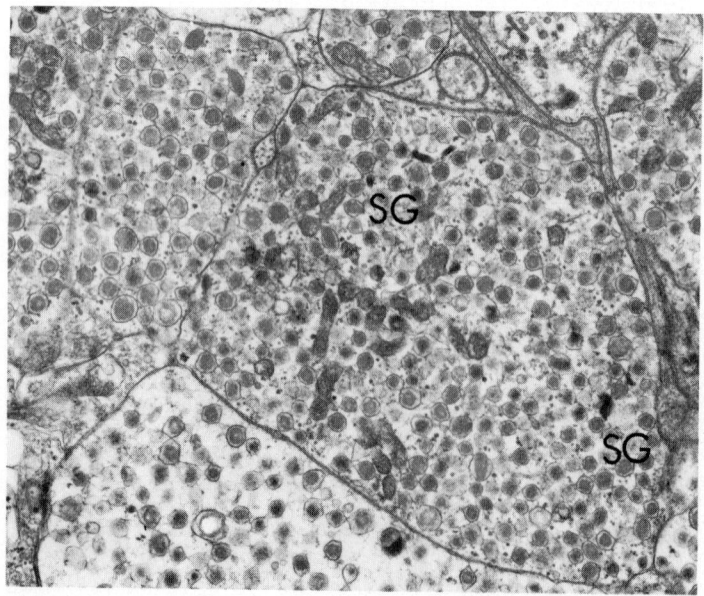

Figure 65–12. Axonal processes in pars nervosa from a normal dog illustrating numerous membrane-bound, ADH-containing secretory granules (SG). ×17,000. From Koestner, A., and Capen, C. C.: Ultrastructural evaluation of the canine hypothalamic-neurohypophyseal system in diabetes insipidus associated with pituitary neoplasms. Pathol. Vet. 4:513, 1967.

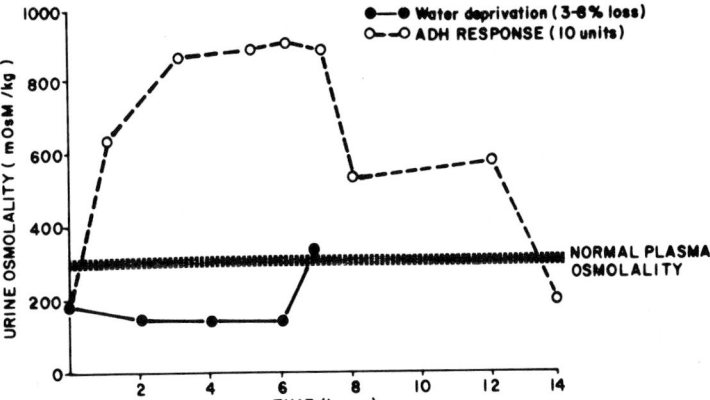

Figure 65–13. Hypophyseal diabetes insipidus in a Great Dane illustrating the decrease in urine osmolality below that of plasma and rapid increase of urine osmolality above normal plasma osmolality in response to exogenous ADH.

central nervous system (Capen, 1978; Gilbert and Willey, 1969; Farrow, 1969). An affected dog often is depressed and has incoordination and other disturbances of balance, weakness, collapse with exercise, and occasionally a change in personality. The animal may become unresponsive to people and develop a tendency to hide at the slightest provocation. In long-standing cases there may be evidence of blindness, with dilated and fixed pupils due to compression and disruption of optic nerves by dorsal extension of the pituitary tumor (Fig. 65–15). Affected dogs often have a progressive loss of weight ("pituitary cachexia"), with muscle atrophy due to a lack of protein anabolic effects of growth hormone (Fig. 65–16). Compression of the cells that secrete gonadotropic hormones or the corresponding releasing hormone results in atrophy of the gonads. They appear to be dehydrated, as evidenced by a lusterless dry haircoat, and the owner may have noticed increased consumption of water.

A consistent finding in dogs and cats with large nonfunctional pituitary tumors is excretion of large volumes of dilute urine with a low specific gravity (approximately 1.007 or lower). Water intake is increased correspondingly and the owner complains that the dog, previously housebroken, urinates frequently in the house. Disturbances of water balance are the result of interference with the synthesis of antidiuretic hormone in the supraoptic nucleus or release of the hormone into capillaries of the pars nervosa (Koestner and Capen, 1967). The posterior lobe, infundibular stalk, and hypothalamus are compressed or disrupted by neoplastic cells. This interrupts the nonmyelinated axons that transport antidiuretic hormone from its site of production, primarily in the supraoptic nucleus of the hypothalamus, to the site of release in the capillary plexus of the pars nervosa. Compression of neurosecretory neurons in the supraoptic nucleus of the hypothalamus by the dorsally expanding neoplasm also may result in decreased antidiuretic hormone synthesis.

Clinical signs in dogs and cats with non-

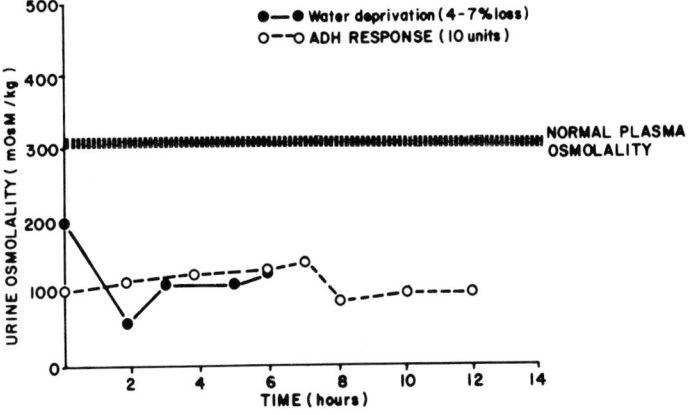

Figure 65–14. Nephrogenic diabetes in a poodle illustrating the decrease in urine osmolality below plasma and lack of response both to hyperosmotic stimuli provided by water deprivation and to the administration of exogenous ADH. Redrawn from Richards (1970).

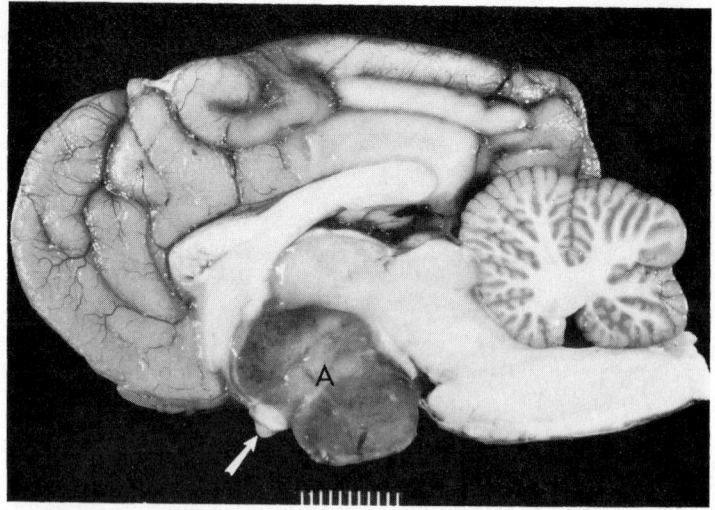

Figure 65–15. Large pituitary adenoma (A) in a dog extending dorsally out of the sella turcica into the overlying brain. The optic chiasm (white arrow) is severely compressed by the large adenoma. The adenohypophysis, neurohypophysis, and hypothalamus are incorporated and destroyed by the neoplasm, resulting in clinical disturbances of panhypopituitarism and diabetes insipidus.

functional pituitary adenomas and hypopituitarism are not highly specific and could be confused with other disorders of the central nervous system such as brain tumors and encephalitis, or chronic renal disease. Hypopituitarism caused by pituitary tumors should be included in the differential diagnosis of diseases characterized by incoordination, depression, polyuria, blindness, and a sudden change in personality in adult or old animals. Because the blindness is central in origin, ophthalmoscopic examination usually fails to reveal significant lesions. There is no effect on body stature associated with compression of the pars distalis and probable interference with growth hormone secretion, because these neoplasms usually arise in adult dogs that have already completed their growth. The atrophy of the skin and loss of muscle

mass may be related to a lack of protein anabolic effects of growth hormone in an adult dog or cat. Interference in the secretion of pituitary tropic hormones often results in gonadal atrophy resulting in either decreased libido or anestrus, reduced basal metabolic rate due to diminished thyrotropin secretion, and hypoglycemia from tropic atrophy of the adrenal cortex.

Endocrinologically inactive pituitary adenomas usually reach considerable size before they cause obvious signs or kill the animal (Fig. 65–15). The proliferating tumor cells incorporate the remaining structures of the adenohypophysis and infundibular stalk. The neoplasms are firmly attached to the base of the sella turcica, but there usually is no evidence of erosion of the sphenoid bone owing to the incomplete diaphragma sellae and dorsal growth of the

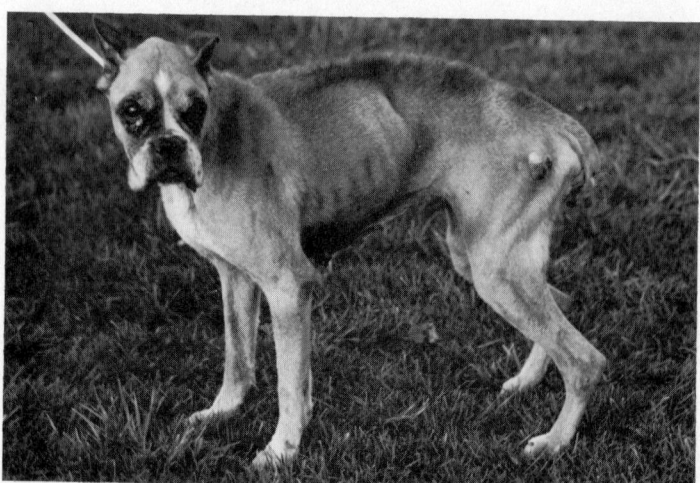

Figure 65–16. Pituitary cachexia in a dog with a large endocrinologically inactive pituitary adenoma resulting in adult-onset panhypopituitarism.

adenoma along lines of least resistance. The entire hypothalamus may be compressed and replaced by the tumor.

The adrenal glands of dogs and cats with large nonfunctional pituitary adenomas are small and consist primarily of medullary tissue surrounded by a narrow zone of cortex (Fig. 65–17). The adrenal cortex is a thin yellow-brown rim composed of a moderately thickened capsule and secretory cells of the outer zona glomerulosa, which are not predominately under the control of adrenocorticotropin. The zona fasciculata and reticularis are severely atrophied compared with these zones in normal adrenal glands. Thyroid glands in dogs and cats with large pituitary adenomas often are smaller than normal, though to a much lesser degree than the adrenal cortex (Fig. 65–17). The majority of the atrophic thyroid follicles are large, lined by a flattened cuboidal epithelium, and have few endocytotic vacuoles near the interface between the colloid and luminal aspect of the follicular cells. The thyroid lesion is due to lack of thyrotropic hormone–induced endocytosis of colloid. Seminiferous tubules of the testes are small and show little evidence of active spermatogenesis.

The cells comprising nonfunctional pituitary adenomas are cuboidal to polyhedral and are either arranged in diffuse sheets or subdivided into small packets by fine connective tissue septa. Special histochemical techniques for pituitary cytology fail to demonstrate specific secretory granules within the cytoplasm of tumor cells. The histogenesis of nonfunctional chromophobe adenomas in dogs is uncertain, but they appear to be derived from pituitary cells that are unable to either store or secrete an excess of a specific hypophyseal tropic hormone.

Functional Corticotroph Adenomas of the Adenohypophysis Associated with Hypercortisolism

Functional tumors arising in the pituitary gland are derived from corticotroph (ACTH-secreting) cells either in the pars distalis or in the pars intermedia. They cause a clinical syndrome of corticol excess (Cushing-like disease). These neoplasms are encountered most frequently in dogs and rarely in other animal species. They develop in adult to aged dogs and have been reported in a number of breeds (Capen et al., 1967; Clarkson et al., 1959; Coffin and Munson, 1953; Hare, 1935; Rijnberk et al., 1967, 1969; White, 1938). Boxers, Boston terriers, and dachshunds appear to have a higher incidence of functional (ACTH-secreting) pituitary tumors than other breeds of dogs. The spectrum of dramatic clinical manifestations and lesions that develop is primarily the result of long-term overproduction of cortisol by hyperplastic adrenal cortices. These changes are the result of the combined gluconeogenic, lipolytic, protein catabolic, and anti-inflammatory action of glucocorticoid hormones on many organ systems of the body.

A number of distinctive clinical and functional alterations develop in dogs with corticotroph (ACTH-secreting) adenomas, resulting in the syndrome of cortisol excess (Capen and Martin, 1975; Capen et al.,

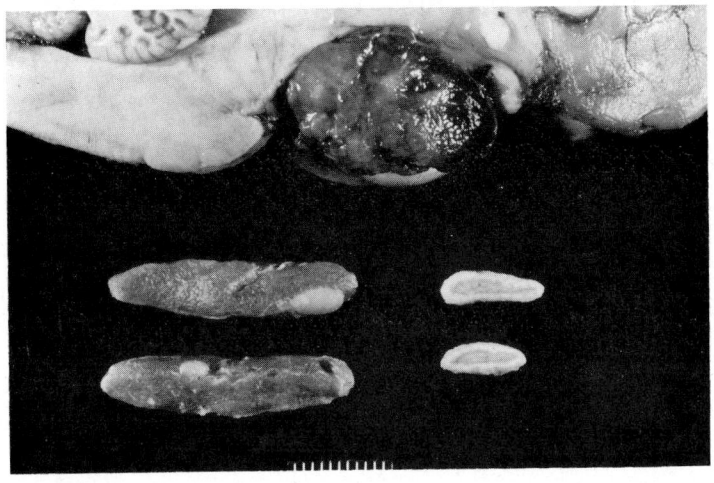

Figure 65–17. Large, endocrinologically inactive, chromophobe adenoma from a dog with extension into the hypothalamus. There is severe tropic atrophy and reduction in size of the adrenal glands (right) due to loss of cells in the zona fasciculata and reticularis from the subnormal secretion of ACTH. The thyroid glands (left) are approximately normal size due to the distension of follicles with colloid in the absence of thyrotropin secretion. The scale at the bottom represents 1 cm.

1967; Lubberink et al., 1971; Siegel et al., 1970). Centripetal redistribution of adipose tissue leads to prominent fat pads on the dorsal midline of the neck, giving the neck and shoulders a thick appearance. Appetite and intake of food may be increased or ravenous, either as a direct stimulation of the appetite center by the cortisol excess or as a result of destruction of the "satiety center" in the ventral medial nucleus of the hypothalamus by the dorsally expanding adenoma. Muscles of the extremities and abdomen are weakened and atrophied. The loss of tone of abdominal muscles and muscles of the abaxial skeleton results in gradual abdominal enlargement ("pot belly"), lordosis, muscle trembling, and a straight-legged skeletal-braced posture to support the body weight. Profound atrophy of the temporal muscles may result in obvious concave indentations and readily palpable prominences of the underlying skull bones. Hepatomegaly due in part to increased fat and glycogen deposition and vacuolation of liver cells may contribute to the development of the distended, often pendulous, abdomen. For a description of additional clinical signs associated with ACTH-secreting pituitary neoplasms, refer to the section on cortisol excess in Adrenal Gland Diseases, Chapter 69.

The pituitary gland is consistently enlarged in dogs with corticotroph adenomas (Fig. 65–18). Neither the occurrence nor the severity of functional disturbances appears to be directly related to the size of the neoplasm. Small adenomas are as likely to be endocrinologically active as are larger neoplasms. The larger adenomas often are firmly attached to the base of the sella turcica without evidence of erosion of the sphenoid bone. In the animal species most likely to develop pituitary neoplasms (e.g., dog and horse), the diaphragma sellae is incomplete. The line of least resistance therefore favors dorsal expansion of the gradually enlarging pituitary mass and invagination into the infundibular cavity; dilation of the infundibular recess and 3rd ventricle; and eventual compression and replacement of the hypothalamus, and extension into the thalamus.

Dorsal expansion of larger corticotroph adenomas results in either a broad-based indentation and compression of the overlying hypothalamus (Fig. 65–18) or an extension into and replacement of the parenchyma of the hypothalamus and occasionally the thalamus (Fig. 65–19). In the larger neoplasms there are often focal areas of hemorrhage, necrosis, mineralization, and liquefaction. In addition, growth of the pituitary tumor along the basilar aspects of the brain may result in incorporation of the second, third, and fourth cranial nerves leading to functional disturbances from a disruption of their function (Fig. 65–20).

There is bilateral enlargement of the adrenal glands in dogs with functional corticotroph adenomas (Fig. 65–18). This enlargement often is striking and is due entirely to increased cortical parenchyma, primarily in

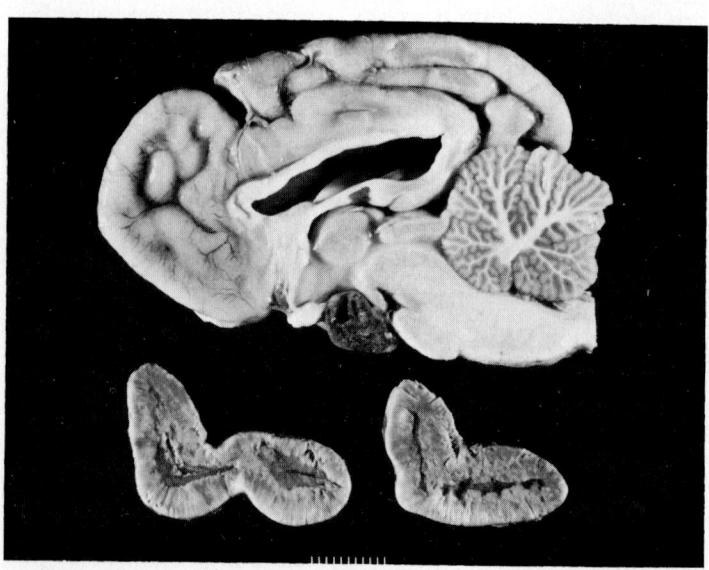

Figure 65–18. Corticotropic hormone (ACTH)–secreting chromophobe adenoma in the pituitary gland from a dog with bilateral enlargement of the adrenal glands. The long-term secretion of ACTH results in hypertrophy and hyperplasia of secretory cells of the zona fasciculata and reticularis in the adrenal gland and an excessive secretion of cortisol. The scale at the bottom represents 1 cm.

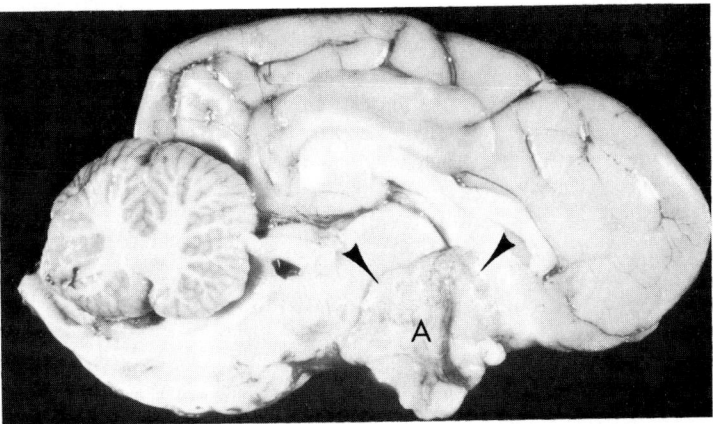

Figure 65–19. Large corticotroph adenoma (A) extending dorsally through the hypothalamus and into the thalamus. The pituitary adenoma is sharply demarcated (arrowheads) from the compressed brain and has completely incorporated the adenohypophysis and neurohypophysis.

the zona fasciculata and reticularis. Nodules of yellow-orange cortical tissue often are found outside the capsule in the periadrenal fat as well as extending down into the adrenal medulla. The cortico-medullary junction is irregular and the medulla is compressed. The secretion of excess cortisol in these dogs can be diminished by the administration of the adrenocytotoxic drugs, such as ortho,para'-DDD (Schechter et al., 1973; Hart et al., 1973).

Pituitary adenomas are composed of well-differentiated secretory cells supported by

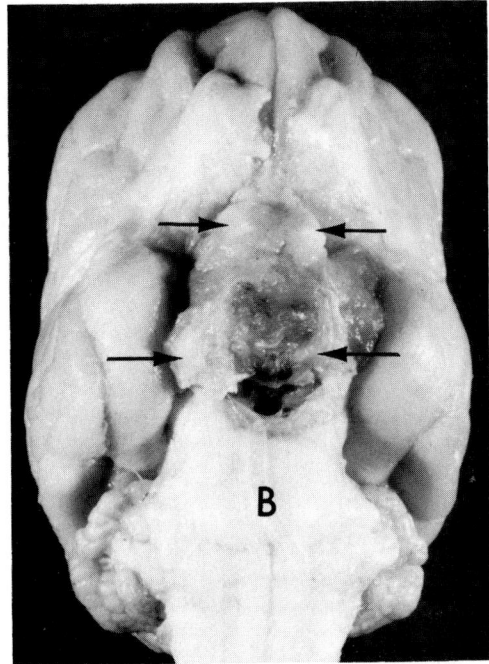

Figure 65–20. Corticotroph adenoma arising in the pituitary gland, with ventral extension along the brain (arrows) with the incorporation of cranial nerves. B, basilar artery.

fine connective tissue septa. Corticotroph adenomas are subclassified into sinusoidal and diffuse types on the basis of the predominant pattern of cellular architecture. They are composed of either large or small chromophobic cells. The cytoplasm of the tumor cells is devoid of secretory granules detectable by specific histochemical procedures used for pituitary cytology. However, pituitary adenomas arising in both the pars distalis and the pars intermedia associated with the syndrome of cortisol excess in dogs are composed of polyhedral cells that immunocytochemically stain selectively for ACTH and MSH (El Etreby et al., 1980). Nodules of focal hyperplasia and microadenomas, composed of similar ACTH/MSH cells, are also present in both lobes of the adenohypophysis.

Although remnants of the pars distalis can be identified near the periphery of the adenomas, the demarcation is not distinct between the neoplasm and pars distalis. The pars distalis is either partly replaced by the neoplasm or severely compressed. The pars nervosa and infundibular stalk are either infiltrated and disrupted by tumor cells or completely incorporated within the larger neoplasms.

Cells comprising functional corticotroph adenomas in dogs have definite ultrastructural evidence of secretory activity (Capen and Koestner, 1967). Organelles concerned with protein synthesis (endoplasmic reticulum) and packaging of secretory products (Golgi apparatus) are well developed in tumor cells. Hormone-containing secretory granules can be demonstrated by electron microscopy in cells comprising functional corticotroph adenomas. This is in contrast to the absence of demonstrable secretory granules within neoplastic cells observed by light microscopy following application of special histochemical procedures. The granules vary in number from cell to cell, are roughly spherical, and are surrounded by a delicate limiting membrane. They are small (mean diameter of 170 mμ), electron-dense, and have a prominent submembranous space.

Adenomas composed of chromophobic cells also have been reported in humans. These tumors possessed secretory activity and were accompanied by increased secretion of ACTH (Nelson et al., 1958; Engel and Kahana, 1963). Although Cushing's disease was first described in association with basophil adenomas of the hypophysis, present evidence suggests that ACTH is secreted by a special population of chromophobic cells in the adenohypophysis of humans and most animal species (Capen and Martin, 1975).

Adenoma of the Pars Intermedia

Adenomas derived from corticotroph cells of the pars intermedia are the second most common type of pituitary neoplasm in dogs. They develop more often in non-brachycephalic breeds of dogs than in brachycephalic breeds (Capen et al., 1967).

Adenomas of the pars intermedia in dogs are either (1) endocrinologically inactive and accompanied by varying degrees of hypopituitarism and diabetes insipidus or (2) associated with the secretion of excessive adrenocorticotropin (ACTH), leading to bilateral adrenocortical hyperplasia and the syndrome of cortisol excess. The clinical signs in dogs with functional corticotroph adenomas arising in the pars intermedia are similar to those arising in the pars distalis and the neoplastic cells stained immunocytochemically for ACTH and MSH (El Etreby et al., 1980).

Adenomas of the pars intermedia in dogs produce only a moderate enlargement of the pituitary gland. The pars distalis is readily identified and sharply demarcated from the anterior margin of the neoplasm. The tumor may extend across the residual hypophyseal lumen and cause compression atrophy, but it usually does not invade the parenchyma of the pars distalis. Though the posterior lobe is incorporated within the tumor, the infundibular stalk is intact. Degenerative changes within the neoplasm are minimal.

Adenomas of the pars intermedia in dogs appear to arise from the lining epithelium of the residual hypophyseal lumen covering the infundibular process. They are relatively small, more strictly localized than chromophobe adenomas arising in the pars distalis, and extend across the residual hypophyseal lumen to compress the pars distalis (Fig. 65–21). They are sharply demarcated from the pars distalis, usually by an incomplete layer of condensed reticulum; however, they are not encapsulated. The histopathologic appearance is strikingly different from adenomas arising in the pars distalis in that there are numerous large, colloid-filled follicles interspersed between nests of chromophobic cells (Fig. 65–21). The neoplastic cells compress and frequent-

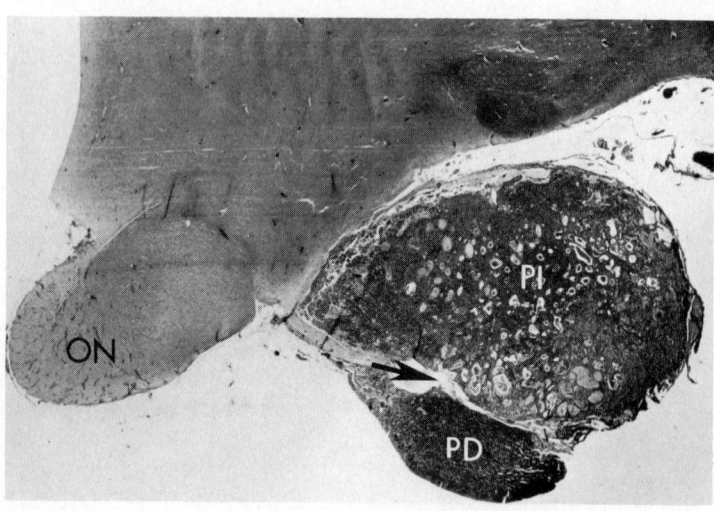

Figure 65–21. Adenoma arising in the pars intermedia of a dog. The neoplasm (PI) is sharply demarcated from the compressed pars distalis (PD). The arrow indicates the residual hypophyseal lumen. There are numerous colloid-filled follicles interspersed between the large nests of chromophobic cells within the adenoma. ON, optic nerve.

ly invade the pars nervosa and infundibular stalk, resulting in disturbances of water metabolism early in the course of development of the tumor (Capen and Koestner, 1967).

Acidophil Adenoma of Pars Distalis

Neoplasms derived from granulated acidophils are relatively uncommon, but acidophil adenomas and an adenocarcinoma have been reported in the dog (Capen et al., 1967a; Hottendorf et al., 1966; King et al., 1962; Lucksch, 1923). Acidophil tumors have been reported in dogs that had thickened cranial bones (Lucksch, 1923) and metahypophyseal diabetes (King et al., 1962) with fewer pancreatic islets than in normal dogs. A large, rapidly growing acidophilic adenoma was reported by Jubb (1962) in a ten-year-old Boston terrier. The tumor had extended out of the sella turcica and compressed the hypothalamus and several cranial nerves. Clinical signs were related to loss of normal hypophyseal function, because the large neoplasm had compressed the pars distalis.

Acidophil adenomas moderately enlarge the pituitary gland and indent the overlying hypothalamus. The enlarged hypophysis is composed of irregular columns of neoplastic acidophils interspersed among numerous large, blood-filled sinusoids. Although the degree of cytoplasmic granulation of acidophils varies from cell to cell, the predominating cells usually contain many secretory granules.

Two types of acidophils occur within pituitary acidophil tumors in dogs (Capen et al., 1967a) and cats. The predominating cell is smaller and contains many secretory granules (Fig. 65–22). The Golgi apparatus is comparatively small and has few presecretory granules. The rough endoplasmic reticulum is composed of flattened membranous sacs. Acidophils of this type are interpreted to be in the "storage phase" of the secretory cycle. The less common type of neoplastic acidophil has a greater cytoplasmic and nuclear area, and the cytoplasm contains numerous organelles but few mature secretory granules (Fig. 65–22). The rough endoplasmic reticulum consists of lamellar arrays and the Golgi apparatus is prominent. These hypertrophied acidophils are interpreted to be in the actively synthesizing phase of the secretory cycle.

Craniopharyngioma Associated with Hypopituitarism

This is a benign tumor derived from epithelial remnants of the oropharyngeal ectoderm of the craniopharyngeal duct (Rathke's pouch). Compared with all other types of pituitary neoplasms, craniopharyngiomas occur in younger dogs, and they are present in either a suprasellar or infrasellar location. They cause panhypopituitarism and dwarfism in young dogs through subnormal secretion of somatotropin and other tropic hormones beginning at an early age, prior to closure of the growth plates. Craniopharyngiomas have alternating solid and cystic areas (White, 1928). The solid areas are composed of nests of epithelial cells (cuboidal, columnar, or squamous) with focal areas of mineralization. The cystic spaces either are lined by columnar or squa-

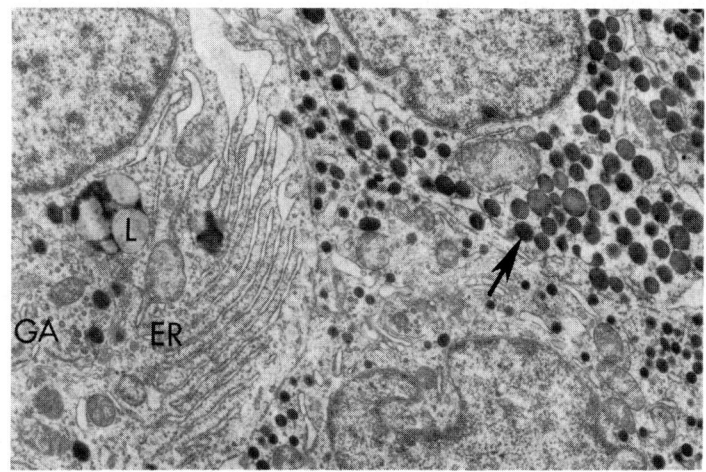

Figure 65–22. Electron micrograph illustrating cells in an acidophil adenoma arising in the adenohypophysis from a dog. The predominating type of neoplastic acidophil contains many large secretory granules (arrow), but organelles concerned with hormonal synthesis are poorly developed. Acidophils of this type were interpreted to be in the storage phase of the secretory cycle. The second type of neoplastic acidophil had few mature secretory granules but extensive profiles of endoplasmic reticulum (ER) and a prominent Golgi apparatus (GA). These acidophils were interpreted to be in the actively synthesizing phase of the secretory cycle. × 12,000.

mous cells and contain keratin debris and colloid.

Craniopharyngiomas in young dogs often are large and grow along the ventral aspect of the brain, where they can incorporate several cranial nerves. In addition, they extend dorsally into the hypothalamus and thalamus (Fig. 65–23). The clinical signs resulting from this type of pituitary tumor often are a combination of (1) lack of secretion of pituitary tropic hormones, resulting in tropic atrophy and subnormal function of the adrenal cortex and thyroid (Fig. 65–23), gonadal atrophy, and failure to attain somatic maturation owing to a lack of growth hormone; (2) disturbances in water metabolism (polyuria, polydipsia, and low urine specific gravity and osmolality) from an interference in the release and synthesis of antidiuretic hormone by the large tumor (Saunders and Rickard, 1952); (3) deficits in cranial nerve function; and (4) central nervous system dysfunction due to extension of the tumor into the overlying brain.

Pituitary Chromophobe Carcinoma

Pituitary carcinomas are much less common than adenomas and are found in older dogs. They usually are endocrinologically inactive but may cause significant functional disturbances by destroying the pars distalis and neurohypophyseal system, leading to panhypopituitarism and diabetes insipidus.

Pituitary carcinomas are large and they invade the brain and sphenoid bone of the sella turcica. Metastases may occur to distant sites such as the spleen or liver. Malignant tumors of pituitary chromophobes are highly cellular and often have large areas of hemorrhage and necrosis. Giant cells, nuclear pleomorphism, and mitotic figures are encountered more frequently in pituitary carcinomas than in adenomas.

Basophil Adenoma of Pars Distalis

Tumors composed of granulated basophils are among the most uncommon pituitary tumors in dogs. Cushing's disease in humans was initially attributed to hypersecretion of ACTH by small basophilic adenomas in the pars distalis. Current evidence indicates that they are a cause of only a small percentage of patients with Cushing's disease (Daughaday, 1974). Several of the early reports on corticotropin-secreting pituitary tumors in dogs with hyperadrenocorticism reflected this concept, and the neoplasms were reported to be basophil adenomas (Coffin and Munson, 1953; Diener and Langham, 1961; Belmonte, 1934; Dämrich, 1959; Spaar and Wille, 1959). Corticotroph (chromophobe) adenomas arising in the pars distalis and pars intermedia are the most common pituitary neoplasms associated with Cushing-like disease of cortisol excess in dogs (Capen et al., 1967; Schechter et al., 1973).

Metastatic (Secondary) Tumors of the Pituitary Gland

The pituitary gland is occasionally either partially or completely destroyed by tumors metastasizing from distant sites or invading

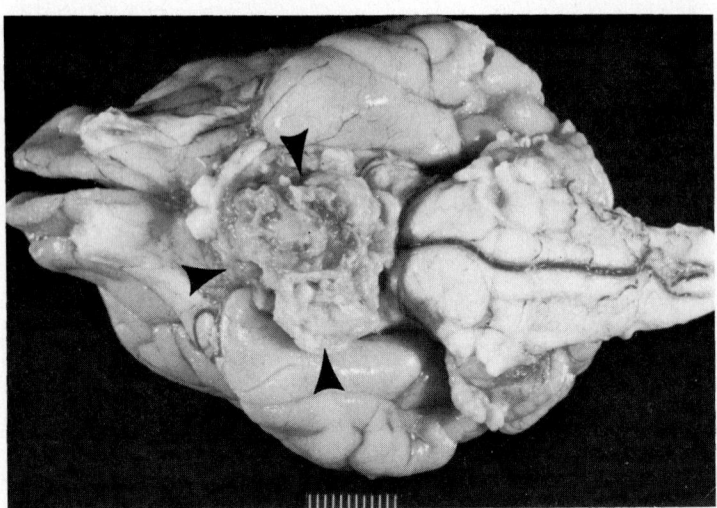

Figure 65–23. Large craniopharyngioma (black arrowheads) growing along the ventral aspect of the brain with incorporation of cranial nerves. The scale at the bottom represents 1 cm.

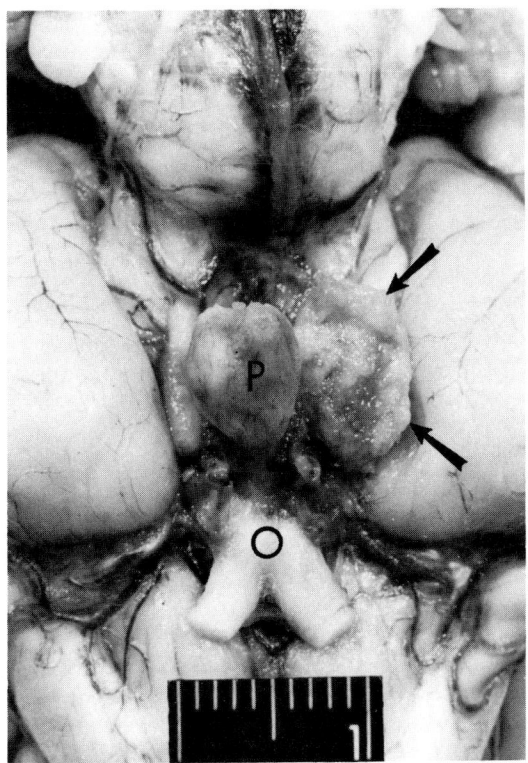

Figure 65–24. Meningioma (arrows) arising on the ventral aspect of the brain near the pituitary gland (P). Tumors of nonpituitary origin may interfere with function of the gland by exerting pressure on the portal system, infundibular stalk, or by incorporating the pituitary gland. O, optic chiasm. The scale at the bottom represents 1 cm.

from adjacent structures. Several examples include malignant lymphoma, malignant melanoma, and adenocarcinoma of the mammary gland in dogs. In addition, the pituitary, portal system, and infundibular stalk may be compressed or destroyed by local infiltration of an osteosarcoma arising in the sphenoid bone; ependymomas arising in the infundibular recess of the third ventricle; benign (Fig. 65–24) and malignant meningiomas arising on the ventral surface of the brain near the pituitary; gliomas ("infundibulomas") of the infundibular stalk (Saunders et al., 1951); and neurofibromas of cranial (e.g., trigeminal) nerves (Fig. 65–25). Small isolated metastatic foci usually are not associated with clinical disturbances of pituitary function. Larger metastatic tumors that disrupt a major function of the hypophysis may result in panhypopituitarism and diabetes insipidus.

CYSTS OF THE CRANIOPHARYNGEAL DUCT

Cysts may develop from remnants of the distal craniopharyngeal duct, which normally disappears by birth in most animal species. The cysts are lined by ciliated cuboidal to columnar epithelium and contain mucin (Rao and Bhat, 1971). In dogs, especially brachycephalic breeds, cysts from these remnants are frequently found at the periphery of the pars tuberalis and the pars distalis. Cystic remnants of the craniopharyngeal duct in one survey were found in 53 per cent of dogs of several breeds (Schiefer and Hänichen, 1967).

Craniopharyngeal duct cysts occasionally become large enough to exert pressure on the infundibular stalk and hypophyseal por-

Figure 65–25. Neurofibroma arising from the covering of the trigeminal nerve resulting in compression of the ventral aspect of the brain (arrows) in a dog. The tumor has extended into the region of the pituitary gland (P). O, optic chiasm. The scale at the bottom represents 1 cm.

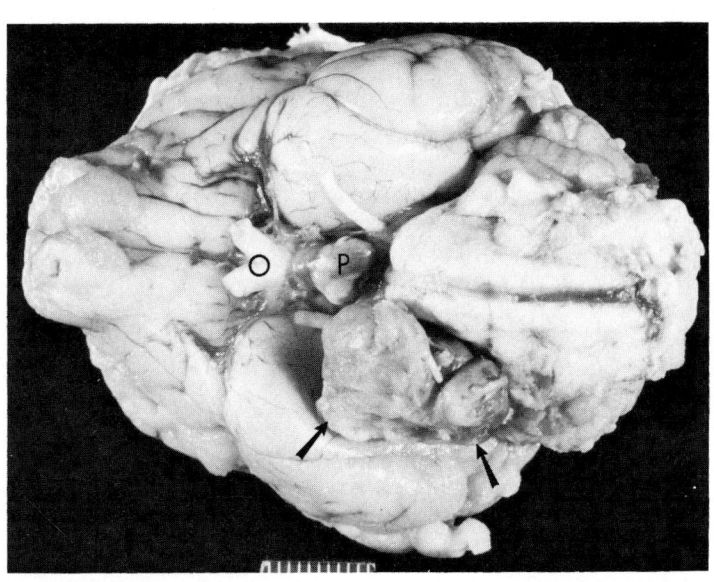

tal system, median eminence, or pars distalis. Structures adjacent to the cysts atrophy to varying degrees, owing to compression and interference with the blood supply. Disruption of a large cyst with escape of the proteinic contents into adjacent tissues may incite an intense, local inflammation with subsequent fibrosis that interferes with pituitary function. Clinical signs may include visual difficulties due to pressure on the optic chiasma, diabetes insipidus, obesity, and hypofunction of the adenohypophysis (gonadal atrophy, decreased basal metabolic rate, and hypoglycemia).

CYSTS DERIVED FROM THE PHARYNGEAL HYPOPHYSIS

The proximal portion of the adenohypophyseal anlage may persist in the dorsal aspect of the oral cavity in adults as undifferentiated remnants of cells along the craniopharyngeal canal or as differentiated cells similar to those of the definitive adenohypophysis. These remnants, called the pharyngeal hypophysis, have been described in dogs, cats, other animal species, and human beings (McGrath, 1974; Cohrs and Nieberle, 1967). In dogs, the pharyngeal hypophysis is physically separated from the sellar adenohypophysis, but in cats it may be continuous, owing to persistence of the craniopharyngeal canal.

The pharyngeal hypophysis of the dog is seen most frequently in brachycephalic breeds. It is a tubular structure lined with ciliated columnar epithelium. It is located on the midline of the nasopharynx and is frequently continuous with a multilocular cyst that is lined with squamous, ciliated cuboidal or columnar epithelium. The cyst contains a colloid-like material and cellular debris. A mass of differentiated acidophilic, basophilic, and chromophobic cells similar to those of the sellar adenohypophysis usually extends from the cyst wall.

Cysts (up to several cm in diameter) may be derived from the oropharyngeal end of the craniopharyngeal duct in dogs and project as a space-occupying mass into the nasopharynx. The predominant clinical sign may be related to respiratory distress due to ventral displacement of the soft palate and occlusion of the posterior nares (Slatter et al., 1976). The cyst wall may be hard on palpation from the presence of partially mineralized woven bone. The contents of the cyst often are yellow-gray and caseous, owing to the accumulation of keratin and desquamated epithelial cells from the cyst lining. The squamous epithelial lining of the cyst appears to be derived from metaplastic transformation of the remnants of the primitive oropharyngeal epithelium.

JUVENILE PANHYPOPITUITARISM ("PITUITARY DWARFISM")

Juvenile panhypopituitarism occurs most frequently in German shepherd dogs, but it has also been reported in other breeds, such as the spitz, toy pinscher, and Carelian bear dogs from Denmark (Alexander, 1962; Andresen et al., 1974; Baker, 1955; Jensen, 1959; Krook, 1969; Moch and Haase, 1953; Willeberg et al., 1975; Andresen and Willeberg, 1976). Pituitary dwarfism in German shepherd dogs usually is associated with a failure of the oropharyngeal ectoderm of Rathke's pouch to differentiate into tropic hormone–secreting cells of the pars distalis. This results in progressively enlarging, multiloculated cysts in the sella turcica and an absence of the adenohypophysis. The cyst(s) are lined by pseudostratified, often ciliated, columnar epithelium with interspersed mucin-secreting goblet cells. The mucin-filled cysts eventually occupy the entire pituitary area in the sella turcica and severely compress the pars nervosa and infundibular stalk (Fig. 65–26). Few differentiated, tropic hormone–secreting chromophils are present in the pituitary region of dwarf pups that immunocytochemically stain for the specific tropic hormones. An occasional small nest or rosette of poorly differentiated epithelial cells are interspersed between the multiloculated cysts, but their cytoplasm usually is devoid of hormone-containing secretory granules.

The dwarf pups appear normal or are indistinguishable from littermates at birth and up to about two months of age. Subsequently the slower growth rate than the littermates, retention of puppy haircoat, and lack of primary guard hairs gradually become evident in dwarf pups (Fig. 65–27). German shepherd dogs with pituitary dwarfism appear coyote- or fox-like owing to their diminutive size and soft woolly hair coat (Muller and Jones, 1973; Muller, 1979). A bilaterally symmetric alopecia develops gradually and often progresses to complete alopecia except for the head and tufts of

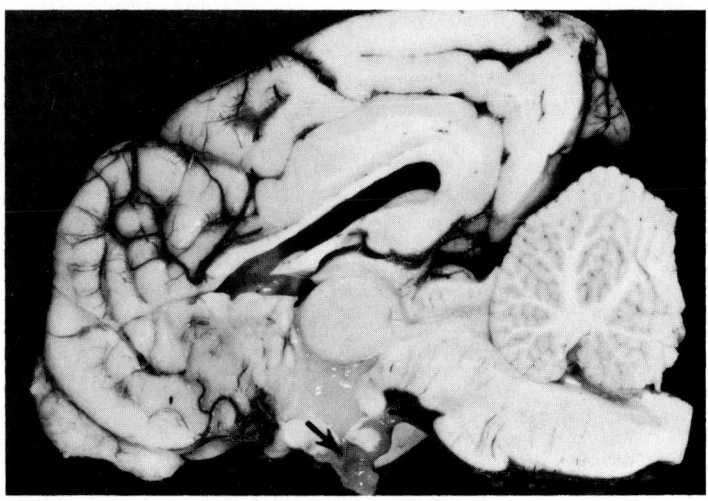

Figure 65–26. Panhypopituitarism ("pituitary dwarfism") in a dog associated with failure of the embryonic oropharyngeal epithelium of Rathke's pouch to differentiate into secretory cells of the adenohypophysis. Longitudinal section of the pituitary region and brain to illustrate the large multiloculated cyst. The pars nervosa was formed normally but was compressed by the mucin-filled cyst (arrow).

hair on the legs. There is progressive hyperpigmentation of the skin until it is uniformly brown-black over most of the body. Adult German shepherd dogs with panhypopituitarism vary in size from as tiny as four lbs up to nearly half the normal size, apparently depending upon whether the failure of formation of the adenohypophysis is nearly complete or only partial.

Permanent dentition is delayed or completely absent. Closure of epiphyses is delayed as long as four years, depending on the severity of hormonal insufficiency. There are few trabeculae in the primary and secondary spongiosa of the metaphysis of long bones, and osteoblasts are decreased in dwarf pups, as compared with normal littermates. The external genitalia usually remain infantile. The testes and penis are small, calcification of the os penis is delayed or incomplete, and the penile sheath is flaccid. In females the ovarian cortex is hypoplastic and estrus irregular or absent. The shortened lifespan in these dogs results not only from the panhypopituitarism but also from the resulting secondary endocrine dysfunction, such as hypothyroidism and hypoadrenocorticism. The increase in blood thyroxine and cortisol levels in response to challenge by exogenous thyrotropin and adrenocorticotropin are subnormal, owing to the hypoplasia of the thyroid gland and adrenal cortex (Scott et al., 1978). The variation in severity and onset of the lesions in pituitary dwarfism appears to be related to the degree that the oropharyngeal epithelium fails to differentiate and the rapidity with which the mucin-filled cysts enlarge and exert pressure on adjacent structures (Allan et al., 1978).

Other useful diagnostic aids include comparison of height with littermates, radiographs of open epiphyseal lines, thyroid function tests, and skin biopsy. Cutaneous

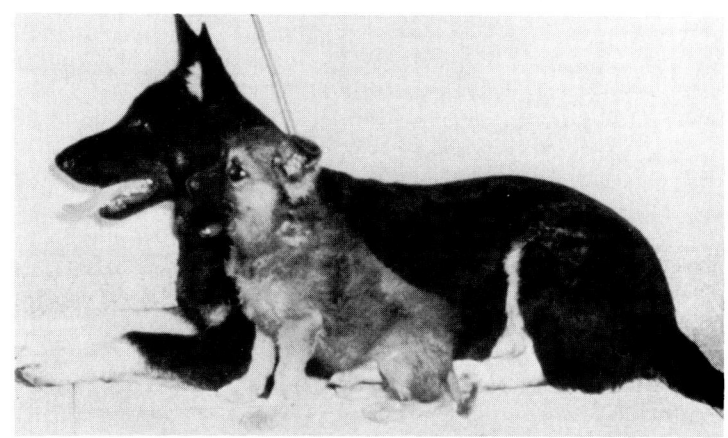

Figure 65–27. Panhypopituitarism ("pituitary dwarfism") in a 5-month-old German shepherd. An unaffected littermate weighed 60 pounds and the dwarf, 8.8 pounds. Note the retention of the puppy hair coat on the dwarf. Courtesy of Dr. J. Alexander and the Canadian Veterinary Journal (1962).

lesions include hyperkeratosis, follicular keratosis, hyperpigmentation, adnexal atrophy and a loss of elastin fibers, and the loose network of collagen fibers in the dermis. Hair shafts are absent and hair follicles are primarily in the telogen (resting) phase of the growth cycle (Muller and Jones, 1973; Cassel, 1978; Allan et al., 1978; Jones, 1979).

Panhypopituitarism in German shepherd dogs often occurs in littermates and related litters, suggesting a simple autosomal recessive mode of inheritance (Andresen and Willeberg, 1976; Andresen et al., 1974; Lund-Larsen and Grondalen, 1976; Willeberg et al., 1975; Nicholas, 1978). The activity of somatomedin (a cartilage growth– promoting peptide whose production in the liver and plasma activity is controlled by somatotropin) is low in dwarf dogs (Lund-Larsen and Grondalen, 1976). Intermediate somatomedin activity is present in the phenotypically normal ancestors suspected to be heterozygous carriers. Assays for somatomedin (a non–species-specific, somatotropin-dependent peptide) provide an indirect measurement of circulating growth hormone activity in dogs with suspected pituitary dwarfism (Willeberg et al., 1975; Van Wyk et al., 1974). Basal levels of circulating canine growth hormone are reported to be detectable but low (normal range: 1.75 ± 0.17 ng/ml) (Hampshire et al., 1975) in pituitary dwarfs and fail to increase following a provocative test for growth hormone secretion provided by clonidine injection (30 μg/kg, intravenous) as in normal dogs (Scott et al., 1978). Insulin hypersensitivity has been demonstrated in pituitary dwarf dogs, probably due to a change in insulin receptor numbers or affinity of binding in response to the low growth hormone levels (Scott et al., 1978). Dwarf dogs developed hypoglycemia of greater magnitude in response to an insulin injection (0.025 U/kg) than that in normal dogs but similar to that in experimentally hypophysectomized dogs.

In affected Carelian bear dogs there is low somatomedin activity. A simple autosomal recessive pattern of inheritance appears likely in these dogs, which were heavily crossbred with German shepherd dogs and apparently acquired the gene for dwarfism (Andresen and Willeberg, 1976).

The interesting dwarf German shepherd dog reported by Müller-Peddinghaus et al. (1980) with a cystic pituitary had surprisingly high (4.1 ng/ml) serum growth hormone levels (normal range 1.8 to 3.8 ng/ml) but an abnormally low (0.13 unit/ml) serum somatomedin level (normal for dog more than 0.50 unit/ml, as determined by ^{35}S incorporation into piglet rib cartilage). These changes in growth hormone and somatomedin levels resemble those found in Laron's syndrome of dwarfism in human infants, in which there is a peripheral resistance to the action of somatotropin. In this dog the adenohypophysis apparently had developed but subsequently underwent pressure atrophy from the multiple cysts in the pituitary gland derived from the craniopharyngeal duct. Only remnants of the adenohypophysis remained with compressed, immunocytochemically stained, tropic hormone–secreting cells.

Roth et al. (1980) investigated the pathogenesis of retarded growth in an inbred colony of Weimaraner dogs. Affected pups developed a wasting disease characterized by unthriftiness, emaciation, chronic anemia, stunted growth, and persistent infections. The thymus was small owing to a markedly diminished cortex. In pups that developed the wasting syndrome there was a lack of lymphocytes in paracortical areas of lymph nodes and around periarteriolar lymphoid sheaths of splenic white pulp. One pup that survived the wasting syndrome had a depressed lymphocyte blastogenic response to phytohemagglutinin compared with that of its surviving littermates. Pups with this syndrome also lacked the increase in plasma growth hormone concentration that occurs in normal dogs after injection of clonidine hydrochloride.

IATROGENIC ACROMEGALY

Acromegaly is a disease characterized by an overgrowth of connective tissue, increased appositional growth of bone, coarsening of facial features, and enlargement of viscera due to a chronic excessive secretion of growth hormone (somatotropin). Under experimental conditions, acromegalic characteristics have been induced in dogs by the long-term injection of anterior pituitary extracts (Putnam et al., 1929; Evans et al., 1933). Recently, Harris and Heaney (1969) increased skeletal mass of adult dogs of both sexes by the exogenous administration of bovine growth hormone (0.5 mg/kg/day) without inducing acromegaly or diabetes.

Although growth hormone–secreting acidophils are one of the major cell types in the adenohypophysis of dogs, the development of adenomas and primary hyperplasia derived from this population of acidophils is of infrequent occurrence in dogs. Lucksch (1923) reported an acidophil adenoma in a dog with thickened cranial bones. An acidophil tumor reported by King et al. (1962) was accompanied by metahypophyseal diabetes with fewer pancreatic islets than seen in normal dogs.

Rijnberk et al. (1980) detected the development of acromegalic features in a six-year-old female Belgian shepherd that had been frequently administered large doses of a progestational drug to prevent estrus. Initial clinical signs included polyphagia, exercise intolerance, intolerance to warmth (frequent panting, preference for cool places to sleep), exaggerated growth of the hair coat, slight exophthalmos, increase in abdominal size, mucometra, and inspiratory stridor. Subsequently, the body weight increased, and there was a disproportionate increase in the size of the head and limbs. The interdental spaces between incisors was considerably widened, owing to the proliferation of connective tissue (Fig. 65–28). The hair coat was thick and curly, and large skin folds were present on the ventral surface of the trunk and neck. Radiographically, there was spondylosis of the lumbar vertebrae and widening of the metaphalangeal bones, with a slight periosteal reaction.

Plasma growth hormone levels, determined by radioimmunoassay, were initially high (over 45 ng/ml) compared with 1.75 ng/ml ± 0.17 for clinically normal dogs (Hampshire et al., 1975) but progressively decreased toward normal over a period of about one year. The dog did not receive additional injections of medroxyprogesterone acetate during the interval of declining growth hormone levels. An oral glucose load resulted in a prolonged elevation of the blood glucose concentration, exaggerated insulin response with a prolonged elevation of plasma insulin levels, and a lack of suppression of the high immunoreactive growth hormone levels in the blood (Rijnberk et al., 1980).

During the interval of declining growth hormone levels, signs of respiratory distress and exercise intolerance progressively disappeared. The increased connective tissue mass appeared to regress, but the skeletal abnormalities remained unchanged. The glucose tolerance curve, insulin response to a glucose load, and growth hormone levels returned to normal over the three-year period of observation.

A stimulation of growth hormone–secreting acidophils in the adenohypophysis by progestational agents has also been reported under experimental conditions in the dog (El Etreby and Fath El Bab, 1978a; El Etreby et al., 1979 and 1979a). El Etreby and Fath El Bab (1978) observed increased numbers of somatotrophs after the administration of progesterone and cyproterone acetate. Diabetes mellitus has been observed in experimental dogs following the administration of medroxyprogesterone acetate

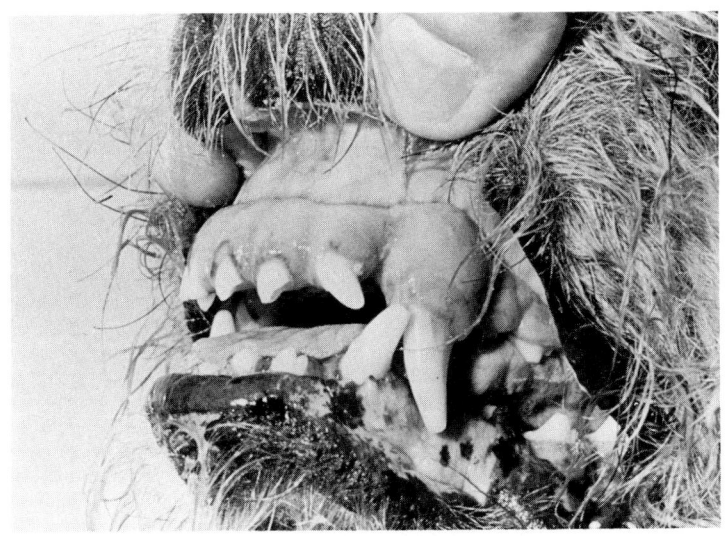

Figure 65–28. Iatrogenic acromegaly in a dog illustrating widening of the interdental spaces between the incisors due to the proliferation of connective tissue. The increased growth hormone secretion was stimulated by the administration of medroxyprogesterone acetate. From Rijnberk *et al.* (1980), Small Animal Clinic, Faculty of Veterinary Medicine, State University of Utrecht, The Netherlands.

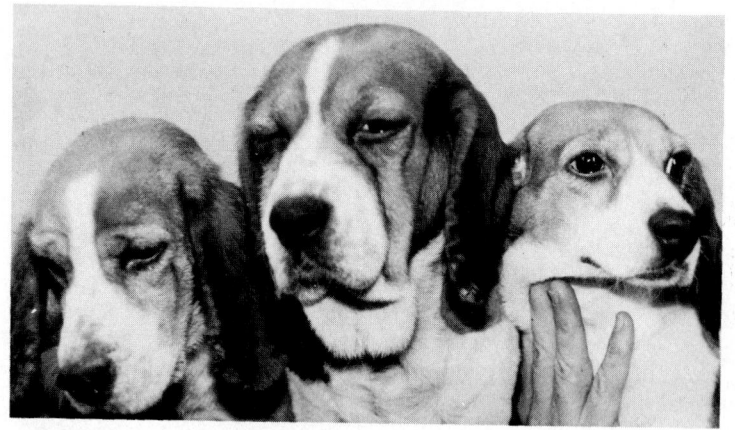

Figure 65–29. Iatrogenic acromegaly in a beagle (center) compared to unaffected littermates (left and right). Note the coarseness of facial features and marked thickening and folding of the skin of the face. Courtesy of Dr. P. Concannon, Department of Physical Biology, New York State College of Veterinary Medicine, Cornell University.

(Hansel et al., 1977) and megestrol acetate (Weikel and Nelson, 1977). The stimulation of growth hormone release in dogs by progestogens differs from the situation in human beings, in whom high prolactin levels result from treatment with these drugs.

Concannon et al. (1980) evaluated changes in plasma growth hormone, prolactin, cortisol, and progesterone levels in beagle bitches following intramuscular injection of medroxyprogesterone acetate (6α-methyl-17-acetoxyprogesterone) (75 mg/kg) every three months for 17 months. Circulating hormone levels were correlated with the development of acromegalic features (Fig. 65–29) and mammary nodules. The extent of acromegalic-like appearance was scored from 0 to 4 according to the following criteria: *0* — normal; *1* — coarse hair with slightly thickened and folded skin on the face, shoulders, back, and flank; *2* — in addition to 1, enlargement of the feet, thickening and folding of the skin on the forelegs; *3* — in addition to 1 and 2, prominent folds of thick skin on and about the face; *4* — in addition to all of the foregoing, more prominent facial changes and folds of thick skin extending over the body to the hind legs (Fig. 65–30).

Medroxyprogesterone acetate increased mean growth hormone levels, incidence of acromegaly-like changes, and frequency of palpable mammary nodules in beagles under controlled conditions (Table 65–1). Growth hormone levels were elevated (2.5 ng/ml and above) in all bitches with acromegalic features (mean 12.8 ng/ml) compared with placebo controls and dogs receiving crystalline progesterone implants. All bitches with elevated growth hormone levels

had multiple mammary nodules that averaged 9.5 ± 2.2 mm in diameter. The elevation in growth hormone levels and development of acromegalic features was greater in older (mean: 65.4 ± 6.9 months) than in younger (mean: 42.0 ± 1.7 months) bitches. Preliminary studies indicated that initial elevations of growth hormone occurred after eight months of medroxyprogesterone acetate treatment. Serum prolactin levels were not changed by either medroxyprogesterone acetate or crystalline progesterone implants, but serum cortisol levels were suppressed significantly compared with those in controls (Table 65–1). The latter probably was the result of

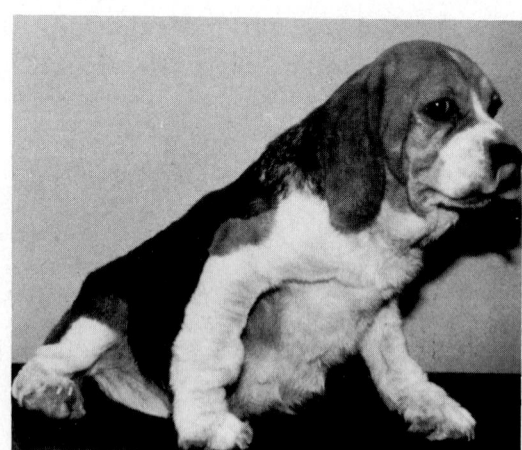

Figure 65–30. Iatrogenic acromegaly in a beagle caused by chronic stimulation of growth hormone secretion following the administration of medroxyprogesterone acetate (75 mg/kg every 3 months for 17 months). The skin of the face, trunk, and forelegs is coarsely thickened and folded. Courtesy of Dr. P. Concannon, Department of Physical Biology, New York State College of Veterinary Medicine, Cornell University.

Table 65–1. Effects of Medroxyprogesterone Acetate (MPA) (75 mg/kg Every Three Months for 17 Months) and Progesterone on Beagle Dogs

	Placebo Controls	MPA (75 mg/kg × 3 mo)	Progesterone Implants[a]
Serum Growth Hormone (ng/ml)	0.4 ± 0.1	9.5 ± 2.8†**	0.6 ± 0.2
Serum Prolactin (ng/ml)	12.6 ± 1.2	13.7 ± 2.8	13.6 ± 2.1
Serum Cortisol (ng/ml)	13.7 ± 1.4	1.7 ± 0.2†**	14.9 ± 1.2
Serum Progesterone (ng/ml)	5.3 ± 3.1	0.2 ± 0.02†**	13.8 ± 2.1*
Mammary Nodules: Numbers	2	35	8
Mean (mm) Diameter (range)	2.0 ± 0.0	7.9 (2-75)	3.7 (206)
Acromegaly Score	0 ± 0.0	1.3 ± 0.4**	0.3 ± 0.3

Different from placebo controls:
  *(P < 0.05)
  †(P < 0.01)
Different from progesterone implants:
  **(P < 0.05-0.01)

[a]Subcutaneous implants crystalline progesterone.

From Concannon, P., et al.: Growth hormone, prolactin, and cortisol in dogs developing mammary nodules and an acromegaly-like appearance during treatment with medroxyprogesterone acetate. Endocrinology *106*:1173, 1980.

medroxyprogesterone-induced suppression of pituitary adrenocorticotropin secretion and corresponding decrease in cortisol synthesis by the adrenal cortex (Concannon et al., 1980; El Etreby and Fath El Bab, 1978a; El Etreby et al., 1979a; El Etreby, 1979).

Growth hormone levels also have been reported to be elevated in dogs with spontaneous mammary tumors, and somatotrophs have cytologic evidence of increased secretory activity (El Etreby et al., 1980a).

REFERENCES

Alexander, J. E.: Anomaly of craniopharyngeal duct and hypophysis. Can. Vet. J. *3*:83, 1962.

Allan, G. S., Huxtable, C. R. R., Howlett, C. R., Baxter, R. C., Duff, B., and Farrow, B. R. H.: Pituitary dwarfism in German shepherd dogs. Small Anim. Pract. *19*:711, 1978.

Andresen, E., and Willeberg, P.: Pituitary dwarfism in Carelian bear-dogs: evidence of simple, autosomal recessive inheritance. Hereditas *84*:232, 1976.

Andresen, E., and Willeberg, P.: Pituitary dwarfism in German shepherd dogs. Additional evidence of simple, autosomal recessive inheritance. Nord. Vet. Med. *28*:481, 1976.

Andresen, E., Willeberg, P., and Rasmussen, P. G.: Pituitary dwarfism in German shepherd dogs. Nord. Vet. Med. *26*:692, 1974.

Baker, E.: Congenital hypoplasia of the pituitary and pancreas glands in the dog. J.A.V.M.A. *126*:468, 1955.

Belmonte, V.: Un caso de adenoma de la hipofisis en el perro. Rev. Hig. Sanidad. Pec. *24*:773, 1934.

Capen, C. C.: Tumors of the endocrine glands. *In* Moulton, J. E. (ed.): Tumors in Domestic Animals. 2nd ed. University of California Press, Berkeley and Los Angeles, 1978.

Capen, C. C., and Koestner, A.: Functional chromophobe adenomas of the canine adenohypophysis. An ultrastructural evaluation of a neoplasm of pituitary corticotrophs. Pathol. Vet. *4*:326, 1967.

Capen, C. C., and Martin, S. L.: Hyperadrenocorticism in dogs. An animal model for Cushing's syndrome in man. Am. J. Pathol. *81*:459, 1975.

Capen, C. C., Martin, S. L., and Koestner, A.: Neo-

plasms in the adenohypophysis of dogs. A clinical and pathologic study. Pathol. Vet. *4*:301, 1967.

Capen, C. C., Martin, S. L., and Koestner, A.: The ultrastructure and histopathology of an acidophil adenoma of the canine adenohypophysis. Pathol. Vet. *4*:348, 1967a.

Cassel, S. E.: Ovarian imbalance in a German Shepherd dwarf. V.M.S.A.C. *73(2)*:162, 1978.

Clarkson, T. B., Netsky, M. G., and de la Torre, E.: Chromophobe adenoma in a dog: Angiographic and anatomic study. J. Neuropathol. Exp. Neurol. *18*:559, 1959.

Coffin, D. L., and Munson, T. O.: Endocrine diseases of the dog associated with hair loss. J.A.V.M.A. *123*:402, 1953.

Cohrs, P., and Nieberle, K.: Textbook of Special Pathological Anatomy of Domestic Animals. 1st English ed. Pergamon Press, New York, 1967.

Concannon, P., Altszuler, N., Hampshire, J., Butler, W. R., and Hansel, W.: Growth hormone, prolactin, and cortisol in dogs developing mammary nodules and an acromegaly-like appearance during treatment with medroxyprogesterone acetate. Endocrinology *106*:1173, 1980.

Dämrich, K.: Ein polymorphzelliges basophiles adenom der hypophyse beim hund. Berl. Münch tierarztl. Wschr. *24*:109, 1959.

Daughaday, W. H.: The adenohypophysis. *In* Williams, R. H. (ed.): Textbook of Endocrinology. W. B. Saunders Co., Philadelphia, 1974.

Diener, R., and Langham, R.: Cushing's disease in the canine. Small Anim. Clin., *1*:274, 1961.

Dousa, T. P.: Cellular action of antidiuretic hormone in

nephrogenic diabetes insipidus. Mayo Clin. Proc. *49*:188, 1974.

El Etreby, M. F.: Effect of cyproterone acetate, levonorgestrel and progesterone on adrenal glands and reproductive organs in the beagle bitch. Cell Tissue Res. *200*:229, 1979.

El Etreby, M. F., and Dubois, M. P.: The utility of antisera to different synthetic adrenocorticotrophins (ACTH) and melanotrophins (MSH) for immunocytochemical staining of the dog pituitary gland. Histochemistry *66*:245, 1980.

El Etreby M. F., and Fath El Bab, M. R.: The utility of antisera to canine growth hormone and canine prolactin for immunocytochemical staining of the dog pituitary gland. Histochemistry *53*:1, 1977.

El Etreby, M. F., and Fath El Bab, M. R.: Effect of cyproterone acetate, d-norgestrel and progesterone on cells of the pars distalis of the adenohypophysis in the beagle bitch. Cell Tissue Res. *191*:205, 1978.

El Etreby, M. F., and Fath El Bab, M. R.: Effect of 17 β-estradiol on cells stained for FSH$^\beta$ and/or LH$^\beta$ in the dog pituitary gland. Cell Tissue Res. *193*:211, 1978a.

El Etreby, M. F., and Fath El Bab, M. R.: Localization of thyrotropin (TSH) in the dog pituitary gland. A study using immunoenzyme histochemistry and chemical staining. Cell Tissue Res. *186*:399, 1978b.

El Etreby, M. F., Friedreich, E., Hasan, S. H., Mahrous, A. T., Schwarz, K., Senge, T., Tunn, U., and Neumann, F.: Role of the pituitary gland in experimental hormonal induction and prevention of benign prostatic hyperplasia in the dog. Cell Tissue Res. *204*:367, 1979.

El Etreby, M. F., Gräf, K. J., Günzel, P., and Neumann, F.: Evaluation of effects of sexual steroids on the hypothalamic-pituitary system of animals and man. Arch. Toxicol., Suppl. *2*:11, 1979a.

El Etreby, M. F., Müller-Peddinghaus, R., Bhargava, A. S., and Trautwein, G.: Functional morphology of spontaneous hyperplastic and neoplastic lesions in the canine pituitary gland. Vet. Pathol. *17*:109, 1980.

El Etreby, M. F., Müller-Peddinghaus, R., Bhargava, A. S., Fath El Bab, M. R., Gräf, K. J., and Trautwein, G.: The role of the pituitary gland in spontaneous canine mammary tumorigenesis. Vet. Pathol. *17*:2, 1980a.

Engel, F. L., and Kahana, L.: Cushing's syndrome with malignant corticotrophin-producing tumor. Am. J. Med. *34*:726, 1963.

Evans, H. M., Meijer, K., and Simpson, M. E.: The growth- and gonad-stimulating hormone of the anterior hypophysis. *In* Memoirs of The University of California. University of California Press, Berkeley, 1933.

Farrow, B. R. H.: Chromophobe adenoma of the pituitary in a dog. Vet. Rec. *84*:609, 1969.

Feldman, E. C.: Effect of functional adrenocortical tumors on plasma cortisol and corticotropin concentrations in dogs. J.A.V.M.A. *178*:823, 1981.

Feldman, E. C., Bohannon, N. V., and Tyrrell, J. B.: Plasma adrenocorticotropin levels in normal dogs. Am. J. Vet. Res. *38(10)*:1643, 1977.

Gilbert, G. J., and Willey, E. N.: Pituitary chromophobe adenoma in the bulldog. J.A.V.M.A. *154*:1071, 1969.

Green, R. A., and Farrow, C. S.: Diabetes insipidus in a cat. J.A.V.M.A. *164*:524, 1974.

Halmi, N. S., Peterson, M. E., Colurso, G. J., Liotta, A.

S., and Krieger, D. T.: Pituitary intermediate lobe in dog: Two cell types and high bioactive adrenocorticotropin content. Science *211*:72, 1981.

Hampshire, J., Altszuler, N., Steele, R., and Greene, L. J.: Radioimmunoassay of canine growth hormone: Enzymatic radioiodination. Endocrinology *96*:822, 1975.

Hansel, W., Concannon, P. W., and McEntee, K.: Plasma hormone profiles and pathological observations in medroxy-progesterone acetate treated beagle bitches. *In* Garattini, S., and Berendes, H. W. (eds.): Pharmacology of Steroid Contraceptive Drugs. Raven Press, New York, 1977.

Hare, T.: Chromophobe cell adenoma of the pituitary gland associated with dystrophia adiposogenitalis in a maiden bitch. Proc. Roy. Soc.Med. *25*:1493, 1935.

Harris, W. H., and Heaney, R. P.: Effect of growth hormone on skeletal mass in adult dogs. Nature *223*:403, 1969.

Hart, M. M., Reagan, R. L., and Adamson, R. H.: The effect of isomers of DDD on the ACTH-induced steroid output, histology and ultrastructure of the dog adrenal cortex. Toxicol. Appl. Pharm. *24*:101, 1973.

Hottendorf, G. H., Nielsen, S. W., and Lieberman, L. L.: Acidophil adenoma of the pituitary gland and other neoplasms in a boxer. J.A.V.M.A. *148*:1046, 1966.

Howe, A.: The mammalian pars intermedia: A review of its structure and function. J. Endocrinol. *59*:385, 1973.

Jensen, E. C.: Hypopituitarism associated with cystic Rathke's cleft in a dog. J.A.V.M.A. *135*:572, 1959.

Jones, S. R.: Panhypopituitary dwarfism. *In* Andrews, E. J., Ward, B. C., and Altman, N. H. (eds.): Spontaneous Animal Models of Human Disease. Academic Press, New York, 1979.

Jubb, K. V.: The hypophysis. *In* Innes, J. R. M., and Saunders, L. Z. (eds.): Comparative Neuropathology. Academic Press, New York, 1962.

Kalimo, H., and Rinne, U. K.: Ultrastructural studies on the hypothalamic neurosecretory neurons of the rat. II. The hypothalamo-neurohypophysial system in rats with hereditary hypothalamic diabetes insipidus. Z. Zellforsch. Mikrask. Anat. *134*:205–225, 1972.

King, J. M., Kavanaugh, J. F., and Bentinck-Smith, J.: Diabetes mellitus with pituitary neoplasms in a horse and a dog. Cornell Vet. *52*:133, 1962.

Koestner, A., and Capen, C. C.: Ultrastructural evaluation of the canine hypothalamic-neurohypophyseal system in diabetes insipidus associated with pituitary neoplasms. Pathol. Vet. *4*:513, 1967.

Krook, L.: Metabolic bone diseases of endocrine origin: Hypopituitarism. *In* Dobberstein, J., Pallaske, G., and Stunzi, H. (eds.): Handbook of the Special Pathological Anatomy of Domestic Animals. Paul Parcy Verlag, Berlin, 1969.

Lage, A. L.: Nephrogenic diabetes insipidus in a dog. J.A.V.M.A. *163*:251, 1973.

Lubberink, A. A. M. E., Rijnberk, A., der Kinderen, P. J., and Thijssen, J. H. H.: Hyperfunction of the adrenal cortex: A review. Aust. Vet. J. *47*:504, 1971.

Lucksch, F.: Uber hypophysentumoren beim hunde. Tierarztl. Arch. *3*:1, 1923.

Lund-Larsen, T. R., and Grondalen, J.: Ateliotic dwarfism in the German shepherd dog: Low somatomedin activity associated with apparently normal pituitary function (2 cases) and with panadenopituitary dysfunction (1 case). Acta Vet. Scand. *17*:293, 1976.

McGrath, P.: The pharyngeal hypophysis in some laboratory animals. J. Anat. *117*:95, 1974.

Meijer, J. C.: An investigation of the pathogenesis of pituitary-dependent hyperadrenocorticism in the dog. Utrecht, The Netherlands, 1980.

Moch, R., and Haase, G.: Hypofunction der adenohypophyse eins hundes. Tierarztl. Umsch. *8*:242, 1953.

Muelheims, G. H., Kinsella, R. A., Jr., and Francis, F. E.: Maturity of the pituitary-adrenal axis in the newborn dog. Proc. Soc. Exp. Biol. Med. *143*:1197, 1973.

Muller, G. H.: Pituitary dwarfism: Cutaneous manifestations of an endocrine disorder. Vet. Clin. North Am. *9*:41, 1979.

Muller, G. H., and Jones, S. R.: Pituitary dwarfism and alopecia in a German shepherd with a cystic Rathke's cleft. J.A.A.H.A. *9*:567, 1973.

Müller-Peddinghaus, R., El Etreby, M. F., Siebert, J., and Ranke, M.: Hypophysärer Zwergwuchs beim Deutschen Schäferhund. Vet. Pathol. *17*:406, 1980.

Nelson, D. H., Meakin, J. W., Dealy, J. B., Matson, D. D., Emerson, K., and Thorn, G. W.: ACTH-producing tumor of the pituitary gland. New Engl. J. Med. *259*:161, 1958.

Nicholas, F.: Pituitary dwarfism in German shepherd dogs: a genetic analysis of some Australian data. Small Anim. Pract. *19*:167, 1978.

Papkoff, H.: Canine pituitary prolactin: Isolation and partial characterization. Proc. Soc. Exp. Biol. Med. *153*:498, 1976.

Putnam, T. J., Benedict, F. B., and Teel, H. M.: Studies in acromegaly, VIII. Experimental canine acromegaly produced by injection of anterior lobe pituitary extract. Arch. Surg. *18*:1708, 1929.

Quinlan, W. J., and Michaelson, S.: Homologous radioimmunoassay for canine thyrotropin: Response of normal and x-irradiated dogs to propylthiouracil. Endocrinology *108*:937, 1981.

Rao, R. R., and Bhat, N. G.: Incidence of cysts in pars distalis of mongrel dogs. Indian Vet. J. *48*:128, 1971.

Ricci, V., and Russolo, M.: Immunocytological observations on the localization of ACTH in the hypophysis of the dog. Acta Anat. *84*:10, 1973.

Richards, M. A.: Polydipsia in the dog. The differential diagnosis of polyuric syndromes in the dog. J. Small Anim. Pract. *10*:651, 1970.

Rijnberk, A., der Kinderen, P. J., and Thijssen, J. H. H.: "Cushing's syndrome" (spontaneous hyperadrenocorticism) in the dog. J. Endocrinol. *37*:Proceedings ii, 1967.

Rijnberk, A., der Kinderen, P. J., and Thijssen, J. H. H.: Canine Cushing's syndrome. Zentralbl. Veterinaermed. *16*:13, 1969.

Rijnberk, A., Eigenmann, J. E., Belshaw, B. E., Hampshire, J., and Altszuler, N.: Acromegaly associated with transient overproduction of growth hormone in a dog. J.A.V.M.A. *177*:534, 1980.

Rogers, W. G., Valdez, H., Anderson, B. C., and Cornella, C.: Partial deficiency of antidiuretic hormone in a cat. J.A.V.M.A. *170*:545, 1977.

Roth, J.: Introduction to session. *In* Beers, R. F., Jr., and Bassett, E. G. (eds.): Cell Membrane Receptors for Viruses, Antigens and Antibiotics, Polypeptide Hormones, and Small Molecules. Raven Press, New York, 1976.

Roth, J.: Receptors for peptide hormones. *In* DeGroot, L., and Cahill, G., Jr. (eds.): Endocrinology. Vol. III. Grune and Stratton, New York, 1979.

Roth, J. A., Lomax, L. G., Altszuler, N., Hampshire, J., Kaeherle, M. L., Shelton, M., Draper, D. D., and Ledet, A. E.: Thymic abnormalities and growth hormone deficiency in dogs. Am. J. Vet. Res. *41*:1256, 1980.

Saunders, L. Z., and Rickard, C. G.: Craniopharyngioma in a dog with apparent adiposogenital syndrome and diabetes insipidus. Cornell Vet. *42*:490, 1952.

Saunders, L. Z., Stephenson, H. C., and McEntee, K.: Diabetes insipidus and adiposogenital syndrome in a dog due to an infundibuloma. Cornell Vet. *41*:445, 1951.

Schally, A. V.: Aspects of hypothalamic regulation of the pituitary gland. Its implications for the control of reproductive processes. Science *202*:18, 1978.

Schechter, R. D., Stabenfeldt, G. H., Gribble, D. H., and Ling, G. V.: Treatment of Cushing's syndrome in the dog with an adrenocorticolytic agent (o,p'DDD). J.A.V.M.A. *162*:629, 1973.

Schiefer, B., and Hänichen, T.: Zur Kenntnis und möglichen Bedeutung von Hypophysencysten beim Hund. Acta Neuropath. *7*:232, 1967.

Scott, D. W., Kirk, R. W., Hampshire, J., and Altszuler, N.: Clinicopathological findings in a German shepherd with pituitary dwarfism. J.A.A.H.A. *14*:183, 1978.

Siegel, E. T., Kelly, D. F., and Berg, P.: Cushing's syndrome in the dog. J.A.V.M.A. *157*:2081, 1970.

Slatter, D. H., Schirmer, R. G., and Krehbiel, J. D.: Surgical correction of cystic Rathke's cleft in a dog. J. Am. Anim. Hosp. Assn. *12*:641, 1976.

Sloan, J. M., and Oliver, I. M.: Progestagen-induced diabetes in the dog. Diabetes *24*:337, 1975.

Sokol, H. W., and Valtin, H.: Morphology of the neurosecretory system in rats homozygous and heterozygous for hypothalamic diabetes insipidus (Brattleboro strain). Endocrinology *77*:692, 1965.

Spaar, F. W., and Wille, J.: Zur verleichenden Pathologie der Hypophysenadenome der Tiere. Zentralbl. Veterinaermed. *6*:925, 1959.

Turner, C. D., and Bagnara, J. T.: General Endocrinology. 5th ed. W. B. Saunders Co., Philadelphia, 1971.

Van Wyk, J. J., Underwood, L. E., Hintz, R. L., Clemmons, D. R., Viona, S. J., and Weaver, R. P.: The somatomedins: A family of insulin-like hormones under growth hormone control. *In* Recent Progress in Hormone Research, Academic Press, New York, *30*:259, 1974.

Weikel, J. H., and Nelson, L. W.: Problems in evaluating chronic toxicity of contraceptive steroids in dogs. J. Toxicol. Environ. Health *3*:167, 1977.

White, E. G.: A suprasellar tumor in a dog. J. Pathol. Bact. *47*:323, 1938.

Wilhelmi, A. E.: Canine growth hormone. Yale J. Biol. Med. *41*:199, 1968.

Willeberg, P., Kastrup, K. W., and Andresen, E.: Pituitary dwarfism in German shepherd dogs: Studies on somatomedin activity. Nord. Vet. Med. *27*:448, 1975.

CHAPTER 66

Calcium-Regulating Hormones and Diseases of the Parathyroid Glands

CHARLES C. CAPEN
and SHARRON L. MARTIN

The total blood calcium of mammals is approximately 10 mg/dl, with some variation due to species, age, dietary intake of calcium, and analytical method used to quantitate blood levels. The calcium concentration in the blood is composed of protein-bound and diffusible fractions (Fig. 66–1). Diffusible calcium consists of calcium complexed to anions such as phosphate and citrate plus the biologically active, "free" (ionic) calcium.

Calcium ion plays a key role in many fundamental biologic processes, including muscle contraction, blood coagulation, enzyme activity, neural excitability, hormone release, and membrane permeability; in addition, it is an essential structural component of the skeleton. Therefore, the precise control of calcium ion in extracellular fluids is vital to the health of humans and animals. To maintain a constant concentration of blood calcium despite marked variations in intake and excretion, endocrine control mechanisms have evolved that consist primarily of the interactions of three major hormones. Although the direct roles of parathyroid hormone (PTH), calcitonin (CT), and vitamin D frequently are emphasized in the control of blood calcium, other hormones such as adrenal corticosteroids, estrogens, thyroxine, somatotropin, and glucagon may contribute to the maintenance of calcium homeostasis under certain conditions.

CALCIUM-REGULATING HORMONES

PARATHYROID HORMONE

Anatomy and Embryology. Parathyroid glands are present in all air-breathing verte-brates. In the dog and cat, both the external and internal parathyroids are in close proximity to the thyroid gland. The external parathyroid (III) in the dog is from two to five millimeters in length and found in the loose connective tissue cranial and slightly lateral to the anterior pole of the thyroid. The internal parathyroid (IV) is smaller, flatter, and situated on the dorsal medial surface of the thyroid beneath the fibrous capsule. The blood supplies of the two pairs of parathyroid glands in the dog are separate, the external parathyroid being supplied by a branch from the cranial thyroid artery and the internal parathyroid by minute ramifications of the arterial supply to the thyroid (Smithcors, 1964).

Functional Cytology of Parathyroid Chief Cells. Present evidence indicates that the parathyroid gland contains a single basic type of secretory cell concerned with the elaboration of one hormone (Capen and Roth, 1973). The parathyroids of man and animals are composed of chief cells in different stages of secretory activity and in transition to oxyphil cells in certain species (Capen, 1975). Chief cells interpreted as being in an inactive (resting or involuted) stage of their secretory cycle predominate in the parathyroid glands of humans and of most animal species. Active chief cells occur less frequently in the parathyroids of most species under normal conditions. The cytoplasm of active chief cells has an increased density, owing to the close proximity of organelles, numerous secretion granules, overall density of the cytoplasmic matrix, and loss of glycogen particles and lipid bodies (Roth and Capen, 1974).

Biosynthesis of Parathyroid Hormone. Recent evidence suggests that a larger bio-

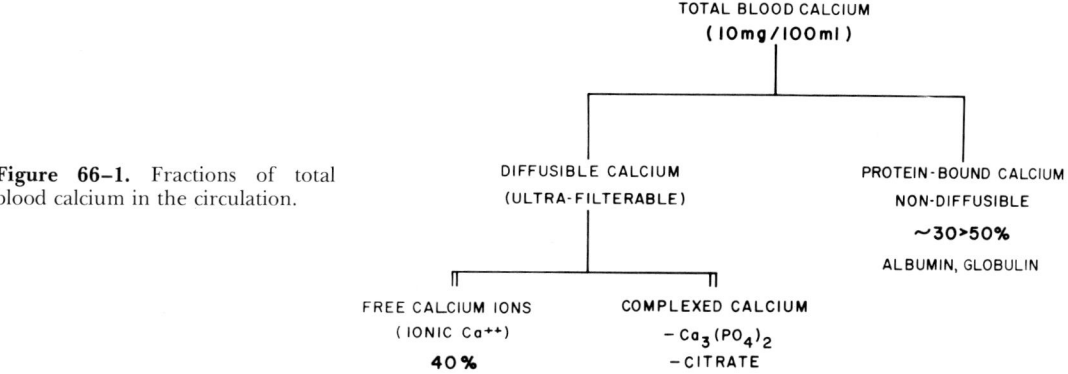

Figure 66–1. Fractions of total blood calcium in the circulation.

synthetic precursor is first synthesized on ribosomes of the rough endoplasmic reticulum in chief cells (Arnaud et al., 1971; Cohen et al., 1974; Habener et al., 1971; Kemper et al., 1972; MacGregor et al., 1973; Potts, 1976; Sherwood et al., 1970; Habener and Kronenberg, 1978; Habener and Potts, 1978). Pre-proparathyroid hormone (pre-proPTH) is the initial translational product

synthesized on ribosomes. It is composed of 115 amino acids and contains a hydrophobic signal or leader sequence of 25 amino acid residues that may facilitate the penetration and subsequent vectorial discharge of the nascent peptide into the cisternal space of the rough endoplasmic reticulum (Habener, 1976; Habener and Potts, 1978) (Fig. 66–2). Preproparathyroid hor-

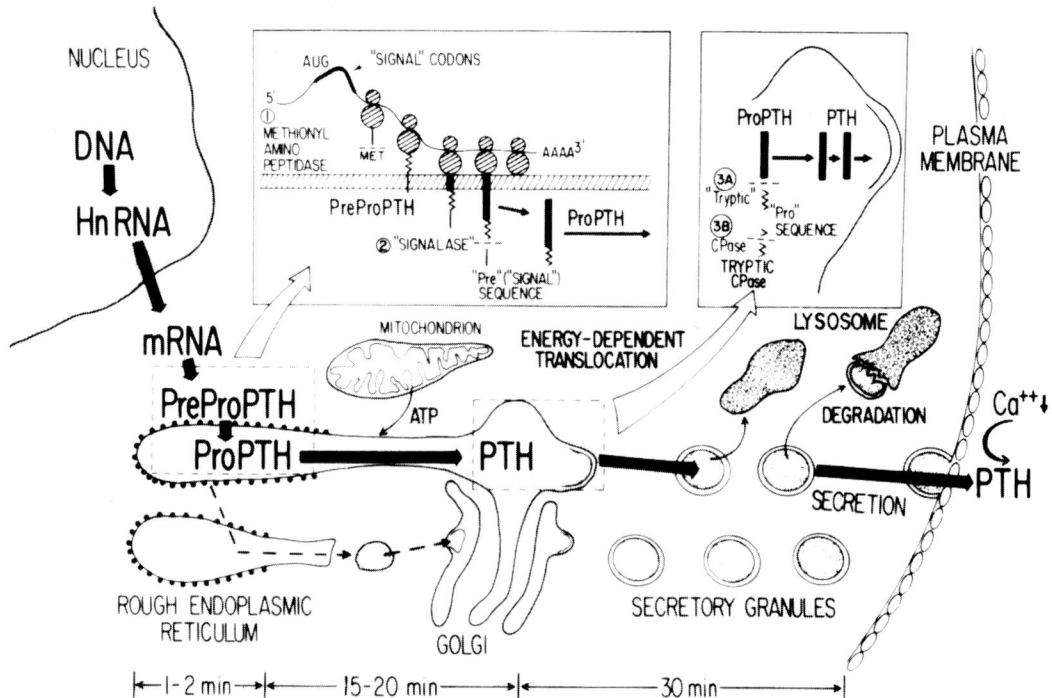

Figure 66–2. Subcellular compartmentalization, transport, and cleavage of precursors of parathyroid hormone (PTH). Pre-proparathyroid hormone (pre-pro-PTH) is the initial translation product from ribosomes of the rough endoplasmic reticulum, which is rapidly converted to pro-parathyroid hormone (pro-PTH). The hydrophobic precursor sequence on the amino-terminal end of the pre-pro-PTH facilitates penetration of the leading portion of the nascent peptide into the lumen of the endoplasmic reticulum. Pro-PTH is transported to the Golgi apparatus, where it is converted enzymatically by a carboxypeptidase (CPase) to biologically active PTH. A major portion of the biosynthetic precursors and active PTH is degraded by lysosomal enzymes and not secreted by chief cells. Parathyroid secretory protein (PSP) may function as a binding protein for PTH during intracellular storage in secretion granules and be released into the extracellular space. (From Habener, J. F., and Potts, J. T., Jr.: Biosynthesis of parathyroid hormone. New Engl. J. Med. *299*:580, 1978.)

mone is rapidly converted (within one minute or less of its synthesis) to proparathyroid hormone (proPTH) by proteolytic cleavage of the NH$_2$-terminal sequence of 25 amino acids (Fig. 66–3) (Habener and Potts, 1979).

The intermediate precursor, proPTH, is composed of 90 amino acids and moves within membranous channels of the endoplasmic reticulum to the Golgi apparatus (Fig. 66–2). Enzymes with trypsin- and carboxypeptidase B–like activity within membranes of the Golgi apparatus cleave a hexapeptide from the NH$_2$-terminal (biologically active) end of the molecule, forming active parathyroid hormone (PTH) (Fig. 66–3) (Habener et al., 1976; Habener and Kemper, 1978; Habener and Potts, 1976; MacGregor et al., 1978). Active PTH is packaged into membrane-limited, macromolecular aggregates in the Golgi apparatus for subsequent storage in chief cells. Under certain conditions of increased demand, PTH may bypass packaging in the Golgi apparatus and be released directly from chief cells.

Biologically active parathyroid hormone secreted by chief cells is a straight chain polypeptide, consisting of 84 amino acid residues with a molecular weight of approximately 9500 (Brewer et al., 1974). Molecular fragments (C- and N-terminal) of PTH are formed in the peripheral circulation, at the target cells of the hormone, and possibly within chief cells. The immunoheterogeneity created by the multiple circulating fragments of PTH has caused significant problems in the development and application of highly specific radioimmunoassays to clinical diagnostic problems (Arnaud, 1973).

Current evidence suggests it is in the Golgi apparatus that PTH (1 to 84 amino acid sequence) is cleaved enzymatically from proparathyroid hormone and packaged into mature secretory or storage granules (Fischer et al., 1972; Cohn et al., 1974). As the Golgi apparatus subsequently involutes, acid phosphatase activity appears in its membranes and acid phosphatase–positive lysosomal bodies are formed in the Golgi complex (Shannon and Roth, 1971). During the involuting phase the parathyroid hormone (1 to 84 amino acid sequence), packaged in granules, moves from the Golgi region and is stored in the cytoplasm prior to secretion from chief cells. Low ambient calcium speeds up the rate of secretion of PTH and shortens the resting phase of chief cells; conversely, high ambient calcium suppresses the rate of hormone secretion and lengthens the resting phase of the secretory cycle.

Storage and Secretion of Parathyroid Hormone. Secretory ("storage") granules have been demonstrated readily at the level of

CHEMISTRY OF PARATHYROID HORMONE AND RELATED PEPTIDES

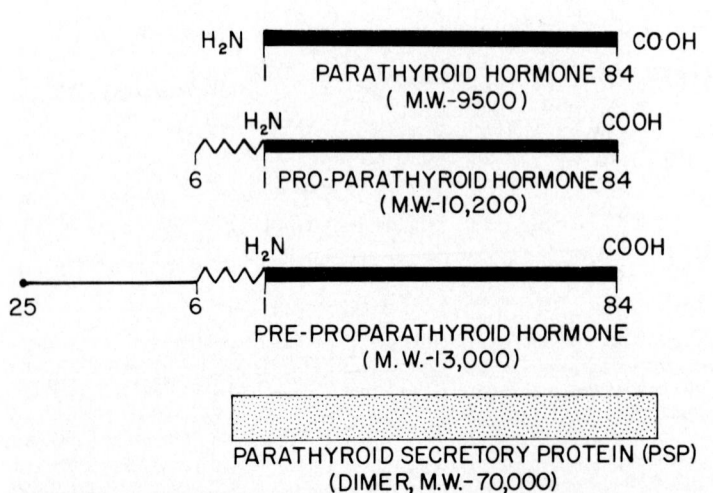

Figure 66–3. Chemistry of parathyroid hormone and related peptides synthesized by chief cells. Active parathyroid hormone is first synthesized as part of large biosynthetic precursor molecules. Pre-proparathyroid hormone (115 amino acids) is the initial translational product from ribosomes and is rapidly converted to pro-parathyroid hormone in the rough endoplasmic reticulum. Pro-parathyroid hormone (90 amino acids) is converted enzymatically to active parathyroid hormone (84 amino acids) in the Golgi apparatus as the hormone is packaged into secretory (storage) granules. Parathyroid secretory protein is a high molecular weight molecule synthesized by chief cells, incorporated into storage granules with active parathyroid hormone, and secreted in parallel with active hormone in response to changes in blood calcium. It probably functions as a binding protein during intracellular transport and secretion into the extracellular space.

ultrastructure within chief cells of the parathyroid glands in man and all animal species examined (Altenähr, 1972; Capen and Roth, 1973; Roth and Capen, 1974). Roth et al. (1974) localized PTH within chief cells of bovine parathyroids to the small membrane-limited secretory granules by immunocytochemical techniques using rabbit antiserum and peroxidase-labeled goat anti-rabbit globulin. The rabbit antiserum used in these studies recognized multiple antigenic determinants of bovine PTH, including the biologically active N-terminal of the molecule. Reaction product was not deposited over the larger acid phosphatase–positive lysosomal bodies in chief cells.

Secretory granules in chief cells also contain a parathyroid secretory protein (PSP) in addition to parathyroid hormone (Fig. 66–3). Kemper et al. (1974) reported that bovine parathyroids incubated *in vitro* secrete a protein that is distinct from both proPTH and PTH. It is a large protein (two or more subunits of molecular weight 70,000) and comprises about 50 per cent of the total protein secreted by the parathyroid. PSP may accompany PTH in the intracellular transport pathway through cytoplasmic organelles and is associated predominantly with the particulate fraction of chief cells (Habener and Potts, 1979). Secretion of PSP is stimulated or inhibited in parallel with that of PTH by varying the concentration of calcium in the incubation medium. The coordinated secretion of PSP and PTH in response to changes in ambient calcium suggests that both molecules are present in the membrane-limited secretion granules in chief cells (Fig. 66–2). Although the function of PSP is uncertain at present, it appears to represent a "binding protein" for parathyroid hormone and may be analogous in function to the neurophysins secreted with oxytocin and vasopressin by the neurohypophyseal system (Fawcett et al., 1968).

The secretory granules migrate peripherally in chief cells, and their limiting membrane appears to fuse with the plasma membrane of the cell. An internal cytoskeleton composed of microtubules and contractile filaments has been reported to be important in the control of the peripheral movement of secretory granules and the liberation of secretory products from other endocrine cells (e.g., beta cells of the pancreatic islets) (Lacy et al., 1968). The presence of peripheral microfilaments in chief

cells as well as the attachment of granules to the plasma membrane by stalklike condensations of cytoplasmic material in some species suggests that a similar secretory mechanism exists in parathyroid glands (Youshak and Capen, 1970).

Secretory granules appear to be extruded from chief cells by exocytosis within cytoplasmic projections into perivascular spaces (Fetter and Capen, 1968). The stalk of these cytoplasmic protuberances constricts and detaches from chief cells (Capen, 1971; Fetter and Capen, 1970). In addition, numerous small spherules of similar size have been observed protruding from secretory surfaces of chief cells into perivascular spaces by scanning electron microscopy (Fig. 66–4) (Capen, 1971). Thiele and Wermbter (1974) used freeze fracture techniques to demonstrate secretory granules being discharged from chief cells by exocytosis in the human parathyroid gland.

Control of Parathyroid Hormone Secretion. Secretory cells in the parathyroids store relatively small amounts of preformed hormone but are capable of responding to minor fluctuations in calcium ion concentration rapidly by altering the rate of hormonal secretion (Potts et al., 1971) and more slowly by altering the rate of hormonal synthesis (Roth and Raisz, 1964). In contrast to most endocrine organs, which are under complex controls, the parathyroids have a unique

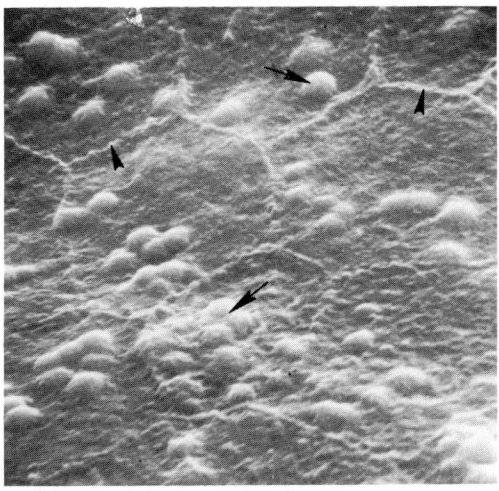

Figure 66–4. Scanning electron micrograph of canine parathyroid gland showing many small spherules (arrows) with hormone-containing secretion granules projecting from the secretory surface of chief cells. Chief cells are polyhedral and distinct cell boundaries can be visualized (arrowheads). × 7500.

feedback control system, controlled primarily by the concentration of calcium (and to a lesser extent magnesium) ion in serum (Targovnik et al., 1976).

If the blood calcium is elevated by the intravenous infusion of calcium, there is a rapid and pronounced reduction in circulating levels of immunoreactive parathyroid hormone (iPTH). Conversely, if the blood calcium level is lowered by EDTA (ethylenediaminetetraacetic acid) there is a brisk and substantial increase in iPTH levels (Oldham et al., 1971). The concentration of blood phosphorus has no direct regulatory influence on the synthesis and secretion of PTH; however, certain disease conditions with hyperphosphatemia in both animals and humans are associated clinically with hyperparathyroidism. An elevated blood phosphorus level may lead indirectly to parathyroid stimulation by virtue of its ability to lower blood calcium according to the mass-law equation when the serum is saturated with respect to these two ions (Krook and Lowe, 1964). If the blood phosphorus level is elevated significantly by an infusion of phosphate and calcium administered simultaneously in amounts to prevent the accompanying reduction of blood calcium, plasma iPTH levels remain within the normal range.

Magnesium ion has an effect on parathyroid secretory rate similar to that of calcium, but its effect is not equipotent to that of calcium (Mayer, 1974; Mayer and Hurst, 1978; Morrissey and Cohn, 1978). The more potent effects of calcium ion in the control of PTH secretion together with its preponderance over magnesium in the extracellular fluid suggest a secondary role for magnesium in parathyroid control.

Calcium ion controls not only the rate of biosynthesis and secretion of parathyroid hormone but also other metabolic and intracellular degradative processes within chief cells (Chu et al., 1973). An increased calcium ion in extracellular fluids rapidly inhibits the uptake of amino acids by chief cells, synthesis of proPTH and conversion to PTH, and secretion of stored PTH (Fig. 66–5). The shifting of the per cent of flow of proPTH from the degradative pathways to the synthetic route represents a key adaptive response of the parathyroid gland to a low calcium diet (Fig. 66–6) (Chu et al., 1973a). Parathyroids from rats fed a low calcium (0.02 per cent) diet convert approximately 40 per cent of proPTH into PTH, compared to a 20 per cent conversion in rats fed a control diet. During periods of long-term calcium restriction, the enhanced synthesis and secretion of PTH would be accomplished by an increased capacity of the entire pathway in individual chief cells and through hyperplasia of active chief cells (Fig. 66–6) (Cohn et al., 1974). Degradation of "mature PTH" by lysosomal enzymes occurs after prolonged exposure of chief cells to a high calcium environment.

Biologic Action of Parathyroid Hormone. Parathyroid hormone is the principal hormone involved in the minute-to-minute fine regulation of blood calcium in mammals. It exerts its biologic actions by directly influencing the function of target cells primarily in bone and kidney, and possibly in the intestine, to maintain plasma calcium at a level sufficient to ensure the optimal functioning of a wide variety of body cells.

PTH acts on bone to mobilize calcium from skeletal reserves into extracellular fluids (Fig. 66–7). The administration of PTH causes an initial decline, followed by a

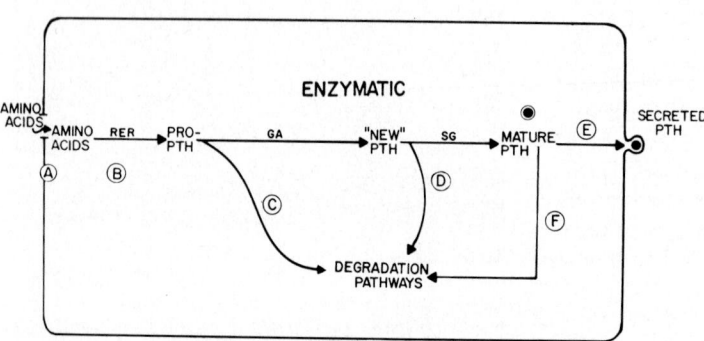

Figure 66–5. Multiple sites of control by calcium ion of parathyroid hormone biosynthesis and secretion in chief cells. (From Chu, L. L. H., et al.: Biosynthesis of proparathyroid hormone and parathyroid hormone by human parathyroid glands. J. Clin. Invest. 52:3089, 1973b.)

MULTIPLE SITES OF CONTROL BY CA⁺⁺

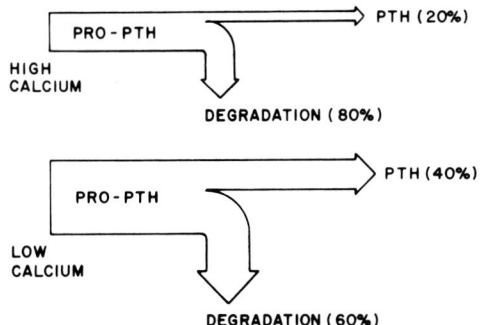

Figure 66–6. Adaptive responses of parathyroid gland to low or high dietary calcium intake initially by increasing the efficiency of conversion of pro-PTH to PTH and secretion of PTH from chief cells. Hyperplasia of chief cells in response to long-term low calcium increases the overall capacity of the parathyroid to synthesize pro-PTH.

sustained increase in circulating levels of calcium. This transitory decrease in blood calcium is considered to be the result of a sequestration of calcium phosphate in bone and soft tissues (Parsons and Robinson, 1971). The subsequent increase in blood calcium results from an interaction of parathyroid hormone with osteoclasts and osteocytes in bone (Fig. 66–7).

The response of bone to PTH is biphasic. The immediate effects are the result of increasing the activity of existing osteoclasts and osteocytes present in bone. This rapid effect of PTH depends upon the continuous presence of hormone and results in an increased flow of calcium from deep in bone to bone surfaces through the coordinated action of osteocytes and endosteal lining cells (inactive osteoblasts) (Fig. 66–7). This osteocyte-osteoblast "pump" is concerned with movement of calcium from the bone fluid to the extracellular fluid compartment (Fig. 66–8).

The late effects of PTH on bone are potentially of a greater magnitude of response and not dependent upon the continuous presence of hormone. Osteoclasts appear to be primarily responsible for the long-term action of PTH on increasing bone resorption and overall bone remodeling. If the increase in PTH is sustained, the active osteoclast pool in bone is increased by activation of osteoprogenitor cells in the endosteal and other bone-cell envelopes (Rasmussen and Bordier, 1974). The plasma membrane of osteoclasts in intimate contact with the resorbing bone surface is modified to form a series of membranous projections referred to as the brush border (Fig. 66–9). This area of active bone resorption is isolated from the extracellular fluids by adjacent transitional ("sealing") zones, thereby localizing the lysosomal enzymes and acidic

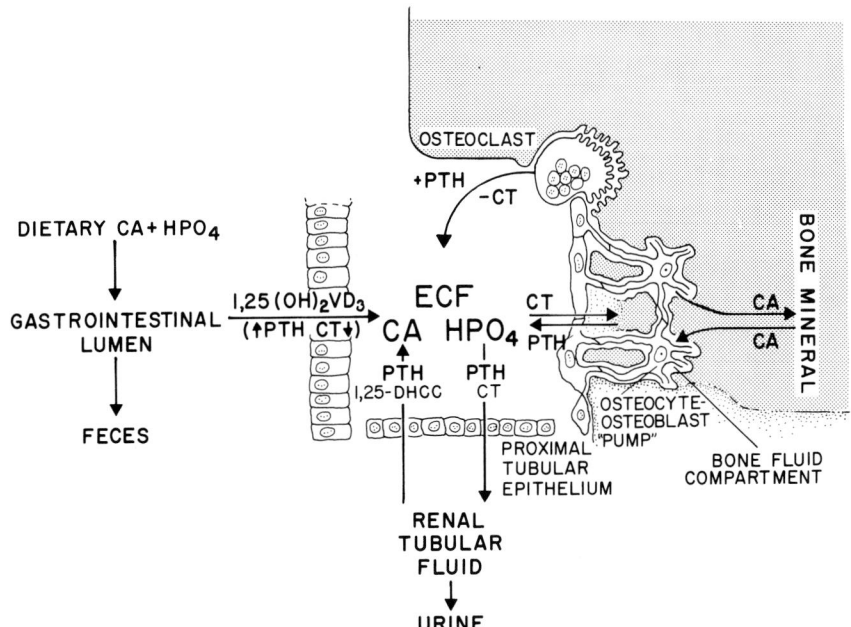

Figure 66–7. Interrelation of parathyroid hormone (PTH), calcitonin (CT), and 1,25-dihydroxycholecalciferol (1,25-(OH)$_2$VD$_3$) in the hormonal regulation of calcium and phosphorus in extracellular fluids.

OSTEOCYTE-OSTEOBLAST PUMP

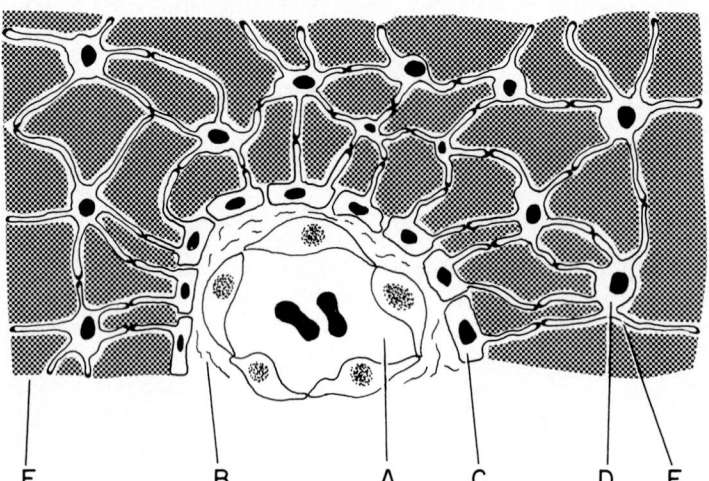

F   B   A   C   D   E

Figure 66–8. Osteocyte-osteoblast "pump" is formed by the fusion of processes of endosteal lining cells (C) (inactive osteoblast) and osteocytes (D) embedded in cortical bone (F). This functional cellular syncytium provides a mechanism for transcellular transport of calcium from the bone-fluid compartment around osteocytes (E) to the extracellular fluid compartment (B) and capillaries (A).

environment to the immediate area undergoing dissolution. The mineral and organic components (e.g., hydroxyproline) released from bone are phagocytized by osteoclasts and transported across the cell in transport vesicles to be released into the extracellular fluid compartment (Fig. 66–9).

A long-term increase in PTH secretion also may result in the formation of greater numbers of osteoblasts, with a resultant increase in bone formation as well as resorption. Resorption is usually greater than formation, however, leading to a net negative skeletal balance.

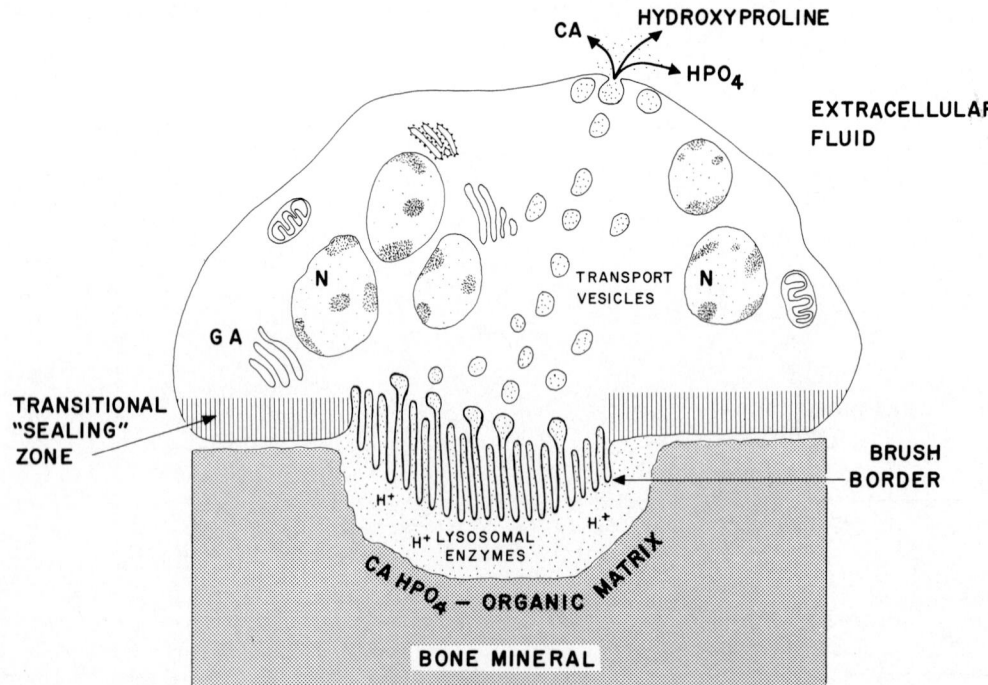

Figure 66–9. Osteoclastic osteolysis on a bone surface with release of calcium, phosphorus, and hydroxyproline (from the organic matrix of bone) into extracellular fluids. The brush border is a specialized area of the plasma membrane of osteoclasts that is in intimate contact with the underlying bone mineral. Adjacent transitional zones isolate the area undergoing active resorption and provide a mechanism for the concentration of lysosomal enzymes and acidic environment required for the dissolution of bone mineral.

Parathyroid hormone has a rapid (within five to ten minutes) and direct effect on renal tubular function, leading to decreased reabsorption of phosphate and phosphaturia. The site of action of PTH for blocking tubular reabsorption of phosphate has been localized by micropuncture methods to the proximal tubule of the nephron (Fig. 66–10). In addition, PTH leads to an increased urinary excretion of potassium, bicarbonate, sodium, cyclic adenosine monophosphate, and amino acids.

Although the effect of PTH on the tubular reabsorption of phosphate has been considered to be of major importance, recent evidence suggests that the ability of PTH to enhance the renal absorption of calcium is of considerable importance in the maintenance of calcium homeostasis. This effect of PTH upon tubular reabsorption of calcium appears to be due to a direct action on the distal convoluted tubule (Fig. 66–10). The urinary excretion of magnesium, ammonia, and titratable acidity also is decreased by PTH. The other important effect of PTH on the kidney is in the regulation of the conversion of 25-hydroxycholecalciferol to 1,25-dihydroxycholecalciferol and other vitamin D metabolites.

Parathyroid hormone is secreted continuously from chief cells under normal conditions. In the peripheral circulation, liver, and at target cells PTH (1 to 84 amino acid sequence) is cleaved into a smaller (approximately one third of a molecule) amino (N–) terminal fragment (biologically active portion) and a larger carboxyl (C–) terminal fragment (biologically inactive portion) (Hruska et al., 1977). The kidney also is a major organ for the degradation of PTH. Biologically active PTH from peritubular capillaries is degraded by specific proteases on the surface of renal tubular cells. In addition, both biologically active (NH_2 1–34) and inactive (34–84 COOH) fragments may be degraded intracellularly by lysosomal enzymes within renal tubular cells.

Subcellular Mechanism of Action of Parathyroid Hormone. The calcium-mobilizing and phosphaturic activities of PTH appear to be mediated through the intracellular accumulation of 3',5'-adenosine monophosphate (cAMP) and cytosol calcium in target cells (Fig. 66–11) (Rasmussen, 1971). Binding of PTH to specific isoreceptors on target cells results in the activation of adenylate cyclase in the plasma membrane. The adenylate cyclase stimulates the conversion of ATP to cAMP in target cells. Cyclic 3',5'-AMP accumulation in target cells functions as an intracellular mediator or second messenger of PTH action, resulting in an increased permeability for calcium ion. The resultant increase in cytosol calcium content in combination with the cAMP accumulation initiates the synthesis and release of lysosomal enzymes, and triggers other biochemical reactions in osteolytic cells that result eventually in breakdown of both the inorganic and organic phases of bone (Rasmussen, 1972).

In addition, PTH contributes to the regulation of the rate of formation of 1,25-dihydroxycholecalciferol, the principal metabolically active form of vitamin D_3, by kidney mitochondria (DeLuca, 1974). The active metabolite(s) of vitamin D makes bone

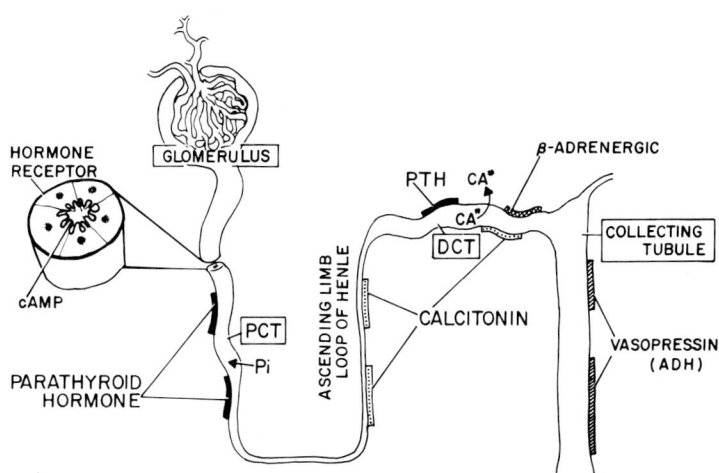

Figure 66–10. Distribution of target cells for parathyroid hormone and calcitonin in the nephron. The parathyroid hormone–mediated diminished tubular reabsorption of phosphorus occurs in the proximal convoluted tubules (PCT), whereas the increased calcium reabsorption occurs in cells located in the distal convoluted tubules (DCT). Cells with receptors for calcitonin situated in the ascending limb of the loop of Henle and in the distal convoluted tubule also diminish tubular reabsorption of phosphorus and cause phosphaturia.

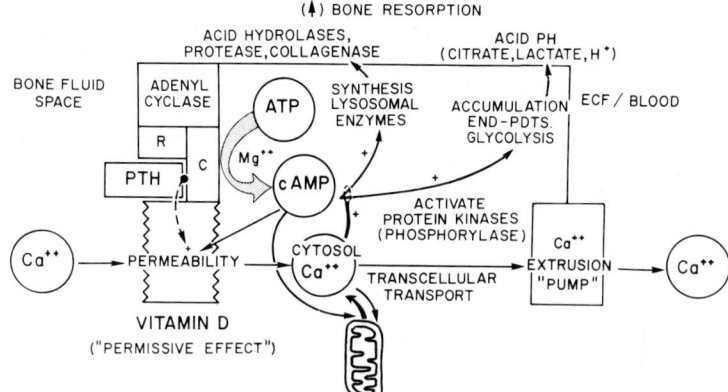

Figure 66–11. Mechanism of action of parathyroid hormone on bone. The accumulation of cyclic adenosine monophosphate and cytosol calcium under the influence of PTH appears to trigger the physiologic reactions within osteolytic cells that result in bone resorption. The local release of lysosomal enzymes and end-products of glycolysis creates an environment that favors the dissolution of bone.

cells more sensitive to the direct effects of PTH ("permissive effect") and greatly enhances the gastrointestinal absorption of calcium, thereby amplifying the effect of PTH upon plasma calcium concentration (Rasmussen and Bordier, 1974).

CALCITONIN

Calcitonin (thyrocalcitonin, CT) was discovered more recently than PTH. Copp et al. (1962), in experiments designed to test the McLean-Urist hypothesis of negative feedback control of blood calcium by PTH, perfused the parathyroid-thyroid complex of dogs with alternating intervals of blood with a low and high calcium concentration and measured the effects on calcium levels in peripheral blood. Two findings from these experiments were difficult to explain based upon the existing concept of a single hormone controlling the concentration of blood calcium. First, the fall in systemic calcium following perfusion of the thyroid-parathyroid complex with high calcium was more rapid and of greater magnitude than expected from only an inhibition of PTH secretion. Second, thyroparathyroidectomy following the last low calcium perfusion resulted in a continued progressive rise in blood calcium level rather than the expected fall after removal of the source of PTH. These and subsequent experiments led to the development of the concept of a second calcium-regulating hormone secreted by the parathyroid-thyroid complex in response to hypercalcemia, which lowered plasma calcium.

C (Parafollicular) Cells in Thyroid. Calcitonin has been shown to be secreted by a second endocrine cell population in the mammalian thyroid gland. C cells are distinct from follicular cells in the thyroid, which secrete thyroxine and triiodothyronine (Kalina and Pearse, 1971). They are situated either within the follicular wall between follicular cells (Fig. 66–12) or as small groups of cells between follicles. C cells do not border the follicular colloid directly, and their secretory polarity is oriented toward the interfollicular capillaries. The distinctive feature of C cells is the presence of numerous small membrane-limited secretory granules in the cytoplasm (Fig. 66–12). Immunocytochemical techniques have localized the CT activity of C cells to these secretory granules (DeGrandi et al., 1971).

Chemistry of Calcitonin. Calcitonin is a polypeptide hormone composed of 32 amino acid residues arranged in a straight chain with a 1 to 7 disulfide linkage (Copp, 1970). It is a smaller molecule than PTH (84 amino acids), and the evidence for the biosynthesis of a larger procalcitonin molecule is less complete at present than with pro-PTH. The complete sequence of 32 amino acids and the disulfide bond are essential for full biologic activity of CT.

Regulation of Calcitonin Secretion. The concentration of calcium ion in plasma and extracellular fluids is the principal physiologic stimulus for the secretion of calcitonin by C cells (Copp, 1970). Calcitonin is secreted continuously under conditions of normocalcemia, but the rate of secretion of calcitonin is increased greatly in response to elevations in blood calcium. Magnesium ion has an effect on CT secretion similar to that of calcium, but these effects are observed only under experimental conditions with nonphysiologic levels of magnesium.

C cells store substantial amounts of CT in their cytoplasm in the form of membrane-

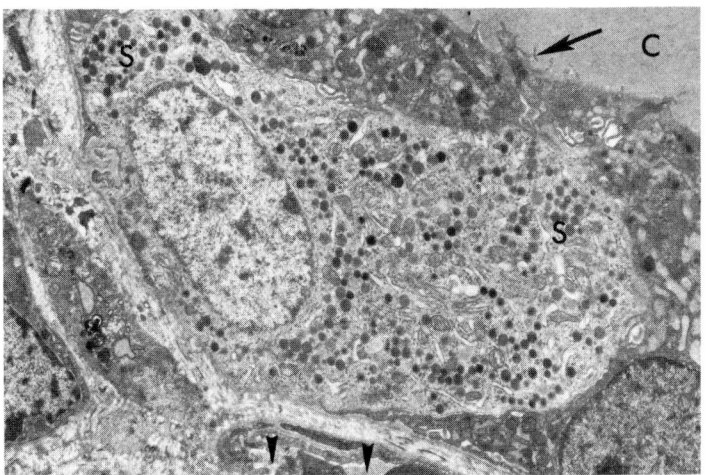

Figure 66–12. C-(parafollicular) cell with numerous secretory granules (S) and moderate development of Golgi apparatuses and rough endoplasmic reticulum. Microvilli from follicular cells (arrow) extend into the colloid in the follicle lumen (C). An interfollicular capillary (arrowheads) with fenestrae and a basement membrane of the thyroid follicle are present.

limited secretory granules (Fig. 66–12). In response to hypercalcemia there is a rapid discharge of stored hormone from C cells into interfollicular capillaries (Fig. 66–13) (Capen and Young, 1969). The hypercalcemic stimulus, if sustained, is followed by an increased development of cytoplasmic organelles concerned with the synthesis and secretion of CT. Hyperplasia of C cells occurs in response to long-term hypercalcemia (Collins et al., 1977; Nunez et al., 1974). When the blood calcium is lowered, the stimulus for CT secretion is diminished and numerous secretory granules accumu-

late in the cytoplasm of C cells (Fig. 66–13). The storage of large amounts of preformed hormone in C cells and rapid release in response to moderate elevations in blood calcium probably are a reflection of the physiologic role of CT as an "emergency" hormone to protect against the development of hypercalcemia.

Calcitonin secretion is increased in response to a high calcium meal, often before a significant rise in plasma calcium can be detected. The cause of this increase in CT secretion could be either a small undetectable rise in plasma ionized calcium or a

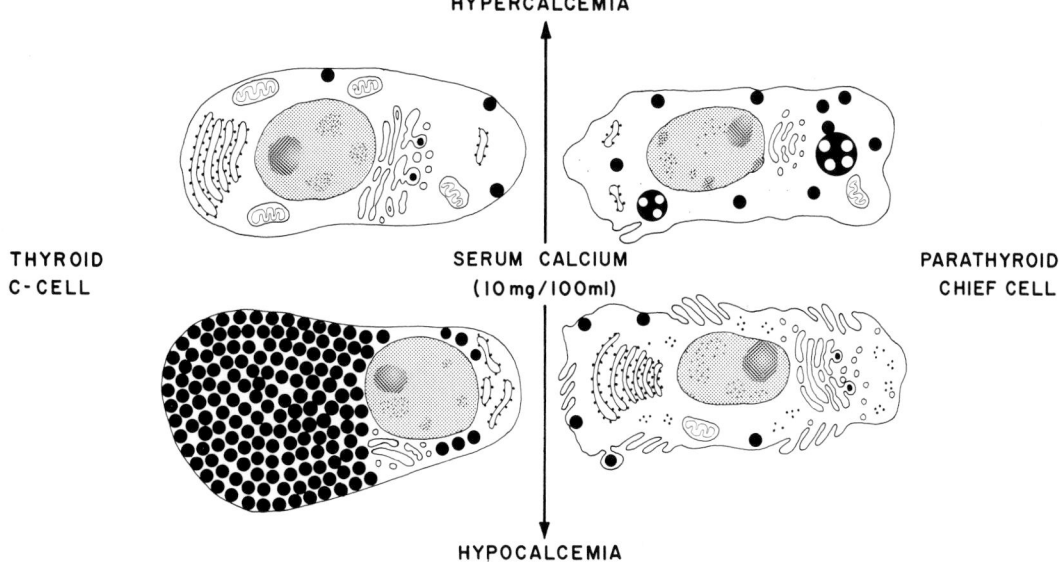

Figure 66–13. Response of thyroid C-cells and parathyroid chief cells to hypercalcemia and hypocalcemia. C-cells accumulate secretory granules in response to hypocalcemia, whereas chief cells are nearly degranulated but have an increased development of synthetic and secretory organelles. In response to hypercalcemia C-cells are degranulated and chief cells are predominantly in the inactive stage of the secretory cycle.

direct stimulation by the oral calcium load of certain gastrointestinal hormones, which in turn act as secretagogues for CT release from the thyroid gland (Fig. 66–14) (Cooper et al., 1972). Gastrin, pancreozymin, and glucagon all have been demonstrated to stimulate CT release under experimental conditions in animals (Care et al., 1970). These findings suggest that gastrointestinal hormones may be important in triggering the early release of CT to prevent the development of hypercalcemia following ingestion of a high calcium meal (Fig. 66–14) (Gray and Ontjes, 1975).

Biologic Action and Physiologic Significance of Calcitonin. The administration of CT or stimulation of endogenous secretion results in the development of varying degrees of hypocalcemia and hypophosphatemia. These effects of CT on plasma calcium and phosphorus are most evident in young animals or older animals with increased rates of skeletal remodeling. Calcitonin exerts its function by interacting with target cells primarily in bone, kidney, and, to a lesser extent, the intestine.

The action of PTH and CT are antagonistic on bone resorption but synergistic on decreasing the renal tubular reabsorption of phosphorus (Fig. 66–7). The hypocalcemic effects of CT are primarily the result of decreased entry of calcium from the skeleton into plasma due to a temporary inhibition of PTH-stimulated bone resorption (Aliapoulios et al., 1966; Friedman et al., 1968). The hypophosphatemia develops from a direct action of CT, increasing the

rate of movement of phosphate out of plasma into soft tissue and bone (Talmage et al., 1972), as well as from the inhibition of bone resorption. The action of CT is not dependent on vitamin D, since it acts both in vitamin D–deficient animals and following the administration of large doses of vitamin D.

The action of CT on inhibiting bone resorption stimulated by PTH and other factors results from blockage of both osteocytic and osteoclastic osteolysis (Fig. 66–7). Specific structural alterations are produced in osteoclasts by CT. Osteoclasts withdraw from resorptive surfaces, and the brush border and transitional zone become atrophic (Kallio et al., 1972; Weisbrode and Capen, 1974). In addition, there is a decrease in the rate of activation of osteoprogenitor cells to preosteoclasts and osteoclasts, resulting in fewer osteoclasts in bone. Although CT can block bone resorption completely, the inhibition is a transitory effect. The continuous administration of CT *in vivo* and *in vitro* in the presence of PTH leads to an "escape phenomenon," whereby the effects of PTH on increasing bone resorption· become manifest in the presence of CT (Friedman et al., 1968).

Both calcitonin and PTH decrease renal tubular reabsorption of phosphate, leading to phosphaturia; however, the adenylate cyclase–linked receptors for CT are found in the ascending limb of the loop of Henle and the distal convoluted tubule (Fig. 66–10). In addition, CT results in diuresis of sodium, chloride, and calcium, whereas PTH in-

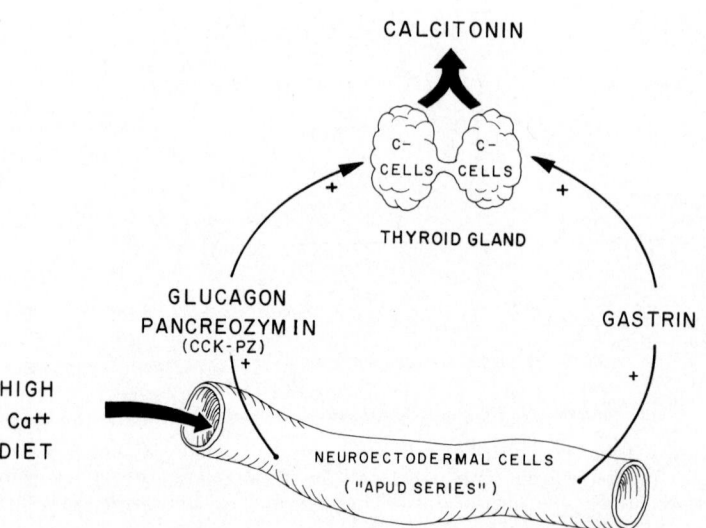

Figure 66–14. Gastrointestinal hormone-thyroid C-cell axis provides a mechanism for the rapid release of calcitonin from the thyroid in response to a high calcium diet before there is a significant elevation in blood calcium.

fusion leads to renal retention of calcium and hydrogen ions (Rasmussen, 1973).

Calcitonin and parathyroid hormone, acting in concert, provide a dual negative feedback control mechanism to maintain the concentration of calcium in extracellular fluids within narrow limits. Present evidence suggests that PTH is the major factor involved in the minute-to-minute regulation of blood calcium under normal conditions. In most higher mammals that live in a relatively low calcium–high phosphorus environment, protection against the development of hypocalcemia by PTH is probably a life-sustaining function. Calcitonin appears to function more as an "emergency" hormone to prevent the development of hypercalcemia during the rapid postprandial absorption of calcium, and to protect against excessive loss of calcium and phosphorus from the maternal skeleton during pregnancy.

CHOLECALCIFEROL (VITAMIN D)

The third major hormone involved in the regulation of calcium metabolism and skeletal remodeling is cholecalciferol, or vitamin D_3. Although this compound has been labeled a vitamin for a long time, recent evidence suggests it can equally be considered a hormone (Kodicek, 1974). Cholecalciferol is ingested in small amounts in the diet and can be synthesized in the epidermis from precursor molecules (e.g., 7-dehydrocholesterol) through a previtamin D_3 intermediate form (Fig. 66–15) (Holick et al., 1980). This reaction is catalyzed by ultraviolet irradiation (wavelength 2900 to 3200 angstroms) from the sun. A high-affinity vitamin D–binding protein transports cholecalciferol from the skin into the blood (Holick and Clark, 1978; Holick et al., 1977).

Metabolic Activation of Vitamin D. It is well established that vitamin D must be metabolically activated before it can produce its known physiologic functions (De-Luca, 1973, 1977; Kodicek et al., 1970). Vitamin D_3 from dietary sources is absorbed by facilitated diffusion and bound to an alpha-2 globulin in the blood for transport. Endogenous cholecalciferol synthesized in the skin from 7-dehydrocholesterol also is bound to an alpha-2 globulin for transport to the liver (Fig. 66–16).

The first step in the metabolic activation of vitamin D is the conversion of cholecalciferol to 25-hydroxycholecalciferol (25-

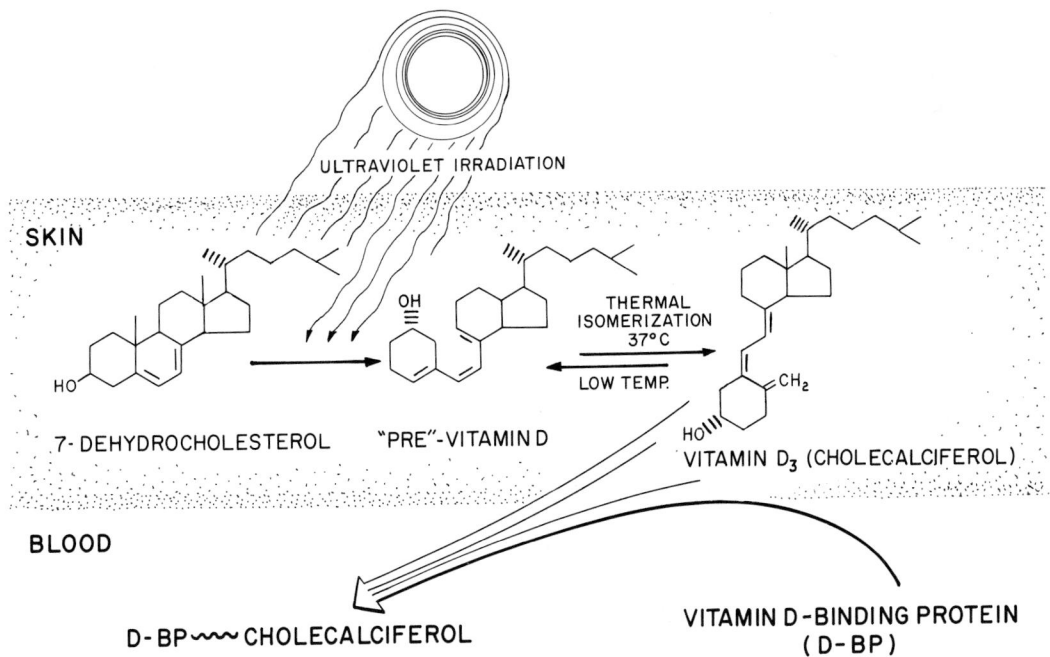

Figure 66–15. Formation of pre-vitamin D in the skin during exposure to sunlight and its subsequent thermal conversion to vitamin D_3 (cholecalciferol). Cholecalciferol is bound subsequently to the vitamin D-binding protein (DBP) in plasma for transport in the circulation. (From Holick, M. F., et al.: Photosynthesis of previtamin D_3 in human skin and the physiologic consequences. Science *210*:203, 1980.)

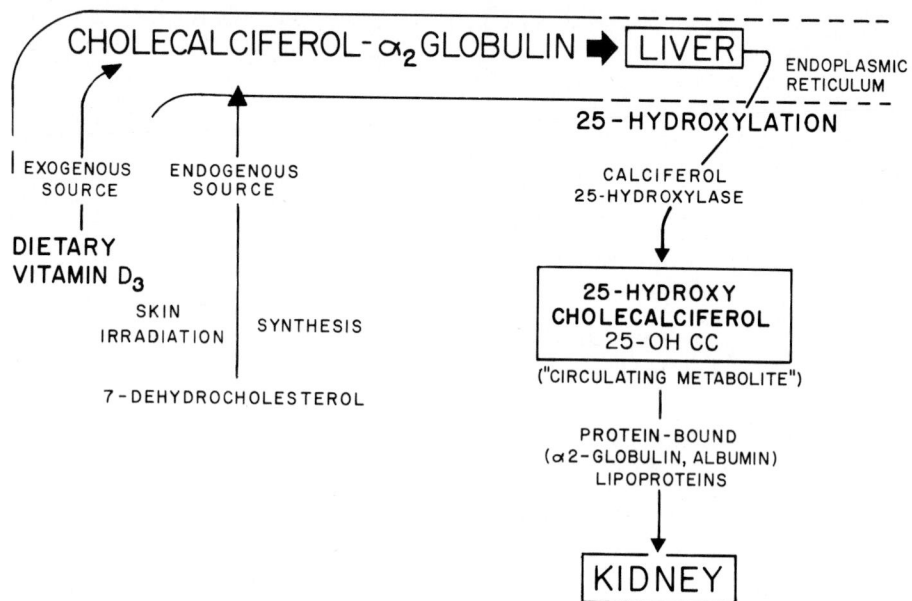

Figure 66–16. Metabolism of vitamin D_3. The initial step of metabolic activation of vitamin D_3 from endogenous and dietary sources is in the liver to form 25-hydroxycholecalciferol.

OH-CC) in the liver (Haussler and McCain, 1977). The enzyme responsible for controlling this reaction is a hepatic microsomal enzyme referred to as calciferol-25-hydroxylase, which is associated with the endoplasmic reticulum (Fig. 66–16) (Bhattacharyya and DeLuca, 1974). Considerably larger amounts of protein-bound 25-OH-CC circulate than with the more hydroxylated metabolites such as 1,25-dihydroxycholecalciferol (1,25-DiOH-CC), which are present in extremely low levels in the blood.

This first metabolite of cholecalciferol (25-OH-CC) is transported to the kidney and undergoes further transformation to a more polar and active metabolite (Haussler et al., 1971) (Fig. 66–17). The principal active metabolite of 25-OH-CC formed in the kidney is 1,25-dihydroxycholecalciferol, but other metabolites are formed, such as 25,26-DiOH-CC and 24,25-DiOH-CC

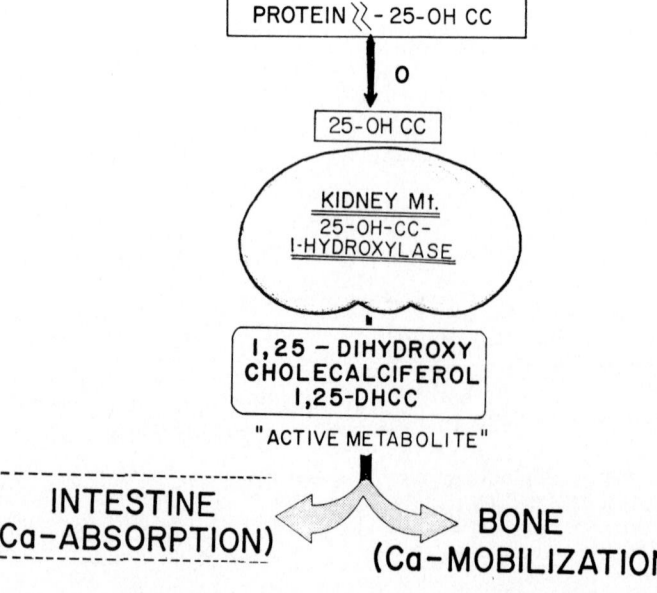

Figure 66–17. Metabolism of vitamin D_3. The final step of metabolic activation of vitamin D_3 is in the kidney, where 25-hydroxycholecalciferol (25-OH-CC) is converted to 1,25-dihydroxycholecalciferol (1,25 DH-CC). 1,25-dihydroxycholecalciferol exerts its function by acting on target cells primarily in the intestine and bone.

(Boyle et al., 1973; DeLuca, 1978; Norman and Henry, 1974; Norman et al., 1976). The formation of 1,25-DiOH-CC is catalyzed by 25-hydroxycholecalciferol-1α-hydroxylase in renal mitochondria, probably in proximal convoluted tubules (Brunette et al., 1978; Midgett et al., 1973). The conversion of 25-OH-CC to 1,25-DiOH-CC is the rate limiting step in vitamin D metabolism and is the primary reason for the delay between vitamin D administration and expression of its biologic effects (Gray et al., 1972).

The control of this final step in the metabolic activation of vitamin D is complex and appears to be regulated in part by the plasma calcium concentration and its influence on the rates of secretion of PTH and CT (Fraser and Kodicek, 1973; Garabedian et al., 1972; Rasmussen et al., 1972) (Fig. 66–18). Parathyroid hormone and conditions that stimulate its secretion increase the transformation of 25-OH-CC to 1,25-DiOH-CC. Low blood phosphorus increases the formation of 1,25-DiOH-CC, whereas high blood phosphorus suppresses the activity of the 1α-hydroxylase (Fig. 66–18).

The rates of synthesis of 24,25-DiOH-CC and 1,25-DiOH-CC appear to be reciprocally related and controlled by similar factors (DeLuca, 1974, 1979; Tanaka and DeLuca, 1974). When 1,25-DiOH-CC synthesis increases, the synthesis of 24,25-DiOH-CC declines, and vice versa (Fig. 66–18). 24,25-dihydroxycholecalciferol may play a role in bone formation (Ornoy et al., 1978) and egg hatchability (Henry and Norman, 1978), and, with 1,25-DiOH-CC, may exert negative feedback control on the parathyroid gland.

Recent evidence suggests that other hormones may increase the activity of renal 1α-hydroxylase and the formation of 1,25-DiOH-CC under certain conditions. Prolactin, estradiol, placental lactogen, and possibly somatotropin enhance 1α-hydroxylase activity (MacIntyre et al., 1973). Increased secretion of these hormones, either alone or in combination, appears to be important in the efficient adaptation to the major calcium demands during life (such as pregnancy and lactation) and during growth.

Chemistry of Cholecalciferol. The chemical structure of cholecalciferol (vitamin D_3) resembles that of other steroid hormones. It is a seco-steroid in which one of the rings of the basic steroid nucleus has undergone fission through breakage of a carbon-carbon bond (Norman and Henry, 1979). Photoactivation by ultraviolet irradiation of 7-dehydrocholesterol in the skin results in a cleavage between the 9 and 10 carbons and unfolding of the B ring of the basic steroid nucleus (Fig. 66–15) (Havinga, 1973). During metabolic activation of cholecalciferol, hydroxyl groups are attached successively to the steroid nucleus by specific hydroxylases at positions 25 and 1 in the liver and kidney to form the hormonal or biologically active form of vitamin D.

There are a number of other sterols closely related to cholecalciferol. Vitamin D_2 is formed by the irradiation of the plant sterol referred to as ergosterol. When irradiated ergosterol is ingested and absorbed from the intestine, it undergoes a series of steps of metabolic activation similar to those described for cholecalciferol. Another related sterol of considerable therapeutic interest is dihydrotachysterol. The A ring of the steroid nucleus in this compound is rotated,

Figure 66–18. Multifactorial control of the final step of metabolic activation of vitamin D in the kidney. Several conditions associated with increased calcium demand result in a stimulation of 1,25-(OH)$_2$-cholecalciferol production from 25-OH-cholecalciferol by increasing the activity of 1α-hydroxylase in mitochondria of renal tubular epithelial cells. Under conditions of decreased calcium demand the production of 1,25-(OH)$_2$-cholecalciferol is diminished but 24,25-(OH)$_2$-cholecalciferol (an inactive metabolite in calcium mobilization) is formed by activation of a 24-hydroxylase.

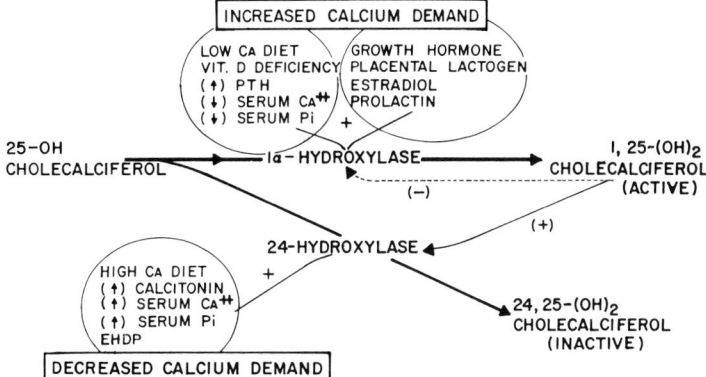

so that the hydroxyl in position 3 occupies a position sterically equivalent to the hydroxyl position of 1 of 1,25-dihydroxycholecalciferol. Current evidence suggests that dihydrotachysterol undergoes metabolic transformation to 25-dihydrotachysterol, but subsequent hydroxylation of position 1 does not occur.

Subcellular Mechanism of Action of Active Vitamin D Metabolites. Vitamin D and its active metabolites function to increase the absorption of calcium and phosphorus from the intestine, thereby maintaining adequate levels of these electrolytes in the extracellular fluids in order to permit the appropriate mineralization of bone matrix (Omdahl and DeLuca, 1973). From a functional point of view, vitamin D can be thought to bring about the retention of sufficient mineral ions to ensure mineralization of bone matrix, whereas PTH maintains the proper ratio of calcium to phosphate in extracellular fluids.

The major target tissue for 1,25-DiOH-CC is the mucosa of the small intestine, where it increases the active transcellular transport of calcium (proximal part) and phosphorus (distal part). Following synthesis in the kidney, 1,25-DiOH-CC is transported in a protein-bound form to specific target cells in the intestine and bone (Fig. 66–17). Free 1,25-DiOH-CC penetrates the plasma membrane of target cells and initially binds to a cytoplasmic receptor in cells of the intestine (Brumbaugh and Haussler, 1973) (Fig. 66–19). Subsequently, the hormone-receptor complex is transferred to the nucleus, and 1,25-DiOH-CC binds to specific receptors in the nuclear chromatin. Here it stimulates gene expression with increased messenger RNA formation, which directs the synthesis of vitamin D–dependent proteins such as calcium-binding protein (CaBP) and calcium-ATPase by intestinal absorptive cells (Haussler et al., 1970; Wasserman and Taylor, 1972).

Intestinal absorptive cells are responsive to 1,25-DiOH-CC and are concerned with the transport of calcium from the lumen to the blood stream. The luminal surface (brush border) of absorptive cells is highly specialized and has numerous microvilli, which greatly increase the intestinal surface area (Fig. 66–20). The microvillar membrane(s) contains vitamin D–dependent enzymes (e.g., CaATPase, alkaline phosphatase) that may be involved in the translocation of calcium from the lumen into absorptive cells (Haussler et al., 1970). In response to 1,25-DiOH-CC, intestinal cells also synthesize a specific CaBP (Taylor and Wasserman, 1970; Wasserman et al., 1968). Calcium-binding protein in mammals has a molecular weight of between 24,000 and 28,000 and has been isolated from several tissues (e.g., small intestine, kidney, para-

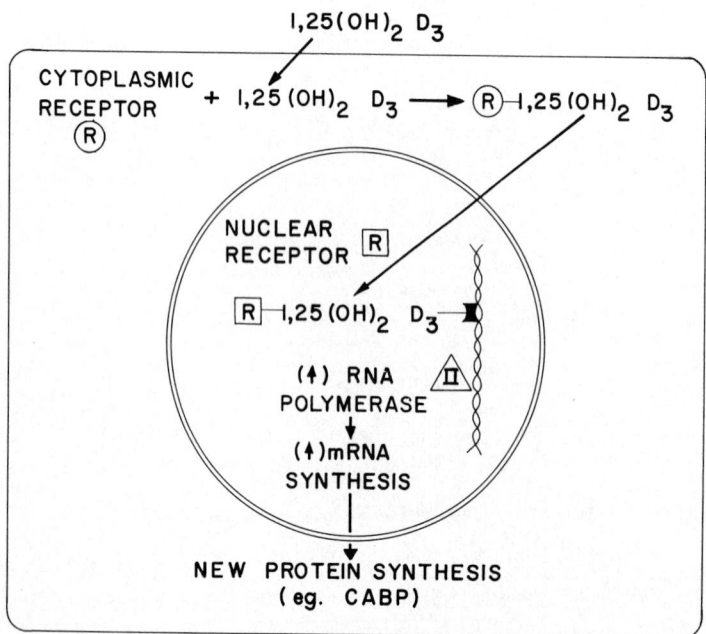

Figure 66–19. Subcellular mechanism of action of the active metabolite of vitamin D ($1,25(OH)_2D_3$) in the intestine. The steroid penetrates the cell membrane, binds to a cytoplasmic receptor, and is transported to the nucleus, where it interacts with the nuclear chromatin to increase the formation of mRNA, which directs new protein synthesis.

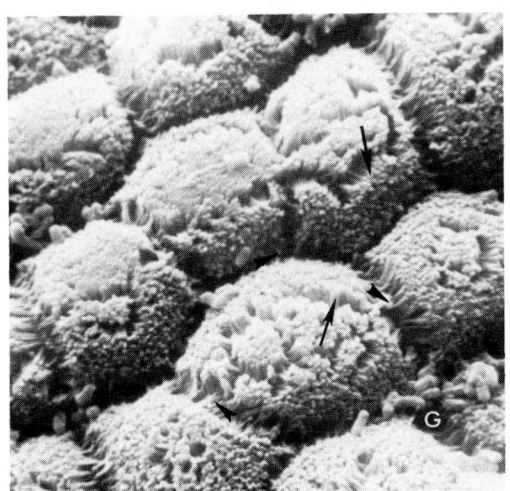

Figure 66–20. Surface architecture of the intestinal villi illustrating junctions between individual absorptive cells (arrowheads) and orifices of goblet cells (G). The luminal surface of absorptive cells is modified by the presence of numerous microvilli (arrows), which greatly increase the intestinal surface area. Scanning electron micrograph, × 3000.

thyroid gland, and the shell gland of laying hens), across which significant amounts of calcium are transported. Recently a vitamin D–dependent CaBP was demonstrated in bone, particularly in the spongiosa and cartilaginous growth plate (Christakos and Norman., 1978).

The absorptive capacity of the intestine for calcium is a direct function of the amount of CaBP present (Ingersoll and Wasserman, 1971; Wasserman and Taylor, 1972). The administration of vitamin D or low calcium diets has been shown to stimulate the synthesis of CaBP, which contributes to the increased intestinal absorption of calcium. The physiologic function of CaBP may be to protect absorptive cells against high cytosolic concentrations of calcium ion during the transcellular transport of calcium from the luminal border to the latero-basilar border of intestinal cells. At the basilar aspect of intestinal absorptive cells, calcium is exchanged for sodium and enters the extracellular fluids.

The active metabolites of cholecalciferol also act on bone (Fig. 66–7) (DeLuca, 1974). In young animals, vitamin D is required for the orderly growth and mineralization of cartilage in the growth plate (Fig. 66–21). Young animals fed diets deficient in vitamin D and housed indoors without exposure to ultraviolet irradiation develop rickets. In the absence of vitamin D, mineral granules do not accumulate within mitochondria of hypertrophied chondrocytes in the growth plates of long bones. Mineralization of the cartilaginous matrix fails to occur, and the formation of woven bone on spicules of cartilage and subsequent remodeling to lamellar bone are blocked in this disease. The epiphyseal plate is irregularly thickened as progressively more primordial cartilaginous matrix accumulates and fails to mineralize. The administration of either cholecalciferol, 25-OH-CC, or 1,25-DiOH-CC leads to reestablishment of a normal calcification front in the osteoid on bone surfaces and at the growth plate, often before there is a change in the mineral ion product of extracellular fluids.

In addition to having this effect on mineralization of bone matrix, vitamin D is necessary for osteoclastic resorption and calcium mobilization from bone in adults. Small amounts of vitamin D or its active metabolite are necessary to permit osteolytic cells to respond to PTH ("permissive effect") under physiologic conditions (Fig. 66–11). Both 25-OH-CC and 1,25-DiOH-CC, and cholecalciferol in pharmacologic doses will stimulate osteoclastic proliferation and the resorption of bone *in vitro* and *in vivo*. 1,25-dihydroxycholecalciferol is about 100 times more potent in stimulating bone resorption *in vitro* than 25-OH-CC on a weight basis (Raisz et al., 1972; Reynolds et al., 1973).

Considerably less is known regarding the action of cholecalciferol and its active metabolite on the kidney. Present evidence suggests that active metabolites of vitamin D stimulate the retention of calcium by increasing renal tubular reabsorption (Fig. 66–7, probably in the distal part of the nephron (Strumpf et al., 1980). The active metabolites of vitamin D may have a direct effect on the parathyroid gland, in addition to its well-characterized action on intestine and bone (Hughes and Haussler, 1978; Wecksler et al., 1977; Capen et al., 1978).

DISORDERS OF CALCIUM METABOLISM

PRIMARY HYPERPARATHYROIDISM

In primary hyperparathyroidism, parathyroid hormone is produced in excess of normal by a functional lesion in the parathyroid gland. This disease is encountered infrequently in older dogs (Carrillo et al.,

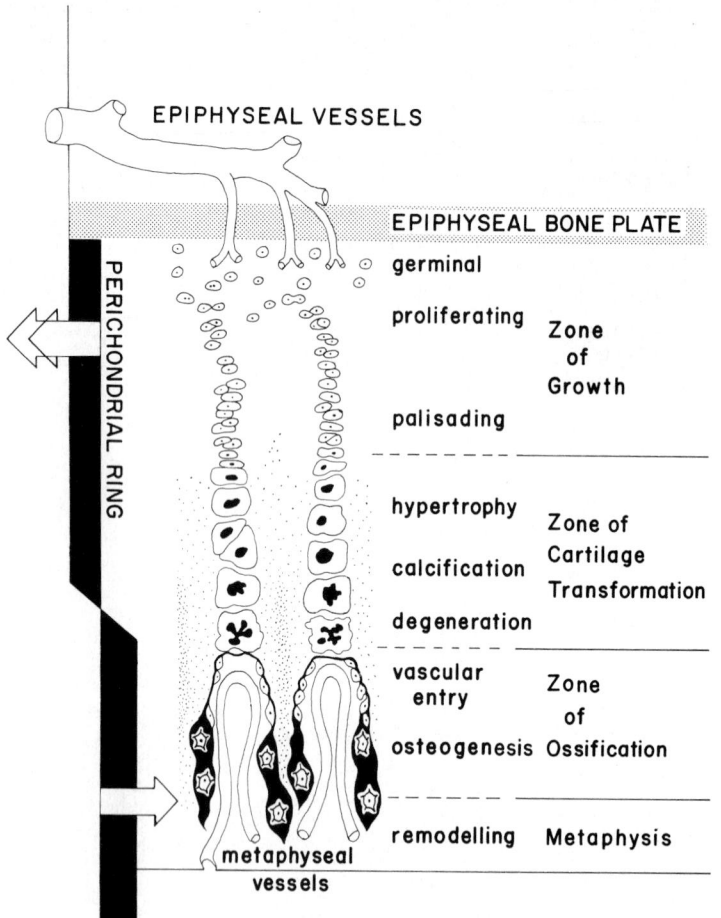

EPIPHYSEAL VESSELS

PERICHONDRIAL RING

EPIPHYSEAL BONE PLATE

germinal

proliferating — Zone of Growth

palisading

hypertrophy — Zone of Cartilage Transformation

calcification

degeneration

vascular entry — Zone of Ossification

osteogenesis

remodelling — Metaphysis

metaphyseal vessels

Figure 66–21. Metaphyseal growth plate from a long bone. Vitamin D provides an adequate concentration of calcium and phosphorus in extracellular fluids to permit the mineralization of cartilaginous matrix, which results in an orderly degeneration of chondrocytes and eventual ingrowth of osteoblasts into the scaffold provided by the degenerating cartilage cells with formation of osteoid.

1979; Goulden and MacKenzie, 1968; Krook, 1957; Legendre et al., 1976; Pearson et al., 1965; Stavrou, 1968). Primary hyperparathyroidism does not appear to be a sequela of long-standing secondary hyperparathyroidism in animals.

Pathophysiology. The normal control mechanisms for PTH secretion by the concentration of blood calcium are lost in primary hyperparathyroidism. Hormone secretion is autonomous, and the parathyroid produces excessive hormone in spite of the increased blood calcium (Arnaud, 1978). PTH acts on cells of the renal tubules initially to promote the excretion of phosphate and retention of calcium. A prolonged increased secretion of PTH results in accelerated osteocytic and osteoclastic bone resorption. Mineral is removed from the skeleton and replaced by immature fibrous connective tissue. The bone lesion of fibrous osteodystrophy is generalized throughout the skeleton but is accentuated in local areas such as in the cancellous bone of the skull.

Parathyroid Lesion. The lesion in the parathyroid gland responsible for the excessive secretion of PTH in dogs usually is an adenoma composed of active chief cells. Adenomas are usually single, light brown-red, and located in the cervical region near the thyroid gland (Fig. 66–22), but may be present in the anterior mediastinum near the base of the heart. Parathyroid neoplasms in the precardial mediastinum are derived from ectopic parathyroid anlage displaced into the thorax with the expanding thymus during embryonic development. Histopathologic demonstration of a rim of normal tissue and fibrous capsule in the biopsy of an enlarged parathyroid suggests a diagnosis of adenoma rather than hyperplasia (Fig. 66–23). Thyroid C cells are markedly hyperplastic in response to the long-term hypercalcemia and appear as small white foci in the thyroid gland (Fig. 66–22). The hyperplastic C cells often displace the colloid-containing follicles lined by follicular cells. Chief cell carcinomas are in-

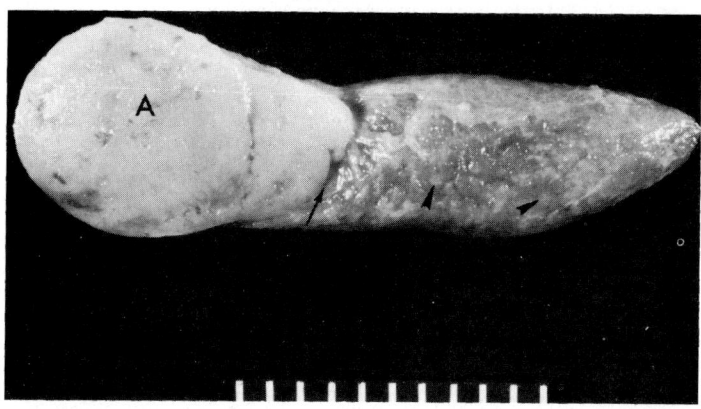

Figure 66–22. Parathyroid adenoma (A) in the external parathyroid gland removed surgically from a dog with persistent hypercalcemia. The chief cell adenoma is sharply demarcated (arrow) from the adjacent thyroid parenchyma. The small light areas in the thyroid represent foci of C-cell hyperplasia (arrowheads), stimulated by the long-term hypercalcemia. (The scale at the bottom represents one cm.)

frequent causes of primary hyperparathyroidism in dogs. Carcinomas tend to be larger than adenomas and fixed to the underlying tissues, owing to local infiltration of neoplastic chief cells.

Clinical Signs. Hypercalcemia results in anorexia, vomiting, constipation, and generalized muscular weakness due to decreased neuromuscular excitability. Other functional disturbances observed are the result of bone weakening through excessive osteoclastic resorption. Lameness due to severe demineralization or fractures of long bones occurs after relatively minor physical trauma. Compression fractures of weakened vertebral bodies may exert pressure on the spinal cord and nerves, resulting in motor and/or sensory dysfunction. Facial hyperostosis with partial obliteration of the nasal cavity by poorly mineralized woven bone and highly vascular fibrous connective

tissue, and loss or loosening of teeth in alveolar sockets have been observed in dogs with primary hyperparathyroidism (Fig. 66–24). The woven bone is composed of spicules of osteoid, numerous capillaries, and immature connective tissue fibers. Active osteoblasts are embedded in the woven bone and are surrounded by abundant collagen fibers of the osteoid but by only occasional initial foci of mineralization. The maxillae and rami of the mandibles are often coarsely thickened by the formation of excessive woven bone (Fig. 66–25). This may interfere with closing of the mouth and may result in pressure ulcerations of the gingival mucosa. Bones of the skull are markedly thinned by the increased osteoclastic resorption and have a characteristic "moth-eaten" appearance radiographically.

Diagnosis. Primary hyperparathyroidism should be included in the differential

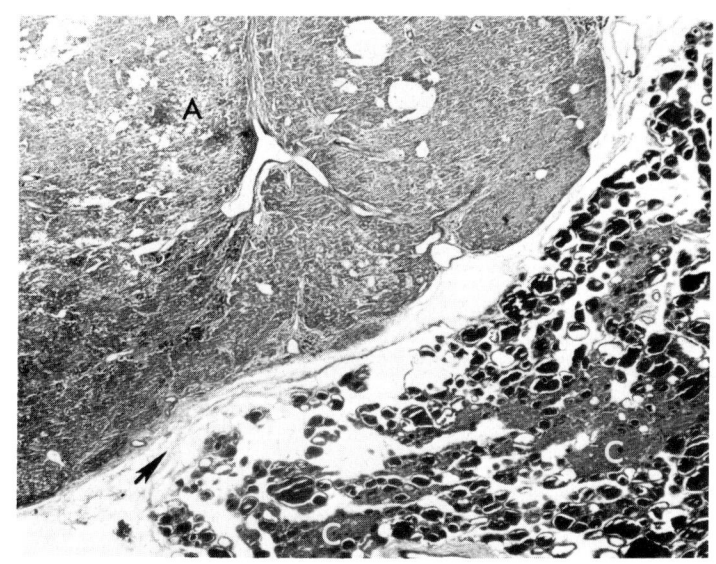

Figure 66–23. Functional chief cell adenoma from a dog with primary hyperparathyroidism. The adenoma (A) is sharply demarcated from the adjacent thyroid by a thin capsule of fibrous connective tissue (arrow). The serum calcium was elevated to 19 mg per 100 ml and the immunoreactive parathyroid hormone level was 822 picograms per ml (three- to four-fold elevation above normal). Prominent areas of C-cell hyperplasia (C) are present between thyroid follicles. Periodic acid-Schiff stain. × 32.

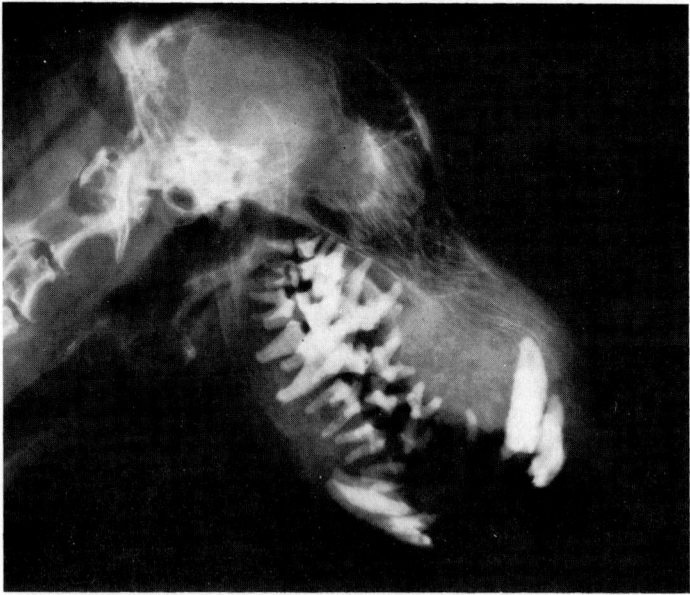

Figure 66–24. Roentgenogram of the skull of a dog with primary hyperparathyroidism. As a result of the chronic hypersecretion of parathyroid hormone, the cancellous bones of the maxilla, mandible, and skull are nearly completely resorbed and replaced by an excessive proliferation of fibrous connective tissue and neocapillaries. Lamina dura dentes and alveolar socket bone are extensively resorbed, and the teeth are loosely embedded in connective tissue.

diagnosis of older dogs with a clinical history of severe, generalized skeletal demineralization and normal renal function. Radiographic evaluation reveals areas of subperiosteal cortical resorption, loss of lamina dura, soft tissue mineralization, bone cysts, a generalized decrease in bone density, and fractures in advanced cases.

The most important and practical laboratory test to aid in establishing the diagnosis of primary hyperparathyroidism is quantitation of total blood calcium (Table 66–1). Although other laboratory findings may be variable, hypercalcemia is a consistent finding and results from accelerated release of calcium from bone. The blood calcium of normal animals is near ten mg per 100 ml with some variation, depending upon the analytic method employed as well as the age and diet of the animal. Calcium values consistently above 11.5 to 12 mg per 100 ml in an adult dog should be considered to be in the hypercalcemic range. Dogs with primary hyperparathyroidism usually have a greatly elevated blood calcium level (12 to 20 mg per 100 ml or above). The blood phosphorus

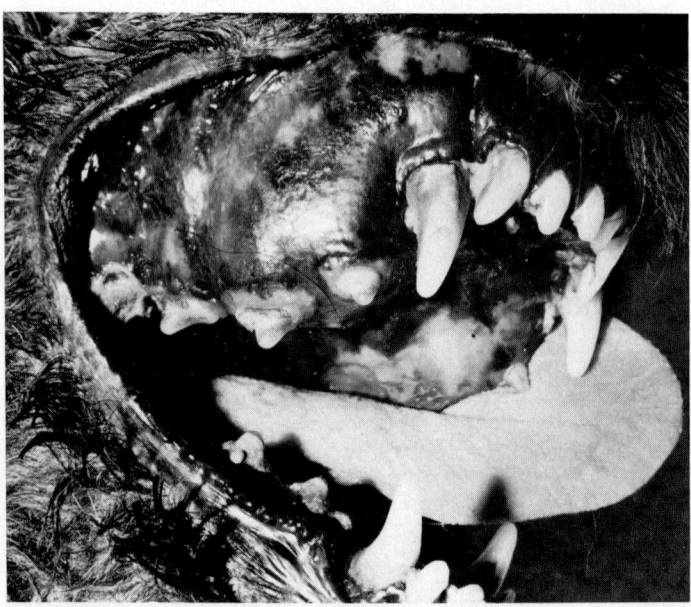

Figure 66–25. Primary hyperparathyroidism in a 12-year-old Scottish terrier with severe hyperostotic fibrous osteodystrophy of the maxilla. The maxilla and mandible were both pliable, and the teeth were loosely embedded in fibrous connective tissue with bone spicules. The dog was unable to close its mouth properly owing to the extensive proliferative reaction in the maxilla.

Table 66–1. Differential Diagnosis of Hypercalcemia in the Dog

Disease	Serum Calcium	Serum Phosphorus	Serum Alkaline Phosphatase	Bone Lesion	Soft Tissue Mineralization	Parathyroid Lesion
Primary hyperparathyroidism	High	Low	Elevated	Severe, generalized	Moderate	Adenoma, carcinoma
Vitamin D intoxication	High	High	Normal	Mild or absent	Severe	Atrophy
Malignant neoplasms with bone metastases	High	Normal or elevated	Moderately elevated	Multifocal	Moderate atrophy	Inactive
Pseudohyperparathyroidism	High	Low	Normal or elevated slightly	Mild	Moderate	Inactive, atrophy

level is low or in the low normal range (four mg per 100 ml or less), because of inhibition of renal tubular reabsorption of phosphorus by excess PTH.

The activity of alkaline phosphatase may be elevated in the serum of animals with overt bone disease. The increased activity of this enzyme is thought to result from a compensatory increase in osteoblasts along the trabeculae as a response to mechanical stress in bones weakened by excessive resorption. The urinary excretion of phosphorus and often calcium is increased and may result in nephrocalcinosis and urolithiasis. Accelerated bone matrix catabolism is reflected in an increased excretion of hydroxyproline in the urine. The detection of elevated circulating levels of PTH by radioimmunoassay in man has greatly facilitated the early diagnosis of hyperparathyroidism.

Differential Diagnosis. Other causes of hypercalcemia that must be considered in differential diagnosis of primary hyperparathyroidism are vitamin D intoxication, malignant neoplasms with osseous metastases, and parathyroid hormone–like activity or the production of other bone resorbing substances by malignant neoplasms of nonparathyroid origin without metastases to bone (Table 66–1). The hypercalcemia of hypervitaminosis D may be of a magnitude similar to that in primary hyperparathyroidism but is accompanied by varying degrees of hyperphosphatemia and normal serum alkaline phosphatase activity. Skeletal disease is usually not present, since the increased concentrations of blood calcium and phosphorus are derived principally from augmented intestinal absorption rather than from bone resorption (Capen et al., 1966; Wasserman, 1978).

Malignant neoplasms with osseous metastases may cause moderate hypercalcemia and hypercalciuria, but the alkaline phosphatase activity and serum phosphorus level are usually normal or slightly elevated. These changes are believed to be due to release of calcium and phosphorus into the blood from areas of bone destruction at rates greater than can be cleared by the kidney and intestine. Bone involvement is more sharply demarcated and localized to the area of metastases. Osteolysis associated with tumor metastases has been shown to be the result of not only a physical disruption of bone by proliferating neoplastic cells but also of the local production of humoral

substances that stimulate bone resorption, such as prostaglandins and osteoclast-activating factor. Multiple myeloma and lymphosarcoma with widespread bone marrow infiltration have been associated with hypercalcemia. Myeloma patients with hypercalcemia may have increased binding of calcium to an abnormal quantity of globulin in addition to the increased amount of ionized calcium from bone dissolution.

Other causes of hypercalcemia include multifocal osteolytic lesions associated with septic emboli, complete immobilization, osteosarcoma, hypoadrenocorticism (Addison-like disease) (Walser et al., 1963; Musselman, 1975), hypocalcitonism due to a destructive thyroid disease, chronic renal disease, hemoconcentration, and hyperproteinemia (Meuten et al., 1982a) (Table 66–2). Metastatic tumors in bone are not commonly encountered in dogs or cats with malignant neoplasms but may be associated with hypercalcemia at certain stages of tumor growth. Primary bone tumors occasionally may be associated with hypercalcemia (Olson and Capen, 1977). Bacterial or fungal osteomyelitis and neonatal septicemia in puppies with septic emboli and lysis of bone are sporadic causes of hypercalcemia. Skeletal radiographs are indicated to document the sites and severity of multifocal bone lesions.

Most cases of chronic renal failure have either a normal or low serum calcium concentration with varying degrees of elevation in blood phosphorus; however, five to ten per cent of dogs with chronic renal failure have serum calcium values of 12.0 mg/dl or greater (Finco and Rowland, 1978; Watson and Canfield, 1979). Pathogenic mechan-

Table 66–2. Diseases Characterized by Hypercalcemia

Pseudohyperparathyroidism
  Lymphosarcoma
  Perirectal apocrine gland carcinoma

Osteolytic lesions
  Primary or metastatic tumors of bone
  Septic osteomyelitis

Primary hyperparathyroidism

Hypervitaminosis D

Primary renal disease
  Chronic renal failure
  Diuretic phase of acute renal failure

Hemoconcentration (hyperproteinemia)

Hypoadrenocorticism (Addison-like disease)

Disuse osteoporosis (immobilization)

Laboratory error

isms that have been suggested to explain the development of hypercalcemia in certain cases of chronic renal failure include (1) decreased excretion of calcium by the diseased kidney, (2) decreased renal tubular degradation of PTH, (3) PTH-induced hypercitricemia with a consequent increase in complexed calcium, (4) autonomous transformation or overcompensation by the parathyroid gland, and (5) an exaggerated response to vitamin D with increased intestinal calcium absorption. In the authors' experience, microscopic evaluation has failed to reveal evidence of "autonomous" or "overcompensated" parathyroid glands in dogs with hypercalcemia associated with chronic renal disease. A transient and mild hypercalcemia has been observed with chronic renal failure in dogs following a precipitous decline in the blood phosphorus value through intestinal binding treatments (e.g., aluminum hydroxide) and fluid therapy. This may be a consequence of a reciprocal movement of calcium from the bone fluid to the extracellular fluid space in response to the rapid lowering of circulating phosphorus levels. Persistent hypercalcemia has been reported in human patients during the diuretic phase of acute renal failure associated with rhabdomyolysis and is thought to be caused by mobilization of calcium from soft tissues, where it was intially deposited during oliguria. The authors have observed dogs recovering from the oliguric phase of acute primary renal failure that developed hypercalcemia during diuresis. The hypercalcemia resolved without specific treatment.

Hypercalcemia may be detected occasionally in dehydrated animals. The magnitude of elevation in blood is usually mild and is attributed to fluid volume contraction that results in hyperproteinemia and an increased relative concentration of ionized and non-ionized calcium. The hypercalcemia rapidly resolves following fluid therapy. The majority of dehydrated animals do not develop hypercalcemia. Prolonged immobilization may lead to hypercalcemia as a consequence of continued bone resorption associated with diminished bone accretion. Hypercalcemia of this type occurs infrequently in animals that cannot move around freely because of extensive musculoskeletal or neurologic injury.

Hypercalcemia is observed in experimentally adrenalectomized dogs and in some cases of naturally occurring Addison-like disease in dogs (Walser et al., 1963; Musselman, 1975). The magnitude of elevation in serum calcium values may exceed 16 mg/dl under experimental conditions, whereas dogs with Addison-like disease evaluated in the authors' hospital have had values up to 15 mg/dl of blood calcium. Experimental evidence suggests that the type of hypercalcemia associated with hypoadrenocorticism is unusual in that the ionized calcium fraction remains normal, whereas the non-ionized calcium fractions increase. If the ionized calcium does indeed remain normal, it follows that this type of hypercalcemia should not be deleterious to the animal. The elevated calcium value rapidly returns to normal following treatment for hypoadrenocorticism.

Treatment. The aim of treatment of primary hyperparathyroidism is to eliminate the source of excessive PTH production. An attempt should be made to identify all four parathyroid glands before excising any tissue. A correlation often exists in man between tumor size and the severity of hypercalcemia and bone disease. Single or multiple adenomas should be removed *in toto*. In case all identifiable glands in the cervical region appear to be of normal or smaller size and a diagnosis has been established with reasonable certainty, surgical exploration of the thorax near the base of the heart may be necessary to localize the neoplasm.

Successful removal of the functional parathyroid lesion results in a rapid decrease in circulating PTH levels, because the half-life of PTH in plasma is approximately 20 minutes. It should be emphasized that plasma calcium levels in patients with overt bone disease may decrease rapidly and be subnormal within 12 to 24 hours postsurgery, resulting in severe hypocalcemic tetany. Hypocalcemia also has been observed in dogs with primary hyperparathyroidism following infarction of a functional chief cell adenoma due to excessive palpation.

Serum calcium levels should be monitored frequently following surgical removal of a parathyroid neoplasm. Postoperative hypocalcemia (five mg per 100 ml and lower) can be the result of (1) depressed secretory activity of chief cells due to long-term suppression by the chronic hypercalcemia or injury to the remaining parathyroid tissue during surgery, (2) abruptly decreased bone resorption due to lowered PTH levels, and (3) accelerated mineralization of osteoid matrix formed by the hyperplastic osteoblasts but previously prevented from undergoing mineralization by the elevated PTH levels. Infusions of calcium gluconate to maintain the serum calcium between 7.5 and 9.0 mg per 100 ml plus providing a high calcium diet and supplemental vitamin D therapy will correct this serious postoperative complication. If hypercalcemia persists for a week or more after surgery or recurs after initial improvement, the presence of a second adenoma or metastases from a carcinoma should be suspected.

Since many of the severe effects of hypercalcemia are accentuated by dehydration, disturbances in fluid balance should be corrected in all instances. Replacement fluids such as isotonic solutions, lactated Ringer's, or 0.9 per cent sodium chloride should be administered intravenously. Calciuresis may be enhanced by administering 0.9 per cent sodium chloride intravenously, because the additional sodium presented to the renal tubules diminishes calcium reabsorption. In cases of hypercalcemic crises, intravenous administration of sodium bicarbonate may be of value in temporarily reducing the toxic effects of elevated ionized calcium concentration. The beneficial effect is related to diminution in the level of ionized calcium associated with alkalosis induced by sodium bicarbonate.

PSEUDOHYPERPARATHYROIDISM

Pseudohyperparathyroidism is a metabolic disorder in which parathyroid hormone (–like) polypeptides or other bone-resorbing substances are secreted in excessive amounts by malignant tumors of nonparathyroid origin. Criteria for the diagnosis of pseudohyperparathyroidism include (1) persistent hypercalcemia and hypophosphatemia, (2) absence of radiographic or pathologic evidence of tumor metastases in bone, (3) atrophy of parathyroid glands and C-cell hyperplasia in the thyroid gland, (4) remission of hypercalcemia when the tumor is destroyed or excised, (5) demonstration of immunologically or biologically active parathyroid (–like) polypeptides or other bone resorbing substances in the tumor tissue, and (6) exacerbation of hypercalcemia if the tumor recurs following therapy. Several hu-

moral substances have been shown to be produced by tumor cells in humans and animals that induce calcium mobilization from bone, including parathyroid hormone (–like) polypeptides (Powell et al., 1973; Singer et al., 1973), prostaglandins (PGE_2) (Galasko and Bennett, 1976; Seyberth et al., 1975; Tashjian, 1978; Voelkel et al., 1975), and osteoclast-activating factor (Mundy et al., 1974, 1974a).

Hypercalcemia and hypophosphatemia develop in dogs and human beings, with several different malignant neoplasms in the absence of bone metastases and functional lesions in the parathyroid glands (Table 66–1). Present evidence suggests that the hypercalcemia is the result of ectopic secretion of bone-resorbing substances by anaplastic tumor cells (Stewart et al., 1980), most likely by the mechanism of genetic derepression (Omen, 1973).

Rijnberk et al. (1970, 1978) originally described a syndrome of pseudohyperparathyroidism in elderly female dogs associated with perirectal adenocarcinomas. The dogs had striking hypercalcemia and hypophosphatemia that returned to normal following surgical excision of the neoplasm in the perirectal area; however, hypercalcemia persisted following removal of the parathyroid glands. Immunoreactive parathyroid hormone levels were within the range of normal for the dog but inappropriately high for the degree of hypercalcemia.

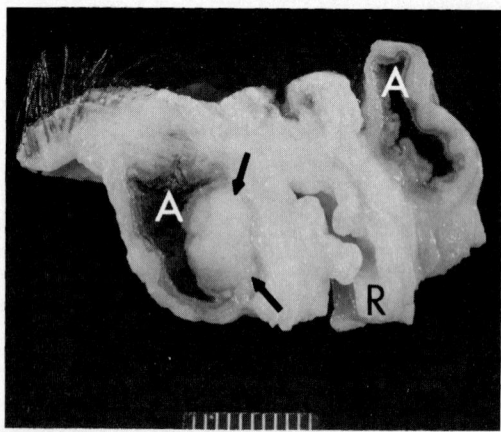

Figure 66–26. Transverse section of perineum from a female dog with hypercalcemia and an adenocarcinoma derived from apocrine glands of the anal sac. Anal sacs (A) are present on both sides of the rectum (R). A tumor nodule (arrows), one cm in diameter, and arising in the wall of the left anal sac, protrudes into its lumen.

Meuten et al. (1981) reported detailed clinical, macroscopic, and histopathologic features of adenocarcinomas arising from the apocrine gland of the anal sac in 36 dogs. This unique syndrome occurred in aged (mean ten years), predominantly female (92 per cent) dogs and was characterized by persistent hypercalcemia (91 per cent) and hypophosphatemia (71 per cent). Serum calcium values ranged from 11.4 to 24.0 mg/dl, with a mean of 16.2 mg/dl. Tumor ablation resulted in a prompt return to normocalcemia, but the hypercalcemia recurred with tumor regrowth, suggesting the neoplastic cells were producing a humoral substance that increased calcium mobilization. All tumors had histopathologic features of malignancy, and 96 per cent had metastasized to iliac and sublumbar lymph nodes.

Clinical Signs and Pathology. Functional disturbances in dogs with pseudohyperparathyroidism include generalized muscular weakness, anorexia, vomiting, bradycardia, depression, polyuria, and polydipsia. These clinical signs are primarily the result of severe hypercalcemia and complicate the problems associated with the malignant neoplasm. Apocrine adenocarcinomas develop as a firm mass (81 per cent unilateral) in the perirectal area, ventrolateral to the anus, in close association with the anal sac, but they are not attached to the overlying skin (Figs. 66–26 and 66–27). This unique neoplasm forms distinctive glandular acini with projections of apical cytoplasm extending into a lumen (Fig. 66–28) and is histologically distinct from the more common perianal (circumanal) gland tumor. The majority of neoplasms were histologically bimorphic, with glandular and solid areas. The solid arrangement of neoplastic cells was characterized by sheets, microlobules, and packets separated by a thin, fibrovascular stroma. Pseudorosettes were common in solid areas adjacent to small blood vessels.

Electron microscopic evaluation has revealed that the tumor cells in adenocarcinomas derived from apocrine glands of the anal sac contain well-developed rough endoplasmic reticulum, clusters of free ribo-

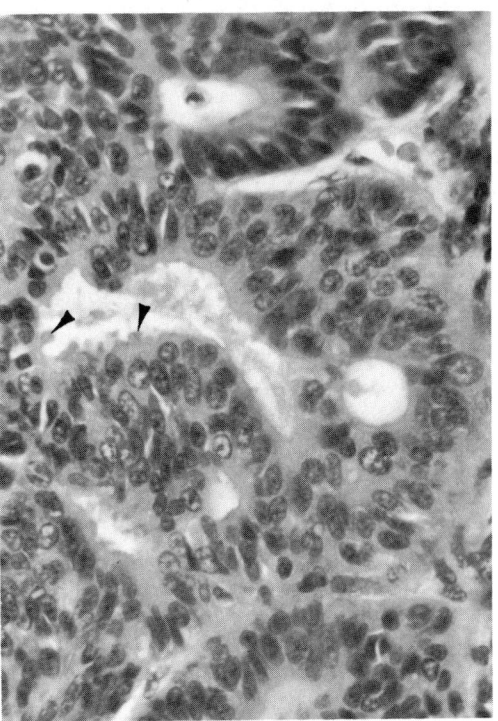

Figure 66–28. Photomicrograph of an adenocarcinoma arising in the anal sac of a dog with pseudohyperparathyroidism and persistent hypercalcemia. The glandular acini are lined by single or multiple layers of columnar neoplastic cells, with apical projections of cytoplasm into the lumen (arrowheads). The acini contained varying amounts of colloid-like material and occasional inflammatory cells. Hematoxylin and eosin, × 315.

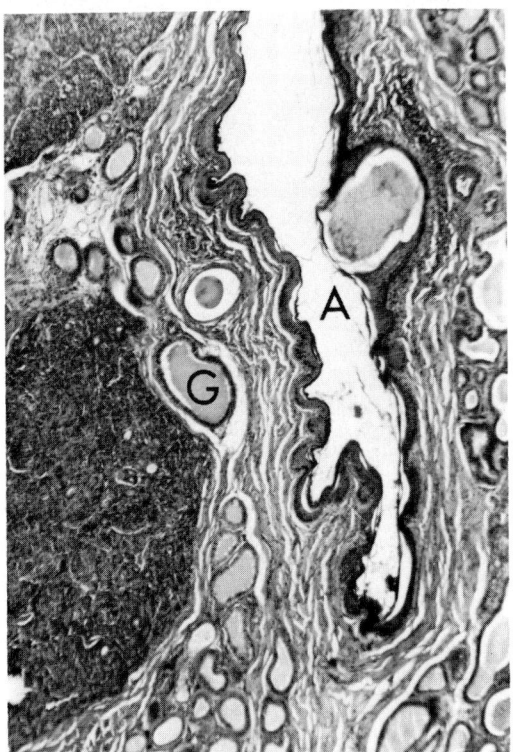

Figure 66–27. Adenocarcinoma (left) derived from apocrine glands (G) of the anal sac in close proximity to the stratified squamous epithelial lining of the anal sac (A). Hematoxylin and eosin, × 32.

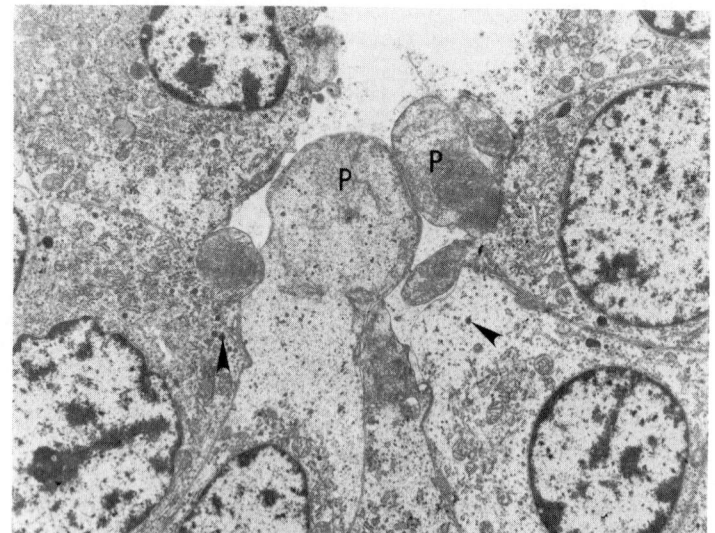

Figure 66–29. Electron micrograph illustrating apical projections (P) of cytoplasm into glandular acini in a dog with persistent hypercalcemia associated with an adenocarcinoma derived from apocrine glands of the anal sac. Small, electron-dense granules (arrowheads) are present in the cytoplasm of the neoplastic cells. These granules are similar morphologically to parathyroid hormone-containing secretory granules in chief cells of the parathyroid gland. × 5000.

somes, large mitochondria, and prominent Golgi apparatuses (Fig. 66–29). Small, membrane-limited, secretory granules often were present in the apical cytoplasm of neoplastic cells. These granules were similar in size and electron density to PTH storage granules in chief cells of normal parathyroid glands; however, additional studies are required to determine if they contain hormonal activity.

The parathyroid glands were small and difficult to locate or not visible macroscopically in 69 per cent of dogs reported by Meuten et al. (1981). Atrophic parathyroid glands in dogs with apocrine adenocarcinomas of the anal sac were characterized by narrow cords of inactive chief cells with an abundant fibrous connective tissue stroma and widened perivascular spaces (Fig. 66–30). The inactive chief cells had a markedly reduced cytoplasmic area and prominent hyperchromatic nuclei, and were closely packed together. These findings were interpreted to suggest that the perirectal adenocarcinomas were not producing a substance that stimulated parathyroid hormone secretion but rather the parathyroid glands were responding to the persistent hypercalcemia by undergoing trophic atrophy. Thyroid parafollicular (C) cells often responded to the persistent elevation in blood calcium by undergoing diffuse or nodular hyperplasia (Meuten et al., 1981).

The degree of skeletal demineralization in dogs with pseudohyperparathyroidism was mild in comparison with other causes of

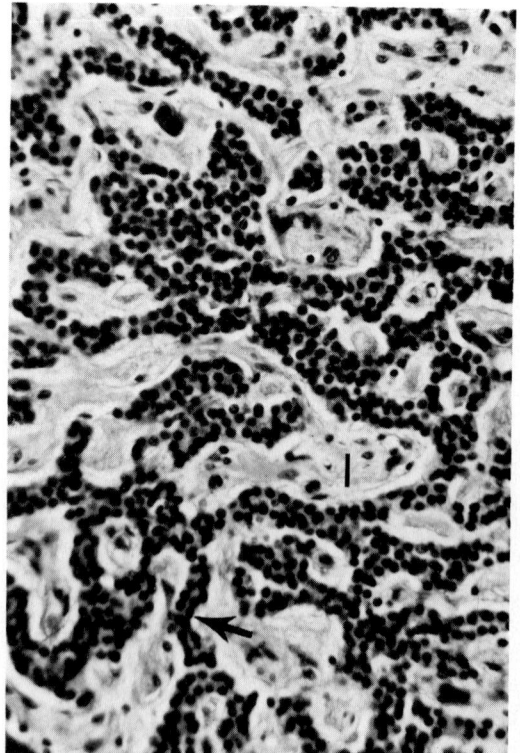

Figure 66–30. Markedly atrophic parathyroid gland from a dog with persistent hypercalcemia associated with an adenocarcinoma derived from the apocrine glands of the anal sac. Narrow cords of inactive chief cells (arrow) with a markedly reduced cytoplasmic area and hyperchromatic nuclei are separated by prominent interstitial spaces (I) with increased fibrous connective tissue. Hematoxylin and Eosin, ×125.

hypercalcemia and usually undetectable by conventional roentgenographic methods (Table 66–1). Neoplastic cells from the perirectal adenocarcinomas rarely metastasized to bone (one of 36 dogs) and caused osteolysis (Meuten et al., 1981). Histomorphometric evaluation revealed that the lumbar vertebrae from hypercalcemic dogs had less trabecular bone, more total resorptive surface, and greater numbers of osteoclasts per millimeter of trabecular bone surface than did lumbar vertebrae from normocalcemic control dogs. Osteocytic osteolysis was not detected microscopically, and the cement lines were smooth and linear (Meuten et al., 1981).

Renal mineralization was detected histologically in 90 per cent of dogs with pseudohyperparathyroidism associated with apocrine adenocarcinomas of the anal sac, particularly when the calcium X phosphorus product was 50 or greater. Tubular mineralization was most pronounced near the cortico-medullary junction but was also present in cortical and deep medullary tubules, Bowman's capsule, and glomerular tuft. Mineralization was present less frequently in the fundic mucosa of the stomach and endocardium (Meuten et al., 1981).

The marked hypercalcemia that occurs in association with apocrine adenocarcinomas derived from the anal sac appears to develop as a result of secretion by the neoplastic cells of a bone-resorbing substance. Preliminary studies reported by Rijnberk et al. (1978) suggested that circulating immunoreactive parathyroid hormone (iPTH) levels were inappropriately high for the degree of elevation in blood calcium levels. Tumor metastases are rarely present in bone, and the blood calcium level returns to normal following removal of this accessible neoplasm in the perirectal area; blood calcium is again elevated, however, if the tumor recurs or metastasizes.

Meuten et al. (1982b) reported that iPTH levels were decreased or undetectable in plasma of dogs with hypercalcemia compared with iPTH levels in control dogs and undetectable in tissue extracts of the adenocarcinoma. There was no increase in plasma concentration of the major metabolite of prostaglandin E_2 in dogs with apocrine adenocarinomas compared with that in normocalcemic tumor controls and clinically normal dogs. Although the serum con-

centration of 1,25-dihydroxycholecalciferol was not significantly different from clinically normal and normocalcemic tumor controls, it was inappropriately high for the degree of hypercalcemia. The humoral factor secreted by the tumor cells in hypercalcemic dogs with apocrine adenocarcinoma of the anal sac (although distinct immunologically from parathyroid hormone) increased osteoclastic bone resorption; increased urinary excretion of calcium, phosphorus, hydroxyproline, and cyclic adenosine monophosphate; and appeared to increase renal 1α-hydroxylase activity to maintain serum 1,25-dihydroxycholecalciferol levels in the presence of the persistent hypercalcemia.

Lymphosarcoma is the most common neoplasm associated with hypercalcemia in dogs and cats (Osborne and Stevens, 1973; Zenoble and Rowland, 1979). Estimates of the prevalence of hypercalcemia in lymphoma dogs vary from ten to 40 per cent. Peripheral lymph node enlargement may or may not be detected, but there usually is evidence of anterior mediastinal or visceral involvement. It is uncertain whether the hypercalcemia develops from the production of humoral substances by neoplastic cells (e.g., PTH-like polypeptides, prostaglandins, osteoclast-activating factor) or from physical disruption of trabecular bone due to frequent marrow involvement, or from both. Heath et al. (1980) recently reported that serum immunoreactive PTH levels were subnormal in hypercalcemic dogs with lymphosarcoma, and that plasma immunoreactive prostaglandin E_2 levels did not differ from controls. Culture media from normal lymphoid tissue and control media had no effect on release of ^{45}Ca from prelabeled fetal mouse forelimb bones; however, media from the tumor tissue increased ^{45}Ca release. These findings suggest that the local production of bone-resorbing factors (e.g., osteoclast-activating factor) is important in stimulating calcium release from bone in certain dogs with lymphosarcoma and hypercalcemia. The 1,25-dihydroxycholecalciferol levels in dogs with persistent hypercalcemia associated with malignant lymphoma, in contrast to those in dogs with apocrine adenocarcinomas of the anal sac, are suppressed relative to those in clinically normal or normocalcemic tumor controls (Meuten et al. 1982b).

RENAL SECONDARY HYPERPARATHYROIDISM

Secondary hyperparathyroidism as a complication of chronic renal failure is a metabolic state characterized by an excessive, but not autonomous, rate of PTH secretion. This disorder is encountered frequently in dogs but also occurs in cats. The secretion of hormone by the hyperplastic parathyroid glands usually remains responsive to fluctuations in blood calcium.

Pathophysiology. The primary etiologic mechanism in this disorder is long-standing, progressive renal disease resulting in severely impaired function. Chronic renal insufficiency in older dogs results from interstitial nephritis, glomerulonephritis, nephrosclerosis, or amyloidosis. Chronic renal disease with periglomerular and interstitial fibrosis in Norwegian elkhounds has been reported to be familial (Finco et al., 1977). Several congenital anomalies such as cortical hypoplasia (Kaufman et al., 1969), polycystic kidneys, and bilateral hydronephrosis may result in renal insufficiency in younger dogs.

When the renal disease progresses to the point at which there is significant reduction in glomerular filtration rate, phosphorus is retained and progressive hyperphosphatemia develops (Fig. 66–31). Although the concentration of blood phosphorus has no direct regulatory influence on the synthesis and secretion of PTH, it may, when elevated, contribute to parathyroid stimulation by virtue of its ability to lower blood calcium levels. Parathyroid stimulation in patients with chronic renal disease can be attributed directly to the hypocalcemia.

Recent evidence suggests that impaired intestinal absorption of calcium due to an acquired defect in vitamin D metabolism plays a significant role in the development of hypocalcemia in chronic renal insufficiency and uremia. Chronic renal disease interferes with the production of 1,25-dihydroxycholecalciferol by the kidney, thereby diminishing intestinal calcium transport and resulting in the development of hypocalcemia.

All parathyroids are considerably enlarged (Fig. 66–32), owing initially to hypertrophy of chief cells, and subsequently to hyperplasia, as compensatory mechanisms to increase hormonal synthesis and secretion in response to the hypocalcemic stimulus. Although the parathyroids are not autonomous, the concentration of PTH in the peripheral blood in human patients with chronic renal failure may exceed that of primary hyperparathyroidism. Parathyroid hormone increases osteoclastic resorption (Weisbrode et al., 1974) and bone remodeling (Norrdin et al., 1977, 1977a; Villafane et al., 1977), resulting in release of stored calcium from bone. The long-standing increase in bone resorption that attempts to return serum calcium to normal eventually results in the metabolic bone disease associated with chronic renal insufficiency. Progressive glomerular and tubular dysfunction with loss of target cells interferes with an expression of the phosphaturic response by the increased circulating PTH in renal disease. Phosphate is retained and the blood concentration continues to rise in spite of the secondary hyperparathyroidism (Fig. 66–31).

Clinical Signs. The predominant clinical signs of vomiting, dehydration, polydipsia, depression, and ammoniacal breath odor are related to progressive renal insuffi-

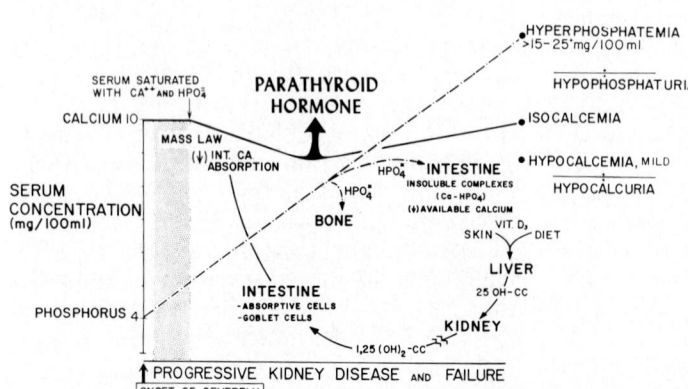

Figure 66–31. Alterations in serum calcium and phosphorus during the pathogenesis of secondary hyperparathyroidism associated with progressive renal failure.

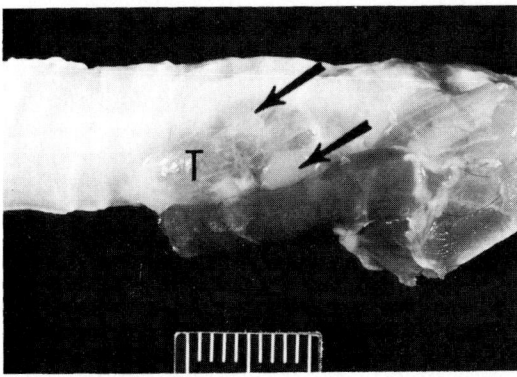

Figure 66–32. Hypertrophy of external and internal parathyroid glands (arrows) in a dog with secondary hyperparathyroidism associated with chronic renal disease. T, adjacent thyroid gland. The scale represents one cm.

ciency and uremia. A spectrum of skeletal lesions of secondary hyperparathyroidism may be present, ranging from minor changes with early (or mild) renal disease to the severe fibrous osteodystrophy of advanced renal failure. Histologic evaluation of the skeleton in dogs with chronic renal disease reveals that a high percentage have generalized fibrous osteodystrophy (Krook, 1957). The volume of affected bones is usually normal (isostotic fibrous osteodystrophy), particularly in older dogs because of the slow onset of renal failure and lower metabolic activity of bones. Hyperostotic bone lesions, such as facial swellings, may be seen in younger dogs (Norrdin, 1975) in which deposition of osteoid by hyperplastic osteoblasts (stimulated by high blood phosphorus) and repair by proliferation of fibrous connective tissue exceed the rate of resorption, resulting in a greater than normal bone volume.

Although skeletal involvement is generalized with hyperparathyroidism, it does not affect all parts uniformly. Lesions become apparent earlier and reach a more advanced stage in certain areas, such as cancellous bone of the skull. In dogs with long-standing renal disease, the increased osteoclastic resorption results in the formation of cystic (radiolucent) areas in bones of the skull, giving a "moth-eaten" appearance similar to that of primary hyperparathyroidism. Resorption of alveolar socket bone and loss of lamina dura dentes occur early and result in loose teeth, which may be dislodged easily and interfere with mastica-

tion. The nasal cavity may be impinged upon, owing to partial collapse of surrounding poorly mineralized bone and displacement of the medial nasal septum. Cancellous bone of the maxilla and mandible also is a site of predilection in hyperparathyroidism. As a result of the accelerated resorption, bones of the mandibles become softened and readily pliable ("rubber jaw disease") (Fig. 66–33), and the jaws fail to close properly. This often results in drooling of saliva and protrusion of the tongue. The severely demineralized mandibles are predisposed to fractures and displacement of teeth from alveolar sockets (Fig. 66–34). Long bones of the abaxial skeleton are less dramatically affected. Lameness, stiff gait, and the occurrence of fractures after relatively minor trauma may result from increased bone resorption.

Diagnosis. Roentgenographically, there is evidence of generalized skeletal demineralization in advanced cases, with localized areas of accentuation and loss of lamina

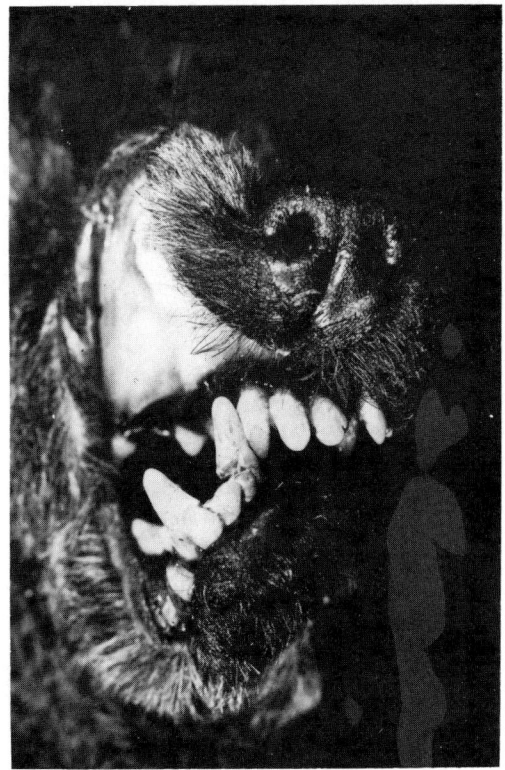

Figure 66–33. Renal secondary hyperparathyroidism in a dog. The extreme pliability of the maxilla and mandible ("rubber jaw") is due to excessive bone resorption stimulated by parathyroid hormone.

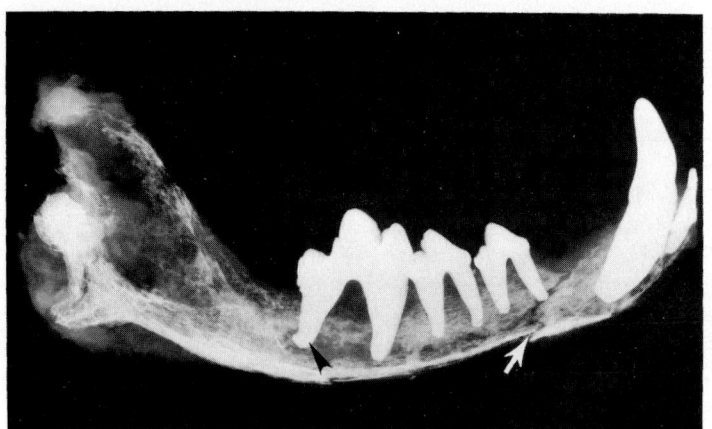

Figure 66–34. Ramus of the mandible from a dog with severe secondary hyperparathyroidism of renal origin. There is diffuse demineralization with loss of lamina dura dentes (black arrowhead), fracture of the distal end of the ramus (white arrow), and extensive resorption of alveolar socket bone.

dura dentes. Several laboratory procedures should be used to establish and assess the extent of renal disease.

Serum should be analyzed for calcium, phosphorus, and alkaline phosphatase. Results of a single determination of these parameters must be interpreted with an appreciation that considerable variation exists, depending upon the stage of the disease, because of the body's compensatory mechanisms (Fig. 66–31). The blood calcium level is variable but is usually in the low normal range because of mobilization of skeletal reserves. A small percentage of dogs with chronic kidney disease will have a moderate hypercalcemia (Finco and Rowland, 1978; Hruska et al., 1975). Alkaline phosphatase activity may be elevated in animals with overt bone disease. Urinary excretion of calcium and phosphorus are decreased.

Treatment. Ideally, the aim of treatment with this disorder would be to interrupt the progression of kidney disease and restore or replace renal function to a semblance of normal. Owing to the stage at which the diagnosis is established in animals and to the progressive nature of the disease, treatment is directed realistically toward reducing the excretory load and providing substances (such as sodium chloride or bicarbonate, water, and so forth) that the failing kidney is unable to conserve. A K/D prescription diet with supplemental calcium (gluconate or lactate) and vitamin D may diminish the severity of hyperparathyroidism and accompanying bone lesions. Recent evidence suggests that 1,25-dihydroxycholecalciferol or 1α-hydroxycholecalciferol have considerable potential in the therapy of impaired intestinal absorption of calcium, hypocalcemia, and osteomalacia associated in human patients with chronic renal disease.

NUTRITIONAL SECONDARY HYPERPARATHYROIDISM

The increased secretion of parathyroid hormone in this metabolic disorder is a compensatory mechanism directed against a disturbance in mineral homeostasis induced by nutritional imbalances. The disease occurs commonly in dogs, cats, certain primates, and laboratory animals, as well as in many farm animals.

Pathophysiology. Dietary mineral imbalances of etiologic importance in the pathogenesis of nutritional secondary hyperparathyroidism are first, a low content of calcium, and second, excessive phosphorus with normal or low calcium levels. The significant end result is hypocalcemia, which results in the parathyroid stimulation (Fig. 66–35). A diet low in calcium fails to supply the daily requirement, even though a greater proportion of ingested calcium is absorbed, and hypocalcemia develops (Rowland et al., 1968; Scott, 1968). Ingestion of excessive phosphorus results in increased intestinal absorption and elevation of blood phosphorus levels. Hyperphosphatemia does not stimulate the parathyroid gland directly but does so indirectly by virtue of its ability to lower blood calcium levels.

In response to the nutritionally induced hypocalcemia, all parathyroid glands undergo cellular hypertrophy and hyperplasia. Since kidney function is normal, the increased levels of PTH result in diminished renal tubular reabsorption of phosphate and increased reabsorption of calcium, returning blood levels toward normal (Fig. 66–35). In addition, osteoclastic bone resorption is accelerated and release of calcium elevates blood calcium levels to the low normal range. Continued ingestion of the unbalanced diet sustains the state of com-

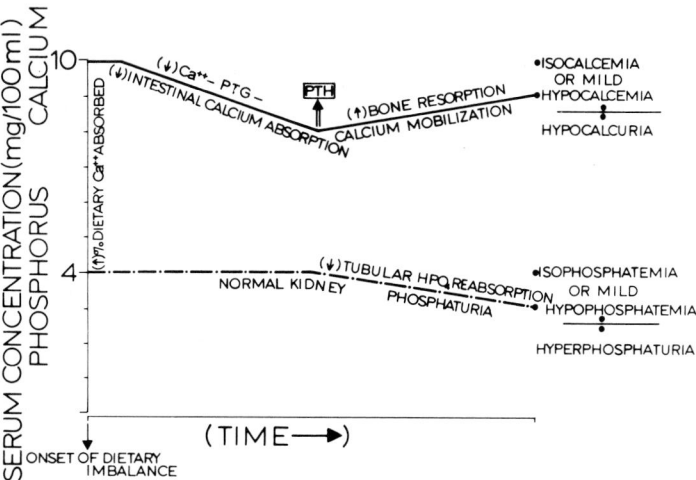

Figure 66–35. Alterations in serum calcium and phosphorus in the pathogenesis of nutritional secondary hyperparathyroidism caused by feeding a diet low in calcium or deficient in cholecalciferol but with normal amounts of phosphorus.

pensatory hyperparathyroidism, leading to progressive development of the metabolic bone disease.

Clinical Signs. The disease develops in young pups and kittens fed a predominantly meat diet. For example, beef heart or liver contains minimal amounts of calcium (seven to nine mg per 100 mg) and has a markedly imbalanced calcium:phosphorus ratio (1:20 to 1:50). The feeding of a monotonous meat diet to dogs of any age results in secondary hyperparathyroidism, with the development of skeletal disease of varying severity. The low calcium content and unfavorable calcium:phosphorus ratio of non-supplemented all-meat diets are unable to fulfill the daily requirements for either growing pups (528 mg of calcium and 440 mg of phosphorus per kg of body weight daily) or adult dogs (264 mg of calcium and 220 mg of phosphorus per kg of body weight daily).

The diet of kittens up to six months of age should supply 200 to 400 mg of calcium and approximately 200 µg of iodine daily, and from 10,000 to 15,000 IU of vitamin A weekly (Scott, 1968). The addition of iodine to all-meat diets prevents the development of thyroid hyperplasia, but not the skeletal disease, in cats.

Kittens that are fed beef heart exclusively develop locomotor disturbances within four weeks. The predominant clinical signs are a reluctance to move, posterior lameness, and an uncoordinated gait. The kittens often assume a standing position with characteristic medial deviation of the paws. The skeletal disease becomes progressively more severe after 5 to 14 weeks. The cortex of long bones is greatly thinned, owing to the increased resorption, and the medullary cavity is widened (Fig. 66–36). The kittens become quiet and reluctant to play. They assume a sitting position or are in sternal recumbency, with the hindlegs abducted at the pelvis. Normal activities may result in sudden onset of severe lameness as a result of incomplete or folding fractures of one or more bones. In kittens that are fed beef heart, the high content of digestible protein (over 50 per cent on a wet basis) and fat promotes rapid growth. These animals appear well nourished and their coat maintains a good luster.

Nutritional secondary hyperparathyroidism has been reported frequently in Siamese and Burmese kittens, but skeletal lesions can be induced readily in other breeds. The indulgence of fussy eating habits with undesirable diets by their owners, rather than a

Figure 66–36. Nutritional hyperparathyroidism in a young cat fed a beef-heart diet for 13 weeks. The cortical bone of the femur is extremely thin (arrow), owing to excessive resorption, and the marrow cavity is widened.

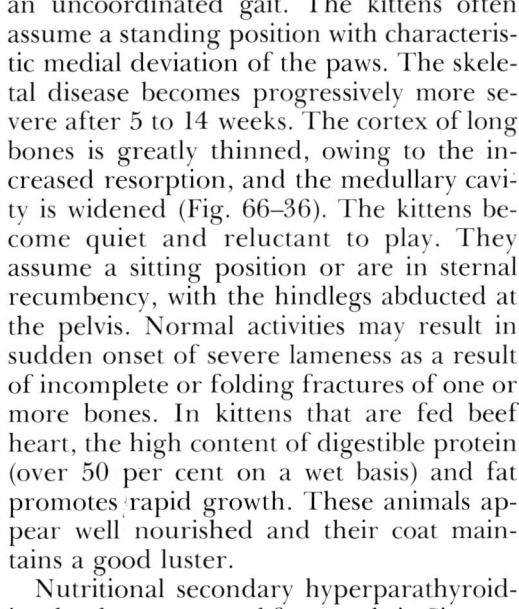

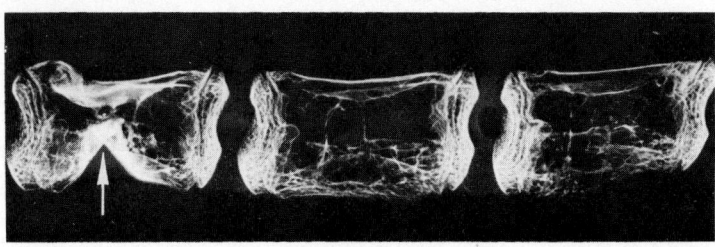

Figure 66–37. Lumbar vertebrae from a cat with nutritional secondary hyperparathyroidism. Note the loss of trabecular bone, thinning of the cortex, and cavitation of the body of the vertebrae (arrow).

genetic predisposition, probably accounts for the higher incidence of the disease in the Siamese and Burmese breeds. Various terms have been used to describe this metabolic disorder in cats, including osteogenesis imperfecta, juvenile osteoporosis, and paper-bone or Siamese cat disease.

In general, kittens are more susceptible to this disorder and develop more severe skeletal lesions than adult cats fed a similar diet. Adult cats fed a beef-heart diet develop osteoporosis slowly after a period of months in response to increased PTH secretion, whereas the skeletons of kittens develop severe generalized osteitis fibrosis within a few weeks. The disease develops rapidly in kittens because the dietary imbalance is wide and their skeletal metabolic rate is high. Resorption proceeds at a faster rate than repair by fibrous connective tissue proliferation and results in a decreased bone volume (hypostotic fibrous osteodystrophy). Vertebral fractures with compression of the spinal cord and paralysis are common in kittens but infrequent in adult cats (Fig. 66–37).

Lameness is the initial functional disturbance in growing dogs (Fig. 66–38) and may vary from a slight limp to complete inability to walk. The bones are painful on palpation, and folding fractures of long bones and vertebrae are not uncommon. Clinical signs are usually related to resorption of jaw bones in adult dogs. Parathyroid hormone–stimulated resorption of alveolar socket bone results in loss of lamina dura dentes, loosening and subsequent loss of teeth from their sockets, and recession of gingivae with partial root exposure in advanced cases.

Diagnosis. The diet should be evaluated for calcium, phosphorus, and vitamin D content in all patients (particularly young and rapidly growing animals) with skeletal disease. In nutritional hyperparathyroidism, there is radiographic evidence of generalized skeletal demineralization, loss of lamina dura dentes, subperiosteal cortical bone resorption, bowing deformities, and multiple folding fractures of long bones due to localized osteoclast proliferation. Laboratory parameters used to assess renal function should be within normal limits in patients with nutritional hyperparathyroidism.

Analysis of the serum for calcium, phosphorus, and alkaline phosphatase should be undertaken with an appreciation that one determination may be of limited diagnostic value. Since the body's compensatory mechanisms with this disease are complex and operational when the animal is seen for the first time, serum calcium and phosphorus levels usually are in a low normal range. Alkaline phosphatase activity often is elevated in animals with overt bone disease. The

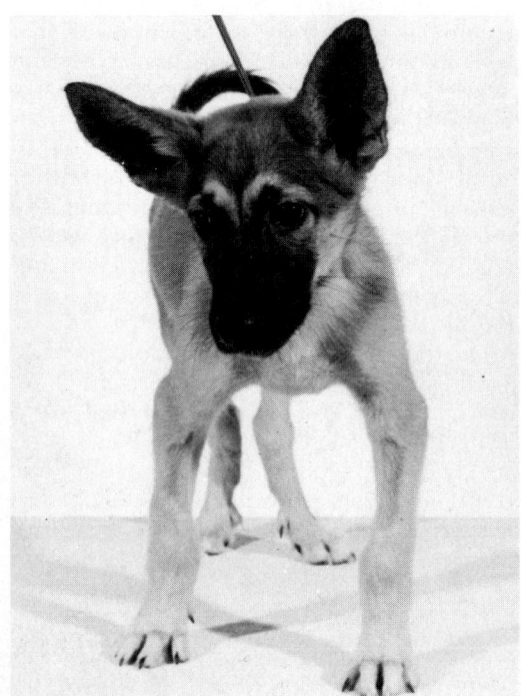

Figure 66–38. Nutritional secondary hyperparathyroidism in a young pup, illustrating severe deformities of the fore- and hindlimbs due to excessive osteoclastic resorption of bone.

increased PTH secretion acts on the normal kidneys to increase phosphate and decrease calcium excretion in the urine.

Treatment. The aim of treatment is to decrease PTH secretion by correcting the dietary mineral imbalance or deficiency. Kittens and pups with the disease should be fed a diet that fulfills their high demand for animal protein and meets the daily requirements for calcium and phosphorus. Calcium gluconate, lactate, or carbonate alone or in combination should be used as dietary supplements to achieve a 2:1 calcium:phosphorus ratio during the healing phase in young animals with severe bone disease. Additional vitamin D is usually not necessary but may be indicated in severely affected animals to increase intestinal absorption of calcium. Calcium gluconate should be given parenterally if the appetite is depressed. The feeding of excessive amounts of calcium for prolonged periods should be avoided both therapeutically and under normal conditions, because it may retard growth and alter remodeling of bone in young dogs.

It is essential to keep affected animals closely confined for at least three weeks after initiation of the supplemental diet. The response to therapy is rapid, and within a week the animals become more active and their attitude improves. Jumping or climbing must be prevented, because the skeleton is still susceptible to fractures. The restrictions need be less rigid after three weeks, but confinement with limited movement is indicated until the skeleton returns to normal. Improvement of the skeleton during dietary supplementation can be followed

radiographically. Fracture calluses become radiodense and the overall mineral density and cortical bone thickness increase progressively with treatment. The skeleton is usually healed after the supplemental diet (calcium:phosphorus ratio of 2:1) has been administered for eight to nine weeks. Subsequently, the diet should supply the total daily requirement of calcium and phosphorus and be balanced at about 1.2:1.0. Even advanced cases respond favorably to dietary supplementation. Good nursing care is essential to prevent complications such as decubital ulcers, constipation, and additional fractures. Healed pelvic fractures may predispose to dystocia and obstipation.

HYPOPARATHYROIDISM

In hypoparathyroidism, either subnormal amounts of PTH are secreted by pathologic parathyroid glands or the hormone secreted is unable to interact normally with target cells. Hypoparathyroidism has been recognized in dogs, particularly in smaller breeds such as schnauzers and terriers (Burk and Schaubhut, 1975; Kornegay et al., 1980; Meyer and Terrell, 1976; Sherding et al., 1980).

Pathophysiology. Several pathogenic mechanisms can result in an inadequate secretion of PTH. The parathyroid glands may be damaged or inadvertently removed during the course of thyroid surgery. If the parathyroid glands or their vascular supply has been damaged, there often is regeneration of adequate functional parenchyma and subsequent disappearance of clinical signs.

Figure 66–39. External parathyroid gland in a dog with lymphocytic parathyroiditis that resulted in hypoparathyroidism and hypocalcemic tetany. There is extensive destruction of chief cells with infiltration of lymphocytes (L) and plasma cells, and nodular hyperplasia of remaining viable chief cells (C). T, thyroid gland, A, arterial branch to external parathyroid. Hematoxylin and Eosin, ×32.

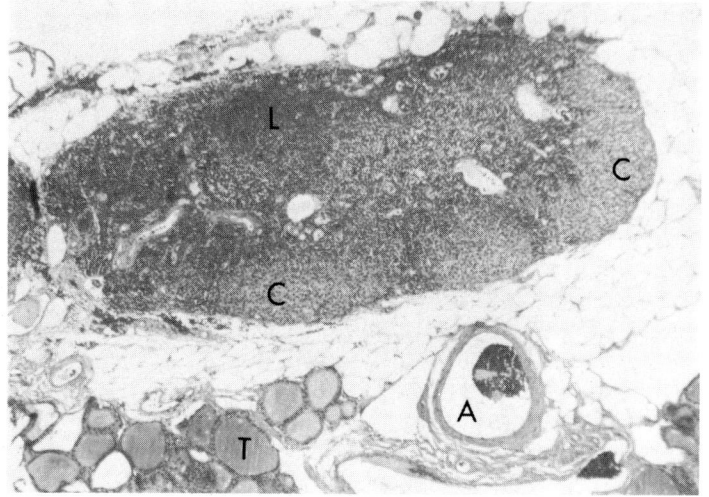

Idiopathic hypoparathyroidism in adult dogs usually is associated with diffuse lymphocytic parathyroiditis resulting in extensive degeneration of chief cells and replacement by fibrous connective tissue. In the early stages of lymphocytic parathyroiditis, there is infiltration of the gland with lymphocytes and plasma cells, and nodular regenerative hyperplasia of remaining chief cells (Fig. 66–39). Later, the parathyroid gland is completely replaced by lymphocytes, fibroblasts, and neocapillaries with only an occasional viable chief cell (Fig. 66–40). The lymphocytic parathyroiditis may develop by means of an autoimmune mechanism, since a similar destruction of secretory parenchyma and lymphocytic infiltration has been produced experimentally in dogs by repeated injections of parathyroid tissue emulsions (Lapelescu et al., 1968).

Other possible causes of hypoparathyroidism include invasion and destruction of parathyroids by primary or metastatic neoplasms in the anterior cervical area and trophic atrophy of parathyroids associated with long-term hypercalcemia. The presence of numerous distemper virus particles in chief cells of the parathyroid gland may contribute to the low blood calcium in certain dogs with this disease (Weisbrode and Krakowka, 1979). Agenesis of both pairs of parathyroids is a rare cause of congenital hypoparathyroidism in pups. Certain cases of idiopathic hypoparathyroidism with histologically normal parathyroids in both animals and man may be due to a lack of the specific enzyme in chief cells that converts the proPTH molecule to the biologically active PTH secreted by the gland (Fig. 66–2).

Pseudohypoparathyroidism is a variant of the syndrome of hypoparathyroidism that has been reported in human beings in which target cells in kidney and bone are unable to respond to the secretion of normal amounts of parathyroid hormone (Birkenhager et al., 1973; Drezner et al., 1973; Farfel et al., 1980). This is due to a lack of the nucleotide regulatory (N–) protein that couples the hormone-receptor complex to the catalytic subunit of adenylate cyclase in the plasma membrane, resulting in an inability to form cyclic AMP in target cells (Fig. 66–41) (Farfel et al., 1980). Severe hypocalcemia develops in patients with pseudohypoparathyroidism even though parathyroid glands are hyperplastic (Roth and Capen, 1974) and immunoreactive parathyroid hormone levels are elevated (Birkenhager et al., 1973).

Clinical Signs. The functional disturbances and clinical manifestations of hypoparathyroidism are primarily the result of increased neuromuscular excitability and tetany. Because of the lack of PTH, bone resorption is decreased and blood calcium levels diminish progressively (four to six mg per 100 ml) (Fig. 66–42). Affected dogs are restless, nervous, and ataxic with weakness and intermittent tremors of individual muscle groups that progress to generalized tetany and convulsive seizures. Concurrently,

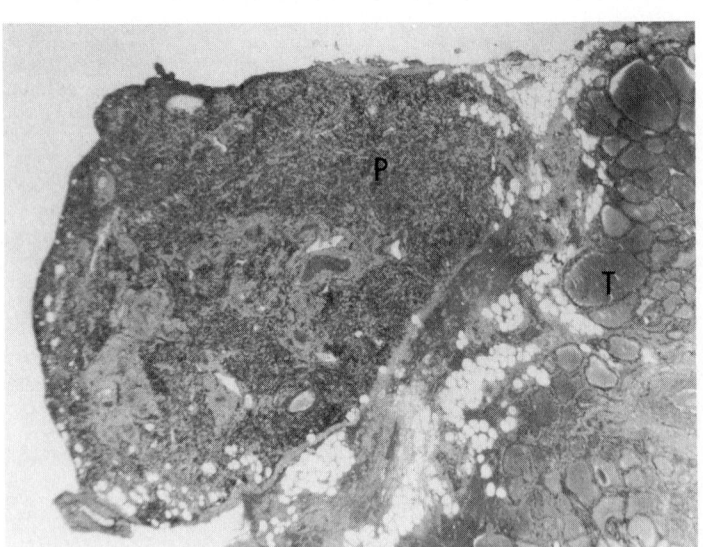

Figure 66–40. Diffuse lymphocytic parathyroiditis (P) in a dog with hypoparathyroidism and hypocalcemia. There is complete replacement of the external parathyroid gland by lymphocytes, plasma cells, fibroblasts, and neocapillaries. T, thyroid gland. Hematoxylin and eosin, ×32.

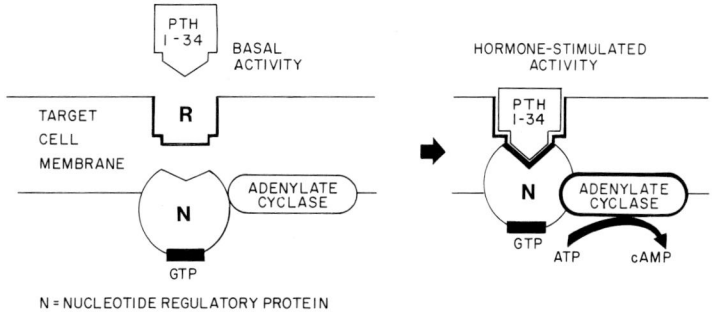

Figure 66–41. Mechanism of parathyroid hormone action. The biologically active end of the hormone (PTH 1–34) binds to specific receptors (R) on the surface of target cells. The receptor-hormone complex is coupled to the catalytic subunit of adenylate cyclase in the cell membrane by a nucleotide regulatory (N–) protein. This results in the intracellular accumulation of cyclic adenosine monophosphate (cAMP), which serves as the "second messenger" for polypeptide hormones such as PTH in target cells and results in expression of the biologic response of the hormone.

blood phosphorus levels are substantially elevated owing to increased renal tubular reabsorption.

Treatment. Tetany should be stopped initially by returning blood calcium levels to near normal through the intravenous administration of organic calcium solutions. Long-term maintenance of blood calcium in the absence of normal PTH secretion should be attempted by feeding diets that are high in calcium and low in phosphorus and that are supplemented with calcium (gluconate or lactate) and vitamin D_3.

Large doses of vitamin D_3 (25,000 to 50,000 or more units per day, depending upon the size of the dog) may be required initially to elevate the blood calcium in hypoparathyroid patients, because the lack of PTH diminishes the rate of formation of the biologically active vitamin D metabolite by the 1α-hydroxylase system in the kidney (Fig. 66–17). In order to prevent the development of hypercalcemia and extensive soft tissue mineralization, the clinician should carefully adjust the dosage of vitamin D by frequently determining the serum calcium levels. After adjusting the dose of vitamin D, a five-day interval should precede the next blood calcium determination in order to fully assess the effects of the change in vitamin D. Once the blood calcium has been returned to the normal range, substantially lower doses of vitamin D are indicated for long-term maintenance of blood electrolyte levels (Fig. 66–43). In some dogs only dietary calcium supplementation is required for long-term stabilization of the blood calcium level (Sherding et al., 1980).

Replacement therapy with either parathyroid extract or PTH derived from heterologous species (such as bovine) is expensive and ineffective on a long-term basis because of the development of antibodies. Synthetic PTH, especially the biologically active amino terminal (1 to 34) end of the molecule, and the active metabolite of vitamin D

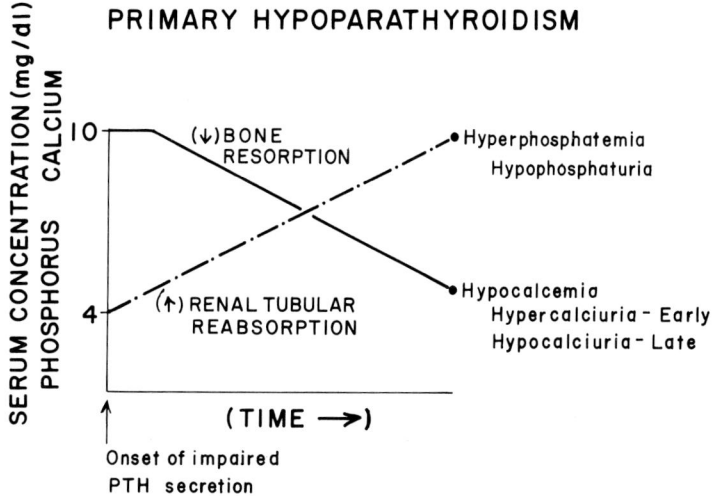

Figure 66–42. Alterations in serum calcium and phosphorus in response to an inadequate secretion of parathyroid hormone. There is a progressive increase in serum phosphorus and marked decline in serum calcium to levels that result in increased neuromuscular excitability and tetany.

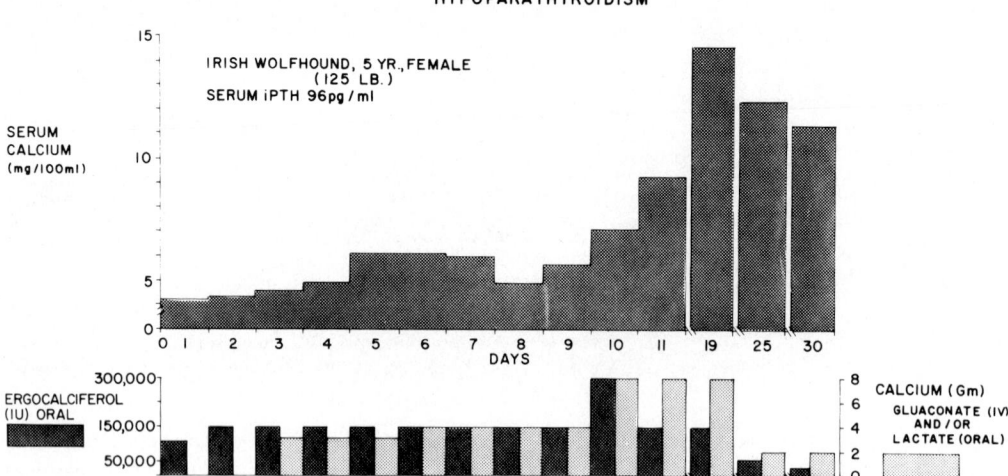

Figure 66–43. Response of serum calcium to varying doses of vitamin D in an Irish wolfhound with hypoparathyroidism. Large daily doses of vitamin D plus oral calcium supplements were required to elevate the serum calcium concentration back to the physiologic range, but considerably smaller doses of vitamin D were required for long-term maintenance.

(1,25-dihydroxycholecalciferol) may be useful in the treatment of hypoparathyroidism of animals in the near future, as has been reported in human patients (Hill et al., 1976).

PUERPERAL TETANY IN THE BITCH

Considerably less is known about the pathogenesis of hypocalcemic syndromes in the dog and cat than is known about their development in the cow (Littledike et al., 1974; Rowland et al., 1972). Puerperal tetany is most frequently encountered in the small, hyperexcitable breeds of dogs and occasionally in the cat (Edney, 1969). The clinical course is rapid and the bitch may proceed from premonitory signs of restlessness, panting, and nervousness to ataxia, trembling, muscular tetany, and convulsive seizures in 8 to 12 hours (Resnick, 1972; Kallfelz, 1968). Hyperthermia frequently is associated with the increased muscular activity, and elevations of body temperature to 107° C are not uncommon.

Pathophysiology. There is little evidence to suggest that puerperal tetany (eclampsia) in heavily lactating bitches is the result of an interference in PTH secretion. Severe hypocalcemia and often hypophosphatemia develop near the time of peak lactation (approximately one to three weeks postpartum), probably as the result of an im-

balance between the rates of inflow and outflow from the extracellular calcium pool (Fig. 66–44). It is well known that feeding high-calcium diets to dairy cows in the prepartum period has a provocative effect on the development of hypocalcemic disorders following parturition because of diminished responsiveness of PTH-mediated bone resorption. The reduced availability of calcium from skeletal sources leads to an excessive reliance on intestinal calcium absorption.

Functional disturbances associated with hypocalcemia in the bitch are primarily the result of neuromuscular tetany (Fig. 66–45),

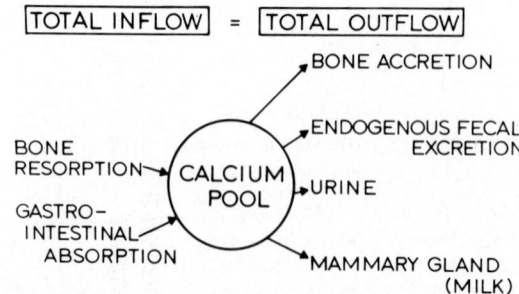

Figure 66–44. Relationship of inflow of calcium into the extracellular pool (from bone resorption and gastrointestinal absorption) and outflow of calcium into milk, urine, feces, and bone. An imbalance between the rates of inflow and outflow from the extracellular fluid calcium pool because of the increased loss into the milk appears to be an important factor in the pathogenesis of puerperal tetany in the bitch.

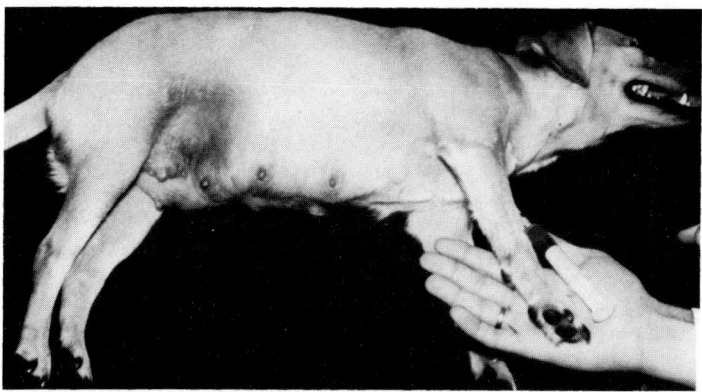

Figure 66–45. Puerperal tetany in a bitch. Increased neuromuscular excitability occurs in the bitch with hypocalcemia, since excitation-secretion coupling is maintained at the motor endplate.

in contrast with those in the cow, in which the clinical sign is mainly paresis. Excitation-secretion coupling is maintained at the neuromuscular junction in the bitch with hypocalcemia. Tetany occurs in the bitch as a result of spontaneous repetitive firing of motor nerve fibers. As a result of the loss of stabilizing membrane-bound calcium, nerve membranes become more permeable to ions and require a stimulus of lesser magnitude to depolarize.

Diagnosis. Clinical diagnosis is based on history, clinical signs, and response to therapy in most cases. If laboratory facilities are readily available, demonstration of hypocalcemia with serum calcium levels less than 7 mg/dl confirms the clinical diagnosis. Serum phosphorus levels often are lowered to a comparable degree. Blood glucose levels are in the low normal range or decreased as a result of the intense muscular activity associated with tetany.

Treatment. The slow intravenous administration of an organic calcium solution such as calcium gluconate should result in rapid clinical improvement and cessation of tetanic spasms within 15 minutes. In most bitches, five to ten ml of ten per cent calcium gluconate will provide sufficient calcium for a bitch weighing between five and ten kg. Intravenous administration should proceed slowly to avoid inducing ventricular fibrillation and cardiac arrest.

Puppies should be removed from the bitch for 24 hours to reduce the lactational drain of calcium. During this period the puppies should be fed a milk substitute or other appropriate diet. If the puppies are mature enough, it is advisable to wean them; otherwise, they should be returned to the bitch after the 24-hour period. Supplemental dietary calcium and vitamin D have

proved useful in preventing relapses in certain bitches with puerperal tetany.

Although some clinicians advocate the use of corticosteroids in addition to calcium and vitamin D to prevent relapses after the original therapy, there is no logical basis for use of these drugs in such treatment regimens. Since corticosteroids may lower serum calcium levels by interfering with intestinal calcium transport, their real value in the treatment of eclampsia is questionable.

Prevention. During gestation a good-quality, balanced diet with a calcium-to-phosphorus ratio of 1:1 or less that provides the required (but not excessive) amounts of calcium may result in a more responsive calcium homeostatic mechanism to meet the markedly increased demands of lactation. Calcium homeostasis in animals fed balanced or relatively low-calcium diets during gestation appears to be under better control by parathyroid hormone secretion with the approach of parturition and initiation of the lactational drain. The higher levels of PTH secreted during the prepartal period by an expanded population of actively synthesizing chief cells appear to result in a larger pool of active bone-resorbing cells to fulfill the increased needs for calcium mobilization at the critical time near parturition and initiation of lactation. These animals appear to be less susceptible to the influence of decreased calcium absorption and flow into the extracellular pool, which can occur in the immediate postpartum period (Yarrington et al., 1977). In contrast, calcium homeostasis in animals fed a high-calcium diet during gestation appears to be maintained principally by intestinal calcium absorption. This greater reliance on intestinal absorption rather than on PTH-stimulated bone resorption probably is a significant factor in

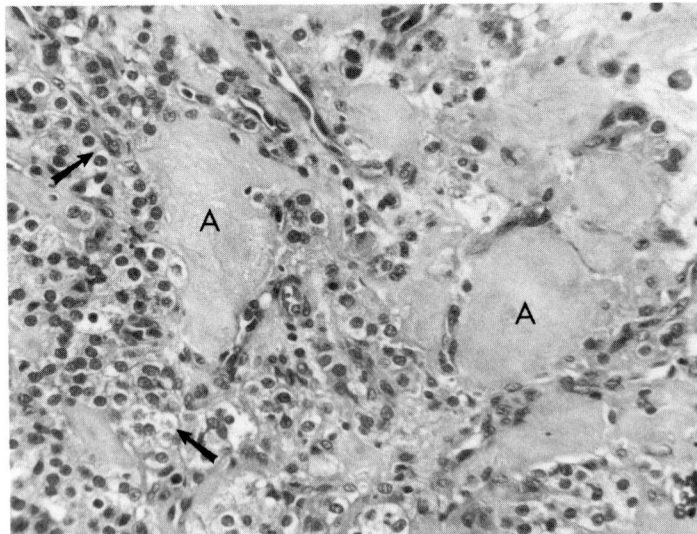

Figure 66–46. Calcitonin-secreting C-cell tumor in the thyroid gland of a dog. The cytoplasmic area of C-cells stains lightly eosinophilic (arrows). The large accumulations of amyloid (A) in the interstitium give this type of thyroid tumor a characteristically firm consistency. Hematoxylin and eosin, × 325.

the more frequent development of hypocalcemia near parturition in animals fed high-calcium diets prepartum (Black et al., 1973, 1973b).

HYPERCALCITONINISM

Clinical syndromes associated with abnormalities in the secretion of calcitonin (CT) are recognized much less frequently than are disorders of parathyroid hormone in both animals and man. A hypersecretion of CT has been reported in human beings (Hazard, 1977; Sipple, 1961), bulls (Black et al., 1973a; Capen et al., 1974), and laboratory rats (Burek, 1978; DeLellis et al., 1979) with medullary (ultimobranchial) thyroid neoplasms derived from C cells. In human beings the syndrome often is familial, with involvement of many individuals in a kindred. A medullary thyroid carcinoma that contained calcitonin was reported recently in a dog with a firm mass in the anterior cervical region and chronic watery diarrhea (Leav et al., 1976). Calcitonin activity was localized to the cytoplasm of tumor cells by immunoenzymatic techniques. Medullary (C cell) carcinomas may secrete humoral substances other than calcitonin, such as prostaglandins, serotonin, and bradykinin, which result in a wide spectrum of clinical manifestations (Melvin et al., 1972).

The incidence of occurrence of C-cell tumors of the thyroid in dogs is uncertain, but they appear to be more common than previously expected. Zarrin (1977) reported that seven of 200 thyroid gland tumors in dogs were derived from C cells. They often are firm on palpation owing to the presence

of large amounts of amyloid in the stroma (Fig. 66–46). Thyroid neoplasms of C-cell origin can be readily differentiated ultrastructurally by the presence of numerous membrane-limited secretory granules in the cytoplasm (Capen, 1978). Small granules of this type are not present in thyroid tumors derived from follicular cells. C-cell tumors in both human beings and animals may be associated with the simultaneous occurrence of pheochromocytoma in the adrenal medulla and neoplasms in other endocrine organs (Sipple, 1961; Yarrington and Capen, 1981).

Serum calcium and phosphorus levels in adults with a chronic excessive secretion of calcitonin either remain in the low normal range owing to the relatively slow turnover rate of bone and compensatory increase in PTH secretion or are significantly decreased below normal (Krook et al., 1971). Osteosclerotic changes have been reported in animals with this syndrome, but the relationship of long-term excessive calcitonin secretion to the pathogenesis of the skeletal lesions and their occurrence in other animal species is uncertain.

HYPOCALCITONINISM

Specific disease syndromes resulting from a lack of calcitonin secretion have not been recognized in either man or animals. However, experimentally thyroidectomized animals are less able than normal animals to handle a high-calcium meal and may develop hypercalcemia (Swaminathan et al., 1972).

REFERENCES

Aliapoulios, M. A., Goldhaber, P., and Munson, P. L.: Thyrocalcitonin inhibition of bone resorption induced by parathyroid hormone in tissue culture. Science 151:330, 1966.

Altenähr, E.: Ultrastructural pathology of parathyroid glands. Curr. Top. Pathol. 56:1, 1972.

Arnaud, C. D.: Parathyroid hormone: Coming of age in clinical medicine. Am. J. Med. 55:577, 1973.

Arnaud, C. D.: Calcium homeostasis: Regulatory elements and their integration. Fed. Proc. 37:2557, 1978.

Arnaud, C. D., Sizemore, G. W., Oldham, S. B., Fischer, J. A., Tsao, H. S., and Littledike, E. T.: Human parathyroid hormone: Glandular and secreted molecular species. Am. J. Med. 50:630, 1971.

Bhattacharyya, M. H., and DeLuca, H. F.: Subcellular location of rat liver calciferol-25-hydroxylase. Arch. Biochem. Biophys. 160:58, 1974.

Bikle, D. D., Morrissey, R. L., and Zolock, D. T.: The mechanism of action of vitamin D in the intestine. Am. J. Clin. Nutr. 32:2322, 1979.

Birkenhager, J. C., Seldenrath, H. J., Hackeng, W. H. L., Schellekens, A. P. M., van der Veer, A. L. J., and Roelfsema, F.: Calcium and phosphorus metabolism, parathyroid hormone, calcitonin and bone histology in pseudohypoparathyroidism. Eur. J. Clin. Invest. 3:27, 1973.

Black, H. E., Capen, C. C., and Arnaud, C. D.: Ultrastructure of parathyroid glands and plasma immunoreactive parathyroid hormone in pregnant cows fed normal and high calcium diets. Lab. Invest. 29:173, 1973.

Black, H. E., Capen, C. C., and Young, D. M.: Ultimobranchial thyroid neoplasms in bulls. A syndrome resembling medullary thyroid carcinoma in man. Cancer 32:865, 1973a.

Black, H. E., Capen, C. C., Yarrington, J. T., and Rowland, G. N.: Effect of a high calcium prepartal diet on calcium homeostatic mechanisms in thyroid glands, bone, and intestine of cows. Lab. Invest. 20:427, 1973b.

Boyle, I. T., Omdahl, J. L., Gray, R. W., and DeLuca, H. F.: The biological activity and metabolism of 24,25-dihydroxyvitamin D_3. J. Biol. Chem. 248:4174, 1973.

Brewer, H. B., Fairwell, T., Rittel, W., Littledike, T., and Arnaud, C. D.: Recent studies on the chemistry of human, bovine, and porcine parathyroid hormone. Am. J. Med. 56:759, 1974.

Brumbaugh, P. F., and Haussler, M. R.: Nuclear and cytoplasmic receptors for 1,25-dihydroxycholecalciferol in intestinal mucosa. Biochem. Biophys. Res. Commun. 51:74, 1973.

Brunette, M. G., Chan, M., Ferriere, C., and Roberts, K. D.: Site of 1,25(OH)₂ vitamin D_3 synthesis in the kidney. Nature 276:287, 1978.

Buckle, R. M., McMillan, M., and Mallinson, C.: Ectopic secretion of parathyroid hormone by a renal adenocarcinoma in a patient with hypercalcemia. Br. Med. J. 4:724, 1970.

Burek, J. D.: Pathology of Aging Rats. CRC Press, West Palm Beach, 1978.

Burk, R. L., and Schaubhut, C. W., Jr.: Spontaneous primary hypoparathyroidism in a dog. J.A.A.H.A. 11:784, 1975.

Capen, C. C.: Fine structural changes of parathyroid glands in response to experimental and spontaneous alterations of extracellular fluid calcium. Am. J. Med. 50:598, 1971.

Capen, C. C.: Functional and Fine Structural Relationships of Parathyroid Glands. In Brandly, C. A., and Cornelius, C. E. (eds.): Advances in Veterinary Sciences and Comparative Medicine. Academic Press, New York, 1975, pp. 219–286.

Capen, C. C.: Tumors of the Endocrine Glands. In Moulton, J. E. (ed.): Tumors in Domestic Animals, 2nd ed. University of California Press, Berkeley and Los Angeles, 1978, pp. 372–429.

Capen, C. C., and Black, H. E.: Calcitonin-secreting ultimobranchial neoplasms of the thyroid gland in bulls: An animal model for medullary thyroid carcinoma in man (Sipple's syndrome). Am. J. Pathol. 74:377, 1974.

Capen, C. C., and Roth, S. I.: Ultrastructural and Functional Relationships of Normal and Pathologic Parathyroid Cells. In Iaochim, H. L. (ed.): Pathobiology Annual, Vol. 3. Appleton-Century-Crofts, New York, 1973.

Capen, C. C., and Young, D. M.: Fine structural alterations in thyroid parafollicular cells of cows in response to experimental hypercalcemia induced by vitamin D. Am. J. Pathol. 57:365, 1969.

Capen, C. C., Cole, C. R., and Hibbs, J. W.: The pathology of hypervitaminosis D in cattle. Pathol. Vet. 3:350, 1966.

Capen, C. C., Henry, H. L., and Norman, A. W.: Fine structural alterations produced by 1,25-dihydroxycholecalciferol, 24R,25-dihydroxycholecalciferol (alone and in combination), and cholecalciferol on the chick parathyroid gland. In Abstracts of the VI Parathyroid Conference, p. 48 (Talmage, R. and Copp, D. H., eds.): Vancouver, Canada, published in Endocrinology of Calcium Metabolism: Proc. VI Parathyroid Conference. Excerpta Medica, Amsterdam, 1978, p. 367.

Care, A. D., Bates, R. F. L., Phillippo, M., Lequin, R. M., Hackeng, W. H. I., Barlet, J. P., and Larvor, P.: Stimulation of calcitonin release from bovine thyroid by calcium and glucagon. J. Endocrinol. 48:667, 1970.

Carrillo, J. M., Burk, R. L., and Bode, C.: Primary hyperparathyroidism in a dog. J.A.V.M.A. 174:67, 1979.

Christakos, S., and Norman, A. W.: Vitamin D₃–induced calcium binding protein in bone tissue. Science 202:70, 1978.

Chu, L. L. H., MacGregor, R. R., Anast, C. S., Hamilton, J. W., and Cohn, D. V.: Studies on the biosynthesis of rat parathyroid hormone and proparathyroid hormone: Adaptation of the parathyroid gland to dietary restriction of calcium. Endocrinology 93:915, 1973a.

Chu, L. L. H., MacGregor, R. R., Liu, P. I., Hamilton, J. W., and Cohn, D. V.: Biosynthesis of proparathyroid hormone and parathyroid hormone by human parathyroid glands. J. Clin. Invest. 52:3089, 1973b.

Cohn, D. V., MacGregor, R. R., Chu, L. I. H., Huang, D. W. Y., Anast, C. S., and Hamilton, J. W.: Biosynthesis of proparathyroid hormone and parathyroid hormone. Chemistry, physiology and role of calcium in regulation. Am. J. Med. 56:767, 1974.

Collins, W. T., Jr., Capen, C. C., Dobereiner, J., and

Tokarnia, C. H.: Ultrastructural evaluation of parathyroid glands and thyroid C cells of cattle fed *Solanum malacoxylon*. Am. J. Pathol. *87*:603, 1977.

Cooper, C. W., Schwesinger, W. H., Ontjes, D. A., Mahgoub, A. M., and Munson, P. I.: Stimulation of secretion of pig thyrocalcitonin by gastrin and related hormonal peptides. Endocrinology *91*:1079, 1972.

Copp, D. H.: Endocrine regulation of calcium metabolism. Ann. Rev. Physiol. *32*:61, 1970.

Copp, D. H., Cameron, E. C., Cheney, B. A., Davidson, A. G. F., and Henze, K. G.: Evidence for calcitonin—a new hormone from the parathyroid that lowers blood calcium. Endocrinology *70*:638, 1962.

DeGrandi, P. B., Kraebenbuhl, J. P., and Campiche, M. A.: Ultrastructural localization of calcitonin in the parafollicular cells of the pig thyroid gland with cytochrome c-labeled antibody fragments. J. Cell. Biol. *50*:446, 1971.

DeLellis, R. A., Nunnemacher, G., Bitman, W. R., Gaggel, R. F., Tashjian, A. H., Blount, M., and Wolfe, H. J.: C-cell hyperplasia and medullary thyroid carcinoma in the rat. Lab. Invest. *40*:140, 1979.

DeLuca, H. F.: The kidney as an endocrine organ for the production of 1,25-dihydroxyvitamin D_3, a calcium-mobilizing hormone. N. Engl. J. Med. *289*:359, 1973.

DeLuca, H. F.: Vitamin D — 1973. Am. J. Med. *56*:871, 1974.

DeLuca, H. F.: Vitamin D as a prohormone. Biochem. Pharmacol. *26*:563, 1977.

DeLuca, H. F.: Vitamin D and calcium transport. Ann. N.Y. Acad. Sci. *307*:356, 1978.

DeLuca, H. F.: Recent advances in our understanding of the vitamin D endocrine system. J. Steroid Biochem. *11*:35, 1979.

DeLuca, H. F.: The vitamin D system in the regulation of calcium and phosphorus metabolism. Nutr. Rev. *37*:161, 1979.

Drezner, M., Neelon, F. A., and Lebovitz, H. E.: Pseudohypoparathyroidism type II. A possible defect in the reception of the cyclic AMP signal. N. Engl. J. Med. *289*:1056, 1973.

Edney, A. T. B.: Lactational tetany in the cat. J. Small Anim. Pract. *10*:231, 1969.

Farfel, Z., Brickman, A., Kaslow, H. R., Brothers, V., and Bourne, H.: Defect of receptor-cyclase coupling protein in pseudohypoparathyroidism. N. Engl. J. Med. *303*:237, 1980.

Fawcett, C. P., Powell, A. E., and Sachs, H.: Biosynthesis and release of neurophysin. Endocrinology *83*:1299, 1968.

Fetter, A. W., and Capen, C. C.: Ultrastructural evaluation of the parathyroid glands of pigs with naturally occurring atrophic rhinitis. Pathol. Vet. *5*:481, 1968.

Fetter, A. W., and Capen, C. C.: The ultrastructure of the parathyroid glands of young pigs. Acta Anat. *75*:359, 1970.

Finco, D. R., and Rowland, G. N.: Hypercalcemia secondary to chronic renal failure in the dog: A report of four cases. J.A.V.M.A. *173*:990, 1978.

Finco, D. R., Duncan, J. R., Crowell, W. A., and Hulsey, M. L.: Familial renal disease in Norwegian elkhound dogs: Morphologic examinations. Am. J. Vet. Res. *38*:941, 1977.

Fischer, J. A., Oldham, S. B., Sizemore, G. W., and Arnaud, C. D.: Calcium-regulated parathyroid hormone peptidase. Proc. Natl. Acad. Sci. U.S.A. *69*:2341, 1972.

Fraser, D. R., and Kodicek, E.: Regulation of 25-hydroxycholecalciferol-1-hydroxylase activity in kidney by parathyroid hormone. Nature (London) *241*:163, 1973.

Friedman, J., Au, W. Y. W., and Raisz, L. G.: Responses of fetal rat bone to thyrocalcitonin in tissue culture. Endocrinology *82*:149, 1968.

Galasko, C. S. B., and Bennett, A.: Relationship of bone destruction in skeletal metastases to osteoclast activation and prostaglandins. Nature *263*:508, 1976.

Garabedian, M., Holick, M. F., DeLuca, H. F., and Boyle, I. T.: Control of 25-hydroxycholecalciferol metabolism by parathyroid glands. Proc. Natl. Acad. Sci. U.S.A. *69*:1673, 1972.

Goulden, B. E., and MacKenzie, C. P.: Suspected primary hyperparathyroidism in the dog. N.Z. Vet. J. *16*:131, 1968.

Gray, R. W., Omdahl, J. L., Ghazarian, J. G., and DeLuca, H. F.: 25-hydroxycholecalciferol-1-hydroxylase: Subcellular location and properties. J. Biol. Chem. *247*:7528, 1972.

Gray, T. K., and Ontjes, D. A.: Clinical aspects of thyrocalcitonin. Clin. Orthop. *111*:238, 1975.

Habener, J. F.: New Concepts in the Formation, Regulation of Release, and Metabolism of Parathyroid Hormone. *In* Polypeptide Hormones: Molecular and Cellular Aspects. Ciba Fnd. Symp 41. Elsevier/Excerpta Medica, Amsterdam, 1976, pp. 197–224.

Habener, J. F., and Kronenberg, H. M.: Parathyroid hormone biosynthesis: structure and function of biosynthetic precursors. Fed. Proc. *37*:2561, 1978.

Habener, J. F., and Potts, J. T., Jr.: Chemistry, Biosynthesis, Secretion and Metabolism of Parathyroid Hormone. *In* Handbook of Physiology, Endocrinology VII — Parathyroid Gland. American Physiology Society, Chapter 13, Washington, D.C., 1976, pp. 313–342.

Habener, J. F., and Potts, J. T., Jr.: Biosynthesis of parathyroid hormone. N. Engl. J. Med. *299*:580, 1978.

Habener, J. F., and Potts, J. T., Jr.: Subcellular distribution of parathyroid hormone, hormonal precursors, and parathyroid secretory protein. Endocrinology *104*:265, 1979.

Habener, J. F., Chang, H. T., and Potts, J. T., Jr.: Enzymatic processing of proparathyroid hormone by cell-free extracts of parathyroid glands. Biochemistry *16*:3910, 1977.

Habener, J. F., Powell, D., Murray, T. M., Mayer, G. P., and Potts, J. T., Jr.: Parathyroid hormone: Secretion and metabolism *in vitro*. Proc. Natl. Acad. Sci. U.S.A. *68*:2986, 1971.

Haussler, M. R., and McCain, T. A.: Basic and clinical concepts related to vitamin D metabolism and action. N. Engl. J. Med. *297*:974, 1977.

Haussler, M. R., Nagode, L. A., and Rasmussen, H.: Induction of intestinal brush border alkaline phosphatase by vitamin D and identity with CA-ATPase. Nature (London) *228*:1199, 1970.

Haussler, M. R., Boyce, D. W., Littledike, E. T., and Rasmussen, H.: A rapidly acting metabolite of vitamin D_3. Proc. Natl. Acad. Sci. U.S.A. *68*:177, 1971.

Havinga, E.: Vitamin D, example and challenge. Experientia *29*:1181, 1973.

Hazard, J. B.: The C cells (parafollicular cells) of the

thyroid gland and medullary thyroid carcinoma. Am. J. Pathol. *88*:214, 1977.

Heath, H., Weller, R. E., and Mundy, G. R.: Canine lymphosarcoma: A model for study of the hypercalcemia of cancer. Calcif. Tissue Int. *30*:127, 1980.

Henry, H. I., and Norman, A. W.: Vitamin D: Two dihydroxylated metabolites are required for normal chicken egg hatchability. Science *201*:835, 1978.

Hill, L. F., Davies, M., Taylor, C. M., and Stanbury, S. W.: Treatment of hypoparathyroidism with 1,25-dihydroxycholecalciferol. Clin. Endocrinol. *5* Suppl: 167, 1976.

Hirshorn, J. E., Vrhovsek, E., and Posen, S.: Carcinoma of the breast associated with hypercalcemia and the presence of parathyroid hormone-like substances in the tumor. J. Clin. Endocrinol. Metab. *48*:217, 1979.

Holick, M. F., and Clark, M. B.: The photobiogenesis and metabolism of vitamin D. Fed. Proc. *37*:2567, 1978.

Holick, M. F., Frommer, J. E., McNeill, S. C., Richtand, N. M., Henley, J. W., and Potts, J. T., Jr.: Photometabolism of 7-dehydrocholesterol to previtamin D_3 in skin. Biochem. Biophys. Res. Commun. *76*:107, 1977.

Holick, M. F., MacLaughlin, J. A., Clark, M. B., Holick, S. A., and Potts, J. T., Jr.: Photosynthesis of previtamin D_3 in human skin and the physiologic consequences. Science *210*:203, 1980.

Hruska, K. A., Kopelman, R., Rutherford, W. E., Klahr, S., and Slatopolsky, E.: Metabolism of immunoreactive parathyroid hormone in the dog. The role of the kidney and the effects of chronic renal disease. J. Clin. Invest. *56*:39, 1975.

Hruska, K. A., Martin, K., Mennes, P., Greenwalt, A., Anderson, C., Klahr, S., and Slatopolsky, E.: Degradation of parathyroid hormone and fragment production by the isolated perfused dog kidney. The effect of glomerular filtration rate and perfusate Ca^{++} concentrations. J. Clin. Invest. *60*:501, 1977.

Hughes, M. R., and Haussler, M. R.: 1,25-dihydroxyvitamin D_3 receptors in parathyroid glands. J. Biol. Chem. *253*:1065, 1978.

Ingersoll, R. J., and Wasserman, R. H.: Vitamin D_3-induced calcium-binding protein. J. Biol. Chem. *246*:2808, 1971.

Kalina, M., and Pearse, A. G. E.: Ultrastructural localization of calcitonin in C-cells of dog thyroid: An immunocytochemical study. Histochemie *26*:1, 1971.

Kallfelz, F. A.: Puerperal Tetany. In Kirk, R. W. (ed.): Current Veterinary Therapy III, W. B. Saunders Co., Philadelphia, 1968.

Kallio, D. M., Garant, P. R., and Minkin, C.: Ultrastructural effects of calcitonin on osteoclasts in tissue culture. J. Ultrastruct. Res. *39*:205, 1972.

Kaufman, C. F., Soirez, R. F., and Tasker, J. P.: Renal cortical hypoplasia with secondary hyperparathyroidism in the dog. J.A.V.M.A. *155*:1679, 1969.

Kemper, B., Habener, J. F., Potts, J. T., Jr., and Rich, A.: Parathyroid hormone: Identification of a biosynthetic precursor to parathyroid hormone. Proc. Natl. Acad. Sci. U.S.A. *69*:643, 1972.

Kemper, B., Habener, J. F., Rich, A., and Potts, J. T., Jr.: Parathyroid secretion: Discovery of a major calcium-dependent protein. Science *184*:167, 1974.

Knill-Jones, R. P., Buckle, R. M., Parsons, V., Calne, R. Y., and Williams, R.: Hypercalcemia and increased parathyroid hormone activity in a primary hepatoma.

Studies before and after hepatic transplantation. N. Engl. J. Med. *282*:704–708, 1970.

Kodicek, E.: The story of vitamin D from vitamin to hormone. Lancet *2*:325, 1974.

Kodicek, E., Lawson, D. E. M., and Wilson, P. W.: Biological activity of a polar metabolite of vitamin D_3. Nature (London) *228*:763, 1970.

Kornegay, J. N., Greene, C. E., Martin, C., Gorgacz, E. J., and Melcon, D. K.: Idiopathic hypocalcemia in four dogs. J.A.A.H.A. *16*:723, 1980.

Krook, L.: Spontaneous hyperparathyroidism in the dog. A pathologic-anatomical study. Acta Pathol. Microbiol. Scand. *41*:(Suppl. 122):1, 1957.

Krook, L., Lutwak, L., McEntee, K., Henrickson, P.-Å., Braun, K., and Roberts, S.: Nutritional hypercalcitoninism in bulls. Cornell Vet. *61*:625, 1971.

Lacy, P. E., Howell, S. I., Young, D. A., and Fink, C. J.: New hypothesis of insulin secretion. Nature (London) *219*:1177, 1968.

Lapelescu, A., Potorac, E., Pop, A., Heitmanek, C., Mercujjev, E., Chisiu, N., Oprisan, R., and Neacsu, C.: Experimental investigation on immunology of the parathyroid gland. Immunology *14*:475, 1968.

Leav, I., Schiller, A. I., Rijnberk, A., Legg, M. A., and der Kinderen, P. J.: Adenomas and carcinomas of the canine and feline thyroid. Am. J. Pathol. *83*:61, 1976.

Legendre, A. M., Merkley, D. F., Carrig, C. B., and Krehbiel, J. D.: Primary hyperparathyroidism in a dog. J.A.V.M.A. *168*:694, 1976.

Littledike, E. T.: Parturient Hypocalcemia, Hypomagnesemia, Mastitis-Metritis-Agalactia Complex of Swine. In Larsen, B., and Smith, V. (eds.): Lactation, Vol. II. Academic Press, New York, 1974, pp. 355–389.

MacGregor, R. R., Hamilton, J. W., and Cohn, D. V.: The mode of conversion of proparathormone to parathormone by a particulate converting enzymic activity of the parathyroid gland. J. Biol. Chem. *253*:2012, 1978.

MacGregor, R. R., Chu, L. L. H., Hamilton, J. W., and Cohn, D. V.: Studies on the subcellular localization of proparathyroid hormone and parathyroid hormone in the bovine parathyroid gland: Separation of newly synthesized from mature forms. Endocrinology *93*:1387, 1973.

MacIntyre, I., Colston, K. W., Szelke, M., and Spanos, E.: A survey of the hormonal factors that control calcium metabolism. Ann. N.Y. Acad. Sci. *307*:345, 1973.

Martin, K. J., Hruska, K. A., Freitag, J. J., Klahr, S., and Slatopolsky, E.: The peripheral metabolism of parathyroid hormone. N. Engl. J. Med. *301*:1092, 1979.

Mayer, G. P.: Relative importance of calcium and magnesium in the control of parathyroid secretion. Abst. 56th Annual Meeting of the Endocrine Society, pp. A–181, 1974.

Mayer, G. P., and Hurst, J. G.: Comparison of the effects of calcium and magnesium on parathyroid hormone secretion rate in calves. Endocrinology *102*:1803, 1978.

Melvin, K. E. W., Tashjian, A. H., Jr., and Miller, H. H.: Studies on familial (medullary) thyroid carcinoma. Recent Prog. Horm. Res. *28*:399, 1972.

Meuten, D. J., Chew, D. J., Capen, C. C., and Kociba, G. J.: Relationship of serum total calcium to serum albumin and total protein concentrations in dogs. J.A.V.M.A. *180*:63, 1982a.

Meuten, D. J., Cooper, B. J., Capen, C. C., Chew, D. J., and Kociba, G. J.: Hypercalcemia associated with an adenocarcinoma derived from the apocrine glands of the anal sac. Vet. Pathol. *18*:454, 1981.

Meuten, D. J., Capen, C. C., Kociba, G. J., and Cooper, B. J.: Animal model of human disease: Hypercalcemia of malignancy. Am. J. Pathol. in press, 1982b.

Meyer, D. J., and Terrell, T. G.: Idiopathic hypoparathyroidism in a dog. J.A.V.M.A. *68*:858, 1976.

Midgett, R. J., Spielvogel, A. M., Coburn, J. W., and Norman, A. W.: Studies on calciferol metabolism. VI. The renal production of the biologically active form of vitamin D, 1,25-dihydroxycholecalciferol: Species, tissue and subcellular distribution. J. Clin. Endocrinol. Metab. *36*:1153, 1973.

Morrissey, J. J., and Cohn, D. V.: The effects of calcium and magnesium on the secretion of parathormone and parathyroid secretory protein by isolated porcine parathyroid cells. Endocrinology *103*:2081, 1978.

Mundy, G. R., Raisz, L. G., Cooper, R. A., Schechter, G. P., and Salmon, S. E.: Evidence for the secretion of an osteoclast stimulating factor in myeloma. N. Engl. J. Med. *291*:1041, 1974.

Mundy, G. R., Laben, R. A., Raisz, L. G., Oppenheim, J. J., and Buell, D. N.: Bone-resorbing activity in supernatants from lymphoid cell lines. N. Engl. J. Med. *290*:867, 1974.

Musselman, E. E.: Electrocardiographic signs of adrenocortical insufficiency with hypercalcemia in the dog. VM SAC *70*:1433, 1975.

Norman, A. W.: Vitamin D metabolism and calcium absorption. Am. J. Med. *67*:989, 1979.

Norman, A. W.: 1,25-(OH)$_2$D$_3$ as a Steroid Hormone. *In* Norman, A. W. (ed.): Vitamin D: Molecular Biology and Clinical Nutrition. Basel, Marcel Dekker, Inc., New York, 1980.

Norman, A. W., and Henry, H.: 1,25-dihydroxycholecalciferol — a hormonally active form of vitamin D$_3$. Recent Prog. Horm. Res. *30*:43, 1974.

Norman, A. W., and Henry, H. L.: Vitamin D to 1,25-dihydroxycholecalciferol: evolution of a steroid hormone. Trends Biochem. Sci. *14*:1979.

Norman, A. W., Johnson, R. L., Osborn, T. W., Procsal, D. A., Carey, S., Hammond, M., Mitra, M., Pirio, M., Rego, A., Wing, R., and Okamura, W.: The chemistry, conformational and biological analysis of vitamin D$_3$, its metabolites and analogues. Clin. Endocrinol. *5*(Suppl):121, 1976.

Norrdin, R. W.: Fibrous osteodystrophy with facial hyperostosis in a dog with renal cortical hypoplasia. Cornell Vet. *65*:173, 1975.

Norrdin, R. W., Bordier, P., and Miller, C. W.: Trabecular bone morphometry in beagles with chronic renal failure. Virchows Arch. [Pathol. Anat.] *375*:169, 1977.

Norrdin, R. W., Phemister, R. D., Jaenke, R. S., and LoPresti, C. A.: Density and composition of trabecular and cortical bone in perinatally irradiated beagles with chronic renal failure. Calcif. Tissue Res. *24*:99, 1977.

Nunez, E. A., Hedhammar, A., Fu-Ming, W., Whalen, J. P., and Krook, L.: Ultrastructure of the parafollicular (C) cells and the parathyroid cells in growing dogs on a high calcium diet. Lab. Invest. *31*:96, 1974.

Oldham, S. B., Fischer, J. A., Capen, C. C., Sizemore, G. W., and Arnaud, C. D.: Dynamics of parathyroid hormone secretion *in vitro*. Am. J. Med. *51*:650, 1971.

Olson, H. M., and Capen, C. C.: Virus-induced animal model of osteosarcoma in the rat. Am. J. Pathol. *86*:437, 1977.

Omdahl, J. L., and DeLuca, H. F.: Regulation of vitamin D metabolism and function. Physiol. Rev. *53*:327, 1973.

Omdahl, J. L., Hunsaker, L. A., Evan, A. P., and Torrez, P.: *In vitro* regulation of kidney 25-hydroxyvitamin D$_3$-hydroxylase enzyme activities by vitamin D$_3$ metabolites. J. Biol. Chem. *255*:7460, 1980.

Omen, G. S.: Pathobiology of Ectopic Hormone Production by Neoplasms in Man. *In* Ioachim, H. L. (ed.): Pathobiology Annual, Vol. 3. Appleton-Century-Crofts, 1973, New York, pp. 177–216.

Ornoy, A., Goodwin, D., Noff, D., and Edelstein, S.: 24,25-dihydroxyvitamin D is a metabolite of vitamin D essential for bone formation. Nature *276*:517, 1978.

Osborne, C. A., and Stevens, J. B.: Pseudohyperparathyroidism in the dog. J.A.V.M.A. *162*:125, 1973.

Parsons, J. A., and Robinson, C. J.: Calcium shift into bone causing transient hypocalcemia after injection of parathyroid hormone. Nature (London) *230*:581, 1971.

Pearson, P. T., Dellman, H. D., Berrier, H. H., Case, A. A., and Collier, B. L.: Primary hyperparathyroidism in a beagle. J.A.V.M.A. *147*:1201, 1965.

Pike, J. W., Gooze, L. L., and Haussler, M. R.: Biochemical evidence for 1,25-dihydroxyvitamin D receptor macromolecules in parathyroid, pancreatic, pituitary, and placental tissues. Life Sci. *26*:407, 1979.

Potts, J. T., Jr.: Chemistry and physiology of parathyroid hormone. Clin. Endocrinol. *5*(Suppl):307, 1976.

Potts, J. T., Jr., Murray, T. M., Peacock, M., Niall, H. D., Tregear, G. W., Kentmann, H. T., Powell, D., and Deftos, L. J.: Parathyroid hormone: Sequence synthesis and immunoassay studies. Am. J. Med. *50*:639, 1971.

Powell, D., Singer, F. R., Murray, T. M., Minkin, C., and Potts, J. T., Jr.: Nonparathyroid humoral hypercalcemia in patients with neoplastic diseases. N. Engl. J. Med. *289*:176, 1973.

Raisz, L. G., Trummel, C. L., Holick, M. F., and DeLuca, H. F.: 1,25-dihydroxycholecalciferol: A potent stimulator of bone resorption in tissue culture. Science *175*:768, 1980.

Rasmussen, H.: Ionic and hormonal control of calcium homeostasis. Am. J. Med. *50*:567, 1971.

Rasmussen, H.: The cellular basis of mammalian calcium homeostasis. Clin. Endocrinol. Metabol. Philadelphia, W. B. Saunders Co., Vol. 1, 1972, pp. 3–20.

Rasmussen, H.: Parathyroid Hormone, Calcitonin, and the Calciferols. *In* Williams, R. H. (ed.): Textbook of Endocrinology, W. B. Saunders Co., Philadelphia, 1973, pp. 660–773.

Rasmussen, H., and Bordier, P.: The Physiological and Cellular Basis of Metabolic Bone Disease. Williams and Wilkins Co., Baltimore, 1974.

Rasmussen, H., Wong, M., Bikle, D., and Goodman, D. B. P.: Hormonal control of the renal conversion of 25-hydroxycholecalciferol to 1,25-dihydroxycholecalciferol. J. Clin. Invest. *51*:2502, 1972.

Resnick, S.: Hypocalcemic tetany in the dog. J.A.V.M.A. *144*:1115, 1964.

Reynolds, J. J., Holick, M. F., and DeLuca, H. F.: The role of vitamin D metabolites in bone resorption. Calcif. Tissue Res. *12*:295, 1973.

Rijnberk, A.: Pseudohyperparathyroidism in the dog. T. Diergeneesk. *95*:515, 1970.

Rijnberk, A., Elsinhorst, Th.A.M., Kolman, J. P., Hacking, W. H. L., and Lequin, R. M.: Pseudohyperparathyroidism associated with perirectal adenocarcinomas in elderly female dogs. T. Diergeneesk. *103*:1069, 1978.

Roth, S. I., and Capen, C. C.: Ultrastructural and Functional Correlations of the Parathyroid Gland. *In* Richter, G. W., and Epstein, M. A. (ed.): International Review of Experimental Pathology, Vol. 13, Academic Press, New York, 1974.

Roth, S. I., and Raisz, L. G.: Effect of calcium concentration on the ultrastructure of rat parathyroid in organ culture. Lab. Invest. *13*:331, 1964.

Roth, S. I., Su, S. P., Segre, G. V., Habener, J. F., and Potts, J. T., Jr.: The immunocytochemical localization of parathyroid hormone in the bovine. Fed. Proc. *33*:241, 1974.

Rowland, G. N., Capen, C. C., and Nagode, L. A.: Experimental hyperparathyroidism in young cats. Pathol. Vet. *5*:504, 1968.

Rowland, G. N., Capen, C. C., Young, D. M., and Black, H. E.: Microradiographic evaluation of bone from cows with experimental hypervitaminosis D, diet-induced hypocalcemia, and naturally occurring parturient paresis. Calcif. Tissue Res. *9*:179, 1972.

Schnoes, H. K., and DeLuca, H. F.: Recent progress in vitamin D metabolism and the chemistry of vitamin D metabolites. Fed. Proc. *39*:2723, 1980.

Scott, P. P.: Special features of nutrition of cats, with observations on wild Felidae nutrition in the London Zoo. Symp. Zool. Soc. (London) *21*:21, 1968.

Seyberth, H. W., Segre, G. V., Morgan, J. L., Sweetman, B. J., Potts, J. T., Jr., and Oates, J. A.: Prostaglandins as mediators of hypercalcemia associated with certain types of cancer. N. Engl. J. Med. *293*:1278, 1975.

Shannon, W. A., and Roth, S. I.: Acid Phosphatase Activity in Mammalian Parathyroid Glands. *In* Arceneaux, C. J. (ed.): 29th Ann. Proc. Electron Microscopy Soc. Amer., Claitor's Publishing, Baton Rouge, 1971, pp. 516–517.

Sherding, R. G., Meuten, D. J., Chew, D. J., Knaack, K. E., and Haupt, K. H.: Primary hypoparathyroidism in the dog. J.A.V.M.A. *176*:439, 1980.

Sherwood, L. M., O'Riordan, J. L. H., Aurbach, G. D., and Potts, J. T., Jr.: Production of parathyroid hormone by nonparathyroid tumors. J. Clin. Endocrinol. *27*:140, 1967.

Sherwood, L. M., Rodman, J. S., and Lundberg, W. B.: Evidence for a precursor to circulating parathyroid hormone. Proc. Natl. Acad. Sci. U.S.A. *67*:1631, 1970.

Singer, F. E., Powell, D., Minkin, C., Bethune, J. E., Brickman, A., and Coburn, J. W.: Hypercalcemia in reticulum cell sarcoma without hyperparathyroidism or skeletal metastases. Ann. Intern. Med. *78*:365, 1973.

Sipple, J. H.: Association of pheochromocytoma with carcinoma of the thyroid gland. Am. J. Med. *31*:163, 1961.

Smithcors, J. F.: The Endocrine System. *In* Miller, M. E., Christensen, G. C., and Evans, H. E. (eds.): Anatomy of the Dog. W. B. Saunders Co., Philadelphia, 1964, pp. 822–826.

Stavrou, V. D.: Beitrag zum Hyperparathyreoidismus des Hundes. Dtsch. Tierärztl. Wochenschr. *75*:117, 1968.

Stevenson, J. C.: The structure and function of calcitonin. Invest. Cell Pathol. *3*:187, 1980.

Stewart, A. F., Horst, R., Deftos, L. J., Cadman, E. C., Lang, R., and Broadus, A. E.: Biochemical evaluation of patients with cancer-associated hypercalcemia. N. Engl. J. Med. *303*:1377, 1980.

Stumpf, W. E., Sar, M., Reid, F. A., Tanaka, Y., and DeLuca, H. F.: Target cells for 1,25-dihydroxyvitamin D_3 in intestinal tract, stomach, kidney, skin, pituitary and parathyroid. Science *206*:1188, 1980.

Swaminathan, R., Bates, R. F. L., and Care, A. D.: Fresh evidence for a physiological role of calcitonin in calcium homeostasis. J. Endocrinol. *54*:525, 1972.

Talmage, R. V., Anderson, J. J. B., and Cooper, C. W.: The influence of calcitonins on the disappearance of radiocalcium and radiophosphorus from plasma. Endocrinology *90*:1185, 1972.

Talmage, R. V., Grubb, S. A., Norimatsu, H., and van der Wiel, C. J.: Evidence for an important physiological role for calcitonin. Proc. Natl. Acad. Sci. U.S.A. *77*:609, 1980.

Tanaka, T., and DeLuca, H. F.: Stimulation of 24,25-dihydroxyvitamin D_3 production by 1,25-dihydroxyvitamin D_3. Science *183*:1198, 1974.

Targovnik, J. H., Rodman, J. S., and Sherwood, L. M.: Regulation of parathyroid hormone secretion *in vitro*: Quantitative aspects of calcium and magnesium ion control. Endocrinology *88*:1477, 1976.

Tashjian, A. H., Jr.: Role of prostaglandins in the production of hypercalcemia by tumors. Cancer Res. *38*:4138, 1978.

Taylor, A. N., and Wasserman, R. H.: Immunofluorescent localization of vitamin D-dependent calcium-binding protein. J. Histochem. Cytochem. *18*:107, 1970.

Thiele, J., and Wermbter, G.: Die Feinstruktur der aktivierten Hauptzelle der menschlichen Parathyroidea. Eine Darstellung mit Hilfe de Gefrieratztechnik. Virchows Arch. (Cell. Pathol.) *15*:251, 1974.

Villafane, F., Norrdin, R. W., Lopresti, C. A., and Kimmel, D.: Bone remodeling in chronic renal failure in perinatally irradiated beagles. Calcif. Tissue Res. *23*:171, 1977.

Voelkel, E. F., Tashjian, A. H., Jr., Franklin, R., Wasserman, E., and Levine, L.: Hypercalcemia and tumor-prostaglandins: The VX2 carcinoma model in the rabbit. Metabolism *24*:973, 1975.

Walser, M., Robinson, B. H. B., and Duckett, J. W., Jr.: The hypercalcemia of adrenal insufficiency. J. Clin. Invest. *42*:456, 1963.

Wasserman, R. H.: Physiological regulation of calcium metabolism. The consequences of excess intake of 1,25-dihydroxycholecalciferol from natural sources. Ann. N.Y. Acad. Sci. *307*:442, 1978.

Wasserman, R. H., and Taylor, A. N.: Metabolic roles of fat-soluble vitamins D, E, and K. Ann. Rev. Biochem. *41*:179, 1972.

Wasserman, R. H., Corradino, R. A., and Taylor, A. N.: Vitamin D-dependent calcium-binding protein. J. Biol. Chem. *243*:3978, 1968.

Watson, A. D. J., and Canfield, P. J.: Renal failure, hyperparathyroidism and hypercalcemia in a dog. Aust. Vet. J. *55*:177, 1979.

Wecksler, W. R., Henry, H. L., and Norman, A. W.: Studies on the mode of action of calciferol: Subcellular localization of 1,25-dihydroxyvitamin D_3 in chicken parathyroid glands. Arch. Biochem. Biophys. *183*:168, 1977.

Wecksler, W. R., Ross, F. P., Mason, R. S., Posen, S., and Norman, A. W.: Biochemical properties of the 1,25-dihydroxyvitamin D_3 cytoplasmic receptors from human and chicken parathyroid glands. Arch. Biochem. Biophys. *201*:95, 1980.

Weisbrode, S. E., and Capen, C. C.: Ultrastructural evaluation of the effects of calcitonin on bone in thyroparathyroidectomized rats administered vitamin D. Am. J. Pathol. *77*:395, 1974.

Weisbrode, S. E., and Krakowka, S.: Canine distemper virus-associated hypocalcemia. Am. J. Vet. Res. *40*:147, 1979.

Yarrington, J. T,, and Capen, C. C.: Ultrastructural and biochemical evaluation of adrenal medullary hyperplasia and pheochromocytoma in aged bulls. Vet. Pathol. *18*:316, 1981.

Yarrington, J. T., Capen, C. C., Black, H. E., and Re, R.: Effects of a low calcium prepartal diet on calcium homeostatic mechanisms in the cow: Morphologic and biochemical studies. J. Nutr. *107*:2244, 1977.

Youshak, M. S., and Capen, C. C.: Fine structural alterations in parathyroid glands of chickens with osteopetrosis. Am. J. Pathol. *60*:257, 1970.

Zarrin, K.: Naturally-occurring parafollicular cell carcinoma of the thyroids in dogs. A histological and ultrastructural study. Vet. Pathol. *14*:556, 1977.

Zenoble, R. D., and Rowland, G. N.: Hypercalcemia and proliferative, myelosclerotic bone reaction associated with feline leukovirus infection in a cat. J.A.V.M.A. *175*:591, 1979.

CHAPTER **67**

Thyroid Diseases

BRUCE E. BELSHAW

ANATOMY AND PHYSIOLOGY

DEVELOPMENT AND ANATOMY

The canine thyroid originates as a thickened plate of epithelium in the floor of the pharynx. In its development, it is intimately related to the aortic sac, and this association leads to the frequent occurrence of accessory thyroids in the mediastinum of the adult dog (Godwin, 1936). Branched cell cords develop from the pharyngeal plate and are temporarily connected to it by a narrow stalk, the thyroglossal duct. The cell cords expand laterally and upward and these extensions form the anteromedial two thirds of the adult lobes. The more medial portion remains close to the aortic sac and forms a transitory isthmus. The ultimobranchial bodies fuse with the lateral extensions and form the caudolateral one third of the adult lobes.

In the adult dog weighing about ten kg, each lobe is about two cm by one cm by one-half cm, and the combined weight of the two lobes is about one gm. The lobes are situated on the lateral surfaces of the trachea, with the right lobe slightly cranial to the left and nearly touching the caudal border of the larynx. Because the lobes are relatively small and are deep to the sternocephalicus muscle, they are not normally palpable. The major blood supply is via the cranial thyroid artery, a branch of the common carotid, and the principal venous drainage is via the caudal thyroid vein, which enters the internal jugular vein.

The follicular cells are four to ten μm in height. Viewed in histologic sections, the follicles range from about 20 to 250 μm in diameter. In random clusters of follicles, the periphery of the colloid is vacuolated. The vacuoles are artifacts resulting from aqueous fixation, but they occur at sites of recent resorption of colloid and thus signify activity mediated by thyroid-stimulating hormone (TSH).

There are few congenital anomalies associated with the canine thyroid. Although an isthmus rarely persists postnatally, microscopic remnants occur along the rich plexus of lymphatics that connect the posterior poles of the two lobes. The most common cyst is of ultimobranchial origin. It may be within or adjacent to the gland and is rarely large enough to be detected in life. A portion of the thyroglossal duct may also persist postnatally to form a cyst, usually on the midline, attached to the base of the tongue by a thin tube or stalk.

Accessory thyroid tissue is quite common in the dog and may be located anywhere from the larynx to the diaphragm. About 50 per cent of adult dogs have accessory thyroids embedded in the fat on the intrapericardial aorta. These nodules are usually one to two mm in greatest dimension and may number from one to five. They are completely lacking in parafollicular cells, which secrete calcitonin, but their follicular structure and function is identical to that of the main thyroid glands (Kameda, 1972). Attempts to induce hypothyroidism in the dog by surgical thyroidectomy are not consistently successful because the accessory thyroids can undergo sufficient hyperplasia to sustain adequate hormone production.

PHYSIOLOGY

Iodine Metabolism. The daily maintenance iodine requirement of the 10- to 15-kg adult dog is about 140 μg (Belshaw et al., 1975). Ad libitum consumption of most commercially manufactured dry dog foods provides the average dog with a daily iodine intake of at least 500 μg, and some foods provide considerably more. Most iodine in the diet is reduced to iodide in the gastrointestinal tract; absorption of iodide begins immediately and is essentially complete within two hours. Iodide is cleared from the plasma by the parotid salivary gland (but not in significant amounts by other salivary glands in the dog) and by the gastric mucosa and is then resorbed. However, a small amount of iodide is normally lost in the feces (about 20 to 25 μg per day at the usual levels of iodine intake), possibly via secretion in the colon.

At the usual levels of iodine intake, the concentration of inorganic iodide in the plasma of the dog is about 5 to 10 μg/100 ml, whereas it is about 0.5 μg/100 ml in man. This difference is due to the dog's higher intake of iodine relative to body weight, proportionately greater recycling of iodide from the thyroid and from peripher-

al degradation of thyroid hormones, and lower fractional clearance by the kidney (Belshaw et al., 1974). In addition to inorganic iodide and iodine in the form of circulating thyroid hormones, canine plasma contains nonhormonal iodine bound to plasma proteins in a concentration of 1 μg or more per 100 ml. Some of the iodination of plasma proteins occurs in the degradation of the thyroid hormones, but most appears to be a direct consequence of the high levels of inorganic iodide in the dog. This nonhormonal iodine bound to plasma proteins accounts for about half of the total protein-bound iodine (PBI) in the dog, and this is the principal reason why the PBI is unsatisfactory as a measurement of circulating thyroid hormone levels in dogs.

Hormone Synthesis and Secretion. Iodide cleared from the plasma is oxidized and then bound to tyrosine residues in the peptide chain of thyroglobulin. The resulting monoiodotyrosine (MIT) and diiodotyrosine (DIT) undergo oxidative coupling to form the iodothyronines, thyroxine (T_4), triiodothyronine (T_3), and reverse triiodothyronine (rT_3). In the normal dog with a thyroid weight of one gram, the thyroid contains about 900 μg of T_4, 75 μg of T_3, and 15 μg of rT_3 (Laurberg, 1978b).

Secretion is initiated by the ingestion of thyroglobulin into the follicular cell in the form of colloid droplets. Ingestion may occur on the surface of the follicular cell by the formation of pseudopods, which enclose a small portion of the colloid (Fig. 67–1), or by micropinocytosis. Pseudopod formation is particularly evident after pharmacologic doses of TSH, but not in resting glands, and it is possible that micropinocytosis is more important in basal secretion. The colloid droplets acquire proteolytic enzymes from lysosomes, probably at the time of formation (Nunez et al., 1972), and then migrate to the base of the cell. The iodothyronines diffuse from the lysosomes and then from the cell into the extracellular space, from which they enter the adjacent capillary. It has recently been shown that there is preferential secretion of T_3 and rT_3 from the canine thyroid, i.e., that the ratios of T_3 and rT_3 to T_4 are higher in the thyroid effluent than in thyroid gland hydrolysates. This appears to be due to enzymatic deiodination of T_4 during the secretory process and is increased by TSH stimulation (Laurberg, 1976, 1978b).

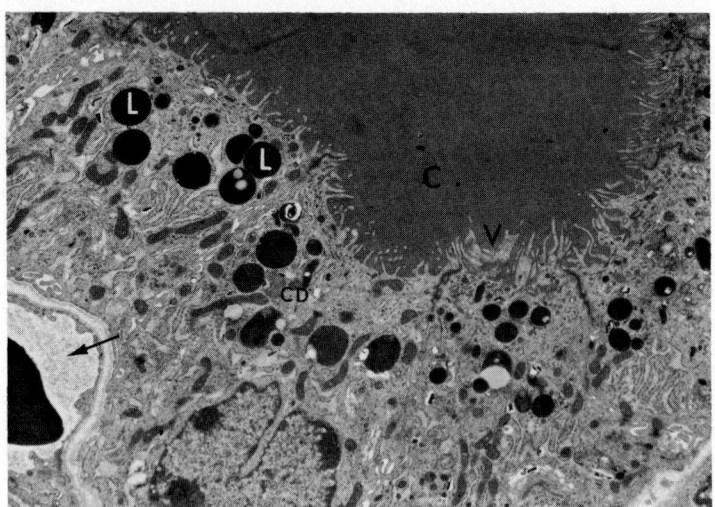

Figure 67–1. Electron micrograph of follicular cells, illustrating long microvilli (V) extending into the luminal colloid (C). Pseudopods from the apical membrane engulf a portion of the colloid to form a colloid droplet (CD). Numerous lysosomes (L) in the apical cytoplasm contribute proteolytic enzymes, which hydrolyze the thyroglobulin and release the thyroid hormones to enter interfollicular capillaries (arrow) at the base of the cell. (Courtesy of Dr. C. C. Capen.)

Uncoupled MIT and DIT in thyroglobulin are also released during proteolysis of the colloid droplets. In man, MIT and DIT are very efficiently deiodinated within the follicular cell, and most of the iodide thus generated is recycled internally to be used again for iodination of tyrosyl groups of thyroglobulin. In the dog, most of the iodotyrosine iodine is released back into the circulation. This nonhormonal iodine release by the canine thyroid represents at least two thirds of the iodine initially trapped and bound to tyrosyl residues. Although only iodide has been identified in the nonhormonal iodine secretion, serum DIT levels have been reported to be higher in the dog than in other species, about four times higher than that in man (Nelson et al., 1975). Hence, it is still not clear whether the substantial loss of nonhormonal iodine from the dog's thyroid is due to inefficient re-utilization of iodide per se or whether there is some limitation of iodotyrosine deiodination and consequent secretion of iodotyrosines. This question needs to be reexamined with radioimmunoassay measurements of the iodinated compounds in the canine thryoid effluent. Regardless of the cause, however, the considerable nonhormonal iodine secretion by the canine thyroid is a major factor in the dog's relatively high iodine requirement, since iodine returned to the circulation is subject to renal clearance and fecal excretion, as well as uptake by the thyroid.

The ratio of T_4 to T_3 in the dog's thyroidal secretion is about 4:1 (Laurberg, 1976), but the total daily production of the two hormones is in a ratio of about 2:1 (about 30 μg of T_4 and 15 μg of T_3 in dogs weighing 10 to 15 kg) (Belshaw et al., 1974). This implies that 50 per cent or more of the dog's daily production of T_3 is via extrathyroidal deiodination of T_4, and production of about 60 per cent of T_3 in this manner is consistent with the results of kinetic analysis of iodine metabolism in dogs. It should be noted that the dog produces more than twice the amount of T_4 and more than three times the amount of T_3 per kilogram of body weight than does man.

Hormone Transport and Metabolism. In canine plasma, T_4 is bound to albumin and three globulin fractions, and T_3 is bound to albumin and one globulin (Refetoff et al., 1970). The overall binding affinity of the plasma proteins for T_4 is lower in the dog than in man. In particular, the dog lacks a paramount high-affinity binding globulin comparable to the inter-α thyroxine-binding globulin (TBG) of man. Partly as a result of weaker binding by plasma proteins, total T_4 concentration is lower, the unbound or free fraction is higher, and hormone turnover is more rapid in the dog than in man. These differences have important consequences in measurements of total and free T_4 in the diagnosis of thyroid disorders in dogs (see below).

In the dog, about 40 per cent of the extrathyroidal T_4 is in the plasma and most of the remainder is taken up by the liver. The total plasma-equivalent space of distribution for T_4 is about 12 per cent of body weight. By comparison T_3 enters peripheral cells more readily than T_4 (partly because it is less firmly bound to plasma proteins) and reaches a total distribution volume equal to 65 per cent of body weight. The ratio of T_4 to T_3 in canine plasma is about 25:1. The equivalent of 115 per cent of extrathyroidal T_4 and 205 per cent of extrathyroidal T_3 is metabolized and replaced each day. About 45 per cent of T_4 turnover is via deiodination and 55 per cent is via fecal excretion; biliary clearance of T_4 is very much higher in the dog than in man. About 70 per cent of T_3 turnover is via deiodination and 30 per cent is via fecal excretion. Both the overall rates of turnover and the losses of hormone in the feces are much higher in the dog than in man. Furthermore, only about 15 per cent of T_4 or T_3 is absorbed from the dog's intestine, while in man about 70 per cent of T_4 and essentially 100 per cent of T_3 is absorbed. One important result of these differences is that the replacement dose of thyroid hormone used in treating hypothyroidism in a ten-kg dog is equivalent to that used in an adult man.

Monodeiodination of the outer ring of T_4 results in the metabolically active hormone T_3, while monodeiodination of the inner ring results in the metabolically inactive rT_3. Many studies have revealed that there are reciprocal changes in T_3 and rT_3 levels in man. In a number of nonthyroidal illnesses and during fasting, fever, and other situations in which it would appear to be advantageous to the organism to limit catabolism, the activating pathway to T_3 is decreased and the inactivating pathway to rT_3 is increased. There is little or no change in plasma T_4 levels, in the overall rate of T_4 turnover, or in plasma TSH levels (indicating that euthyroidism is maintained). The changes in T_3 and rT_3 are reversed during convalescence. The mechanisms controlling the balance between the two pathways of T_4 metabolism are not yet known, but they may be related to energy balance. It is reasonable to expect that similar changes may occur in the dog, and, indeed, plasma T_3 levels are reduced during prolonged fasting and in several nonthyroidal illnesses in dogs, with little or no change in plasma T_4. However, reported data on rT_3 levels in dogs are too limited to permit further comparisons at present.

Metabolic Action. Much of the current interest and research concerning the metabolic action of thyroid hormone is an outgrowth of the extensive work that has been done on the production and metabolism of T_3. If one considers the preferential secretion of T_3 by the canine thyroid (i.e., the intrathyroidal conversion of T_4 to T_3 during secretion) and the extrathyroidal conversion (which accounts for about 60 per cent of daily T_3 production), together with the fact that T_3 is about three times as potent as T_4, one can infer that most of the metabolic effect of thyroid hormone could be provided by T_3. This is similar to the line of reasoning for the action of T_3 in man, which has led to the concept that T_4 may serve chiefly as a circulating reserve or prohormone for conversion to T_3. T_4 is still recognized as having some intrinsic hormone activity and plays a role, albeit a small one, in feedback control of thyroid function.

A unifying explanation of the molecular basis of thyroid hormone action has not yet been fully developed, but probably the most important step was the discovery of specific nuclear binding sites for T_3 (Oppenheimer et al., 1972; Oppenheimer, 1975). Interaction of T_3 with nuclear binding sites may lead to augmented transcription of DNA or modulation of RNA, thus influencing protein synthesis and enzyme action. The attractiveness of this explanation is that it has the potential of dealing with the extremely diverse effects of thyroid hormone, which include the promotion of growth and maturation of tissues, regulation of the production and turnover of many substances, and regulation of many enzymatic reactions. The diversity of effects may be explained not by a multiplicity of actions of the hormone per se but by the presence or absence of specific nuclear binding sites for the hormone. Given the presence of a receptor, determined genetically, binding of the hormone could simply influence the related process via transcription of DNA or modulation of RNA. Much work remains to be done to explore this hypothesis in detail and to elucidate the steps that follow nuclear binding at the molecular level.

Control of Thyroid Function. The principal regulation of thyroid function is by the pituitary gland through TSH. TSH attaches to receptors on the follicular cell, activates adenylate cyclase, and enhances cyclic adenosine monophosphate (cAMP) production. It is likely, but not yet proven in all instances, that cAMP mediates the effects of TSH on follicular cell growth, iodination and thyroid hormone synthesis, and thyroid hormone secretion (van Herle et al., 1979). Within minutes after TSH administration, there is enhancement of iodide binding to protein, iodothyronine synthesis, thyroglobulin secretion into the follicular lumen, and ingestion of colloid via pseudopod formation. Increased trapping of iodide follows after an interval of a few hours. TSH remains attached to the receptors for a long time and secretion continues for some time even if TSH is removed. In the dog, intravenous administration of TSH causes an increase in the release of iodide from the thyroid, followed by increased secretion of thyroid hormone within 15 to 30 minutes. When a relatively large dose of 10 IU of TSH is given, plasma T_4 concentration continues to rise for 8 to 12 hours.

Both the synthesis and release of TSH are stimulated by thyrotropin releasing hormone (TRH), which is a tripeptide amide produced by neurons in the thyrotropic area of the hypothalamus, as well as in other parts of the brain. TRH is released from the neurons in the median eminence and is transported to the pituitary via the portal circulation. It then attaches to receptors on the pituitary thyrotrophs, stimulates the adenyl cyclase–cAMP system, and increases TSH release within minutes.

Negative feedback control of TSH secretion is mediated by thyroid hormone, principally T_3, acting directly on the pituitary thyrotrophs. Small doses of thyroid hormone suppress, and large doses completely abolish, the TRH-induced release of TSH. In contrast to the very rapid stimulatory effect of TRH, the inhibiting effect of thyroid hormone takes several hours, for it involves thyroid hormone-stimulated synthesis of new protein. Cortisol and other glucocorticoids also suppress the TRH-induced release of TSH, and in man it has been shown that the diurnal rhythm in plasma cortisol concentration causes a reciprocal diurnal rhythm in TSH secretion.

In addition to the negative feedback control of thyroid function via inhibition of TSH secretion, there are certain negative control mechanisms acting directly upon the thyroid. In the dog, acetylcholine inhibits the TSH-induced increase in thyroidal cAMP and thyroid hormone secretion (but also mimics TSH activation of thyroid hormone synthesis) (Dumont et al., 1978). A gradual increase in iodide intake (and hence in thyroidal iodide levels) results in a gradual increase in the amount of iodide bound to thyroglobulin, but beyond a certain level binding is progressively inhibited. This is the Wolff-Chaikoff effect (Wolff and Chaikoff, 1948) and it is also induced abruptly by the administration of a single large dose of iodide. The inhibition of iodide binding is transient in normal animals and man, and escape occurs after several hours.

THYROID FUNCTION TESTS

PLASMA T_4

The measurement of plasma T_4 is now generally accessible to veterinarians in most of North America and western Europe via medical and veterinary institutional laboratories and commercial diagnostic laboratories. Most laboratories now use either displacement methodology (often called competitive protein binding assay) or radioimmunoassay. There is an important consideration in the measurement of plasma T_4 in dogs that is not fully appreciated by most veterinarians, namely, that most of the available procedures are not (and are not intended to be) sufficiently sensitive for accurate diagnostic measurements in dogs. In man it is seldom necessary to be able to measure values below 1 μg/100 ml, but it is advantageous to be able to measure values as high as 30 μg/100 ml in undiluted plasma. In the dog it is advantageous to be able to measure values as low as 0.1 μg/100 ml but seldom necessary to measure values above 10 μg/100 ml. Kit procedures for either displacement methods or radioimmunoassay, although very convenient and widely used by smaller laboratories, are simply not flexible enough to be readily adapted for accurate measurement of the low plasma T_4 levels that are encountered in dogs. In some kits the lowest reference standard is 2.0 μg/100 ml, and in at least one it is 5.0 μg/100 ml. Instructions for the kits indicate that the standard curve can be extrapolated to the zero reference value, but the real curve diverges from the extrapolated curve at progressively lower T_4 concentrations, and at some point the assay can no longer distinguish between real values and zero. In general, the higher the upper limit of measurement of an assay, the higher the lower limit of measurement as well. This applies to standard laboratory methods as well as to kit procedures, and assays that are set up to measure T_4 concentrations as high as 20 or 30 $\mu g/100$ ml cannot be expected to be accurate at values below one or even two $\mu g/100$ ml. Such limitations are of little or no importance in most diagnostic measurements in man, but they nullify the use of plasma T_4 measurements in their most frequent application in the dog, namely, in the diagnosis of hypothyroidism.

Radioimmunoassay methods for measuring plasma T_4 (excluding kit procedures) can easily be adapted to provide accurate measurements over a range of T_4 concentrations that is appropriate for most diagnostic purposes in the dog. With one method that has been reported (Belshaw and Rijnberk, 1979) and a good quality antiserum, a basic measurement range of 0.1 to 10 $\mu g/100$ ml is easily obtained, and somewhat wider limits (as low as 0.06 and as high as 16 $\mu g/100$ ml) are often observed. With this assay we have found plasma T_4 values in normal dogs of 1.5 to 3.6 $\mu g/100$ ml. In dogs with primary hypothyroidism, values are consistently below 1.0 $\mu g/100$ ml, and often below 0.1 $\mu g/100$ ml. Maximal T_4 concentrations in normal dogs after TSH stimulation seldom exceed 10 $\mu g/100$ ml, and while higher values are often found in hyperthyroidism in both dogs and cats, this possibility can usually be anticipated on the basis of clinical findings so that the assay can be performed on diluted as well as undiluted plasma. Plasma T_4 values in normal cats are very similar to those in dogs, ranging from about 1.5 to 3.5 $\mu g/100$ ml.

Displacement methods for plasma T_4 can also be modified, but the modifications are difficult or quite impractical with kit procedures for radioimmunoassay. It is, however, disturbing that a greater than fourfold difference among mean plasma T_4 values has been reported in normal dogs by different investigators using displacement methods (Kraft, 1976).

Plasma T_4 concentration in dogs can be moderately to severely depressed by certain drugs (glucocorticoids, diphenylhydantoin, phenobarbital, phenylbutazone, o,p'DDD) and by the glucocorticoid excess of Cushing's disease, regardless of its etiology. In man, glucocorticoids decrease the release of TRH, the TRH-induced release of TSH, and the T_4 binding capacity of TBG. Diphenylhydantoin interferes with binding of T_4 to plasma proteins and increases the conversion of T_4 to T_3. Phenobarbital increases biliary excretion of T_4 and possibly also T_4 deiodination. Phenylbutazone and o,p'DDD both interfere with binding of T_4 to plasma proteins. In dogs receiving any of the aforementioned drugs, both thyroidal trapping activity and responsiveness to TSH remain normal. More than 50 per cent of dogs receiving any one of these drugs and more than 50 per cent of dogs with Cushing's disease (regardless of etiology) have plasma T_4 values below the normal range. Dogs maintained for months or years on any of these drugs do not develop clinical signs of hypothyroidism, however. There have been no detailed studies of the exact mechanism by which each of these drugs affects plasma T_4 concentration in the dog, but the above observations suggest that the effect is chiefly on T_4 binding to plasma proteins and that euthyroidism is maintained by adequate levels of free T_4 and T_3. In general, plasma T_4 concentration gradually returns to normal over a period of two to four weeks after administration of any of these drugs is stopped.

PLASMA T_3

The concentration of T_3 in plasma or serum is measured by radioimmunoassay, and in general, assays that have been set up for measurements in man are quite suitable for use in the dog. We have observed a normal range of about 50 to 150 ng/100 ml (Belshaw and Rijnberk, 1979), which is only slightly lower than the normal range in man (about 100 to 200 ng/100 ml), and most T_3 assays have a sensitivity of 25 or even 10 $\mu g/100$ ml. Although assay procedures set up by laboratories usually include adequate definition of the standard curve, kit procedures usually do not and must be modified by the preparation of additional dilutions of the standard in order to determine the sensitivity in each performance of the assay. Since most kits do not include an excess of the T_3-depleted plasma with which such dilutions should be made, correct modification may not be possible.

We find very few clinical situations in which the measurement of plasma T_3 is a useful addition to the information provided by the measurement of plasma T_4. Measurements of plasma T_4 and T_3 are of about equal value in discriminating between normal dogs and those with primary hypothyroidism, and we have yet to see hyperthyroidism in the dog associated with elevation of plasma T_3 concentration alone. Drugs (and the glucocorticoid excess of Cushing's disease) that lower plasma T_4 concentration usually affect plasma T_3 concentration as well, and plasma T_3 concentration is reduced by nonthyroidal factors that divert T_4 metabolism from T_3 to rT_3. In addition, the plasma T_3 response to TSH stimulation is less helpful than that of plasma T_4 in the diagnosis of hypothyroidism (see following discussion). Further investigation of changes in plasma T_3 concentration in various disorders in the dog is surely warranted, but in the routine evaluation of canine thyroid function in veterinary practice, measurement of plasma T_3 is of doubtful additional value.

Plasma T_3 concentration in normal cats is similar to that in dogs, with a normal range of about 50 to 150 ng/100 ml, and is almost certainly subject to a similar array of nonthyroidal influences. Measurement of both plasma T_4 and T_3 may be somewhat more helpful in cats than in dogs in the diagnosis of hyperthyroidism.

FREE T_4

In man, the measurement of free T_4 concentration in the plasma is specifically useful in determining whether an abnormal total T_4 concentration is due to altered T_4 secretion or altered binding of T_4 by the plasma proteins. When T_4 binding capacity is reduced (owing to TBG deficiency or interference by other substances), total T_4 concentration is reduced but the per cent of free T_4 is increased and their product, free T_4 concentration, is maintained within the normal range. Similarly, when TBG concentration is increased (as by estrogens), total T_4 concentration is increased but the per cent of free T_4 is decreased and hence free T_4 concentration remains normal. In both situations, thyroid homeostasis remains normal and euthyroidism is maintained. In contrast, both total and free T_4 concentrations are reduced in hypothyroidism and elevated in hyperthyroidism. The direct measurement of the per cent free T_4 by dialysis is inconvenient for routine clinical use, and although plasma TBG concentration can be measured by radioimmunoassay, a much more convenient alternative has been found in the determination of the *in vitro* T_3 resin uptake. In man, this is inversely proportional to the available T_4-binding capacity of TBG and correlates very well with the per cent of free T_4. Hence, a free T_4 index (FTI), which is the product of the plasma total T_4 concentration and the T_3 resin uptake value, is widely used as a quite reliable substitute for the direct measurement of free T_4 concentration.

Unfortunately, there is very poor correlation between T_3 resin uptake values and the per cent of free T_4, as measured by dialysis, in the dog. The FTI, therefore, is not a valid index of free T_4 concentration in this species. The per cent of free T_4 is higher in the dog than in man (about .15 per cent versus .05 per cent), as should be expected from the weaker binding of T_4 and the lower total T_4 concentration in the dog. Although the per cent of free T_4 is generally reduced in hypothyroidism in man, it remains unchanged in the dog. T_3 resin uptake values are higher and much less sensitive to changes in plasma T_4 concentration in the dog than in man.

The result of these differences is that we do not have a convenient method of estimating free T_4 concentration in the dog, although the measurement is often needed. Plasma total T_4 concentration lowered by certain drugs or the glucocorticoid excess of Cushing's disease should be distinguished from hypothyroidism by measurement of free T_4, and without the latter we must depend upon the response to TSH stimulation (see following discussion).

THYROIDAL UPTAKE OF RADIOIODINE

The fraction of a tracer dose of radioiodine taken up by the thyroid is dependent upon the functional integrity of the thyroid, the endogenous output of TSH, and the dietary intake of iodine. In canine breeds of European origin, peak uptake of radioiodine normally occurs between 48 and 96 hours after the administration of the tracer, and radioiodine is released from the gland with a half-life of about 8 to 15 days. Peak uptake ranges from about 15 per cent of the dose in dogs whose iodine intake is 500 μg per day (most commercial diets provide this amount of iodine or more), to about 40 per cent when iodine intake is 140 μg per day (for dogs weighing 10 to 15 kg). In the Basenji, peak uptake occurs within 12 to 24 hours and the half-life of disappearance of radioiodine from the gland is about three days. In addition, peak uptake in the Basenji is much lower — about one half that in European breeds at the same level of iodine intake (Nunez et al., 1970).

In dogs with primary hypothyroidism, thyroidal uptake is usually less than five per cent of the tracer dose, but uptake can also be depressed to this degree by dietary levels of iodine above 500 μg per day. If the patient's iodine intake cannot be determined with certainty, a low-iodine diet should be used for one week prior to the measurement (Rijnberk, 1971). This can be accomplished by feeding fresh, cooked meat and vegetables without salt or other additives.

Thyroidal uptake of radioiodine is elevated, and the release of radioiodine from the gland is accelerated in iodine deficiency and in hyperthyroidism due to functional thyroid tumors. Although iodine deficiency is now extremely rare in countries in which commercial dog foods are used, these two conditions can easily be distinguished by measurement of plasma T_4 concentration. In extremely active thyroid tumors, the intrathyroidal iodine pool may be quite small because of the very rapid turnover of iodine, and peak uptake of radioiodine may occur as early as two hours after administration of the tracer.

Measurements of thyroidal uptake and turnover of radioiodine are useful in studying unusual disorders of the thyroid (congenital defects in hormone synthesis) and may be essential in the characterization of certain kinds of defects. However, they are impractical for routine clinical use in the dog because of their disproportionate requirements of time, personnel, equipment, and facilities.

THYROID SCINTIGRAPHY

Scintigraphic imaging of the thyroid by means of a rectilinear scanner or a gamma camera is extremely useful in diagnosis in all of the thyroid disorders of dogs and cats. It is unfortunate that the instruments are so expensive, limiting the use of the technique to those working in veterinary schools and practitioners who are able to make arrangements for scanning in the nuclear medicine departments of human hospitals. Gamma camera imaging is distinctly preferable to rectilinear scanning, because imaging time is so short that sedation of the animal is not

required. Gamma camera images of the thyroids in dogs and cats can be made 30 minutes after an intravenous dose of 2 mCi of pertechnetate ($^{99m}TcO_4^-$), with an imaging time of about one minute. We find the technique useful in identifying and locating functional thyroid tumors and their metastases, in differentiating between hypothyroidism and drug-induced lowering of plasma T_4 concentration, in evaluating thyroidal response to TSH stimulation, in detecting partial thyroidal destruction due to thyroiditis, and in evaluating restoration of function of the remaining thyroid lobe after removal of a unilateral functional thyroid tumor (Fig. 67–2). Gaining experience in interpretation of scintigrams of the thyroid is very much helped by the study of corresponding thyroid biopsies.

TSH STIMULATION

The response of the thyroid to stimulation with exogenous TSH can be evaluated by measurements of thyroidal uptake of radioiodine or plasma T_4 concentration, or by scintigraphic imaging. The most obvious use of TSH stimulation is in differentiating between primary hypothyroidism and secondary (TSH deficiency) or tertiary (TRH deficiency) hypothyroidism. In actual practice, however, our most frequent use of TSH stimulation is in confirming the diagnosis of primary hypothyroidism and thereby ruling out drug-induced lowering of plasma T_4 concentration. This is by no means essential in every case of lowered plasma T_4 concentration if the patient is under the care of a single veterinarian or practice and the record of medications is known with certainty. The decision concerning whether TSH stimulation should be performed cannot be based solely on the plasma T_4 concentration. Although we have not observed basal plasma T_4 values above 1.0 μg/100 ml in dogs with subsequently confirmed primary hypothyroidism, plasma T_4 can be depressed even to as low as 0.2 μg/100 ml in euthyroid dogs under treatment with phenylbutazone or glucocorticoids, as well as in dogs with Cushing's disease. If the possibility of drug-induced lowering of plasma T_4 cannot be excluded, TSH stimulation should be used to confirm the diagnosis of hypothyroidism before treatment is started. Compared with the possibility of unnecessary lifelong treatment with thyroid hormone, the additional expense and effort of a TSH stimulation test is rather insignificant. When it is necessary to confirm the diagnosis of hypothyroidism in a dog already receiving L-thyroxine or desiccated thyroid, the replacement therapy should be stopped for one to two weeks before the TSH stimulation test is performed.

For these routine uses of TSH stimula-

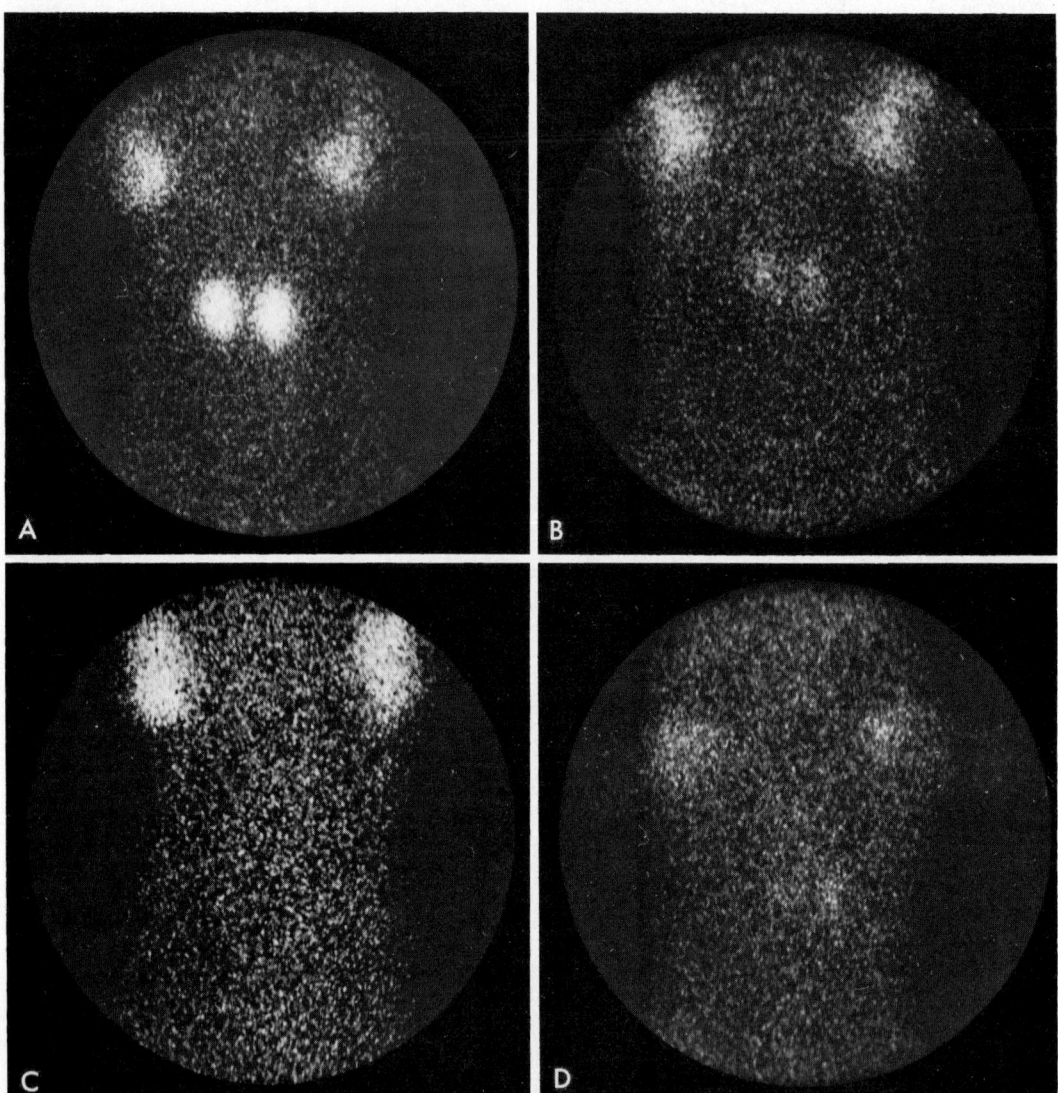

Figure 67–2. Gamma camera images of thyroids. The animals are in dorsal recumbency. The parotid salivary glands are also visualized in dogs, but not in cats. (a) Normal thyroid image in a two-year-old Bouvier. (b) Thyroid atrophy due to chronic lymphocytic thyroiditis in a ten-year-old German Shepherd Dog. (c) Thyroid atrophy (idiopathic follicular atrophy) in a six-year-old Doberman Pinscher. (d) Severe secondary hypothyroidism due to a pituitary tumor in an eight-year-old Chow Chow. Plasma T_4 was 0.34 μg/100 ml but increased to 1.20 μg/100 ml at four hours after 10 IU TSH. (e) Same dog as in (d), after three days of TSH stimulation. (f) Follicular-compact carcinoma of the right thyroid in a nine-year-old Boxer. The tumor had moderate trapping activity, but plasma T_4 and T_3 levels were normal. (g) Reexamination of a 12-year-old Boxer because of recurrence of polydipsia three years after removal of a follicular carcinoma of the left thyroid that had caused hyperthyroidism. This image reveals a normal right thyroid and no recurrence of the tumor; additional studies revealed Cushing's disease. (h) Inoperable bilateral thyroid carcinoma in a nine-year-old Boxer. In spite of intense trapping activity, the tumor did not secrete thyroid hormone and the dog was hypothyroid because of destruction of normal thyroid tissue (plasma T_4 was 0.30 μg/100 ml). (i) Adenocarcinoma of the left thyroid in a seven-year-old Cyprus cat. The tumor has gravitated to the thoracic inlet; the area of activity projected on the image is much larger than the tumor. Plasma T_4 was 26 μg/100 ml and there was severe hyperthyroidism, but surgery and subsequent recovery were uneventful.

Illustration continued on opposite page

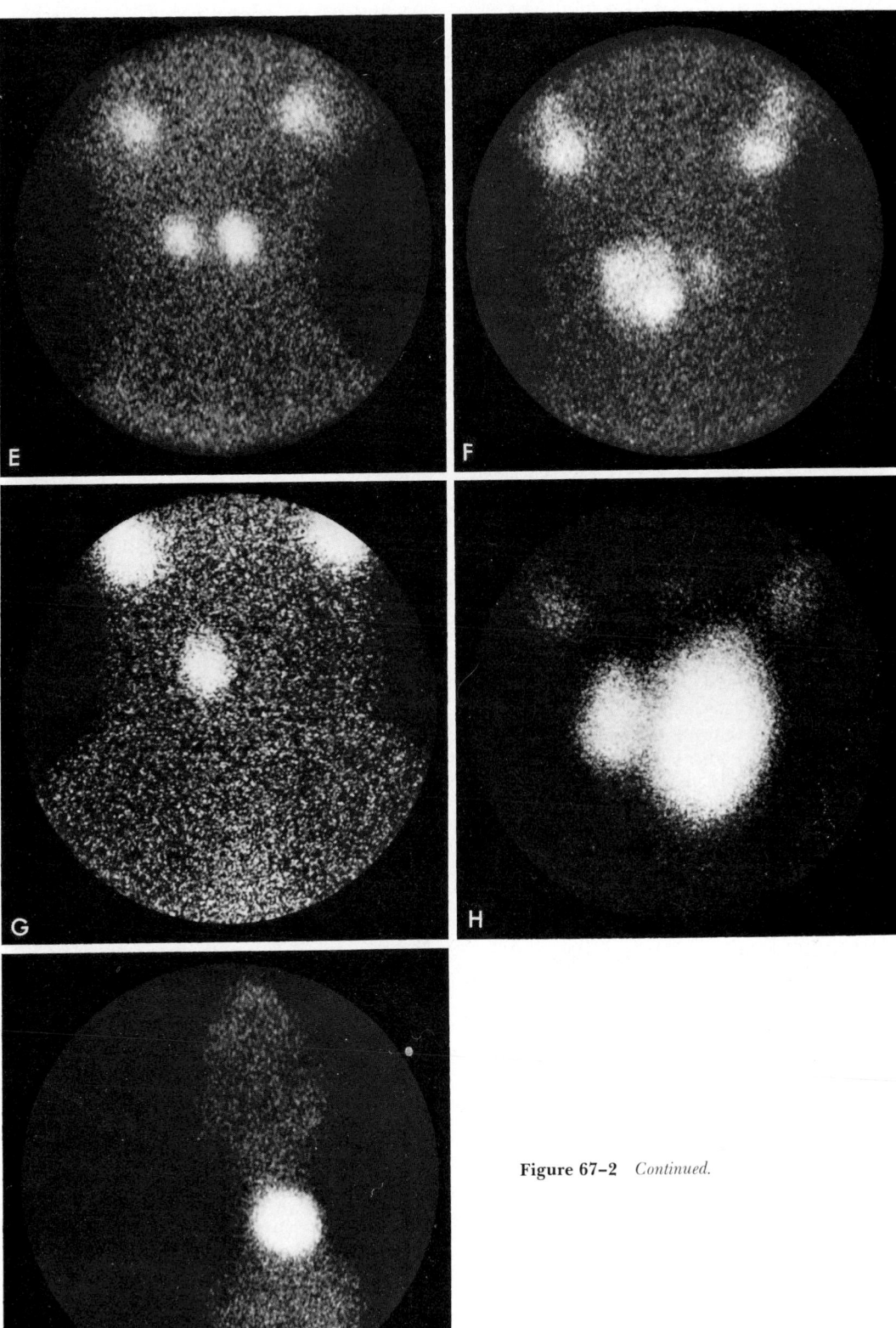

Figure 67-2 *Continued.*

tion, plasma T_4 concentration is measured in samples collected immediately before and four hours after the intravenous administration of 10 IU of bovine TSH. Although the maximal increase in plasma T_4 in normal dogs occurs at 8 to 12 hours after the TSH administration, the response by four hours is sufficient for differential diagnosis. In normal dogs, plasma T_4 concentration increases from the basal range of 1.5 to 3.6 μg/100 ml to values between about 3.0 and 6.5 μg/100 ml. In dogs with primary hypothyroidism, the increase is seldom more than 0.2 μg/100 ml above the basal value. In dogs with drug-induced lowering of plasma T_4, TSH causes an increase that is roughly parallel to that in normal dogs. Hence, T_4 concentration rises from as low as 0.2 μg/100 ml to above 1.0 μg/100 ml, or from 1.0 μg/100 ml to about 3.0 μg/100 ml.

In dogs with secondary or tertiary hypothyroidism, the response to a single dose of TSH is quite variable and probably depends upon the degree and duration of subnormal thyroid activity. In most of our cases a single dose of TSH has caused an increase in plasma T_4 concentration similar to that in dogs with drug-induced lowering of plasma T_4, but in some cases the response to a single dose of TSH has been quite small. In the latter, three consecutive days of TSH stimulation (10 IU daily, subcutaneously) were required to elevate plasma T_4 levels above 1.5 μg/100 ml and simultaneously to produce normal gamma camera images of the thyroid. Three days of TSH stimulation are also used when the response is determined by measurements of thyroidal uptake of radioiodine (Rijnberk, 1971).

TRH STIMULATION

The indication for TRH stimulation is in differentiating between secondary (TSH deficiency) and tertiary (TRH deficiency) hypothyroidism, and hence, it is only required in cases of hypothyroidism in which the thyroid has been shown to respond to exogenous TSH stimulation. Ideally, the response to TRH should be determined by measurements of plasma TSH concentration, but in the dog we are still dependent upon measurement of the thyroidal response to the TRH-induced release of TSH. Plasma T_4 concentration is measured in samples collected immediately before and four hours after the intravenous adminis-

tration of 0.2 mg of TRH. In normal dogs, the increase in plasma T_4 ranges from as little as 0.5 to as much as 2.0 μg/100 ml above the basal concentration. Simultaneously, plasma T_3 concentration increases from 10 to 40 ng/100 ml above the basal level. In some dogs the peak increase in plasma T_3 occurs in two hours. In the hypothyroid dog in which a definite response to TSH has been demonstrated, the additional finding of an increase in plasma T_4 of at least 1.0 μg/100 ml after TRH implies that the underlying cause of the hypothyroidism is a defect in production, release, or transport of TRH. On the other hand, a seemingly negligible increase in plasma T_4 (or T_3) following TRH administration in such a patient should be interpreted with some caution, in view of the rather small response in some normal dogs. In such cases we repeat the test once or twice before accepting the conclusion that the defect lies in the production or release of TSH. The possibility of glucocorticoid suppression of the TRH-induced release of TSH must also be excluded. It is fortunate that TRH stimulation is seldom required (secondary and tertiary forms of the disease account for less than five per cent of all cases of hypothyroidism in dogs), since the measurement of plasma TSH in the dog is not yet available.

THYROID BIOPSY

With the introduction of accurate methods for measuring plasma T_4 in the dog, thyroid biopsy has become needed less frequently in the routine diagnosis of primary hypothyroidism. However, until the measurement of plasma TSH in dogs becomes a practical reality, thyroid biopsy will continue to provide the most conclusive evidence of deficient endogenous TSH stimulation. It is also extremely helpful in the early stages of hypothyroidism due to thyroiditis, when both clinical signs and plasma T_4 sometimes fluctuate.

Either lobe of the thyroid can be exposed via a midline incision extending five to six cm caudally from the caudal border of the larynx. The sternohyoideus muscles are separated on the midline, and blunt dissection between the trachea and the muscles on one side will expose the corresponding lobe of the thyroid. The caudal half or the entire lobe may be removed; it is usually not difficult to leave the anterior parathyroid with an intact blood supply. The thyroid should be handled with care to avoid traumatic artifacts and should be placed directly into Bouin's fixative for four to six hours. Following this it may be cut lengthwise, and if the surface is still slightly pink, fixation can be continued in Bouin's fixative for an additional one to two hours before transferral to ten per cent neutral buffered formalin. Bouin's fixation considerably reduces shrinkage artifacts but results in brittleness if excessive. Sections from paraffin-embedded specimens should be cut at four to six microns and stained with hematoxylin-eosin and with the periodic acid-Schiff reaction.

DISORDERS OF THE THYROID

PRIMARY HYPOTHYROIDISM

Etiology. There are at least two distinct and apparently unrelated forms of thyroid atrophy leading to hypothyroidism in adult dogs. The slightly more prevalent disorder is the progressive destruction of follicles caused by chronic lymphocytic thyroiditis. This disease is similar both histologically and serologically to Hashimoto's thyroiditis in man and it is well known in laboratory colonies of beagles following the histological description by Tucker (1962). Its familial occurrence in beagles was shown by Musser and Graham (1968), and Mizejerski et al. (1971) demonstrated the presence of antibodies against thyroglobulin, a second colloid antigen, and a microsomal antigen, but antibody titers were not found to be correlated with the severity or progression of the histologic lesions in the thyroid. Recently, Gosselin et al. (1980) found circulating antibodies against thyroglobulin in 48 per cent of pet dogs with hypothyroidism, using the chromic chloride passive hemagglutination test and canine thyroglobulin. The earliest histologic evidence of the disease has been found in dogs at seven to eight months of age (Musser and Graham, 1968), but the author has also observed the initial infiltration of lymphocytes in dogs as old as four years. The progressive destruction of follicles leading to hypothyroidism appears to require at least two to three years, and comparison of histologic findings with the results of thyroid function studies in experimental beagles suggests that at least three fourths of the follicles must be destroyed before hypothyroidism ensues. The thy-

roiditis per se is asymptomatic, in that there is no goiter, pain, fever, or difficulty in swallowing, but it is sometimes accompanied by transient polyuria and polydipsia, the pathogenesis of which remains obscure. The characteristic histologic features of the disease — diffuse and nodular infiltration of the gland by lymphocytes and plasma cells, distinct germinal centers in some lymphoid nodules, invasion of individual follicles by lymphocytes and macrophages, and neutrophils usually around only necrotic epithelium — are often considerably diminished by the time hypothyroidism occurs and a thyroid biopsy is obtained. The end-stage lesion that is usually observed consists of a residual infiltrate of lymphocytes and plasma cells, large packets of parafollicular cells that congregate because of the disappearance of follicles and collapse of the stroma, and a few small follicles, most of which contain degenerating epithelium and poorly-staining colloid.

The other common form of thyroid atrophy in the dog is noninflammatory, and its etiology and pathogenesis remain unknown. Since thyroid biopsies are usually obtained only after hypothyroidism has developed, this lesion is also usually observed only in its terminal stage. The atrophy is often so complete that the specimen removed for histologic examination is only a lobe of parathyroid. Histologically, there may be nothing more than parathyroid tissue, adipose tissue, and two or three very small thyroid follicles in an entire section. Examination of multiple sections reveals no inflammatory cells whatsoever and, remarkably, no parafollicular cells, either. In a slightly different and less frequently observed form of idiopathic atrophy, there is also virtually complete disappearance of follicles, but parafollicular cells remain and there is linearly arranged, new connective tissue in addition to the collapsed stroma. There is also some increase in collagen around blood vessels, and very small nests of lymphocytes may be found adjacent to packets of parafollicular cells. It may be questioned whether idiopathic atrophy is really a separate entity (or perhaps two), or whether the absence of inflammatory cells is simply the consequence of the disappearance of follicular epithelium and colloid and hence the antigenic stimulus for their continuing presence. This seems unlikely, inasmuch as a few degenerating follicles can be found without lymphocytes in attendance. Goselin et al. (1981) have also concluded that idiopathic follicular atrophy is a distinct entity in dogs and have given an excellent description of the histologic and ultrastructural features of this lesion and of lymphocytic thyroiditis in dogs.

There are also cases of thyroid atrophy in which there is infiltration of lymphocytes but not in proportion to the loss of follicles and the degeneration of the epithelium in those remaining, and without invasion of the latter by lymphocytes. In these cases it is usually impossible to decide whether the initial lesion was autoimmune thyroiditis or idiopathic atrophy.

Clinical Signs. Primary hypothyroidism usually occurs in middle-aged and older dogs, rarely before the age of two years. It affects males and females about equally. The author has seen primary hypothyroidism neither in toy breeds of dogs (e.g., toy poodles and smaller breeds), nor as a spontaneous disease in cats. It can occur as a transient or even permanent disorder in cats following removal of a unilateral functional thyroid tumor, and insofar as the hypothyroidism progresses before the opposite lobe returns to function or thyroid hormone administration is begun, the clinical signs resemble those in dogs.

The onset of clinical signs is usually very gradual, and since the initial changes are neither very specific nor alarming, some months may pass before the dog is presented for veterinary examination. The most consistent and familiar signs of hypothyroidism are related to a generalized slowing of metabolism. The hypothyroid dog becomes more easily fatigued by its usual exercise and begins sleeping for increasing periods of the day. It has difficulty in maintaining normal body temperature, seeks warmth, and may be distinctly reluctant to go outside in cool weather. As hypothyroidism is extended, mental activity also becomes slowed and the dog becomes less interested in familiar activities and less excited by unusual events. Dogs that have been trained for police work or for sporting activities may remain alert and well motivated but become unable to perform long or strenuous exercise. There is often an increase in body weight, even in spite of restricted food intake and enforced exercise.

Some hypothyroid dogs move rather slowly and stiffly, particularly when they arise after sleeping, and the anteriodorsal surfaces of the front toenails become worn by the inadequate lifting of the feet. Infrequently, there is swelling of the capsule of one or more of the carpal and tarsal joints, with no increase in synovial fluid or radiographic evidence of involvement of the joint surfaces. The swelling can result in slight pain and lameness.

The pulse rate is sometimes slowed, the femoral pulse and apex beat are usually weak, and there may be low voltage on the ECG, sometimes accompanied by inversion of T waves.

The dermatologic effects of hypothyroidism are quite variable. The earliest changes are dryness of the coat and skin, excessive shedding, and retarded growth of hair. Loss of the undercoat may give the impression that the coat has become rather coarse, because of the predominance of guard hairs. Alopecia, sometimes with increased pigmentation of the skin, may occur on the ventral and lateral surfaces of the trunk, the caudal surfaces of the thighs, the ventral surfaces of the neck, and the dorsum of the nose. Histologically, there is atrophy of the sebaceous glands and of the epidermis, with epidermal and follicular hyperkeratosis, but the dermis may be thickened by accumulation of neutral and acid mucopolysaccharides. This occurs particularly on the forehead and face, leading to a puffy appearance and thickened folds of skin above the eyes. Together with slight blepharoptosis, these changes in the face give some hypothyroid dogs a tragic expression (Fig. 67–3). In boxers, retarded shedding of hair on the head, particularly the temporal areas, results in a dense carpet-like coat.

A rather infrequent effect of hypothyroidism is slight weakness of the facial muscles (drooping of the lower eyelid and upper lip) on one side and/or slight lateral tilting of the head. These disturbances are probably caused by myxedematous swelling of the common dural sheath of the facial, vestibular, and cochlear nerves in their passage through the internal acoustic meatus. The changes are reversible, with correction of the hypothyroidism if they have been present for no more than a few months.

Estrus is usually diminished in intensity and duration and may be completely absent. Slight atrophy of the testicles occurs in some male dogs, and the absence of spermatozoa

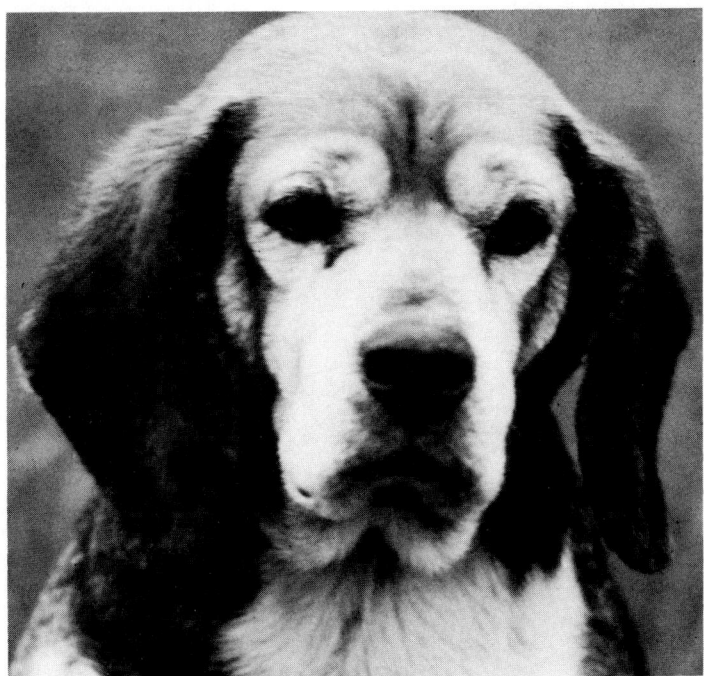

Figure 67–3. Hypothyroid Beagle with the puffy facial appearance, thickened folds of skin above the eyes, and tragic expression of the severely hypothyroid dog. (Courtesy of Dr. C. C. Capen.)

may be noted in examinations of urinary sediment.

Hypothyroid dogs usually have rather dry feces, and intestinal transit time is prolonged. Occasionally there is a history of periodic episodes of mild diarrhea.

Polydipsia, polyuria, and polyphagia are not typically seen in hypothyroidism, and this is a helpful point in clinically differentiating between hypothyroidism and Cushing's disease. Polydipsia and polyuria do occur occasionally in thyroiditis, however, usually well before the onset of clinical signs of hypothyroidism. The problem is transient, lasting but a few weeks, but can be recurrent. The cause of the disorder is not known, but it is not due to transient hyperthyroidism resulting from the thyroiditis, for plasma T_4 and T_3 levels are not elevated.

Hypercholesterolemia is found in about one half of hypothyroid dogs, and occasionally there is elevation of serum creatinine phosphokinase levels; for both substances, the elevation is due primarily to decreased turnover. There may also be hypertriglyceridemia and increases in certain lipoproteins (Rogers et al., 1975). A moderate normochromic, normocytic anemia is not unusual in longstanding cases.

Diagnosis. Diagnosis of hypothyroidism on the basis of clinical findings alone is unreliable, because any one of the changes seen in this disease can have other causes. Diagnosis based on the response to a trial course of treatment with thyroid hormone is also unreliable; for although the hypothyroid dog does indeed improve with treatment, there is nothing to prevent spontaneous improvement, concurrent with the administration of thyroid hormone, in the dog who is not hypothyroid. This possibility may seem far fetched, but experience has shown that it is not. Indeed, the fortuitous improvement that may accompany the administration of thyroid hormone and that is, unfortunately, too often accepted as adequate proof of the diagnosis of hypothyroidism has led to many misconceptions about the disease.

The measurement of plasma T_4 concentration is the most useful screening procedure, if the method of assay meets the requirements of sensitivity noted previously, for plasma T_4 concentration is invariably depressed well below the normal range in primary hypothyroidism. There have been a few reports to the contrary, i.e., of the finding of normal basal plasma T_4 levels but a convincing lack of response to TSH stimulation. In all such reports there has been a notable lack of information about the assay method and its sensitivity and reproducibility. Even with a sufficiently sensitive and accurate assay, however, the measurement of plasma T_4 as a screening procedure for hypothyroidism in dogs is far from ideal, since several nonthyroidial factors can also lower plasma T_4 concentration. Nevertheless, it does distinguish patients in which plasma T_4 concentration is normal and in which the diagnosis of hypothyroidism can therefore be eliminated. The measurement of plasma T_3 concentration is slightly less useful, inasmuch as plasma T_3 is reduced by an even greater number of nonthyroidal factors.

In recent years, it has been suggested that hypothyroidism occurs rather frequently in dogs owing to inadequate peripheral conversion of T_4 to T_3. This idea was intended to explain the finding of subnormal plasma T_3 values together with normal plasma T_4 values in dogs having clinical signs suggestive of hypothyroidism. This line of reasoning also led to the proposition that such dogs cannot be expected to respond to treatment with L-thyroxine and must be treated with L-triiodothyronine. Hence, treatment with L-triiodothyronine has also come into vogue and, not surprisingly, support for the idea has been found in the recovery of some dogs from their illness, concurrent with this treatment. Unfortunately, as Chastain and Zenoble (1979) have pointed out, the concept has been fostered with a remarkable lack of awareness or appreciation of the abundant literature on transient lowering of plasma T_3 concentration in a wide variety of illnesses, via the increase in conversion of T_4 to rT_3. It must be reemphasized that any one of the clinical changes seen in hypothyroidism can have other causes. It is not the least bit surprising that subnormal plasma T_3 values are found in dogs with signs mimicking those of hypothyroidism, nor that spontaneous recovery from transient illnesses may fortuitously accompany the administration of L-triiodothyronine. The notion has grown without any attempt to prove that the dogs in question are indeed *hypothyroid* and with disregard for the appropriate design of clinical studies to evaluate response to therapy. The author hopes that the vogue will quietly disappear.

Only occasionally has the author encountered a dog with such impressive clinical signs of hypothyroidism, and such an extremely low plasma T_4 concentration, that the diagnosis of hypothyroidism seems unquestionable. Nevertheless, it remains questionable until confirmed. While TSH stimulation need not be performed in every patient with a low basal plasma T_4 concentration (since the cause is often found in the record of recent or current medications or in the diagnosis of Cushing's disease), confirmation of the diagnosis of hypothyroidism should always be made before treatment with thyroid hormone is begun. Measurement of the plasma T_4 response to TSH stimulation is the most practicable means of confirmation, but scintigraphic imaging or thyroid biopsy are equally suitable. Measurement of the plasma T_3 response to TSH stimulation is not reliable, for although TSH causes little or no increase in plasma T_3 in dogs with primary hypothyroidism, it also causes little or no increase in some normal dogs, in spite of substantial increase in plasma T_4 (Belshaw and Rijnberk, 1979).

During the last few months of the progression of chronic lymphocytic thyroiditis leading to permanent thyroid insufficiency, there can be intermittent periods of clinical hypothyroidism and fluctuations in plasma T_4 and T_3 between normal and subnormal levels. As noted above, there is occasionally also intermittent polyuria and polydipsia, which, not being typical signs of hypothyroidism per se, add to the uncertainty. Repeated measurements of plasma T_4 and T_3 at follow-up examinations will eventually reveal repeated low values and TSH stimulation, or thyroid scintigraphy or thyroid biopsy will provide the diagnosis. The recent studies of Gosselin et al. (1980) suggest that measurement of antithyroglobulin antibodies would be helpful in earlier recognition of thyroiditis.

Treatment. Hypothyroidism in the dog is treated by the once-daily oral administration of L-thyroxine in a dose of 20 μg per kg of normal body weight. In countries in which L-thyroxine is not readily available or when its cost is prohibitive, the alternative is desiccated thyroid in a once-daily oral dose of 15 to 20 mg per kg of normal body weight. Some desiccated thyroid tablets are extremely hard and are intended to be chewed before swallowing; for administration to dogs, they should be crushed or ground and given in a small amount of food. A small proportion of hypothyroid dogs do not make a fully satisfactory recovery on desiccated thyroid, even when the dose is increased, but respond promptly when treatment is changed to L-thyroxine at the usual dose.

Following oral administration of L-thyroxine, plasma T_4 concentration reaches a peak in about four to five hours in the dog. The peak approaches or slightly exceeds the upper limit of normal plasma T_4 levels, and by the end of 24 hours after administration, plasma T_4 declines to the lower half of the normal range. Measurements of plasma T_4 for the purpose of evaluating replacement dosage are thus made about 24 hours after administration of the daily dose. The rates of disappearance of T_4 and T_3 from the plasma are slowed in hypothyroidism, and plasma T_4 concentration remains elevated during the first four weeks of treatment, but by the end of eight weeks it is well stabilized within the normal range. There are no persuasive arguments for administering L-thyroxine or desiccated thyroid in divided doses. Although the daily rise and fall in plasma T_4 concentration accompanying once-daily administration may be thought undesirable, there are also variations in plasma T_4 during the day, and from day to day, in most normal dogs. There are also no persuasive arguments for administering L-triiodothyronine, either alone or in combination with L-thyroxine, since the conversion mechanism handles the production of T_3 quite adequately, according to metabolic requirements.

A distinct increase in physical and mental activity is usually evident after about ten days of treatment, and there is considerable reversal of most of the signs of hypothyroidism by the first follow-up examination in two months. Full regrowth of hair in areas of alopecia requires four to six months, and there is sometimes pruritis during the first few weeks, associated with the shedding of old hair and exfoliation of excessive keratin. This can be relieved by frequent brushing of the coat and applications of olive oil or other softening agents to extremely dry or crusted areas of the skin.

Follow-up examinations are required only so long as problems remain, and usually only two or three examinations at about two-month intervals are required. Plasma T_4 concentration is measured each time, the dose of L-thyroxine for that day being withheld until after the sample has been collected. We have learned to rely upon the owner's evaluation of the dog's response as much as upon plasma T_4 concentration. The finding of a plasma T_4 concentration slightly below the normal range at 24 hours after L-thyroxine administration does not necessarily warrant an increase in dosage if both the owner and the veterinarian are quite satisfied with the dog's physical and mental improvement. In dogs that have gained weight as a result of hypothyroidism, the initial dose is based on the known or estimated normal weight, since the excess weight is usually lost rather quickly with treatment. Occasionally, adjustment of the dose according to actual weight is required. Overdosage results in the clinical signs of hyperthyroidism: polyuria and polydipsia; restlessness; panting; and, if overdosage is prolonged, weight loss in spite of increasing appetite, tachycardia, and high voltage on the electrocardiogram. The owner should be made aware of these signs when treatment is started and should be instructed to decrease the dose promptly if they appear.

There are very few complications in the treatment of hypothyroidism, but the restoration of the dog's enthusiasm for physical activity may unmask or intensify other problems, such as arthritis of the hip or knee. It should also be recognized that thyroid hormone replacement will not cure simple obesity, and when excessive weight remains a problem after reversal of all other signs of hypothyroidism, restriction of food intake — rather than an increase in the dose of thyroid hormone — is indicated.

So far as the author knows, there are no clinical features that distinguish chronic lymphocytic thyroiditis from idiopathic follicular atrophy; in both disorders, by the time clinical hypothyroidism is recognized, there is too little thyroid tissue remaining to permit restoration of euthyroidism, even if the destructive process could be arrested at that point. Furthermore, even if lymphocytic thyroiditis could be diagnosed at a much earlier stage, e.g., by routine screening for antithyroglobulin antibodies, it is unlikely that one could do more than temporarily retard the disease by corticosteroid therapy (based on experience in man). Long-term suppression of the thyroiditis by continuing corticosteroid therapy, even if successful, would seem to be less desirable than treatment of hypothyroidism. Earlier detection of thyroiditis would, however, permit earlier initiation of thyroid hormone replacement and the avoidance of an intervening period of hypothyroidism.

CONGENITAL PRIMARY HYPOTHYROIDISM

There have been no well-documented published reports of congenital intrathyroidal defects causing hypothyroidism in the dog. In man, defects have been found in iodide transport, iodination of tyrosine, coupling of iodotyrosines to form thyroglobulin, thyroglobulin synthesis, and deiodination of tyrosines following hydrolysis of thyroglobulin. The lack of reports suggests that such disorders must be quite rare in the dog, but they could also be overlooked among other causes of neonatal death in puppies.

SECONDARY AND TERTIARY HYPOTHYROIDISM

Etiology. These disorders account for less than five per cent of all cases of hypothyroidism in the dog, and in lieu of measurements of plasma TSH concentration before and after TRH stimulation, it may be difficult to differentiate between the two with absolute certainty. Secondary hypothyroidism is due to deficiency of TSH secretion caused by a lesion involving the pituitary gland. In the dog it can occur as either a congenital or acquired disorder in association with deficiencies of one or more other pituitary hormones. Congenital secondary hypothyroidism occurs in association with pituitary dwarfism, most notable in the German shepherd, owing to hypoplasia of the pars distalis or replacement by cysts arising from Rathke's pouch or both. Acquired secondary hypothyroidism can occur as a result of compression atrophy or replacement of the pars distalis by pituitary tumor. In both the congenital and acquired forms of secondary hypothyroidism, deficiencies of one or more other pituitary hormones are to be expected.

Tertiary hypothyroidism is due to deficient production or release of TRH. We have seen this in the dog both as a congenital defect of apparently isolated TRH deficiency and as an acquired disorder in adult dogs, occurring alone or in combination with moderate adrenocortical insufficiency. There has been no evidence of space-occupying lesions involving the hypothalamus (or pituitary), and a biochemical defect is presumed.

Clinical Signs. In general, the clinical signs of secondary and tertiary hypothyroidism are not as progressive or as extensive as those of primary hypothyroidism. Lack or loss of physical stamina is usually the most prominent finding and may be the only serious complaint. In congenital secondary hypothyroidism associated with pituitary dwarfism, the effects of the growth hormone deficiency dominate the clinical picture; the moderate hypothyroidism may be distinguished only by studies of thyroid function and may be appreciated only retrospectively, by the response to thyroid hormone administration. In acquired secondary hypothyroidism due to pituitary tumor, the neurologic consequences of the tumor usually dominate the clinical picture (depression, disturbances in locomotion, head pressing, epileptic seizures), and physical changes due to hypothyroidism (gain in weight, alopecia) may be mild or absent. Indeed, the hypothyroidism may be recognized only as a result of routine diagnostic studies, but confirmation of its etiology can be helpful in localizing the tumor. A very illustrative case of secondary hypothyroidism was reported by Chastain et al. (1979).

Congenital tertiary hypothyroidism results in a clinical picture of cretinism similar to that seen in congenital hypothyroidism of any etiology, but without goiter. Mental dullness, retardation of normal behavioral development, and retarded growth are the most impressive clinical findings. The skull may be disproportionately large and broad, and the legs short in relation to the trunk. The slow rate of growth is quite apparent after the first few weeks of life. In man, delay in recognition and treatment of congenital hypothyroidism results in a permanent deficit in mental development and the greater the delay, the greater the retardation. In the dog, there can be rather remarkable improvement in mental alertness and responsiveness, even if treatment is not begun until the animal is several months old. In acquired tertiary hypothyroidism, there is a distinct loss of physical stamina and increased sleeping, but mental alertness and responsiveness are not always so seriously affected and there are few physical changes other than gain in weight and dryness of the skin and coat.

Diagnosis. Plasma T_4 and T_3 concentrations are usually not decreased to the degree that is seen in primary hypothyroidism, as might be anticipated from the less severe clinical signs. In some cases of secondary or tertiary hypothyroidism in adult dogs, plasma T_4 and T_3 levels fluctuate above and below the lower limits of their respective normal ranges. Because of the less severe and less progressive clinical signs, and the fact that several nonthyroidal factors can depress plasma T_4 and/or T_3 levels, the diagnosis of secondary or tertiary hypothyroidism in an adult dog is often elusive and may not be given serious consideration until several other diagnostic possibilities have been eliminated. The opposite is true in the congenital disorders, for the retardation of growth alone prompts the examination of thyroid function, regardless of other findings.

The steps to be taken in differential diagnosis are, first, differentiation from primary hypothyroidism by testing thyroidal responsiveness to stimulation with TSH and, second, differentiation between secondary and tertiary hypothyroidism by testing pituitary responsiveness to stimulation with TRH. In some dogs with secondary or tertiary hypothyroidism, there is a quite distinct elevation in plasma T_4 concentration following a single dose of TSH, while in others three consecutive days of TSH stimulation may be required. It is obviously impractical to pursue the latter course in every dog with hypothyroidism, and the choice usually rests upon some suspicion engendered by the clinical findings (e.g., the rather mild signs of hypothyroidism or the neurologic signs of pituitary tumor or congenital onset). In dogs in which the use of plasma T_4-depressing drugs cannot be excluded, differentiation of primary from secondary or tertiary hypothyroidism may require determining the response to TSH by thyroid scintigraphy or measurement of radioiodine uptake or thyroid biopsy.

Thyroid biopsy provides an unambiguous differential diagnosis in such cases. In acquired primary hypothyroidism, there is an impressive loss of follicles, regardless of whether the cause is idiopathic atrophy or chronic lymphocytic thyroiditis, and there is usually also gross atrophy of the gland. In secondary and tertiary hypothyroidism, there is no apparent loss of follicles but the follicular epithelium is flattened, the follicles are slightly to markedly distended by the continuing accumulation of colloid, and there are very few or no resorption vacuoles at the cell-colloid interface. The reduction in size of the follicular cells is usually more than offset by the increase in colloid, so that the thyroid gland is either grossly normal or slightly increased in size. When plasma T_4 is depressed by drugs, thyroid histology remains, quite simply, normal.

Until measurement of plasma TSH levels in the dog becomes available, pituitary responsiveness to stimulation with TRH must be determined by measurements of plasma T_4 concentration. The reliability of this approach is directly dependent upon the accuracy and reproducibility of the T_4 assay, for the differentiation rests upon discrimination of a change in plasma T_4 concentration of as little as 0.5 μg/100 ml. Furthermore, since the index of response is a change in plasma T_4 concentration mediated by release of endogenous TSH, adequate thyroidal responsiveness to exogenous TSH stimulation must first be demonstrated, and a lack of response to TRH should be confirmed by repeating the TRH test at least once.

The extent to which the differential diagnosis between secondary and tertiary hypothyroidism need be pursued is somewhat dependent upon the clinical findings. Pituitary dwarfism in the German shepherd is well known (Scott et al., 1978, and references therein) and a presumptive diagnosis can usually be made on the basis of the clinical findings. Strictly speaking, in this and other forms of congenital dwarfism without goiter, it is only essential to determine whether there is hypothyroidism (measurements of plasma T_4 concentration usually suffice) and/or secondary glucocorticoid deficiency (by measurement of the plasma cortisol response to ACTH stimulation) to determine appropriate replacement therapy.

In the adult dog, the differential diagnosis has a direct bearing upon the prognosis, since acquired secondary hypothyroidism is almost certain evidence of pituitary tumor, while tertiary hypothyroidism implies a functional (rather than space-occupying) lesion in the hypothalamus. In both cases, measurement of the plasma cortisol response to ACTH stimulation is also useful.

Treatment. Treatment of secondary or tertiary hypothyroidism is identical to the treatment of primary hypothyroidism. When there is concurrent glucocorticoid deficiency (including the finding of normal resting plasma cortisol concentration but a distinctly subnormal response to ACTH), treatment with cortisone acetate is begun at the same time in an oral dose of one half mg per kg of body weight, twice daily.

THYROID TUMORS AND HYPERTHYROIDISM IN DOGS

Clinical and Pathological Aspects. About one third of all primary tumors of the canine thyroid are adenomas and two thirds are adenocarcinomas. However, only about 15 per cent of the adenomas, compared with at least 60 per cent of the carcinomas, are detected clinically, the remainder being discovered only at autopsy. Thus, about 90 per cent of the clinically apparent thyroid tumors in the dog are carcinomas. This designation applies to tumors that have either metastasized or invaded locally, or both, or exhibited substantial histologic evidence of so doing (Leav et al., 1976).

Secondary tumors (i.e., metastases from tumors of other organs) and parathyroid tumors are rare in the dog. Cysts, abscesses, foreign bodies, and carotid body tumors must also be considered in the differential diagnosis, but a firm mass in the ventral cervical region, anywhere between the larynx and the thoracic inlet, should be considered to be a thyroid tumor until proved otherwise.

The adenomas are usually less than two cm in maximum dimension and have a very thin, almost transparent capsule. A few become enlarged by cystic degeneration and internal hemorrhage; these develop a thick fibrous capsule and are usually filled with amber fluid.

In nearly 40 per cent of the cases of adenocarcinoma, metastasis has already occurred by the time the dog is examined clinically, but this follows an average delay of about six months (ranging from one to 30 months) between the owner's detection of the mass and presentation of the dog for examination. Lymphatic extension most frequently involves the retropharyngeal nodes, for the principal lymphatic drainage is from the anterior rather than the posterior pole of the lobe. Malignant thyroid tumors in the dog have a propensity for invading veins within the tumor mass and its capsule, and metastasis to the lungs occurs more frequently and earlier than to lymph nodes.

About 75 to 80 per cent of the adenocarcinomas can be classified histologically as follicular compact tumors, i.e., composed of a mixture of distinct follicles and compact cellular growth. Ten to 15 per cent of the adenocarcinomas are essentially pure follicular tumors; giant cell, papillary, and small-cell tumors together compose the remaining five to ten per cent (Leav et al., 1976). The follicular carcinomas grow more rapidly than do the majority of the follicular-compact tumors. In addition, a tumor that is predominantly compact in its primary site may be predominantly follicular in its metastases. Although the proportion of giant cell tumors is small, these atypical types are usually more malignant than the follicular-compact carcinoma. As a group, thyroid carcinomas occur with about equal frequency in males and females, but they are much more common in the boxer than in any other breed.

The probability of metastasis increases in proportion to the size and duration of the tumor. For example, metastasis was found to have occurred in only 14 per cent of the cases of carcinoma in which the volume of the tumor was less than 21 cc but in 78 per cent of the cases in which the volume was greater (Leav et al., 1976).

Treatment. These data provide some useful guidelines for the clinician. First, if a tumor is large enough to have been detected by the owner, it is more likely to be a carcinoma. If the tumor is small (three cm or less in maximum dimension) and if there has not been an extended delay since its initial detection, the prospects for complete excision without recurrence are reasonably good. If the tumor is large or fixed in position, or if it has grown rapidly within the previous month or two, there is a greater possibility of metastasis. The most ill-advised approach is to wait to see if it does grow rapidly, since 90 per cent of the clinically detected tumors are carcinomas and to delay removal is to increase the risk of metastasis.

Prompt surgical removal should be undertaken in every case unless palpation and radiographic examination reveal that the tumor already encircles the larynx and trachea or there is already dyspnea due to pulmonary metastases. In some cases, the extent of local invasion can be evaluated only after surgical exposure and it is found that the tumor cannot be completely removed because of invasion of the larynx or envelopment of the recurrent laryngeal nerve and carotid artery. Surgery may involve partial excision of cervical muscles and removal of the medial retropharyngeal lymph node. Both lobes of the thyroid are involved in only 15 per cent of the cases of carcinoma, and only occasionally is the tumor in the second lobe so small that it can be excised completely while still preserving at least one parathyroid with an intact blood supply.

No replacement therapy is required following removal of a unilateral thyroid tumor in the dog; even when the function of the contralateral lobe has been suppressed, plasma T_4 concentration returns to normal within two to three weeks. Following bilateral thyroidectomy, L-thyroxine is given in the usual replacement dose of 20 μg per kg, once daily, for life. When total parathyroidectomy is unavoidable, the parathyroid insufficiency should be managed according to the method of Meyer (1980). In our experience, the postoperative management of parathyroid insufficiency requires so much additional effort and concern by the owner that euthanasia of the dog is usually requested within a few weeks or months. Because of this, we tend to discourage surgical intervention in cases of large, bilateral thyroid tumors in which total parathyroidectomy will also obviously be required.

In cases of thyroid tumor with severe hyperthyroidism (see following discussion), it would seem advisable to attempt to diminish the hyperthyroidism before surgery by treatment with iodine or antithyroid drugs. However, the author has encountered no serious complications during or following surgery without such preparation, even in elderly dogs with large tumors requiring considerable dissection. He has never observed a condition comparable to "thyroid storm" in man, i.e., an explosive episode of severe hyperthyroidism due to the sudden and massive release of thyroid hormone, such as that caused by surgical manipulation of an inadequately blocked, hyperfunctioning goiter or tumor. That this hazard does not occur in the dog is probably largely due to the much more rapid rates of deiodination and excretion of both T_4 and T_3 in this animal.

The presence of pulmonary metastases does not necessarily argue against removal of the primary tumor, for it is sometimes possible to retard the growth of metastases or even to induce considerable regression and an extended period of quiescence by suppressing TSH secretion via administration of L-thyroxine. This cannot be expected to succeed if the tumor itself is producing high plasma levels of T_4, and it should not be attempted if the pulmonary metastases are already causing severe dyspnea. With these exceptions, suppression can be attempted following surgery by administering L-thyroxine in a starting dose of 30 μg per kg per day in two or three divided portions to maintain a more uniform plasma T_4 level. The dose is increased in small steps to determine the highest dose that the dog can tolerate comfortably without developing signs of hyperthyroidism; polydipsia and restlessness are the first indications.

Functional Aspects. More than three fourths of the clinically detected thyroid tumors in dogs trap sufficient radioiodine or pertechnetate to be visualized by scintigraphic imaging, and more than one half produce sufficient amounts of hormone to result in partial or complete suppression of trapping by the contralateral lobe. By the time of first clinical examination, however, only about one fourth produce sufficient amounts of thyroid hormone to cause hyperthyroidism. In general, suppression of TSH secretion, and hence of trapping by the contralateral lobe, occurs when plasma T_4 concentration is raised to about 4 $\mu g/100$ ml. Surprisingly, suppression occurs with this increase in plasma T_4 concentration, even though plasma T_3 concentration remains well within its normal range. Indeed, plasma T_4 can be increased to as high as 7 to 8 $\mu g/100$ ml without elevated plasma T_3 levels and without clinical signs of hyperthyroidism. This may be due to the suppression of TSH-dependent intrathyroidal monodeiodination of T_4 to form T_3, as well as to decreased peripheral conversion. Although we have only seen clinical hyperthyroidism in the presence of substantial elevations of both T_4 and T_3 plasma levels, there is no a priori reason to doubt that predominant or even exclusive production of T_3 by some thyroid tumors can occur in the dog, as in man.

Polydipsia is usually the first clinical sign of hyperthyroidism in the dog and it may be gradual or rather abrupt in onset. It appears to be due to interference with the action of antidiuretic hormone on the renal tubule. It is followed by gradual loss of body weight in spite of simultaneous polyphagia. Other signs develop in proportion to the severity and duration of the hyperthyroidism and include a more forceful apex beat and arterial pulse, high voltage on the ECG, excessive panting and preference for a cool environment (although rectal temperature is seldom elevated), restlessness, and fatigue. There are no specific abnormalities in laboratory findings other than the elevation of plasma T_4 and T_3 concentrations.

Hyperthyroidism should always be considered in the differential diagnosis of polydipsia in an adult dog, and the physical examination in connection with this complaint should include careful palpation of the neck from the larynx to the thoracic inlet. In the dog, a thyroid tumor that is large enough to produce hyperthyroidism is large enough to be palpated, unless it is a solitary tumor arising from accessory thyroid tissue at the base of the heart (an apparently rare event). The diagnosis of hyperthyroidism can be confirmed by measurement of plasma T_4 and T_3, but this is not strictly essential once the tumor has been detected. The tumor is a surgical problem, and if hyperthyroidism is also present, its severity is indicated as much by clinical signs as by the elevation of plasma T_4 and T_3 levels.

THYROID TUMORS AND HYPERTHYROIDISM IN CATS

Hyperthyroidism has been recognized as a distinct entity in cats and is now being diagnosed with increasing frequency. The first documented report of the disease was published by Holzworth et al. (1980). As these authors noted, it is not yet clear whether hyperthyroidism in cats has simply been misdiagnosed in the past or whether there has been a recent and substantial increase in the frequency of its occurrence. Clark and Meier (1958), Lucke (1964), and Leav et al. (1976) have described the proliferative lesions in the thyroids of elderly cats, more than 90 per cent of which have been adenomas or adenomatous hyperplasia. In the past, the lesions have been found almost exclusively at autopsy, although retrospective consideration of clinical findings has occasionally suggested the possibility of hyperthyroidism.

Adenomatous hyperplasia is usually bilateral, whereas discrete adenomas and adenocarcinomas are usually unilateral. Metastasis of the histologically malignant tumors is infrequent by the time of clinical diagnosis and surgical removal. In both the benign and the malignant lesions, there can be considerable variation in histology, from compact or solid cellular growth to well-differentiated follicles, even within the same nodule of multinodular lesions.

Clinical and Laboratory Findings. The clinical signs of hyperthyroidism are usually gradual in onset, but as Theran and Holzworth (1980) have aptly pointed out, they are so striking that having once been recognized, they are not likely to be missed or misinterpreted in future cases. They seldom appear before the age of nine years but may also develop beyond the age of 20 years. There appears to be no distinct predilection for either sex. Weight loss and polyphagia are usually the most prominent signs, and in a few cases the appetite is insatiable. Defecation is frequent and the stools are soft and bulky. Polydipsia and polyuria usually develop but are not usually as severe as in hyperthyroidism in the dog. Restlessness, continual walking, and frequent crying are also common, and the cat may neglect its normal grooming habits. The most serious effects of hyperthyroidism in the cat are the disturbances in cardiac function. There can be quite severe tachycardia, with cardiac enlargement, high voltage on the ECG, murmurs, and arrhythmias; congestive heart failure may ensue.

Adenomatous hyperplasia may cause only moderate enlargement of one or both lobes of the thyroid, while adenomas and adenocarcinomas usually result in a more distinct mass. Palpation is facilitated by the wasting of subcutaneous fat, but an enlarged thyroid can be missed by cursory examination. If enlargement of one or both thyroids is not readily palpable, the cat should be lightly sedated with thiamylal or ketamine to permit thorough and undistracted palpation from the larynx to the thoracic inlet. A gentle sliding motion with the fingertip is sometimes more successful than grasping with the finger and thumb. Gamma camera scintigraphy with pertechnetate will invariably reveal hyperfunctioning nodules, as well as otherwise undetected extensions or metastases of functional carcinomas. Gamma camera imaging is somewhat preferable to rectilinear scanning, because the cat does not have to be anesthetized and because the higher resolution of the gamma camera provides much more certain differentiation between unilateral and bilateral involvement prior to surgery.

Both T_4 and T_3 plasma levels are usually elevated in hyperthyroid cats, although Holzworth et al. (1980) reported that one or the other hormone alone was elevated in individual cases. In some cases, plasma T_4 concentration has exceeded 20 μg/100 ml and plasma T_3 has exceeded 400 ng/100 ml. These authors also reported that SGPT, SGOT, and alkaline phosphatase levels are usually elevated.

Treatment. Surgical removal of the enlarged thyroid gland(s) should be given first consideration, not only because this brings the most rapid and certain cessation of the hyperthyroidism, but also because the possibility of a malignant lesion cannot be excluded on the basis of clinical and laboratory findings. In most cases surgery can be undertaken directly, but in cases of severe hyperthyroidism, particularly with serious cardiac complications, it may be advisable or even essential to attempt preoperative treatment of the hyperthyroidism and stabilization of cardiac function. Propylthiouracil, in an oral dose of 50 mg every eight hours, may be effective in lowering plasma T_4 and T_3 concentrations within one to two weeks; its action is to inhibit the iodination of tyrosine. Regular administration on an eight-hour schedule should be emphasized. If the initial response is favorable, continuation of treatment for an additional two to three weeks may result in adequate amelioration of the hyperthyroidism to satisfactorily reduce the risk of surgery. Alternatively, excess iodine can be used to inhibit thyroid hormone secretion for two weeks prior to surgery; in man this has the additional effect of reducing the extreme vascularity of thyroid nodules. Based on experience in man and in the dog, a dose of one to two mg of sodium iodide or potassium iodide administered once daily by mouth (in aqueous solution) should be more than adequate to block thyroid secretion in the cat.

Surgical considerations in the cat differ somewhat from those in the dog, in that bilateral involvement is more frequent and the incidence of carcinoma is much lower. If preoperative thyroid scintigraphy cannot be performed, bilateral involvement can be determined in some cases only by careful inspection at surgery. Since most of the bilateral lesions are adenomatous hyperplasia rather than tumor, there may be a greater possibility than in the dog of preserving the exterior (usually anterior) parathyroid gland on one or both sides.

Following unilateral thyroidectomy, the remaining lobe usually returns to adequate function within two to three weeks; temporary postoperative thyroid hormone replacement is contraindicated, since it will only delay the process by maintaining feedback suppression of TSH secretion. When function of the remaining lobe is not restored or when bilateral thyroidectomy has been performed, lifelong replacement therapy with L-thyroxine is required. We have used the same dose in the cat as in the dog (20 μg per kg of body weight, once daily), with satisfactory clinical response and maintenance of normal plasma T_4 levels.

Theran and Holzworth (1980) have reported that following bilateral thyroidectomy and parathyroidectomy, most cats recover uneventfully and that in the minority of cases in which hypocalcemia occurs, it is a transient problem (two or three days). This is presumably explained by the presence of accessory parathyroid tissue. When parathyroid insufficiency occurs, whether transient or permanent, the discussion by Meyer (1980) of its treatment in the dog will be found helpful.

REFERENCES

Belshaw, B. E., Barandes, M., Becker, D. V., and Berman, M.: A model of iodine kinetics in the dog. Endocrinology 95:1078, 1974.

Belshaw, B. E., Cooper, T. E., and Becker, D. V.: The iodine requirement and influences of iodine intake on iodine metabolism in the adult beagle. Endocrinology 96:1280, 1975.

Belshaw, B. E., and Rijnberk, A.: Radioimmunoassay of plasma T_4 and T_3 in the diagnosis of primary hypothyroidism in dogs. J.A.A.H.A. 15:17, 1979.

Chastain, C. B., and Zenoble, R. D.: Letter to the editor. J. A. A. H. A. 15:533, 1979.

Chastain, C. B., Riedesel, D. H., and Graham, C. L.: Secondary hypothyroidism in a dog. Canine Practice 6:59, 1979.

Clark, S. T., and Meier, H.: A clinico-pathological study of thyroid disease in the dog and cat. Part I: Thyroid pathology. Zentralbl. Veterinaermed. 5:17, 1958.

Dumont, J. E., Boeynaems, J. M., Decoster, C., et al.:

Biochemical mechanisms in the control of thyroid function and growth. Adv. Cyclic Nucleotide Res. 9:723, 1978.

Godwin, M. C.: The early development of the thyroid gland in the dog with especial reference to the origin and position of accessory thyroid tissue within the thoracic cavity. Anat. Rec. 66:233, 1936.

Gosselin, S. J., Capen, C. C., Martin, S. L., and Targowski, S. P.: Biochemical and immunological investigations on hypothyroidism in dogs. Can. J. Comp. Med. 44:158, 1980.

Gosselin, S. J., Capen, C. C., and Martin, S. L.: Histopathologic and ultrastructural evaluation of thyroid lesions associated with hypothyroidism in dogs. Vet. Pathol. 18:299, 1981.

Holzworth, J., Theran, P., Carpenter, J. L., Harpster, N. K., and Todoroff, R. J.: Hyperthyroidism in the cat: Ten cases. J.A.V.M.A. 176:345, 1980.

Kameda, Y.: The accessory thyroid glands of the dog around the intrapericardial aorta. Arch. Histol. Jpn. 34:375, 1972.

Kraft, W.: Schilddrüssenfunktionsstörungen beim Hund (Thyroid function disturbances in the dog). Thesis, Justus Liebig University, Giessen, West Germany, 1976.

Laurberg, P.: T_4 and T_3 release from the perfused canine thyroid isolated in situ. Acta Endocrinol. 83:105, 1976.

Laurberg, P.: Non-parallel variations in the preferential secretion of 3,5,3'-triiodothyroine (T_3) and 3,3',5'-triiodothyronine (rT_3) from dog thyroid. Endocrinology 102:757, 1978a.

Laurberg, P.: Selective inhibition of the secretion of triiodothyronine from the perfused canine thyroid by propylthiouracil. Endocrinology 103:900, 1978b.

Leav, I., Schiller, A. L., Rijnberk, A., et al.: Adenomas and carcinomas of the canine and feline thyroid. Am. J. Pathol. 83:61, 1976.

Lucke, V. M.: An histological study of thyroid abnormalities in the domestic cat. J. Small Anim. Pract. 5:351, 1964.

Meyer, D. J.: Primary Hypoparathyroidism. In Kirk, R. W. (ed.): Current Veterinary Therapy VII. Philadelphia, W. B. Saunders Company, 1980.

Mizejerski, G. J., Baron, J., and Poissant, G.: Immunologic investigations of naturally occurring canine thyroiditis. J. Immunol. 107:1152, 1971.

Musser, E., and Graham, W. A.: Familial occurrence of

thyroiditis in purebred beagles. Lab. Anim. Care 18:58, 1968.

Nelson, J. C., Weiss, R. M., Palmer, F. J., Lewis, J. E., and Wilcox, R. B.: Serum diiodotyrosine. J. Clin. Endocrinol. Metab. 41:1118, 1975.

Nunez, E. A., Becker, D. V., Furth, E. D., Belshaw, B. E., and Scott, J. P.: Breed differences and similarities in thyroid function in purebred dogs. Am. J. Physiol. 218:1337, 1970.

Nunez, E. A., Belshaw, B. E., and Gershon, M. D.: A fine structural study of the highly active thyroid follicular cell of the African basenji dog. Am. J. Anat. 133:463, 1972.

Oppenheimer, J. H.: Initiation of thyroid-hormone action. N. Engl. J. Med. 292:1063, 1975.

Oppenheimer, J. H., Koerner, D., Schwartz, H. L., et al.: Specific nuclear triiodothyronine binding sites in rat liver and kidney. J. Clin. Endocrinol. Metab. 35:330, 1972.

Refetoff, S., Robin, N. I., and Fang, V. S.: Parameters of thyroid function in serum of 16 selected vertebrate species: A study of PBI, serum T_4, free T_4, and the pattern of T_4 and T_3 binding to serum proteins. Endocrinology 86:973, 1970.

Rijnberk, A.: Iodine metabolism and thyroid disease in the dog. Thesis, University of Utrecht, Utrecht, The Netherlands, 1971.

Rogers, W. A., Donovan, E. F., and Kociba, G. J.: Lipids and lipoproteins in normal dogs and in dogs with secondary hyperlipoproteinemia. J.A.V.M.A. 166:1092, 1975.

Scott, D. W., Kirk, R. W., Hampshire, J., and Altszuler, N.: Clinicopathological findings in a German shepherd with pituitary dwarfism. J. A. A. H. A. 14:183, 1978.

Theran, P., and Holzworth, J.: Feline Hyperthyroidism. In Kirk, R. W. (ed.), Current Veterinary Therapy VII. Philadelphia, W. B. Saunders Company, 1980.

Tucker, W. E., Jr.: Thyroiditis in a group of laboratory dogs. Am. J. Clin. Pathol. 38:70, 1962.

Van Herle, A. J., Vassart, G., and Dumont, J. E.: Control of thyroglobulin synthesis and secretion. N. Engl. J. Med. 301:239, 1979.

Wolff, J., and Chaikoff, I. L.: Plasma inorganic iodide as a homeostatic regulator of thyroid function. J. Biol. Chem. 174:555, 1948.

CHAPTER 68

EDWARD C. FELDMAN

Diseases of the Endocrine Pancreas

PHYSIOLOGY

The pancreas aids in the digestion and assimilation of food. The digestion of food is the primary job of the *exocrine* pancreas, which excretes enzymes into the intestinal lumen. Also present in this gland are microscopic islets of Langerhans, which function endocrinologically. At least four proteins with hormonal activity are secreted by the islets of Langerhans. Two of the hormones, *insulin* and *glucagon,* are known to have important roles in the regulation of the intermediary metabolism of carbohydrates, proteins, and fats. A third hormone, *somatostatin,* appears to mediate the release of insulin and glucagon. The role of another pancreatic hormone, *pancreatic polypeptide,* remains to be elucidated. Glucagon and somatostatin are also secreted by cells in the mucosa of the gastrointestinal tract.

Insulin is an anabolic hormone that increases the storage of glucose, amino acids, and fatty acids. Glucagon is a catabolic hormone that mobilizes glucose, amino acids, and fatty acids, bringing about their transfer from storage depots into the bloodstream. Thus, these two major pancreatic hormones are reciprocal in their actions and are reciprocally secreted, in most circumstances. Insulin excess causes hypoglycemia, which results in weakness, convulsions, and death. Insulin deficiency, either relative or absolute, is seen as diabetes mellitus. Glucagon excess worsens the diabetic condition, while glucagon deficiency can result in hypoglycemia. Excess production and secretion of pancreatic somatostatin results in abnormally elevated blood glucose concentrations as well as other manifestations of diabetes mellitus. Carbohydrate metabolism is further regulated by a variety of nonpancreatic hormones (Ganong, 1979).

The cells that compose the islets of Langerhans are divided on the basis of staining properties and morphology. Five distinct cell types have been identified, including A (alpha) cells, which secrete glucagon and account for approximately twenty per cent of the secreting cells; B (beta) cells, which make up more than half the cells and which secrete insulin; and a small number of D (delta) cells, which secrete somatostatin. The fourth cell type consists of pancreatic polypeptide secreting cells, and the function of the fifth cell type is unknown; both of these cell types remain unnamed (Bloom and Fawcett, 1975).

INSULIN

Structure

Insulin is a polypeptide containing two chains of amino acids that are linked by two disulfide bridges. There are minor differences in the amino acid sequence of the polypeptide from species to species (Table 68–1).

The series of six amino acids in the S–S ring of chain A is of special interest because oxytocin and vasopressin are peptides that also contain six amino acids within an S–S bridge. This configuration may be significant in the interaction of peptides and hormone-sensitive cells. It has been suggested that this portion of the insulin molecule is "exposed" and that it may be the site of binding to muscle and other tissues (Williams and Porte, 1974).

Biosynthesis

Insulin is synthesized in the endoplasmic reticulum of the B cells. It is then transported to the Golgi complex, where the insulin is packaged into membrane-bound granules. Fusion of these granules with the cell wall

1615

Table 68–1. Variations in Amino Acid Sequence of Insulins in Common Mammals

Species	A Chain Position			B Chain Position
	8	9	10	30
Human	Thr —	Ser —	Ile	Thr
Rabbit	Thr —	Ser —	Ile	Ser
Cattle, goats	Ala —	Ser —	Val	Ala
Sheep	Ala —	Gly —	Val	Ala
Horse	Ala —	Gly —	Ile	Ala
Pig	Thr —	Ser —	Ile	Ala
Dog	Thr —	Ser —	Ile	Ala

allows for expulsion of the insulin to the exterior by exocytosis after a stimulus for insulin secretion, such as glucose, is applied. This release process has been shown to require calcium. In order to enter the bloodstream, the expelled extracellular insulin must cross the basal lamina of the parent B cell and the basal lamina of a capillary, and pass through the fenestrated endothelium of the capillary.

Insulin is synthesized initially as a long (81 to 86 residue) polypeptide molecule called *preproinsulin*. This insulin folds on itself within the B cell after an amino acid fragment is removed from the C terminal. The folding allows formation of the important disulfide links in the mid-product called *proinsulin*. Proinsulin contains insulin plus a polypeptide that *connects* (C peptide) the A and B chains (Fig. 68–1). C peptide contains 31 amino acids, which are removed by proteolytic cleavage within the granules of B cells prior to exocytosis. The result is reduction of the 9000 molecular weight (m.w.) proinsulin to insulin (6000 m.w.) and C peptide (3000 m.w.). C peptide enters the bloodstream along with insulin when the granule contents are extruded from the cell. This polypeptide, which has not been found to have a specific action, can be measured by radioimmunoassay, and its concentration provides an index of B cell function in humans receiving exogenous insulin (Steiner et al., 1971).

Proinsulin and insulin interact with antibody present in most insulin immunoassays. Since both peptides contain common immunologic determinants, it is difficult to develop an immunoassay for insulin that does not measure some proinsulin. In fasting humans, 5 to 30 per cent of measured insulin is proinsulin.

Regulation of Insulin Secretion

Insulin is the body's most important anabolic hormone, and its secretion control is complex. Many substrates and hormones participate in this regulation. The major control of insulin secretion is the feedback effect of blood glucose concentration directly on the pancreas. Glucose entrance into the islet cells is independent of insulin. When the blood glucose concentration perfusing the pancreas of the rat exceeds 110 mg/dl, insulin secretion in pancreatic venous blood increases. As glucose levels fall below normal, insulin secretion diminishes (Marliss et al., 1977).

When glucose is presented to the islet as a sudden increase in concentration and held constant above 100 mg/dl, there is an immediate insulin response (30 seconds to one minute) that peaks within a few minutes. This short-lived increase in secretion falls and then gradually rises to reach another steady-level (Curry et al., 1968). The magnitude of the initial increase in this biphasic response is dependent upon the amount of insulin stored and immediately available for release. This capability is determined by the species involved as well as by the individual animal's past history, which established the "set" of the B cells.

Insulin is also secreted in the intact animal in the basal state without an exogenous glucose stimulus. Glucose appears to be a partial controller of this insulin secretion, but control is separate from the biphasic

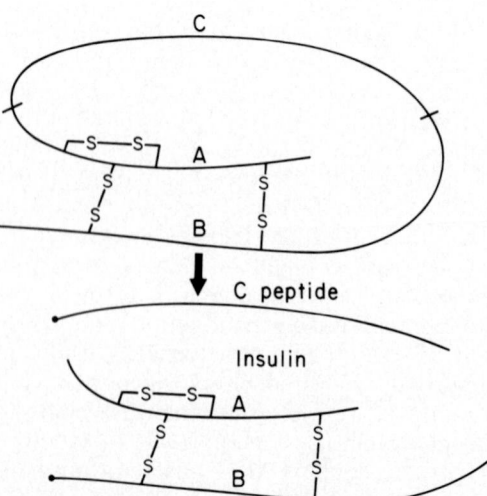

Figure 68–1. Structure of proinsulin and the cleavage that takes place within the pancreatic B cells to produce insulin and C peptide.

response to a glucose load described previously. The basal secretion rate is probably determined by the animal's past history as well as by numerous substances that have the potential for affecting insulin secretion rates (Williams and Porte, 1974).

Glucose has a stimulatory effect on insulin secretion. Fatty acids, ketone bodies, and certain amino acids also have such an effect. There is a wide range of potency of the amino acids, which may be related to the simultaneous stimulation of glucagon and growth hormone (Floyd et al., 1966). The sympathetic and parasympathetic nerves supplying the pancreatic islets are believed important in maintaining normal sensitivity to glucose (Ganong, 1979).

Orally administered glucose or amino acids exert greater insulin-stimulating effects than do intravenously administered agents. It has been shown that glucagon, secretin, cholecystokinin-pancreozymin, gastrin, and gastric inhibitory peptide are intestinal hormones that are secreted in response to oral glucose or amino acids; these substances, in turn, increase insulin secretion. Intravenous loading of glucose or amino acids bypass these important hormones. It appears that the main physiologic action of gastric inhibitory peptide is its glucose-dependent insulinotropic effect. It is the primary gut factor that stimulates insulin secretion (Brown, 1977; Said and Zfass, 1978).

Glucagon increases insulin secretion, even in very small amounts, as a direct B-cell effect. Although glucose regulates insulin and glucagon reciprocally, so that as one rises the other tends to fall, amino acids stimulate both simultaneously. Therefore, in this situation, glucagon may potentiate the insulin-stimulatory properties of amino acids. Glucagon also prevents the uptake and storage of glucose by the liver, allowing for the storage of amino acids in peripheral muscles in response to secreted insulin while protecting the cerebral cortex from hypoglycemia at the same time (Williams and Porte, 1974).

Several other hormones increase insulin concentrations by increasing peripheral tissue resistance to insulin. These antagonistic hormones include growth hormone, glucocorticoids, progesterone, and estrogen. Under the influence of these hormones, hyperinsulinism is observed as a compensation for the insulin resistance. It is unknown whether the hormones directly stimulate the islets or whether this is an indirect effect (Williams and Porte, 1974).

Transport and Binding

Insulin does not appear to be bound to plasma protein after it is secreted. Insulin is fixed to many cells, but red blood cells and most of the cells in the brain do not bind it. Large amounts are bound in the liver and kidneys.

The half-life of insulin in the circulation is about five minutes (Ganong, 1979). It appears that insulin, once secreted by the pancreas, is either bound to liver, kidney, fat, or muscle tissue or lost from the circulation by excretion into the bile, lymph, and to a lesser degree, the urine.

The insulin receptor that accounts for insulin binding is a glycoprotein with a molecular weight of approximately 300,000. This specific insulin binding protein is located in the plasma membrane of cells. The binding of insulin to its receptor does not appear to result in inactivation or other chemical changes in either; rather, this complex appears to be a simple dissociable combination. Bound insulin is not displaced during fasting by glucocorticoids or by peptides such as growth hormone, glucagon, or ACTH. The number of insulin receptors on cells varies, and there is evidence that the number is decreased when plasma insulin is increased and vice versa. Obese individuals have relatively few receptors, and this accounts for their resistance to the effects of insulin (Ganong, 1979; Cuatrecasas, 1972; Freychet et al., 1971).

Principal Actions of Insulin

Adipose Tissue. The body's highest concentration of calories and, therefore, its primary reservoir of energy, is adipose tissue. The concentrations of free fatty acids, glucose, and single amino acids are relatively low in fat. In response to need, adipose tissue can liberate large quantities of free fatty acids and some amino acids. Insulin, however, is the primary hormone for promoting storage of nutrients in adipose tissue and it prevents fat breakdown. After binding, insulin stimulates intracellular synthesis of glycogen, fat, protein, and nucleic acids. It increases glucose oxidation and markedly increases formation of triglyceride by increasing formation of fatty acids within fat cells (Williams and Porte, 1974).

As insulin promotes production, it decreases breakdown, that is, glycogenolysis, lipolysis, and proteolysis. Numerous compounds appear to stimulate lipolysis and are, therefore, insulin antagonists. These include glucocorticoids, growth hormone, glucagon, and others (Williams and Porte, 1974).

Muscle. Insulin's effect on muscle is mainly anabolic, which is similar to the actions it has on adipose tissue. In muscle, however, it stimulates greater protein, nucleotide, and glycogen synthesis, but diminishes triglyceride formation.

Insulin decreases catabolic processes such as glycogenolysis, proteolysis, lipolysis, and fatty acid oxidation. As in adipocytes, insulin promotes transmembrane passage of certain sugars and amino acids, as well as potassium and magnesium ions. It has also been suggested that insulin may play a role in changing electrical membrane potentials of muscle cells, thus causing a net increase in intracellular potassium and a decrease in sodium. These alterations in membrane potential may also play a role in other transport functions of the cell wall.

Liver. The cells of muscle and adipose tissue contain a specific transport system that is catalyzed by insulin. Liver cells, on the other hand, are freely permeable to glucose. Once glucose enters the hepatocyte, the initial reaction is phosphorylation, with the formation of glucose-6-phosphate. The formation of this substance is catalyzed by two enzymes, hexokinase and glucokinase. There is evidence that glucokinase is an inducible enzyme, with insulin, rather than glucose, serving as the inducer. It appears that insulin exerts long-term control over the amount of enzyme present, while short-term regulation is determined by the sensitivity of the enzyme to changes in glucose concentration. Insulin also exerts a marked stimulating effect on glycogen synthetase, which is a key enzyme in the synthesis of glycogen.

Normally, as the blood sugar rises above approximately 120 mg/dl, release of glucose from the liver is markedly inhibited as glucose uptake by hepatocytes increases; these changes are catalyzed by insulin. The opposite reaction — glucose release by the liver — is seen as blood sugar falls and is associated with increases in lipolysis and gluconeogene-

sis, which are stimulated by growth hormone, glucocorticoids, epinephrine, and glucagon.

Table 68–2 summarizes the principal actions of insulin. It must be remembered that insulin increases the entry of glucose into many tissues (increased tissue utilization) and decreases net release of glucose from the liver. These actions prevent hyperglycemia and increase utilization of metabolic substrates.

GLUCAGON

Structure

Glucagon is a product of the A cells of the pancreatic islets of Langerhans and of similar cells in the wall of the stomach and duodenum. Porcine and human glucagon are identical small, linear polypeptides containing 29 amino acids. Evidence suggests that glucagon is formed from a larger polypeptide precursor (proglucagon) in the A cells.

Metabolism

Glucagon has a plasma half-life of five to ten minutes and is primarily degraded by

Table 68–2. Principal Actions of Insulin

Adipose tissue
1. Increased glucose entry
2. Increased fatty acid synthesis
3. Increased glycerol phosphate synthesis
4. Increased triglyceride deposition
5. Activation of lipoprotein lipase
6. Inhibition of hormone-sensitive lipase
7. Increased K^+ uptake

Muscle
1. Increased glucose entry
2. Increased glycogen synthesis
3. Increased amino acid uptake
4. Increased protein synthesis in ribosomes
5. Decreased protein catabolism
6. Decreased release of gluconeogenic amino acids
7. Increased ketone uptake
8. Increased K^+ uptake

Liver
1. Decreased cyclic AMP
2. Decreased ketogenesis
3. Increased protein synthesis
4. Increased lipid synthesis
5. Decreased glucose output due to decreased gluconeogenesis and increased glycogen synthesis

the liver. Peripheral circulatory concentrations of glucagon are low relative to the levels found in the portal vein. This discrepancy is explained by the liver's capacity to utilize and remove glucagon from the portal blood.

Action

Glucagon and insulin have opposite metabolic effects. Insulin is glucogenic, antigluconeogenic, and antilipolytic in its actions; it is a hormone of energy storage. Glucagon, however, is a hormone of energy release; it is a glycogenolytic and ketogenic hormone. Glucagon stimulates hepatic breakdown of glycogen via activation of adenylate cyclase, which leads to an increase in phosphorylase. It increases gluconeogenesis from available amino acids in the liver and elevates the metabolic rate.

Regulation of Secretion

Glucagon secretion is decreased by a rise in plasma glucose levels, an effect that requires the presence of insulin. Thus, the A cells of the islet can be characterized as insulin-dependent tissue. Secretion of glucagon is also responsive to the sympathetic nerves of the pancreas, as is insulin. Stimulation of beta-adrenergic receptors increases secretion, and stimulation of alpha-adrenergic receptors inhibits secretion of glucagon. The overall pancreatic A cell response to sympathetic stimulation, however, is increased secretion of glucagon; thus, the beta-receptors appear to predominate. The sympathetic nerves are important mediators, at least in part, of the response to stresses such as those of infection, trauma, and exercise.

Both intake of a protein-containing meal and infusions of various amino acids increase glucagon secretion. Under the influence of glucagon, the liver converts the glucogenic amino acids to glucose. The increased glucagon secretion following a protein meal is an important protective measure of the pancreas. Since amino acids and/or protein stimulate insulin secretion, hypoglycemia would follow a protein meal if glucagon were not secreted to maintain homeostasis.

Glucagon secretion increases during fasting. These concentrations decline as fatty acids and ketones become the major source of energy. The gastrointestinal mucosa plays a role in glucagon secretion by releasing cholecystokinin-pancreozymin and gastrin, both of which stimulate the A cells.

Glucagon secretion is inhibited by somatostatin, free fatty acids, and ketones. However, the inhibitory effects of the latter two may be overriden, as is seen in diabetic ketoacidosis.

HYPOINSULINISM (DIABETES MELLITUS)

PATHOPHYSIOLOGY

In the state of a relative or absolute deficiency in insulin, glucose obtained from the diet or via hepatic gluconeogenesis is not efficiently or normally utilized by muscle, adipose tissue, or the liver itself. Consequently, glucose accumulates in the blood (hyperglycemia), and as its concentration exceeds the renal tubular maximum transport threshold, glucose spills into the urine (glycosuria). The renal threshold for glucose in the dog is usually between 175 and 220 mg/dl. Glycosuria creates an osmotic diuresis, causing polyuria and, thus, obligatory polydipsia. Polyphagia occurs because the body is literally starving in spite of hyperglycemia. In response to this starvation caused by insulin deficiency, fat and muscle enter a catabolic state to provide energy for needy tissues. As polydipsia, polyuria, polyphagia, and weight loss become obvious to an owner, the pet is brought to the veterinarian for care.

Unfortunately, some cats and dogs are not identified by their owners as having symptoms of disease, and these untreated diabetics may ultimately develop ketoacidosis. As discussed previously, insulin deficiency alone will result in increased lipolysis. The nonesterified fatty acids released from adipose tissue are assimilated by the liver at a rate dependent on their plasma concentration and are also used extrahepatically as oxidative fuels. With insulin present, fatty acids are incorporated into triglycerides, but when insulin is lacking these fatty acids are converted into the CoA derivative called acyl CoA, which is oxidized to acetyl CoA (Fig. 68–2) (Alberti and Hockaday, 1977). In severe diabetes this acetyl CoA is diverted almost entirely to ketone body formation with the formation of acetoacetyl CoA and hence to acetoacetic acid. Acetoacetic acid is further metabolized to beta-hydroxybutyric

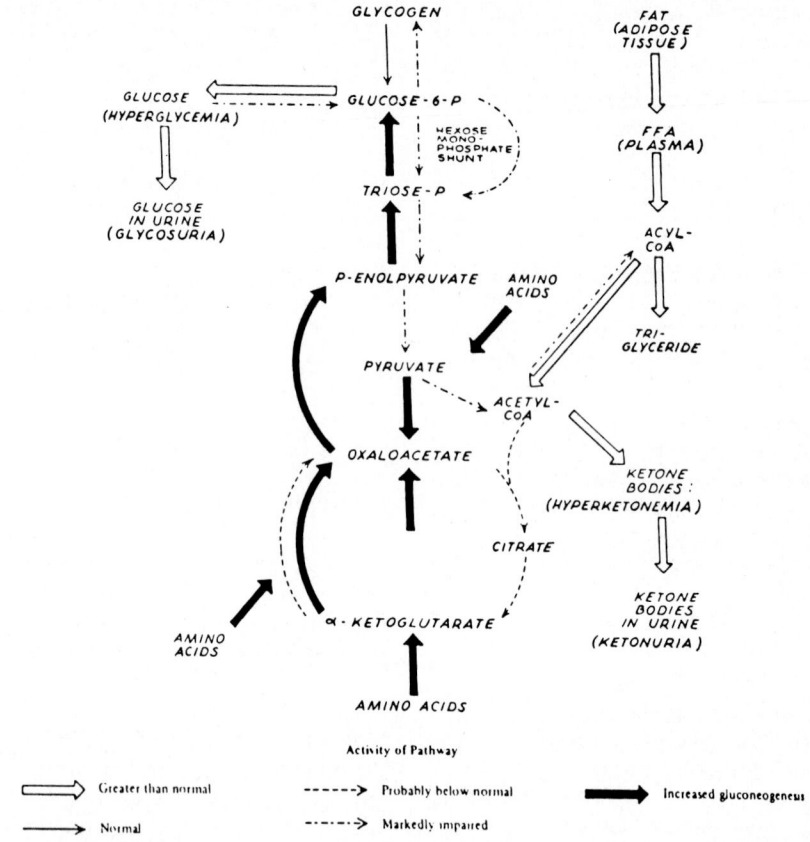

Figure 68–2. Metabolic abnormalities in the liver in uncontrolled diabetes.

acid, and a third physiologic ketone body, acetone, arises by spontaneous decarboxylation of acetoacetate. These ketone bodies — acetoacetic acid, beta-hydroxybutyric acid, and acetone — result in the ketosis and acidosis of ketoacidosis.

In a short-term situation, the conversion of free fatty acids to ketone bodies is actually a positive process. The condition of diabetes mellitus is interpreted physiologically as being a state of starvation. In the face of starvation, ketone bodies can be used in place of sugar by many tissues; thus, the production of ketone bodies is a safety measure by the body. However, the liver has tremendous potential for producing large quantities of ketone bodies. The rate of ketogenesis is linked to the rate of gluconeogenesis; the more rapid the latter, the more rapid is ketone production (Alberti and Hockaday, 1977). Inhibition of ketogenesis has been demonstrated to follow inhibition of gluconeogenesis (Blackshear et al., 1975). Linking of the two processes may explain why ketogenesis is more active in uncon-

trolled diabetes than in starvation, since gluconeogenesis is more rapid in diabetes owing to insulin deficiency. Concentrations of ketones in the extracellular space are further increased, because owing to insulin deficiency, the peripheral tissues are less able to utilize ketones (Balasse and Neef, 1975). These ketones can overwhelm the body's buffering system, causing an increase in arterial hydrogen ion concentration and a decrease in serum bicarbonate. As ketones accumulate in the extracellular space, they surpass the renal threshold and eventually spill into the urine, contributing to an osmotic diuresis (Fig. 68–2). In the short term the production of ketones can be life preserving, but in the long term the severe metabolic consequences of ketone production, which include acidosis, osmotic diuresis, dehydration, vomiting, and obtundation, can ultimately be fatal.

In addition to ketone production, the other major metabolic disturbance of diabetic ketoacidosis is hyperglycemia. The relative or absolute deficiency of insulin that results in the development of ketosis also contributes to the underutilization or lack of utilization of sugar. Glycosuria concomitant with hyperglycemia is a potent osmotic diuretic that causes not only a loss of water but also depletion of sodium, potassium, and chloride. Further loss of water and electrolytes will occur as a result of repeated bouts of vomiting or diarrhea, which often are associated with diabetic ketoacidosis. Overproduction of glucose by the liver compounds this metabolic disease state.

Insulin deficiency causes a marked increase first in glycogenolysis, with total depletion of glycogen stores, and then in gluconeogenesis (Alberti and Hockaday, 1977). The enhanced rate of fatty acid oxidation enables gluconeogenesis to proceed more quickly (Blackshear, 1974) as the enhanced gluconeogenesis increases ketogenesis. In addition, ingested glucose, no longer utilized by the liver (Felig, 1975; Johnston and Alberti, 1976), passes entirely into the peripheral circulation and brings about a rapid, large rise in blood glucose concentration (Alberti et al., 1975). A further rise in blood glucose concentration is the result of decreased transport and metabolism of glucose into nonhepatic, insulin-dependent tissues (Fig. 68–3). Glucose metabolism may also be inhibited by the rise in peripheral fatty acid and ketone concentrations (Randle et al., 1963; Newsholme, 1976).

The hyperglycemia, osmotic diuresis, and prerenal uremia that occur in these dogs often result in moderate to severe hyperosmolarity of the extracellular fluid.

Glucagon, Epinephrine, Cortisol, and Growth Hormone

The previous discussion on the pathogenesis of diabetes mellitus and ketoacidosis is based primarily on a unihormone theory that all of the metabolic aberrations of severe diabetes are the direct consequence of insulin deficiency. Over the past several years it has become increasingly evident that certain of the metabolic abnormalities formerly attributed solely to insulin deficiency are invariably associated with a relative or absolute increase in the stress hormones glucagon, epinephrine, cortisol, and growth hormone. Studies negating a simple role for insulin deficiency in ketoacidosis reveal the normal plasma insulin concentration in the majority of ketoacidotic cases (Schade and Eaton, 1979), as well as the delayed onset of ketoacidosis after insulin withdrawal from diabetics (Muller et al., 1973). Further support of the influence of other hormones in the development of ketoacidosis is the lack of hypolipolytic and hypoketonemic effects of insulin without prior stress hormone adipocyte and hepatocyte stimulation (Mahler et al., 1964).

Evidence that stress hormones (glucagon, catecholamines, cortisol, and growth hormone) contribute to the metabolic decompensation of ketoacidosis materialized when

Figure 68–3. Disordered blood glucose homeostasis in insulin deficiency. The heavy arrows indicate reactions that are accentuated. The rectangles across arrows indicate reactions that are blocked.

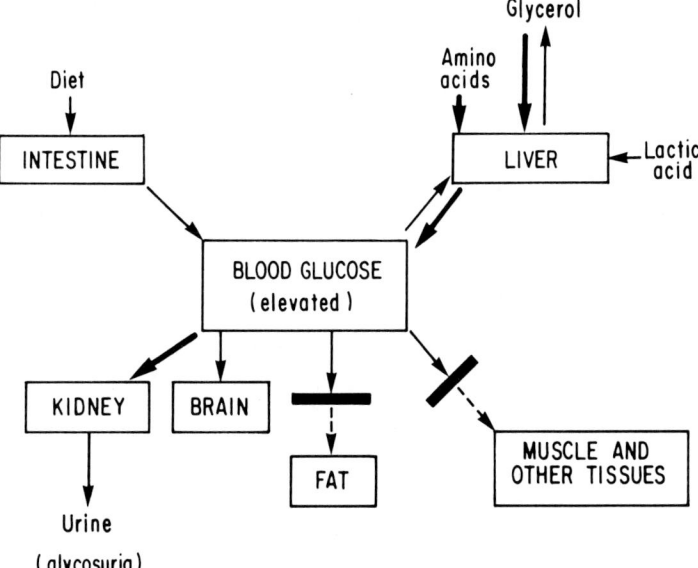

measurement of plasma hormone concentrations became feasible after 1960. In every case of diabetic ketoacidosis in which these hormones were measured, their concentrations were elevated (Schade and Eaton, 1979). The only exception to this generalization was the concentration of plasma growth hormone. It is now suggested that the diabetogenic effects of growth hormone may be expressed at a time when the concentration of this hormone has returned to the normal range (Schade et al., 1978).

Further evidence that stress hormones play a role in the pathogenesis of diabetic ketoacidosis follows: (1) Pharmacologic blockade of each of the stress hormones reduces the rate and/or frequency of metabolic decompensation, such as the use of somastatin to suppress glucagon (Gerich, 1976; Dobbs et al., 1977); (2) removal of the pituitary and/or the adrenal glands, which eliminates the source of some stress hormones, completely prevents the development of ketoacidosis after insulin withdrawal in diabetic animals; and (3) administration of each of the four stress hormones under appropriate conditions induces metabolic decompensation in diabetes with "normal" circulating concentrations of plasma insulin (Schade and Eaton, 1979). This information has important clinical application. Infection, the most common precipitating factor in diabetic ketoacidosis, causes a marked increase in secretion of both cortisol (Beisel et al., 1967) and glucagon (Rocha et al., 1973). This may explain the association between infection and ketoacidosis. Other common precipitating factors include heart disease and trauma, both of which are associated with increased circulating levels of glucagon and catecholamines (Alberti and Hockaday, 1977).

Diabetic ketoacidosis is a heterogenous syndrome in which many factors may participate in a pathogenic role. The major hormonal abnormalities include a relative deficiency of insulin and a concurrent excess of stress hormones (Fig. 68–4). Since the clinical cause of diabetic ketoacidosis is characteristically a stress, rather than insulin withdrawal, future research may provide safe and effective pharmacologic methods of blocking the diabetogenic effects of excess stress hormone secretion.

Classification of Diabetes

Classification of animal diabetics has not been used in a clinical setting. With the development of the insulin radioimmunoassay, however, recent comparisons between canine and human stages of diabetes have been proposed. The comparisons are based on reports that juvenile human diabetics have minimal or undetectable endogenous insulin concentrations, while the stable, adult-onset diabetics have normal or elevated concentrations (Berson and Yalow, 1965). One early study of spontaneous canine diabetics revealed low endogenous insulin concentrations in six of seven patients. These were believed to be consistent with juvenile human diabetes. One dog, however, had normal insulin concentrations (Manns and Martin, 1972). In a subsequent study by Hendriks et al. (1976), overtly diabetic dogs were compared with normal dogs and those with latent diabetes. Insulin and glucose concentrations as well as glucose tolerance tests were compared. The widely varying results in endogenous insulin concentrations were comparable to the classifications used in humans.

A series of 22 diabetic dogs were studied by Kaneko et al. (1977). On the basis of fasting plasma glucose and insulin concentrations, plus glucose tolerance tests, these animals were separated into three distinct groups. These included a type I diabetic comparable to the juvenile (absolute insulin

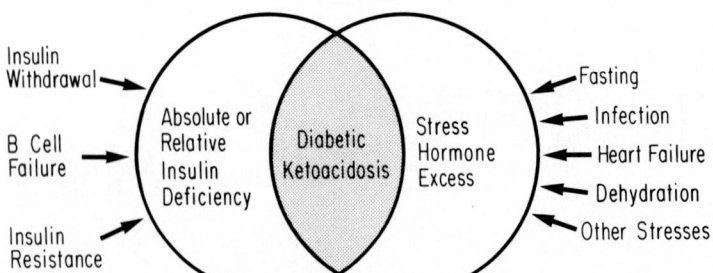

Figure 68–4. The hormonal pathogenesis of diabetic ketoacidosis, illustrating the interaction of insulin deficiency and stress hormone excess necessary in the development of the ketoacidotic state.

deficiency) form of human diabetes, a type II diabetic comparable to maturity onset (relative insulin deficiency) form of human diabetes, and a type III that was compared with chemical (subclinical) diabetes in man. It was suggested that these different types represent stages in the natural history of the development of diabetes mellitus in dogs. Whether this classification scheme will ultimately be shown to have a clinical application, as has been suggested (Kaneko, 1979) remains to be seen.

Diabetogenic Factors

Factors that increase the chance of an animal's developing diabetes mellitus include genetic predisposition, diet and/or obesity, hormone abnormalities, islet cell destruction, and stress. The ultimate development of diabetes is difficult to predict.

Dogs or cats with a family history of diabetes are uncommon (Gershwin, 1975; Kramer, 1977), although this may be a result of a lack of family history for most pet dogs. Familial tendency to develop diabetes probably exists and awaits detailed study. In a recent epidemiologic study on diabetes mellitus in dogs, a number of common dog breeds including cocker spaniels, German shepherds, collies, Pekingese, and boxers appeared to be at relatively low risk. This indicates a possible genetic resistance of these breeds to diabetes or precursor diseases. Puliks, Cairn terriers, and miniature pinschers are breeds at higher risk than explained by breed popularity, which reflects a definite probability of genetic predisposition (Marmor et al., 1982).

A strong association exists between obesity and diabetes mellitus. In most instances, there is also a strong association between dietary intake and obesity. Obese human diabetics tend to have a *relative* deficiency of insulin secretion. This is further complicated by the reversible insulin resistance seen in obesity.

A close association is seen between the development of diabetes mellitus and the use of various pharmaceuticals. The most commonly used drugs that have been implicated as causing diabetes include glucocorticoids and progestogens. Many other hormones can be related to this disease. Although steroid diabetes is most often observed when adrenal corticosteroids are used systemically, in rare instances such side effects follow the topical application of steroids in the treatment of dermatologic disorders (Kershbaum, 1963). The diminished carbohydrate tolerance is the result of several mechanisms. The principal mechanism is the increase of glucose production by the liver as a result of gluconeogenesis. Other mechanisms are the mobilization of fatty acids from tissue stores, an antagonism to insulin action at the receptor level, and decreased utilization of glucose by the tissues (Alberti and Hockaday, 1977). In most instances, steroid diabetes is reversed when the drug is discontinued, although iatrogenic diabetes in a previously normal dog or cat may be indicative of subclinical diabetes mellitus. Progesterone therapy, especially in the feline, has been shown to cause a reversible diabetic state. Other administered hormones (ACTH, glucagon, estrogen, epinephrine) have been associated with a diabetes-like state in dogs. Numerous nonsteroidal agents, including chlorpromazine, diphenylhydantoin, furosemide, and thiazides (Williams and Porte, 1974), have been implicated in affecting glucose tolerance by causing hyperglycemia in man.

Endogenous hormone excess or alteration may also be associated with a diabetic state. This includes hyperadrenocorticism, which, in the author's experience, is complicated by overt diabetes in five to ten per cent of canine cases. In a recent review of 71 dogs with hyperadrenocorticism, seven had overt diabetes mellitus (Lubberink, 1977); in another, 57 per cent of the dogs had above-normal fasting blood glucose values (Ling et al., 1979). Hyperadrenocorticism is uncommon in the feline. However, all three cases seen by the author and all reported cases have involved diabetics that have been difficult to control (Fox and Beatty, 1975; Meijer et al., 1978; Swift and Brown, 1976).

The estrous cycle of the bitch is a second example of endogenously produced hormones that deleteriously affect glucose tolerance. Estrogen and, more importantly, progesterone appear to decrease peripheral sensitivity to insulin (Gebhardt and Garnett, 1975). Several reviews of canine diabetes have revealed that the intact bitch is most prone to develop diabetes mellitus and that she is likely to first show symptoms during estrus or diestrus (Joshua, 1963; Wilkinson, 1960; Gartner et al., 1968; Foster, 1975).

Destruction of the B cells of the pancreatic islets is an obvious diabetogenic factor;

rarely, this is attributed to trauma, surgical manipulation, or growing neoplasms. Pancreatitis, however, is a common problem in today's well-fed pet population. In a recent survey of diabetic dogs, eight of 33 necropsied dogs had evidence of previous episodes of pancreatitis. Also, 29 of the 33 dogs had reduced numbers or absence of islet cells together with degeneration, hyalinization, or vacuolation of these cells (Ling et al., 1977). In a study of ten cats with spontaneous diabetes, nine had congophilic protein deposits in the islets, which were believed to be the cause of the disease. One cat showed primary atrophy, degranulation, and hydropic degeneration of the islets as seen in diabetic dogs or young human cases (Loppnow and Gemhardt, 1976).

Stress may be an important factor in causing the latent diabetic to become overt in symptomatology. Stress may include injury, infection, pregnancy, or any acute illness. Again, the relation between these stresses and overt diabetes may rest with the interplay of certain hormones (cortisol, glucagon, growth hormone, epinephrine) in a patient suffering from a relative or absolute insulin deficiency.

CLINICAL FEATURES

Age, Sex, and Breed

The age and sex distributions of dogs with diabetes mellitus in several series reveal that most affected dogs are 4 to 14 years old, with a peak incidence at 7 to 9 years of age (Marmor et al., 1982). Females are affected about twice as frequently as males. The disease has been recognized in puppies, but this has not been found to be common. The breeds most often mentioned in a recent review include dachshunds and poodles (Marmor et al., 1982). In cats, the disease is most common in the domestic shorthair older than five years of age. No significant sex predilection was determined in cats, although 67 per cent of the cases reported were males (Schaer, 1976).

Anamnesis

The anamnesis in virtually all diabetics includes the classic alterations of polydipsia, polyuria, polyphagia, and weight loss. Owners will often bring previously housebroken pets to the veterinarian because they notice the dog or cat urinating in the home.

The other symptoms are established by further questioning of the owner. A complete anamnesis is extremely important even in the so-called "obvious diabetic," because the clinician must be aware of any complicating or concurrent problem in the patient. Since these dogs are usually older animals, all the potential disorders of any geriatric animal must be evaluated. In addition, the clinician must ask, "Why has the patient shown symptoms now?" In many instances these are believed to be borderline or latent diabetics that develop overt diabetes secondary to drug therapy, pancreatitis, congestive heart failure, estrous cycle, or a myriad of other potential causes.

Physical Examination

There are no classic physical examination findings typical of the nonketotic diabetic. Most dogs and cats are obese but are otherwise in good physical condition. Dogs with prolonged untreated diabetes may lose a good deal of weight but are rarely thin. Weight loss is due to lack of glucose utilization, plus the catabolic processes involving muscle and adipose tissue. Secondary to mobilization of fats is the development of hepatic lipidosis, and therefore, hepatomegaly is one of the clinical findings in diabetic dogs. As will be further explained, cataracts are another common clinical finding in these patients.

Diagnosis

Diabetes mellitus is suspected whenever there is a history of polydipsia, polyuria, polyphagia, and weight loss. The diagnosis is confirmed by the finding of persistent fasting hyperglycemia. The normal fasting blood glucose concentration in the dog is 70 to 110 mg/dl, and the repeated finding of *fasting* values greater than 150 mg/dl is usually considered diagnostic of overt diabetes in the absence of complicating factors. Complicating factors include hyperglycemia induced by stress (which can be quite dramatic in the feline), postprandial hyperglycemia (which should be less that 120 mg/dl), or hyperglycemia in an animal receiving diabetogenic medications (Feldman, 1980).

When the blood glucose concentration exceeds the renal threshold, glycosuria results; this is easily detected with Diastix paper strips or Clinitest tablets. Glycosuria without hyperglycemia can be caused by primary renal disease (most often noted in the Norwegian elkhound and basenji) (see Chapter 26) (Finco et al., 1970).

It must be emphasized that in the nonketotic feline, the anamnesis is of paramount importance. The hyperglycemic, fractious cat without the classic symptoms of polydipsia, polyuria, polyphagia, and weight loss is usually not diabetic but simply quite stressed. In the dog, however, persistent fasting hyperglycemia with concomitant glycosuria is diagnostic of diabetes mellitus. Factors such as hyperadrenocorticism, estrus, drugs, and so forth may be the primary insult, but many of these patients require therapy for the diabetes mellitus, at least until the causative factor has been removed.

Carbohydrate Tolerance Test. In the dog or cat with overt diabetes mellitus, carbohydrate tolerance testing is unnecessary in establishing a diagnosis. With our present knowledge, information gained from a glucose tolerance test (GTT) would not alter therapy or prognosis. However, circumstances do exist in which a GTT is indicated. The major indication for a GTT is the animal with borderline hyperglycemia (120 to 175 mg/dl) without concomitant glycosuria. Other instances that would possibly dictate running such a test would be the animal that has glycosuria without diagnostic hyperglycemia or the pet with a family history of diabetes mellitus that does not have symptoms or chemistry alterations itself. In the author's clinical practice, the GTT is rarely performed.

The drawback of any GTT is that while it is a sensitive study, the test is not necessarily specific for determining pancreatic B cell function. In other words, the GTT is influenced by diet, drugs, nonpancreatic disease, fear, and other variables that may or may not be controlled or obvious. In man, specific diets and activity plans are recommended for several days prior to the test. Also, all nonessential medications are discontinued prior to testing. Glucose tolerance deteriorates later in the day, and therefore, standard tests are done in the morning (Prout, 1975). The dangers of performing a GTT are very small. Even patients with undiagnosed elevated blood glucose values that inadvertently are given a loading dose of glucose for testing purposes are not likely to be harmed (Prout, 1975).

There appears to be general agreement in the human literature that the *oral* GTT provides the most reliable information. Intravenous (IV) GTT is reserved for patients in whom oral glucose administration might yield equivocal data, such as patients who have had a subtotal gastrectomy (Prout, 1975).

The protocol for an oral GTT would be to administer glucose at a dose of 1.75 gm per kilogram of ideal body weight as a 25 per

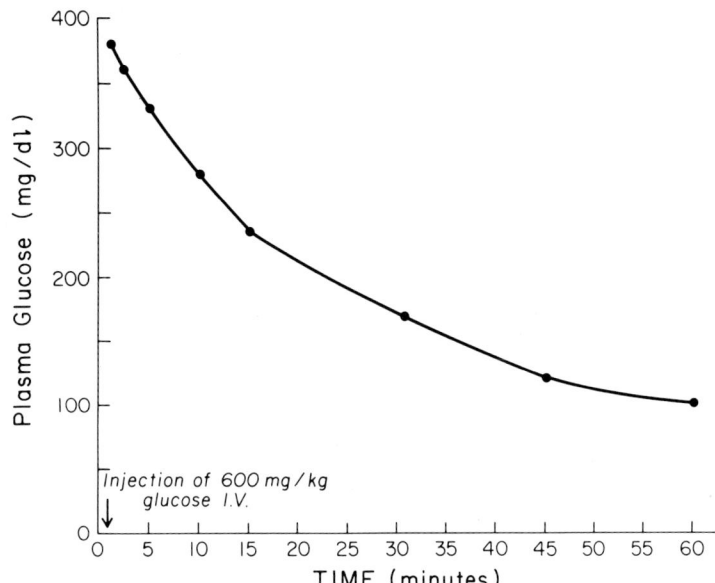

Figure 68–5. Intravenous glucose tolerance test curve in the normal dog.

cent solution. Allow several minutes to administer the fluid, since vomiting will result if it is given too rapidly. A pretest blood glucose is obtained, as well as 30-, 60-, 90-, 120-, and 180-minute samples. In the normal dog, the plasma glucose concentration should return to the normal range within 60 to 90 minutes of glucose loading.

Kaneko (1979) has recommended the intravenous GTT with concurrent measurement of both glucose and insulin concentrations. After an overnight fast, glucose is administered at the dose of 600 mg per kilogram of body weight as a 50 per cent solution (Rottiers et al., 1981). This infusion is injected over a 30-second time period. Using another vein, samples are obtained prior to the glucose injection and at 5, 15, 25, 35, 45, and 60 minutes after administration. Here, the blood glucose should return to normal by 60 minutes (Fig. 68–5). Using this technique, dogs have been separated into the three categories described above. Unfortunately, glucose and insulin determinations on multiple samples are expensive. More importantly, such data gathering is not necessary to aid in the diagnosis or treatment of the overt diabetic. Continuing research may aid in putting this information to prognostic or therapeutic use.

Clinicopathology. A thorough laboratory and radiographic evaluation is recommended for any suspected or known diabetic. The clinician must be aware of any disease that might be causing or contributing to the carbohydrate intolerance, such as hyperadrenocorticism, infection, pancreatitis, congestive heart failure, liver or renal disease, and many others. Finally, the practitioner should be searching for abnormalities caused by the diabetic state, such as prerenal uremia, urinary tract infection, or ketoacidosis.

The minimum laboratory evaluations in any candidate for long-term insulin therapy should include a urinalysis, fasting blood glucose, complete blood count (CBC), renal function test (BUN or creatinine), total serum protein, serum albumin, serum glutamic pyruvic transaminase (SGPT), and serum alkaline phosphatase. Dogs suffering from vomiting, diarrhea, anorexia, and dehydration should be evaluated for pancreatitis as well as electrolyte and acid-base balance. Stool testing for trypsin activity should be considered. The thorax and abdomen should be examined radiographically. After obtaining the anamnesis and completing the physical examination, other tests may be warranted.

Since most veterinarians utilize clinical laboratories that offer panels of tests rather than individual tests, the common alterations that occur secondary to diabetes mellitus will be reviewed. Obvious lipemia is frequently encountered in the untreated diabetic. In uncontrolled diabetes, there is an increase in the plasma concentration of triglycerides, cholesterol, lipoproteins, chylomicrons, and free fatty acids. These factors contribute to the development of lipemic plasma. The rise in these constituents is due mainly to decreased removal of triglycerides into the fat depots. The enzyme lipoprotein lipase aids in the metabolism of very low-density lipoprotein (VLDL) and chylomicrons. Without insulin, lipoprotein lipase fails to be produced and the lipemia mentioned above is produced. With insulin therapy, the triglyceride-rich VLDL and chylomicrons are metabolized and triglyceride concentrations will be reduced. Low-density lipoprotein, which is high in cholesterol, is a by-product of chylomicron metabolism. Therefore, the treated diabetic often is seen to have reducing serum triglyceride concentrations and elevated serum cholesterol concentrations. This alteration may persist for months (Karam, 1980).

In diabetes, the plasma cholesterol concentration is usually elevated, and this may play a role in the accelerated development of the arteriosclerotic vascular disease, which is a major long-term complication of diabetes in humans. There is evidence that in severe diabetes, cholesterol synthesis is decreased. Part of the rise in plasma cholesterol is due to an increase in the cholesterol containing very low-density and low-density beta-lipoproteins secondary to the great increase in circulating triglycerides. Another factor may be a decline in hepatic degradation of cholesterol (Ganong, 1979).

Serum enzyme analyses are frequently used. The serum glutamic pyruvic transaminase (SGPT) and alkaline phosphatase levels are commonly elevated in association with the fatty infiltration of the liver that accompanies the tremendous mobilization of fats seen in the diabetic. In addition, the BSP retention time will also be prolonged in some diabetic dogs. Because of these expected secondary abnormal liver tests, the diagnosis of concurrent liver disease in the animal with diabetes mellitus is difficult.

Both chronic and acute pancreatitis may be the cause of the diabetic condition of a dog or cat (Ling et al., 1977; Cotton et al., 1971). With this possible correlation, those diabetics with concurrent pancreatitis will commonly have elevated serum lipase concentrations. Chronic pancreatitis may ultimately result in the diabetic state. In most chronic pancreatitis cases the serum lipase concentrations will be normal. In dogs or cats with symptoms of both diabetes mellitus and exocrine pancreatic insufficiency, suitable diagnostic studies should be pursued (see Chapter 61).

The complete blood count and blood urea nitrogen (BUN) concentrations are usually normal in the uncomplicated diabetic. Elevation of the white blood count may be caused by an infectious process, which should be identified. An elevated BUN may be caused by primary renal disease or prerenal uremia secondary to dehydration.

The urinalysis provides extremely valuable information. The uncomplicated diabetic should have glycosuria without ketonuria. In addition, proteinuria may be the result of urinary tract infection or glomerular damage secondary to the disruption of the basement membrane associated with diabetes mellitus (Feldman and Feldman, 1977). A careful inspection of the urine sediment for changes consistent with infection (white blood cells, red blood cells, protein, bacteria) must be made, because infection is common (Ling et al., 1977). Whenever possible, urine obtained by cystocentesis using aseptic techniques should be submitted for culture and sensitivity if evidence of urinary tract infection is found.

Radiographically, the common finding in diabetic dogs and cats is hepatomegaly. This is a common alteration seen in diabetes mellitus due to fatty infiltration of the liver. With proper therapy the liver size will slowly return toward normal. Other uncommon changes on radiographs of diabetic dogs and cats include the intramural and intraluminal emphysema of the urinary bladder, which is associated with urinary tract infection. In addition, right-sided cranial abdominal indistinctness may be a clue to the presence of pancreatitis in some diabetics (Ticer, 1977).

Glycosylated hemoglobin (HbA$_{1C}$) appears to be formed by a nonenzymatic, post-translational modification of the hemoglobin molecule. The rate of glycosylation is dependent on the nature and concentration of carbohydrate in the red blood cell. Because red blood cells are insulin-independent, hyperglycemia for long periods of time causes increased production of HbA$_{1C}$. Therefore, measurement of this hemoglobin may aid in determining the success of any particular insulin regimen, since good diabetic control should result in normal or near normal HbA$_{1C}$ concentrations. Poor diabetic control would result in elevated levels (Wood and Smith, 1980).

TREATMENT

Oral Hypoglycemic Agents. These drugs have commonly been used in humans with adult-onset diabetes mellitus, but they have rarely been employed in veterinary practice. Diabetic dogs and cats are almost consistently absolute insulin-deficient animals; they require insulin to control their diabetes. Therefore, we believe that the Type II and Type III diabetics described by Kaneko et al. (1977) need further definition. Such dogs often are found to have hyperadrenocorticism or to be in the luteal phase of an estrus cycle. Insulin-antagonistic drug therapy must also be ruled out.

Insulin. By the time diabetes mellitus is diagnosed in the dog or cat, daily injections of insulin are usually required to control the disease. NPH insulin is currently the most widely used form of insulin.

All insulins should be kept from extremes of heat or cold, and the contents of the bottle must be mixed thoroughly (not shaken) before each dose is given. Following subcutaneous administration of NPH insulin, the onset of action in dogs is approximately one to three hours; peak blood levels occur in four to eight hours, and the total duration of effect is twelve to twenty-four hours. PZI insulin is thought to be less potent and longer acting (Table 68–3). As the effect of insulin reaches its maximum, blood glucose concentration falls. To avoid the induction of possible hypoglycemic reactions, feeding must be timed to correspond with the period prior to insulin's greatest activity (Fig. 68–6).

In a recent study by Comerci et al. (1980), questions were raised concerning the half-life of NPH insulin after administration in

Table 68–3. Effects of Commonly Used Insulin Preparations in the Canine

Type	Form	Route	Hours After Injection		
			Effects Begin	*Maximum Action*	*Duration of Effects*
Regular	Solution	IM	1/4	1 to 3	4 to 8
Regular	Solution	SQ	1/2	2 to 4	6 to 8
NPH	Crystalline	SQ	1 to 3	4 to 8	12 to 20
PZI	Amorphous	SQ	3 to 4	14 to 20	24 to 36

the dog. They found the biological half-life to be 53.2 ± 8.7 minutes. Unfortunately, this insulin was injected intramuscularly, not via the recommended subcutaneous route. Further studies are needed to determine if the biologic activity of various insulins in dogs and cats are radically different from that in the human.

NPH and PZI insulin, 100 units per ml (U100), are the preparations available to most veterinarians. Since cats and small dogs often require small doses, the insulin can be diluted with saline to make administration of the correct amount easier for the owner. A 1:10 dilution is prepared, so that a full 100 unit syringe contains only ten units of insulin. Many pharmacists are reluctant to dilute insulin because diluted insulin is

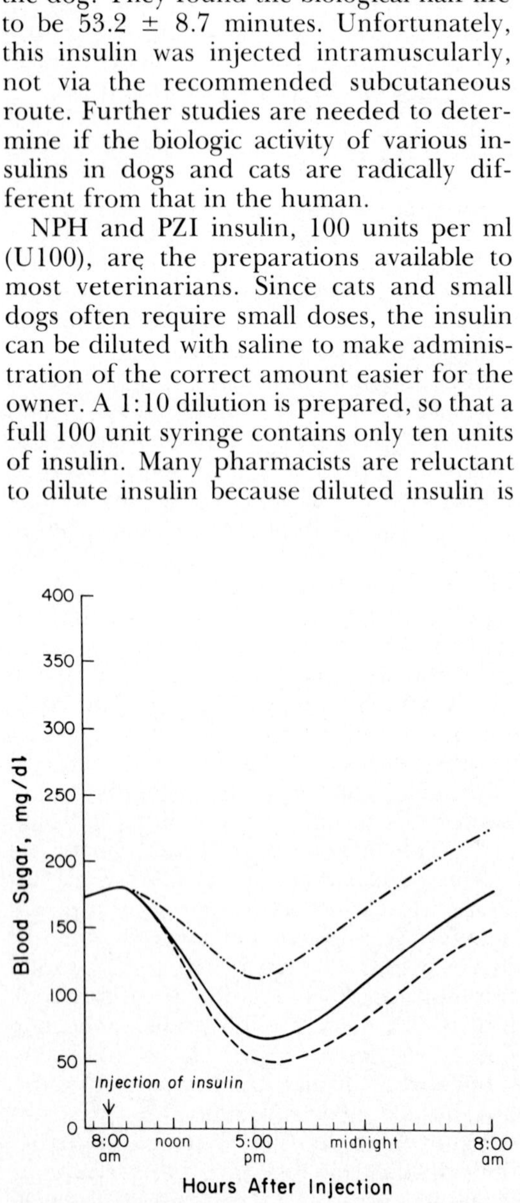

Figure 68–6. Ideal blood glucose concentrations over a 24-hour period after NPH insulin administration (_____). Also illustrated is the ideal response to excess insulin dose (........) as well as an insufficient dose of insulin (__ .. __ .. __).

reported to be unstable. However, the author has found dilute insulin to be stable over a period of two to three months. Nevertheless, it is wise to remember that this insulin has been altered. If problems arise in regulating a patient on diluted insulin, the clinician should realize that the insulin may be at fault.

Client Instruction. Diabetes mellitus is a serious disease and its treatment requires capable and willing owners. These owners must accept the responsibility for giving daily injections and feeding their pets at the proper time of day. Even though such a pet requires much more care than normal, it is unusual in this author's experience to have a client reject the responsibility and choose euthanasia.

This responsibility is important because of the serious consequences of improper care. Acute insulin *overdosage* can result in a hypoglycemic episode, which may be seen as weakness and lethargy, changed behavior, or loss of consciousness and convulsions. Chronic *underdosage* can result in the cascade of metabolic changes that lead to a return of polydipsia, polyuria, polyphagia, and weight loss. Ultimately, ketoacidosis can occur. *Cataracts are a common sequela to mild insulin underdosage and persistent hyperglycemia* (see Cataracts, later in this chapter). The time period between development of hyperglycemia and development of cataracts is unpredictable.

Daily monitoring of urine glucose and ketone levels by the owner is suggested in the care of diabetic dogs. The goal of careful monitoring is to aid in making insulin dose adjustments in order to maintain the blood glucose concentration as close to normal for as much of each 24-hour period as possible. The reported incidence of cataract development and blindness in poorly monitored diabetic dogs (Ling et al., 1977) is quite high. The incidence of cataract development is lower in the author's patients, for which daily urine monitoring is imperative. This point should be emphasized to the owner/client. Day-to-day caloric intake and exercise are unavoidably variable and will affect the daily insulin requirement. Hence, the owner must understand that adjustments in insulin dosage must be based on the results of daily urine monitoring. These adjustments are made in concert with occasional blood glucose measurements by the veterinarian.

The owner is also instructed to maintain a daily diary to aid the veterinarian and to make the treatment easier. This should include the results of morning urine glucose and ketone measurements, the dose of insulin, the time the patient ate (in the morning and/or evening), and the site of insulin injection (which should vary).

Method of Treatment. Exogenous insulin replacement is not as physiologic a process as one would hope. In contrast with the sensitively regulated endogenous secretion of insulin into the portal vein, exogenous insulin is given subcutaneously in one or two large doses. It is then absorbed slowly throughout the day. Food must be ingested at certain times and in specific amounts to avoid hyperglycemia or hypoglycemia. Each diabetic should be hospitalized until its metabolic condition is stabilized. The initial dose of insulin in the dog is approximately 0.5 to 1 unit (U)/kg body weight, subcutaneously. In the cat, which is more sensitive to exogenous insulin, the initial dose is 0.25 U/kg, subcutaneously. It is preferable to begin therapy at a low dose, since it is easier to adjust for hyperglycemia than to deal with an acute hypoglycemic crisis. In the hospital and at home a simple schedule is followed for monitoring and treating the diabetic (Table 68–4).

Each morning the urine is tested for glucose and ketone levels, with Keto-Diastix. The *corrected* dose of NPH or PZI insulin (see following discussion) is then administered subcutaneously, and the patient is given 10 to 25 per cent of its daily food intake. The main meal is given approximately 5 to 12 hours later, to coincide with the peak in insulin action. Once the diabetic is stable and well in the home environment, the morning meal is slowly tapered and the evening meal increased. Most of our diabetic dogs eventually receive only an evening meal, no snacks, and *no morning meal.*

During the initial in-hospital period, the

Table 68–4. Recommended Initial Treatment Schedule for Diabetic Dogs and Cats*

8:00 AM	Collect urine sample and determine level of glycosuria.
8:15 AM	Administer insulin dose.
8:30 AM	Feed 1/8 to 1/4 of the total daily food requirement.
4:00 to 5:00 PM	Feed 3/4 of the total daily food requirement.

*Note: For some animals that are stable, the morning meal may be further reduced or eliminated. Timing of the main meal may be improved by serial blood glucose determinations throughout a 12- or 24-hour period.

afternoon blood glucose concentration must also be monitored seven to nine hours after insulin is administered. Such a determination allows the clinician to directly assess insulin's effect and time of action in each patient. The ideal afternoon blood glucose, prior to the afternoon feeding, is approximately 70 to 110 mg/dl. A series of blood glucose measurements should also be obtained at least once during the initial hospitalization, two, four, six, eight, ten, and 12 hours after insulin administration. This is done to document individual variability in patient sensitivity to and metabolism of insulin (see Complications). Serial blood glucose determinations are the most important tool we have, as veterinarians, in understanding individual diabetic dogs and cats.

All blood glucose determinations should be performed prior to the evening meal. When animals are rechecked after their initial hospitalization, they must be seen at a time corresponding with the major insulin effects prior to their evening meal, to best assess their response to insulin. It must be emphasized that any single blood glucose determination reflects only one brief moment in daily carbohydrate metabolism. It is usually difficult to predict whether the blood glucose was declining, rising, or stable when the blood sample is obtained. Therefore, blood glucose determinations are *aids* in therapy but do not always reflect precisely the effect of insulin on a given animal. One major variable is the time at which insulin action peaks, which differs from individual to individual in the dog and cat. This can only be assessed with serial blood glucose determinations.

The basic objective of insulin therapy is to maintain the patient 1/10 to ¼ per cent (trace to +) glycosuria in the *morning,* because one cannot obtain afternoon blood sugars once the animal is sent home. This goal avoids the precipitation of a severe hypoglycemic episode prior to the *evening* meal. No snacks are allowed. If the animal appears to be weak prior to the evening meal (suggesting hypoglycemia), the meal should be given earlier in the day.

The phrase *daily corrected insulin dose* refers to the change in insulin dosage determined by the morning urinalysis. Slightly too much insulin should decrease the glycosuria the following morning, while too little will increase it (Fig. 68–6). The urine glucose should be negative most of each day, ideally being positive only between approximately 4 to 10 AM. The dosage adjustments (Table 68–5) are appropriate for a ten-kg dog. They should be reduced somewhat for cats or smaller dogs and increased for large dogs. When a urine specimen cannot be obtained, the previous day's dose should be repeated. Both Tables 68–4 and 68–5 are included as client handouts when the pet is first returned to the owner after hospitalization.

Occasional ketonuria that is noticed by the owner on the Keto-Diastix test is not worrisome if the dog is alert, eating, and not vomiting. Ketonuria on two consecutive days or the appearance of illness in the animal may signal the need for specific therapy for ketoacidosis, and in such cases the veterinarian should be notified.

Complications of Insulin Therapy. The accepted renal threshold for glucose is 175 to 225 mg/dl; successful urine monitoring is dependent on this fact. Variable renal thresholds outside this range do occur, however. If a patient is not reacting as expected during therapy, one can attempt to determine the renal threshold by comparing several urine and blood glucose concentrations. A urine glucose level will be accurate if the bladder is emptied 15 to 30 minutes prior to obtaining the test sample. This procedure prevents misleading readings caused by urine mixing in the bladder over a period of time.

Occasionally, marked glycosuria is observed each morning, even with increasing doses of insulin and proper renal thresholds for glucose. When the dose of insulin approaches 1.0 unit/lb. of body weight (2.2 U/kg), there is an increased risk of significant hypoglycemia later in the day. Hence, the veterinarian must be consulted whenever high doses appear to be needed, and serial blood glucose determinations considered.

The most common causes for an apparent increase in the dose requirement are (1) improper administration of the insulin by the owner, (2) inadequate mixing of the insulin prior to its withdrawal from the vial, (3) use of insulin that is outdated or inactivated by improper storage, and (4) use of inaccurate Keto-Diastix. Endogenous or exogenous diabetogenic hormone excess (hyperadrenocorticism, female estrous, etc.)

Table 68–5. Daily Insulin Dose Adjustment for the Average Ten-Kilogram Dog

Glycosuria*	Adjustment
2%	Increase 1 unit
1%, 0.5%	Increase 1/2 unit
0.1 to 0.25%	Repeat previous day's dosage
Negative	Decrease 1 unit

*Keto-Diastix determinations.

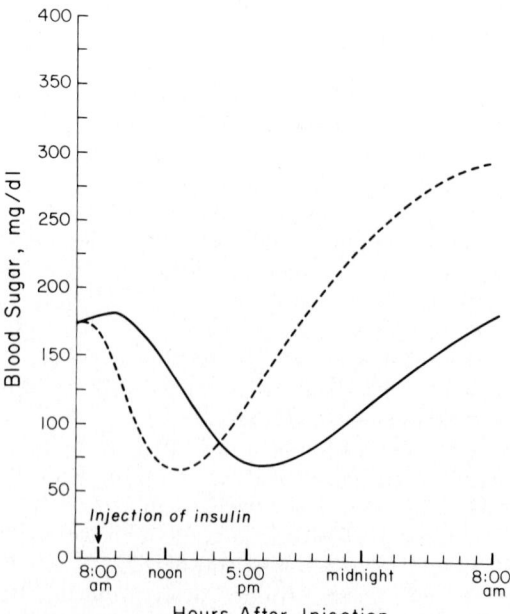

Figure 68–7. The ideal blood glucose concentrations over a 24-hour period after NPH insulin administration (———). Also illustrated is the alteration in blood glucose if insulin is metabolized in too short a period of time in an individual canine (- - - - - -).

must be considered. Described below in greater detail are additional potential causes for an apparent rise in insulin requirement.

Transient Insulin Activity. If the above causes of morning glycosuria are eliminated, the possibility that the administered insulin is being metabolized too rapidly must be considered. When insulin levels in the blood are inadequate or absent for a majority of the day, blood glucose levels rise and glycosuria occurs, resulting in the presence of large amounts of glucose in the morning urine specimen (see Fig. 68–7). This problem may be resolved by the use of PZI insulin, which appears to have a slightly longer duration of effect (see Table 68–3). Thus, the early morning absence of insulin in the blood could be eliminated and improved control can be achieved. This problem has occurred more frequently in the cat than in the dog, and therefore, cats are routinely treated with PZI insulin. In some cases, administering insulin twice daily has been successful in controlling such cases (Schaer, 1976). PZI insulin administered once daily would be easier for owners.

Insulin-Induced Posthypoglycemic Hyper-glycemia: The Somogyi Overswing. The phenomenon of administering too much insulin to a patient, causing subclinical but significant hypoglycemia, which is followed by severe hyperglycemia, has been recognized in humans almost as long as insulin has been used clinically. Joslin et al. (1922) referred to this problem and suggested that efforts be taken to prevent wide fluctuations in blood sugar. The phenomenon was further documented when Somogyi studied a group of diabetic patients difficult to manage and concluded that overinsulinization was the cause of the "brittleness" of their diabetic control (Somogyi et al., 1938; Somogyi, 1953, 1959).

The occurrence of insulin-induced hypoglycemia will evoke the compensatory homeostatic mechanisms. This prevents the hypoglycemic loss of consciousness or convulsions by producing rapid hepatic glucose mobilization and hyperglycemia. These mechanisms probably include the release of the stress hormones glucagon, growth hormone, cortisol, and epinephrine (Ganong, 1979). In the nondiabetic subject, the hyperglycemic response to hypoglycemia would be moderated by additional B cell insulin release, so that very high or very low blood glucose concentrations do

not occur (Foa et al., 1949). However, in the insulin-dependent diabetic patient — that is to say most diabetic dogs and cats — such compensatory insulin secretion is not present, and there would be no hindrance to the rapid, hormone-induced increase in blood glucose. The wide fluctuation in blood glucose concentrations observed in these patients (Fig. 68–8) is thus explained, because a rapid increase in blood glucose is usually not observed during simple insulin deficiency (Bloom et al., 1969).

The "Somogyi overswing" is one of the primary complications seen with urine monitoring for diabetic control. Figure 68–8 illustrates graphically the confusion that can result from administration of too much insulin. Such animals have high concentrations of glucose in the urine on the morning following the overdosage. This is easily interpreted as a result of insulin underdosage because (1) morning glycosuria is noted, (2) signs of previous hypoglycemia may not be seen, (3) return of polydipsia and polyuria often occurs, and (4) occasional polyphagia is also present. Good warning signals include persistent glycosuria as well as insulin doses that approach 2.2 U/kg of body weight. Only close monitoring by owner and veter-

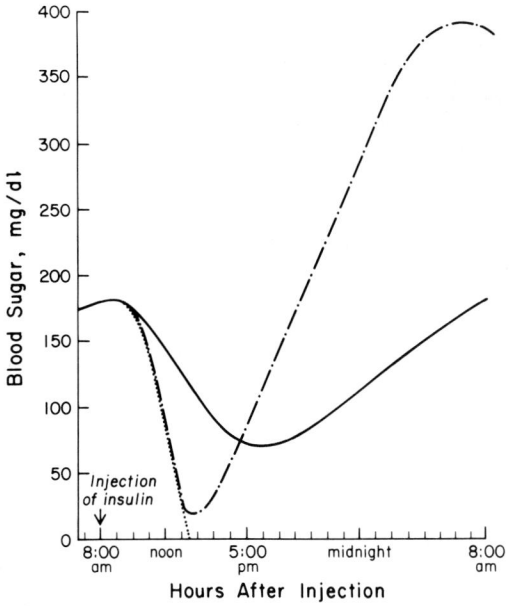

Figure 68–8. Proposed changes in blood glucose concentration after insulin injection to a well-controlled diabetic (———————) and when insulin is overdosed, resulting in a Somogyi overswing (—.—.—.—.). Also illustrated is insulin overdosage with severe hypoglycemia (. . . .).

inarian, avoiding inordinately high insulin doses, will avoid such a complication.

Insulin Antibodies. Because injected insulin is a "foreign" protein it consistently causes production of antibodies to insulin in man. Fortunately, production of antibodies sufficient to interfere with treatment is rare. Insulin products are constantly being made more pure, reducing unwanted antigenic protein. However, some patients develop insulin resistance because of insulin-binding antibodies (which can be measured in man). This condition sometimes improves in the dog with the substitution of pork insulin for beef insulin, because pork insulin appears to be less antigenic.

Hypoglycemic Reactions. The owner should be instructed to have a glucose-containing syrup, such as Karo syrup, available at all times. If the animal appears to be weak or unusually tired, the syrup should be administered orally immediately. This most commonly occurs between three and seven hours after insulin administration (Fig. 68–8). If convulsions occur, the owner should pour the syrup over his fingers and this syrup should be rubbed into the buccal mucosa, *not* poured into the mouth. The owner should be instructed to do this *immediately,* even before notifying the veterinarian. Hypoglycemia can produce coma as well as seizures.

Whenever a known diabetic is presented to the veterinarian because of an acute generalized central nervous system disturbance, a blood sample should be obtained for blood glucose determination and then a minimum of five to ten ml of intravenous 50 per cent dextrose should be given immediately unless ketoacidosis is obvious.

Special Considerations

Diet. Once diabetes mellitus has been diagnosed, the patient's diet must be constant. The amount of food ingested will directly affect the amount of insulin required to maintain stability. Ideally, a palatable commercial canned food should be found, because they have a relatively constant caloric value. Semi-moist commercial foods are avoided because of their simple sugar content.

The patient should be fed according to its ideal body weight. A small dog should receive approximately 75 kcal/kg body weight, and large dogs should receive approximate-

ly 55 kcal/kg. If weight loss is deemed necessary to reach ideal body weight, total daily caloric intake should be reduced. The reducing diabetic must be monitored closely at home, since the daily insulin requirement often will decrease as body weight decreases.

Recently, a new concept has been put forth regarding diet and diabetes mellitus. Studies using high vs. low fiber and high vs. low carbohydrate diets in diabetics have been reported. It has been found that high fiber and high carbohydrate diets were beneficial in lowering blood glucose concentrations in some diabetic patients, and therefore, decreased exogenous insulin requirements were seen as well (Miranda and Horwitz, 1978; Anderson and Ward, 1978).

Exercise. The amount of daily exercise will greatly affect the daily insulin requirement and should therefore be as constant as possible. Working dogs require *less* insulin on working days. Although the cause is not well understood, the entry of glucose into skeletal muscle is facilitated during exercise even in the absence of insulin. Hence, diabetes is more difficult to manage in the working dog and requires close communication between the owner and the veterinarian. In the author's experience, dogs exercise more at home than in the hospital, but they also consume more food at home, so insulin requirement usually increases after the animal is released from the hospital.

Nonspayed Bitches. Estrus and pregnancy complicate the management of diabetes. The hormones produced during pregnancy and in normal proestrus, estrus, and diestrus antagonize the effects of insulin. Insulin is destroyed by an insulinase produced by the placenta. The increased energy needs associated with estrus and pregnancy often result in the onset of ketosis secondary to the bitch's chronic hyperglycemia, which in turn stimulates fetal growth hormone. Abortion is common. Fetuses of diabetic bitches tend to be large. In the neonate there is an increased risk of a hypoglycemic crisis due to beta-cell hyperplasia, which results from chronic stimulation by high blood glucose concentrations *in utero.* Thus, ovariohysterectomy should be performed soon after a female diabetic's condition is stabilized.

Elective Surgery. A simple protocol should be followed when any operation is performed on the diabetic dog or cat. Ketosis, hyperglycemia, and hypoglycemia must be prevented during and immediately after surgery. Elective major operations should be delayed until the patient's clinical condition is stable.

The day prior to surgery the patient receives the normal dose of insulin and is fed as usual. No food is given after midnight. On the morning of the operation, half of the calculated dose of insulin for that day is given. During surgery the patient is maintained on an IV drip of five per cent dextrose in water or five per cent dextrose in saline until oral intake is reestablished. The IV dextrose drip is important, because it provides carbohydrate for response to the stress of surgery. Insulin must also be administered, so that the diabetic animal can utilize the dextrose. A lower insulin dosage is administered, since the normal amount of food may not be consumed that day. It is easier to correct hyperglycemia than to treat a hypoglycemic crisis.

During and after surgery, total urine output, urine ketones, and urine glucose must be monitored at frequent intervals. Measurements of blood glucose may also be required postoperatively. If hyperglycemia and glycosuria occur, small amounts of regular insulin can be given at four- to six-hour intervals. The dose of regular insulin in this situation is approximately 20 per cent of the total daily dose of NPH insulin for 4+ glycosuria or for blood glucose greater than 300 mg/dl. The dose is reduced further for lesser degrees of glycosuria or if long-acting insulin is expected to peak during the period of significant hyperglycemia.

On the day after surgery the diabetic can usually be returned to the routine schedule of insulin administration and feeding. A patient that is not eating can be maintained on IV dextrose and saline. Since the carbohydrate load in this situation is continuous, it is desirable to maintain a continuous supply of insulin. This is accomplished by giving half the usual dose subcutaneously at 12-hour intervals until the animal is eating regularly and can be returned to the normal schedule.

Cataracts

Occasionally in diabetes mellitus the initial presentation of the animal is not for the systemic manifestations of polyuria, polydipsia, polyphagia, and weight loss. Some owners seek veterinary care because their pet has become blind owing to cataract formation or because they notice the cataracts forming before blindness occurs.

Incidence of cataracts in diabetic dogs is quite high because such patients have significant hyperglycemia. Indeed, the majority of canine patients are maintained on insulin doses that result in a mild hyperglycemia and glycosuria. The rate of onset of diabetic cataracts in rats has been demonstrated to be inversely related to the degree of hyperglycemia (Bellows, 1975).

The pathogenesis of diabetic cataract formation is thought to be related to altered osmotic relationships in the lens. Glucose enters the lens from the aqueous humor by facilitated transport. In the normal lens, glucose concentration is approximately ten per cent of the blood glucose and is converted to lactic acid via the anaerobic glycolytic pathway. In the presence of elevated glucose concentrations, the glycolytic enzymes become saturated. Glucose is then metabolized through the sorbitol pathway, with glucose being converted to sorbitol by the action of aldose reductase. Sorbitol is unable to exit from the lens and is a potent hydrophilic agent. As a result, there is an influx of water, which leads to swelling and rupture of the lens fibers and is responsible for cataract development.

The development of cataracts can occur quite rapidly. Clinically, dogs may progress from having normal vision to blindness over a period of weeks or even days. The owner of a diabetic pet should be made aware of the high probability of cataract formation. Good diabetes control may decrease the likelihood of cataracts. If such an animal does become blind, cataract surgery will usually restore vision (Peiffer et al., 1977).

DIABETIC KETOACIDOSIS

Before the availability of insulin, diabetic ketoacidosis was a uniformly fatal catastrophe. With years of experience in therapy, controversy still exists as to the best treatment regimen in this serious disease condition in both humans and animals. Successful treatment depends in large measure on individualization of therapy and intensive patient care. The following is a guide for the formation of a treatment regimen in dogs, rather than a simple step-by-step protocol.

Anamnesis

The length of severe illness as described by the owners of ketoacidotic dogs is usually of one to seven days' duration. Such dogs are frequently anorexic, severely depressed, vomiting, and diarrhetic, and will not drink water. If the owner is questioned closely with regard to past history, however, the changes noted before severe illness set in include the classic history for diabetes mellitus, i.e., polydipsia, polyuria, polyphagia, and weight loss. These signs can be seen in other diseases, including pyometra and renal failure. When a severely ill animal is presented to the veterinarian, the owner will often omit signs that were present prior to those most obvious and worrisome at the moment. It requires a careful historian to obtain this information from a distressed owner.

Clinical Signs

The symptoms detected by the veterinarian include dehydration, depression, weakness, tachypnea, vomiting, and often a strong odor of acetone on the breath. The initial physical examination should focus on an evaluation of the status of hydration, on the extent of central nervous system (CNS) depression, and also on a careful search for any possible initiating cause for the ketoacidosis. It must be remembered that many animals tolerate a borderline or overt case of diabetes mellitus for prolonged periods of time without becoming ketotic. Therefore, it is important to search for any disease process that could cause the diabetic to decompensate.

There are correlations between vague processes such as infection and the pathogenesis of ketoacidosis via the stress hormones (Fig. 68–4). The common disease processes to be ruled out include pneumonia, pyometra, prostatitis, pancreatitis, or congestive heart failure. To evaluate these patients completely requires various blood, urine, and radiographic studies. These are expensive procedures, and the owner must be made aware of the costs of treating such pets. In addition, in-hospital testing can be quite stressful to the patient. The patient's welfare must be considered, and the usefulness of any diagnostic test weighed against the possibility of worsening a critical situation. In certain instances, therapy takes precedence over diagnostics.

Initial Evaluation

If diabetic ketoacidosis is suspected, a urine sample should be obtained first. If the urine sample is positive for ketones and glucose, therapy for ketoacidosis should commence. However, to aid in development of a treatment protocol, a *ketoacidosis profile* must be performed. Without this evaluation, a clinician cannot adequately assess a patient's biochemical status and, therefore, cannot be expected to begin therapy with sufficient knowledge of the specific abnormalities to be corrected. The minimum required tests include urinalysis, determination of blood glucose, venous total CO_2 or arterial acid-base evaluation, BUN or serum creatinine, serum electrolytes (including sodium and potassium), and an electrocardiogram. If evidence of ketones in the urine cannot be found, Acetest tablets may be used: a drop of either serum or plasma on a crushed tablet determines whether ketones are present. If present, the ketones may not have reached the renal threshold that would result in ketonuria. The tablets do not detect one of the most important acids in the development of ketoacidosis, beta-hydroxybutyric acid.

These studies are needed for the immediate diagnosis and care of the patient. Knowing the results of the above tests allows for proper choice of fluid therapy as well as corrections that must be made with respect to electrolyte alterations, acidosis, and renal function. Other data, such as radiographs or further clinical pathology, may be needed for complete understanding of any individual animal; however, the ketoacidosis profile provides the information necessary to begin proper emergency therapy.

Treatment

The goals in treatment are (1) to provide adequate insulin to normalize intermediary metabolism, (2) to restore water and electrolyte losses, (3) to correct acidosis, (4) to identify precipitating factors in this disease process, and (5) to provide a carbohydrate substrate when required by the treatment. Proper therapy does not imply as rapid a return to normal as possible. Because osmotic and biochemical disequilibria are created, rapid changes in various vital parameters can be as harmful as, or more harmful than, no change at all. If all abnormal parameters can be *slowly* returned toward normal, there is better likelihood of success in therapy.

The precipitating factor must be sought out and treated. Since infection is the most important of these (Alberti and Nattrass, 1978), culture of the urine, trachea, or blood may be warranted. A broad spectrum antibiotic may be used, ideally after obtaining the necessary cultures. Given the impaired leukocyte function that is generally present in ketoacidosis and the use of intravenous and urinary catheters, one is probably justified in initiating antibiotic treatment before receiving culture results (Alberti and Nattrass, 1978).

If facilities do not exist that allow the veterinarian to properly treat this difficult medical emergency, it is strongly recommended that the owner be so advised. The willing owner and pet can then be referred to a colleague or teaching hospital that is equipped for treating such cases.

Fluid Therapy. Replacement of fluids is accomplished with an indwelling intravenous jugular or cephalic catheter. The volume and rate administered for the initial period are determined by calculating the dehydration deficit and maintenance requirements. Maintenance requirements primarily involve replacement of excessive fluid lost as urine, as well as that lost from the gastrointestinal tract (including fluid loss due to vomiting and/or diarrhea). When possible, central venous pressure determinations should be made.

The second important procedure that should be performed is catheterization of the bladder. The catheter should be connected in a "closed-system" aseptic method of collection to reduce the chance of iatrogenic infection. This allows the clinician to monitor urine output and to precisely determine whether the animal is polyuric, oliguric, or anuric. Administration of fluids becomes more precise and safer for the

animal if known requirements, rather than estimated requirements, are replaced. The polyuric animal may require large fluid loads, while the anuric animal requires additional immediate therapy. The urinary catheter will also allow the practitioner to monitor the urine glucose and ketone levels.

Since dehydration is a consequence of osmotic diuresis, the loss of water is relatively greater than that of salt. When an extremely ill patient is presented in diabetic ketoacidosis, it is usually hyperosmotic as well. For this reason, half strength (0.45 per cent) saline has been recommended for the initial one to two hours of therapy (Feldman, 1980). The author's practice at present is to use isotonic (0.9 per cent) saline, because in most cases the initial plasma sodium concentration is low (Table 68–6) and an infusion of isotonic saline should help support plasma sodium concentrations. More importantly, isotonic infusions prevent too rapid a fall in extracellular osmolality, which will occur as blood glucose and plasma urea concentrations return toward normal. Simultaneous increase in the serum sodium concentration will dampen this effect and decrease the likelihood of cerebral edema (Duck et al., 1976; Arieff and Kleeman, 1974).

In the ensuing hours of treatment, the intravenous infusion should be changed to five per cent dextrose in water or saline. This prevents hypoglycemia and reduces the likelihood of cerebral edema, which can accompany rapid, insulin-induced reductions in blood glucose at levels below 250 mg per 100 ml.

The development of cerebral edema is related to an enzyme reaction similar to that described in the formation of diabetic cataracts. Glucose saturates the Embden-Meyerhof pathway and is then metabolized through polyol pathway via the enzyme aldose reductase within brain cells. The most

Table 68–6. Initial Chemistry Values in Twenty Dogs With Severe Diabetic Ketoacidosis

	Venous or Arterial Bicarbonate (mEq/L)	Blood Glucose (mg/dl)	Serum Chloride (mEq/L)	Serum Sodium (mEq/L)	Serum Potassium (mEq/L)	Blood Urea Nitrogen (mg/dl)
Mean	8.1	520	89.1	131.5	3.8	59.4
Range	03 to 12	320 to 915	58 to 112	118 to 145	1.9 to 5.6	13 to 159
Normal Values	18 to 27	65 to 140	105 to 118	141 to 155	3.5 to 5.1	11 to 22

important polyol is sorbitol. With hyperglycemia, the brain cell has the potential to produce large quantities of sorbitol. Sorbitol, once formed, is osmotically active until metabolized, since no mechanism facilitates its transport across cell membranes. Thus, this substance will pull water into the cell to balance intracellular and extracellular osmolality. When the animal is dehydrated and, therefore, hyperosmotic extracellularly, sorbitol production in brain cells is not a problem. With vigorous exogenous insulin therapy, however, a rapid reduction in blood sugar results in a rapid reduction in extracellular osmolality. Water can therefore move into the sorbitol-induced hyperosmotic brain cells. In this manner, a rapid fall in blood glucose can result in cerebral edema and worsening CNS function (Clements et al., 1968, 1971). For this reason, the veterinarian must be aware of the CNS function prior to initiation of therapy. If the patient becomes depressed or obtunded with treatment, it may be the result of rapidly falling blood glucose levels and/or cerebral edema.

Insulin Therapy. Each dog with diabetes mellitus has different insulin requirements. It is therefore difficult to know what insulin dose to administer to the dog with diabetic ketoacidosis. In this situation, the patient needs an insulin that acts quickly, and the veterinarian needs a short-acting insulin that will allow for rapid correction if the dose given is too much or too little. Rapid-acting, regular insulin meets the above criteria and is the only insulin to be used in the emergency situation (Table 68–3).

It is recommended that regular insulin be given at an initial dosage of one unit per kg body weight. Twenty-five per cent of this dose is given intravenously, as a bolus. The remaining 75 per cent is given intramuscularly. Intravenously, the half-life of insulin is only three to five minutes, and it falls to less than one per cent of the initial peak after 25 minutes. Intramuscularly, the onset of action of insulin is 5 to 15 minutes and it peaks in one to three hours. The duration of action is approximately four hours.

Insulin is given intramuscularly rather than by the usual subcutaneous route because absorption from an intramuscular injection is less affected by dehydration and shock than is absorption from subcutaneous sites. By administering insulin in this fashion (some IV and some IM), immediate and continuous effects of insulin can be obtained to correct the metabolic abnormalities present in the individual patient. As the intravenous insulin is wearing off, the insulin given intramuscularly will begin to act. Adequate blood levels of insulin can thus be achieved from the time treatment is begun until approximately four hours after the dose is given.

After the insulin is administered to each patient, the urinary catheter is used to monitor the presence of glucose and ketones in the urine. The bladder must be totally drained at least once every hour or, ideally, every 30 minutes. This frequent bladder drainage is recommended because mixing of urine that contains different concentrations of glucose can be quite misleading. In addition, dogs that present to the hospital with "++++" glycosuria (two per cent) on a Keto-Diastix often have a much higher percentage of sugar present in the urine. As an example, if the animal receives the correct dose of insulin, the urine that initially had a "++++" glycosuria may be reduced after one hour to, perhaps, "+++" glycosuria; after two hours it will be reduced to "++" glycosuria; after three hours, to a trace or "+" glycosuria; and after four hours the amount of sugar in the urine may be negative on a Keto-Diastix. If these different urines being produced by the kidneys over a period of four hours are mixed in the bladder, an assessment of the level of glycosuria after this time period will be incorrect. The urine sample after four hours will probably read as "+++" or "++++." This can be confusing because the urine actually produced by the kidneys after four hours is negative for sugar. This will not only cause confusion with the second dose of insulin, but can also confuse the timing of conversion of the intravenous infusion from saline to five per cent dextrose in water. By checking the urine every hour, the intravenous fluids can be changed from saline to the five per cent dextrose in water whenever the urine sugar falls below "++," regardless of the time that this occurs. If blood glucose determinations are available, this method would be more precise than urine glucose. As the blood glucose approaches 250 mg/dl, the intravenous fluids should be changed to five per cent dextrose in water.

Insulin is administered every four hours and the level of urine sugar and ketones at the four-hour intervals will determine any change in dose. Table 68–7 indicates the insulin dose adjustments based on changes in urine glucose and ketones. The patient is believed to be stable when the blood sugar is in the range of 150 to 250 mg/dl and the patient is no longer acidotic. Additionally, when the pet is alert and eating, longer acting insulin can be safely used. The longer acting insulin of choice is NPH insulin. If a ketoacidotic patient is presented at noon of day one and is treated for diabetic ketoacidosis for the following 20 hours (8:00 AM the next morning), and the dog is looking much brighter, is more alert, and is able to eat, NPH insulin should be administered.

NPH insulin is assumed to have its peak effect four to eight hours after subcutaneous administration and a duration of 12 to 24 hours. Since the patient should be under some direct observation when NPH insulin is peaking, it is recommended that the initial injection be given between 7:00 and 9:00 AM. If a patient being treated for ketoacidosis appears stable at 2:00 PM, rather than switch to a new, untested insulin at this time, it would be safer to continue regular insulin subcutaneously every six hours until the following morning. The clinician should be comfortable with regular insulin after administering several doses to an animal. However, the initial NPH insulin dose will again be new and untested. There is always potential for an over- or underdosage when this insulin is first started. Therefore, the clinician must be certain that the animal is in stable condition and that it can be checked visually and by blood or urinalysis as the new insulin takes effect.

This method of insulin treatment has proved to be quite successful. It is recommended here as the approach that is most familiar to the author.

Alternate Insulin Therapies. Several therapeutic plans are described in the literature in addition to that just discussed. In one recent study, a low-dose intramuscular insulin therapy for ketoacidotic diabetic dogs was used. Dosages employed were two units of regular insulin IM initially, followed by one unit per hour IM for dogs with body weights below ten kilograms. Dogs weighing more than ten kilograms were given an initial IM dose of 0.25 Units per kilogram of body weight followed by hourly injections of 0.1 Unit per kilogram of body weight. Blood glucose was monitored hourly. Blood monitoring and insulin administration continued hourly until the blood glucose fell below 250 mg/dl, at which time the regular insulin was administered subcutaneously every eight hours (Chastain and Nichols, 1981). This treatment protocol was successful in seven dogs described. It would be difficult, unfortunately, for many private practitioners to monitor blood glucose concentrations hourly. However, monitoring urine glucose concentration, although less satisfactory, may provide the required information.

Use of continuous intravenous insulin infusions has also been described for the dog (Schall and Cornelius, 1980). In this protocol, insulin is administered intravenously at a rate of 0.5 to 1.0 Unit per hour, diluted in lactated Ringer's solution. Blood glucose concentration determination is recommended every two hours, until the blood glucose falls to 200 mg/dl. This fall in blood glucose was described as requiring six to eight hours. An intermittent intravenous bolus of insulin has also been described (Schall and Cornelius, 1980).

Bicarbonate Treatment. Much controversy surrounds the use of bicarbonate in this disease condition. It must be remem-

Table 68–7. Insulin Adjustments in a Ten-Kilogram Ketoacidotic Diabetic Dog

Urine Glucose*	Urine Ketones*	Insulin Adjustment (add or subtract from previous dose)	Route	IV Fluids
2%, 1%, 0.5%	Large, moderate	Increase 2 U	IM	0.9% saline
0.25%, 0.1%, Negative	Large, moderate	No change	IM	5% dextrose in water
2%, 1%, 0.5%	Small	Increase 1 U	SC	0.9% saline
0.25%, 0.1%, Negative	Small	No change	SC	5% dextrose in water
2%	Negative	Increase 1 U	SC	0.9% saline
1%, 0.5%	Negative	Increase 1/2 U	SC	0.9% saline
0.25%, 0.1%	Negative	No change	SC	5% dextrose in water
Negative	Negative	Decrease 2 U	SC	5% dextrose in water

*Keto-Diastix determinations.

bered that acetoacetic acid and betahydroxybutyric acid are usable anions. With insulin therapy, the production of ketoacids will dramatically diminish, and therefore, serum bicarbonate will return toward normal without using alkali containing solutions. Thus, it is recommended that animals with a serum bicarbonate level (or a total venous CO_2 concentration) greater than 12 mEq/L not be treated with bicarbonate because these animals will not need alkali to correct the state of acidosis. Many diabetic ketoacidotic dogs are severely acidotic, however (Table 68–6). Therefore, when the bicarbonate level is 12 mEq/L or less (the total venous CO_2 is below 12), it is recommended that one fourth of the dosage of bicarbonate, as determined by calculations from the following formula, should be given over the first four to six hours. The bicarbonate deficit, i.e., the milliequivalents of bicarbonate needed to correct acidosis, is calculated as follows:

$$\text{mEq bicarbonate} = \text{body weight (kg)} \times 0.4 \times \text{base deficit}$$

The base deficit is the difference between the patient's serum bicarbonate concentration and the normal value of approximately 24 mEq/L. The factor 0.4 corrects for the space in which bicarbonate is distributed (40 per cent of body weight). One fourth of this dose of bicarbonate should be added to the intravenous infusion (thus given slowly, over a longer period of time) and should not be given by bolus. After six hours of therapy, the acid-base status should be rechecked, and the above calculations repeated.

Objections to bicarbonate therapy have been that (1) therapy with alkali may result in metabolic alkalosis, which is potentially as serious as metabolic acidosis; (2) any alkalinization can cause a shift to the left of the oxygen dissociation curve, thereby limiting tissue oxygen delivery; and (3) a rapid elevation in arterial pH may be accompanied by an exaggerated fall in the cerebrospinal fluid (CSF) pH with resultant worsening of CNS function (Kaye, 1975).

The reason for the paradoxical fall in CSF pH is that hydrogen ions and bicarbonate move slowly across the blood-brain barrier. Carbon dioxide, however, diffuses almost immediately across this barrier. If peripheral serum acidosis is corrected rapidly, the serum CO_2 increases. While most of this CO_2 can be removed through the lungs, significant amounts of CO_2 will diffuse across the barrier. This will, by virtue of the following equation, increase the spinal fluid hydrogen ion concentration and, therefore, decrease the pH. The result is CNS acidosis. The equation is:

$$H_2O + CO_2 \leftrightarrows H_2CO_3 \rightleftarrows H^+ + HCO_3^-$$

It has been known that in man and in dogs the state of CNS depression related to acidosis is primarily dependent on the pH of the CSF, and not that of the peripheral circulation. A patient that presents with a severely depressed peripheral pH, but is bright and alert, probably has a normal or near normal pH in the CNS. However, a patient that presents to the hospital with severe depression and severe peripheral acidosis may have severe central nervous system acidosis. These are difficult patients to treat, and the only safe therapy is to *slowly* correct the metabolic acidosis in the peripheral circulation, thereby slowly altering the pH of the CSF at the same time (Posner and Plum, 1967). Since blood lactate levels tend to be elevated in many ketoacidotic patients, there is no justification for the infusion of sodium lactate in preference to bicarbonate (Felig, 1974).

Potassium. As a consequence of the metabolic acidosis, osmotic diuresis, diarrhea, and vomiting present in diabetic ketoacidosis, body potassium stores are often depleted by five to ten mEq/kg body weight (Felig, 1974). Nevertheless, the serum potassium concentration may be low, normal, or elevated (Table 68–6). Normal or elevated concentrations are due to the shift in potassium from intracellular to extracellular fluid compartments associated with acidosis and hyperglycemia. With the correction of acidosis and the stimulation of cellular uptake of glucose with insulin, serum potassium levels decline as potassium enters the intracellular space. Accordingly, the administration of potassium chloride or phosphate is usually necessary one to four hours after the initiation of therapy for ketoacidosis. This time interval is necessary for patients with serum potassium concentrations above 4.0 mEq/L in order to be certain that these patients are not anuric or oliguric and to avoid complicating any hyperkalemia that may be present initially. If a patient initially has a low normal or low serum potassium level (less than 4.0 mEq/L) and is not anuric or oliguric, it should be treated immediately with potassium-containing fluids. In either situation, it is recommended that the initial potassium therapy consist of adding ten mEq of potassium to each 250 ml of intravenous fluids. With this method, the amount of potassium delivered is determined by the dog's body weight, urine output, and total fluid requirements rather than based simply on body weight. This dose of potassium can then be increased or decreased depending on continued monitoring of serum concentrations or the electrocardiogram.

Since abnormalities in serum potassium are common both before and during therapy, an electrocardiogram was recommended as part of the initial evaluation of these animals. If an electrocardiogram and a serum potassium are obtained prior to therapy, the electrocardiogram becomes an important tool for monitoring potassium levels as therapy is continued. Ideally, serum potassium levels should be monitored every two to four hours. However, laboratory facilities for these tests are not often available, especially in the evening hours. When such facilities are available, continuing to monitor serum electrolyte levels can become extremely expensive. For this reason, monitoring the electrocardiogram can be a safe, relatively reliable, inexpensive, and easy procedure. The electrocardiogram is not reliable in detecting subtle changes from normal in the potassium level. It is reliable when the potassium level is below 2 mEq/L and above 6.5 mEq/L (Feldman and Ettinger, 1977).

It must be remembered that both hyperkalemia and hypokalemia can occur as a result of therapy. At the same time, continued loss of potassium through vomiting, diarrhea, or urination is possible. The most important electrocardiographic sign of hypokalemia is prolongation of the QT interval. The other, more subtle changes are depression of the ST segment, low or inverted P waves, and depressed T waves. If potassium overdosage is occurring, the initial signs of hyperkalemia are shortening of the QT interval, as well as peaking of the T waves and prolongation of the PR interval and QRS complexes (Feldman and Ettinger, 1977).

Treatment Failure. Despite all precautions and diligent therapy, a fatal outcome

Table 68–8. Treatment of Diabetic Ketoacidosis

A. Initial Therapy
1. Fluids: 0.9% NaCl
2. Insulin: Regular only, 1 U/kg body weight divided (25% IV and 75% IM)
3. Bicarbonate: 25% of calculated dose by intravenous infusion over first 6 hours
4. Broad spectrum antibiotics
5. If initial serum potassium is less than 4.0 mEq/L add 7 mEq of KCl to each 250 ml of infusion solution

B. Guidelines
1. Repeat plasma electrolytes, CO_2, and blood glucose at four-hour intervals until normal levels are approached
2. Drain all urine from bladder every 30 minutes and note amount recovered as well as levels of glycosuria and ketonuria
3. Monitor central venous pressure and EKG

C. Subsequent Therapy
1. Fluids: Change intravenous infusion to 5% dextrose in water (0.45% NaCl and 5% dextrose in water can be combined for long-term maintenance)
2. Insulin: Regular insulin every four hours at adjusted doses until NPH insulin is instituted
3. Bicarbonate: Adjust dose depending on subsequent blood CO_2 levels
4. Potassium: If animal is not anuric and the initial serum potassium was normal or elevated, add potassium to intravenous infusion after two to four hours of therapy

cannot be avoided in some cases. This could be the result of a severe underlying illness, such as renal failure, overwhelming sepsis, severe acute pancreatitis, shock, hypokalemia, or cerebral edema (Alberti and Nattrass, 1978). In addition, disseminated intravascular coagulation (DIC) is increasingly recognized as a serious complication of diabetic ketoacidosis in man. DIC may be related to cell damage secondary to acidemia with release of tissue thromboplastins. Platelet function may also be impaired (Nobis et al., 1975). With logical therapy, however, the mortality rate can be dramatically reduced. A summary of the treatment protocol is provided in Table 68–8.

HYPEROSMOLAR NONKETOTIC DIABETES

Diabetic hyperosmolar nonketotic syndrome (DHNS) is an uncommon complication of diabetes mellitus in the dog and cat (Schaer et al., 1974; Schaer, 1975). This syndrome is characterized by (1) severe hyperglycemia (blood glucose concentration greater than 600 mg/dl), (2) hyperosmolarity (greater than 350 mOsm/kg), (3) severe clinical dehydration, (4) lack of urine or serum ketone bodies, (5) no or mild metabolic acidosis, and (6) some central nervous system depression, at least to the point of lethargy (Podolsky, 1978). As with ketoacidosis, a precipitating condition such as renal disease, pneumonia, certain drug therapies, or other severe stress is associated with DHNS.

The pathogenesis of DHNS begins with decreased utilization and increased production of glucose. As the blood glucose increases, the extracellular osmolarity increases, and this further stimulates water intake. It is believed, however, that at some critical point the increasing osmolarity begins to impair the function of the central nervous system, which interferes with continued ability to meet fluid intake requirements. As the extracellular space becomes contracted, tissue perfusion diminishes, resulting in a decreased glomerular filtration rate that in turn causes azotemia and worsening hyperglycemia due to glucose retention. Azotemia and glucose retention further increase serum osmolarity, and thus, a vicious circle begins to repeat itself. The absence of ketosis is not well understood. In humans with adult-onset type diabetes mellitus, endogenous insulin secretion is present and should be anti-ketogenic. Furthermore, the stimulus for lipolysis is reduced because of low concentrations of growth hormone, cortisol, and glucagon in these patients, as compared with ketoacidotic patients. The free fatty acid levels are lower in DHNS than in ketoacidosis (Gerich et al., 1971). In contrast to the short time course of developing ketoacidosis, the DHNS may be gradual and prolonged (Gerich, 1976).

Owners report progressive polyuria and polydipsia initially, with later progressive development of weakness, anorexia, and vomiting. Physical examination reveals an animal that is usually extremely depressed, dehydrated, and hypothermic with slow mucous membrane refill time.

Blood glucose concentrations in DHNS are often extremely elevated. Virtually all patients with DHNS present with azotemia, which may be renal or prerenal in origin. These patients all have considerably depleted body potassium stores, despite the fact that serum potassium concentrations can be high, normal, or low (Podolsky et al., 1974). Serum sodium concentrations are also variable. The serum concentrations of sodium and potassium are of no value in estimating the magnitude of net ion losses, except for the fact that initial hypokalemia indicates *severe* potassium loss (Podolsky, 1978).

Serum osmolarity, which is quite elevated in DHNS, may be measured by determination of its freezing point with an osmometer, or it may be calculated by the following formula:

$$\text{mOsm per kg} = 2\times \text{(serum Na} + \text{K)} + \text{blood glucose}/18 + \text{BUN}/2.8$$

The normal canine serum osmolarity is approximately 300 mOsm/kg.

Therapy of DHNS is directed toward (1) correction of the extreme degree of volume depletion, (2) correction of the hyperosmolar state, and (3) detection and correction of any underlying precipitating cause, such as illness or drug administration.

The key to adequate therapy of DHNS is vigorous hypotonic fluid replacement. The fluid of choice is 0.45 per cent (half-strength) saline. Half of the estimated dehydration deficit plus maintenance requirements should be replaced in the first 12 hours, and the remainder in the next 24 hours. Balance studies have suggested that the fluid lost in the syndrome contains about 60 mEq/L sodium plus potassium, which closely approximates half-normal saline (Arieff and Carroll, 1972).

The replacement doses of insulin and potassium are the same as those outlined for diabetic ketoacidosis (Table 68–8). Monitoring of urine output, electrocardiogram, central venous pressure, serum electrolytes, BUN, and urine glucose is imperative. As with ketoacidosis, the clinician must attempt to steadily (not precipitously) correct the hyperosmolarity, hyperglycemia, and dehydration, while stimulating diuresis to lower the BUN. These patients are critically ill and require close supervision.

The prognosis for recovery is guarded to poor. The major cause of death in the author's patients is renal failure.

HYPERINSULINISM

The insulinoma syndrome in man was firmly established with the report of eight cases (Whipple and Frantz, 1935). It is of interest to note that the first case of hypoglycemia associated with a pancreatic B cell tumor in a dog was also in 1935 (Slye and Wells, 1935). Since this report, numerous single case reports have appeared in the veterinary literature and these were recently reviewed (Hill et al., 1974). In addition, an accumulative study involving the cases seen at eleven veterinary colleges has also appeared (Priester, 1974). With the advent of the radioimmunoassay for insulin as well as an increased awareness of this condition by veterinarians, diagnosis of hyperinsulinism has become more common. Hyperinsulinism remains, however, a syndrome rare in the dog and even less frequent in the cat (Priester, 1974).

Hyperinsulinism is caused by a functional tumor of the B cells of the pancreatic islets of Langerhans. Such tumors produce and secrete excessive amounts of biologically active insulin.

PATHOPHYSIOLOGY

Glucose is the only fuel normally used in appreciable quantities by the brain. The carbohydrate reserves in neural tissue are quite limited, and normal function depends upon a continuous glucose supply. As the blood glucose concentration falls, the cortex and other brain areas with high metabolic rates are affected first, followed by the more metabolically slower vegetative centers below the cerebral cortex. Thus, early cortical symptoms of disorientation, weakness, and hunger are followed by convulsions and coma. If the hypoglycemia is prolonged, irreversible changes develop in the same sequence, i.e., the cerebral cortex first and the lower centers later. Death is caused by depression of the respiratory center (Ganong, 1979).

Hypoglycemia is a potent stimulus to sympathetic discharge and increased secretion of catecholamines, particularly epinephrine. The tremors and nervousness in hypoglycemia are probably due to sympathetic overactivity. The increase in adrenal medullary secretion is accompanied by increased cortisol, glucagon, and growth hormone secretion. These hormones mediate compensation for hypoglycemia.

The blood glucose concentration at which symptoms of hypoglycemia appear is variable. Normal canines rarely have fasting blood glucose concentrations as low as 40 mg/dl. Some patients with insulin-secreting tumors adapt to blood glucose concentrations of 20 to 30 mg/dl. The mechanisms responsible for this adaptation are unknown.

CLINICAL FEATURES

Age, Sex, and Breed

Hyperinsulinism in the dog usually occurs in the age range of 5 to 15 years. It is most common in dogs 8 to 12 years of age. There is no sex predilection (Hill et al., 1974). Various breeds have been implicated as having a higher incidence of insulin-producing tumors than would be predicted by simple breed popularity. These breeds include the standard poodle, boxer, and fox terrier (Priester, 1974; Hill et al., 1974; Caywood and Wilson, 1980). A functional pancreatic B cell tumor has also been reported in a 15-year-old female Persian cat (Priester, 1974).

Anamnesis

The symptoms seen by the owner of a dog with hyperinsulinism are usually purely related to low blood glucose concentrations. These symptoms are typically intermittent. Stimuli such as fasting, excitement, or exercise may produce hypoglycemia and thus result in obvious clinical signs. Insulin-producing tumors, both adenomas and carcinomas, appear to be glucose responsive. For this reason, eating may cause symptoms of hypoglycemia by raising blood glucose concentrations; this in turn causes exaggerated secretion of insulin from the neoplastic cells with the development of postprandial hypoglycemia. In the author's experience, the postprandial decreases in blood glucose occur one to four hours after the intake of a meal.

Affected dogs that are fed once daily are susceptible to becoming hypoglycemic during long periods between meals. The basal insulin secretion rates in these dogs may be normal to quite elevated. Without eating, blood glucose and insulin should fall. If the insulin-producing tumor causes a continuing utilization of glucose beyond what the compensatory mechanisms can support, symptoms will develop. Exercise increases glucose utilization via a mechanism that does not depend on increased secretion of insulin. In normal dogs the secretion of insulin is inhibited during exercise by activation of the sympathetic nervous system, while glucose utilization is balanced by its increased output by the liver (Williams and Porte, 1974). In patients with hyperinsulinism the utilization of glucose increases during exercise but secretion of insulin is not inhibited, thus creating the potential for hypoglycemia. Prolonged excitement is assumed to have a similar mechanism of action.

Owners report having seen symptoms of hypoglycemia for varying periods of time before seeking veterinary attention. In the author's patients, the duration of signs varied from one day to as long as three years. Most dogs, however, have symptoms for less than six months. One report describes symptoms being present in one dog as long as 72 months before the diagnosis was made (Johnson, 1977).

General (grand mal) seizures are the most common symptom seen in dogs with insulin-secreting tumors. Seizures may occur intermittently throughout the course of the disease or they may appear only late in the course of the illness. Virtually all dogs with hyperinsulinism exhibit some symptoms other than seizures, all of which appear intermittently. Correlation between time of meals and clinical signs is often not apparent. Common owner reports include episodic incoordination, ataxia, generalized weakness, posterior paresis, muscle twitching or fasciculations, syncope, blindness, nervousness, depression, hyperactivity, and polyphagia. Other reported symptoms include running and barking, hysteria with loss of bowel and bladder control, and yelping as if in pain (Johnson, 1977).

Hypoglycemic episodes characteristically become more frequent and severe during the course of the disease. Since some dogs experience greater hunger correlating with progression of the disease, owners often inadvertently treat their dogs by attempting to satisfy the pet's desire to eat. We have had dogs that were being fed as infrequently as once daily and others that were being fed as often as every two to three hours.

Insulin-producing tumors are usually small. Rarely, they are microscopic or diffuse in nature and not readily apparent to the veterinary surgeon; most tumors, however, are easily seen or palpated within the pancreas at laparotomy. Symptoms of pancreatitis, adjacent organ compression, or malignant cachexia are not common (Johnson, 1977).

Physical Examination

The physical examination of a dog with hyperinsulinism is usually not helpful in making a diagnosis. Most dogs are free of significant abnormalities. Five of 25 cases seen at the University of California since 1977 were obese. One dog had persistent polyneuropathy and was unable to stand or walk. The polyneuropathy was believed to be related to the carcinoma, but this was not confirmed. Obvious persistent brain damage is an uncommon but potential sequela to profound, untreated hypoglycemia.

Differential Diagnosis of Seizures or Episodic Weakness

Seizure disorders are relatively common in veterinary practice. All diseases of the central nervous system (CNS) as well as illnesses outside the CNS that may cause CNS signs should be ruled out before instituting chronic anticonvulsant therapy (see Chapter 10). Common categories of diseases that result in *episodic weakness* include metabolic, cardiovascular, and neuromuscular disorders (Lorenz, 1977) (see Chapter 9). Numerous disorders can be attributed to cases that are brought to the veterinarian with an anamnesis that includes seizures, episodic weakness, or incoordination; such animals therefore require further diagnostic work if a diagnosis is to be established.

DIAGNOSTIC EVALUATION

Routine Studies

Radiographs, hemograms, and most blood chemistry analyses are normal in insulinoma patients. In a recent review of a series of insulinoma dogs, abnormalities were detected in the serum albumin, phosphorus, alkaline phosphatase, and alanine aminotransferase (GPT) concentrations (Feldman and Feldman, 1977). These alterations were not consistent and are nonspecific. However, normal test results do aid the clinician in ruling out other causes of the clinical symptoms described herein.

The blood glucose concentration in a routine, nonfasting blood sample is often below normal (less than 70 mg/dl) and may be quite low (less than 50 mg/dl). A single normal, nonfasting blood glucose level does not eliminate hypoglycemia as a cause of episodic symptoms of weakness or seizure.

Careful discussions with an owner are mandatory before arbitrarily fasting a dog for a number of hours. The clinician can assess the current feeding schedule and the timing of clinical symptoms. Fasting prior to blood sampling can thus be suited to the individual dog in question.

In 1935, Whipple and Frantz established criteria to aid in the diagnosis of insulinoma or hyperinsulinism. These criteria have come to be called "Whipple's Triad" and involve (1) patients with symptoms occurring after fasting or exercise; (2) serum glucose levels at 50 mg/dl or less at the time of symptoms; and (3) relief of symptoms with the administration of glucose. While these criteria were timely, they have proved to be rather nonspecific and may be found in other conditions that result in hypoglycemia (Kaplan and Lee, 1979). The differential diagnosis of hypoglycemia is presented in Table 68-9.

Amended Insulin:Glucose Ratio

The measurement of plasma insulin concentration by radioimmunoassay has been extremely useful in the diagnosis of insulin-secreting tumors. The diagnosis is made primarily by demonstrating inappropriately elevated concentrations of circulating insulin, especially at a time of hypoglycemia. Dogs that are suspected of suffering from hyperinsulinism are approached with a simple protocol. The dog is fed at 7:00 AM by the owner or in the hospital. At 9:00 AM a

Table 68-9. Differential Diagnosis of Hypoglycemia

Hyperinsulinism

Hepatic Dysfunction
  a) inherited: glycogen storage disease, vascular shunts, etc.
  b) acquired: inflammation, fibrosis, neoplasia.

Adrenal cortical insufficiency

Hypopituitarism

Large extrapancreatic neoplasm

Starvation: puppy hypoglycemia

Sepsis
Iatrogenic
Artifact

blood glucose is obtained. Blood is drawn every two to three hours during the day until the glucose concentration is noted to have fallen below 60 mg/dl. In all our hyperinsulinism cases, this degree of hypoglycemia has been achieved within eight hours, and in some, within two to three hours of fasting. Others have commented on needing 24- or even 48-hour fasts in certain individual dogs to bring about significant hypoglycemia (Johnson, 1977). Once the blood glucose falls below 60 mg/dl, a blood sample is submitted to the laboratory for both glucose and insulin assays and the patient is then fed.

Using the results of this simple test, a diagnosis can be confirmed in most cases. Normally, a direct relationship does exist between serum concentrations of glucose and insulin. As the serum glucose falls, the serum insulin also falls. Normally, serum insulin concentrations are near zero when the glucose concentration approximates 30 mg/dl (Turner et al., 1971, 1973). Based on this observation, an amended insulin:glucose ratio (AIGR) has been used in man to discriminate patients with hyperinsulinism from those with other causes of hypoglycemia (Turner et al., 1973; Kaplan and Lee, 1979). This AIGR is obtained using the following formula:

$$\frac{\text{Serum insulin } (\mu\text{U/ml} \times 100)}{\text{Serum glucose (mg/dl)} - 30} = \text{AIGR}$$

The AIGR has been recently reported as an aid in confirming the diagnosis of hypoinsulinism in dogs (Mattheeuws et al., 1976; Caywood et al., 1979). Normal values were shown to be 15.6 ± 4.14 in a study of four normal dogs (Caywood et al., 1979), while in a review of 18 normal dogs, the author found similar results (13.9 ± 4.60). Diagnostic results are AIGR levels greater than 30 (Turner et al., 1971; Caywood et al., 1979). In a series of 23 dogs with insulin secreting tumors, the AIGR ranged from 16 to 7000. Borderline or unexpected normal results should be repeated.

Use of fasting serum insulin and glucose concentrations have been applied to other criteria in attempting to separate hyperinsulinism dogs from dogs that do not have islet cell tumors. The glucose:insulin ratio, insulin:glucose ratio, and fasting serum insulin concentration alone were shown to be less reliable than the AIGR (Caywood et al.,

1979; Caywood and Wilson, 1980). The author considers the withholding of food and the assessment of insulin and glucose concentrations, plus the AIGR, to be safe, reliable, and inexpensive. The post-testing meal should be small and food should be given several times over a period of two hours. This aids in avoiding postprandial reactive hypoglycemia, should the dog truly have hyperinsulinism.

Provocative Testing

In addition to the AIGR, a test that also has found popularity in veterinary practice is the glucagon tolerance test. Intravenous glucagon causes rapid elevation in the blood glucose concentration, which stimulates insulin release. The insulin concentration will often dramatically elevate in the blood of hyperinsulinism dogs, illustrating that these tumors (carcinomas or adenomas) are not autonomous but, rather, are responsive to changes in the blood glucose concentration as well as being directly responsive to glucagon. The excessive concentrations of insulin are reflected in the depressed blood glucose concentrations seen throughout the study (Figs. 68–9 and 68–10). As with the AIGR, the test should begin with a fasting blood glucose of less than 60 mg/dl. Glucagon, U.S.P., is injected intravenously at a dose of 0.03 mg/kg of body weight. Serum samples for analysis of both glucose and insulin (if possible) should be obtained at 0, 1, 3, 5, 15, 30, 45, 60, 90, and 120 minutes (Johnson, 1977).

The diagnostic criteria for hyperinsulinism with the glucagon tolerance test are (1) a peak blood glucose throughout the test of less than 135 mg/dl; (2) hypoglycemia (blood glucose less than 60 mg/dl) returning within two hours of the intravenous infusion; (3) plasma insulin concentration above 50 μU/ml one minute after infusion of glucagon; (4) a decrease in blood glucose concentration one or two minutes after injection, which is assumed to be associated with a rapid rise in serum insulin concentrations; and (5) an insulin:glucose ratio one minute after infusion of glucagon that is greater than 75 (Johnson, 1977).

Other tests that have been used in veterinary medicine include the intravenous glucose tolerance test (Caywood and Wilson, 1980), the oral glucose tolerance test (Hill et al., 1974), the leucine tolerance test, and the tolbutamide tolerance test (Johnson, 1977).

PATHOLOGIC CHARACTERISTICS

In our series of dogs with insulin-secreting tumors, 11 were found in the right lobe of the pancreas, 9 in the left lobe, 1 in

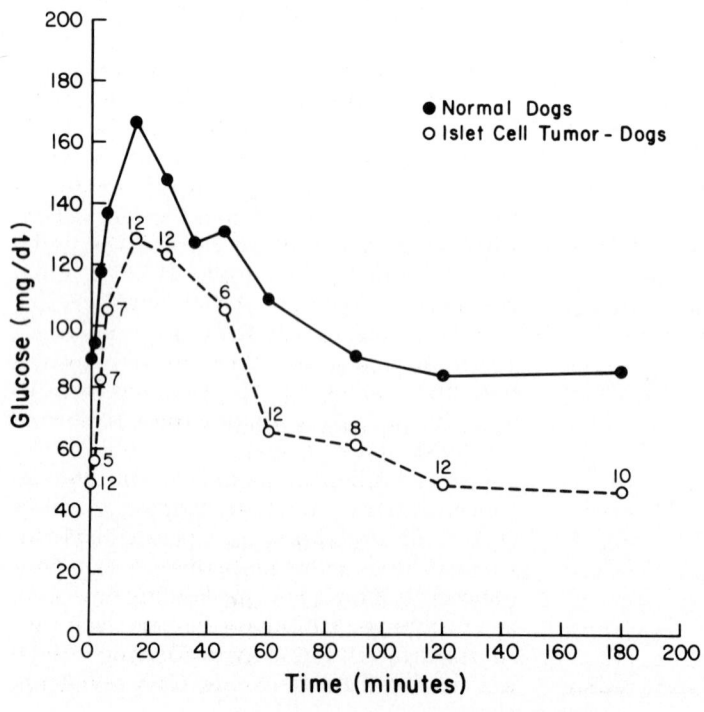

Figure 68–9. Plasma glucose concentrations during glucagon tolerance testing in normal dogs and dogs with functioning pancreatic islet cell tumors.

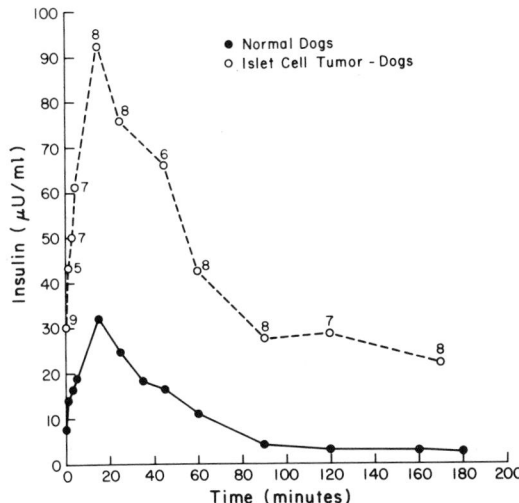

Figure 68-10. Plasma immunoreactive insulin concentrations during glucagon tolerance testing in normal dogs and dogs with functioning pancreatic islet cell tumors.

the body, and 2 were diffuse in nature (Kruth et al., in press). In dogs these tumors are usually visible to the surgeon. Occasionally, however, they are difficult to see or are microscopic. Multiple pancreatic tumors have not been described in the dog. A review of reported cases revealed that 69 per cent were malignant in one series, and 82 per cent in another (Johnson, 1977; Capen, 1969). In our series of 20 cases, in which the pathologist distinguished malignant from benign tumors, 19 (95 per cent) were malignant.

MANAGEMENT OF SERUM GLUCOSE CONCENTRATION

Hypoglycemic Crisis. Any patient brought to the veterinarian acutely comatose or in status epilepticus should have, among the various diagnostic studies performed, blood obtained for glucose determination. Dogs with recurrent single seizures or other transient hypoglycemic symptoms usually have minimal neuronal damage. Such dogs quickly respond to intravenous glucose or, when possible, to feeding. Over the phone, owners are instructed to rub Karo syrup into the buccal mucosa of dogs known to suffer hypoglycemic reactions. Such dogs usually respond to therapy within 30 to 60 seconds. In a crisis, intravenous glucose is administered slowly as 50 per cent dextrose, to effect. Prolonged, untreated hypoglycemia may re-

sult in irreversible cerebral lesions (Krook and Kenny, 1962; Capen and Martin, 1969). This is believed to be hypoxic damage due to prolonged, decreased metabolism. Lack of amelioration of symptoms in response to glucose therapy may be indicative of both cerebral hypoxia and edema. The therapy for such patients includes intravenous dextrose, diazepam, mannitol, glucocorticoids, and local hypothermia (Johnson, 1977).

Preoperative Preparation. After an insulin-secreting tumor is diagnosed, it is important that the pet be protected from the dangers of hypoglycemia until surgery is performed. This can be accomplished in most patients by frequent feedings. On the evening prior to surgery the patient is allowed no food. An intravenous glucose solution (five per cent dextrose in water) should therefore be administered.

Intraoperative Management. The author has found that a blood glucose immediately prior to surgery, as well as one or two during surgery, are helpful. Dogs with any anesthetic or intraoperative complications need to have potential glucose abnormalities monitored. Thus, in an emergency, one can know whether or not the problems can be the result of hypoglycemia. Problems due to hypoglycemia in surgery are not common, but they do occur.

Surgery. In veterinary medicine, no test is available to predict widespread metastasis or prognosis. Dogs with biochemically confirmed hyperinsulinism have a guarded to poor prognosis. However, exploratory celiotomy is recommended as the best diagnostic and prognostic tool available. If a dog is to be cured, surgery provides the best chance for the pet. Surgical preparation is no different for suspected hyperinsulinism patients than for any other, except for the fluid therapy described previously.

A complete exploratory surgery should be performed prior to examination of the pancreas. The entire pancreas must be carefully palpated for masses, even after one mass is discovered. It is important to examine the liver and local lymph nodes carefully for metastases. If possible, any pancreatic mass and abnormal lymph tissue should be surgically excised. With obvious widespread metastases to liver or abdominal contents, the lesions are considered operatively uncorrectable. If no insulin-secreting tumor can be found in a patient with good evidence of such a tumor, surgical removal of the left lobe of the pancreas is recommended, because surgeons find this lobe to be most difficult to examine visually. The removed portion of pancreas must be carefully and completely examined histologically for neoplasia.

Postoperative Management. Pancreatitis has been described as a common sequela to surgery (Johnson, 1977). The author has not had significant clinical postoperative problems. These dogs are kept off oral food and water for 36 to 48 hours routinely. Intravenous fluids are given to maintain a normal homeostasis of glucose, fluid, and electrolyte balance. Usually, dogs are eating by day three and are no longer receiving intravenous fluids by day four or five.

We do not recommend euthanasia if malignancy is discovered. Many dogs with proper therapy remain asymptomatic for prolonged periods of time even with good evidence of metastasis. Therefore, we monitor blood glucose and symptoms after surgery. Approximately 25 per cent of our dogs experienced transient (days to six months duration) diabetes mellitus. It is believed that the tumor production of insulin may cause atrophy of normal pancreatic B cells. Within days to months the diabetic state will dissipate. Therapy for diabetes mellitus with insulin is initiated only if blood glucose concentrations are consistently above 250 mg/dl and glycosuria is found consistently over several days.

No medication is given postoperatively in nondiabetic dogs. Such dogs are monitored for hypoglycemia in the hospital for five to seven days postoperatively. If symptoms of hypoglycemia are observed, a blood glucose is obtained. Hypoglycemia in the hospital, or clinical symptoms noted by the owner, dictates the necessity of frequent feedings. This is also strong evidence of metastasis of functional insulin-secreting tumor cells.

When frequent feedings fail to control symptoms or if an owner cannot feed the pet frequently enough to avoid problems, medication is begun. Arbitrarily, the author has chosen glucocorticoids as the first therapy to support the blood glucose. These are the least expensive drugs with the fewest side effects. Prednisone is given orally at a dose of 0.25 to 0.5 mg/kg body weight in divided doses daily. Success has been variable. Some dogs have been helped for as long as two years, while others improve for

only a matter of weeks. Long-term maintenance dosage is determined from a compromise of eliminating clinical symptoms and attempting to avoid the common glucocorticoid side effects, which include polydipsia, polyuria, polyphagia, hair loss, and infection.

If glucocorticoids no longer control symptomatology, diazoxide is the drug the author uses next. Diazoxide is chemically related to the thiazide diuretics and can increase blood glucose by several mechanisms. In large doses, it causes adrenal medullary release of epinephrine. It also inhibits the release of insulin. In the presence of adequate glycogen stores, however, it can produce an increase in plasma glucose and free fatty acid levels in pancreatectomized and adrenalectomized animals. In the intact animal, diazoxide increases hepatic release of glucose, inhibits glucose utilization in the periphery, and increases the rate of mobilization of free fatty acids. Little is known about its metabolism (Meyers et al., 1970; Schein et al., 1973).

Side effects of this drug include nausea, vomiting, and edema formation. Edema has not been seen in dogs. Nausea and vomiting are decreased by feeding at the time of drug administration and by continuing glucocorticoid medication. The author has used a dose of 10 to 20 mg/kg body weight in divided doses. This dose has been used for as long as a year in some patients before the endogenous insulin production appeared to be nonsuppressible. Increased toxicity in dogs has been noted when diazoxide was given concomitantly with trichlormethiazide, a thiazide diuretic.

Propranolol has been used in man as a hyperglycemic agent. This drug is commonly used in canines with cardiomyopathy and is inexpensive and readily available, and has few side effects (Blum et al., 1975).

Streptozotocin is an anticancer agent that is a naturally occurring nitrosourea isolated from the fermentation cultures of *Streptomyces achromogenes* (Herr et al., 1967). This drug has had some excellent results in man (Broder and Carter, 1973; Schein et al., 1973). There are, unfortunately, severe potential side effects. Renal tubular damage is the most common serious drug toxicity (Sadoff, 1970). This drug has only been used in the treatment of two dogs, both of which developed renal tubular defects (Meyer, 1976; Meyer, 1977).

Prognosis. Insulin-secreting tumors in the dog are rarely totally excised. These cancers commonly metastasize prior to veterinary intervention. Death usually results from hypoglycemia, metastatic problems, or an owner's inability to tolerate the symptoms. We recommend medical management in dogs after the first attempt at surgery, should spread of the cancer be evident. There are reports of excellent survival times in such dogs when monitored closely and treated as necessary (Caywood and Wilson, 1980).

REFERENCES

Physiology

Bloom, W. F.: Review of Medical Physiology. Lange Medical Publications, Los Altos, Ca., 1979.

Brown, J. C.: GIP: Gastric inhibitory polypeptide or glucose-dependent insulinotropic polypeptide? Guidelines to Metabolic Therapy 6:1, 1977.

Cuatrecasas, P.: The insulin receptor. Diabetes 21(Suppl. 2):396–402, 1972.

Curry, D. L., Bennett, L. L., and Grodsky, G. M.: Dynamics of insulin secretion by the perfused rat pancreas. Endocrinology 83:572–584, 1968.

Floyd, J. C., Fajans, S. S., Conn, J. W., Knopf, R. F., and Rull, J.: Stimulation of insulin secretions by amino acids. J. Clin. Invest. 45:1487–1502, 1966.

Freychet, P., Roth, J., and Neville, D. M.: Insulin receptors in the liver: Specific binding of (I-125) insulin to the plasma membrane and its relation to insulin bioactivity. Proc. Nat. Acad. Sci. 68:1833–1837, 1971.

Ganong, W. F.: Review of Medical Physiology. Lange Medical Publications, Los Altos, Ca., 1979.

Marliss, E. B., Murray, F. T., Stokes, E. F., et al.: Normalization of glycemia in diabetes during meals with insulin and glucagon delivery by the artificial pancreas. Diabetes 26:663, 1977.

Muller, W. A., Faloona, F. R., and Unger, R. H.: Hyperglucagonemia in diabetic ketoacidosis. Am. J. Med. 54:52–57, 1973.

Said, S. I., and Zfass, A. M.: Gastrointestinal Hormones, Disease-A-Month, Year Book Medical Publishers, Inc., Chicago, 1978.

Schade, D. S., and Eaton, R. P.: Pathogenesis of diabetic ketoacidosis: A reappraisal. Diabetes Care 2:296–306, 1979.

Schade, D. S., Eaton, R. P., and Peake, G. T.: The regulation of plasma ketone body concentration by counterregulatory hormones in man. II. Effects of growth hormone in diabetic man. Diabetes 27:916–924, 1978.

Steiner, D. F., Oyer, P., Cho, S., Melani, F., and Rubenstien, A. H.: Structural and Immunological Studies on Human Proinsulin. *In* Rodriguez, R. R., and Vallance-Owen, J. (eds.): Fed. Excerpta Medica Foundation, Amsterdam, 1971, pp. 281–291.

Swift, G. A., and Brown, R. H.: Surgical treatment of Cushing's syndrome in the cat. Vet. Rec. 99:374, 1976.

Williams, R. H., and Porte, D.: The pancreas. *In* Williams, R. H. (ed.): Textbook of Endocrinology, W. B. Saunders Co., Philadelphia, 1974, pp. 502–626.

Hypoinsulinism

Alberti, K. G. M. M., Christensen, N. J., Iverson, J., et al.: Role of glucagon and other hormones in development of diabetic ketoacidosis. Lancet 1:1307–1311, 1975.

Alberti, K. G. M. M., and Hockaday, T. D. R.: Diabetic coma. Clin. Endocrinol. Metab. 6:421–425, 1977.

Alberti, K. G. M. M., and Nattrass, M.: Severe diabetic ketoacidosis. Med. Clin. North Am. 62:799–814, 1978.

Anderson, J. W., and Ward, K.: Long-term effects of high-carbohydrate, high-fiber diets on glucose and lipid metabolism: A preliminary report on patients with diabetes. Diabetes Care 1:77–82, 1978.

Arieff, A. I., and Carroll, H. J.: Nonketotic hyperosmolar coma with hyperglycemia: Clinical features, pathophysiology, renal function, acid-base balance, plasma-cerebrospinal fluid equilibria and the effects of therapy in 37 cases. Medicine (Balt.) 51:73–94, 1972.

Arieff, A. I., and Kleeman, C. R.: Cerebral edema in diabetic comas. II. Effects of hyperosmolarity, hyperglycemia and insulin in diabetic rabbits. J. Clin. Endocrinol. Metab. 38:1057–1067, 1974.

Balasse, E. O., and Neef, M. A.: Isotopic studies in the ketosis of fasting and diabetes in man. Diabetologia 11:331, 1975.

Beisel, W. R., Sawyer, W. D., Ryll, E. D., et al.: Metabolic effects of intracellular infections in man. Ann. Intern. Med. 67:744–779, 1967.

Bellows, J. G.: Cataract and Abnormalities of the Lens. Grune and Stratton, New York, 1975, pp. 97–125.

Berson, S. A., and Yalow, R. S.: Some current controversies in diabetes research. Diabetes 14:549–572, 1965.

Blackshear, P. B.: Metabolic studies in experimental diabetic ketoacidosis. D. Phil. Thesis, University of Oxford, 1974.

Blackshear, P. B., Holloway, P. A. H., and Alberti, K. G. M. M.: The effects of inhibition of gluconeogenesis on ketogenesis in starved and diabetic rats. Biochem. J. 148:353–362, 1975.

Bloom, M. E., Mintz, D. H., and Field, J. B.: Insulin-induced posthypoglycemic hyperglycemia as a cause of "brittle" diabetes. Am. J. Med. 47:891–903, 1969.

Chastain, C. B., and Nichols, C. E.: Low-dose intramuscular insulin therapy for diabetic ketoacidosis in dogs. J.A.V.M.A. 178:561–564, 1981.

Clements, R. S., Jr., Prockop, L. D., and Winegrad, A. I.: Acute cerebral edema during treatment of hyperglycemia. An experimental model. Lancet 2:384–386, 1968.

Clements, R. S., Jr., Blumenthal, S. A., and Morrison, A. D.: Increased cerebrospinal-fluid pressure during treatment of diabetic ketosis. Lancet 2:671–675, 1971.

Comerci, C. A., Wyckoff, J. T., Rotch, J., Ravis, W. R.,

Spano, J. S., Dillon, A. R., and Ganjam, V. K.: Immunoassayable Levels of Insulin; and Studies on Biological Half-Life of Administered NPH-Insulin to Both Normal and Diabetic Dogs. Abstract *in* American College of Veterinary Internal Medicine Scientific Proceedings. Washington, D.C., July 21, 1980.

Cotton, R. B., Cornelius, L. M., and Theran, P.: Diabetes mellitus in the dog: A clinicopathologic study. J.A.V.M.A. *159*:863–870, 1971.

Dobbs, R., Schusdziarra, V., Rivier, J., et al.: Somatostatin analogs as glucagon suppressants in diabetes. Diabetes *26*(Suppl. 1):360, 1977.

Duck, S. C., Weldon, V. V., Pagiana, A. S., et al.: Cerebral oedema complicating therapy for ketoacidosis. Diabetes *25*:111–115, 1976.

Feldman, B. F., and Feldman, E. C.: Routine laboratory diagnosis in endocrine disease. Vet. Clin. North Am. 7:443, 1977.

Feldman, E. C.: Diabetic ketoacidosis in dogs. Comp. Cont. Ed. *11*:456–463, 1980.

Feldman, E. C., and Ettinger, S. J.: Electrocardiographic changes associated with electrolyte disturbances. Vet. Clin. North Am. 7:3, 1977.

Felig, P.: Diabetic ketoacidosis. N. Engl. J. Med. *290*:1360–1362, 1974.

Felig, P.: The liver in glucose homeostasis in normal man and in diabetes. *In* Vallance-Owen, J. (ed.): Diabetes: Its Physiological and Biochemical Basis. Lancaster Medical and Technical Publishers, Berkeley, Ca., 1975, pp. 93–124.

Finco, D. R., Kurtz, H. J., Low, D. G., and Perman, V.: Familial renal disease in Norwegian elkhound dogs. J.A.V.M.A. *156*:747–760, 1970.

Foa, P. P., Weinstein, H. R., and Smith, J. A.: Secretion of insulin and of a hyperglycemic substance studied by means of pancreatic-femoral gross-circulation experiments. Am. J. Physiol. *157*:197–204, 1949.

Foster, S. J.: Diabetes mellitus — A study of the disease in the dog and cat in Kent. J. Small Anim. Pract. *16*:295–315, 1975.

Fox, J. G., and Beatty, J. O.: A case report of complicated diabetes mellitus in a cat. J.A.A.H.A. *11*:129–134, 1975.

Ganong, W. F.: The Pancreas. *In* Review of Medical Physiology. Lange Medical Publications, Los Altos, Ca., 1979, pp. 257–277.

Gartner, K., Kirschner, M. A., and Mandl, I.: Untersuchungen zur Disposition der Hundin fur Diabetes Mellitus. Zentralbl. Veterinaermed. *15*:517–526, 1968.

Gebhardt, M. C., and Garnett, W. R.: Drugs Affecting Carbohydrate Metabolism. *In* Sussman, K. E., and Metz, R. J. S. (eds.): Diabetes Mellitus, 4th ed. American Diabetes Association, New York, 1975, pp. 271–276.

Gerich, J. E., Martin, M. M., and Recant, L.: Clinical and metabolic characteristics of hyperosmolar nonketotic coma. Diabetes *20*:228–238, 1971.

Gerich, J. E.: Metabolic effects of long-term somatostatin infusion in man. Metabolism *25*(Suppl. 1):1505–1507, 1976.

Gershwin, L. J.: Familial canine diabetes mellitus. J.A.V.M.A. *167*:479–480, 1975.

Hendricks, H. J., Teunissen, G. H. B., Schopman, W., Hackeng, W. H. L., and Antonisse, H. W.: Studies on glucose and insulin levels in the blood of normal and diabetic dogs. Zentralbl. Veterinaermed. *23*:206–216, 1976.

Johnston, D. G., and Alberti, K. G. M. M.: Carbohy-

drate metabolism in liver disease. Clin. Endocrinol. Metabol. *5*:675–702, 1976.

Joshua, J. O.: Some clinical aspects of diabetes mellitus in the dog and cat. J. Small Anim. Pract. *4*:275–280, 1963.

Joslin, E. P., Gray, H., and Root, H. L.: Insulin in the hospital and at home. J. Metab. Res. *2*:651, 1922.

Kaneko, J. J.: New perspectives in canine diabetes mellitus. California Veterinarian, pg. 24, October, 1979.

Kaneko, J. J., Mattheeuws, D., Rottiers, R. P., and Vermeulen, A.: Glucose tolerance and insulin response in diabetes mellitus of dogs. J. Sm. Anim. Pract. *18*:85–94, 1977.

Karam, J.: Personal Communication, 1980.

Kaye, R.: Diabetic ketoacidosis — the bicarbonate controversy. J. Pediatr. *87*:156–159, 1975.

Kershbaum, A.: Diabetogenic effect of fluorine containing steroids. Br. Med. J. *2*:253–257, 1963.

Kramer, J. W.: Inherited early onset canine diabetes mellitus — A new model of human diabetes mellitus. Fed. Am. Soc. Exp. Biol. *36*:279–285, 1977.

Ling, G. V., Lowenstine, L. J., Pulley, T., and Kaneko, J. J.: Diabetes mellitus in dogs: A review of initial evaluation, immediate and long-term management and outcome. J.A.V.M.A. *170*:521–530, 1977.

Ling, G. V., Stabenfeldt, G. H., Comer, K. M., Gribble, D. H., and Schechter, R. D.: Canine Hyperadrenocorticism: pretreatment clinical and laboratory evaluation of 117 cases. J.A.V.M.A. *174*:1211–1215, 1979.

Loppnow, H., and Gembardt, C.: Zur pathogenese des spontanen diabetes mellitus der katze. Berl. Muench. Tieraerztl. Wochenschr. *89*:79–83, 1976.

Lubberink, A. A. N. A.: Diagnosis and Treatment of Canine Cushing's Syndrome. Ph.D. Thesis, University of Utrecht, The Netherlands, 1977.

Mahler, R., Stafford, W. S., and Tarrant, M. E.: The effect of insulin on lipolysis. Diabetes *13*:297–302, 1964.

Manns, J. G., and Martin, C. L.: Plasma insulin, glucagon and nonesterified fatty acids in dogs with diabetes mellitus. Am. J. Vet. Res. *33*:981–985, 1972.

Marmor, M., Willeberg, P., Glickman, L. T., Priester, W. A., Cypess, R. H., and Hurvitz, A.: Epidemiologic patterns of diabetes mellitus in dogs. Am. J. Vet. Res. *43*:465–470, 1982.

Meijer, J. C., Mulder, G. H., Rijnberk, A., and Croughs, R. J. M.: Hypothalamic corticotrophin releasing factor activity in dogs with pituitary-dependent hyperadrenocorticism. J. Endocrinol. *79*:209–213, 1978.

Miranda, P. M., and Horwitz, D. L.: High-fiber diets in the treatment of diabetic mellitus. Ann. Intern. Med. *88*:482–486, 1978.

Newsholme, E. A.: Carbohydrate metabolism in vivo: regulation of the blood glucose level. Clin. Endocrinol. Metab. *5*:543–578, 1979.

Nobis, H., Bruneder, H., and Falkensammer, C.: Untersuchungen der blutgerrinnung in coma diabeticum. Intensivmedizin *12*:52–60, 1975.

Peiffer, R. L., Gelatt, K. N., and Gwin, R. M.: Diabetic cataracts in the dog. Canine Pract. *4*:18–22, April, 1977.

Podolsky, S.: Hyperosmolar nonketotic coma in the elderly diabetic. Med. Clin. North Am. *62*:815–828, 1978.

Podolsky, S., Melissinos, C., and Burrows, B. A.: Potassium depletion in fatal diabetic ketoacidosis: High serum potassium with low body potassium and similar skeletal and myocardial potassium values. Diabetes *23*:381, 1974.

Posner, J. B., and Plum, F.: Spinal-fluid pH and neurologic symptoms in systemic acidosis. N. Engl. J. Med. *277*:605–613, 1966.

Prout, T. E.: The Use of Screening and Diagnostic Procedures: The Oral Glucose Tolerance Test. *In* Sussman, K. E., and Metz, R. J. S. (eds.): Diabetes Mellitus. 4th ed. American Diabetes Association, Inc., New York, 1975, pp. 57–67.

Randle, P. J., Garland, P. B., Hales, C. N., and Newsholme, E. A.: The glucose fatty-acid cycle. Its role in insulin sensitivity and the metabolic disturbances of diabetes mellitus. Lancet *1*:785–789, 1963.

Rocha, D. M., Santeusanio, F., Faloona, G. R., et al.: Abnormal pancreatic alpha-cell function in bacterial infections. N. Engl. J. Med. *288*:700–703, 1973.

Rottiers, R., Mattheeuws, D., Kaneko, J. J., and Vermeulen, A.: Glucose uptake and insulin secretory responses to intravenous glucose loads in the dog. Am. J. Vet. Res. *42*:155–158, 1981.

Schaer, M.: Diabetic hyperosmolar nonketotic syndrome in a cat. J.A.A.H.A. *11*:42–46, 1975.

Schaer, M.: Transient insulin response in dogs and cats with diabetes mellitus. J.A.V.M.A. *168*:417–418, 1976.

Schaer, M., Scott, R., Wilkins, R., Kay, W., Calvert, C., and Wolland, M.: Hyperosmolar syndrome in the non-ketoacidotic diabetic dog. J.A.A.H.A. *10*:357–361, 1974.

Schall, W. D., and Cornelius, L. M.: Diabetic Ketoacidosis. *In* Kirk, R. W. (ed.): Current Veterinary Therapy, VII. W. B. Saunders Co., Philadelphia, 1980, pp. 1016–1019.

Somogyi, M.: Diabetogenic effects of insulin hypoglycemia. Bull. Jewish Hosp. *3*:1–15, 1953.

Somogyi, M.: Exacerbation of diabetes by excess insulin action. Am. J. Med. *26*:169–173, 1959.

Somogyi, M., Kirstein, M. G., and Freidewald, W. F.: Symposium on the management of unstable, severe, diabetic patients. Weekly Bull. St. Louis Med. Soc. *32*:498, 1938.

Ticer, J. W.: Roentgen signs of endocrine disease. Vet. Clin. North Am. 7:465, 1977.

Wilkinson, J. S.: Spontaneous diabetes mellitus. Vet. Res. 72:548–555, 1960.

Wood, P. A., and Smith, J. E.: Glycosylated hemoglobin and canine diabetes mellitus. J.A.V.M.A. *176*:1267–1268, 1980.

Hyperinsulinism

Blum, I., Doron, M., Laron, Z., and Atsmon, A.: Prevention of hypoglycemic attacks by propanolol in a patient suffering from insulinoma. Diabetes *24*:535–537, 1975.

Broder, L. E., and Carter, S. K.: Pancreatic islet cell carcinoma. Clinical features of 52 patients. Ann. Intern. Med. *79*:101–107, 1973.

Capen, C. C., and Martin, S. L.: Hyperinsulinism in dogs with neoplasia of the pancreatic islets. A clinical, pathologic and ultrastructural study. Pathol. Vet. *6*:309–341, 1969.

Caywood, D. D., and Wilson, J. W.: Functional Pancreatic Islet Cell Adenocarcinoma in the Dog. *In* Kirk, R. W. (ed.): Current Veterinary Therapy, VII. W. B. Saunders Co., Philadelphia, 1980, pp. 1020–1023.

Caywood, D. D., Wilson, J. W., Hardy, R. M., and

Shull, R. M.: Pancreatic islet cell adenocarcinoma: Clinical and diagnostic features of six cases. J.A.V.M.A. *174*:714–717, 1979.

Feldman, B. F., and Feldman, E. C.: Routine laboratory diagnosis in endocrine disease. Vet. Clin. North Am. 7:443–464, 1977.

Ganong, W. F.: Endocrine Functions of the Pancreas and the Regulation of Carbohydrate Metabolism. *In* Medical Physiology. Lange Medical Publications, Los Altos, Ca., 1979, p. 276.

Herr, R. R., Jahnke, H. K., and Argondelis, A. S.: Structure of streptozotocin. J. Am. Chem. Soc. *89*:4808–4809, 1967.

Hill, F. W. G., Pearson, H., Kelly, D. F., and Weaver, B. M. Q.: Functional islet cell turnover in the dog. J. Small Anim. Pract. *15*:119–127, 1974.

Johnson, R. K.: Insulinoma in the dog. Vet. Clin. North Am. 7:629–636, 1977.

Kaplan, E. L., and Lee, C.: Diagnosis and treatment of insulinomas. Surg. Clin. North Am. *59*:119–129, 1979.

Krook, L., and Kenny, R. M.: Central nervous system lesions in dogs with metastasizing islet cell carcinoma. Cornell Vet. *52*:385–415, 1962.

Lorenz, M. D.: Episodic Weakness in the Dog. *In* Kirk, R. W. (ed.): Current Veterinary Therapy, VI. W. B. Saunders Co., Philadelphia, 1977, pp. 818–822.

Mattheeuws, D., Rottiers, R., DeRijcke, J., et al.: Hyperinsulinism in the dog due to pancreatic islet cell tumor: A report of three cases. J. Small Anim. Pract. 7:313–318, 1976.

Meyer, D. J.: A pancreatic islet cell carcinoma in a dog treated with streptozotocin. Am. J. Vet. Res. *37*:1221–1223, 1976.

Meyer, D. J.: Temporary remission of hypoglycemia in a dog with an insulinoma after treatment with streptozotocin. Am. J. Vet. Res. *38*:1201–1204, 1977.

Meyers, F. H., Jawetz, E., and Goldfein, A.: Insulin, Glucagon, Oral Antidiabetic Drugs, and Hyperglycemic Agents. *In* Medical Pharmacology. Lange Medical Publications, Los Altos, Ca., 1970, pp. 334–346.

Priester, W. A.: Pancreatic islet cell tumors in domestic animals. Data from 11 colleges of veterinary medicine in the United States and Canada. J. Nat. Cancer Institute *53*:227–229, 1974.

Sadoff, L.: Nephrotoxicity of streptozotocin (NSC-85998). Cancer Chemother. Rep. *54*:457–459, 1970.

Schein, P. S., DeLellis, R. A., Kahn, C. R., Gordon, P., and Kraft, A. R.: Islet cell tumors: Current concepts and management. Ann. Intern. Med. *79*:239–257, 1973.

Slye, M., and Wells, H. G.: Tumor of islet tissue with hyperinsulinism in a dog. Arch. Pathol. *19*:537–542, 1935.

Turner, R. C., Oakley, N. W., and Nabarro, J. D. N.: Control of basal insulin secretion, with special reference to diagnosis of insulinomas. Br. Med. J. *2*:132–135, 1971.

Turner, R. C., Oakley, N. W., and Nabarro, J. D. N.: Changes in plasma insulin during ethanol-induced hypoglycemia. Metabolism *22*:111–121, 1973.

Whipple, A. O., and Frantz, V. K.: Adenoma of islet cells with hyperinsulinism. A review. Ann. Surg. *101*:1299, 1935.

Williams, R. H., and Portem, D.: The Pancreas. *In* Williams, R. H. (ed.): Textbook of Endocrinology. W. B. Saunders Co., Philadelphia, 1974, pp. 502–626.

CHAPTER 69

The Adrenal Cortex

EDWARD C. FELDMAN

The adrenal glands are bilateral structures located on the superomedial aspect of the kidneys. They consist of the cortex and medulla, which are embryologically and functionally separate endocrine glands. The cortex is derived from splanchnic mesodermal cells and is capable of synthesizing hormones early in fetal life. Hormones produced by this pair of small endocrine glands are vital, and under- or over-secretion of these products results in disease states that present a diagnostic challenge to the veterinarian. Proper diagnosis and therapy can return an extremely ill, debilitated animal to the owner in good health.

BIOSYNTHESIS AND METABOLISM OF ADRENOCORTICAL STEROIDS

INTRODUCTION

Terminology

All adrenocortical hormones are steroids. The term *steroid* is used to designate those compounds containing a four-ring structure, the cyclopentanoperhydrophenanthrene nucleus (Fig. 69–1). The steroids differ from each other in the atoms attached to this central nucleus; relatively slight changes in these attachments sometimes result in major differences in biological activity. For example, the difference between the major androgen (testosterone) and the major estrogen (estradiol) is but one methyl group and one hydrogen atom.

Although numerous steroids have been isolated from the mammalian adrenal cortex (Bethune, 1974), only a few are normally secreted into the blood and provide significant biologic activity. The significant hormones are classified into three groups, based on their predominant role in body physiology. Those adrenal steroids having their main effect on intermediary metabolism are called *glucocorticoids* (cortisol and corticosterone), those with their main effect on salt and water metabolism are called *mineralocorticoids* (aldosterone), and those with an effect like testosterone are called adrenal *androgens*. Generally speaking, they are the sugar, salt, and sex hormones, respectively.

Biosynthesis

The production of steroids, such as cortisol, involves a complex interaction between intracellular organelles, as seen in Figure 69–2 (Popjak and Cornforth, 1966). Control of the quantity of hormone secreted is determined outside the cell. In the case of glucocorticoids, isolated adrenocortical tissues secrete at a low rate, and pituitary corticotrophin (ACTH) is required to effect normal secretory rate and to increase adrenocortical output in times of stress. The precise mechanism by which ACTH induces steroid synthesis and release is unknown. It probably initiates intracellular events by acting directly on the cell membrane, thereby activating adenylcyclase on the inner membrane of the cell wall (Fig. 69–3).

Adrenal steroids are synthesized in the cell via cholesterol formation from acetate. In addition, cholesterol is extracted from circulating blood and assimilated by the adrenal synthesizing cell. The common biosynthetic pathway from cholesterol is via pregnenolone, the stem precursor for the three major groups of adrenal steroids (Fig. 69–4). Aldosterone is produced in the zona glomerulosa of the adrenal cortex, cortisol is produced primarily in the zona fasciculata, and androgens are produced in the zona reticularis.

Binding of Adrenal Steroids for Transport

The adrenal steroids are secreted into the blood and are then circulated to all parts of

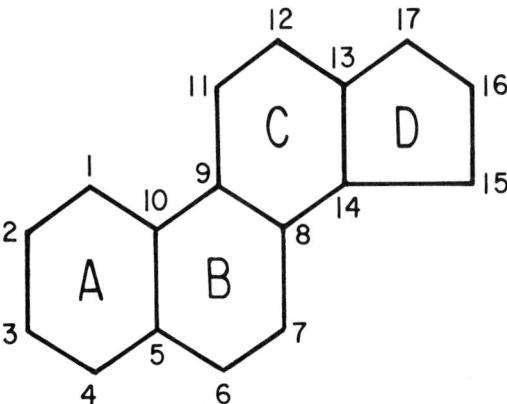

Figure 69–1. Structural formula of the steroid nucleus, cyclopentanoperhydrophenanthrene.

the body. The steroids do not exist in the blood purely in solution; to a large extent, the body has solubilized these hormones by binding them with plasma proteins. These proteins act as an efficient transport system as well as constituting a ready source of preformed circulating steroid. Cortisol is reversibly bound in the plasma to two proteins, a specific binding high affinity α_2-globulin called *transcortin or corticosteroid binding globulin (CBG)* and *albumin*, which has a nonspecific low affinity for binding steroids. At body temperature, 94 per cent of circulating cortisol is bound firmly to CBG and 6 per cent is free or very loosely bound to albumin. As free steroid is used up by peripheral tissues, it is directly replaced from this large "protein-bound bank," which is replenished by adrenal secretions.

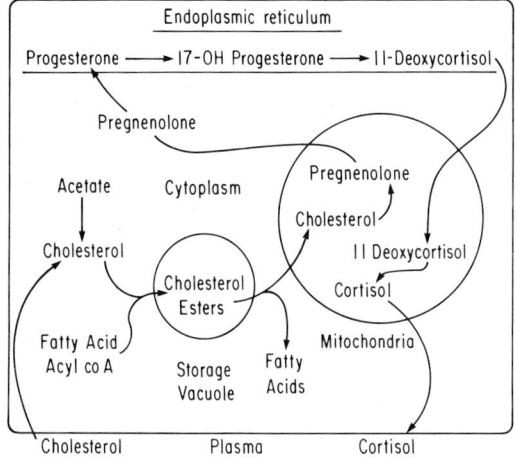

Figure 69–2. Pathway of cortisol synthesis within the cell of the zona fasciculata of the adrenal cortex.

Now that the episodic nature of the secretion of steroid hormones has been recognized (James et al., 1978), the importance of the buffering provided by protein binding of steroids becomes evident. CBG insures a steady and readily available supply of cortisol at the tissue level, despite fluctuations in secretion or removal rates. Globulin-bound steroid is not biologically active. However, cortisol bound to CBG is reversible and can become free cortisol if it is needed. Generally, the free steroid plasma concentration is maintained in a normal range by ACTH secretion.

Aldosterone is much less tightly bound and is mainly associated with albumin. Since aldosterone is not bound tightly to specific proteins in the plasma, it is more readily available for metabolism and it has a short half-life. The effect of CBG is to decrease the amount of cortisol that can be metabolized in a given time period, so that its biological half-life is approximately 80 minutes (Peterson, 1971).

Metabolism of Adrenal Steroids

Metabolism of adrenal steroids occurs primarily in the liver. The rate of removal of adrenocortical steroids by the liver, together with the adrenal secretory rate and the plasma concentration of CBG, determines their plasma concentration. In the presence of severe liver disease, the clearance of adrenocortical steroids may be decreased, but since steroid production adjusts to this by negative feedback from plasma cortisol or aldosterone, high blood levels do not occur (Peterson, 1971).

Biochemical Assays for Adrenocortical Steroids

Cortisol is the major glucocorticoid normally circulating in canine and feline plasma. The ratio of cortisol to corticosterone (the second major glucocorticoid) in dog plasma varies (Hechter et al., 1955) but is usually between 5:1 (Van der Vies, 1961) and 3.39:1 (Halliwell et al., 1971). Plasma glucocorticoid (cortisol) can be measured using one of three methods to detect total plasma cortisol. The extraction procedures remove both free and protein bound steroid. No method commonly available is sufficiently sensitive to measure only free plasma cortisol.

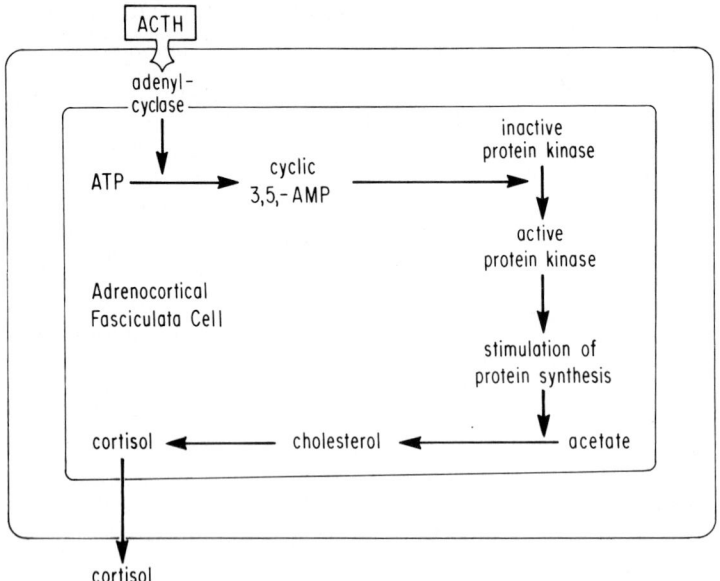

Figure 69–3. A proposed group of molecular events leading to the secretion of cortisol through the action of ACTH.

Fluorescent Cortisol. In the presence of sulphuric acid, cortisol fluoresces readily. This fluorescence is given by steroids possessing an 11-hydroxyl group. It is a simple assay to perform and very sensitive (Mattingly, 1962), but it is liable to interference by drugs, dirty reaction tubes, and nonspecific fluorescence found in some plasma samples. It also measures corticosterone. Such an assay, despite its limitations, has been found to be reliable in veterinary medicine (Feldman and Tyrrell, 1977).

Competitive Protein Binding Cortisol (CPG). Cortisol already bound to CBG can be displaced by adding more cortisol to the solution containing the CBG-cortisol complex. If known amounts of radioactive cortisol are added to a constant amount of CBG in a test tube, later addition of increasing amounts of "cold" cortisol will displace increasing counts of this "hot" cortisol from the CBG. Measurement of the amount of radioactivity displaced is proportional to the amount of cold cortisol added, and a stan-

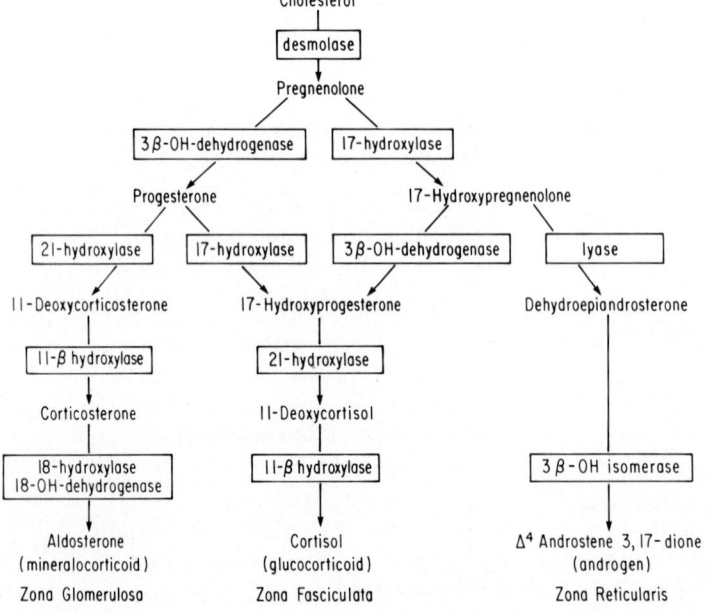

Figure 69–4. The three principal pathways of steroid biosynthesis in the adrenal cortex.

dard curve of this may be constructed. If plasma is extracted to elute the cortisol from the donor's CBG and then continued through this procedure, an extremely accurate estimate of cortisol in the plasma sample can be made. This method is simple, and neither drugs nor nonspecific fluorescent material interfere with it (Bassett and Hinks, 1969).

Radioimmunoassay

Radioimmunoassays for cortisol have been developed and applied to both plasma and urine. Given the availability of antiserum, they provide some technical advantages over both fluorescent and CPB assays. The principle of this assay system is similar to that of CPB, except that the binder is an antibody instead of CBG. Slightly lower and perhaps more specific plasma values have been found with radioimmunoassay (Cryer, 1976; Johnston and Mather, 1978).

These three systems have each been employed successfully in veterinary medicine. Each will be of value if there are established normal values for the species and test in question.

TISSUE EFFECT OF GLUCOCORTICOIDS

Mechanism of Action of Glucocorticoids

Steroid hormones freely cross the cell membrane and enter the cytoplasm. Once inside the cell, corticosteroid molecules bind to cytoplasmic protein receptors with high affinity for corticosteroids (Munck, 1971). Evidence implies that the glucocorticoid-specific receptor interaction is necessary for a glucorticoid response (Rousseau et al., 1972). Subsequent to binding in the cytoplasm, the steroid molecule–receptor complex leaves the cytoplasm and binds reversibly to specific sites on the chromatin of the cell nucleus. Interaction of the steroid-receptor complex with the nucleus may play a role either directly or indirectly in the amount or activity of specific messenger RNAs, which, in turn, code for enzymes or other proteins to produce the observed hormonal effects (Baxter et al., 1972).

It is important to realize that corticosteroids exert their effect by modifying the expression of the genetic information already manifest in a specific cell. Thus, by the single mechanism of stimulating protein synthesis, these hormones may elicit completely different responses from different cells.

Time Course of Glucocorticoid Effects

Most glucocorticoid-induced tissue responses can be detected within two hours and some within 10 to 30 minutes. *In vitro* studies indicate that specific nuclear binding of steroids can be detected within five minutes (Munck, 1971). The time interval between the nuclear binding and the response is presumed to be that necessary for intracellular processes to occur. Some responses do take longer than others. For this reason, the time required for steroid disappearance from plasma does not always indicate the duration of steroid action but depends on the time required for cessation of each stop in the individual process (Baxter and Forsham, 1972). The plasma half-life in dogs varies from 30 to 120 minutes, but the duration of action of a corticosteroid may persist for some time after the plasma level declines (Ritschel, 1972).

The plasma half-life of a particular corticosteroid is also markedly influenced by the preparation used. Therefore, the duration of action for a given corticosteroid, as measured by suppression of hypothalamic-pituitary activity, may be altered by the vehicle in which it is administered. Short-acting corticosteroids (hydrocortisone) have a duration of action of less than 12 hours, while intermediate-acting steroids (prednisolone, prednisone, and triamcinolone) last 12 to 13 hours. Long-acting corticosteroids such as flumethasone or dexamethasone have a duration of action of 36 to 72 hours (Enos, 1980). The relation between the steroid ester present in a preparation and its absorption period and duration of action may vary significantly. Sodium succinate esters may have a duration of action lasting hours, while pivalate esters may persist in action for weeks (Enos, 1980).

Metabolic Effects of Glucocorticoids

General. Table 69–1 summarizes the catabolic and anabolic biologic responses to corticosteroids. Muscle, skin, lymphoid, adipose, and connective tissues show some or all of the following catabolic processes: de-

Table 69–1. Some Biologic Responses
to Corticosteroids

Hepatic effects
  Increased glycogen stores
  Increased gluconeogenesis
  Induction of certain enzymes

Protein wasting
  Muscle
  Bone
  Skin
  Connective tissue

Hematologic effects
  Erythrocytosis
  Decrease in circulating lymphocytes
  Decrease in circulating eosinophils
  Increase in circulating neutrophils

Renal effects (predominantly mineralocorticoids)
  Decreased sodium excretion
  Increased hydrogen and potassium excretion

Suppression of ACTH secretion

Diminished inflammatory response

Suppression of delayed hypersensitivity

Increased urinary calcium excretion

Enhanced response of adipocytes to certain
lipolytic hormones

Facilitation of "free water" excretion

Maintenance of normal blood pressure

creased synthesis and increased degradation of protein, fat, RNA, and DNA, and decreased uptake of glucose and amino acids. Conversely, the liver responds anabolically to glucocorticoids with increased production of protein, RNA, and glucose.

The action of glucocorticoids on carbohydrate, protein, and lipid metabolism is the sparing of glucose and a tendency to glucose production and hyperglycemia. Within minutes of an infusion of glucocorticoid there is a decrease in glucose uptake in various peripheral tissues, such as adipose tissue and skin, as well as increased catabolism in these and other areas. The catabolism provides amino acids for hepatic gluconeogenesis and, to a lesser degree, for kidney gluconeogenesis. Further, there is decreased lipogenesis and increased lipolysis in adipose tissue, which results in the release of glycerol and free fatty acids. Glycerol provides an additional substrate for gluconeogenesis, and the free fatty acids may inhibit glucose uptake and utilization. These serve as an energy source to further conserve glucose and increase gluconeogenesis by generating NADH (Munck, 1971; Cahill, 1971).

This increase in blood glucose causes a secondary hyperinsulinism that counters and sometimes normalizes glucocorticoid action not only on glucose uptake but also on fat and protein metabolism. The end result in the normal animal is a balance between glucocorticoid action and opposing factors. This complex interplay between hormones and tissues may account for some variability in the clinical manifestations of both hyper- and hypoadrenocorticism (Baxter and Forsham, 1972).

Immune System and Inflammatory Response. Glucocorticoids are among the most important drugs used clinically in suppressing the immune systems. This suppression is helpful in preventing fibrosis and controlling various disease states, but there is the disadvantage of reducing resistance to a number of bacterial, viral, fungal, and even parasitic diseases. Glucocorticoids (endogenous as well as exogenous) may impair the immune response at various stages, from the initial interactions and processing of antigens by cells of the reticuloendothelial system, through induction and proliferation of immunocompetent lymphocytes and antibodies. They also suppress inflammatory reactions, wound healing, and scar formation (Cope, 1972).

Liver. In addition to processes already mentioned that take place in the liver, the specific deposition of glycogen represents a cardinal manifestation of glucocorticoids on hepatic metabolism. Several mechanisms are probably involved. First, glucocorticoids indirectly activate glycogen synthetase; second, glycogen deposition is increased indirectly via glucocorticoid-induced hyperglycemia itself; and third, glycogen is deposited secondary to hyperinsulinism caused by the increased blood glucose (De Wulf, 1971).

Among the many enzymes that are increased or induced by glucocorticoids is a unique alkaline phosphatase in the canine. This will be discussed in Canine Hyperadrenocorticism.

Adipose Tissue. Glucocorticoids increase lipolysis, which results in the release of free fatty acids and glycerol. Insulin is the counter-regulatory hormone that inhibits lipolysis and stimulates lipogenesis. Since glucocorticoids inhibit glucose uptake and lipogenesis, emaciation can be seen in some hyperadrenocorticoid animals. The redistribution of fat to the abdomen and back of the neck in dogs with excess levels of glucocorticoids may be due to the fact that the insulin response predominates in regions of increased fat, and steroid response predominates in the areas of fat loss (Rudman and DiGirolamo, 1971).

Muscle. In general the catabolic actions of glucocorticoids on muscle result in wasting and myopathy, which are common abnormalities seen with canine hyperadrenocorticism (Duncan et al., 1977; Griffiths and Duncan, 1973). The effects of glucocorticoids on muscle are both catabolic *and* antianabolic, since there is evidence for both an increased egress of amino acids into the circulation from muscle and a decreased incorporation of labeled amino acids into muscle proteins (Cahill, 1971).

Blood. Cortisol leads to an increase in circulating neutrophils and thrombocytes. Granulocytosis is probably due to an increased influx of cells from bone marrow, as well as to a decrease in the rate of egress of cells from the blood (Bishop et al., 1968). Steroids decrease circulating lymphocyte numbers by induction of cytolysis of the short-lived lymphocyte population (Craddock et al., 1967). The decreased numbers of circulating eosinophils are most likely the result of processes similar to the effects on lymphocytes. Increased erythrocytes and polycythemia are noted with glucocorticoid therapy, but the mechanism is unclear (Baxter and Forsham, 1972).

Skeleton and Bone. Several mechanisms account for the osteoporosis and the associated negative nitrogen and calcium balance caused by glucocorticoids. Tissue catabolism occurs in the bone matrix, which interferes with ossification by decreasing the surface on which bone mineral can be deposited. Glucocorticoids also reduce the intestinal absorption of calcium by inhibiting the action of vitamin D. This is achieved by inhibiting the transformation of relatively inactive calciferol to the active 25-hydroxycalciferol. Calcium clearance through the kidneys is increased by steroids as the result of a direct tubular action as well as increased glomerular filtration rates (Baxter and Forsham, 1972).

Stomach. Subjectively, oral glucocorticoids do cause gastric irritation, as well as gastrointestinal bleeding, in some dogs. This may be the result of enhanced cholinergic stimulation of hydrochloric acid secretion, which is observed in the basal state but is particularly evident with pharmacologic doses. The protective gastric mucus is also thinned by these hormones, which may contribute to the deleterious side effects (Toombs et al., 1980; David et al., 1970).

Regulation of Glucocorticoid Release

Secretion by the adrenal cortex of cortisol and/or corticosterone is subject to multiple controls and stimuli. In the normal dog, a regular daily release with diurnal variation is maintained to support a number of metabolic reactions that would otherwise not function adequately (Rijnberk et al., 1968). The major regulator of adrenal glucocorticoid synthesis and secretion is the 39-amino acid molecule adrenocorticotrophic hormone (ACTH) from the anterior pituitary (Jones, 1979). The secretion rate of ACTH is determined by a number of factors that are difficult to separate. The rate of synthesis, amount of storage, degree of release, and length of half-life all contribute to the measurable circulating level of ACTH.

Corticotrophin-Releasing Factor (CRF). Since the early descriptions of portal circulation connecting the hypothalamus and the pituitary, it has been recognized that the hypothalamus exerts control over secretion of ACTH by the anterior pituitary. The factor responsible for the control was identified as CRF. There is good evidence that CRF controls ACTH *release*, but it does not increase synthesis of the hormone. There is probably also a feedback control by ACTH on CRF secretion. This internal or "short-loop" feedback system is directly controlled by the blood level of ACTH at the hypothalamic level (Upton et al., 1973). There is a question as to the role vasopressin (ADH) plays in the control of ACTH secretion. It is likely that ADH may be released during certain stresses and that it potentiates the action of CRF (Jones, 1979).

Physiologic factors that influence the secretions of ACTH can conveniently be divided into two main groups, those that are under control of the diurnal mechanism and those resulting from stress. Although there is no evidence proving that there are two different corticotrophin-releasing hor-

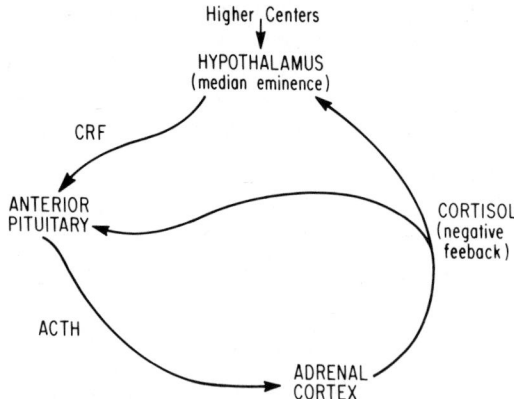

Figure 69–5. Interactions involving the hypothalamic-pituitary-adrenal axis.

mones, or two different pathways by which CRF acts, this division is a convenient one and is corroborated by much experimental data (Nelson, 1980). When considering these two control systems, one must also take into account the simple negative-feedback loop involving the adrenals and the pituitary.

Simple Negative Feedback Loop. In the resting state, ACTH and cortisol bear a reciprocal control relationship to one another (Fig. 69–5). ACTH release produces a rise in plasma cortisol, which in turn acts on receptors in the hypothalamus to decrease CRF secretion and thus reduce ACTH release. As the effective level of glucocorticoid diminishes, CRF secretion increases and then the cycle is complete. This simple mechanism can be overridden by other stimuli originating in other centers of the central nervous system, however. This alter-

ation from the simple negative feedback control may be seen both in the diurnal pattern of cortisol secretion and in times of stress.

DIURNAL VARIATION. The diurnal variation in glucocorticoid secretion is characterized by high levels of circulating cortisol in the early morning hours (at approximately sunrise) and low levels in the late evening. In most mammals the secretion of ACTH appears to be episodic in nature. Oscillating patterns of secretion of cortisol have been established (Fig. 69–6). Thus, in interpreting plasma corticosteroid determinations in clinical situations, a single determination may be misleading. If cortisol concentration levels reflect "bursts" of ACTH secretion, the plasma cortisol value depends on the moment of venous sampling relative to the timing of the adrenal burst of hormone release.

The circadian rhythm in plasma ACTH and cortisol is usually absent in human patients with hyperadrenocorticism. The normal rhythm in ACTH concentrations, however, is present in hypoadrenocorticism, although owing to the lack of the normal corticosteroid feedback to the pituitary gland, all concentrations are elevated. Thus the periodicity of the circadian rhythm is independent of the negative feedback effects of corticosteroids. The absence of a rhythm in hyperadrenocorticism is assumed to be an associated dysfunction at either the adrenal, pituitary, or hypothalamic level (Jones, 1979).

There is a circadian rhythm in the ability of natural and synthetic exogenous corticosteroids to suppress ACTH secretion. In

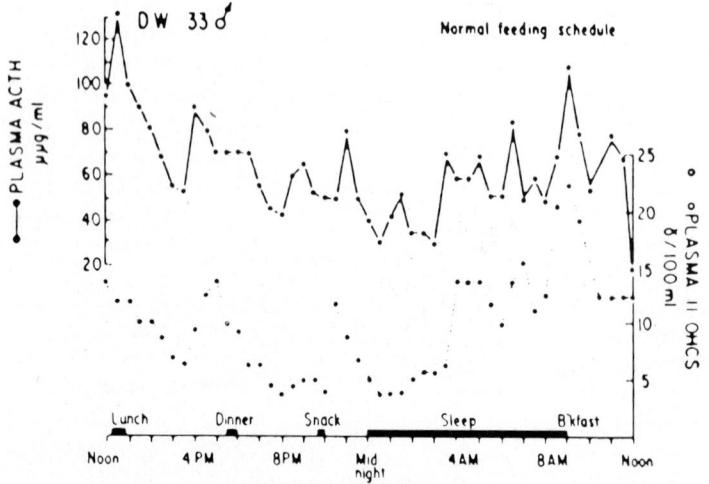

Figure 69–6. Variations in plasma ACTH and plasma 11-OHCS determined at half-hourly intervals in the study by Krieger et al. This figure demonstrates not only the higher levels in the early morning as opposed to late evening but also that ACTH secretion does not follow a smooth curve. There is a periodic release of ACTH resulting in stimulation of corticosteroid secretion at irregular intervals.

man and the rat the maximum inhibitory effect is exerted when these substances are administered four to eight hours before the circadian peak (Retiene et al., 1968). There is, therefore, a good argument for restricting corticosteroid administration in veterinary patients to the morning only (when possible), thereby limiting the dangers of pituitary suppression (Jones, 1979).

STRESS. Under normal circumstances, mammals respond to a variety of stressful situations, both physical and psychological, by increased secretion of ACTH. Studies have demonstrated the importance of the nervous system in the mediation of these responses (Mangli et al., 1966), illustrated by the marked increase in ACTH secretion after severe trauma to a limb. Denervation of the involved limb decreases the response, because the stimulus travels via peripheral nerves to central locations in the median eminence of the hypothalamus, where it stimulates secretion of CRF. The hypothalamic transmitter is carried by the hypophyseal portal circulation to the anterior pituitary, where it stimulates production of ACTH. CRF produced in this response cannot easily be suppressed by corticosteroids. This mechanism is necessary to prevent stress-induced increases in corticosteroids from immediately suppressing further ACTH production, thereby blocking the additional surge of corticosteroids needed to combat the stressful situation. In severe and prolonged stress, corticosteroid levels rise and continue at very high levels over extended periods of time (Hume et al., 1956).

ACTH secretion in response to stress is also episodic. The secretory spike frequency increases under stress, since average spike frequency in the morning and in the evening is statistically lower under nonstressed conditions than during stress (Nelson, 1980).

CONTROL OF ALDOSTERONE SECRETION

Aldosterone is synthesized and released from the zona glomerulosa of the adrenal cortex. As aldosterone has little direct influence on its own production from the adrenal cortex, or on release of renin by the kidney, it is clear that feedback is mediated by the effects of salt metabolism. This contrasts with the direct role of circulating cortisol levels in ACTH release. The secretion of aldosterone is influenced primarily by renin-angiotensin system and levels of potassium in the blood. ACTH and levels of sodium in the blood play a less significant role.

Renin-Angiotensin System

The renin-angiotensin system is a major physiologic mechanism controlling body fluid volume by regulating aldosterone secretions. Its function is closely related to that of the juxtaglomerular apparatus, which consists of the juxtaglomerular cells surrounding the afferent arterioles of renal cortical glomeruli and a group of special staining cells, the macula densa, situated in the distal convoluted tubule. The juxtaglomerular cells are specialized myoepithelial cells cuffing the afferent arterioles and acting as miniature pressure tranducers. They monitor renal perfusion pressure by perceiving pressure changes as distortions of the existing stretch on the arteriolar walls. Therefore, volume depletion caused by events such as hemorrhage, diuretic administration, and salt restriction would be perceived by the juxtaglomerular cells as a decreased stretch. These cells would then release an increased quantity of renin, which ultimately would result in increased aldosterone release by the adrenals. Aldosterone in increased levels would cause increased sodium retention, expansion of the extracellular fluid volume, increased renal perfusion, and a dampening out of the initiating signal for renin release (Liddle, 1971).

Potassium

Aldosterone secretion can be regulated independently of the renin-angiotensin system as a function of plasma potassium concentrations. When a solution of potassium ions is injected into adrenal arteries, there is an immediate increase in adrenal venous aldosterone concentration (Fundor et al., 1969). It appears that potassium has a direct stimulatory effect on the adrenocortical production of aldosterone, presumably through a transmembrane effect (Boyd et al., 1973). This potassium-mediated aldosterone control system operates in parallel with the renin-angiotensin system and can be of comparable potency.

Role of ACTH and Sodium

ACTH can stimulate the release of aldosterone, but it is not the dominant drive in secretion by the zona glomerulosa. Apparently ACTH is not an important control mechanism in most physiologic conditions, but it appears to exert a "permissive" influence over aldosterone secretion (Liddle, 1971). The renin-angiotensin system is probably the main stimulus to aldosterone secretion under conditions of sodium depletion via reduced blood pressure and poor renal perfusion (Jones, 1979).

MINERALOCORTICOID ACTION

Aldosterone stimulates active sodium reabsorption and sodium-potassium transport across the membranes of many epithelial tissues specialized for this function. These include the intestinal mucosa, salivary glands, sweat glands, and, of course, the kidneys. The action appears to be exerted chiefly on the renal tubules to produce proximal convoluted tubular absorption of chloride and sodium, and distal convoluted tubular absorption of sodium by exchange with potassium. This is the primary action of aldosterone (Nelson, 1980).

In excess amounts, aldosterone sharply increases renal sodium retention. Water retention and weight gain are seen in humans receiving excess mineralocorticoids. Before edema occurs, however, an "escape" from the sodium-retaining effect of this hormone occurs, and water losses return to approximate fluid intake. This escape phenomenon is not present in disease states such as congestive heart failure, nephrosis, and ascites, so that these patients continue to retain fluid and salt with resultant massive edema. At the same time, potassium excretion is increased, with the potential of potassium depletion, alkalosis, bicarbonate retention, and muscle weakness.

The escape is presumably due to inhibition of proximal tubular sodium resorption. The factor responsible for the inhibition is not yet understood (Bethune, 1974).

ADRENOCORTICAL INSUFFICIENCY

CAUSES OF ADRENOCORTICAL INSUFFICIENCY

Primary Causes. Hypoadrenocorticism (Addison's disease) is the result of primary adrenocortical failure. The etiology of primary adrenocortical failure is usually not known. Idiopathic atrophy, in which all the layers of the adrenal cortex are involved and usually markedly reduced in thickness, is the most frequently observed lesion in dogs (Capen et al., 1975). True cases of idiopathic adrenocortical atrophy have no pituitary lesions and are believed to result from an autoimmune process. Less common causes of canine adrenocortical insufficiency include destruction of the adrenal cortices by granulomatous disease such as histoplasmosis, blastomycosis, or tuberculosis; hemorrhagic infarctions; metastasis of cancer to the adrenal glands; and amyloidosis of the adrenal cortices (Capen et al., 1975). The adrenocorticolytic drug 1,1-Dichloro-2,2-bis(*p*-chlorophenyl)ethane (*o,p'*-DDD) inhibits steroid biosynthesis in the canine by destroying the adrenal cortex (Nelson and Woodward, 1949; Kirk et al., 1974; Kirk and Jensen, 1975) and thus has the potential for causing primary adrenocortical failure.

Secondary Causes. In addition to disease processes affecting the adrenal gland primarily, reduced secretion of ACTH will lead to decreased synthesis and secretion of adrenocortical hormones and hence to adrenal insufficiency (Bethune, 1974; Cryer, 1976). Abnormally depressed ACTH concentrations are usually the result of destructive lesions in the pituitary or the hypothalamus. Decreased ACTH concentrations can also be produced iatrogenically as a consequence of long-term treatment with corticosteroids (Scott and Greene, 1974) and can follow chronic injectable, oral, or topical application. Adrenal insufficiency secondary to corticosteroid therapy occurs in all patients receiving sufficient quantities of corticosteroids to suppress ACTH secretion. Although estimates of the relative biologic effectiveness of the clinical analogs vary, recent studies have shown dexamethasone to be 50 to 150 times more potent in its ability to suppress ACTH secretion than cortisol (Meikle and Tyler, 1977). Thus, very small quantities of this potent synthetic corticosteroid may be sufficient to produce adrenal atrophy. Dogs with iatrogenic adrenal atrophy may appear normal in the resting state but fail to increase corticosteroid secretion in response to stress, owing to lack of adrenal reserve. These animals need tapering glucocorticoid support to allow their pituitary-adrenal axis to return to normal, before such medication can be discontinued.

CLINICAL FEATURES OF ADRENOCORTICAL INSUFFICIENCY

Age, Sex, and Breed

Hypoadrenocorticism is uncommon in the canine and has not been reported in the feline (Capen et al., 1975; Feldman et al., 1977; Keeton et al., 1972; Mulnix, 1971). It is more common in females,·as is typical of most autoimmune disorders (Mulnix, 1971). Hypoadrenocorticism also appears to be a disease of young and middle-aged dogs. The author's series of cases includes dogs from six months to seven and a half years of age (Feldman and Tyrrell 1977a), while Peterson (1980) has described hypoadrenal dogs 2 to 12 years of age. No breed predilection has been described and canine Addison's disease appears to affect animals regardless of body size.

Pathogenesis

Destruction of the adrenal cortex, regardless of the underlying etiology, results in Addison's disease. The major clinical manifestations are attributable to deficiencies of both aldosterone and cortisol. Development of adrenal cortical insufficiency is believed to require destruction of at least 90 per cent of the adrenal cortex (Tyrrell and Forsham, 1974). In most instances destruction of the glands is a gradual process, first leading to a partial syndrome of adrenal insufficiency characterized by inadequate adrenal reserve, with symptoms manifested only during times of stress (associated with surgery, trauma, infection, or even psychological distress, such as times when dogs are placed in boarding kennels). Basal hormone secretion in the unstressed state may be adequate; the diagnosis can be confirmed only with tests that assess adrenal cortical reserve. As destruction of the adrenal glands progresses, hormone secretion becomes inadequate even under basal conditions and a true metabolic crisis results.

Lack of aldosterone results in impaired ability to conserve sodium and excrete potassium. With adequate sodium intake, a deficiency of aldosterone may have few, if any, consequences. If the sodium intake diminishes, however, or if sodium loss is increased because the dog experiences anorexia, vomiting, or diarrhea, the animal's condition may quickly deteriorate. Excretion of sodium rapidly exceeds its intake. Deficiency in aldosterone (sodium) results in

decreased circulating blood volume (hypovolemia), which is soon associated with hypotension. Subsequent to these changes is a reduction in cardiac output and heart size that ultimately causes reduced perfusion of the kidneys as well as other tissues. The decreased glomerular filtration causes prerenal azotemia, increased renin production, and mild metabolic acidosis. Weight loss, weakness, and depression are common.

Lack of aldosterone also results in the development of severe hyperkalemia, owing to diminished glomerular filtration rate and diminished cation exchange by the distal convoluted tubules. The most prominent manifestations of hyperkalemia are seen in the heart, where they consist of a decrease in myocardial excitability, an increase in the refractory period of the myocardium, and a slowing of conduction. Hypoxia also contributes to increased myocardial irritability. The mild acidosis is the result of an inability to retain bicarbonate and chloride ions as well as failure to excrete metabolic waste products and hydrogen ions (Ganong, 1969; Liddle, 1974).

Lack of cortisol may result in the gastrointestinal signs of anorexia, vomiting, abdominal pain, and weight loss. Mental changes such as diminished vigor and lethargy are noted. Energy metabolism is diminished owing to impaired gluconeogenesis, impaired fat metabolism and utilization, and liver glycogen depletion with the potential for fasting hypoglycemia. Impaired ability to excrete water free of sodium, which in turn results in hyponatremia, is possible. An unrestrained secretion of ACTH from the pituitary also occurs. One of the hallmark symptoms of Addison's disease is impaired tolerance to stress, and any of the above manifestations might become more pronounced if the animal is stressed.

Hypoadrenocorticism produced iatrogenically with the adrenocorticolytic drug o,p'-DDD could produce similar physiologic changes in dogs. One study (Kirk and Jensen, 1975) used this drug at the accepted daily dose (Schechter, 1974; Schechter et al., 1973) for long periods of time (36 to 150 days) in ten normal adult mongrels. Eight of the ten dogs appeared healthy and normal during the duration of treatment (Kirk and Jensen, 1975). One dog died after becoming weak following 124 days of treatment and the other dog appeared weak during the final two weeks of the 147 day treatment period. In our experience, however, dogs with Cushing's syndrome are much more sensitive to the effects of *o,p'*-DDD than is suggested in the previous paper (see pp. 1690).

In adrenal insufficiency secondary to pituitary or hypothalamic disease, which results in inadequate ACTH secretion, the renin-angiotensin-aldosterone system is preserved, and therefore, normal serum electrolyte concentrations are maintained. The same is true in dogs chronically treated with corticosteroids when medication administration is acutely discontinued. The iatrogenic corticosteroids inhibit ACTH secretion through negative feedback, which results in secondary adrenal cortical atrophy and spares the zona glomerulosa (Scott and Greene, 1974).

ANAMNESIS

History

The diagnosis of canine Addison's disease can only be made after the clinician suspects that a dog may be suffering from this disorder. Discussing with owners the various abnormalities they have seen should provide the basis for further diagnostic work. One of the most telling clues is the description of a "waxing-waning" or "episodic" course of illness. In many spontaneous hypoadrenal animals, the owners note episodic illness, weaknesss, and depression for brief periods of time during the previous 2 to 52 weeks. These dogs vacillate between appearing normal for periods and appearing quite ill, either suddenly or following a gradual downhill course. The periods of apparent good health often follow veterinary therapy consisting of corticosteroid medication or parenteral fluid administration.

The anamnesis (Table 69–2) commonly includes the description of a dog that is or has been depressed, lethargic, weak, and anorexic during the episodes of illness. The etiology of shivering in these patients is unknown although it is believed to be an expression of muscle weakness. Unfortunately, owner observations are vague and compatible not only with hypoadrenocorticism but also with more common renal and gastrointestinal diseases. Also, the severity of each abnormality noted in the history is highly variable from dog to dog.

If one accepts that acute adrenal insufficiency is the result of hemorrhage or acute

Table 69–2. Possible Indications of Addison's Disease

Historical Abnormalities	Occurrence (%)
Depression/lethargy	93
Waxing-waning course	91
Weakness	86
Anorexia	79
Shaking or shivering	57
Diarrhea	57
Weight loss	50
Vomiting	43
Abdominal pain	29
Polydipsia/polyuria	21
Reluctance to walk	21

necrosis (Tyrrell and Forsham, 1974) and that this form of the illness is "rapidly progressive over a number of hours" (Irvine and Barnes, 1972), then it appears that most dogs with hypoadrenocorticism have chronic rather than simple acute disease. The period of time over which owners note such abnormalities, be they progressive or episodic, is often two weeks or longer. This is not to say that these dogs did not present in crisis from naturally occurring disease, but that they developed acute adrenal crisis secondary to progressive untreated chronic adrenal or pituitary disease. One must remember that a dog presented with several of the vague complaints mentioned herein is potentially an addisonian, unless another malady is diagnosed or Addison's disease has been proven not to be at fault.

The history from owners whose dogs were presented to the hospital in acute crisis is similar to that provided when the dog is mildly ill. The only difference is in the degree of depression, weakness, or other signs described. Some dogs are so weak that they have to be carried.

Physical Examination

As can be seen in Table 69–3, depression was the only stand-out abnormality noted on physical examinations of the author's patients. The often-noted alterations of weak femoral pulse, generalized muscle weakness, bradycardia, dehydration, abdominal pain, and hypothermia (Keeton et al., 1972; Mulnix and Smith, 1975; Mulnix, 1971; Wolland, 1974; Lorenz, 1979) were seen, but in a surprisingly low percentage of the patients. This points out the importance of obtaining and evaluating a good medical

Table 69–3. Findings on Physical Examination Indicating Addison's Disease

Physical Examination Abnormalities	Occurrence (%)
Depression	93
Weakness	64
Weak pulse	43
Dehydrated	36
Slow mucous membrane refill time	21
Bradycardia	14
Abdominal pain	14

history, as well as carefully choosing one's diagnostic studies.

CLINICAL PATHOLOGY

Erythrocyte Parameters

In adrenal insufficiency, a normocytic, normochromic anemia accompanied by little or no reticulocyte response secondary to bone marrow suppression is common (Keeton et al., 1972). If an animal becomes hemoconcentrated secondary to dehydration, however, the underlying anemia will be masked. Once rehydrated, these dogs will exhibit the typical mild anemia of hypoadrenocorticism (Feldman and Feldman, 1977).

Leukocyte Counts

In a recent review, white blood counts in addisonian dogs varied between 7400 and 28,700 (Feldman and Tyrrell, 1977a). No definite pattern was noted among the total cell counts. The elevated white blood cell counts may have reflected a granulocytic response to an intercurrent infection.

The presence of an absolute eosinophilia in hypoadrenal dogs appears to be in dispute in the veterinary literature, with some having noted it consistently (Capen et al., 1975; Siegel and Belshaw, 1968) and others finding it to be an inconsistent feature (Keeton et al., 1972; Mulnix and Smith, 1975; Mulnix, 1971; Wolland, 1974). Eosinophils were lacking on admission CBCs in 3 of 22 dogs seen by the author, while three dogs had elevated eosinophil counts. The remaining 16 dogs all had eosinophil counts that were within the normal range, both on relative and absolute tabulations. The finding of a normal absolute eosinophil count in

an ill canine is significant, because a stress pattern with no or few eosinophils would have been expected in dogs of similar clinical status with normal plasma glucocorticoid concentrations. The finding of a normal eosinophil count in a stressed dog should be viewed with a suspicion of hypoadrenocorticism.

Lymphocytosis has previously been reported to be fairly common in canine adrenocortical insufficiency (Capen et al., 1975; Siegel and Belshaw, 1968). Others have found lymphocytosis to be an inconstant parameter (Keeton et al., 1972; Mulnix, 1971; Feldman and Tyrrell, 1977a). Normal lymphocyte levels in an ill dog are unusual, since the normal stressed dog with adequate glucocorticoids would be expected to exhibit lymphopenia. Hypoadrenocorticism should be suspected as a possible cause when normal and elevated lymphocyte counts are present in ill dogs.

Blood Urea Nitrogen (BUN) and Urinalysis

Prerenal azotemia with an increased BUN occurs secondary to reduced renal perfusion and an associated decrease in glomerular filtration rate. The decreased blood flow to the kidneys is a result of the hypovolemia resulting from chronic fluid loss through the kidneys, vomiting and/or diarrhea, reduced cardiac output, and eventually a severe drop in blood pressure. The BUN level in hypoadrenal dogs varied from a mild increase of 28 to severe increases of 124 and 154 mg per cent (Feldman and Tyrrell, 1977a). With rehydration and return of an adequate blood vascular volume, the BUN should return to a normal level. In rare cases, however, this may not occur, indicating inadequate fluid therapy or perhaps primary renal involvement following chronic decreased renal vascular perfusion. The initial elevated BUN level in a dog described by the owner as having clinical signs consistent with renal disease can be misleading to the veterinary practitioner. This may be further perplexing, in trying to diagnose hypoadrenocorticism, when the BUN fails to fall as rapidly as has been reported (Lorenz and Cornelius, 1976). It is urged therefore that practitioners use electrolyte concentrations and urinalysis in conjunction with renal function tests. The urine specific gravity in an animal with prerenal uremia should be elevated, while that in an animal with primary renal disease often is isosthenuric. The serum creatinine levels were found to correlate well with the BUN levels. Ultimately, hormone assay is required to confirm the presence or absence of adrenal disease.

Blood Glucose and Calcium

Fasting hypoglycemia is an unusual finding in hypoadrenal canines (Keeton et al., 1972; Lorenz and Cornelius, 1976; Mulnix and Smith, 1975; Mulnix, 1971), although hypoglycemia (blood sugar less than 60 mg per cent) was seen in two recently reported cases (Feldman and Tyrrell, 1977a). Both of these animals were presented in states of extreme depression, which certainly had been made more severe by their hypoglycemia. Serum calcium concentrations are occasionally elevated in hypoadrenal dogs that are in crisis.

Serum Electrolytes

The classic electrolyte changes in an addisonian involve the hyponatremia, hypochloremia, and hyperkalemia that would be expected when mineralocorticoids are lacking. These electrolyte alterations result from the loss of sodium and chloride into the urine and the simultaneous failure of the kidneys to excrete potassium. In the author's series, the serum sodiums ranged from a normal value of 145 to an extremely low 106 mEq/L, while serum potassium elevations varied from a slight increase of 5.0 to concentrations as high as 10.2 mEq/L.

The sodium-potassium ratio has frequently been used as a diagnostic tool to clarify potentially vague results. The normal ratio varies between 27:1 and 40:1 in the author's laboratory. Values are often below 27 and may be found below 20. Determination of serum electrolyte concentrations on dogs suspected of having adrenal insufficiency is of paramount importance. The finding of hyperkalemia with or without alterations in the serum sodium or chloride should prompt immediate therapy. The assumption that one is treating an addisonian is well warranted and, in fact, may be life saving.

The limitations of serum electrolyte determination, however, must be realized. Reliance on electrolytes as the sole factor in diagnosing adrenal insufficiency can be misleading if three factors are not kept in mind: First and most important is the slow, progressive nature in the development of primary adrenal insufficiency; second is that dogs with pituitary failure can normally secrete aldosterone; and third is that hyperkalemia may not always be associated with adrenal insufficiency.

Adrenal insufficiency is usually insidious in onset and gradually progressive, although acute adrenal crisis may be precipitated by intercurrent stress. The results of any diagnostic studies performed will depend on when clinical signs first develop or when a clinician first suspects that a dog may be suffering from this disease. If it presents when ill, a serum electrolyte determination may well reveal the diagnosis, while stable animals may have normal electrolyte concentrations. The diagnosis in these patients must be confirmed with tests that measure adrenal cortical reserve.

Electrolyte alterations are attributed to inadequate mineralocorticoids. Therefore, an animal that has pituitary deficiency of ACTH may have a clinical syndrome that reflects only glucocorticoid deficiency. Since aldosterone is only minimally effected by ACTH, such an animal will maintain normal electrolyte concentrations. The gastrointestinal, mental, and metabolic changes typical of hypocortisolemia may become obvious to the owner and veterinarian, while those changes ascribed to hypoaldosteronism are absent. Electrolyte alterations in such a patient may never be seen. Therefore, serum electrolytes should not be used as the sole diagnostic criterion for the diagnosis of hypoadrenocorticism in the dog. ACTH deficiency may occur as a result of a primary pituitary problem (trauma, infection, cancer) or secondary to long-term corticosteroid medication that is acutely discontinued. Clinically, these dogs may be indistinguishable from true addisonian dogs as well as dogs with common renal and gastrointestinal problems. Only a thorough medical history will alert the veterinarian to the possibility of secondary adrenal disease.

Dogs with nonadrenal causes of hyperkalemia must be distinguished from those with hypoadrenocorticism. Although the acute management of hyperkalemia is similar regardless of its cause, one must be certain of a diagnosis before pursuing lifelong therapy. The most common nonadrenal causes of hyperkalemia are some severe gastrointestinal diseases and acute renal failure. Hyperkalemia is uncommon in chronic renal failure unless the patient is terminally anuric or oliguric. Rapid cellular release of potassium and hyperkalemia result from severe acidosis or increased tissue breakdown (following surgery, crush injury, extensive infection, or massive hemolysis). These conditions may also be associated with impaired renal excretion of potassium. Exogenous potassium is an uncommon cause of hyperkalemia except in patients with renal insufficiency. The use of potassium-sparing diuretics has the potential of causing mild hyperkalemia.

Artifactual elevation in serum potassium concentration may be associated with significant elevations of the platelet count if the blood sample is hemolyzed or refrigerated, or if separation of red blood cells from the plasma is delayed.

Any cause of hyponatremia can alter the serum sodium-potassium ratio. Other than hypoadrenocorticism, conditions in which hyponatremia is manifest include renal tubular disease, diuretic sodium loss, and sodium loss in diabetes mellitus due to osmotic diuresis. Hyponatremia may also result from inadequate sodium intake, vomiting, or diarrhea. Lipemia will cause a false depression of sodium. Lipemia displaces a significant amount of the aqueous phase of plasma in which sodium ions are found. When lipemic plasma is sampled, less aqueous phase will be obtained, resulting in an erroneous depression in sodium concentration. If sodium concentration is expressed as plasma water rather than whole plasma, the sodium concentration will probably be normal. Hyponatremia may also result from the osmotic effect of hyperglycemia, causing movement of water from the cells to the interstitial fluid with dilution of extracellular sodium (Feldman and Feldman, 1977).

It can be seen that electrolyte panels in dogs suspected of having hypoadrenocorticism are extremely valuable. They can be used to support one's tentative diagnosis and are tremendously useful as tools in treatment. However, a definitive diagnosis is made by the measurement of plasma hormone levels, as will be described in a later section.

Serum CO_2

Mild to moderate acidosis is a frequent finding with hypoadrenocorticism. The use of venous total CO_2 or arterial blood gas analysis is an adequate method of deter-

mining a patient's acid-base status (Ganong, 1969). The venous CO_2 or bicarbonate level in normal dogs is 18 to 24 mEq/L, with metabolic acidosis being revealed as levels below 18 mEq/L.

Radiographs

Dogs with a shock-like syndrome occurring secondary to hypoadrenocorticism often have radiographic signs of decreased heart size caused by hypovolemia. This is usually accompanied by a flattening and decreased diameter of the descending aortic arch, as seen in lateral projection and a small or thin posterior vena cava. Similar signs may be seen in some dogs with more insidious signs such as depression, lethargy, and weakness. This finding not only lends credence to one's tentative diagnosis but also is a crude tool for evaluating the degree of hypovolemia present. It must be remembered that microcardia is a sign of hypovolemia or shock that may occur in any state of vascular collapse.

Caution is needed in interpreting lateral thoracic radiographs of dogs with a deep thorax, such as the Irish wolfhound and the borzoi, since the normal heart is frequently not long enough for the apex to contact the sternum, and it thus mimics decreased heart size.

Two of the author's hypoadrenal dogs, interestingly, had radiographic and fluoroscopic evidence of an aperistaltic esophageal dilatation. This abnormality disappeared with treatment for the hypoadrenalism and may have been a reflection of generalized muscle weakness.

Electrocardiogram (ECG)

For those practitioners with ECG machines, hyperkalemia becomes a rapidly recognizable aberration (see Fig. 69–7). The most prominent manifestations of hyperkalemia are found in the ECG, which is a vital tool for estimating the functional severity of the disease. The veterinarian must always keep in mind that hypoadrenocorticism is only one of several potential causes of hyperkalemia. Once hyperkalemia is diagnosed, however, potentially life-saving measures can be initiated. No in-hospital screening test is as simple and rapid as an ECG, and none is as easily used in monitoring a patient during treatment.

The earliest electrocardiographic alter-

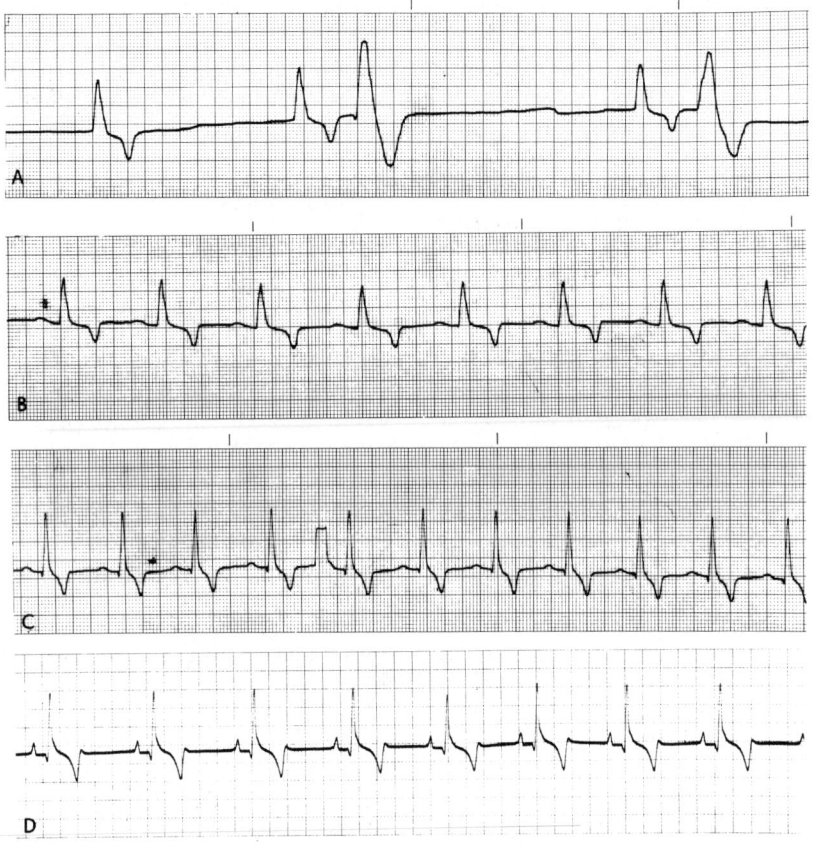

Figure 69–7. *A,* EKG segment from an addisonian dog with a serum potassium of 8.6 mEq per liter. Note the lack of visible P waves, the short-wide QRS complexes, and the tall but *not* "spiked" T waves. *B,* Same dog one hour after institution of intravenous normal saline as the only treatment with a serum potassium of 7.6 mEq per liter. Note the reappearance of wide P waves, prolonged P-R interval. QRS complexes which are shorter in duration than in *A,* and T waves which appear more "spiked" *C.* The serum potassium is 6.2 mEq per liter, and the P, P-R, QRS and T waves are of shorter duration. The R wave is taller. *D,* EKG with a serum potassium of 1.6 mEq per liter. Note the Q-T interval is shorter in *C* than in *B* or *D.*

ation is peaking of the T wave, which occurs when the serum potassium concentration exceeds 5.5 mEq/L. This change is frequently associated with shortening of the Q–T interval. The characteristic tall and narrow T waves occur before the ECG shows any measurable alteration of the QRS complex. T wave changes are *not* seen in all cases of mild hyperkalemia. As the serum potassium concentration rises about 7.0 mEq/L, the T wave may lose its classic "peaked" shape, if present, because abnormalities that take place secondary to intraventricular conduction disturbances obscure the primary T wave changes.

Slowing of the intraventricular impulse conduction is responsible for the QRS complex alterations that occur as the serum potassium concentration exceeds 6.5 mEq/L. At this juncture the T wave abnor-

malities and the uniformly widened QRS complex allow the presumptive diagnosis to be made. With increasing serum potassium concentrations, the QRS duration increases progressively. Thus, a rough correlation between duration of the QRS complex and the degree of hyperpotassemia can be made.

As the serum potassium concentration rises above 7 mEq/L, the P wave amplitude decreases and its duration becomes prolonged secondary to slowed impulse conduction through the atria. The P–R interval also increases in duration as a result of slower atrioventricular transmission. When serum potassium concentrations exceed 8.5 mEq/L the P wave frequently becomes invisible. When P waves are absent, an erroneous diagnosis of atrial fibrillation may be made, particularly when the ventricular rate is irregular.

Continued elevation of serum potassium can be associated with deviation from the baseline of the S–T segment. When potassium concentrations reach the magnitude of 11 to 14 mEq/L, the electrocardiographer may see ventricular asystole or ventricular fibrillation.

The early diagnosis, provided in many cases with the ECG, allows rapid institution of therapy, so that one need not await the results of the serum electrolytes. Regardless of its cause, marked hyperkalemia is an emergency situation demanding quick therapeutic response from the practitioner.

HORMONE STUDIES

Plasma Cortisol Levels

Various methods have been described to assess the function of the adrenal cortex in dogs. One of the most accurate is the measurement of urinary 17 hydroxycorticosteroids (Rijnberk et al., 1968a; Siegel et al., 1970; Wilson et al., 1967), but obtaining the necessary 24-hour urine samples from housebroken pets in metabolism cages can be awkward, if not impossible, for the veterinarian. Measurement of *plasma* cortisol (cortisol and corticosterone in most methods) before and after stimulation with ACTH has been used commonly in the diagnosis of canine Cushing's syndrome (Capen et al., 1975; Martin et al., 1971; Rijnberk et al., 1969; Rijnberk et al., 1968b) and, more recently, in canine Addison's disease (Baarchers et al., 1975; Feldman and Tyrrell, 1977a; Lorenz, 1979). Naturally occurring ACTH (animal extract) has been the traditional agent for adrenal stimulation studies in dogs to assess adrenal cortical reserve of glucocorticoids. The use of synthetic ACTH is also gaining acceptance (Table 69–4). Synthetic ACTH, called tetra-

cosactrin, has now been shown to be an excellent agent for assessment of canine adrenocortical reserve. Its uptake from an intramuscular injection site is rapid and its action transient (Campbell and Watts, 1973; Feldman and Tyrrell, 1977b; Feldman et al., 1977).

The ACTH stimulation study is equally practical for outpatient and inpatient use, since it requires little time (one or two hours) and only two venipunctures. The advantage of the synthetic preparation is that a 0.25-mg dosage (one vial) of synthetic corticotrophin is adequate for adrenal stimulation, regardless of the dog's weight, age, or sex (Feldman and Tyrrell, 1977b). The drug's potency is consistent because its purity can be assayed by weight (Landon et al., 1964; Wood et al., 1965), in contrast with the less precise bioassay of animal-extract ACTH.

The procedure for a stimulation study using either synthetic or natural ACTH is quite simple. When possible, the test is begun between 8:00 and 10:00 AM to avoid any confusion in the test results caused by circadian rhythm (Besser et al., 1971), although such stimulation has been reported to be reliable at any time of day (Irvine and Barnes, 1972). The author recommends the method of Schechter et al. (1973) or Feldman et al. (1977). A baseline sample of venous blood (three to five cc) is obtained and then ACTH is administered (Table 69–4). The venous blood is drawn into heparinized syringes and centrifuged immediately; the plasma is then transferred to a storage vial and frozen. Sixty or 120 minutes after the injection, the post-stimulation venous sample is obtained. In a patient suspected to be in hypoadrenal crisis, the test is performed upon admission to the hospital, regardless of the time of day.

Practitioners are urged to follow instruc-

Table 69–4. Corticotrophin Stimulation Test Recommendations

Author	ACTH Preparation	Dose	Route of Administration	Timing of Post-ACTH Administration Plasma Cortisol
Capen et al., 1975	Aqueous ACTH	0.25 IU	IV	1 and 3 hours
Mulnix and Smith, 1975	ACTH gel	10.0 IU	IM	1 hour
Scott and Green, 1974	ACTH gel	40.0 IU	IM	2 hours
Schechter et al., 1973	ACTH gel	20.0 IU	IM	2 hours
Schechter et al., 1973	ACTH gel	1.0 IU/lb BW	IM	2 hours
Feldman et al., 1977	Tetracosactin	0.25 mg	IM	1 hour
Lubberink, 1977	Tetracosactin	0.25 mg	IV	1/2, 1, 1 1/2 hours
Ling et al., 1979	ACTH gel	1.0 IU/lb BW	IM	2 hours
Lorenz, 1980	ACTH gel	2.0 IU/kg BW	IM	2 hours

tions provided by their laboratory concerning the amount of plasma needed and its handling. Cortisol in canine plasma can be determined with fluorometric assay, competitive protein binding (CPB), and radioimmunoassay (RIA). All three methods are reliable. One must use normal dogs to determine the normal range of baseline and post-stimulation plasma cortisols using one's own laboratory. Because of the measurement of corticosterone and nonspecific substances, the fluorometrically determined plasma cortisol concentrations tend to yield values that are higher than the results seen with CPB or RIA (Besser and Edwards, 1972; Feldman and Tyrrell, 1977b; Feldman et al., 1977).

Three criteria should be established in using plasma cortisol concentrations to differentiate dogs with hypoadrenocorticism from normals: the basal plasma cortisol concentration, the post-exogenous-ACTH plasma cortisol concentration, and the increment of change between the two above determinations.

All three criteria should be normal before the response to ACTH is regarded as normal. A normal response excludes the diagnosis of adrenal insufficiency, while an impaired response confirms the diagnosis. Borderline results should be repeated. This test, in the author's experience (Feldman and Tyrrell, 1977b), will *not* separate dogs with primary adrenal disease from those with secondary insufficiency due to pituitary failure or chronic iatrogenic corticosteroid administration, as has been suggested (Schaer, 1980).

Dogs with primary or secondary adrenal failure have plasma cortisol concentrations that were either normal or below normal. The post-stimulation plasma cortisols were *all* below normal and in some of the dogs the 60-minute concentration was actually less than the baseline. In each case the increment of change was also below normal. These dogs failed to meet two, and in some cases all three, of the criteria for normal adrenal cortical reserve. The difference between normal and hypoadrenal animals is also visualized in Figure 69–8, where the aforementioned results in hypoadrenal dogs are compared with results in 21 normal dogs. These studies also revealed the failure of adrenocortical response to ACTH administration in dogs (Feldman et al., 1977; Flukinger, 1960; Freudiger, 1965)

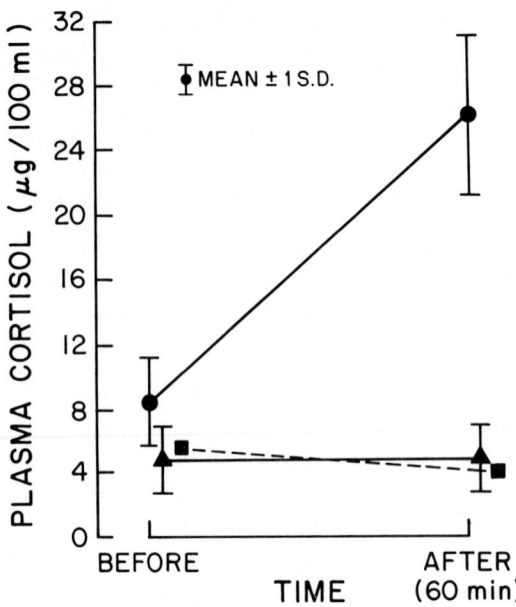

Figure 69–8. Baseline "plasma-cortisols" (mean ± 1 standard deviation) of 21 normal dogs and 7 addisonian dogs, as well as the effects of synthetic corticotrophin administration to these two groups of dogs. Normal = ●; addisonian = ▲.

having pituitary failure of ACTH and secondary hypoadrenocorticism.

Plasma Endogenous ACTH

Endogenous ACTH tests are still relatively expensive; however, such a test, when more readily available, will not only provide the practitioner with conclusive evidence confirming the presence of the disease, but can also provide information regarding the site of failure within the pituitary-adrenal axis. In other words, as seen in Figure 69–9, a dog with primary adrenocortical failure provides little negative feedback to the pituitary, which should result in increased ACTH release. The same is true of dogs treated with the adrenocorticolytic drug *o,p'*-DDD. A dog with secondary adrenal atrophy caused by pituitary disease (Fig. 69–9), however, should have less than normal ACTH being secreted, which would result in the adrenal failure. This would also be seen in a patient iatrogenically and chronically overtreated with corticosteroids (Fig. 69–9).

Plasma ACTH values have been determined in the dog by using a modification of the radioimmunoassay of Rees et al. (1971). It appears to be useful in the plasma of man,

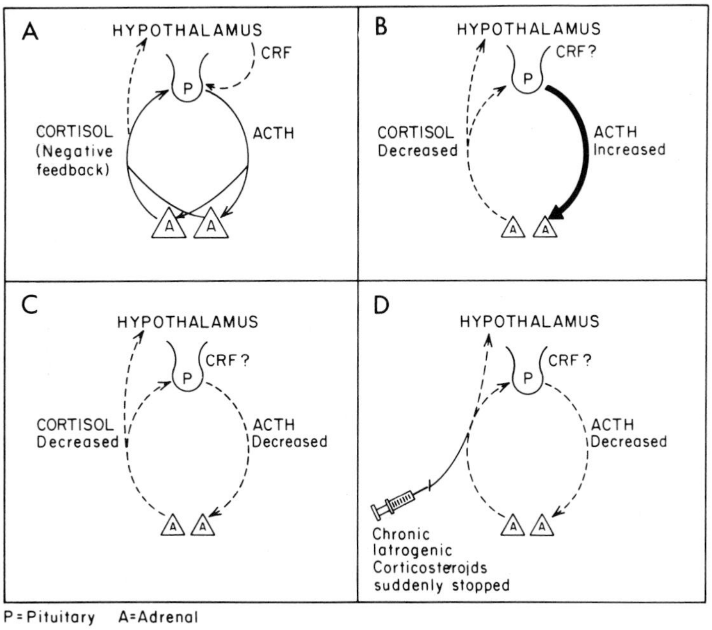

Figure 69–9. The pituitary adrenal axis in normal dogs (A), in dogs with primary adrenal insufficiency (B), pituitary failure to secrete ACTH (C), and iatrogenic adrenal and pituitary insufficiency (D). A = adrenal, P = pituitary.

Table 69–5. Plasma Cortisol Concentrations Before and After Exogenous ACTH Stimulation and Endogenous Plasma ACTH Concentration in Hypoadrenal Dogs*

Dog No.	Plasma-Cortisol Levels (gm/100 ml)			Plasma ACTH (pg/ml)	
	Before	After 60 Minutes	Increment	Before Treatment	After Treatment
1	4.3	2.8	−1.5	2170	5
2	5.7	4.7	−1.0	3610	205
3	8.5	7.7	−0.8	1220	
4	5.0	6.3	1.3	2750	62
5	5.3	6.0	0.7	846	119
6	3.5	5.0	1.5	1205	39
7	2.0	2.0	0	2228	
8	7.2	4.1	−3.1	548	240
9	2.3	11.0	8.7	675	15
10	3.7	4.0	0.3	565	
11	0.4†	0.4†	0	607	
12	3.0	4.5	1.5	2630	
13	2.0	2.0	0	1760	
14	0.3†	0.3†	0	572	
15	2.0	2.0	0	1115	
16	1.9	1.7	−0.2	1345	
17	2.3	8.2	5.9	373	
18	0.1†	0.1†	0	1457	
19	1.6†	0.7†	−0.9	1840	
20	3.8	2.8	−1.0	8	
21	2.0	5.5	3.5	18	
22	2.0	3.1	1.1	5	
Normal Range	3.8–13.5	18.5–35.0	11.0–24.8	17–98	
Normal Mean	8.33	26.20	17.99	45.77	
Normal Range†	0–8.1	4.9–19.7			
Normal Mean†	3.3	12.3			

*Dogs 1–19 had primary adrenal failure. Dogs 20–22 had secondary adrenal failure. All cortisol concentrations are fluorometric assay results except (†), which are competitive protein binding results.

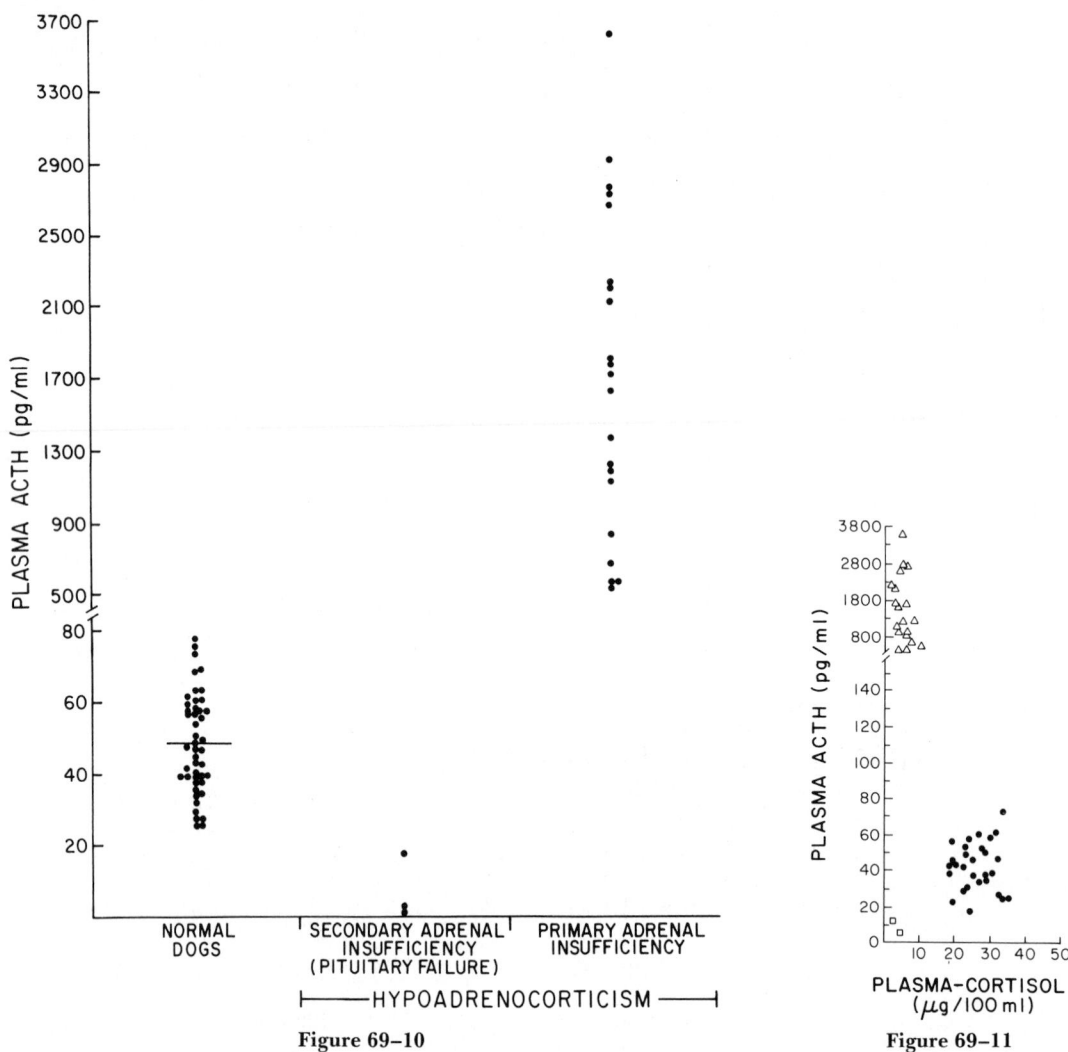

Figure 69–10

Figure 69–11

Figure 69–10. Plasma endogenous ACTH concentrations in normal dogs, dogs with secondary adrenal failure, and dogs with primary adrenal failure.

Figure 69–11. Plasma-cortisol determination post synthetic ACTH administration vs. endogenous plasma ACTH level in normal (●), primary adrenal insufficiency (△), and adrenal insufficiency secondary to pituitary failure to release ACTH (□).

rat, sheep, rabbit, guinea pig, and rhesus monkey as well as the dog (Wood et al., 1981). An N-terminal antibody is prepared for the ACTH assay in rabbits using corticotrophin zinc[a] as antigen. This antibody reacts most strongly with the 19 to 24 amino acid sequence of bovine, ovine, porcine, and human ACTH.

Blood for the radioimmunoassay of ACTH must be handled with urgency, because the disappearance rate of ACTH from fresh whole blood is rapid, the biologic half-life being approximately 25 minutes (Steinbeck and Theile, 1974). In order to avoid erroneously low values, blood specimens should not be allowed to stand at room temperature for even short periods of time. Contact with glass must be avoided during collection, separation, and storage, since it is known that plasma ACTH adheres to glass (Yalow et al., 1964). Plasma ACTH levels can be effectively preserved by processing blood samples in plastic containers and storing them at low temperatures (Demura et al., 1966). The mean resting level in one study, measured between 9:00 and 9:30 AM, was 45.77 ± 16.85 pg/ml with a range of 17.0 to 98.0 pg/ml (Feldman et al., 1977). As

Table 69–6. Treatment of Acute Addison's Disease

Initial Therapy
1. Fluids: Sodium chloride injection, U.S.P. (normal saline)
2. Baseline cortisol and post-ACTH stimulation cortisol
3. Glucocorticoid
   a. Prednisolone sodium succinate 2 to 10 mg/lb IV
   b. Dexamethasone 1 to 2 mg/lb into infusion bottle
4. Mineralocorticoid: Desoxycorticosterone acetate (DOCA Acetate) 1 to 2 mg/10 lb IM
5. Consider IV glucose and insulin to rapidly lower serum potassium (if serum K is above 8.5 mEq/L)
6. Acidosis: Bicarbonate; 25% of calculated dose intravenously during first six hours of therapy

Guidelines
1. Repeat serum electrolytes and CO_2 at 4-hour intervals
2. Monitor urine production
3. Monitor EKG, if possible
4. Observe central venous pressure, if possible

Subsequent Therapy
1. Fluids: Maintain until oral alimentation is possible
2. Glucocorticoids: Injectable dexamethasone should be used until oral prednisone (usually low dose) can be initiated
3. Mineralocorticoid: DOCA acetate should be utilized once every 24 hours until oral fludrocortisone can be given
4. Bicarbonate: Adjust dose depending on subsequent blood CO_2 levels

can be seen in Table 69–5, the endogenous plasma ACTH levels in dogs 1 through 19 are all significantly elevated when compared with the normal range of 17 to 98 pg/ml. This lends credence to the supposition that the canine adrenal cortex is controlled by pituitary ACTH and that these 19 dogs had extremely high ACTH levels because of primary adrenal cortical disease, failure of negative feedback to the pituitary, and an unrestrained secretion of pituitary ACTH (Figure 69–9). Dogs 20, 21, and 22 (Table 69–5), however, had an endogenous plasma ACTH well below normal (Fig. 69–10). Since these dogs had never received corticosteroid medication prior to testing, it can be assumed that the patient is suffering from pituitary failure to release ACTH (Fig. 69–9). Since ACTH has only a mild effect on the renin-angiotensin-aldosterone system, this explains why the serum electrolytes were normal in dogs 20, 21, and 22, while they suffered many of the consequences of glucocorticoid deficiency.

One of the easiest methods of separating a normal from a hypoadrenal dog is to plot the post-stimulation plasma cortisol level against the baseline endogenous ACTH value. As can be seen in Figure 69–11, the hypoadrenal dogs are obviously distinct from the normals. Since treatment for hy-

poadrenocorticism should lower the extremely elevated ACTH level in dogs with Addison's disease, values were checked in some dogs several months after treatment was begun. As expected, in each case, the endogenous ACTH level had fallen dramatically owing to negative feedback to the pituitary from the medication each dog had received.

TREATMENT

Rapid institution of therapy is extremely important in dogs known or suspected of being in hypoadrenal crisis. If serum electrolytes, electrocardiogram, or the anamnesis is strongly suggestive of hyperkalemia or Addison's disease, treatment should be based on an assumption of the presence of Addison's disease until this diagnosis is refuted. Treatment in acute Addison's disease is directed toward (1) correcting hypotension and hypovolemia, (2) improving vascular integrity and providing an immediate source of glucocorticoid, (3) correcting electrolyte imbalances, and (4) correcting acidosis (Table 69–6).

Hypovolemia

Since death in this syndrome is often attributed to irreversible shock, rapid correction of hypovolemia is of first priority. An indwelling intravenous catheter is placed in the jugular or cephalic vein. In an attempt to both treat the patient and ultimately obtain a diagnosis, a blood sample is taken for serum electrolytes as well as plasma cortisol concentration once the catheter is in place. Tetracosactrin, 0.25 mg in one ml of saline, is given intramuscularly. 0.9 per cent normal saline is rapidly administered intravenously during the first hour, at a rate of 10 to 40 ml/lb of body weight. Total fluid replacement is determined from the dehydration deficit, urinary output, and insensible fluid loss. The urinary bladder should be catheterized and emptied. When possible, central venous pressure should be monitored. After one hour, the poststimulation plasma cortisol sample can be obtained and the urinary bladder should be drained again to be assured that the dog is not anuric. At this time additional hormone therapy can be instituted.

Normal saline is felt to be the intravenous

fluid of choice because it will aid in correcting hypovolemia, hyponatremia, and hypochloremia. Hyperkalemia may be reduced by simple dilution, since saline contains no potassium. Any fluid containing potassium would be contraindicated. If the dog is anuric, diuretics such as Lasix would be indicated.

If hypoglycemia is suspected or known to be present, a five per cent glucose solution should be administered or a stronger dextrose solution may be given to effect. This fluid should be used in conjunction with normal saline in order to prevent dilution of the already deficient sodium and chloride ions. It must be emphasized that normal saline alone, given intravenously, is the *most important* portion of the therapeutic regimen.

Vascular Integrity and Glucocorticoids

In order to improve vascular integrity and provide glucocorticoids to the hypoadrenal animal, prednisolone sodium-succinate should be administered intravenously over two to four minutes. The dosage is 2 to 10 mg/lb body weight and this may be repeated in two to six hours. Rather than repeat the administration of this rapid-acting, water soluble glucocorticoid, one may elect to add dexamethasone (1 to 2 mg/lb) to the intravenous infusion. This should provide an adequate and continuous source of glucocorticoid for the dog until oral medication can be safely begun.

Electrolyte Imbalance

The most rapid method of determining the presence of hyperkalemia (the most dangerous electrolyte alteration) is with the ECG, as discussed previously. Therapy need not be over-zealous when potassium concentrations are below 6.5 mEq/L, whereas intensive therapy must be instituted in animals with serum potassium concentrations greater than 8.0 mEq/L. With marked hyperpotassemia, rapid institution of treatment may be life-saving. Intravenous normal saline is a reliable treatment when one is attempting to lower the serum potassium concentration. However, if this is not successful and death from hyperkalemia is believed to be imminent, lowering of the serum potassium can be further aided by the intravenous infusion of a ten per cent glucose solution. Two to five ml/lb body weight should be given in the first 30 to 60 minutes, and this fluid may be added to the saline infusion. Glucose uptake by the cells is accompanied by potassium from the vascular department. Subcutaneous or intravenous infusions of regular insulin at a dose of .125 to .5 Unit/lb body weight will enhance the cellular uptake of glucose. For each unit of regular insulin, one should administer at least 20 cc of ten per cent glucose to avoid precipitating hypoglycemia.

Regardless of the use of glucose and insulin, mineralocorticoids must be given to the dog to maintain improved electrolyte balance. Desoxycorticosterone acetate (DOCA) in oil is the initial mineralocorticoid of choice at a dose of one to two mg/10 lbs of body weight. This drug must be mixed thoroughly before administration, and it is given once every 24 hours.

The author has never needed glucose and insulin therapy for hypoadrenal animals. In fact, rapid intravenous infusion of saline alone over the first hour of therapy has uniformly resulted in marked improvement of each dog's clinical status by lowering serum potassium concentration with concomitant return towards a normal ECG. The serum potassium level declines because of the dilutional effect of the saline and improved renal perfusion. This increased renal blood flow allows further excretion of potassium into the urine. Sodium bicarbonate therapy also aids in shifting potassium into the intracellular space.

Acidosis

Acidosis is most directly corrected with an infusion of sodium bicarbonate. In a severely ill patient, a base deficit of ten mEq/L can be arbitrarily chosen rather than awaiting laboratory results. When arterial blood gas analysis is not available, venous CO_2 can be used to estimate base deficit by subtracting the patient's venous CO_2 level from the normal venous CO_2 (approximately 22 mEq/L.). The number of milliequivalents of bicarbonate needed to correct acidosis is then determined from the following equation:

Deficit in milliequivalents=(Body weight in kg)(.5)(Base deficit)

Rarely do patients require complete bicarbonate replacement dosage. It is therefore recommended that 25 per cent of the calculated dose be administered in the intravenous fluids during the initial six to eight hours of therapy. At the end of this time the acid-base status of the animal should be reassessed.

MAINTENANCE THERAPY

Primary Hypoadrenal Dogs

Maintenance therapy can be initiated as soon as a patient is stable and under control with parenteral medication. This assumes that the dog has a good appetite and that vomiting, diarrhea, weakness, and depression are no longer problems. The veterinary practitioner has several alternatives when choosing long-term mineralocorticoid medications, including subcutaneous implants, intramuscular injections, and oral therapy.

Implants. Desoxycorticosterone acetate pellets (125 mg) have been used successfully in the treatment of adrenocortical insufficiency (Mulnix, 1975). These pellets must be surgically placed under the skin, with strict attention to asepsis to avoid wound contamination. It is recommended that one DOCA pellet be used for each 0.5 mg of daily DOCA injection required to maintain normal serum electrolyte concentrations. It has been suggested that each pellet releases mineralocorticoid for at least ten months (Mulnix, 1975), and overdosage with development of hypokalemia has been reported (Schaer, 1980). Every ten months the remaining pellet material should be removed and new material should be implanted.

The author feels that implants are the least reliable and most expensive mode of therapy. Tremendous individual variability has been seen with pellets both in day to day control of the disease and in length of action. Pellets are not recommended, because this regimen is not amenable to simple correction of dose and adequate patient control.

Intramuscular. Desoxycorticosterone (mineralocorticoid) is available in a pivalate form (DOCP) that slowly releases the hormone at a rate of 1 mg per day per 25 mg suspension. Therefore, a dog initially controlled with a daily intramuscular injection of 1 mg DOCA would require 25 mg of DOCP every 25 days. The average 20-kg dog would require 50 mg of DOCP, with

doses in most dogs varying between 12.5 mg and 100 mg, proportional to body weight. Good success has been achieved using monthly injections. The major drawback of this therapy is the inconvenience and expense of monthly visits to the veterinarian.

Oral. Fludrocortisone acetate is commonly used in the treatment of humans with Addison's disease (Nelson, 1980) and is recommended for the treatment of canine hypoadrenocorticism (Feldman and Tyrrell, 1977a). The tablet contains 0.1 mg of mineralocorticoid, with one tablet approximately equivalent to 1 mg DOCA. The average 20-kg dog requires two to four tablets daily. The dose varies, depending on body size, between one half and nine tablets daily (usually divided b.i.d.).

The major advantage of tablet administration is the ease of diagnosing and correcting an incorrect dose, i.e., daily administration is easily altered. Daily therapy also serves as a constant reminder to the dog owner that his animal is afflicted with a serious, life-threatening disease and that it is dependent on the owner for survival. It appears that less reliable owners are best told to administer daily oral medication, since failure to give one or two oral doses is usually not serious, whereas failure to remember a monthly injection or a 6-8-10 month implant can have major deleterious consequences. This mode of therapy is the least expensive approach to management.

Initially the serum electrolytes should be monitored every one to two weeks until the patient is known to be stable. Rechecks, consisting of physical examination, progress report, and a serum analysis of the sodium, potassium, and BUN (used in a crude evaluation of blood volume and tissue perfusion) are recommended every three months. Using oral therapy, it has been our experience that the dose of fludrocortisone acetate increases during the first six months to a year and a half of therapy. This may reflect continuing destruction of the adrenal glands. After this period, the dose usually plateaus and remains relatively stable. Similar experience has been noted with monthly injections. This dose increase constitutes another drawback to the use of subcutaneous implants.

The major drawbacks to oral therapy have been the development of polydipsia and polyuria in some dogs, as well as extremely high doses needed in others. Dogs with increased urine output have been satisfactorily treated with monthly injections of DOCP and discontinuation of oral medication. Unusually high doses of oral medications have responded to oral salt and fewer tablets of fludrocortisone.

Glucocorticoid. Approximately 50 per cent of the author's patients require no glucocorticoid medication in addition to the mineralocorticoids. However, a dog may be reported not to be in perfect health yet have normal serum electrolyte concentrations. In this situation, a moderate dose of prednisone or prednisolone (2.5 to 10.0 mg daily) often improves the dog's well being. Owners quickly note improvement, and this medication is inexpensive.

Salt Supplementation. This author has needed to use salt tablets or salting of food only rarely to aid in controlling a patient's hypoadrenocorticism or hyponatremia. The use of salt supplementation is reported to be beneficial by others (Lorenz, 1979; Schaer, 1980). Salt supplementation may be used to offset unusually high doses of fludrocortisone.

Secondary Hypoadrenal Dogs

Animals with secondary hypoadrenocorticism do not have mineralocorticoid deficiency. Therefore, daily doses of glucocorticoids, as described previously, are usually sufficient to control the symptoms associated with this disease. The veterinarian must monitor serum electrolyte concentrations, however, since some animals that are believed to be pituitary-deficient ultimately are found to have primary adrenal insufficiency.

Dogs that have developed signs after *o,p'*-DDD therapy usually can be controlled with glucocorticoids only. Mineralocorticoid deficiency has been reported, however, and must be ruled out using serum electrolyte concentrations (Feldman and Tyrrell, 1977a).

Iatrogenic hypocortisolism caused by the use or overuse of glucocorticoids must be treated conservatively. Usually such animals are treated with slowly tapering doses of prednisone. Initially one must attempt to achieve an alternate day dosage schedule

and ultimately wean dogs off all medication (Scott and Green, 1974).

PROGNOSIS

The prognosis in dogs afflicted with hypoadrenocorticism has been excellent when oral therapy has been used. Such dogs have led normal lives, with few if any restrictions. The most important factor in canine response to therapy is owner education. This disease must be carefully described and owners warned of the consequences of apparent mild illnesses. All owners should have glucocorticoid available to administer to their dogs in times of stress. Some owners have learned how to give injections and keep parenteral glucocorticoids on hand should the need arise. Veterinarians should be aware of the increased glucocorticoid requirements of hypoadrenal dogs that undergo surgery or are ill with a nonadrenal related disease.

HYPERADRENOCORTICISM
PATHOPHYSIOLOGY

In 1932 Dr. Harvey Cushing described 12 human cases of a disorder that he suggested was the result of "pituitary-basophilism." Since a careful study of these and later cases in humans suggests multiple causes of the syndrome, the eponym "Cushing's syndrome" is an inclusive term now used to refer to the constellation of clinical and chemical abnormalities resulting from a chronic excess of glucocorticoids. The eponym "Cushing's disease" is applied to those cases of Cushing's syndrome in which hypercortisolism is secondary to inappropriate secretion of ACTH by the pituitary, i.e., pituitary-dependent hyperadrenocorticism (PDH). Canine Cushing's syndrome (CCS) also has various pathophysiologic origins, but all have one common denominator, which is increased concentrations of circulating cortisol.

A pathophysiologic classification of the causes of CCS would include adrenocortical hyperplasia due to excess pituitary ACTH, or excess ACTH from ectopic nonendocrine tumors; adrenal tumor due to adrenal cortical adenoma, or adrenal cortical carcinoma; and iatrogenic causes due to exces-

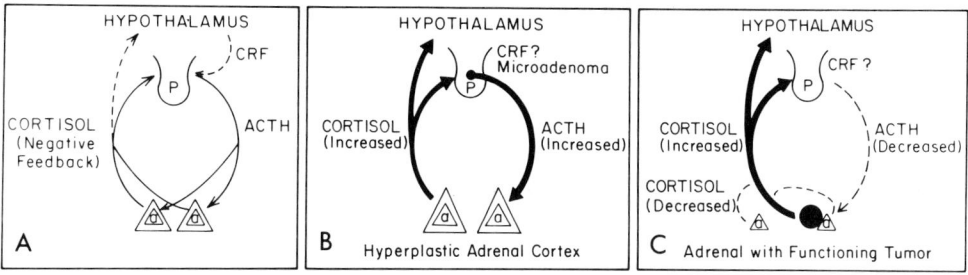

Figure 69–12. The pituitary-adrenal axis in normal dogs (A), dogs with pituitary dependent hyperadrenocorticism (B), and dogs with functional adrenal tumor (C). a = adrenal, P = pituitary.

sive ACTH administration (rare) or excessive glucocorticoid medication (common).

Adrenal Neoplasia

CCS is one of the common endocrine disorders diagnosed by veterinary practitioners. In one recent study involving 94 cases of CCS, seven dogs with adrenal tumors were diagnosed. These included five carcinomas and two adenomas (Lubberink, 1977). In another study, 14 dogs with histologically confirmed adrenal tumors were diagnosed in 107 cases of CCS, and these adrenal tumors included seven adenomas and seven carcinomas (Peterson, 1980). In the author's experience, there have been 11 cases of adrenal tumors in 76 CCS patients, seven having adenomas and four carcinomas (Feldman, 1980 and Feldman, 1981). Adrenal tumors, therefore, account for 7 to 15 per cent of the spontaneously occurring cases of hyperadrenocorticism. These tumors have all been unilateral, although bilateral adrenal neoplasia has been diagnosed in one dog seen by the author. Adrenal tumors are autonomous in character, which is illustrated by the atrophy seen in the nontumorous adrenocortical tissue in Figure 69–12 (Feldman, 1980).

Pituitary-Dependent Hyperadrenocorticism (PDH)

Pituitary-dependent hyperadrenocorticism is the result of an excessive secretion of ACTH by the pituitary gland and is associated with bilateral adrenocortical hyperplasia. One group has found pituitary tumors in approximately 20 per cent of their cases of canine pituitary-dependent hyperadrenocorticism (Meijer, 1980). The pituitary glands were closely studied in eight dogs with CCS in another study. All these dogs were found to have chromophobe adenomas, and evidence was noted on electronmicroscopy that suggested the secretory nature of these tumors (Capen and Koestner, 1967). Careful microdissection is necessary in many cases to find these microscopic tumors. In a study of 26 pituitary glands from dogs with PDH, no abnormalities were seen in 16 glands, while diffuse or nodular hyperplasia was noted to involve either basophils alone or both basophils and chromophobes (Lubberink, 1977). These functional tumors may arise from the pars distalis or the pars intermedia of the canine pituitary gland (Capen et al., 1975).

In Harvey Cushing's original paper, seven cases with pituitary adenomas were reported from the nine cases examined at postmortem. In addition, Tyrrell and coworkers (Tyrrell et al., 1978) recently published the results of microsurgery in 20 consecutive patients with Cushing's disease. They found pituitary adenomas that were three to ten mm in diameter in 18 patients (confirmed histologically in 15), despite the fact that in all patients the plain pituitary radiographs were considered normal.

The role of the hypothalamus in PDH is unknown, but for many years it had been held that the increased ACTH secretion that is known to occur was the result of increased corticotrophin releasing factor (CRF) activity (Daughaday, 1978). Thus the preservation of certain control mechanisms for the secretion of ACTH — e.g., the suppressive effect of exogenous corticosteroids (albeit in high dose) — suggested that pituitary function was not autonomous and that an abnormality in the hypothalamus was involved in the development of this disease state (Krieger, 1978). However, as has been pointed out, such theories remain speculative (Liddle, 1977). At present it is not known if pituitary adenomas arise as a result of prolonged overstimulation by the hypothalamus or if they will recur after removal.

Unfortunately, neither the nature of corticotrophin releasing factor (CRF) nor the pharmacological basis for its control are fully understood. CRF assays for peripheral plasma do not yet exist, and the role of the hypothalamus in PDH will remain obscure until they do. Similarly, attempts to define the neuropharmacologic mechanisms involved in ACTH release have led to a confusing mass of data, some of which are conflicting (Jeffcoate and Edwards, 1979). It may well be that there are at least two etiologies of PDH, namely pituitary and hypothalamic. If this is so, it would obviously be helpful if these could be distinguished clinically, so as to properly decide on appropriate therapy. Undoubtedly the clinical entity or entities known as PDH will have increased secretion of ACTH by the pituitary gland as a final common pathway.

In the dog, there appears to be no correlation between the amount of adrenal hyperplasia and the size of the pituitary tumor or the severity of the clinical signs (Owens and Drucker, 1977). It is believed that the pituitary tumor growth rate is slow and that in many dogs these tumors remain quite small. This is despite evidence that the animal has had PDH for as long as five to six years before a diagnosis is made. Since there is no restricting diaphragma sellae in the dog, when the growth is extensive it tends to be dorsal, rather than ventral or lateral as in man, and therefore does not commonly result in bony changes to the sella turcica (Capen et al., 1975). Such tumor expansion can interfere, however, with the vascular and nervous connections between the hypothalamus and the pituitary gland. This compression may also have some direct effect on the hypothalamus, optic chiasm, and other areas of the brain (Owens and Drucker, 1977). The resulting clinical signs depend on the location and extent of the tumor growth.

CRF activity has been determined in five dogs with hyperadrenocorticism. This hypothalamic CRF activity was low or undetectable in four dogs with PDH and was reduced in one dog with functional adrenocortical tumor. These findings supply the first evidence that PDH is primarily a pituitary disease. The results, however, are not conclusive (Meijer et al., 1978). As discussed above, conclusive evidence must await specific assays for CRF.

Ectopic ACTH Syndrome

This syndrome has not yet been diagnosed in the dog. These comprise a varying group of tumors in humans which are capable of producing and secreting ACTH and ultimately cause adrenal hyperplasia with hypercortisolism.

PATHOGENIC MECHANISMS

The elevated circulating glucocorticoid concentrations that account for CCS are the result of three major processes in the canine (Fig. 69–12). Spontaneous causes include PDH, which is associated with the elevated and/or noncircadian rhythm of pituitary ACTH that results in bilateral adrenal hyperplasia and hypercortisolism. The less common, spontaneous, "autonomous" adrenal tumor results in hypercortisolism and suppression of pituitary ACTH secretion and thus causes atrophy of all remaining non-neoplastic adrenocortical tissue. Iatrogenic overuse of glucocorticoid administration will suppress pituitary secretion of ACTH and possibly cause atrophy of these pituitary gland cells, and atrophy of all adrenocortical tissue as well (Fig. 69–90).

CLINICAL FEATURES

Age, Sex, and Breed

The age at the time of diagnosis of hyperadrenocorticism varies between two and 16 years (Ling et al., 1979). The author has seen one dog less than one year of age at the time of diagnosis (Fig. 69–13); it is generally agreed, however, that PDH is a disease of middle-aged and older dogs, usually six years of age and older, with a median between seven and nine years (Lubberink, 1977). Dogs with hyperadrenocorticism caused by functional adrenocortical tumors tend to be older, however, with the median

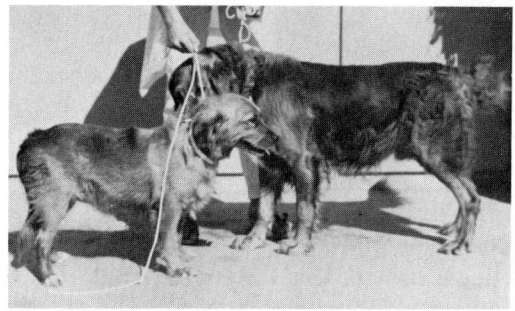

Figure 69–13. A 1-year-old cushingoid dog (left) and a normal adult. Note the short stature and immature hair coat in the young dog with Cushing's syndrome.

Table 69–6. Initial History for Dogs with Hyper-adrenocorticism

Polydipsia/polyuria
Polyphagia
Abdominal enlargement
Decreased exercise tolerance (muscle weakness)
Increased panting
Lethargy
Obesity
Alopecia (skin atrophy)
Calcinosis cutis
Anestrus (♀)
Heat tolerance
Acne (skin infection)
Cutaneous hyperpigmentation

age at the time of diagnosis being 10 to 11 years (Meijer, 1980). In another study, the ages varied between 9 and 13 years (Feldman, 1981).

Dogs with hyperadrenocorticism did not have a significant difference in sex distribution (Ling et al., 1979), nor was one sex believed to be more at risk in the PDH group reviewed. Females, however, were found to be three times more frequently affected by adrenal tumors than males (Meijer, 1980).

No breed preference was seen in dogs with adrenal tumors (Meijer, 1980), while poodles, dachshunds, and boxers were found to be at increased risk to develop PDH when compared with the general population of canine patients at one hospital (Ling et al., 1979). The Boston terrier has also been mentioned to be at increased risk (Capen et al., 1975). PDH has been diagnosed in numerous breeds.

History

As a result of the chronic relative or absolute elevations in plasma glucocorticoids, affected dogs usually develop a classic combination of dramatic clinical signs and lesions. These are the sequelae of the combined gluconeogenic, lipolytic, protein catabolic, anti-inflammatory, and immunosuppressive effects of glucocorticoid hormones on many organ systems.

The course of the disease is insidious and slowly progressive. Owners typically report the presence of some alterations typical of hyperadrenocorticism for one to six years before the diagnosis is made (Table 69–6). They also note a similar time period before seeking veterinary attention, since these changes are quite gradual in onset and are often believed by the client to be simple "aging" by the pet. It is only when the signs become intolerable or after they are specifically pointed out by people who have seen the pet infrequently (therefore noting obvious changes that have developed so slowly the owners themselves don't observe them), that professional opinions are sought. The most common reasons that owners give for finally seeking veterinary help are usually polydipsia and polyuria, polyphagia, lethargy and hair coat changes.

Signs and Symptoms

Polydipsia and Polyuria. These are extremely common symptoms of CCS and represent perhaps the major reason the owner brings the pet to the veterinarian. Previously housebroken animals are no longer able to endure the night without urinating. The pet pesters the owner to be let outside or urinates indoors, and the situation quickly becomes intolerable for the client. Polydipsia and polyuria are seen in 85 to 97 per cent of dogs with CCS (Lubberink, 1977; Owens and Drucker, 1977; Ling et al., 1977; Meijer, 1980).

The polydipsia is most assuredly secondary to polyuria and the tremendous fluid losses that may occur. Using a normal water intake for the average canine of approximately 20 ml per pound of body weight per day (Osbourne et al., 1972), owners will usually report the water intake in polydipsic hyperadrenal dogs to vary between two and ten times normal. The cause of the polyuria remains obscure. Some believe the polyuria to be the result of interference by cortisol with the action of antidiuretic hormone at the level of the renal collecting tubules (Meijer, 1980). It has been proposed that cortisol may increase the glomerular filtration rate, thus initiating a diuresis (Owens and Drucker, 1977). In man, however, cortisol raises the responsive threshold of osmoreceptors (Aubry et al., 1965). A direct depression of renal tubular permeability to water has been noted in normal dogs (Sadowski et al., 1972), and large doses of glucocorticoids prevented increased release of vasopressin from the pituitary in adrenalectomized dogs under certain acute stressful conditions (Share and Travis, 1971). It seems unlikely that direct compression of the posterior pituitary gland by an anterior pituitary tumor or compression of the hypothalamus or hypothalamic stalk as suggested (Capen et al., 1975) would cause the polyuria in most cases of CCS, since these patients usually have quite small *micro*-tumors.

Polyphagia. Increased appetite may be troublesome to some owners, because the canine with CCS may resort to stealing food, eating garbage, begging continuously, and occasionally aggressively attacking or protecting food. In most instances, however, it is a dog's continued excellent appetite in the face of other abnormalities that convinces an owner that their pet is healthy and does not require veterinary attention. Increased appetite is assumed to be a direct effect of glucocorticoids, but this has not been proven. It is possible that glucocorticoid-anti-insulin effect produces a subclinical (sometimes overtly clinical) case of diabetes mellitus in which various cells are unable to utilize glucose. This could result in an increased appetite as the patient attempts to compensate for "starvation." Polyphagia was present in 77 to 87 per cent of CCS patients (Lubberink, 1977; Owens and Drucker, 1977; and Meijer, 1980).

Abdominal Enlargement. The pot-bellied appearance in hyperadrenocorticism is a classic symptom in man and is present in 93 to 95 per cent of dogs (Lubberink, 1977; Owens and Drucker, 1977; Meijer, 1980). This pendulous abdomen is believed to be the result of the redistribution of fat from various storage areas to the abdomen. The abdominal fat stores in many of these dogs is remarkable. This mobilization of fat also

results in increased hepatic glycogen deposition and, therefore, hepatomegaly. The mechanism responsible for this redistribution of fat is not understood (Walton and Ney, 1975) but accounts for a significant increase in the weight of abdominal contents as a whole. When this is coupled with the second factor, muscle wasting, a pendulous abdomen results. Protein catabolism accounts for muscle wasting and, therefore, muscle weakness (Walton and Ney, 1975). The abdominal contents are held up by abdominal muscles, which when weakened by glucocorticoid effects, simply cannot prevent the bulging noted in Figure 69–14.

Muscle Weakness and Lethargy. This symptom is rarely a major owner concern. Patients with CCS are usually quite capable of rising from a prone position and of going for walks. The only major symptom of muscle weakness in these dogs is an inability to climb stairs, although they can often come down stairs without hesitation. Owners may also note an inability to jump onto furniture, which returns with successful therapy. Infrequently, muscle weakness is more profound. Exercise tolerance is often reduced, while CCS dogs can walk without problem, normal running may cause undue fatigue. As with abdominal distension, muscle weakness is the result of muscle wasting caused by protein catabolism. It has been noted in 74 to 82 per cent of CCS patients (Lubberink, 1977; Owens and Drucker, 1977; Meijer, 1980).

Myotonia has been diagnosed in five cases of CCS with the aid of the electromyograph. Myotonia was defined as the continued active contraction of a muscle that persists after the cessation of voluntary effort or stimulation. These animals have signs of stiffness of the limbs; one dog's rear legs, for example, were described as being in permanent extension. The cause of the myotonia, and therefore the abnormal electromyographic findings, was not known (Griffiths and Duncan, 1973; Duncan et al., 1977).

Lethargy is probably an expression of muscle weakness and muscle wasting. Hyperadrenal dogs are normally alert, but they are usually not active. As mentioned above, this is a vague symptom and certainly one which most clients attribute to simple aging.

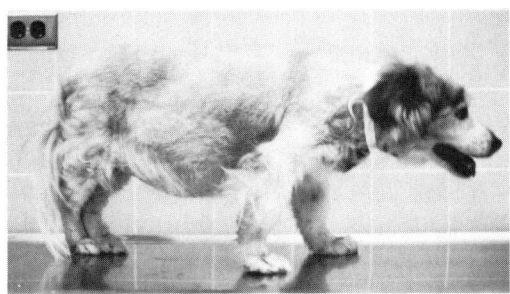

Figure 69–14. This dog with pituitary-dependent hyperadrenocorticism illustrates the "pot-bellied" appearance seen in CCS. The dog's hair was clipped by the owner one year previously; note the lack of regrowth.

Alopecia, Skin Atrophy, Thin skin, and Acne. Endocrine alopecia is commonly associated with thyroid, ovarian, testicular, and growth hormone disturbances, as well as with hypercortisolism. This is typically a bilaterally symmetric alopecia, which may be severe (Figs. 69–15 and 69–16), mild (Fig. 69–17) or involve a poor and abnormal hair coat (Figs. 69–18 and 69–19). Bilaterally symmetric alopecia has also been noted in cats with hyperadrenocorticism (Fig. 69–20).

The hair loss associated with CCS is one of the major concerns of an owner, since it is one of the most obvious symptoms of the disease. As with other symptoms, this is a slow and progressive problem that begins with hair loss at points of wear (such as bony prominences) and eventually involves the flanks, perineum, and belly. The end result (Fig. 69–15) is severe alopecia with only the head and distal extremities retaining coat. Compare this with a picture of the same dog after successful o,p'-DDD therapy (Fig. 69–16). Bilaterally symmetrical alopecia can

be mild (Fig. 69–17). The pinna and base of the ears are often alopecic. This endocrine alopecia has been recognized in 55 to 90 per cent of the cases reported (Lubberink, 1977; Owens and Drucker, 1977; and Meijer, 1980).

The skin of animals with hyperadrenocorticism is thin and easily wrinkled. Often one can view subcutaneous blood vessels with ease. In addition, keratin-plugged follicles are often found around the nipples and along the dorsal midline, although they may be present anywhere on the trunk.

Prolonged exposure to elevated glucocorticoids will result in atrophy of the skin in a majority of patients. Also involved is atrophy of hair follicles and the pilosebaceous apparatus, with keratin accumulation within the atrophic hair follicle being common. This disrupts the attachment of hair shaft to follicle, causing hair loss and lack of hair regrowth. If the hair is shaved, regrowth is poor or nonexistent (Figs. 69–14, 69–18 and 69–19), and any new hair is brittle, sparse, and fine (Owens and Drucker, 1977). The abnormal hair follicles and thin skin are quite susceptible to infection, and localized or diffuse pyoderma is a common sequela with this damaged skin. The suppressed immune system associated with hyperadrenocorticism exaggerates the problem. Hyperadrenocorticism has been diagnosed in the cat, which may also have the classic bilaterally symmetrical alopecia seen in dogs (Fig. 69–20).

Obesity. Owners commonly are unconcerned about an apparent weight gain in their pets. In fact, dogs with hyperadrenocorticism do not gain a large amount of weight; rather, they have fat redistribution, as mentioned previously, and a pot-bellied

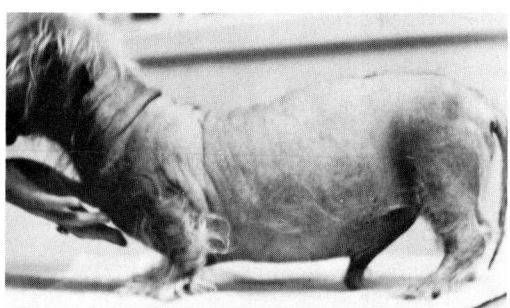

Figure 69–15. Dachshund with PDH illustrating severe bilaterally symmetrical alopecia. Note also the skin infection present along the dorsal midline.

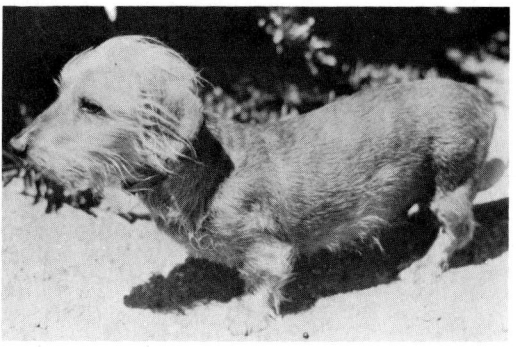

Figure 69–16. Same dog as in Figure 69–15, two months after therapy with o,p -DDD.

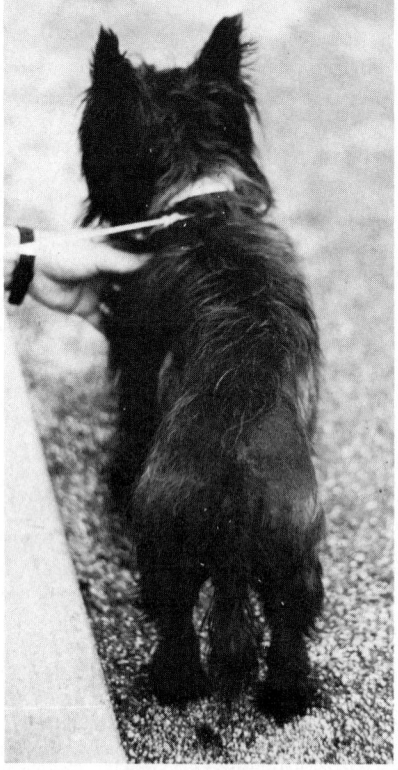

Figure 69–17. This dog illustrates bilaterally symmetrical alopecia and hyperpigmentation of the flanks and thighs.

appearance, which exaggerates the true weight. Truncal obesity is a classic symptom in humans with Cushing's syndrome. In dogs and humans this truncal obesity appears to occur at the expense of muscle and fat wasting from the extremities; true obesity is present in less than half the cases.

Increased Panting. Dogs with CCS are often noted to be short of breath or to have a rapid respiratory rate while at rest. These animals have increased fat deposition over the thorax, muscle wasting and weakness of the muscles involved in respiration, and increased abdominal pressure from adipose tissue. All these factors might be expected to disturb ventilatory mechanics. Nocturnal cough is not a common owner complaint, however. The signs of mild respiratory distress are believed to be exaggerated by a marked reduction in expiratory reserve volume and a decreased chest wall compliance, which increase the work of breathing. If such a dog also has a collapsing trachea, the combination of expiratory distress associated with the tracheal problem and the changes seen with obesity can cause marked signs of respiratory disease. Similar problems can easily be appreciated if the obese dog also has chronic mitral and/or tricuspid valvular fibrosis. Signs become further exaggerated with the stress of excitement, exercise, and trauma. The author has seen, and the veterinary literature has alluded to, a syndrome of marked obesity, alveolar hypoventilation, cyanosis, secondary polycythemia, and heart failure. In humans, this is called the "pickwickian" syndrome, and changes suggestive of this syndrome are not uncommon in the hyperadrenal dog.

Panting in a few CCS dogs has progressed to severe dyspnea. This may be the result of congestive heart failure or, as described more recently, pulmonary thromboembolic disease (see p. 887) (Burns et al., 1981).

Physical Examination

The veterinarian will note on physical examination of the dog with hyperadrenocorticism many of the symptoms seen by

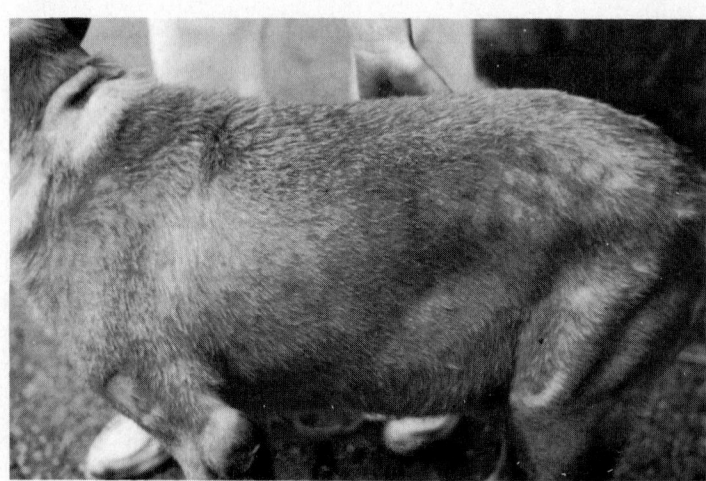

Figure 69–18. This Labrador retriever, which had hyperadrenocorticism caused by a functional adrenal tumor, illustrates alopecia and a poor haircoat secondary to hyperadrenocorticism. Note the "pot-belly" as well.

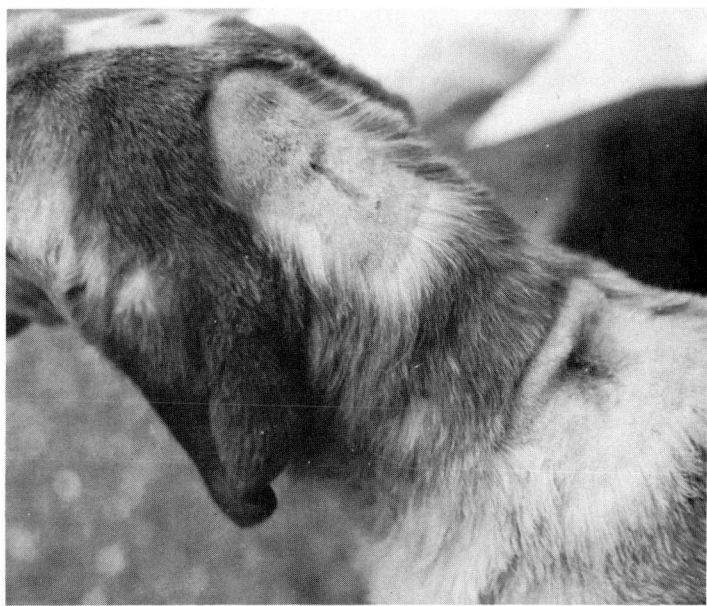

Figure 69–19. Close-up of dog in Figure 69–18. Areas had been shaved 8 months earlier by referring veterinarian prior to removing small skin tumors. Note the failure of the hair to grow back as well as the obvious scars from the surgeries. These scars are the result of poor wound healing with resultant "striae" formation.

owners. The obvious symptoms include abdominal enlargement, increased panting, truncal obesity, bilaterally symmetric alopecia, skin infections, and comedones (hair follicles filled with keratin and debris, usually black in color and easily expressed). In addition, hyperpigmentation, ectopic calcification, testicular atrophy, clitoral hypertrophy, hepatomegaly, and easy bruisability are common.

Hyperpigmentation. Hyperpigmentation may be diffuse or focal (Fig. 69–15). Histologically, there are increased numbers of melanocytes in the stratum corneum, basal epidermis, and dermal tissues (Capen et al., 1975). It appears that hyperpigmentation is more common in humans (and canines) with PDH than in patients with adrenal tumors (Nelson, 1980). As increased evidence has accumulated concerning the source of the pigmentation associated with Cushing's disease, it appears that most tumors produce not only ACTH but a larger molecule, β-lipotropin, which also has melanocyte-stimulating activity. It is unlikely that any of the small peptide β-MSH is directly secreted by the gland or the tumor (Bachelot et al., 1977). Amounts of the larger peptide sufficient to produce pigmentation are present in varying quantities but are roughly proportionate to the size of the tumor and the amount of ACTH being secreted.

Hepatomegaly. The enlarged liver seen in CCS contributes to the abdominal enlargement previously discussed. This hepatic enlargement is usually the result of fat mobilization and redistribution, and development of a liver with large glycogen deposits and vacuolization.

Testicular Atrophy, Anestrus, Clitoral Hy-

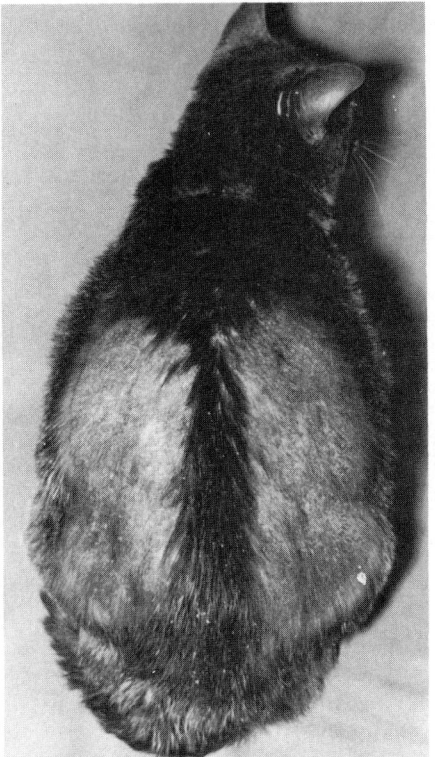

Figure 69–20. This feline had pituitary-dependent hyperadrenocorticism and illustrates the resulting bilaterally symmetrical alopecia.

pertrophy. The hypercortisolism of CCS results in decreased pituitary gonadotrophin release. This suppression of FSH and LH secretion is believed to be the cause of long interestrous periods, or lack of estrus, in females. In addition, it explains the testicular atrophy seen in males. The clitoral hypertrophy noted in many females with CCS is thought to be the result of excess androgens produced by the hyperplastic or neoplastic adrenal cortex.

Ectopic Calcification. Calcium deposition in the dermis and subcutis is a common symptom of CCS. On examination these areas feel like firm plaques in or under the skin, almost as if a collar-stay was inserted into these areas. The common locations of this calcium deposition, called *calcinosis cutis,* include the temporal area of the head, the dorsal midline, neck, ventral abdominal, and inguinal areas. Ectopic calcification is also seen involving the tracheal rings and bronchial walls, the kidneys, and, rarely, major arteries and veins. This calcification may only be noted histologically on some dogs but occasionally will be visible radiographically if it was not noted on physical examination. The exact pathogenesis is not known.

Bruisability. Easy bruisability is common following venipuncture in the dog with CCS. An unusually bad bruise may result from any trauma. This is a reflection of the poor wound healing associated with suppressed tissue granulation secondary to glucocorticoid excess.

In-Hospital Evaluation

Any dog or cat suspected of having hyperadrenocorticism should be thoroughly evaluated before specific diagnostic procedures are undertaken. These initial tests should include clinicopathologic studies (complete blood count, urinalysis, and SMA-12, including liver enzymes, renal function tests, calcium, phosphorus, cholesterol, blood glucose, total plasma protein, plasma albumin, and total bilirubin). The finding of a large percentage of initial screening tests consistent with a diagnosis of hyperadrenocorticism allows the veterinarian to establish a presumptive diagnosis of CCS. The more expensive and sophisticated studies needed to confirm a diagnosis and an etiology of the syndrome can then be

suggested to the client. The initial results not only assure that the veterinarian is pursuing the correct diagnosis but also will alert the clinician to any concomitant medical problems in the patient. Such problems may be common in CCS or unexpected but in either case should not be ignored, since seemingly minor disturbances may be of medical importance to the hyperadrenal dog.

Complete Blood Count (CBC). Excessive production of cortisol results in a neutrophilia and monocytosis due to steroid-produced capillary demargination of these cells and the subsequent prevention of normal egress of the cells from the vascular system. Lymphopenia is most likely the result of steroid lympholysis, and eosinopenia results from bone marrow sequestration of eosinophils (Feldman and Feldman, 1977). The foregoing condition is seen as a stress response in the white blood cell differential. Eighty per cent of CCS patients had depressed lymphocyte and eosinophil counts in one recent study, with elevated white blood cell counts seen in 24 per cent of the cases (Ling et al., 1979). The red blood cell count is usually normal, although occasionally mild polycythemia has been noted. Polycythemia may be secondary to ventilatory problems associated with obesity or caused by androgen excess with resultant stimulation of the bone marrow.

Blood Glucose. CCS frequently results in elevated fasting plasma glucose concentrations and less commonly in overt diabetes mellitus (Peterson et al., 1981; Katherman et al., 1980). Fifty-seven per cent of CCS patients had an elevated plasma glucose value in one study (Ling et al., 1979). Presumably, glucocorticoids increase gluconeogenesis and decrease peripheral utilization of glucose by antagonizing the effects of insulin. Glycosuria may be manifest if the renal threshold for plasma glucose (175 to 225 mg/dl) is exceeded (Feldman, 1977). A suspicion of CCS should be raised in any diabetic dog encountered with high daily insulin requirements or difficulty in lowering blood glucose.

Blood Urea Nitrogen (BUN). With the diuresis stimulated by glucocorticoids, the kidneys appear to constantly flush the system of urea nitrogen. This diuresis is secondary to several mechanisms described herein. The BUN was below normal in 56 per cent of dogs tested in one review (Ling et al., 1979), with a mean half that of normal dogs in another (Feldman and Feldman, 1977). The serum creatinine concentrations also tend to be normal or low.

Serum Glutamic Pyruvic Transaminase (SGPT). The SGPT (alanine aminotransferase) is quite commonly elevated in CCS. This is usually a mild elevation believed to occur secondary to liver damage caused by hepatic glycogen accumulation (Feldman and Feldman, 1977; Ling et al., 1979).

Alkaline Phosphatase. The alkaline phosphatases are a group of enzymes that catalyze the hydrolysis of phosphate esters. The main sources of serum alkaline phosphatase are liver, bone, and in some cases, intestine (Kaplan, 1972). As a result of hepatic glycogen deposition and vacuolization impinging on the biliary tract in CCS, the alkaline phosphatase production rate is increased. This partially accounts for the elevated concentrations of the enzyme in the serum. However, the major increase of serum alkaline phosphatase in hyperadrenocorticism has been shown to be caused by glucocorticoid induction of a specific hepatic isoenzyme of alkaline phosphatase distinct from that seen in normal dogs and those with nonsteroid related illness (Dorner et al., 1974). An elevated serum alkaline phosphatase is perhaps one of the most reliable indicators of hyperadrenocorticism. It is reported to be elevated in 90 per cent of cases by one group (Meijer, 1980) and 76 per cent by another (Ling et al., 1979). This elevation is commonly 5 to 40 times above the normal mean.

Cholesterol and Lipemia. Glucocorticoid stimulation of excessive peripheral lipolysis is recognized. Concomitantly, an increase in blood lipid and cholesterol results. Ninety per cent of 71 CCS cases were noted to have elevated plasma cholesterol concentrations (Ling et al., 1979). Lipemia is at least as frequent. An important factor is that lipemia itself will cause other testing inaccuracies. Affected parameters include red cell counts, hemoglobin, red cell indices, total plasma proteins, albumin, total bilirubin, alkaline phosphatase, amylase, lipase, sodium, and BSP retention studies (Feldman and Feldman, 1977).

Sulfobromophthalein Dye Retention (BSP). The BSP retention test is a recognized and excellent liver function test. This study is frequently employed by veterinarians attempting to assess the degree of liver damage in the canine. It has been shown to be frequently abnormal in CCS owing to vascular disease or liver damage caused by glycogen accumulation. These abnormalities may be mild to quite severe and are reversible with successful treatment of the syndrome.

Serum Electrolytes. Although of little diagnostic or chemical significance, mild abnormalities in the serum sodium (elevation) and potassium (depression) concentrations are seen in approximately half of patients with CCS (Ling et al., 1979). These analyses are not recommended in the routine evaluation of CCS. Such studies become extremely important if such a dog develops anorexia, vomiting, or diarrhea, because exaggeration of these abnormal electrolyte concentrations may become life-threatening.

Amylase and Lipase. Dogs with CCS rarely develop pancreatitis. This may occur secondary to the elevated circulating glucocorticoid concentrations or lipemia or because such polyphagic dogs eat garbage or large quantities of fat, and so forth. In these instances the amylase and lipase levels are elevated and are important diagnostic aids.

Urinalysis. This is perhaps one of the most important initial studies to be performed. It is strongly recommended that owners obtain a urine sample by catch prior to bringing the pet to the hospital or that a sample be collected immediately following initial examination. The most frequent abnormality is the finding of dilute urine (specific gravity below 1.007), which occurs in 85 per cent of the author's cases. Others (Ling et al., 1979) have found dilute urine less frequently, because samples are often obtained after the dog has been hospitalized for hours or even days. Hyperadrenal dogs often do *not* consume water in a foreign environment as they would at home. Some animals consume much less, with the specific gravity reflecting this reduction in intake. It is therefore unreliable to measure water intake in the hospital, and this practice is discouraged.

The urine concentrating ability of water-deprived hyperadrenal dogs has been well documented. Such animals can concentrate the urine osmolality well above plasma osmolality, although usually this concentrating ability is less than normal (Joles and Mulnix, 1977). Having the owner bring in a urine sample certainly aids in finding low specific gravity, which confirms the client's belief that the pet is polydipsic and polyuric and adds evidence to support the suspicion of CCS.

In addition to determining specific gravity, the veterinarian can assess the urine sample for the presence of glycosuria. Such a finding has been noted in ten per cent of one series of cases (Meijer, 1980) and indicates that overt diabetes mellitus is present and that therapy is required for this condition in addition to that undertaken for CCS. The clinician must also be aware that uncomplicated diabetes mellitus is one of the differential diagnoses in a dog with clinical signs of hyperadrenocorticism. The finding of hyperglycemia and glycosuria is diagnostic of diabetes mellitus, which may or may not be secondary to CCS.

Since urinary tract infection is a common sequela to CCS (Ling et al., 1979), the urine obtained should be analyzed for the presence of infection. If infection is suspected, cystocentesis with culture and sensitivity testing of the urine sample is strongly recommended.

Blood Pressure. Blood pressure is often elevated in humans with Cushing's syndrome. The elevation is moderate and sustained, caused by expansion of the vascular volume (Nelson, 1980). This hypervolemia is most likely a consequence of enhanced renal tubular sodium reabsorption and secondary fluid retention (Walton and Ney, 1975). Eleven hyperadrenal dogs had blood pressure determinations prior to therapy. In nine of these dogs both systolic and diastolic pressures were elevated (Lubberink, 1977).

Radiographs. Radiographs of the chest and abdomen should be examined in suspected or proven cases of hyperadrenocorticism. In addition to the possible changes mentioned later, the veterinarian should remember that most dogs with CCS are older animals. Such patients may have concurrent (perhaps subclinical) diseases that may be revealed radiographically and are possibly important in the overall management of the case. Radiographs of the skull are not recommended, as they are usually normal and such studies require an anesthetized patient. Changes seen in the human sella turcica (Nelson, 1980) are not expected to be seen in the canine (Owens and Drucker, 1977).

ABDOMINAL RADIOGRAPHS. Radiographs of the abdomen can be useful in establishing a presumptive diagnosis of CCS as well as rarely helping to define the cause. Abdominal contents should be seen with good contrast radiographically, because of the large amounts of fat distributed into the abdomen. The pot-bellied appearance and hepatomegaly are usually obvious. Occasionally, one may have the impression that osteoporosis involving the lumbar spine is present. It is probable that the catabolic effects of corticosteroids are exerted on bone matrix. Furthermore, cortisol increases urinary calcium excretion as well as inhibiting gastrointestinal absorption of calcium by interfering with the action of vitamin D. Thus, the depletion of matrix accompanied by loss of mineral may result in osteoporosis (Walton and Ney, 1975). Calcinosis cutis and subcutaneous calcification are occasionally observed and are usually focal in appearance.

One may see a grossly distended urinary bladder radiographically. Since CCS patients are house pets, they are usually housebroken. These animals probably attempt to avoid urinating indoors, and it is the author's subjective opinion that many such dogs develop secondary mild-to-moderate atonic bladders. Thus, such dogs may not be capable of totally emptying their bladder. If these animals were allowed to urinate on their own prior to obtaining abdominal radiographs, one may still see a large, partially filled bladder.

Perhaps the most important but least common finding on abdominal radiographs would be unilateral calcification in the area of an adrenal gland (Fig. 69–21). Such a finding would be suggestive of an adrenal tumor, although this is not always true (Hoeldtke, et al., 1980). Unfortunately, most adrenal tumors, whether they are adenomas or carcinomas, are not calcified (Feldman, 1980). It is also possible that the adrenal tumor may be large enough to displace the kidneys or other abdominal organs.

THORACIC RADIOGRAPHS. Several changes may be observed on the thoracic radiographs of a hyperadrenal dog. One should be aware of the "pickwickian" syndrome (see p. 896). Ectopic calcification is frequently seen radiographically, involving the tracheal rings and bronchial and bronchiolar walls. Osteoporosis may be suspected from the appearance of the thoracic vertebrae. Any evidence of metastasis of a malignant adrenal tumor must be investigated when examining the lung fields.

Thyroid Function Tests. Plasma thyroxine (T_4) concentration is often subnormal in

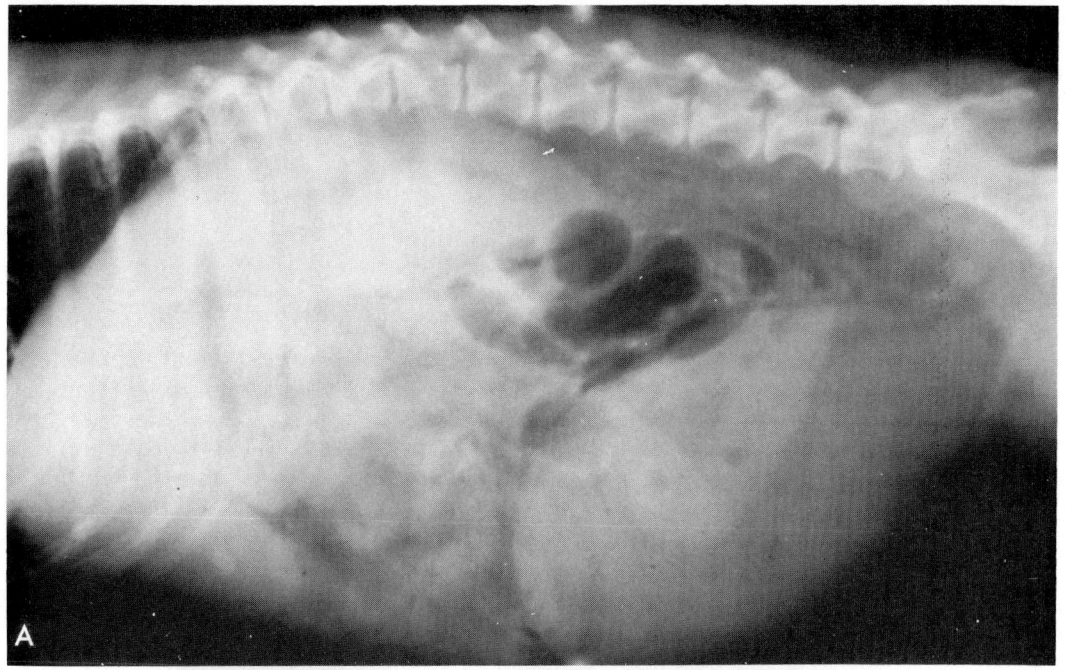

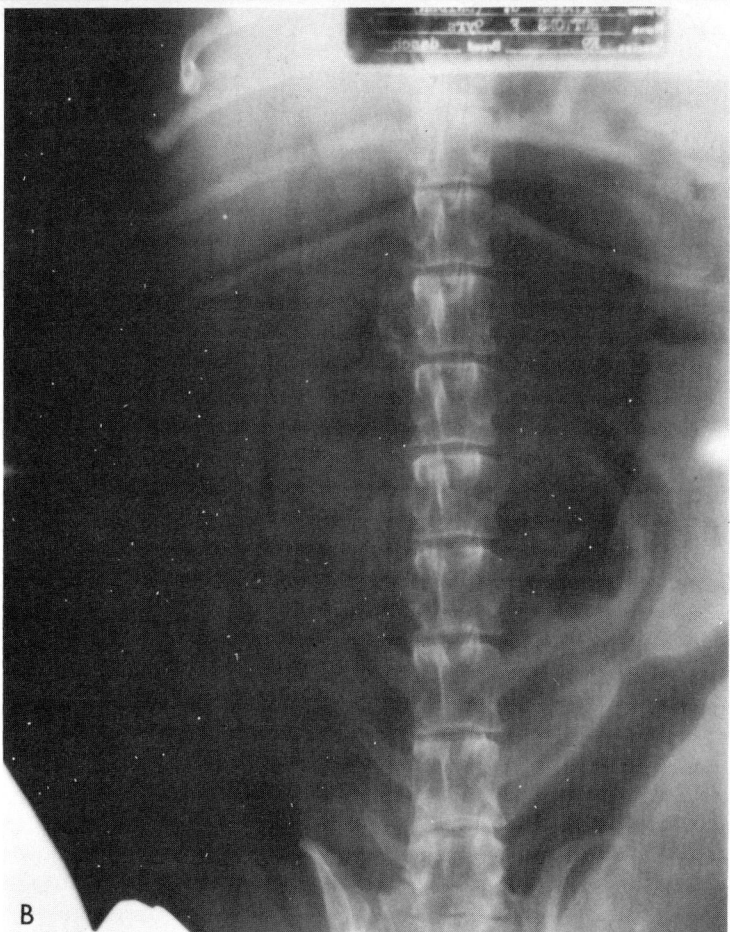

Figure 69–21A,B. Lateral and ventro-dorsal radiographs of a dog with a functional adrenal tumor causing hyperadrenocorticism. Note the calcified adrenal tumor, hepatomegaly, distended (atonic) bladder, and excellent contrast due to fat mobilization.

dogs with hyperadrenocorticism, as are the thyroxine determinations after administration of TSH. This is important because of the overlap in symptomatology between canines with hypothyroidism and those with CCS. Treatment of a hyperadrenal dog with thyroid replacement medication does not have any deleterious effect. In fact, many such dogs become more active. Since the primary disease is not being treated, however, symptoms will continue to develop, which would alert the veterinarian that simple hypothyroidism is not the total explanation of a dog's problems. Various clinical and biochemical features of CCS would not likely be found in hypothyroidism.

Insulin Assay. The use of a plasma insulin assay to diagnose questionable cases of CCS has been suggested (Ling et al., 1979). In assessing 30 consecutive CCS patients with fasting insulin concentrations, the author has found abnormally elevated concentrations in less than half the patients. Those with elevated insulin concentrations occasionally have markedly high values, however; this may be explained by the insulin antagonism caused by glucocorticoids. The pancreas in this situation is secreting increased amounts of insulin in an attempt to bring about carbohydrate tolerance. The use of an insulin assay in the diagnostic evaluation of CCS needs further evaluation before recommendations can be made.

Liver Biopsy. Elevations in liver enzymes and liver function tests are common in CCS. For this reason, patients with vague clinical features of hyperadrenocorticism may be thought to be suffering from primary liver disease. With the increasing use of liver biopsies, this procedure may often be performed on hyperadrenal dogs. Canines with endogenous hyperadrenocorticism or those given exogenous glucocorticoids will likely have histologic evidence of glucocorticoid-induced hepatopathy. This hepatopathy is histologically characterized by centrilobular vacuolization, perivacuolar glycogen accumulation within hepatocytes, and focal centrilobular necrosis. (Rogers and Ruebner, 1977). Any dog with these findings on liver biopsy should be evaluated for CCS.

DIFFERENTIAL DIAGNOSIS

The preceding history and physical examination is surprisingly definitive of hyperadrenocorticism. As with any illness, however, dogs with vague signs are seen and a differential diagnosis must be established. Among the diseases that may be considered are diabetes mellitus, diabetes insipidus, renal failure, liver disease, pyometra, hypothyroidism, Sertoli cell tumor, and hypercalcemia.

FELINE HYPERADRENOCORTICISM

As seen in Figure 69–20, cats may develop hyperadrenocorticism. These animals have the typical symptoms described for dogs, and clinicopathologic parameters are usually not as remarkable as those in CCS. The exception to this is the blood glucose, which has revealed diabetes mellitus in each of the hyperadrenal cats seen by this author. ACTH stimulation may be used in confirming a diagnosis. Plasma cortisol concentrations in normal cats appear to be lower than those seen in dogs. The author has treated cats by bilateral adrenalectomy to date. Both pituitary-dependent hyperadrenocorticism and functional adrenal tumors have been described in cats (Fox and Beatty, 1975; Meijer et al., 1978; Swift and Brown, 1976).

COMPLICATIONS OF HYPERADRENOCORTICISM

Several life-threatening problems may occur in dogs afflicted with CCS. Although most hyperadrenal dogs are surprisingly healthy and vital, the long term effects of elevated glucocorticoids can be catastrophic in certain circumstances.

Pyelonephritis

As discussed above, urinary tract infections are common in CCS, and such infections can ascend to the kidneys. The result is severe and chronic infection plus, in some cases, renal failure. Suspicion of pyelonephritis should be raised if a urinary tract infection cannot be cleared, even after proper antibiotic therapy chosen in light of the results of culture and sensitivity on a urine sample obtained by cystocentesis. Pyelonephritis is best diagnosed by contrast dye studies of the kidneys or by renal biopsy.

Congestive Heart Failure

One of the sequelae of excess glucocorticoids is hypertension secondary to hypervolemia. This increases the work load of the myocardium and results in myocardial hypertrophy. Congestive heart failure may occur as hypertension and fluid retention becomes severe. CCS frequently affects middle aged and older dogs of breeds commonly known to have chronic mitral and tricuspid valvular fibrosis. The combined effect of valvular insufficiency and CCS is a definite strain on the myocardium. Overt congestive heart failure is not unusual in such a setting. Radiographs of the thorax often reveal cardiomegaly associated with a prominent left ventricle and sometimes vascular congestion. Electrocardiographically, left ventricular hypertrophy is a frequent finding. These animals respond poorly to therapy consisting of digitalization and sodium restriction. In dogs that are polydipsic and polyuric from their primary disease, diuretic therapy should be used with caution, since it can easily lead to hypokalemia and/or alkalosis. Treatment of the congestive heart failure and hypertension is best accomplished by focusing on the underlying cause of these disorders. With the appropriate diagnosis and treatment, CCS dogs may be rendered normotensive, leading to control of the cardiovascular complications of this disease (Feldman, 1980).

Pulmonary Thromboembolism

Three cases have recently been described with CCS respiratory distress, orthopnea, and a jugular pulse. Radiographs of the thorax revealed pleural effusion, increased diameter and blunting of the pulmonary arteries, lack of perfusion of the obstructed pulmonary vasculature, and over-perfusion of the unobstructed pulmonary vasculature. Thrombosis was confirmed by nonselective angiocardiography in each case (Burns et al., 1981).

Central Nervous System Signs

Although uncommon, occasionally CCS is the result of a large pituitary tumor. Such a mass with dorsal expansion may compress the optic chiasm and hypothalamus, invaginate the stalk, and dilate the infundibular recess and third ventricle (Capen et al., 1975). Clinical signs as a result of this damage include seizures, somnolence, aimless wandering, head pressing, ataxia, blindness, anisocoria, and Horner's syndrome (Owens and Drucker, 1977).

DIRECT EVALUATION OF THE PITUITARY-ADRENOCORTICAL AXIS

After establishing a presumptive diagnosis of canine or feline hyperadrenocorticism, one must proceed to confirm such a diagnosis and, if possible, to determine the etiology of the disorder. The mainstay of these diagnostic procedures is the measurement of plasma cortisol concentrations. As previously described, assays for these hormone values include fluorometric (FL), competitive-protein-binding (CPB), and radioimmunoassay (RIA) methods. In the author's experience all three assay systems are adequate; however, CPB and RIA are more precise and provide generally lower values.

Blood collected for cortisol determination is placed in a tube containing heparin as the anticoagulant. Other anticoagulants are not recommended simply to eliminate potential confusion if nondiagnostic results are obtained. This heparinized blood should be centrifuged soon after obtaining the sample, with the separated plasma placed in a clean vial and frozen. Cortisol concentrations in frozen plasma are stable for long periods (at least months and perhaps years) (Lester et al., 1981). A minimum of one ml of plasma should be sent to the laboratory for each sample, which will provide more than adequate volumes if duplicate assays are to be performed; however, one should follow individual laboratory recommendations.

The measurement of urinary excretion of glucocorticoids and their metabolites has been reviewed (Capen et al., 1975). Since these procedures are rarely employed by veterinarians, interested readers are referred to the first edition of this text.

Resting Plasma Cortisol Concentrations

Basal morning plasma cortisol determination is, by itself, of little diagnostic value when one is attempting to distinguish normal dogs from those with CCS. The mean resting plasma cortisol concentration in CCS is significantly above the normal mean; however, most dogs with hyperadrenocorticism have normal resting plasma cortisol concentrations, that is, there is an overlap in value (Fig. 69–22) when the normal mean ± two standard deviations (SD) is compared with the actual concentrations of plasma cortisol in individual dogs with CCS (Schechter, 1977). Several recent reports disagree with

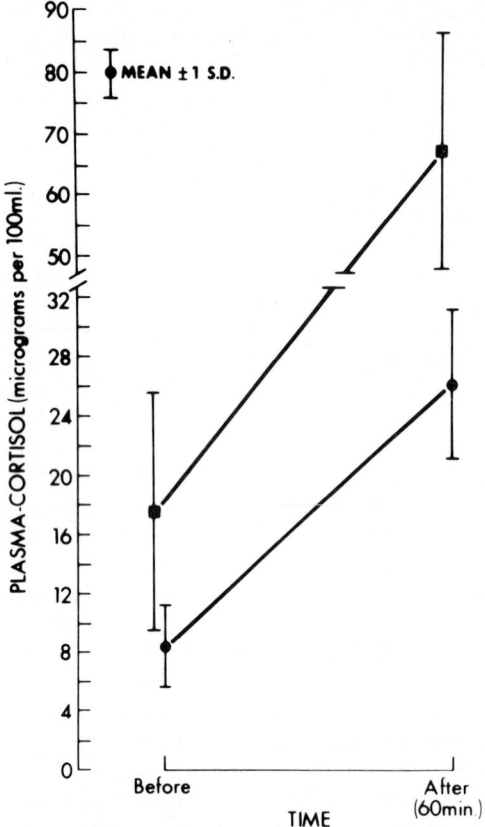

Figure 69–22. Baseline "plasma-cortisols" (mean ± 1 standard deviation) of normal dogs (●) and dogs with pituitary-dependent hyperadrenocorticism (■). Also shown is the effect of intramuscular synthetic corticotrophin on these two groups of dogs.

the percentage of resting plasma cortisol concentrations that has been abnormally elevated in a series of dogs with CCS. Ling et al. (1979) report seven per cent, and Lubberink (1977) reports 64 per cent.

It must be questioned why an animal with a normal plasma cortisol concentration would ever develop clinical features of hyperadrenocorticism. In humans with Cushing's syndrome this is explained by noting a failure of normal circadian rhythm in cortisol concentrations. The morning cortisol values should be the day's highest, with much lower concentrations found at night. A simple chronic failure in this rhythm will result in signs of hyperadrenocorticism. This is based on the knowledge that most humans with Cushing's syndrome have morning plasma cortisol concentrations that are normal, and that throughout the day these values fail to decrease. Rather, they remain at the morning concentration constantly.

When such a lack of rhythm occurs over months to years, the person becomes "cushingoid" (Nelson, 1980). This same pathogenesis is believed to occur in most dogs with CCS.

Investigators have had difficulty demonstrating diurnal variation in plasma cortisol concentrations in dogs. As noted in one such study, "the stresses of handling, venipuncture, and disruption of both light-dark and sleep-wake cycles during sampling" affect cortisol secretion (Johnston and Mather, 1978). Studies to confirm the presence of circadian rhythm will require avoidance of these factors, which is difficult in the canine.

The ACTH Stimulation Test

The ACTH stimulation test has proved to be a reliable study in the diagnosis of CCS (Halliwell et al., 1971; Siegel et al., 1970; Rijnberk et al., 1969; Schechter et al., 1973). In this test, the secretory ability, or "adrenal reserve," is assessed by determining the adrenal response to the administrations of a supraphysiologic dose of exogenous ACTH. The test has recently been shown, however, *not* to be reliable in the diagnosis of Cushing's syndrome caused by functional adrenal tumors (Lubberink, 1977; Feldman, 1980). Its use is recommended for the diagnosis of pituitary-dependent hyperadrenocorticism (PDH), because it appears reliable in approximately 90 per cent of dogs with PDH. Since the adrenals of dogs with PDH have been chronically overstimulated by ACTH, these glands have greater capacity to secrete cortisol in response to an injection of ACTH than normal glands have.

The ACTH preparation used and its dose have varied (Table 69–4). Most authors observe a good separation between normal dogs and dogs with hyperadrenocorticism in the results of the ACTH stimulation test.

It is recommended that patients suspected of having CCS be hospitalized at least 24 hours before conducting the stimulation study to aid in the animal's adaptation to the hospital environment and its personnel. These studies can also be easily performed on an outpatient basis. Test results are extremely important to the animal's future and could be affected by exposure to new people and the hospital environment. However, one study did not reveal significant alteration in adrenocortical response to ACTH stimulation caused by change in environment (Vial et al., 1979).

The protocol in ACTH stimulation studies is as follows: (1) obtain a baseline plasma sample for cortisol concentration between 8:00 AM and 10:00 AM; (2) administer ACTH IM; the author uses 0.25 mg of synthetic ACTH, which is alpha 1–24 corticotrophin (consult Table 69–4 for other doses); (3) obtain post-stimulation plasma for cortisol determination one hour later. If ACTH gel is used, a two-hour post-stimulation cortisol is recommended.

In order to interpret the results of such a study, one must know the normal values for both baseline and post-stimulation plasma cortisol concentrations. Figure 69–22 illustrates what is expected with pituitary hyperadrenocorticism.

The use of ACTH stimulation has not been found to be a reliable test in the diagnosis of hyperadrenocorticism caused by a functional adrenocortical tumor. A recent report demonstrated that stimulation tests failed to distinguish normal dogs from those with adrenal tumors and also failed to separate PDH from dogs with adrenal tu-

mors. In addition, it was shown that stimulation tests in individual dogs with functional adrenal tumors resulted in widely fluctuating results (Fig. 69–23) when such tests were repeated (Feldman, 1981). Similar data were obtained in two other reports (Meijer et al., 1979; Peterson et al., 1982).

Dexamethasone Suppression Tests

Dexamethasone suppression tests have been used in the diagnosis and etiology of human Cushing's syndrome for many years (Nelson, 1980). Similar studies in the dog are now being used. Dexamethasone will depress pituitary secretion of ACTH by the negative feedback principle, and perhaps suppresses release of CRF from the hypothalamus as well. Animals with PDH require higher doses of dexamethasone to suppress pituitary ACTH secretion than do normal dogs. In both normal animals and animals with PDH, plasma cortisol concentrations decline after an increased dosage of dexamethasone because of decreased ACTH release and lack of adrenal cortical stimulation. Functional adrenal tumors *do not* usually de-

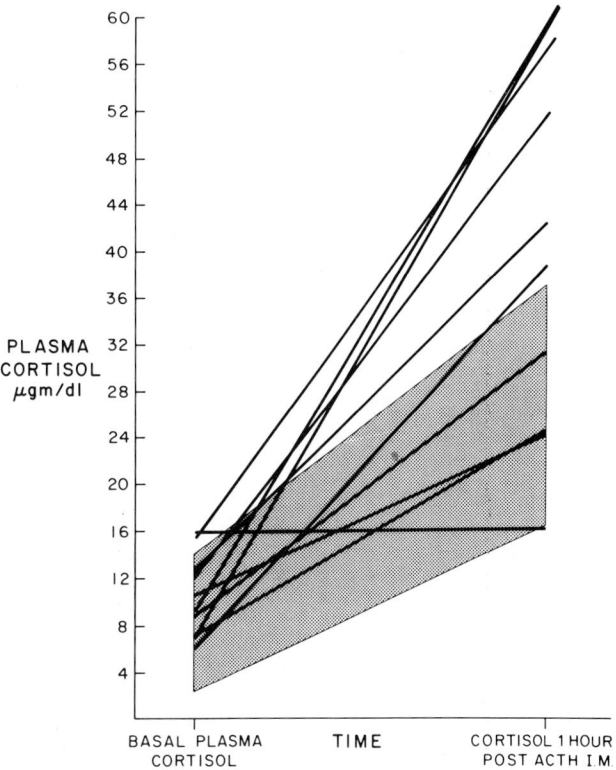

Figure 69–23. Basal and post-exogenous-ACTH-stimulation plasma cortisol concentrations in dogs with functional adrenal tumors. The shaded area is the "normal" mean ± 2 SD for fluorometric basal and post-stimulation plasma cortisol concentrations. This illustrates the variability seen in using stimulation tests to aid in the diagnosis of canine hypoadrenocorticism.

crease cortisol secretion after the dexamethasone dose, which *will* decrease cortisol release in normal patients and in those with PDH. Therefore, protocols have been designed that recommend a dose of dexamethasone to suppress cortisol release in normal dogs but not in those with CCS (Low Dose Dexamethasone Test, LDDT). Dose regimens are also being established to suppress PDH but not animals with functional adrenal tumors (High Dose Dexamethasone Test, HDDT). Dexamethasone is the glucocorticoid used in the above studies because it is not assayed, after administration, by conventional plasma cortisol assays (Nelson, 1980).

Low-Dose Dexamethasone Suppression Test. As described previously, this test should differentiate normal dogs from those with CCS, regardless of cause. Presently, the recommended protocol is to obtain a morning baseline plasma sample for cortisol determination and follow this with administration of 0.01 mg of dexamethasone per kilogram of body weight intravenously. Samples should then be taken eight hours later for cortisol determination (Meijer, 1980). Plasma should be frozen until sent to the laboratory for analysis.

The interpretation must first be aided by a series of normal suppression tests. In the author's laboratory, using the preceding protocol, normal dogs have less than 1.4 μg/dl of cortisol eight hours after dexamethasone administration. Dogs with hyperadrenocorticism have cortisol concentrations above 1.4 μg/dl on the eight-hour sample. In a recent review, it was suggested that a cortisol concentration less than half of baseline at three hours but greater than 1.5 mg/dl at eight hours was most likely PDH, while a concentration greater than one half of the baseline concentration at three hours and greater than 1.5 mg/dl at eight hours could be PDH or an adrenal tumor (Meijer, 1980). Again, a single group of tests is never one hundred per cent reliable, and results that do not correspond to what is expected may need to be repeated. Although such an approach is expensive, it allows for a more reasonable interpretation of data.

High-Dose Dexamethasone Suppression Test. This study should differentiate dogs with PDH from those with functional adrenal tumors. Dexamethasone doses recommended for this procedure do vary, 0.1 mg/kg of body weight IV (Meijer, 1980) and 1.0 mg/kg of body weight IM (Peterson et al., 1980) being most common. The rationale is to establish a dose of dexamethasone that will consistently suppress ACTH release in dogs with PDH but will not affect cortisol secretion by an adrenal tumor. It would appear from our data that the former (0.1 mg/kg of body weight IV) dose is inadequate, but further testing is necessary.

Oral Dexamethasone Suppression Test. Meijer (1980) has developed this oral test for dogs with inconclusive or confusing results from the intravenous suppression test. A dog is given 1.0, 1.5, or 2.0 mg of dexamethasone (dose determined by body size) three times daily for three consecutive days. Cortisol concentration is determined once each morning. Suppression on the fourth morning of cortisol concentration to less than half of the initial baseline cortisol is suggestive of PDH, while lack of such suppression is indicative of an adrenal tumor. Again, these tests are not presently considered completely reliable, but they may aid in the diagnosis of the disease.

Endogenous ACTH Determinations

As is seen in Figure 69–12, the ability to measure circulating endogenous ACTH concentrations should be extremely helpful in the diagnosis of CCS and in the differentiation of PDH from functional adrenal tumors. As discussed in the section on hypoadrenocorticism, such assays are presently available for use in dogs. The handling of samples and pertinent material concerning the assay are also presented.

Dogs with PDH would be expected to have elevated endogenous ACTH concentrations, while those with adrenal tumors should have depressed levels. As seen in Figure 69–24, the mean normal plasma ACTH concentration measured between 9:00 and 9:30 AM is 45.77 ± 16.85 (1 SD) pg/ml, with a range of 17.0 to 98.0 pg/ml (Feldman et al, 1977).

The foregoing results are to be contrasted with those from 52 dogs with PDH. There was an overlap with normal dogs but the mean plasma endogenous ACTH concentration was 119.7 ± 85.8 (SD), with a range of 38 to 394 pg/ml. In one recent study in humans using the same assay reported here, the normal range for morning ACTH concentrations was 20 to 100 pg/ml; patients with PDH had concentrations between 37 and 345 pg/ml, whereas those with adrenal tumors had concentrations below 20 pg/ml

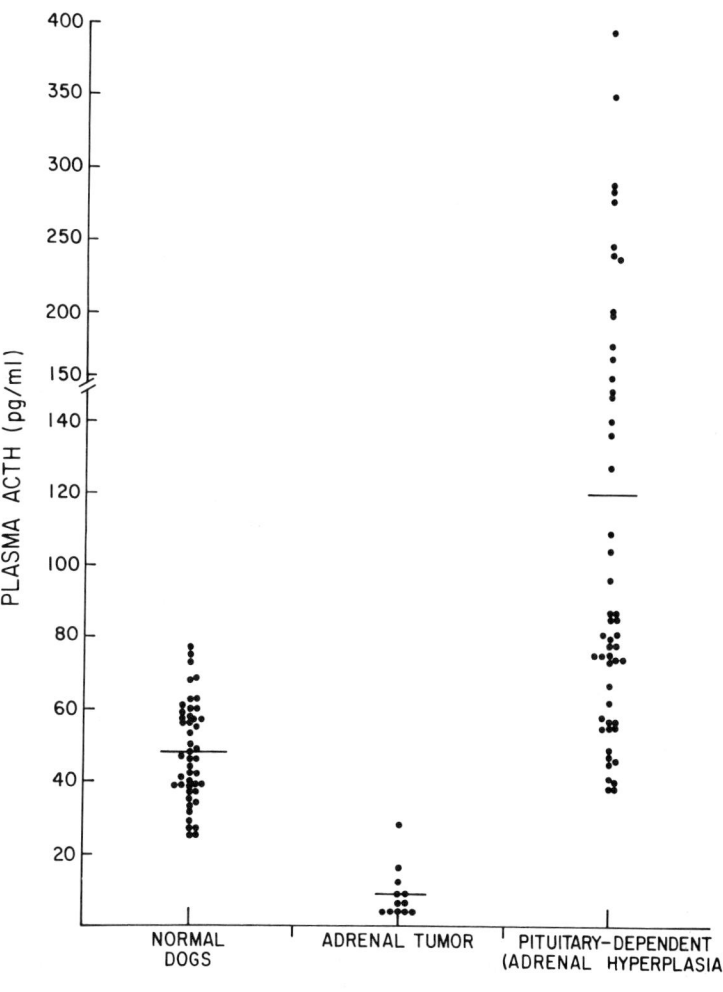

Figure 69–24. Endogenous plasma ACTH concentrations in normal dogs and in dogs with pituitary-dependent and functional adrenal tumors causing hyperadrenocorticism.

(Tyrrell et al., 1978). These data illustrate the similarity between canine and human hyperadrenocorticism.

The cost of these assays is becoming reasonable for many dog owners. The ACTH concentration provides valuable information concerning the etiology of CCS, especially when used in conjunction with ACTH stimulation studies (Fig. 69–25). The major drawback in the clinical use of this assay is the necessity of using a cold centrifuge and avoiding glass equipment.

Within the pituitary, ACTH is synthesized as part of a larger polypeptide, termed pro-ACTH. This large precursor contains the sequence of other peptides, including lipotropic hormone and the opioid-like endorphins. These peptides have been shown to be secreted concurrently with ACTH, and the changes in plasma concentrations of these peptides parallel each other, both in normal dogs and in those with various pituitary and adrenal disorders (Peterson, 1981).

Additional Studies

Other testing procedures in the diagnosis of CCS have been investigated, including metyrapone and lysine-vasopressin. Such procedures do not appear to have contributed to better understanding. Adrenal gland imaging (using the intravenous injection of radiolabeled cholesterol) has permitted visualization of the adrenal glands and thereby the distinguishing of bilateral hyperplasia from unilateral tumors. This technique requires sophisticated equipment (Mulnix et al., 1976).

TREATMENT

As discussed previously, approximately 80 to 85 per cent of dogs with CCS have

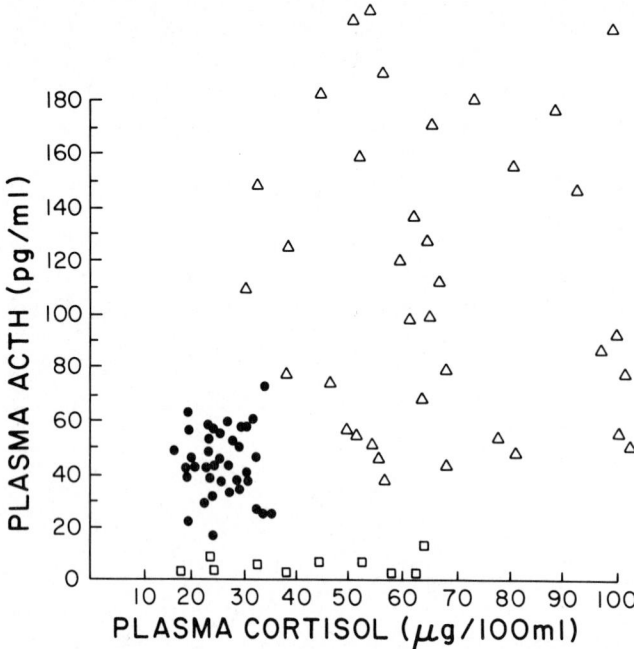

Figure 69–25. Plasma cortisol determination post synthetic ACTH administration vs. endogenous plasma ACTH level in normal ●, and in pituitary Cushings ▲, and primary adrenal adenomas □.

PDH, while the remainder suffer from functional adrenal tumors. Therapy is dependent on the cause of CCS as well as on the veterinarian's surgical experience. Several therapeutic options are available, including sophisticated surgery as well as medical treatment.

An excellent rapport between veterinarian and owner is necessary for the long-term management of these animals. The surgical and medical options should be discussed in detail, including what is expected of the owner. One hopes to return such dogs to a normal endocrine state, but this is not always possible and all complications must be discussed. These dogs may have endocrine excesses or deficiencies after treatment, and the prepared owner can accept these setbacks. Time spent in explaining the pathophysiology in lay terms is well worth the effort to improve client understanding and to establish a good basis for communication.

Pituitary-Dependent Hyperadrenocorticism (PDH)

Hypophysectomy. Surgery to remove the pituitary gland, and thus the source of ACTH in PDH has been successfully performed in the dog. The procedure has been described (Lubberink, 1980) and should be performed by surgeons with considerable experience. If successful, the dog will lose all the features of CCS. These patients also lose all ability to secrete ACTH, however, and will therefore require glucocorticoid therapy for life. Such animals also develop transient or permanent diabetes insipidus as well as hypothyroidism. With an experienced surgeon, hypophysectomy is the ideal treatment. Such animals will not suffer from the growth of pituitary tumors, nor will they face the risks associated with chemotherapy or adrenalectomy.

Adrenalectomy. PDH results in bilateral adrenocortical hyperplasia. Removal of both adrenals will result in a disappearance of the symptoms of CCS. This surgery involves the risk of putting an ill animal with a compromised immune system and poor wound healing through a difficult surgical procedure. As with hypophysectomy, in experienced hands (using the flank approach), the risks can be minimized (Johnston, 1977). However, such dogs must be treated for hypoadrenocorticism for the rest of their lives, and they always have the potential for developing a hypoadrenal crisis.

Chemotherapy using o,p'-DDD (initial). Since the treatment protocol first suggested by Schechter et al. (1973), chemotherapy has been the major therapeutic approach in CCS.

When finished with the in-hospital diagnostic studies in dogs with CCS, polydipsic animals are returned to the owners for water intake monitoring. If an owner has more than one pet, the intake of the non-cushingoid pets is determined while the suspect dog is in the hospital. In this manner, the dog with CCS can be returned to its normal environment for water intake monitoring, knowing how much to subtract from the total to determine its intake. Water intake is determined for 24 consecutive hours over a minimum of five days to eliminate errors in measuring and to achieve a reliable average figure from which therapy can begin. Most owners are capable of, and enjoy taking, an active part in their dog's therapy. Given proper instructions, owners usually provide reliable information. Any measuring device can be used, but we recommend a measuring cup or spoon measuring in ounces because these are common kitchen tools and they provide quantities of fluid that are easy to handle (1 cup = 240 ml; 1 ounce = 30 ml).

Therapy is begun *at home* with the owner giving 25 mg/kg bodyweight of *o,p'*-DDD twice daily. The daily medication is continued until the water intake approaches 60 ml per kg of body weight per day. Daily *communication between owner and veterinarian is imperative.* The author has seen water intake in dogs fall into the normal range in as few as two days and as long as 28 days. Owners must continue to monitor the water intake daily until it falls below 60 ml per kg body weight per day.

A small percentage of dogs will demonstrate mild gastric irritation from the drug three to four days after medication has been started. If this occurs, dividing the dose further may be helpful or discontinuing the medication for a few days may be necessary. Also, some dogs develop profound weakness, lethargy, and anorexia within three to four days of beginning this therapy. In the author's experience this is quite uncommon, but it is recommended that daily treatment be initiated on a Saturday so that if illness develops after three days, the veterinarian should be available and in a regular workweek, rather than on a week-end.

Before therapy it is wise to obtain blood for BUN, sodium, and potassium concentrations. These parameters are rechecked every seven to ten days during the daily treatment. Although *o,p'*-DDD is reported to spare the zona glomerulosa (Nelson and Woodard, 1949) and therefore mineralocorticoid secretion, cases of complete adrenocortical failure have developed. Dogs that develop signs of weakness, anorexia, vomiting, and so on, without electrolyte imbalance, require immediate glucocorticoid

therapy. Dogs with electrolyte disturbances suggestive of deficient mineralocorticoids have been produced iatrogenically with *o,p'*-DDD and require both glucocorticoid and mineralocorticoid therapy.

When water intake reaches 60 ml per kg per day, daily medication is stopped and maintenance therapy is begun. It is impossible to predict how long an individual dog will take to return to normal. The average length of initial therapy is 7 to 12 consecutive days of treatment. When compared with hypophysectomy or adrenalectomy, this treatment protocol is simple and inexpensive. Some veterinarians administer glucocorticoids daily while giving *o,p'*-DDD (Lubberink, 1980). The author has not found this to be necessary, although such additional therapy should not be deleterious. It has also been suggested that an ACTH stimulation test be performed to determine the endpoint of daily therapy (Peterson and Drucker, 1980). The stimulation test with adequate therapy should reveal a normal response or a response consistent with hypoadrenocorticism. This is an extremely reliable alternative to water monitoring, but additional expense is involved.

In dogs with diabetes mellitus and CCS, it is important to begin insulin treatment as soon as possible for the diabetes mellitus. Once the dog is stabilized on insulin, treatment for CCS is initiated. Occasionally it is difficult to achieve good control of a dog with both diabetes and CCS. In this instance, insulin doses adequate to prevent severe hyperglycemia are recommended. In the diabetic, the author recommends a dose of 25 to 30 mg/kg *o,p'*-DDD *once* daily for CCS. Some such animals, after *o,p'*-DDD therapy, require lower insulin doses and, rarely, no insulin at all in controlling hyperglycemia. Therefore, all dogs with diabetes mellitus and CCS require close monitoring of the blood glucose during daily *o,p'*-DDD treatment. With reduction in glucocorticoid concentrations, both endogenous and exogenous insulin have less antagonism at the receptor sites.

Dogs that are not polydipsic are usually treated for seven to ten consecutive days and then placed on maintenance treatment. Repeated ACTH stimulation studies can be used to determine the end-point in therapy. Eosinophil or lymphocyte numbers have not been found to be reliable indicators for use in the treatment protocol. These dogs are usually treated in the veterinary hospital in order to allow veterinarians to closely monitor them for side effects.

Chemotherapy using o,p'-DDD (maintenance). Maintenance of medication is required, because use of *o,p'*-DDD has no effect on the pituitary nor does it cause irreversible damage to the adrenal cortices in most dogs. Therefore, if dogs with CCS are left untreated following initial *o,p'*-DDD therapy, the elevated ACTH concentration will cause redevelopment of bilateral adrenal hyperplasia and all the symptoms of CCS within six months to two years of cessation of the drug. A dose of *o,p'*-DDD every 7 to 14 days, however, appears to be sufficient to prevent recurrence of the disease.

Dogs are commonly placed on this medication at the same dose (50 mg/kg), except that this is administered once every 7 to 14 days. Occasionally the medication causes gastrointestinal upset. Owners have also reported that their dogs will act strangely for 24 hours after receiving medication; behavior changes include severe restlessness or pacing, panting, staring at walls, and incessant barking. These signs are usually relieved by giving half the dose on consecutive days.

It is recommended that the owners observe their pets for return of polydipsia, polyuria, polyphagia, or hair coat changes. If alterations occur that suggest return of CCS, daily medication may be needed again. If a patient fails to respond to re-treatment, other therapy must be considered.

Dogs should be rechecked by the veterinarian every three to four months; the evaluation should include a history and physical examination as well as blood drawn for CBC, BUN, sodium and potassium concentrations. Such studies may be indicative of *o,p'*-DDD overdosage or return of CCS.

Dogs that respond well to treatment experience rapid reduction in urine output and polyphagia, which correlates with the reducing water consumption. Within weeks dogs become more playful and active, and there is a reduction in size of pot belly. The hair coat usually continues to be dry and the alopecia commonly worsens, as the skin becomes quite flaky and scaly. After one to three months, new hair growth is seen and the coat usually becomes thick with normal skin texture. It is extremely important to warn owners that new hair growth may be thicker and a different color from the original coat.

Chemotherapy: Cyproheptidine, Bromocriptine, and Trilostane. These drugs have been used in humans to treat hyperadrenocorticism. Cyproheptidine has also been used in the dog in a small number of cases (Peterson, 1980). All of these drugs need to be investigated further before recommendations can be made concerning their use in the dog or cat.

Functioning Adrenocortical Tumor (FAT)

The dogs diagnosed as having FAT should have the tumor surgically removed, with histopathology performed on all tissue resected. Eleven dogs so treated by this author have done extremely well and are alive one to three years after surgery. The flank approach is recommended. If the adrenal tumor is not calcified, usually one must guess at which side to approach first. If the tumor is not on the side chosen, the dog will require a second surgery over the opposite flank to find the tumor.

The protocol followed in such dogs is quite simple. At the time of anesthesia these dogs are placed on intravenous fluids (saline or lactated Ringer's solution). When the adrenal tumor is recognized by the surgeon, dexamethasone is placed in the intravenous infusion bottle at a dose of 0.50 mg per kg of body weight. This is to be given over a six-hour period and will be repeated. When the tumor is excised, desoxycorticosterone acetate is administered at a dose of 0.10 to 0.20 mg per 5 kg of body weight IM. These dogs are then closely watched for blood pressure, BUN, and serum electrolyte and glucose concentrations. Adrenal tumors, it must be remembered, cause decreased secretion of pituitary ACTH, and this causes atrophy of all normal adrenocortical tissue. When an adrenal tumor is excised, an acute hypoadrenal patient has been created.

After successful recovery from surgery, dogs are continued on glucocorticoid and mineralocorticoid medications using the treatment protocol described for hypoadrenocorticism. During a period of three to six months these medication dosages should be gradually reduced. Ideally, dogs should be on alternate day therapy within four to eight weeks of surgery and off all medication by six months. This time period and tapering of medication should allow sufficient time for return of normal pituitary-adrenal function. ACTH stimulation tests can be used as an adjunct to therapy in determining when to discontinue medication.

PROGNOSIS

The prognosis in dogs with CCS caused by resectable benign adrenal tumors is excellent. Dogs with malignant adrenal tumors may develop metastasis and carry a guarded prognosis. Dogs with CCS caused by PDH also carry a guarded prognosis. In chemotherapy there are risks associated with a growing pituitary tumor, overdosage of medication, side effects of medication, or return of CCS due to underdosage or poor response to the drug. Problems associated with adrenalectomy include the risk of surgery as well as the long-term complications of hypoadrenocorticism and constant need of medication. Dogs with PDH have perhaps the best prognosis after successful hypophysectomy.

Despite the above drawbacks, a good percentage of the author's canine patients live several years on *o,p'*-DDD and have relatively normal lives. Owners are strongly encouraged to treat their pets, as a significant number respond well to therapy.

REFERENCES

Adrenocortical Physiology

Bassett, J. M., and Hinks, N. T.: Microdetermination of corticosteroids in ovine peripheral plasma. J. Endocrinol. 44:387, 1969.

Baxter, J. D., and Forsham, P. H.: Tissue effects of glucocorticoids. Am. J. Med. 53:573, 1972.

Baxter, J. D., Rousseau, G. G., Benson, M. C., Garcea, R. L., Ito, J., and Tomkins, G. M.: Role of DNA and specific cytoplasmic receptors in glucocorticoid action. Proc. Natl. Acad. Sci. 69:1892, 1972.

Bethune, J. E.: The Adrenal Cortex. Scope Monograph, 1974.

Bishop, C. R., Athens, J. W., Boggs, D. R., Warner, H. R., Cartwright, G. E., and Wintrobe, M. M.: Leukokinetic studies, XIII. J. Clin. Invest. 47:249, 1968.

Boyd, J. E., Mubrow, P. J., Palmore, W. P., and Silva, P.: Importance of potassium in the regulation of aldosterone production. Circ. Res. (Suppl 1) 32:1, 1973.

Cahill, G. F.: Action of Adrenal Cortical Steroids on Carbohydrate Metabolism. In Christy, N. P. (ed.): The Human Adrenal Cortex. Harper and Row, New York, 1971, p. 205.

Cope, C. L.: Adrenal Steroids and Disease. J. B. Lippincott Co., Philadelphia, 1972.

Craddock, C. G., Winkelstein, A., Matsuyuki, Y., and Lawrence, J. S.: The immune response to foreign red blood cells and the participation of short-lived lymphocytes. J. Exp. Med. 125:1149, 1967.

Cryer, P. E.: The Adrenal Cortex. In Diagnostic Endocrinology. Oxford University Press, New York, 1976, p. 61.

David, D. S., Greico, M. H., and Cushman, P.: Adrenal glucocorticoids after twenty years. A review of their clinically relevant consequences. J. Chronic Dis. 22:637, 1970.

De Wulf, H.: The Control of Glycogen Metabolism in the Liver. Université Catholique de Louvain Faculté de Médecine, Louvain, Vander:1, 1971.

Duncan, I. D., Griffiths, I. R., and Nash, A. S.: Myotonia in canine Cushing's disease. Vet. Rec. 100:30, 1977.

Enos, L. R.: Corticosteroid preparations. Pharmacy Bulletin, VMTH, University of California, Davis 1:1, 1980.

Feldman, E. C., and Tyrrell, J. B.: Adrenocorticotropic effects of a synthetic polypeptide alpha 1-24 corticotropin — in normal dogs. J.A.A.H.A. 13:494, 1977.

Fundor, J. W., Blair-West, J. R., Coglan, J. P., Denton, D. A., Scoggins, B. A., and Wright, R. D.: Effect on K+ on the secretion of aldosterone. Endocrinology 85:381, 1969.

Griffiths, I. R., and Duncan, I. D.: Myotonia in the dog: a report of four cases. Vet. Rec. 93:184, 1973.

Halliwell, R. E. W., Schwartzman, R. M., Hopkins, L., and McEvoy, D.: The value of plasma corticosteroid assays in the diagnosis of Cushing's disease in the dog. J. Small Anim. Pract. 12:453–462, 1971.

Hechter, O., Macchi, I. A., Korrman, H., Frank, E. D., and Frank, H. A.: Quantitative variations in the adrenocortical secretion of dogs. Am. J. Physiol. 182:29, 1955.

Hume, D. M., Nelson, D. H., and Nutter, D. W.: Blood and urinary 17-hydroxycorticosteroids in patients with severe burns. Ann. Surg. 143:316, 1956.

James, V. H. T., Tunbridge, R. D. G., Wilson, G. A., Hutton, J., Jacobs, H. S., and Rippon, A. E.: Steroid Profiling: A Technique for Exploring Adrenocortical Physiology. In James, V. H. T., Serio, M., Guisti, G., and Martini, L. (eds.): The Endocrine Function of the Human, 1978.

Johnston, S. D., and Mather, E. C.: Canine plasma cortisol measured by radioimmunoassay: clinical absence of diurnal variation and results of ACTH stimulation and dexamethasone suppression tests. Am. J. Vet. Res., 39:1766, 1978.

Jones, M. T.: Control of Adrenocorticol Hormone Secretion. In James, V. H. T. (ed.): The Adrenal Gland. Raven Press, New York, 1979.

Liddle, G. W.: The Physiology of Adrenal Cortical Function. In Clinician I, The Adrenal Gland. Medcom, Inc. 1, 1971.

Mangli, G., Motta, M., and Martini, L.: Control of Adrenocorticotropic Hormone Secretion. In Martini, L., and Ganong, W. F. (eds.): Neuroendocrinology. Academic Press, New York, 1966, p. 298.

Mattingly, D.: Simple fluorometric method for the estimation of free 11-hydroxycorticoids in human plasma. J. Clin. Pathol. 15:374, 1962.

Munck, A.: Glucocorticoid inhibition of glucose intake by peripheral tissues: Old and new evidence, molecular mechanism, and physiological significance. Perspect. Biol. Med. 265, 1971.

Nelson, D. H.: Mechanism of Corticosteroid Action. *In* The Adrenal Cortex. W. B. Saunders Co., Philadelphia, 1980, p. 240.

Peterson, R. E.: Metabolism of Adrenal Cortical Steroids. *In* Cristy, N. P. (ed.): The Human Adrenal Cortex. Harper and Row, New York, 1971, p. 87.

Peterson, R. E., and Pierce, C. E.: The metabolism of corticosterone in man. J. Clin. Invest. *39*:741, 1960.

Popjak, G., and Cornforth, J. W.: Substrate stereochemistry in squalene biosynthesis. Biochem. J., *101*:553, 1966.

Retiene, K., Zimmerman, E., Schindler, W. J., Neuenschwander, J., and Lipscomb, H. S.: A correlative study of endocrine rhythms in rats. Acta Endocrinol. *57*:615, 1968.

Rijnberk, A., der Kinderen, P. J., and Thijssen, J. H. H.: Investigations on the adrenocortical function of normal dogs. J. Endocrinol. *41*:387, 1968.

Ritschel, W. A: Biological Half-Lives and Their Clinical Applications. *In* Franke, D. E., and Whitney, H. A. K., Jr. (eds.): Perspectives in Clinical Pharmacy, Drug Intelligence Publications, Hamilton, Ill., 1972, p. 286.

Rousseau, G. G., Baxter, J. D., and Tomkins, G. M.: Glucocorticoid receptors: Relations between steroid binding and biological effects. J. Mol. Biol. *67*:99, 1972.

Rudman, D., and DiGirolamo, M.: Effect of Adrenal Cortical Steroids on Lipid Metabolism. *In* Christy, N. P. (ed.): The Human Adrenal Cortex. Harper and Row, New York, 1971, p. 241.

Toombs, J. P., Caywood, D. D., Lipowitz, A. J., and Stevens, J. B.: Colonic perforation following neurosurgical procedures and corticosteroid therapy in four dogs. J.A.V.M.A. *177*:68, 1980.

Upton, G. V., Corbin, A., Mabry, C. C., and Hollingsworth, D. R.: Evidence for the internal feedback phenomenon in human subjects: effects of ACTH on plasma CRF. Acata Endocrinol *73*:437, 1973.

Van der Vies, J.: Individual determination of cortisol and corticosterone in a single sample of peripheral blood. J. Acta Endocrinol. *38*:399, 1961.

Hypoadrenocorticism

Baarchers, J. J., Hommes, U. E., and Poll, P. H. A.: A case of Addison's disease in a dog. Tijdschr. Diergeneeskd. *100*:894, 1975.

Besser, G. M., and Edwards, C. R. W.: Cushing's syndrome. Clin. Endocrinol. Metab. *1*:451, 1972.

Besser, G. M., Cullen, D. R., Irvine, W. J., Ratcliffe, J. G., and Landon, J.: Immunoreactive corticotropin levels in adrenocortical insufficiency. Br. Med. J. *13*:374, 1971.

Bethune, J. E.: The Adrenal Cortex. Scope Monograph, 1974.

Breznock, E. M., and McQueen, R. D.: Rapid fluorometric analysis of plasma corticosteroids as a test of adrenocortical function in the dog. Am. J. Vet. Res. *30*:1523, 1969.

Campbell, J. R., and Watts, C.: Assessment of adrenal function in dogs. Br. Vet. J. *129*:134, 1973.

Capen, C. C., Belshaw, B. E., and Martin, S. L.: Endocrine Disorders. *In* Ettinger, S. J. (ed.): Textbook of Veterinary Internal Medicine. 1st ed. W. B. Saunders Co., Philadelphia, 1975.

Cryer, P. E.: Diagnostic Endocrinology. Oxford University Press, London, 1976.

Demura, H., West, C. D., Nugent, C. A., Nakagawa, K., and Tyler, F. H.: A sensitive radioimmunoassay for plasma ACTH levels. J. Clin. Endocrinol. *26*:1297, 1966.

Feldman, B. F., and Feldman, E. C.: Routine laboratory abnormalities in endocrine disease. Vet. Clin. North Am. 7:443, 1977.

Feldman, E. C., and Tyrrell, J. B.: Hypoadrenocorticism. Vet. Clin. North Am. 7:555, 1977a.

Feldman, E. C., and Tyrrell, J. B.: Adrenocorticotropic effects of a synthetic polypeptide — alpha 1-24 corticotropin — in normal dogs. J.A.A.H.A. *13*:494, 1977b.

Feldman, E. C., Bohannon, N. V., and Tyrrell, J. B.: Plasma adrenocorticotropin (ACTH) levels in normal dogs. Am. J. Vet. Res. *38*:1643, 1977.

Feldman, E. C., Tyrrell, J. B., and Bohannon, N. V.: The synthetic ACTH stimulation test and measurement of endogenous plasma ACTH levels: useful diagnostic indicators for adrenal disease in dogs. J.A.A.H.A. *14*:524, 1978.

Flukinger, E. W.: Die biologische aktivitat von syntetischem alpha-MSH. Acta Endocrinol. (Kbh) *35*,51:333, 1960.

Freudiger, Von U.: Die Nebennierenrinden-Insuffizienzen beim Hund. Dsch. Tierarztl. Wochenschr. *72*:60, 1965.

Ganong, W. F.: Review of Medical Physiology. Lang Medical Publications, Los Altos, Ca., 1969.

Irvine, W. J., and Barnes, E. W.: Adrenocortical insufficiency. *In* Mason, A. S. (ed.): Clin. Endocrinol. Metab. W. B. Saunders Co., *1*:549, 1972.

Keeton, K. S., Schechter, R. D., and Schalm, O. W.: Adrenocortical insufficiency in dogs. Mod. Vet. Pract. 25, 1972.

Kirk, G. R., and Jensen, H. E.: Toxic effects of *o,p'*-DDD in the normal dog. J.A.A.H.A. *11*:765, 1975.

Kirk, G. R., Boyer, S., and Hutcheson, D. P.: Effects of *o,p'*-DDD on plasma cortisol levels and histology of the adrenal gland in the normal dog. J.A.A.H.A. *10*:179, 1974.

Landon, J., James, V. H. T., Cryer, R. J., Wynn, V., and Frankland, A. W.: Adrenocorticotic effects of a synthetic polypeptide — beta 1-24 corticotropin — in man. J. Clin. Endocrinol. Metab. *24*:1206, 1964.

Liddle, G. W.: The Adrenal Cortex. *In* Williams, R. H. (ed.): Textbook of Endocrinology. W. B. Saunders Co., Philadelphia, 1974.

Lorenz, M. D.: Canine hyperadrenocorticism: diagnosis and treatment. Comp. Cont. Educ. *1*:315, 1979.

Lorenz, M. D., and Cornelius, L. M.: Laboratory Diagnosis of Endocrinological Disease. *In* Tasker, J. B. (ed.): Vet. Clin. North Am. *4*:687, 1976.

Martin, S. L., Murdick, P. W., and Capen, C. C.: Laboratory Evaluation of Adrenocortical Function in Dogs. *In* Kirk, R. W. (ed.): Current Veterinary Therapy IV. W. B. Saunders Co., Philadelphia, 1971, p. 589.

Meikle, A. W., and Tyler, F. H. Potency and duration of action of glucocorticoids. Effects of hydrocortisone, prednisone, and dexamethasone on human pituitary-adrenal function. Am. J. Med. *63*:200, 1977.

Mulnix, J. A.: Hypoadrenocorticism in the dog. J.A.A.H.A. 7:220, 1971.

Mulnix, J. A., and Smith, K. W.: Hyperadrenocorticism in a dog: a case report. J. Small Anim. Pract. *16*:193, 1975.

Nelson, A. A., and Woodard, G.: Severe cortical atrophy (cytotoxic) and hepatic damage produced in dogs by feeding 2,2-bis(parachlorophenyl)-1,1-dichloroethane (DDD or TDE). Arch. Pathol. *48*:387, 1949.

Nelson, D. H.: The Adrenal Cortex. Physiological Function and Disease. W. B. Saunders Co., Philadelphia, 1980, p. 113.

Peterson, M. E., and Drucker, W. D.: Biochemical Characterization and Treatment of Spontaneous Canine Cushing's Syndrome. Sci. Proc. Am. Coll. Vet. Intern. Med., 1980. (abstract)

Rees, L. H., Cook, D. M., Kendall, J. W., Allen, C. F., Kramer, R. M., Ratcliffe, J. G., and Knight, R. A.: A radioimmunoassay for rat plasma ACTH. Endocrinology 89:254, 1971.

Rijnberk, A., der Kinderen, P. J., and Thijssen, J. H. H.: Investigation on the adrenocortical function of normal dogs. J. Endocrinol. 41:387, 1968a.

Rijnberk, A., der Kinderen, P. J., and Thijssen, J. H. H.: Spontaneous hyperadrenocorticism in the dog. J. Endocrinol. 41:397, 1968b.

Rijnberk, A., der Kinderen, P. J., and Thijssen, J. H. H.: Canine Cushing's syndrome. Zentralbl Veterinaermed. 16:13, 1969.

Schaer, M.: Hypoadrenocorticism. In Kirk, R. W. (ed.): Current Veterinary Therapy VII. W. B. Saunders Co., Philadelphia, 1980, p. 983.

Schechter, R. D.: Hyperadrenocorticism. In Kirk, R. W. (ed.): Current Veterinary Therapy. V. W. B. Saunders Co., Philadelphia, 1974, p. 783.

Schechter, R. D., Stabenfeldt, G. H., Gribble, D. G., and Ling, G. V.: Treatment of Cushing's syndrome in the dog with an adrenocorticolytic agent (o,p'-DDD). J.A.V.M.A. 162:629, 1973.

Scott, D. W., and Greene, C. E.: Iatrogenic secondary adrenocortical insufficiency in dogs. J.A.A.H.A. 10:555, 1974.

Siegel, E. T., and Belshaw, B. E.: Laboratory Evaluation of Adrenocortical and Thyroid Functions in the Dog. In Kirk, R. W. (ed.): Current Veterinary Therapy, III. W. B. Saunders Co., Philadelphia, 1968, p. 545.

Siegel, E. T., Kelly, D. F., and Berg, P.: Cushing's syndrome in the dog. J.A.V.M.A. 157:2081, 1970.

Steinbeck, A. W., and Theile, H. M.: The Adrenal Cortex. In Bayliss, R. I. S. (ed.): Clin. Endocrinol. Metab. 3:557, 1974.

Tyrrell, J. B., and Forsham, P. H.: Chronic Adrenal Cortical Insufficiency. In Conn, H. F., and Conn, R. B., Jr. (eds.): Current Diagnosis 4. W. B. Saunders Co., Philadelphia, 1974, p. 742.

Wilson, R. B., Kleine, L. J., Clarke, T. J., Hendricks, E. C., and Grossman, M. S.: Response of dogs to corticotropin measured by 17-hydroxycorticosteroid excretion. Am. J. Vet. Res. 28:313, 1967.

Wolland, M.: Primary Adrenocortical Insufficiency. In: Kirk, R. W. (ed.): Current Veterinary Therapy V. W. B. Saunders Co., Philadelphia, 1974, p. 789.

Wood, J. B., James, V. H. T., Frankland, A. W., and Landon, I.: A rapid test of adrenocortical function. Lancet 1:243, 1965.

Yalow, R. S., Glick, S. M., Roth, J., and Berson, S. A.: Radioimmunoassay of human plasma ACTH. J. Clin. Endocrinol. 24:1219, 1964.

Hyperadrenocorticism

Aubry, R. H., Nankin, H. R., Moses, A. M., and Streeten, D. H. P.: Measurement of the osmotic threshold for vasopressin release in human subjects, and its modification by cortisol. J. Clin. Endocrinol. Metab. 25:1481, 1965.

Azzopardi, J. G., and Williams, E. D.: Pathology of "non-endocrine" tumors. Cancer 22:274, 1968.

Bachelot, I., Wolfson, A. R., and Odell, W. B.: Pituitary and plasma lipotropins: demonstration of the artifactual nature of b-MSH. J. Clin. Endocrinol. Metab. 44:939, 1977.

Burns, M. G., Kelly, A. B., Hornof, W. J., and Howerth, E. W.: Pulmonary artery thrombosis in three dogs with hyperadrenocorticism. J.A.V.M.A. 178:388, 1981.

Capen, C. C., and Koestner, A.: Functional chromophobe adenomas of the canine adenohypophysis: an ultrastructural evaluation of a neoplasm of pituitary corticotrophs. Pathol. Vet. 4:326, 1967.

Capen, C. C., Belshaw, B. E., and Martin, S. L.: Endocrine Diseases. In Ettinger, S. J. (ed.): Textbook of Veterinary Internal Medicine. W. B. Saunders Co., Philadelphia, 1975, p. 1395.

Cushing, H.: The basophil adenomas of the pituitary body and their clinical manifestations (pituitary basophilism). Bull. Johns Hopkins Hosp. 50:127, 1932.

Daughaday, W. M.: Cushing's disease and basophilic miaoadenomas. N. Engl. J. Med. 298:793, 1978.

Dorner, J. L., Hoffman, W. E., and Long, G. B.: Corticosteroid inducation of an isoenzyme of alkaline phosphatase in the dog. Am. J. Vet. Res. 35:1457, 1974.

Duncan, I. D., Griffiths, I. R., and Nash, A. S.: Myotonia in canine Cushing's disease. Vet. Rec. 100:30, 1977.

Feldman, B. F., and Feldman, E. C.: Routine laboratory abnormalities in endocrine disease. Vet. Clin. North Am. 7:443, 1977.

Feldman, E. C.: Diabetes Mellitus. In Kirk, R. W. (ed.): Current Veterinary Therapy VI. W. B. Saunders Co., Philadelphia, 1977, p. 1001.

Feldman, E. C.: Influence of Non-cardiac Disease on the Heart. In Kirk, R. W. (ed.): Current Veterinary Therapy VII. W. B. Saunders Co., Philadelphia, 1980, p. 340.

Feldman, E. C.: The effect of functional adrenocortical tumors on plasma cortisol and corticotropin concentrations in dogs. J.A.V.M.A., 178:823, 1981.

Feldman, E. C., and Tyrrell, J. B.: Endogenous corticotrophin (ACTH) levels in dogs with hyperfunctioning adrenocortical tumors. Sci. Proc. Am. Coll. Vet. Intern. Med., 1980, p. 115.

Feldman, E. C., Bohannon, N. V., and Tyrrell, J. B.: Plasma adrenocorticotropin levels in normal dogs. Am. J. Vet. Res. 38:1643, 1977.

Feldman, E. C., Tyrrell, J. B., and Ettinger, S. J.: Cushing's syndrome: Case report and discussion. Mod. Vet. Pract. 58:995, 1977.

Fox, J. G., and Beatty, J. O.: A case report of complicated diabetes mellitus in a cat. J.A.A.H.A. 11:129, 1975.

Griffiths, I. R., and Duncan, I. D.: Myotonia in the dog: a report of four cases. Vet. Rec. 93:184, 1973.

Halliwell, R. E. W., Schwartzman, R. M., and Hopkins, L.: The value of plasma corticosteroid assays in the diagnosis of Cushing's disease in the dog. J. Small Anim. Pract. 12:453, 1971.

Hoeldtke, R. D., Donald, R. A., and Nichols, M. G.: Functional significance of idiopathic adrenal calcification in the adult. Clin. Endocrinol. 12:319, 1980.

Jeffcoate, J., and Edwards, C. R. W.: Cushing's Syndrome: Pathogenesis, Diagnosis, and Treatment. In James, V. H. T. (ed.): The Adrenal Gland. Raven Press, New York, 1979, p. 165.

Johnston, D. E.: Adrenalectomy via retroperitoneal approach in dogs. J.A.V.M.A. 170:1092, 1977.

Johnston, S. D., and Mather, E. C.: Canine plasma cortisol (hydrocortisone) measured by radioimmunoassay: Clinical absence of durinal variation and results of ACTH stimulation and dexamethasone suppression tests. Am. J. Vet. Res. *39*:1766, 1978.

Joles, J. A., and Mulnix, J. A.: Polyuria and Polydipsia. *In* Kirk, R. W. (ed.): Current Veterinary Therapy VI. W. B. Saunders Co., Philadelphia, 1977, p. 1050.

Kaplan, M. M.: Alkaline phosphatase. N. Engl. J. Med. *286*:200, 1972.

Katherman, K. A., O'Leary, T. P., Richardson, R. C., Polzin, D. J., and Kaufman, G. M.: Hyperadrenalcorticism and diabetes in the dog. J.A.A.H.A. *16*:705, 1980.

Krieger, D. T.: Circadian Rhythms of ACTH and Adrenal Corticosteroids: Treatment of ACTH Hypersecretion in Cushing's Disease. *In* James, V. H. T., Serio, M., Guisti, G., and Martini, L. (eds.): The Endocrine Function of the Human Adrenal Cortex. Academic Press, London, 1978, p. 193.

Krieger, D. T., Amorsa, M. D., and Linick, F.: Cyproheptidine-induced remission of Cushing's disease. N. Engl. J. Med. *293*:893, 1975.

Lamberts, S., Tummermans, H., De Jong, F., and Birkenhager, J.: The role of dopaminergic depletion in the pathogenesis of Cushing's disease and the possible consequences for medical therapy. Clin. Endocrinol. 7:185, 1977.

Lester, S., Bellamy, J. E. C., MacWilliams, P. S., and Feldman, E. C.: A rapid radioimmunoassay method for the evaluation of plasma cortisol levels and adrenal function in the dog. J.A.A.H.A. *17*:121, 1981.

Liddle, G. W.: Cushing's syndrome. Ann. N.Y. Acad. Sci. *297*:594, 1977.

Liddle, G. W., and Melmon, K. L.: The Adrenals. *In* Williams, R. H. (ed.): Textbook of Endocrinology. W. B. Saunders Co., Philadelphia, 1974, p. 232.

Ling, G. V., Stabenfeldt, G. H., Comer, K. M., Gribble, D. H., and Schechter, R. D.: Canine hyperadrenocorticism: Pretreatment clinical and laboratory evaluation of 117 cases. J.A.V.M.A. *174*:1211, 1979.

Lubberink, A. A. M. E.: Diagnosis and Treatment of Canine Cushing's Syndrome. Ph.D. Thesis, University of Utrecht, The Netherlands, 1977.

Lubberink, A. A. M. E.: Therapy for Spontaneous Hyperadrenocorticism. *In* Kirk, R. W. (ed.): Current Veterinary Therapy VII. W. B. Saunders Co., Philadelphia, 1980, p. 979.

Meijer, J. C.: Canine Hyperadrenocorticism. *In* Kirk, R. W. (ed.): Current Veterinary Therapy VII. W. B. Saunders Co., Philadelphia, 1980. p. 975.

Meijer, J. C., Mulder, G. H., Rijnberk, A., and Groughs, R. J. M.: Hypothalamic corticotrophin releasing factor activity in dogs with pituitary-dependent hyperadrenocorticism. J. Endocrinol. *79*:209, 1978.

Meijer, J. C., Lubberink, A. A. M. E., and Gruys, E.: Cushing's syndrome due to adrenocortical adenoma in a cat. Tijdschr. Diergeneeskd. *103*:1048, 1978.

Meijer, J. C., Lubberink, A. A. M. E., Rijnberk, A., and Groughs, R. J. M.: Adrenocortical function tests in dogs with hyperfunctioning adrenocortical tumors. J. Endocrinol. *80*:315, 1979.

Mulnix, J. A., Van den Brom, W. E., and Lubberink, A. A. M.E.: Gamma camera imaging of bilateral adrenocortical hyperplasia and adrenal tumors in the dog. Am. J. Vet. Res. *37*:1467, 1976.

Nelson, A. A., and Woodard, G.: Severe adrenal cortical atrophy (cytotoxic) and hepatic damage produced in dogs by feeding 2,2-bis (parachlorophenyl)-1,1-cichloroethane (DDD or TDE). Arch. Pathol. *48*:387, 1949.

Osborne, C. A., Low, D. G., and Finco, D. R.: Canine

and Feline Urology. W. B. Saunders Co., Philadelphia, 1972.

Owens, J. M., and Drucker, W. D.: Hyperadrenocorticism in the dog: Canine Cushing's syndrome. Vet. Clin. North Am. 7:583, 1977.

Pearse, A. G. E., and Polak, J. M.: Neural crest origin of the endocrine polypeptide (APUD) cells of the gastrointestinal tract and pancreas. Gut *12*:783, 1971.

Pearse, A. G. E., and Welbourn, R. B.: The Apudomas. Br. J. Hosp. Med. *10*:617, 1973.

Peterson, M.: personal communication, 1981.

Peterson, M. E., and Drucker, W. D.: Biochemical Characterization and Treatment of Spontaneous Canine Cushing's Syndrome. Sci. Proc. Am. Coll. Vet. Intern. Med. 1980.

Peterson, M. E., Gilbertson, S. R., and Drucker, W. D.: Plasma corticol response to exogenous ACTH in 22 dogs with hyperadrenocorticism caused by an adrenocortical neoplasia. J.A.V.M.A. *180*:542–544, 1982.

Peterson, M. E., Nesbitt, G. H., and Schaer, M.: Diagnosis and management of concurrent diabetes mellitus and hyperadrenocorticism in thirty dogs. J.A.V.M.A. *178*:66, 1981.

Rijnberk, A., der Kinderen, P. J., and Thijssen, J. H.: Canine Cushing's syndrome. Zentralbl. Veterinaermed. *16*:13, 1969.

Rogers, W. A., and Ruebner, B. H.: A retrospective study of probable glucocorticoid-induced hepatopathy in dogs. J.A.V.M.A. *170*:603, 1977.

Sadowski, J., Nazar, K., and Szczepanska-Sadowska, E.: Reduced urine concentration in dogs exposed to cold: relation to plasma ADH and 17-OHCS. Am. J. Physiol. *222*:607, 1972.

Schechter, R. D.: Hyperadrenocorticism. *In* Kirk, R. W. (ed.): Current Veterinary Therapy VI. W. B. Saunders Co., Philadelphia, 1977, p. 1027.

Schechter, R. D., Stabenfeldt, G. H., Gribble, D. H., and Ling, G. V.: Treatment of Cushing's syndrome in the dog with an adrenocorticolytic agent (*o,p'*-DDD). J.A.V.M.A. *162*:629, 1973.

Share, L., and Travis, R. H.: Interrelations between the adrenal cortex and the posterior pituitary. Fed. Proc. *30*:1378, 1971.

Siegel, E. T., Kelly, D. F., and Berg, P.: Cushing's syndrome in the dog. J.A.V.M.A. *157*:2081, 1970.

Swift, G. A., and Brown, R. H.: Surgical treatment of Cushing's syndrome in the cat. Vet. Rec. *99*:374, 1976.

Tyrrell, J. B., Brooks, R. M., Fitzgerald, P. A., Cofoid, P. B., Forsham, P. H., and Wilson, C. B.: Cushing's disease — selective transphenoidal resection of pituitary microadenomas. N. Engl. J. Med. *298*:753, 1978.

Vial, G. C., Stabenfeldt, G. H., Franti, C. E., and Ling, G. V.: Influence of environment on adrenal cortical response to ACTH stimulation in clinically normal dogs. Am. J. Vet. Res. *40*:919, 1979.

Walton, J., and Ney, R. L.: Current concepts of corticosteroids, uses and abuses. Disease-a-Month, Year Book Medical Publishers, Inc., Chicago, June, 1975.

Wilber, J. F., and Utiger, R. D.: The effect of glucocorticoids on thyrotropin secretion. J. Clin. Invest. *48*:2096, 1969.

Wood, C. E., Shinsako, J., Keil, L. C., Ramsey, D. J., and Dallman, M. F.: Hormonal and hemodynamic responses to 15 ml/kg hemorrhage in conscious dogs: responses correlate to body temperature. Soc. Exp. Biol. Med. *167*:15–19, 1981.

The Reproductive System

CHAPTER 70

Reproductive Physiology of Dogs and Cats

TERRY M. NETT
and PATRICIA N. S. OLSON

REPRODUCTIVE ANATOMY AND PHYSIOLOGY

MALE DOGS AND CATS*

Anatomy of the Reproductive Organs

The reproductive tract of male dogs and cats consists of a scrotum, two testes, the epididymides, the ductus deferentes, the prostate gland, the penis, and the urethra. In addition, the tom cat has a pair of bulbourethral glands. Vesicular glands are absent in both species (Fig. 70–1).

The scrotum of dogs is located about midway between the inguinal region and the anus. In cats, it is located caudal to the thighs and caudoventral to the ischiatic arch. The scrotum is divided into two cavities by a median septum, and each cavity is occupied by a testis, epididymis, and the distal portion of the spermatic cord. Testes of healthy animals are ovoid and firm. The mediastinum testis gives rise to connective tissue septae, which divide the testis into incomplete lobules. The lobules contain the seminiferous tubules, which drain into the rete testis, which in turn empties into the efferent ducts. The efferent ducts unite to form the head of the epididymis.

In both dogs and cats, the head of the epididymis begins on the medial surface of the testis but courses around the cranial end to attain a lateral position. The body of the epididymis is extremely convoluted and is closely attached to the dorsolateral surface of the testis. The tail of the epididymis is attached to the caudal end of the testis and continues craniodorsally through the spermatic cord as the ductus deferens.

The spermatic cord extends from the inguinal ring, where its constituent parts converge through the inguinal canal to the attached border of the testicle. It consists of the testicular artery, the testicular veins (forming the pampiniform plexus around the artery), the lymphatics, the autonomic nerves of the testis, the ductus deferens, smooth muscle tissue (former cremaster internus) about the vessels, and the visceral layer of the vaginal tunic.

The ductus deferens is a continuation of the tail of the epididymis. It extends from the tail of the epididymis through the spermatic cord and into the abdominal cavity to enter the craniodorsal surface of the prostate, where it fuses with the urethra. The ductus deferens has a narrow, aglandular ampulla in the dog; no ampullary region has been described in the cat.

In the dog, the prostate is a large, dense structure located at or near the cranial border of the pubis. The gland is subject to much variation in size and is often enlarged in older animals. It is composed of two lobes that surround the neck of the bladder and the urethra. In contrast to the dog, the prostate gland of the cat is located two to three cm caudal to the bladder and consists of two distinct lobes that are joined only on the dorsal surface of the urethra.

Bulbourethral glands (present only in the cat) are paired glands that lie at the posterior rim of the pelvis. Each is about the size of a pea and opens into the urethra at the root of the penis.

The penis of dogs and cats has several distinct features. In the caudal portion there are two distinct corpora cavernosa separat-

---

*Specific measurements used to describe the anatomy of the reproductive tract refer to values for a 10- to 12-kg male dog and a four-kg tom cat.

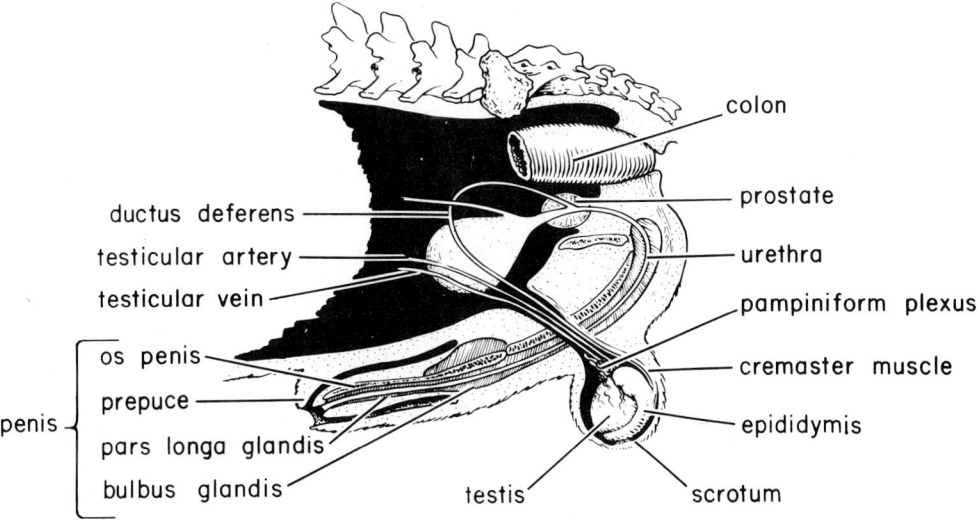

Figure 70–1. Anatomy of the reproductive tract of the male dog.

ed by a medial septum. In the cranial portion there is a bone, the os penis, considered to be a part of the corpus cavernosum that has ossified. Ventrally, the os penis is grooved for the urethra. The glans is quite long, extending over the entire length of the os penis. In the cat it contains a number of small spines. The cranial part of the glans, the pars longa glandis, is cylindrical and narrows to a pointed end; the caudal portion of the glans is the bulbus glandis. Both of these structures are composed of erectile tissue. The prepuce forms a complete sheath around the cranial part of the non-erect penis and covers the pars longa glandis and part of the bulbus glandis (Ellenport, 1975; Christensen, 1979).

Spermatogenesis and Semen Formation

Little information concerning spermatogenesis and formation of semen in dogs and cats is available. The duration of the cycle of the seminiferous epithelium of the mature beagle is 13.6 days (Foote et al., 1972). Similar information is not available for the cat. Spermatozoa first appear in the ejaculate of dogs between 6 and 12 months of age, compared to 8 to 12 months for cats.

Detailed studies concerning formation of seminal fluid have not been reported for dogs or cats. In the dog, prostatic secretion is rich in sodium and chloride ions, but the concentration of citrate is low. The normal pH of canine prostatic fluid is approximately 6.8. Prostate function appears to be regulated by circulating androgens. Semen from both dogs and cats has very low concentrations of fructose, possibly due to the absence of vesicular glands in these species.

In the dog, semen is ejaculated in three fractions. The first fraction is a clear, sperm-free fluid that is released before complete erection is attained. The second fraction is released during the intense ejaculatory reaction and is the sperm-rich fraction. The third fraction is emitted while the animals are "locked" together and is a clear fluid. The volume of an ejaculate from dogs averages six ml (range 2 to 15 ml) and contains approximately 500×10^6 sperm (Boucher, 1957).

In the cat, ejaculation is extremely rapid, and therefore, it is difficult to determine if semen is ejaculated in more than one fraction. During electroejaculation, two distinct fractions of semen have been noted. The volume of semen per ejaculate averages 0.05 ml (range 0.01 to 0.2 ml), with approximately 57×10^6 sperm.

Endocrine Regulation of Reproduction

Hypothalamic-Pituitary-Gonadal Axis. Although hypothalamic content of gonadotropin-releasing hormone (GnRH) has not been studied in male dogs and cats, it is undoubtedly involved in the regulation of follicle-stimulating hormone (FSH) and luteinizing hormone (LH) secretion by the anterior pituitary gland. GnRH does stimulate release of LH and FSH when administered to dogs (Jones and Boyns, 1974, 1976; Jones et al., 1976; Reimers et al., 1978).

In normal adult male dogs, circulating concentrations of LH have been examined and LH appears to be released in a pulsatile manner. The interval between peaks of LH was approximately 110 minutes and there was no diurnal variation in either frequency or height of the peaks (DePalatis et al., 1978). Circulating concentrations of FSH have not been reported in male dogs. LH stimulates secretion of testosterone by the Leydig cells of the testis; hence, serum concentrations of testosterone follow a pattern similar to those observed for LH but have a lag phase of approximately 50 minutes (DePalatis et al., 1978). This lag phase is longer than that reported for other species, and the physiologic significance of the long lag phase is unknown. The testis also produces estradiol-17β, but there have been no detailed studies concerning its secretion.

Both testosterone and estradiol-17β inhibit secretion of LH (and presumably FSH) in the dog by exerting a negative feedback at the hypothalamus or pituitary gland or both. Administration of testosterone to castrated male dogs maintains serum concentrations of LH at baseline (Vincent et al., 1979). However, treatment of dogs with testosterone did not diminish release of LH in response to a GnRH challenge (Jones and Boyns, 1974). These data indicate that the negative feedback effect of testosterone on release of LH is probably exerted on the hypothalamus.

Administration of estradiol-17β to male dogs suppressed basal concentrations of LH and blocked secretion of LH in response to an intravenous injection of GnRH (Jones and Boyns, 1974). Therefore, it appears that estradiol-17β can exert a negative feedback effect on secretion of LH at the level of the pituitary; however, an additional effect at the hypothalamus has not been ruled out.

It is likely that both testosterone and estradiol-17β are involved in regulation of FSH secretion in dogs; however, this remains to be proved. Secretion of pituitary gonadotropins and testicular steroids has not been examined in the tom cat.

Considering the growth-promoting properties of androgens, pet owners may be tempted to administer such compounds to dogs. Such treatments should be used with extreme caution. The androgens used to promote growth will most likely decrease secretion of gonadotropins by exerting a negative feedback on the hypothalamo-hypophyseal axis. This will result in decreased synthesis of testosterone by the testis, ultimately resulting in decreased sperm production and possible sterility.

FEMALE DOGS AND CATS*

Anatomy of the Reproductive Organs

Anatomic relationships between various components of the reproductive system of the bitch are illustrated in Fig. 70–2. Ovaries of bitches and queens are small, oval structures. In the bitch, the average length is approximately two cm compared to about one cm in the queen. The ovaries are located about halfway between the last rib and the crest of the ilium. The right ovary is commonly located slightly more cranially than the left. As a female ages and undergoes numerous pregnancies, both ovaries migrate ventrocaudally. In dogs, each ovary is entirely closed in a peritoneal pouch, the ovarian bursa. The ovarian bursa of the queen is less confining than that of the bitch, and it is possible to visualize the ovaries. The peritoneal layers that form the bursa continue to the horn of the uterus, thus constituting the mesosalpinx and the proper ligament of the ovary. The ovarian bursa is also attached to one of the last two ribs by the suspensory ligament of the ovary.

The oviduct (uterine tube or fallopian tube) transports oocytes from the ovary to the uterus. Each tube passes cranially in the lateral part of the ovarian bursa, turns caudad in the anterior portion of the bursa, and runs caudally through the medial part to join the anterior end of the uterine horns. At the ovarian end, the oviduct ends as a funnel-shaped infundibulum that opens near the slit in the ovarian bursa. The extremity of the infundibulum is lined with fimbria, fingerlike processes of smooth muscle that create currents to pull newly ovulated ova into the oviduct.

The uterus of dogs and cats has a relatively short body and long, narrow horns. In an average size bitch, the body of the uterus is two to three cm long, whereas the horns are 12 to 15 cm long. The proper ligament of

---

*Specific measurements used to describe the anatomy of the reproductive tract refer to values for a ten-kg bitch and a three-kg queen.

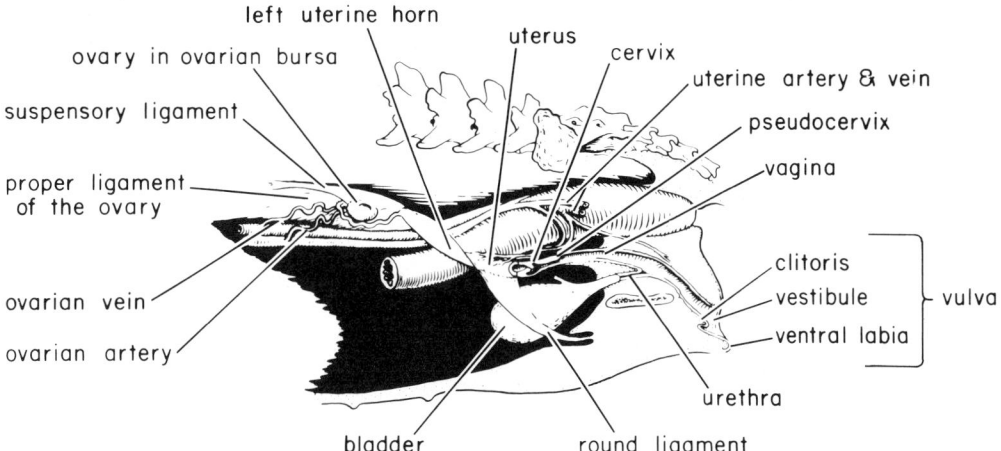

left uterine horn
ovary in ovarian bursa
uterus
cervix
suspensory ligament
uterine artery & vein
pseudocervix
proper ligament of the ovary
vagina
ovarian vein
clitoris
vestibule
ovarian artery
ventral labia
vulva
urethra
bladder
round ligament

Figure 70–2. Anatomy of the reproductive tract of the bitch.

the ovary is a caudal extension of the supensory ligament and connects the ovary to the uterine horns. The cervix lies between the body of the uterus and the vagina. The cervical canal is directed caudoventrally. Thus, the internal orifice of the cervical canal opens almost directly dorsally, whereas the external cervical orifice is directed towards the ventral wall of the vagina. There is also a prominent ventral fornix. In the bitch, the external orifice of the cervix opens on a hillock just beneath the dorsal median postcervical fold of the vagina. This fold has been termed a pseudocervix (Pineda et al., 1973). The presence of a pseudocervix, a prominent fornix, and a caudoventral orientation of the cervical canal makes cannulation of the uterus a very difficult procedure.

The vagina extends from the cervix to the vulva, ending just cranial to the urethral orifice. It is a musculomembranous structure that can increase greatly in both width and length during copulation, pregnancy, and parturition. The structure of its lining is highly dependent on circulating concentrations of ovarian steroids and can be used to determine stages of the reproductive cycle (see following discussion).

The vulva, or external genitalia, is composed of the vestibule, the clitoris, and the labia. The vestibule is the space connecting the vagina with the external genital opening. There is no definite hymen marking the vaginovestibular junction. The urethral tubercle is a ridgelike projection on the ventral floor of the vestibule and contains the external urethral orifice. The labia, or lips,

form the external boundary of the vulva and are homologous to the scrotum of the male. They are composed of fibroelastic connective tissue, smooth muscle fibers, and an abundance of adipose tissue, so they are soft and pliable. The labia are fused dorsally and ventrally to form commissures. The clitoris is located just inside the ventral commissure. It has a body that is infiltrated with fat and is not erectile, and a glans that is composed of erectile tissue. The glans is located in a fossa. A fold of mucous membrane extends caudally over the glans and the fossa, and a central projection of this fold can be mistaken for the glans.

Blood is supplied to the female reproductive system by three major pairs of arteries. The ovarian arteries originate from the dorsal aorta caudal to the renal arteries. In addition to the ovaries, these arteries supply the uterine tubes and the tips of the uterine horns. Just prior to reaching the ovary, each artery gives off a caudal branch that anastomoses with the uterine artery. It may, therefore, be possible for the ovaries to receive supplemental blood from the uterine arteries via retrograde flow through this anastomosis, although there is some controversy concerning the existence of the anastomosis (Del Campo and Ginther, 1974). The uterine arteries arise from the urogenital arteries and course cranially on either side of the uterine body and horns. These provide the primary blood supply for the uterus. The vaginal arteries originate from the urogenital arteries and supply blood to the vagina and external genitalia. The external genitalia are also supplied in part by branches of external and internal pudendal arteries (Ellenport, 1975; Christensen, 1979).

ESTROUS CYCLE, PSEUDOPREGNANCY, AND REPRODUCTIVE ENDOCRINOLOGY

THE CANINE ESTROUS CYCLE

Proestrus. In dogs, proestrus has been defined as that stage of the reproductive cycle characterized by a bright red or sanguinous discharge from the vulva. The average duration of proestrus is 9 days, but it can range from 2 to 15 days. It appears that hormonal events leading to the onset of proestrus may begin several weeks earlier. Plasma concentrations of estradiol-17β rise slightly about five weeks before the onset of estrus (Edqvist et al., 1975) and then remain relatively stable until the onset of proestrus. During the first six or seven days of proestrus there was a more rapid rise in concentrations of estradiol-17β. Most investigators agree that peak concentrations of estradiol-17β occur one to two days before the end of proestrus and are declining when acceptance is first observed (Concannon et al., 1975; Nett et al., 1975; Wildt et al., 1979). Serum concentrations of progesterone remain low prior to and during the first few days of proestrus (Edqvist et al., 1975); however, during the two to three days prior to acceptance there is a slight increase in concentrations of progesterone (Wildt et al., 1979). This increase appears to be correlated with pre-ovulatory luteinization of ovarian follicles (Wildt et al., 1978). Serum concentrations of LH remain near baseline during most of proestrus; however, approximately 50 per cent of bitches appear to have a small surge of LH three to ten days prior to acceptance. The significance of this early peak in LH is uncertain, but it may be associated with preovulatory luteinization of the follicle. Serum concentrations of FSH appear to be at their lowest during late proestrus (Reimers et al., 1978).

Estrus. Estrus is that period of the reproductive cycle characterized by the bitch's acceptance of the male. This period normally lasts for about 9 days but can range in length from 1 to 15 days. The bitch appears to become receptive to the male after serum concentrations of estradiol-17β are beginning to fall and concentrations of progesterone are beginning to rise (Concannon et al., 1977a). This hypothesis is supported by data obtained after administration of estradiol-17β alone or followed by progesterone to ovariectomized bitches. Behavioral estrus was not displayed until after administration of the estradiol-17β was halted, and the onset of estrous behavior was more synchronous when progesterone was administered at the time of estrogen withdrawal (Concannon et al., 1979a). Similarly, release of the pre-ovulatory surge of LH appears to be mediated by the decline in serum concentrations of estradiol-17β with a concomitant rise in concentrations of progesterone (Concannon et al., 1979b). Some investigators have reported that the preovulatory surge of LH occurs on the first day of estrus (Nett et al., 1975; Reimers et al., 1978). Others have found no correlation between the preovulatory surge of LH and the onset of estrus (Concannon et al., 1975; Wildt et al., 1978). The preovulatory surge of LH in the bitch is prolonged compared with that of many other species. Duration of the LH surge appears to range from 48 to 96 hours in bitches, with concentrations of LH increasing from baseline to peak in approximately 24 hours and then returning to baseline in the next 30 to 60 hours (Nett et al., 1975; Wildt et al., 1978). There is a surge in serum concentrations of FSH that occurs coincidentally with the preovulatory LH surge; however, it appears that a longer time is required for FSH to return to baseline (Reimers et al., 1978).

Ovulation in the bitch can occur from 0 to 96 hours after the LH peak, although most ovulations occur between 24 and 72 hours after maximum serum concentrations of LH are noted (Phemister et al., 1973; Wildt et al., 1978). Whether ovulations occur only after the onset of estrus, or whether some can occur during late proestrus, has not been resolved. The wide variation in time of ovulation in relation to the LH peak may be due to the long duration of the LH peak.

As mentioned previously, serum concentrations of progesterone begin rising during late proestrus. This gradual rise continues until after the LH surge, when serum concentrations of progesterone undergo a more rapid increase for approximately ten days (Christie et al., 1971; Smith and McDonald, 1974; Nett et al., 1975; Mellin et al., 1976; Wildt et al., 1979). The bitch appears to be unique in that behavioral estrus is exhibited in the face of high concentrations of progesterone. There is no corpus hemorrhagicum formed in the bitch at ovulation, possibly owing to the rather extensive luteinization prior to ovulation. Unlike most other species, the bitch ovulates a primary oocyte, rather than a secondary oocyte. The first meiotic division begins about one day after ovulation, usually in the mid-portion of the oviduct. Oocyte maturation is complete within three days after ovulation. Once maturation is complete, the viable lifespan of the secondary oocyte is approximately 24 hours.

Serum concentrations of estradiol-17β slowly return to baseline during the six to eight days following the LH peak (Nett et al., 1975; Wildt et al., 1979). Although not yet examined in detail, it appears that superficial epithelial cells may disappear from the vaginal smear about the same time serum concentrations of estradiol-17β reach their baseline. On the average, this occurs about three days prior to the end of the behavioral estrus (Holst and Phemister, 1974).

Diestrus. Behaviorally, onset of diestrus is defined as the first day after a period of estrus that a bitch refuses a male. As noted above, there is a sharp decline in superficial cells from the vaginal epithelium about three days prior to the end of estrus. It has been suggested that the onset of diestrus be defined by this event rather than by behavior. There is some merit to this suggestion, since the LH peak, ovulation, oocyte maturation, and other events can be timed more accurately using the disappearance of superficial cells from the vaginal epithelium as a marker (Holst and Phemister, 1974, 1975) rather than using breeding or the end of behavioral estrus.

During early diestrus, serum concentrations of progesterone continue to increase, reaching a maximum 10 to 20 days after the LH peak (Smith and McDonald, 1974; Concannon et al., 1975). This plateau is maintained until about day 20 of diestrus, at which time serum concentrations of progesterone begin a gradual decrease that continues for five to six weeks. Serum concentrations of LH, FSH, estradiol-17β, and prolactin remain relatively stable throughout diestrus (Concannon et al., 1975; Nett et al., 1975; Edqvist et al., 1975; Reimers et al., 1978). The endocrine changes observed during the estrous cycle of the bitch are summarized in Figure 70–3.

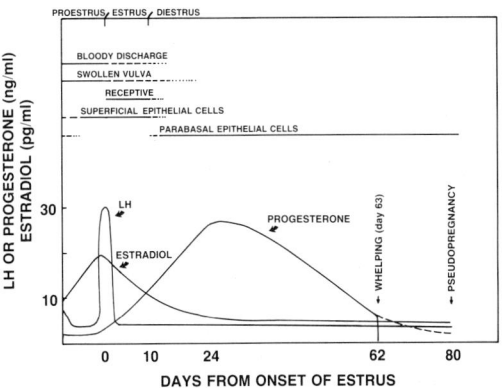

Figure 70–3. Peripheral concentrations of reproductive hormones, estrual activity and changes in vaginal epithelial cells during the estrous cycle of the bitch.

During diestrus there is a slight decrease in hematocrit from 48 per cent to 44 per cent (Concannon et al., 1975; Tietz et al., 1967). No change in concentrations of serum corticoids occurs during the estrous cycle of the nonpregnant bitch.

Anestrus. Following a reproductive cycle, the bitch enters a period of ovarian quiescence called anestrus. This phase can last from two to ten months. Very little is known about this phase of the canine reproductive cycle. Although it is quite difficult to induce ovulation and fertile estrus consistently by using exogenous gonadotropins during this period, this is the easiest time of the cycle to induce ovulation. Clearly, this is one area of canine reproduction requiring more study.

VAGINAL CYTOLOGY IN THE DOG

The vaginal epithelium is one of the target tissues for ovarian hormones. Changes in exfoliated vaginal epithelial cells occur as a result of changing secretory patterns of ovarian hormones. Daily evaluation of exfoliated vaginal epithelial cells can be helpful in analyzing phases of the estrous cycle and in determining optimum breeding times.

The cell types found in vaginal smears taken during the estrous cycle have been described by a number of authors (Roszel, 1975, 1977; Dahlgren, 1979; Gier, 1960; Fletch, 1973; Holst and Phemister, 1974; Christie and Bell, 1972; Dore, 1978). The terms "cornified" and "noncornified," frequently used to describe the cells on a vaginal smear, are not adequate. It seems more appropriate to name them in the epithelium at the time of maximal cornification, beginning with the deepest vaginal layer and progessing to the layer nearest the lumen, as follows.

Basal cells ultimately give rise to all the epithelial cell types observed in a vaginal smear. These cells line the basement membrane of the vagina and are not normally exfoliated.

Parabasal cells are the smallest epithelial cells in the vaginal smear. They are round and have a large nucleus (Fig. 70–4,*A*).

Intermediate cells vary in size but are generally about twice the size of the parabasal cells. They have a round nucleus and are located between the parabasal and superficial cell layers (Fig. 70–4,*B*) (Roszel, 1977).

Superficial vaginal epithelial cells are the largest epithelial cells in the vaginal smear. The nuclei, if present, are small, dark, and centrally located (Roszel, 1977). These cells line the luminal surface of the estrogen-stimulated vagina and have borders that appear flat or folded (Fig. 70–4,*C*).

"Metestrum" cells have been defined as parabasal cells that appear to contain a neutrophil in their cytoplasm (Schutte, 1967). These cells are not seen during estrus but may be observed whenever neutrophils are present (Fig. 70–4,*D*).

"Foam" cells are parabasal cells that contain cytoplasmic vacuoles (Fig. 70–4,*E*) (Schutte, 1967).

Erythrocytes, neutrophils, and bacteria are also frequently present in vaginal smears. The appearance and/or disappearance of various cell types during the reproductive cycle of the bitch is now considered.

PROESTRUS. During proestrus, serum concentrations of estradiol rise as ovarian follicles mature. This results in proliferation of the vaginal epithelium and diapedesis of red blood cells through uterine capillaries.

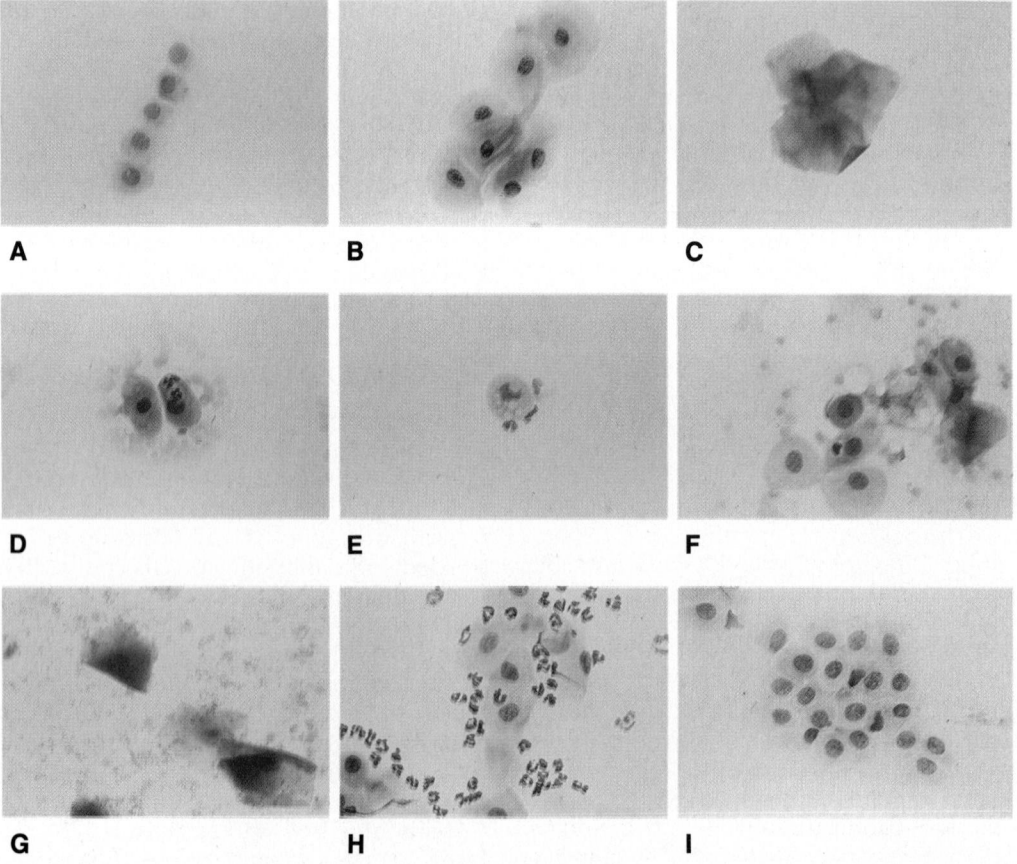

Figure 70–4. Canine vaginal cytology. *A*, parabasal cells, *B*, intermediate cells. *C*, superficial vaginal epithelial cells. *D*, metestrum cell. *E*, foam cell. *F*, proestrous smear. *G*, estrous smear. *H*, diestrous smear, and *I*, anestrous smear.

Vaginal proliferation and uterine diapedesis accounts for the red blood cells and superficial vaginal epithelial cells seen in vaginal smears taken during proestrus.

In early proestrus, neutrophils as well as parabasal and intermediate cells may be present (Fig. 70–4,*F*). By mid-proestrus, the neutrophils decrease in number and are usually absent in smears taken during late proestrus. Erythrocytes are usually abundant in smears taken in mid- or late proestrus, and epithelial cells are of the superficial type. Bacteria are often abundant but may be found in vaginal smears throughout the estrous cycle.

ESTRUS. Vaginal smears taken during estrus usually contain no neutrophils, and red blood cells diminish in number, although a few may be observed throughout estrus and in early diestrus in some dogs. Large numbers of bacteria are often observed in the background without a leukocytic response (Fig. 70–4,*G*). In beagle bitches, superficial epithelial cells were reported to be intact with well-defined borders two days before the onset of diestrus. One day before the onset of diestrus, superficial cells were usually in clumps or large sheets with poorly defined cytoplasmic borders (Holst and Phemister, 1974).

DIESTRUS. Cytologically, an abrupt change in relative numbers of epithelial cell types has been reported to signal the onset of diestrus in the beagle bitch (Holst and Phemister, 1974). The number of superficial cells decreased by at least 20 per cent; the number of parabasal cells and intermediate cells, which were previously either absent or less than five per cent of the total, increased to more than ten per cent and often to greater than 50 per cent (Fig. 70–4,*H*). Neutrophils appear in variable numbers and usually coincide with the increased numbers of parabasal and intermediate cells, but they occasionally precede or lag behind these changes. On the first day of diestrus, many of the superficial cells appear torn, folded, or smudged (Holst and Phemister, 1974). The amount of cytolysis (presence of nuclear shadows without any surrounding cytoplasm) seen in epithelial cells has been reported to be less during the first month than during the remainder of diestrus (Dore, 1978). Although Dore speculates that these cytologic changes may be due to lactobacilli acting on noncornified surface epithelial cells, *Lactobacillus sp.* was

isolated from the posterior vagina less than two per cent of the time in 81 normal postpuberal bitches (Olson and Mather, 1978). "Metestrum" cells and "foam" cells may also be seen throughout diestrus (Roszel, 1977).

ANESTRUS. Serum concentrations of progesterone and estradiol are lowest during anestrus. Parabasal cells and intermediate cells are the predominant cell types present in vaginal smears taken during this period (Fig. 70–4,*I*). Neutrophils may be present or absent but are generally fewer in number than during early diestrus.

THE FELINE ESTROUS CYCLE

The principal difference between reproduction in dogs and cats is that cats are induced ovulators. Therefore, if mating does not occur, queens will continue to demonstrate estrus at regular intervals for several months, depending on the breed, time of year, and environmental conditions.

Proestrus. Queens have a short period of proestrus, usually one or two days in duration. There is no sanguinous discharge from the vulva of the queen at this time. Often this stage is not recognized in the queen (Schille et al., 1979).

Estrus. In the absence of a male, queens will generally show estrus at intervals of 14 to 28 days. Estrus usually lasts for nine to ten days and appears to be related to elevated concentrations of estradiol-17β in the circulation (Verhage et al., 1976). When concentrations of estradiol-17β decrease, the queen stops exhibiting estrus. Concentrations of estradiol-17β usually rise again in one to two weeks, and the queen returns to estrus. Serum concentrations of progesterone remain at their baseline throughout periods of polyestrus (Fig. 70–5).

Pseudopregnancy. If queens are induced to ovulate by a sterile mating, injection of ovulating agents, vaginal stimulation with a glass rod, or other means, pseudopregnancy will result. Corpora lutea are formed, and an increase in circulating concentrations of progesterone are noted within two days after ovulation. Concentrations of progesterone continue to increase until day 10 to 20 of pseudopregnancy and then return to baseline approximately 40 days postovulation (Paape et al., 1975; Verhage et al., 1976). Concentrations of estradiol-17β re-

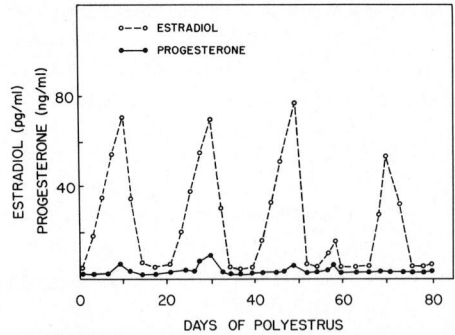

Figure 70–5. Peripheral concentrations of estradiol-17β and progesterone during a period of polyestrus in the cat. (Adapted from Verhage et al., 1976.)

main at their baseline throughout pseudo-pregnancy (Fig. 70–6).

Anestrus. Anestrus, or the nonbreeding season, is a period of ovarian quiescence lasting for more than 30 days. This usually occurs between September and January in the northern hemisphere. Occurrence of anestrus also may be related to the breed of cat. Approximately 90 per cent of long-haired breeds had a nonbreeding season, whereas only 40 per cent of short-haired breeds displayed anestrus (Jemmet and Evans, 1977). Concentrations of reproductive hormones have not been quantified during anestrus in the cat.

VAGINAL CYTOLOGY IN THE CAT

Epithelial cell types found in vaginal smears from the cat are similar to those found in canine vaginal smears. The interpretation of vaginal smears during the feline estrous cycle has been reported (Herron, 1977; Cline et al., 1980; Mowrer et al., 1975).

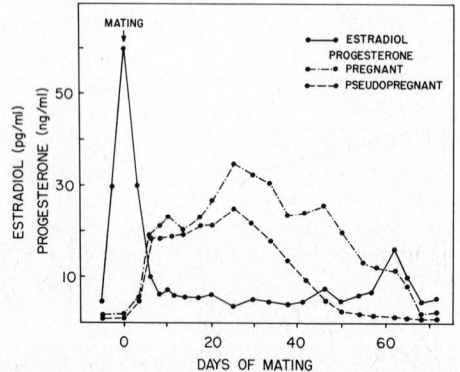

Figure 70–6. Peripheral concentrations of estradiol-17β and progesterone during pregnancy and pseudo-pregnancy in the queen. (Adapted from Verhage et al., 1976.)

PROESTRUS. During proestrus few parabasal cells are seen. The number of intermediate cells increases, and superficial cells generally constitute 60 per cent or more of the cell count by the time behavioral signs of estrus are observed (Herron, 1977). Unlike the dog, red blood cells are not a characteristic finding in vaginal smears taken from a cat during proestrus.

ESTRUS. Vaginal smears taken during estrus have predominantly superficial epithelial cells. Parabasal cells and neutrophils are absent. Maximum receptivity was consistently identified when mature superficial cells, devoid of nuclei, became equal to that of the previously dominant cell type, superficial cells with pyknotic nuclei (Mowrer et al., 1975; Schille et al., 1979).

DIESTRUS. In early pregnancy or pseudopregnancy, parabasal and intermediate cell types reappear. The superficial epithelial cells that were abundant during estrus rapidly decrease in number. The end of estrus or onset of diestrus was defined by the appearance of large masses or sheets of mature cells (Mowrer, et al., 1975).

ANESTRUS. The predominant epithelial cell type in vaginal smears taken during anestrus is the parabasal cell. Intermediate epithelial cells may also be seen. Neutrophils may be present, but few superficial epithelial cells are observed.

PREGNANCY IN DOGS

Fertilization and Embryonic Development. As noted earlier, ovulation in the bitch usually occurs between 24 and 72 hours after the LH peak. Considering the variability in occurrence of the LH peak as related to the onset of estrus, it is extremely difficult to recommend a "best" time to breed a bitch to obtain maximum likelihood of conception. Fortunately, canine spermatozoa can survive in the female reproductive tract for periods of up to seven days after mating (Doak et al., 1967).

Since bitches ovulate a primary oocyte, the egg is not ready for fertilization until about three days after ovulation. Once the secondary oocyte forms, fertilization can be completed. High fertility can be attained from a single breeding that occurs any time during the interval from four days prior to ovulation until three days after ovulation. Fertilization usually occurs in the distal one third of the oviduct. Pronuclei are evident about 24 hours after fertilization, and after an additional 24 hours the first cleavage has occurred. Cleavage continues while the eggs are in the oviduct, and morulae of 16 cells or more enter the uterus six to seven days after fertilization, on day two to day three of diestrus (Holst and Phemister, 1971, 1975). Shortly after entering the uterus the morulae become blastocysts and they remain free-floating in the uterus for approximately one week. During this time they migrate through the uterus and become rather evenly spaced.

Implantation. Implantation in the bitch occurs about day 11 or 12 of diestrus, or about 15 or 16 days after fertilization. It is first marked by endometrial edema. At this point the blastocysts are no longer free-floating; they shed their zona pellucidae, and the differentiation of the embryonic disc into the primitive streak begins (Holst and Phemister, 1971).

The placenta in dogs is endotheliochorial in nature. Only a central zone of the placenta actually implants into the endometrium, thus the zonary classification. Information concerning fetal development after implantation is sketchy. Interested readers should see the article by Evans (1979) on this subject.

Endocrine Patterns During Pregnancy. Circulating concentrations of reproductive hormones in the pregnant bitch are similar to those observed during diestrus and cannot be used as a pregnancy test. Smith and McDonald (1974) suggested that serum concentrations of progesterone in pregnant bitches were higher at 20 to 25 days after the LH peak than in nonpregnant bitches. Similarly, Concannon et al. (1975) observed secondary increases in progesterone between days 20 and 40 in 75 per cent of pregnant bitches. Other investigators have failed to substantiate these findings (Parkes et al., 1972; Edqvist et al., 1975; Nett et al., 1975). Serum concentrations of progesterone return to baseline at the time of parturition (day 62) in pregnant bitches but may remain above baseline until day 80 in nonpregnant bitches (Smith and McDonald, 1974; Concannon et al., 1975). Concentrations of estradiol-17β and LH remain at basal values throughout gestation. Concentrations of prolactin were reported to increase slightly about day 40 of pregnancy and return to baseline by day 50 (Knight et al., 1977); however, only two bitches were used in this study. Reimers et al. (1978) reported increased concentrations of both prolactin and FSH on days 28 and 57 of pregnancy, but again the data were from only two bitches and sampling was infrequent.

Pregnancy can be diagnosed by abdominal palpation after approximately day 21 in some bitches. Following implantation there is a progessive decrease in hematocrit from about 45 per cent to 31 per cent. The decrease in hematocrit is inversely correlated with body weight, which increases 36 per cent during gestation (Concannon et al., 1970).

The bitch requires an ovarian source of progesterone throughout pregnancy. Ovariectomy as late as day 55 results in premature delivery of the pups (Sokolowski, 1971).

Parturition. The exact stimulus responsible for initiation of parturition in the bitch has not been identified. Unlike several other species, an increase in circulating concentrations of estradiol-17β has not been detected prior to delivery. Concentrations of progesterone decrease slowly from approximately day 30 until the end of gestation, but during the last two days prior to parturition the decrease is much more rapid. Following the decrease in progesterone by approximately 12 hours is a decrease in body temperature of the bitch from 38°C to 37°C (101.3°F to 98.8°F). Coincident with or slightly preceding the decline in progesterone is a rise in concentrations of corticoids in the bitch (Concannon et al., 1977b). It has not been determined whether the rise in corticoids is due to secretion from maternal adrenal glands or whether it is of fetal origin, as appears to be the case in other species (Fig. 70–7).

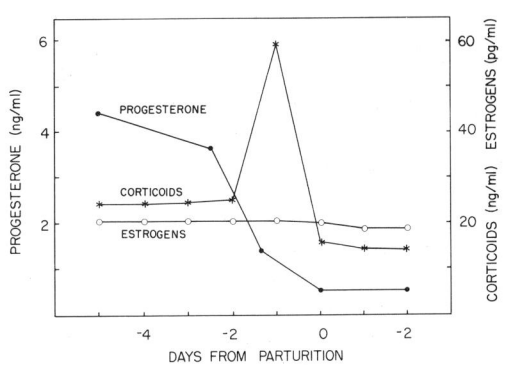

Figure 70–7. Changes in peripheral concentrations of estradiol-17β, progesterone and cortisol prior to whelping in the bitch. (Adapted from Concannon et al., 1977b.)

Just prior to delivery, nesting behavior is intensified. At this time the vulva becomes relaxed and some clear mucus may be passed. When uterine contractions are first initiated, bitches become restless and exhibit an increased panting rate. When the head of a fetus begins its passage through the pelvic canal, abdominal contractions are initiated.

PREGNANCY IN CATS

Fertilization and Implantation. Ovulation in cats is induced by mating. The mating stimulus induces release of LH; however, one copulation may not be sufficient to sustain the release of LH long enough to induce ovulation. Two to three matings in one day are generally recommended to insure ovulation. Ovulation normally occurs 24 to 48 hours after mating (Greulich, 1934; Sojka et al., 1970). If fertilization occurs, the fertilized eggs reach the uterus in about five days and implantation occurs 13 to 14 days after mating.

Endocrine Patterns During Pregnancy. After mating, the circulating concentration of estradiol-17β declines and remains at baseline until just prior to parturition, when it increases. Serum concentrations of progesterone remain low the first two or three days after mating, then rise rapidly to reach a plateau about day ten. This is a brief plateau, followed by another rise to a second peak about day 20 (Verhage et al., 1976). The secondary rise in progesterone is more dramatic in pregnant queens than in pseudopregnant queens (Fig. 70–3). Circulating concentrations of progesterone begin a gradual decline about 20 days after mating and return to baseline just prior to parturition, or about 65 days after mating. Unlike the bitch, the rate of decrease in concentrations of progesterone is more rapid in the pseudopregnant queen (basal concentrations of progesterone are reached approximately 40 days postovulation) than in the pregnant queen.

Parturition. Parturition in cats has not been the subject of detailed examinations. As in the bitch, there appears to be a decrease in body temperature one to two days prior to delivery. The signs of labor and rates of delivery of the kittens are similar to those described for the bitch.

Other Endocrine Glands. Normal rates of production and secretion of hormones from other endocrine glands, although not directly responsible for regulating the reproductive system, are necessary for optimal reproductive efficiency of both males and females. Certainly, those animals with endocrine imbalances (hyper- or hypothyroidism, Addison's disease, Cushing's disease, diabetes, and others) have reduced reproductive efficiency.

SEXUAL BEHAVIOR IN DOGS AND CATS

Puberty. Puberty usually occurs between 6 and 12 months of age in dogs, with females reaching sexual maturity a few weeks before males (McDonald, 1975). Puberty is generally reached within a few weeks of the time when dogs reach their adult body weight (Anderson and Wooten, 1959). In general, smaller breeds reach adult body size earlier than larger breeds, so it follows that the smaller breeds also reach puberty at an earlier age (Hancock and Rowlands, 1949).

Recently, Chakraborty et al. (1980) compared hormonal changes during the first and second estrous cycles in Labrador retriever bitches. They found that during proestrus of the first cycle, serum concentrations of estradiol-17β, progesterone, and LH were lower than during proestrus of the second cycle. In addition, the LH peak was of lesser magnitude during the first cycle than during the second. These investigators also noted that proestrous-estrous period was shorter during the first cycle than during the second. They suggested that lower concentrations of LH during the week prior to the LH surge of the pubertal estrus were not sufficient to stimulate preovulatory follicular luteinization. Therefore, circulating concentrations of progesterone were lower prior to ovulation. Since rising progesterone is associated with the onset of estrus in the bitch, display of sexual receptivity was delayed until after ovulation. This could reduce the chances of mating and pregnancy during the pubertal estrus in the bitch.

The age at which cats reach puberty may vary from 4 to 21 months, depending on the breed and the time of year when the cat was born (Povey, 1978). Kittens born from late October to December in the northern hemisphere may not reach sexual maturity by the onset of the breeding season in January. These kittens may not have their first estrus until the second breeding season. Thus, the large range in age at puberty in female cats may be related more to seasonality than to sexual maturity. Male cats generally reach puberty between 9 and 12 months of age (Beaver, 1977).

Seasonality. Although many breeders feel that there are two breeding seasons a year for dogs, examination of breeding records indicates a lack of seasonality (Asdell, 1964; Christie and Bell, 1971; Stabenfeldt and Schille, 1976). An exception to this occurs in basenjis, which show only one estrous cycle per year, usually in the fall. This trait appears to be hereditary.

Some investigators have reported a seasonal incidence of breeding in cats (Scott and Lloyd-Jacob, 1959; Robinson and Cox, 1970). In general, it is stated that cats show a seasonal incidence of breeding, with two peaks noted, one in January to February and one in May to June. More recently, Jemmett and Evans (1977) observed that only 40 per cent of short-haired cats showed a season of anestrus, whereas 90 per cent of the long-haired breeds showed a seasonal nonbreeding period. In those cats having a seasonal anestrus it occurred most often from October through January.

REFERENCES

Anderson, A. C., and Wooten, E.: The Estrous Cycle of the Dog. *In* Cole, H. H., and Cupps, P. T. (eds.): Reproduction in Domestic Animals. Academic Press, New York, 1959, p. 359.

Asdell, S. A.: Carnivora and Pinnipedia. *In* Asdell, S. A. (ed.): Patterns of Mammalian Reproduction. Cornell University Press, Ithaca, New York, 1964, p. 425.

Beaver, B. V.: Mating behavior in the cat. Vet. Clin. North Am. 7:729, 1977.

Boucher, J. H.: Evaluation of semen quality in the dog and effects of frequency of ejaculation upon semen quality, libido, and restoration of sperm reserves. M.S. Thesis, Cornell University, Ithaca, New York, 1957.

Chakraborty, P. K., Panko, W. B., and Fletcher, W. S.: Serum hormone concentrations and their relationships to sexual behavior at the first and second estrous cycles of the Labrador bitch. Biol. Reprod. 22:227, 1980.

Christensen, G. C.: The Urogenital Apparatus. *In* Evans, H. E., and Christensen, G. C. (eds.): Miller's Anatomy of the Dog. W. B. Saunders Co., Philadelphia, p. 544, 1979.

Christie, D. W., and Bell, E. T.: Some observations on the seasonal incidence and frequency of oestrus in breeding bitches in Britain. J. Small Anim. Pract. 12:159, 1971.

Christie, D. W., Bell, E. T., Horth, C. E., and Palmer, R. F.: Peripheral plasma progesterone levels during the canine oestrous cycle. Acta Endocrinol. 68:543, 1971.

Christie, D. W., Bailey, J. B., and Bell, E. T.: Classification of cell types in vaginal smears during the canine oestrous cycle. Br. Vet. J. 128:301, 1972.

Cline, E. M., Jennings, L. L., and Sojka, N. J.: Analysis of the feline vaginal epithelial cycle. Feline Pract. 10:47, 1980.

Concannon, P. W., Hansel, W., and Visek, W. J.: The ovarian cycle of the bitch. Plasma estrogen, LH and progesterone. Biol. Reprod. 13:112, 1975.

Concannon, P. W., Hansel, W., and McEntee, K.: Changes in LH, progesterone and sexual behavior associated with preovulatory luteinization in the bitch. Biol. Reprod. 17:604, 1977a.

Concannon, P. W., Powers, M. E., Holder, W., and Hansel, W.: Pregnancy and parturition in the bitch. Biol. Reprod. 16:517, 1977b.

Concannon, P. W., Weigand, N., Wilson, S., and Hansel, W.: Sexual behavior in ovariectomized bitches in response to estrogen and progesterone treatments. Biol. Reprod. 20:799, 1979a.

Concannon, P. W., Cowan, R., and Hansel, W.: LH release in ovariectomized dogs in response to estrogen withdrawal and its facilitation by progesterone. Biol. Reprod. 20:523, 1979b.

Dahlgren, R. R.: Vaginal Cytology of the Dog. Ralston Purina Company, St. Louis, Mo., GP 2738 A 7607, 1979.

Del Campo, C. H., and Ginther, O. J.: Arteries and veins of uterus and ovaries in dogs and cats. Am. J. Vet. Res. 35:409, 1974.

DePalatis, L., Moore, J., and Falvo, R. E.: Plasma concentrations of testosterone and LH in the male dog. J. Reprod. Fertil. 53:201, 1978.

Doak, R. L., Hall, A., and Dale, H. E.: Longevity of spermatozoa in the reproductive tract of the bitch. J. Reprod. Fertil. 13:51, 1967.

Dore, M. A.: The role of the vaginal smear in the detection of metoestrus and anoestrus in the bitch. J. Small Anim. Pract. 19:561, 1978.

Edqvist, L. E., Johansson, E. D. B., Kasstrom, H., Olsson, S. E., and Richkind, M.: Blood plasma levels of progesterone and oestradiol in the dog during the oestrous cycle and pregnancy. Acta Endocrinol. 78:554, 1975.

Ellenport, C. R.: Carnivore Urogenital Apparatus. *In* Getty, R. (ed.): Sisson and Grossman's The Anatomy of the Domestic Animals. W. B. Saunders Co., Philadelphia, 1975, p. 1576.

Evans, H. E.: Reproduction and Prenatal Development. *In* Evans, H. E., and Christensen, G. C. (eds.): Miller's Anatomy of the Dog. W. B. Saunders Co., Philadelphia, 1979, p. 13.

Fletch, S. M.: Canine vaginal cytology — comments and review. (Abstracts) Meeting of Am. Soc. Vet. Clin. Pathol., Sunnybrook Hospital, Univ. Toronto, 1973.

Foote, R. H., Swierstra, E. E., and Hunt, W. L.: Spermatogenesis in the dog. Anat. Rec. 173:341, 1972.

Gier, H. T.: Estrous cycle in the bitch; vaginal fluids. Vet. Scope 5:2, 1960.

Greulich, W. W.: Artificially induced ovulation in the cat (*Felis domestica*). Anat. Rec. 58:217, 1934.

Hancock, J. L., and Rolands, I. W.: The physiology of reproduction in the dog. Vet. Rec. *61*:771, 1949.

Herron, M. A.: Feline vaginal cytologic examination. Feline Pract. *7*:36, 1977.

Holst, P. A., and Phemister, R. D.: The prenatal development of the dog. Preimplantation events. Biol. Reprod. *5*:194, 1971.

Holst, P. A., and Phemister, R. D.: Onset of diestrus in the beagle bitch. Definition and significance. Am. J. Vet. Res. *35*:401, 1974.

Holst, P. A., and Phemister, R. D.: Temporal sequence of events in the estrous cycle of the bitch. Am. J. Vet. Res. *36*:705, 1975.

Jemmet, J. E., and Evans, J. M.: A survey of sexual behaviour and reproduction of female cats. J. Small Anim. Pract. *18*:31, 1977.

Jones, G. E., and Boyns, A. R.: Effect of gonadal steroids on the pituitary responsiveness to synthetic luteinizing hormone releasing hormone in the male dog. J. Endocrinol. *61*:123, 1974.

Jones, G. E., and Boyns, A. R.: Inhibition by oestradiol of the pituitary response to luteinizing hormone releasing hormone in the dog. J. Endocrinol. *68*:475, 1976.

Jones, G. E., Baker, K., Fahmy, D. R., and Boyns, A. R.: Effect of luteinizing hormone releasing hormone on plasma levels of luteinizing hormone, oestradiol and testosterone in the male dog. J. Endocrinol. *68*:469, 1976.

Knight, P. J., and Hamilton, J. M.: Serum prolactin during pregnancy and lactation in the beagle bitch. Vet. Rec. *101*:202, 1977.

McDonald, L. E.: Reproductive Patterns of Dogs. *In* McDonald, L. E. (ed.): Veterinary Endocrinology and Reproduction, Lea and Febiger, Philadelphia, 1975, p. 377.

Mellin, T. N., Orczyk, G. P., Hichens, M., and Behrman, H. R.: Serum profiles of luteinizing hormone, progesterone and total estrogens during the canine estrous cycle. Theriogenology *5*:175, 1976.

Mowrer, R. T., Conti, P. A., and Rossow, C. F.: Vaginal cytology, an approach to improvement of cat breeding. Vet. Med. Small Anim. Clin. *70*:691, 1975.

Nett, T. M., Akbar, A. M., Phemister, R. D., Holst, P. A., Reichert, L. E., and Niswender, G. D.: Levels of luteinizing hormone, estradiol and progesterone in serum during the estrous cycle and pregnancy in the beagle bitch. Proc. Soc. Exp. Biol. Med. *148*:134, 1975.

Olson, P. N. S., and Mather, E. C.: Canine vaginal and uterine bacterial flora. J.A.V.M.A. *172*:708, 1978.

Paape, S. R., Shille, V. M., Seto, H., and Stabenfeldt, G. H.: Luteal activity in the pseudopregnant cat. Biol. Reprod. *13*:470, 1975.

Parkes, M. F., Bell, E. T., and Christie, D. W.: Plasma progesterone levels during pregnancy in the beagle bitch. Br. Vet. J. *128*:15, 1972.

Phemister, R. D., Holst, P. A., Spano, J. S., and Hopwood, M. L.: Time of ovulation in the beagle bitch. Biol. Reprod. *8*:74, 1973.

Pineda, M. H., Kainer, R. A., and Faulkner, L. C.: Dorsal median postcervical fold in the canine vagina. Am. J. Vet. Res. *34*:1487, 1973.

Povey, R. C.: Reproduction in the pedigree female cat. A survey of breeders. Can. Vet. J. *19*:207, 1978.

Reimers, T. J., Phemister, R. D., and Niswender, G. D.: Radioimmunological measurement of follicle stimulating hormone and prolactin in the dog. Biol. Reprod. *19*:673, 1978.

Robinson, R., and Cox, H. W.: Reproductive performance in a cat colony over a 10-year period. Lab. Anim. *4*:99, 1970.

Roszel, J. F.: Genital cytology of the bitch. Vet. Scope *19*:2, 1975.

Roszel, J. F.: Normal canine vaginal cytology. Vet. Clin. North Am. *7*:667, 1977.

Schille, V. M., Lundstrom, K. E., and Stabenfeldt, G. H.: Follicular function in domestic cats as determined by estradiol-17β concentrations in plasma. Relation to estrous behavior and cornification of exfoliated vaginal epithelium. Biol. Reprod. *21*:953, 1979.

Schutte, A. P.: Canine vaginal cytology. I. Technique and cytological morphology. J. Small Anim. Pract. *8*:301, 1967.

Schutte, A. P.: Canine vaginal cytology. II. Cyclic changes. J. Small Anim. Pract. *8*:307, 1967.

Scott, P. P., and Lloyd-Jacob, M. A.: Reduction in the anestrus period of laboratory cats by increased illumination. Nature (London) *184*:2022, 1959.

Smith, M. S., and McDonald, L. E.: Serum levels of luteinizing hormone and progesterone during the estrous cycle, pseudopregnancy, and pregnancy in the dog. Endocrinology *94*:404, 1974.

Sojka, N. J., Jennings, L. L., and Hammer, C. E.: Artificial insemination in the cat (*Felis catus*). Lab. Anim. Care *20*:198, 1970.

Sokolowski, J. H.: The effects of ovariectomy on pregnancy maintenance in the bitch. Lab. Anim. Sci. *21*:696, 1971.

Stabenfeldt, G. H., and Shille, V. M.: Reproduction in the Dog and Cat. *In* Cole, H. H., and Cupps, P. T. (eds.): Reproduction in Domestic Animals. 3rd ed., Academic Press, New York, 1977, p. 499.

Tietz, W. J., Benjamin, M. M., and Angleton, G. M.: Anemia and cholesterolemia during estrus and pregnancy in the beagle. Am. J. Physiol. *212*:693, 1967.

Verhage, H. G., Beamer, N. B., and Brenner, R. M.: Plasma levels of estradiol and progesterone in the cat during polyestrus, pregnancy, and pseudopregnancy. Biol. Reprod. *14*:579, 1976.

Vincent, D. L., Kepic, T. A., Toenjes, A., Pirmann, J., and Falvo, R. E.: Maintenance of physiologic concentrations of plasma testosterone in the castrated male dog, using testosterone-filled polydimethylsiloxane capsules. Am. J. Vet. Res. *40*:705, 1979.

Wildt, D. E., Chakraborty, P. K., Panko, W. B., and Seager, S. W. J.: Relationship of reproductive behavior, serum luteinizing hormone and time of ovulation in the bitch. Biol. Reprod. *18*:561, 1978.

Wildt, D. E., Panko, W. B., Chakraborty, P. K., and Seager, S. W. J.: Relationship of serum estrone, estradiol-17β and progesterone to LH, sexual behavior and time of ovulation in the bitch. Biol. Reprod. *20*:648, 1979.

CHAPTER 71

THOMAS J. BURKE

Reproductive Disorders

DATA BASE

The genital system is the most varied of all the major body systems of mammals and it is one of the few systems whose total dysfunction is neither life-threatening nor disfiguring. Functional disruption of other organ systems often results in reproductive failure, but infertility can also be a result of disease of the genital system alone.

The dog and the cat have reproductive physiologies that vary markedly from those of other animals normally found in close association with man. Often a prolonged period of time will pass while one awaits the appropriate phase or phases of the estrous cycle that need to be studied. A data base is mandatory to approach the diagnosis, treatment, and prognosis of reproductive·failure with any degree of accuracy.

The mandatory parts of the data base for infertility in the dog and cat are: history, physical examination, thyroid function testing, *Brucella canis* testing (dog only), semen evaluation, culture, feline leukemia testing (cat only), and toxoplasmosis testing (cat only). Studying these points will uncover the vast majority of causes of infertility in a minimum of time in most cases.

This enables one to rationally approach therapy and prognosis in a majority of cases, based upon accurate diagnosis. Obviously, certain cases will require further, less commonly employed diagnostic procedures. It is also possible that one may never arrive at a precise diagnosis, regardless of the extent and expense of the diagnostic efforts.

HISTORY

The objective is to acquire as much information about the patient and his or her sexual partner(s) as possible. The clinician should strive to obtain the owner's observations — *not* interpretations — of the patient, with special attention to the reproductive system.

A complete general history is recommended in order to look for clues to any seemingly unrelated disorder that could alter the patient's health sufficiently to impair fertility. Questions about the female reproductive tract should concern age at first estrus (heat), dates of subsequent heats, dates of breeding, natural or artificial inseminations and dates, dates of whelping or queening, dystocia, rearing success, pregnancy testing (any form), history of false pregnancies, success of partner(s) before and after mating(s) in question, diagnostic tests performed, drugs (especially hormones) administered, and overall impression of the owner about the quality of estrus and breedings. In the male, one should be concerned about age at first breeding, libido, history of trauma during breeding, success of partner(s) before and after mating(s) in question, history of any severe or febrile illness, general breeding management, and other matters involving drug therapy and previous diagnostic tests, as for the female.

PHYSICAL EXAMINATION

Females. As with the history, a complete physical examination to detect other systemic disease should be performed. Most of the female genital system cannot be examined directly on an outpatient basis. However, the retrorenal areas should be palpated for masses associated with the ovaries. General abdominal palpation of the cervix, uterine body, and horns is usually possible. Size, location, consistency, and relationship to other organs should be noted. Excellent descriptions of the changes associated with the normal estrous cycle and pregnancy are available in the literature.

The vulva, vestibule, and clitoral fossa may be examined visually. Palpation of the vulvar lips is advisable. Digital palpation of the vestibule and lower (posterior) vagina is advisable in virgin bitches, those with a history of pain at breeding or inability of the male to achieve intromission (tie), and those presented for bleeding not in association with proestrus. Digital palpation is not possible in domestic cats.

Vaginoscopy often requires sedation, especially in cats. A sterile speculum of suitable size (otoscope cone to proctoscope) should be advanced to the level of the anterior vaginal cul-de-sac or until resistance is met and the entire vaginal canal visualized upon withdrawal of the instrument. Insufflation with air is helpful.

Males. Physical examination should include careful palpation of the testes, epididymides, vasa, and prostate (dog only). This may require sedation in the cat. Attention should be paid to size, symmetry, and consistency of each organ. Unusual sensitivity to pain may indicate inflammation. The penis should be prolapsed to the preputial reflection and examined.

DIAGNOSTIC PROCEDURES

Cytologic Studies. Vaginal cytology may aid in the diagnosis of abnormal cycles, infection, or neoplasia. Either swabs or plastic pipettes may be used to obtain samples. A speculum is used in anestral and metestral bitches to avoid sampling the vulva and vestibule. Only water or saline is used as a lubricant. For cats in estrus the author uses a medicine dropper containing a small amount of normal saline to obtain specimens, as insertion of a swab may induce ovulation. The tip of the dropper is inserted one half to one cm into the vulva. The bulb is squeezed several times and the recovered fluid is spread on a slide. Any good cytologic stain may be used. The use of special stains to display keratin is time consuming and not often indicated.

Interpretation requires a knowledge of the normal estrous cycle and the changes induced by estrogens. One should pay attention to the morphology of the epithelial cells, the appearance and disappearance of WBC, and the appearance of RBC (Figs. 71–1 through 71–4). Bizarre, primitive cells may indicate neoplasia. Serial evaluations may be necessary, since it is seldom possible to ascertain a normal cycle with one smear. Several reviews of normal canine and feline vaginal cytology have been published (Bell and Christie, 1971; Burke, 1976; Christie et al., 1972; Gier, 1960; Herron, 1977; Roszel, 1975; Schutte, 1967; Shille et al., 1974; Sokolowski, 1973).

Biopsy. Biopsy of the vulva is usually accomplished by an excisional wedge technique. The vagina may be biopsied with standard colon or uterine punch forceps. The uterus and ovaries may be biopsied via laparotomy. Serial uterine biopsies in normal bitches have resulted in naturally resolving cystic endometrial hyperplasia when done in the period of peak follicular activity and early luteal formation. These bitches showed a cloudy vaginal (uterine) discharge. Single biopsies taken during the luteal phase may result in localized "pseudopregnant" swellings. Untoward effects of vulvar, vaginal, or ovarian biopsies have not been reported. All biopsies are done with the patient under general anesthesia, as local infiltration may interfere with interpretation.

Testicular biopsy requires a procedure with minimum disruption of architecture. Aspiration and cutting needle techniques are inferior to excisional wedges. Using an antescrotal midline incision, the testis is positioned so that the epididymis is away from the incision. The tunics are cut with a scalpel until parenchyma is encountered, then a sterile razor blade is used to remove a small amount of tissue with a scooping motion (Figs. 71–5 and 71–6). The tunics and skin are closed in routine fashion, taking care to insure that the testis resumes a normal scrotal position. This method is preferred to scrotal incision because it presents fewer healing problems and less hemorrhage at the time of surgery.

Radiographic Studies. Radiographic examination of the genital tract demonstrates pregnancy, an enlarged uterus, ovarian masses, and neoplasia. Both routine and special contrast studies have been employed, including pneumovaginography and positive contrast hysterosalpingography. The latter requires deposition of the dye under pressure into the mid to anterior vagina. The cervix must be patent. The cervix of the bitch is virtually impossible to see or cannulate, except during parturition, so the dye must be forced through it from the vagina with positive pressure.

The major use of radiography in the male is for assessment of the prostate gland. The reader is referred to Chapter 63 for a more

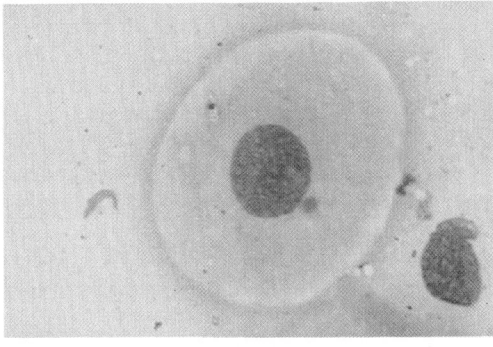

Figure 71-1.

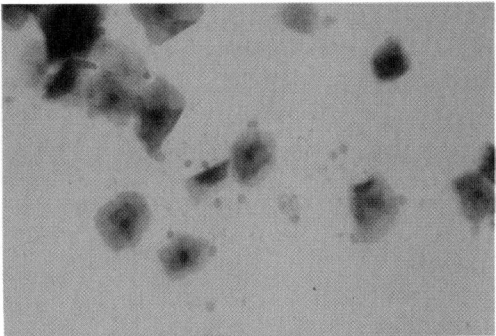

Figure 71-2.

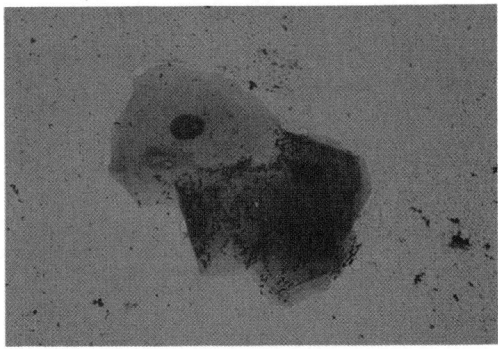

Figure 71-3.

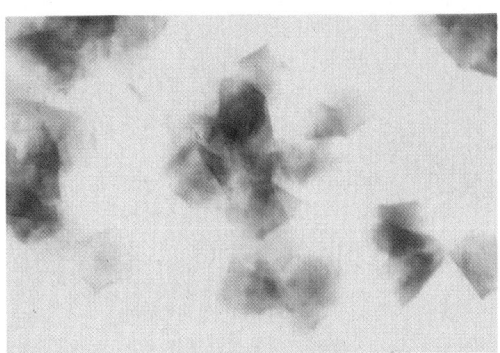

Figure 71-4.

Figure 71-1. Normal noncornified or parabasal vaginal epithelial cell from a bitch in anestrus. **Figure 71-2.** Typical canine vaginal cytology in proestrus. All epithelial cells are angular; some are anuclear while others have pyknotic nuclei. Note presence of RBC and absence of WBC. **Figure 71-3.** Canine vaginal epithelial cells from bitch in proestrus. Cells on left and top right have pyknotic nucleus; those in bottom center are anuclear. **Figure 71-4.** Canine vaginal epithelial cells from bitch in standing heat. Virtually all are anuclear.

complete discussion. Fractures of the os penis have been reported and are diagnosed radiographically. Excretory urethrography may be useful in patients with a history of urolithiasis or trauma if there is an inability to ejaculate correctly or to maintain erection. This is especially true in tomcats.

Cultures. All cultures should be taken prior to the onset of any local or systemic antibacterial therapy. Cultures of the vagina may be taken at any time using a short sterile speculum (chemical or "cold" sterilization is unacceptable). Media suitable for recovering both aerobes and anaerobes should be inoculated as soon as possible. Transport media must be employed if the sample is to be sent out to a laboratory. Some organisms (e.g., *Mycoplasma*) require special enriched media for best results. Virus isolations, requiring special transport media, may be attempted for cases such as suspected herpes virus infection.

Culture of uterine contents may be done via laparotomy at any time or, more practically, by sampling the anterior vagina (pericervical area) during proestrus, estrus, or at other times when the cervix is open. This requires a suitably long swab. Routine culture swabs may be used in cats and small dogs. For most bitches the author uses disposable guarded equine culture instruments. In either case a speculum is used to bypass the lower vagina and vulva.

Semen may be cultured by free-catch during ejaculation. Prostatic fluid for culture may be obtained in this manner or by placement of a urinary catheter in the prostatic urethra followed by prostatic massage per rectum. Cultures of ejaculate are frequently contaminated by bacteria from the prepuce and glans penis. It is advisable to also culture the glans penis at the time of semen culture as an aid in interpreting the results. Testicular parenchyma may be cultured at biopsy.

Hormone Assays. Hormone assays for

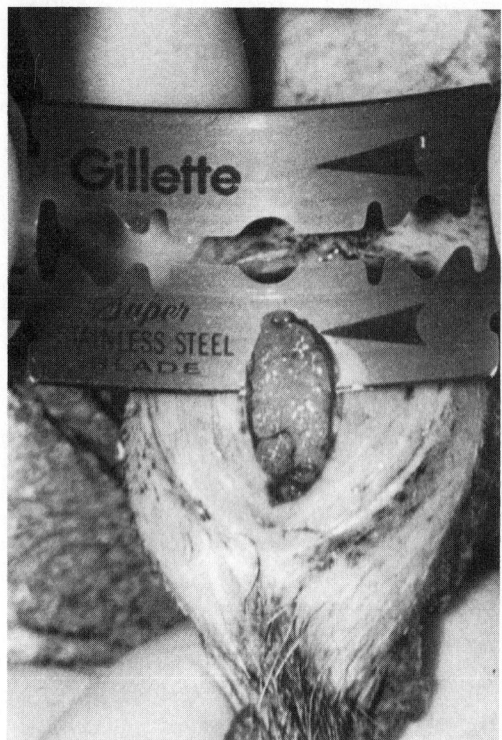

Figure 71–5. Technique of testicular biopsy using razor blade scoop method.

progesterone and estrogen (17 B estradiol) are widely available. A few university laboratories are able to perform gonadotropin assays. Normal values have been established for the various portions of the estrous cycle of the bitch and queen. Actual levels vary with the laboratory, and the clinician should judge the results with the normals for the particular laboratory. The same is true for testosterone levels in the dog and cat. Hormone assays may aid in the diagnosis of ovarian cysts, neoplasia, abnormal cycles, and decreased libido.

Serologic Testing. Serologic testing for *Brucella canis* is widely available. An in-office rapid slide agglutination test using *Brucella ovis* antigen provides rapid presumptive diagnostic information. Positive reactors to this test should undergo further tests to confirm the diagnosis. Tube agglutination tests incorporating 2-mercaptoethanol are highly specific and are widely available.

The reader is referred to Chapter 27 for discussion of serologic testing for the major feline infectious diseases that may affect fertility.

Semen Analysis. Semen for analysis may be collected by manual or electro-ejaculation. The latter requires anesthesia but is rewarding when other methods fail, especially in the cat. Manual collection may require the presence of a teaser bitch. Some males require the bitch to be in natural or drug-induced estrus, while others will ejaculate if any dog is placed in front of them. Semen should be collected in a sterile container that has been rinsed free of *any* chemical agents (soaps and so forth) to a predetermined volume. The author routinely collects five ml of fluid if a total analysis is to be performed. The sample is analyzed for motility immediately. Several slides for live:dead ratio and sperm morphology are prepared as soon after collec-

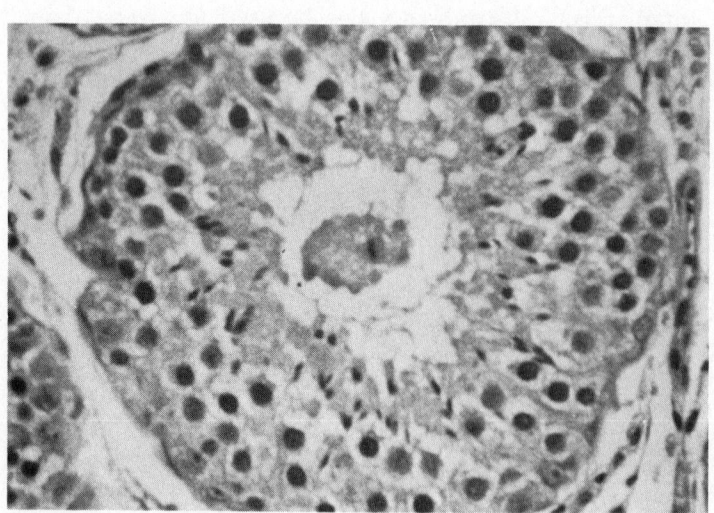

Figure 71–6. Normal canine seminiferous tubule from biopsy sample taken in Figure 71–5. Note lack of compression artifacts. Hematoxylin and eosin stain.

tion as possible. One drop of aqueous two per cent eosin is mixed with one drop of semen; one drop of one per cent nigrosin is added for background, and the entire mixture spread onto glass slides and heat fixed immediately. Counting is done using standard red blood cell methods. White blood cells and abnormal epithelial cells may be seen with routine hematologic stains.

SPECIFIC DISORDERS OF MALES AND FEMALES

Brucellosis. *Brucella canis* infection in the dog was first described in 1966, when it produced abortion in beagle bitches. A gram-negative coccobacillus, the organism has since been recovered from a vast number of breeds and from mongrels. Its distribution is virtually worldwide. Incidence rates for infection in the general dog population vary as high as five per cent, but one per cent is more likely in most areas of the United States. While cats have been shown to be experimentally infected, the naturally occurring clinical disease has not been reported. Humans also may become infected with *B. canis.* Although the number of cases is small, this is a zoonosis; nearly half of the human cases have been in laboratory workers.

In bitches, the classic symptom is abortion in the last trimester, most often between 45 and 55 days. Early fetal death and resorption or term litters of weak and/or stillborn puppies occur less frequently. Lymphadenopathy may or may not be noted on physical examination. The only clue to brucellosis may be a history of apparent infertility.

In the male, brucellosis classically produces epididymitis, which often leads to excessive licking of the scrotum (possibly due to pain) and to a secondary scrotitis-orchitis. Orchitis also may accompany brucellosis as a primary lesion. Testicular atrophy and chronic epididymitis are common sequelae. The organism usually sequesters in the prostate but seems to produce little reaction there.

Infected dogs become infertile for prolonged periods; most become permanently infertile. While the sperm count may remain in the normal range, there is a preponderance of primary defects (up to 90 per cent) and decreased motility, as well as detached heads. Head-to-head agglutination of sperm also is frequently seen.

Diagnosis employs both serologic and bacteriologic testing. One should be as absolute in this diagnosis as possible because of the gravity of the outcome for the patient and its owners. The rapid slide agglutination test (Pitman-Moore) provides presumptive diagnosis if positive. If negative, the animal either is negative or has not been infected long enough to have a significant titer. It is important to note that false positive tests do occur, so this test is *only* presumptive.

Tube agglutination tests (TATs) are widely available. The addition of 2-mercaptoethanol (2-ME) reduces nonspecific reactions but also reduces the titer. Interpretation of TATs thus depends upon the method and, to a degree, the laboratory. TAT titers of 1:200 or greater usually signify active infection. 2-ME-TAT titers are usually considered significant at 1:100 or greater.

Whenever possible the diagnosis should be confirmed by organism identification. Qualified laboratories are required, since the organism is best isolated on certain enriched media. *B. canis* does not require CO_2. Uterine fluid, aborted uterine contents, and semen are excellent sources of the organism. Blood cultures may be positive for more than two years after infection.

There is no uniformly successful treatment for brucellosis. Spontaneous recovery has occurred in a few dogs. The two regimes most likely to produce eradication of *B. canis* from the patient's body are

1. Tetracycline HCl per os for three weeks; discontinue for three to four weeks; re-treat for another three weeks with the addition of streptomycin intramuscularly (IM) for the first week.

2. Minocycline HCl per os (25 mg/lb bid) for 14 days with streptomycin IM for the first seven days.

Routine doses of both tetracycline and streptomycin are used; neither treatment is 100 per cent successful. Treated animals must be kept isolated and rigorously monitored. If possible, affected bitches should be spayed and affected males castrated. If not, until more is known about the long-term "recovery" of these animals, the author suggests only artificial insemination. Since tetracyclines do not reach effective levels in the prostate, it is questionable if treatment will work in the male at all. The testicular and epididymal changes often are permanent.

The author leans very heavily toward euthanasia for all positive animals. It is hoped that position will change with the use of newer tetracyclines and publication of long-term follow-up studies of treated cases.

There currently is no immunization procedure for *B. canis.* Control of brucellosis in kennels can be accomplished most readily by a test-and-slaughter approach. Only under extraordinary circumstances should positive animals be allowed to survive, and they should be isolated throughout the treatment period. All animals in an infected kennel should be tested monthly. Animals with three consecutive negative tests may be considered "clean." The same procedure should be followed for animals added to a "clean" kennel. Prevention cannot be overemphasized to dog owners. Stud dogs should be tested periodically and never bred to a bitch that has not had a negative *Brucella* test within the past 30 days.

Kennel disinfection is important, as are routine sanitary measures for kennel personnel and visitors. Roccal and Wescodyne solutions have been shown to kill *B. canis* organisms.

Hypothyroidism. Inappropriate function of the thyroid gland frequently results in impaired fertility in both bitches and dogs. In females there is usually some degree of obvious estral distortion (prolonged anestrus or weak estrus, for example), but some patients present with only an apparent inability to conceive. Males may show decreased libido and/or decreased sperm production. In some cases the testes are smaller and softer than normal, although many patients have no detectable physical abnormalities. Other signs of hypothyroidism may or may not be present (see Chapter 67).

Laboratory tests are usually unrewarding. Some patients have a mild normochromic-normocytic anemia and hypercholesterolemia. When obtainable, semenograms show decreased count and motility. Sperm abnormalities are usually within acceptable limits. Precise hormone testing, including TSH challenge, is necessary for accurate diagnosis (see Chapter 67).

Return to normal fertility following replacement therapy may require several months. Obese patients may remain functionally infertile until satisfactory weight loss has been achieved.

Hypogonadism. Congenital or acquired gonadal atrophy as a result of inappropriate gonadotropin secretion probably occurs in dogs, but precise etiology almost always remains unknown. The author has seen gonadal atrophy in cases of hypothalamic neoplasia.

In the male, both follicle stimulating hormone (FSH) and luteinizing hormone (LH) appear to be necessary for complete spermiogenesis. Presumably, deficiency of one or both may lead to infertility. Affected patients have small, soft testes. Libido is often reported as normal. When obtainable, semenograms show either no sperm (azoospermia) or drastically reduced count (oligospermia) with reduced motility. Until gonadotropin assays become commonplace, testicular biopsy can be used to give clues to the possible cause. Tubular atrophy without inflammation suggests a lack of FSH, while a paucity of interstitial cells would suggest an LH deficiency. The latter may be associated with decreased libido.

In the bitch, the major sign is prolonged anestrus. This is observed when the onset of puberty is delayed beyond 24 months of age (congenital) or when more than twice the normal interestrus period for the patient has passed (acquired). There are many causes of acquired prolonged anestrus, and the patient should have a thorough work-up prior to the initiation of gonadotropin therapy, especially for other endocrinopathies, ovarian cysts, and neoplasia. In cats, the cause may be as simple as inappropriate exposure to daylight. Exposure to 50-plus foot-candles of illumination for 12 to 14 hours (per 24-hour cycle) may be curative. There is no known effect of prolonged darkness on the canine estrous cycle. Also, prior to hormonal therapy the patient should be housed with another female in estrus. In many cases this will bring about a natural estrus, presumably a result of the effect of pheromones from the animal in heat on the neurohormonal system of the patient.

Treatment in the bitch consists of injections of FSH as FSH-P Burns-Biotec), 0.75 mg/kg/day IM for ten days. Luteinizing hormone, as human chorionic gonadotropin, is given on the 10th to 12th days at 100 IU/kg/day IM or IV. The dog is allowed to mate naturally, any time from the 10th to the 20th day from the start of treatment.

Some treated bitches will conceive; others will become cyclic on their own and conceive at a later date.

In queens, the treatment consists of injections of FSH-P at a dose of 2 mg/cat/day for five days. Ovulation can be induced with HCG at 250 to 500 IU/cat/day for two days while in standing heat or GnRH at a dose of 25 mcg/cat on day two of standing heat. All injections are given IM.

In males therapy has been unrewarding; however, a few have responded temporarily to gonadotropin therapy. Empirically, FSH-P at 1.0 mg/kg IM every other day for 10 to 15 doses has helped a few dogs. Decreased libido can often be improved with oral methyltestosterone, 0.1 mg/kg/day.

Gonadal Agenesis. Congenital lack of one gonad (ovary or testis) does not result in impaired fertility. In the female it usually is a serendipitous discovery at the time of ovariohysterectomy. In the male, it may be confused with unilateral cryptorchidism, as it is often impossible to tell if an atrophied remnant is present or if there was true agenesis. The genetics of agenesis have not been reported, but it is possible that it is not a genetically transmitted condition and that affected males could safely be used as sires.

Bilateral agenesis in either sex leads to infertility. There is no treatment.

SPECIFIC DISORDERS OF THE FEMALE

Metritis-Pyometritis. Severe bacterial infection of the luteal phase (metestral) uterus, usually following whelping, is the hallmark of this disease. The literature is most confusing on terminology, and to enter into such a discussion is beyond the scope and intention of this chapter. It should be sufficient to say that this is an acute to subacute, severe infection characterized by purulent to sanguinopurulent vaginal discharge. The affected animal is clinically ill with depression, fever to hypothermia, dehydration, and other constitutional signs characteristic of toxemia or bacteremia.

Laboratory blood work-ups showing a neutrophilic left shift or a degenerative neutropenia and hemoconcentration are most commonly found. Serum chemistry alterations depend upon the involvement of other organs (e.g., kidney or liver).

The treatment of choice is surgical removal of the infected uterus, with appropriate systemic antibiotics, fluid therapy if indicated, and other appropriate nursing care. The author prefers to institute therapy with gentamicin until culture and sensitivity results are available. Dose and administration interval are appropriately reduced in the face of azotemia. Carbenicillin is added if the patient is critically ill. In cases where the uterus must be preserved, the use of prostaglandin $F_{2\alpha}$($PGF_{2\alpha}$) has been beneficial. The author currently uses a dose of 250 mcg/kg given by subcutaneous (SQ) injection once daily until there is virtually no discharge and the patient responds clinically. Treatment has required from three to ten days. At this dose, $PGF_{2\alpha}$ (1) produces uterine contraction, thus promoting drainage of infected contents; (2) increases uterine blood flow, thus improving the efficacy of the antibiotics; and (3) maintains cervical patency. It is *not* luteolytic at this dose; thus, recurrent infection or a closed pyometra may occur. Side effects of $PGF_{2\alpha}$ treatment are frequent but transitory. They include vomiting, loose (cow-pie) stool, hypersalivation, staggering, collapse, and tachypnea. Only one case of vomiting has required symptomatic therapy.

Treated cases are cultured at the next proestrus for evidence of lingering infection. Several treated animals have been successfully bred.

The treatment of a closed bacterial infection of the uterus (closed pyometra) parallels that outlined above. Diagnosis of this condition may be a bit more difficult, and the pathogenesis is not as clear-cut. Though it may take a slower, more gradual course, it is more life-threatening to the patient. Both conditions will cause high mortality if left untreated, however.

Endometritis. Low-grade uterine infection (defined here as endometritis) is, in the author's experience, the most common cause of acquired infertility in the bitch; it is also very common in the queen. The patient is clinically normal and generally has no clinical pathologic abnormalities. The only historical abnormality is inability to conceive when mated to fertile males. Vaginal cytology is nearly always normal. A few patients may have leukocytes present during estrus when they should normally be absent.

The diagnosis is based upon culture of the pericervical area during proestrus or estrus by the method formerly described. The only reliable correlation between culture results and disease has been in the quantity of organisms recovered. This interpretation should not be based upon organism identification or its antibiogram but rather on the degree of growth. Moderate to heavy growth, regardless of the organism, should be considered as evidence of significant infection, and treatment is required. A light growth suggests the absence of active infection; it does not, however, preclude the possibility of significant inflammation in the endometrium or post-inflammatory fibrosis.

As we are unable to readily view or biopsy the endometrium, as is commonly done in cattle and horses, the natural history and staging of this disease is virtually unknown. Anatomic and financial limitations make it unlikely that we will ever know.

Treatment consists of appropriate systemic antibiotic therapy for three to four weeks. Bacteriocidal agents are used whenever possible. Douches also may be used until the cervix closes, especially in cases of very heavy growth. The question of breeding while undergoing treatment poses the problem of antibiotic-induced teratogenesis. The author has treated many bitches and several queens with semisynthetic penicillins and cephalosporins without producing fetal anomalies in litters conceived while the dam was being treated. Tetracycline has been incriminated in teratogenesis, and chloramphenicol is not used because of its immunosuppressive activity. Douches, because of their spermacidal nature, must be stopped 48 hours prior to breeding.

One course of treatment may clear a female of infection for long periods, but many bitches will have significant cultures at each estrus. Here one must take the risk of treatment during mating and early embryogenesis if breeding success is to be achieved.

Some females will not conceive in spite of repeated vigorous therapy. A few of these have been biopsied and found to have significant fibrosis and chronic inflammatory changes. These animals are presumed to be permanently infertile.

Vaginitis. Inflammation of the vagina is a common clinical disease. Most often it is a result of bacterial or possibly viral infection. Physical and chemical insults and certain hormones (especially androgens) also can produce vaginitis. As the lower (posterior) vagina usually harbors some bacteria, the etiologic diagnosis may be difficult. Mixed cultures are not uncommon.

Clinical signs include purulent discharge, licking at the vulva, and congestion of the vaginal mucosa. The color of the discharge may reflect the bacteria present. It is common for prepuberal bitches to have a white discharge; *Staphylococcus albus* is frequently isolated.

Juvenile vaginitis may not require any therapy. If the infection causes housekeeping or training problems for the owner, then local treatment with a mild douche is instituted and repeated as needed. Most cases of juvenile vaginitis regress spontaneously after the first estrus or spaying, which suggests that it is an age-related phenomenon.

Vaginitis in the adult can become a therapeutic challenge and is often a recurrent medical problem. Periodic local therapy often controls the condition, but a long-term cure may be impossible for some.

Diagnostic methods to be employed to rule out other conditions include vaginoscopy of the *entire* vaginal canal (with the patient anesthetized if necessary), culture, biopsy, and exfoliative cytology.

Necessary treatment usually consists only of a mild douche administered via bulb syringe b.i.d. Tamed iodine (0.5 per cent) or chlorhexidine (0.05 per cent) is satisfactory. In cases where the mid to anterior vagina is involved, systemic antibacterials may be used. Severe vaginitis may cause infertility, presumably as a result of the spermicidal effects of bacteria. Ascending infection also may result. Such cases should be treated prior to mating, but treatment should cease 48 hours prior to insemination. The procedure of culturing all bitches' vaginas prior to breeding is a highly questionable practice in the author's opinion.

Owners of affected animals must realize that chronic flare-ups may occur and that a cure may not be possible. Vaginitis is not, in itself, a fatal disease.

Mummification-Stillbirth-Abortion (MSA). The MSA complex in queens presents a diagnostic challenge. There are many known causes and others remain unknown, since precise diagnosis is reached in only a fraction of the cases. Prophylaxis is equally difficult, and some cases are at present insoluble.

Nutrition and parasitism should be considered as causes but are less common today than in the past. From those cases of MSA that are solved, infectious agents appear to be the most common cause. These include upper respiratory viruses, especially herpes virus; *Chlamydia; Toxoplasma*; leukemia virus; feline infectious peritonitis; and a variety of bacteria. The role of chronic stress and environmental insults (especially thermal) remains unknown. A diagnostic work-up should endeavor to rule out infectious causes first. When identified, appropriate prophylaxis should be applied with the knowledge that untreatable carrier states exist for many of these diseases.

Nymphomania. Constant estrus or estrus-like behavior in the bitch and queen is usually a result of chronic estrogen stimulation from cystic ovaries. If a bitch is in behavioral estrus for more than 21 days, she probably has cystic ovaries. Medical treatment consists of HCG, 100 IU/lb/day IM for three days, repeated in one week if necessary. Surgery may be required if two treatments fail. Aspiration of the cysts may be done with infusion of each cyst with 25 IU of HCG. This failing, spaying is curative. Successfully treated bitches will often have a normal fertile estrus shortly after therapy; others may wait an appropriate interestrus period.

Premature Luteolysis. Luteal function is necessary for pregnancy maintenance in the bitch and for most of pregnancy in the queen. Early luteolysis results in nonseptic abortion. Some animals become habitual aborters with no other demonstrable cause. The diagnosis is usually based upon history and lack of any other cause. Serum progesterone levels measured at the time of abortion should be subnormal.

Treatment consists of progesterone in oil, 1 mg/lb IM weekly, beginning a week prior to the anticipated (based upon history) abortion and stopping at least a week prior to calculated delivery. Even with treatment, some will experience prolonged gestation and require cesarean sections. The literature suggests that progesterone masculinizes female fetuses, but this has not occurred in the author's experience. Nonetheless, the owner should be warned of this possible consequence.

Anatomic Causes. Among the common noninfectious causes of infertility are anatomic defects that prevent either copulation or fertilization. Vaginal strictures, single or multiple, render copulation painful for either or both partners and thereby prevent successful mating. Such strictures may be congenital or acquired, and most are found by digital palpation of the vagina. The most common site in the bitch is the vulvovestibular junction. The treatment is surgical, episioplasty often being sufficient.

Bilateral blockage of the uterine horns or oviducts is uncommon but, when present, will lead to infertility. Diagnosis based upon dye or saline infusion depends upon location of the blockages at laparotomy. Successful repair is rare.

Neoplasia. Tumors of the female genital tract are less common than those in the male and are generally benign; about 10 to 15 per cent of ovarian tumors are malignant. Most ovarian tumors produce prolonged anestrus or other aberrations of the estrous cycle. Many produce hormones, either progesterone or estrogens. The incidence of ovarian neoplasia increases with age in both dogs and cats. Many cases involve a palpable mass in the region of the ovary. Treatment is usually surgical. Reasonable care should be exercised, as serosal seeding of tumor cells may occur. Chemotherapy of ovarian tumors has not been thoroughly investigated.

Neoplasia of the tubular genitalia is uncommon. Most tumors are benign leiomyomas. Uterine tumors may produce no symptoms other than abdominal enlargement and a palpable mass. Vaginal tumors may ulcerate and bleed and may prevent intromission by the male. Tumors of the vulva may present as diffuse swellings that are ill-defined even by careful palpation or as isolated nodules. Diagnosis is made by excisional or wedge biopsy. Treatment usually involves surgery and, depending upon cell type, other forms of cancer therapy (see Chapters 30 to 32).

Transmissible venereal sarcoma is uncommon in the United States. It is spread by transplantation during copulation and is found most often in young dogs. The gross appearance of the tumor varies from papular to ulcerated lobulated masses (Fig. 71–7). Metastasis has been reported. Combination chemotherapy, surgical excision, radiation

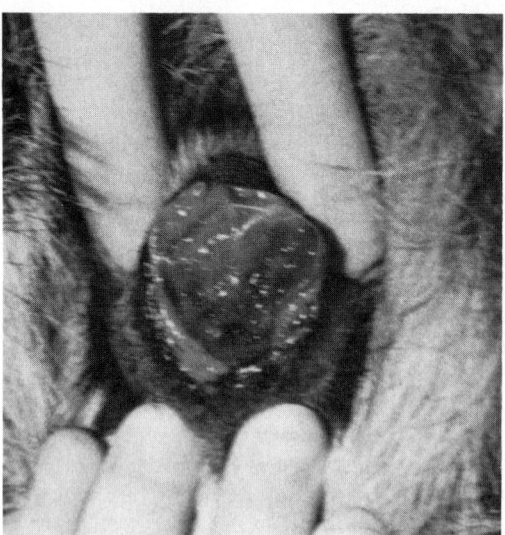

Figure 71–7. Ulcerated, sessile form of transmissible venereal tumor in the vulva of a bitch.

therapy, and immunotherapy have all been reported as successful treatments. Recovered animals are said to be immune to further infection.

Drug-Induced Causes. Many compounds have been shown to interfere with the estrous cycle. Some obviously are used for just that purpose, especially progestogens and androgens. Estrogens may cause signs of estrus but will *not* produce a fertile heat and may interfere with ovulation if given during proestrus.

Drugs that produce luteolysis or fetal death can cause nonseptic abortions. A safe, reliable abortifacient has yet to be developed for dogs. Prostaglandin $F_{2\alpha}$ at a dose of 60 mcg/kg divided into two or three doses SQ for three days produced abortion in four of seven bitches between 33 and 53 days of pregnancy. In cats, $PGF_{2\alpha}$ reliably produced abortion at doses of 0.5 to 1.0 mg/kg SQ in one or two daily doses, if the cats were 40 or more days pregnant.

Diethylcarbamazine has been incriminated anecdotally as causing infertility in bitches. To date there is no scientific evidence to support this claim when the drug is given at doses sufficient to prevent heartworm infection. Several kennels that the author is familiar with have experienced no decrease in fertility after several years of continual treatment.

SPECIFIC DISORDERS OF THE MALE

Orchitis. Severe inflammation of the testes is usually the result of infection or trauma. Usually it is painful enough that the owner becomes quite concerned. If there is any chance of maintaining fertility, orchitis should be handled as an emergency. In an infectious case, the heat of inflammation may produce irreversible testicular damage in a short time. Trauma may allow exposure of sperm and/or tubule antigens to the body and thus lead to the development of autoantibodies and subsequent infertility.

A severely traumatized testicle should be removed. Salvage should be undertaken only in dogs whose primary purpose is for show, as the American Kennel Club will not permit dogs with only one testis to compete. Infertility is a common sequel, and the owner should be informed of this fact.

Medical therapy of orchitis should include anti-inflammatory therapy and local hypothermia. Antibacterial drugs are appropriate in infectious cases. Regardless of therapy, the prognosis will always be guarded.

Constrictive foreign bodies ("the nasty child" or "pervert syndrome") are usually presented too late for fertility to be preserved. If the pain has subsided and the scrotum is cool to the touch, then castration and scrotal ablation should be performed.

Prostatitis. Bacterial prostatitis may cause infertility, presumably as a result of death of sperm caused by bacterial toxins. Libido is usually good unless the prostate is acutely inflamed. The sperm count remains normal, but virtually all sperm are dead. Large numbers of secondary sperm abnormalities, especially tailless heads, may be seen.

Diagnosis and treatment of prostatitis are covered in Chapter 63. The author prefers long-term therapy with oral trimethoprim-potentiated sulfas. This failing, subtotal prostatectomy preserving the vasa deferentia has returned several males to normal fertility.

Prostate disease is apparently rare in cats and so will not be covered here. The reason for this extreme species difference is unknown but may have some basis in the fact that approximately seven times as many cats are castrated in the United States as dogs.

Difficulty in examining the feline prostate may also play a role in underdiagnosis.

Anatomic Defects. Incomplete closure of the urethra (hypospadias) produces a disruption in the normal flow of urethral contents and thus leads to infertility. In addition, affected males, even after natural or surgical closure of the defect, may have adhesions that result in inability to prolapse the penis from the sheath (phimosis). Hypospadias is uncommon in dogs and its heritability is unknown. Even if corrected, affected males should probably not be used as breeding stock, since there may be a hereditable component.

Penile frenulums prevent normal erection. These are readily found by physical examination (Fig. 71–8) and are easily corrected by simple surgical transection. The heritability is unknown.

Phimosis may be congenital or acquired. In some instances the preputial orifice is hypoplastic from birth. In acquired cases there is usually a history of preputial pyoderma, chemical or physical trauma, or masturbation that leads to local edema or subsequent scarring. In any case the orifice is too small to permit erection and mating. Appropriate medical therapy should be instituted in acute cases; chronic or congenital cases may require reconstructive surgery.

Phimosis as a result of penis-prepuce adhesions is rare unless there is history of urethral surgery. Treatment involves reduction of the adhesions.

Paraphimosis is most often a result of inability of an erect penis to detumesce. It usually results from the rolling inward of

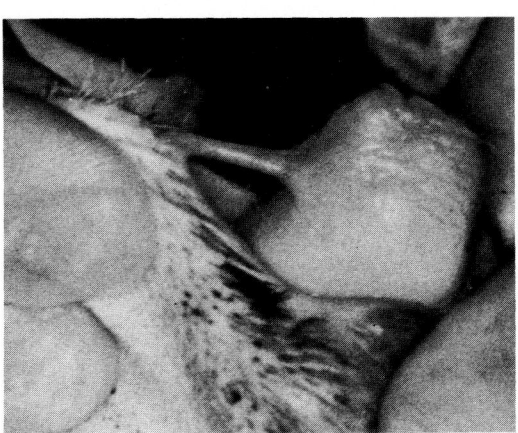

Figure 71–8. Penile frenulum in a dog.

the tip of the prepuce, with the long hairs located there becoming a restrictive band. This condition constitutes an emergency, since irreversible gangrene can occur in a matter of hours. Immediate surgical intervention may save the penis, but after one day penile amputation is routinely required. These patients cannot achieve erection but may be electroejaculated and serve as semen donors for artificial insemination. Prevention involves good post-breeding management and routine trimming of the preputial hair.

Cryptorchidism may be unilateral or bilateral. Unilaterally affected animals are usually fertile. Nonscrotal testes are nonfunctional, presumably as a result of constant exposure to body temperature. By the time the scrotum has developed in the neonate, both testes should be in a scrotal position. Testes that seem to be scrotal at times and nonscrotal at other times almost invariably become permanently nonscrotal. Medical therapy using LH and/or testosterone is routinely unsuccessful. Since this condition is heritable, orchiopexy is considered unethical.

Retained testes are at a significantly greater risk of developing neoplasms. In unilaterally affected dogs, the scrotal testis also has a higher rate of neoplasia than in normal males. For this reason, and the fact that this is a heritable defect, bilateral castration is recommended.

Intersex. Intersex states seen in dogs have included true hermaphroditism, male pseudohermaphroditism (masculine and feminine types), and female pseudohermaphroditism. All are infertile except rare hermaphrodites in cocker spaniels that have whelped. The external genitalia varies widely and the diagnosis is based upon gonadal biopsy.

Several cases of masculine-type male pseudohermaphrodites have developed Sertoli cell tumors and cystic uterus masculinus (Fig. 71–9). Those with a "uterus" have developed pyometra (Fig. 7–10), necessitating surgical removal of the infected organ.

Some intersex patients may require cosmetic surgery to make them esthetically acceptable to their owners.

Inappropriate Body Length. Male cats grasp the queen by the back of the neck with their teeth during copulation. If the male's

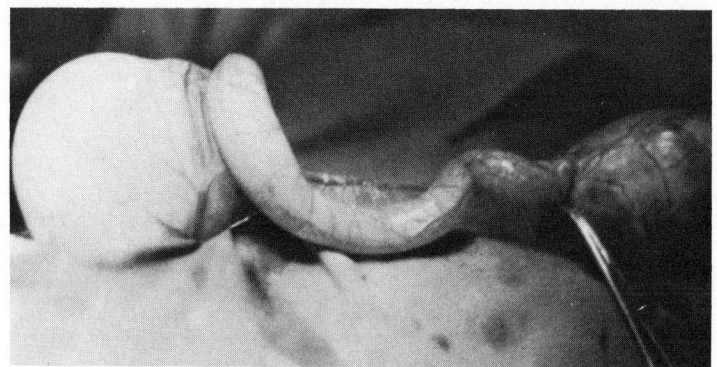

Figure 71–9. Cystic uterus masculinus (left) in a pseudohermaphrodite miniature schnauzer dog with Sertoli cell tumor of retained testis (right).

body length is significantly shorter than that of the female, he may not be able to achieve intromission. Both owners and clinicians should be aware of this possible physical unsuitability for mating.

Penile Hair Rings. Male cats, especially long-haired breeds, can develop rings of hair at the base of the glans penis. These have been noted to prevent copulation. Removal by snipping with suture scissors is simple but may require sedation of the patient.

Neoplasia. Tumors of the penis and prepuce may physically prevent mating. They are rare in both dogs and cats, but of those reported, many were malignant squamous cell carcinomas. Treatment consists of surgical excision and radiation therapy when indicated. Transmissible venereal tumor has been covered in the discussion of the female but is more worrisome in males, since they can potentially infect a greater number of females.

Testicular neoplasms are common in male dogs, being exceeded in incidence only by tumors of the skin and connective tissue. The incidence in cats appears to be quite low, but this also may be related to the high proportion of castrated cats in the general population (about 50 per cent).

Seminomas, Sertoli cell tumors, and interstitial cell tumors all may cause reduced fertility by compression of adjacent tissue or by production of hormones. An immune-mediated phenomenon also may occur, as it is not unusual for dogs to remain sterile after the removal of a unilateral tumor. Estrogen-secreting tumors may produce feminizing syndromes, alopecia, dermal hyperpigmentation, and prostatic disease. A firm abnormal mass is usually palpable, although some tumors may be quite small and escape detection, especially interstitial cell tumors. Diagnosis and treatment is surgical in nature.

Abnormal Karyotype. Sex chromosome

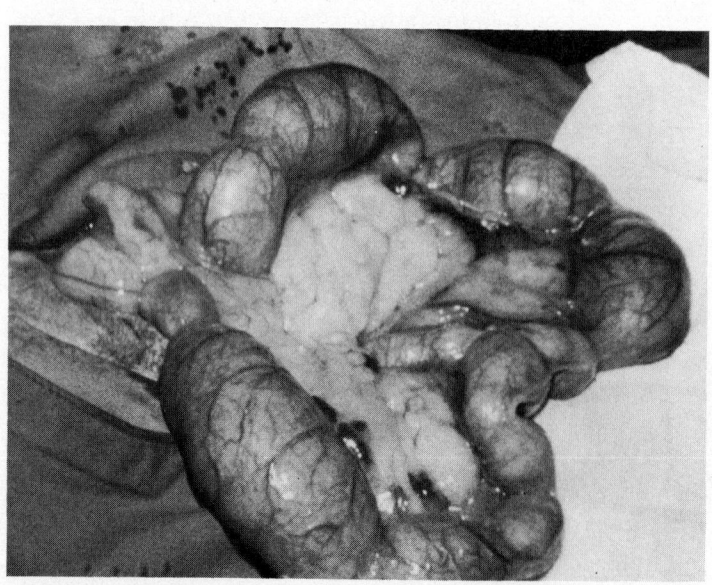

Figure 71–10. Infected uterus (pyometra) in a pseudohermaphrodite miniature schnauzer dog.

abnormalities of the XXY type have been diagnosed in male dogs and cats. This has produced testicular hypoplasia and, in cats, is associated with the sterile tortoise shell coloration. A German short-haired pointer with this defect also had a congenital heart defect. In cats, no other abnormalities have been consistently associated with XXY karyotype. There is no treatment.

Trauma. Trauma, especially bite wounds, to the prepuce and/or glans penis may produce sufficient inflammation and infection to interfere with normal breeding. Such wounds are far more common in cats than in dogs. Because of the potential for serious sequelae (urethral stenosis, preputial adhesions), vigorous treatment is required, including reconstructive surgery when indicated. Maintenance of urine flow is obviously of primary concern.

Drug-Induced Infertility. Many drugs including many routinely used in cancer chemotherapy (cyclophosphamide, vinblastine, chlorambucil), have testicular cytotoxic effects. This leads one to seriously consider this mode of therapy in stud dogs with neoplasia of other body systems. In some instances therapy may not be initiated if the owner desires quality semen from the patient (for one last litter). The perfection of techniques for successfully freezing dog and cat semen has mitigated these decisions, however.

Diethylcarbamazine (DEC) has been incriminated by anecdotal evidence as a cause of infertility. Controlled laboratory studies have refuted these claims. In addition, testicular biopsies from medicated infertile animals have failed to show any consistent lesion. In the author's opinion, DEC at doses used to prevent canine dirofilariasis has no effect on fertility.

Psychologic and Environmental Causes. Some apparently healthy male dogs seem prone to temporary sterility when under stress. Germinal epithelial changes have been reported in dogs placed in new environments, but these reversed within six months.

Sterility may also result from exposure to high environmental temperatures. Precise duration-temperature data on this phenomenon are not available. Potentially, its damage is irreversible. Good kennel management should prevent this, but the practitioner should be aware that summer temperatures in some parts of the country may produce lowered sperm counts. Reassessment during the cooler months often reveals a normal count.

Unwillingness to mate may have a basis in psychologic dysfunction. Proper socialization of the puppy and early training as a stud dog usually obviate these causes. The clinician generally is unable to do anything other than recommend a good stud dog trainer or artificial insemination if the dog can be ejaculated. Testosterone therapy is virtually without benefit.

Exogenous Hormone Therapy. Estrogens will produce infertility in male dogs. Testicular atrophy (usually irreversible) may be expected with chronic administration, and libido is low. In addition, irreversible adenomyosis of the epididymides may be produced, resulting in infertility.

Testosterone in high doses may cause oligospermia, presumably via negative feedback on gonadotropin release. This condition is potentially reversible. Physiologic doses of testosterone in the dog are in the range of 0.1 to 0.2 mg/kg/day.

Progestogens will reduce willingness to mate and may interfere with spermatogenesis after chronic use. The former is thought to be a direct, centrally mediated effect, especially in cats. The latter may result from inhibition of gonadotropin release.

The effects of glucocorticoids are not known in dogs or cats but presumably could, because of their steroid nature, also inhibit gonadotropin release or alter their effect on target tissues.

The potential side effects should warn one to approach the administration of exogenous hormones to breeding animals with caution. One must be absolutely certain that they are indicated and are administered at the lowest possible effective dose.

REFERENCES

Bell, E. T., and Christie, D. W.: Erythrocytes and leucocytes in the vaginal smear of the beagle bitch. Vet. Rec. *88*:546, 1971.

Brodey, R. S., and Roszel, J. F.: Neoplasms of the canine uterus, vagina and vulva: a clinicopathologic survey of 90 cases. J.A.V.M.A. *151*:1294, 1967.

Brodey, R. S., and Martin, J. E.: Sertoli cell neoplasms in the dog. J.A.V.M.A. *133*:249, 1958.

Brown, N. O., Calvert, C., and MacEwen, E. G.: Chemotherapeutic management of transmissible venereal tumors in 30 dogs. J.A.V.M.A. *176*:983, 1980.

Brown, T. T., Burek, J. D., and McEntee, K.: Male pseudohermaphroditism, cryptorchism, and Sertoli cell neoplasia in three miniature schnauzers. J.A.V.M.A. *169*:821, 1976.

Burke, T. J.: Feline reproduction. Vet. Clin. North Am. *6*:317, 1976.

Burke, T. J.: Post-parturient problems in the bitch. Vet. Clin. North Am. *7*:693, 1977.

Carmichael, L. E.: Canine brucellosis. *In* Morrow, D. A. (ed.): Current Therapy in Theriogenology. W. B. Saunders Co., Philadelphia, 1980.

Carmichael, L. E.: Canine brucellosis: an annotated review with selected cautionary comments. Theriogenology *6*:105, 1976.

Carmichael, L. E., and Kenney, R. M.: Canine abortion caused by Brucella canis. J.A.V.M.A. *152*:605, 1968.

Christie, D. W., Bailey, J. B., and Bell, E. T.: Classification of cell types in vaginal smears during the canine oestrous cycle. Br. Vet. J. *128*:301, 1972.

Clough, E., Pyle, R. L., Hare, W. D., Kelly, D. F., and Patterson, D. F.: An XXY sex-chromosome constitution in a dog with testicular hypoplasia and congenital heart disease. Cytogenetics *9*:71, 1970.

Cobb, L. M.: The radiographic outline of the genital system of the bitch. Vet. Rec. *71*:66, 1959.

Cobb, L. M., and Archibald, J.: The radiographic appearance of certain pathological conditions of the canine uterus. J.A.V.M.A. *134*:393, 1959.

Concannon, P. W., and Hansel, W.: Prostaglandin $F_{2\alpha}$-induced luteolysis, hypothermia, and abortions in beagle bitches. Prostaglandins *13*:533, 1977.

Cotchin, E.: Canine ovarian neoplasms. Res. Vet. Sci. *2*:133, 1961.

Cotchin, E.: Testicular neoplasms in dogs. J. Comp. Pathol. *72*:232, 1960.

Crow, S. E.: Neoplasms of the reproductive organs and mammary glands of the dog. *In* Morrow, D. A. (ed.): Current Therapy in Theriogenology. W. B. Saunders Co., Philadelphia, 1980.

Curtis, E. M., and Grant, R. P.: Masculinization of female pups by progestogens. J.A.V.M.A. *144*:395, 1964.

Dain, A. R., and Walker, R. G.: Two intersex dogs with mosaicism. J. Reprod. Fert. *56*:239, 1979.

Dow, C.: Ovarian abnormalities in the bitch. J. Comp. Pathol. *70*:59, 1960.

Dow, C.: Testicular tumors in the dog. J. Comp. Pathol. *72*:247, 1962.

Durfee, P. T., Jr.: Surgical treatment of postparturient metritis in the bitch. J.A.V.M.A. *153*:40, 1968.

Gier, H. T.: Estrous cycle in the bitch: vaginal fluids. Vet. Scope *5*:2, 1960.

Hadley, J. C.: The development of cystic endometrial hyperplasia in the bitch following serial uterine biopsies. J. Small Anim. Pract. *16*:249, 1975.

Hardy, R. M., and Osborne, C. A.: Canine pyometra: pathophysiology, diagnosis and treatment of uterine and extrauterine lesions. J.A.A.H.A. *10*:245, 1974.

Hare, W. C. D.: Cytogenetics. *In* Morrow, D. A. (ed.): Current Therapy in Theriogenology. W. B. Saunders Co., Philadelphia, 1980.

Hart, B. L., and Peterson, D. M.: Penile hair rings in male cats may prevent mating. Lab. Anim. Sci. *21*:422, 1971.

Herron, M. A.: Feline vaginal cytologic examination. Feline Pract. *7*:36, 1977.

Herron, M. A., and Boehringer, B. T.: Male pseudohermaphroditism in a cat. Feline Pract. *5*:30, 1975.

Herron, M. A., and Stein, B.: Prognosis and management of feline infertility. *In* Kirk, R. W. (ed.): Current Veterinary Therapy, VII. W. B. Saunders Co., Philadelphia, 1980.

Hirsh, D. C., and Wiger, N.: The bacterial flora of the normal canine vagina compared with that of vaginal exudates. J. Small Anim. Pract. *18*:1977.

House, C.: Laboratory diagnosis of canine brucellosis. Pract. Vet. *46*:7, 1974.

Hubbert, N. L., Bech-Nielsen, S., and Barta, O.: Canine brucellosis: comparison of clinical manifestations with serologic test results. J.A.V.M.A. *177*:168, 1980.

Jackson, D. A.: Pseudohermaphroditism. *In* Kirk, R. W. (ed.): Current Veterinary Therapy, VII. W. B. Saunders Co., Philadelphia, 1980.

Jackson, D. A., Osborne, C. A., Brasmer, T. H., and Jessen, C. R.: Nonneurogenic urinary incontinence in a canine female pseudohermaphrodite. J.A.V.M.A. *172*:926, 1978.

Johnston, S. D.: Diagnostic and therapeutic approach to infertility in the bitch. J.A.V.M.A. *176*:1335, 1980.

Johnston, S. D.: Use of prostaglandins in reproduction. D.V.M. Magazine *10*:18, 1979.

Joshua, J. O.: Feline reproduction: the problem of infertility in purebred queens. Feline Pract. *5*:52, 1975.

Kelly, D. F., Long, S. E., and Strohmenger, G. D.: Testicular neoplasia in an intersex dog. J. Small Anim. Pract. *17*:247, 1976.

Larsen, R. E.: Infertility in the male dog. *In* Morrow, D. A. (ed.): Current Therapy in Theriogenology. W. B. Saunders Co., Philadelphia, 1980.

Larsen, R. E., and Johnston, S. D.: Management of canine infertility. *In* Kirk, R. W. (ed.): Current Veterinary Therapy, VII. W. B. Saunders Co., Philadelphia, 1980.

Lauderdale, J. W.: Distribution and biological effects of prostaglandins. J. Anim. Sci. Suppl. I *38*:22, 1974.

Leighton, R. L.: Ablation of the penis and castration in a male pseudohermaphrodite dog. J.A.A.H.A. *12*:664, 1976.

Lindberg, R., Jonsson, O. J., and Kasström, H.: Sertoli cell tumors associated with feminization, prostatitis and squamous metaplasia of the renal tubular epithelium in a dog. J. Small Anim. Pract. *17*:451, 1976.

Lipowitz, A. J., and Larsen, R. E.: Acute metritis. *In* Kirk, R. W. (ed.): Current Veterinary Therapy VII. W. B. Saunders Co., Philadelphia, 1980.

McEntee, K.: Fertility problems of the male dog. *In* Kirk, R. W. (ed.): Current Veterinary Therapy, III. W. B. Saunders Co., Philadelphia, 1968.

McFeely, R. A., and Biggers, J. D.: A rare case of female pseudohermaphroditism in the dog. Vet. Rec. 77:696, 1965.

Murti, G. S., Gilbert, D. L., and Borgmann, A. R.: Canine intersex states. J.A.V.M.A. *149*:1183, 1966.

Nachreiner, R. F., and Marple, D. N.: Termination of pregnancy in cats with prostaglandin $F_{2\alpha}$. Prostaglandins *7*:303, 1974.

Oduye, O. O., Ikede, B. O., Esuruoso, G. O., and Akpokodje, J. U.: Metastatic transmissible venereal tumour in dogs. J. Small Anim. Pract. *14*:625, 1973.

Olson, P. N. S.: Canine vaginitis. *In* Kirk, R. W. (ed.): Current Veterinary Therapy, VII. W. B. Saunders Co., Philadelphia, 1980.

Olson, P. S.: Canine vaginitis. *In* Morrow, D. A. (ed.): Current Therapy in Theriogenology. W. B. Saunders Co., Philadelphia, 1980.

Olson, P. N. S., and Mather, E. C.: Canine vaginal and uterine bacterial flora. J.A.V.M.A. *172*:708, 1978.

Platz, C. C., Jr., and Seager, S. W. J.: Semen collection by electro-ejaculation in the domestic cat. J.A.V.M.A. *173*:1353, 1978.

Pollock, R. V. H.: Canine brucellosis: current status. Compend. Cont. Educ. *1*:255, 1979.

Poste, G., and King, N.: Isolation of a herpes virus from the canine genital tract: association with infertility, abortion and still births. Vet. Rec. *88*:229, 1971.

Pullen, C. M.: True bilateral hermaphroditism in a beagle: A case report. Am. J. Vet. Res. *31*:1113, 1970.

Reid, J. S., and Frank, R. J.: Double contrast hysterogram in the diagnosis of retained placentae in the bitch: a case report. J.A.A.H.A. *9*:367, 1973.

Reif, J. S., and Brodey, R. S.: The relationship between cryptorchidism and canine testicular neoplasia. J.A.V.M.A. *155*:2005, 1969.

Roszel, J. F.: Genital cytology of the bitch. Vet. Scope *19*:3, 1975.

Schoeb, T. R., and Morton, R.: Scrotal and testicular changes in canine brucellosis: a case report. J.A.V.M.A. *172*:598, 1978.

Schutte, A. P.: Canine vaginal cytology — I technique and cytological morphology. J. Small Anim. Pract. *8*:301, 1967.

Schutte, A. P.: Canine vaginal cytology — II cyclic changes. J. Small Anim. Pract. *8*:307, 1967.

Selden, J. R.: The intersex dog: classification, clinical presentation, and etiology. Compend. Cont. Educ. *1*:435, 1979.

Senior, D. F.: Infertility in the cycling bitch. Compend. Cont. Educ. *1*:17, 1979.

Shille, V. M., Stabenfeldt, G. H., and Andersen, A. C.: The estrous cycle of the bitch. Canine Pract. *1*:29, 1974.

Sokolowksy, J. H.: Prostaglandin $F_{2\alpha}$-THAM for medical treatment of endometritis, metritis, and pyometritis in the bitch. J.A.A.H.A. *16*:119, 1980.

Sokolowski, J. H.: Reproductive features and patterns in the bitch. J.A.A.H.A. *9*:71, 1973.

Sokolowski, J. H.: The effects of ovariectomy on pregnancy maintenance in the bitch. Lab. Anim. Sci. *21*:696, 1971.

Sokolowski, J. H., and Geng, S.: Effects of prostaglandin $F_{2\alpha}$-THAM in the bitch. J.A.V.M.A. *170*:536, 1977.

Spence, J. A., Holt, P. E., Sayer, P. D., Rottcher, D., and Cooper, J. E.: Metastasis of a transmissible venereal tumour to the pituitary. J. Small Anim. Pract. *19*:175, 1978.

Stein, B. S.: The genital system. *In* Catcott, E. J. (ed.): Feline Medicine and Surgery. American Veterinary Publications, Inc., Santa Barbara, 1975.

Todoroff, R. J.: Congenital urogenital anomalies. Compend. Cont. Educ. *1*:780, 1979.

Wallace, L. J., and Cox, V. S.: Canine cryptorchidism. *In* Kirk, R. W. (ed.): Current Veterinary Therapy, VII. W. B. Saunders Co., Philadelphia, 1980.

Weaver, A. D., Harvey, M. J., Munro, C. D., Rogerson, P., and McDonald, M.: Phenotypic intersex (female pseudohermaphroditism) in a dachshund dog. Vet. Rec. *105*:230, 1979.

Wensing, C. J. G.: Developmental defects, including cryptorchidism. *In* Morrow, D. A. (ed.): Current Therapy in Theriogenology. W. B. Saunders Co., Philadelphia, 1980.

CHAPTER **72**

PATRICIA N. S. OLSON
and TERRY M. NETT

Small Animal Contraceptives

INTRODUCTION

Uncontrolled dogs and cats continue to challenge city and rural governments to discover ways to limit the pet population. The exact number of controlled and uncontrolled dogs and cats in the United States is unknown. There is a general impression in cities and rural areas that feral animals are common, but in fact, most urban and rural uncontrolled dogs are stray pets (Beck,

1974). No official estimate of the United States pet population has been published by the Census Bureau, but based on the results of a survey conducted by the Upjohn Company in 1976, the total dog population that year was estimated at 48,846,000, with almost half (48 per cent) of all households in the U.S. owning at least one dog (Bush, 1978). Uncontrolled pets present numerous problems throughout the U.S. Unrestricted dogs can prey on sheep, cattle, and deer and often do not eat their kills. Instead, uncontrolled dogs and cats eat garbage, resulting in overturned trash cans and spilled garbage, which increases the cost of refuse removal. Removal of animal feces presents problems for many city governments. Furthermore, zoonotic diseases are difficult to control in roaming animal populations, and people bitten by stray pets must decide whether or not to begin prophylactic treatment for rabies.

The population of the United States increased by 11.7 per cent from 1960 to 1970; from 1964 to 1971 the pet population increased by 23.3 per cent (Phillips, 1974). That many of these animals are free-roaming (or unwanted) is attested to by the fact that approximately 13.5 million dogs and cats are euthanatized annually. Therefore, it seems that improved laws for control of companion animals are needed. Veterinarians must also acquaint the public (particularly pet owners) with the fact that free-roaming dogs and cats are primarily lost or abandoned pets.

Finally, with the animal population still increasing at a rapid pace, it seems imperative to continue to search for better methods of contraception, since those currently available have not alleviated the tremendous overpopulation of uncontrolled pets.

METHODS OF FEMALE CONTRACEPTION

SURGICAL CONTROL

Surgical removal of the gonads and/or part of the reproductive tract is the most effective way to prevent pregnancy in the bitch or queen. Although ovariohysterectomy is the most common method of surgical contraception for dogs and cats, hysterectomy, tubal ligation, or salpingectomy is also effective. Ovariohysterectomy has the advantage of eliminating estrous cycles and the attraction of male animals to a female in heat. If performed early in life, it also decreases the incidence of mammary tumors. Either ovariohysterectomy or hysterectomy will also eliminate the possibility of later uterine disease. With the availability of laparoscopic equipment, tubal ligation or salpingectomy can now be performed with minimal difficulty. Animals with tubal ligation or salpingectomy will continue to have reproductive cycles and will also retain the potential for uterine disease.

Surgical contraception has not been a satisfactory means of controlling the pet population in the United States. Even in communities implementing public clinics for spaying, the problem of overpopulation continues. Although most veterinarians state that complications following ovariohysterectomy are minimal, others report that post-surgical sequelae in dogs may be as high as 31.5 per cent (Dorn and Swist, 1977). Whether such complications would deter owners from subjecting another pet to the procedure is unknown. Cost is a definite consideration for pet owners and frequently may deter them from utilizing surgical means of contraception or may delay their decision until after the bitch or queen has been mated. Surgical contraception as currently practiced by veterinarians is permanent and does not permit a temporary means of contraception for owners wanting to breed their animals at a later date. It is the opinion of some that the majority of spays and castrations may in fact be performed for esthetic reasons and not for birth control or disease prevention (Burke, 1979).

MECHANICAL CONTROL

Intravaginal devices have been available for bitches in the past but are no longer marketed. Perforation of the vaginal wall, loss of the device, and persistent vaginitis contributed to poor public acceptance of this method of contraception.

Intrauterine devices in the dog or cat should inhibit fertility. However, inserting a device via the vagina and through the cervix would be extremely difficult, so the method is impractical for these species.

PHARMACOLOGIC CONTROL

Canine pharmacologic contraceptives are now available to the public, but there is currently no pharmacologic contraceptive approved for use in the cat. Many steroid compounds can inhibit fertility, but because of the undesirable side effects seen with some steroids, pharmaceutical companies have had to be extremely cautious in attempting to market contraceptives that will prove safe and that will not render the animal permanently sterile.

A good pharmacologic contraceptive must satisfy several criteria: it must prevent pregnancy, it must be safe and not contribute to pathologic conditions of the reproductive tract or other body systems, it should prevent estrous behavior, it should be easily administered by the owner or veterinarian at convenient time intervals, and it should be reversible.

The results of several common laboratory tests are affected in humans taking oral contraceptives (Abramowicz, 1979). Although comparable information is lacking for the dog, the veterinarian should be aware that certain laboratory test results may be altered in an animal receiving oral contraceptives. For example, liver enzymes are reportedly elevated in some dogs receiving mibolerone (Sokolowski, 1978a).

Progestins

Several progestational compounds have been used experimentally and shown to be effective contraceptives (Christie and Bell, 1970; Goyings et al., 1977; Van Os and Oldenkamp, 1978; Bigbee and Hennessey, 1977; Burke and Reynolds, 1975). Although many progestins are efficacious as contraceptives, they may have undesirable side effects. These include stimulation of the canine endometrium (Sokolowski and Zimbelman, 1973), increased incidence of uterine disease (Dow, 1959); Cox, 1970; Lauderdale et al., 1977), increased mammary tumor formation (Briggs, 1977; Weikel and Nelson, 1977; Geil and Lamar, 1977), increased numbers of prolactin-producing cells in the anterior pituitary gland (Attia and Zayed, 1979), increased morphologic features suggesting high secretory activity in growth hormone–producing cells (El Etreby and Fath El Bab, 1978), pancreatic changes typical of diabetes mellitus (Weikel and Nelson, 1977), and masculinization of female puppies (Sokolowski, 1979).

The only progestational contraceptive currently approved for use in dogs in the United States is megestrol acetate. It is a potent, orally active synthetic progestogen, which in the dog is excreted mainly by the liver with about 10 per cent renal excretion (Burke and Reynolds, 1975). The mechanism of action is reportedly suppression of estrus or ovulation through inhibition of gonadotropin release.

The dosage of megestrol acetate administered to bitches depends on the stage of the reproductive cycle. If the dog is in early proestrus, estrus can be postponed when megestrol acetate is given orally at a dosage of 2.2 mg/kg/day for eight consecutive days. It is important that animals be started as close to the first day of proestrus as possible to ensure efficacy of the product and to minimize side effects. According to the manufacturer, when given as recommended, the incidence of pyometra should be comparable to or lower than that in non-treated animals.

In anestrous bitches, megestrol acetate can be used in a 32-day administration schedule of 0.55 mg/kg/day orally. For suppression of estrus, the drug must be initiated at least seven days prior to the expected onset of proestrus.

Results of one study suggest that megestrol acetate is safe and effective in first-heat bitches when the onset of proestrus can be accurately determined (Bigbee and Hennessey, 1977). It is not approved for use in postponing estrus in first-heat bitches, however, because early research showed considerable variation in the initial appearance of proestrous bleeding and/or vulvular swelling in relation to the first ovulation in young females.

Dogs with mammary tumors should not be given this contraceptive, since some canine mammary tumors may be stimulated by exogenous progestogens. Megestrol acetate is also contraindicated in dogs with uterine disease. Occasionally, transient progestational side effects such as mammary enlargement, lactation, listlessness, increased appetite, and temperament change were noted in clinical studies. Confirmed cases of pyometra occurred in 0.6 per cent of the cases, which was similar to or lower than the incidence of pyometra in control animals.

The next estrus may occur one to seven months after cessation of treatment of animals administered megestrol acetate during proestrus or anestrus (Burke and Reynolds, 1975). If estrus occurs within 30 days of cessation of treatment, the manufacturers recommend that mating not be allowed. In clinical studies, most dogs returned to estrus in four to six months.

In cats, a hyperglycemic-glucosuric syndrome (Pukay, 1979), increased incidence of pyometra (Remfry, 1978), and mammary hypertrophy (Nimmo-Wilkie, 1979) have been noted following progestogen therapy. A detailed study of the potential side effects following progestogen therapy in the cat is needed.

Androgens

Androgenic compounds have also been studied for their potential uses as contraceptives in the bitch (Simmons and Hamner, 1973; Sokolowski, 1978b; Sokolowski and Kasson, 1978; Sokolowski and Shu Geng, 1977; Krzeminski et al., 1978). Androgenic compounds apparently act to inhibit release of pituitary gonadotropins, thus preventing estrus and ovulation. Side effects reported with testosterone implants are clitoral enlargement and intermittent, nonodorous, low volume vaginal discharge (Simmons and Hamner, 1973). The only currently approved androgenic compound for canine contraception in the United States in mibolerone.

Mibolerone is a steroid that has anabolic, androgenic, and antigonadotropic activity. Primary and secondary follicular development can occur in the ovaries of animals receiving this drug, but these follicles do not mature to ovulatory size. Because the preovulatory surge of luteinizing hormone (LH) is supposedly blocked, ovulation should not occur. Ovulation and corpora lutea formation, therefore, should be prevented for as long as mibolerone is administered. Metabolites of mibolerone are excreted in approximately equal quantities in the urine and feces.

Mibolerone drops are administered orally once a day by adding the dose to a small portion of food or directly into the dog's mouth. Dosages recommended by the manufacturer of mibolerone for heat prevention range from 30 μg/dog/day for bitches 25 pounds and under to 180 μg/dog/day for bitches over 100 pounds. German shepherd bitches must receive 180 μg/day, regardless of body weight. Mibolerone can be used continuously for 24 months. Administration of the drug should be initiated at least 30 days prior to an expected estrus. If estrus occurs during the first 30 days of treatment, breeding should not be allowed. Care should be taken not to administer mibolerone to pregnant bitches, since the drug can masculinize female fetuses. The masculinization can be manifested as alterations in the patency of the vagina, multiple urethral openings into the vagina, a phallus-like structure in place of the clitoris, accumulations of fluid in the vagina or uterus, and development of testeslike structures. Gross effects have not been observed in male off-spring.

Mibolerone should not be administered to any animal with a prior history of liver or kidney disease. Increased concentrations of serum glutamic-pyruvic transaminase (SGPT) may be encountered in bitches receiving this drug and should be determined at six-month intervals. If increased concentrations of SGPT are noted, the attending veterinarian should use discretion in recommending discontinuance of the drug. Additionally, mibolerone should not be administered to prepubertal bitches, because steroids with androgenic activity can induce early epiphyseal closure. Occasionally, clitoral hypertrophy, vaginitis, and epiphora have been reported in dogs receiving the drug. Toxicologic studies over several years suggest that mibolerone, even at dosages much higher than those needed to suppress estrus, is relatively safe.

The efficacy of the drug in prevention of estrus is reported to be 90 per cent. After mibolerone treatment is discontinued, the animal may have the next estrus as soon as seven days or as long as 200 days after the last treatment. The average time to the next anticipated estrus is approximately 70 days. Mibolerone is not approved for use in cats, since hepatotoxicity and/or thyrotoxicity have been noted after chronic administration (Burke, 1978).

Estrogens

Estrogenic compounds are not used as canine or feline contraceptives but have been used in clinical practice for years in the form of "mismate shots." Injectable estradiol cypionate (ECP) and diethylstilbestrol

(DES) have both been used for terminating unwanted pregnancies in dogs and cats. These compounds should be administered only during estrus. Overdosage can produce life-threatening bone marrow suppression; underdosage may render the therapy ineffective. Unfortunately the range between overdosage and underdosage is small. In addition, some clinicians feel there is an increased incidence of pyometra following treatment, particularly if the estrogen is administered during diestrus. Owners should be made aware of these potential dangers, and injectable estrogens should never be given more than once per estrous cycle. A total dose of 0.1 mg ECP is used to abort a toy breed bitch, and up to, but never exceeding, 1.0 mg ECP is used to abort giant breed bitches.

Prostaglandins

Prostaglandin $F_{2\alpha}$ has been used experimentally to abort bitches but is not approved for clinical use. The effective luteolytic dose (ED_{50}) following a single injection of $PGF_{2\alpha}$ is near the lethal dose (LD_{50}). When given experimentally during the mid- or late-luteal phase of the cycle (day 25 to 58) at a dose of 20 μg/kg every eight hours or 30 μg/kg every 12 hours, four of seven bitches aborted. Luteolysis did not occur in two bitches treated in the early luteal phase (prior to day 20) (Concannon and Hansel, 1977).

POTENTIAL CONTRACEPTIVES FOR DOGS

Immunologic Means of Birth Control

Anti-Luteinizing Hormone (anti-LH). Immunizing dogs with bovine and ovine LH has been attempted as a means of rendering the animals infertile (Faulkner et al., 1975; Faulkner, 1980). Because the interestrous interval of the bitch is several months long, the research was done primarily on male dogs. Within three weeks after immunization, most dogs developed antibodies to LH and became azoospermic. Although the males did develop antibodies to LH that cross-reacted with extracts of canine anterior pituitary gland, the duration of antibody titers sufficient to maintain infertility was variable and unpredictable.

Immunizing dogs with human chorionic gonadotropin (hCG) failed to inhibit reproduction in male and female dogs. This was attributed to the lack of cross-reactivity between canine pituitary gonadotropins and antibodies to hCG. This fact may be clinically significant, suggesting that giving repeated injections of hCG to a dog might not produce antibodies capable of cross-reacting with the animal's own LH.

Anti–Gonadotropin-Releasing Hormone (anti-GnRH). Research has been done in an attempt to develop a means to sterilize animals by immunizing them against gonadotropin-releasing hormone (GnRH). GnRH is a decapeptide and therefore not highly immunogenic unless conjugated to another molecule such as albumin. Fraser et al. (1975) have studied an immunologic contraceptive for dogs using GnRH as the antigen. Immunizing dogs with this immunogen resulted in inhibition of reproductive cycles in the bitch and sterility in the male. Subsequent work in rats has shown that animals with the highest antibody titers to GnRH have the least follicular development (Fraser and Baker, 1978). While antibodies to GnRH seem to have a contraceptive effect in some species, it is interesting to note that superactive analogs of GnRH may also inhibit maturational development of Leydig cell function (Sharpe and Fraser, 1979). Whether such analogs will prove to be useful clinically as contraceptives is to date only speculative, but research is currently under way to test that hypothesis.

Anti–Zona Pellucida (anti-ZP). Antibodies to porcine zona pellucida inhibit binding of spermatozoa and fertilization of human ova (Trounson et al., 1980). Studies are currently being conducted on active immunization of baboons, marmosets, and dogs with porcine zona antigens (Shivers et al., 1981). Strong cross-reactivity between canine and porcine antigens has been demonstrated. The availability of large quantities of pig zonae provides the basis for using pig zona antigens for active immunization of the dog (Shivers et al., 1981). Mahi and Yanagimachi (1979) have demonstrated that antibodies to canine ovary will inhibit *in vitro* fertilization of canine oocytes, thereby suggesting the plausibility of an anti–zona pellucida vaccine for birth control in the bitch. Antibodies to the zona pellucida would have at least two focal points for inhibiting fertility: first, by preventing spermatozoal attachment and penetration through the zona (provided the oocyte is exposed to antibody before fertilization), and second, by blocking implantation by interfering with zona shedding if fertilization does occur (Shivers, 1975). Passive immunizations might potentially be used as an alternative to mismate shots if implantation can be prevented by antibodies that inhibit zona shedding.

METHODS OF MALE CONTRACEPTION

SURGICAL CONTROL

Surgical removal of the gonads (castration) is an effective way to inhibit fertility in the male. By removing the major source of androgens as well as the sperm cells, castration may also attenuate male behavior such as roaming, aggressiveness, or undesirable urination patterns in the dog and cat.

Male dogs and cats can be easily vasectomized, offering an alternative to the client who does not want a male castrated. Vasectomized animals will still maintain their male behavior patterns, since the androgen-producing cells have not been altered. Spermatozoa may still be present in ejaculates from male dogs 21 days postvasectomy (Pineda et al., 1976). Male cats may have spermatozoa in ejaculates obtained via electroejaculation up to 21 days postvasectomy. We recommend that vasectomized males be evaluated six weeks postvasectomy for spermatozoa in the ejaculates. Prior to that time we suggest owners confine vasectomized males to prevent the possibility of a fertile mating.

PHARMACOLOGIC CONTROL

Several potential oral contraceptives have been evaluated for efficacy in the human male, and many have been discarded owing to their depressant action on libido. This might actually be a desirable effect in male dogs and cats. Relatively few studies have been done to evaluate the effect of steroidal compounds on fertility of male companion animals. Such studies seem warranted, not only to develop a male contraceptive but also to evaluate the effects on male fertility of various steroidal drugs used routinely in clinical medicine.

A method for chemical vasectomy in the male dog has been developed and is currently being tested (Pineda et al., 1977; Pineda, 1978). Injection of a sclerosing agent into the caudae of the epididymides of adult and prepubertal dogs induces a long-lasting and probably irreversible azoospermia (Pineda et al., 1977). Male dogs can be administered the sclerosing agent on an outpatient basis, as the cauda of the epididymis is easily palpated in most dogs and the injection causes minimal discomfort for the animal. Ejaculates are evaluated six weeks post-injection for the presence of spermatozoa. The sclerosing agent currently being tested is 4.5 per cent chlorhexidine digluconate. Currently, studies are also being conducted to determine the effectiveness of an epididymal sclerosing agent in cats.

REFERENCES

Abramowicz, M. (ed): Effects of oral contraceptives on laboratory tests. The Medical Letter 21:54, 1979.

Attia, M. A., and Yayed, I.: Cytological study on the anterior pituitary of beagle bitches treated subcutaneously with progesterone for 13 weeks. Arch. Toxicol. 42:147, 1979.

Beck, A. M.: Proceedings of the National Conference on the Ecology of the Surplus Dog and Cat Problem, May 21–23, 1974, p. 31.

Bigbee, H. G., and Hennessey, P. W.: Megestrol acetate for postponing estrus in first-heat bitches. VM SAC 72:1727, 1977.

Briggs, M.: Minireview: The beagle dog and contraceptive steroids. Life Sci. 21:275, 1977.

Burke, T. J.: Birth control for dogs. D.V.M. 10:6:9, 1979.

Burke, T. J.: Mibolerone studies in the cat. Proceedings of the Symposium on Cheque^R for canine estrus prevention. Brook Lodge, Augusta, MI, March 13–15, 1978.

Burke, T. J., and Reynolds, H. A.: Megestrol acetate for estrus postponement in the bitch. J.A.V.M.A. 167:285, 1975.

Bush, R. R.: Proceedings of the Symposium on Cheque^R for Canine Estrus Prevention. Brook Lodge, Augusta, Michigan, March 13–15, 1978, p. 77.

Christie, D. W., and Bell, E. T.: The use of progestogens to control reproductive function in the bitch. Commonwealth Bureau of Animal Breeding and Genetics, Reprint No. 83, reprinted from Animal Breeding Abstr. 38:1, 1970.

Concannon, P. W., and Hansel, W.: Prostaglandin $F_{2\alpha}$ induced luteolysis, hypothermia, and abortion in beagle bitches. Prostaglandins 13:533, 1977.

Cox, J. E.: Progestogens in bitches: a review. J. Small Anim. Pract. *11*:759, 1970.

Dorn, A. S., and Swist, R. A.: Complications of canine ovariohysterectomy. J.A.A.H.A. *13*:720, 1977.

Dow, C.: Experimental reproduction of the cystic hyperplasia-pyometra complex in the bitch. J. Pathol. Bacteriol. *78*:267, 1959.

El Etreby, M. F., and Fath, El Bab, M. R.: Effect of cyproterone acetate, d-norgestrel, and progesterone on cells of the pars distalis of the adenohypophysis in the beagle bitch. Cell Tissue Res. *191*:205, 1978.

Faulkner, L. C.: Immunological Control of Fertility in Dogs. *In* Morrow, D A. (ed.): Current Therapy in Theriogenology, W. B. Saunders Co., Philadelphia, 1980, p. 677.

Faulkner, L. C., Pineda, M. H., and Reimers, T. J.: Immunization against gonadotropins in dogs. *In* Nieschlag, E. (ed.): Immunization with Hormones in Reproduction Research, 1975. North-Holland Publishing Co., Amsterdam, The Netherlands, p. 199.

Fraser, H. M., and Baker, T. G.: Changes in the ovaries of rats after immunization against luteinizing hormone releasing hormone. J. Endocrinol. *77*:85, 1978.

Fraser, H. M., Borthwick, R., and Fraser, A. F.: Sterilising by immunisation (correspondence). Vet. Rec., April 5, 1975, p. 323.

Geil, R. G., and Lamar, J. K.: FDA studies of estrogen, progestogens, and estrogen/progestogen combinations in the dog and monkey. J. Toxicol. Environ. Health *3*:179, 1977.

Goyings, L. S., Sokolowski, J. H., Zimbelman, R. G., and Geng, S.: Clinical, morphologic, and clinicopathologic findings in beagles treated for two years with melengestrol acetate. Am. J. Vet. Res. *38*:1923, 1977.

Krzeminski, L. F., Sokolowski, J. H., Dunn, G. H., Van Ravenswaay, F., and Pineda, M.: Serum concentrations of mibolerone in beagle bitches as influenced by time, dosage form and geographic location. Am. J. Vet. Res. *39*:567, 1978.

Lauderdale, J. W., Goyings, L. S., Krzeminski, L. F., and Zimbelman, R. G.: Studies of a progestogen (MGA) as related to residues and human consumption. J. Toxicol. Environ. Health *3*:5, 1977.

Mahi, C. A., and Yanagimachi, R.: Prevention of in vitro fertilization of canine oocytes by anti-ovary antisera: A potential approach to fertility control in the bitch. J. Exp. Zool. *210*:129, 1979.

Nimmo-Wilkie, J. S.: Progesterone therapy for cats (a letter). Can. Vet. J. *20*:164, 1979.

Phillips, R. T.: Proceedings of the National Conference on the Ecology of the Surplus Dog and Cat Problem, May 21–23, 1974, p. 49.

Pineda, M. H.: Chemical vasectomy in dogs. Canine Practice *5*:34, 1978.

Pineda, M. H., Reimers, T. J., and Faulkner, L. C.: Disappearance of spermatozoa from the ejaculates of vasectomized dogs. J.A.V.M.A. *168*:502, 1976.

Pineda, M. H., Reimers, T. J., Faulkner, L. C., Hopwood, M. L., and Seidel, G. E., Jr.: Azoospermia in dogs induced by injection of sclerosing agents into the caudae of the epididymis. Am. J. Vet. Res. *38*:831, 1977.

Pukay, B. P.: A hyperglycemia-glucosuria syndrome in cats following megestrol acetate therapy (letter). Can. Vet. J. *20*:117, 1979.

Remfry, J.: Control of feral cat population by long-term administration of megestrol acetate. Vet. Rec. *103*:403, 1978.

Sharpe, R. M., and Fraser, H. M.: Inhibition of maturational changes in Leydig cell function after treatment of rats with an agonist of luteinizing hormone releasing hormone. Proc. Soc. Endocrinol. in J. Endocrinol. *81*:159, 1979.

Shivers, C. A.: Antigens of the ovum as a potential basis for the development of contraceptive vaccine. Development of vaccines for fertility regulation. WHO session: 3rd Int. Symp. on Immunology of Reproduction, Varna, Bulgaria, 21–25 September, 1975.

Shivers, C. A., Sieg, P. M., and Kitchen, H. Pregnancy prevention in the dog: Potential for an immunological approach. J.A.A.H.A. *17*:823, 1981.

Simmons, J. G., and Hamner, C. E.: Inhibition of estrus in the dog with testosterone implants. Am. J. Vet. Res. *34*:1409, 1973.

Sokolowski, J. H.: A view of practical teratogenesis. Canine Practice *6*:16, 1979.

Sokolowski, J. H.: Evaluation of the safety of mibolerone for the canine. Proc. Symp. on Cheque[R] for Canine Estrus Prevention. Brook Lodge, Augusta, MI, March 13–15, 1978a.

Sokolowski, J. H.: Evaluation of estrous activity in bitches treated with mibolerone and exposed to adult male dogs. J.A.V.M.A. *173*:983, 1978b.

Sokolowski, J. H., and Kasson, C. W.: Effects of mibolerone on conception, pregnancy, parturition, and offspring in the beagle. Am. J. Vet. Res. *39*:837, 1978.

Sokolowski, J. H., and Shu Geng: Biological evaluation of mibolerone in the female beagle. Am. J. Vet. Res. *38*:1371, 1977.

Sokolowski, J. H., and Zimbelman, R. G.: Canine reproduction: effects of a single injection of medroxyprogesterone acetate on the reproductive organs of the bitch. Am. J. Vet. Res. *34*:1493, 1973.

Trounson, A. O., Shivers, C. A., McMaster, R., and Lopata, A.: Inhibition of sperm binding and fertilization of human ova by antibody to porcine zona pellucida and human sera. Arch. Androl. *4*:29, 1980.

Van Os, J. L., and Oldenkamp, E. P.: Oestrus control in bitches with proligestone, a new progestational compound. J. Small Anim. Pract. *19*:521, 1978.

Weikel, J. H., and Nelson, L. W.: Problems in evaluating chronic toxicity of contraceptive steroids in dogs. J. Toxicol. Environ. Health *3*:167, 1977.

SECTION XIII

Diseases
of the
Urinary
System

CHAPTER 73

CARL A. OSBORNE
DELMAR R. FINCO
and DONALD G. LOW

Pathophysiology of Renal Disease, Renal Failure, and Uremia

APPLIED ANATOMY AND PHYSIOLOGY WITH CLINICAL CORRELATIONS

INTRODUCTION

Conceptual understanding of nephrology is inseparably linked to familiarity with the structure and function of the kidney. The explosion of scientific information concerning structural and functional interrelationships of the kidney in the past decade has produced a vast wealth of knowledge of great clinical significance. Since the scope of this chapter precludes in-depth discussion of many significant morphologic, physiologic, biochemical, and therapeutic discoveries the following discussion will touch upon those aspects most likely to aid the clinician in establishing diagnoses and formulating meaningful prognoses and effective therapy. For in-depth discussions about interrelationships between structure and function of the kidney, consult appropriate reference material (Beeuwkes, 1980; Brenner and Beeuwkes, 1978; Brenner and Rector, 1981; Bulger, 1979; Finco, 1980; Stein and Faden, 1978; Tisher, 1981).

STRUCTURAL ORGANIZATION

The cut surface of the bisected kidney may be grossly separated into a superficial dark colored cortex that completely surrounds an inner light-colored medulla. As will be discussed, it is helpful to consider the kidneys in terms of glomerular, tubular, interstitial, or vascular components when evaluating structure and function. With the exception of a few ectopic pelvic glomeruli (Fourman and Moffat, 1971), all glomeruli are located within the renal cortex. This anatomic fact is of considerable significance in proper procurement of renal biopsy samples. Unlike some species, there are no glomeruli within a wide peripheral zone of the outer cortical surface of dog kidneys (Bulger et al., 1979; Sherwood, 1969). Both cortex and medulla contain renal tubules, vessels, and interstitial tissue.

The Nephron

The anatomic and functional unit of the kidney is called the nephron. Differences in size of kidneys of various species are related to the numbers of the nephrons they contain. There are approximately 190,000 glomeruli (and presumably nephrons) per kidney in the cat and 400,000 in the dog, (Finco and Duncan, 1972; Kunkel, 1930; Rytand, 1938; Sellwood, 1955; McFarlene, 1976). The normal canine renal cortex contains sufficient glomeruli to expect an average of 25 glomeruli per punch biopsy sample obtained with a Franklin-Silverman biopsy needle (Osborne and Low, 1971).

Classically, nephrons have been divided into several components on the basis of certain histologic and functional characteristics. These segments are renal (or malpighian) corpuscles, composed of a tuft of highly branched capillaries (glomerulus) surrounded by a capsule (Bowman's capsule); proximal tubule; loop of Henle; distal convoluted tubule; and collecting duct. The space between the glomerulus and Bowman's capsule that collects glomerular filtrate is called the urinary space (or Bowman's space).

Heterogenicity of Nephrons. Although

nephrons are qualitatively similar in structure and function, they are quantitatively dissimilar (Finco, 1980). For example, nephrons whose glomeruli are located in outer portions of the renal cortex have relatively short loops of Henle, while nephrons whose glomeruli are located adjacent to the renal medulla (so-called juxtamedullary glomeruli) have relatively long loops of Henle that extend deep into the renal medulla. Other differences between nephrons include those related to glomerular size, efferent arteriolar perfusion pattern, and intracellular enzyme composition, distribution, and quantity (Finco, 1980). Knowledge of heterogenicity of nephrons within each kidney is of importance in evaluation of normal and abnormal structure and function.

Glomeruli. Glomeruli contain capillary endothelial cells, visceral and parietal epithelial cells, mesangial cells and mesangial matrix, and capillary basement membranes (Osborne et al., 1977) (Fig. 73–1). Glomeruli produce large quantities of an ultrafiltrate of plasma, only a small portion of which ultimately is voided from the body as urine.

Glomerular capillary endothelial cells are similar to endothelial cells lining capillaries in other parts of the body, except that their cytoplasm contains numerous large pores (or fenestrae, Fig. 73–1). The functional significance of these pores is as yet unknown. They are too large to inhibit filtration of macromolecules with a molecular weight similar to that of plasma albumin (MW = 68,000 daltons). At one time endothelial cells were considered to be an insignificant barrier to all macromolecules; however, it has since been established that the negative charge imparted by sialoproteins coating the endothelial cells plays a vital role in repelling the passage of negatively charged macromolecules, including albumin (Fig. 73–2) (Brenner and Beeuwkes,

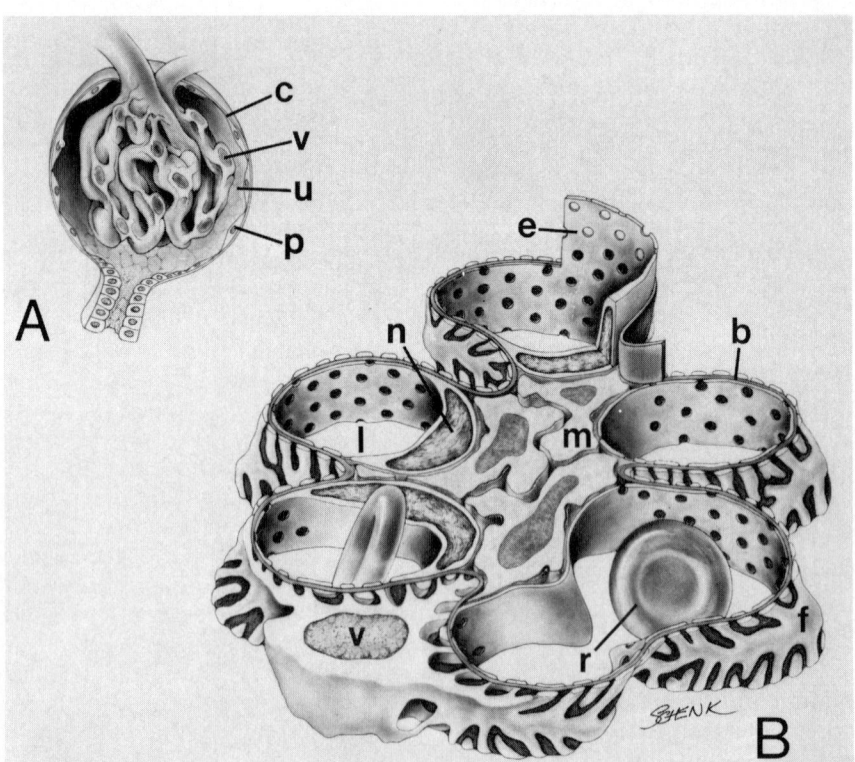

Figure 73–1. A, Renal corpuscle with glomerular tuft, urinary space, and Bowman's capsule. B, Cross section of a portion of a glomerulus. c, Bowman's capsule; u, urinary space; p, parietal epithelial cell; v, nucleus of visceral epithelial cell; f, foot processes of visceral epithelial cell; n, nucleus of capillary endothelial cell; e, cytoplasm of capillary endothelial cell containing large pores; m, mesangial cells; I, capillary lumen; r, red blood cell. (From Osborne, C. A.: Glomerulonephropathy and the nephrotic syndrome. *In* Kirk, R. W. (ed.): Current Veterinary Therapy, VI. W. B. Saunders Co., Philadelphia, PA, 1977.)

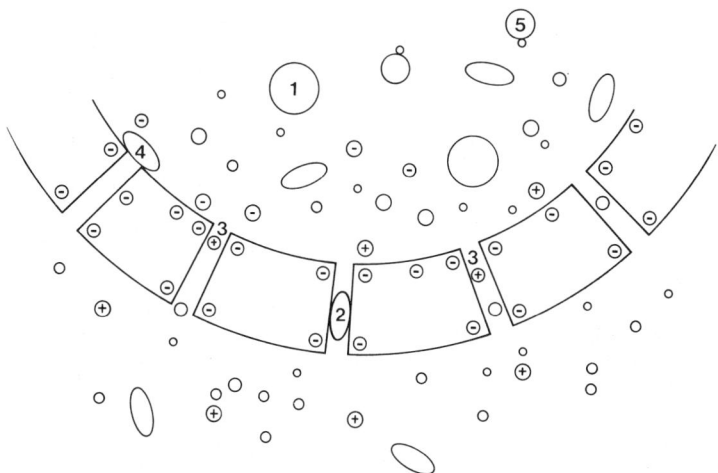

Figure 73–2. Schematic illustration of factors influencing the selective permeability of glomerular capillary walls to filtration of protein molecules. 1, Large size molecule; 2, viscous drag associated with friction caused by passage of protein molecule through glomerular pore; 3, repulsion of negatively charged (so-called electrical hindrance) and attraction of positively charged molecules by negatively charged glomerular capillary wall; 4, steric hindrance caused by malalignment of elongated protein molecule with glomerular pore; 5, increased size associated with binding of small and large protein molecules. (Modified from Heinemann, H. O., Maack, T. M., and Sherman, R. L.: Proteinuria. Amer. J. Med. 56:71–82, 1974.)

1978). Thus, plasma proteins with a size that would readily pass through electrically neutral glomerular capillary endothelium are restricted from passage if they are negatively charged.

The *glomerular basement membrane* (GBM) is located between endothelial cells and visceral epithelial cells in peripheral portions of capillaries, and between mesangial cells and visceral epithelial cells in other portions of the glomerular tuft (Fig. 73–1). The GBM does not surround the entire capillary lumen, as is the case with other capillaries in the body, but covers the glomerular tuft in a fashion somewhat analogous to that of the serosa of the abdominal cavity. It is not located between endothelial cells and mesangial cells. Like endothelial cells and visceral epithelial cells, the GBM contains fixed negatively charged sites that may influence the filtration of electrically charged macromolecules (Caufield et al., 1976). The GBM also appears to serve as a primary filtration barrier to large, high molecular weight macromolecules present in plasma that are neutral. It apparently does not prevent filtration of smaller noncharged molecules, however. Special structures (called slit-pore membranes) associated with the cytoplasm of visceral epithelial cells are thought to act as the filtration barrier for smaller substances (Fig. 73–3).

Glomerular capillaries are covered with *visceral epithelial cells* (commonly called podocytes), characterized by an elaborate layer of primary, secondary, and tertiary cytoplasmic processes that extend to the GBM (Figs. 73–1 and 73–3). Immediately adjacent foot processes originate from different visceral epithelial cells (Fig. 73–4). The spaces between the epithelial foot processes are called filtration slits or slit pores. Ultrastructural studies have revealed the presence of thin membranes (slit-pore membranes) that close the spaces between the foot processes. It is presumed that filtration occurs at these sites. The visceral epithelium is also covered with negatively charged sialoprotein, which tends to inhibit passage of negatively charged macromolecules (Fig. 73–3). In contrast, the negative charge of glomerular capillary walls appears to enhance filtration of positively charged molecules. The visceral epithelium is thought to produce one or more components of the GBM (Osborne et al., 1977).

Mesangial cells typically have an irregular shape caused by elongated cytoplasmic processes (Fig. 73–1). They occupy a space between capillaries and are separated from capillary lumina by endothelial cytoplasm and mesangial matrix rather than by the GBM. Mesangial cells are separated from visceral epithelial cells by the GBM (Fig. 73–1). These cells are able to phagocytose material in a fashion similar to that of reticuloendothelial cells. The cells extend cytoplasmic processes between capillary endothelial cells and the GBM, where they remove filtration residues that might other-

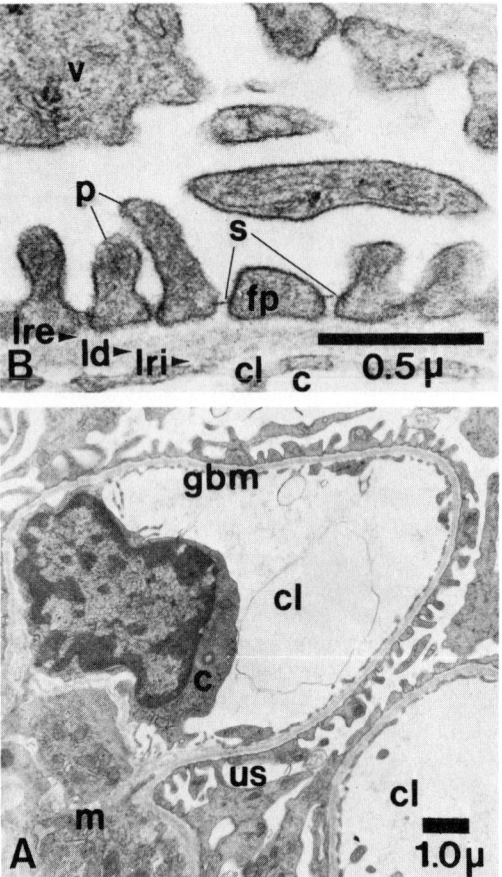

Figure 73–3. Electron micrograph of a normal adult dog glomerulus. A, Low-power magnification illustrating patent capillary lumens (cl) surrounded by fenestrated endothelial cytoplasm (c), glomerular basement membrane (gbm), and foot processes of visceral epithelial cytoplasm; m, mesangium; us, urinary space. B, Higher magnification of glomerular capillary wall consisting of fenestrated endothelial cytoplasm (c), glomerular basement membrane composed of three layers (lri, lamina rara internia; ld, lamina densa; lre, lamina rara externa), and foot processes (fp) of visceral epithelial cytoplasm. Slit pore membranes (s) are located between foot processes in the slit pores. Foot processes are covered with glomerular polyanion (p); v, cytoplasm of visceral epithelial cell. (From Osborne, C. A., et al.: The glomerulus in health and disease. Adv. Vet. Sci. Comp. Med. *21*:207–285, 1977.)

and renewal of the GBM. Demonstration of contractile elements in the mesangium and contractile response of glomerular cells to angiotensin II have led to the hypothesis that the mesangium may also play a role in modulation of glomerular filtration (Beeuwkes et al., 1981). Changes in mesangial cells (hypercellularity) and mesangial matrix (increased accumulation) reflect much of the injury to glomeruli associated with inflammation, and these areas appear to be the sites where hyaline material accumulates in patients with diabetes mellitus and amyloidosis.

The components of glomeruli function as a unit. Filtration of plasma through glomerular capillaries is influenced by several factors, including the size, shape, molecular configuration and charge of molecules, and the architecture of glomerular capillary walls (Fig. 73–2). Negatively charged sialoproteins that coat endothelial cells and visceral epithelial cells facilitate passage of cationic macromolecules and impede passage of anionic macromolecules. The glomerular basement membrane appears to impede passage of larger uncharged macromolecules, while slit pore membranes impede passage of somewhat smaller molecules. Visceral epithelial cells may also recover proteins that leak through the filters. The mesangium reconditions and unclogs the filtration barriers by removing and dispos-

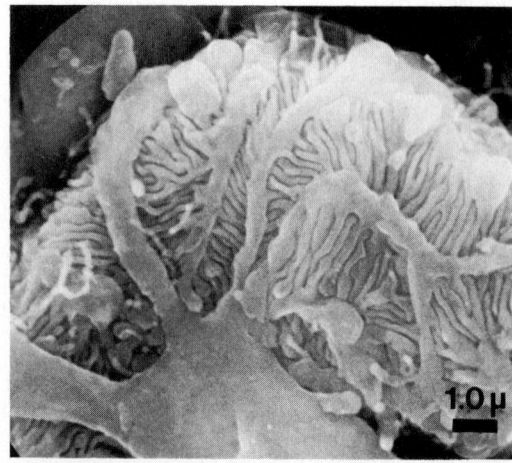

Figure 73–4. Scanning electron micrograph of glomerulus obtained from an adult dog illustrating interdigitating relationship of foot processes of visceral epithelial cells. (From Osborne, C. A. et al.: The glomerulus in health and disease. Adv. Vet. Sci. Comp. Med. *21*:207–285, 1977.)

wise interfere with filtration or damage the GBM. Mesangial cells also help to anchor (or support) the GBM, which does not completely surround glomerular capillary lumina. Mesangial cells are separated from each other by a variable quantity of dense basement-membrane-like material called mesangial matrix. It has been suggested that mesangial matrix is formed in part from deposition of "old" GBM following turnover

ing of filtration residues that accumulate on the endothelial side of the GBM.

Loss of the negative charge of glomerular capillary walls or damage to the GBM or slit pore membranes as a result of various disease processes may alter the selective semi-permeability of glomeruli and result in varying degrees of proteinuria. Disorders that result in proliferation and hypertrophy of mesangial cells and/or an increase in mesangial matrix may result in their encroachment on glomerular capillary lumen size. If generalized and severe, an increase in the mesangium may lead to reduced perfusion of glomerular capillaries, reduction in glomerular filtration rate, and retention of metabolites normally filtered by glomeruli (urea, creatinine, phosphorus, and so forth).

Bowman's Capsule. Bowman's capsule is composed of a collagenous membrane lined by flattened squamous epithelium called parietal epithelium (Figs. 73–1 and 73–5). Bowman's capsule has generally been assumed to function as a passive container for glomerular filtrate, which is then passed on to proximal tubules. Although passage of material through Bowman's capsule may be of little quantitative significance under physiologic conditions, it may become functionally significant under pathologic conditions (Osborne et al., 1977).

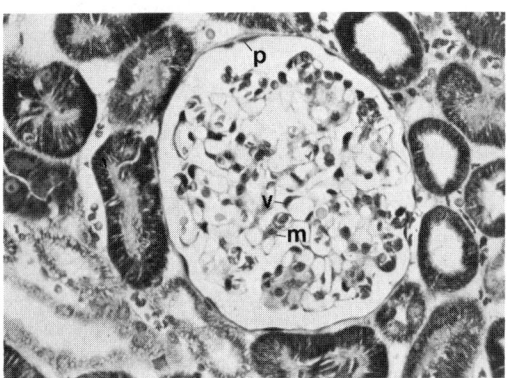

Figure 73–5. Photomicrograph of a normal glomerulus obtained from an adult dog. Bowman's capsule is lined by flattened parietal epithelial cells (p). Visceral epithelial cells (v) are adjacent to the glomerular basement membrane, which is of uniform thickness. Mesangial cells (m) are surrounded by glomerular capillary lumens. The glomerulus is surrounded by tubules. Tubules are surrounded by a sparse amount of interstitial tissue. PAS stain; 2 micron section; 100× = original magnification. (From Osborne, C. A., et al.: The glomerulus in health and disease. Adv. Vet. Sci. Comp. Med. *21*:207–285, 1977.)

Proliferation of parietal epithelial cells may result in formation of multiple layers of cells surrounded by varying quantities of collagen-like material that protrudes into Bowman's space (Fig. 73–6). Because proliferation of these cells results in concentric layers of cells and intracellular material, they are commonly called *crescents*. Progressive enlargement of crescents may encroach on the glomerulus and ultimately lead to adhesions and eventual tuft collapse. The consensus is that crescents represent a reaction of parietal epithelium to macromolecules that have escaped into the urinary space as a result of severe damage to glomerular capillary walls (Osborne et al., 1977). When present in large numbers in renal biopsy samples, crescents indicate severe and often irreversible glomerular damage.

Proximal Tubules. Proximal tubules collect glomerular filtrate from Bowman's space. The beginning portion of the proximal tubule has a convoluted configuration (pars convoluta) that pursues a meandering path through the renal cortex before a straight portion (pars recta) descends toward the renal medulla. Proximal tubules are lined by a single layer of columnar to cuboidal epithelial cells that contain subcellular organelles designed to permit active and passive reabsorption of almost 75 per cent of the glomerular filtrate (Table 73–1). The luminal borders of proximal tubular epithelial cells are completely covered with a well developed "brush-border" of numerous elongated microvilli. These microvilli increase the luminal reabsorptive surface area (by a factor greater than 35× in rabbits) of proximal tubules in a fashion analogous to the microvilli in the small intestine (Welling and Welling, 1975).

Loops of Henle. Filtrate modified by proximal tubules drains into loops of Henle, tubular structures that traverse a hairpin pathway as they move toward and then away from the renal pelvis (Fig. 73–7) (Bulger et al., 1979). The descending and ascending limbs of the loops of Henle run in opposite directions but in close proximity to each other.

As will be discussed, the loops of Henle play a major role in generating a gradient of solute concentration within the medullary interstitium that is substantially in excess of the solute concentration in plasma. The lengths of Henle's loops are dependent on

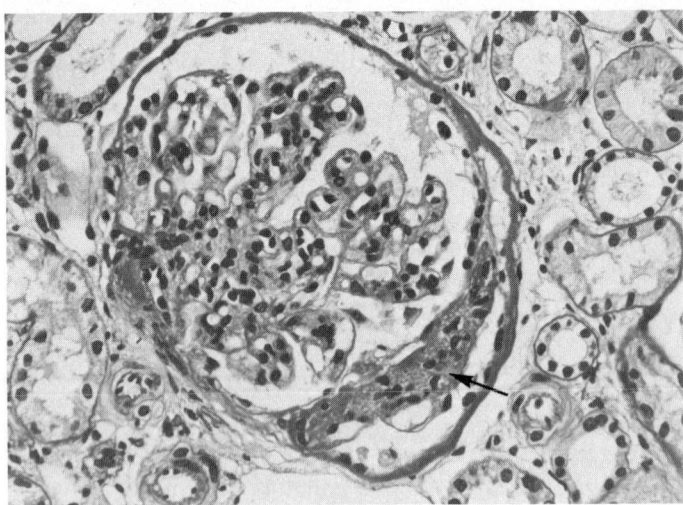

Figure 73–6. Photomicrograph of a renal biopsy specimen obtained from a proteinuric, uremic 11-year-old male German shorthair pointer dog illustrating membranoproliferative glomerulonephritis. A fibrocellular crescent protrudes into Bowman's space (arrow). PAS stain; 2 micron section; 100× = original magnification.

the location of corresponding glomeruli within the renal cortex. Nephrons with glomeruli in the outer cortex have the shortest loops of Henle, whereas nephrons with glomeruli located near the corticomedullary junction have the longest loops of Henle. Varying ability of different species to maximally concentrate urine (man = ±1.035; dog = ±1.060; cat = ±1.080) may be related, at least in part, to the ratio of shorter to

Table 73–1. Localization of Altered Glomerular Filtration and Azotemia

Cause	Localization of Azotemia
Decreased blood volume	Prerenal
Decreased blood pressure	Prerenal
Decreased colloidal osmotic pressure	Prerenal
Decreased number of patent vessels	Primary renal
Decreased glomerular permeability	Primary renal
Increased renal interstitial pressure	Primary renal
Increased intratubular pressure	Primary renal (tubular obstruction)
Increased intratubular pressure	Postrenal (obstruction of ureters, bladder, urethra)

longer loops, and to the actual length of loops (Schmidt-Nielsen and O'Dell, 1961; Tisher, 1981). Other factors may also be involved (Schmidt-Nielsen, 1979).

Distal Convoluted Tubules and Collecting Ducts. The thick ascending limbs of loops of Henle return in close proximity to the afferent arterioles and glomeruli from which they are attached. The distal tubule becomes somewhat dilated in the vicinity of its own glomerulus, and cells in that part of the tubule adjacent to juxtaglomerular cells of afferent arterioles become narrower and taller. These specialized tubular epithelial cells form the *macula densa,* a component of the juxtaglomerular apparatus. The macula densa arbitrarily marks the beginning of the distal convoluted tubule. Cells lining remaining portions of distal tubules are lower than those of proximal tubules and contain only a few luminal microvilli.

Distal convoluted tubules drain into collecting ducts, which progressively increase in size as they approach the renal pelvis. Portions of collecting ducts that enter the renal pelvis are often called papillary ducts.

Cells lining Henle's loops, distal tubules, and collecting ducts have been shown by immunofluorescent techniques to have the capacity to locally secrete a mucoprotein called Tamm-Horsfall (T-H) mucoprotein (Hoyer and Seiler, 1979). For reasons that remain poorly defined, precipitation of T-H mucoprotein within tubular lumens of these sites results in the formation of structures that conform to the shape of tubular

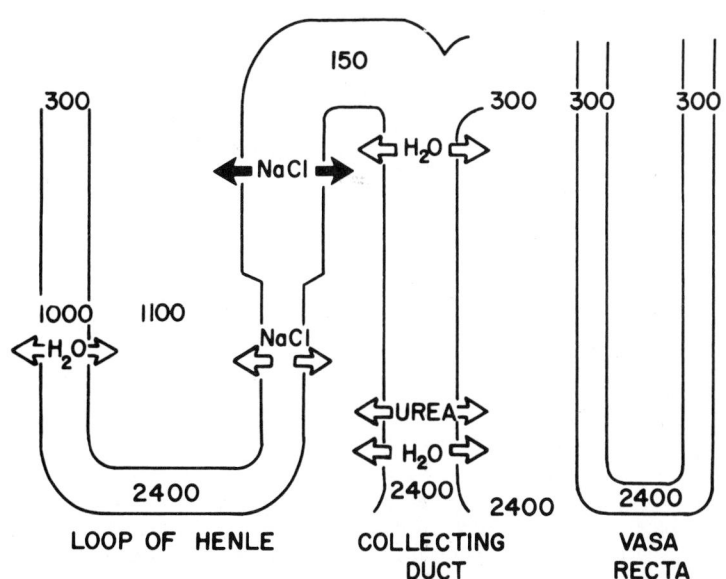

Figure 73–7. Schematic representation of a popular theory of the urine-concentrating mechanism in the renal medulla. Numbers represent milliosmoles per liter. Solute in the descending loop of Henle is concentrated by passive movement of water into the hyperosmolar interstitium. The ascending limb is impermeable to water, but NaCl moves into the interstitium passively (open arrows) in the inner medulla and by active transport (opaque arrow) in the outer medulla, creating dilute urine in the distal tubule (150 mOsm/ liter). Water may be reabsorbed in both the outer and inner medulla if collecting duct cells are rendered water permeable by ADH. Urea passively reabsorbed in the inner medulla in the presence of ADH contributes to interstitial hyperosmolarity. The vasa recta provide nutrition to the medulla and remove quantities of solute and solvent beyond that necessary to maintain normal interstitial volume and osmolality.

lumens. They are called *tubular casts.* Although the mechanism(s) responsible for precipitation of T-H mucoprotein is not understood, cast formation in these areas of nephrons is thought to be related (at least in part) to a summation of the following factors: secretion of T-H mucoprotein is limited to these sites, and urine has the potential of reaching maximum concentration and acidity at these sites (Hoyer and Seiler, 1979). Casts composed primarily of T-H mucoprotein are called hyaline casts (Schumann et al., 1978). If any material or object is present within the lumens of tubules at the time T-H mucoprotein gels, it may be incorporated into the casts. Entrapment of cells and other structures within the precipitated mucoprotein matrix has been likened to entrapment of fruit and vegetables in gelatin salads. Based on their morphologic appearance, casts may be classified as hyaline, epithelial cell, granular, waxy, fatty, red blood cell, white cell, hemoglobin, broad, or mixed casts (Stevens and Osborne, 1978). Since casts are formed in Henle's loops, distal tubules, and collecting ducts, detection of significant numbers of them in urine sediment indicates tubular involvement in an active pathologic process. Absence of casts does not rule out tubular disease, however, Casts are not a reliable index of the severity, duration, or reversibility of the underlying disease. They should

never be relied upon as an index of tubular function.

Interstitial Tissue. Interstitial tissue surrounds glomeruli, tubules, vessels, and nerves. It normally is scanty in quantity, but progressively increases from the cortex to the medulla (Fig. 73–5). Normal interstitial tissue is composed of fibroblasts, collagen, and a few mononuclear cells.

The predominant interstitial cell type in the renal medulla contains lipid (Tisher, 1981). Because the renal medulla is known to be a rich source of prostaglandins (a family of 20 carbon chain unsaturated fatty acids derived from arachidonic acid), these cells were considered to be the likely site of their production. Recent studies have cast considerable doubt on this hypothesis, however (Tisher, 1981). Unlike classical hormones, prostaglandins exert their biologic activity close to their site(s) of synthesis. Prostaglandin E_2 and $F_2\alpha$ appear to have a variety of biological activities that affect renal function, including their ability to suppress antidiuretic hormone activity and cause vasodilation, natriuresis, and renin release (Lifschitz and Stein, 1981).

Vascular Supply

Macrocirculation. Each kidney is usually supplied by one main renal artery. The left renal artery is a completely double structure in approximately 13 per cent of dogs (Barber, 1975; Reis and Tepe, 1956; Shiveley, 1978); double renal arteries occur in 10 per cent of cats (Rieck and Reis, 1953). The primary renal artery divides into two branches, each of which subdivides into so-called interlobar arteries (Fourman and Moffat, 1971).

Following penetration of the renal parenchyma at the level of the corticomedullary junction, interlobar arteries give rise to arcuate arteries. These in turn branch into interlobular arteries and eventually afferent arterioles (Beeuwkes, 1980). Afferent arterioles provide comparatively little resistance to blood flow and thus transmit blood at relatively high hydrostatic pressure to glomeruli. Afferent arterioles divide into numerous capillaries to form glomeruli, the sites of filtration of blood. Glomerular capillaries subsequently reunite to form one or more high resistance efferent arterioles (Fourman and Moffat, 1971). Coordination of vasomotor activity and vascular resistance to blood flow in afferent and efferent arterioles maintains renal blood flow at a relatively stable and high hydrostatic pressure despite wide variations in mean systemic arterial pressure (80 to 180 mmHg) (Pitts, 1974). This phenomenon tends to stabilize renal blood flow and filtration rate despite changes in renal arterial pressure. It is called *autoregulation* because renal blood flow is relatively independent of arterial pressure in denervated and isolated perfused kidneys. Therefore this autoregulatory control system must reside entirely within the kidney and must be independent of extrinsic nerves or bloodborne hormones.

Multiple renal veins are common in cats (Rieck and Reis, 1953), but are rare in dogs (Reis and Tepe, 1956). In both species, venous vessels anastomose at several levels. Both dogs and cats have well developed cortical venous systems (Beeuwkes, 1971; Beeuwkes et al., 1981). The cortical veins in cats form a prominent subcapsular network that extends around the surface of the kidney to join the renal vein at the hilus (Nissen and Galskov, 1972).

Renal arteries are considered to be "end arteries" without significant collateral blood supply. The clinical relevance of this observation is that sudden occlusion of any portion of the renal arterial tree by thrombosis or embolism would be followed by infarction of parenchyma perfused by the vessel distal to the obstructed site. Studies recently performed in normal and experimental dogs have revealed collateral arterial connections between interlobular or arcuate arteries and extrarenal arteries (i.e., phrenicoabdominal, spermatic, deep circumflex iliac, ureteral, caudal mesenteric, lumbar, and adrenal arteries) (Christie, 1980). In diseases associated with gradual occlusion of the main renal artery or its major branches, these collateral arterial connections may undergo sufficient hypertrophy to maintain significant renal function.

Microcirculation. The structure and function of glomeruli have been described under the section entitled The Nephron.

The microcirculation of the renal cortex differs greatly from that of the medulla. The efferent arterioles divide into capillaries of different structure and function, depending on their location within the renal cortex (Beeuwkes, 1981). Efferent arterioles derived from glomeruli in outer portions of the cortex form a peritubular capillary network that perfuses tubules and interstitial tissue primarily in the renal cortex. An association between efferent arterioles and corresponding tubules of the same nephron only exists for proximal tubules of the superficial cortex (Beeuwkes, 1981). There is perfusion of corticomedullary tubules originating from glomeruli located deeper in the cortex that are dissociated from post-efferent vessels of the same nephron, in that these capillaries may be derived from vessels originating from several unrelated nephrons (Beeuwkes, 1971; Beeuwkes and Bonaventure, 1975). Whereas superficial cortical microcirculation patterns can be highly localized, perfusion patterns of the juxtamedullary cortex and medulla are derived from several sources. This microvascular organization provides a plausible explanation for the patchy and seemingly unpredictable pattern of tubular epithelial cell and basement membrane destruction commonly associated with acute ischemic renal failure (Beeuwkes et al., 1981).

Efferent arterioles that arise from glomeruli located adjacent to the medulla form vessels (*vasa recta*) that loop deep into the renal medulla before returning to the cortex (Fig. 73–7). Multiple vasa recta arise from a single efferent arteriole (Fourman and Moffat, 1971). Their hairpin configuration is similar to that of the loops of

Henle. Vasa recta play a vital role in the so-called countercurrent system by removing water from the medullary interstitium that would otherwise reduce the concentration of solute trapped there.

High resistance efferent arterioles reduce the hydrostatic pressure in peritubular capillaries to a value significantly below that in glomerular capillaries. Whereas the high hydrostatic pressure in glomerular capillaries favors glomerular filtration, the much reduced hydrostatic pressure in peritubular capillaries favors reabsorption of solute and water from tubular lumens (Brenner and Beeuwkes, 1978).

Blood perfusing peritubular capillaries must first pass through glomeruli. Knowledge of this vascular pattern arranged in series is of clinical significance, because it provides a plausible explanation of one mechanism whereby diseases of glomeruli may result in secondary diseases of tubulo-interstitial structures. Interruption in blood flow through glomeruli will result in a corresponding reduction in perfusion of peritubular capillaries. The potential consequence is ischemic atrophy and/or necrosis of tubulo-interstitial structures.

In a review of "the renal circulations" by Brenner and Beeuwkes, renal circulation was described as a composite of several microcirculations, each having a specialized role (Brenner and Beeuwkes, 1978). While nephrons compose the accepted functional units of the kidney, they cannot function independently of vascular perfusion. The microcirculation in each different region of the kidney has a structural organization and vascular properties uniquely suited to specific exchange processes at the capillary level that will provide the final ureteral urine of required volume and composition. The glomerular circulation is specialized for filtration, the first step in urine formation; the cortical peritubular capillary network is specialized for reabsorption of fluid and solutes from tubules; the medullary circulation is specialized to facilitate urine concentration and dilution. Abnormalities of these specialized microcirculations play important roles in the pathophysiology of renal disease. Selective damage to glomerular capillaries leads to decreased glomerular filtration rate and/or proteinuria. Similarly, destruction of medullary microcirculations impairs urine concentration and/or dilution.

URINE FORMATION

Basic Mechanisms

The urinary system plays a major role in maintaining homeostasis by eliminating waste products from the body in soluble form. In the process the kidneys are intimately involved in the control and maintenance of body balance (i.e., maintenance of a constant amount) of water, electrolytes, acid-base metabolites, and some hormones. Conceptual understanding of renal functions is an essential prerequisite to comprehension of fundamentally different mechanisms that may cause renal disorders and to formulation of therapy to correct them.

Formation of urine by nephrons results from three basic processes: glomerular filtration, tubular reabsorption, and tubular secretion. Viewed from a slightly different perspective, the kidney processes some substances primarily by glomerular filtration (creatinine), some primarily by glomerular filtration and tubular reabsorption (glucose, sodium, amino acids, and so forth), some by filtration, reabsorption and secretion (potassium), and some primarily by tubular secretion (hydrogen ion and ammonia). The combined effect of these functions on the removal of a substance from plasma and excretion of that substance in urine is often referred to as *clearance* of the substance. Clearance of a filtered substance is only equal to glomerular filtration rate when the substance is not reabsorbed or secreted by renal tubules.

Glomerular Filtration

Mechanism. The initial phase of urine formation consists of production of a large quantity of an acellular low-protein ultrafiltrate of blood "filtered" through glomeruli. Formation of filtrate from blood (or plasma) is a passive (non-energy requiring) process for the kidneys. Energy required for glomerular filtration is derived from blood pressure generated by contraction of the left ventricle and the elasticity of vascular walls. The rate at which kidneys form glomerular filtrate from plasma is called the *glomerular filtration rate* (GFR).

Factors that influence the quantity and quality of glomerular filtrate include (1) hydrostatic (blood) pressure, (2) volume of blood in glomerular capillaries, (3) colloidal osmotic (or oncotic) pressure of blood in glomerular capillaries, (4) the number of patent renal vessels and glomerular capillaries, (5) the permeability of glomerular capillaries, (6) renal interstitial pressure, and (7) renal intratubular hydrostatic pressure (Table 73–1). The quantity of protein in glomerular filtrate contained in Bowman's space is normally so small that the resulting osmotic effect is not significant enough to enhance glomerular filtration. Arterial hydrostatic pressure is the major force favoring glomerular filtration. Forces that oppose glomerular filtration include colloidal osmotic pressure (which arises primarily from non-filtered protein molecules, especially albumin, in glomerular capillary plasma), renal intratubular and interstitial pressure, and the selective permeability of glomerular capillary walls.

The major function of glomeruli is to behave as a sieve that increasingly restricts passage of macromolecules of increasing diameter and molecular weight. Most substances in glomerular filtrate have a molecular weight of less than 68,000 daltons (Table 73–2). Since cells, most proteins (and therefore molecules bound to proteins), and most lipoproteins are too large to pass through glomerular capillary walls, they are retained within the vascular compartment and are not present in glomerular filtrate in significant quantities.

Although the ability of many substances to traverse glomerular capillary walls is related to their molecular weight, electrical charge is also an extremely important variable that influences the degree to which some charged macromolecules are filtered. The negative charge of glomerular capillary walls impedes the passage of negatively charged (anionic) macromolecules (such as albumin) that otherwise would be small enough to be filtered (at least to some degree). In contrast, the negatively charged glomerular capillary wall enhances filtration of some positively charged (cationic) macromolecules. The shape (or configuration) of macromolecules may also influence their ability to traverse glomerular capillary walls (Fig. 73–2).

Glomerular filtrate is qualitatively similar to plasma with respect to its concentration of electrolytes and macromolecules of relatively low molecular weight. Glomerular filtrate contains the majority (but not all) of the solutes and water that must be eliminated from the body, but often in quantities far in excess of those that ultimately appear in urine. It also contains a large quantity of vital metabolites that must be retrieved prior to elimination in urine if body homeostasis is to be maintained. At first impression the composition of glomerular filtrate might appear to be paradoxic, since one might expect the glomerular "filter" to retain vital metabolites in plasma and to permit only waste products to escape into the urinary space. Glomeruli effectively restrict passage of vital blood components such as cells and most proteins but are unable to discriminate between vital and waste metabolites that are similar in structure and electrical charge. The common denominator of substances that appear in glomerular filtrate appears to be related, not to their potential value to the body, but to their molecular characteristics (size, shape, and electrical charge). In order for the kidneys to regulate body fluid, electrolyte, and acid-base balance, it is essential that both beneficial and worthless metabolites with similar characteristics be subjected to potential loss in urine.

Table 73–2. Comparison of Molecular Weights of Substances Included in, and Excluded from, Glomerular Filtrate

Substance	Molecular Weight	Presence in Glomerular Filtrate
Water	18	+
Potassium	19	+
Urea	60	+
Phosphate	96	+
Creatinine	113	+
Glucose	180	+
Lysozyme	14,000	+
Myoglobin	17,000	+
Bence Jones monomers	22,000	+
Bence Jones dimers	44,000	+
Amylase	50,000	+
Hemoglobin*	68,000	±
Albumin	69,000	±
Immunoglobulin-G	160,000	−
Immunoglobulin-A (dimer)	300,000	−
Fibrinogen	400,000	−
Alpha-2-macroglobulin	840,000	−
Immunoglobulin-M	900,000	−

*Probably excreted as a dimer with a molecular weight of approximately 32,000.

Clinical Correlation. It is conceptually useful to view the consequences of glomerular dysfunction as impaired excretion of unwanted metabolites such as urea and creatinine and/or unwanted excretion of vital metabolites, primarily plasma proteins.

Abnormal retention of nonprotein nitrogenous waste products such as urea and creatinine as a result of reduced glomerular filtration is one form of azotemia. As will be discussed, azotemia that results from decreased GFR may be categorized (or localized) as prerenal, primary renal, and postrenal (Table 73–1).

Most forms of glomerular damage, especially immune mediated glomerulonephropathy and canine renal amyloidosis, are associated with a variable degree of increased permeability of glomerular capillary walls to protein molecules (Table 73–3). A characteristic and occasionally the only clinical indication of glomerular dysfunction is persistent proteinuria, which is often unassociated with significant hematuria or pyuria. Albumin is the principal protein found in the urine of such patients, allegedly because of its size (Table 73–2). Depending on the severity of damage to glomerular capillary walls, varying quantities of plasma proteins with higher molecular weights may also be excreted. Because plasma proteins tend to reduce the solubility of Tamm-Horsfall mucoprotein, hyaline or granular casts may also be observed. Prolonged and/or severe proteinuria that occurs secondary to damage to glomerular capillary walls may initiate physiologic, metabolic, and nutritional defects associated with the nephrotic syndrome (Osborne et al., 1977). The nephrotic syndrome is characterized by proteinuria, hypoproteinemia, hypoalbuminemia, hypercholesterolemia, and frequently edema. It may or may not be associated with decreased glomerular filtration rate and azotemia.

If the proteinuria that occurs secondary to damage to the filtration barriers of glomerular capillary walls is persistent and severe, urine protein (especially albumin) loss may exceed the capacity of the liver to maintain normal plasma protein concentration. In uremic patients, increase in the rate of endogenous catabolism of albumin and decreased dietary intake of protein may also contribute to hypoalbuminemia. Since albumin molecules account for approximately 77 per cent of plasma colloidal osmotic pressure, progressive hypoalbuminemia is associated with a proportionate decrease in plasma colloidal osmotic pressure. According to the Starling-Landis cycle of capillary-interstitial fluid exchange, a marked decrease in colloidal osmotic pressure will initiate an abnormal shift of fluid from the vascular compartment to the extravascular compartment, resulting in hypovolemia and edema. Nonpainful pitting edema is usually most severe in dependent portions of the

Table 73–3. **Magnitude of Proteinuria Commonly Associated with Selected Urinary and Nonurinary Disorders**

Disorder	Reaction of Urine to Strip Tests or Sulfosalicylic Acid			
	Trace to 100 mg	*100–500 mg*	*500–1000 mg*	*>1000 mg*
Nonurinary				
Strenuous exercise	±			
Fever	±			
Hyperproteinemia (>10 grams/dl)	±	±	Uncommon	
Congestive heart failure	±			
Inflammatory or hemorrhagic diseases of the genital system	+	+	±	
Urinary: Renal				
Glomerular	+	+	+	+
Tubular	+	±		
Inflammatory	+	+	+	
Hemorrhagic	+	+	+	
Urinary: Ureter, Bladder, Urethra				
Inflammatory	+	+	+	
Hemorrhagic	+	+	+	

body (ventral midline, limbs) because venous hydrostatic pressure is greatest in these locations. In severe cases, ascites and hydrothorax may develop.

Tubular Reabsorption and Secretion. Some filtered substances (creatinine and allantoin) cannot be reutilized by the body and are not reabsorbed by tubules. Other filtered substances (amino acids, vitamins, glucose) are essential for body homeostasis and are almost completely reabsorbed by energy-requiring, active tubular transport mechanisms. The body's requirement for water, electrolytes, and some other filtered substances is variable, being dependent on intake, metabolism, and loss of these substances via nonrenal routes. Nephrons regulate conservation and excretion of these substances by active or passive tubular reabsorption. Still other metabolites (hydrogen ion, ammonia, and potassium) gain entrance into urine primarily by tubular secretion. Thus, as glomerular filtrate passes through the tubules, it rapidly loses its original identity as tubular reabsorption and tubular secretion selectively modify it according to body need. Whereas formation of glomerular filtrate is a passive process for the kidneys, modification of glomerular filtrate by the tubules appears to demand the majority of energy expended by the kidneys.

Approximately 75 per cent of the total volume of glomerular filtrate is recovered by proximal tubular reabsorption. While proximal tubular reabsorption of water is passive, proximal tubular reabsorption of many substances (amino acids, calcium, glucose, and others) is an active process that requires energy (Table 73–4). Reabsorption of many metabolites is influenced by hormones.

Some metabolites (including glucose, amino acids, and water soluble vitamins) are called *threshold substances,* because the capacity of tubules to reabsorb them is not unlimited. They are almost totally reabsorbed from glomerular filtrate, provided their concen-

Table 73–4. Summary of Physiologic Activities in Nephrons and Collecting Ducts During Formation of Urine

Component of Nephron	Physiologic Process	
Glomerulus	Passive formation of ultrafiltrate of plasma devoid of most protein	
Bowman's capsule	Collection of glomerular filtrate	
Proximal tubule	*Active Reabsorption of:* Glucose, proteins & amino acids, vitamins, ascorbic acid, acetoacetate, hydroxybutyrate, uric acid, sodium, potassium, calcium ($\uparrow$ by PTH), phosphate ($\downarrow$ by PTH), sulfate, bicarbonate	
	Passive Reabsorption of: Chloride, water, urea	*Active Secretion of:* Hydrogen ion
Henle's loop	Generation of medullary hyperosmolality	
Descending limb	*Passive Reabsorption of:* Water	*Passive Secretion of:* Sodium, urea
Thin ascending limb	*Passive Reabsorption of:* Urea, sodium impermeable to water	
Thick ascending limb	*Active Reabsorption of:* Chloride, calcium	*Passive Reabsorption of:* Sodium, impermeable to water, potassium
Distal tubule	*Active Reabsorption of:* Sodium ($\uparrow$ by aldosterone), calcium, HCO_3^- small amounts of glucose	*Passive Reabsorption of:* Chloride, water ($\uparrow$ by ADH)
	Active Secretion of: Hydrogen ion, ammonia, uric acid	*Passive Secretion of:* Potassium
Collecting ducts	*Active Reabsorption of:* Sodium ($\uparrow$ by aldosterone)	*Passive Reabsorption of:* Chloride, water ($\uparrow$ by ADH)
	Active Secretion of: Hydrogen ion	*Passive Secretion of:* Potassium

tration is not excessive. If their concentration in blood, and thus glomerular filtrate, exceeds the capacity of tubular transport mechanisms, however, a "threshold" concentration is reached, above which they spill into urine. Thus, hyperglycemic glucosuria occurs when venous blood glucose concentrations exceed approximately 180 mg/dl. The maximal rate at which an active transport system can reabsorb a particular solute is called its *transport maximum* (abbreviated T_m). The amount of a particular solute transported is proportionate to the amount present in tubular filtrate up to the T_m for the solute. At higher concentrations, the transport mechanism is saturated and there is no appreciable increment in the amount transported.

Filtrate also undergoes considerable modification by tubular reabsorptive and secretory processes in the distal tubules and collecting ducts. Some events of clinical significance that occur in distal nephrons include hydrogen ion secretion, ammonia secretion, potassium excretion, bicarbonate and sodium reabsorption, and urine concentration or dilution (Table 73–4). Antidiuretic hormone significantly influences water reabsorption in distal nephrons by increasing tubular epithelial cell permeability.

Clinical Correlation. Impairment of tubular reabsorption may lead to unwanted loss of varying quantities of metabolites (calcium, bicarbonate, water soluble vitamins, and so forth), while impairment of tubular secretion may result in retention of some unwanted metabolites (hydrogen ion, potassium, and so on). If severe, systemic excesses and/or deficits in fluid, electrolyte, and acid-base balance may induce polysystemic disease. Correction of systemic water, electrolyte, and acid-base imbalances caused by glomerular and/or tubular dysfunction is a primary goal of symptomatic and supportive management of patients with primary renal failure and uremia.

Relationship to Hormones

Hormonal Influence on Renal Function. Glomerular filtration, tubular reabsorption, and tubular secretion are modified and integrated by several hormones and other bioactive agents, including renin-angiotensin, catecholamines, antidiuretic hormone, aldosterone, parathormone, glucagon, growth hormone, prohormone (vitamin) D, prostaglandins, calcitonin, thyroxin, and probably a natriuretic factor (Katz and Lindheimer, 1977; Klahr and Rodriguez, 1975; Stein, 1979). In this context, nephrons may be viewed as end organs for multifaceted biological control systems. It is not surprising, therefore, that endocrinopathies frequently adversely affect body homeostasis by altering renal function. Notable examples include pituitary and renal diabetes insipidus, inappropriate secretion of antidiuretic hormone, hyperadrenocorticism, hypoadrenocorticism, diabetes mellitus, hyperthyroidism, primary hyperparathyroidism, and pseudohyperparathyroidism.

The Kidney as an Endocrine Organ. In addition to being influenced by various extrarenal hormones, the kidneys produce hormones that act on other target organs. The kidneys are involved in regulation of red cell production by way of synthesis and release of erythropoietin when the oxygen tension of blood perfusing the kidneys is reduced (Fisher, 1979; Fried, 1975; Spivak and Graber, 1980). The site(s) of production of erythropoietin within the kidneys is unknown, but the juxtaglomerular apparatus, glomeruli, and renal medulla have been proposed (Anagnostou et al., 1981; Busuttil et al., 1972). Although there are extrarenal sites of erythropoietin production in some species, the kidneys are apparently the sole site of its production in dogs (Fisher, 1972; Murphy et al., 1970). The carotid bodies have been reported to be an extrarenal site of erythropoietin production in cats (Tramezzani et al., 1971). Erythropoietin stimulates stem cells in bone marrow to form sufficient red cells to correct hypoxemia.

Impaired production of erythropoietin contributes to nonregenerative anemia, a well-known complication of chronic uremia. Administration of erythropoietin would logically appear to be of value in the treatment of uremic anemia, but quantities in excess of those normally released by the kidneys might be required, since bone marrow cells are less responsive to erythropoietin in a uremic environment (Naetz, 1975; Stone and Max, 1979). Because of contamination with endotoxins, commercially produced erythropoietin is not currently available. To date, androgenic anabolic hormones (testosterone and synthetic derivatives of testosterone) appear to be the most useful nonspecific stimulus of red cell production in uremic patients (Osborne and Polzin, 1979).

In contrast to the nonregenerative anemia associated with impaired production of erythropoietin in patients with chronic primary renal failure, secondary erythrocytosis may be caused by excessive production of erythropoietin as a result of local (rather than systemic) renal hypoxia. Disorders incriminated in secondary erythrocytosis include constriction of renal arteries, intrarenal vascular lesions, hydronephrosis, renal cysts, and vasoactive agents (Osborne and Johnston, 1977). Renal neoplasms, especially renal cell carcinomas, may produce excessive quantities of erythropoietin and induce erythrocytosis irrespective of systemic blood oxygen tension (Scott and Patnaik, 1972).

The kidneys influence calcium and phosphorus homeostasis by metabolizing vitamin (prohormone) D (25-hydroxycholecalciferol), which is formed in the liver, to its most metabolically active form (1,25-dihydroxycholecalciferol) (Deluca, 1973; Schoolwerth, 1975). Intracellular phosphorus concentration influences production of 1.25-vitamin D (i.e., a low intracellular phosphorus concentration enhances its production). Since intracellular phosphorus concentration in renal tubular epithelial cells is influenced by parathormone, parathormone influences 1,25-vitamin D synthesis. Some important roles of vitamin D include stimulation of calcium absorption from the small intestines (an action that is augmented by parathormone) and mobilization of calcium and phosphorus from bone in conjunction with parathormone. Because 1,25-dihydroxycholecalciferol is synthesized by the kidneys and acts on distant target organs (bones and intestines), it has recently been classified as a hormone.

Clinical and experimental evidence indicate that renal secondary hyperparathyroidism is a frequent complication of chronic renal failure and begins early during the course of renal failure (Coburn and Slatopolsky, 1981; Osborne and Polzin, 1979). Reduced renal clearance of phosphorus resulting in hyperphosphatemia plays a major role in initiating renal secondary hyperpara-

thyroidism. Hyperphosphatemia leads to a reciprocal decrease in serum calcium concentration (hypocalcemia), which in turn causes increased production of parathormone (hyperparathormonemia). Impaired renal synthesis of 1,25-vitamin D plays a significant role in perpetuating and augmenting the severity of renal secondary hyperparathyroidism, and may be caused by generalized renal lesions and/or increased production of parathormone. Administration of 1,25-vitamin D or a vitamin D analogue in conjunction with therapy to minimize hyperphosphatemia to human beings with naturally occurring chronic renal failure, and dogs with experimentally induced chronic renal failure, has been of benefit in controlling renal secondary hyperparathyroidism and associated abnormalities (Fiaschi et al., 1978; Rutherford et al., 1977).

Renal Degradation of Hormones. The kidneys also degrade and/or excrete several hormones including parathormone, growth hormone, secretin, cholecystokinin, glucagon, gastrin, prolactin, circulating insulin, thyrotropic hormone, and antidiuretic hormone (Avioli, 1978; Bonomini et al., 1979; Onyang et al., 1979; Knochel and Seldin, 1981). Failure to degrade hormones as a consequence of renal failure plays an important role in the etiopathogenesis of the uremic syndrome. Excessive quantities of hormones normally degraded by the kidneys have been added to the impressively long list of so-called "uremic toxins" (Table 73–5).

The Juxtaglomerular Apparatus and Tubuloglomerular Feedback Structure. Specialized myoepithelial cells called juxtaglomerular cells are located in the walls of the afferent and efferent arterioles adjacent to corresponding glomeruli. These cells contain renin and other biologically active substances important in regulation of renal and systemic blood pressure and blood flow.

The distal portions of the thick ascending limbs of the loops of Henle pass in close proximity to the juxtaglomerular cells of afferent arterioles of corresponding nephrons. At this site, modified tubular epithelial cells, collectively called the macula densa, can be identified. The macula densa has arbitrarily been designated as the point where loops of Henle end and distal tubules begin.

Juxtaglomerular cells of the afferent and

Table 73–5. Some Metabolites Which Have Been Incriminated as Uremic Toxins

Acetoin	Hippuric acid
Amines	Hyperosmolality
Aliphatic	Indole and its derivatives
Aromatic	Lipochromes
Polyamines	Middle molecules
Ammonia	Monoamine oxidase
Calcitonin	Myoinositol
Creatinine	Natriuretic hormone
Cyanate	Oxalic acid
Cyclic AMP	Parathormone
Excesses of electrolytes	Phenol and its derivatives
Gastrin	Pseudouridine
Glucagon	Renin
Glucuronic acid	Sulfates
Growth hormone	Urea
Guanadine and its derivatives	Uric acid
Guanidinoacetic acid	
Guanidinosuccinic acid	
Methylguanidine	

efferent arterioles, the macula densa of distal tubules, and granular cells (also called lacis cells) located between these two structures are collectively called the *juxtaglomerular apparatus.*

FUNCTION. The juxtaglomerular apparatus plays an important role in modifying systemic hemodynamics and local renal hemodynamics. As reviewed in detail elsewhere, stimuli that decrease extracellular fluid volume, reduce mean renal perfusion pressure, and/or stimulate sympathetic activity result in release of a proteolytic enzyme called renin, primarily from afferent arterioles, and to a lesser extent from efferent arterioles and lacis cells (Lifschitz and Stein, 1981). Renin converts a circulating inactive plasma protein called angiotensin, which is produced in the liver, to angiotensin I. Angiotensin I is subsequently converted to a potent vasoconstrictor called angiotensin II by so-called "converting" enzymes located primarily in the lung. Converting enzymes are also present in other tissues, including the kidneys. In addition to its effect on vascular tone, angiotensin II stimulates the release of aldosterone from the adrenal cortex. Aldosterone in turn promotes tubular reabsorption of sodium (and water) and tubular secretion of potassium. Local production of angiotensin II by the kidneys affects renal vasomotor activity, while local production of angiotensin II in the brain stimulates thirst (Severs and Daniels-Severs, 1973).

Angiotensin II has an extremely short biological half-life (less than one minute under normal conditions) (Lifschitz and Stein, 1981). It is apparently inactivated by several organs, including the kidneys.

The juxtaglomerular apparatus appears to play a significant role in modifying intrarenal hemodynamics in response to stimuli originating from the renal tubules (Lifschitz and Stein, 1981). There is a consensus that events related to tubular modification of glomerular filtrate are detected and relayed by macula densa cells to juxtaglomerular cells, which in turn affect glomerular filtration rate by inducing dilation or constriction of afferent arterioles. Available data suggest that as glomerular filtration rate increases, flooding of proximal tubular transport sites results in an increase in the rate and volume of tubular filtrate (including chloride ion) at the site of the macula densa. As a result, an increased quantity of chloride is reabsorbed by the macula densa (Thurau et al., 1972). Increased quantities of chloride in juxtaglomerular cells are followed by generation and/or release of biologically active substances (renin-angiotensin, prostaglandins, and/or cyclic AMP), which reduce glomerular filtration rate by causing vasoconstriction of afferent arterioles. This tubuloglomerular feedback mechanism helps to coordinate glomerular filtration and tubular reabsorption, even though both mechanisms are dependent on different energy sources.

Clinical Correlation. Disorders that cause reduced renal perfusion pressure and/or reduced tension of afferent arteriolar walls may stimulate release of renin and activation of angiotensin. Increased angiotensin activity increases vascular tone and stimulates aldosterone-mediated tubular reabsorption of sodium and water. Hypertension and/or edema may result. Examples of disorders that may be associated with these events include renal artery stenosis (so-called renovascular hypertension) and congestive heart failure.

Tubuloglomerular feedback has been hypothesized to play a protective role in some forms of acute renal failure associated with generalized damage to tubules by initiating a phase of oliguria (Thurau and Boylan, 1976). The need for oliguria can be emphasized by the fact that the circulating volume of plasma is filtered and reabsorbed by the kidneys approximately twice each hour.

When nephrotoxic agents or renal ischemia cause generalized acute tubular necrosis, impaired tubular reabsorption of glomerular filtrate could lead to rapid death from profound loss of fluid and metabolites. An appropriate compensatory response to a signal indicating reabsorptive failure is reduction in glomerular filtration rate. It has been suggested that marked increase in the concentration of chloride ions at the site of the macula densa as a consequence of impaired tubular reabsorption in proximal portions of nephrons stimulates local production and release of angiotensin, which in turn causes intense constriction of afferent arterioles. Profound reduction in GFR results in oliguria, which in turn prevents rapid depletion of fluid and electrolytes from the body. Thus life can be sustained for a longer period. In this situation, glomeruli have assumed the volume-conserving function normally handled by the tubules. The trade-off for indiscriminate renal conservation of fluid and metabolites, however, is retention of metabolic wastes normally cleared from plasma by filtration. The immediate threat to life is averted, but at the expense of regulation of body fluid composition. Azotemia, hyperkalemia, hyperphosphatemia, acidemia, and other metabolic imbalances associated with acute oliguric renal failure are the consequence. If allowed to progress, death from uremia will ultimately occur. According to this hypothesis, if the patient survives long enough to permit sufficient regeneration and repair of underlying lesions so that the tubules regain some ability to reabsorb filtrate, glomerular filtration rate will improve. Because restoration of GFR often does not correspond to restoration of tubular reabsorption, however, a secondary phase of polyuria often occurs. When adequate regeneration, repair, and compensatory changes have occurred, tubuloglomerular balance and urine volume return to normal.

Concentration and Dilution of Urine

The kidneys play a vital role in maintaining fluid balance by regulating the excretion of water. They may conserve (or concentrate) water in times of need, and eliminate (or dilute) urine when the body contains excessive water. The fact that transport of water from one area to another is passive, following gradients established by hydrostatic and osmotic forces, is of fundamental importance in comprehending urine concentration and dilution (Table 73–6). Knowledge that concentration and dilution of urine excreted into the renal pelvis are terms comparing final urine composition to glomerular filtrate is also of fundamental importance. Urine concentration is associated with tubular conservation of water in excess of solute; urine dilution is associated with conservation of solute in excess of water.

Urine Concentration. Of the approximately 60 liters of glomerular filtrate formed by a 20-lb adult dog each day, less than one per cent (approximately 0.5 liter) is normally eliminated as urine. Almost 75 per cent of the water is passively reabsorbed by proximal tubules following active reabsorption of solutes such as sodium, calcium, phosphorus, glucose and others (Table 73–4). Since the relative quantities of water and solute reabsorbed by proximal tubules are more or less equal, the osmolality and specific gravity of modified filtrate at their

---

Table 73–6. Some Facts About Urine Concentration

1. Water cannot be actively transported across tubular basement membranes. It passively follows osmotic gradients created by movement or accumulation of solute.

2. Final concentration of urine characterized by removal of more water than solute occurs in the distal tubules and collecting ducts.

3. Concentration of urine is dependent on hyperosmolality of renal medullary interstitial tissue.

4. Renal medullary hyperosmolality is generated and maintained by the counter-current system.

5. Urine concentration is dependent on increased permeability of epithelial cells in the distal tubules and collecting ducts mediated by antidiuretic hormone.

terminal portions is roughly the same as that of glomerular filtrate (SG = ± 1.008 to 1.012; mOsm/L = ± 300). Proximal tubular reabsorption of water is often referred to as "obligatory water reabsorption," since it is not influenced by mechanisms specifically directed toward modulation of fluid balance. Even though proximal tubules do not play a primary role in water balance, they may affect the volume and concentration of final urine if pharmacologic (osmotic diuretics) or pathologic (hyperglycemic glucosuria, Fanconi syndrome, and so forth) mechanisms impede the usual quantity of solute (and therefore water) from being reabsorbed. Interference with proximal tubular reabsorption may overwhelm the reabsorptive capacity of distal portions of nephrons. The mechanism of the resultant pharmacologic or pathologic polyuria is commonly referred to as osmotic diuresis (in contrast to water diuresis) (Gennard and Kassirer, 1974; Osborne et al., 1975).

The descending and beginning portions of the ascending limbs of Henle's loops are lined by flattened attenuated cells, whereas the terminal portions of the ascending limbs are lined by thicker cells (and thus they are called the thick ascending limb of Henle's loops). Differences in morphology in various segments of Henle's loops are related to differences in their ability to actively transport solute (Table 73–4). Chloride is actively (and sodium, passively) transported out of lumens of thick ascending limbs of Henle's loops, which are impermeable to water.

The quantity of water removed from modified filtrate by the distal nephron is influenced by body water balance. Recall that the loops of Henle and vasa recta have a structure that is responsible for a gradient of increasing solute concentration (especially sodium, chloride, and urea) from the outer portion (adjacent to the cortex) to the inner portion (adjacent to the renal pelvis). The anatomic configuration and function of medullary tubules (loops of Henle, distal tubules, and collecting ducts) and vessels (vasa recta) responsible for hyperosmolality of renal medullary interstitial tissue are collectively called the "countercurrent system." The structure and function of this system have been described in detail (Hay, 1976; Jamison and Maffley, 1976; Jamison, 1981) but are beyond the scope of this chapter. Conceptual understanding of this system, however, is a fundamental prerequisite to meaningful evaluation of patients with disorders of urine concentration and dilution. The name "countercurrent system" depicts the fact that the hairpin shape of the loops of Henle and vasa recta allow filtrate inflow to run parallel to, in close proximity to, and in an opposite direction to that of filtrate outflow (Fig. 73–7). The anatomic arrangement of Henle's loop multiplies the osmotic gradient actively generated by this structure as it moves toward the renal pelvis. Vasa recta are often called "countercurrent exchangers." In addition to providing nutrients to structures in the renal medulla, they remove water and excess solute reabsorbed by the distal tubules and collecting ducts. Because of the relatively slow rate of blood flow in the vasa recta, solutes passively diffuse out of portions of vessels leaving the medulla and into portions of vessels traveling toward the renal pelvis. Conversely, water passively diffuses out of descending vessels and into ascending vessels. Hyperosmolality is maintained because solutes tend to circulate in the medulla, whereas water tends to bypass it.

In the thin descending limb of the loops of Henle, water passively leaves the tubular lumens, attracted by the ever-increasing gradient of solutes in medullary interstitial tissue generated by the countercurrent system. As a result, intraluminal solute increases in concentration. At the turn of the loop, tubular filtrate is almost as hyperosmotic as the adjacent medullary interstitium, because water has been removed in excess of solute (in dogs SG = ± 1.060 and mOsm/L = ± 2400; in cats SG = ± 1.080 and mOsm/L = ± 3000). Solute (sodium chloride) is actively transported out of the thick ascending portion of Henle's loop, but an equivalent amount of water cannot passively follow (Table 73–4). Separation of sodium chloride and water at this site is important in establishment of medullary interstitial hyperosmolality. Because solute is removed from tubular lumens in excess of water, the fluid that enters the distal tubular lumens of dogs is hypo-osmotic (Clapp and Robinson, 1966), and the fluid that enters the distal tubular lumens of cats is iso-osmotic (Finco, 1980), compared with glomerular filtrate (and plasma). In the process of moving through loops of Henle, an additional five per cent of the original volume of

Table 73–7. Some Facts About Antidiuretic Hormone*

1. ADH (also called vasopressin) is formed in the supraoptic and paraventricular nuclei of the hypothalamus.

2. Dogs and most other mammals (except pigs) form arginine vasopressin.

3. ADH flows in transport granules via axons in the hypothalamoneurohypophyseal tract to the posterior pituitary gland, where it is stored.

4. Stimulation of osmoreceptors located in the anterior hypothalamus by an increase (approximately 2% or greater) in plasma osmolality will increase the rate of neuronal discharge and result in release of ADH in the systemic circulation.

5. ADH increases the permeability of distal tubular and collecting duct epithelium to water.

6. The biologic half-life of ADH is relatively short (approximately 30 to 45 minutes). It is thought to be inactivated by the kidney and liver.

7. Factors other than an increase in plasma osmolality may result in the release of ADH, including reduction in blood volume, angiotensin II, pain, surgical stress, morphine, nicotine, and barbiturates.

*Adapted from Forsling, M. L.: Antidiuretic hormone. Ann. Res. Rev. *4*:1–164, 1979; Hays, R. M.: Antidiuretic hormone. N. Engl. J. Med. *295*:659–665, 1976.

glomerular filtrate is removed. So-called loop or saluretic diuretics (furosemide and ethacrynic acid) induce diuresis (at least in part) by inhibiting active chloride transport by the thick ascending limbs of Henle's loops.

Antidiuretic hormone (ADH) is an important component of the urine concentrating mechanism, because it influences the permeability of distal tubular and collecting duct epithelium to water (Table 73–7). Provided there is sufficient medullary solute concentration to create an osmotic gradient between the interstitium and tubular lumens, and provided there is sufficient ADH to increase the permeability of epithelial cells of the distal nephrons to water, more water than solute will migrate from tubular lumens to the medullary interstitium (Table 73–8). Consequently, the remaining tubular fluid will contain more solute than water in comparison with glomerular filtrate. Following passage

through the loops of Henle, 80 per cent of the glomerular filtrate has been reabsorbed. Of the remaining 20 per cent of the volume of original glomerular filtrate, approximately 15 per cent is reabsorbed by the distal tubules and more than four per cent is reabsorbed by collecting ducts. During states of maximum water conservation (or antidiuresis), the specific gravity of final urine of dogs may equal or slightly exceed 1.060 (± 2400 mOsm/L). Maximum antidiuresis in cats may be associated with formation of final urine with a specific gravity equal to or slightly greater than 1.080 (± 3000 mOsm/L). The fact that cats have a greater capacity to maximally concentrate urine than dogs is commonly attributed to the hypothesis that their countercurrent system has the ability to generate a higher medullary solute concentration than dogs. Other factors may also be involved, however (Schmidt-Nielsen, 1979).

Urine Dilution. In the absence of an-

Table 73–8. Factors Promoting Maximum Urine Concentration*

1. Adequate reabsorption of solute and water by proximal tubules to prevent flooding of the distal nephron.

2. Active reabsorption of NaCl by the thick ascending limb of Henle's loops.

3. Availability of adequate urea to contribute to medullary hyperosmolality.

4. Distal nephron response to adequate circulating ADH.

5. Maintenance of relatively slow medullary blood flow.

*From Finco, D. R.: Kidney Function. *In* Kaneko, J. J. (ed.): Clinical Biochemistry of Domestic Animals. 3rd ed. Academic Press, New York, 1980.

tidiuretic hormone, relatively little water is removed from the lumens of distal tubules and collecting ducts. Active transport of solutes (such as sodium) from lumens of distal nephrons is not impaired, however, and consequently more solute is removed from tubular lumens than water; such urine is said to be dilute (or hyposthenuric), compared with glomerular filtrate (and plasma). The rate at which water is excreted without solute during production of hypotonic urine is called *"free water clearance."* The specific gravity (and osmolality) of dilute urine (SG = 1.001 to ± 1.006; mOsm/ L = 50 to ± 275) would be less than that of glomerular filtrate. Pharmacologic agents (ethanol, morphine, and so forth) or pathologic disorders (pituitary diabetes insipidus, renal diabetes insipidus) that interfere with the production, release, or action of ADH on distal nephrons are commonly associated with profound polyuria. This form of diuresis is commonly called obligatory water diuresis (in contrast to osmotic diuresis) (Osborne et al., 1975) A compensatory water diuresis may occur in association with so-called psychogenic (or primary) polydipsia.

Clinical Correlations. The purpose of the countercurrent system is to generate and maintain a sufficiently high concentration of solutes (primarily sodium, chloride, and urea) in the renal medullary interstitium to attract water from a region of lower solute concentration (distal tubular and collecting duct lumens). The importance of urea in the countercurrent system is illustrated by the fact that dogs fed a high protein diet are better able to maximally concentrate urine than dogs fed a low protein diet (Jolliffe and Smith, 1931). Impaired synthesis of urea resulting from some forms of generalized hepatic disease (cirrhosis and portal vascular shunts) may be responsible, at least in part, for the polyuria commonly associated with these disorders. Likewise, excessive loss of sodium chloride from the medullary interstitium (so-called medullary solute washout) would be associated with impaired ability to concentrate urine. It seems logical that excessive loss of sodium in urine as a consequence of hypoadrenocorticism may reduce renal medullary solute concentration sufficiently to account (at least in part) for the impaired

ability to concentrate urine commonly observed in association with this endocrinopathy. Likewise, impaired function of a sufficient population of nephrons as a consequence of primary glomerular, tubular, interstitial, or vascular disorders will interfere with generation of renal medullary hyperosmolality by loops of Henle. Obligatory polyuria and compensatory polydipsia are well known consequences.

Generalized renal disease of sufficient severity to impair approximately two thirds or more of nephron function impairs urine concentration and dilution. If damage to nephrons is extensive, the specific gravity may become "fixed" at approximately 1.008 to 1.012 (so-called isosthenuria). Although the specific gravity of urine is similar to that of glomerular filtrate in such patients, one should not infer that the tubules have completely lost the ability to modify it. The vast majority of water and metabolites filtered by the glomeruli of such patients must be recovered if life is to be sustained. Lack of detectable glucose in the urine of most patients with primary renal failure and isosthenuria illustrates the point. Consider also the fact that polyuria takes place in azotemic patients with glomerular filtration that is 25 per cent or less of normal, an occurrence that is sometimes viewed as a paradox. Shouldn't the volume of urine formed also be 25 per cent or less of normal? The confusion can readily be resolved by comparing the daily volume of glomerular filtrate in a 20-lb dog (60 liters) with that formed by a patient with primary polyuric renal failure (25% of 60 liters, or 15 liters), and the daily volume of urine produced by a normal individual (approximately 0.5 liter) with that produced by the patient with polyuric renal failure (approximately two liters). Even though the volume of glomerular filtrate formed as a consequence of renal failure is 25 per cent of normal (15 liters), impaired ability of the tubules to modify the filtrate results in polyuria characterized by a fourfold increase in urine volume.

TERMS AND CONCEPTS RELATED TO RENAL DISEASE, RENAL FAILURE, AZOTEMIA, AND UREMIA

Confusion caused by the use of the terms renal disease, renal failure, azotemia, and uremia synonymously may result in mis-diagnosis and formulation of inappropriate or even contraindicated therapy.

RENAL DISEASE

Because of the tremendous reserve capacity of the kidneys, renal disease should not be used synonymously with renal failure or uremia, unless it is described as generalized renal disease. Depending on the quantity of renal parenchyma affected and the severity and duration of lesions, renal disease(s) may or may not cause renal failure or uremia. The clinical relevancy of the difference between renal disease and renal failure is emphasized by the fact that symptomatic and supportive therapy designed to correct fluid, electrolyte, acid-base, nutrient, and endocrine imbalances in patients with renal failure are not appropriate for patients with renal disease without renal dysfunction!

Some renal diseases may be associated with dysfunction (some forms of nephrogenic diabetes insipidus) or biochemical abnormalities (cystinuria) without detectable morphologic alterations. Renal lesions (anomalies, infection, endogenous or exogenous toxins, obstruction to urine outflow, neoplasms, and others) associated with morphologic renal disease may occur in one or both kidneys. The specific cause(s) of renal disease(s) may or may not be known; however, quantitative information about renal function (or dysfunction) is not defined. Renal diseases may affect glomeruli, tubules, interstitial tissue, and/or vessels. The disease may regress, persist, or advance. Unfortunately, many renal diseases escape detection until they become so generalized that they induce clinical signs as a result of serious impairment of renal function.

RENAL FAILURE

Failure is defined as an inability to perform. Renal failure (or renal insufficiency) implies that two thirds to three fourths or more of the functional capacity of the nephrons of both kidneys has been impaired. It often is used to connote a less severe state of renal dysfunction (or renal insufficiency) that is not (yet) associated with polysystemic clinical manifestations (i.e.,

uremia). In dogs, impaired ability to concentrate and dilute urine caused by primary renal disease cannot be readily detected by evaluation of urine specific gravity or urine osmolality until the functional capacity of about two thirds of the nephrons of both kidneys has been surgically extrapolated (Osborne et al., 1969). Although the serum concentrations of urea nitrogen and creatinine vary inversely with glomerular filtration rate, primary renal azotemia and retention of other metabolites normally excreted by the kidneys are usually not recognized until the functional capacity of 70 to 75 per cent of the nephrons is affected (Table 73–9).

Renal function *adequate* for homeostasis does not require that *all* nephrons be functional. The concept that adequate renal function is not synonymous with total renal function is of importance in understanding the difference between renal disease and renal failure, formulating meaningful prognoses, and formulating specific, supportive and symptomatic therapy.

The term renal failure is analogous to liver failure or heart failure in that a level of organ dysfunction is described rather than a specific disease entity. The kidneys perform multiple functions, including selective elimination of waste products of metabolism from the body, synthesis of a variety of hormones, and degradation of a variety of hormones. Failure to perform these functions may not be an "all or none phenomenon" (Table 73–9). For example, in slowly progressive renal diseases, failure of the ability to concentrate or dilute urine according to body need typically precedes failure to eliminate waste products of metabolism of such magnitude that it causes clinically apparent azotemia. In turn, laboratory detection of impaired ability to eliminate waste products of metabolism (such as urea and creatinine), and to maintain electrolyte and nonelectrolyte solute balance within normal limits, typically precedes onset of polysystemic signs of renal dysfunction.

Clinical signs of polysystemic disorders caused by abnormalities of water, electrolyte, acid-base, endocrine, and nutrient balance are not invariably present in patients with primary renal failure (i.e., not all patients with primary renal failure are uremic). This is related, at least in part, to the reserve capacity of the kidneys and the

Table 73–9. Comparison of Level of Nephron Function Associated with Typical Manifestations of Renal Failure

Impaired Function	Degree of Nephron Dysfunction (%)
Altered glomerular capillary permeability to plasma proteins	Variable*
Impaired tubular concentration or dilution of glomerular filtrate	≥66
Azotemia and hyperphosphatemia due to impaired glomerular filtration rate	≥75
Impaired synthesis of erythropoietin and 1,25- vitamin D	>75
Polysystemic signs of uremia	>75

*Glomerular proteinuria may occur in patients with normal glomerular filtration rate, normal tubular reabsorption, and normal tubular secretion. It may also occur when these functions are mildly or severely altered.

ability of unaffected nephrons to undergo compensatory hypertrophy and hyperplasia. Polysystemic signs of renal failure (e.g., uremia), including vomiting, diarrhea, depression, anorexia, dehydration, and weight loss, usually do not occur until approximately three quarters or more of the total nephron population have been functionally impaired.

Although compensatory mechanisms of the body maintain a state of biochemical homeostasis despite significant renal dysfunction, a price is paid for loss of functional renal reserve capacity. Patients with presymptomatic primary renal failure have reduced capacity to respond to physiologic and pathologic stresses. As renal failure progresses, patients are forced to live in a narrowed state of physiologic activity. A uremic crisis may be suddenly precipitated by decreased intake of water or nutrients, development of concomitant but unrelated diseases, and/or inappropriate administration of certain drugs.

AZOTEMIA

Azotemia is defined as an abnormal concentration of urea, creatinine, and other nonprotein nitrogenous substances in blood, plasma, or serum. Azotemia is a laboratory finding (unlike uremia, which is a clinical syndrome) with fundamentally different causes. Since nonprotein nitrogenous compounds (including urea and creatinine) are endogenous substances, abnormally elevated concentrations in serum may be caused by an increased rate of production (by the liver for urea; by muscles for creatinine) or a decreased rate of loss (primarily by the kidneys). Because azotemia may be caused by factors that are not directly related to the urinary system, and by abnormalities of the lower urinary tract not directly related to the kidney, azotemia should not be used as a synonym for renal failure or uremia.

Azotemia may occur when renal structure and function is normal; renal structure is normal, but renal function is abnormal; and/or renal structure and function are abnormal. Determination of the underlying cause(s) of azotemia is of great clinical significance, since this information will significantly influence prognosis and therapy. Failure to do so may lead to formulation of ineffective and even contraindicated therapy.

Because azotemia by definition is dependent on accumulation of nonprotein nitrogenous substances produced by the body in blood, plasma, or serum, the underlying mechanisms of azotemia must be related to an increased rate of production, a decreased rate of excretion, or both of these mechanisms. Increased rates of production of urea nitrogen and creatinine may cause a mild degree of azotemia. If the normal endogenous rate of production of urea nitrogen and creatinine are constant, however, azotemia occurs as a result of reduction in glomerular filtration rate. Reduction in glomerular filtration may be caused by alterations in blood volume, blood pressure, colloidal osmotic pressure, the number of patent renal arteries and glomerular capillaries, the permeability of glomerular capillaries, renal interstitial pressure, and/or renal intratubular pressure (Table 73–1). Thus, glomerular filtration is dependent on prerenal components (blood volume, blood pressure, colloidal osmotic pressure), renal components (patency of renal arteries and glomerular capillaries, permeability of glomerular capillaries, renal interstitial pressure, renal intratubular pressure), and postrenal components (influence of patency of ureters, bladder, and urethra on intratubular pressure). Therefore, the cause(s) of reduction in glomerular filtration may be categorized as prerenal, primary renal, and postrenal. Because of clinically significant differences in pathogenesis, prognosis, and treatment, it is recommended that causes of decreased glomerular filtration associated with azotemia always be localized according to this classification (Table 73–1). The fact that different forms of azotemia may coexist should also be considered. Consult Chapters 21 and 74 for further information about the pathophysiology and localization of azotemia.

UREMIA

Uremia is defined as abnormal quantities of urine constituents in blood caused by primary *generalized* renal disease and as the *polysystemic* toxic syndrome that occurs as a result of abnormal renal function. When the structural and functional integrity of both kidneys has been compromised to such a degree that polysystemic signs of renal failure become manifest clinically, the relatively predictable symptom complex called uremia appears, regardless of underlying cause. In some instances, uremic crises may suddenly be precipitated by prerenal disorders (i.e., congestive heart failure, acute pancreatitis, hypoadrenocorticism), or less commonly, by postrenal disorders (urethral obstruction, displacement of the urinary bladder into a perineal hernia, and so forth), in patients with previously compensated primary renal failure.

Uremia is characterized by multiple physiologic and metabolic alterations that result from renal insufficiency. Renal insufficiency may be caused by a large number of disease processes that have in common impairment of at least three quarters of the nephrons of both kidneys. Depending on the biological behavior of the disease in question, primary renal failure may be reversible or irreversible, acute or chronic, and oliguric and/or polyuric. Consult sections under these titles for further details.

RENAL DISEASE VS. RENAL FAILURE

Differentiation between renal disease and renal failure (with or without uremia) may be facilitated by the knowledge that not all diagnostic procedures used to detect disorders of the urinary system provide information about renal functional capacity, nor is it always possible to differentiate inflammatory diseases of the lower urinary tract from those affecting the upper urinary tract (Table 73–10). For example, detection of a significant number of casts in urine sediment provides reliable evidence of renal tubular involvement, because casts form in the loops of Henle, distal tubules, and collection ducts. One cannot infer that detection of large numbers of casts is indicative of renal failure, however, because their presence or absence cannot be correlated with the degree of renal dysfunction (if any).

Differentiation between renal disease and renal failure is of great clinical significance when gastrointestinal, endocrine, pancreatic, and hepatic diseases causing clinical signs similar to those associated with uremia (e.g., vomiting, diarrhea, polydipsia, dehydration, depression, anorexia, and weight loss) secondarily induce prerenal azotemia and ischemic tubular disease characterized by formation of variable numbers of epithelial, granular, and waxy casts. Although extrarenal fluid loss and subsequent reduction in renal perfusion may be of sufficient magnitude to damage some nephrons and cause prerenal azotemia, detection of concentrated urine (SG > 1.030 in dogs or > 1.035 in cats) indicates an adequate population of functioning nephrons to prevent signs caused by primary renal failure. Every effort should be made to restore renal perfusion, however, since progressive destruction of nephrons caused by prerenal factors may induce primary ischemic renal failure.

Table 73–10. Diagnostic Procedures Commonly Used to Detect and Localize Disorders of the Urinary System

Method	Renal Function	Localize to Kidney	Localize to Urinary System
Urea nitrogen (serum or plasma)	GFR	No*	No
Creatinine (serum or plasma)	GFR	No*	No
Specific gravity (urine)	Tubular reabsorption	No*	No
Osmolality (urine)	Tubular reabsorption	No*	No
Phenolsulfonphthalein (urine excretion)	RBF; tubular secretion	No*	No
Sodium sulfonilate (plasma retention)	GFR	No*	No
Intravenous urography	Crude index of RBF and GFR	Yes	Yes
Water deprivation and vasopressin response tests	Tubular function	No*	No
Renal tubular epithelial cells	No	No†	—
Urinary casts	No	Yes	—
Renal biopsy	No	Yes	—
Significant bacteriuria	No	No	Yes‡
Proteinuria	No	No§	No
Pyuria	No	No‖	Yes‡
Hematuria	No	No‖	Yes‡

*Alterations in renal function are not always caused by diseases localized to the kidneys.
†Renal tubular epithelial cells cannot be consistently differentiated from other types of cells in urine sediment.
‡Assuming urine is not contaminated by genital tract.
§Large quantities of protein in absence of RBC and WBC suggest glomerular disease.
‖Unless present in urinary casts.
GFR = glomerular filtration rate; RBF = renal blood flow.

TERMS AND CONCEPTS RELATED TO URINE OSMOLALITY AND SPECIFIC GRAVITY AND THEIR INTERPRETATION

OSMOLALITY

Dissolution of one or more substances (or solutes) in a solvent (water) changes four mathematically interrelated physical characteristics (known as colligative properties): osmotic pressure, freezing point, vapor pressure, and boiling point. These properties are all directly related to the total number of solute particles within the solution and are independent of the homogenicity or nonhomogenicity of molecular species, molecular weight, and molecular size. As solute is added to solvent osmotic pressure increases, freezing point decreases, vapor pressure decreases, and boiling point increases. Changes in these colligative properties are dependent on the number of particles of solute in solution and not on other characteristics, such as molecular weight, electrical charge, chemical nature, or shape of dissolved particles. In clinical medicine, the osmotic concentration of solutions is usually measured with instruments that determine freezing point (freezing point osmometer) or vapor pressure (vapor pressure osmometer).

The unit of osmotic concentration is the osmole. Since the osmole represents a large mass of solute, the milliosmole (mOsm) has been developed for clinical use. One mOsm = 0.001 osmole. Sodium, chloride, and bicarbonate account for approximately 90 per cent of the osmotic activity in extracellular fluid. The osmotic concentration of plasma, serum, interstitial fluid, and intracellular fluid is approximately 300 mOsm/kg of water. Sodium, chloride, and urea account for the majority of osmotic activity in urine. Normally the osmotic concentration of urine is variable, being dependent on the fluid and electrolyte balance of the body and the nitrogen and electrolyte content of the diet. Species differences in the ability to concentrate urine are significant (Table 73–11).

The ratio of urine osmolality (U_{osm}) to plasma osmolality (P_{osm}) is a good clinical index of the ability of the kidneys to concen-

Table 73–11. Osmolality and Specific Gravity Values for Adult Dog, Cat, and Human Urine

Factor	Species		
	Dog	*Cat*	*Human*
Range of normal SG	1.001 to ± 1.065+	1.001 to ± 1.080+	1.001 to ± 1.035+
Usual SG—normal hydration	1.015 to 1.045	1.035 to 1.060	1.015 to 1.025
Range of normal osmolality (mOsm/kg)	50 to 2500+	50 to 3000+	50 to 1500+

trate or dilute glomerular filtrate (Bovee, 1969). A U/P_{osm} ratio above one indicates that the kidneys are concentrating urine above plasma and glomerular filtrate. Following water deprivation, the U/P_{osm} of normal dogs may be seven or higher (Hardy and Osborne, 1979). A U/P_{osm} ratio of approximately one indicates that water and solute are being excreted in a state that is iso-osmotic with plasma. A U/P_{osm} ratio significantly below one indicates that the tubules are capable of reabsorbing solute in excess of water (i.e., they are diluting glomerular filtrate).

SPECIFIC GRAVITY

Urine specific gravity is a measurement of the density of urine compared with pure water. Stated in another way, urine specific gravity is the ratio of the weight of urine to the weight of an equal volume of water, both measured at the same temperature $\left(SG = \frac{\text{wt. of urine}}{\text{wt. of water}}\right)$. Since specific gravity represents a ratio, it has no units. The specific gravity of water is 1.000. Urine is more dense than water, because it is composed of water and various solutes of different densities.

There is only an approximate relationship between specific gravity and total solute concentration. In addition to the number of molecules of solute, specific gravity is influenced by other factors, including molecular size and molecular weight of solutes. Each species of solute has its own characteristic effect on the specific gravity of urine. Urine samples having equivalent numbers of solute molecules per unit volume may have different specific gravity values if different mixtures of solutes are present. Equal numbers of molecules of urea, sodium, chloride, albumin, globulin, fibrinogen, and glucose have a different quantitative

effect on specific gravity. Thus urine specific gravity is a direct, but not necessarily proportional, index of the number of solute particles in urine. It provides only an estimate of osmolality, because of the variability in quantity of heterogeneous solutes in urine. Measurement of urine specific gravity is useful as a screening procedure but may be unsuitable in some circumstances requiring more precise evaluation of renal tubular concentrating and diluting capacity.

Interpretation of urine SG values of randomly obtained samples is dependent on knowledge of the patient's hydration status, the plasma or serum concentration of urea nitrogen or creatinine, and knowledge of drugs or fluids that have been administered to the patient. Knowledge of urine volume and water consumption may also be helpful. In some instances, interpretation may require knowledge of urine and plasma osmolality.

HYPERSTHENURIA, ISOSTHENURIA, AND HYPOSTHENURIA

Hypersthenuria (also called baruria) depicts urine of high specific gravity and osmolality. *Isosthenuria* depicts urine with a specific gravity and osmolality similar to that of plasma and glomerular filtrate. Loss of ability to concentrate or dilute glomerular filtrate according to body need is sometimes referred to as "fixed specific gravity." Hyposthenuria depicts urine with a *specific gravity* and osmolality that is significantly lower than that of plasma and glomerular filtrate.

The SG of urine of normal dogs and cats is variable, being dependent on the fluid and electrolyte balance of the body, the nitrogen and electrolyte content of the diet, and other variables related to species and individuals (Table 73–11). The urine SG often fluctuates widely from day to day, and within the same day. Urine specific gravity may range from 1.001 to 1.060 or greater in adult normal dogs, and from 1.001 to 1.080 or greater in adult normal cats. Depending on the requirements of the body for water and/or solutes, any specific gravity value within these ranges may be normal. Therefore, the concept of an average normal specific gravity is misleading, because it implies that values above or below the average may not be normal. Randomly collected urine samples from normal adult dogs and cats often have a specific gravity that encompasses a narrower range than that just mentioned (approximately 1.015 to 1.045 for dogs, and 1.035 to 1.060 for cats) (Table 73–11), but an individual urine sample with a specific gravity outside these values is not reliable evidence of renal dysfunction.

Maximum, minimum, and typical urine specific gravity values for infant and immature dogs and cats have not been extensively evaluated. The urine specific gravity of canine fetuses ten days prior to birth ranged from 1.008 to 1.025 (Rahill and Subramanian, 1973). Randomly collected urine samples collected from dogs two days old had an osmolality approximately twice that of plasma, but the urine osmolality was approximately seven times that of plasma when the pups were 77 days old (Horster and Valtin, 1971). These observations have been interpreted to suggest that the kidneys of newborn puppies can concentrate urine to some degree, and that concentrating capacity improves with age (Finco, 1980). It is emphasized that appropriate caution must be used when interpreting urine specific gravity and osmolality values of immature animals, since they probably have different average, minimum, and maximum values than those of mature animals. Similar caution is appropriate when comparing normal adult and infant levels of glomerular filtration and tubular reabsorption (Nash and Edelmann, 1973).

A urine specific gravity that is similar to that of glomerular filtrate (1.008 to 1.012) may be observed in individuals with normal renal function, since the ability of normal kidneys to influence specific gravity encompasses these values. Since such values may be normal or abnormal, they should be viewed as presumptive evidence of an abnormality. Further data will be required, however, to prove or disprove this presumption.

SIGNIFICANCE OF U_{SG} = 1.025 IN MAN, DOGS, AND CATS

The ability of patients to excrete urine with a specific gravity significantly above that of glomerular filtrate (1.008 to 1.012) is dependent on an intact system for production and release of antidiuretic hormone, a sufficient population of functional nephrons to generate and maintain a high solute concentration in the renal medulla, and a sufficient population of functional tubules to respond to antidiuretic hormone. Data obtained from experimental studies in dogs suggest that only about one third of the nephrons of both kidneys are required to concentrate urine to 1.025 or greater (Hayman et al., 1939). Stated in another way, significant impairment of the kidneys' ability to concentrate (or dilute) urine is usually not detected until at least two thirds of the total renal functional parenchyma has been impaired.

The ability of dogs to concentrate urine to a specific gravity of 1.025 has been generally accepted as evidence of "adequate" renal concentrating capacity to maintain homeostasis and to prevent clinical signs of primary renal failure. It appears that the urine specific gravity end point of 1.025 used by many veterinarians has been extrapolated from human data. Since human beings can concentrate their urine to a maximum of 1.035 to 1.040, whereas values for dogs may reach 1.060 or more and values for cats may reach 1.080 or more, concentration of urine to 1.025 probably implies better renal tubular function in man than in cats or dogs (Table 73–11).

Uncontrolled clinical observations in dogs indicate that detection of a urine specific gravity ≥ 1.025 indicates an adequate population of nephrons to prevent clinical signs associated with primary renal failure. A significant degree of renal disease may exist in dogs able to concentrate their urine to a specific gravity of 1.025, however. In one study, the maximal urine specific gravities of three partially nephrectomized dogs (two thirds of total nephrons removed) subjected to 48 hours of water deprivation were 1.023, 1.018, and 1.027 (Hayman et al., 1939).

Experimental studies performed on cats at the University of Georgia revealed that animals with less than 25 per cent of functional nephrons could concentrate their urine significantly higher than SG = 1.025 (Ross and Finco, 1980). Further studies in cats are required to determine the urine SG value that indicates an adequate population of functional nephrons to prevent clinical signs associated with primary renal failure.

Since metabolic work is required to dilute glomerular filtrate by removing solute in excess of water, a urine SG significantly below 1.008 indicates that a sufficient number of functional nephrons (commonly estimated to be at least one third of the total population) are present to prevent clinical signs associated with primary renal failure.

ABNORMAL VALUES

Consult the section on definitions of terms and concepts for information related to renal disease, renal function, azotemia, and uremia.

Relationship to Renal Failure

Varying degrees of impaired ability to concentrate or dilute glomerular filtrate is a consistent finding in all forms of primary renal failure. Because the kidneys have tremendous reserve capacity, impairment of their ability to concentrate or dilute urine may not be detected until at least two thirds (dogs) or more (cats) of the total population of nephrons have been damaged. Complete inability of the nephrons to modify glomerular filtrate typically results in formation of urine with a specific gravity that is similar to that of glomerular filtrate. Total loss of the ability to concentrate and dilute urine (SG = 1.008 to 1.012) often does not occur as a sudden event but may develop gradually. For this reason urine specific gravity values between approximately 1.007 and 1.029 in dogs, and between 1.007 and 1.034 in cats associated with clinical dehydration and/or azotemia are highly suggestive of primary renal failure (Table 73–12). Contrary to statements widely publicized at one time, acute renal diseases of sufficient severity to cause primary renal failure are not associated with marked elevation in urine specific gravity values. Azotemia associated with hypersthenuria should prompt a high index of suspicion of prerenal azotemia.

Table 73–12. Characteristic Urine Volumes and Urine Specific Gravity Associated With Different Types of Azotemia in Dogs and Cats

Prerenal Azotemia
Physiologic oliguria
  Dogs: $U_{SG} > 1.030$
  Cats: $U_{SG} > 1.035$

Primary Acute Ischemic or Nephrotoxic Azotemia
Initial oliguric
  Dogs: $U_{SG} = 1.007$ to 1.029
  Cats: $U_{SG} = 1.007$ to 1.034
Secondary polyuric phase
  Dogs: $U_{SG} = 1.007$ to 1.029
  Cats: $U_{SG} = 1.007$ to 1.034

Obstructive Postrenal Azotemia
Initial oliguria or anuria. Diuresis and polyuria following relief of obstruction.

Primary Chronic Azotemia
Polyuria
  Dogs: 1.007 to 1.029
  Cats: 1.007 to 1.034*
Terminal oliguric phase
  $U_{SG} = 1.008$ to 1.012
Reversible oliguria may be caused by onset of nonrenal disorder that induces prerenal azotemia.
  Dogs: $U_{SG} = 1.007$ to 1.029
  Cats: $U_{SG} = 1.007$ to 1.034

*Urine specific gravity may become fixed between approximately 1.008 and 1.012 if sufficient nephron function is altered. The specific gravity of glomerular filtrate is approximately 1.008 to 1.012.

Once urine specific gravity reflects impaired ability to concentrate or dilute urine (1.007 to 1.029 in dogs), it is more of a general index of nephron function than a specific index of distal tubular and collecting duct function, since in addition to generalized tubular lesions, this abnormality is related to other factors. These factors include (1) increased clearance and decreased fractional tubular reabsorption of solutes retained in plasma (urea, creatinine, phosphorus, sodium, etc.) by viable nephrons. These phenomena induce an obligatory osmotic diuresis; and (2) reduction in the number of functioning nephrons, resulting in impaired ability to maintain the high osmotic gradient normally present in the renal medulla.

Once the ability to concentrate or dilute urine has been premanently destroyed, repeated evaluation of specific gravity will not be of aid in evaluation of progressive deterioration of renal function. Therefore, serial evaluation of urine specific gravity is of the greatest aid in detecting functional changes earlier during the course of primary renal failure, or in monitoring functional recovery associated with reversible renal diseases.

If sufficient clinical evidence is present to warrant examination of the patient's renal function by determining the serum concentration of creatinine or blood urea nitrogen, the urine specific gravity (or osmolality) should be evaluated at the same time. As emphasized previously, a concentrated urine sample associated with an abnormal elevation in serum creatinine or urea nitrogen concentration suggests the probability of *prerenal azotemia* (Table 73–12). Azotemia associated with specific gravity of 1.007 to ± 1.029 (dogs) or 1.034 (cats) indicates the probability of primary renal failure, although on occasion hypoadrenocorticism may induce similar findings. If nonazotemic patients have impaired ability to concentrate urine, causes of pathologic polyuria should be explored. Determination of urine specific gravity or osmolality may allow one to determine whether a disorder characterized by water (1.001 to ± 1.006) or solute (± 1.008 or greater) diuresis is probable (Osborne et al., 1975). See Polyuric Versus Oliguric Primary Renal Failure for further information. Water deprivation and vasopressin response tests may also be required (Breitschwerdt, 1981; Finco, 1980; Hardy and Osborne, 1980).

PROGNOSTIC AND THERAPEUTIC SIGNIFICANCE OF REVERSIBLE AND IRREVERSIBLE RENAL FAILURE

SIGNIFICANCE

Renal failure may be reversible or irreversible (Table 73–13) (Osborne et al., 1969). Antemortem differentiation of potentially reversible from progressive irreversible primary renal failure is an essential prerequisite to establishment of a meaningful prognosis and formulation of effective therapy. Whereas detection of renal diseases that are potentially reversible is often justification for aggressive use of therapeutic regimens, progressive irreversible renal failure may not warrant such effort and expense. Unfortunately, distinction between potentially reversible and irreversible failure on the basis of clinical and laboratory findings is often difficult because of the nonspecificity of associated clinical and biochemical abnormalities.

In order to differentiate potentially reversible primary renal failure from irreversible renal failure in the living patient, it is important to have a conceptual understanding of basic morphologic and functional changes that occur in kidneys as a result of various types of injury, and the relationship of the latter to clinical manifestations of abnormal function. This knowledge and the intelligent use and interpretation of radiographic findings, laboratory data, and information obtained by biopsy are the most reliable means with which to consistently make such a decision. The magnitude of renal dysfunction is itself an unreliable index of potential reversibility.

DEFINITION

The definition of reversibility is of great clinical significance. The concept of reversibility may be applied to underlying renal lesions; the degree of renal dysfunction; and/or the effect of specific, supportive, and symptomatic therapy. Renal function *adequate* to sustain homeostasis is not synonymous with *total* renal function. Even in the presence of irreversible renal lesions, if an adequate population of nephrons remain to maintain homeostasis, signs of renal dysfunction will not develop. As discussed in a preceding section of this chapter, this concept is the basis for distinguishing renal disease from renal failure. Similarly, if a patient has irreversible generalized lesions of sufficient magnitude to cause renal dysfunction, the polysystemic manifestations of renal failure may be minimized by appropriate symptomatic and supportive therapy. Irreversibility of renal lesions is not synonymous with irreversibility of clinical and biochemical sequelae.

Irreversible lesions may be progressive or nonprogressive. Examples of nonprogressive irreversible lesions include those caused by ischemia or hypercalcemia, the underlying cause of which has been corrected. Examples of progressive irreversible lesions include renal amyloidosis (Osborne et al., 1970), renal neoplasia (Caywood et al., 1980), untreated bacterial pyelonephritis,

Table 73–13. Checklist of Some Potentially Reversible Causes of Azotemia

Prerenal	Primary Renal	Postrenal
Catabolic States	*Acute Tubular Necrosis*	*Rent in Excretory Pathway*
1. Catabolic drugs	1. Ischemia	*Obstruction*

a. Glucocorticoids
   b. Tetracyclines?
   c. Thyroid preps
	2. Nephrotoxins	1. Calculi

	a. Ethylene Glycol b. Arsenicals	2. Operable neoplasms

2. Anorexia	c. Amphotericin-B
	   d. Aminoglycoside
	     antibiotics
		3. Herniated bladder

3. Extensive tissue necrosis	e. Others	4. Blood clots
Decreased Renal Perfusion	*Immune Disorders*	
1. Dehydration due to:	*Hypercalcemia*	

a. Vomiting
   b. Diarrhea
   c. Diuretics
   d. Limited water consumption
	Pyelonephritis	

	Drug Reactions	
2. Hypovolemia due to hemorrhage	*Heatstroke*	
3. Heart failure	*Leptospirosis*	
4. Severe hypoalbuminemia	*Some Forms of*	
5. Hypoadrenocorticism	*Glomerulonephropathy*	
6. Diuretics		
7. Anesthetics		
Increased NPN Production		
1. High protein diets		
2. Gastrointestinal hemorrhage		

and many immune-mediated glomerular diseases (Osborne et al., 1977).

RENAL RESERVE CAPACITY

The functional reserve capacity of many organs of the body, including the kidneys, is well known. An entire kidney can be destroyed by disease, or removed for the purpose of transplantation, without causing alteration in homeostasis (Allen, 1974; Hayslett, 1979). Impairment of the urine concentrating capacity of canine kidneys cannot be detected by conventional clinical laboratory techniques until approximately two thirds of the total renal parenchyma is surgically extirpated (Hayman et al., 1939; Osborne et al., 1972). Although the serum concentrations of urea nitrogen and creatin-

ine vary inversely with glomerular filtration rate, approximately three quarters of the nephrons of both kidneys must be functionally impaired before unequivocal azotemia develops. Because of the large functional reserve capacity of the kidneys, detection of renal disease before the occurrence of serious impairment of renal function is difficult (Tables 73–9 and 73–10).

RENAL RESPONSE TO INJURY

Although the kidneys have a large functional reserve capacity in terms of numbers of nephrons necessary to maintain homeostasis, the ability of nephrons to regenerate following destruction by disease is somewhat limited. Formation of nephrons (nephrogenesis) continues for approximately three weeks following birth in dogs; subsequently the kidneys cannot produce additional nephrons (Horster et al., 1971; Nash and Edelman, 1973). Although renal function and renal size continue to increase following the third week of life, increases are primarily related to growth of renal tubules (Horster et al., 1971).

Glomeruli

Glomeruli have good capacity to repair acute inflammatory lesions (Wright et al., 1973), but repair of persistent, severe, or chronic lesions seldom results in normal glomeruli (Osborne et al., 1977). Amyloid and diffuse epithelial crescents are usually irreversible lesions. Progressive irreversible lesions initially localized to glomeruli are eventually responsible for the development of lesions in the remaining but initially unaffected portions of nephrons, and ultimately for healing by replacement fibrosis and scarring.

These generalities should not be interpreted to indicate that all glomerular diseases are clinically irreversible. For example, mixed membranoproliferative glomerulonephropathy in dogs with pyometra may be associated with complete functional recovery (Obel et al., 1964; Hardy and Osborne, 1974). Others may be associated with irreversible but nonprogressive lesions. For example, membranous glomerulonephropathy associated with the nephrotic syndrome in a four-year-old dog was associated with complete spontaneous functional recovery despite persistent nonprogressive glomerular lesions of more than three years' duration (Osborne et al., 1976). Functional recovery may be complete, even when considerable nephron destruction has occurred, since remaining viable nephrons may increase their functional capacity by compensatory hypertrophy.

Tubules

Nephrons damaged as a result of ischemia or nephrotoxins may regain structural and functional competence, provided the basement membranes of tubules are not severely damaged and provided a sufficient number of tubular epithelial cells have escaped injury, so they can proliferate and reline denuded renal tubules. At first, newly regenerated tubular epithelial cells develop cytoplasmic organelles necessary for protein synthesis, regeneration, and replication. At this stage the tubules are unable to concentrate or dilute urine. When necrotic epithelial cells have been replaced by newly regenerated epithelium, cytoplasmic organelles necessary for tubular reabsorption and secretion develop, and the ability to concentrate and dilute urine may eventually be regained.

Although renal failure caused by ischemia is clinically indistinguishable from renal failure caused by nephrotoxins, each produces a different type of tubular lesion. Microscopic and microdissection studies of kidneys of dogs have revealed that structural damage induced by severe renal ischemia is characterized by irregular or patchy distribution of lesions throughout the tubules (Balint, 1968; Ben-Ishay, 1967; Levinsky et al., 1981; Oliver et al., 1951). The lesions consist of varying degrees of disruption, fragmentation, or dissolution of tubular basement membranes and necrosis of tubular epithelial cells. Variable numbers of nephrons are damaged, but rarely is an entire nephron damaged. With the possible exception of a paucity of red blood cells in glomerular capillaries and the presence of platelet thrombi, the glomeruli of affected kidneys are morphologically normal. This variable pattern of distribution of lesions can be explained on the basis of the fact that capillaries originating from the efferent arteriole of one nephron may (superficial cortex) or may not (remainder of kidney) perfuse the tubules of the same nephron. The tubules are the major site of pathologic alterations, because the high metabolic activity of tubular epithelial cells makes them more susceptible to the effects of ischemia than glomeruli, blood vessels, and interstitial tissue. Thus, the quantitatively most important alteration, tubular necrosis, is considered to be a consequence of primary ischemia, not the result of renal functional impairment caused by tubular casts.

In contrast with renal ischemia, structural damage induced by nephrotoxic nephrosis in pure form is characterized by cellular degeneration and necrosis that is primarily confined to the epithelium of the proximal portions of all of the tubules. Unlike renal ischemia, all of the nephrons may be affected, and basement membranes of damaged portions of renal tubules are not significantly altered (Balint, 1968; Oliver et al., 1951). Explanation of the distribution of lesions caused by nephrotoxins may be related to the fact that nephrotoxins can be filtered by all glomeruli and thus can be concentrated by renal tubular cells in sufficient quantity to cause cell death. Since most nephrotoxins cause damage to cells of other organs, they may also cause renal ischemia and associated tubular basement membrane lesions as a result of generalized fluid loss and hypotension.

Intact tubular basement membranes are an essential prerequisite to tubular regeneration, because they provide a framework that permits the orderly reconstruction of the tubule by regenerating epithelial cells. Once fragmentation or dissolution of tubular basement membranes occurs, the lack of continuous supporting scaffold may result in the lack of orderly re-epithelialization of the tubule or the obstruction of the tubular lumen as a result of ingrowth of granulation tissue from the interstitial tissue. Extensive proliferation of tubular epithelium still may occur, but failure of restoration of a patent tubular lumen destroys the excretory and conservatory capacity of the nephron. The end result of such injury is usually replacement of affected nephrons by connective tissue. Because of the nature of the renal lesions they produce, the potential for nephron repair may be greater following injury by nephrotoxins than by ischemia.

Interstitial Tissue

Lesions of interstitial tissue may be reversible or irreversible, depending on the etiopathogenesis of the disease in question. For example, generalized interstitial edema would be expected to produce a profound alteration of renal function as a result of increased interstitial pressure, but the changes would be expected to be reversible if the predisposing cause could be rapidly eliminated. Experimentally induced canine leptospirosis causes an acute interstitial nephritis that is potentially reversible if patients do not succumb during initial phases of the disease (Low et al., 1967). Chronic bacterial infection of the interstitium (i.e., pyelonephritis) often results in progressive inflammation and interstitial fibrosis that irreversibly damage the renal microcircula-

tion and renal tubules. The renal medulla is far more susceptible to bacterial infection than is the renal cortex (Osborne et al., 1979).

Vessels

Complete occlusion of renal arteries (end-arteries) will result in infarction of the renal parenchyma supplied by occluded vessels. Healing subsequently occurs by replacement with collagenous connective tissue.

Chronic Generalized Nephropathy (Nephritis)

Three important phenomena are related to the evolution of progressive renal diseases: (1) various components of nephrons (glomeruli, tubules, peritubular capillaries, and interstitial tissue) are functionally interdependent; (2) morphologic and functional abnormalities of the kidneys can be manifested clinically in only a limited number of ways, irrespective of underlying cause; and (3) following maturation, new nephrons cannot be formed to replace others irreversibly destroyed by disease. If any portion of the nephron is irreversibly destroyed, the function of the remaining portions is also damaged. Progressive, irreversible lesions initially localized to the renal vascular system, glomeruli, tubules, or interstitial tissue are eventually responsible for development of lesions in the remaining, but initially unaffected, portions of nephrons. For example, progressive lesions (such as amyloid) confined initially to glomeruli will decrease peritubular capillary perfusion of tubules and thus induce tubular cell atrophy, degeneration, and necrosis. Ultimately, nephron destruction initiated by progressive glomerular disease will stimulate repair by fibrosis (Osborne et al., 1970). Likewise, generalized progressive pyelonephritis will damage or destroy tubules and glomeruli, and stimulate repair by replacement fibrosis. If the majority of nephrons have been destroyed, these events will be associated with reduction in renal size, capsular adhesions, and generalized pitting of the capsular surface of the cortex.

Because of structural and functional interdependence of various components of nephrons, antemortem and postmortem differentiation of various generalized, progressive renal diseases that have reached an advanced stage may be difficult. Varying types of functional and structural change prominent during earlier phases of progressive generalized renal diseases may permit identification of a specific cause and/or localization of the initial lesion to one or more components of the nephrons (glomerulonephropathy, acute tubular necrosis, acute interstitial nephritis, tubulo-interstitial disease, and so forth). With time, however, destructive changes of varying severity (atrophy, inflammation, fibrosis, and mineralization of disease nephrons), which are superimposed on compensatory and adaptive changes (hypertrophy and hyperplasia) of partially and totally viable nephrons, provide a gross and microscopic similarity to these diseases. As a generality, the greater the degree of destruction of nephrons by progressive irreversible renal diseases, the less obvious are differences in parameters of their functional capacity and in their gross and microscopic appearance. The important point is that primary irreversible progressive diseases of glomeruli, tubules, vessels, and interstitial tissue may lead to chronic generalized nephropathy. The underlying cause of chronic generalized nephropathy may (e.g., amyloidosis) or may not be detected.

At one time, poor understanding of renal response to injury and lack of laboratory and biopsy techniques with which to detect antemortem lesions at an early stage of development led to the widespread but erroneous assumption that the vast majority of "chronic *generalized* nephritis" was caused by a specific disease entity called "chronic *interstitial* nephritis" (so-called CIN). Because leptospirosis was a well-documented cause of acute interstitial nephritis, the hypothesis (which was never proved) was dogmatically advanced that leptospirosis was also the most common cause of CIN (Bloom, 1954). Primary irreversible progressive diseases of the renal interstitium (chronic interstitial nephritis) can cause chronic generalized nephropathy (nephritis) characterized by reduction in renal size. Although it may occur elsewhere in the world (Spencer and Wright, 1981), leptospirosis is apparently an extremely uncommon cause of CIN (and therefore an uncommon cause of chronic generalized nephritis) in the United States.

Interstitial nephritis, whether it be acute or chronic, is a valid descriptive term. When used as a morphologic diagnosis, however, it suggests that the underlying disorder is characterized by morphologic and functional abnormalities of interstitial tissue, which if progressive may induce changes in the renal tubules, glomeruli, and vessels. Interstitial nephritis is distinguished from other types of primary renal disease (e.g., glomerulonephropathy, acute tubular necrosis) by changes that initially and predominantly affect interstitial tissue. Unfortunately, many chronic generalized diseases of the kidney that originated in vessels, glomeruli, or tubules are associated with a marked degree of interstitial inflammation and fibrosis.

The term "end-stage" kidney implies the presence of renal diseases that are generalized, progressive, irreversible, and at an extremely advanced or "end" stage of development. "End-stage" kidneys are one step beyond chronic generalized nephropathy (nephritis), and the term applies to all cases in which the antecedent cause of renal destruction cannot be identified or localized to any particular portion of the nephron.

Self-Perpetuation of Renal Destruction

Empirical clinical observations and results of experimental studies in a variety of species suggest that loss of a critical mass of functional renal tissue may result in further self-perpetuating deterioration of renal function that culminates in uremia and death, despite absence of the initial cause of nephron destruction. The underlying mechanisms that cause progressive self-perpetuating destruction of renal parenchyma have not been clearly defined. Hypertension appears to be an important cause in man (Alfrey, 1981) and has been implicated in dogs (Anderson and Fisher, 1968).

Recent studies in rats with experimentally induced renal failure suggest that dietary restriction of phosphate may prevent progressive deterioration of renal function by minimizing renal secondary hyperparathyroidism (Ibels et al., 1978). When rats with renal failure induced by ligation of renal arteries (so-called remnant kidney model) were fed a diet high in phosphorus, they developed secondary hyperparathyroidism and lesions in remaining portions of the remnant kidney characterized by interstitial mineralization, inflammation, and fibrosis. There was a corresponding progressive reduction in renal function and, therefore, perpetuation of hyperphosphatemia. When control rats with a similar degree of surgically induced renal dysfunction were fed a low phosphorus diet, remnant kidneys were microscopically normal and renal function remained stable. Similar morphologic findings have been observed in cats studied in an almost identical fashion (Ross and Finco, 1980). Consult the section Renal Secondary Hyperparathyroidism for further details about the mechanisms that cause precipitation of calcium phosphate salts in various body tissues as a result of renal failure.

These preliminary results, if subsequently proved to be valid, are of tremendous clinical importance, since they suggest that therapeutic manipulations designed to control hyperphosphatemia not only may improve the quality of life by reducing the wide variety of manifestations associated with renal secondary hyperparathyroidism, but also may actually prolong life. A clinical study in humans indicated that maintenance of serum phosphorus concentration in the range of 2 to 3 mg/dl was associated with reduction in the rate of progression of renal dysfunction in many patients (Walser et al., 1979).

Methods currently available that may be of value in controlling hyperphosphatemia include enhancing glomerular filtration rate by correcting dehydration and maintaining sodium and water balance, reducing dietary phosphorus by feeding diets low in phosphorus, and enhancing gastrointestinal loss of phosphorus by administration of nonabsorbable phosphorus-binding agents (Osborne and Polzin, 1979).

MORPHOLOGIC AND FUNCTIONAL ADAPTATION OF KIDNEYS TO INJURY

Compensatory Phenomena

Although the kidneys cannot produce additional nephrons once maturation has occurred or effectively repair nephrons severely damaged as a result of various disease processes, compensatory hyperplasia (increase in cell number) and compensatory hypertrophy (increase in cell size) are highly effective adaptive mechanisms by which the functional capacity and size of all portions of surviving nephrons are increased (Bricker and Fine, 1981; Hayslett, 1979). Functional elimination of the majority of nephrons (by surgery, partial infarction, and/or ligation of ureters) is immediately followed by an increase in the function of nephrons in the intact contralateral or remnant kidney (Allen, 1974; Bricker and Fine, 1981; Hayslett, 1979; Rous and Wakim, 1967). Compensatory changes that continue to occur for the next several months include an increase in viable nephron size and further increases in viable nephron function.

Whether there is a gross increase in the overall size of the kidneys of patients with nephron damage depends on the number of nephrons that remain intact. Provided the vast majority of nephrons remain viable in one kidney following destruction or ablation of its mate, the size of the functioning contralateral kidney will perceptibly increase. Compensatory hyperplasia and hypertrophy also increase the size and functional capacity of viable nephrons in patients with chronic generalized disease. Microdissection of viable nephrons from dogs with chronic generalized renal disease revealed that proximal convoluted tubular (PCT) length had tripled, PCT volume had doubled, PCT thickness had increased by approximately one half, and glomerular surface had approximately doubled (Bloom, 1954). Despite compensatory size increase in viable nephrons, however, the overall size of the kidneys was reduced, because the majority of nephrons had been destroyed and replaced with collagenous connective tissue.

The number of functional nephrons required to maintain homeostasis is dependent upon the rapidity with which the remainder are destroyed. Acute removal of more than 75 per cent of the renal mass from normal dogs is often associated with signs of renal failure and sometimes death, whereas staging removal of renal parenchyma may permit survival with a far greater reduction in renal mass. These observations provide insight into the fact that progressive renal diseases that destroy renal parenchyma at a relatively slow rate allow viable nephrons more time to undergo structural and functional transformation. Thus, a large number of nephrons may be destroyed before renal function is reduced to such a degree that functional abnormalities become clinically detectable. Acute generalized renal diseases are often associated with clinical signs of uremia following destruction of fewer nephrons than in chronic progressive renal failure, since viable nephrons have not had the opportunity to adapt by hypertrophy and hyperplasia. These observations may account for the significant variability between the magnitude of renal dysfunction and the severity of clinical signs of uremia. Patients with acute renal failure often have severe polysystemic illness, even though their serum concentration of urea or creatinine is lower than that observed in asymptomatic patients with polyuric chronic renal failure. If a uremic patient with acute renal failure associated with irreversible but nonprogressive lesions can be kept alive with appropriate therapy, recovery of *adequate* function to sustain life without continued intensive therapy may be associated with compensatory adaptation of remaining viable nephrons.

Nephrogenesis

New nephrons cannot be formed to replace damaged ones following cessation of nephrogenesis. The period of nephrogenesis varies with species and may influence renal response to injury. This knowledge is of clinical relevance to congenital renal disorders and acquired diseases that affect newborn infants. If a unilateral nephrectomy is performed in a newborn species of animal that maintains nephrogenesis following birth (rats, mice, and dogs), additional nephrons will form in the contralateral kidney (Bonvalet, 1978). In those species in which nephrogenesis is completed prior to birth (guinea pigs and humans), however, unilateral nephrectomy shortly following birth will not stimulate compensatory nephrogenesis (Bonvalet, 1978; Osathanondh and Potter, 1963). The duration of nephrogenesis in cats has apparently not been determined.

Time Required for Completion of Compensation

The time required for completion of the compensatory process following destruction of renal parenchyma has been poorly defined, but it is apparently species dependent

(Allen, 1974). It has been estimated to require two to three months following unilateral nephrectomy in dogs (Levy and Blalock, 1938; Rous and Wakim, 1967). This information is of clinical relevance with respect to the prognosis of acute and chronic generalized renal disease. In patients with acute renal failure, parenchymal regeneration has not yet had an opportunity to occur, and compensatory and adaptive mechanisms of viable nephrons have not yet been expended. If the patient is kept alive with the aid of appropriate therapy for a sufficient period for these processes to occur, the kidneys may regain an adequate quantity of function to maintain homeostasis. In chronic renal failure, however, compensatory and adaptive nephron changes have usually been exhausted, and parenchymal regeneration has had an opportunity to occur. The fact that signs of renal failure are present indicates that regenerative and compensatory processes have been overwhelmed.

As will be discussed, irreversibility of renal lesions is not synonymous with irreversibility of clinical signs and biochemical abnormalities associated with renal failure and uremia. Therapy designed to minimize abnormalities in fluid, electrolyte, acid-base, endocrine, and nutrient balance, and to minimize retention of metabolic waste products, may permit the patient to regain a comfortable state of existence, despite the presence of irreversible generalized disease.

Causes of Compensatory Adaptation

The basic mechanism(s) that are responsible for compensatory renal hyperplasia and hypertrophy have not, as yet, been clearly defined. A large body of evidence, however, indicates that nondialyzable, heat-labile, organ-specific humoral factors (so-called renotropins) produced by the kidneys and inactivated by the liver are involved (Allen, 1974; Bricker and Fine, 1981). The rate of compensatory growth may be stimulated by a number of additional factors including a high protein diet, amino acids, administration of ammonium chloride, and several endogenous hormones (Allen, 1974; Malt, 1969). Conversely, starvation, protein depletion, and endocrine abnormalities appear to retard compensatory renal growth

(Allen, 1974; Hayslett, 1979; Polzin et al., 1981). Age is also an important factor. The capacity for compensatory renal adaptation is far greater in immature animals than in adults, and greater in younger adults than in older adults (Allen et al., 1974; Aschinberg et al., 1978; Bricker and Fine, 1981; Galla et al., 1974).

The Intact Nephron Hypothesis

The fact that compensatory changes in the structure and function of partially or totally viable nephrons occur in an orderly and predictable fashion supports the popular "intact nephron hypothesis" proposed by Bricker and his colleagues (Bricker, 1969; Bricker and Fine, 1981). The same fundamental principle is embraced by the "adaptive nephron hypothesis" (Gottschalk, 1971). Despite progressive reduction in the population of functional nephrons by a wide variety of diverse diseases with differing etiopathogenic mechanisms that cause a heterogeneous group of morphologic alterations, remaining viable nephrons retain homogenicity of glomerulotubular balance. The balance between intake of water and nutrients (phosphorus, sodium, and so forth) and their excretion by the kidneys may be maintained without therapy during early phases of renal failure by the same biologic control mechanisms operative in normal patients. For example, even though dietary intake of phosphorus and sodium remain unchanged during progressive destruction of nephrons, augmented filtration of these solutes by viable nephrons and proportional reduction in fractional tubular reabsorption of these solutes mediated by regulatory hormones allow dietary intake to be balanced by urinary output. Likewise, continued consumption of the same quantity of dietary potassium during progressive polyuric renal failure does not result in hyperkalemia, because of a proportional increase in the rate of secretion of potassium by viable nephrons.

In order for these events to occur, each surviving nephron must accept a greater proportion of overall nephron function (perhaps 10 to 30 times greater than normal). As overall glomerular filtration rate decreases, the excretory response of each surviving nephron must increase to a degree that is inversely proportional to the number of surviving nephrons. This phenomenon has been called the "magnification phenomenon" of chronic progressive renal disease, and it represents further refinement of the intact nephron hypothesis (Bricker et al., 1978; Bricker and Fine, 1981).

The intact nephron hypothesis and magnification phenomenon are based on the observation that partially and totally viable nephrons in diseased kidneys function as though they were structurally and functionally intact. The well known clinical and biochemical signs of renal dysfunction only develop when the population of viable nephrons falls below that required to maintain homeostasis. The intact nephron hypothesis has great clinical significance, because it permits use of meaningful generalities based on well established physiologic principles to (1) formulate a unifying concept of the pathophysiology of chronic renal failure and (2) formulate supportive and symptomatic therapy for renal failure caused by a variety of diverse disease entities.

SUMMARY

In summary, renal diseases may be reversible, irreversible and nonprogressive, or irreversible and progressive. Renal diseases may not be associated with renal dysfunction, because the large functional reserve capacity of the kidneys is often associated with adequate function to maintain homeostasis, despite the presence of renal disease.

Repair of various components of nephrons may occur but is, in general, somewhat limited. Unfortunately, new nephrons cannot be formed to replace those destroyed by disease. Fortunately, adaptation of remaining viable nephrons is good. The adaptive process is not always immediate, however, and is not unlimited.

In general, the metabolic sequelae (e.g., uremia) of renal dysfunction are predictable. There is a significant conceptual difference between irreversibility of damage to nephrons and the potential reversibility of the metabolic sequelae of renal dysfunction. Supportive and symptomatic therapy designed to minimize or correct fluid, electrolyte, acid-base, endocrine, and nutritional imbalances that occur as a consequence of persistent renal dysfunction may permit amelioration of clinical signs and survival for months and even years.

ACUTE VERSUS CHRONIC RENAL FAILURE AND UREMIA

SIGNIFICANCE

Although renal failure and uremia have been classically classified as acute and chronic, vague definitions of these terms add little to the understanding of their etiology and pathophysiology, because there is considerable overlap in cause, lesions, and biologic behavior. Classification of renal failure as potentially reversible or irreversible is likely to be of greater benefit in formulating a prognosis. Likewise, determination of whether renal failure is associated with polyuria or oliguria is of far greater importance in formulating therapy than knowledge of whether the underlying process is of acute or chronic duration.

Nonetheless, distinction between acute and chronic renal failure may be of value. In general, a favorable long-term prognosis is more often justified for patients with acute primary renal failure (ARF) than for those with chronic primary renal failure (CRF). Unfortunately, at the present, most chronic generalized renal diseases of dogs and cats are held to be progressive and irreversible. In this discussion, acute renal failure will be used in the context of days to a few weeks, whereas chronic renal failure implies a duration of months to years.

SIMILARITIES

An acute onset of polysystemic clinical and biochemical abnormalities caused by an acute destruction of nephrons often mimics the acute onset of polysystemic and bio-

Table 73–14. Similarities and Differences Between Most Patients with Acute and Chronic Primary Renal Failure

Factor	Acute Renal Failure	Chronic Renal Failure
Clinical Signs		
Urine volume	Initial oliguria; subsequent polyuria	Polyuria; potential oliguria
Weight loss	Primarily due to fluid loss	Due to tissue and fluid loss
Kidney size	Normal to ↑	Normal to ↓ ; ± ↑
Erosions and ulcerations of GI mucosa	Variable	Variable
Urinalysis		
Impaired ability to concentrate or dilute urine	Yes	Yes
Pyuria	Variable	Variable
Hematuria	Variable	Variable
Proteinuria	Variable	Variable
Tubular casts	Frequent	Less common
Hemogram		
PCV and Hb	May be normal, ↑ or ↓	Normal to ↓
Leukocytosis	Variable	Typically mild to moderate mature neutrophilia
Blood Chemistry		
Serum urea nitrogen	Increased	Increased
Serum creatinine	Increased	Increased
Serum osmolality	Increased	Increased
Serum potassium	Increased if oliguric; normal if polyuric	Normal if polyuric; increased if oliguric
Blood pH	Normal to ↓	Normal to ↓
Plasma bicarbonate	Decreased	Decreased
Serum calcium	Usually normal; may be ↑ or ↓	Usually normal to ↓ ; may be ↑
Serum phosphorus	Increased	Increased
Radiography		
Osteodystrophy	Absent	Present
Calcification of kidneys	Uncommon	Uncommon

chemical abnormalities caused by chronic and progressive destruction of nephrons (Table 73–14). Of great clinical significance is the recognition of the difference between (1) an acute onset of clinical signs caused by acute generalized renal disease, (2) an acute onset of clinical signs caused by chronic progressive generalized renal disease, and (3) an acute onset of clinical signs caused by a combination of extrarenal and primary renal factors. Sudden appearance of uremic signs does not necessarily imply sudden destruction of a large number of nephrons, since it may be the culmination of gradual destruction of nephrons. Likewise, sudden onset of uremic signs does not necessarily imply continued gradual destruction of nephrons, since it may be precipitated by extrarenal factors.

Clinical findings associated with acute and chronic primary renal failure are more similar than dissimilar, because functional and morphologic abnormalities of kidneys can be clinically manifested in only a limited number of ways. Weakness, depression, anorexia, stomatitis, gastrointestinal disturbances, and central nervous system disturbances may occur in acute or chronic, reversible or irreversible uremia (Tables 73–12 and 73–14). Detection of these signs does indicate generalized functional impairment, since approximately three quarters or more of the nephrons of both kidneys must be functionally impaired before clinical signs of uremia develop. Likewise reduction in glomerular filtration rate (characterized by azotemia and reduced clearance of creatinine, sodium sulfanilate, or inulin), hyperphosphatemia, metabolic acidosis, increased serum osmolality, reduced urinary excretion of phenosulfonphthalein (PSP) dye, and impaired ability to concentrate or dilute glomerular filtrate may be associated with acute or chronic renal failure (Table 73–14). Although severe hypercalcemia appears to be a more common cause than complication of renal failure, it may occur in acute or chronic forms (Finco and Rowland, 1978; Osborne and Stevens, 1977). Hyperkalemia, a manifestation of oliguric renal failure, most often is observed in association with acute renal failure but may occur in association with chronic renal failure.

DIFFERENCES

Chronic Renal Failure

Chronic renal failure in dogs and cats may be caused by a variety of primary glomerular, tubular, interstitial, or vascular disorders, which may be congenital or acquired (Table 73–15). Etiologic agents encompass immune-complex disorders, amyloidosis, infectious pyelonephritis, neo-

Table 73–15. Examples of Renal Diseases According to Primary Site of Involvement

Glomeruli	Tubules	Interstitium	Vessels
1. Amyloidosis	1. Congenital disorders	1. Amyloid (cats)	1. Atherosclerosis (uncommon)
2. Diabetic glomerulopathy (?)	2. Hypercalcemia	2. Drugs	
3. Disseminated intravascular coagulation	3. Immune-complex and anti-tubular basement membrane disorders (?)	3. Heavy metals	2. Embolic disorders
4. Embolic disorders	4. Ischemia	4. Immune disorders (?)	3. Polyarteritis nodosa (uncommon)
5. Immune-complex disorders	5. Nephrotoxins	5. Leptospirosis	4. Others
a. Bacterial endocarditis (?)	a. Drugs	6. Pyelonephritis	
b. *Dirofilaria immitis*	b. Heavy metals	7. Systemic mycoses	
c. Drugs (haptens)	6. Neoplasia	8. Others	
d. Feline leukemia			
e. Lupus erythematosus	7. Obstructive disorders		
f. Neoplasia	8. Tubular transport disorders		
g. Pyometra (?)	a. Fanconi syndrome		
h. Idiopathic forms	b. Renal tubular acidosis		
6. Antiglomerular basement membrane disorders	c. Primary renal glucosuria		
a. *Dirofilaria immitis* (?)	9. Others		
b. Idiopathic forms			
7. Others			

plasia, obstruction to urine outflow (hydronephrosis), and hypercalcemia. A large number of idiopathic disorders of various components of nephrons may also cause chronic renal failure.

Nonregenerative anemia, radiographic evidence of renal osteodystrophy, bilateral reduction in renal size, and an accurate history of progressive clinical signs (weight loss, polyuria-polydipsia, anorexia) are usually reliable indices of chronic renal failure (Table 73–14). Hypocalcemia is usually a manifestation of advanced chronic renal failure. Chronicity may be inferred from the fact that all of these clinical signs require time to develop. The generalized nature of the underlying disease may be inferred from the fact that at least two thirds (polyuria-polydipsia) to three quarters or more of the renal parenchyma must be functionally impaired before clinical signs develop.

Acute Renal Failure

Nephrotoxins (ethylene glycol, therapeutic arsenicals, nephrotoxic antimicrobial agents) represent the most common cause of acute renal failure in dogs and cats in America. Ischemia is a potential cause of acute tubular necrosis and acute renal failure in these species, but it occurs much less commonly in animals than in man. Thromboembolism of major renal vessels is a potential cause of acute renal failure in cats with aortic thromboembolism. It may also occur in dogs but is uncommon. The authors have observed acute renal failure in three dogs caused by rapidly progressive glomerular amyloidosis. Acute generalized interstitial lesions caused by leptospirosis is a well-documented cause of acute renal failure in dogs but currently is extremely uncommon in America. Urinary tract infection in the face of partial or complete outflow obstruction may cause acute renal failure in dogs; it is very uncommon in cats.

An accurate history of exposure to nephrotoxins or sudden development of vascular collapse supports the existence of acute renal failure. Likewise, documentation of sudden obstruction to urine outflow associated with urinary tract infection, fever, and neutrophilic leukocytosis is indicative of ARF caused by pyelonephritis.

Renal pain may also be suggestive of acute renal failure. Studies in man have revealed that renal pain is caused by stretching or compression of the peripelvic renal capsule and renal pelvis, by traction of the renal pedicle containing the renal artery and vein, and by intrarenal or extrarenal obstruction to urine outflow (DeWolf and Fraley, 1975; Ray and Neill, 1947). Portions of the renal capsule covering the greater curvature of the kidneys and the renal parenchyma itself apparently do not transmit sensations of pain. Presumably a similar situation occurs in animals. It is known that renal pain is not associated with chronic generalized renal diseases, slowly growing neoplasms, chronic hydronephrosis, or polycystic disease of dogs and cats (Osborne et al., 1980). Since pain associated with renal disease occurs only when there is acute stretching or distention of the renal capsule, it would be expected to occur in association with acute obstruction to urine outflow at the level of the ureters or renal pelves, and with acute generalized nephritis or nephrosis. When possible, the presence of renal pain should be confirmed by palpation of the kidneys rather than by palpation of the lumbar muscles or vertebral column. Since pain localized to the area normally occupied by the kidneys can be caused by nonrenal disorders (spinal cord disorders, bone diseases, intervertebral disc disease, gastrointestinal disorders), its significance should be evaluated by laboratory and/or radiographic techniques.

Examination of renal biopsy samples is a reliable method of differentiating acute from chronic renal failure. Renal lesions associated with acute renal failure are often characterized by acute tubular necrosis. The morphology of biopsy samples obtained from patients with acute renal failure caused by ischemia or nephrotoxins may appear remarkably normal even though renal function tests are abnormal. Lesions typical of chronic renal failure are characterized by destructive changes (atrophy, inflammation, fibrosis, and mineralization of diseased nephrons) that are superimposed on compensatory and adaptive changes of partially and totally viable nephrons.

EXCEPTIONS TO GENERALITIES

There are significant exceptions to these generalities, however. Polyuria, nocturia, and polydipsia are cardinal signs of chronic generalized disease, but they also occur during the polyuric phase of acute renal failure caused by nephrotoxins and ischemia (Table 73–12). Knowledge of the duration of polyuria and polydipsia may be of value in distinguishing between acute and chronic renal failure. Oliguria is the cardinal sign of the initial phase of acute renal failure caused by generalized ischemic or nephrotoxic tubular disease; however, it may also occur if a prerenal cause of reduced perfusion is superimposed on chronic renal failure, or as a terminal event in chronic renal failure (Table 73–12). Anemia may result from a combination of events in patients with acute renal failure, including blood loss caused by impaired coagulation, and hemolysis (Levinsky et al., 1981). Although absence of anemia does not rule out earlier stages of chronic renal failure, when patients with severe polysystemic signs of renal failure are not anemic (appropriate consideration being given to dehydration), acute renal failure should be considered.

Absence of other signs associated with chronic renal failure does not consistently exclude its presence. Progressive renal diseases that destroy renal parenchyma at a relatively slow rate allow partially and totally viable nephrons to undergo structural and functional adaptation. Thus, a numerically greater number of nephrons may be destroyed before renal function is reduced to such a degree that abnormalities become clinically detectable.

POLYURIC VERSUS OLIGURIC PRIMARY RENAL FAILURE

SIGNIFICANCE

Because there are significant differences in the type and magnitude of excesses and deficits associated with fluid, electrolyte, acid-base, nutrient, and endocrine imbalances in patients with oliguric and nonoliguric primary renal failure, it is imperative to divide candidates for therapy of renal failure into two groups: those with oliguria and those with polyuria (Tables 73–12 and 73–16). Primary polyuric renal failure tends to be associated with greater deficits caused by impaired tubular modification of glomerular filtrate. Primary oliguric renal failure tends to be associated with greater excesses caused by profound reduction in renal blood flow and glomerular filtration.

Biochemical trends associated with pathologic oliguria include (1) excesses in water, potassium, hydrogen ion, sodium, chloride, phosphates, sulfates, and nitrogenous wastes, and (2) deficits in calories, amino acids, and vitamins. Negative body water balance may be a result of severe vomiting and/or diarrhea. Although uncommon, severe vomiting may cause metabolic alkalosis instead of the more common metabolic acidosis.

Biochemical trends associated with primary polyuric renal failure include (1) deficits in water, sodium, chloride, bicarbonate, calcium, vitamins, erythropoietin, amino acids, and calories, and (2) excesses in phospho-

Table 73–16. Biochemical Similarities and Differences in Patients with Polyuric and Oliguric Primary Renal Failure

Factor	Polyuria	Oliguria
Urine S.G.	1.007 to 1.029 (dog) 1.007 to 1.034 (cat)	1.007 to 1.029 (dog) 1.007 to 1.034 (cat)
Urea nitrogen (serum)	Increased	Increased
Creatinine (serum)	Increased	Increased
Sodium (serum)	Usually normal	Variable
Sodium (total body)	Variable	Variable
Potassium (serum)	Usually normal	Increased
pH (blood)	Normal to decreased	Marked decrease
Phosphorus (serum)	Usually increased	Usually increased
Calcium (serum)	Usually normal to decreased*†	Usually normal to decreased*†

*Unless renal failure is caused by hypercalcemia.
†Occasionally hypercalcemia occurs in patients as a sequela to primary renal failure.

rus, sulfates, hydrogen ion (nonvolatile acids), parathormone, and nitrogenous wastes. Although polyuric patients are usually normokalemic, they may become hypokalemic or hyperkalemic.

NORMAL URINE VOLUME

Normal urine volume is influenced by several variables, including species, body weight and size, diet (especially salt and water content), fluid intake, physical activity, and environmental factors such as temperature and humidity. It has been estimated that normal adult dogs in a normal environment will produce approximately 12 to 20 ml of urine per pound of body weight per 24 hours. In one study, normal dogs in a controlled environment produced 3.9 to 23.3 ml of urine per kg body weight per 24 hours (DiBartola et al., 1980). In another study, cats fed dry, semi-moist, and moist diets produced approximately 8 to 13 ml of urine per pound of body weight per 24 hours (Lawler, 1981).

Production of at least 0.5 to 1.0 ml of urine per kg body weight per hour is commonly used to indicate adequate perfusion of canine kidneys during fluid therapy (Kolata et al., 1980). This value represents an empirical clinical observation, as yet uncorroborated by controlled studies, in which renal blood flow and glomerular filtration rate were compared with the volume of urine produced.

POLYURIA

Polyuria is defined as the formation and elimination of large quantities of urine. Depending on the body's need to conserve or eliminate water and/or solutes, polyuria may be normal (physiologic) or abnormal (pharmacologic or pathologic). The significance of polyuria, and establishment of whether it is an obligatory or adaptive phenomenon, cannot be determined without additional information (history, physical examination, results of urinalyses, water deprivation test, and so forth).

Physiologic Polyuria

The most common form of polyuria is physiologic polyuria. It usually occurs as a compensatory response to increased fluid intake. Owing to the drinking habits of these animals, compensatory polyuria caused by excessive water consumption is far less common in dogs and especially cats than in man. Proper evaluation of a patient with physiologic polyuria often requires a water deprivation or vasopressin response test (Finco, 1980; Hardy and Osborne, 1980).

Pharmacologic Polyuria

Pharmacologic polyuria may occur following ingestion of sufficient quantities of salt to increase thirst, following administration of various diuretic agents and parenteral administration of fluids. It commonly occurs in dogs following administration of glucocorticoids. The cause(s) of glucocorticoid-induced polyuria in dogs is not known, but solute diuresis caused by gluconeogenesis (Osbaldiston, 1971) and alteration of the permeability of the distal nephrons to water (Levi et al., 1972) have been incriminated.

Pathologic Polyuria

Pathologic polyuria may be localized to mechanisms associated with *water diuresis* or *solute diuresis* on the basis of evaluation of urine specific gravity and osmolality, water deprivation tests, and vasopressin response tests. Pathologic polyuria may result from several primary disorders of other body systems, in addition to diseases of the kidney. It is beyond the scope of this chapter to discuss the pathophysiology of these mechanisms in detail. Conceptual understanding of them is essential, however, to prevent misdiagnosis of renal failure.

Water Diuresis. In general, water diuresis (hyposthenuria) is characterized by a urine specific gravity and osmolality (SG = 1.001 to ± 1.006; Osm = 50 to ± 250) below that of glomerular filtrate (SG = ± 1.008 to 1.012). Pathophysiologic mechanisms for patients with water diuresis include (1) deficiency of ADH (partial or total central diabetes insipidus, drugs that inhibit ADH), (2) unresponsiveness to adequate quantities of ADH (nephrogenic diabetes insipidus, medullary solute washout), and (3) inhibition of ADH (glucocorticoids, hypercalcemia, hypokalemia, primary polydipsia and others) (Breitschwerdt, 1981; Finco, 1980; Hardy and Osborne, 1980; Osborne et al., 1975).

Solute Diuresis. In general, solute diuresis is characterized by formation of urine with a specific gravity and osmolality equal to, or greater than, that of glomerular filtrate. Solute diuresis results from excretion of solute in excess of tubular capacity to reabsorb it, impaired tubular reabsorption of one or more solutes, and/or abnormal reduction in medullary solute concentration that impairs the countercurrent system. As a result, the kidneys have reduced capacity to control water excretion independent of solute excretion. In addition to primary polyuric renal failure (Tables 73–12 and 73–16), disorders associated with pathologic polyuria and solute diuresis include diabetes mellitus, post-obstructive diuresis, tubular reabsorptive disorders (Fanconi-like syndrome, etc.), and some cases of hepatic failure (Breitschwerdt, 1981; Finco, 1980; Hardy and Osborne, 1980; Osborne et al., 1975). The mechanisms responsible for pathologic polyuria associated with canine hyperadrenocorticism may include a combination of water and solute diuresis.

Solute diuresis associated with chronic primary renal failure appears to be related to at least two mechanisms: (1) loss of the functional capacity of a sufficient population of nephrons, which damages the countercurrent system and reduces the medullary solute gradient, and (2) obligatory solute diuresis. The obligatory solute diuresis is due to the fact that a small number of viable nephrons are required to excrete a daily solute load similar to that present when renal function was normal. Increased glomerular filtration of solutes retained in plasma (urea, creatine, sodium, and so forth) by remaining functional nephrons impairs tubular reabsorption of water. In addition to these mechanisms, the polyuric phase of acute renal failure may be associated with generalized damage to tubular epithelial cells.

Compensatory Polydipsia. The body compensates for obligatory polyuria by an appropriate degree of polydipsia. If there is inadequate water intake (e.g., vomiting in patients with polyuric primary renal failure), water required for obligatory polyuria will be derived from various body fluid compartments. Dehydration will occur as a result. If dehydration becomes severe, reduction in renal perfusion may cause reduction in glomerular filtration and oliguria. Unlike the situation with prerenal azotemia in patients with normal kidneys, however, superimposition of prerenal azotemia on primary renal azotemia will cause oliguria characterized by a relatively low specific gravity and osmolality.

OLIGURIA

Oliguria is defined as a decrease in the rate of formation and/or elimination of urine. It may be prerenal (physiological), primary renal, or postrenal. Pathologic oliguria presumably exists if urine volume is too low to excrete metabolic waste products without concomitant alteration in body fluid balance and composition. In humans, it is typically associated with production of less than 400 ml of urine per day (Levinsky et al., 1981). Comparable data are not available for dogs and cats.

Prerenal Oliguria

Prerenal (physiologic) oliguria is a compensatory response by normal kidneys to conserve water in excess of solute in order to maintain or restore normal body fluid balance. It is associated with formation of a reduced volume of highly concentrated urine with a low sodium concentration. It may be associated with azotemia if there is a concomitant reduction in renal blood flow and glomerular filtration.

Primary Renal Oliguria

Pathologic primary renal oliguria may occur during the early phase of acute primary renal failure due to generalized ischemic or nephrotoxic tubular disease (Table 73–12). Although an initial phase of oliguria is a common event in humans with acute renal failure (Levinsky et al., 1981), the incidence of oliguria associated with the initial phases of acute renal failure in dogs and cats is unknown. The exact sequence of events involved in production of oliguria in patients with acute renal failure has not been established, but experimental studies performed in dogs and other animals suggest that different mechanisms may be associated with different causes, and that more than one mechanism may occur concomitantly (Levinsky et al., 1981). Available clinical and experimental evidence has been interpreted to suggest that persistent renal vasoconstriction (vasomotor theory) is an important factor (refer to the section on the juxtaglomerular apparatus for additional information) (Thurau and Boylan, 1976). Obstruction of tubular lumens with casts and necrotic debris, abnormal reabsorption of filtrate through damaged tubular walls (passive backflow theory), and/or reduction in permeability of glomerular capillary walls (reduced glomerular ultrafiltration coefficient) may also be involved in some cases (Levinsky et al., 1981).

Primary renal oliguria may persist for hours to days, but in some instances its duration may be so transient that it is not detected. In such a situation, the patient may be nonoliguric or polyuric. The specific gravity and osmolality of urine (regardless of volume) obtained from patients with acute oliguric primary renal failure will reflect impaired tubular capacity to concentrate or dilute glomerular filtrate. If a sufficient number of nephrons have been damaged, it may be isosthenuric.

Oliguria may occur in patients with primary polyuric renal failure if some prerenal abnormality (such as vomiting, decreased water consumption, or cardiac decompensation) develops (Table 73–12). If the prerenal cause of reduced renal perfusion is removed, if additional ischemic nephron damage has not occurred, and/or if proper fluid balance is restored, polyuria will resume. Primary renal oliguria may also develop as a terminal event in patients with chronic progressive, generalized renal disease.

Postrenal Oliguria

Oliguria associated with elimination of a decreased volume of urine from the body may occur in association with diseases of the lower urinary system (ureters, urinary bladder, and/or urethra) that impair flow of urine through the excretory pathway. Examples of diseases that impair urine outflow include neoplasms, strictures, or calculi that partially occlude the urethral lumen, and herniation of the urinary bladder that partially obstructs urine outflow through the urethra and/or urine inflow from the ureters.

ANURIA

The term anuria has been used to indicate lack of urine formation by the kidneys and lack of elimination of urine from the body. Although it is possible that anuria could occur as a result of complete shutdown of renal function due to lack of renal perfusion or primary renal failure, it is usually associated with obstructive uropathy or rents in the lower urinary tract.

THE UREMIC SYNDROME

The literal translation of uremia is urine in blood. The terming of intoxication as "uremic poisoning" by lay people is conceptually accurate. The "poisons" may be endogenous waste products or exogenous drugs, the metabolism of which has been impaired by renal dysfunction. Virtually every cell of the body may suffer the consequence of severe impairment in renal function. See Terms and Concepts Related to Renal Disease, Renal Failure, Azotemia and Uremia for further details about the uremic syndrome.

Conceptual understanding of current knowledge of uremic syndrome pathophysiology is of diagnostic, therapeutic, and prognostic significance. Recent advances in the understanding of uremia have provided better insight into formulation of therapy to correct or reduce the severity of clinical signs and biochemical abnormalities. Although a variety of useful therapeutic procedures may be utilized, most are directed toward elimination of the underlying cause (specific therapy), correction of deficits and excesses of metabolites caused by renal dysfunction (supportive therapy), and amelioration of clinical signs (symptomatic therapy) (Osborne and Polzin, 1979).

COMMON DENOMINATOR OF CLINICAL MANIFESTATIONS

Although the clinical findings associated with the uremic syndrome may vary from patient to patient and from time to time within individual patients, they are the result of three basic underlying phenomena. The first and most obvious involves signs caused by generalized renal lesions that are directly referable to the kidneys (renal pain, alteration in renal size, silent hematuria, etc.). The second phenomenon represents polysystemic signs associated with autointoxication caused by a reduction of renal function below that required to clear

Table 73–17.   Interaction of Multiple Factors Contributing to Polysystemic Manifestations of Uremia

Abnormalities	Sequelae
Electrolyte Imbalances	
Sodium deficit	Dehydration
Sodium excess	Overhydration
Potassium deficit	Muscular weakness;
	Decreased urine concentration
Potassium excess	Cardiotoxicity
Calcium deficit	Osteodystrophy, tetany
Calcium excess	Calcium nephropathy, muscular atony
Acid-Base Imbalances	
Hydrogen ion retention	Metabolic acidosis
Increased bicarbonate utilization	Metabolic acidosis
Increased bicarbonate loss in urine	Metabolic acidosis
Decreased renal tubular production of ammonia	Metabolic acidosis
Fluid Imbalance	
Polyuria; vomiting; diarrhea	Dehydration
Oliguria; anuria	Predisposition to overhydration
Endocrine Imbalance	
Decreased erythrocyte–stimulating factor production	Anemia
Decreased production of 1,25-dihydroxycholecalciferol	Hypocalcemia
Decreased degradation of parathormone	Bone demineralization, osteodystrophy, hyperbicarbonaturia, others
Decreased degradation and clearance of insulin	Increased sensitivity to exogenous insulin
Caloric Imbalance	
Anorexia, vomiting, diarrhea	Weight Loss
Metabolic Waste Imbalance	
Decreased clearance of urea, creatinine, guanidines, phenols, and others	GI disorders, neurologic disorders, bleeding, immunologic disturbances, others

plasma of metabolic waste products, an impaired ability of tubules to conserve vital metabolites in glomerular filtrate, and reduced synthesis and reduced degradation and/or elimination of hormones (Table 73–17). The third phenomenon consists of the body's compensatory responses to the metabolic deficits and excesses caused by these abnormalities in an attempt to maintain homeostasis (Table 73–18). The common denominator underlying the polysystemic clinical and laboratory manifestations of uremia is the summation of the results of deficits and excesses in fluid balance, electrolyte balance, acid-base balance, endocrine balance, nutrient and caloric balance, and metabolic waste products. Each individual component encompassed in these categories may be insufficient to cause a severe disturbance, but collectively they are capa-

Table 73–18.   Examples of Body's Compensatory Reactions to Renal Dysfunction

Disorder	Compensation
Polyuria	Polydipsia
Hypocalcemia	Hyperparathyroidism
Severe metabolic acidosis	Elimination of CO_2 by increased rate and depth of respiration
Retention of metabolic waste products	Vomiting = ?
Nephron destruction	Hypertrophy, hyperplasia, and increased function of viable nephrons

ble of inducing profound alterations in homeostasis and even death.

PERSPECTIVE OF UREMIC TOXINS

A variety of toxins have been incriminated as underlying causes of polysystemic signs characteristic of uremia (Bovee 1976; Giovannetti and Barsolti, 1975; Knochel and Seldon, 1981; Schreiner and Maher, 1961) (see Table 73–5). While a direct cause-and-effect relationship has not always been proved, it is generally accepted that many so-called "uremic-toxins" are intermediary or end products of protein and nucleoprotein metabolism that accumulate in blood as a result of impaired renal clearance. In addition to nitrogenous substances, proteinaceous foods contribute significant quantities of hydrogen ions, sulfur, potassium, and phosphorus. Some uremic toxins are products of intestinal bacterial degradation and intestinal putrefaction (Giovannetti and Barsolti, 1975). Others are excessive quantities of hormones normally produced by the body (Knochel and Seldon, 1981). Some uremic toxins attain high extracellular concentrations, while others appear to attain highly intracellular concentrations. It has been hypothesized that some of these toxic metabolites induce abnormalities by inhibiting intracellular enzymes (Bergstrom and Bittar, 1969; Knochel and Seldon, 1981).

Uremic toxins are not the sole cause for uremia, however, as evidenced by the inability to identify a substance that can induce a similar syndrome when administered to experimental animals. This observation, along with the fact that the uremia syndrome has variable clinical manifestations, suggests that it is mediated by the *summation* of toxic metabolites in addition to fluid, acid-base, electrolyte, endocrine, nutrient, and enzymatic imbalances.

Deficits due to loss of water and electrolytes in patients with renal failure are caused by one or a combination of the following: generalized nephron damage, polyuria, anorexia, vomiting, and diarrhea. These abnormalities have the potential to induce varying degrees of dehydration and negative body balance of several metabolites including sodium, chloride, calcium, and bicarbonate ions.

Excesses due to retention of water, electrolytes, and non-electrolytes in patients with renal failure are caused by a reduction in renal clearance due to generalized nephron damage. This abnormality has the potential to induce varying degrees of edema (uncommon, and when present usually associated with generalized glomerular disease), hyperkalemia, hyperphosphatemia, retention of dietary nonvolatile acids, and retention of catabolic waste products (urea, creatinine, guanidines, phenols, indoles, and others).

METABOLIC DISTURBANCES

The onset and spectrum of clinical signs of uremia may vary from patient to patient, depending on the nature, severity, duration (acute or chronic), rate of progression of the underlying disease, presence or absence of coexistent but unrelated disease(s), and administration of therapeutic agents. The volume of urine produced (oliguria or polyuria) is also an important variable. In most instances, however, uremia is the clinical state toward which all progressive generalized renal diseases ultimately converge, and associated signs are more similar than dissimilar. In addition to manifestations of impaired renal function (azotemia, metabolic acidosis, oliguria or polyuria, hyponatremia, hypokalemia or hyperkalemia, hypocalcemia, and hyperphosphatemia), one may observe signs indicative of variable involvement of the gastrointestinal, cardiovascular, pulmonary, neuromuscular, skeletal, hemopoietic, immune, genital, and endocrine systems, as well as of coagulation defects.

Body Water Balance

In the dog and cat, dehydration may be a cause or an effect of renal failure. Dehydration may cause prerenal azotemia. Dehydration may occur secondary to acute or chronic generalized renal disease as a result of impairment of the renal concentrating mechanisms. Polyuria unaccompanied by compensatory polydipsia or complicated by vomiting and diarrhea also will result in dehydration. Thus, prerenal azotemia due to dehydration may be superimposed on primary renal azotemia. Dehydration equivalent to a loss of 12 to 15 per cent body weight will result in death from hypovolemic shock. Vigorous fluid therapy is indicated in the dehydrated uremic patient.

Primary renal failure and uremia is uncommonly associated with overhydration in the dog and cat. When encountered, however, it usually is assocated with hypoproteinemia and the nephrotic syndrome, or parenteral administration of large quantities of fluids to uremic patients with oliguria or anuria. Death due to overhydration of uremic dogs and cats is unlikely to occur, since the patients usually refuse to drink and often are vomiting. Death due to iatrogenic overhydration of an oliguric patient is more likely.

Serum and Body Sodium Balance

The question of sodium balance in patients with renal failure is extremely important, since negative sodium balance would result in negative water balance, contraction of extracellular fluid volume, reduction in renal blood flow, and ultimately reduction in glomerular filtration rate. The resulting prerenal azotemia would aggravate the reduction in renal function caused by generalized renal lesions. In contrast, positive sodium balance would lead to positive water balance, expansion of fluid volume in various body compartments, and a variety of undesirable sequelae (hypertension, edema, release of potentially toxic quantities of biologic substances to maintain sodium balance, etc.).

In past years, it was generally accepted that patients with polyuric renal failure lose or "waste" sodium to varying degrees. Carefully performed clinical studies in dogs and cats that document this assumption have not been performed, however. The problem is compounded by the fact that knowledge of the serum concentration of sodium is not a reliable index of total body sodium concentration. Measurement of the quantity of sodium lost in urine compared with sodium intake would help to solve this problem (Yium, 1973).

Experimental studies performed in dogs have suggested that increased excretion of sodium in urine by functioning nephrons may represent an adaptive rather than an obligatory phenomenon (Bricker and Fine, 1981; Schmidt et al., 1974). If oral intake of a solute normally excreted in urine (such as sodium) remains unaltered while renal function declines, body balance can be maintained only if fractional excretion of the solute increases in proportion to reduc-

tion in nephron numbers. A biologically active substance that induces natriuresis in rats and inhibits sodium transport by the frog skin and toad bladder has been identified .in the serum of uremic dogs and humans (Fine et al., 1976). A factor with the same characteristics has been found in the urine of uremic humans; its natriuretic action appears to be related to concurrent patterns of sodium excretion (Bricker et al., 1975). It has been hypothesized that this factor is a "natriuretic hormone" that serves as a modulator for sodium excretion.

Care must be used in the evaluation of urine sodium excretion in uremic animals or man following reduction of sodium intake. Abrupt reductions of sodium intake caused sodium wasting in human patients with severe renal insufficiency, whereas gradual reduction of sodium intake resulted in much-improved adjustment of sodium excretion to equal intake (Danovitch et al., 1977). Proportional reduction of salt intake to match proportional reduction in nephrons in dogs allowed sodium balance to be maintained without a detectable rise in natriuretic factor (Schmidt et al., 1974).

Further studies are required before such generalities are allowed to influence the formulation of therapeutic maneuvers for maintaining sodium homeostasis in patients with renal failure and uremia. It seems logical that sodium balance in patients with primary renal failure would vary with location(s) of lesions within nephrons, volume of urine produced (oliguria or polyuria), severity and extent of nephron dysfunction, and each individual patient. Patients with primary tubulo-interstitial forms of renal failure are more likely to have impaired renal conservation of sodium than patients with primary glomerular forms of renal failure (Wilson, 1972).

Metabolic Acidosis

Patients with oliguric or polyuric primary renal failure develop varying degrees of metabolic acidosis. Several mechanisms may contribute to the metabolic acidosis of renal failure and uremia, including (1) impaired tubular reabsorption of bicarbonate (and perhaps other buffer ions) resulting from hyperparathormonemia and renal tubular dysfunction, (2) catabolism of exogenous (dietary) or endogenous (body) protein for energy, (3) impaired production of ammonia by renal tubular epithelial cells, and/or (4) impaired tubular secretion of hydrogen ion (Cogan et al., 1981; Hayslett, 1979).

A major factor involved in uremic acidosis is reduction of hydrogen ion secretion by tubular cells. This reduction is related, at least in part, to impaired renal tubular production of ammonia. Normally, lipid-soluble ammonia (NH_3) produced by tubular cells diffuses through cell walls into tubular fluid. There it acts as a buffer by combining with hydrogen ions to form ammonium ions (NH_4). Since ammonium ions are not lipid soluble, they cannot return to tubular cells and are excreted in urine. The maximal hydrogen ion gradient against which tubular transport mechanisms can secrete hydrogen ions corresponds to a pH of about 4.5 to 5.0. When tubular production of ammonia is impaired and other buffers in urine are saturated with hydrogen ion, this pH is rapidly attained and tubular secretion of hydrogen ions is inhibited.

If the buffer systems of the body are capable of compensating for the acidosis, the pH of the blood will remain within normal limits (approximately 7.3 to 7.45). When the blood pH is within the normal range, compensated acidosis may be recognized in an abnormally low concentration of bicarbonate. If the buffer systems cannot completely compensate for metabolic acidosis, both bicarbonate concentration and the pH of blood will be abnormally low.

On occasion, metabolic alkalosis may develop in patients with primary renal failure as a consequence of severe vomiting. This is the exception rather than the rule, however.

The role of acidosis in contributing to death in uremic patients depends on its severity. Blood pH values below 6.8 are almost invariably incompatible with life, regardless of cause. Even uremic dogs in which acidosis has been corrected by treatment do not consistently recover. Furthermore, some dogs die of uremia without developing acidosis of sufficient magnitude to be incompatible with life. There is no direct relationship between the concentration of BUN or creatinine and the degree of acidosis. The preceding observations indicate that when the blood pH of a uremic patient approaches 6.8, death is probable, and that a less severe state of acidosis may contribute to the death of a uremic patient but is not the sole cause.

Renal Secondary Hyperparathyroidism, Serum Phosphorus, and Serum Calcium

Conceptual understanding of the interrelationships of calcium, phosphorus, vitamin D, and parathormone is important in comprehending the genesis and perpetuation of renal secondary hyperparathyroidism.

Applied Biochemistry. Dietary phosphorus absorption occurs primarily in the small intestine, especially in the jejunum and duodenum. It is influenced by vitamin D. Approximately 70 per cent of the ingested phosphorus is eliminated by the kidneys, while approximately 30 per cent is eliminated in the feces. Approximately 80 to 85 per cent of the phosphorus in the body is contained within the skeleton, while approximately 10 to 15 per cent is in muscle. Despite random variations in phosphorus ingestion, serum phosphorus concentration is normally maintained within relatively narrow limits (2.8 to 4.5 mg/dl). Much higher concentrations of phosphorus are present within cells, however. Approximately 95 per cent of the inorganic phosphorus in serum is filtered by glomeruli. Tubular reabsorption of filtered phosphorus is influenced by parathormone, which plays an important role in regulating serum phosphorus concentration.

1,25-Dihydroxycholecalciferol (1,25-vitamin D) appears to be the most biologically active form of vitamin D. It is synthesized by the kidneys from 25-hydroxycholecalciferol, which is formed in the liver (Deluca, 1973; Schoolwerth, 1975). Reduced intracellular phosphorus concentration in renal tubules is thought to stimulate production of 1,25-vitamin D. Since parathormone impairs tubular reabsorption of phosphorus, increased production of parathormone in response to hypocalcemia indirectly stimulates synthesis of 1,25-vitamin D. Some important biologic roles of vitamin D include stimulation of calcium absorption from the small intestines (an action that is augmented by parathormone) and mobilization of calcium and phosphorus from bone in conjunction with parathormone. Generalized renal disease is associated with reduced production of 1,25-vitamin D.

Parathormone (PTH) promotes active calcium reabsorption from the duodenum in cooperation with 1,25-vitamin D (Slatopolsky et al., 1977). While some intestinal absorption of calcium can occur in the absence of PTH, none can occur in the absence of vitamin D. Parathormone also promotes calcium and phosphorus reabsorption from bone in cooperation with 1,25-vitamin D. PTH blocks reabsorption of phosphorus from the proximal and distal renal tubules but promotes renal tubular reabsorption of calcium.

Pathophysiology of Renal Secondary Hyperparathyroidism. Increased production of parathormone as a consequence of renal failure is associated with hypocalcemia. Hypocalcemia associated with renal failure develops as a result of several mechanisms (Albers, 1978; Coburn, 1980; Massry and Ritz, 1978; Schoolwerth and Engle, 1975), including (1) hyperphosphatemia caused by decreased clearance of phosphorus and tissue catabolism. Hyperphosphatemia results in induction of a reciprocal decrease in serum ionized calcium concentration; (2) impaired renal production of 1,25-vitamin D; (3) impaired tubular reabsorption of filtered calcium caused by lesions in nephrons; (4) skeletal resistance to parathormone; and (5) reduced consumption of dietary calcium.

Hypocalcemia mediated by hyperphosphatemia requires further explanation. The relationship between calcium and phosphate ions in body fluid is governed by physiochemical solubility laws. If the product of serum calcium times serum phosphorus concentration exceeds a solubility limit (commonly estimated to be approximately 60 in man), calcium and phosphorus precipitate as an insoluble salt in soft tissues (Barber and Rowland, 1979; Hubert et al., 1966; Slatopolsky et al., 1971; Slatopolsky and Bricker, 1973; Kaplan et al., 1978). Primary renal diseases that progressively reduce glomerular filtration rate cause varying degrees of hyperphosphatemia, which may induce precipitation of calcium and phosphorus. The result rapidly reduces the magnitude of hyperphosphatemia but as a result leads to hypocalcemia. At this point, the magnitude of hypocalcemia cannot be detected by routine laboratory methods, but is detected by the parathyroid glands. Hypocalcemia leads to increased production of parathormone. The stimulus for release of PTH occurs early in chronic progressive

nephron destruction, long before the onset of azotemia (Finco, 1980). Parathormone restores serum calcium concentration to normal by enhancing calcium absorption from the duodenum, promoting calcium (and phosphorus) reabsorption from bone, and enhancing calcium reabsorption by the renal tubules (Slatopolsky et al., 1977). Parathormone decreases fractional renal tubular reabsorption of phosphorus in proportion to the number of nephrons that have been damaged. Serum phosphorus and calcium concentrations can be maintained within normal limits despite a persistent reduction of glomerular filtration rate, provided hyperparathormonemia is sustained. This mechanism is so efficient that detectable rises in serum phosphorus concentration cannot usually be detected until the glomerular filtration rate is reduced to approximately 25 per cent of normal. This degree of reduction in GFR coincides with the onset of azotemia. Serum calcium concentration is usually maintained within normal limits until GFR is reduced to a much greater degree. When GFR drops below 25 per cent of normal, however, the increased production and release of parathormone is unable to overcome the effects of impaired filtration of phosphorus. Despite persistent hyperparathormonemia, hyperphosphatemia persists and may become more severe. With progressive reduction of renal function, varying degrees of measurable hypocalcemia also develop.

As previously mentioned, impaired intestinal absorption of calcium as a consequence of impaired renal synthesis of 1,25-vitamin D is also a significant cause of abnormal calcium metabolism in patients with severe uremia. Although it is not known when during the course of progressive chronic generalized renal disease that intestinal malabsorption begins, it cannot be detected in human patients with mild renal failure (Coburn, 1980). Administration of small quantities of 1,25-dihydroxycholecalciferol to acutely uremic rats (Wrong et al., 1972) and to human beings with chronic renal failure (Brickman et al., 1972) stimulated intestinal calcium transport and augmented calcium mobilization from bone. Vitamin D analogues have also been shown to improve intestinal calcium absorption from uremic human beings (Vergne-Marini et al., 1976). Although it has not been determined whether or not altered vitamin D metabolism is a significant factor during early phases of renal insufficiency, impaired synthesis of 1,25-vitamin D plays an important role in reduced intestinal absorption of calcium (and phosphorus) during later stages of renal failure (Coburn, 1980).

Persistent hyperparathormonemia, which occurs as a result of hypocalcemia in patients with primary renal failure, plays an important role in the polysystemic manifestations of uremia. Parathormone has been incriminated as a uremic toxin because it may play a role in causing the following abnormalities (Avram et al., 1978; Coburn, 1980; Coburn and Slatopolsky, 1981; Crumb et al., 1974; Goldstein et al., 1978; Massry and Goldstein, 1978; Puschett and Zurbach, 1976): (1) decreased renal tubular reabsorption of bicarbonate, which aggravates metabolic acidosis; (2) decreased renal tubular reabsorption of amino acids; (3) decreased renal tubular reabsorption of sodium; (4) renal osteodystrophy; (5) metastatic calcification; (6) neuromuscular disturbance; (7) pruritis; (8) pancytopenia (via myelofibrosis); and (9) sexual dysfunction. Consult the discussions about the effects of uremia on various body systems in this section for additional information.

Trade-Off Hypothesis. Development of long-term sequelae of hyperparathormonemia have been likened to "trading-off" an immediate problem that threatens homeostasis (i.e., hypocalcemia) for longer term ones that are not an immediate threat to homeostasis or life (Bricker and Fine, 1978; Bricker and Fine, 1981). Because of the vast store of calcium in bone, it is a ready reserve for deficits of calcium elsewhere in the body. As renal failure progresses, however, the animal is forced to live in a narrowed state of physiologic adaptivity. A price must be paid for life-saving adaptations in nephron function. Ultimately the bony reserve can be depleted to such a degree that the function of the skeletal system becomes impaired (i.e., renal osteodystrophy). The "trade-off hypothesis" represents an important concept in explaining the pathophysiology of renal secondary hyperparathyroidism, as well as other components of the uremic syndrome, such as how body sodium balance is maintained by increased production of natriuretic factor.

Hypercalcemia. Severe hypercalcemia is more often a cause than a consequence of primary renal failure (Osborne and Stevens, 1977). Although dogs and cats with chronic renal failure typically have normal to reduced serum calcium concentrations, on occasion they may be elevated (so-called tertiary hyperparathyroidism) (Finco and Rowland, 1978). The underlying mechanism(s) of hypercalcemia that occurs as a sequela remains unknown; however, the following abnormalities may be involved: reduced renal degradation of parathormone, reduced renal degradation of prostaglandins, overproduction of parathormone, hypercitricemia, and/or retention of calcium as a consequence of reduced glomerular filtration.

Serum Potassium Concentration

Alterations in the serum concentration of potassium are especially important, since relatively small changes in serum concentration can produce hazardous clinical changes. The clinical signs of hyperkalemia or hypokalemia are primarily related to the serum concentration of potassium, despite the large quantity of potassium in intracellular fluid.

Normally, potassium filtered through glomeruli is removed from tubular fluid by active reabsorption by the proximal tubules and is secreted into tubular fluid by distal tubular cells. The amount of potassium excreted in urine is approximately equal to potassium intake and absorption, and potassium balance is maintained. Since the kidneys are the primary route of excretion of potassium, patients with oliguria or anuria will ultimately develop hyperkalemia.

The toxic effect of hyperkalemia on the heart is one of the major factors that contribute to the death of patients with uncorrected or irreversible oliguric or anuric renal failure (Hiatt and Sheinkopf, 1971). Clinical signs of hyperkalemia usually appear when the serum concentration of potassium is between 7 and 10 mEq per liter and are characterized by cardiac conduction disturbances (arrhythmias, bradycardia, and heart block) and, in some instances, muscular weakness. Death from cardiac arrest commonly occurs when the serum concentration of potassium exceeds 10 mEq per liter. Acidosis tends to perpetuate the severity of hyperkalemia, because the kidneys tend to conserve potassium ions and excrete hydrogen ions. In addition, acidosis is associated with movement of hydrogen ions into cells and potassium ions out of cells.

If patients with renal failure can maintain an adequate urine volume, the serum concentration of potassium tends to remain within physiologic limits. While hyperkalemia is a common finding in oliguric renal failure, it is not a feature of polyuric renal failure, since viable nephrons undergo compensatory adaptation and renal tubules are capable of secreting a sufficient quantity of potassium to prevent clinically significant hyperkalemia (Schultz et al., 1971). Just as phosphorus and sodium balance appear to be maintained by decreased fractional tubular reabsorption as nephron destruction progresses, potassium balance is maintained by a proportional increase in renal tubular potassium secretion. Control of serum potassium concentration by a kaliuretic hormone has been hypothesized (Bricker and Fine, 1981).

Hyperglycemia

Until recently, knowledge of the effect of chronic renal failure on glucose and insulin metabolism has been limited to two seemingly paradoxical clinical observations in man. One is that hyperglycemia occasionally developed in patients with chronic renal failure, and the other was that insulin requirements of patients with diabetes mellitus decreased with the onset of renal insufficiency.

Glucose intolerance in patients with primary renal failure is sometimes called azotemic pseudodiabetes, because they have a diabetic-like glucose tolerance curve. In contrast to diabetes mellitus, however, azotemic pseudodiabetes is not associated with severe hyperglycemia, glucosuria, ketonuria, ketonemia, or severe metabolic acidosis. Glucose intolerance in uremic patients is characterized by mild prolongation of hyperglycemia following oral or intravenous administration of glucose (Reaven et al., 1974). Fasting blood glucose concentrations in uremic dogs are usually normal and, when elevated, do not exceed 150 mg/dl (Bovee, 1976). The degree of glucose intolerance is proportional to the degree of azotemia.

There is no evidence to suggest that glucose intolerance associated with azotemia is associated with a primary defect in insulin secretion. In fact, an increase in plasma insulin concentration usually occurs (Knochel and Seldon, 1980). It has been hypothesized that peripheral resistance to insulin-mediated uptake of glucose by tissues is the cause of azotemic glucose intolerance (Defronzo and Alvestrand, 1980; Merrill and Hampers, 1970). This hypothesis is supported by studies that indicate that the ability of exogenous insulin to lower plasma glucose concentration is impaired in uremic humans and dogs (Reaven et al., 1974). Although it appears that peripheral insulin resistance occurs in uremia, the underlying cause is obscure. Metabolic acidosis has been incriminated but has been found to play only a minor role in dogs with experimentally induced renal failure (Bovee, 1976; Reaven et al., 1974). Abnormal glucose tolerance curves have been induced in dogs with urea but not methylguanidine (Balestri et al., 1970). A defect in intracellular metabolism or in the glucose transport system has been hypothesized (Defronzo and Alvestrand, 1980).

Studies in dogs indicate that a profound effect of renal insufficiency on glucose and insulin metabolism is marked reduction in removal of insulin from plasma as a result of loss of functional renal parenchyma (Reaven et al., 1974). Dog kidneys remove approximately two thirds of the insulin that reaches the general circulation (Swenson et al., 1971). Since only a small amount of the insulin removed by the kidneys is excreted in urine, the kidneys appear to be an important site of insulin degradation.

The modest rise in serum creatinine concentration that occurs immediately following bilateral nephrectomy in dogs is associated with a marked reduction in the rate of loss of insulin from plasma (Reaven et al., 1974). However, the onset of severe uremia several days following nephrectomy is not associated with further reduction in the half-life of insulin. These observations indicate that uremia per se has little effect on the rate of insulin removal from plasma, and that loss of renal parenchyma is primarily responsible for prolongation of the half-life of insulin in dogs with renal insufficiency. Impaired renal degradation of insulin is the best available explanation of the observation that uremic human beings with diabetes mellitus require less insulin than do nonuremic diabetics.

Studies in dogs also indicate that the net

amount of insulin entering the general circulation decreases after nephrectomy (Reaven et al., 1974). It appears that the dog responds to impaired renal degradation of insulin by secreting less insulin.

With the exception of the obvious need to differentiate azotemic pseudodiabetes from diabetes mellitus complicated by uremia, the clinical implications of abnormal glucose tolerance in uremia are not yet known. Peritoneal dialysate solutions with high concentrations of glucose should be used with caution.

Hyperamylasemia

Hyperamylasemia associated with naturally occurring primary renal failure has been observed in man (Salt and Schenker, 1976) and dogs (Finco and Stevens, 1969) without other clinical evidence of concomitant pancreatitis. Increased serum amylase activity has also been observed in dogs with experimentally induced renal failure (Meroney et al., 1956). Hyperamylasemia associated with primary renal failure is thought to occur, at least in part, as a result of impaired clearance of amylase by glomerular filtration. In one study of 28 days with spontaneously occurring primary renal failure, mean serum amylase activity was approximately 2.5 times normal, as compared with amylase values of approximately seven times normal in dogs with histologically confirmed acute pancreatitis (Finco and Stevens, 1969). The mean serum amylase activity of dogs with probable acute pancreatitis was 2.5 times normal.

Although it is generally agreed that primary renal insufficiency may result in hyperamylasemia, the degree of elevation that may be attributed solely to renal malfunction is unclear. No obvious relationship existed between the degree of azotemia and the degree of hyperamylasemia in uremic dogs (Stevens and Finco, 1969). Detection of lesions in the pancreas of uremic humans and dogs has prompted speculation that uremia-induced pancreatitis may contribute to the magnitude of azotemic hyperamylasemia in some cases (Bagenstoss, 1948; Bartos et al., 1970). To date, however, the function of the exocrine pancreas has not been investigated in man or animals with renal failure, and involvement of the pancreas in uremia is at best only a histologic entity.

Studies in dogs indicate that amylase may be eliminated from the circulation via the liver as well as by renal clearance (Hiatt and Bonorris, 1966). In man, it has been estimated that only about 24 per cent of the serum amylase is excreted in urine (Salt and Schenker, 1976). The fact that amylase may be removed from the circulation by extrarenal routes may explain why only modest increases in serum amylase activity occur in association with primary renal failure. This hypothesis is supported by the lack of correlation between serum and urine amylase activity in dogs with experimentally produced pancreatitis (Brobst et al., 1970).

Hyperlipasemia has been observed in uremic humans and rats but has not been carefully investigated in dogs or cats (Sommer et al., 1975). Pilot studies of naturally occurring renal failure in dogs suggest that hyperlipasemia may occur, but this is not a consistent finding (Osborne et al., 1980).

Serum Lipid Concentration

Hypercholesterolemia is a common finding in dogs and cats with protein-losing glomerulopathy and the nephrotic syndrome (Osborne et al., 1977). The underlying mechanism(s) is obscure. Clinical investigation of the nephrotic syndrome in man has revealed that serum-lipid and serum-albumin concentrations typically have an inverse relationship (Glassock et al., 1981). The observation that the concentration of serum lipids, including cholesterol, decreases following parenteral administration of albumin or dextran suggests that plasma colloidal osmotic pressure may be involved in the pathogenesis of the disorder.

Non-nephrotic human beings with chronic renal failure often develop hypertriglyceridemia, an event linked to the high incidence of atherosclerosis in this species (Knochel and Seldon, 1981). The serum cholesterol concentration in such patients is normal or reduced. Although the precise pathogenesis of uremic hyperlipidemia has not yet been defined, it appears to be related to a defect in removal of very low density lipoproteins (including triglycerides) from plasma by peripheral tissues (Reavan et al., 1980). Increased hepatic synthesis of triglycerides has also been incriminated. Lipoprotein metabolism in uremic dogs and cats has not been well documented. It is of interest, however, that atherosclerosis is not a common manifestation of uremia in these species.

Negative Caloric Balance

Uremia is a catabolic syndrome. Because it is associated with varying degrees of vomiting, diarrhea, and anorexia, a negative caloric balance develops. Glucose intolerance, intestinal malabsorption, elevated serum insulin and glucagon concentrations, and other pathophysiologic disturbances associated with uremia may alter carbohydrate and fat metabolism, and caloric balance. As a result, the body must catabolize its own tissues for energy. Catabolism of proteins perpetuates abnormalities in acid-base and electrolyte balance, because protein catabolism is associated with release of intracellular potassium and phosphorus, and production of protein waste products including nonprotein nitrogenous substances and nonvolatile acids. A negative caloric balance may also be aggravated by proteinuria.

Uremia is associated with altered metabolism of protein (Finco, 1980; Polzin and Osborne, 1979). Available evidence suggests that the type and quantity of essential amino acids required during renal failure may be different from normal. These factors must be considered when evaluating the nutritional requirements of uremic dogs and cats.

POLYSYSTEMIC MANIFESTATIONS OF UREMIA

Nonspecific Signs

Nonspecific signs that may accompany uremia include depression, anorexia, lethargy, and weight loss. Studies in dogs indicate that the anorexia is associated, at least in part, with stimulation of the medullary emetic hemoreceptor trigger zone by circulatory toxins such as guanidines (Barsotti et al., 1975; Borison and Herbertson, 1959; Giovanetti et al., 1969). Ablation of the medullary emetic chemoreceptor trigger zone in nephrectomized dogs suppressed the onset of anorexia.

During recent years defects in intestinal absorption of calcium, proteins, and carbohydrates have been identified in uremic humans and animals. In addition to varying degrees of anorexia, vomiting, and diar-

rhea, it appears that these defects in intestinal function contribute to a low-grade malabsorption syndrome (Denneberg et al., 1974; Gulyassay, 1970).

Endocrine System

As reviewed in the section on applied anatomy and physiology, renal function is regulated by a variety of hormones. In addition, the kidneys form and degrade a variety of hormones. Therefore, it is not surprising that endocrine imbalances are a major contributor to various manifestations of uremia. For example, excessive production and decreased degradation of parathormone has been incriminated in the pathophysiology of uremic disorders of the central nervous system, in addition to soft tissue necrosis, soft tissue calcification, pruritis, osteodystrophy, anemia, hyperlipidemia, and sexual dysfunction (Massry and Goldstein, 1978). Additional metabolic-hormonal derangements associated with uremia include anemia, hypertension, glucose intolerance, thyroid dysfunction, altered gastrointestinal dysfunction, and infertility (Avioli, 1978; Bonomini et al., 1979; Owyang et al., 1979). Specific details related to many polysystemic consequences of uremic endocrinopathies are discussed under other headings in this section.

Gastrointestinal System

Uremic Stomatitis. Dogs and cats with acute or chronic renal failure occasionally develop oral ulcers, brownish discoloration of the dorsal surface of the tongue, and fetor of breath. The mucous membranes may also become dry (xerostoma). These abnormalities, singly or collectively, are commonly called uremic stomatitis.

Experimental studies performed in dogs and clinical studies in humans incriminate the local caustic action of ammonia generated by bacterial decomposition of abnormally high concentrations of salivary urea as the cause of oral ulcers (Bliss, 1937; Gruskin, 1970). In one study, tartar scraped from the teeth of normal and nephrectomized dogs hydrolyzed urea to ammonia in a few minutes, suggesting that dental tartar contained urease (Bliss, 1937; Gruskin, 1970). It is probable that urease-producing bacteria were present in the tartar. Ulcerations of the buccal mucosa and tongue of nephrectomized dogs occurred adjacent to teeth and could be prevented by removal of dental tartar from nephrectomized azotemic dogs (Bliss, 1937). The fact that uremic stomatitis has been observed in completely edentulous humans indicates that urease does not solely originate from dental tartar, or that urease is not the only cause of uremic stomatitis (Gruskin, 1970). The observation that there is no consistent relationship between serum urea nitrogen concentration and stomatitis also suggests the involvement of other factors (Johnson et al., 1972). Several species of bacteria produce urease, some of which are present in the normal oral flora in man. It is probable that a similar situation occurs in animals. Variations of the normal flora among different species, and among individuals within species, may explain the sporadic occurrence of uremic stomatitis (Osborne et al., 1980).

The cause of the brownish discoloration of the tongue associated with uremia is unknown. Xerostoma may be caused by reduction in production of saliva by dehydration, and compensatory hyperventilation associated with metabolic acidosis. Uremic fetor of breath may be caused by stomatitis and escape of volatile compounds that accumulate in the body as a result of renal failure. Studies in man indicate that dimethylamine and trimethylamine are involved (Simenhoff et al., 1977).

Vomiting. Vomiting is a well known but inconsistent sign associated with uremia. The severity of vomiting is not a reliable index of the severity or reversibility of uremia. Vomiting associated with renal failure may be associated with any one or combination of the following causes: stimulation of the medullary emetic chemoreceptor trigger zone by circulating toxins (Barsoti, 1975; Borison and Herbertson, 1959), gastritis, attempts to induce oral food or fluids, and intolerance to medications (such as antibiotics and cardiac glycosides).

Although vomiting might be considered a compensatory response that aids in the elimination of uremic toxins and minimizes the severity of metabolic acidosis, it appears to aggravate the uremic syndrome. In addition to the loss of gastric juices that augment imbalances in fluid and electrolytes, inhibition of compensatory polydipsia in patients with obligatory polyuria results in severe volume depletion and further reduction in

glomerular filtration. Catabolism of body proteins for energy as a result of insufficient consumption of nutrients contributes to further retention of protein catabolic byproducts in the body. Aspiration pneumonia may further complicate the patient's precarious balance between life and death.

Hemorrhagic and ulcerative gastritis has been commonly observed in dogs and cats with severe primary renal failure. In dogs, lesions commonly affect the body of the stomach and the fundic zone. Results of gross, microscopic, and ultrastructural evaluation of lesions have been interpreted to suggest that canine uremic gastritis is primarily a disease of the lamina propria characterized by arteriopathy, hemorrhage from capillary lesions, edema, mastocytosis, mucosubstance deposition, fibroplasia, and mineralization (Cheville, 1979). Even though gastric lesions are collectively described as gastritis, there is often a conspicuous absence of inflammatory cells.

The pathogenesis of uremic gastritis is unknown. Popular hypotheses of their cause include local irritation by ammonia produced from urea, alteration of the protective surface layer of mucus, uremic vasculitis, and/or coagulopathies (Osborne et al., 1980). On the basis of evaluation of the stomachs of four uremic dogs by light and electron microscopy, and comparing results with normal canine stomachs, it was suggested that uremic gastropathy is a disease of the mucosal lamina propria caused by parietal cell dysfunction, and anoxia induced by vascular injury (Cheville, 1979). Release of histamine from mastocytes, acidosis, hypergastrinemia, impaired coagulation, and altered plasma concentrations of calcium, phosphorus, and magnesium appear to be involved in its pathogenesis.

Diarrhea. Diarrhea is not a constant finding associated with uremia. In fact, dehydrated animals without a significant degree of enterocolitis may become constipated. The latter is thought to occur in response to conservation of intestinal fluids by the body in an attempt to restore fluid balance. In man, uremia may be associated wth ileus.

Enterocolitis, manifested clinically as diarrhea, may occur in severely uremic dogs and cats but is usually less severe than hemorrhagic gastritis. The lesions are similar to those observed in the stomach, except for lack of calcification of intestinal mucosa. Intussusceptions have frequently been reported in dogs with experimentally produced uremia, and we have observed them in dogs with naturally occurring uremia (Osborne et al., 1980).

The etiology of hemorrhagic and ulcerative lesions in the large and small intestine, like that of gastric lesions, is unknown. Several hypotheses have been proposed, including caustic action of ammonia, increased susceptibility of intestinal mucosa to pancreatic and bacterial enzymes, and abnormal coagulation (Osborne, et al., 1980).

Musculoskeletal System

Progressive uremia induces abnormalities of the musculoskeletal system, collectively called renal osteodystrophy. The term renal osteodystrophy encompasses a variety of lesions, including osteomalacia, osteitis fibrosa, osteosclerosis, and osteopenia.

Radiographic evidence of skeletal demineralization may be detected in patients with chronic uremia, especially if they have not reached physical maturity. It has been estimated that 30 to 50 per cent of bone mineral must be lost to be visible radiographically (Agus and Goldberg, 1972; Shapiro, 1972). Skeletal changes associated with secondary renal hyperparathyroidism tend to be more severe in immature dogs, because their bones are in an active state of growth. For an unexplained reason, the bones of the skull are most severely affected. Occasionally the first evidence of chronic progressive renal failure in dogs (especially when immature) owned by unobservant clients is demineralization of the skull associated with loosening of the teeth. This abnormality, sometimes called "rubber jaw," may be associated with distortion of facial bones by extensive proliferation of connective tissue (fibrous osteodystrophy). In general, renal osteodystrophy of sufficient severity to cause pathologic fractures or signs clearly referrable to bone pain is uncommon in dogs and cats with naturally occurring uremia.

The etiopathogenesis of renal osteodystrophy is not completely understood, but it may include varying combinations and interactions of hyperphosphatemia, hypocalcemia, hypermagnesemia, parathyroid hyperplasia, elevated concentrations of serum parathormone, decreased renal degrada-

tion of parathormone, skeletal resistance to the action of parathormone, metabolic acidosis, abnormal vitamin D metabolism, and defective intestinal absorption of calcium (Coburn, 1980; Norrdin et al., 1977; Slatopolsky et al, 1978; Villafane, 1977). Some of these pathogenic factors become operative months or even years before patients manifest overt disease during late stages of advanced renal failure. As discussed in a previous section, persistent hyperparathormonemia and skeletal lesions represent a "trade-off" for maintenance of serum phosphorus concentration during early stages of renal failure and prolonged maintenance of serum ionized calcium concentration (Bricker, 1979; Bricker and Fine, 1981).

Cardiovascular System

Abnormalities in cardiac rate and conduction may occur as a result of potassium retention in oliguric or anuric uremic patients. Auscultation and electrocardiograms may reveal varying degrees of bradycardia, arrhythmias, and heart block.

The heart rate may be accelerated in advanced chronic renal failure as a result, at least in part, of the anemia that is frequently present. Left ventricular hypertrophy has been observed in dogs with chronic generalized renal disease. Although its exact cause is unknown, it may be associated with anemia or hypertension. Uremic pericarditis, a well documented lesion in uremic humans, has been rarely encountered in uremic dogs and cats.

Hypertension is a well documented sequela of experimentally produced renal ischemia in dogs and other animals, and of naturally occurring renal ischemia in man (so-called renovascular hypertension) (Spangler et al., 1977; Schambelan and Perloff, 1981). It may also occur as a result of bilateral nephrectomy (so-called renoprival hypertension) (Grollman et al., 1949). Hypertension is also a well documented phenomenon in human patients with a variety of renal parenchymal lesions (Schambelan and Perloff, 1981). The limited amount of information available also suggests that a variable degree of hypertension may occur in dogs with naturally occurring generalized renal disease and renal failure. In one study of 20 dogs with advanced renal failure due to a diversity of causes, hypertension (systolic/diastolic blood pressure > 180/90 mm Hg) was detected by the indirect Doppler method of blood pressure measurement in 75 per cent of the cases (Weiser et al., 1977).

The pathophysiology of hypertension associated with renal disorders has not yet been precisely defined. Several factors have been incriminated, including inappropriate activation of the renin-angiotensin system, decreased production of prostaglandins by the renal medulla, and retention of sodium and water as a result of decreased renal clearance (Dollery, 1979). Determining whether the underlying renal lesions are unilateral or bilateral and where they are located (renal artery versus renal parenchyma) is important in formulating prognoses and management in human beings (Schambelan and Perloff, 1981).

In man, lesions of the renal arteries may cause hypertension, and in turn, hypertension may cause vascular lesions in the kidney and elsewhere (Dollery, 1979; Schambelan and Perloff, 1981). Renal vascular lesions have been observed in dogs with renal failure, but their relationship to hypertension has not been well documented (Anderson and Fischer, 1968; Weiser et al., 1977).

Respiratory System

Major involvement of the respiratory system is not a consistent finding in uremia. Patients with severe uremia may develop an increased respiratory rate in order to compensate for anemia, metabolic acidosis, or uncommonly, pulmonary edema. Patients with advanced uremia may also develop varying degrees of bronchopneumonia, presumably as a result of immunodeficiency.

Hemic System

Red Blood Cells. Anemia, which is typically nonregenerative, is a common manifestation of chronic uremia. It may also occur in patients with acute uremia, however. Causes of anemia associated with primary renal failure and uremia include (1) decreased production of erythropoietin by damaged kidneys; (2) inhibition of erythroblasts in bone marrow by toxic substances in uremic serum; (3) shortened red blood cell survival; (4) iron deficiency caused by chronic blood loss, impaired gastrointestinal absorption, and repeated blood sampling; (5) myelofibrosis secondary to renal osteodystrophy; and (6) chronic infection and malnutrition (Anagnostou et al., 1981; Lamperi et al., 1974; Moel, 1978; Naets, 1975; Wallner et al., 1978; Weinberg et al., 1977). Because multiple etiologic factors may underlie the anemia of uremia, the potential significance of each should be considered when formulating therapy to correct it.

White Blood Cells. As a generality, primary inflammatory diseases of the kidneys of dogs and cats are not associated with marked alteration in leukocytes. Because the total quantity of tissue involved is relatively small when compared with the body as a whole, it is hypothesized that the stimulus for bone-marrow production of leukocytes is correspondingly small.

Pyonephrosis, generalized acute pyelonephritis, and large abscesses involving one or both kidneys are exceptions to this generality, since they often are associated with leukocytosis and immature neutrophilia. Polysystemic diseases, such as pyometra, bacterial endocarditis, or leptospirosis, which affect the kidneys in addition to other bodily organs and tissues, are also often associated with immature neutrophilia. Varying degrees of leukocytosis may also occur as a result of secondary bacterial infection of various body systems in immunodeficient uremic patients.

Chronic generalized renal diseases that cause renal failure are commonly associated with mature neutrophilia and lymphopenia. This response is probably caused by an increased output of adrenocortical hormones, which occurs as a result of stress.

Coagulation Factors. Studies performed in uremic dogs and humans have revealed a major coagulopathy associated with an acquired, reversible qualitative defect in thrombocyte function (Anagnostou et al., 1981; Johnson et al., 1972). Platelet numbers were not altered. This abnormality undoubtedly contributes to insidious but significant blood loss from the gastrointestinal tract. It may be associated with bloody diarrhea, less frequently gingival hemorrhage, and rarely hematemesis. The platelet dysfunction is characterized by diminished activation of platelet factor 3, decreased platelet adhesiveness and aggregation, and impaired prothrombin consumption. Studies in dogs with experimentally induced uremia revealed that the severity of abnormal coagulation was related to the severity of uremia (Larrain and Langell, 1956). Current evidence implicates circulating uremic toxins, especially guanidinosuccinic acid and hydroxyphenolacetic acid, in the etiopathogenesis of uremic platelet dysfunction (Anagnostou et al., 1981). Recent studies in man have implicated prostacyclin, a prostaglandin that inhibits platelet aggregation, in the pathophysiology of the bleeding tendency associated with renal failure (Remuzzi et al., 1979). Despite the potential for platelet dysfunction in uremic patients, bleeding has not been a significant problem in dogs and cats following needle-punch biopsy of the kidney.

In human beings with some forms of glomerulonephropathy, activation of the clotting mechanism by immune reactants has been incriminated in the genesis of glomerular lesions (Alfrey, 1981). Dogs with glomerulonephropathy and severe hypoproteinemia (nephrotic syndrome) may also develop thromboembolism of major vessels (DiBartola and Meuten, 1980; Jeraj and Osborne, 1977; Osborne et al., 1976; Slauson and Gribble, 1971). Pulmonary thrombosis is commonly encountered, although thrombi have also been observed in the abdominal aorta and in coronary, splenic, renal, mesenteric, iliac, and/or brachial arteries. Clinical signs (sudden dyspnea, sudden death, progressive limb dysfunction, etc.) are referable to the affected system. A deficiency of antithrombin III caused by excessive urinary loss has been incriminated in the etiopathogenesis of thromboembolism in nephrotic patients. Thromboembolism has recently been observed in dogs with uremia experimentally induced by ligation of renal arteries and contralateral nephrectomy (Polzin et al., 1981). The underlying cause was not determined.

IMMUNE SYSTEM

Humoral and especially cellular components of the immune system have been found to be suppressed in experimental animals and human patients with renal failure and uremia (Anagnostou et al., 1981; Kunori et al., 1980, Mansell and Grimes, 1979). Although the precise underlying mechanism(s) that induce immunodeficiency as a result of uremia have not been defined, uremic serum factors have been incriminated (Anagnostou et al., 1981; Raska et al., 1980). Lymphopenia in varying degrees is a common finding in uremic dogs and cats, and also occurs in uremic humans. In uremic humans, both B and T circulating lymphocytes are decreased (Anagnostou et al., 1981). The concentration of serum immunoglobulins may be normal or abnormal. Activation of complement and granulocyte function may be impaired.

Despite the potential for immunosuppression, experience with dogs and cats with experimentally induced or naturally occurring primary renal failure indicates that secondary bacterial infections are uncommon until advanced stages of uremia. The likelihood of immunosuppression warrants appropriate caution with use of urinary catheters, however. Because the magnitude of immunosuppression appears to be insufficient to predispose to frequent occurrence of secondary bacterial infections in all but terminally uremic dogs and cats, and because of the increased potential for adverse drug reactions in patients with renal failure, antimicrobial agents should not be included as a prophylactic maneuver in the supportive and symptomatic therapy of renal failure and uremia.

Nervous System

Uremic encephalopathy and uremic neuropathy are common manifestations of uremia in man, irrespective of the underlying cause of renal failure (Arieff, 1981). Signs that may develop during stages of uremia include impaired mental activity characterized by impaired memory, inability to concentrate, slurred speech, apathy, and lethargy. As uremia becomes more severe, neurologic signs may encompass abnormalities of gait, action tremors, multifocal myoclonus, and asterixis. Signs referable to cranial nerve dysfunction may also occur (e.g., blindness, deafness, and nystagmus). Advanced stages of uremia may be associated with seizures and eventually coma. Clinical signs of peripheral neuropathy are uncommon unless patients have been maintained by chronic dialysis. They include the so-called restless leg syndrome, which is characterized by sensations of crawling, prickling, and pruritis of the lower extremities. Muscle fatigability, weakness, atrophy, and cramps may also occur.

With the exception of lethargy and depression, neurologic disturbances have not been well documented in uremic dogs and cats. In one study of three young (less than one-year-old) dogs with chronic uremia, the owner's complaint consisted chiefly of abnormal behavior, tremors, and/or seizures (Wolf, 1980). Lack of information pertaining to peripheral neuropathies may be related to difficulty in their detection and to the fact that the vast majority of dogs and cats with uremia are not maintained by chronic dialysis.

Proposed mechanisms in the pathophysiology of neurologic disturbances associated with uremia have been reviewed (Arieff, 1981). The results of clinical studies in uremic humans and experimental studies in dogs indicate that hyperparathormonemia and calcium deposition in the brain are significant factors (Arieff, 1981; Goldstein et al., 1978; Goldstein and Massry, 1978; Guisado et al., 1975).

Tetanic convulsions presumably caused by hypocalcemia may occur, but they are uncommon. This is related to the fact that ionized serum calcium concentration usually does not decrease to dangerous levels. In addition, concomitant metabolic acidosis tends to prevent hypocalcemic tetany by conversion of nonionized calcium to the biologically active ionized form. As a result, neurologic manifestations of hypocalcemia may not develop even though the serum concentration of calcium is approximately 6 to 7 mg/dl.

Integumentary System

Dehydration is often present in vomiting patients during a uremic crisis, especially if they have obligatory polyuria. Dehydration is manifested clinically by varying degrees of loss of skin pliability. Uremic frost, a crystalline, white material that may accumulate on the skin of uremic human beings, does not occur in the dog and cat.

Nonpainful, pitting edema of the subcutaneous tissue of the dependent portions of the body may occur in hypoproteinemic patients with protein-losing glomerular diseases (amyloidosis, glomerulonephropathy, and so forth).

Genital System

Atrophy of germinal epithelium of the testicles of uremic dogs, and presumably cats, results in infertility. Infertility is also a common complication of uremia in men and women (Knochel, and Seldon, 1981). Primary lesions of the gonads and derangement of hormones that influence gonad function are related to the problem. In one study, 70 per cent of 40 dogs developed permanent erections following parathyroidectomy and nephrectomy (Massry and Goldstein, 1978).

REFERENCES

Agus, Z. S., and Goldberg, M.: Pathogenesis of uremic osteodystrophy. Radiol. Clin. North Am. *10*:545–556, 1972.

Albers, C.: Diet in uremia. Calcium and phosphorus. A review. CRN News *3*:3–4, 1978.

Alfrey, A. C.: The Renal Response to Vascular Injury. *In* Brenner, B. M., and Rector, F. C. (eds.): The Kidney, Vol. 2. 2nd ed. W. B. Saunders Co., Philadelphia, 1981.

Allen, T. D.: Compensatory Renal Hypertrophy. *In* Johnston, J. H., and Goodwin, W. E. (eds.): Reviews in Pediatric Urology. Excerpta Medica, Amsterdam, 1974.

Anagnostou, A., Fried, W., and Kurtzman, N. A.: Hematologic Consequences of Renal Failure. *In* Brenner, B. M., and Rector, F. C. (eds.): The Kidney, Vol. 2. 2nd ed. W. B. Saunders Co., Philadelphia, 1981.

Anderson, L. J., and Fisher, E. W.: The blood pressure in canine interstitial nephritis. Res. Vet. Sci. *9*:304–313, 1968.

Arieff, A. I.: Neurological Complications of Uremia. *In* Brenner, B. M., and Rector, F. C. (eds.): The Kidney, Vol. 2. 2nd ed. W. B. Saunders Co., Philadelphia, 1981.

Aschinberg, L. C.: Koskimies, O., Bernstein, J., Nash, M., Edelmann, C. M., and Spitzer, A.: The influence of age on the response to renal parenchymal loss (dogs). Yale J. Biol. Med. *51*:341–345, 1978.

Avioli, L. V.: Pathogenesis and significance of hormonal-metabolic derangements in uremia. Am. J. Clin. Nutr. *31*:1554–1560, 1978.

Avram, M. M., Feinfeld, D. A., and Huaturo, A. H.: Decreased motor nerve conduction velocity and elevated parathyroid hormone in uremia. N. Engl. J. Med. *298*:1000–1003, 1978.

Bagenstoss, A. H.: The pancreas in uremia: a histopathologic study. Am. J. Pathol. *24*:1003–1011, 1948.

Balestri, P. L., Biagini, M., Rindi, P., and Giovanetti, S.: Uremic toxins. Arch. Int. Med. *126*:843–845, 1970.

Balint, P.: Pathogenesis of mercuric chloride induced renal failure in the dog. Acta Med. Acad. Sci. Hung. *25*:287–297, 1968.

Barber, D. L.: Renal angiography in veterinary medicine. J. Am. Vet. Rad. Soc. *16*:187–205, 1975.

Barber, D. L., and Rowland, G. N.: Radiographically detectable soft tissue calcification in chronic renal failure. Vet. Radiol. *20*:117–123, 1979.

Barsotti, G., Bevilacqua, G., Morelli, E., Cappelli, P., Balestri, P. L., and Giovanetti, S.: Toxicity arising from guanidine compounds: role of methylguanidine as uremic toxin. Kidney Int. 7:S-299 to S-301, 1975.

Bartos, V., Melichar, J., and Erben, J.: The function of the exocrine pancreas in chronic renal failure. Digestion *3*:33–40, 1970.

Beeuwkes, R.: The vascular organization of the kidney. Ann. Rev. Physiol. *42*:531–542, 1980.

Beeuwkes, R.: Efferent vascular patterns and early vascular-tubular relations in the dog kidney. Am. J. Physiol. *221*:1361–1374, 1971.

Beeuwkes, R., and Bonaventure, J. V.: Tubular organization and vascular tubular relations in the dog kidney. Am. J. Physiol. *229*:695–713, 1975.

Beeuwkes, R., Ichikawa, I., and Brenner, B. M.: The renal circulations. *In* Brenner, B. M., and Rector, F. C. (eds.): The Kidney, Vol. 1. 2nd ed. W. B. Saunders Co., Philadelphia, 1981.

Ben-Ishay, A., Wiener, J., Sweeting, J., Bradley, S. E., and Spiro, D.: Fine structural alterations in the canine kidney during hemorrhagic hypotension. Effects of osmotic diuresis. Lab. Invest. *17*:190–210, 1967.

Bergstrom, J., and Biltar, E. E.: The Basis of Uremic Toxicity. *In* Biltar, E. E., and Biltar, N. (eds.): The Biologic Basis of Medicine. Vol. 6. Academic Press, New York, 1969.

Bliss, S.: The cause of sore mouth in nephritis. J. Biol. Chem. *121*:425–427, 1937.

Bloom, F.: Pathology of the dog and cat. The genitourinary system, with clinical considerations. American Vet. Publ. Inc., Evanston, Ill., 1954.

Bonomini, V., Orsoni, G., Stefoni, S., and Vangelista, A.: Hormonal changes in uremia. Clin. Nephrol. *11*:275–280, 1979.

Bonvalet, J. P.: Evidence of induction of new nephrons in immature kidneys undergoing hypertrophy. Yale J. Biol. Med. *51*:315–319, 1978.

Borison, H. L., and Herbertson, L. M.: Role of medullary emetic chemoreceptor trigger zone in postnephrectomy vomiting dogs. Am. J. Physiol. *197*:850–852, 1959.

Bovee, K. C.: The uremic syndrome. J.A.A.H.A. *12*:189–197, 1976.

Breitschwerdt, E. B.: Clinical abnormalities of urinary concentration and dilution. Comp. Cont. Ed. *3*:414–421, 1981.

Brenner, B. M., and Beeuwkes, R.: The renal circulations. Hosp. Pract. *13*:35–46, 1978.

Bricker, N. S.: On the meaning of the intact nephron hypothesis. Am. J. Med. *46*:1–11, 1969.

Bricker, N. S., and Fine, L. G.: The renal response to progressive nephron loss. *In* Brenner, B. M., and Rector, F. C., The Kidney, Vol. 1. 2nd ed. W. B. Saunders Co., Philadelphia, 1981.

Bricker, N. S., and Fine, L. G.: The trade-off hypothesis: current status. Kidney Int. *13*:S-5 to S-8, 1978.

Bricker, N. S., Fine, L. G., Kaplan, M., Epstein, M., Bourgoigne, J. J., and Light, A.: Magnification phenomenon in chronic renal disease. N. Engl. J. Med. *299*:1287–1293, 1978.

Bricker, N. S., Schmidt, R. W., Favre, H., Fine, L., and Bourgoigne, J. J.: On the biology of sodium excretion: the search for a natriuretic hormone. Yale J. Biol. Med. *48*:293–303, 1975.

Brickman, A. S., Coburn, J. W., and Norman, A. W.: Action of 1,25-dihydroxycholecalciferol, a potent kidney-produced metabolite of vitamin D_3, in uremic man. N. Engl. J. Med. *287*:891–895, 1972.

Brobst, D., Ferguson, A. B., and Carter, J. M.: Evaluation of serum amylase and lipase activity in experimentally induced pancreatitis in the dog. J.A.V.M.A. *157*:1697–1702, 1970.

Busuttil, R. W., Roh, B. L., and Fisher, J. W.: Localization of erythropoietin in the glomerulus of the hypoxic dog kidney using a fluorescent antibody technique. Acta Haematol. *47*:238–242, 1972.

Caulfield, J. P., and Farquhar, M. G.: Distribution of anionic sites in glomerular basement membranes: Their possible role in filtration and attachment. Proc. Nat'l Acad. Sci. *73*:1646, 1976.

Caywood, D. D., Osborne, C. A., and Johnston, G. R.: Neoplasms of the canine and feline urinary tracts. *In* Kirk, R. W. (ed.): Current Veterinary Therapy. 7th ed. W. B. Saunders Co., Philadelphia, 1980.

Cheville, N. F.: Uremic gastropathy in the dog. Vet. Pathol. *16*:292–309, 1979.

Christie, B. A.: Collateral arterial blood supply to the normal and ischemic canine kidney. Am. J. Vet. Res. *41*:1519–1525, 1980.

Clapp, J. R., and Robinson, R. R.: Osmolality of distal tubular fluid in the dog. J. Clin. Invest. *45*:1847–1853, 1966.

Coburn, J. W.: Renal osteodystrophy. Kidney Int. *17*:677–693, 1980.

Coburn, J. W., and Slatopolsky, E.: Vitamin D, parathyroid hormone, and renal osteodystrophy. *In* Brenner, B. M., and Rector, F. C. (eds.): The Kidney, Vol. 2. 2nd ed. W. B. Saunders Co., Philadelphia, 1981.

Cogan, M. G., Rector, F. C., and Seldin, D. W.: Acid-base disorders. *In* Brenner, B. M., and Rector, F. C. (eds.): The Kidney, Vol 1. 2nd ed. W. B. Saunders Co., Philadelphia, 1981.

Crumb, C. K., Martinez-Maldonado, M., Eknoyan, G. E., and Suki, W. N.: Effects of volume expansion, purified parathyroid extract, and calcium on renal bicarbonate absorption in the dog. J. Clin. Invest. *54*:1287–1294, 1974.

Danovitch, G. M., Bourgoigne, J., and Bricker, N. S.: Reversibility of the "salt-losing" tendency of chronic renal failure. N. Engl. J. Med. *296*:14–19, 1977.

DeFronzo, R. A., and Alvestrand, A.: Glucose intolerance in uremia: site and mechanism. Am. J. Clin. Nutr. *33*:1438–1445, 1980.

DeLuca, H. F.: The kidney as an endocrine organ involved in calcium homeostasis. Kidney Int. *4*:80–88, 1973.

Denneberg, T., Lindbein, T., Berg, N. O., and Dahlquist, A.: Morphology, dipeptidases and disaccharidases of small intestinal mucosa in chronic renal failure. Acta Med. Scand. *195*:465, 1974.

DeWolf, W. C., and Fraley, E. E.: Renal pain. Urology *6*:403–408, 1975.

DiBartola, S. P., and Meuten, D. J.: Renal amyloidosis

in two dogs presented for thromboembolic phenomena. J.A.A.H.A. *16*:129–135, 1980.

DiBartola, S. P., Chew, D. J., and Jacobs, G.: Quantitative urinalysis including 24-hour protein excretion in the dog. J.A.A.H.A. *16*:537–546, 1980.

Dollery, C. T.: Arterial hypertension. *In* Beeson, P. B., et al. (ed.): Cecil Textbook of Medicine. 15th ed. W. B. Saunders Co., Philadelphia, 1979.

Fiaschi, E., Maschio, G., D'Angelo, A., Bonucci, E., Tessitored, N., and Messa, P.: Low protein diets and bone disease in chronic renal failure. Kidney Int. *13*:579–582, 1978.

Finco, D. R.: Kidney Function. *In* Kaneko, J. J. (ed.): Clinical Biochemistry of Domestic Animals. 3rd ed. Academic Press, New York, 1980.

Finco, D. R., and Duncan, J. R.: Evaluation of blood urea nitrogen and serum creatinine as indicators of renal dysfunction: A study of 111 cases and a review of related literature. J.A.V.M.A. *168*:593–601, 1976.

Finco, D. R., and Duncan, J. R.: Relationship of glomerular number and diameter to body size of the dog. Am. J. Vet. Res. *33*:2447–2450, 1972.

Finco, D. R., and Rowland, G. N.: Hypercalcemia secondary to renal failure in the dog: a report of 4 cases. J.A.V.M.A. *173*:990–994, 1978.

Finco, D. R., and Stevens, J. B.: Clinical significance of serum amylase activity in the dog. J.A.V.M.A. *155*:1686–1691, 1969.

Fine, L. G., Bourgoigne, J. J., Kwang, K. H., and Bricker, N. S.: On the influence of the natriuretic factor from patients with chronic uremia on the bioelectric properties and sodium transport of the isolated mammalian collecting duct. J. Clin. Invest. *58*:590–597, 1976.

Fisher, J. W.: Erythropoietin: pharmacology, biogenesis, and control of production. Pharmacol. Rev. *24*:459–508, 1972.

Fisher, J. W.: Extrarenal erythropoietin production. J. Lab. Clin. Med. *93*:695–699, 1972.

Forsling, M. L.: Antidiuretic hormone. Ann. Res. Rev. *4*:1–164, 1979.

Fourman, J., and Moffat, D. B.: The Blood Vessels of the Kidney. Blackwell Scientific Publications. F. A. Davis, Co., Philadelphia, 1971.

Fried, W.: Erythropoietin and the kidney. Nephron *15*:327–349, 1975.

Galla, J. H., Klein-Robenhaar, T., and Hayslett, J. P.: Influence of age on the compensatory response in growth and function to unilateral nephrectomy. Yale J. Biol. Med. *47*:218–226, 1974.

Gennard, F. J., and Kassirer, J. P.: Osmotic diuresis. N. Engl. J. Med. *291*:714–720, 1974.

Giovanetti, S., Biagini, M., Balestri, P. L., et al.: Uremia-like syndrome in dogs chronically intoxicated with methylguanidine and creatinine. Clin. Sci. *36*:445–452, 1969.

Glassock, R. J., Cohen, A. H., Bennett, C. M., and Martinez-Maldonado, M.: Primary glomerular disease. *In* Brenner, B. M., and Rector, F. C. (eds.): The Kidney, Vol. 2. 2nd ed. W. B. Saunders Co., Philadelphia, 1981.

Goldstein, D. A., and Massry, S. G.: Effect of parathyroid hormone and its withdrawal on brain calcium and electroencephalogram. Min. Elect. Metab. *1*:84–91, 1978.

Goldstein, D. A., Chul, L. A., and Massry, S. G.: Effect of parathyroid hormone and uremia on peripheral nerve calcium and motor nerve conduction velocity. J. Clin. Invest. *62*:88–93, 1978.

Gottschalk, C. W.: Function of the chronically diseased kidney. The adaptive nephron. Circ. Res. *28*:1–13, 1971.

Grollman, A., Muirhead, E. E., and Vanatta, J.: Role of the kidney in the pathogenesis of hypertension as determined by a study of the effects of bilateral nephrectomy and other experimental procedures on the blood pressure of the dog. Am. J. Physiol. *157*:21–30, 1949.

Gruskin, S. E., Tolman, D. E., and Wagoner, R. D.: Oral manifestations of uremia. Minn. Med. *53*:495–499, 1970.

Guisado, R., Arieff, A. I., and Massry, S. G.: Changes in the electroencephalogram in acute uremia: Effects of parathyroid hormone and brain electrolytes. J. Clin. Invest. *55*:738–745, 1975.

Gulyassay, P. F., Aviram, A., and Peters, J. H.: Evaluation of amino acid and protein requirements in chronic uremia. Arch. Int. Med. *126*:855, 1970.

Hardy, R. M., and Osborne, C. A.: Water deprivation and vasopressin concentration tests in the differentiation of polyuric syndromes. *In* Kirk, R. W. (ed.): Current Veterinary Therapy. Vol. 8. W. B. Saunders Co., Philadelphia, 1980.

Hardy, R. M., and Osborne, C. A.: Water deprivation test in the dog: Maximal normal values. J.A.V.M.A. *174*:479–483, 1979.

Hardy, R. M., and Osborne, C. A.: Canine pyometra: Pathophysiology, diagnosis and treatment of uterine and extra-uterine lesions. J.A.A.H.A. *10*:245–268, 1974.

Hayman, J. M., Shumway, N. P., Dumky, R., and Miller, M.: Experimental hyposthenuria. J. Clin. Invest. *18*:195–212, 1939.

Hays, R. M.: Antidiuretic hormone. N. Engl. J. Med. *295*:659–665, 1976.

Hayslett, J. P.: Functional adaptation to reduction in renal mass. Physiol. Rev. *59*:137–164, 1979.

Hiatt, N., and Bonorris, G.: Removal of serum amylase in dogs and the influence of reticuloendothelial blockade. Am. J. Physiol. *210*:133–138, 1966.

Hiatt, N., and Sheinkopf, J. A.: Treatment of experimental hyperkalemia with large doses of insulin. Surg. Gynecol. Obstet. *133*:833–836, 1971.

Horster, M., and Valtin, H.: Postnatal development of renal function: Micropuncture and clearance studies in the dog. J. Clin. Invest. *50*:779–795, 1971.

Horster, M., Kemler, B. J., and Valtin, H.: Intracortical distribution of number and volume of glomeruli during postnatal maturation in the dog. J. Clin. Invest. *50*:796–800, 1971.

Hoyer, J. R., and Seiler, M. W.: Pathophysiology of Tamm-Horsfall protein. Kidney Int. *16*:279–289, 1979.

Hubert, L. A., Lemann, J., Petersen, J. R., and Lennon, E. J.: Studies of the mechanisms by which phosphate infusion lowers serum calcium concentration. J. Clin. Invest. *45*:1886–1894, 1966.

Ibels, L., Alfrey, A. C., Haut, L., and Huffer, W. E.: Preservation of function in experimental renal disease by dietary restriction of phosphate. N. Engl. J. Med. *298*:122–126, 1978.

Jamison, R. L.: Urine concentration and dilution. *In* Brenner, B. M., and Rector, F. C. (eds.): The Kidney, Vol. 1. 2nd ed. W. B. Saunders Co., Philadelphia, 1981.

Jamison, R. L., and Maffly, R. H.: The urinary concentrating mechanism. N. Engl. J. Med. *295*:1059–1067, 1976.

Jeraj, K., and Osborne, C. A.: Renal Amyloidosis. *In*

Kirk, R. W. (ed.): Current Veterinary Therapy. Vol. VI. W. B. Saunders Co., Philadelphia, 1977.

Johnson, W. L., Hagge, W. W., Wagoner, R. D., Dinapoli, R. P., and Rosevear, J. W.: Effects of urea loading in patients with far-advanced renal failure. Mayo Clinic Proc. 47:21–29, 1972.

Jolliffe, N., and Smith, H. W.: The excretion of urine in the dog. Am. J. Physiol. 98:572–577, 1931.

Kaplan, M. A., Canterbury, J. M., Gavellas, G., Jaffe, D., Bourgoigne, J. J., Reiss, E., and Bricker, N. S.: Interreactions between phosphorus, calcium, parathyroid hormone, and renal phosphate excretion in response to an oral phosphorus load in normal and uremic dogs. Kidney Int. 14:207–214, 1978.

Katz, A. I., and Lindheimer, M. D.: Actions of hormones on the kidney. Ann. Rev. Physiol. 39:97–134, 1977.

Kjellstrand, C. M.: The clinical significance of middle molecules. Dial. Transpl. 8:860–865, 1979.

Klahr, S., and Rodriguez, H. J.: Natriuretic hormone. Nephron 15: 387–408, 1975.

Knochel, J. P., and Seldin, D. W.: The pathophysiology of uremia. In Brenner, B. M., and Rector, F. C. (eds.): The Kidney, Vol. 2. 2nd ed. W. B. Saunders Co., Philadelphia, 1981.

Kolata, R. J., Burrows, C. F., and Soma, L. R.: Shock: pathophysiology and management. In Kirk, R. W. (ed.): Current Veterinary Therapy. Vol. 7. W. B. Saunders Co., Philadelphia, 1980.

Kunkel, P. A.: The number and size of glomeruli in the kidney of several mammals. Bull. Johns Hopkins Hosp. 47:285–291, 1930.

Kunori, T., Fehrman, I., Ringden, O., and Moller, E.: In vitro characterization of immunologic responsiveness of uremic patients. Nephron 26:234–239, 1980.

Lamperi, S., Bandiana, G., Fiorio, P., Muttini, P., and Scaringi, G.: Effect of some substances retained in uremia on erythropoiesis: The effect on bone marrow cell cultures. Nephron 13:278–287, 1974.

Larrain, C., and Langell, R. D.: The hemostatic defect of uremia. II. Investigation of dogs with experimentally produced acute urinary retention. Blood 11:1067–1972, 1956.

Lawler, D. F.: Unpublished data. Ralston Purina Co., Checkerboard Square, St. Louis, Missouri, 1981.

Levi, J., Massry, S. G., and Kleeman, C. R.: The requirement of cortisol for the inhibitory effect of norepinephrine on the antidiuretic action of vasopressin. Clin. Res. 20:200, 1972.

Levinsky, N. G., Alexander, E. A., and Venkatachalam, M. A.: Acute renal failure. In Brenner, B. M., and Rector, F. C. (eds.): The Kidney, Vol. 1. 2nd ed. W. B. Saunders Co., Philadelphia, 1981.

Levy, S. E., and Blalock, A.: The effects of unilateral nephrectomy on the renal blood flow and oxygen consumption of unanesthetized dogs. Am. J. Physiol. 122:609–613, 1938.

Lifschitz, M. D., and Stein, J. H.: Renal vasoactive hormones. In Brenner, B. M., and Rector, F. C. (eds.): The Kidney, Vol. 1. 2nd ed. W. B. Saunders Co., Philadelphia, 1981.

Low, D. G., Mather, G. W., Finco, D. R., and Anderson, N. V.: Long-term studies of renal function in canine leptospirosis. Am. J. Vet. Res. 28:731–739, 1967.

Macfarlane, W. V.: Water and electrolytes in domestic animals. In Phillis, J. W. (ed.): Veterinary Physiology. W. B. Saunders Co., Philadelphia, 1976.

Malt, R. A.: Compensatory renal growth of the kidney. N. Engl. J. Med. 280:1446–1458, 1969.

Mansell, M., and Grimes, A. J.: Red and white cell abnormalities in chronic renal failure. Br. J. Hematol. 42:169–174, 1979.

Massry, S. G., and Goldstein, D. A.: Role of parathyroid hormone in uremic toxicity. Kidney Int. 13:39–42, 1978.

Massry, S. G., and Ritz, E.: The pathogenesis of secondary hyperparathyroidism of renal failure. Is there a controversy? Arch. Int. Med. 138:853–856, 1978.

Meroney, W. H., Lawson, N. L., Rubini, M. E., and Carbone, J. V.: Some observations of the behavior of amylase in relation to acute renal insufficiency. N. Engl. J. Med. 255:315–320, 1956.

Merrill, J. P., and Hampers, C. L.: Uremia. N. Engl. J. Med. 282:953–961; 1014–1021, 1970.

Moel, D. I.: The conservative management of uremia in childhood. In Friedman, E. A. (ed.): Strategy in Renal Failure. Wiley Medical Publications, New York, 1978.

Murphy, G. P., Mirand, E. A., Kenny, G. M., Niemat, S., and Staubitz, W. J.: Extrarenal and renal erythropoietin levels in human beings and experimental animals in intact, anephric and renal allotransplanted state. J. Urol. 103:686, 1970.

Naets, J. P.: Hematologic disorders in renal failure. Nephron 14:181–194, 1975.

Nash, M. A., and Edelmann, C. M. Jr.: The developing kidney. Immature function or inappropriate standard. Nephron 11:71–90, 1973.

Nisser, O. I., and Galskov, A.: Direct measurement of the superficial and deep venous flow in the cat kidney. Circ. Res. 30:82–96, 1972.

Norrdin, R. W., Bordier, P., and Miller, C. W.: Trabecular bone morphometry in beagles with chronic renal failure. Virchows Arch. A. Pathol. Anat. Histol. 375:169–183, 1977.

Oliver, J., MacDowell, M., and Tracy, A.: The pathogenesis of acute renal failure associated with traumatic and toxic injury. Renal ischemia, nephrotoxic damage, and the ischemuric episode. J. Clin. Invest. 30:1307, 1439, 1951.

Osathanondh, V., and Potter, E. L.: Development of human kidney as shown by microdissection. III. Formation and interrelationship of collecting tubules and nephrons. Arch. Pathol. 76:290–302, 1963.

Osboldiston, G. W.: Renal effects of long term administration of triamcinolone acetonide in normal dogs. Canad. J. Comp. Med. 35:28–35, 1971.

Osborne, C. A., and Johnston, S.D.: Ectopic hormone production by nonendocrine neoplasms. In Kirk, R. W. (ed.): Current Veterinary Therapy. Vol 7. W. B. Saunders Co., Philadelphia, 1977.

Osborne, C. A., and Low, D. G.: Size, adequacy and artifacts of canine renal biopsy samples. Am. J. Vet. Res. 32:1865–1871, 1971.

Osborne, C. A., and Polzin, D. J.: Strategy in the diagnosis, prognosis and management of renal disease, renal failure, and uremia. Proc. 46th Ann. Mtg. Am. Anim. Hosp. Assoc., South Bend, Ind., 1979, pp. 559–630.

Osborne, C. A., and Stevens, J. B.: Hypercalcemic nephropathy. In Kirk, R. W. (ed.): Current Veterinary Therapy. Vol 6. W. B. Saunders Co., Philadelphia, 1977.

Osborne, C. A., Finco, D. R., and Scott, R. C.: Problem

oriented diagnosis of diseases of the urinary system: I. The kidney. Scientific Proc., 42nd AAHA Annual Meeting, South Bend, Indiana, 1975.

Osborne, C. A., Hammer, R. F., Resnick, J. S., Stevens, J. B., Yano, B. L., and Vernier, R. L.: Natural remission of nephrotic syndrome in a dog with immune complex glomerular disease. J.A.V.M.A. *168*:129–137, 1976.

Osborne, C. A., Hammer, R. F., Stevens, J. B., O'Leary, T. P., and Resnick, J. S.: Immunologic aspects of glomerular disease in the dog and cat. *In* 26th Gaines Vet. Symposium, Gaines Dog Research Center, White Plains, N.Y., 1976.

Osborne, C. A., Hammer, R. F., Stevens, J. B., Resnick, J. S., and Michael, A. F.: The glomerulus in health and disease: Review of domestic animals and man. Adv. Vet. Sci. Comp. Med. *21*:207–285, 1977.

Osborne, C. A., Johnson, K. H., Perman, V., Fangmann, G. M., and Riis, R. C.: Clinicopathologic progression of renal amyloidosis in a dog. J.A.V.M.A. *157*:203–219, 1970.

Osborne, C. A., Klausner, J. S., and Lees, G. E.: Urinary tract infections: Normal and abnormal host defense mechanisms. Vet. Clin. North Am., *9*:587–609, 1979.

Osborne, C. A., Low, D. G., and Finco, D. R.: Reversible versus irreversible renal disease in the dog. J.A.V.M.A. *155*:2062–2078, 1969.

Osborne, C. A., Low, D. G., and Finco, D. R.: Canine and Feline Urology. W. B. Saunders Co., Philadelphia, 1972.

Osborne, C. A., Stevens, J. B., and Polzin, D. J.: Gastrointestinal manifestations of urinary diseases. *In* Anderson, N. V. (ed.): Veterinary Gastroenterology. Lea and Febiger, Philadelphia, 1980.

Owyana, C., Miller, L. J., Dimagno, E. P., Brennan, L. A., and Go, V. L. W.: Gastrointestinal hormone profile in renal insufficiency. Mayo Clin. Proc. *54*:769–773, 1979.

Peraino, R. A.: The effect of parathyroid hormone infusion on renal bicarbonate absorption in the presence of carbonic anhydrase inhibition. Mineral Elect. Metab. *1*:65–73, 1978.

Pitts, R. F.: Physiology of kidney and body fluids. 3rd ed. Year Book Medical Publ. Inc., Chicago, Ill., 1974.

Polzin, D. J., and Osborne, C. A.: Unpublished observations. College Vet. Med., University of Minnesota, St. Paul, 1981.

Polzin, D. J., and Osborne, C. A.: Management of chronic primary polyuric renal failure with modified protein diets: Concepts, questions and controversies. *In* 29th Gaines Veterinary Symposium. Gaines Dog Research Center, White Plains, N.Y., 1979, pp. 24–35.

Polzin, D. J., Osborne, C. A., Hayden, D. W., and Stevens, J. B.: Experimental evaluation of reduced protein diets in the management of primary polyuric renal failure. Preliminary findings and their clinical significance. Minnesota Vet., *21*:16–29, 1981.

Puschett, J. B., and Zurbach, P.: Acute effects of parathyroid hormone on proximal bicarbonate transport in the dog. Kidney Int. *9*:501–510, 1976.

Rahill, W. J., and Subramanian, S.: The use of fetal animals to investigate renal development. Lab. Anim. Sci. *23*:92–96, 1973.

Raska, K., Morrison, A. B., and Raskova, J.: Humoral inhibitors of the immune response in uremia. Lab. Invest. *42*:636–642, 1980.

Ray, B. S., and Neil, C. L.: Abdominal visceral sensation in man. Ann. Surg. *126*:709–724, 1947.

Reaven, G. M., Swenson, R. S., and Sanfelippo, M. L.: An inquiry into the mechanism of hypertriglyceridemia in patients with chronic renal failure. Amer. J. Clin. Nutr. *33*:1476–1484, 1980.

Reaven, G. M., Weisinger, J. R., and Swenson, R. S.: Insulin and glucose metabolism in renal insufficiency. Kidney Int. Suppl. *6*:S-62 to S-69, 1974.

Reis, R. H., and Tepe, P.: Variations in the patterns of renal vessels and their relation to the type of posterior vena cava in the dog. Am. J. Anat. *99*:1–55, 1956.

Remuzzi, G., Marchesi, D., Cavenaghi, A. E., Livio, M., Donati, M. B., Degaetano, G., and Mecca, G.: Bleeding in renal failure. A possible role of vascular prostacycline (PG12). Clin. Nephrol. *12*:127–131, 1979.

Rieck, A. F., and Reis, R. H.: Variations in patterns of renal vessels and their relation to the type of posterior vena cava in the cat. Am. J. Anat. *93*:457–474, 1953.

Ross, L. A., and Finco, D. R.: Unpublished data. Dept. Physiology, College Vet. Med., Univ. Georgia, Athens, Georgia, 1980.

Rous, S. N., and Wakin, K. G.: Kidney function before, during and after compensatory hypertrophy. J. Urol. *98*:30–35, 1967.

Rutherford, W. E., Bordier, P., Marie, P., Hruska, K., Harter, H., Greenwall, A., Blondin, J., Haddah, J., Bricker, N. S., and Slatopolsky, E.: Phosphate control and 25-hydroxycholecalciferol administration in preventing renal osteodystrophy in the dog. J. Clin. Invest. *60*:332–341, 1977.

Rytand, D. A.: The number and size of mammalian glomeruli as related to kidney and to body weight, and methods for their enumeration and measurement. Am. J. Anat. *62*:507–520, 1938.

Salt, W. B., and Schenker, S.: Amylase — its clinical significance. A review of the literature. Medicine *55*:269–289, 1976.

Schambelan, M., and Perloff, D.: Renovascular and renal parenchymal hypertension. *In* Brenner, B. M., and Rector, F. C. (eds.): The Kidney, Vol. 2. 2nd ed. W. B. Saunders Co., Philadelphia, 1981.

Schmidt, R. W., Bourgoigne, J., and Bricker, N. S.: On the adaptation in sodium excretion in chronic uremia: the effects of "proportional reductions" of sodium intake. J. Clin. Invest. *53*:1736–1741, 1974.

Schmidt-Nielsen, B.: Urinary concentrating processes in vertebrates. Yale J. Biol. Med. *52*:545–561, 1979.

Schmidt-Nielsen, B., and O'Dell, R.: Structure and concentrating mechanism in the mammalian kidney. Am. J. Physiol. *200*:1119–1124, 1961.

Schoolwerth, A. C., and Engle, J. E.: Calcium and phosphorus in diet therapy of uremia. J. Am. Diab. Assoc. *66*:460–464, 1975.

Schultze, R. G., Taggart, D. D., Shapiro, H., Pennell, J. P., Gaglar, S., and Bricker, N. S.: On the adaptation in potassium excretion associated with nephron reduction in the dog. J. Clin. Invest. *50*:1061–1068, 1971.

Schumann, G. B., Harris, S., and Henry, J. B.: An improved technique for examining urinary casts and a review of their significance. Am. J. Clin. Pathol. *69*:18–23, 1978.

Scott, R. C., and Patnaik, A. K.: Renal carcinoma with secondary polycythemia in the dog. J.A.A.H.A. *8*:275–283, 1972.

Sellwood, R. V., and Verney, E. B.: Enumeration of glomeruli in the kidney of the dog. J. Anat. *89*:63–68, 1955.

Seveis, W. B., and Daniels-Seveis, A. E.: Effects of angiotension on the central nervous system. Pharmacol. Rev. #3, *25*:415–449, 1973.

Shapiro, R.: Radiologic aspects of renal osteodystrophy. Radiol. Clin. North Am. *10*:557–568, 1972.

Shively, M. J.: Origin and branching of renal arteries in the dog. J.A.V.M.A. *173*:986–989, 1978.

Simenhoff, M. L., Burke, J. F., Saukkonen, J. J., Ordinario, A. T., and Doty, R.: Biochemical profile of uremic breath. N. Engl. J. Med. *297*:132–135, 1977.

Slatopolsky, E., and Bricker, N. S.: The role of phosphorus restriction in the prevention of secondary hyperparathyroidism in chronic renal disease. Kidney Int. *4*:141–145, 1973.

Slatopolsky, E., Caglar, S., Pennell, J. P., Taggart, D. D., Canterbury, J. M., Reiss, E., and Bricker, N. S.: On the pathogenesis of hyperparathyroidism in chronic experimental renal insufficiency in the dog. J. Clin. Invest. *50*:492–499, 1971.

Slatopolsky, E., Rutherford, E., Hruska, K., Martin, K., and Klahr, S.: How important is phosphate in the pathogenesis of renal osteodystrophy. Arch. Int. Med. *138*:848–852, 1978.

Slatopolsky, E., Rutherford, W. E., Rosenbaum, R., Martin, K., and Hruska, K.: Hyperphosphatemia. Clin. Nephrol. *7*:138–146, 1977.

Slauson, D. O., and Gribble, D. H.: Thrombosis complicating renal amyloidosis in dogs. Vet. Path. *8*:352–362, 1971.

Sommer, H., Kasper, H., and Fosel, T.: Serum lipase activity in chronic renal failure. Acta Hepato-Gastroenterol. *22*:248–252, 1975.

Spangler, W. L., Gribble, D. H., and Weiser, M. G.: Canine hypertension. A review. J.A.V.M.A. *170*:995–998, 1977.

Spencer, A. J., and Wright, N. G.: Chronic interstitial nephritis in the dog: an immunofluorescence and elution study. Res. Vet. Sci. *30*:226–232, 1981.

Spivak, J. L., and Graber, S. E.: Erythropoietin and the regulation of erythropoiesis. Johns Hopkins Med. J. *146*:311–320, 1980.

Stein, J. H.: Hormones and the kidney. Hosp. Pract. *14*:91–105, 1979.

Stein, J. H., and Fadem, S. Z.: The renal circulation. J.A.M.A. *239*:1308–1312, 1978.

Stevens, J. B., and Osborne, C. A.: Urinary casts: What are their significance? Minn. Vet. *18*:11–18, 1978.

Swenson, R. S., Silvers, A., Peterson, D. T., Kohatsu, S., and Reaven, G. M.: Effect of nephrectomy and acute uremia on plasma insulin IZ5-I removal rate. J. Lab. Clin. Med. *72*:829, 1971.

Thurau, K., and Boylan, J. W.: Acute renal success. The unexpected logic of oliguria in acute renal failure. Am. J. Med. *61*:308–315, 1976.

Tisher, C. C.: Anatomy of the kidney. *In* Brenner, B. M., and Rector, F. C. (eds.): The Kidney, Vol. 1. 2nd ed. W. B. Saunders Co., Philadelphia, 1981.

Tramezzani, J. H., Morita, E., and Chiocchio, S. R.: The carotid body as a neuroendocrine organ involved in control of erythropoiesis. Proc. Nat. Acad. Sci. *68*:52–55, 1971.

Van Stone, J. C., and Max, P.: Effect of erythropoietin on anemia of peritoneally dialyzed anephric rats. Kidney Int. *15*:370–375, 1979.

Vergne-Marini, P., Parker, T. F., Pak, C. Y. C., Hull, A. R., Deluca, H. F., and Fordtran, J. S.: Jejunal and ileal calcium absorption in patients with chronic renal disease: effect of 1α-hydroxycholecalciferol. J. Clin. Invest. *57*:861–866, 1976.

Villafine, F., Norrdin, R. W., Lopresit, C. A., and Kimmel, D.: Bone remodelling in chronic renal failure in perinatally irradiated beagles. Calcif. Tiss. Res. *23*:171–178, 1977.

Wallner, S. F., Kurnick, J. E., Vautrin, R., and Ward, H. P.: The effect of serum from uremic patients on erythropoietin. Am. J. Hematol. *3*:45–55, 1977.

Walser, M., Mitch, W. E., and Collier, V. U.: The effect of nutritional therapy on the course of chronic renal failure. Clin. Nephrol. *11*:66–70, 1979.

Weinberg, S. G., Lubin, A., Wiener, S. N., et al.: Myelofibrosis and renal osteodystrophy. Am. J. Med. *63*:755–764, 1977.

Weiser, M. G., Spangler, W. L., and Gribble, D. H.: Blood pressure measurement in the dog. J.A.V.M.A. *171*:364–368, 1977.

Welling, L. W., and Welling, D. J.: Surface areas of brush border and lateral cell walls in the rabbit proximal nephron. Kidney Int. *8*:343–348, 1975.

Wilson, D. R.: The effect of papillectomy on renal function in the rat during hydropenia and after an acute saline load. J. Physiol. Pharmacol. *50*:662–673, 1972.

Wolf, A. M.: Canine uremic encephalopathy. J.A.A.H.A. *16*:735–738, 1980.

Wrong, R. G., Norman, A. W., and Reddy, C. R.: Biologic effects of 1,25-dihydroxycholecalciferol in acutely uremic rats. J. Clin. Invest. *51*:1287–1291, 1972.

Yium, J. J.: Determination of diet orders by analysis of lab values. Texas Med. *69*:71–74, 1973.

CHAPTER 74

LARRY D. COWGILL

Diseases of the Kidney

Every clinician has seen animals that live asymptomatically with a solitary kidney or morphologic disease that affects both kidneys. The ability of the remnant renal mass to assume the functional capabilities of normal kidneys is testimony to the reserve capacity and adaptive potential of the renal parenchyma. Renal disease causes a finite loss of functional parenchyma, and simultaneously a complex and incompletely understood series of adaptive changes begins. Renal injury that proceeds faster than adaptive responses can occur will produce more profound clinical signs than a comparable degree of renal insufficiency produced at a more insidious rate. Some renal insults, on the other hand, produce profound clinical signs without substantial alterations in renal excretory function. The remainder of this chapter will address the spectrum of these renal injuries and the resulting disease syndromes that are recognized in the dog and cat. Renal insufficiency leading to renal failure is the common final pathway for the expression of most of these insults; these topics, therefore, will be developed in detail and followed by discussions of more specific subjects. This approach, the author hopes, will illustrate the dynamics of renal injury and help to distinguish the differences between renal disease and renal failure. The reader is encouraged to review the adaptive and compensatory changes in renal growth, blood flow and glomerular filtration rate (GFR), solute excretion, metabolism, and endocrine functions that occur in response to progressive nephron loss (see Chapter 73).

RENAL INSUFFICIENCY AND RENAL FAILURE

ETIOLOGY

Renal failure, or uremia, is the clinical state wherein functional renal mass has deteriorated to such a degree that it can no longer compensate for the lost capacity: metabolic waste products cannot be cleared completely, endocrine and metabolic functions are impaired, and secondary systemic disturbances are created by the attempted compensations. The clinician must distinguish between renal disease (or injury) and renal failure. Many animals will have significant renal disease but will not manifest renal failure.

Because of the close physiologic ties between the kidney and other organ systems, there is multisystemic involvement in renal failure. Renal failure can result from a single insult or from a combination of insults to which the kidney is subjected; common insults include immune-mediated inflammation, infection, ischemia, toxins, congenital or inherited abnormalities, trauma, obstruction, and neoplasia. In many cases, the clinician will view the patient for the first time at an "end stage" of the disease and will be unable to discern the primary cause or causes of the uremia. At this point, therapeutic efforts are necessarily palliative to minimize the spectrum and severity of the clinical signs and to halt progressive renal injury.

Renal disease, on the other hand, represents any degree of parenchymal involvement, whether focal or diffuse, localized or generalized, morphologic or functional, and is not necessarily associated with clinically detectable renal failure. Renal disease may be entirely reversible, if mild and limited in degree, or it may be extensive and progressive, culminating in renal failure.

There is no readily available information regarding the incidence of the various causes of renal insufficiency in the dog or cat. "Chronic interstitial nephritis" should not be regarded as an etiology of chronic renal failure, as has been generally suggested in the past. The term as used clinically represents only a morphologic description of the pathologic response of the kidney to a variety of insults. It is now recognized that distinctly different pathophysiologic entities (i.e., glomerulonephritis, congenital nephropathy, ischemia, and pyelonephritis) may be difficult or impossible to distinguish clinically and morphologically when advanced to this chronic stage (Wright et al., 1976). For these reasons, it is more acceptable to refer to small, fibrotic, irreversibly failing kidneys as "end-stage kidneys," a term that does not infer an etiologic pathologic process (Bovee, 1971; Low, 1977; Osborne and Johnson, 1970).

CLINICAL PRESENTATION AND PATIENT EVALUATION

The clinical manifestations of renal failure are, to a considerable degree, stereotyped and consistent from one patient to another. Despite the uniform clinical manifestations, the diagnosis of renal failure is made difficult by the vague and nonspecific character of the clinical signs. Furthermore, the overt manifestations of uremia may appear suddenly as a patient deteriorates from a tenuous state of functional compensation to overt decompensation. The presentation may also be obscured or modified by the presence of concurrent diseases (congestive heart failure, sepsis, diabetes mellitus or therapeutic manipulations). The clinician, therefore, must be on guard to recognize the pattern and consistencies of the historical and clinical manifestations characteristic of renal failure.

Renal failure is not limited to any particular age, sex, or breed. It is more prevalent in middle-aged to aged animals, but a significant incidence of renal disease secondary to congenital or inherited renal anomalies is found in animals during the first few years of life. In a survey of 170 canine and 36 feline cases of end-stage renal failure presented to the Veterinary Medical Teaching Hospital of the University of California, the mean age was 6.95 years for dogs and 7.42 years for cats. Richards and Hoe (1967) report a similar value of 6.5 years in a review of 119 cases in the dog. In 157 experimental dogs whose renal function was evaluated for an average of 13.25 years, fatal uremia was recognized in only eight dogs (5.10 per cent), with a mean onset at 11.34 years of age (Cowgill and Spangler, 1981). Azotemia was recognized in only

18.47 per cent of these dogs and is therefore a sign of renal insufficiency in the minority of the canine population.

The presenting signs in patients with renal insufficiency are often nonspecific and nonlocalizing. Weight loss, depression, listlessness, anorexia, and poor growth are frequently noted. Vomiting, diarrhea, fetid breath, pallor, polydipsia, polyuria, nocturia, and lingual ulceration are typical of advanced stages.

It is important to explore these problems with a careful and thorough history. Questions should elicit quantitative responses concerning the duration of both overt and subtle manifestations of the illness, including the magnitude of any weight loss and the validity of true changes in urine volume (as opposed to a change in the frequency of urination). Changes in the character of the urine and alterations in the pattern of urination should be explored. Is the urine notably different in color or odor? Has the frequency or time of urination changed, i.e., nocturia? These questions help to focus on urinary tract disease and to distinguish between renal disease and renal failure.

Because of differences in therapeutic approach, treatment cost, and prognosis, it is important to distinguish between acute and chronic uremia at an early stage. From the client's perspective, overt manifestation of disease may not have developed until several days before presentation, implying an acute onset, whereas identification by the clinician of preexisting or progressive polydipsia, polyuria, nocturia, intermittent vomiting, anorexia, anemia, or a fetid breath suggests a longer term of progression.

PHYSICAL FINDINGS

The physical findings will vary with the degree of renal insufficiency, the rapidity of onset, the type of renal injury, and the nature of previous therapy, if any. Compensated renal insufficiency causes few clinical signs; therefore, most patients are presented for the evaluation of advanced renal insufficiency and uremia.

A notable loss of body condition associated with a historical or detectable loss of body weight is common, but animals who were overweight prior to the onset of disease may now have a normal body conformation when examined. The hair coat is often coarse and lusterless and may be fecal or bile stained. The overall appearance is that of an unthrifty or ill-kept animal.

Skin turgor may be reduced in association with dehydration. Alternatively, generalized edema due to glomerular diseases associated with profound proteinuria and hypoproteinemia may be detected. Pallor of the mucous membranes and gingivitis or gingival ulcerations may be evident. Gingival lesions (thought to result from excessive bacterial production of ammonia from salivary urea) are especially noticeable on the upper arcade above and adjacent to the canine teeth, premolars, and molars.

A fetid or ammoniacal odor is also often detectable on the breath. On occasion, with profound uremia, the tip or anterior-lateral margins of the tongue appear darkened and devitalized, and slough owing to localized infarction of the lingual arteries. The necrosis may spread posteriorly to the level of the frenum. In young animals or in older animals with long-standing renal insufficiency, the teeth may become loose and movable or, in severe cases, the facial bones will be pliable and enlarged subsequent to renal osteodystrophy (Fig. 74–1). Marked conjunctival and scleral injection and hyperemia are commonly noted.

Thoracic examination is usually unre-

markable. In advanced uremia with fluid and electrolyte disturbances, a variety of arrhythmias may be detectable, including bradycardia associated with hyperkalemia. Evidence of pulmonary congestion and edema may be recognized as auscultable fluid rales. This is an important finding in animals receiving supportive fluid or intensive fluid diuresis. In an effort to compensate for metabolic acidosis, tachypnea characterized by deep inspiratory and expiratory components can be noted (Kussmaul respiration).

The left kidney of most small dogs and both kidneys in cats can be evaluated by abdominal palpation. In large breeds or deep-chested dogs, only the caudal pole of the left kidney may be palpable. The palpable character of the kidney is dependent on the underlying nature, severity, and duration of the renal injury. Typically in end-stage renal disease, regardless of cause, the kidneys are bilaterally small and firm, and have an irregular surface. If the disease is active, the kidneys may be painful to palpation. This is particularly evident in suppurative disorders or nephrosis. Renal pain may be expressed by "hunching" of the back, stiff-legged gait, and resentment of palpation. These findings are valuable localizing signs when present; in the author's experi-

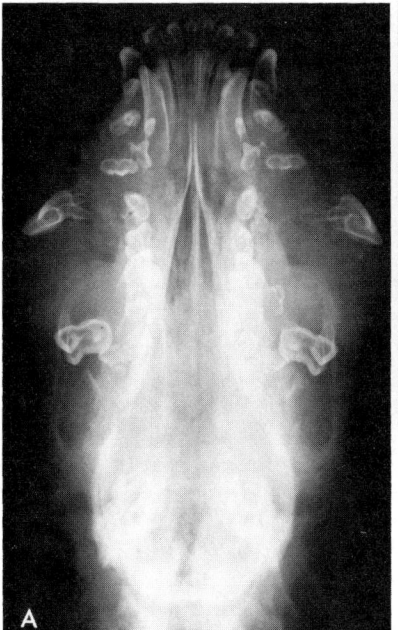
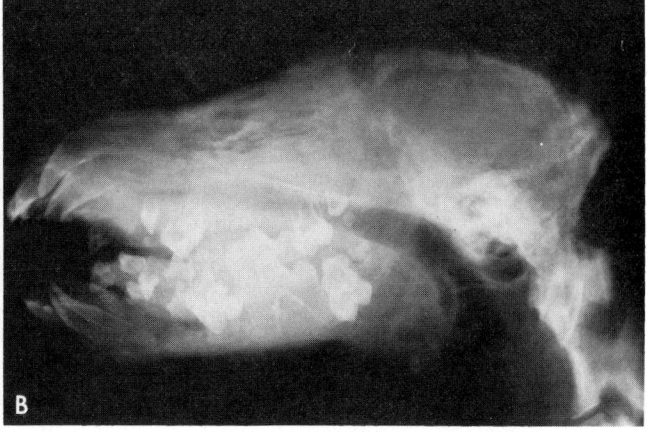

Figure 74–1. Lateral and ventrodorsal skull radiographs of a five-month-old Airedale with renal failure and advanced renal osteodystrophy. Osseous development is markedly abnormal. The mandible and maxilla are grossly enlarged and bone density is decreased. Multiple teeth are displaced and the lamina dura is absent. The dorsum of the cranium demonstrates decreased osseous density and an irregular "moth-eaten" periosteal response.

ence, however, they are uncommon and overemphasized, and must be distinguished from other causes of lumbar pain. Identification of an enlarged, irregular renal structure is consistent with neoplasia, cystic disease, or hydronephrosis. Cystic renal disease is often bilateral and may cause huge renal masses with little functional capacity. Normal or bilaterally enlarged kidneys with a firm consistency and smooth surface are recognized in early renal amyloidosis, bilateral infarction, nephrosis, and neoplastic infiltration, e.g., lymphosarcoma.

LABORATORY EVALUATION

The laboratory evaluation of renal function is the cornerstone of clinical detection and evaluation of progressive renal injury. Fortunately, only a few key parameters need to be measured. For specific circumstances, more precise and detailed evaluations of discrete renal processes are necessary, including renal plasma flow rate, transport maximum, plasma threshold, ammonia production, and others. These studies are generally beyond the requirements for patient management and will be mentioned only where necessary to describe a specific disease process.

Hematology

Blood is characteristically and uniformly altered by advancing renal insufficiency. The hallmark of the hematologic disturbance is a progressive normocytic, normochromic, nonregenerative anemia that is highly correlated with the degree of azotemia (Erslev and Shapiro, 1979; Kasanen and Kelliomaki, 1957; Loge et al., 1958). Red blood cell (RBC) count, hemoglobin concentration, and packed cell volume are all depressed in moderate and advanced states of renal insufficiency. The anemia is characterized by a reduced mass of mature erythrocytes; thus, the erythrocytic indices — mean corpuscular volume (MCV), mean corpuscular hemoglobin (MCH), and mean corpuscular hemoglobin concentration (MCHC) — are generally within normal limits.

The early pluripotent stem cell and erythroid progenitor cell compartments of the bone marrow are hypoproliferative, which causes the deficit of reticulocytes or nucleated RBCs seen in responsive anemias. Serum iron values are generally normal, but iron use is significantly decreased in advanced uremia (Joske et al., 1956; Loge et al., 1958).

Detection of nonregenerative anemia is considerably helpful in differentiating acute and chronic uremic states and in staging the severity of chronic renal insufficiency. It is important, however, to distinguish the anemia of chronic diseases, including infection and neoplasia, from that of advanced renal insufficiency (Madewell and Feldman, 1980; Wallner et al., 1976). Dehydration may mask the anemia of chronic renal failure by falsely increasing the hematocrit and hemoglobin concentrations. Overhydration or excessive fluid administration, on the other hand, can cause hydremia and underestimation of erythron mass.

The anemia of renal failure has multiple causes (Fisher, 1980). The life span of RBCs is markedly shortened in uremic plasma as a result of morphologic and metabolic disturbances of the RBCs and alterations in the erythrocyte membrane. The degree of shortening correlates with the degree of uremia (Giovannetti et al., 1968; Joske et al., 1956; Loge et al., 1958; Shaw, 1967). Working in concert with the decreased erythrocyte lifespan is a marked reduction in erythrocyte production and heme synthesis (Fisher, 1980; Ohno et al., 1978; Ohno and Fisher, 1977; Wallner and Vautrin, 1978; Wallner et al., 1975), lack of appropriate erythropoietin production (Fisher, 1980), and vitamin and iron deficiencies. External blood loss from hemorrhage into the gastrointestinal tract is an additional contributor to the anemia. These losses may be clinically inapparent or manifested by bloody vomitus or bloody stools.

Alterations in platelet-mediated hematostasis can significantly contribute to the external blood loss (Eschbach et al., 1976; Horowitz et al., 1970; Rabiner, 1976) and are recognized by prolonged bleeding and clot retraction times and decreased prothrombin time. The defective release of platelet factor III promotes diminished *in vivo* platelet adhesiveness and platelet aggregation (Castaldi et al., 1966). These alterations in platelet function are generally responsible for the bleeding disorders of uremia and are associated with the plasma accumulations of guanidinosuccinic acid and hydroxyphenylacetic acid. Dialysis or dietary therapy that diminishes these compounds can reverse these disorders and restore normal coagulation profiles.

Abnormalities in the remainder of the hemogram depend largely on the underlying or concurrent diseases or stress. Leukocytosis may be feature of acute, fulminating, or progressive renal injuries such as leptospirosis or pyelonephritis, but is atypical of chronic, end-stage renal disease. Lymphopenia, on the other hand, is a frequent finding in either acute or chronic uremia, and appears to be a manifestation of a specific uremic effect on lymphoid tissue.

Red blood cell morphology may be characterized by bizarre shapes, including crenation, helmet cells, and burr cells. Because anemia is such a consistent and important manifestation of advanced renal insufficiency, a complete blood count is important in the evaluation of uremia.

Glomerular Function

Glomerular filtration is the initial step in the formation of urine and modulates the kidney's excretory capabilities. Glomerular filtration rate (GFR) is the volume of plasma water that undergoes ultrafiltration per unit of time and is directly proportional to the number of functioning glomeruli. The normal canine kidneys contain approximately 800,000 glomeruli (Rytand, 1938) and produce approximately 86 liters of glomerular filtrate per day in a 15 kg dog. After destruction of half these glomeruli, the remaining 400,000 would be initially capable of producing only 43 liters of filtrate. Direct or indirect assessments of GFR, therefore, provide a useful index of functional renal mass and the severity of renal disease. Direct methods to estimate GFR use the renal clearance of solutes like inulin or creatinine, whose clearances serve as markers of the filtration process. Although clearance procedures are valuable in clinical settings, they are inconvenient for routine diagnostic purposes. Similar but less precise information can be obtained indirectly by measuring the steady-state plasma concentration of creatinine or urea nitrogen.

Creatinine. Serum creatinine has long been used as an index of renal function in man and in animals. Creatinine is produced primarily in muscle tissue from the spontaneous degradation of creatine to creatinine.

The release of creatinine from muscle is a nonregulated process that proceeds at a uniform and constant daily rate (Bloch et al., 1941). In general, the day-to-day production of creatinine in individual animals is reasonably constant.

Glomerular filtration, therefore, is the major variable that determines the excretion and steady-state plasma concentration of creatinine. Decreases in GFR increase plasma creatinine concentration until a new steady-state is reached and the amount produced is again matched by the amount excreted. The amount of creatinine excreted is the product of the higher plasma concentration and the lower glomerular filtration rate and is equal to the steady state production. It is evident, therefore, that the serum concentration of creatinine serves as a rough index of the level of renal function (see Fig. 74–2). A 75 per cent reduction in GFR or renal mass will produce quadrupling of the serum creatinine concentration, and so on; thus, reasonable estimates of the degree of renal impairment can be quickly determined by its measurement. A patient with a creatinine concentration of 10 mg/dl would have an estimated GFR ten per cent of normal. The relationship between GFR and serum creatinine as shown in Figure 74–2 is not linear and predicts that small changes in serum creatinine at the low end of the creatinine scale are associated with much greater losses of renal function than are similar absolute changes in creatinine at modestly or severely elevated levels. Careful interpretation of serum creatinine in the 1.0 to 2.0 mg/dl range is tremendously important in the early detection of renal injury. Unfortunately, this critical range is considered "normal" by most references and clinical laboratories. If 2.0 mg/dl is routinely used as the upper limit of normal for the dog, many patients will have significant but unrecognized reductions in renal function (Bovee and Joyce, 1979). It is perhaps more appropriate to consider 1.2 mg/dl as the upper limit of normal and suspiciously evaluate patients with increases from this baseline. Because of the more linear nature of the creatinine-GFR relationship at moderately elevated creatinine levels, changes in the plasma value above the 3.5 mg/dl can, in most clinical settings, be correlated with proportional alterations in renal function.

The degree of tubular secretion of creat-

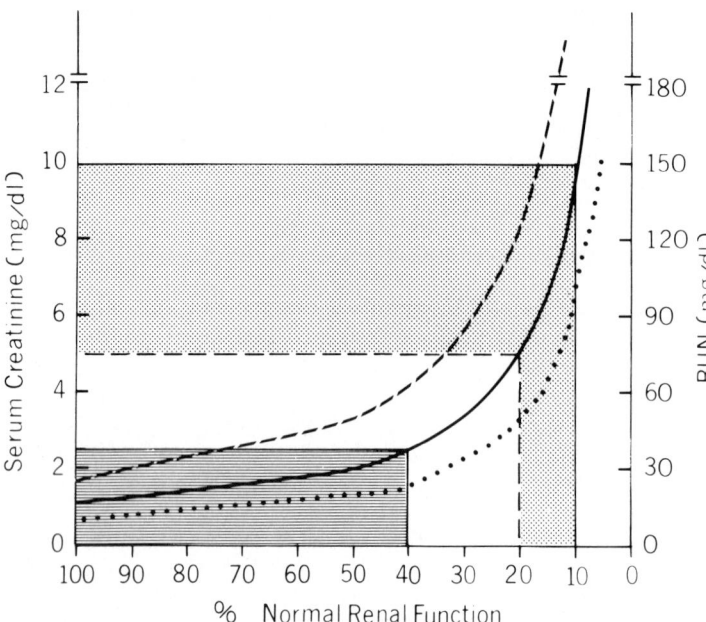

Figure 74–2. Theoretical relations for changes in serum creatinine (solid line) and BUN (all lines) with change in renal function. The blocked areas represent mild (hatched), moderate (clear, center), and severe (stippled) stages of renal insufficiency. The curved lines predict the influence of different protein intakes on BUN (as predicted by the BUN/creatinine ratio; see text) as renal function is changed. BUN/creatinine ratio = 10 (dotted line); BUN/creatinine ratio = 15 (solid line, also creatinine vs. renal function curve); BUN/creatinine ratio = 25 (dashed line).

inine that exists in male dogs is a possible limitation for the use of creatinine as an index of renal function (O'Connell et al., 1962; Robinson et al., 1974; Swanson and Hakim, 1962). The degree of tubular secretion is proportional to the elevation of serum creatinine, so at markedly elevated serum concentrations the enhanced renal excretion will provide an underestimation of the true glomerular filtration rate. This characteristic, however, rarely alters clinical interpretations or the evaluation of the patient. A second, relative limitation involves the method of creatinine analysis. The alkaline picrate (Jaffe) method is used most often. This method, in addition to determining creatinine, detects other non-creatinine chromogens that exist in plasma. At normal plasma concentrations, non-creatinine chromogens can represent a significant percentage of the total reactable chromogens and give an inappropriately high determination. More specific methods use Lloyd's reagent, which separates creatinine from the other chromogens. The Jaffe alkaline picrate method is widely used by commercial laboratories, and this relative imprecision will rarely affect clinical judgment and becomes less significant as the serum creatinine becomes elevated in renal insufficiency. True serum creatinine is most important in the determination of endogenous creatinine clearance, which is a more precise index of GFR.

Endogenous Creatinine Clearance. The renal clearance of endogenously produced creatinine can be used to provide an approximation of GFR by virtue of its relatively constant rate of production and plasma concentration, its complete filterability at the glomerulus, and its lack of tubular reabsorption. The small secretory component that exists in male dogs slightly overestimates GFR, but in most clinical circumstances the endogenous creatinine clearance provides a useful and sensitive evaluation of renal function.

The test requires timed urine collections of variable length and creatinine determinations on the collected urine and plasma. These values are arranged in the standard renal clearance formula, and the solution is expressed in ml/min or standardized for the kilogram body weight or body surface area to provide ml/min/kg or ml/min/m², respectively (Low, 1978).

Clearance of creatinine

$$= \frac{\text{urine creatinine concentration} \times \text{urine flow rate}}{\text{plasma creatinine concentration} \times \text{kg body weight or m}^2 \text{ body surface area}}$$

Normal values for the dog are reported to be between 2.8 and 3.7 ml/min/kg body weight, or approximately 60.0 ml/min/m² body surface area (Bovee and Joyce, 1979; Finco, 1971, 1980; Low, 1978). These values are consistent with the author's experience and provide a basis for estimating the percentage of remaining renal function in patients with renal insufficiency. To obtain meaningful results, urine collection must be quantitative, particularly when using short collection periods. Normal values are not established as yet for cats, but the techniques should be applicable if carefully performed.

Other tests using the plasma disappearance or urinary excretion of radiolabeled compounds or chemicals have been described for the estimation of renal function. The phenosulfonphthalein excretion test (Finco, 1971) and sodium sulfanilate tests (Carlson and Kaneko, 1971; 1971a) are the most clinically applicable to patients with renal insufficiency but provide less specific information about GFR than the endogenous creatinine clearance.

Urea. The blood, plasma, or serum urea concentration has been used as an index of renal insufficiency for decades. The accumulation of urea in the blood of patients with renal failure was recognized early and presumed to be the primary toxin in uremia. Although urea is now considered only a minor uremia toxin, it remains an important and universal biochemical parameter for the clinical assessment of renal function. The steady-state concentration of blood urea nitrogen (BUN) or serum urea nitrogen (SUN) is a function of the relationship between urea production and its excretion via glomerular filtration. In normal individuals, urea is primarily produced in the liver as an excretory compound derived from endogenous and dietary protein metabolism. The rate of urea synthesis is dependent upon the rate at which protein nitrogen is delivered to the liver for metabolism in the urea cycle.

BUN varies in direct proportion to the quantity of ingested protein or amino acids. Increases in urea formation can be detected within hours of a protein meal and have a significant effect on the measured concentration (Anderson and Edney, 1969; Bovee et al., 1979a,c; Simmons, 1972; Street et al., 1968). The rate of amino acid release from tissues during catabolism of body proteins additionally modulates the production of urea. Enhanced tissue catabolism is associated with fever, infection, and corticosteroid administration. Intestinal bleeding increases urea production from the bacterial breakdown of hemoglobin to ammonia, which is

subsequently incorporated into urea. Alternatively, the production rate of urea can be lowered by reducing dietary protein, through the administration of anabolic hormones and by marked hepatic insufficiency (when the capacity to synthesize urea is impaired).

Once synthesized, urea equilibrates throughout all body water by simple diffusion from blood. The kidneys represent the major excretory route for urea, and as with creatinine, glomerular filtration is the major determinant of renal excretion. Unlike creatinine, however, urea undergoes a variable degree of reabsorption that is highly dependent upon solute and water reabsorption and urine flow rate. States associated with enhanced tubular reabsorption of salt and water characteristically enhance urea reabsorption, and states characterized by salt and water diuresis are attended by reduced rates of urea reabsorption and a higher renal clearance.

Under steady state conditions in which the production of urea and urine flow are constant, the blood or serum concentration of urea will vary inversely with the glomerular filtration rate. A rapid decline in renal function will be associated with an increase in BUN until excretion at the elevated concentration and reduced GFR can once again balance the endogenous production of urea. Blood, plasma, or serum urea nitrogen will, therefore, serve as a crude index of glomerular filtration rate and functional renal mass. BUN, however, is significantly influenced by a variety of nonrenal parameters that must be considered in its interpretation.

The comparative value of serum creatinine or BUN as a reliable index of renal function is subject to considerable individual preference. From the preceding discussion it is apparent that BUN is not as precise an index of glomerular filtration as is serum creatinine. BUN is substantially influenced by diet, concurrent disease, state of hydration, and drugs, all of which commonly fluctuate in the patient with renal insufficiency. Nevertheless, if carefully interpreted, BUN is a valuable clinical tool in the assessment of renal insufficiency.

An elevation of BUN to the range of 50 to 100 mg/dl is substantially beyond the range of influence of extrarenal factors and can be construed as reasonable evidence of renal insufficiency. BUN concentrations above this range are assuredly associated with significant impairments of renal function. BUN concentrations generally vary between 30 and 80 mg/dl with prerenal disorders and will rarely exceed 120 mg/dl. In postrenal azotemia, on the other hand, BUN and creatinine concentrations rise in proportion to the duration and completeness of the urinary obstruction, and may approach 250 mg/dl and 20 mg/dl, respectively. Animals with intrinsic parenchymal failure will cover a spectrum of azotemia, depending on the severity of parenchymal loss, associated diseases, and the duration of the illness. BUN is commonly between 100 and 250 mg/dl and plasma creatinine will range from 4 to 13 mg/dl. This degree of azotemia is not specific for acute parenchymal failure but will usually distinguish dogs with prerenal abnormalities. A drawback in the use of BUN as an index of renal function is found in the mildly elevated range from 20 to 50 mg/dl. Within this range, a 20 to 30 mg/dl increase could represent either a significant loss of functional renal mass or enhanced urea production secondary to nonrenal factors and a normal GFR. To an extent, this evaluation can be improved by sampling animals only in the fasted state and carefully screening for nonrenal influences in the history. The use of urea, like creatinine, is hampered by the marked variability and broad range reported for normal animals. A BUN of 20 mg/dl might represent a normal value for a given diet or may represent a twofold elevation in the patient whose basal BUN is 10 mg/dl.

In human patients considerable attention is given to the BUN/creatinine ratio in the differential diagnosis of azotemia. Finco and Duncan (1976) evaluated the usefulness of the BUN/creatinine ratio in the diagnosis of azotemia in the dog and cat. Despite observed differences in the ratio in animals with prerenal compared to renal parenchymal or postrenal abnormalities, no predictable localizing value could be given to the site of the abnormality. They additionally concluded that no predictive value exists for differentiating acute from chronic azotemia. The BUN/creatinine ratio for dogs in stable chronic renal insufficiency varied between 25 and 30 (Finco and Duncan, 1976). This ratio, however, is significantly influenced by the dietary protein intake (Fig. 74–3), which must be considered in its inter-

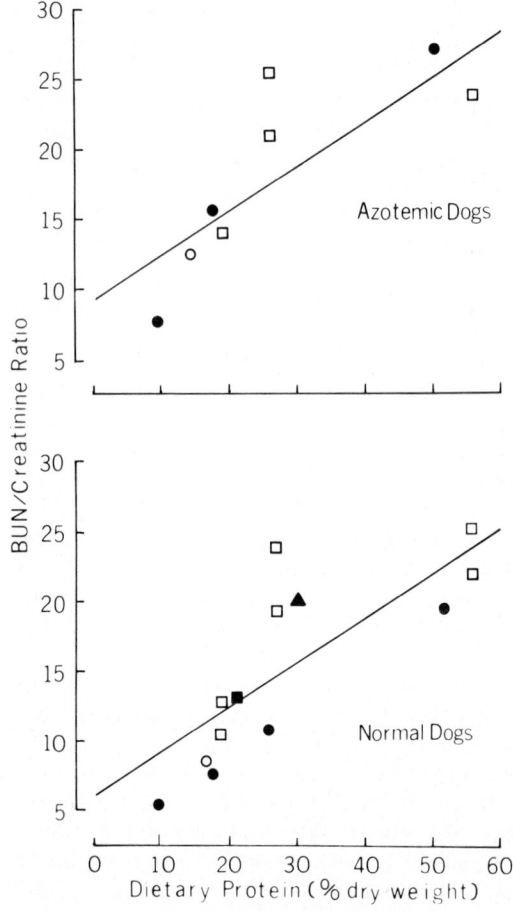

Figure 74–3. The relationship between dietary protein and BUN/creatinine ratio for normal dogs and dogs with renal insufficiency. The straight line is the regression analysis (r = 0.824 and 0.762 for azotemic and normal dogs, respectively) for data derived from literature sources and personal observations. The graph predicts an appropriate dietary protein content for a desired BUN/creatinine ratio (see text). Solid circles (azotemic), Polzin and Osborne, 1979; solid circles (normal), Morris and Doering, 1978; open squares, Bovee et al., 1979a, c; open circles, closed triangles and squares, Cowgill, personal observations.

pretation (discussed later). Marked elevations from this ratio have been detected in dogs with prerenal abnormalities or rupture of the urinary tract (Burrows and Bovee, 1974).

The BUN/creatinine ratio can also be used to monitor patients with chronic renal failure who are maintained on protein restricted diets (Kopple and Coburn, 1974). The ratio can be used to select an appropriate level of dietary protein to ameliorate the clinical signs of uremia and serve as an early indicator of concurrent catabolic processes in patients stabilized on restrictive protein intakes (Kopple and Coburn, 1974; see under management of renal insufficiency).

Serum Electrolytes

The evaluation of serum electrolytes is becoming more commonplace in veterinary diagnostics with the advent of multichannel biochemical panels. The kidneys have a major role in the overall management of body fluids and electrolytes, and their evaluation should be considered a routine part of the biochemical data base in azotemic patients. Disorders of serum electrolytes arise from alterations in the total body content for the particular ionic species, fluctuations in the volume of distribution for an electrolyte, or a combined disturbance of both these factors. The electrolytes of primary clinical importance in renal disease include sodium, potassium, chloride, calcium, phosphorus, and hydrogen. Additional electrolyte disturbances, including hyper- and hypomagnesemia, are also recognized (Coburn et al., 1969).

Sodium. Serum sodium is highly regulated by the kidneys in health and disease in an effort to control precisely the volume of the extracellular fluid compartment. External balance for sodium is generally maintained during the progression of renal insufficiency, and gross alterations in the serum concentration of sodium are usually absent. Alterations in sodium concentration are more likely to reflect the hydration status of the patient than the altered renal sodium conservation. In individual patients, however, discrete dysnatremias may develop. A severely compromised kidney may be unable to adapt to sudden sodium loads associated with parenteral fluid administration or dietary alteration resulting in transient hypernatremia. On the other hand, improper diuretic use, sudden reductions in dietary salt, excessive administration of hyponatric fluids, or excessive urinary salt losses could promote hyponatremia. The sodium status of the patient is better determined by clinical parameters (presence or absence of edema, dehydration, central venous pressure, blood pressure, and skin turgor) than by changes in serum sodium concentration. In acute renal insufficiency, however, alterations in serum sodium are

more common. In this setting, the dysnatremia is often related to the etiology of the acute renal failure and usually reflects the overall volume of the extracellular fluid compartment. Hypernatremia is seen in heat prostration or excessive administration of hypernatric fluid to diurese the patient. Hyponatremia suggests excessive ingestion of water or the administration of hyponatric fluids in animals unable to excrete the excessive water load. Exorbitant losses of sodium with or without commensurate water losses can occur with vomiting, diarrhea, and diuretic administration. These disturbances of fluid and sodium should be identified in the history and physical examination and evaluated further with serum electrolyte measurements.

Chloride. Chloride is the major extracellular anion and will generally mirror the sodium concentration. Specific chloride deficits should be anticipated in patients with prolonged and severe vomiting, in which hypochloremic metabolic alkalosis is commonly recognized. Patients receiving isotonic saline without regard for insensible freewater losses may experience hyperchloremia and hypernatremia.

Potassium. As for sodium, urine is the major excretory route for dietary potassium, and there exists a highly regulated and functionally adaptive system for the maintenance of external potassium balance (Hayslett, 1979). Patients with moderate, or even severe, chronic renal insufficiency are able to maintain potassium balance and a normal serum potassium concentration. This situation is quite distinct from acute uremia, in which potassium homeostasis is markedly imbalanced and characteristically there is an elevation in serum potassium concentration. Serum potassium, therefore, can be used to help differentiate acute from chronic forms of uremia. For BUN and creatinine concentrations below 150 mg/dl and 9.0 mg/dl., respectively, an increase in serum potassium suggests an acute disorder. In chronic renal failure, potassium balance and serum potassium are maintained by the residual nephron population through adaptive increases in potassium secretion. In some cases, the excretory rate for potassium may exceed the load filtered at the glomerulus (Schultze et al., 1971).

Increased fecal potassium excretion is identified in advanced uremia, and undoubtedly contributes to potassium homeostasis. As renal failure advances to a critical level (less than five to ten per cent of normal function), these adaptations are exhausted and potassium retention and hyperkalemia occur. This hyperkalemia is a serious and life-threatening electrolyte disturbance because of its adverse effects on cardiac function.

Hyperkalemia is an early and serious manifestation of acute uremia and must be routinely evaluated and managed. In lieu of direct determinations of serum potassium, its cardiotoxicity can be frequently identified with an electrocardiogram. The characteristic electrocardiographic signs of hyperkalemia include slowing of atrial conduction, diminution of the P-wave, prolongation of the Q-T interval, peaking and narrowing of the T-wave, or biphasic T-waves (Ettinger and Suter, 1970; Surawicz, 1967). The electrocardiographic abnormalities are demonstrated inconsistently and should not be substituted for direct measurement of serum potassium. An inappropriate hyperkalemia may develop in dogs with chronic renal failure with severe restriction of dietary sodium, salt depletion from gastric or intestinal losses, the administration of potassium-sparing diuretics, or secondary to metabolic acidosis.

Hypokalemia may be identified in the early stages of chronic renal disease and is generally a consequence of reduced potassium intake due to inadequate nutrition, anorexia, or as a result of excessive diuretic use.

Calcium. Serum calcium in patients with stable renal insufficiency is quite variable. As a rule, calcium is maintained in the normal range until terminal phases of uremia, when either hypercalcemia or hypocalcemia may be evident. The maintenance of normocalcemia during the progression of chronic renal disease is a result of extensive physiologic adaptations of the remnant renal mass and the development of hyperparathyroidism. There is a tendency for a subtle hypocalcemia with advancing renal insufficiency as a consequence of phosphate retention, alterations in vitamin D activation, intestinal malabsorption of calcium, and decreased calcium mobilization from bone. Hyperparathyroidism develops in response to this tendency and reestablishes external balance for calcium and phosphate

and corrects the hypocalcemia. In advanced renal failure, either hypercalcemia subsequent to excessive and uncontrollable hyperparathyroidism or hypocalcemia secondary to extreme phosphate retention and calcium malabsorption may be demonstrated. It is important to recognize that approximately 50 per cent of total serum calcium is bound to plasma albumin. Serum calcium concentrations should therefore be interpreted with reference to the concurrent serum albumin concentration. Hypoalbuminemia is often associated with a decrease in total serum calcium, which is often below normal limits. The protein-induced changes in total serum calcium are generally not associated, however, with elevations or reductions in ionized calcium, which is the physiologically active species.

In acute renal failure, the sudden retention of phosphorus and rapid development of hyperphosphatemia is often associated with significant hypocalcemia. In this circumstance the adaptive potentials of the kidney and parathyroid glands are too sluggish to maintain normocalcemia and may serve to distinguish the acute uremia.

In high concentrations, calcium can be a potent nephrotoxin and should be screened as a possible cause of renal injury and azotemia. The recognition of moderate to severe hypercalcemia in association with normal or hypophosphatemia should alert the clinician to the possibility of hypercalcemic nephrotomy (Chew and Capen, 1980). Hypercalcemia should be expected in mature animals when the serum calcium concentration is greater than 12.0 mg/dl. In younger, growing animals, a higher upper limit of normal is to be anticipated and should not create undue alarm. Early identification of hypercalcemia and its correction is important in order to prevent the continuous renal injury promoted by sustained elevations.

Phosphorus. Renal excretion of phosphate is primarily a function of glomerular filtration and a variable degree of tubular reabsorption. Five to 15 per cent of filtered phosphate is normally excreted each day. The renal capacity to excrete phosphate is tremendously adaptable through alterations in tubular reabsorption. A hallmark of renal injury is a transient retention of phosphate subsequent to reduced glomerular filtration. External balance, however, is maintained in steady state by reductions in its tubular reabsorption and the establishment of hyperparathyroidism. The serum phosphate concentration is thus maintained in the normal range until the adaptive capability of the remnant nephron mass is diminished and external balance is achieved only by an elevation of serum phosphate. The serum phosphate concentration, therefore, becomes an important and useful indicator of functional renal mass and provides significant diagnostic and prognostic information. In chronic renal disease serum phosphate concentration will remain within normal limits until approximately two thirds of functional renal capacity has been lost. It will progressively increase with reductions of renal function from this point. When serum phosphate exceeds 5.5 mg/dl, the clinician can predict that at best, one third of normal renal function remains. A normal serum phosphate in the presence of moderate azotemia provides assurance that a significant remnant renal mass is intact and an aggressive therapeutic program may prove beneficial. Phosphate concentrations greater than 7 mg/dl predict more significant and extensive renal insufficiency and indicate a more guarded prognosis.

The serum phosphate of young animals is normally higher than that of adults and should not be construed to indicate renal disease (Fig. 74–4). These general guidelines, therefore, are inappropriate for animals less than one year of age.

In acute prerenal, renal parenchymal, and postrenal disorders, serum phosphate increases in proportion to the decrement in renal function and serves as an indirect index of GFR similar to creatinine and BUN. Since insufficient time is available for compensatory mechanisms to regulate the serum phosphate, the increases with acute azotemia do not necessarily indicate irreversible renal injury as previously described, nor do they necessarily predict an unfavorable response to therapy. In chronic renal failure, increases in fasting serum phosphate are not generally recognized until serum creatinine approaches 4 to 5 mg/dl, after which it rises progressively with further decrements in renal function. In acute uremia, increases will be seen when creatinine concentrations are lower and serum phosphate will be higher at comparable levels of chronic azotemia.

Acid-base. Moderate renal insufficiency is generally attended by disturbances of acid-base balance. Nonvolatile acid metabolites must be excreted by the kidney. It can be anticipated, therefore, that a positive hydrogen ion balance will result with progressive renal failure. Compensatory mechanisms are operative in early stages of renal insufficiency to enhance acid excretion by the residual renal tissue; but as renal function declines, compensatory mechanisms fail, promoting the induction of metabolic acidosis. Metabolic acidosis is readily detected by the determination of serum bicarbonate with a complete blood gas analysis or by measurement of total plasma CO_2 content.

As a rule, patients with modest to moderate reductions in renal function have a re-

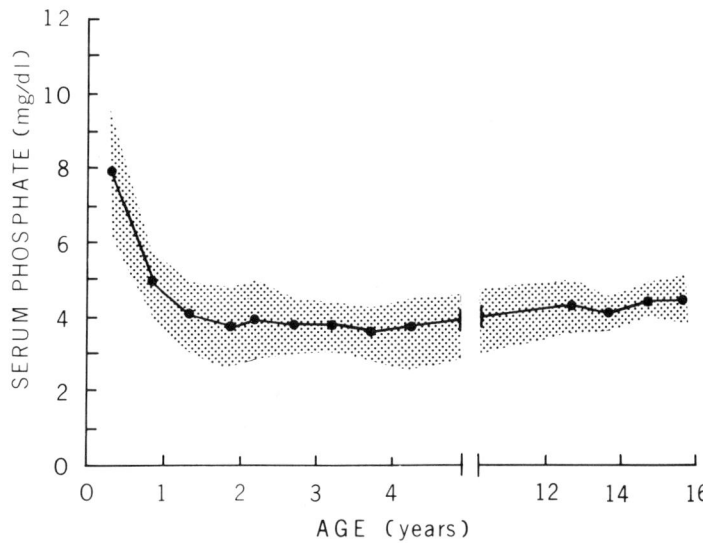

Figure 74–4. Serum phosphate as a function of age in normal beagles. Each point represents the mean value for successive 0.5-year intervals for up to 201 dogs. The stippled area is one standard deviation from the mean. The dogs represent a control population maintained at the Laboratory for Energy Related Health Research at the University of California, Davis.

duced serum bicarbonate. Bicarbonate concentration is generally maintained above 19 mEq/L in compensated chronic renal failure. As renal disease progresses to an advanced or uncompensated state, metabolic acidosis becomes more profound and serum pH falls as a result of greater hydrogen ion retention and inadequate respiratory compensation. Profuse vomiting may cause metabolic alkalosis, despite severe renal failure, and represents an important exception to the previous generalization.

Acute renal failure is generally characterized by metabolic acidosis directly proportional to the severity of the azotemia. Precise correlations between the degree of azotemia and metabolic acidosis are lacking for dogs and cats, but for clinical purposes, mild, moderate, and severe degrees of renal insufficiency are consistently associated with bicarbonate deficits of 5, 10, and 15 mEq/L, respectively (Osborne et al., 1975). Other primary or mixed acid-base imbalances (metabolic and respiratory acidosis, metabolic alkalosis, and respiratory alkalosis) may also exist, depending on the nature of the illness.

Serum Enzymes

Serum Alkaline Phosphatase. Alkaline phosphatase is liberated as isoenzymes from liver, bone, intestine, or kidney, and serum levels are variably elevated in patients with renal failure. In man, alkaline phosphatase of skeletal origin may be increased as a result of the osteoblastic and osteoclastic osteolysis associated with secondary hyperparathyroidism. Although this remains a possibility for veterinary patients, little information is available and other causes for an elevation should be pursued diagnostically.

Serum Amylase and Lipase. In the dog, mild increases in serum amylase and lipase are consistently associated with azotemia (Osborne et al., 1980). In contrast to man, there is no identifiable renal component to the normal disappearance of these enzymes from plasma. Consequently, it is unlikely that reduced renal clearance of these enzymes is responsible for detectable elevations (Hudson and Strombeck, 1978). Uremia must therefore promote an enhanced production of these enzymes from pancreatic or nonpancreatic sources.

Urinalysis

A complete, precise, and systematic evaluation of the urine is essential for the minimum data base for ill patients and will help elucidate occult or clinically silent renal disease. To be meaningful, urine samples must be collected and handled in a precise fashion and the analysis should be performed soon after collection.

The method of urine collection is dictated by clinical circumstances and personal preferences. For the evaluation of renal disorders, the ease of sample collection, and the greater interpretative potential, the author prefers the use of antipubic cystocentesis (Ling, 1976; Ling and Kaneko, 1976). This method is of particular importance in the diagnosis of urinary tract infection. Attention must be given to voided or catheterized urine samples to properly interpret the presence of bacteria and the cellularity of the sediment, since these samples are subject to contamination by the lower urogenital tract.

Once the sample is obtained, it should be refrigerated immediately unless the analysis is performed within 30 to 45 minutes. If improperly handled after collection or left to stand at room temperature, alterations in both the chemical and cellular composition occur. This may lead to misinterpretation and may compromise diagnostic efforts. Refrigerated urine should be analyzed as soon as possible and may be unsuitable for evaluation as soon as four hours after collection.

A complete urinalysis should include an evaluation of the visual and physical characteristics, chemical composition of the supernatant, and microscopic examination of the centrifuged sediment. Visually, the color and clarity are noted. The intensity of the yellow color is a function of the urochrome concentration of the urine. Urine may become abnormally colored by the excretory products of many drugs or chemicals or by the abnormal excretion of heme pigments (Stevens and Osborne, 1974). Abnormally colored urine is not necessarily pathologic, but it warrants a careful clinical and historical evaluation to uncover the cause. Turbidity most commonly results from an increase in formed elements, including white and red blood cells, epithelial cells, neoplastic cells, microorganisms, crystals, amorphous urates, or sperm. Concentrated urine will generally be more turbid than dilute urine because of the higher density of formed elements. Bacterial contamination or overgrowth, crystal precipitation, and changes in pH may promote turbidity if the sample is improperly handled. Concentrated urine is more subject to reduced clarity when allowed to stand because of the greater likelihood for urine solutes to precipitate.

Once collected and visually evaluated, a standard volume (generally five to ten ml) is centrifuged at 1000 to 2000 RPM for five minutes to sediment suspended formed elements. The supernatant fraction is chemically analyzed to identify a variety of solutes that have diagnostic value. The sediment is used to determine the quality and quantity of the formed elements of the urine. As a minimum, the supernatant fraction should be evaluated for the following parameters: specific gravity and/or osmolality, pH, protein, glucose, ketones, bilirubin, blood, and urobilinogen. The specific gravity, pH, protein, glucose, and blood can provide information relevant to the diagnosis of renal disease.

Specific Gravity. Urine specific gravity is an index of solute concentration of the urine and therefore serves as a crude indicator of the concentrating or diluting capacity of the kidney. Specific gravity provides only an approximate evaluation of urine solute concentration because it is dependent on the amount of dissolved solutes as well as on their molecular size and weight. A more precise evaluation of urine concentration can be obtained with osmolality, which is influenced only by the number of dissolved solute particles. For clinical purposes, however, specific gravity is a helpful indicator of urinary concentrating ability. The normal urinary specific gravity in the dog may vary from 1.001 to 1.060 or higher as physiologic conditions dictate (Hardy and Osborne, 1979; Stevens and Osborne, 1974). In the cat, the normal range can vary from 1.001 to 1.080 or higher (Dunkan and Prasse, 1976; Stevens and Osborne, 1974). Urine is considered dilute or concentrated when the specific gravity is less or greater than that of the glomerular ultrafiltrate (1.008 to 1.012), respectively.

The specific gravity obtained on a particular urine collection depends upon the level of activity and the age of the animal, the environmental temperature, the fluid and electrolyte balance, and the protein content of the diet. Randomly obtained urine samples from normal animals will generally demonstrate urinary concentration in the more restricted ranges of 1.015 to 1.045 (for the dog) and 1.035 to 1.060 (for the cat). Random values outside this range should not be construed as necessarily indicating renal disease, however.

The diagnostic importance of urinary specific gravity is in its capacity to reflect the adequacy of functional renal mass. Despite its relative insensitivity to alterations of renal function, the inability to maximally concentrate urine may be an early indicator of reduced renal capacity in the absence of gross alterations in serum chemistries. Hardy and Osborne (1979) suggest that dogs who produce urine specific gravities of 1.040 or greater have normal urine concentrating abilities. As renal mass is reduced, the ability to maximally concentrate urine is likewise restricted. Bovee and coworkers (1979c) have recently demonstrated a limitation of concentrating capabilities in experimental dogs undergoing 40 to 50 per cent reduction in GFR. Despite this magnitude of renal impairment, dogs with experimentally induced pyelonephritis or subtotal nephrectomy were still able to concentrate urine to as high as 1400 mOsm/kg of water following water deprivation. The limited defect associated with such substantial reductions of renal function can be readily appreciated. Osborne and colleagues (1975) have suggested that animals capable of forming a urine specific gravity greater than 1.025 will generally have renal function sufficient, albeit reduced, to prevent the biochemical and clinical manifestation of renal insufficiency. Significant degrees of renal insufficiency can exist, however, in the presence of higher urine specific gravities.

As renal function progressively deteriorates, the ability either to concentrate or to dilute urine will be lost and specific gravity will approximate the glomerular filtrate at 1.008 to 1.012. At this point, the specific gravity is considered to be "fixed" or isosthenuric and reflects a substantial impairment of renal function. Isosthenuria is particularly significant in the presence of dehydration, azotemia, or the external manifestation of uremia. Other diseases, including diabetes insipidus, pyometra, hypercalcemia, hyperadrenocorticism, and excessive water consumption, are also capable of impairing renal concentrating ability. Thus, alterations in renal concentrating capacity do not necessarily signify the presence of intrinsic renal parenchymal disease.

The demonstration of a concentrated urine in the face of azotemia is indicative of a prerenal disorder causing primarily a reduction in renal blood flow and GFR. The early stages of glomerular injury are an exception in which significant reductions in glomerular filtration may coexist with disproportionately intact tubular function and renal concentrating ability. As the disease progresses, however, the disparity between glomerular and tubular function will be narrowed and concentrative capability will diminish.

Urine specific gravities between 1.001 and 1.007 indicate the formation of a dilute urine. The ability to form a dilute urine is adequately maintained until renal reserve is severely diminished (Hayslett, 1979). The pathological causes of hyposthenuria are extensive and are considered in other sections of this text.

pH. The pH of the urine provides little specific information on the nature or presence of renal disease. Urine pH is dependent upon the dietary acid load and is generally acidic on diets containing animal protein and slightly alkaline on diets composed of vegetable constituents. Urine pH will also become more alkaline upon standing secondary to bacterial metabolism of urea. The pH of the urine from normal dogs and cats on normal diets ranges from 5.5 to 8.0. More alkaline urines are often associated with infection of the urinary tract or the administration of alkalinizing drugs. Because of the multiple variables that regulate renal acid excretion, urinary pH should not be used as a reliable index of systemic acid-base status.

Protein. Persistent proteinuria is an important indicator of urinary tract disease. The renal metabolism of protein is complex and involves molecular selectivity at the glomerulus, tubular reabsorption, and net addition to the urine. The interpretation of persistent proteinuria therefore requires careful clinical and laboratory evaluation to define renal or extrarenal causes for this abnormality. Very little protein appears in urine of normal animals. The protein concentration of randomly collected urine is generally below the qualitative detection limits of routine clinical and dipstick methodologies. Persistently positive urine protein reactions signify urinary disease in the absence of fever, icterus, and congestive heart failure.

Barsanti and Finco (1979) consider protein concentrations below 65 mg/dl as normal for dogs, regardless of the urinary specific gravity. In samples with a specific gravity greater than 1.030, 200 mg/dl can be considered the upper limit of normal. Quantitation of daily protein excretion provides a more specific index of the significance of proteinuria. Twenty-four hour urinary protein excretion has been variously reported. The results in normal dogs are influenced considerably by the method of analysis but are generally less than 200 mg/24 hours (Barsanti and Finco, 1979; Bovee et al., 1979c; DiBartola et al., 1980a). Greater excretion rates have been reported (DiBartola et al., 1980a; Stuart et al., 1975), but for clinical purposes excretion rates of less than 300 mg/24 hours can generally be presumed normal. Daily protein excretion appears to be highly correlated with body size (DiBartola et al., 1980a), however, and an adjustment that factors for body size should provide a more precise expression for clinical evaluation. By this criterion, the average excretion for a small sampling of normal dogs was approximately 14 mg/kg body weight/day (DiBartola et al., 1980a).

Glomerular proteinuria is frequently associated with detectable hyaline, and granular or waxy casts, as well as red blood cells and inflammatory cells in the urinary sediment. A major quantity of filtered protein is routinely reabsorbed by the proximal tubule. Protein may therefore be associated with the escape of proximal tubular protein secondary to intrinsic renal tubular injury, hypoxia, or toxin exposure. Dogs with generalized or selective proximal tubular transport disorders may not, however, demonstrate proteinuria (Bovee et al., 1979b), even though it is often identified in humans. Renal proteinuria may also result from the inflammatory products of hemorrhage concurrent with infectious, inflammatory, or neoplastic disorders of the kidney.

Nonrenal proteinuria can similarly be associated with inflammatory or hemorrhagic lesions of the lower urinary tract. Lower urinary proteinuria is usually associated with the presence of inflammatory cells or hemorrhage and the absence of tubular casts. Thus, it becomes critically important to review carefully the urinary sediment when attempting to localize the origin of urine protein. The larger protein losses that result from glomerular injury may help to distinguish renal from extrarenal causes of proteinuria.

The clinical evaluation of proteinuria should attempt to distinguish transient from persistent, extraurinary from urinary, and renal from extrarenal causes of proteinuria. These distinctions can be made with a careful clinical evaluation and appropriate laboratory procedures, which should include quantitation of daily excretion.

Glucose. The tubular maximum for glucose transport is normally in excess of the filtered glucose load, so that urinary excretion is negligible and undetectable. Clinical conditions characterized by either an increase in plasma glucose above the renal threshold or a reduction in the reabsorptive capacity cause glucose to appear in the urine. Glucosuria is usually associated with elevations of the filtered load as seen in diabetes mellitus or exogenous glucose infusion. Less commonly, it results from a marked reduction in the tubular transport capacity as a consequence of transport defects (Bovee et al., 1978; Bovee et al., 1979b), specific tubular toxins, generalized proximal tubular injury, or ischemia (Krane, 1979). These conditions are termed "renal glycosuria." Differentiation among these disorders can be made by measuring the plasma glucose concentration. High load states will always have an elevated plasma glucose, whereas renal glycosuria will occur in the presence of a normal or reduced glucose concentration.

Small quantities of glucose may be detectable in the urine of dogs with acute tubular necrosis. Filtered glucose will be incompletely reabsorbed by the damaged epithelium and appear in final urine (Westinfelder et al., 1980). This finding can be of particular importance in distinguishing acute from chronic renal failure. In chronic renal failure, the surviving nephron population will generally have normal glucose transport and glycosuria is not generally demonstrated (Bricker et al., 1960).

It is important to recognize the specificity and limitations of the analytic methods used to evaluate glycosuria. Copper reduction methods measure a variety of reducing substances, including fructose, pentoses, formalin, ascorbic acid, and a variety of pharmacologic agents, which can give false positive reactions. The glucose oxidase method is more specific for detecting glucose but may be influenced by ascorbic acid, which is normally found in canine and feline urine (Stevens and Osborne, 1974).

Hemoglobin and Occult Blood. Tests for the detection of occult blood are very sensitive and indicate the presence of hematuria, hemoglobinuria, and myoglobinuria. They are measures only of free hemoglobin or myoglobin and will not detect hematuria unless sufficient lysis of red blood cells has occurred. Hemoglobinuria in the absence of RBCs may be identified, particularly in dilute urine, if red blood cells undergo rapid lysis. The presence of hematuria is highly suggestive of disease intrinsic to the urogenital system. It may occur secondary to inflammation, infection, neoplasia, parasites, structural abnormalities, trauma, ischemia, coagulopathies, or calculi. A detailed evaluation of the clinical interpretation and causes of hematuria in the dog and cat has been recently reviewed (Lage, 1978). In male dogs, hematuria may also occur with prostatic disease if the urine is contaminated by blood. Hematuria may be visible grossly or by microscopic finding on examination of the sediment.

The evaluation of hematuric diseases should attempt to localize the disorder to the kidney, or to the lower urinary or genital sites, or both. Often the origin of blood can be inferred from historical information relating the appearance of blood in the voided stream and the presence of pain or dysuria. Although inconsistent, the recognition of blood at the beginning or end of the urinary stream in association with painful voiding is suggestive of prostatic or bladder disease, respectively. The presence of red cell casts or mixed cellular casts is suggestive of upper tract disease.

Hemoglobinuria results from hematuria and subsequent red cell lysis or intravascular hemolysis and filtration of the free hemoglobin. Myoglobinuria develops with muscle necrosis and subsequent filtration of the released myoglobin. It is important to distinguish myoglobinuria disorders from those that cause bleeding and hemoglobinuria.

Urinary Sediment Exam. Sediment examination is performed to identify bacteria, WBCs, RBCs, casts, crystals, epithelial cells, spermatozoa, yeast, fungi, and parasitic ova. Bacteria may be visualized in either stained or unstained urine, provided they occur in sufficient quantity. Cocci and rod-shaped bacteria must usually exist at concentrations of 10^4 to 10^5 or greater in order to be seen microscopically. Rod-shaped bacteria are generally easier to identify, and a Gram stain can be used for a more definitive evaluation. The urine collection method will influence the interpretation of visualized bacteria. Catheterized or mid-stream samples will often contain contaminating bacteria from the urethra, vagina, or prepuce that are unassociated with significant urinary infection. Improperly refrigerated samples may have erroneously high bacterial counts from postcollection bacterial growth.

WHITE BLOOD CELLS (PYURIA). Ling and Kaneko (1976) report that 0 to 3 WBCs per high dry field and 0 to 8 WBCs per high dry field are normal for urine collected by cystocentesis or catheterization and mid-stream voiding, respectively. Increases above this range are suggestive of urinary tract infection or inflammation and should be pursued diagnostically. Prostatic secretion or exudate may contaminate the urine and increase the white blood cell counts. Pyuria occurs commonly in association with increased red blood cell numbers and proteinuria. Excessive numbers of white blood cells in the urine indicates an abnormality in the urogenital tract that necessitates further evaluation.

RED BLOOD CELLS (HEMATURIA). The number of red blood cells normally found in urine is variable and, to an extent, dependent upon the method of urine collection. Traumatic catheterization and cystocentesis can create a significant hematuria. Zero to five RBC per high dry field are probably insignificant and considered to be normal for atraumatic collection techniques.

CASTS. Casts are formed within the tubular lumina, shed into the urine, and therefore are reliable indicators of renal injury. They are composed of precipitates of mucoprotein or plasma protein with or without formed cellular elements. Casts are extremely sensitive to urine pH and may dissolve in alkaline urine. Urinary casts are classified according to their material content and state of decomposition. Hyaline casts are composed of mucoproteins or plasma proteins without accompanying formed cellular elements or inclusions and are characteristically identified in diseases associated with glomerular proteinuria. Epithelial, granular, fatty, and waxy casts represent different evolutionary stages of cast formation and degeneration. The epithelial cast is composed of desquamated tubular epithelial cells incorporated in a mucoprotein matrix. As the cellular components degenerate, fatty cytoplasmic changes become visible, denoting fatty casts. With further degeneration of cellular organelles and nuclear protein, coarse and fine granules are formed that designate these casts, respectively. Complete degeneration of all inclusion particles and granules creates a highly refractive and homogeneous structure, termed a "waxy cast."

Casts of various descriptions and stages of formation can be seen simultaneously and signify the presence of tubular or epithelial damage. Red blood cell casts occur in association with tubular hemorrhage and glomerulonephritis in man. These casts are exceedingly delicate and rarely observed in canine or feline urine; when seen, however, they signify renal damage and should prompt suspicion of glomerular injury. The occasional identification of a hyaline or granular cast may not necessarily signal renal injury; however, the consistent presence of one, two, or more casts of any description per high dry field, and in particular in a dilute urine sample, is definite evidence of renal disease.

The number of casts identified in a urine sample is not necessarily predictive of the extent or duration of renal injury. Patients with extensive glomerular atrophy may shed only an occasional hyaline or granular cast. Extensive cylindruria, however, is generally indicative of active generalized renal injury. Tubular casts must be carefully distinguished from mucous threads, which are long, irregular noncylindric structures of a density similar to that of hyaline casts.

Mucous threads are derived from lower urogenital loci and are not indicative of renal injury.

CRYSTALS. Many varieties of crystals are found in the sediment of canine and feline urine but are rarely of diagnostic or pathologic signficance. Calcium, magnesium, and ammonium phosphate are the most common. Calcium carbonate, uric acid, cystine, and hippuric acid crystals may likewise be present. Cystine crystals, when present in large numbers in the urine of male dachshunds, Scottish terriers, or Irish terriers, are suggestive of canine cystinuria. Oxalate crystals may be causally associated with ethylene glycol poisoning in dogs and cats, but small numbers of oxalate crystals may be present in normal urine or histologic sections of normal kidney.

Additional identifiable formed elements include renal, transitional, squamous epithelial, or neoplastic epithelial cells, as well as spermatozoa, fungi, yeast, lipid droplets (normal finding in feline urine), and the ova of the metazoan parasites *Capillaria plica* and *Dictaphyma renale*. Fungi, yeast, parasite ova, and neoplastic cells have obvious pathological signficance, whereas small numbers of normal squamous epithelia, spermatozoa, and lipid droplets have no particular diagnostic significance.

Radiologic Evaluation

Survey Radiographic Evaluation. In normal dogs and cats, the kidneys are usually located in the extraperitoneal space of the cranial abdomen. The right kidney is positioned more cranially than the left, and its cranial pole is often obscured by abdominal viscera. The left kidney is generally visible on both lateral and ventrodorsal radiographic projections and can be examined for size and shape. In the dog, the kidneys occupy an abdominal region that corresponds to the thirteenth thoracic through the third lumbar vertebrae. Because canine kidneys are reasonably anchored to other abdominal structures, deviations from this position should be investigated. In the cat, the kidneys are more pendulous and assume variable positions within the abdomen. Unlike the dog, however, both kidneys are routinely visible on radiographs in both the ventrodorsal and lateral projections (Bartels, 1973). In the cat, the right kidney generally occupies a region at the level of the first to the fourth lumbar vertebrae and the left kidney occupies a level corresponding to the second to fifth lumbar vertebrae. Failure to identify either kidney in the cat should be considered abnormal and pursued with contrast radiography.

Survey radiographs mainly provide a morphologic evaluation of kidney size, shape, and density. Normal dog kidneys vary in length from 2.5 to 3.5 times the length of the second lumbar vertebra (Finco et al., 1971). In the cat, this same parameter is 2.4 to 3 times the length of the second lumbar vertebra (Barrett and Kneller, 1972). Uniform renal enlargement on survey radiographs may suggest such abnormalities as compensatory hypertrophy, acute inflammation, hydronephrosis, generalized interstitial neoplasia, urinary tract obstruction, intracapsular hemorrhage, or cystic disease of the kidney. Precise differentiation of the preceding disorders may be evident from the history or physical examination or may require contrast radiography for further clarification. The size of one kidney should be carefully compared with the contralateral kidney whenever possible. Dissymmetry is suggestive of unilateral renal disease, whereas symmetric enlargements or reductions could signify bilateral and uniform renal involvement.

Radiographically, small kidneys are indicative of reduced renal mass and are commonly associated with end-stage fibrotic kidneys, congenital hypoplasia, chronic inflammation, or chronic infection. The renal image is an index of actual kidney size and is dependent upon abdominal positioning and the magnification factor of the radiographic technique. For this reason, subtle differences between kidneys may not be significant or suggest lateralization of disease.

SHAPE. Normal kidneys have a characteristic bean shape with smooth and regular borders. Marked irregularities in renal shape or contour are significant radiologic findings. Focal or uniformly irregular borders in kidneys of normal or smaller size most commonly indicate previous infarction or scarring. Neoplasia, renal cysts, or congenital abnormalities may also cause irregularities in renal shape and enlargement of the image. Variations in radiographic shape of normal kidneys may result from differences in abdominal positioning, angulation,

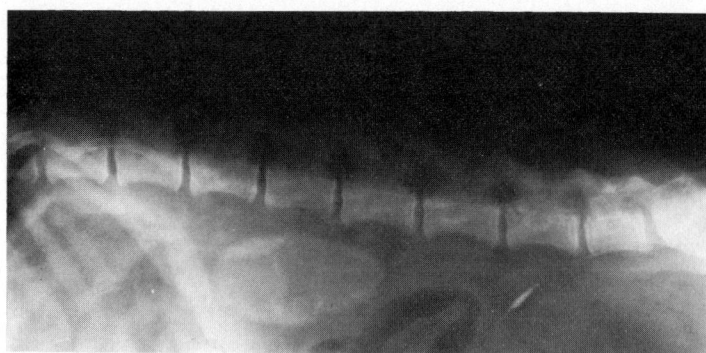

Figure 74–5. Lateral abdominal radiograph of a five-month-old Airedale with renal failure and advanced renal osteodystrophy. The radiograph demonstrates extensive calcification of the kidneys (especially the cortical rim), which considerably enhances their radiographic density. The serum phosphate was 23.3 mg/dl and the serum calcium was 13.6 mg/dl.

or image projection. Irregularities on the renal border are usually underestimated on the radiograph and therefore become significant findings.

RADIOGRAPHIC DENSITY. Normal kidneys have a soft-tissue or fluid radiographic density. They are particularly evident in animals with sufficient extraperitoneal or perirenal fat to contrast other organ densities. An enhancement of the radiographic density occurs with the deposition of calcium in the interstitium and with nephrocalcinosis (Fig. 74–5). This lesion is seen in advanced renal failure, dystrophic calcification subsequent to renal infection or neoplasia, and nonrenal disorders characterized by enhanced calcium mobilization from bone or urinary excretion (hyperadrenocorticism, hypercalcemia of malignancy, hypervitaminosis D, or primary hyperparathyroidism). In longstanding chronic renal insufficiency, calcification of nonrenal viscera, including major arteries, pulmonary parenchyma, and periarticular soft tissues may be seen (Fig. 74–6).

Renal Contrast Radiography. Additional information on the position, size, or shape of the kidneys or nonvisualized kidneys on survey radiographs can be obtained by contrast radiography. Many contrast procedures have been described to provide a better radiographic evaluation of the kidneys, including intravenous urography, renal arteriography, percutaneous nephropyelocentesis, retrograde pyelography, and intraperitoneal gas insufflation. Intravenous urography and renal arteriography are the most commonly used and the most useful. Patients should be properly prepared for contrast examinations to maximize radiographic quality and interpretation. Proper preparation generally requires overnight fasting and the cleansing of the intestinal tract with laxatives and enemas.

INTRAVENOUS UROGRAPHY. Intravenous urography is indicated for the evaluation of mass lesions in the region of the kidney, nonvisualization of the kidneys on the survey radiographs, anatomic characterization of either large or small kidneys, evaluation of the diverticular and the pelvic collecting systems, diagnosis of pyelonephritis, or investigation of renal trauma. It is often considered a function study, but is not expressly

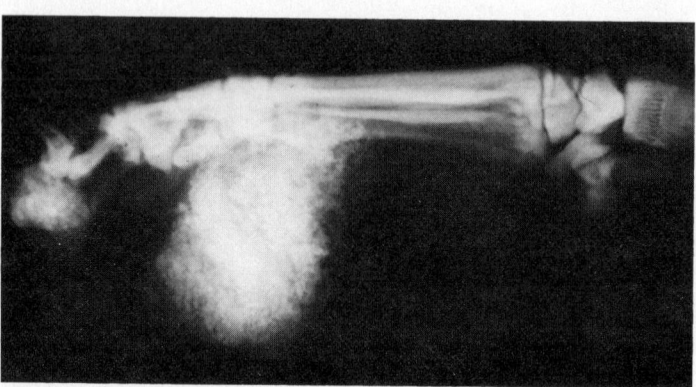

Figure 74–6. Radiograph of the foot of a dog with chronic renal failure. Note the extensive soft tissue mineralization of the metacarpal pad.

indicated for this purpose and will provide, at best, only a crude, qualitative evaluation of glomerular filtration rate.

Intravenous urography is performed by injecting a variety of triiodinated compounds (meglumine or sodium salts of diatrizoate or iothalamate), which are primarily excreted by glomerular filtration. These agents selectively accumulate and concentrate within the kidney and enhance the radiographic density of the urinary tract. There are no specific contraindications for excretory urography except previous hypersensitivity or allergy to the contrast agents. Anaphylactic reactions are uncommon in both man and animals but may occur. Side effects to excretory urography are also few and usually of little clinical consequence. Acute renal failure following the contrast procedure is the major complication in man. Most incidences, however, are associated with dehydration of the patient prior to beginning the study. As a precaution, it is important to insure the patient is properly hydrated and subsequently to monitor for early indications of oliguria. Reflex vomiting following contrast injection is the most common side effect in the dog. Extravasation of the contrast material will cause pain and localized cellulitis, which should be managed with regional infiltration of sterile saline and local anesthetic agents.

The techniques of excretory urography are adequately described in several recent reviews (Ackerman, 1979; Biery, 1978; Kneller, 1974; Osborne et al., 1979). Patients should be fasted overnight and the gastrointestinal tract cleansed with warm water enemas and/or laxatives prior to the procedure. Survey abdominal radiographs should be obtained when the colon has been thoroughly evacuated prior to initiating the contrast study. An initial dose of 0.5 ml of contrast agent per kg body weight is routinely administered and is generally satisfactory for a thorough evaluation. Ventrodorsal and lateral radiographs are obtained immediately following contrast administration and at 5, 10, 15, and 30 minutes postinjection. If renal opacification is unsatisfactory with the initial dosage, an additional 0.5 ml per kg body weight can be administered. Doses as large as 1.5 ml/kg body weight have been used but rarely increase the diagnostic yield.

If diagnostically indicated, a better evaluation of the diverticula, pelvis, or proximal ureter can be obtained with posterior abdominal compression applied with an elastic bandage. Sufficient pressure must be applied to prevent ureteral peristaltic flow and to dilate and distend the proximal collecting system. Additional radiographs are obtained following five minutes of abdominal compression and, if satisfactory information is obtained, the compression is relieved and the study completed.

The excretory urogram is functionally evaluated in two phases. The first, or nephrogram, phase occurs immediately following contrast injection as the medium is transiting the proximal nephron subsequent to glomerular filtration. This phase is captured on the first film of the sequence and is characterized by a marked and generally uniform increase in renal opacification. The nephrogram is best suited for evaluation of renal size, shape, and position. The density of the nephrogram is variable and dependent upon the quantity of contrast administered, the glomerular filtration rate, and the degree of contrast dilution in the tubules. In animals with severely compromised renal function, the nephrogram may be faint and unsuitable for proper evaluation. The second phase, called the pyelogram phase, is best suited for demonstrating pyelonephritis, calculi, and defects of the pelvis and proximal ureter.

MISCELLANEOUS. It is often helpful to radiograph nonrenal structures when evaluating renal disease. A characteristic abnormality is renal osteodystrophy or "rubber jaw," which represents a fibrous dysplasia of the mandible, and, most noticeably, the maxilla. In severe cases, these bones become ostensibly replaced with fibrous connective tissue, so that the facial bones become pliable or rubbery and the teeth become loosened and movable, and fall out (Fig. 74–1). The lamina dura is frequently absent, and the skeleton may become extensively demineralized and lose trabeculation. Holmes (1957) has described radiographic changes in the terminal phalanges in dogs with and without simultaneous mandibular lesions. Typically there is marked erosion of the tufts of the terminal phalanges and subperiosteal erosion of the middle and proximal phalanges. These lesions are inconsistent but characteristic of the radiographic lesions that occur with hyperparathyroidism in man (Avioli and Teitelbaum, 1979). In severe cases, there may be generalized osteoporosis and pathologic fractures of highly stressed bones.

Renal osteodystrophy in the dog is most noticeable in young animals with congenital or acquired renal failure or in protracted cases of chronic renal insufficiency when sufficient time has allowed complete development of osseous lesions. Soft tissue calcification is an additional feature of renal osteodystrophy (Figs. 74–5 and 74–6). The calcific densities develop in a variety of forms, including large tumoral masses of mineral around articular surfaces or interstitial calcium deposition in gastric mucosa, tracheal and bronchial walls, arteries, lung, kidney, and heart (Figs. 74–5 and 74–6).

In young animals, renal rickets may be seen radiographically by a widening and lucency of the physis and metaphysis. Rickets is associated with short stature and bone length, or bowing deformities of the limbs.

Renal arteriography is a specialized procedure used to outline the renal vasculature radiographically. It requires the selective or nonselective retrograde passage of a catheter into the renal arteries or aorta adjacent to the renal arteries, respectively. Renal arteriography is useful for the evaluation of kidneys that fail to visualize on survey radiographs or excretory urography, differentiation of renal tumors, or renal vascular disease. Because of the specialized equipment required for the procedure and the invasive nature of the catheterization, it remains unsuitable for routine evaluations in private practice. On selected patients, however, its diagnostic potential is important and may warrant referral to a center where it can be performed (Fig. 74–7).

Renal ultrasonography offers an exciting, new, and noninvasive approach to the evaluation of renal morphology and the diagnosis of specific disorders including hydronephrosis, nephrolithiasis, neoplasia, and cysts (Cartee et al., 1980) (Fig. 74–8). This diagnostic capability also requires expensive equipment and will not play an important role in private practice in the immediate future.

Nuclear imaging is another field showing rapid development and promise in specialized centers of veterinary practice. These techniques are also outside the scope of private veterinary practice but are becoming increasingly available in university practices (Fig. 74–9).

MEDICAL MANAGEMENT OF RENAL INSUFFICIENCY

The manifestations of uremia are polysystemic and diverse in clinical expression. It is therefore unrealistic to conceive that simple, one-step therapeutic approaches will have measurable benefits. Therapy for renal in-

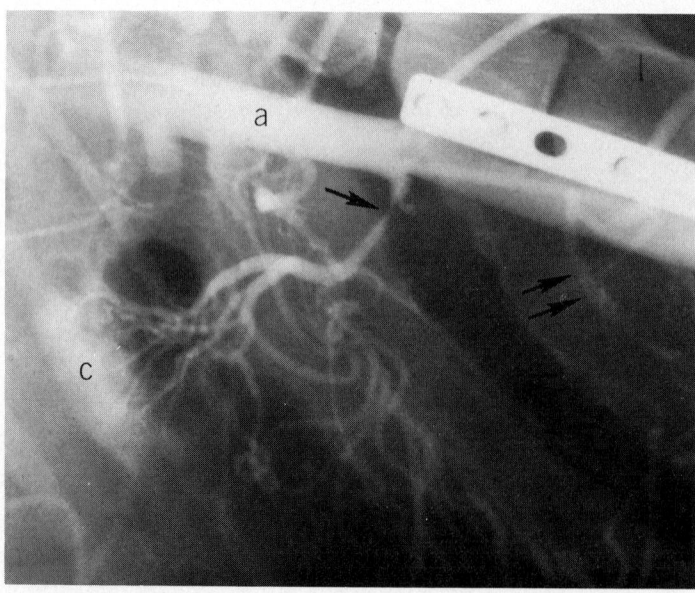

Figure 74–7. Nonselective renal arteriogram in a dog with acute oliguric renal failure following automobile trauma, a dorsal laminectomy, and repair of a fractured spine. Both kidneys failed to visualize following an excretory urogram. The arteriogram demonstrates an area of marked stenosis and irregularity at the origin of the right renal artery (arrow). The cranial and caudal poles of the right kidney are infarcted, leaving only a small segment of perfused parenchyma in the center of the kidney (c). The left kidney, at the level of the spinal fracture, is completely infarcted and nonvisualized. A portion of the left renal artery is seen but terminates abruptly (double arrow). a, Aorta.

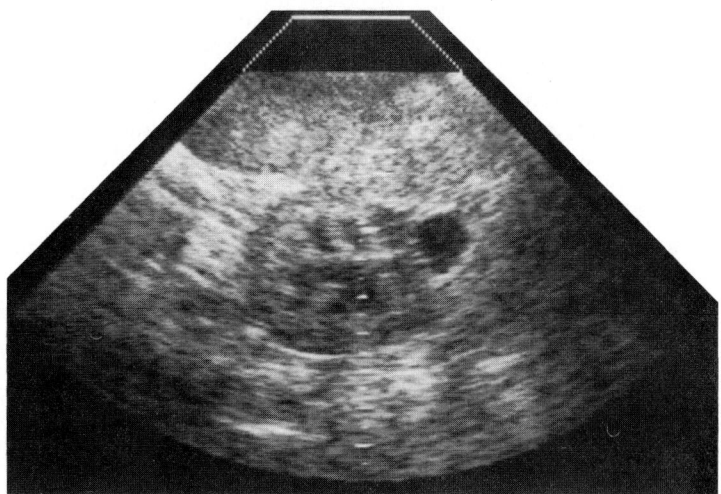

Figure 74–8. Ultrasonic image of a canine kidney with a large cyst in the parenchyma of the caudal pole. The renal pelvis and diverticula are also visualized. (Courtesy of Dr. Thomas Nyland.)

sufficiency must be tailored to the individual patient and comprehensive enough to address all recognized or anticipated clinical disorders. In veterinary medicine, renal transplantation or chronic maintenance dialysis is impractical (Cowgill and Bovee, 1977; Cowgill, 1980), and conservative medical management is the only therapy currently available. This encompasses all therapeutic measures that must be instituted to ameliorate established or ongoing biochemical and endocrine imbalances and fluid, electrolyte, and acid-base derangements. Because the biochemical, physiologic, and clinical manifestations of uremia are generally predictable and stereotyped, the principles of conservative therapy are the same regardless of the underlying cause of the renal failure. Such therapy is primarily indicated to reduce clinical symptomatology and will rarely reverse established renal dysfunction. When a definite etiology can be established, specific therapy can be combined with supportive measures to halt the progression of renal injury. The timely institution of symptomatic treatment may also play a significant role in protecting the remnant renal mass from progressive injury.

Specific guidelines for the management of renal insufficiency must be formulated in relation to the degree of renal dysfunction, and they should address the following clinical, biochemical, or physiologic disturbances characteristic of renal insufficiency: (1) nutritional imbalances, (2) retained "uremia toxins," (3) disorders of acid-base homeostasis, (4) disorders of electrolyte metabolism, (5) alterations in divalent ion metabolism, (6) anemia, and (7), fluid imbalances.

DIET THERAPY: CONTROL OF ALTERED NITROGEN METABOLISM

Dietary manipulations are of paramount importance in the conservative management of renal insufficiency. The goal of dietary therapy is to minimize the signs of

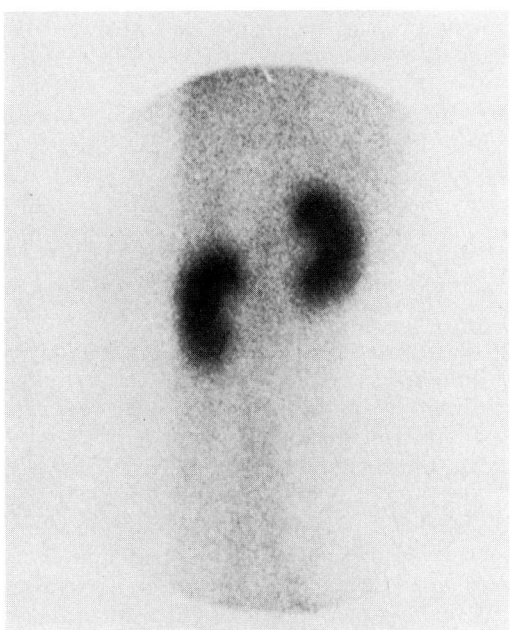

Figure 74–9. Delayed image of normal canine kidneys as visualized during a renal scan using Tc 99m DTPA. (Courtesy of Dr. William Hornof.)

uremia and metabolic disorders while maintaining good nutrition. Uremia is associated with weight loss, muscle wasting, retarded growth, and alterations in the profiles of plasma proteins and amino acids. Nutritional intake is reduced through nausea, anorexia and vomiting, and alterations in intestinal absorption (Gulyassy et al., 1970). It is well established in human patients that these nutritional disturbances directly contribute to uremic signs (Kopple, 1976).

In addition to obvious deficiencies in the intake or the absorption of essential nutrients, there exists a long-standing clinical premise and experimental data to implicate alterations in the assimilation, excretion, degradation, or synthesis of dietary constituents in the production of many clinical signs of uremia (Kopple, 1976). The accumulation of dietary metabolites, or "uremia toxins," can be demonstrated in uremic sera and shown to alter the biologic activity of numerous metabolic functions and are thought to contribute to the manifestations of renal failure (Bergstrom and Furst, 1978). Of the substances that accumulate in uremia, the metabolic products of proteins and amino acids are generally regarded as the most significant. In contrast to fats or carbohydrates, which can be completely oxidized to carbon dioxide and water and are eliminated from the body, proteins and amino acids are incompletely oxidized and produce nonvolatile or nondiffusible metabolites that require renal excretion. The list of nitrogenous metabolites that accumulate in uremia includes urea, aromatic acids, aliphatic amines, aromatic amines, guanidines, indoles, nucleic acid derivatives, phenols, proteins, peptides, "middle molecules," and pyridine derivatives (Bergstrom and Furst, 1978; Kopple, 1976; Kopple et al., 1978).

Urea is quantitatively the most significant of these nitrogenous products. The contributions of urea to uremic signs are unclear, but accumulating evidence suggests that it may contribute to the development of excessive salivation, vomiting, diarrhea, tremors, twitching, convulsions, coma, hemorrhagic gastroenterocolitis (Grollman and Grollman, 1959; Leiter, 1921), abnormalities of the electroencephalogram, weakness, drowsiness, hypothermia, and glucose intolerance (Balestri et al., 1972; Kopple et al., 1976; Perkoff et al., 1958). Many of these abnormalities develop at only markedly elevated blood urea nitrogen concentrations, whereas others occur at concentrations below 200 mg per dl and are frequently encountered in clinical disease. Urea is therefore classified as a mild uremic toxin, but more importantly, its plasma concentration serves as an index of the accumulation of other nitrogenous compounds that are more toxic. The generation of urea and nitrogenous toxins is directly related to the turnover of dietary and body proteins. Dietary restriction of the precursor nitrogen should therefore reduce the appearance of nitrogenous products and ameliorate many signs of uremia.

Proteins ingested in excess of the minimum requirements for structural protein synthesis and turnover are metabolized for energy, and their nitrogen moiety is incorporated into urea for renal excretion. During periods of inadequate caloric intake or catabolism (sepsis, fever, starvation, chronic wasting, diabetes mellitus, and corticosteroid administration), body proteins are metabolized for energy, and their nitrogen moiety is converted to urea. If sufficient calories are provided, dietary protein restriction will result in decreased formation of urea and a reduced urea load for renal excretion. For any degree of renal function, therefore, the steady-state serum urea concentration will be proportional to the dietary protein intake and the utilization of body proteins. In anabolic states, more of the dietary nitrogen is directed to protein synthesis and less is available for urea formation and renal excretion.

Clinical Guidelines for Dietary Protein Management of Chronic Renal Insufficiency

The institution of a protein-restricted diet is generally correlated with a reduction in clinical signs and restoration of a more normal clinical status in veterinary patients as in humans with uremia (Bovee, 1972; Edney, 1970; Polzin and Osborne, 1979; Richards and Hoe, 1967). Despite these observations the precise role of dietary therapy, and of protein restriction in particular, has been controversial. As a result, precise guidelines and a clear perspective for the practicing veterinarian have been obscured on such key questions as when in the course of renal failure to initiate protein limitations and the degree to which protein intake should be reduced. There is little substantive information in the dog or cat to provide guidelines on these issues. Therapeutic decisions must be made on clinical judgment, personal experience, and observations in man or laboratory animals, in which these issues have been better resolved.

There is general consensus that dietary protein restriction helps to ameliorate many clinical aspects of uremia, but to date there has been little consensus regarding the stage of renal failure when dietary protein should be limited. Although this remains a matter of personal judgment, general but differing guidelines have been advocated by various authors (Bovee, 1972; Bovee and Kronfeld, 1981; Morris, 1980; Morris and Doering, 1978; Polzin and Osborne, 1979).

The considerable benefits of dietary protein restriction on survival in established renal insufficiency have been dramatically demonstrated in the rat (Ibels et al., 1978; Kleinknecht et al., 1979; Ritz et al., 1978; Swenseid et al., 1975). These investigations illustrate the importance of restricting dietary protein when uremic symptomatology becomes evident. Other investigations failed to demonstrate any change in longevity or health in moderately uremic dogs maintained on normal protein intakes (Bovee et al., 1979a). Dogs maintained on higher protein intakes tended to have a higher incidence of glomerulosclerosis, interstitial lymphoid infiltration and fibrosis, and chronic pyelitis. These changes, however, appeared to have negligible effects on long-term renal function (Bovee et al., 1979a).

Another controversy involves the degree to which protein intake should be limited when restriction is clinically indicated. Observations have been recently described in dogs with moderate renal insufficiency maintained on diets containing 5.4 per cent and 2.4 per cent protein on an as-fed basis (Polzin and Osborne, 1979). These protein-restricted diets generated lower BUN concentrations and promoted better clinical well-being and coat quality than similar animals maintained on a ten per cent commercial diet. Similarly, Edney (1970) reported clinical improvement in 27 out of 30 dogs with renal insufficiency receiving a five per cent protein diet. Despite the clinical improvement, dogs maintained on a 2.4 per cent protein diet demonstrated reduced

serum albumin concentrations suggestive of protein malnutrition (Polzin and Osborne, 1979). Protein restriction will also lower important renal function parameters' like GFR and renal plasma flow (Bovee et al., 1979a,c; Bovee and Kronfeld, 1981; Polzin and Osborne, 1979).

The precise definition of the minimum protein requirements for uremic animals is of vital interest if these complications are to be addressed. Considerable individual variation is likely to prevail as a result of environmental and dietary factors, superimposed diseases, and metabolic disturbances. Patients given protein in excess of the amount required for maintenance at reduced levels of renal function will manifest increased retention of nitrogenous metabolites and an exacerbation of uremic signs. Patients maintained on a protein intake below individual minimum requirements will become protein-depleted, characterized by reductions in body weight, lean muscle mass, plasma proteins, immunoglobulins and complement, alterations in the composition of plasma amino acids, changes in the binding characteristics of drugs, and a marked negative nitrogen balance. Protein depletion will cause excessive tissue catabolism and an enhancement of azotemia from endogenous nitrogen (Kopple, 1976).

Despite the controversies, it seems reasonable to use the available information on nitrogen metabolism in uremia to formulate a workable scheme for the management of patients with renal insufficiency. In general, protein restriction should be initiated to control the clinical signs of uremia, and the degree of restriction should promote neither protein malnutrition nor protein overload. Most patients with stable chronic renal insufficiency are free of significant clinical signs until the BUN is greater than 80 to 90 mg/dl. Therefore, dietary therapy should maintain the BUN concentration below this symptomatic range. To achieve this goal it is necessary to reduce protein intake in proportion to the reduction in functional renal mass. Nitrogen balance can thus be maintained at a constant BUN concentration. For example, a normal dog that ingests 40 grams of protein on an all-meat diet would maintain a constant BUN if the dietary protein were reduced to 20 grams per day concomitantly with a 50 per cent reduction in renal mass.

In dogs, as in humans, a direct relationship exists between the BUN/serum creatinine ratio and dietary protein (Kopple and Coburn, 1974; Fig. 74–3). BUN is influenced by the dietary protein intake and the rate of endogenous protein breakdown, as well as the level of renal function. Serum creatinine concentration, on the other hand, is dependent primarily on the steady-state level of renal function and minimally influenced by diet or extrarenal parameters. Consequently, factoring the BUN concentration by serum creatinine normalizes the BUN for the influences of renal function and accentuates extrarenal influences.

The BUN/creatinine ratio is useful, therefore, as a guide for selecting an appropriate protein intake for dogs with renal insufficiency. If it is desirable to maintain the BUN at a level below 80 mg per dl, which will generally ameliorate the overt manifestation of azotemia, the necessary protein content can be estimated by the determination of the desired BUN/creatinine ratio (Figs. 74–3 and 74–10). To maintain the BUN at 60 mg per dl in a dog with a serum creatinine of 4.0 mg per dl (BUN/creatinine ratio = $60 \div 4.0 = 15$), a diet containing a maximum of 18 per cent protein on a dry matter basis is required (Figs. 74–3 and 74–10). Diets providing a greater percentage of protein promote excessive urea generation and elevation of the BUN above 60 mg/dl. A diet that is more protein-restrictive at this level of renal insufficiency is undesirable on the basis of reduced palatability, reduction of renal hemodynamics, and the potential for specific nutritional deficiencies. Progressive decline of renal function will require further adjustment of protein intake to maintain an acceptable BUN.

With this scheme, it is also possible to adopt guidelines for timing the institution of protein restriction. Renal insufficiency can be roughly divided into mild, moderate, severe, and terminal stages. Each stage can be reasonably correlated with creatinine clearance or serum creatinine concentration (Fig. 74–2).

Mild Renal Insufficiency. This category arbitrarily includes patients with glomerular filtration rates between 100 per cent and 40 per cent of normal and serum creatinine concentrations up to 2.5 mg/dl (see Fig. 74–2). Animals with this degree of renal insufficiency rarely require protein limitations and can be maintained on standard

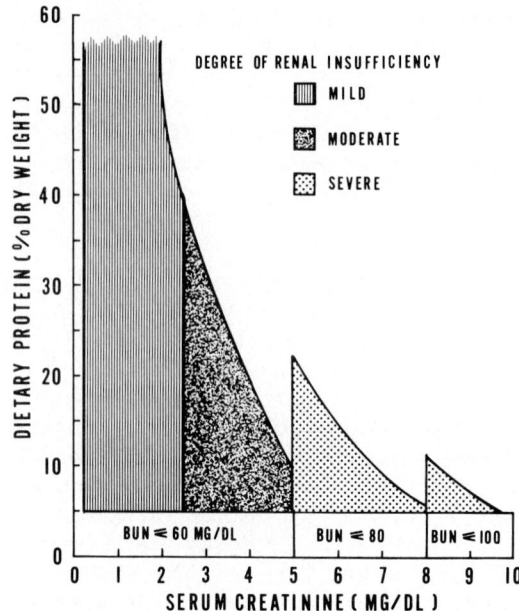

Figure 74–10. Approximate maximal dietary protein required at varying serum creatinine concentrations to maintain BUN at or below the indicated levels. Values for dietary protein are derived from the relationship for dietary protein and the BUN/creatinine ratio for azotemic dogs (see Fig. 74–3). Five per cent protein (dry weight) is taken as the minimal metabolizable protein requirement for maintenance of normal adult dogs. The protein content (dry matter basis) of representative commercial dog foods are as follows: canned, all meat — 50.3 per cent; canned, mixed — 36.7 per cent; dry, high protein — 30.9 per cent; dry cereal — 25.8 per cent; semimoist — 29.3 per cent (Kronfeld, 1975). The protein content of specialty diets G/d, K/d, and U/d (Hills, Topeka, Kansas) are 18.7, 14.1 and 9.1 per cent, respectively. (From Cowgill, L. D., and Spangler, W. L.: Renal insufficiency in geriatric dogs. Vet. Clin. North Am. *11*:727, 1981.)

commercial diets, providing that they are not sufficiently high in protein to raise the BUN above 60 to 80 mg/dl or promote clinical signs. In the latter situation, selection of an alternate commercial diet with a lower protein content should reduce the BUN without nutritional or functional compromise.

Moderate Renal Insufficiency. Moderate renal insufficiency is staged by GFRs between 40 per cent and 20 per cent of normal and associated serum creatinine concentrations between 2.5 and 5.0 mg/dl respectively. To maintain a BUN below 60 mg/dl in the creatinine range between 2.5 and 4.0 mg/dl (BUN/creatinine ratio between 24 and 15), commercial dog foods or specialty diets with protein contents between 40 per cent and 20 per cent (dry matter), respectively, will be satisfactory (Figs. 74–3 and 74–10). In the creatinine range between 4.0 and 5.0 mg/dl, commercial dog foods will not provide the necessary protein limitation, and moderately restricted diets (20 per cent to 12 per cent protein dry matter basis) will be required. Such a diet can be formulated by modification of a commercial dog food to which the patient is accustomed, formulation of a homemade diet, or institution of selected prescription dietary products. The diet should be palatable and highly digestible, provide protein of high biologic value, and meet caloric requirements.

Severe Renal Insufficiency. Severe renal insufficiency develops when renal disease has progressed to such a degree that alterations in renal function can no longer compensate for reductions in renal mass. At this point, uremia becomes clinically apparent. Severe renal insufficiency is characterized by GFRs between 20 per cent and 10 per cent of normal, and serum creatinine concentrations between 5 and 10 mg/dl, respectively. As the creatinine concentration approaches 10 mg/dl, strict dietary management becomes of utmost importance. Protein intake must be limited to the minimum requirements and the diet must be formulated so that the supplied nitrogen is most efficiently utilized.

A major drawback in formulating an appropriate diet is the uncertainty of the minimum protein requirements of renal-insufficient dogs. Because such information is unavailable, minimum protein requirements for normal dogs are generally adopted as a guideline. Studies in humans support this recommendation, since no consistent differences in the protein requirements of uremic patients and normal subjects have been demonstrated (Ford et al., 1969). There is no single minimum protein requirement for dogs, but 1.25 to 1.5 gm of high biologic protein per kg body weight per day (0.57 to 0.68 gm per lb per day) is generally recommended (Bovee, 1972, 1979a; Cunha et al., 1974; Morris and Doering, 1978; Polzin and Osborne, 1979).

The type of protein used in the diet is of equal importance to the amount supplied. In the dog, tryptophan, threonine, histidine, lycine, leucine, isoleucine, methionine, valine, and phenylalanine are regarded as essential amino acids and must, therefore, be supplied by dietary sources. Nonessential amino acids, on the other hand, can be synthesized from carbohydrates and protein or nonprotein nitrogen precursors. Provision of essential amino acids in a proportion similar to their requirements for protein turnover is critical for efficient use of dietary nitrogen without excessive production of nitrogenous metabolites.

The nutritional quality of protein is assessed as its ability to be used efficiently and is semi-quantitated by the term "biological value." Proteins with a high biological value contain a majority of essential amino acids in proportion to their metabolic requirements. Proteins with low biological values are limited in some or all essential amino acids, and are less efficiently used and inappropriate in the management of chronic renal insufficiency.

For the greatest benefit, uremic animals placed on restricted nitrogen intake should be supplied with proteins of high biological value. Egg protein is considered a reference standard, but milk, milk byproducts, and muscle meats also have relatively high biological values and should comprise the majority of the supplied protein. Generally, vegetable proteins are limited in some essential amino acids, which restricts their usefulness.

Severely restricted protein diets are generally unpalatable and unacceptable to the uremic patient, which is often inappetant or vomiting. It is often difficult to initiate protein restriction during this stage of renal insufficiency.

The following recommendations are guidelines for the development of protein-restricted diets for severely uremic dogs. More specific guidelines will be forthcoming only when the dietary management of chronic renal insufficiency is investigated in experimental or carefully controlled clinical trials. These guidelines are the author's synthesis of the available information as it can be most practically employed in clinical situations. Table 74–1 lists the recommended intake of quality protein for uremic dogs that require strict protein limitation, assuming that the minimum metabolizable protein requirements of adult uremic dogs are similar to the maintenance requirements of normal dogs (Cunha et al., 1974). These requirements must be adjusted upward to accommodate protein losses in the urine or

Table 74–1. Recommended Dietary Protein and Caloric Maintenance Requirements of Severely Uremic Adult Dogs

Weight		Dietary Protein Requirements (gm/day)	Dietary Energy Requirements (Kcal/day)
Kg	Pounds		
1	2.20	1.80	158
2	4.41	3.03	264
5	11.02	6.02	528
7	15.43	7.75	678
10	22.05	10.12	889
15	33.07	13.72	1204
20	44.09	17.02	1494
25	55.12	20.12	1766
30	66.14	23.07	2025
40	88.18	28.63	2513
50	110.23	33.85	2971

Derived from the apparent metabolizable protein and apparent metabolizable energy requirements of adult dogs of 1.5 gm/kg$^{0.75}$ per day and 132 Kcal/kg$^{0.75}$ per day (Cunha et al., 1974) and adjusted to an 80 per cent digestible diet (see text).

increased catabolism. In proteinuric dogs, it is desirable to quantitate the daily protein excretion and supplement the dietary requirements by the measured loss. Urine protein losses can be easily determined by analyzing the protein content of a quantitative 12- or 24-hour urine collection. An endogenous creatinine clearance can be performed on the same urine collection to better evaluate the patient's renal function.

The quantity of protein from sources that provide high biological value (such as eggs, milk, meat, and so on) can be calculated from standard nutrition tables. Such a table has been suggested by Bovee (1972).

Diets for severely uremic dogs should contain 15 per cent to 5 per cent protein on a dry matter basis when serum creatinine ranges from 5.5 to 8.0 mg/dl, respectively (Fig. 74–10). Diets that approach 5 per cent protein are likely to promote signs of protein malnutrition. A diet that supplies 8 to 10 per cent protein is less likely to cause malnutrition but will generate a slightly higher BUN. With more advanced renal failure, BUN concentrations will exceed 80 gm/dl at the lowest permissible protein intake. Only one commercially available diet for dogs will provide the degree of protein limitation required at the lower extremes of renal function. With this exception, it is necessary to formulate a homemade diet according to the previous recommendations. The available commercial product (Prescription Diet U/d) is formulated to provide a protein intake of 1.49 gm per kg per day (Morris and Doering, 1978) and will provide BUN/creatinine ratios of 5 to 8 in normal and azotemic dogs, respectively (Morris and Doering, 1978; Polzin and Osborne, 1979; Fig. 74–3). In moderately uremic animals this diet is reported to improve clinical condition, but it also reduced serum albumin concentrations when compared to similarly studied dogs at higher protein intakes (Polzin and Osborne, 1979). This finding may indicate that uremic dogs have a higher protein requirement than do normal dogs, which is the requirement currently recommended for the management of uremia.

Homemade diets suffer the disadvantages of inconvenience, variability of composition, and difficulty of formulation, although they provide the option of individualization of the diet to meet specific needs and may provide a more palatable diet. There is little information, however, to compare the efficacy of homemade diets to commercial formulations.

In suddenly decompensated chronic uremic dogs, dietary therapy alone cannot be expected to ameliorate the acute acceleration of clinical signs and debilitation. It may be necessary to institute either osmotic diuresis therapy or dialysis to establish a more physiologic baseline before these dietary principles can be implemented.

Recent studies in human uremic patients who were ingesting the minimum daily protein requirements of 0.6 gm per kg body weight suggests that standard dietary proteins are used too inefficiently to promote zero or positive nitrogen balance. Supplementation of these diets with additional nitrogen in the form of essential amino acids dramatically enhances nitrogen balance, reduces urea appearance, lowers the BUN, and reduces uremic toxicity. A new concept that may hold considerable importance for the management of uremic dogs is the supplementation of the minimum nitrogen requirement with the keto acid precursors of some essential amino acids (Kopple and Swendseid, 1977; Walser, 1981). By providing the carbon skeleton of essential amino acids, endogenous nitrogen can be used for the synthesis of essential amino acids and the promotion of positive balance nitrogen. Although considerable research is needed in this area, recent investigations demonstrate that keto-analogue therapy may promote better nutrition and minimize uremic toxicity in human patients who cannot be managed on dialysis or with renal transplantation.

Caloric Requirements. The provision of an adequate caloric intake is as critical to the management of uremia as is the limitation of dietary protein. If insufficient calories are provided with nonprotein sources, dietary and endogenous proteins will be used for the deficit energy needs. Nitrogen turnover as well as urea generation will thus accelerate, and nitrogen balance and clinical well-being will deteriorate. The caloric requirements must be carefully calculated and provided as carbohydrates or fats.

The energy requirements of the dog are best determined on the basis of metabolic body size. On a body weight basis, the requirements of a one kg dog will differ markedly from a dog weighing 60 kg. The metabolizable maintenance energy requirements of normal adult dogs are estimated to be 132 kcal per kg body weight$^{0.75}$ (Cunha et al., 1974; see Table 74–1). This figure serves as a baseline requirement but may vary with age, body condition, activity, environment, temperature, and body conformation. Energy requirements may also vary with concurrent diseases and must be adjusted upward for infection, fever, growth, metabolic disturbances, or unusual physical activity.

The bulk of energy intake should be supplied as nonprotein calories selected from normal dietary sources or commercial caloric supplements (Table 74–2). Nutrition tables can be used to determine the amount of selected foods required to provide the recommended caloric intake.

With these considerations, it is necessary to select the food substances most acceptable to the patient and calculate the amounts required to provide the minimum protein, energy, and fat requirements. Sample diets and selected foods have been published for guidelines (Bovee, 1972; Morris, 1980).

Once a protein-restricted diet has been formulated and administered, it is necessary to monitor changes in body weight, plasma protein concentration, and body conformation as a guide to the adequacy of the protein and caloric inputs.

Nutritional Requirements for Severely Uremic Cats. Clinical experience with uremic cats is limited. It is therefore necessary to blindly adopt the recommendations established for dogs and man as acceptable for the cat until additional information is available. A formulated diet should provide a minimum of 80 kcal per kg body weight per day as the metabolizable energy requirement (Ullrey et al., 1978). The maintenance protein requirement of adult cats is not precisely defined. Available evidence indicates that 19 per cent of the metabolizable calories as quality protein (i.e., mammalian, avian, or fish muscle) is adequate. This requirement is the equivalent of a 21 per cent protein diet, which provides 4.5 calories of metabolizable energy per gram of dry matter, or 3.73 grams of metabolizable protein per kg body weight per day (Ullrey et al., 1978).

The relatively high protein requirement of cats makes them less than ideal for the conservative management of chronic renal failure. Cats are reluctant to consume low protein diets or to adapt to subtle alterations in established dietary habits. These factors,

Table 74–2. Caloric Supplements for Uremic Diets*

	Controlyte (Doyle)	Polycose (Ross)	Sumacal (Organon)
Pro, gm	Trace	0	0
Fat, gm	48	0	0
CHO, gm	143	250	250
Na, mEq	0.85	12	4.34
K, mEq	0.20	2.5	2.94
For 1000 Kcal	198 gm dry wt	263 gm dry wt	1000 ml liquid
Type	low protein, low electrolyte	oligosaccharides	CHO source

*Values per 1000 Kcal.

in combination with the inappetence and depression characteristic of uremia, provide formidable obstacles for effective application of dietary principles. Nevertheless, individual patients may be responsive to dietary therapy, which should be selectively applied and evaluated whenever possible.

Water Intake. Water intake of uremic patients varies greatly, depending on the diet, degree of renal insufficiency, environmental temperature and humidity, and concurrent diseases. Uremic animals can generally regulate water balance until they become severely compromised, so that intentional restriction of water is not required. It is generally sufficient to supply an unlimited source of fresh water. Accidental or deliberate limitation of water intake could promote chronic dehydration and progression of existing renal injury. Adulteration of the water supply with drugs or supplements should be avoided if this affects fluid consumption.

Vitamin Therapy. Water soluble vitamins are not stored within the body and must be supplied as an integral part of the diet. Inappetence and modifications in dietary constituents increase the tendency for vitamin deficiencies. Water soluble vitamins should be routinely administered to insure adequate supplies. Vitamin A can accumulate to toxic levels in humans with uremia and should not be supplemented. With the exception of Vitamin D (see following discussion), additional fat soluble vitamin supplementation is unnecessary.

Salt and Sodium Bicarbonate Requirements in Renal Insufficiency

Recommendations for the management of sodium and bicarbonate are ill-defined. The use of sodium chloride in the management of chronic renal insufficiency has evolved from the premise that uremic dogs have an obligatory loss of sodium in the urine and are prone to negative sodium balance (Bovee, 1972; Osborne et al., 1972c, 1975). Therapeutically, liberal dietary supplementation of sodium chloride and sodium bicarbonate has been recommended to obviate this presumed imbalance. In recent years, the adaptations to progressive renal insufficiency have become more clearly defined, and this recommendation needs reevaluation. Investigation in dogs as well as in man indicate that the increase in salt excretion per unit of surviving renal mass is a physiologic adaptation to maintain salt balance (Danovitch et al., 1977; Schmidt et al., 1974; Schultze et al., 1969).

Human patients and dogs on a normal salt intake remain in external balance for salt during steady state despite moderate or severe reductions in functional renal mass. There is neither net retention of salt (i.e., dietary or parenteral inputs greater than urinary outputs) nor net depletion of salt (inputs less than outputs). Each nephron, therefore, must excrete a greater proportion of its sodium load in renal insufficiency than in health. The observed increase in salt excretion per unit of surviving renal mass is a physiologic response to maintain salt balance and is not an obligatory event. The exact events that regulate this adaptive natriuresis are unknown but appear to involve the interplay of many factors whose individual importance are dependent upon the experimental or clinical circumstances.

Dogs in varying degrees of renal failure can regulate sodium excretion and maintain sodium balance within the normal range of dietary intake, but the capacity to adjust sodium excretion rapidly to accommodate sudden changes in intake becomes severely limited as renal insufficiency advances. Sudden reductions in sodium intake can promote salt wasting, decreases in total body sodium, and dehydration. Acute increases in sodium intake can increase total body sodium and expand extracellular fluid volume (ECFV).

The physiologic or clinical consequences of these adaptations in sodium excretion are important considerations in the management of chronic renal failure (Bricker, 1972; Bricker and Fine, 1978; Bricker et al., 1975). Expansion of ECFV, hypertension, and edema are potential clinical consequences in uremic dogs that have been maintained on normal or high salt diets.

Hypertension has been virtually ignored as a clinical entity in veterinary medicine, yet the incidence of hypertension is substantial in dogs with renal disease. It may also be a substantial contributor to the progression of renal injury in the dog, as in humans (Spangler et al., 1980a).

Blood pressure has been variably reported for normal dogs, depending on the recording method and the physiologic state of

Table 74–3. Arterial Blood Pressure in 35 Dogs with Renal Disease

	Per Cent	Systolic	Diastolic (mmHg)	Mean
Normotensive (14)	40	149.1 ± 14.4	85.6 ± 9.8	105.1 ± 9.6
P		<.001	<.001	<.001
Hypertensive (21)	60	195.1 ± 27.2	123.5 ± 23.4	148.3 ± 26.8

the animal. In conscious or slightly sedated dogs, systolic pressure of 130 to 180 mmHg and a diastolic pressure of 60 to 95 mmHg is representive (Anderson and Fisher, 1968; Hamilton et al., 1940; Spangler et al., 1980a; Stamler et al., 1949; Weiser et al., 1977), although slightly higher values have been reported (Freundlich et al., 1972; Valtonen and Oksanen, 1972).

The lack of convenient and accurate non-invasive methods to measure blood pressure in dogs and cats is undoubtedly a major consideration in the infrequent attention given to this disorder. The ultrasonic Doppler principle has been recently used for noninvasive measurements of systemic blood pressure in conscious dogs without vascular invasion or pain (Freundlich et al., 1972; Garner et al., 1975; Weiser et al., 1977). Direct percutaneous punctures of the femoral artery can also be easily performed with minimal patient discomfort or risk, and this is the author's preference if recording equipment is available.

The incidence of spontaneous hypertension in the dog is low but not clearly established. In a survey of 1000 research dogs in controlled environments, the incidence was less than one per cent (Katz et al., 1954). In separate studies containing 200 and 400 dogs, 0.5 per cent maintained a consistent mean arterial pressure greater than 150 mmHg (McCubbin and Corcoran, 1953; Walkerlin, 1943), and in a fourth study of 115 dogs, two per cent had pressures exceeding the reported normal values (Hamil-

ton et al., 1940). The incidence of hypertension in dogs with renal disease is notable, however, and has been reported to occur in 58 to 93 per cent of patients (Anderson and Fisher, 1968; Hamilton et al., 1940; Wieser et al., 1977; Table 74–3). In cocker spaniels with renal cortical hypoplasia, Persson and coworkers (1961a) found no evidence of hypertension, but in general it is a significant and consistent pathologic abnormality in dogs with a variety of renal abnormalities (Tables 74–3 and 74–4).

Of major concern is the clinical significance of hypertension in the manifestations, development, or progression of renal insufficiency in dogs. A direct and consistent correlation exists between renal insufficiency, hypertension, and the development of renal vascular pathology. Necrosis, fibrinoid lesions, sclerosis, hyalinization, and capillary occlusion are described in the glomeruli of hypertensive dogs (Anderson and Fisher, 1968; Platt, 1952). Fibrinoid lesions, hyalinization and myoarteritis are demonstrated in arterioles as well as tubular degeneration and fibrous replacement of the parenchyma (Anderson and Fisher, 1968; McGill et al., 1958; Muirhead et al., 1951; Platt, 1952). These hypertension-induced degenerative changes are thought to create atrophy and sclerosis of the renal cortex, renal ischemia, and progressive parenchymal loss (Freis et al., 1967; Freis et al., 1970; Weiser et al., 1977).

Left ventricular hypertrophy is also attributed to hypertension and is a consistent

Table 74–4. Effects of Salt Intake On Arterial Blood Pressure In Dogs with Renal Disease

	Systolic	Diastolic (mmHg)	Mean
Normal Salt (Commerical diet) (15)	178.2 ± 28.3	109.3 ± 21.8	131.7 ± 24.2
P	<.05	N.S.	<.05
Restricted Salt (Prescription diet) (6)	153.9 ± 18.0	100.8 ± 19.1	108.3 ± 13.9

feature of renal insufficiency in dogs (Weiser et al., 1977; Platt, 1952; Mueller et al., 1978). The cardiovascular stress induced by hypertension may progress to ventricular dilatation and cardiac failure. It may reduce the cardiac reserve and predispose the myocardium to ischemia (Mueller et al., 1978).

There are no conclusive studies in the dog that definitively demonstrate the importance of hypertension in the progression of renal injury, the erosion of residual renal function, or the development of other systemic disturbances. In one study in dogs with moderate degrees of spontaneous hypertension, renal function was stable when serially evaluated for periods up to 64 weeks. Necropsy findings were consistent with the histologic alterations characteristic of established hypertension (Stamler et al., 1949). Until more definitive information is available that correlates alterations in renal morphology with changes in renal function, it is reasonable to regard hypertension as a detrimental force and the resultant arteriolosclerosis, glomerular and tubular atrophy, and nephrosclerosis as significant factors in the reduction of residual renal mass. In man, a clear association exists between hypertension and morbid alterations in the heart, brain, and kidneys (Freis et al., 1967; Freis et al., 1970).

The pathogenesis of renal hypertension involves a variety of factors that are imprecisely defined and act singularly or in combination to deregulate pressor and volume homeostatic mechanisms. Arterial hypertension develops either from an increased flow of blood and increased cardiac output or from increased resistance to blood flow secondary to enhanced peripheral vascular resistance, or from a combination of both.

Major factors initiating or sustaining the hypertensive state include (1) failure to excrete a normal salt or fluid volume load at normotensive pressures, causing expansion of total body water and circulatory congestion; (2) stiffening of the venous capacitance system; (3) alterations of adrenergic activity; (4) activation of the renin-angiotensin-aldosterone axis, leading to increased vascular resistance and salt retention; (5) stimulation of renopressor systems; or (6) suppression of renodepressors or prostaglandins (Fronlich, 1977; Brod, 1978).

The treatment of renal hypertension consists of nonpharmacologic controls and a hierarchy of drugs commensurate with the severity of the hypertension. Restriction of salt intake is the mainstay of nondrug therapy to counteract the tendency for positive sodium and water balance.

Sodium should be reduced to 0.1 to 0.3 per cent of the diet, which provides approximately 200 to 600 mg daily to a 15 kg dog. Supplementation of sodium to renal insufficient dogs with hypertension to promote an increase in water turnover is contraindicated. Drug therapy consists of diuretics, sympatholytic agents, and vasodilators that are administered as required for pressor control.

Specific protocols have not been formulated or tested for the management of hypertension in dogs. The similarities in pathogenesis, however, warrant a treatment program similar to that used for man (Himori et al., 1978). Drug therapy should be initiated with a thiazide diuretic (or furosemide, if renal function is greatly diminished). If arterial pressure is not normalized by sodium restriction alone or in combination with diuretics, propranolol, a β-adrenergic blocking agent can be instituted at 5 to 20 mg, two to three times daily as a sympatholytic. A vasodilator like hydralazine (1 to 2 mg per kg every 8 to 12 hours) or prazosin hydrochloride (0.5 to 1.0 mg twice daily initially) and should be combined with the previous therapy failing an adequate response. Arterial pressure should be monitored with direct or indirect techniques at two-week intervals so the therapy can be adjusted for proper pressor control.

In the author's experience with a limited population of dogs, most are ineffectively controlled with diuretic or sympatholytic therapy alone and require addition of a vasodilator.

What effects dietary salt has on the development of metabolic acidosis in uremia is an important but unresolved question. Rats maintained on normal salt intakes were shown to develop reduced serum bicarbonate levels, lower bicarbonate thresholds, and lower maximal reabsorptive capacities for bicarbonate than were uremic rats maintained on salt-limited diets (Espinel, 1975). Human patients also have a reduced plasma bicarbonate concentration while subjected to sodium loading (van Assendelft and Mees, 1970). Opposite results have been demonstrated in the dog. Uremic dogs were shown to have a higher bicarbonate reabsorptive capacity than were normal animals, even though plasma bicarbonate levels were comparable (Arruda et al., 1976). Uremic dogs on salt-limited diets demonstrated a lower reabsorptive capacity for bicarbonate than dogs maintained on normal salt-containing diets (Schmidt and Gavellos, 1977). The resolution of these problems will have a major influence on the future recommendations for dietary salt intake in uremia and the management of metabolic acidosis.

Disregarding the complications of hypertension, a subtle increase in extracellular fluid volume may measurably increase glomerular filtration rate and urea clearance, and lower plasma urea concentrations (Husted et al., 1975; Landis et al., 1935; van Assendelft and Mees, 1970). Salt supplementation has been recommended for uremic dogs on the basis of these presumptions and clinical experiences (Bovee, 1972, 1979; Osborne et al., 1972c, 1975; Osborne and Polzin, 1979).

The objective of salt therapy is to supply a level of dietary sodium that will promote clinical benefits without producing overt clinical complications and progressive renal damage. Recommendations must be based on clinical experiences, a clear understanding of the pathophysiology of sodium metabolism in uremia, and knowledge of the risks and benefits of manipulations in dietary sodium. Changes in dietary sodium should not be made suddenly unless the changes are small or the renal insufficiency is mild. The kidney is adapted to a level of sodium excretion equal to the existing sodium intake and may not be able to accommodate sudden adjustments in dietary load. If a dietary alteration is made, the sodium content of the new diet should be initially adjusted to the estimated previous intake. After the new diet is established the sodium content should be formulated to accommodate concurrent conditions, including cardiovascular disease, edema, or hypertension. The transition from one diet to another with differing sodium contents can be accomplished by initially mixing the two diets and gradually tapering the former diet over a two- to four-week period. Congestive heart failure and pulmonary edema represent states of serious sodium imbalance and require more rapid limitation of the sodium load and/or diuretic administration. Sodium depletion states, hypotension, and rare sodium-losing states, on the other hand, require aggressive sodium supplementation to correct the existing and ongoing deficits.

Nephrotic syndrome and compensated valvular heart disease are characterized by positive sodium balance and diminished cardiac reserve, respectively. Sodium supplementation in these conditions perpetuates or aggravates the tenuous balance and is contraindicated. Sodium restriction and/or diuretic therapy is more appropriate. Diuretics should be used cautiously in patients with profound hypoalbuminemia to prevent hypotension, hypovolemia, and reduced renal perfusion.

Acid-Base Management

Moderate to severe metabolic acidosis is a consistent finding in advanced renal insufficiency. Respiratory and renal compensation delay the onset of acidosis until renal function falls below 20 per cent of normal. Acidosis becomes more prevalent as renal function deteriorates beyond this point or as additional metabolic or dietary stresses are imposed. At what point metabolic acidosis should be therapeutically managed is debatable. Serum pH is generally normal in stable uremic dogs, and the acidosis is recognized only by a low serum bicarbonate concentration, low P_{CO_2}, or increased anion gap [(Na + K) − (HCO$_3$ + Cl)]. Chronic metabolic acidosis should be treated with oral sodium bicarbonate at incremental doses necessary to maintain the serum bicarbonate between 18 to 24 mEq/L. The dosage is variable and depends upon the degree of acidosis and dietary acid load, and the severity of renal insufficiency. An initial dosage of 25 to 35 mg per kg per day can be modified to normalize serum bicarbonate concentration on the basis of subsequent bicarbonate determinations.

The sodium load provided by sodium bicarbonate therapy should be calculated as part of the total dietary sodium intake. In sodium retention states, sodium bicarbonate must be provided in lieu of an equivalent amount of sodium chloride. In this regard, sodium bicarbonate is better tolerated in patients with uremia and is less likely to produce hypertension or salt retention (Husted et al., 1975). Parathyroid hormone has been implicated in the alterations in renal bicarbonate absorption. The mechanism of this effect is not known but amelioration of the hyperparathyroidism enhances bicarbonate reabsorptive capacity in dogs. The increased bicarbonate reabsorption is associated with elevations in serum bicarbonate. A combination of phosphate restriction and sodium bicarbonate administration should be effective to regulate the acid-base status of uremic animals (Schmidt and Garvellas, 1977).

Androgen Therapy

Anemia is a characteristic and morbid feature of chronic renal insufficiency. In most cases, uremic patients have adequate iron stores and are unresponsive to hematinics, including folic acid and iron. The lack of erythropoietin has hindered the management of anemia in uremic patients, although oral and parenteral androgen preparations have been shown to promote the generation of erythropoietin and erythrocyte production in uremic animals and humans (Cattran et al., 1977; Doane et al., 1975; Hendler et al., 1974; Shahidi, 1973; Williams et al., 1974; Zanjani and Banisadre, 1979). Increased hematocrit, hemoglobin concentration, and red blood cell mass; decreased transfusion requirements; and increased levels of 2,3-diphosphoglycerate have resulted from androgen therapy. Demonstrated clinical benefits in human patients include increased weight gain, improved strength, increased skeletal mass, and decreases in BUN. Preparations with a high anabolic-to-androgenic activity allow effective stimulation of erythropoiesis with minimal side effects associated with virilism. Increases in serum transaminase activity and serum triglyceride concentrations are reported side effects. Virilization should be a minimal contraindication in dogs and cats.

Guidelines for the administration of anabolic agents to veterinary patients have not been established. Nandrolone decanoate, testosterone enanthate, and fluoxymesterone stimulate renal and extrarenal erythropoietin production and the transformation of undifferentiated stem cells into the erythroid sequence independently of erythropoietin. Other androgens, including oxymethalone and stanozolol (Winstrol) have only the erythropoietin-stimulating properties and are less effective in the absence of renal parenchyma. In view of the demonstrated efficacy of nandrolone decanoate and testosterone (Doane et al., 1975; Cottran, 1977; Gorshein et al., 1973) and the reduced potency and lack of hematopoietic benefits of oxymetholone (Gorshein et al., 1973; Davis et al., 1972), the use of the former agents seems more appropriate.

Timing for the administration of anabolic therapy is a matter of clinical discretion. In view of their demonstrated effects on hematopoiesis, clinical well-being, weight gain, and nitrogen balance, these agents should be implemented upon detection of nonresponsive anemia. Attempts should be made to maintain hematocrits above 30 per cent and hemoglobin concentrations above 10.0 gm/dl. A dosage of 1 to 5 mg per kg per week of nandrolone decanoate with a maximum dosage of 200 mg has been suggested for the dog (Low, 1980; Schall and Perman, 1975; Barsanti, 1979). Hematologic responses may not be evident for several weeks.

Major side effects of androgenic steroids include masculinization, which should be of minimal concern in veterinary patients. In young animals, androgens may promote premature epiphyseal closure and a failure to obtain normal stature. Patients receiving anabolic steroids should be monitored for evidence of salt and fluid retention, and liver transaminases should be periodically monitored to detect hepatotoxic effects. Adjunctive therapy should include the routine administration of multiple vitamin preparations to provide B-complex and folate. Unless chronic subtle bleeding is present, most patients will have adequate iron stores and will rarely need iron supplementation.

Renal Osteodystrophy. Renal osteodystrophy and extraosseous mineralization are serious consequences of chronic renal insufficiency in human patients (Avioli and Teitelbaum, 1979). The development of sensitive hormone assays for parathyroid hormone (PTH) and vitamin D metabolites has provided a greater awareness and understanding of these disorders. The clinical manifestations of altered mineral metabolism associated with renal insufficiency has received only spotty recognition in the veterinary literature (Brody et al., 1961; Burk and Barton, 1978; Cordy, 1967; Hogg, 1948; Holmes, 1975; Kaufman et al., 1957;

Norrdin et al., 1977). It is evident that many of these manifestations are present biochemically and histologically in the early development of renal failure and appear to play prominent roles in the symptomatology and development of the uremic state.

Renal osteodystrophy is a uremic complication with a multifactorial pathogenesis and variable clinical expression (see discussion in Chapter 73). In the dog it is most often manifested in aged animals with protracted chronic uremia and in young patients with congenital or early acquired renal insufficiency. Renal osteodystrophy has been discussed under a variety of names, including "rubber jaw," "renal osteitis fibrosa cystica," and "renal rickets" (Brodey et al., 1961). Clinical signs may include firm bilateral swelling of the maxillary and mandibular bones (Fig. 74–1); skeletal pliability; osseous pain; loosening, loss, or irregular positioning of the teeth; stunted axial and apendicular growth; and bowing deformities of the limbs. These findings are variable but will be demonstrated along with other physical signs of uremia. The radiographic features are described under Radiologic Evaluation.

Histologically, the osseous lesions are characteristic of hyperparathyroidism. Fibrous tissue replacement of the normal cortical and tubecular bone, excessive osteoid volume and surface area, proliferation of osteoclast numbers, and enhanced osteoclastic resorption surface are typical changes.

Extraosseous Calcification. Soft tissue mineralization is a more common sequela of disordered mineral metabolism. Excessive mineral deposition is seen in periarticular, visceral, and vascular tissues (Figs. 74–5 and 74–6). Large tumoral calcific masses may develop around tendon sheaths and in foot pads (Fig. 74–6). As these masses develop, they cause pain, dysfunction, and disfigurement (Barber and Rowland, 1979; Cordy, 1967; Legendre and Dade, 1974). They may fluctuate in size and location as the uremia progresses.

Visceral and vascular calcification is an early and consistent developmental lesion of uremia. The mineral content of these tissues becomes dramatically increased with the progression of renal insufficiency (Alfrey et al., 1976; Kraikitpanitch et al., 1978). Areas of predilection include gastric mucosa, bronchial walls, myocardium, endocardium,

renal interstitium, glomeruli, lung, intercostal muscle, and the posterior capsule of the eye. Visceral and vascular calcification may be radiographically recognized when it is extensive in the gastric mucosa, kidney, lungs, trachea, aorta, and peripheral arteries (Fig. 74–5).

The extraosseous and vascular mineral is deposited as brushite and is subsequently transformed to an apatite structure. The visceral deposits, on the other hand, are a unique amorphous mineral that has a high magnesium and pyrophosphate content (Alfrey et al., 1976; Avioli and Teitelbaum, 1979).

The development of these extraosseous mineral disturbances is not well defined. The mineral deposition may result from dystrophy or metastasis, or it may occur by an as yet undefined process (Avioli and Tietelbaum, 1979; Haut et al., 1980; Alfrey et al., 1976). As the plasma concentrations of phosphate and calcium exceed their solubility product, metastatic mineral deposition can occur in "apparently healthy" tissue. Alternatively, dystrophic calcification can occur in the presence of unaltered plasma mineral concentrations in tissues damaged by the presence of disease. The recent observations that the pattern, tissue specificity, and composition of mineral deposits change as uremia progresses suggests that additional mechanisms and mineral disturbances are involved (Haut et al., 1980). Abnormalities in magnesium metabolism and high plasma magnesium and pyrophosphate concentrations characteristic of uremia are suggested to modify and promote visceral mineralization (Alfrey et al, 1976).

Treatment of Renal Osteodystrophy and Extraosseous Calcification. It is apparent that these disorders are consistent consequences of renal insufficiency in man as well as in dogs, and appear in some species to have a profound effect on the propagation of renal damage (Gimenez et al., 1981; Haut et al., 1980; Ibels et al., 1978). Therapeutic recommendations for these disorders must be formulated from theoretical considerations and from observations in human patients in the absence of direct experience in the dog and cat. The diagnostic tools to assess skeletal or soft tissue damage or the alterations in hormone status are unfortunately not readily available for veterinary practitioners.

The development of renal osteodystrophy, however, can be divided into stages comparable to those depicted in Figure 74–2, and the therapeutic requirements developed according to the onset and severity of the clinical and biochemical abnormalities. In the early stages of renal insufficiency, compensatory mechanisms are operative to maintain the integrity of external mineral balance at the expense of hyperparathyroidism (Bricker, 1972; Bricker and Fine, 1978; Slatopolsky et al., 1971). This early stage of hyperparathyroidism can be prevented in experimental dogs and human patients and reversed by a reduction of phosphate intake proportional to the decrease in renal function (Kaplan et al., 1979; Maschio et al., 1980; Rutherford et al., 1977; Slatopolsky et al., 1971, 1972). Phosphate restriction alone, however, may not entirely prevent the long-term development of subtle hyperparathyroidism and bone demineralization (Rutherford et al., 1977). Combined early phosphate restriction and vitamin D supplementation will effectively control both the hyperparathyroidism and metabolic bone disease in experimental dogs (Rutherford et al., 1977).

In the remnant kidney model in rats, proportional phosphate restriction will prevent the nephrocalcinosis, accelerated renal destruction, and uremia that occurs in animals maintained on a normal phosphate intake (Haut et al., 1980; Ibels et al., 1978).

In mild renal insufficiency (serum creatinine between 1.5 and 3.5 mg/dl) (see Fig. 74–2), even though serum calcium and phosphate concentrations are normal, a subtle degree of hyperparathyroidism and renal osteodystrophy are present in all likelihood. Therapy at this stage includes moderate (30 to 50 per cent) restriction of dietary phosphate and supplementation of dietary calcium (Maschio et al., 1980). Dietary phosphate is difficult to restrict when feeding commercial foods, since most contain similar amounts of phosphate on a dry matter basis (Kronfeld, 1975; Morris, 1980). Selected dietary products contain substantially less phosphate than do commercial foods and would seemingly be beneficial for this stage of disease. Since little protein restriction is necessary, Prescription diet G/d or Cadillac N, which contains a lower phosphate content, may be used effectively, depending on the degree of renal insufficiency. Without the availability of

PTH assays or quantitative bone histology, the benefits of this recommendation are difficult to assess clinically or biochemically.

With moderate to severe renal insufficiency (serum creatinine concentrations between 3.5 and 10.0 mg/dl), the levels of plasma phosphate progressively increase. Intestinal absorption of calcium is reduced by decreased food consumption and diminished production of 1,25-dihydroxycholecalciferol $(1,25(OH)_2D_3)$. Renal osteodystrophy and soft tissue calcification will be substantial, albeit clinically occult. Treatment is palliative and directed at healing the metabolic bone disease and halting the hyperparathyroidism and extraosseous calcification. Phosphate intake should be limited by rigid restriction of dietary protein and phosphate. Absorption of phosphate can be reduced with intestinal phosphate binders such as aluminum hydroxide and aluminum carbonate, which are available in capsule, tablet, and liquid forms. The dosage of phosphate binders is adjusted when combined with restriction of dietary phosphate to promote a stable plasma phosphate between 4.0 and 4.5 mg/dl. An initial dosage of 300 to 500 mg of aluminum carbonate three times daily should be adjusted according to serial evaluations of the plasma phosphate. The dosage should be monitored biweekly during the initial phases of therapy to insure efficacy and to avoid hypophosphatemia and depletion of phosphate. Constipation is a common side effect that may necessitate administration of laxatives.

Dietary calcium and vitamin D supplementation should be avoided in the presence of hyperphosphatemia to minimize soft tissue mineralization. Once serum phosphate is strictly controlled, calcium and/or vitamin D (or its synthetic metabolites) can be administered to control the hyperparathyroidism, hypocalcemia, bone disease, and calcium malabsorption. The dosage of vitamin D for use in chronic renal failure is individualized to the patient's responsiveness. An initial dose of 5000 to 10,000 IU per day must be monitored at regular and frequent intervals. If plasma calcium remains below 10.0 to 10.5 mg/dl or if alkaline phosphatase levels remain elevated in the face of strict phosphate control, the daily dose can be cautiously increased or a more potent vitamin D metabolite can be used.

Dehydrotachysterole, 25-hydroxycholecalciferol, or 1-α-hydroxycholecalciferol have been used to correct the calcium malabsorption, hyperparathyroidism, and hypocalcemia, as well as the histologic, radiographic, and clinical bone disease in human patients (Avioli and Teitelbraum, 1979; Massry, 1980). With the exception of 25-hydroxycholecalciferol, there is a limited experience with these preparations in the dog. These hormones are extremely potent and promote frequent hypercalcemic episodes. Dosage guidelines have recently been outlined and may be useful as initial recommendations (Osborne and Polzin, 1979).

Cimetidine, a histamine H_2-receptor antagonist, has recently been shown to dramatically reduce the level of circulating parathyroid hormone in both uremic humans (Jacob et al., 1980) and uremic dogs (Jacob et al., 1981). In the dog, cimetidine causes decreased secretion of parathyroid hormone, decreased bone resorption, decreased serum phosphate, increased levels of serum calcium and $1,25(OH)_2D_3$, and a positive calcium balance. This drug may offer promise in the future for control of renal osteodystrophy.

Modification of the periarticular, visceral, and vascular soft tissue calcifications has also been demonstrated in humans and rats with inhibitors of calcium crystal formation (Gimenez et al., 1981; Haut et al., 1980; Russel et al., 1975; Zuccehelli et al., 1978). The further development of these concepts may allow future resolution of these deleterious consequences of uremia. The management of renal failure in the dog or cat requires a multifaceted approach proportional to the degree of renal insufficiency and the appearance of clinical signs. Each clinician should resist overtreatment but should be committed to an aggressive approach when appropriate to manage all the signs and functional disorders associated with the loss of renal function.

GLOMERULAR DISEASE

The canine and feline glomerulus is subject to a variety of pathophysiologic alterations that have profound clinical manifestations. Extensive progressive, or unresolved glomerular injuries can initiate morphologic and functional alterations of the tubular epithelium, vasculature, and interstitium, and can establish end-stage disease indistinguishable from other causes of interstitital scarring.

PREVALENCE

Glomerular disease was rarely recognized as a significant form of renal injury in dogs and cats in the past (Monlux, 1953). The present awareness is largely due to the application of percutaneous renal biopsy techniques in animals with renal disease. Despite its heightened recognition, the actual prevalence of glomerular disease in dogs or cats is still in question. Murray and Wright (1974) reported an incidence of 3.7 per cent in 1136 necropsy specimens in dogs. Their study, however, excluded a variety of clinically significant glomerular lesions. Stuart et al. (1975) reported a 25 per cent incidence of proteinuria in a colony of research dogs and described in detail 13 of 218 (5.0 per cent) dogs with glomerulonephritis. Rouse and Lewis (1975) identified by histologic criteria an 18 per cent (12 of 65) incidence in nonselected dogs submitted for euthanasia. At the extreme, Muller-Peddinghaus and Trautwein (1977) morphologically identified glomerulonephritis in 90 per cent of 101 necropsied dogs that were unselected for renal disease. It is apparent from recent reports that glomerular disease represents an important component of the spectrum in renal injury.

ETIOLOGY

Glomerulonephropathies have a pronounced immunologic basis, but the precise cause for the immune activation is not always known. Recognized causes have a diverse basis, despite similar clinical manifestations. A bacterial etiopathology associated with infections by specific types of Group A hemolytic streptococci (Glassock, 1979; Kashgarian et al., 1974), as well as with a variety of other primary bacterial diseases (Fish and Michael, 1979), is clearly established in man. The specificity for streptococci has not been established for veterinary patients, but the association with bacterial infections is well documented in canine pyometra (Asheim, 1965; Obel et al., 1964; Sandholm et al., 1975) and is suggested for bacterial endocarditis (Highman et al., 1958).

Concurrent viral infections and glomerulonephritis are well documented in a variety of animal species (Osborne et al., 1977; Slauson and Lewis, 1979). In experimental dogs, canine adenovirus causes an immune complex, proliferative glomerulonephritis (Wright et al., 1974). Circulating immune complexes from the serum of infected dogs will localize in the glomerular basement membrane after passive transfer to a murine intermediate (Morrison and Wright, 1976).

Glomerulonephritis is a classical but inconsistent feature of systemic lupus erythematosus (SLE) in the dog (Lewis, 1974; Lewis et al., 1973; Osborne et al., 1973). Although details of the etiopathology are incomplete, the involvement of a replicating agent or virus has been suggested (Lewis, 1974; Lewis et al., 1973).

A strong association with a viral etiology is also found in cats concomitant with FeLV infection or lymphosarcoma. This relationship is analogous to the membranous glomerulonephritis produced in mice subsequent to infection by species-specific oncornaviruses. The reported incidence of glomerulonephritis in cats with lymphoma or FeLV-related disease is between 14 per cent (Anderson and Jarrett, 1971) and 32 per cent (Francis et al., 1980; Glick et al., 1978). In one survey, renal lesions were recognized with all histologic types of lymphoma and were absent in cases free of FeLV group–specific antigens in the blood (Glick et al., 1978). More recently, however, Wright et al. (1981) reported 11 cases of membranous nephropathy in cats with no evidence of FeLV infection. The glomerular lesion is an immune-complex type and will manifest in FeLV-infected cats without identifiable neoplastic involvement (Glick et al., 1978; Thornburg et al., 1979; Mackey, 1975; Cotter et al., 1975). In a few cases, group-specific FeLV antigen-antibody complexes were identified in glomerular basement membranes of FeLV-infected cats, which further strengthens the viral etiology of this disorder (Hardy, 1974).

In the dog, a glomerulopathy has been demonstrated in natural and experimental infections with *Dirofilaria immitis* (Casey and Splitter, 1975; Simpson et al., 1974). A strong association with active heartworm infection remains a consistent finding.

Glomerulonephritis is a prominent disorder in dogs and cats with extrarenal neoplasia. In a survey of 42 cases of glomerulonephritis in dogs, approximately 40 per cent had associated malignant neoplasia (Murray and Wright, 1974). Sixty-nine per cent of dogs with mastocytoma demonstrated glomerular pathology (Hottendorf and Neilsen, 1968). In more recent evaluations, 33 per cent (7 of 21, Di Bartola et al., 1980b; 21 of 63, Muller-Peddinghaus and Trautwein, 1977) of dogs with glomerulonephritis demonstrated malignant neoplasia as prominent extrarenal lesions. These findings exemplify the close and frequent association of the two disorders and demonstrate the necessity to thoroughly evaluate proteinuric patients for occult neoplasia.

Hepatocellular degeneration and nodular hyperplasia, rheumatoid arthritis, pancreatic necrosis, and a variety of infectious processes have been associated with glomerular diseases in dogs and cats, but a causal relationship cannot be defined. It is likely that any process (infectious, inflammatory, or degenerative) capable of generating a sustained antigenic stimulation can potentially induce immune-mediated glomerular injury.

PATHOGENESIS OF GLOMERULAR INJURY

Immunologic mechanisms have long been suspected of participating in the establishment and progression of glomerular injury. It has been only recently, however, that developments in immunologic technology have provided clear insights into the pathogenesis of renal injury. The immunopathogenesis of glomerular injury is classically divided into antigen-antibody complex (immune complex) disease and anti-glomerular basement membrane (anti-GMB) nephritis. These topics have been extensively reviewed and will only be summarized below (Fish and Michael, 1979; Merrill, 1974; Wilson and Dixon, 1981).

Immune-Complex Glomerulonephritis

The interaction of soluble antigen with specific antibody in the circulation creates a reaction product that initiates immune-complex glomerulonephritis. The nephritogenicity of this product is highly dependent on the quantity and characteristics of the individual antigen and antibody reactants.

The relative proportion of antigen to specific antibody is of considerable importance in the susceptibility and localization of glomerular deposition. This ratio determines the ultimate size and solubility of the complexes. Large complexes, formed in antibody excess, are less likely to circulate and be trapped in the glomerulus. Small complexes, characteristic of antigen excess, are relatively soluble, circulate freely, and are more likely to be cleared by filtration or to localize in the periphery of capillary loops. Intermediate-sized complexes formed near antigen-antibody equivalence are most likely to promote mesangial or glomerular capillary deposition and immune-mediated renal injury (Germuth and Rodriguez, 1973). In certain situations, the immune complex might be formed *in situ* as a result of circulating antibodies reacting with non-renal antigens previously localized in the GBM.

The nature and extent of the renal damage induced by immune complex deposition is highly variable and dependent on a multitude of host and antigen characteristics. The kidneys are uniquely susceptible to the development of immune complex injury. Collectively, they receive approximately 25 per cent of the cardiac output and are therefore substantially exposed to circulating immune complexes. The glomerulus is an efficient ultrafilter and is therefore most susceptible to particle deposition. This feature is enhanced when the glomerulus is exposed to endogenous vasoactive substances, such as histamine, serotonin, epinephrine, or kinins that enhance glomerular permeability and immune complex deposition. Vasoactive substances may be released either systemically or locally in response to the immune reaction. The thickness of the GBM makes it additionally prone to entrapment of filtered immune complexes. Factors that influence the rate of renal plasma flow or glomerular filtration have profound influences on the nature and extent of immune complex deposition and renal injury (Germuth et al., 1967).

The antibody response of the host is a major factor influencing the matching or mismatching of antibody level to antigen load. An active antibody former is relatively protected (antibody excess) from small antigen loads yet susceptible to nephritogenic immune complexes (antibody-antigen equivalence) with large antigenic loads. The avidity of the antibody class and the integrity of the reticuloendothelial system are thought to influence the development, size, and disposition of immune complexes.

The size, load, and physical characteristics of the antigen are influential in the ultimate nephritogenicity of immune complexes. With limited exposure to an antigen, renal reactivity will resolve as the antigen load is removed. If the disease is not fatal, its manifestations will be clinically acute and nonprogressive, and will resolve with variable degrees of parenchymal loss. With sustained antigenic exposure, the glomerular damage will be ongoing and a chronic progressive glomerulonephritis will be recognized clinically (Germuth and Rodriguez, 1973).

The physical damage and functional disturbances that result from immune-complex deposition in the glomerulus are primarily dependent on the activation of one or several host defense mechanisms, which translate the immune complex entrapment into the inflammatory reaction and tissue destruction. The involvement of complement was initially suspected because of its depletion from the serum during the active phases of experimental and naturally-occurring immune-complex nephritis (Ellis and Walton, 1958; Germuth and Rodriguez, 1973). The subsequent detection of complement components in diseased glomeruli by immunofluorescent microscopy has confirmed a role for this system in the dog and cat (Kurtz et al., 1972; Murray and Wright, 1974; Osborne et al., 1973, 1976; Wright et al., 1973, 1981) as well as in man and experimental animals (Schreiber and Muller-Eberhard, 1979; Valenzuela and Deodhar, 1980). The biologic effects of complement activation are directly responsible for much of the tissue damage and inflammation that occur in glomerulonephritis. This is demonstrated by the protective effects of complement depletion in certain forms of experimental glomerulonephritis. Specific cleavage products of complement components can stimulate the release of vasoactive amines and promote leukocyte chemotaxis and immune adherence. Vasoactive amines enhance capillary permeability, proteinuria, and further complex deposition. The chemotactic influx of polymorphonuclear leukocytes promotes the release of proteolytic enzymes, displacement of the endothelium from the GBM, tissue necrosis, digestion of the glomerular basement membrane, and adherence and aggregation of platelets, which obstruct the capillary lumen (Dixon and Cochrane, 1970; Wilson and Dixon, 1981).

Through Hageman factor, the complement system is linked with the coagulation and kallikrein systems. This results in the potential deposition of fibrin in areas of immunologic injury and in the production of bradykinin. Fibrin deposition in glomerular capillaries and capsule are important mediators of glomerular injury and may promote glomerulosclerosis. Other mechanisms independent of complement and polymorphonuclear leukocytes probably contribute to the pathophysiologic and clinical expression of immune renal injury. Studies in experimental animals demonstrate that certain glomerulopathies can be manifested in complement- and leukocyte-depleted states (Cochrane, 1979). However, the exact mechanisms mediating the disease in these situations are unclarified. In man, however, the majority of information suggests that immune-mediated renal injury involves classical pathway-of-complement activation and complement-mediated tissue injury (Schriber and Muller-Eberhard, 1979). A similar situation is likely to occur in the dog and cat but the confirmation is less precise.

Anti-Glomerular Basement Membrane (Anti-GBM) Nephritis

A less common form of glomerular injury occurs in man when autologous antibodies bind to intrinsic glomerular basement membrane antigens. This form of disease differs from immune-complex nephritis in that the antigen is intrinsic to the host glomerulus and the humoral component represents autoantibodies to host tissue. Anti-GBM nephritis accounts for five to ten per cent of human glomerulopathies and has only recently been suspected in the dog (Di Bartola et al., 1980a; Osborne et al., 1976) and the horse (Banks and Henson, 1972).

The dog is used extensively, however, to study experimental anti-GBM disease. In the experimental disease, heterologous anti-GBM antibodies are generated in different species after exposure to dog kidney homogenates. The nephrotoxic antiserum is subsequently injected into a canine host, where it rapidly binds to specific glomerular antigens (heterologous phase), fixes complement, and initiates proteinuria and tissue injury. As the disease progresses, the canine host produces antibody to the glomerular-bound heterologous immunoglobulin, which stimulates secondary and delayed immunologic injury (autologous phase). In some animals, autoimmune anti-GBM nephritis can be experimentally induced by immunization with GBM-enriched materials (Wilson and Dixon, 1979).

Experimentally as well as in natural anti-GBM nephritis, antigenically similar basement membranes of other organs may be simultaneously damaged. Alveolar basement membrane is particularly susceptible. Concomitant immunologic involvement of glomerular and pulmonary basement membranes produces a disease complex in man called Goodpasture's syndrome. The immunopathological fingerprint of anti-GBM nephritis is the smooth, continuous, linear disposition of IgG and complement observed on the surface of the GBM with immunofluorescent microscopy. This is in contrast to the random, granular disposition of IgG noted in immune-complex disease.

The chemical nature of the nephrogenic GBM antigen is unknown. The GBM consists of a network of fibrils that are embedded in an amorphorus matrix composed of collagenous and noncollagenous glycoproteins. Evidence suggests that the nephrogenic antigen is a noncollagenous, macromolecular glycoprotein (Wilson and Dixon, 1979). The stimulus for the production of anti-GBM antibodies is unknown, but regardless of the mechanism, the immunologic consequences are similar to those of immune-complex disease.

Amyloid Deposition

The progressive accumulation of amyloid proteins can also cause destruction of glomerular architecture and disruption of normal function (Fig. 74–11). Subendothelial amyloid deposition occurs as a late development in a variety of chronic suppurative, granulomatous, neoplastic, or inflammatory diseases and is designated "secondary or reactive systemic amyloidosis." Alternatively, it may occur in patients without discernible preexisting illness and is termed "pri-

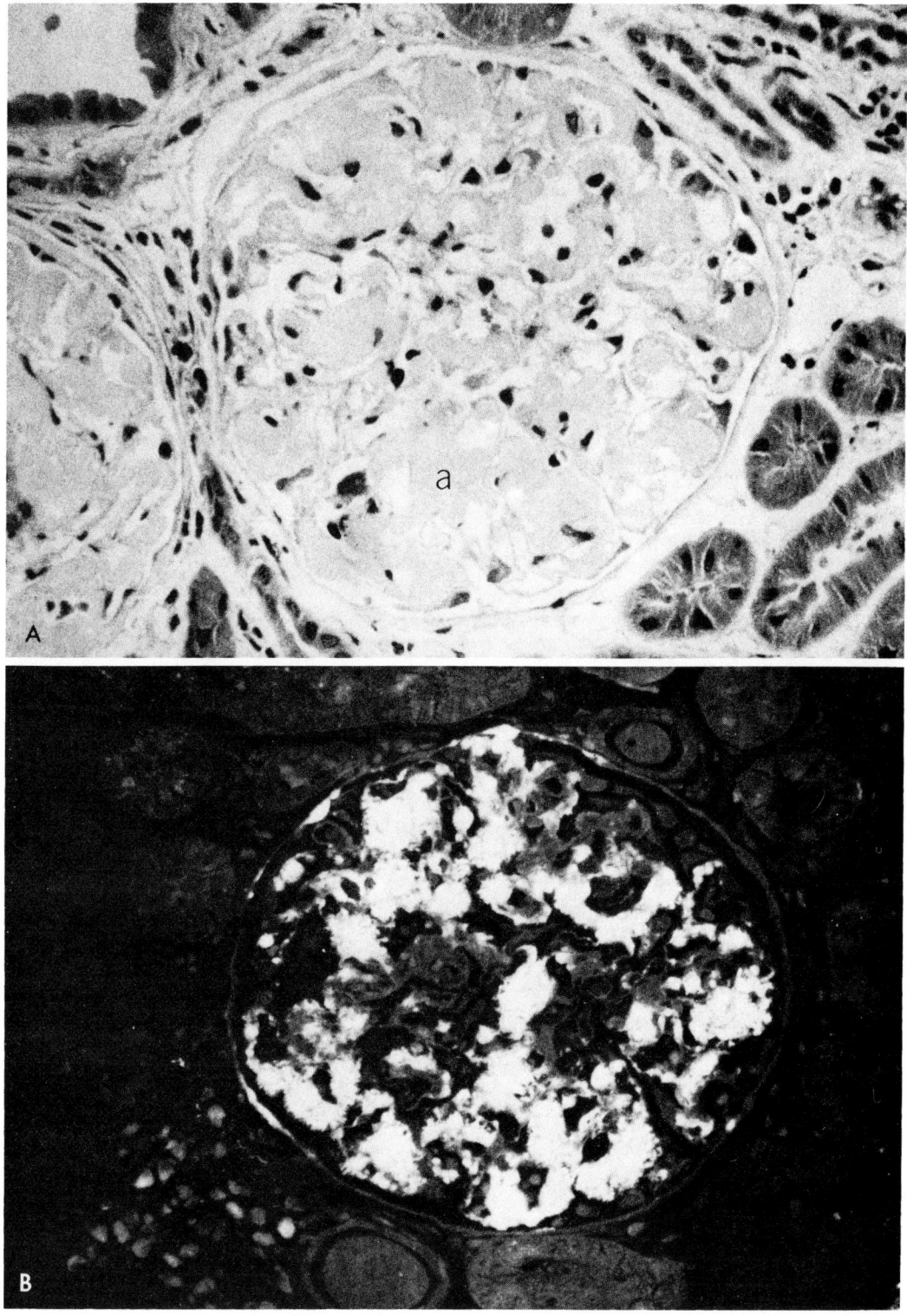

Figure 74–11. Primary renal amyloidosis in a 10-year-old Brittany spaniel. *A*, Photomicrograph of a glomerulus showing extensive deposition of amyloid (a) in the glomerular capillaries, causing obliteration of the capillary lumen. Note the absence of cellular response. Hematoxylin and eosin stain. ×285.

B, Photomicrograph of glomerulus stained with thioflavin-T. The amyloid deposits are identified by the bright fluorescence under ultraviolet light. ×285.

Illustration continued on following page

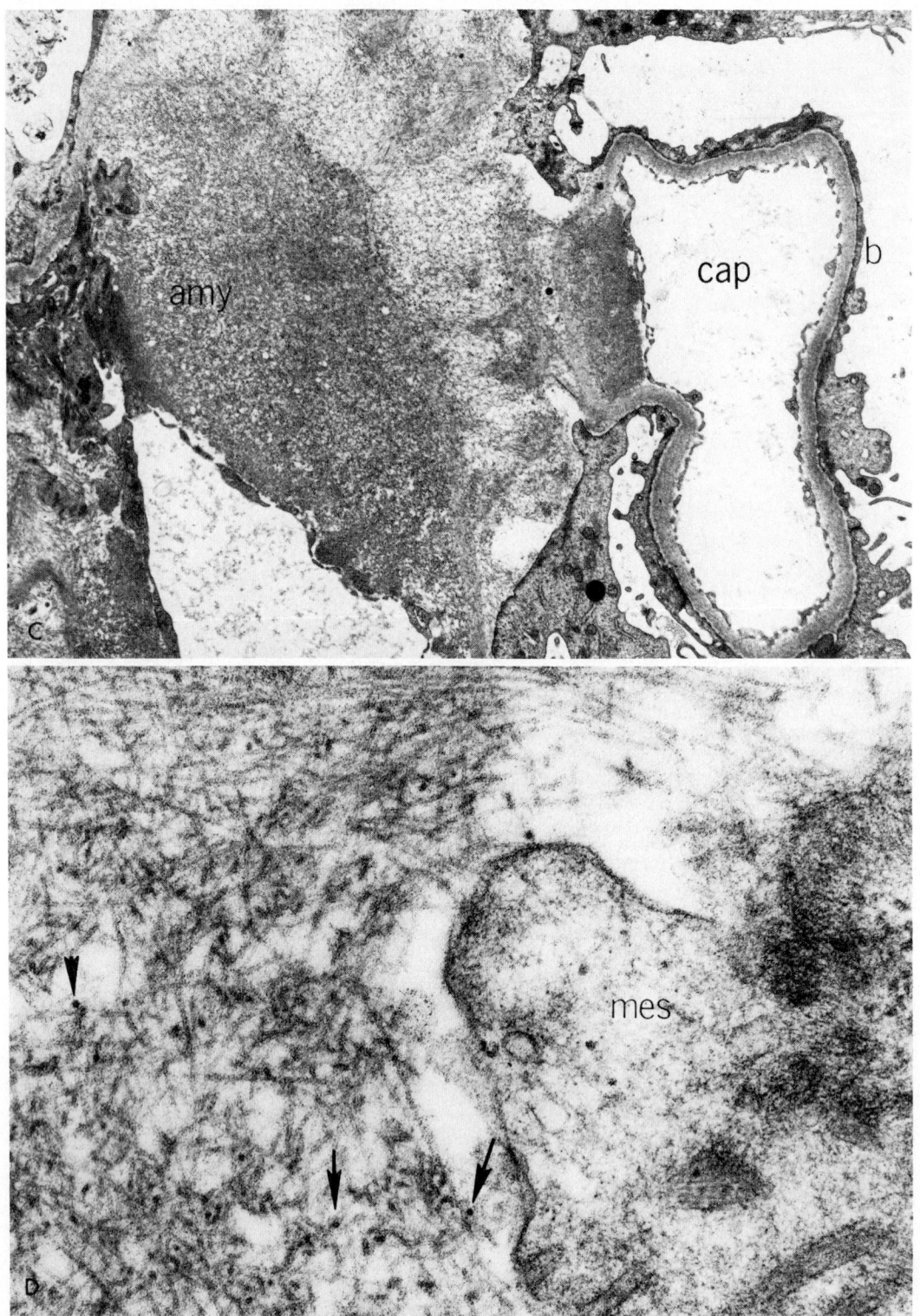

Figure 74–11 *Continued.*   *C,* Electron photomicrograph showing a peripheral capillary (cap). The peripheral basement membrane (b) is of normal thickness and has uniform staining density. The capillary is distorted by a large expanding amyloid deposit (amy). ×7100.

   D, Electron photomicrograph at higher magnification showing a small portion of a mesangial cell (mes) surrounded by amyloid fibrils. These fibers have an estimated diameter of 100Å and when cut in cross section have a circular profile (arrows). ×66,500. All photographs courtesy Dr. Charles Gamble.)

mary amyloidosis." In man, there is a significant association with multiple myeloma and immunocyte-derived dyscrasias.

The protein deposits present in these distinct forms of amyloidosis have a unique β-pleated structure and are indistinguishable by histologic or electron microscopic techniques. They are distinguishable, however, by chemical and immunologic criteria into two major protein types. The amyloid protein, most often found in primary amyloidosis or multiple myeloma of man, is characteristic of light-chain fragments of immunoglobulin and is most likely the protein product of an immunocyte clone (Glenner, 1980; Glenner et al., 1972; Walker and Solez, 1979). The deposits in secondary amyloidosis appear to be from nonimmunoglobulin precursors and are of obscure origin. Whether or not similar distinctions occur in veterinary patients is unknown. Regardless of their origins, amyloid proteins, presumably from plasma, are deposited in glomerular capillaries, and produce the glomerular injury by physical encroachment. Glomerular inflammation is characteristically absent from the pathogenesis, and the functional disturbances result from disruption of the GBM and filtration surface (Fig. 74–11).

Systemic Hypertension

Hypertension can induce progressive pathologic and functional alterations in renal vasculature and glomeruli. The nature and extent of the glomerular lesions are related to the severity of the hypertensive state and range from ischemic obsolescence and glomerular atrophy to proliferative glomerulitis and fibrinoid necrosis (Spargo et al., 1980). Proteinuria and immunoglobulin deposition often accompany these lesions.

CLINICAL CONSEQUENCES OF GLOMERULONEPHRITIS

Alterations in Renal Plasma Flow and GFR

Renal plasma flow (RPF) may be increased, unchanged, or decreased during the pathogenesis of glomerular inflammation. RPF is highly dependent upon com-

pensatory factors, as well as the severity and chronicity of the disease (Earle et al., 1951).

The kidney has intrinsic mechanisms to initially compensate for increases in capillary resistance due to glomerular injury or capillary obstruction. The early changes in vascular resistance are complement-dependent and may result from release of vasoconstrictor substances (Blantz et al., 1979). Compensatory decreases in afferent arteriolar tone protect renal plasma flow in the early and mild stages of disease. With progressive glomerular capillary damage total renal blood flow declines and the kidneys become hypoperfused. In more fulminating forms of disease, renal plasma flow will decline markedly from capillary damage, endothelial swelling, and arteriolar vasoconstriction (Blantz et al., 1978; Blantz and Wilson, 1976).

As glomerular injury progresses, initial compensatory mechanisms will fail and renal perfusion will decrease. The decreased renal blood flow promotes variable degrees of tubular ischemia, tubular necrosis and fibrosis, and the eventual loss of the entire nephron.

The glomerular filtration rate is similarly protected in the initial, or in mild stages of glomerular damage. Patients with notable glomerular injury as detected by proteinuria, hematuria, sodium retention, and edema may show normal or only mild alteration of serum creatinine, BUN, or creatinine clearance. Of the three major determinants of glomerular ultrafiltration — hydrostatic pressure, renal plasma flow, and capillary permeability coefficient — the latter two are primarily affected (Allison et al., 1974; Blantz and Wilson, 1976; Rocha et al., 1973). In both clinical and experimental settings, the blunted reduction of GFR is often a consequence of hypertension and increased effective filtration pressure.

Sodium and Fluid Retention

Sodium and fluid retention are consistent features of glomerulonephropathies, particularly the acute forms, and are often accompanied by edema and hypertension. In chronic glomerulonephritis, the capacity to excrete a salt load may be enhanced owing to adaptive mechanisms (Wignild and Gutmann, 1976), but the potential for salt retention remains prominent. The renal mechanisms that promote an enhanced and inappropriate reabsorption of salt and water are not entirely understood. It seems, however, that the altered regulation occurs at sites other than the proximal tubule, since glomerulotubular balance is generally maintained. Salt retention in the early phases of glomerulonephritis is therefore the result of reduced glomerular filtration rate or enhanced reabsorption in the distal nephron due to undefined hormonal, hemodynamic, or physical factors.

In the nephrotic syndrome, renal salt retention is further influenced by the reduction in plasma volume and stimulation of the renin-angiotensin-aldosterone system (Earley and Forland, 1979).

Proteinuria

Proteinuria is the hallmark of glomerular injury. A small amount of protein is normally excreted in the urine but is undetectable by routine tests. Following glomerular insults, the normal selective permeability of the glomeruli are compromised and abnormal quantities of plasma proteins pass into the ultrafiltrate. When the amount of filtered protein exceeds the proximal tubular reabsorptive capacity, detectable quantities will appear in the urine. Proteinuria can also result from nonglomerular diseases of the kidney, but these are generally associated with limited excretion of inflammatory proteins or globulins rather than albumin.

Glomerular permeability to plasma proteins is dependent upon the integrity of the filtration barrier, the molecular characteristics of the protein, and renal hemodynamics. *In vivo* studies in animals including dogs, using well defined macromolecules, have demonstrated that molecular size is one of the major barriers to the filtration of proteins. Increases in the molecular radius are associated with corresponding reductions in glomerular permeation. Molecules with molecular dimensions similar to that of albumin are minimally filtered by the normal glomerulus (Brenner et al., 1977; 1978; Deen et al., 1979). Size restriction appears to be a function of the GBM, and diseases that increase GBM pore radius promote filtration of larger macromolecules.

Electrical charge, in addition to molecular size and shape, is also an important determinant of macromolecular filtration. Glomerular charge selectivity results from the electrostatic hindrance created by fixed negative charges associated with structural elements of the filtration apparatus. The glomerular epithelial cells, slit diaphragm (final permeability barrier), and endothelial cells are coated with sialoproteins that are highly negatively charged. As a result, circulating negatively charged plasma proteins, such as albumin, are repelled from the GBM and filtration channels. The surface negativity of the epithelial cells appears also to maintain the morphologic integrity of the foot processes and slit diaphragm. Neutralization or destruction of these surface charges promotes an enhanced transit of polyanionic proteins across the glomerulus and morphologic fusion of the epithelial foot processes. Disrupting these fixed negative charges may also promote immune complex deposition in the GBM and mesangium and enhance the production of mesangial matrix.

Massive quantities of protein may be lost in the urine in the absence of a clinically detectable reduction in GFR or changes in serum creatinine, BUN, or urinary concentrating ability. The degree of proteinuria is often poorly correlated with the extent of histologic abnormalities or the degree of renal insufficiency (Di Bartola et al., 1980b). The selectivity of the proteinuria is perhaps more reflective of the extent of histologic damage in that less proliferative disorders tend to be more protein selective. These correlations are crude, however, and should not surpass evaluation by renal biopsy.

The degree of proteinuria can markedly influence the clinical course. If urinary losses are moderate, enhanced hepatic synthesis may fully compensate. In markedly proteinuric conditions, however, hepatic synthesis may fail to match urinary losses, and hypoalbuminemia, negative nitrogen balance, and nephrotic syndrome may result.

Nephrotic Syndrome

Nephrotic syndrome describes a complex of clinical and laboratory signs that include proteinuria, hypoalbuminemia, hyperlipoproteinemia (generally recognized as hypercholesterolemia), and edema. Nephrotic syndrome can manifest in any glomerular disorder wherein the urinary loss of protein is sufficient to produce severe hypoproteinemia. Because of the greater magnitude of proteinuria in renal amyloidosis and membranous glomerulonephritis, these diseases are more commonly associated with nephrotic syndrome (De Schepper et al., 1974; Di Bartola et al., 1980a, 1980b; Larken et al., 1972; Osborne et al., 1973, 1976). The syndrome may appear in either azotemic or nonazotemic patients, but should alert the clinician to the presence of significant renal damage, even if BUN and serum creatinine concentrations are normal.

Peripheral edema or ascitic fluid accumulates because of the disturbance in physical forces that regulate the distribution of plasma water across capillary beds. The marked hypoalbuminemia reduces plasma oncotic pressure to such a degree that capillary filtration exceeds reabsorption. Extravascular fluid will accumulate until tissue hydrostatic pressure equalizes the filtration forces or until increased lymphatic drainage can compensate. Fluid loss into the interstitium creates a state of intravascular volume depletion, which in turn activates ill-defined hormonal, hemodynamic, or intrarenal mechanisms to promote sodium and water conservation. The retained salt and water could serve to restore the intravascular deficit, but the inability to effectively retain fluid within this compartment creates further extravascular expansion and edema formation (Earley and Forland, 1979).

Hypercholesterolemia is a well recognized component of nephrotic syndrome in animals, but further characterization of the extent and spectrum of such hyperlipoproteinemia is lacking. Evidence in man with nephrotic syndrome indicates that the nature of the lipoproteins changes from low density lipoproteins to very low density lipoproteins, which are triglyceride-rich, as the hypoproteinemia progresses (Earley and Forland, 1979). The abnormal accumulations of lipoproteins are the apparent result of decreased peripheral utilization and enhanced hepatic synthesis. In man, severe and longstanding hyperlipoproteinemia may contribute to atherosclerotic disease, but the risk of this complication in companion animals is presently unknown.

Coagulation Disorders

Abnormalities in both coagulation and fibrinolytic factors have been well character-

ized in association with the glomerulopathies in man. These disorders tend to promote a state of hypercoagulability and thrombosis. Increases in plasma fibrinogen as well as factors V, VII, VIII, and X are most common. Similar dyscrasias have been recognized in the canine nephrotic syndrome. Hyperfibrinogenemia, which is inversely proportional to the plasma albumin, is the most frequently identified disorder in dogs (unpublished observations). Although the clinical consequences of these biochemical abnormalities are not known for dogs and cats, they may contribute or predispose to the thrombosis recognized with renal amyloidosis (Slauson and Gribble, 1971).

CLINICAL FEATURES

With few exceptions, the clinical signs of patients with generalized glomerular disease are nonspecific and nonlocalizing. Affected animals will usually evidence weight loss, anorexia, depression, and weakness or listlessness. There is no apparent breed or sex predisposition. All ages are affected, but the incidence increases in dogs over five years of age and the nature of the glomerular injury differs in younger, as compared to older, dogs (Muller-Peddinghaus and Trautwein, 1977; Lewis, 1976). The general manifestations will, however, be influenced by the chronicity and severity of the glomerular disease. If associated with advanced renal insufficiency, vomiting, diarrhea, polydipsia, polyuria, nocturia, and oral ulceration may be prominent clinical features. Clinical signs that are suggestive, but by no means diagnostic, of glomerular injury include peripheral, ventral, or facial edema; ascites; or pleural effusion.

Abdominal palpation may demonstrate kidneys of normal or abnormal size. Amyloidosis and acute glomerulonephritis are often associated with renal enlargement, while chronic glomerulonephritis or glomerulosclerosis cause fibrosis and a shrunken renal mass.

The clinical diagnosis of glomerulopathy is supported on routine urinalysis by the demonstration of persistent proteinuria. The urine sediment may also demonstrate cylinduria (hyaline, RBC, and granular casts) and microscopic hematuria but is generally free of significant numbers of inflammatory cells and cellular debris. The significance and origin of routinely determined proteinuria must be carefully evaluated to distinguish glomerular origin protein from that derived from other renal or lower genitourinary sites (see urinalysis).

A precise determination of the urinary protein loss is best obtained by quantitating daily protein excretion (see urinalysis). Less than 450 mg of protein will normally appear in the urine per 24 hours (Bovee et al., 1979c; Barsanti and Finco, 1979; Stuart et al., 1975). Greater quantities are pathologic and justify an extensive clinical evaluation. The excretion of greater than 1.5 grams of protein per day is unlikely to be caused by genital or lower urinary tract disease and suggests significant glomerular abnormalities. Lesser losses, on the other hand, require careful differentiation. Severely affected patients may lose more than 20 grams of protein per 24 hours, which promotes marked negative nitrogen balance and extreme debilitation.

Once suspected in a patient, glomerular disease warrants a comprehensive biochemical, pathological, and immunologic assessment, the extent of which is dictated by available diagnostic capabilities and client commitment. The following approach outlines a framework that can be modified or expanded to meet individual circumstances.

The minimum laboratory data base should include a complete blood count (CBC), urinalysis and sediment examination, and a biochemical profile. The CBC is examined for abnormalities suggestive of underlying or causal conditions including hematopoetic neoplasia, chronic infection, pyometra, systemic lupus erythematosus, and heartworm disease. The hemogram may reflect a nonregenerative anemia in the face of chronic uremia.

Biochemically, plasma protein and plasma albumin should be determined to evaluate the significance of the urinary losses and to monitor trends in the disease. Hypoproteinemia is a variable finding subject to the quantity of renal losses, hepatic compensation, and nutritional intake. Edema is also a variable feature and rarely develops until plasma albumin falls below 1.5 gm/dl. A more precise characterization of the plasma and urine protein abnormalities can be determined with electrophoretic analysis.

A complete biochemical evaluation of renal function should be routinely performed. BUN and plasma creatinine may be normal or variably elevated, depending upon the impairment of GFR. Patients may be markedly proteinuric yet demonstrate no, or only subtle, alterations of these parameters. An endogenous creatinine clearance test can be performed simultaneously with urine protein quantitation tests to provide a more precise estimate of GFR. Serum phosphorus is elevated in advanced renal insufficiency and provides clues to the chronicity of the disease. In animals less than eight to ten months old, phosphorus concentrations are physiologically higher than adult values and should be interpreted accordingly (Fig. 74–4). Serum calcium concentrations are influenced directly by plasma albumin. Mild hypocalcemia, therefore, is an expected finding in patients manifesting hypoalbuminemia, but hypoalbuminemia is not associated with reductions in ionized calcium or clinical signs of hypocalcemia. Serum electrolytes are generally normal but should be included as part of the data base. Nephrotic patients may demonstrate variable degrees of hyponatremia despite an obvious excess of total body sodium. Plasma cholesterol or triglycerides are commonly elevated with hypoproteinemia and are components of the nephrotic syndrome. Additional serum biochemistries should be determined as dictated by the presenting clinical signs or progression of the disease.

Radiographic examinations generally provide little specific information, since renal dimensions vary according to the nature and chronicity of the condition. Radiography may be of value to identify renal tumors that cause proteinuria and hematuria; to characterize extrarenal disease manifestations; or to differentiate nonrenal causes of proteinuria, hypoproteinemia, subcutaneous edema, or ascites. Abdominal radiographs or urinary contrast studies may be included in the routine evaluation of glomerulopathies but should receive proper priority in terms of diagnostic dollars.

Immunologic diagnostics are becoming more widely available and sophisticated, and constitute an important aspect of patient evaluation. Testing should include LE cell identification, serum antinuclear antibody titer, FeLV antigen detection in cats, and occult heartworm titer in suspect dogs. Immunofluorescent pathology should be a routine part of renal biopsy examination. These studies provide information about potential causes of the glomerular injury as well as insights into their pathophysiology.

Renal histopathology provides the most specific information on the nature, extent, and prognosis of glomerulopathies. A renal biopsy should be obtained by either open or percutaneous methods to provide tissue for light and immunofluorescent microscopy. Electron microscopy will provide additional information for classification of the lesions but is not routinely available. Tissue submitted for immunofluorescent microscopy should be evaluated for the deposition of IgG, IgM, IgA, and complement.

Immune-complex glomerular disease is identified with immunofluorescent microscopy by the characteristic deposition of immunoglobulin and complement in an irregular, interrupted, and granular pattern along the basement membrane or in the mesangium. Immune complex disease can also be identified by the presence of electron-dense deposits in an epimembranous, intramembranous, or subendothelial location with electron microscopy (Fig. 74–12). Anti-GBM nephritis is distinguished by immunoglobin deposition in a smooth, continuous, and linear pattern by immunofluorescent microscopy (Fish and Michael, 1979; Valenzuela and Deodhar, 1980). Care

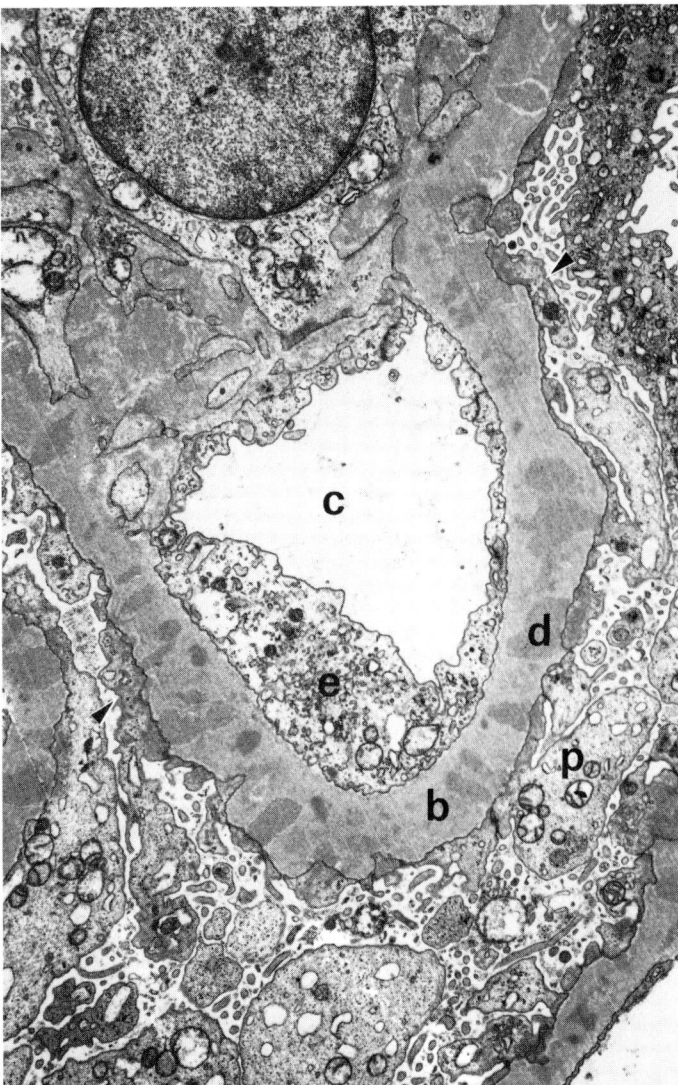

Figure 74–12. Electron photomicrograph of membranous glomerulonephritis. The basement membrane (b) of the capillary is markedly thickened and surrounds several dense subepithelial deposits (d). Podocyte foot processes are fused into large continuous cytoplasmic processes (arrows). Podocyte (p), capillary lumen (c), endothelial cell (e). ×9800. (Courtesy Dr. Brad Barr.)

should be exercised, however, to distinguish truly linear fluorescence from confluent, small granular deposits that mimic a linear pattern. Careful examination at high-power magnification will uncover these pseudolinear situations. In human patients who demonstrate linear fluorescence, circulating anti-GBM antibodies may often be detected in serum by indirect immunofluorescence techniques. These methods are not routinely available in private practice but may be requested at some university hospitals.

In comparison with the complex classification schemes for glomerulonephritis that exist in human medicine, the veterinary classification is embryonic and based largely on necropsy specimens and terminology extrapolated from human nephrology. In the dog and cat, glomerulonephritis is usually divided into four major categories — membranous, proliferative, membranoproliferative, and sclerosing — plus a variety of combinations, depending on the characteristics of the histologic reactions (Slauson and Lewis, 1979; Murray and Wright, 1974;

Muller-Peddinghaus and Trautwein, 1977a; Stuart et al., 1975; Osborne et al., 1977). Each reaction can be further described as "generalized" if the disease involves all glomeruli examined, "focal" if only some glomeruli are involved and others are spared, "diffuse" if all portions of affected glomeruli are uniformally involved, and "segmental" if the reaction is localized to certain portions or lobules of a glomerulus and absent from other portions.

Membranous Nephropathy. Membranous nephropathy is identified histologically by diffuse and irregular thickening of the basement membrane and variable increases in mesangeal matrix (Figs. 74–12 and 74–13). The glomeruli are often enlarged, but there is no increase in glomerular cellularity. Capillary diameters will vary from widely patent to closed, depending on the extent and chronicity of the disease. A characteristic "spike" appearance on the epithelial side of the GBM can be identified with silver stains in more advanced cases (Heptinstall, 1974; Slauson and Lewis, 1979; Wright et

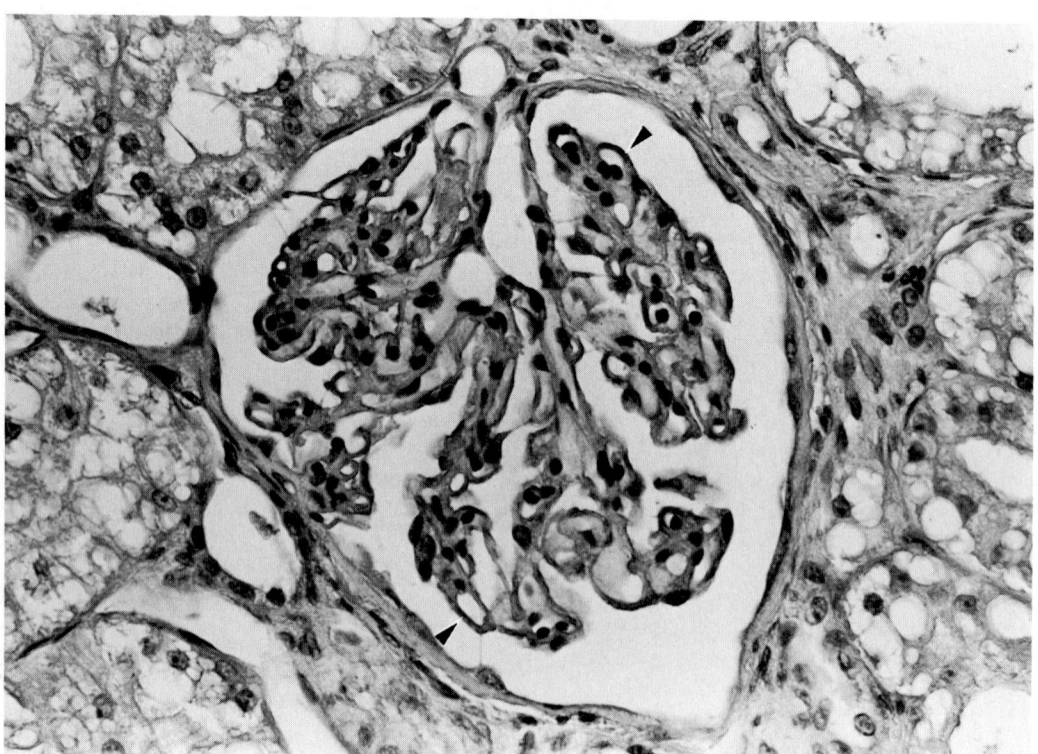

Figure 74–13. Light photomicrograph of membranous glomerulonephritis in a cat. Note the uniform thickening of peripheral capillary loops (arrows). Cellular density is normal. Hematoxylin and eosin stain. ×400 (Courtesy of Dr. Brad Barr.)

al., 1981) and represents remodeling of the GBM around epimembranous immune-complex deposits. Immunofluorescent microscopy reveals a diffuse granular deposition of IgG and C_3. Electronmicroscopically, the GBM is markedly irregular and thickened by electron-dense deposits in an epimembranous or intramembranous location or in the mesangium (Fig. 74–12). The epithelial foot-processes are swollen and fused (Murray and Wright, 1974; Wright et al., 1981).

Clinically, membranous nephropathy is associated with heavy proteinuria and frequently an insidiously progressive course leading to renal failure (Wright et al., 1981). It is a common cause of the nephrotic syndrome and is the most common form of glomerular disease in cats (Anderson and Jarrett, 1971; Farrow et al., 1969; Nash et al., 1979; Slauson et al., 1971; Slauson and Lewis, 1979; Thornburg et al., 1979; Wright et al., 1981).

Proliferative Glomerulonephritis. This disease is recognized with light microscopy by marked swelling and hypercellularity of glomeruli. The cellular prominence is the result of reactive hyperplasia of epithelial, mesangial, or endothelial cells or an influx of inflammatory cells into or around the glomeruli.

Progressive proliferative reactions of the endothelial or mesangial cells may produce capillary lumen obliteration or compression of the glomerular tuft. Severe proliferative reactions may be associated with the formation of "crescents" and a rapidly progressive clinical course. The proliferation may be focal or generalized throughout the kidney and diffuse or segmental in the glomerulus (Murray and Wright, 1974).

Inflammatory cell infiltrates may be seen in the kidney in the early acute stages as well as in the urine along with inflammatory debris. Proliferative diseases have a tendency to be fulminating and progressive. Immunofluorescent microscopy generally demonstrates immunoglobin and complement as granular deposits in the mesangium and along capillary walls. Ultrastructurally, electron-dense deposits are identified in or on the surfaces of the basement membrane and within the mesangium. Foot process fusion is common near the dense deposits.

Membranoproliferative (Mesangiocapillary) Glomerulonephritis. This type of glomerular injury is the most commonly recog-nized glomerulopathy in the dog (Muller-Peddinghaus and Trautwein, 1977a; Murray and Wright, 1974; Slauson and Lewis, 1979; Stuart et al., 1975). Histologically, it is recognized by cellular proliferation and diffuse thickening of the glomerular basement membrane. Mesangial proliferation is predominant and accompanied by increased mesangial matrix (Fig. 74–14).

Glomerulosclerosis. Glomerulosclerosis is an end-stage of chronic inflammatory disease in which glomerular elements are replaced or infiltrated with hyaline or fibrotic material. Glomerulosclerosis is also recognized as an aging or degenerative change of dogs. Periglomerular fibrosis, fibrous adhesions of the capillary tuft to Bowman's capsule, and glomerular obsolescence may be coexistent. Glomerulosclerosis is also present as a degenerative change in perinatally irradiated puppies (Phemister et al., 1973).

Miscellaneous. In early renal amyloidosis, the kidneys are normal in size or slightly enlarged, firm, and pale tan in color. Amyloid deposits are often grossly identifiable by their dark brown staining characteristics with iodine solutions. Histologically, amyloid is diagnosed as a homogenous eosinophilic deposit with hematoxylin and eosin stain localized in the glomerular capillary or mesangium (Fig. 74–11,*A*). Deposits may also be found in vascular walls, the renal interstitium, and around collecting tubules (particularly in the cat). When stained with congo red and viewed with polarized light, the amyloid deposits demonstrate a diagnostic birefringence. An apple green fluorescence is seen when amyloid deposits are stained with thioflavine-T and viewed under ultraviolet light (Fig. 74–11,*B*). Ultrastructurally, the deposits are revealed in the mesangial region and along the basement membrane, separating it from the endothelium. Amyloid may be seen to disrupt and fragment the GBM. Epithelial foot-process fusion may be noted as well as the characteristic fibrillar appearance of the amyloid protein (Fig. 74–11,*C,D*). Varying degrees of tubular vacuolization, degeneration, and atrophy can be identified, depending on the severity of the glomerular involvement.

THERAPY OF GLOMERULAR DISEASE

The clinical management of glomerular disease can be separated into specific thera-

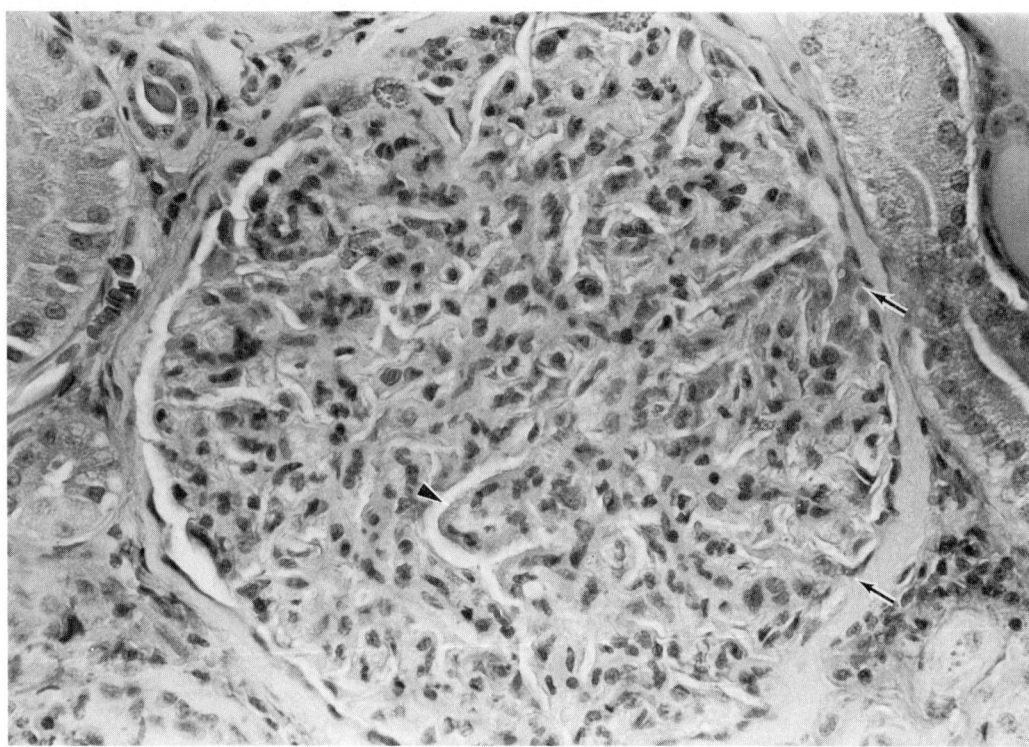

Figure 74–14. Light photomicrograph of chronic membranoproliferative glomerulonephritis in a dog. The striking feature is the increased glomerular cellularity and mesangial thickening. Individual capillary loops are difficult to discern, but occasional thickened loops can be seen (arrowhead). Bowman's capsule is thickened and there are multiple adhesions between the capsule and tuft (small arrows). Hematoxylin and eosin stain. ×400. (Courtesy Dr. Brad Barr.)

py to alter the nature or course of the disease and supportive measures aimed at symptomatic relief. At present, a lack of understanding of the pathogenesis of most glomerulopathies in the dog and cat precludes outlining any truly specific treatment program. Few correlations between disease classification, biologic behavior, and response to specific therapy have been established in veterinary medicine; therapeutic recommendations are largely empirical; and therapeutic responses are primarily anecdotal. In human nephrology, specific therapies have also evolved from empirical considerations and in many cases have only recently been supported or refuted by controlled therapeutic trials. Hopefully, in time, sufficient clinical material will be available from veterinary patients to provide sound foundations for therapeutic recommendations.

At present, three courses of action are available for the specific management of glomerular disease. Firstly, specific therapy may be withheld entirely to avoid potential or real harm in the face of uncertain efficacy (Osborne and Jeraj, 1980; Osborne et al., 1976). Secondly, traditionally empirical therapy may be administered with the uncertainty that resulting benefits or complications are treatment-specific (Bown, 1977). Thirdly, observations and recommendations obtained in other species can be adapted and transferred to veterinary patients in the hope that similar morphologic and pathophysiologic criteria will elicit similar and predictable therapeutic responses.

The acceptance of one or a combination of these options must rest with the assessment of the clinical circumstances and the experience of the clinician. It must be recognized, however, that proteinuric disorders that appear clinically stereotyped are distinctly heterogeneous in their biologic behavior and prognosis and will not likely respond in a uniform manner to a stereotypic therapeutic plan.

SPECIFIC THERAPEUTIC RECOMMENDATIONS

The most specific and possibly the most effective form of therapy for glomerulonephritis is to identify and eliminate the source of antigenic stimulation. This is difficult to implement in most circumstances, since the antigen is generally obscure or impossible to eliminate (i.e., neoplasia, SLE, FeLV, glomerular basement membrane). If the glomerular damage is associated with recognizable problems such as pyometra, *Dirofilaria immitis,* bacterial endocarditis, or chronic sepsis, treatment directed at these primary disorders will often resolve the active glomerular inflammation (Osborne and Jaraj, 1980; Obel et al., 1964; Germuth and Rodriguez, 1973).

The use of anti-inflammatory agents and corticosteroids in active glomerulonephritis has been questioned for decades. Certain glomerulopathies, e.g., lipoid nephrosis of man, seem exquisitely responsive to corticosteroids while in other glomerular diseases it is uncertain if the benefits of corticosteroids outweigh the hazards. It seems empirically sound that drugs that alter immune balance, inflammation, and coagulation — the mediators of glomerulonephritis — should have a role in the management of glomerular disease.

The differences in the biologic behavior of morphologically distinct glomerulopathies require that their management be analyzed on an individual basis. To an extent, these analyses have been reported for human diseases and may provide a basis for the management of veterinary patients.

Membranous Nephropathy

It is difficult to evaluate therapeutic efficacy in membranous nephropathy because of its typically insidious progression and the frequency of spontaneous remissions in both animals and man (Osborne et al., 1976; Earley and Forland, 1979; Row et al., 1975; Wright et al., 1981). In controlled therapeutic trials, the results of prednisolone or combined prednisolone and cytotoxic therapy have been mixed.

Early controlled studies in man used daily low-dosage programs and failed to demonstrate any benefits of steroid therapy on the magnitude of proteinuria, even though it may have delayed progression of renal insufficiency (Black et al., 1970; Rose, 1976; Row et al., 1975). More recently, however, controlled and uncontrolled studies using a high-dose, alternate day regimen for short intervals have generated more favorable results (Brodehl and Krohn, 1976; Coggins, 1979). Treatment with corticosteroids caused a greater incidence of complete or partial remission of proteinuria and significantly delayed deterioration of renal function when compared with untreated controls. These benefits were obtained without evidence of significant drug toxicity (Coggins, 1979).

Azathioprine and cyclophosphamide, on the other hand, appear to offer no therapeutic benefits alone or in combination with corticosteroids to warrant their administration (Abramowicz et al., 1970; Donadio et al., 1978; Rose, 1976; Simon and Rosenberg, 1978).

Limited information is available on the management of dogs with membranous nephropathy (Osborne et al., 1973; Larkin et al., 1972). In light of these recent findings, it seems reasonable to recommend the administration of prednisolone (or prednisone) at a high dose (1.5 to 2.0 mg/kg body weight) on alternate mornings for a restricted period of time (Coggins, 1979; Scott, 1980). If no response is demonstrated after eight weeks of therapy, the drug should be tapered during the subsequent four weeks. If complete remission or considerable improvement in proteinuria or renal function is recognized, the drug should be tapered over eight weeks. Relapses following a complete or partial remission should be managed by returning to the original dosage level for an additional month with subsequent tapering. The benefits of more prolonged therapy are unknown but are encouraging in man (Hopper, 1973). It should be emphasized that this recommendation is extrapolated from controlled clinical trials in human patients and has not as yet been tested for efficacy in veterinary medicine. It does, however, offer the potential for control with a minimum of risk or long-term side effects.

Proliferative and Mesangiocapillary Glomerulonephritis

Proliferative lesions as a rule are both clinically and pathologically progressive and unlikely to undergo spontaneous remission. The usual clinical course is variably progressive to renal failure. In general, therapeutic trials with corticosteroid or cytotoxic drugs, alone or in combination, fail to demonstrate definitive benefits (Glassock, 1979; Earley and Forland, 1979; German Glomerulonephritis Research Group, 1976; Kincaid-Smith, 1972; Simon and Rosenberg, 1978). In one report, long-term, alternate day prednisone therapy provided marked improvement in glomerular histology and preservation of renal function for 5 to 11.5 years in children (McAdams et al., 1975). Patients with diffuse proliferative lupus nephritis have fewer and milder recurrences if initially treated with combined prednisone and cyclophosphamide, but progression of the disease mortality and preservation of renal function are not influenced by the addition of cyclophosphamide to the treatment program (Donadio et al., 1978). The combination therapy of cyclophosphamide, dipyridamole (an antiplatelet agent), and anticoagulants has provided the most impressive and encouraging benefits in human patients (Kincaid-Smith, 1972; Cameron, 1978). With this approach, a retrospective analysis revealed a highly significant improvement in survival, resolution of morphologic glomerular changes, and disappearance of proteinuria for as long as 30 months of evaluation. The demonstrated benefits of such therapy must be carefully weighed against the risks of the employed drugs, however. Controlled studies are currently in progress in man to better document the efficacy of this "cocktail" therapy.

On the basis of present experience it is impossible to state specific treatment recommendations for these diseases. Such patients are probably best managed with supportive therapeutics to control hypertension, edema, hypoproteinemia, and uremia. The future may provide better insights.

Glomeruloslcerosis

Scarring and sclerosis of the glomerular capillaries represent an obviously chronic and irreversible lesion. Hypertension should be controlled (see section on management of hypertension) to preserve marginally affected glomeruli and prevent tubular ischemia. Patients with chronic glomerulosclerosis should be managed symptomatically for uremia, hypertension, and nephrotic syndrome.

Renal amyloidosis is characterized by a relentlessly progressive course without demonstrated therapeutic responsiveness (Crowell et al., 1972; Osborne et al., 1968, 1969). Because of the varied and uncertain pathogenesis and the resistance of amyloid proteins to phagocytosis and dissolution, few specific approaches have been successful. In reactive or secondary amyloidosis, isolated case reports document resolution of the proteinuria and improvement in renal function and histology following treatment of the primary disorder (Lowenstein and Gallo, 1970). The prognosis of secondary amyloidosis in man is considered better than immunocytic amyloidosis, so aggressive management of predisposing conditions is warranted (Glenner, 1980). Administration of cytotoxic drugs to diminish immunoglobulin synthesis has been variably successful in controlling amyloidosis associated with immunocyte dyscrasias (Glenner, 1980; Cohen et al., 1975). Because of the generally poor prognosis in this disorder, a trial course of single or combined cytotoxic agents (cyclophosphamide, melphalan) is recommended for those patients with primary amyloidosis, even when an immunocyte dyscrasia or multiple myeloma is not identifiable (Glenner, 1980; Walker and Solez, 1979). This type of therapy is obviously contraindicated in secondary amyloidosis where an infectious or inflammatory etiology would be aggravated. Corticosteroids alone or in combination have proved to be ineffective and have no therapeutic role.

Some reports have documented the efficacy of colchicine therapy in preventing or improving renal amyloidosis in experimental animals and in human patients with predisposing familial disease (Dinarello et al., 1974; Shirahama and Cohen, 1974). Dimethyl sulfoxide (DMSO) has also been studied as a possible therapeutic agent for amyloidosis. Its action is unknown, but it may be of value in reducing amyloid deposits or blocking amyloid protein synthesis (Isobe and Asserman, 1976; Ravid et al.,

1977; van Rijswijk et al., 1979). In a limited trial, 10 per cent DMSO (125 mg/kg body weight) administered orally twice daily resulted in marked improvement in BUN, creatinine, phosphate, creatinine clearance, and clinical condition during nine months of therapy in a dog with severe generalized renal amyloidosis (Fig. 74–11). DMSO therapy was minimally effective in correcting the marked proteinuria, however. Cyclophosphamide was ineffective when administered during a two-month trial in the same dog. At present, the benefits of drug therapy in renal amyloidosis are purely speculative in the dog and cat but deserve further investigation. The efficacy of DMSO is particularly attractive and may prove to be of value when evaluated more extensively. Supportive therapy for uremia, edema, pulmonary embolism, hypertension, and other complicating disorders should be provided.

NONSPECIFIC AND SUPPORTIVE THERAPY

In general, supportive therapy has no effect on the primary renal insult and should be applied to the individual patient as clinical circumstances dictate.

Diet

Weight loss is a major problem associated with the excessive excretion of urinary protein. It may be coupled with hypoproteinemia and negative protein balance. In the absence of specific measures to reduce the proteinuria, it is necessary to insure that dietary protein is sufficient to accommodate both the maintenance requirements and urinary losses. These losses are best defined by quantitating the daily excretion. When the excretion is excessive enough to cause weight loss, edema, or hypoproteinemia, the diet should be changed or supplemented to provide a higher protein density (Blainey, 1954; Keutman and Bassett, 1935; Osborne and Jeraj, 1980). Dietary protein should be of sufficiently high biologic value to allow efficient synthesis of albumin and structural proteins. Care should be taken, however, to avoid increases in sodium intake during the dietary manipulations. This often arises as patients are changed from kibble to high protein canned foods. The response to therapy can be monitored by changes in plasma albumin concentrations. Anabolic steroids may be beneficial in promoting more efficient conversion of dietary nitrogen into structural proteins.

Patients with proteinuria and uremia require special dietary considerations. As renal function declines, proteinuria may decline as well and reduce protein requirements. To ameliorate the signs of uremia, it is necessary to restrict protein intake to minimize the production and accumulation of nitrogenous metabolites (see management of renal insufficiency). The dietary intake, however, must supply the urinary protein losses in addition to fulfilling the other protein needs of the patient. Failure to compensate for actual renal losses when restricting protein will potentially promote negative nitrogen balance and protein malnutrition. Other recommendations for the management of uremia should be instituted simultaneously with dietary controls.

Edema

In addition to having an excess of total body sodium, nephrotic patients are hypoalbuminemic and require a dual therapeutic approach. The hypoalbuminemia should be corrected by dietary protein repletion while attempts are made to reduce renal protein loss. Increased plasma albumin will improve intravascular oncotic pressure and the diminished intravascular volume.

The positive sodium balance should be controlled by reducing sodium intake and promoting renal sodium excretion. In most instances it is advisable to restrict dietary salt. In practice, however, this is often difficult to accomplish while the patient is eating commercial foods, and diuretics are usually necessary. The reduced acceptability of low-salt diets may also limit the usefulness of this form of therapy. Sodium-restricted prescription diets, however, may be beneficial for this purpose. Salty treats and processed food should be avoided and care should be exercised when the animal is changed from kibble to high-protein canned or semi-moist preparations.

In patients with advanced renal insufficiency, fractional salt excretion may be high, despite the edema from the functional adaptations to nephron loss (Wignild and Gutmann, 1976). Acute or drastic salt restriction might, in this circumstance, induce volume depletion and further renal injury.

Gradual limitation of salt and conservative diuretic administration is therefore advisable.

Pharmacologic control of sodium balance with diuretics is the basis of therapy for edema. Diuretics induce a negative sodium balance and effectively drain off excessive body sodium and fluid. Diuretics acting at the loop of Henle have the greatest potency and are the most useful in the nephrotic syndrome. Furosemide is the diuretic of choice and is generally administered at two to four mg/kg body weight one to four times daily until the edema is clinically resolved. A maintenance level may be necessary until salt intake is restricted or the hypoalbuminemia corrected. In edematous patients with severe hypoproteinemia, intravascular volume may be severely reduced and diuretics should be used with caution to prevent further hypovolemia and hypotension. Animals with advanced renal failure may have a blunted response to diuretic therapy but should be carefully protected from hypovolemia, hypotension, and acute renal failure. Dosage modification, selection of a less potent diuretic, or dietary salt control should be considered at the first sign of these complications. Long-term use of diuretics in combination with salt restriction carries the potential for sodium depletion, which should be monitored at regular intervals. Hypokalemia is a potential complication of long-term furosemide therapy but is uncommon in dogs.

Hypertension

Hypertension is a consistent finding in dogs with either acute or chronic glomerulonephritis. Specific therapy with salt restriction, diuretics, β-adrenergic blocking agents, and vasodilators is discussed under Management of Renal Insufficiency in this chapter, and elsewhere (Gantt, 1978).

PROGNOSIS

Insufficient long-term evaluations of veterinary patients with different types of glomerular injury are available to make specific statements regarding the prognosis and natural course. Actuarial analysis in human patients suggests that progression to death or renal failure is influenced by age, morphology of the disease, and pathogenic mechanisms. Generally, glomerulonephritis

associated with pyometra or heartworm disease will resolve following removal of the underlying disease (Obel et al., 1964). Membranous nephropathy is often an insidiously progressive disease but is associated with frequent spontaneous remissions (Osborne et al., 1976; Row et al., 1975; De Schepper et al., 1974). Proliferative and membrano-proliferative glomerulonephritis and renal amyloidosis generally have more precipitous courses and are consistently progressive.

Progressive glomerular inflammation ultimately results in functional deterioration, capillary obliteration, glomerular fibrosis, or glomerular atrophy. The long-term prognosis in immune-mediated glomerulonephritis is generally guarded but not invariably hopeless. Each patient should be evaluated individually. Compensatory renal mechanisms and proper supportive care can effectively extend patient survival.

ACUTE RENAL FAILURE

Acute renal failure (ARF), a clinical state encountered in the emergency room, results from trauma, some drugs, or poisoning or from critical complications in surgical or medical patients. It is characterized most frequently by rapid onset of oliguria or anuria, reduced renal blood flow (RBF) and glomerular filtration rate, and the biochemical and clinical consequences of a reduced GFR. Rapid increases in BUN, serum creatinine, potassium, and phosphate, and disturbances of acid-base metabolism are evidence of the excretory failure. ARF is a tenuously reversible state and must be quickly diagnosed and aggressively treated. Failure to initiate appropriate therapy quickly results in irreversible parenchymal damage and death from the metabolic consequences of uremia. The incidence of ARF in veterinary practice is substantially lower than that of chronic renal insufficiency. The presentations may be confusingly similar, however, and the clinician must distinguish between these conditions to direct the proper course of therapy. ARF must also be recognized as a component of more overt surgical or medical disease states.

CLINICAL PRESENTATION

Despite a somewhat stereotyped clinical presentation, the signs of ARF are nonspecific and may overlap the clinical expression of concomitant or predisposing disorders. Depression, anorexia, vomiting, inappetance, and diarrhea of recent onset are characteristic. Other signs include dehydration, fetid breath, oral erosions or ulceration, scleral injection, and cranial lumbar pain. In the absence of obvious or overwhelming sepsis, most patients are normothermic or hypothermic.

Oliguria and, less frequently, anuria are hallmarks of ARF. English (1979) has arbitrarily defined oliguria in the dog and cat as the daily urine production of less than 6.5 ml/kg body weight (0.27 ml/kg/hour) and anuria as less than 2.0 ml/kg (0.08 ml/kg/hour). However, nonoliguric forms of ARF are increasingly recognized in human patients (Anderson et al., 1977, 1980) and dogs (personal observations). Nonoliguric ARF is more frequently recognized because of the greater awareness and earlier recognition of ARF; the widespread use of intravenous fluids and osmotic and chemical diuretics in acute uremia; and the more widespread use of nephrotoxic antimicrobials that may induce this form of renal injury. The mere quantitation of urine output, therefore, may be insufficient to identify many dogs with acute uremia.

CLASSIFICATION AND ETIOLOGY

Acute oliguric states are traditionally categorized into three basic groups — prerenal, renal parenchymal, and postrenal — that anatomically and functionally define the focus of the renal insult.

Prerenal Azotemia

The kidney depends upon an adequate circulation for its function. Capillary hydrostatic pressure is the major determinant of glomerular filtration, which in turn is dependent upon systemic blood pressure, circulating blood volume, and peripheral vascular resistance. Within moderate alterations of these parameters, the kidney effectively autoregulates its blood flow and capillary filtration pressure, so that GFR remains relatively constant. Severe reductions in these circulatory parameters exhaust the kidney's adaptive capability. Renal blood flow as well as solute and water excretion will decrease proportionally, attended by the chemical and clinical consequences of renal insufficiency. Identifiable characteristics of prerenal disease include mild to moderate azotemia, substantial reductions in urine flow and sodium excretion, and alterations in the direct and indirect indices of glomerular filtration rate, i.e., BUN, serum creatinine, or creatinine clearance. The factors that initiate renal hypoperfusion will generally stimulate the secretion of antidiuretic hormone and concomitant concentration of the urine.

Prerenal azotemia can occur in any clinical situation characterized by cardiovascular instability sufficient to produce renal hypoperfusion or ischemia. Common settings include hemorrhagic, septic, or cardiogenic shock; surgical stress; hypoadrenocorticism; trauma; and dehydration. It should be clearly understood that prerenal azotemia represents a functional disorder of the kidney. Early recognition and treatment of the hemodynamic disturbances will completely restore renal function without parenchymal damage or loss. Failure to effectively manage prerenal oliguria in its earliest stages may result in its eventual irreversibility and the initiation of substantial parenchymal injury. The pathogenesis of the continuum from functional disturbance to organic damage is not precisely understood. It is clear, however, that early and appropriate management is effective in preventing the progression from functional to structural injury.

Postrenal Azotemia

Postrenal azotemia may result from any process that obstructs urine flow or causes extravasation of urine into body compartments other than the urinary bladder. Postrenal azotemia generally ensues from bilateral compromise of renal function, since unilateral disease rarely causes azotemia. In the early phases of obstruction, the kidneys remain structurally intact and the uremic consequences are totally reversible. If allowed to persist, increases in hydrostatic pressure cause dilation of the ureters and renal pelvis, which leads to hydronephrosis and renal parenchymal atrophy. Uncorrected postrenal obstruction or rupture of the urinary conduits causes uremia and death within days.

Common causes of postrenal azotemia

include urolithiasis, feline urologic syndrome, and traumatic rupture of the urinary bladder. If the cause of postrenal azotemia is effectively and rapidly corrected, the impairments in renal functions should resolve.

Primary Acute Renal Parenchymal Failure (ARF)

Unlike prerenal oliguria, the functional and morphologic damage characteristic of ARF is not amenable to rapid or simple therapeutic resolution. Long-term survival is possible only if sufficient renal mass is preserved through repair, hypertrophy, or functional compensations when healing is complete. The causes of ARF are varied and can be broadly described as (1) hemodynamically mediated, (2) nephrotoxic, and (3) miscellaneous, which includes vascular disease and intrinsic nephritis.

Hemodynamically Mediated ARF. Renal ischemia or hypoperfusion is a major factor associated with the induction of acute parenchymal failure. The causes of hemodynamically mediated ARF are the same as those which predispose to prerenal azotemia. In the former situation, however, the hypoperfused state is overlooked and persistent, or is of such profound intensity that it cannot be readily reversed. In this setting, the functional disturbances that are characteristic of prerenal azotemia progress to the extensive structural changes that are commonly associated with tubular necrosis. The term "acute tubular necrosis" has been popularized for many decades but incompletely describes this condition, which may be manifested in the absence of overt pathologic

evidence of necrosis (Stein et al., 1978; Finn, 1979).

It should be emphasized again that any condition that predisposes the animal to hypotension, hypovolemia, circulatory collapse, or insufficient renal perfusion has the potential of initiating ARF (Table 74–5). It is of utmost importance for the clinician to recognize these predisposing situations and to critically evaluate renal function in their presence. Animals suffering from hemorrhage, trauma, extensive surgery, prolonged anesthesia, or poor cardiovascular integrity are at increased risk. Age and preexisting renal disease are additional risk factors to consider. The geriatric kidney undergoes a substantial decline in weight, volume, and glomerular numbers (Goldman, 1977; Lowenstein, 1978) and demonstrates a blunted hypertrophic capacity when compared with more youthful kidneys (Kaufman et al., 1975). As a result of this reduced renal reserve, older animals are more sensitive to subtle or overt renal insults and will generally suffer more permanent functional losses (Levinsky, 1981). Risk statistics are not available for the aged dog and cat, but azotemia and morphologic changes are recognized in the kidneys of older dogs (Cowgill and Spangler, 1981). It is likely, therefore, that age and preexisting renal disease represent additional risk factors for dogs as well.

Hypoperfusion may also result from renal infarcts, disseminated intravascular coagulation, incompatible blood transfusions, or septic thrombi. Vasculitis, peritonitis, hypoproteinemia, and gastric torsion are clinical states associated with the contraction of intravascular volume and renal function

---

Table 74–5. Causes of Acute Renal Failure

Hemodynamically Mediated
Hypotension ⎫
Hypovolemia ⎪ Hemorrhagic, septic, or cardiogenic shock; adrenal insufficiency; heat prostration;
Circulatory collapse ⎬ prolonged anesthesia; DIC; peritonitis; thromboembolism
Renal hypoperfusion ⎭
Nephrotoxic
Heavy metals: arsenic, mercury, lead, uranium, thallium
Organic compounds and solvents: ethylene glycol, carbon tetrachloride
Antimicrobials: aminoglycosides, amphotericin B
Miscellaneous: radiographic contrast agents, heme pigments, intrinsic renal diseases
Miscellaneous
Acute glomerulonephritis ⎫
Leptospirosis ⎬ Malignant lymphoma, hyperparathyroidism, hypervitaminosis D
Hypercalcemia ⎭

should be carefully monitored when these conditions are present.

Nephrotoxins. Nephrotoxins are the second major cause of acute renal failure. The spectrum of potential toxins is extensive and includes a variety of heavy metals, organic compounds, solvents, antimicrobials, miscellaneous drugs, and endogenous solutes (Table 74–5) (Maher, 1976; Porter and Bennett, 1980; Thornhill, 1980). Heavy metal nephrotoxicity is rarely encountered in clinical practice but is extensively used for investigational purposes. Inorganic and organic arsenic, lead, thallium, bismuth, mercury, and uranium are all potent nephrotoxic agents. Despite legal restrictions and careful regulation, poisonings with thallium or arsenic rodenticides are still recognized sporadically. Industrial herbicides likewise provide a potential source of arsenic intoxication.

Ethylene glycol and diethylene glycol are common organic nephrotoxins in dogs (Beckett and Shields, 1971; Ettinger and Feldman, 1977; Kersting and Nielsen, 1965; Jonsson and Rubarth, 1967). Automobile antifreeze is the usual source of ethylene glycol, and histories of dogs ingesting radiator fluid prior to a sudden onset of illness are frequently obtained. Glycols are also components of lacquers, cosmetics, and flavoring extracts. Oxalic acid, a major metabolic product of ethylene glycol, is considered to be a primary toxic intermediate. Oxalic acid readily produces necrosis of epithelial cells and intratubular obstruction subsequent to calcium oxalate crystal deposition (Fig. 74–15). Besides renal involvement, ethylene glycol affects the central nervous system and heart. Stupor, convulsions, coma, and metabolic acidosis inappropriate for the degree of azotemia, will commonly accompany this intoxication. Because of the marked intratubular obstruction and tubular necrosis, intoxicated dogs usually manifest profound oliguria or anuria. Chloroform, carbon tetrachloride, and tetrachlorethane are also associated with ARF in man (Maher, 1976). Since these industrial solvents are widely available, they serve as potential sources of intoxication for dogs.

Antimicrobials are important nephrotoxic agents for dogs as well as for man (Porter and Bennett, 1980; Thornhill, 1980; Appel and Neu, 1977, 1977a). The aminoglycoside antimicrobials, in particular, are increasingly implicated in the production of ARF (Appel and Neu, 1978). For many of these drugs the kidney is the major excretory pathway. When coupled with a large renal blood flow, exposure of the renal epithelium to toxic doses is enhanced and makes it particularly vulnerable to toxic insult. An additional risk factor is the clinical setting in which antimicrobials are administered. Dogs and cats are often conditioned for renal damage by preexisting renal disease, reduced regenerative capabilities, disorders of fluid and electrolyte balance, and concomitant drug therapy. Antibiotics may initiate ARF through hypersensitivity or anaphylactic reactions or by immune-mediated glomerular damage. The aminoglycoside antibiotics appear to disrupt cellular function, thereby causing cellular death (Appel and Neu, 1978; Adelman et al., 1979; Spangler et al., 1980). Gentamicin, in addition, has been shown to impair glomerular ultrafiltration in the rat, which may add to the morphologic abnormalities it causes (Baylis et al., 1977).

The sulfonamides may precipitate in the tubular lumen of man, causing tubular obstruction or epithelial necrosis. The advent of modern sulfonamides with greater urine solubility has essentially eliminated this nephropathy. Clinical experience has also failed to demonstrate serious nephrotoxicity from the antimicrobic combination trimethoprim sulfamethoxazole, which is currently the most widely used agent in this category (Porter and Bennett, 1980). Sulfonamide nephrotoxicity is not an apparent problem in dogs or cats, however.

Amphotericin B is a polyene with serious nephrotoxic side effects. The administration of this agent will invariably cause renal damage in a dose-related fashion. In clinical settings that require high doses or multiple courses of therapy, permanent renal damage may result. The nephrotoxicity is due to renal vasoconstriction and direct toxic effects on the tubular epithelium (Appel and Neu, 1977a; Porter and Bennett, 1980). Amphotericin B is primarily reserved for the treatment of life-threatening fungal diseases in which a limited degree of renal toxicity may be an acceptable compromise. Patients should be closely monitored and attempts made to reduce its nephrotoxicity by detecting early azotemia and maintaining good hydration. Hellebusch et al. (1972)

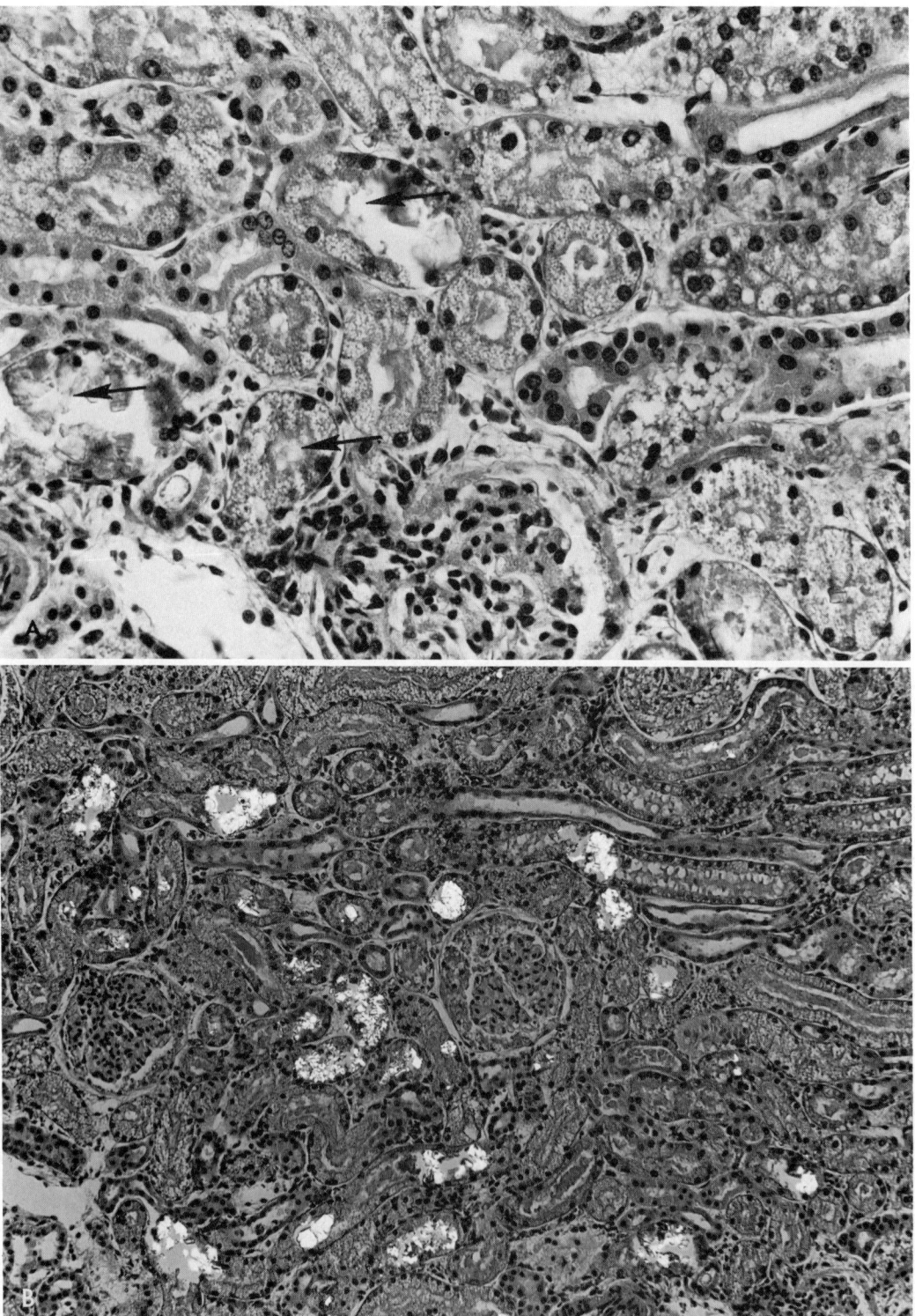

Figure 74–15. Photomicrograph of canine kidney during the oliguric stage of ethylene glycol–induced renal failure. *A,* The parenchyma is characterized by widespread necrosis of the tubular epithelium, tubular dilation, and impaction of the tubule with necrotic debris and calcium oxalate crystals (arrows). Hematoxylin and eosin stain, ×250. *B,* The same kidney when visualized under polarized light. The highly refractile areas are intratubular deposits of calcium oxalate crystals.

have shown that the concomitant use of mannitol with amphotericin B in dogs will reduce its nephrotoxicity. Mixed results have been observed in man, however (Bullock et al., 1976; Olivero et al., 1975).

The aminoglycosides are the most widely used nephrotoxic antimicrobials in veterinary therapeutics, owing to the large number of commonly used drugs within this category and the important role they play in the therapy of serious infections. Neomycin is the most nephrotoxic, but despite its poor intestinal absorption, patients receiving massive doses can accumulate toxic levels and sustain significant kidney damage. Gentamicin is the aminoglycoside most frequently used and therefore most commonly associated with acute nephrotoxicity. Its nephrotoxicity lies between that of neomycin and streptomycin and causes renal damage in a dose-related fashion. Acidosis, dehydration, sodium depletion, methoxyflurane anesthesia, and concomitant cephalothin or furosemide therapy reportedly enhance its nephrotoxicity in man as well as animals, including dogs (Porter and Bennett, 1980; Appel and Neu, 1978; Adelman et al., 1979). Gentamicin is excreted primarily by glomerular filtration; therefore, preexisting renal disease will enhance its plasma concentration and nephrotoxicity, unless dosage schedules are appropriately adjusted (Bennett et al., 1979, 1980; Chan et al., 1972; Reiner et al., 1978). Cloudy swelling of the tubular epithelium, proximal tubular necrosis, vacuolization, and myeloid body formation occur in a dose-related fashion. Enzymuria, proteinuria, cylindruria, progressive azotemia, and oliguria or polyuria attend the toxicity.

Kanamycin, cephaloridine, polymixin B, vancomycin, and colistimethate are additional antimicrobics with significant nephrotoxic potential at therapeutic dosage levels.

Miscellaneous Causes of ARF. A variety of anesthetic agents, methoxyflurane in particular, cause nephrotoxicity in man. Methoxyflurane is not associated with comparable nephrotoxicity in dogs or cats, although sporadic cases have been cited (Haskins, 1979). Despite the rarity of direct nephrotoxic effects, any anesthesia may cause periods of prolonged hypotension, renal vasoconstriction, redistribution of renal blood flow, stimulation of the sympathetic nervous system and cardiovascular depression (Hart, 1981). Anesthesia will predictably depress renal function on a temporary basis, and in diseased animals or those with compromised renal function, it may promote ARF (Hart, 1981).

Radiographic contrast media are a frequent cause of acute azotemia in man. The nephrotoxicity is dose related and enhanced by high-dose techniques, volume depletion, preexisting renal insufficiency or vascular disease (Carvallo et al., 1978; Porter and Bennett, 1980). Multiple myeloma and diabetes mellitus appear to predispose human patients to contrast media risks, but similar experiences have not been reported in dogs. Contrast media nephropathy is generally an oliguric disorder that is responsive to therapy.

PIGMENT NEPHROPATHY. Oliguria is an important but variable complication of hemolytic episodes, transfusion reaction, or severe rhabdomyolysis following heat stroke or crush injuries (Levinsky, 1981). Heme-pigment nephropathy is an infrequent cause of ARF in companion animals but should be anticipated in association with blood transfusions, marked intravascular hemolysis, heat prostration, or extensive muscle injury.

INTRINSIC PARENCHYMAL DISEASE. Immune-mediated glomerulonephritis, systemic lupus erythematosus, or hypersensitivity angiitis may cause sufficient injury to create acute oliguria. Miscellaneous disorders include renal artery occlusion, renal vein thrombosis, accelerated hypertension, and hypercalcemic nephropathy.

Hypercalcemic nephropathy has been diagnosed with increased frequency in the dog (Chew and Capen, 1980; Osborne and Stevens, 1973, 1977; MacEwen and Siegel, 1977). Hypercalcemia may occur from primary hyperparathyroidism, hypervitaminosis D, malignant lymphoma, perianal adenocarcinoma, or excessive oral or parenteral intake of calcium. The elevated plasma calcium concentrations damage the tubular epithelium and glomeruli and induce arteriolar constriction and ischemia (Spangler et al., 1979). Epithelial degeneration, necrosis, and intracellular and interstitial calcification highlight the renal lesions.

Leptospirosis, although uncommon, is a recognized cause of ARF and should be considered in any differential diagnosis involving acute parenchymal failure (Monlux, 1953). Other bacteria, including *E. coli*, streptococci, staphylococci, *Proteus spp.*, and

Klebsiella spp., may cause an acute nephritis following retrograde or blood-borne infection.

DIAGNOSTIC METHODS

The importance of early therapy necessitates that the diagnosis of ARF be confirmed as rapidly as possible. Many dogs with compensated and asymptomatic renal insufficiency will manifest a seemingly acute uremic crisis following subtle insults, including fever, concomitant disease, vomiting, diarrhea, congestive heart failure, change of environment, and dietary indiscretion. A distinction must therefore be made between acute and chronic renal failure. It is also important to distinguish pre- and postrenal causes of oliguria from intrinsic renal parenchymal disease.

A complete history of the illness is helpful in establishing the duration of the disease. Historical clues may help to pinpoint the etiology or to distinguish patients with chronic renal failure. Dogs are generally oliguric with prerenal azotemia; oliguric or anuric with renal parenchymal disease; and typically anuric with postrenal disorders, cortical necrosis or bilateral renal infarction. Polyuria may occur in ARF and is characteristic of the recovery stage. On the other hand, it is a consistent feature of chronic renal insufficiency and may be a distinguishing feature. A history of recent pelvic or urethral surgery or previous episodes of urolithiasis is indicative of postrenal problems. A combination of prerenal, acute parenchymal, or chronic parenchymal disease may coexist in the patient and cause a confusing presentation.

Physical Examination

Acutely uremic animals are generally depressed, dehydrated, and hypothermic. Their respiratory rate is often elevated as a result of metabolic acidosis. Heart rate may be slow and irregular, and the pulse pressure weak. Vomiting, diarrhea, and retching are commonly seen in severe cases. Convulsions may occur in the terminal stages of the disease or as a consequence of specific nephrotoxins. The kidneys in ARF may be normal in size or enlarged and firm on palpation, while small, irregularly shaped kidneys suggest chronic disease. A greatly distended urinary bladder, the detection of urethral calculi, or the presence of free urine in the abdomen will generally identify postrenal disorders. Advanced chronic renal failure is typically associated with poor body condition and hair coat and pallor of the mucous membranes. Dogs with ARF may, on the other hand, be distinguished by normal body and coat condition.

Arterial blood pressure can be assessed by a variety of direct and indirect methods to determine if prerenal factors are contributing to the acute oliguria (Spangler et al., 1980a). Oliguria and azotemia associated with hypotension or dehydration is consistent with prerenal disorders, while oliguria in a normotensive and well-hydrated dog is suggestive of intrinsic parenchymal failure.

Laboratory Studies

The data base for ARF should include a complete blood count, serum creatinine and/or BUN, electrolytes (including sodium, potassium, chloride, calcium, phosphate), a urinalysis, and evaluation of the acid-base status (see section on laboratory evaluation).

In man, evaluation of urine composition is routine for the differentiation of prerenal azotemia from acute parenchymal failure (Espinel and Gregory, 1980; Mathew et al., 1980; Miller et al., 1978). Table 74–6 outlines anticipated alterations in urine sodium, specific gravity, urine to plasma urea ratio, and urine to plasma creatinine ratio with prerenal and renal parenchymal diseases of man. Considerable overlap exists, however, and may lead to confusion or misdiagnosis (Bastl et al., 1980; Espinel and Gregory, 1980; Miller et al., 1978; Mathew et al., 1980). To reduce the incidence of overlap, the fractional excretion of sodium (FE_{Na}) has been utilized to distinguish acute tubular necrosis (oliguric and nonoliguric) and urinary tract obstruction from prerenal azotemia or acute glomerulonephritis (Espinel and Gregory, 1980; Espinel, 1976). The value for FE_{Na} can be simply calculated from determinations of creatinine and sodium in plasma (P) and untimed urine collections (U) according to the formula,

$$FE_{Na} = (U/P)_{Na} \div (U/P)\text{creatinine} \times 100.$$

With acute tubular necrosis or urinary obstruction FE_{Na} is greater than one, and in

Table 74–6. Urine Composition and Renal Function Indices in Acute Oliguria in Man

	Prerenal	Parenchymal
Sodium (mEq/L)	<10	>25
Specific gravity	>1.025	1.007–1.015
U/P urea	>20/1	<10/1
U/P creatinine	40/1 ⩽ 20/1	<20/1
FE_{Na}	>1	<1

prerenal azotemia or acute glomerulonephritis the FE_{Na} is typically less than one. It should be recognized that these parameters have not been adequately examined in dogs or cats but should be quantitatively similar in comparable clinical settings.

The laboratory status of the acutely uremic dog is dynamic and subject to considerable variation, depending upon the severity of the disease and the response to therapy. Accordingly, many or all of the parameters elaborated previously will require at least daily surveillance to identify trends, response to therapy, and the appearance of concurrent diseases and complications.

Excretory urography, contrast cystography, urethrography, and/or renal arteriography are required if further information is necessary to distinguish parenchymal from postrenal disorders or to distinguish dogs with chronic failure from those with ARF. (See Radiographic Evaluation.)

Few diagnostic procedures can surpass the value of kidney biopsy in the evaluation of acute uremia. The potential reversibility or irreversibility, chronicity, and the specific pathologic basis of the disease can generally be obtained with needle biopsies. Histopathology is invaluable in helping to establish the diagnosis and prognosis and may help to establish the etiology and therapeutic plan. The prognosis is particularly important when expense and effort must be justified in relationship to the potential reversibility of the renal insult. Percutaneous needle biopsy can be readily performed in most uremic dogs with a minimum of effort and patient risk. It is particularly valuable if coupled with frozen section techniques that allow a rapid histologic evaluation. The techniques, indications, and contraindications of renal biopsy have been thoroughly reviewed (Osborne et al., 1972, 1974, 1975).

PATHOPHYSIOLOGY

Acute renal failure can be divided sequentially into four functional stages: (1) the initiation stage, (2) the oliguric or maintenance stage, (3) the diuretic stage, and (4) recovery or death. The initiation stage is the period during which the renal insult establishes a reduction in glomerular filtration and urine output. This period is variable in length but is generally less than one or two days in duration. The maintenance stage is the period during which the reduction in GFR or the oliguria is sustained and may persist for weeks. The onset of the diuretic phase is signaled by a progressive increase in urine output and usually indicates the return of function. Urine volume may increase several fold and must be carefully balanced with fluid therapy to prevent dehydration (Fig. 74–16). The recovery phase has neither a clearly defined beginning nor end. In animals that survive the previous stages there is a progressive increase in renal function that may return to normal or plateau at a clinically stable level (Fig. 74–16).

Initiation and Maintenance Stages

The initiation and the maintenance stages have received considerable attention in an attempt to establish the pathophysiologic mechanisms responsible for the reduced GFR and urine flow. A precise understanding of these events has been sought in an attempt to therapeutically thwart the responsible mechanisms and alleviate the oliguria. Many experimental models have been evaluated in dogs and other animals using a broad array of scientific methods. No single model is totally compatible with the events and clinical behavior of ARF in humans or dogs; when taken in total, however, they have provided many insights into the natural condition. Although a clear and undisputed scheme has not been forthcoming, four major mechanisms are presently considered to participate in the initiation and maintenance of acute oliguria (Fig. 74–17). However, the events that initiate ARF are not necessarily the same as those factors which perpetuate the oliguria.

Reduced Renal Blood Flow. Reduced renal blood flow and renal vasoconstriction have long been considered primary factors

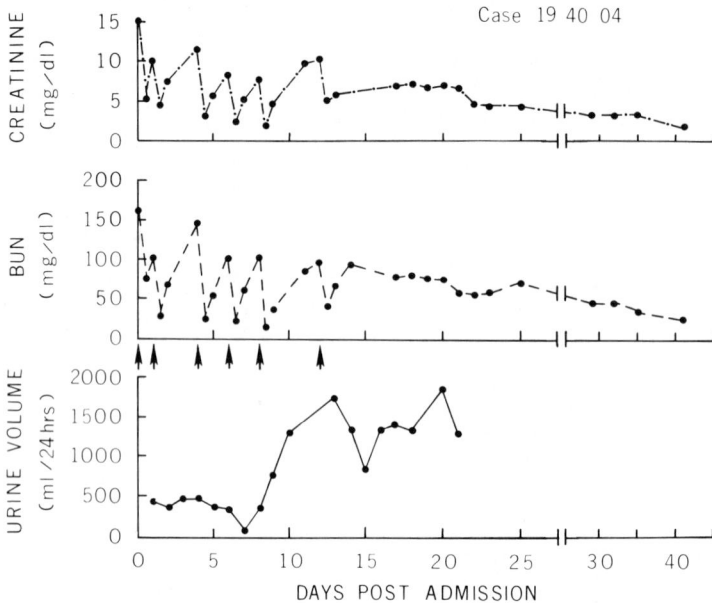

Figure 74–16. Clinical course of a four-year-old, mix-breed female with acute oliguric renal failure of undetermined cause. The graphs depict changes in plasma creatinine (upper panel), BUN (middle panel), and urine output (lower panel) during the course of therapy. Arrows indicate hemodialysis treatments. The graphs clearly demonstrate the transition from the oliguric phase to the diuretic phase at day 7 and the extended recovery period with the onset of diuresis. The fall in urine volume at day 13 was in response to a thrombocytopenic hemorrhagic episode. (From Cowgill, L. D.: Acute Renal Failure. *In* Bovee, K. C. (ed.): Canine Nephrology. Year Book Medical Publishers, Chicago, 1982, in press.)

in the initiation of ARF. They generally participate in the early stages of clinical or experimental models of both hemodynamic or nephrotoxic ARF (Conger and Schrier, 1980; Hostetter et al., 1980; Smolens and Stein, 1980; Stein et al., 1978). The initial reduction in renal blood flow is secondary to intrarenal alterations in vascular resistance, but the precise nature and mechanisms of the increased resistance are unclear. The renin-angiotensin system, through a stimulated tubuloglomerular feedback mechanism (Flamenbaum et al., 1976; Mason, 1976; Mason et al., 1978), altered renal prostaglandin activity (Conger and Schrier, 1980; Oken, 1975), epithelial cell swelling (Flores et al., 1972; Summers and Jamison, 1971), and intrarenal coagulation, has been evaluated in this disorder (Conger and Schrier, 1980). In addition to the reduction of total renal blood flow, there is often a preferential redistribution of blood away from the outer cortex to deeper cortical and medullary areas (Flamenbaum,

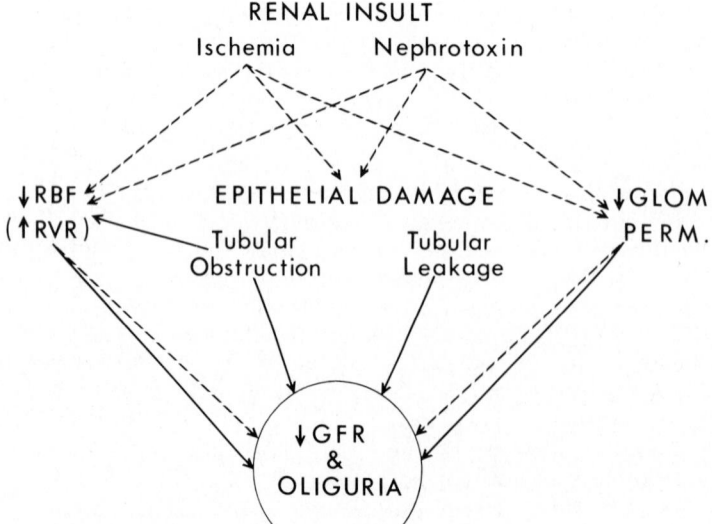

Figure 74–17. Schematic representation of the multiple factors that participate in the initiation (broken lines) and maintenance (solid lines) stages of experimental acute renal failure. The relative contributions of individual factors will vary, depending on the ischemic model or nephrotoxin utilized. (From Cowgill, L. D.: Acute Renal Failure. *In* Bovee, K. C. (ed.): Canine Nephrology. Year Book Medical Publishers, Chicago, 1982, in press.)

1972). Since a majority of renal blood flow is normally distributed to cortical glomeruli, this selective redistribution may have an impact on the development of functional and morphologic lesions and reduced glomerular filtration (Flamenbaum, 1972; Smolens and Stein, 1980; Flamenbaum et al., 1974).

The renin-angiotensin system has been circumstantially linked to the pathogenesis of ARF for decades (Flamenbaum, 1973, 1977). Other investigations, however, have disassociated the two events and have failed to support a causal role for renin or angiotensin in the induction stages of ARF (Carvalho and Page, 1978; Sasaki et al., 1978; Baranwuski et al., 1978; Oken et al., 1975; Bidani et al., 1979).

There is ample experimental evidence in the dog that demonstrates altered renal hemodynamics in the initiation stage of norepinephrine-induced (Cox et al., 1974; Mauk et al., 1977; Burke et al., 1980; Taguma et al., 1980), nephrotoxic (Baehler et al., 1977; Flamenbaum et al., 1972; Stein et al., 1975), and hypotensive (Powers, 1970) models of ARF. Renal hemodynamics, however, can be shown to remain normal or to increase to control levels or above in the dog (Flamenbaum et al., 1972; Baehler et al., 1977; Cox et al., 1974; Kurtz and Hsu, 1978) as well as the rat and rabbit at a time when urine flow and GFR are greatly diminished. This disassociation of renal hemodynamics from the induction and maintenance stages of some forms of ARF make doubtful the primacy of these factors in the establishment or maintenance of acute oliguria. Vascular alteration may, however, contribute to and superimpose on other mechanisms to further affect GFR and urine formation.

Because renal hemodynamics seem to play little causal role in the perpetuation of most experimental forms of ARF, initial therapeutic efforts to replace fluid deficits or expand ECF volume may effectively reestablish renal blood flow without measurable benefit in improving renal function or urine formation.

Intratubular Obstruction. Intratubular obstruction is a significant pathophysiologic mechanism in ischemic models of ARF in the dog (Cronin et al., 1978; Donohoe et al., 1978; Patak et al., 1979; Toguma et al., 1980) as well as in the rat and in clinical settings in man. The obstruction results from desquamated epithelial debris in both the initiation and maintenance stages of oliguria. Tubular obstruction is an obvious pathogenic mechanism in heme-pigment nephropathy (Hostetter et al., 1980; Wada et al., 1977), sulfonamide nephrotoxicity (Apple and Neu, 1977; Wada et al., 1977) and ethylene glycol–induced oxalate precipitation (Parry and Wallach, 1974) (Fig. 74–15).

Intratubular obstruction causes tubular dilatation and distention of Bowman's space, increases in intratubular pressure, and decreases in the net ultrafiltration pressure and GFR in the absence of hemodynamic alterations. It may additionally increase afferent arteriolar resistance and concomitantly decrease renal blood flow (Arendshorst et al., 1975). Return of urine flow and restoration of glomerular filtration will depend upon resolution of the tubular obstruction.

Tubular obstruction appears to play little or no role in the initiation stage of experimental nephrotoxic ARF in dogs but may contribute to the later maintenance stage (Flamenbaum et al., 1972; Mason et al., 1977; Hostetter et al., 1980). Functional confirmation of tubular obstruction may be masked, however, by reductions in GFR and back leakage of the tubular fluid characteristic of nephrotoxic ARF.

Tubular Leakage. A third factor that has been thought to participate in the initiation and maintenance of acute oliguria is "back-leakage" of filtrate across the damaged tubular epithelium. Examination of histologic sections from ischemic or nephrotoxic damaged kidneys demonstrates large areas of epithelial necrosis (Fig. 74–15). The permeability characteristics of the tubule to fluid and large molecules and the integrity of the epithelial surface are lost after such damage. Numerous experimental studies have demonstrated the leakage of dyes, enzymes, or chemicals, confirming the enhanced permeability characteristics of the damaged epithelium (Donohoe et al., 1976; Sudo et al., 1980; Hostetter et al., 1980). Through this mechanism, and particularly when coupled with tubular obstruction, filtrate is shunted directly to the peritubular capillaries and urine flow remains diminished. The contribution of back leakage in a given experimental circumstance is variable and difficult to quantitate, but there appears little doubt that it contributes to the maintenance of the oliguric state.

Glomerular Permeability. Both direct and indirect evidence indicate that decreases in glomerular permeability may participate in the establishment of nephrotoxic and vasoconstrictor models of ARF. In dogs, swelling of podocyte cell bodies, primary and secondary foot processes, obliteration of the foot process structure, and increased villi formation are demonstrated with transmission and scanning electron microscopy in mercuric chloride (Baehler et al., 1977), two-hour norepinephrine (Cox et al., 1974), and uranyl nitrate induced ARF (Stein et al., 1975). In other studies, however, no ultrastructural abnormalities were recognized with either transmission or scanning electron microscopy (Cronin et al., 1978; Taguma et al., 1980; Schrier et al., 1978). Decreases in glomerular permeability and ultrafiltration coefficient have also been measured directly subsequent to ischemia (Savin et al., 1979), aminonucleoside toxicity (Avasthi and Evans, 1979), uranyl nitrate (Blantz, 1975), and aminoglycoside toxicity (Baylis et al., 1977). Reductions in the diameter, density, and area of glomerular fenestrae as well as constriction and obstruction of glomerular capillaries may thus contribute to the altered permeability and filtrate formation (Avasthi et al., 1979, 1980; Avasthi and Evans, 1979; Dach and Kurtzman, 1976). These abnormalities have thus far been identified only in the initiation stage of ARF, and their presence or significance in later stages is undefined.

The mechanisms that underlie the alterations in glomerular morphology or the ultrafiltration coefficient are presently unknown. Nephrotoxins or ischemia may directly damage the glomerular cells to produce the morphologic changes that secondarily reduce hydraulic permeability or glomerular surface area. The changes in permeability may also be a secondary response to a variety of hormones or vasoactive substances that alter glomerular circulatory dynamics and reduce filtration area. Circumstantial evidence for the involvement of angiotensin II in this mechanism has been identified, but direct correlations are lacking (Dach and Kurtzman, 1976; Hostetter et al., 1980).

Therapeutically, the reestablishment of normal renal blood flow with fluid administration and volume expansion may have little influence on the resumption of urine production or renal function if filtration failure is continued by this mechanism in the maintenance phase of the disease.

The initiation and maintenance of acute oliguria results from a single or combination of events that interact to impair formation of the glomerular ultrafiltrate and/or its delivery out of the nephron (Fig. 74–17). The perturbations of one stage are not necessarily contributory to the functional disturbances of subsequent or preceding stages. In nephrotoxic forms of ARF, direct toxic alterations in the function or structure of renal tubules and glomeruli are paramount with hemodynamic factors appearing to contribute only secondarily. In ischemic forms of ARF, vasoconstriction appears to initiate the reduced renal blood flow, filtrate formation, and urine output. In the maintenance stage, antecedent hemodynamic factors, tubular obstruction, backleak or altered glomerular permeability variably perpetuate the oliguria, depending on the duration and severity of the ischemic events.

Diuretic Stage

The diuretic stage is signaled by a progressive increase in daily urine production. The increase may occur suddenly or gradually (Fig. 74–16), and the onset of diuresis is variable but occurs in most dogs within two to three weeks from the onset of disease. The diuretic stage generally indicates renal repair and the onset of recovery but should not be regarded as a state of improved renal function. On the contrary, GFR will generally remain depressed in the early phase of diuresis along with persistently elevated or increasing BUN and serum creatinine concentrations (Fig. 74–16). Tubular regulatory processes are rarely intact, and the potential for serious losses of water and electrolytes exists. Careful surveillance and support of fluid and electrolyte balance is necessary to avoid hypovolemia, hypokalemia, and dysnatremia. Urine output may increase to several times the normal fluid requirements and requires comparable fluid replacement; efforts to keep up with urine losses, however, may perpetuate the diuretic state. When the course of the disease appears stabilized, judicious reductions in the administered fluid will be necessary to taper the diuresis. The relative load of sodium and fluid prior to the onset of diuresis will also influence the magnitude of the diuretic response. Tubular functions progressively return after the onset of diuresis, so derangement of fluid and electrolytes is minimized in the later phases.

Recovery Stage

The recovery stage lasts weeks to months, during which lesions are repaired and renal function improves. There are no studies in dogs that correlate return to renal function with the extent of the oliguric phase or the methods of treatment. Observations in man are nonconclusive, but age appears to significantly influence the adaptation to acute renal injury.

MANAGEMENT

The treatment of acute oliguria must be tailored to the individual patient and requires identification of the nature and site of the underlying disorder. In prerenal disorders, reestablishment of extracellular fluid volume (ECFV) and correction of predisposing factors restore renal hemodynamics, glomerular filtration, and urine formation. Similarly, in the postrenal disorders, early correction of the underlying abnormality reestablishes the normalcy of renal function and alleviates the uremic crisis. Acute renal parenchymal damage, on the other hand, is attended by both structural and functional changes in the kidney that do not respond readily to these simple therapeutic maneuvers.

The management of ARF is functionally divided into conservative therapy and dialysis. Conservative therapy is formulated to remedy the disturbances of greatest consequence, which include (1) alterations in the ECFV, (2) hyperkalemia, (3) acid-base imbalances, and (4) the retention of nitrogenous waste and "uremia toxins." The aims of such therapy are to pharmacologically correct renal hemodynamics and alleviate the fluid and biochemical abnormalities until the kidneys repair. As first priority, known causes for the oliguric state should be eliminated. The fluid status of the patient must be assessed and monitored at regular

intervals to direct the initial course of therapy and to prevent extremes of fluid balance during the course of disease. The fluid status can be evaluated by skin turgor, presence or absence of edema, prominence of jugular veins, central venous pressure, hematocrit, total serum solids, and blood pressure. Of utmost importance is the accurate and regular measurement of body weight and urine volume. Urine output is best evaluated with an indwelling urinary catheter attached to a closed, sterile drainage system.

Volume Status

Animals with ARF are characteristically hypovolemic and dehydrated. The volume deficit should be estimated and a replacement volume calculated on the basis of body weight (Cornelius, 1980; Cowgill, 1980a; Michell, 1979; Osborne and Low, 1972; Short, 1980). Volume deficits result primarily from ionic fluid losses through vomiting and diarrhea and should be replaced intravenously with balanced electrolyte solutions within the first two to six hours of therapy. Five per cent dextrose in water is not an adequate replacement solution and should be reserved for insensible maintenance losses.

Correction of fluid deficits generally requires an intravenous infusion rate of 5 to 15 ml/kg/hr, but faster rates may be used in patients with severe dehydration or hypotension. At faster infusion rates, or in the presence of compromised cardiovascular function, central venous pressure is a useful indicator of volume expansion and the ability of the heart to accept the fluid load. In the case of severe hemorrhage, more rapid correction of the vascular volume or the administration of compatible whole blood is indicated. In oliguric or anuric renal failure with initial fluid retention, all fluids must be restricted and volume therapy directed toward the production of an intensive diuresis to prevent congestive heart failure and pulmonary edema.

The establishment of a urine flow between 0.5 to 2.0 ml/kg/hr with volume replacement suggests a significant prerenal component to the oliguric state. Failure to induce a significant diuresis after volume replacement indicates that either the parenchymal damage is severe or the fluid deficit was underestimated. Additional fluid may be administered, if care is taken to prevent overhydration. The body weight after restoration of fluid balance should be used as the baseline for comparison to future changes. Gross fluctuations generally represent alterations in fluid volume and reflect dehydration or overhydration. Inappetent dogs whose fluid requirements are being adequately met should sustain an approximate 0.5 to 1.0 per cent loss in body weight per day as a reflection of tissue catabolism (Parker, 1981). After the initial fluid and electrolyte deficits are corrected, subsequently administered fluid must reflect the maintenance requirements and ongoing losses. Maintenance fluid should be limited to five or ten per cent dextrose in water to replace insensible losses (20 to 25 ml/kg/day) and balanced electrolyte solutions to replace measured urine output and gastrointestinal losses. Commercially available maintenance solutions may be used at an appropriately calculated volume. Evaporative losses substantially increase in hyperthermic animals or in hot, low humidity environments. Appropriate adjustments should be made to prevent dehydration and hypernatremia.

Overhydration or hypervolemia can be as detrimental to the oliguric dog as hypovolemia. Hypervolemia occurs with overzealous fluid therapy or improper monitoring of fluid balance. It may lead to peripheral and pulmonary edema, congestive heart failure, and hypertension. Once administered, an excessive fluid load represents a serious therapeutic error that is difficult to resolve.

In nonoliguric animals or during the diuretic stage, urine flow may exceed the normal rate of 1 to 2 ml/kg/hr, and substantial losses of sodium, potassium, and water may attend this diuresis. It is important, therefore, to adjust fluid requirements to meet urinary losses and to prevent hypovolemia, sodium depletion, and further renal injury.

Diuretics

Osmotic (hypertonic mannitol or glucose) or potent loop diuretics (furosemide, ethacrynic acid) have been advocated for the management of oliguric renal failure when volume replacement fails to initiate significant urine production (English, 1974; Gourley, 1970; Osborne et al., 1972, 1975; Parker, 1980). In large part, this advocation

stems from their demonstrated effectiveness to protect renal function in experimental ARF (Flores et al., 1972; De Torrente et al., 1978; Patak et al., 1979; Schrier et al., 1978).

The protective effects of diuretics correlate with their ability to reduce renal vascular resistance, increase renal blood flow, and promote an increase in solute excretion. Despite the benefits of hyperosmotic agents or diuretics in the prophylaxis of ARF, they are often of little benefit in the maintenance stages of greater than 20 hours duration.

Mannitol has been extensively evaluated in the protection and treatment of acute renal failure. In human patients it improves survival and renal function subsequent to traumatic, surgical, or myoglobinuric acute renal shutdown (Levinsky et al., 1981). In the dog mannitol will improve GFR, RBF, urine output, and survival when administered prior to or shortly following the induction of ARF by hemorrhage, intrarenal epinephrine or norepinephrine (Cronin et al., 1978; Burke et al., 1980; Hatcher et al., 1959), dehydration (Balint et al., 1975), ischemia (De Torrente et al., 1978; Abbott and Austen, 1974), or amphotericin B when administered simultaneously (Hellebusch et al., 1972).

The mechanism of action of mannitol in the prevention or treatment of ARF is unknown. An earlier belief that its major effect was to improve renal hemodynamics by reducing endothelial cell swelling (Flores et al., 1972; Summers and Jamison, 1971) is no longer as tenable (Frega et al., 1979; Levinsky et al., 1981). The disassociation between improved GFR, vascular resistance, and urine formation from simultaneous improvements in RBF suggests that effects on renal hemodynamics are not a major action of mannitol (Cronin et al., 1978). Recent studies in the dog agree that the protective effects of mannitol are best correlated with induced increases in osmolar clearance (Cronin et al., 1978; Patak et al., 1979; Schrier et al., 1978). The partial improvement and protection afforded by other hypertonic solutions may occur by a similar mechanism. The preservation of tubular flow and the development of high intratubular hydrostatic pressures appear to prevent obstruction, which, in combination with hemodynamic improvements, may mediate its effectiveness.

Controlled evaluations of the efficacy of

mannitol administration in the treatment of clinical forms of ARF in dogs are not available. In view of its demonstrated efficacy to protect and modify the early stages of experimental ARF in many species, including dogs, a trial course of therapy seems justified and offers minimal risk. In posttraumatic or surgical patients or in nephrotoxin exposure when the onset of oliguria is early and clearly established, osmotic diuretics may be beneficial (De Torrente et al., 1978; Flores et al., 1972; Patak et al., 1979; Gourley, 1970; Cronin et al., 1978). In these settings, a trial infusion of mannitol (as a 20 to 25 per cent solution) at 0.25 to 0.5 gm/kg body weight can be administered to fluidrepleted patients. If a significant diuresis results, a maintenance infusion of eight to ten per cent mannitol can be continued to promote the diuresis for the next 12 to 24 hours. If diuresis is not established within one hour of the trial infusion, additional doses should be withheld to avoid vascular overload and the potential for pulmonary edema. Unless the patient is hypervolemic at the initiation of diuretic therapy, urine output must be precisely replaced to prevent hypovolemia.

Hypertonic glucose has been advocated in lieu of mannitol for osmotic diuresis in dogs (English, 1974; Osborne et al., 1975; Osborne and Low, 1972; Finco and Low, 1980). Although clinical experience has justified its use in promoting diuresis, there is little experimental data to compare its efficacy in preventing acute oliguria or in modifying glomerular dynamics, GFR, RBF, urine production, intrarenal hormone induction, or patient survival in response to acute renal injury. Hyperglycemia has been demonstrated, however, to preserve urine production (and probably GFR) during hemorrhagic hypotension in dogs (Coelho and Bradley, 1964). The use of glucose as a caloric supplement is highly beneficial but is not recommended in amounts required to provide osmotic diuresis.

Loop diuretics are purported to cause diuresis in oliguric human patients and have protected or moderated some experimental models of ARF in dogs (Patak et al., 1979; Schrier et al., 1978; De Torrente et al., 1978). In other models, however, their efficacy is inconclusive (Lindner et al., 1979; Mohring and Madsen, 1973; Chandrankunnel et al., 1980). In general, loop diuretics are less consistently effective than mannitol

in improving renal function following experimental renal injury, and their diuretic response may not be associated with simultaneous improvements in GFR or in renal morphology (Papadimitriou et al., 1978).

The mechanism underlying the effects of loop diuretics is not known with certainty. In vasoconstrictor models, renal protection appears to correlate with the induction of a solute diuresis. The enhanced tubular flow may promote relief of the tubular obstruction that is recognized in this model. The vasodilatory effects of these agents may likewise contribute but cannot account for their actions entirely (Levinsky et al., 1981). These mechanisms are similar to those proposed for mannitol, and the differences in efficacy may relate to the sites of action of the two agents in the nephron. Mannitol exerts its diuretic effects along the entire nephron and therefore has a direct action on the proximal convoluted tubule, whereas furosemide only influences distal nephron sites. The potential for osmotic agents to expand ECFV and prevent cell swelling may be additional distinctions.

Evidence for the efficacy of loop diuretics in the management of established ARF is scanty (Levinsky et al., 1981). In the early stages of some forms of acute oliguria, loop diuretics may be beneficial to promote an increase in urine flow and solute excretion. Measurable benefits in modifying the clinical course, morbidity, or mortality, and demonstrated improvements in renal function are inconsistent. The conversion of acute oliguric renal failure to a nonoliguric state often facilitates the management of fluid and electrolyte disturbances; if improperly monitored, however, the induced diuresis may promote hypovolemia, electrolyte disturbances, and deterioration of existing renal function.

Because of the limited risks of a single therapeutic trial, furosemide administration has been routinely advocated in human patients and animals that fail to diurese with fluid repletion (Osborne et al., 1972, 1975, 1979; Osborne and Polzin, 1979; Parker, 1981; Levinsky et al., 1981). It is administered intravenously at 2 to 4 mg/kg body weight. This dose may be doubled or tripled if the initial trial fails to induce a diuretic response within 30 minutes. Parker (1981) has recently suggested that dopamine infused at 2 to 5 μg/kg body weight/min in a five per cent dextrose solution may be beneficial in dogs unresponsive to loop diuretics alone. Lindner and coworkers (1979) used dopamine plus furosemide to synergistically prevent the hemodynamic and physiologic alteration associated with nephrotoxic ARF in the dog.

It is the author's experience that the duration of oliguria or anuria is sufficiently long by the time most animals are presented for evaluation that diuretic agents are generally ineffective. In lieu of their theoretical benefits, they form no substitute for the application of proper fluid and electrolyte therapy and strict clinical supervision. If a diuretic regimen fails to promote a significant diuresis, continued administration is pointless and dialysis must be considered as an alternative therapy. If, on the other hand, fluid repletion or diuretic therapy is effective, the increased urine production may facilitate the regulation of fluid volume, serum potassium, and hydrogen, and the concentration of "uremia toxins." If these parameters can be kept under control until the kidneys repair, dialysis will be unnecessary.

Hyperkalemia

Hyperkalemia is a serious complication of acute oliguric renal failure by virtue of its potential to disrupt myocardial depolarization and conduction. These disturbances are responsible for the early mortality of acute oliguria and must rapidly be corrected (Hoff et al., 1941).

The management of hyperkalemia depends on the degree of potassium elevation and the severity of the cardiac disturbances. When the potassium concentration is greater than 8 mEq/L and the ECG disturbances are profound, parenteral calcium is the treatment of choice. As a specific antagonist to its cardiotoxicity, ten per cent calcium gluconate (approximately 0.5 to 1.0 ml/kg body weight) should be administered as a slow intravenous bolus in sufficient quantity to correct the ECG abnormalities. The effects of calcium infusion on the ECG are immediate but dissipate within 10 to 15 minutes and have no influence in altering the plasma potassium concentration. For these reasons, it is administered primarily to correct life-threatening situations until other controls are initiated.

Moderate hyperkalemia (serum potassium between 5.5 and 8.0 mEq/L) is managed by promoting the movement of extracellular potassium to the intracellular compartment, where it is clinically silent. In nonalkalemic or non–volume-loaded animals, sodium bicarbonate is administered intravenously at 0.5 to 1.0 mEq/kg body weight. Alternately, a 20 to 30 per cent glucose solution may be administered intravenously with or without regular insulin (1/8 to 1/4 unit/kg body weight) to promote the potassium transfer (Osborne and Polzin, 1979). The benefits of the exogenously administered insulin may be questionable, however, compared with those of glucose therapy alone (Hiatt and Sheinkopf, 1971). The effects of both glucose and bicarbonate occur within minutes and may last for several hours. For prolonged control, the cationic exchange resin, sodium polystyrene sulphonate, can be administered orally at 2 gm/kg body weight/day in three divided doses, but the most effective long-term control is obtained with peritoneal dialysis or hemodialysis. Potassium inputs must be strictly limited, and potassium laden parenteral fluids, medications, or foods should be withheld until a diuresis can be established.

Acidosis

Most animals with acute oliguric renal failure develop metabolic acidosis proportional to the severity of the uremia. A variety of simple or mixed acid-base disturbances can be detected, however. For this reason, it is desirable to measure the bicarbonate deficit or to perform a complete blood gas analysis before treating empirically. If the bicarbonate deficit is known, the required sodium bicarbonate replacement can be calculated from the formula, bicarbonate replacement (mEq) = body weight (kg) × 0.3 × bicarbonate deficit. If the bicarbonate deficit is not determined, an estimate based on the clinical status of the patient can be used. Mild uremic states are often characterized by a bicarbonate deficit of 5 mEq/L, whereas the deficit in moderate and advanced uremia is typically 10 to 15, respectively. Bicarbonate should not be administered in an attempt to correct the acidosis quickly. Half the calculated replacement should be given in the first hour, and the remainder during the subsequent five to six hours. The acid-base status should be reevaluated at six hours the first day and at least daily thereafter, in order to monitor the adequacy of replacement therapy and to detect changes or ongoing disturbances. Sodium bicarbonate should be used to manage only the metabolic component of the acid-base disorder and could be inappropriate or contraindicated if other disturbances are present.

Miscellaneous Conservative Measures

The maintenance of adequate nutrition is an extremely important but generally neglected aspect of therapy. When the caloric intake is insufficient from inappetence or withholding of food, the uremic animal uses endogenous proteins for calories, which contributes to the excretory nitrogen burden. The daily caloric requirements must be supplied as high-caloric-density fats and carbohydrates to prevent marked tissue catabolism and toxin accumulation. The problem is further complicated by anorexia and vomiting, which preclude oral administration of protein-restricted diets. Alternatively, the nutrient requirements must be supplied parenterally with combinations of hypertonic dextrose, lipid emulsions and protein hydrolysates (Finco, 1980).

Parenteral nutrition and therapy with essential amino acid mixtures offers considerable promise in the management of acute uremia (Finco, 1980; Toback, 1980). Damaged renal tissue undergoes an accelerated rate of synthesis and regeneration following an insult. Within days, new epithelial cells replace necrotic epithelium. Cellular regeneration is accompanied by increased synthesis of protein, nucleic acids, and phospholipids, despite the generalized catabolism characteristic of acute uremia (Toback, 1980). The administration of amino acids can dramatically enhance the rate of these synthetic processes in experimental models of ARF, and thus augment the rate of renal regeneration and tissue repair (Simpson et al., 1977; Toback, 1980).

In anephric dogs the administration of hypertonic dextrose or combined hypertonic dextrose and essential amino acids can double survival time compared with dogs receiving either oral nutrition or five per cent dextrose in water (Van Buren et al., 1972). Dextrose plus amino acid therapy blunts the rise in BUN, despite similar increases in creatinine seen in dogs receiving hypertonic or isotonic glucose or oral nutrition (Van Buren et al., 1972). The benefits of amino acid therapy outweigh and are independent of the benefits of hypertonic glucose, since they promote positive nitrogen balance, diminish weight loss, improve wound healing, moderate uremic signs, and ameliorate hyperkalemia and hyperphosphatemia (Toback, 1980).

Guidelines for parenteral nutrition therapy cannot be precisely formulated, although the theoretical advantages are clear. There is presently no information on the exact nitrogen or caloric requirements, the correct amino acid composition, or the role of nonessential amino acids or α–keto analogs of essential amino acids in the management of acute uremia in animals. Empirically, the normal caloric requirements of 132 kcal/$kg^{0.75}$/day (Cunha et al., 1974) should be provided as a minimum with augmentation to match excessively catabolic states (see Table 74–1). The caloric requirements can be provided by 20 to 30 per cent dextrose solutions or lipid emulsions (Intralipid) suitable for intravenous administration (Finco, 1980). Hypertonic solutions must be delivered via central venous catheters in volumes and at rates that avoid overhydration or hyperosmolality. Lipid emulsions provide the advantages of high caloric density, low volume, isotonicity, and peripheral vein administration. They suffer the disadvantage of considerable expense.

Amino acids can be provided as protein hydrolysate or as purified amino acid mixtures. The relative merits of these preparations have not been determined for animals, but amino acid mixtures with a high essential amino acid content should provide the most benefits with the least nitrogen load. The empirical administration of 0.3 to 0.53 gm/kg body weight daily has been recommended (Finco, 1980; Van Buren et al., 1972). Parenteral nutrition supplemented with essential amino acids may provide an important boost to the conservative therapy of ARF in dogs in the general absence of dialysis capabilities.

Care must be taken when administering drugs to uremic dogs. Renal excretion represents the major clearance route for many pharmacologic agents including antibiotics, cardiac glycosides, and some analgesics. Furthermore, some drugs have direct nephrotoxic effects and must be avoided. Modified dosage schedules have been established for many drugs in varying degrees of renal insufficiency in man (Bennett et al., 1980) and dogs (Davis, 1980; Osborne and Klausner, 1977). Drugs should be used discriminatingly, and only those with specific indications and known metabolic fates and toxicities should be administered.

Dialysis

The principal veterinary indication for either peritoneal dialysis or hemodialysis is acute reversible renal failure in patients whose fluid, electrolyte, and metabolic disturbances are unresponsive or unmanageable by conservative, supportive measures. It provides a means to effectively remove the metabolic waste products that contribute to the signs of renal failure.

Peritoneal dialysis uses the peritoneum as a semipermeable exchange surface against which a solution, the dialysate, corrects abnormalities of plasma volume and composition by mass transfer. Peritoneal dialysis is a technically straightforward procedure and within the scope of modern veterinary hospitals (Osborne and Polzin, 1979; Parker, 1980). Even though this procedure is feasible, it should never be performed on whim by unknowledgeable or untrained personnel. Once instituted on acutely uremic animals, peritoneal dialysis becomes a major undertaking with rigid time demands if it is to be either useful or successful.

Hemodialysis is similar in principle to peritoneal dialysis. Alterations in the volume and composition of the ECF are adjusted by regulating osmotic and diffusion gradients between the plasma and dialysate across a selective cellulose membrane. The artificial membrane allows a more efficient exchange of solutes and water between the blood and the dialysate than does the peritoneum. Because the exchange occurs outside the patient's body, an extracorporeal circulation of blood is required. The combination of a large surface area in the dialyser, thin and highly permeable exchange membranes, and a high extracorporeal blood flow accounts for the greater efficiency of hemodialysis (Fig. 74–16). The comparatively short treatment periods minimize patient fatigue and manipulation, and dialysis requires fewer dietary and drug restrictions.

Because of economic considerations and the need for specialized technical personnel, a versatile clinical laboratory, and intensive care facilities, hemodialysis is limited at present to veterinary teaching hospitals. In the future, however, hemodialysis should become more readily available to service the needs of clinical practice.

Prognosis

A good recovery can be anticipated in patients with prerenal oliguria. The prognosis for animals with acute parenchymal failure, however, is guarded to unfavorable. The duration of oliguria, concurrent medical or surgical problems, and the extent of nephron destruction affect the response to therapy. The establishment of a sustained diuresis can be considered a favorable response. Failure to sustain a diuresis with conservative therapeutics indicates severe or advanced disease and suggests an unfavorable outcome.

INTERSTITIAL DISEASE

Interstitial disease has been considered a common cause of chronic renal injury in the dog. This belief was primarily based on the gross and histologic appearance of the kidneys at the terminus of disease when small, contracted, fibrotic kidneys were identified grossly, and sparse, atrophic tubules and interstitial fibrosis were seen histologically. It has been subsequently recognized that these gross and microscopic findings are not unique to chronic interstitial inflammation but are recognized as an end-stage of a variety of renal injuries (Krohn et al., 1971; Osborne and Johnson, 1970; Wright et al., 1976). Primary interstitial or tubulo-interstitial disease does occur with regularity in companion animals, but the temptation to classify all end-stage kidney as "chronic interstitial nephritis" should be avoided.

In human nephrology, a broad spectrum of discrete interstitial diseases have been recognized (Freedman, 1979). A similar complement undoubtedly exists in companion animals, but as yet only a few categories have been described and well characterized. Interstitial inflammation can generally be categorized as suppurative or nonsuppurative according to morphologic criteria. Acute or chronic, focal or diffuse, or other appropriate modifiers can be used when appropriate for finer distinctions.

SUPPURATIVE INTERSTITIAL INFLAMMATION

Pyelonephritis is an acute or chronic suppurative inflammation of the tubulo-interstitium caused by bacterial infection. The true prevalence of pyelonephritis in companion animals is unknown because of the difficulty in recognizing and confirming this disease by routine clinical methods. In an evaluation of autopsy material from dogs and cats, Gribble (unpublished observations) identified pyelonephritis by histologic criteria in 12 out of 541 (2.2 per cent) and 6 out of 226 (2.7 per cent) cases, respectively. Crowell and Finco (1975), however, reported an incidence of pyelitis between 6 and 25 per cent in nonselected populations of young and adult dogs. In a preliminary investigation in which the presence and locus of urinary infection was established with cystocentesis and nephropyelocentesis, Ling (unpublished data, 1982) identified asymptomatic bacteriuria in 10 of 125 (8 per cent) clinically normal dogs. Five (50 per cent) of the bacteriuric dogs also had positive cultures in urine collected directly from the renal pelves. In addition to the lack of overt clinical manifestations, renal infection may occur as a transient but recurrent disorder in the presence of persistent or recurrent lower urinary tract infection. In dogs in which pyelonephritis was established and monitored by nephropyelocentesis, renal infection could be demonstrated to manifest and disappear intermittently during the course of a year's observation (Ling, unpublished data, 1982). These observations suggest that pyelonephritis may not necessarily lead to progressive renal injury when untreated, and that host and environmental factors must modify the clinical expression of the disease.

The most common route for infection of the kidney is by retrograde passage of bacteria from the lower urinary tract along the ureter. Although this is counter to the normal direction of urine flow, retrograde passage of urine can occur from the bladder by vesicoureteral reflux (Christie, 1971; Newman et al., 1973; see Chapter 75). In the absence of infection, vesicoureteral reflux does not generally cause morphologic change in the kidneys (Newman et al., 1974); in the presence of infection in the bladder, however, reflux has a profound influence on the establishment of renal infection and pyelonephritis (Crowell and Finco, 1975). This fact is exemplified in a recent study of 20 dogs in which one kidney was infected by nephropyelocentesis. Within two weeks, the contralateral kidney became infected in 14 of the dogs (70 per cent) (Ling, unpublished data, 1982).

The renal medulla has an enhanced susceptibility to infection by virtue of the high osmolality and ammonia concentration that exist at this site (Freedman and Beeson, 1968; Freedman, 1979; Osborne et al., 1979a). It is also predisposed to infection by urinary obstruction, renal trauma, anatomic abnormalities, urinary tract instrumentation, and extrarenal diseases that impair host defenses or enhance bacterial growth in the urine (e.g., canine Cushing's syndrome, diabetes mellitus).

Pyelonephritis is infrequently established by hematogenous bacteria. Chronic or acute bacteremia, discospondylitis, or bacterial endocarditis may cause secondary renal infection. Identical organisms can frequently be cultured from both the blood and urine in septicemic diseases. Morphologic and progressive lesions characteristic of chronic pyelonephritis may develop in the absence of viable microorganisms, and immunologic mechanisms initiated by previous infection or persistent bacterial antigens are thought to be involved (Aoki et al., 1969; Glassock et al., 1974). The precise role of immune mechanisms in the establishment of pyelonephritis remains controversial, however.

The major consequence of pyelonephritis is renal insufficiency following suppurative destruction of renal mass. Glomeruli are initially spared but are eventually replaced by a fibrous tissue following the tissue necrosis and vascular aberrations initiated by the infection. Pyelonephritis also alters renal concentrating ability (Finco et al., 1979; Martinez-Maldonado and Opava-Stitzer, 1977). This can be used in a limited manner to help localize the site of renal infection, since lower tract infections have no influence on urine concentration. Pyelonephritis is also associated with the formation of nephrolithiasis. The major urolith in the dog is composed of struvite and is strongly associated with the presence of urease-producing bacteria, such as *Staphylococcus* or *Proteus spp* (Klausner and Osborne, 1979).

The diagnosis of pyelonephritis requires a high index of suspicion because of its typically silent clinical manifestations. Fever, lumbar or renal pain, leukocytosis, and a "hunched-back" stance are classic signs but are infrequently expressed in either acute or chronic pyelonephritis (Finco et al., 1979). Polyuria may be evident but must be differentiated from a variety of diseases manifesting this sign.

The urinalysis may support a presumptive diagnosis of pyelonephritis but is often nonspecific and nonlocalizing. The supernatant of centrifuged urine will generally demonstrate a positive protein reaction, variable occult blood and pH, and a positive nitrite test. The urine specific gravity obtained in patients with pyelonephritis is often low when compared with that in patients with lower urinary infection and may be the most localizing characteristic (Finco et al., 1979). The sediment may contain WBCs in moderate to high numbers, with a variable degree of microscopic hematuria. Inflammatory cell casts provide good evidence of pyelonephritis but are not often demonstrated. If bacteria are present in sufficient numbers, they may be visualized in stained or unstained preparations. To be visualized, rod-shaped bacteria and cocci must be present in numbers greater than 10^4 and 10^5 per ml of urine, respectively (Ling et al., 1979). Gram staining can be used to differentiate gram-negative and gram-positive bacteria, but the failure to identify organisms in the urinary sediment should not be equated with the absence of bacterial infection.

Urine culture is the most definitive way to document urinary tract infection. The methods and interpretation of urinary microbiology are beyond the scope of this discussion but have been recently reviewed (Ling et al., 1979). No data are available to document the frequency of bacterial isolates from naturally occurring cases of pyelonephritis in animals. However, renal infections usually arise from the lower tract and are therefore associated with *E. coli*, *Staphylococcus aureus*, *Proteus mirabilis*, *Streptococci spp*, *Klebsiella pneumoniae*, *Pseudomonas aeruginosa*, and *Enterobacter spp*, in descending order of frequency in dogs (Ling et al., 1979).

Radiographic signs can support the diagnosis of pyelonephritis but are variable in expression. Identifiable radiographic lesions include an irregular renal contour, decreased renal size, and cortical atrophy and asymmetry. Excretory urography may reveal dilation, blunting, asymmetry, or distortion of the diverticuli and pelvis. The ureters are also frequently dilated (Biery, 1978; Finco and Barsanti, 1979). Documented, long-standing renal infections may, however, produce no identifiable radiographic lesions (Ling, unpublished data).

Although a vast spectrum of techniques (ureteral catheterization, bladder washout, antibody-coated bacteria, enzymuria, and nephropyelocentesis) have been evaluated to localize bacteriuria, to date no tests have proved clinically useful or reliable for this purpose (Finco and Barsanti, 1979; Freedman, 1979). The diagnosis of pyelonephritis must therefore be based on sound clinical assessments.

TREATMENT OF PYELONEPHRITIS

The treatment of pyelonephritis logically begins with the identification of the infecting organisms by bacterial culture and selection of an antimicrobial that will sterilize the kidney and urine as efficiently and economically as possible. Pyelonephritis is an interstitial disease, and the selected antimicrobial agent must be available at the appropriate concentration in interstitial fluid. The heterogeneity of regional blood flow, pH, osmolality, and anatomy within the kidney make selection of an effective drug difficult at best. Differences in host defenses to bacteria may reduce the efficacy of antimicrobics that are effective at other sites of infection. Indiscriminate and inappropriate antimicrobial usage may lead to the induction of plasmid resistance, particularly with the use of sulfonamides, penicillins, tetracycline, streptomycin, kanamycin, and chloramphenicol (Ling, 1979).

Knowledge of the minimum inhibitory urine concentrations (MIC) of antimicrobics to the infecting organism aids selection of an appropriate drug (Stamey et al., 1974; Ling, 1979). The treatment of pyelonephritis may be compromised by the impaired renal concentrating ability, which reduces achievable urinary antimicrobic concentrations. In many circumstances, urine levels may be similar or only several times greater than blood concentrations, in which case inhibitory concentrations become of utmost importance in the selection of an antimicrobial.

In instances in which minimum inhibitory concentrations for an isolate cannot be readily obtained, Ling has outlined a workable scheme of antimicrobial selection based on an extensive series of clinical and experimental trials with common urinary tract isolates (Ling, 1979). Essentially all urinary infections with streptococcal and staphylococcal organisms can be effectively managed with penicillin G (approximately 40,000 U/kg body weight three times daily, orally) or ampicillin (approximately 26 mg/kg body weight three times daily, orally).

For *E. coli* isolates, approximately 80 per cent will be susceptible to trimethoprim/sulfa at an oral dosage of 2.2 mg/kg body weight based on the trimethoprim fraction twice daily. *Proteus mirabilis* and *Pseudomonas spp* can be successfully treated in 80 per cent of cases with oral penicillin or ampicillin (dosage given previously) or oral tetracycline (18 to 20 mg/kg body weight three times daily), respectively. The susceptibility of *Klebsiella pneumoniae* is not predictable and is best determined with MIC assay. Alternatively, a broad-spectrum agent such as gentamicin or tobramycin may be used.

Urinary tract infections with multiple organisms may be managed by the use of a single antimicrobial if all isolates are susceptible (e.g., broad-spectrum aminoglycosides) or by the use of sequential antimicrobials to which the individual isolates are susceptible. With few exceptions, simultaneous combinations of antimicrobials should be avoided.

Once selected, an antimicrobial should be administered for a two- to four-week treatment period. Regular, long-term follow-up to ensure sterility of the urine is a critical requirement for the management of pyelonephritis. Patients should be monitored for 6 to 12 months at one- to three-month intervals. Monthly cultures should be taken by cystocentesis until the urine is sterile on three consecutive cultures, at which time culture intervals can be lengthened to three months. Caution should be taken to avoid instrumentation or catheterization of the bladder, which might reinfect the urinary tract.

If reinfection occurs in the absence of instrumentation, a thorough search for the source of infection should be undertaken. In male dogs, the prostate gland is an important and common site of residual infection. Anatomic abnormalities, obstruction, patent urethrostomy, or immune deficiencies predispose to reinfection and should be identified and corrected. Persistent infections in the presence of specific antimicrobials could indicate intestinal malabsorption or impaired renal excretion of the therapeutic agents. In patients with a predilection for recurrent urinary tract infections, long-term suppressive doses of an antimicrobial agent may be instituted for prolonged control (Freedman, 1979). Trimethoprim-sulfa or nitrofurantoin and penicillin derivatives have been effective when given at one fourth to one third the total daily dose as a single evening administration following the last voided urine for predisposing gram-negative and gram-positive organisms, respectively (Ling, 1979). This treatment is instituted for six months, with appropriate follow-up cultures. If the urine remains sterile during this interval, the drug is discontinued. Subsequent bacteriuric episodes should be treated aggressively with specific antimicrobials and reinstitution of the low dose regimen when the urine is again sterile.

The dosage of any antimicrobial agent should be modified appropriately in patients with renal insufficiency (Bennett et al., 1980). Many antimicrobials are excreted primarily in the urine and may achieve toxic concentrations on normal dose schedules. Nephrotoxic agents should be used with extreme caution.

CONGENITAL AND INHERITED DISORDERS

Congenital and inherited abnormalities in renal morphology, development, or function are recognized sporadically as young animals are surveyed for renal disease. In recent years, a variety of disorders have been well characterized in specific breeds of dog, which suggests their inheritability.

DEVELOPMENTAL MALFORMATIONS

Agenesis is the complete absence of a kidney and can occur unilaterally or bilaterally. The unilateral condition is usually an incidental finding and not typically associated with clinical signs unless accompanied by additional developmental defects or infection. Unilateral agenesis is recognized more commonly in the cat and is associated with hypertrophy of the intact kidney (Finco, 1979b; Osborne et al., 1972a). Bilateral agenesis is obviously fatal and is a recognized cause of neonatal death.

Renal hypoplasia denotes a marked reduction in the developmental size or mass of the kidneys in the absence of acquired disease. It is often misused to describe renal disorders of young animals with a distinct pathogenesis but similar morphologic consequences (Finco, 1979c). Renal cortical hypoplasia has been described in a variety of breeds, including the cocker spaniel (Persson et al., 1961; English and Winter, 1979), malamute (Kaufman et al., 1969), Yorkshire terrier (Klopfer et al., 1978), German shepherd dog, Doberman pinscher, and dachshund (Kaufman et al., 1969). Whether or not each report represents renal cortical hypoplasia in the strictest sense is unknown; each disease, however, has morphologic features that are consistent with hypoplasia.

Renal cortical hypoplasia is recognized by the development of chronic renal insufficiency, if the involvement is bilateral, but may be unaccompanied by signs if the involvement is unilateral or mild. Affected animals variably demonstrate polydipsia and polyuria, stunted growth, weight loss, pale mucous membranes, azotemia, and renal osteodystrophy at an early age. Some animals will also demonstrate proteinuria and glycosuria. Signs develop from several months to several years of age and frequently progress to fatal uremia. The diagnosis is suggested by the detection of uremia in young animals with palpable or radiographically shrunken kidneys. Marked reductions in the number of glomeruli, glomerular atrophy, nephrosclerosis, and nephrocalcinosis typify the renal histology.

In addition to the developmental defects, progression of the uremia may be caused by secondary factors (i.e., hypertension and renal mineralization) that erode the residual renal mass.

Other, but less common, developmental disorders include polycystic disease (Osborne et al., 1972a), in which the renal parenchyma is disrupted by a variable number of fluid-filled cysts. The cysts range in size from minute to massive and may

predispose the kidneys to infection or cause renal failure. Horseshoe kidney is a result of early embryonic fusion of the kidneys but is rarely identified in cats and dogs. Renal ectopia is described in both the cat and dog (Johnson, 1979; Webb, 1974). The ectopic kidney is frequently located in the pelvic area, where it must be differentiated from other abdominal masses. Few functional abnormalities should develop, unless the ectopia is accompanied by other developmental abnormalities or infection. O'Handley and colleagues (1979) reported a case of renal and ureteral duplication in a dog that manifested intermittent hermaturia, bacteriuria, urinary incontinence, and cystic calculi. Developmental abnormalities, although frequently benign, can predispose the kidneys to secondary complications, including infection, obstruction, or vesicoureteral reflux, and the subsequent development of recognizable disease.

FAMILIAL PROGRESSIVE RENAL INSUFFICIENCY

An apparently inherited disorder that progresses to morphologically end-stage kidneys and uremia has been characterized in several breeds of dog. Whether or not these diseases represent a similar genetic deficiency or pathogenesis is not known, but their clinical presentations are frequently similar.

Familial Nephropathy of Lhasa Apso and Shih Tzu Dogs

A disproportionate incidence of morbidity and mortality from chronic renal failure is recognized in young dogs of the Lhasa Apso and Shih Tzu breeds (Finco, 1979a). Both sexes are affected equally. Many affected animals will die of uremia within months of birth, while in others the disease will be occult until three to four years of age. The typical signs include reduced growth, poor conditioning, polydipsia, polyuria, and malaise in young animals. Laboratory findings are consistent with chronic renal insufficiency. The kidneys are bilaterally small and misshapen when examined grossly. They often appear coarsely nodular from irregular, deep scarring, finely granular, or they demonstrate focal areas with numerous cortical cysts. They may show discrete, dense bands or a diffuse distribution of connective tissue radiating through the cortex and medulla. The parenchyma can be intermittently normal, hyperplastic, atrophic, or completely collapsed about the intervening connective tissue when examined histologically. The glomeruli are randomly small, collapsed, immature, and unperfused. More normally developed glomeruli frequently demonstrate glomerulosclerosis and epithelial or endothelial cell proliferation.

The pathogenesis of these lesions is unknown; however, the pattern and the associated hyaline and hypertrophic arteriolarsclerotic pathology are consistent with a vascular etiology (Finco, 1979a). During nephrogenesis, the glomeruli often fail to mature and atrophy with their tubular constituents, thus promoting the observed fibrosis. Although the inheritability of this disorder seems certain, the exact pattern of inheritance is unknown. It appears to be complex and multifactorial. Affected animals should be treated symptomatically for the manifestations of uremia that develop. No recommendation can be presently offered regarding modifications of existing breeding programs. The carrier state is often well masked and may surface after an extensive and uneventful breeding program.

Familial Renal Disease of Norwegian Elkhound Dogs

A progressive familial renal disease has been identified and well characterized in the Norwegian elkhound breed of dogs (Finco, 1976; Finco et al., 1970, 1977). Both sexes are affected and the disease is recognized by the development of renal insufficiency and azotemia between the ages of three months and five years. The exact etiology is unknown, but nephrogenesis appears to be abnormal, as indicated by the reduced glomerular counts, cortical thickness, and renal size.

Morphologically, the affected kidneys demonstrate periglomerular fibrosis, which proceeds to interstitial fibrosis, and cortical collapse, diffuse epithelial proliferation, mesangial thickening and variable glomerular atrophy. In advanced stages, focal cortical and medullary fibrosis, tubular atrophy, and mononuclear cell infiltration into the superficial cortex, cortico-medullary junc-

tion, and pelvis can be seen (Finco et al., 1977). The disease is diagnosed by breed predisposition, clinical and laboratory signs of renal insufficiency, and renal biopsy. Glycosuria and aminoaciduria are recognized in some dogs.

Treatment is purely symptomatic, and no genetic markers are available to define the mode of inheritance (Finco, 1973). The prognosis is guarded and dependent on the rate of progression and severity of the renal fibrosis.

Miscellaneous Familial Diseases

Familial tendencies for progressive renal insufficiency have been reported for other breeds but are insufficiently evaluated to describe their pathogenesis or inheritance. A hereditary nephritis has been described in five related Samoyed dogs that died between 7 and 11 months of age. It was characterized by diffuse, segmental glomerulosclerosis, and proteinuria. Males appeared to be more frequently and more severely affected (Bernard and Valli, 1977).

Renal cortical hypoplasia is recognized as an inherited disorder in the cocker spaniel (Krook, 1957; Kaufman et al., 1969; English and Winter, 1979). Questions concerning whether or not this disease represents true hypoplasia have been raised (Finco, 1973, 1979c), but regardless, the juvenile expression of a progressive renal failure is present in this breed and probably represents an inherited abnormality.

Progressive renal fibrosis, glomerular drop-out, and early progressive renal failure appear in the basenji breed in association with the inherited metabolic and transport defects (Easley and Breitschwerdt, 1976; Bovee et al., 1978, 1979b).

FUNCTIONAL RENAL ABNORMALITIES

Discrete metabolic and functional abnormalities make up an additional category of inherited renal disorders, but their recognition and description in companion animals has been limited.

Canine Cystinuria

The excessive urinary excretion of cystine may predispose to the formation of cystine calculi in the kidney or elsewhere in the urinary tract. Cystine calculi have been reported in male dogs of several breeds and mixed breeds, but is most common in the dachshund (Bovee et al., 1974; Holtzapple et al., 1969; Lage, 1980). A detailed discussion of this disorder can be found in Chapter 76.

Canine Fanconi Syndrome

A disorder resembling Fanconi syndrome of children has been reported in the dog and appears to be inherited in the basenji. The canine disease represents a generalized reabsorptive defect that is probably localized to the proximal nephron. It is characterized by glycosuria, aminoaciduria, proteinuria, phosphaturia, hypophosphatemia, renal tubular acidosis, and reabsorptive abnormalities for sodium, potassium, and urate (Bovee et al., 1978, 1979b). It is distinguished from the human disorder by the lack of metabolic bone disease, by growth disturbances and dwarfing, and by urolithiasis.

Clinical signs include polydipsia, polyuria, weight loss, dehydration, and progressive renal insufficiency. The diagnosis is confirmed by breed predilection and the demonstration of the associated renal transport defects. The renal glycosuria is documented by the detection of heavy glycosuria in the presence of a normal or slightly reduced plasma glucose concentration; thus, it is the simplest abnormality to detect. Documentation of other transport defects is beyond the scope of routine diagnostics, but hypokalemia, hypophosphatemia, and metabolic acidosis may be evident in severely affected dogs.

A variable degree of renal insufficiency is common and contributes to the overall clinical picture (Bovee et al., 1979b). No specific treatment is available to reverse the tubular defects. Therapy is symptomatically directed to clinically detectable abnormalities, including renal insufficiency, acidosis, hypophosphatemia, and hypokalemia.

Primary Renal Glycosuria

Renal glycosuria is recognized as a component of the generalized tubular defects seen in canine Fanconi syndrome but may also occur as a specific and singular transport abnormality (Krane, 1979). The hallmark of renal glycosuria is significant urinary glucose excretion in the presence of a normal plasma glucose concentration and the absence of diabetes mellitus. Affected animals have marked reductions in both the transport maximum and plasma threshold for glucose and may excrete gram quantities of glucose in daily urine. Primary renal glycosuria can be identified sporadically in various breeds of dog but recently has been recognized and characterized as an inherited disorder in the Norwegian elkhound (Cowgill et al., 1982). It occurs as an incidental clinical finding and is not associated with recognizable disease or morphologic injury. It is important, however, to distinguish this disorder from diabetes mellitus and to screen affected dogs for urinary tract infection.

PRIMARY TUMORS OF THE KIDNEY

Renal neoplasia is infrequently diagnosed in companion animals. The incidence in the dog is variably reported to be between 0.6 and 1.7 per cent of all canine tumors (Baskin and de Paoli, 1977; Theilen and Madewell, 1979; Hays and Fraumeni, 1977). The adenocarcinoma and uncharacterized carcinoma are the most commonly reported renal tumors, but embryonal nephroma, fibrosarcoma, adenoma, hemangiosarcoma, fibroma, and lipoma are also seen. In the renal pelvis, the transitional cell carcinoma, squamous cell carcinoma, undifferentiated carcinoma, and fibrosarcoma can be recognized.

No breed predilection has been recognized for renal tumors (Hays and Fraumeni, 1977; Lucke and Kelley, 1976). With the exception of embryonal nephroma, renal tumors are usually found in dogs between the ages 7 and 8.5 years. Embryonal nephromas are most commonly recognized in dogs less than one year of age. The incidence in male dogs is twice as great as that in females, as is true in humans. The majority of renal tumors are malignant, with the lungs and regional lymph nodes common sites of metastasis.

Clinical Signs and Diagnosis

The signs associated with renal neoplasia are usually nonspecific and include weight loss, anorexia, depression, and fever. Findings suggestive of urinary disease are often lacking. Hematuria is variably reported, despite its frequent association with renal neoplasia in man. The hematuria is usually microscopic and only recognized on urine sediment examination. The deterioration of body condition is usually insidious but may be compounded acutely with ureteral obstruction and progressive pain.

A presumptive diagnosis of renal neoplasia is made by palpation of the mass in the cranial abdomen. Malignant tumors tend to be large when ultimately discovered. Clinical suspicions can be confirmed by excretory urography, renal arteriography, or renal ultrasonography. Renal tumors must be differentiated from renal cysts, abscesses, hematomas, hydronephrosis, and functional hypertrophy, which are also associated with renal enlargement.

Renal function may be only mildly altered because of the insidious encroachment and compression of the normal parenchyma and hypertrophy of the contralateral kidney. The urinalysis may reveal gross or microscopic hematuria, atypical renal cells, proteinuria, and superimposed urinary infection. Polycythemia is rarely reported and is presumably secondary to stimulation of erythropoietin. Thoracic radiographs should be evaluated to detect pulmonary or bronchial lymph node metastasis. Differentiation of the lesion may be determined by fine needle aspiration and cytology or by needle or surgical biopsy of the mass.

Treatment

The therapy of renal neoplasia requires initial surgical removal of the mass. A unilateral nephrectomy is usually indicated, but partial nephrectomy may be performed with benign renal tumors or if renal function is severely compromised. Veterinary experience with adjuvant chemotherapy is too limited to allow specific recommendations for any histologic classification of renal neoplasm. Radiotherapy is being used increasingly in veterinary patients and may prove useful with further testing. Management of renal lymphosarcoma by combination chemotherapy seems justified and will often promote an acute resolution of urinary signs and renal enlargement (Madewell, 1975; MacEwen, 1980).

The behavior of renal carcinomas is variable. Some cases have survived for years post-nephrectomy (Lucke and Kelly, 1976). This would warrant an aggressive surgical approach despite the overall unfavorable prognosis.

In both the dog and cat, malignant lymphoma is frequently metastatic to the kidneys and may represent the sole site of clinical expression.

RENAL PARASITES

Dioctophyma renale and *Capillaria plica* are the major parasites of the dog kidney. Both parasites undergo a complicated life cycle in an intermediate host before infection and development in the kidneys of the definitive host. The reported incidence of renal parasites in North America is low, but individual cases or outbreaks may be identified sporadically (Osborne et al., 1969; Senior et al., 1980, 1980a).

For *D. renale,* the dog is infected by ingesting uncooked fish or frogs that contain encysted and infective larvae (Osborne et al., 1969). After infection, the larvae migrate to a variety of locations but are most commonly identified free in the peritoneal cavity or within the parenchyma of the kidney. The life cycle of *C. plica* is unclear but appears to require, in part, passage through earthworms as an intermediate host, which may also be infective (Senior, 1980).

Clinical signs may be inapparent, or hematuria or pollakiuria may be recognized. Renal insufficiency may become evident if the uninfected kidney becomes secondarily diseased or if both kidneys are parasitized.

Renal parasites are usually diagnosed inadvertently by the detection of parasitic ova in the urine or by the identification of adult stages during surgical exploration of the abdomen. Renal enlargement may be demonstrated clinically or radiographically with *D. renale* infections and must be differentiated from other causes of renal enlargement or hydronephrosis.

Nephrectomy or nephrotomy and parasite removal are the only available treatments at present. Because of the potential for widespread infection with *C. plica* in kennel environments, management modification should be recommended in epizootic outbreaks to prevent soil contamination with ova and host exposure (Senior, 1980).

REFERENCES

Abbott, W. M., and Austen, W. G.: The reversal of renal cortical ischemia during aortic occlusion by mannitol. J. Surg. Res. *16*:482, 1974.

Ackerman, N.: Excretory urogram — technique. Calif. Vet. *33*(10):10, 1979.

Adelman, R. D., Spangler, W. L., Beasom, F., Ishizaki, G., and Conzelman, G. M.: Furosemide enhancement of experimental gentamicin nephrotoxicity: Comparison of functional and morphological changes with activities of urinary enzymes. J. Infect. Dis. *140*:342, 1979.

Alfrey, A. C., Solomons, C. C., Ciricillo, J., and Miller, N. L.: Extraosseous calcification: Evidence for abnormal pyrophosphate metabolism in uremia. J. Clin. Invest. *57*:692, 1976.

Allison, M. E. M., Wilson, C. B., and Gottschalk, C. W.: Pathophysiology of experimental glomerulonephritis in rats. J. Clin. Invest. *53*:1402, 1974.

Abramowicz, M., Barnett, H. L., Edelmann, C. M., Griefer, I., Kobayashi, Q., Arneil, G. C., Barron, B. A., Gordillo, P. G., Hallmann, N., and Tiddens, H. A.: Controlled trial of azathioprine in children with nephrotic syndrome. Lancet *1*:959, 1970.

Anderson, L. J., and Fisher, E. W.: The blood pressure in canine interstitial nephritis. Res. Vet. Sci. *9*:304, 1968.

Anderson, L. J., and Jarrett, W. F. H.: Membranous glomerulonephritis associated with leukaemia in cats. Res. Vet. Sci. *12*:179, 1971.

Anderson, R. J., and Schrier, R. W.: Clinical Spectrum of Oliguric and Nonoliguric Acute Renal Failure. *In* Brenner, B. M., and Stein, J. H. (eds.): Contemporary Issues in Nephrology. Vol. 6. Acute Renal Failure. Churchill Livingstone, New York, 1980.

Anderson, R. J., Linas, S. L., Berns, A. S., Henrich, W. L., Miller, T. R., Gabow, P. A., and Schrier, R. W.: Nonoliguric acute renal failure. N. Engl. J. Med. *296*:1134, 1977.

Anderson, R. S., and Edney, A. T. B.: Protein intake and blood urea in the dog. Vet. Rec. *84*:348, 1969.

Aoki, S., Imamura, S., Aoki, M., and McCabe, W. R.: "Abacterial" and bacterial pyelonephritis. Immunofluorescent localization of bacterial antigen. N. Engl. J. Med. *281*:1375, 1969.

Appel, G. B., and Neu, H. C.: The nephrotoxicity of antimicrobial agents. N. Engl. J. Med. *296*:722, 1977.

Appel, G. B., and Neu, H. C.: The nephrotoxicity of antimicrobial agents. N. Engl. J. Med. *296*:784, 1977a.

Appel, G. B., and Neu, H. C.: Gentamicin in 1978. Ann. Intern. Med. *89*:528, 1978.

Arendshorst, W. J., Finn, W. F., and Gottschalk, C. W.: Pathogenesis of acute renal failure following temporary renal ischemia in the rat. Circulation Res. *37*:558, 1975.

Arruda, J. A. L., Carrasquillo, T., Cubria, A., Rademacher, D. R., and Kurtzman, N. A.: Bicarbonate reabsorption in chronic renal failure. Kidney Int. *9*:481, 1976.

Asheim, A.: Pathogenesis of renal damage and polydipsia in dogs with pyometra. J.A.V.M.A. *147*:736, 1965.

Avasthi, P. S., and Evan, A. P.: Glomerular permeability in aminonucleoside-induced nephrosis in rats. A proposed role of endothelial cells. J. Lab. Clin. Med. *93*:266, 1979.

Avasthi, P. S., Evan, A. P., and Hay, D.: Glomerular endothelial cells in uranyl nitrate-induced acute renal failure in rats. J. Clin. Invest. *65*:121, 1980.

Avasthi, P. S., Huser, J., and Evan, A. P.: Glomerular endothelial cells in gentamicin-induced acute renal failure in rats. Kidney Int. *16*:771, 1979.

Avioli, L. V., and Teitelbaum, S. L.: Renal Osteodystrophy. *In* Earley, L. E., and Gottschalk, C. W. (eds.): Strauss and Welt's Diseases of the Kidney., Vol. 1. 3rd ed. Little, Brown and Company, Boston, 1979.

Baehler, R. W., Kotchen, T. A., Burke, J. A., Galla, J. H., and Bhathena, D.: Considerations on the pathophysiology of mercuric chloride-induced acute renal failure. J. Lab. Clin. Med. *90*:330, 1977.

Balestri, P. L., Rindi, P., Biagini, M., and Giovannetti, S.: Effects of uraemic serum, urea, creatinine and methylguanidine on glucose metabolism. Clin. Sci. *42*:395, 1972.

Balint, P., Laszlo, K., Szocs, E., and Tarjan, E.: Renal haemodynamics in dogs with dehydration azotaemia. Acta Med. Acad. Sci. Hungaricae *32*:193, 1975.

Banks, K. L., and Henson, J. B.: Immunologically mediated glomerulitis of horses. II. Antiglomerular basement membrane antibody and other mechanisms in spontaneous disease. Lab. Invest. *26*:708, 1972.

Baranowski, R. L., Westenfelder, C., and Kurtzman, N. A.: Intrarenal renin and angiotensins in glycerol-induced acute renal failure. Kidney Int. *14*:576, 1978.

Barber, D. L., and Rowland, G. N.: Radiographically detectable soft tissue calcification in chronic renal failure. Vet. Radiol. *20*:117, 1979.

Barrett, R. B., and Kneller, S. K.: Feline kidney mensuration. Acta Radiol. Suppl. *319*:279, 1972.

Barsanti, J. A.: Treatment of aplastic anemia with androgens. Scientific Presentations of the 46th Annual Meeting American Animal Hospital Association, New Orleans, Louisiana, 1979, p. 233.

Barsanti, J. A., and Finco, D. R.: Protein concentration in urine of normal dogs. Am. J. Vet. Res. *40*:1583, 1979.

Bartels, J. E.: Feline intravenous urography. J.A.A.H.A. *9*:349, 1973.

Baskin, G. B., and De Paoli, A.: Primary renal neoplasms of the dog. Vet. Pathol. *14*:591, 1977.

Bastl, C. P., Rudnick, M. R., and Narins, R. G.: Diagnostic Approaches to Acute Renal Failure. *In* Brenner, B. M., and Stein, J. H. (eds.): Contemporary Issues in Nephrology. Vol. 6. Acute Renal Failure. Churchill Livingstone, New York, 1980, p. 17.

Baylis, C., Rennke, H. R., and Brenner, B. M.: Mechanisms of the defect in glomerular ultrafiltration associated with gentamicin administration. Kidney Int. *12*:344, 1977.

Beckett, S. D., and Shields, R. P.: Treatment of acute ethylene glycol (antifreeze) toxicosis in the dog. J.A.V.M.A. *158*:472, 1971.

Bennett, W. M., Muther, R. S., Parker, R. A., Feig, P., Morrison, G., Golper, T. A., and Singer, I.: Drug therapy in renal failure: Dosing guidelines for adults. Part 1: Antimicrobial agents, analgesics. Ann. Intern. Med. *93*:62, 1980.

Bennett, W. M., Plamp, C. E., Gilbert, D. N., Parker, R. A., and Porter, G. A.: The influence of dosage regimen on experimental gentamicin nephrotoxicity: Dissociation of peak serum levels from renal failure. J. Infect. Dis. *140*:576, 1979.

Bergstrom, J., and Furst, P.: Uremic toxins. Kidney Int. *13*(suppl. 8):S–9, 1978.

Bernard, M. A., and Valli, V. E.: Familial renal disease in Samoyed dogs. Can. Vet. J. *18*:181, 1977.

Bidani, A., Churchill, P., and Fleischmann, L.: Sodium-chloride-induced protection in nephrotoxic acute renal failure: Independence from renin. Kidney Int. *16*:481, 1979.

Biery, D. N.: Upper Urinary Tract. *In* O'Brien, T. R. (ed.): Radiographic Diagnosis of Abdominal Disorders in the Dog and Cat. W. B. Saunders Co., Philadelphia, 1978.

Black, D. A. K., Rose, G., and Brewer, D. B.: Controlled trial of prednisone in adult patients with the nephrotic syndrome. Br. Med. J. *3*:421, 1970.

Blainey, J. D.: High protein diets in the treatment of the nephrotic syndrome. Clin. Sci. *13*:567, 1954.

Blantz, R. C.: The mechanism of acute renal failure after uranyl nitrate. J. Clin. Invest. *55*:621, 1975.

Blantz, R. C., and Wilson, C. B.: Acute effects of antiglomerular basement membrane antibody on the process of glomerular filtration in the rat. J. Clin. Invest. *58*:899, 1976.

Blantz, R. C., Hostetter, T. H., and Brenner, B. M.: Functional Adaptations of the Kidney to Immunological Injury. *In* Wilson, C. B., Brenner, B. M., and Stein, J. H. (eds.): Contemporary Issues in Nephrology, Vol. 3. Immunologic Mechanisms of Renal Disease. Churchill Livingstone, New York, 1979, p. 122.

Blantz, R. C., Tucker, B. J., and Wilson, C. B.: The acute effects of antiglomerular basement membrane antibody upon glomerular filtration in the rat. The influence of dose and complement depletion. J. Clin. Invest. *61*:910, 1978.

Bloch, K., Schoenheimer, R., and Rittenberg, D.: Rate of formation and disappearance of body creatinine in normal animals. J. Biol. Chem. *138*:155, 1941.

Bovee, K. C.: The uremic syndrome: Patient evaluation and treatment. Comp. Cont. Ed. Pract. Vet. *1*:279, 1979.

Bovee, K. C.: Relationship of dietary protein to renal function in dogs. Scientific Proceedings, American College of Veterinary Internal Medicine, Seattle, Washington, July 23, 1979a, p. 83.

Bovee, K. C.: What constitutes a low protein diet for dogs with chronic renal failure? J.A.A.H.A. *8*:246, 1972.

Bovee, K. C.: Chronic Interstitial Nephritis. *In* Kirk, R. W. (ed.): Current Veterinary Therapy IV. W. B. Saunders Co., Philadelphia, 1971, p. 719.

Bovee, K. C., and Joyce, T.: Clinical evaluation of glomerular function: 24-hour creatinine clearance in dogs. J.A.V.M.A. *174*:488, 1979.

Bovee, K. C., and Kronfeld, D. S.: Reduction of renal hemodynamics in uremic dogs fed reduced protein diets. J.A.A.H.A. *17*:277, 1981.

Bovee, K. C., Abt, D. A., and Kronfeld, D. S.: The effects of dietary protein intake on renal function in dogs with experimentally reduced renal function. J.A.A.H.A. *15*:9, 1979a.

Bovee, K. C., Joyce, T., Blazer-Yost, B., Goldschmidt, M. S., and Segal, S.: Characterization of renal defects in dogs with a syndrome similar to the Fanconi syndrome in man. J.A.V.M.A. *174*:1094, 1979b.

Bovee, K. C., Kronfeld, D. S., Ramberg, C., and Goldschmidt, M.: Long-term measurement of renal function in partially nephrectomized dogs fed 56, 27, or 19% protein. Invest. Urol. *16*:378, 1979c.

Bovee, K. C., Joyce, T., Reynolds, R., and Segal, S.: Spontaneous Fanconi syndrome in the dog. Metabolism *27*:45, 1978.

Bovee, K. C., Thier, S. O., Rea, C., and Segal, S.: Renal clearance of amino acids in canine cystinuria. Metabolism *23*:51, 1974.

Bown, P.: Glomerulonephritis in the dog: a clinical review. J. Small Anim. Pract. *18*:93, 1977.

Brenner, B. M., Bohrer, M. P., Baylis, C., and Deen, W. M.: Determinants of glomerular permselectivity: Insights derived from observations *in vivo*. Kidney Int. *12*:229, 1977.

Brenner, B. M., Hostetter, T. H., and Humes, H. D.: Molecular basis of proteinuria of glomerular origin. N. Engl. J. Med. *298*:826, 1978.

Bricker, N. S.: On the pathogenesis of the uremic state. An exposition of the "trade-off hypothesis." N. Engl. J. Med. *286*:1093, 1972.

Bricker, N. S., and Fine, L. A.: The trade-off hypothesis: Current status. Kidney Int., *13*(Suppl. 8):S–5, 1978.

Bricker, N. S., Orlowski, T., Kime, S. W., Jr., and Morrin, P. A. F.: Observations on the functional homogeneity of the nephron population in the chronically diseased kidney of the dog. J. Clin. Invest. *39*:1771, 1960.

Bricker, N. S., Schmidt, R. W., Favre, H., Fine, L., and Bourgoignie, J. J.: On the biology of sodium excretion: The search for a natriuretic hormone. Yale J. Biol. Med. *48*:293, 1975.

Brod, J.: Hypertension and renal parenchymal disease: Mechanisms and management. Cardiovasc. Clin. *9*:137, 1978.

Brodehl, J., and Krohn, H. P.: Steroid Trial in Frequently Relapsing Nephrotic Syndrome in Children. *In* Kluthe, R., Vogt, A., and Batsford, S. R. (eds.): Glomerulonephritis. International Conference on Pathogenesis, Pathology and Treatment. Georg Thieme Publishers, Stuttgart, 1976, p. 210.

Brodey, R. S., Medway, W., and Marshak, R. R.: Renal osteodystrophy in the dog. J.A.V.M.A. *139*:329, 1961.

Bullock, W. E., Luke, R. G., Nuttall, C. E., and Bhathena, D.: Can mannitol reduce amphotericin B nephrotoxicity? Double-blind study and description of a new vascular lesion in kidneys. Antimicrob. Agents Chemother. *10*:555, 1976.

Burk, R. L., and Barton, C. L.: Renal failure and hyperparathyroidism in an Alaska Malamute pup. J.A.V.M.A. *172*:69, 1978.

Burke, T. J., Cronin, R. E., Duchin, K. L., Peterson, L. N., and Schrier, R. W.: Ischemia and tubule obstruction during acute renal failure in dogs: mannitol in protection. Am. J. Physiol. *238*:F305, 1980.

Burrows, C. F., and Bovee, K. C.: Metabolic changes due to experimentally induced rupture of the canine urinary bladder. Am. J. Vet. Res. *35*:1083, 1974.

Cameron, J. S.: The Treatment of Severe Glomerulonephritis with Combined Immunosuppression and Anticoagulation. *In* Barcelo, R., et al. (eds.): Proc., Seventh International Congress of Nephrology. Basel, S. Karegar, Montreal, Canada, 1978, p. 419.

Carlson, G. P., and Kaneko, J. J.: Simultaneous estimation of renal function in dogs, using sodium sulfanilate and sodium iodohippurate [131]I. J.A.V.M.A. 158:1229, 1971.

Carlson, G. P., and Kaneko, J. J.: Sulfanilate clearance in clinical renal disease in the dog. J.A.V.M.A. 158:1235, 1971a.

Cartee, R. E., Selcer, B. A., and Patton, C. S.: Ultrasonographic diagnosis of renal disease in small animals. J.A.V.M.A. 176:426, 1980.

Carvalho, J. S., and Page, L. B.: Serial studies of the renin system in rats with glycerol-induced renal failure. Nephron 20:47, 1978.

Carvallo, A., Rakowski, T. A., Argy, W. P., and Schreiner, G. E.: Acute renal failure following drip infusion pyelography. Am. J. Med. 65:38, 1978.

Casey, H. W., and Splitter, G. A.: Membranous glomerulonephritis in dogs infected with Dirofilaria immitis. Vet. Pathol. 12:111, 1975.

Castaldi, P. A., Rozenberg, M. C., and Stewart, J. H.: The bleeding disorder of uraemia. A qualitiative platelet defect. Lancet 2:66, 1966.

Cattran, D. C., Fenton, S. S. A., Wilson, D. R., Oreopoulos, D., Shimizu, A., and Richardson, R. M.: A controlled trial on nandrolone decanoate in the treatment of uremic anemia. Kidney Int. 12:430, 1977.

Chan, R. A., Benner, E. J., and Hoeprich, P. D.: Gentamicin therapy in renal failure: A nomogram for dosage. Ann. Int. Med. 76:773, 1972.

Chandrankunnel, J. M., Saxanoff, S., Moss, S. W., Rosenzweig, P., Snyder, M., and Eisinger, R. P.: Effect of furosemide on acute renal failure in dogs. Induced by mercuric chloride. N. Y. State J. Med. 80:19, 1980.

Chew, D. J., and Capen, C. C.: Hypercalcemic Nephropathy and Associated Disorders. In Kirk, R. W. (ed.): Current Veterinary Therapy VII. Philadelphia, W. B. Saunders Co., 1980, p. 1067.

Christie, B. A.: Incidence and etiology of vesicoureteral reflux in apparently normal dogs. Invest. Urol. 9:184, 1971.

Coburn, J. W., Popvtzer, M. M., Massry, S. G., and Kleeman, C. R.: The physiochemical state and renal handling of divalent ions in chronic renal failure. Arch. Intern. Med. 124:302, 1969.

Cochrane, C. G.: Mediation Systems in Neutrophil-Independent Immunologic Injury of the Glomerulus. In Wilson, C. B., Brenner, B. M., and Stein, J. H. (eds.): Contemporary Issues in Nephrology, Vol. 3. Immunologic Mechanisms of Renal Disease. Churchill Livingstone, New York, 1979.

Coelho, J. B., and Bradley, S. E.: Function of the nephron population during hemorrhagic hypotension in the dog, with special reference to the effects of osmotic diuresis. J. Clin. Invest. 43:386, 1964.

Coggins, C. H.: A controlled study of short-term prednisone treatment in adults with membranous nephropathy. Collaborative study of the adult idiopathic nephrotic syndrome. N. Engl. J. Med. 301:1301, 1979.

Cohen, H. J., Lessin, L. S., Hallal, J., and Burkholder, P.: Resolution of primary amyloidosis during chemotherapy. Studies in a patient with nephrotic syndrome. Ann. Intern. Med. 82:466, 1975.

Conger, J. D., and Schrier, R. W.: Renal hemodynamics in acute renal failure. Ann. Rev. Physiol. 43:603, 1980.

Cordy, D. R.: Apocrine cystic calcinosis in dogs and its relationship to chronic renal disease. Cornell Vet. 57:107, 1967.

Cornelius, L. M.: Fluid therapy in small animal practice. J.A.V.M.A. 176:110, 1980.

Cotter, S. M., Hardy, W. D., and Essex, M.: Association of feline leukemia virus with lymphosarcoma and other disorders in the cat. J.A.V.M.A. 166:449, 1975.

Cowgill, L. D.: Acute Renal Failure. In Bovee, K. C. (ed.): Canine Nephrology. Year Book Medical Publishers, Chicago, 1982 (in press).

Cowgill, L. D.: Management of Oliguric and Anuric Renal Failure. In Kirk, R. W. (ed.): Current Veterinary Therapy VII. W. B. Saunders Co., Philadelphia, 1980a, p. 1087.

Cowgill, L. D.: Current Status of Veterinary Hemodialysis. In Kirk, R. W. (ed.): Current Veterinary Therapy VII. W. B. Saunders Co., Philadelphia, 1980, p. 1111.

Cowgill, L. D., and Bovee, K. C.: Current Status of Hemodialysis and Renal Transplantation. In Kirk, R. W. (ed.): Current Veterinary Therapy VI. W. B. Saunders Co., Philadelphia, 1977, p. 1149.

Cowgill, L. D., and Spangler, W. L.: Renal insufficiency in geriatric dogs. Vet. Clin. North Am. 11:727, 1981.

Cowgill, L. D., Clyma, A. B., and Johnson, D. L.: Renal glucosuria: An inherited disorder in the Norwegian Elkhound dog. In preparation, 1982.

Cox, J. W., Baehler, R. W., Sharma, H., O'Dorisio, T., Osgood, R. W., Stein, J. H., and Ferris, T. F.: Studies on the mechanisms of oliguria in a model of unilateral acute renal failure. J. Clin. Invest. 53:1546, 1974.

Cronin, R. E., de Torrente, A., Miller, P. D., Bulger, R. E., Burke, T. J., and Schrier, R. W.: Pathogenic mechanisms in early norepinephrine-induced acute renal failure: Functional and histological correlates of protection. Kidney Int. 14:115, 1978.

Crowell, W. A., and Finco, D. R.: Frequency of pyelitis, pyelonephritis, renal perivasculitis, and renal infarction in dogs. Am. J. Vet. Res. 36:111, 1975.

Crowell, W. A., Goldston, R. T., Schall, W. D., and Finco, D. R.: Generalized amyloidosis in a cat. J.A.V.M.A. 161:1127, 1972.

Cunha, T. J., et al.: Nutrient requirements of dogs, No. 8. Washington, D.C., National Academy of Sciences, 1974.

Dach, J. L., and Kurtzman, N. A.: A scanning electron microscopic study of the glycerol model of acute renal failure. Lab. Invest. 34:406, 1976.

Danovitch, G. M., Bourgoignie, J., and Bricker, N. S.: Reversibility of the "salt-losing" tendency of chronic renal failure. N. Engl. J. Med. 296:14, 1977.

Davis, L. E.: Drug Therapy in Renal Disorders. In Kirk, R. W. (ed.): Current Veterinary Therapy VII. W. B. Saunders Co., Philadelphia, 1980, p. 1114.

Deen, W. M., Brohrer, M. P., and Brenner, B. M.: Macromolecule transport across glomerular capillaries: Application of pore theory. Kidney Int. 16:353, 1979.

de Schepper, J., Hoorens, J., Mattheeuws, D., and Van Der Stock, J.: Glomerulo-nephritis and the nephrotic syndrome in a dog. Vet. Rec. 95:434, 1974.

De Torrente, A., Miller, P. D., Cronin, R. E., Paulsen, P. E., Erickson, A. L., and Schrier, R. W.: Effects of furosemide and acetylcholine in norepinephrine-induced acute renal failure. Am. J. Physiol. 235:F131, 1978.

DiBartola, S. P., Chew, D. J., and Jacobs, G.: Quantitative urinalysis including 24-hour protein excretion in the dog. J.A.A.H.A. *16*:537, 1980a.

DiBartola, S. P., Spaulding, G. L., Chew, D. J., and Lewis, R. M.: Urinary protein excretion and immunopathologic findings in dogs with glomerular disease. J.A.V.M.A. *177*:73, 1980b.

Dinarello, C. A., Wolf, S. M., Goldfinger, S. E., Dale, D. C., and Alling, D. W.: Colchicine therapy for familial Mediterranean fever. A double-blind trial. N. Engl. J. Med. *291*:934, 1974.

Dixon, F. J., and Cochrane, C. G.: The pathogenicity of antigen-antibody complexes. Pathol. Ann. *5*:355, 1970.

Doane, B. D., Fried, W., and Schwartz, F.: Response of uremic patients to nandrolone decanoate. Arch. Intern. Med. *135*:972, 1975.

Donadio, J. V., Holley, K. E., Ferguson, R. H., and Ilstrup, D. M.: Treatment of diffuse proliferative lupus nephritis with prednisone and combined prednisone and cyclophosphamide. N. Engl. J. Med. *299*:1151, 1978.

Donohoe, J. F., Venkatachalam, M. A., Bernard, D. B., and Levinsky, N. G.: Tubular leakage and obstruction in acute ischemic renal failure. Kidney Int. *10*:567, 1978.

Dossetor, J. B.: Creatininemia versus uremia. The relative significance of blood urea nitrogen and serum creatinine concentrations in azotemia. Ann. Intern. Med. *65*:1287, 1966.

Duncan, J. R., and Prasse, K. W.: Clinical examination of the urine. Vet. Clin. North Am. *6*:647, 1976.

Earle, D. P., Farber, S. J., Alexander, J. D., and Pellgrino, E. D.: Renal function and electrolyte metabolism in acute glomerulonephritis. J. Clin. Invest. *30*:421, 1951.

Earley, L. E., and Forland, M.: Nephrotic Syndrome. *In* Earley, L. E., and Gottschalk, C. W. (eds.): Strauss and Welt's Diseases of the Kidney, Third Ed., Vol. 1. Little, Brown and Company, Boston, 1979.

Easley, J. R., and Breitschwerdt, E. B.: Glucosuria associated with renal tubular dysfunction in three Basenji dogs. J.A.V.M.A. *168*:938, 1976.

Edney, A. T. B.: Observations on the effects of feeding a low protein diet to dogs with nephritis. J. Small Anim. Pract. *11*:281, 1970.

Ellis, H. A., and Walton, K. W.: Variations in serum complement in the nephrotic syndrome and other forms of renal disease. Immunology *1*:234, 1958.

English, P. B.: Acute renal failure in the dog and cat. Aust. Vet. J. *50*:384, 1974.

English, P. B., and Winter, H.: Renal cortical hypoplasia in a dog. Aust. Vet. J. *55*:181, 1979.

Erslev, A. J., and Shapiro, S. S.: Hematologic Aspects of Renal Failure. *In* Earley, L. E., and Gottschalk, C. W. (eds.): Strauss and Welt's Diseases of the Kidney, Vol. I, Third Ed. Little, Brown and Company, Boston, 1979.

Eschback, J. W., Harker, L. A., and Dale, D. C.: The Hematological Consequences of Renal Failure. *In* Brenner, B. M., and Rector, F. C. (eds.): The Kidney, Vol. II. W. B. Saunders Co., Philadelphia, 1976.

Espinel, C. H.: The FE_{Na} test. Use in the differential diagnosis of acute renal failure. J.A.M.A. *236*:579, 1976.

Espinel, C. H.: The influence of salt intake on the metabolic acidosis of chronic renal failure. J. Clin. Invest. *56*:286, 1975.

Espinel, C. H., and Gregory, A. W.: Differential diagnosis of acute renal failure. Clin. Nephrol. *13*:73, 1980.

Ettinger, S. J., and Feldman, E. C.: Ethylene glycol poisoning in a dog. Mod. Vet. Pract. *58*:237, 1977.

Ettinger, S. J., and Suter, P. F.: Canine Cardiology. W. B. Saunders Co., Philadelphia, 1970.

Farrow, B. R. H., Huxtable, C. R., and McGovern, V. J.: Nephrotic syndrome in the cat due to diffuse membranous glomerulonephritis. Pathology *1*:67, 1969.

Finco, D. R.: Simultaneous determination of phenolsulfonphthalein excretion and endogenous creatinine clearance in the normal dog. J.A.V.M.A. *159*:336, 1971.

Finco, D. R.: Congenital and inherited renal disease. J.A.A.H.A. *9*:301, 1973.

Finco, D. R.: Familial renal disease in Norwegian Elkhound dogs: Physiologic and biochemical examinations. Am. J. Vet. Res. *37*:87, 1976.

Finco, D. R.: Familial or Hereditary Chronic Nephritis. *In* Andrews, E. J., Ward, B. C., and Altman, N. H. (eds.): Spontaneous Animal Models of Human Disease, Vol. II. Academic Press, New York, 1979a, p. 274.

Finco, D. R.: Renal Agenesis. *In* Andrews, E. J., Ward, B. C., and Altman, N. H. (eds.): Spontaneous Animal Models of Human Disease, Vol. II. Academic Press, New York, 1979b, p. 267.

Finco, D. R.: Renal Hypoplasia. *In* Andrews, E. J., Ward, B. C., and Altman, N. H. (eds.): Spontaneous Animal Models of Human Disease, Vol. II. Academic Press, New York, 1979c, p. 273.

Finco, D. R.: Nutrition During the Uremic Crisis. *In* Kirk, R. W. (ed.): Current Veterinary Therapy VII. W. B. Saunders Co., Philadelphia, 1980, p. 1104.

Finco, D. R., and Barsanti, J. A.: Localization of urinary tract infection in the dog. Vet. Clin. North Am. *9*:775, 1979.

Finco, D. R., and Duncan, J. R.: Evaluation of blood urea nitrogen and serum creatinine concentrations as indicators of renal dysfunction: A study of 111 cases and a review of related literature. J.A.V.M.A. *168*:593, 1976.

Finco, D. R., and Low, D. G.: Intensive diuresis in polyuric renal failure. *In* Kirk, R. W. (ed.): Current Veterinary Therapy VII. W. B. Saunders Co., Philadelphia, 1980, p. 1091.

Finco, D. R., Duncan, J. R., Crowell, W. A., and Hulsey, M. L.: Familial renal disease in Norwegian Elkhound dogs: Morphologic examinations. Am. J. Vet. Res. *38*:941, 1977.

Finco, D. R., Stiles, N. S., Kneller, S. K., Lewis, R. E., and Barrett, R. B.: Radiologic estimation of kidney size of the dog. J.A.V.M.A. *159*:995, 1971.

Finco, D. R., Kurtz, H. J., Low, D. G., and Perman, V.: Familial renal disease in Norwegian Elkhound dogs. J.A.V.M.A. *156*:747, 1970.

Finco, D. R., Shotts, E. B., and Crowell, W. A.: Evaluation of methods for localization of urinary tract infection in the female dog. Am. J. Vet. Res. *40*:707, 1979.

Finn, W. F.: Acute Renal Failure. *In* Earley, L. E., and Gottschalk, C. W. (eds.): Strauss and Welt's Diseases of the Kidney. Third Edition, Vol. I. Little, Brown and Company, Boston, 1979, p. 167.

Fish, A. J., and Michael, A. F.: Immunopathogenesis of Renal Disease. *In* Earley, L. E., and Gottschalk, C. W. (eds.): Strauss and Welt's Diseases of the Kidney, Third Edition, Vol. I, Little, Brown and Company, Boston, 1979, p. 541.

Fisher, J. W.: Mechanism of the anemia of chronic renal failure. Nephron *25*:106, 1980.

Flamenbaum, W.: Pathophysiology of acute renal failure. Arch. Intern. Med. *131*:911, 1973.

Flamenbaum, W.: Pathophysiology of Acute Renal Failure. *In* Kurtzman, N. A., and Martinez-Maldonado, M. (eds.): Pathophysiology of the Kidney. Charles C Thomas, Springfield, Ill. 1977, p. 795.

Flamenbaum, W., Hamburger, R., and Kaufman, J.: Distal tubule [Na⁺] and juxtaglomerular apparatus renin activity in uranyl nitrate induced acute renal failure in the rat. An evaluation of the role of tubuloglomerular feedback. Pfluegers. Arch. *364*:209, 1976.

Flamenbaum, W., Huddleston, M. L., McNeil, J. S., and Hamburger, R. J.: Uranyl nitrate-induced acute renal failure in the rat: Micropuncture and renal hemodynamic studies. Kidney Int. *6*:408, 1974.

Flamenbaum, W., NcNeil, J. S., Kotchen, T. A., and Saladino, A. J.: Experimental acute renal failure induced by uranyl nitrate in the dog. Circ. Res. *31*:682, 1972.

Flores, J., DiBona, D. R., Beck, C. H., and Leaf, A.: The role of cell swelling in ischemic renal damage and the protective effect of hypertonic solute. J. Clin. Invest. *51*:118, 1972.

Ford, J., Phillips, M. E., Toye, F. E., Luck, V. A., and de Wardener, H. E.: Nitrogen balance in patients with chronic renal failure on diets containing varying quantities of protein. Br. Med. J. *1*:735, 1969.

Francis, D. P., Essex, M., Jakowski, R. M., Cotter, S. M., Lerer, T. J., and Hardy, W. D.: Increased risk for lymphoma and glomerulonephritis in a closed population of cats exposed to feline leukemia virus. Am. J. Epidemiol. *111*:337, 1980.

Freedman, L. R.: Interstitial Renal Inflammation, Including Pyelonephritis and Urinary Tract Infection. *In* Earley, L. E., and Gottschalk, C. W. (eds.): Strauss and Welt's Diseases of the Kidney. Third Edition Vol. II. Little, Brown and Company, Boston, 1979, p. 817.

Freedman, L. R., and Beeson, P. B.: Experimental pyelonephritis: IV. Observations on infections resulting from direct inoculation of bacteria in different zones of the kidney. Yale J. Biol. Med. *30*:406, 1958.

Frega, N. S., DiBona, D. R., and Leaf, A.: The protection of renal function from ischemic injury in the rat. Pfluegers Arch. *381* :159, 1979.

Freis, E. D., et al.: Effects of treatment on morbidity in hypertension. Results in patients with diastolic blood pressures averaging 115 through 129 mmHg. J.A.M.A. *202*:1028, 1967.

Freis, E. D., et al.: Effects of treatment on morbidity in hypertension. II. Results in patients with diastolic blood pressure averaging 90 through 114 mmHg. J.A.M.A. *213*:1143, 1970.

Freundlich, J. J., Detweiler, D. K., and Hance, H. E.: Indirect blood pressure determination by the ultrasonic Doppler technique in dogs. Curr. Ther. Res. *14*:73, 1972.

Fronlich, E. D.: Pathophysiology of Hypertension. *In* Kurtzman, N. A., and Martinez-Maldonado, M. (eds.): Pathophysiology of the Kidney. Charles C Thomas, Springfield, Ill., 1977, p. 881.

Gantt, C. L.: Drug therapy of hypertension. Med. Clin. North Am. *62*:1273, 1978.

Garner, H. E., Hahn, A. W., Hartley, J. W., Hutcheson, D. P., and Coffman, J. R.: Indirect blood pressure measurement in the dog. Lab. Anim. Sci. *25*:197, 1975.

German Glomerulonephritis Research Group. *In* Kluthe, R., Vogt, A., and Batsford, S. R. (eds.): Glomerulonephritis. International Conference on Pathogenesis, Pathology and Treatment. Freiburg, June 1976. Georg Thieme Publishers, Stuttgart, 1976, p. 174.

Germuth, F. G., and Rodriguez, E: *Immunopathology of the Renal Glomerulus.* Little, Brown and Co., Boston, 1973.

Germuth, F. G., Keleman, W. A., and Pollack, A. D.: Immune complex disease II. The role of circulatory dynamics and glomerular filtration in the development of experimental glomerulonephritis. Johns Hopkins Med. J. *120*:252, 1967.

Gimenez, L., Tew, W., Hermann, J., and Walker, W. G.: Prevention of phosphate induced nephrocalcinosis in experimental renal insufficiency by phosphocitrate. Kidney Int. *19*:110, 1981.

Giovannetti, S., and Maggiore, Q.: A low-nitrogen diet with proteins of high biological value for severe chronic uraemia. Lancet *1*:1000, 1964.

Giovannetti, S., Cioni, L., Balestri, P. L., and Biagini, M.: Evidence that guanidines and some related compounds cause haemolysis in chronic uraemia. Clin. Sci. *34*:141, 1968.

Glassock, R. J.: Clinical Aspects of Acute, Rapidly Progressive, and Chronic Glomerulonephritis. *In* Earley, L. E., and Gottschalk, C. W. (eds.): Strauss and Welt's Diseases of the Kidney. Third ed. Vol. I. Little, Brown and Company, Boston, 1979, p. 691.

Glassock, R. J., Kalmanson, G. M., and Guze, L. B.: Pyelonephritis. XVIII. Effect of treatment on the pathology of enterococcal pyelonephritis in the rat. Am. J. Pathol. *76*:49, 1974.

Glenner, G. G.: Amyloid deposits and amyloidosis. The β-fibrilloses. (First of two parts). N. Engl. J. Med. *302*:1283, 1980.

Glenner, G. G., Ein, D., and Terry, W. D.: The immunoglobin origin of amyloid. Am. J. Med. *52*:141, 1972.

Glick, A. D., Horn, R. G., and Holscher, M.: Characterization of feline glomerulonephritis associated with viral-induced hematopoietic neoplasms. Am. J. Pathol. *92*:321, 1978.

Goldman, R.: Aging of the Excretory System: Kidney and Bladder. *In* Finch, E. E., and Hayflick, L. (eds.): Handbook of the Biology of Aging. Van Nostrand Reinhold Co., New York, 1977.

Gorshein, D., Murphy, S., and Gardner, F. H.: Comparative study on the erythropoietic effects of androgens and their mode of action. J. Appl. Physiol. *35*:376, 1973.

Gourley, I. M. G.: Prevention and treatment of acute renal failure in the canine surgical patient. J.A.V.M.A. *157*:1722, 1970.

Grollman, E. F., and Grollman, A.: Toxicity of urea and its role in the pathogenesis of uremia. J. Clin. Invest. *38*:749, 1959.

Gulyassy, P. F., Avirman, A., and Peters, J. H.: Evaluation of amino acid and protein requirements in chronic uremia. Arch. Intern. Med. *126*:855, 1970.

Hamilton, W. F., Pund, E. R., Slaughter, R. F., Simpson, W. A., Colson, G. M., Coleman, H. W., and Bateman, W. H.: Blood pressure values in street dogs. Am. J. Physiol. *128*:233, 1940.

Hardy, R. M., and Osborne, C. A.: Water deprivation

test in the dog: Maximal normal values. J.A.V.M.A. *174*:479, 1979.

Hardy, W. D.: Immunology of oncornaviruses. Vet. Clin. North Am. *4*:133, 1974.

Hart, R.: Anesthesia for the Patient in Renal Failure. *In* Sattler, F. P., Knowles, R. P., and Whittick, W. G. (eds.): Veterinary Critical Care. Lea & Febiger, Philadelphia, 1981, p. 228.

Haskins, S. C.: Anesthetic management for the end-stage renal failure patient. Calif. Vet. *33*(6):13, 1979.

Hatcher, C. R., Gagnon, J. A., and Clarke, R. W.: The effects of hydration on epinephrine-induced renal shutdown in dogs. Surgical Forum *9*:106, 1958.

Haut, L. L., Alfrey, A. C., Guggenheim, S., Buddington, B., and Schrier, N.: Renal toxicity of phosphate in rats. Kidney Int. *17*:722, 1980.

Hayes, H. M., and Fraumeni, J. F., Jr.: Epidemiological features of canine renal neoplasms. Cancer Res. *37*:2553, 1977.

Hayslett, J. P.: Functional adaptation to reduction in renal mass. Physiol. Rev. *59*:137, 1979.

Hellebusch, A. A., Salama, F., and Eadie, E.: The use of mannitol to reduce the nephrotoxicity of amphotericin B. Surg. Gynecol. Obst. *134*:241, 1972.

Heller, J., Horecek, V., and Hollyova, J.: Comparison of inulin and creatinine clearance in dogs after unilateral nephrectomy. Nephron *25*:299, 1980.

Hendler, E. D., Goffinet, J. A., Ross, S., Longnecker, R. E., and Bakovic, V.: Controlled study of androgen therapy in anemia of patients on maintenance hemodialysis. N. Engl. J. Med. *291*:1046, 1974.

Heptinstall, R. H.: Idiopathic Membranous, Membranoproliferative, and Lobular Glomerulonephritis. *In* Heptinstall, R. H. (ed.): Pathology of the Kidney. 2nd Ed. Vol. 1. Little, Brown and Company, Boston, 1974, p. 393.

Hiatt, N., and Sheinkopf, J. A.: Treatment of experimental hyperkalemia with large dosages of insulin. Surg. Gynecol. Obstet. *133*:833, 1971.

Highman, B., Roshe, J., and Altand, P. D.: Endocarditis and glomerulonephritis in dogs with aortic insufficiency. Production by a single bacterial inoculation and effect of cortisone. Arch. Pathol. *65*:388, 1958.

Himori, N., Ishimori, T., Izumi, A., Hisatomi, M., and Hayakawa, S.: Antihypertensive effects of a combination of a diuretic and a β-adrenoceptor blocking agent in conscious, renal hypertensive dogs. Jpn. J. Pharmacol. *28*:811, 1978.

Hoff, H. E., Smith, P. K., and Winkler, A. W.: The cause of death in experimental anuria. J. Clin. Invest. *20*:607, 1941.

Hogg, A. H.: Osteodystrophic disease in the dog, with special reference to rubber jaw (renal osteodystrophy) and its comparison with renal rickets in the human. Vet. Rec. *60*:117, 1948.

Holmes, J. R.: A radiological study of the digits in renal osteodystrophy in the dog. Vet. Rec. *69*:642, 1957.

Holtzapple, P. G., Bovee, K. C., Rea, C. F., and Segal, S.: Amino acid uptake by kidney and jejunal tissue from dogs with cystine stones. Science *166*:1525, 1969.

Hopper, J., Jr.: Membranous glomerulonephritis. Ann. Intern. Med. *79*:285, 1973.

Horowitz, H. I., Stein, I. M., Cohen, B. D., and White, J. G.: Further studies on the platelet-inhibitory effect of guanidinosuccinic acid and its role in uremic bleeding. Am. J. Med. *49*:336, 1970.

Hostetter, T. H., Wilkes, B. M., and Brenner, B. M.: Mechanisms of Impaired Glomerular Filtration in Acute Renal Failure. *In* Brenner, B. M., and Stein, J. H. (eds.): Contemporary Issues in Nephrology, Vol. 6. Acute Renal Failure. Churchill Livingstone, New York, 1980, p. 52.

Hottendorf, G. H., and Nielsen, S. W.: Pathologic report of 29 necropsies on dogs with mastocytoma. Pathol. Vet. *5*:102, 1968.

Hudson, E. B., and Strombeck, D. R.: Effects of functional nephrectomy on the disappearance rates of canine serum amylase and lipase. Am. J. Vet. Res. *39*:1316, 1978.

Husted, F. C., Kolph, K. D., and Maher, J. F.: $NaHCO_3$ and NaCl tolerance in chronic renal failure. J. Clin. Invest. *56*:414, 1975.

Ibels, L. S., Alfrey, A. C., Haut, L., and Huffer, W. E.: Preservation of function in experimental renal disease by dietary restriction of phosphate. N. Engl. J. Med. *298*:122, 1978.

Isobe, T., and Osserman, E. F.: Effects of Dimethyl Sulfoxide (DMSO) on Bence Jones Proteins, Amyloid Fibrils and Casein-Induced Amyloidosis. *In* Wegelius, O., and Pasternack, A. (eds.): Amyloidosis. Proceedings of the Fifth Sigrid Juselius Foundation Symposium. Academic Press, London, 1976.

Jacob, A. I., Lambert, P. W., Canterbury, J. M., Gavellas, G., and Bourgoignie, J. J.: Further studies with cimetidine in uremic dogs. Kidney Int. *19*:111, 1981.

Jacob, A. I., Lanier, D., Canterbury, J., and Bourgoignie, J. J.: Reduction by cimetidine of serum parathyroid hormone levels in uremic patients. N. Engl. J. Med. *302*:671, 1980.

Jakob, W.: Spontaneous amyloidosis of mammals. Vet. Pathol. *8*:292, 1971.

Johnson, C. A.: Renal ectopia in a cat: A case report and literature review. J.A.A.H.A. *15*:599, 1979.

Jonsson, L., and Rubarth, S.: Ethylene glycol poisoning in dogs and cats. Nord. Vet. Med. *19*:265, 1967.

Joske, R. A., McAlister, J. M., and Prankerd, T. A. J.: Isotope investigations of red cell production and destruction in chronic renal disease. Clin. Sci. *15*:511, 1956.

Kaplan, M. A., Canterbury, J. M., Bourgoignie, J. J., Veliz, G., Gavellas, G., Reiss, E., and Bricker, N. S.: Reversal of hyperparathyroidism in response to dietary phosphorus restriction in the uremic dog. Kidney Int. *15*:43, 1979.

Kasanen, A., and Kalliomaki, J. L.: Correlation of some kidney function tests with hemoglobin in chronic nephropathies. Acta Med. Scand. *158*:213, 1957.

Kashgarian, M., Hayslett, J. P., and Spargo, B. H.: Renal disease. Am. J. Pathol. *89*:187, 1977.

Kassirer, J. P.: Clinical evaluation of kidney function and glomerular function. N. Engl. J. Med. *285*:385, 1971.

Katz, J. I., Skom, J. H., and Wakerlin, G. E.: Pathogenesis of spontaneous and pyelonephritic hypertension in the dog. Circ. Res. *5*:137, 1957.

Kaufman, C. F., Soirez, R. F., and Tasker, J. P.: Renal cortical hypoplasia with secondary hyperparathyroidism in the dog. J.A.V.M.A. *155*:1679, 1969.

Kaufman, J. M., Hardy, R., and Hayslett, J. P.: Age-dependent characteristics of compensatory renal growth. Kidney Int. *8*:21, 1975.

Kersting, E. J., and Nielsen, S. W.: Ethylene glycol poisoning in small animals. J.A.V.M.A. *146*:113, 1965.

Keutmann, E. H., and Bassett, S. H.: Dietary protein in

hemorrhagic Bright's disease. II. The effect of diet on serum proteins, proteinuria and tissue proteins. J. Clin. Invest. *14*:871, 1935.

Kincaid-Smith, P.: The treatment of chronic mesangiocapillary (membranoproliferative) glomerulonephritis with impaired renal function. Med. J. Aust. *59*(2):587, 1972.

Klopfer, U., Nobel, T. A., and Kaminski, R.: A nephropathy similar to renal cortical hypoplasia in a Yorkshire terrier. VM SAC *73*:327, 1978.

Klausner, J. S., and Osborne, C. A.: Urinary tract infection and urolithiasis. Vet. Clin. North Am. *9*:701, 1979.

Kleinknecht, C., Salusky, I., Broyer, M., and Gubler, M. C.: Effect of various protein diets on growth, renal function, and survival of uremic rats. Kidney Int. *15*:534, 1979.

Kneller, S. K.: Role of excretory urogram in the diagnosis of renal and ureteral disease. Vet. Clin. North Am. *4*:843, 1974.

Kopple, J. D.: Nutritional management of chronic renal failure. Post Grad. Med. *64*(5):135, 1978.

Kopple, J. D.: Nitrogen Metabolism. *In* Massry, S. A., and Sellers, A. L. (eds.): Clinical Aspects of Uremia and Dialysis. Charles C Thomas, Springfield, Ill., 1976.

Kopple, J. D., and Coburn, J. W.: Evaluation of chronic uremia. Importance of serum urea nitrogen, serum creatinine, and their ratio. J.A.M.A. *227*:41, 1974.

Kopple, J. D., and Swendseid, M. E.: Amino acid and keto acid diets for therapy in renal failure. Nephron *18*:1, 1977.

Kraikitpanitch, S., Lindeman, R. D., Yunice, A. A., Baxter, D. J., Haygood, C. C., and Blue, M. M.: Effects of azotemia on the myocardial accumulation of calcium. Mineral Electrolyte Metab. *1*:12, 1978.

Krakowka, S.: Glomerulonephritis in dogs and cats. Vet. Clin. North Am. *8*:629, 1978.

Krane, S. M.: Renal Glycosuria. *In* Stanbury, J. B., Wyngaarden, J. B., and Fredrickson, D. S. (eds.): The Metabolic Basis of Inherited Disease, 4th Edition. McGraw-Hill Book Company, New York, 1979.

Krohn, K., Mero, M., Oksanen, A., and Sandholm, M.: Immunologic observations in canine interstitial nephritis. Am. J. Pathol. *65*:157, 1971.

Kronfeld, D. S.: Nature and Use of Commercial Dog Foods. *In* Kronfeld, D. S., and Low, D. G. (eds.): Diet and Disease in Dogs. Proceedings of the Second Conference on Canine Nutrition, University of California, Irvine, California. November, 1975, p. 20.

Krook, L.: The pathology of renal cortical hypoplasia in the dog. Nord. Vet. Med. *9*:161, 1957.

Kurtz, J. M., Russell, S. W., Lee, J. C., Slauson, D. O., and Schechter, R. D.: Naturally occurring canine glomerulonephritis. Am. J. Pathol. *67*:471, 1972.

Kurtz, T. W., and Hsu, C. H.: Systemic hemodynamics in nephrotoxic acute renal failure. Nephron *21*:100, 1978.

Lage, A. L.: Cystinuria and Cystine Urolithiasis. *In* Kirk, R. W. (ed.): Current Veterinary Therapy VII. W. B. Saunders Co., Philadelphia, 1980.

Lage, A. L.: Hematuria, a clinical approach: Its meaning and differential diagnosis in the dog and cat. Small Animal Vet. Med. Update series. No. 15, 1978.

Landis, E. M., Elsom, K. A., Bott, P. A., and Shiels, E.: Observations on sodium chloride restriction and urea clearance in renal insufficiency. J. Clin. Invest. *14*:525, 1935.

Larkin, H. A., Lucke, V. M., and Kidder, D. E.:

Nephrotic syndrome in a dog. J. Small Anim. Pract. *13*:333, 1972.

Legendre, A. M., and Dade, A. W.: Calcinosis circumscripta in a dog. J.A.V.M.A. *164*:1192, 1974.

Leiter, L.: Observations on the relationship of urea to uremia. Arch. Intern. Med. *28*:331, 1921.

Levinsky, N. G., Alexander, E. A., and Venkatachalam, M. A.: Acute Renal Failure. *In* Brenner, B. M., and Rector, F. C. (eds.): The Kidney, 2nd ed. Vol. 1. W. B. Saunders Co., Philadelphia, 1981.

Lewis, R. J.: Canine glomerulonephritis: Results from a microscopic evaluation of fifty cases. Can. Vet. J. *17*:171, 1976.

Lewis, R. L.: Spontaneous Autoimmune Diseases of Domestic Animals. *In* Richter, G. W., and Epstein, M. A. (eds.): International Review of Experimental Pathology. Vol. 13. New York, Academic Press, 1974.

Lewis, R. M., Andre-Schwartz, J., Harris, G. S., Hirsch, M. S., Black, P. H., and Schwartz, R. S.: Canine systemic lupus erythematosus. Transmission of serologic abnormalities by cell-free filtrates. J. Clin. Invest. *52*:1893, 1973.

Lindner, A., Cutler, R. E., and Goodman, W. G.: Synergism of dopamine plus furosemide in preventing acute renal failure in the dog. Kidney Int. *16*:158, 1979.

Ling, G. V.: Treatment of urinary tract infections. Vet. Clin. North Am. *9*:795, 1979.

Ling, G. V.: Antipubic cystocentesis in the dog: An aseptic technique for routine collection of urine. Calif. Vet. *30*(8):50, 1976.

Ling, G. V., and Kaneko, J. J.: Microscopic examination of canine urine sediment. Calif. Vet. *30*(10):14, 1976.

Ling, G. V., Biberstein, E. L., and Hirsh, D. C.: Bacterial pathogens associated with urinary tract infections. Vet. Clin. North Am. *9*:617, 1979.

Loge, J. P., Lange, R. D., and Moore, C. V.: Characterization of the anemia associated with chronic renal insufficiency. Am. J. Med. *24*:4, 1958.

Low, D. G.: Medical Management of Polyuric Renal Failure: Anabolic Agents. *In* Kirk, R. W. (ed.): Current Veterinary Therapy VII. W. B. Saunders Co., Philadelphia, 1980, p. 1102.

Low, D. G.: Creatinine clearance as an estimation of glomerular filtration rate. Calif. Vet. *32*(7):8, 1978.

Low, D. G.: Chronic Interstitial Nephritis. *In* Kirk, R. W. (ed.): Current Veterinary Therapy VI. W. B. Saunders Co., Philadelphia, 1977, p. 1129.

Lowenstein, J., and Gallo, G.: Remission of the nephrotic syndrome in renal amyloidosis. N. Engl. J. Med. *282*:128, 1970.

Lowenstein, L. M.: The rat as a model for aging in the kidney. *In* Gibson, D. C., Adelman, R. C., and Finch, C. (eds.): Development of the Rodent as a Model System of Aging. U.S. Department of Health, Education and Welfare, Washington, D.C., 1978, p. 233.

Lucke, V. M., and Kelly, D. F.: Renal carcinoma in the dog. Vet. Pathol. *13*:264, 1976.

MacEwen, E. G.: Canine Lymphosarcoma. *In* Kirk, R. W. (ed.): Current Veterinary Therapy VII. W. B. Saunders Co., Philadelphia, 1980, p. 419.

MacEwen, E. G., and Siegel, S. D.: Hypercalcemia: A paraneoplastic disease. Vet. Clin. North Am. 7:187, 1977.

Mackey, L.: Feline leukaemia virus and its clinical effects in cats. Vet. Rec. *96*:5, 1975.

Madewell, B. R.: Chemotherapy for canine lymphosarcoma. Am. J. Vet. Res. *36*:1525, 1975.

Madewell, B. R., and Feldman, B. F.: Characterization

of anemias associated with neoplasia in small animals. J.A.V.M.A. *176*:419, 1980.

Maher, J. F.: Toxin Nephropathy. *In* Brenner, B. M., and Rector, F. C. (eds.): The Kidney. 2nd ed. Vol. II. W. B. Saunders Co., Philadelphia, 1976.

Martinez-Maldonado, M., and Opava-Stitzer, S.: Pathophysiology of Clinical Disorders of Urine Concentration and Dilution. *In* Kurtzman, N. A., and Martinez-Maldonado, M. (eds.): Pathophysiology of the Kidney. Charles C Thomas, Springfield, Ill., 1977, p. 992.

Maschio, G., Tessitore, N., D'Angelo, A., Bonnucci, E., Lupo, A., Valvo, E., Loschiavo, C., Fabris, A., Morachiello, P., Previato, G., and Fiaschi, E.: Early dietary phosphorus restriction and calcium supplementation in the prevention of renal osteodystrophy. Am. J. Clin. Nutr. *33*:1546, 1980.

Mason, J.: Tubulo-glomerular feedback in the early states of experimental acute renal failure. Kidney Int. *10*:S–106, 1976.

Mason, J., Olbricht, C., Takabatake, T., and Thruau, K.: The early phase of experimental acute renal failure. I. Intratubular pressure and obstruction. Pfluegers Arch. *370*:155, 1977.

Mason, J., Takabatake, T., Olbricht, C., and Thruau, K.: The early phase of experimental acute renal failure. III. Tubuloglomerular feedback. Pfluegers Arch. *373*:69, 1978.

Massry, S. G.: Requirements of vitamin D metabolites in patients with renal disease. Am. J. Clin. Nutr. *33*:1530, 1980.

Mathew, O. P., Jones, A. S., James, E., Bland, H., and Groshong, T.: Neonatal renal failure: Usefulness of diagnostic indices. Pediatrics *65*:57, 1980.

Mauk, R. H., Patak, R. V., Fadem, S. Z., Lifschitz, M. D., and Stein, J. H.: Effect of prostaglandin E administration in a nephrotoxic and vasoconstrictor model of acute renal failure. Kidney Int. *12*:122, 1977.

McAdams, A. J., McEnery, P. T., and West, C. D.: Mesangiocapillary glomerulonephritis: Changes in glomerular morphology with long-term alternate-day prednisone therapy. J. Pediatr. *86*:23, 1975.

McCubbin, J. W., and Corcoran, A. C.: Arterial pressures in street dogs: Incidence and significance of hypertension. Soc. Exp. Biol. Med. *84*:130, 1953.

McGill, H. C., Geer, J. C., Strong, J. P., and Holman, L. L.: Two forms of necrotizing arteritis in dogs related to diet and renal insufficiency. Arch. Pathol. *65*:66, 1958.

Merrill, J. P.: Glomerulonephritis (first of three parts). N. Engl. J. Med. *290*:257, 1974.

Michell, A. R.: The pathophysiological basis of fluid therapy in small animals. Vet. Rec. *104*:542, 1979.

Miller, T. R., Anderson, R. J., Linas, S. L., Henrich, W. L., Berns, A. S., Gabow, P. A., and Schrier, R. W.: Urinary diagnostic indices in acute renal failure. A prospective study. Ann. Int. Med. *89*:47, 1978.

Mohring, K., and Madsen, P. O.: The effect of dextrans, furosemide, and heparin on renal function changes caused by hemolysis in the dog. Invest. Urol. *10*:404, 1973.

Monlux, A. W.: The histopathology of nephritis of the dog. I. Introduction; II. Inflammatory interstitial diseases. Am. J. Vet. Res. *14*:425, 1953.

Morris, M. L.: Feeding tips for sick pets. Scientific Proceedings, 47th Annual Meeting of the American Animal Hospital Association, Los Angeles, California, April 19–25, 1980, p. 293.

Morris, M. L.: Phosphorus: The deadly element in renal failure. Scientific Proceedings, 47th annual meeting of the American Animal Hospital Association, Los Angeles, California, April 19–25, 1980, p. 171.

Morris, M. L., and Doering, G. G.: Dietary management of chronic renal failure in dogs. Canine Practice *5*(1):46, 1978.

Morrison, W. I., Nash, A. S., and Wright, N. G.: Glomerular deposition of immune complexes in dogs following natural infection with canine adenovirus. Vet. Rec. *96*:522, 1975.

Morrison, W. I., and Wright, N. G.: Detection of immune complexes in the serum of dogs infected with canine adenovirus. Res. Vet. Sci. *21*:119, 1976.

Mueller, T. M., Marcus, M. L., Kerber, R. E., Young, J. A., Barnes, R. W., and Abboud, F. M.: Effect of renal hypertension and left ventricular hypertrophy on the coronary circulation in dogs. Circ. Res. *42*:543, 1978.

Muirhead, E. E., Turner, L. B., and Grollman, A.: Hypertensive cardiovascular disease. (Nature and pathogenesis of the arteriolar sclerosis induced by bilateral nephrectomy as revealed by a study of its tinctorial characteristics.) Arch. Pathol. *52*:266, 1951.

Muller-Peddinghaus, R., and Trautwein, G.: Spontaneous glomerulonephritis in dogs. II. Correlation of glomerulonephritis with age, chronic interstitial nephritis and extrarenal lesions. Vet. Pathol. *14*:121, 1977.

Muller-Peddinghaus, R., and Trautwein, G.: Spontaneous glomerulonephritis in dogs. I. Classification and immunopathology. Vet. Pathol. *14*:1, 1977a.

Murray, M., and Wright, N. G.: A morphologic study of canine glomerulonephritis. Lab. Invest. *30*:213, 1974.

Nash, A. S., Wright, N. G., Spencer, A. J., Thompson, H., and Fisher, E. W.: Membranous nephropathy in the cat: A clinical and pathological study. Vet. Rec. *105*:71, 1979.

Newman, L. B., Bucy, J. G., and McAlister, W. H.: Incidence of naturally occurring vesicoureteral reflux in mongrel dogs. Invest. Radiol. *8*:354, 1973.

Newman, L. B., Schulman, C. C., and Bucy, J. G.: Vesicoureteral reflux in the dog. A histologic and radiologic evaluation. Invest. Urol. *11*:496, 1974.

Norrdin, R. W., Phemister, R. D., Jaenke, R. S., and Lo Presti, C. A.: Density and composition of trabecular and cortical bone in perinatally irradiated beagles with chronic renal failure. Calcif. Tis. Res. *24*:99, 1977.

Obel, A-L., Nicander, L., and Asheim, A.: Light and electron microscopical studies of the renal lesion in dogs with pyometra. Acta Vet. Scand. *5*:146, 1964.

O'Connell, J. M. B., Romeo, J. A., and Mudge, G. A.: Renal tubular secretion of creatinine in the dog. Am. J. Physiol. *203*:985, 1962.

O'Handley, P., Carrig, C. B., and Walshaw, R.: Renal and ureteral duplication in a dog. J.A.V.M.A. *174*:484, 1979.

Ohno, Y., and Fisher, J. W.: Inhibition of bone marrow erythroid colony forming cells (CFU-E) by serum from chronic anemic uremic rabbits. Proc. Soc. Exp. Biol. Med. *156*:56, 1977.

Oken, D. E.: Role of prostaglandins in the pathogenesis of acute renal failure. Lancet *1*:1319, 1975.

Oken, D. E., Cotes, S. C., Flamenbaum, W., Powell-Jackson, J. D., and Lever, A.: Active and passive immunization to angiotensin in experimental acute renal failure. Kidney Int. 7:12, 1975.

Olivero, J. J., Lozano-Mendez, J., Ghafary, E. M., Eknoyan, G., and Suki, W. N.: Mitigation of amphotericin B nephrotoxicity by mannitol. Brit. Med. J. 8:181, 1975.

Osborne, C. A., and Jeraj, K.: Glomerulonephropathy and the Nephrotic Syndrome. In Kirk, R. W. (ed.): Current Veterinary Therapy VII. W. B. Saunders Co., Philadelphia, 1980.

Osborne, C. A., and Johnson, K. H.: End-stage kidneys in dogs and cats. J.A.A.H.A. 6:174, 1970.

Osborne, C. A., and Klausner, J. S.: Adverse Drug Reactions in Uremic Patients. In Kirk, R. W. (ed.): Current Veterinary Therapy VI. W. B. Saunders Co., Philadelphia, 1977.

Osborne, C. A., and Low, D. G.: The application of principles of fluid and electrolyte therapy to patients with renal failure. J.A.A.H.A. 8:181, 1972.

Osborne, C. A., and Polzin, D. J.: Strategy in the diagnosis, prognosis and management of renal disease, renal failure, and uremia. Scientific proceedings of the 46th Annual Meeting of the American Animal Hospital Association, New Orleans, Louisiana, April 21–27, 1979, pp. 559–619.

Osborne, C. A., and Stevens, J. B.: Pseudohyperparathyroidism in the dog. J.A.V.M.A. 162:125, 1973.

Osborne, C. A., and Stevens, J. B.: Hypercalcemic Nephropathy. In Kirk, R. W. (ed.): Current Veterinary Therapy VI. W. B. Saunders Co., Philadelphia, 1977.

Osborne, C. A., Finco, D. R., and Low, D. G.: Renal Failure: Diagnosis, Treatment and Prognosis. In Ettinger, S. J. (ed.): Textbook of Veterinary Internal Medicine: Disease of the Dog and Cat, Vol. 2, First Ed. W. B. Saunders Co., Philadelphia, 1975.

Osborne, C. A., Hammer, R. F., Stevens, J. B., O'Leary, T. P., and Resnick, J. S.: Immunologic aspects of glomerular disease in the dog and cat. Proc., 26th Gaines Veterinary Symposium, Columbus, Ohio, Oct. 27, 1976.

Osborne, C. A., Hammer, R. F., Stevens, J. B., Resnick, J. S., and Michael, A. F.: The glomerulus in health and disease: A comparative review of domestic animals and man. Adv. Vet. Sci. Comp. Med. 21:207, 1977.

Osborne, C. A., Klausner, J. S., and Lees, G. E.: Urinary tract infections: Normal and abnormal host defense mechanisms. Vet. Clin. North Am. 9:587, 1979a.

Osborne, C. A., Johnson, K. H., and Perman, V.: Amyloid nephrotic syndrome in the dog. J.A.V.M.A. 154:1545, 1969a.

Osborne, C. A., Johnson, K. H., Perman, V., and Schall, W. D.: Renal amyloidosis in the dog. J.A.V.M.A. 153:669, 1968.

Osborne, C. A., Johnston, G. R., and Feeney, D. A.: A compendium of survey and contrast uroradiography. Proceedings, 46th Annual Meeting of the American Animal Hospital Association, New Orleans, Louisiana, 1979.

Osborne, C. A., Low, D. G., and Finco, D. R.: Congenital and Inherited Renal Disease. In Canine and Feline Urology. W. B. Saunders Co., Philadelphia, 1972a.

Osborne, C. A., Low, D. G., and Finco, D. R.: Percutaneous Renal Biopsy. In Canine and Feline Urology. W. B. Saunders Co., Philadelphia, 1972b.

Osborne, C. A., Low, D. G., and Finco, D. R.: Treatment of Renal Failure. In Canine and Feline Urology. W. B. Saunders Co., Philadelphia, 1972c.

Osborne, C. A., Stevens, J. B., Hanlon, G. F., Rosin, E., and Bemrick, W. J.: Dioctophyma renale in the dog. J.A.V.M.A. 155:605, 1969.

Osborne, C. A., Stevens, J. B., and Perman, V. L.: Kidney biopsy. Vet. Clin. North Am. 4:351, 1974.

Osborne, C. A., Stevens, J. B., and Polzin, D. J.: Gastrointestinal manifestations of urinary disease. In Anderson, N. V. (ed.): Veterinary Gastroenterology. Lea and Febiger, Philadelphia, 1980.

Osborne, C. A., Stevens, J. B., McClean, R., and Vernier, R. L.: Membranous lupus glomerulonephritis in a dog. J.A.A.H.A. 9:295, 1973.

Papadimitriou, M., Milionis, A., Sakellariou, G., and Metaxas, P.: Effect of furosemide on acute ischemic renal failure in the dog. Nephron 20:157, 1978.

Parker, H. R.: Evaluation and Management of Acute Renal Failure in the Emergency Patient. In Salter, F., Knowles, R., and Whittich, W. (eds.): Veterinary Critical Care. Lea and Febiger, Philadelphia, 1981.

Parker, H. R.: Current Status of Peritoneal Dialysis. In Kirk, R. W. (ed.): Current Veterinary Therapy VII. W. B. Saunders Co., Philadelphia, 1980, p. 1106.

Parry, M. F., and Wallach, R.: Ethylene glycol poisoning. Am. J. Med. 57:143, 1974.

Patak, R. V., Fadem, S. Z., Lifschitz, M. D., and Stein, J. H.: Study of factors which modify the development of norepinephrine-induced acute renal failure in the dog. Kidney Int. 15:227, 1979.

Perkoff, G. T., Thomas, C. L., Newton, J. D., Sellman, J. C., and Tyler, F. H.: Mechanism of impaired glucose tolerance in uremia and experimental hyperazotemia. Diabetes 7:375, 1958.

Persson, F., Persson, S., and Asheim, A.: Renal cortical hypoplasia in dogs. A clinical study in uraemia and secondary hyperparathyroidism. Acta Vet. Scand. 2:68, 1961.

Persson, F., Persson, S., and Asheim, A.: Blood-pressure in dogs with renal cortical hypoplasia. Act. Vet. Scand. 2:129, 1961a.

Phemister, R. D., Thomassen, R. W., Norrdin, R. W., and Jaenke, R. S.: Renal failure in perinatally irradiated beagles. Radiol. Res. 55:399, 1973.

Platt, H.: Morphological changes in the cardiovascular system associated with nephritis in dogs. J. Pathol. Bacteriol. 64:539, 1952.

Polzin, D. J., and Osborne, C. A.: Conservative Management of Polyuric Primary Renal Failure: Diet Therapy. In Kirk, R. W. (ed.): Current Veterinary Therapy VII. W. B. Saunders Co., Philadelphia, 1980, p. 1097.

Polzin, D. J., and Osborne, C. A.: Management of chronic primary polyuric renal failure with modified protein diets: Concepts, questions, and controversies. Proc. 29th Gaines Vet. Symp., Gaines Dog Research Center, White Plains, N.Y. 1979, p. 24.

Porter, G. A., and Bennett, W. M.: Nephrotoxin-Induced Acute Renal Failure. In Brenner, B. M., and Stein, J. H. (eds.): Contemporary Issues in Nephrology. Vol. 6. Acute Renal Failure. Churchill Livingstone, New York, 1980, p. 123.

Powers, S. R.: The maintenance of renal function following massive trauma. J. Trauma 10:554, 1970.

Rabiner, S. F.: Bleeding Abnormalities. In Massry, S. G., and Sellers, A. L., (eds.): Clinical Aspects of Uremia and Dialysis. Charles C Thomas, Springfield, Ill., 1976, p. 179.

Ravid, M., Kedar, I., and Sohar, E.: Effect of a single dose of dimethyl sulphoxide on renal amyloidosis. Lancet *1*:730, 1977.

Reiner, N. E., Bloxham, D. D., and Thompson, W. L.: Nephrotoxicity of gentamicin and tobramycin given once daily or continuously in dogs. J. Antimicrob. Chemother. *4*(Suppl. A):85, 1978.

Richards, M. A., and Hoe, C. M.: A long-term study of renal disease in the dog. Vet. Rec. *80*:640, 1967.

Ritz, E., Mehls, O., Gilli, G., and Heuck, C. C.: Protein restriction in the conservative management of uremia. Am. J. Clin. Nutr. *31*:1703, 1978.

Robinson, T., Harbison, M., and Bovee, K. C.: Influence of reduced renal mass on tubular secretion of creatinine in the dog. Am. J. Vet. Res. *35*:487, 1974.

Rocha, A., Marcondes, M., and Malnic, G.: Micropuncture study in rats with experimental glomerulonephritis. Kidney Int. *3*:14, 1973.

Rose, G.: Medical Research Council Trials. *In* Kluthe, R., Vogt, A., and Batsford, S. R. (eds.): Glomerulonephritis. International Conference on Pathogenesis, Pathology and Treatment. Freiburg, June 1976. Georg Thieme Publishers, Stuttgart, 1976, p. 174.

Rouse, B. T., and Lewis, R. J.: Canine glomerulonephritis: Prevalence in dogs submitted at random for euthanasia. Can. J. Comp. Med. *39*:365, 1975.

Row, P. G., Cameron, J. S., Turner, D. R., Evans, D. J., White, R. H. R., Ogg, C. S., Chantler, C., and Brown, C. S.: Membranous nephropathy. Long-term follow-up and association with neoplasia. Q. J. Med. *44*:207, 1975.

Russell, J. E., Termine, J. D., and Avioli, L. V.: Experimental renal osteodystrophy. The response to 25-hydroxycholecalciferol and dicholomethylene diphosphate therapy. J. Clin. Invest. *56*:548, 1975.

Rutherford, W. E., Bordier, P., Marie, P., Hruska, K., Harter, H., Greenwalt, A., Blondin, J., Haddad, J., Bricker, N., and Slatopolsky, E.: Phosphate control and 25-hydroxycholecalciferol administration in preventing experimental renal osteodystrophy in the dog. J. Clin. Invest. *60*:332, 1977.

Rytand, D. A.: The number and size of mammalian glomeruli as related to kidney and to body weight with methods for their enumeration and measurement. Amer. J. Anat. *62*:507, 1938.

Sandholm, M., Vasenius, H., and Kivisto, A-K.: Pathogenesis of canine pyometra. J.A.V.M.A. *167*:1006, 1975.

Sasaki, Y., Michimata, Y., Minai, K., Shioji, R., Furuyama, T., and Yoshinaga, K.: Plasma renin activity in acute renal failure induced by norepinephrine infusion in unilaterally nephrectomized dogs. Contrib. Nephrol. *9*:35, 1978.

Savin, V. J., Patak, R. V., and Marr, G.: Glomerular filtration in ischemic renal failure. Kidney Int. *16*:776, 1979.

Schall, W. D., and Perman, V.: Diseases of the Red Blood Cells. *In* Ettinger, S. J. (ed.): Textbook of Veterinary Internal Medicine. W. B. Saunders Co., Philadelphia, 1975, p. 1581.

Schmidt, R. W., and Gavellas, G.: Bicarbonate reabsorption in experimental renal disease: Effects of proportional reduction of sodium or phosphate intake. Kidney Int. *12*:393, 1977.

Schmidt, R. W., Bourgoignie, J. J., and Bricker, N. S.: On the adaptation in sodium excretion in chronic uremia. The effects of "proportional reduction" of sodium intake. J. Clin. Invest. *53*:1736, 1974.

Schreiber, R. D., and Muller-Eberhard, H. J.: Complement and Renal Disease. *In* Wilson, C. B., Brenner, B. M., and Stein, J. H. (eds.): Contemporary Issues in Nephrology. Vol. 3. Immunologic Mechanisms of Renal Disease. Churchill Livingstone, New York, 1979, p. 67.

Schrier, R. W., Cronin, R. E., Miller, P., De Torrento, A., Burke, T., and Bulger, R.: Role of solute excretion in prevention of norepinephrine-induced acute renal failure. Yale J. Biol. Med. *51*:355, 1978.

Schultze, R. G., Shapiro, H. S., and Bricker, N. S.: Studies on the control of sodium excretion in experimental uremia. J. Clin. Invest. *48*:869, 1969.

Schultze, R. G., Taggart, D. D., Shapiro, H., Pennell, J. P., Caglar, S., and Bricker, N. S.: On the adaptation in potassium excretion associated with nephron reduction in the dog. J. Clin. Invest. *50*:1061, 1971.

Scott, D. W.: Systemic Glucocorticoid Therapy. *In* Kirk, R. W. (ed.): Current Veterinary Therapy VII. W. B. Saunders Co., Philadelphia, 1980, p. 988.

Senior, D. F.: Parasites of the Canine Urinary Tract. *In* Kirk, R. W. (ed.): Current Veterinary Therapy VII. W. B. Saunders Co., Philadelphia, 1980, p. 1141.

Senior, D. F., Solomon, G. B., Goldschmidt, M. H., Joyce, T., and Bovee, K. C.: *Capillaria plica* infection in dogs. J.A.V.M.A. *176*:901, 1980a.

Shahidi, N. T.: Androgens and erythropoiesis. N. Engl. J. Med. *289*:72, 1973.

Shaw, A. B.: Haemolysis in chronic renal failure. Br. Med. J. *2*:213, 1967.

Shirahama, T., and Cohen, A. S.: Blockage of amyloid induction by colchicine in an animal model. J. Exp. Med. *140*:1102, 1974.

Short, C. E.: Fluid and Electrolyte Therapy. *In* Kirk, R. W. (ed.): Current Veterinary Therapy VII. W. B. Saunders Co., Philadelphia, 1980, p. 49.

Simmons, W. K.: Urinary urea nitrogen/creatinine ratio as indicator of recent protein intake in field studies. Am. J. Clin. Nutr. *25*:539, 1972.

Simon, N. M., and Rosenberg, M. J.: Medical treatment of glomerular disease. Med. Clin. North Am. *62*:1157, 1978.

Simpson, C. F., Gebhardt, B. M., Bradley, R. E., and Jackson, R. F.: Glomerulosclerosis in canine heartworm infection. Vet. Pathol. *11*:506, 1974.

Simpson, E. H., Brasel, J., and Heird, W. C.: Effect of amino acids and glucose on recovery from acute renal ischemia. Pediatr. Res. *11*:558, 1977.

Slatopolsky, E., Caglar, S., Gradowska, L., Canterbury, J., Reiss, E., and Bricker, N. S.: On the prevention of secondary hyperparathyroidism in experimental chronic renal disease using "proportional reduction" of dietary phosphorus intake. Kidney Int. *2*:147, 1972.

Slatopolsky, E., Calgar, S., Pennell, J. P., et al.: On the pathogenesis of hyperparathyroidism in chronic experimental renal insufficiency in the dog. J. Clin. Invest. *50*:492, 1971.

Slauson, D. O., and Gribble, D. H.: Thrombosis complicating renal amyloidosis in dogs. Vet. Pathol. *8*:352, 1971.

Slauson, D. O., and Lewis, R. M.: Comparative pathology of glomerulonephritis in animals. Vet. Pathol. *16*:135, 1979.

Slauson, D. O., Russell, S. W., and Schechter, R. D.: Naturally occurring immune-complex glomerulonephritis in the cat. J. Pathol. *103*:131, 1971.

Smolens, P., and Stein, J. H.: Hemodynamic Factors in Acute Renal Failure: Pathophysiologic and Therapeutic Implications. *In* Brenner, B. M., and Stein, J. H. (eds.): Contemporary Issues in Nephrology. Vol. 6. Acute Renal Failure. Churchill Livingstone, New York, 1980, p. 180.

Spangler, W. L., Adelman, R. D., Conzelman, G. M., and Ishizaki, G.: Gentamicin nephrotoxicity in the dog: Sequential light and electron microscopy. Vet. Pathol. *17*:206, 1980.

Spangler, W. L., Gribble, D. H., and Lee, T. C.: Vitamin D intoxication and the pathogenesis of vitamin D nephropathy in the dog. Am. J. Vet. Res. *40*:73, 1979.

Spangler, W. L., Gribble, D. H., and Weiser, M. G.: Canine hypertension: A review. J.A.V.M.A. *170*:995, 1980a.

Spargo, B. H., Seymour, A. E., and Ordonez, N. G.: Renal Biopsy Pathology with Diagnostic and Therapeutic Implications. John Wiley and Sons, New York, 1980.

Stamey, T. A., Fair, W. R., Timothy, M. M., Millar, M. A., Mihara, G., and Lowery, Y.: Serum versus urinary antimicrobial concentrations in cure of urinary tract infections. N. Engl. Med. *291*:1159, 1974.

Stamler, J., Katz, L. N., and Rodbard, S.: Serial renal clearances in dogs with nephrogenic and spontaneous hypertension. J. Exp. Med. *90*:511, 1949.

Stein, J. H., Lifschitz, M. D., and Barnes, L. D.: Current concepts on the pathophysiology of acute renal failure. Am. J. Physiol. *234*:F171, 1978.

Stein, J. H., Gottshall, J., Osgood, R. W., and Farris, T. F.: Pathophysiology of a nephrotoxic model of acute renal failure. Kidney Int. *8*:27, 1975.

Stevens, J. B., and Osborne, C. A.: Urinalysis: Indications, methodology, and interpretation. Scientific Presentations and Seminar Synopses, 41st Annual Meeting, Am. Anim. Hosp. Assoc., South Bend, Indiana, 1974.

Street, A. E., Chesterman, H., Smith, G. K. A., and Quinton, R. M.: Prolonged blood urea elevation observed in the beagle after feeding. Toxicol. Appl. Pharmacol. *13*:363, 1968.

Stuart, B. P., Phemister, R. D., and Thomassen, R. W.: Glomerular lesions associated with proteinuria in clinically healthy dogs. Vet. Pathol. *12*:125, 1975.

Sudo, M., Honda, N., Hishida, Akira, A., and Nagase, M.: Renal hemodynamics in oliguric and nonoliguric acute renal failure of rabbits. Nephron *25*:144, 1980.

Summers, W. K., and Jamison, R. L.: The no reflow phenomenon in renal ischemia. Lab. Invest. *25*:635, 1971.

Surawicz, B.: Relationship between electrocardiogram and electrolytes. Am. Heart J. *73*:814, 1967.

Swanson, R. E., and Hakim, A. A.: Stop-flow analysis of creatinine excretion in the dog. Am. J. Physiol. *203*:980, 1962.

Swendseid, M. E., Wang, M., Vyhmeister, I., Chan, W., Siassi, F., Tam, C. F., and Kopple, J. D.: Amino acid metabolism in chronically uremic rats. Clin. Nephrol. *3*:240, 1975.

Taguma, Y., Sasaki, Y., Kyogoku, Y., Arakawa, M., Shioji, R., Furuyama, T., and Yoshinaga, K.: Morphological changes in an early phase of norepinephrine-induced acute renal failure in unilaterally nephrectomized dogs. J. Lab. Clin. Med. *96*:616, 1980.

Theilen, G. H., and Madewell, B. R.: Tumors of the Urogenital Tract. *In* Theilen, G. H., and Madewell, B. R. (eds.): Veterinary Cancer Medicine. Lea and Febiger, Philadelphia, 1979, p. 357.

Thornburg, L. P., Kinden, D., and Digilio, K.: Immune glomerulitis in a cat. Vet. Pathol. *16*:604, 1979.

Thornhill, J. A.: Toxic Nephropathy. *In* Kirk, R. W. (ed.): Current Veterinary Therapy VII. W. B. Saunders Co., Philadelphia, 1980, p. 1047.

Toback, F. G.: Amino Acid Treatment of Acute Renal Failure. *In* Brenner, B. M., and Stein, J. H. (eds.): Contemporary Issues in Nephrology. Vol. 6. Acute Renal Failure. Churchill Livingstone, New York, 1980, p. 202.

Ullrey, D. E., Kealy, R. D., Mehring, J. S., and Smith, R. E.: Nutrient Requirements of Cats. National Research Council, National Academy of Sciences, Washington, D.C., 1978.

Valenzuela, R., and Deodhar, S. D.: Interpretations of immunofluorescent patterns in renal disease. Pathol. Ann. *10*:183, 1980.

Valtonen, M. H., and Oksanen, A.: Cardiovascular disease and nephritis in dogs. J. Small Anim. Pract. *13*:687, 1972.

van Assendelft, P. M. B., and Mees, E. J. D.: Urea metabolism in patients with chronic renal failure: Influence of sodium bicarbonate or sodium chloride administration. Metabolism *19*:1053, 1970.

Van Buren, C. T., Dudrick, S. J., Dworkin, L., Baumbauer, E., and Long, J. M.: Effects of intravenous essential L-amino acids and hypertonic dextrose on anephric beagles. Surg. Forum *23*:83, 1972.

van Rijswijk, M. A., Donker, A. J. M., Ruinen, L., and Marrink, J.: Treatment of renal amyloidosis with dimethylsulfoxide (DMSO). Proc. Europ. Dial. Transplant. Assoc. *16*:500, 1979.

Wada, T., Kan, K., Aizawa, K., Kuroda, S., Ino, Y., Inamoto, H., Kitamoto, K., Ogawa, M., and Yamayoshi, W.: Morphologic demonstration of tubular obstruction in acute renal failure. Am. J. Pathol. *87*:323, 1977.

Walker, W. G., and Solez, K.: Dysproteinemias: Renal Involvement in Multiple Myeloma and Amyloidosis. *In* Earley, L. E., and Gottschalk, C. W. (eds.): Strauss and Welt's Diseases of the Kidney. Third ed. Vol. II. Little, Brown and Company, Boston, 1979, p. 1241.

Wakerlin, G. E.: Normotension and hypertension in the dog. J.A.V.M.A. *102*:346, 1943.

Wallner, S. F., and Vautrin, R. M.: The anemia of chronic renal failure: studies of the effect of organic solvent extraction of serum. J. Lab. Clin. Med. *92*:363, 1978.

Wallner, S. F., Kurnick, J. E., Ward, H. P., Vautrin, R., and Alfrey, A. C.: The anemia of chronic renal failure and chronic diseases: *In vitro* studies of erythropoiesis. Blood *47*:561, 1976.

Wallner, S. F., Ward, H. P., Vautrin, R., Alfrey, A. C., and Mishell, J.: The anemia of renal failure: *In vitro* response of bone marrow to erythropoietin. Proc. Soc. Exp. Biol. Med. *149*:939, 1975.

Walser, M.: Conservative management of the uremic patient. *In* Brenner, B. M., and Rector, F. C. (eds.): The Kidney. W. B. Saunders Co., Philadelphia, 1981.

Webb, A. I.: Renal ectopia in a dog. Aus. Vet. J. *50*:519, 1974.

Weiser, M. G., Spangler, W. L., and Gribble, D. H.:

Blood pressure measurement in the dog. J.A.V.M.A. *171*:364, 1977.

Westenfelder, C., Arevalo, G. J., Crawford, P. W., Zerwer, P., Baranowski, R. L., Birch, F. M., Earnest, W. R., Hamburger, R. K., Coleman, R. D., and Kurtzman, N. A.: Renal tubular function in glycerol-induced acute renal failure. Kidney Int. *18*:432, 1980.

Wignild, J. P., and Gutmann, F. D.: Functional adaptation of nephrons in dogs with acute progressing to chronic experimental glomerulonephritis. J. Clin. Invest. *57*:1575, 1976.

Williams, J. S., Stein, J. H., and Ferris, T. F.: Nandrolone decanoate therapy for patients receiving hemodialysis. A controlled study. Arch. Intern. Med. *134*:289, 1974.

Wilson, C. B., and Dixon, F. J.: The renal response to immunological injury. *In* Brenner, B. M., and Rector, F. C. (eds.): The Kidney. W. B. Saunders Co., Philadelphia, 1981.

Wilson, C. B., and Dixon, F. J.: Renal Injury from Immune Reactions Involving Antigens in or of the Kidney. *In* Wilson, C. B., Brenner, B. M., and Stein, J. H. (eds.): Contemporary Issues in Nephrology, Vol. 3. Immunologic Mechanisms of Renal Disease. Churchill Livingstone, New York, 1979, p. 35.

Wright, N. G., Fisher, E. W., Morrison, W. I., Thomson, W. B., and Nash, A. S.: Chronic renal failure in dogs: A comparative clinical and morphological study of chronic glomerulonephritis and chronic interstitial nephritis. Vet. Rec. *98*:288, 1976.

Wright, N. G., Morrison, W. I., Thompson, H., and Cornwell, H. J. C.: Messangial localization of immune complexes in experimental canine adenovirus glomerulonephritis. Br. J. Exp. Pathol. *55*:458, 1974.

Wright, N. G., Nash, A. S., Thompson, H., and Fisher, E. W.: Membranous nephropathy in the cat and dog. A renal biopsy and follow-up study of sixteen cases. Lab. Invest. *45*:269, 1981.

Wright, N. G., Thompson, H., Cornwell, H. J. C., and Morrison, W. I.: Ultrastructure of the kidney and urinary excretion of renal antigens in experimental canine adenovirus infection. Res. Vet. Sci. *14*:376, 1973.

Zanjani, E. D., and Banisadre, M.: Hormonal stimulation of erythropoietin production and erythropoiesis in anephric sheep fetuses. J. Clin. Invest. *64*:1181, 1979.

Zucchelli, P., Fusaroli, M., Fabbri, L., Pavlica, P., Casanova, S., Viglietta, G., and Sasdelli, M.: Treatment of ectopic calcification in uremia. Kidney Int. *13*(suppl. 8):S–86, 1978.

CHAPTER 75

BOYD R. JONES

Diseases of the Ureters

Primary diseases of the ureter are uncommon in dogs and cats. When the ureters are involved in disease processes, the kidneys, bladder, or urethra are usually involved also. For this reason clinical signs of ureteral disease cannot be distinguished from clinical signs related to concurrent disease of other parts of the urinary tract. Since urinary tract disease is now usually investigated with contrast radiography, ureteral diseases have become more frequently recognized.

ANATOMY AND PHYSIOLOGY

The ureters actively transport urine produced in the kidney and the renal pelvis to the bladder. Urine that accumulates in the renal pelvis initiates peristalsis in the pelvic smooth muscle and then ureteral smooth muscle, so that boluses of urine are propelled along the ureteral lumen to the bladder (Veerecken, 1976).

The ureter in the canine possesses three layers of muscle, an inner and outer longitudinal layer and a middle layer of fibers whose orientation varies from circular in the middle portion of the ureter to oblique in the upper and lower portions. At high rates of urine flow, the middle and lower segments act independently of each other in the manner of two reservoirs in series, the middle segment being distended to a certain critical pressure before discharging (Bannigan, 1975). On entry to the bladder, the ureters run an oblique course through the bladder wall and at the trigone form a flap valve that normally prevents retrograde flow of urine from the bladder (Christie, 1971a).

CONGENITAL DISEASES

URETERAL DUPLICATION

Ureteral duplication can result either from the premature bifurcation of a single ureteric bud or from the development of more than one ureteric bud during embryologic differentiation. Complete duplication occurs from the separate development of two buds, each of which induces the development of renal tissue that fuses to form two parts of a complete duplex kidney.

This condition, which is a common congenital condition of the ureter in man, has been reported only once in the dog (O'Handley et al., 1979). The 18-month-old male bulldog had a history of urinary incontinence and hematuria since six months of age and was shown by excretory urography to have a normal left kidney and ureter but a right kidney that had two collecting systems and two functional ureters.

CONGENITAL URETERAL VALVES

Ureteral valves are transverse folds of ureteral mucosa that can be demonstrated by excretory urography as transverse filling defects of the ureter, which may also be dilated. Other conditions can cause transverse filling defects of the ureter; therefore, histologic demonstration of smooth muscle in the fold is the only sure way of confirming the presence of ureteral valves. In man, folds often disappear by the fourth month of life, but persisting valves may cause obstruction. The condition is usually unilateral. Pollock and Schoen (1971) reported this condition in a six-month-old female collie that had shown urinary incontinence since eight weeks of age. The urinary incontinence responded to ureteronephrectomy; however, the mechanism by which the ureteral valves caused incontinence was not demonstrated. This condition is rare but should be considered in young animals with urinary incontinence or radiographic evidence of ureteral obstruction and dilation.

URETERAL ECTOPIA

Ureteral ectopia is a congenital condition in which one or both ureters do not drain into the bladder lumen but instead terminate in the urethra or genital tract.

Etiology

Ureteral ectopia may be bilateral or unilateral and is the result of faulty differentiation of the mesonephric and metanephric ducts during embryogenesis. Owen (1973a) discussed aspects of embryologic development of the urinary tract and provided explanations for how ectopic ureters might arise in both male and female animals. At the time of this review there was no evidence to suggest that ectopic ureter was an inherited condition. Since that time, however, a definite breed incidence has been found and a genetic etiology is suspected (Hayes, 1974; Osborne and Oliver, 1977; Lennox, 1978). Breeding experiments with affected golden retrievers have shown that the condition is inherited in this breed (Jones, 1980a). Ectopic ureters have been produced experimentally in the offspring of pregnant rats by altering their diet during certain stages of gestation, but there is no evidence for a similar etiology in the dog or cat.

Incidence

Breed Incidence. Hayes (1974) showed that Siberian huskies, West Highland white terriers, fox terriers, and miniature and toy poodles had a higher risk for ectopic ureter than other breeds of dog. Black Labrador retrievers (Osborne and Oliver, 1977) and golden retrievers (Jones, 1980a) also have a higher than expected incidence of the condition.

Age. Ureteral ectopia is one of the most common causes of urinary incontinence in bitches, and since it is a congenital anomaly the incidence in young dogs is high. In one survey (Hayes, 1974), 58 per cent of female dogs with this condition were diagnosed before they were one year old.

Sex. The incidence of ectopic ureters is not known, although it is recognized more frequently in females than in males. When ureteral ectopia is present in the female it is almost always associated with urinary incontinence (Owen, 1973a), but ectopic ureters can be present without any sign of urinary incontinence (Osborne and Oliver, 1977; Jones, 1980b). In the male, when a ureter empties into the urethra, the urine can flow back into the lumen of the bladder because the proximal urethra is less resistant to urine flow than are the more distal portions. Two golden retriever stud dogs in whose female progeny ureteral ectopia was present were found to have bilateral ectopic ureters with urethral termination. Urine flowed from the urethra back into the bladder in each case, and they did not show signs of urinary incontinence until they were four and five years of age. Both dogs had been used extensively as stud dogs before ureteral ectopia was diagnosed (Jones, 1980b). In male dogs with ectopic ureters, urinary incontinence may be seen (Osborne et al., 1975; Lennox, 1978).

Location. Owen (1973b), in his review of published literature, found that when an ectopic ureter was present unilateral ectopia (80 per cent) was found more frequently than bilateral ectopia (20 per cent) and that the vagina (70 per cent) was the most common site of ureteral termination followed by the urethra (20 per cent), the neck of the bladder (8 per cent), and the uterus (2 per cent).

Cats. Four cases of ectopic ureter have been reported in young cats (Bebco et al., 1977; Biewenga et al., 1978; Orr, 1979). Three of the four cases diagnosed were male, and in each case urinary incontinence was present.

Associated Conditions

Ectopic ureters are often associated with other congenital anomalies of the urinary system and with diseases that develop as a sequel to ureteral ectopia.

Megaureter is a common finding and is characterized by dilation of the ureteral lumen and abnormal peristalsis. The cause of the dilation is not known; there is seldom evidence of mechanical obstruction. Impaired peristalsis may cause a functional obstruction, which results in megaureter because of decreased emptying of the affected ureter. Urinary tract infection is often present in dogs with ectopic ureters. In dogs studied at Massey University, the greatest degree of megaureter was always found when concurrent infection was present. Urinary tract infection caused by *E. coli* is known to inhibit ureteral peristalsis in the dog (Grana et al., 1968).

Hypoplasia of the bladder may be observed (Owen, 1973b), particularly in cases of bilateral ureteral ectopia. The reduction in size is probably due to disuse rather than to embryologic causes and is therefore potentially reversible. Hypoplasia of the kidney and hydronephrosis have also been observed. The reduction in renal size may be due, not to abnormalities of embryologic development, but to chronic pyelonephritis.

Urethral abnormalities have been observed in dogs with ectopic ureters (Osborne and Oliver, 1977), and female dogs may have a persistent hymen (Jones, 1980b).

Clinical Findings

Affected female dogs usually have a history of persistent urinary incontinence since birth or weaning. If only one ureter is ectopic, the bitch can urinate normally, but if both ureters are ectopic, normal micturition will not be observed. Urine may drip from the vulva to soil the perineal area or pool in the vagina and pass out in large volumes as the dog changes body position. Affected bitches often do not grow as rapidly or are not as active as their normal litter mates, particularly when the complication of bacterial urinary tract infection is present (Fig. 75–1).

In male dogs, urinary incontinence is the most common presenting sign; however, the

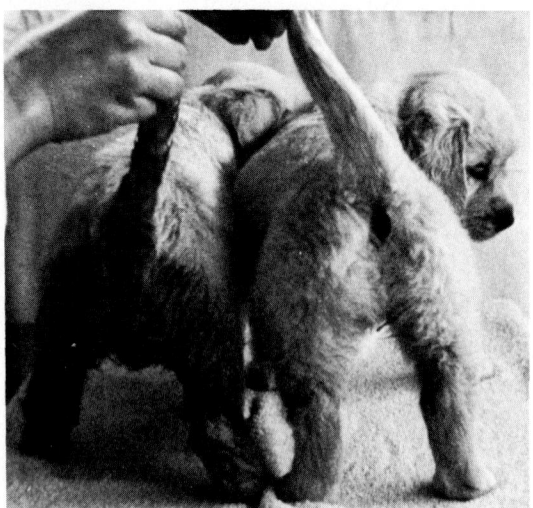

Figure 75–1. Two six week old female Golden Retriever littermates. The smaller puppy (left) shows soiling of the perineal area from urinary incontinence due to ureteral ectopia.

condition may be asymptomatic or signs may not develop until the dog becomes an adult (Lennox, 1978; Jones, 1980b).

Diagnosis

Endoscopy. Opening of one or both ureters into the vagina can be detected by vaginal endoscopy; however, the ureteral openings can be difficult to find. A vaginoscope that gives a satisfactory view of the entire vaginal mucosa must be used. To do this, distension of the vaginal wall is essential. Fiber optoscopes, pediatric proctoscopes, or a pyrex test tube from which the bottom has been removed and the end polished are all satisfactory for endoscopy (Osborne and Oliver, 1977). It should be remembered that female dogs with ectopic ureters often have a persistent hymen, which may prevent endoscopy, or the opening between the hymen and the vaginal wall can be mistaken for the ectopic ureteral orifice. If an abnormal orifice is detected by vaginal endoscopy, it should be catheterized with a flexible, radiopaque catheter, followed by retrograde ureteropyelography to establish a definite diagnosis. Catheterization can be technically difficult to perform, however.

Radiology. EXCRETORY UROGRAPHY. Excretory urography provides evaluation of the whole urinary tract and also helps to de-termine if ectopic ureter(s) are present (Owen, 1973b). Excretory urography is an important diagnostic aid, but the exact site of termination of the distal ureters is often impossible to determine. Accumulation of contrast agent in the bladder may obscure the distal ureter. An ectopic ureter often enters the bladder in the normal position and passes submucosally to the urethra. Insufficient contrast agent in the lumen of the distal ureter will give non-diagnostic films, and renal damage may cause an insufficient amount of contrast agent to be excreted to outline the ureter.

In normal dogs the dose of contrast agent administered was shown to influence many of the measurements, both linear and density in the excretory urogram (Feeney et al., 1979). The use of high-dose urography (Osborne et al., 1972) in dogs with a suspected ectopic ureter can overcome the problem of poor definition, and in addition, megaureter and dilated renal pelves are more likely to be demonstrated. Osborne and Oliver (1977) reported that megaureter was a more consistent finding in cases evaluated by high dose urography than in other studies. With this method, the enlarged ureters were filled with contrast agent over their entire length. They were often more tortuous and their diameter in some areas was greater than normal, while the normal ureter was not distended or filled with contrast agent over its entire length. If definite confirmation of ureteral ectopia by excretory urography cannot be made, the presence of megaureter, pyelectasis, and reduction in renal size provides strong supportive evidence.

Technique. Patient preparation is very important if successful excretory urography is to be achieved. Food should be withheld for 24 hours and a thorough enema given. It is important not only that all fecal material is removed but also that air administered with the enema be excreted. Plain survey radiographs should be taken immediately prior to the procedure to ensure that the gastrointestinal tract is empty of feces and air. The dog is anesthetized and placed in dorsal recumbency. The dosage of contrast agent is calculated in milligrams of iodine per kilogram of body weight. A dose of from 800 to 1200 mg Iodine/kg of one of the mixtures of sodium and meglumine diatrizoates or iothalamates is administered rapidly intravenously. Alternatively, the same volume of agent can be given in an equal volume of 5 per cent dextrose saline and infused more slowly over a ten-minute period. Care should be taken to prevent perivascular extravasation of contrast material, as it is irritating and may produce a slough. At the end of infusion, lateral and ventrodorsal radiographs are taken of the abdomen and again at 5, 10 and, if necessary, up to 20 minutes later. Not only should ventrodorsal and lateral abdominal radiographs be taken, but also right and left ventro-dorsal oblique views of the trigone should be obtained to try to show the exact site of termination of the ureters.

VAGINOGRAPHY. In bitches in which a vaginal ectopic ureter is suspected but the ureteral opening cannot be seen, or in bitches too small to examine by endoscopy, retrograde vaginography is a suitable method for confirming a diagnosis. The bitch should be anesthetized and placed in dorsal recumbency. Sufficient contrast agent (any diatrizoate or iothalamate media diluted to 10 per cent iodine W/V may be used) is injected into the vagina through an inflated Foley or Swan-Ganz balloon catheter to distend the vagina. The inflated balloon of the catheter prevents the escape of contrast agent from the vulva, and as the vagina distends contrast agent will pass into the ectopic ureter (see Fig. 75–2).

URETHROGRAPHY. In male dogs in which urethral termination of the ureter is most likely, and when this is suspected in bitches, retrograde urethrography should be performed (Johnston et al., 1977).

The patient should be fasted overnight and given an enema before being anesthetized or sedated. Water soluble organic iodides are the contrast material of choice and should be diluted to approximately 10 to 15 per cent final concentration. Application of a local anesthetic agent (2 to 5 ml of lidocaine) to the urethra prior to urethrography is advisable to reduce urethral pain, irritation, and spasm. Balloon catheters (Swan-Ganz or Foley) are recommended. The tip of the catheter is positioned distal to the os penis and the balloon inflated. Inject 10 to 20 ml of contrast medium slowly to fill and distend the urethra, and expose the film just prior to completion of the injection. Lateral and oblique views may be required to detect termination of one or both ureters into the proximal urethra.

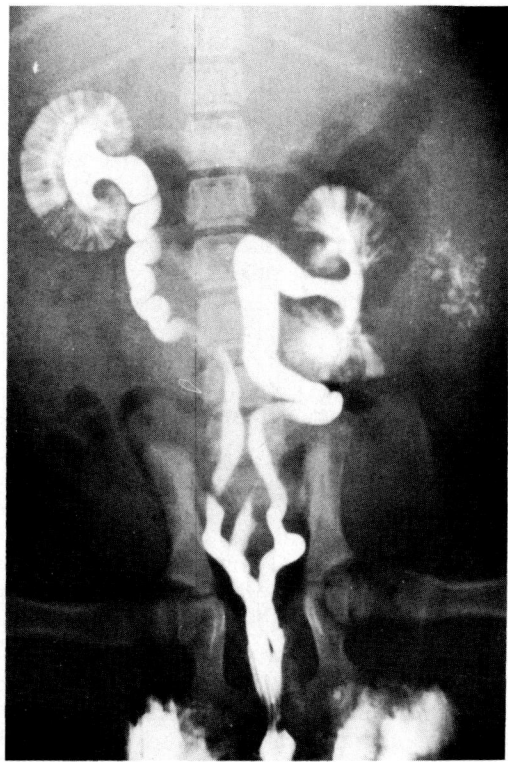

Figure 75–2. Vaginogram of six week old Golden Retriever with urinary incontinence. This shows bilateral ureteral ectopia and megaureter.

OTHER INVESTIGATIONS. Exploratory laparotomy should be completed if endoscopy and radiography fail to confirm the presence of an ectopic ureter. The site of termination of the ureters can be observed, and the diagnosis confirmed. Ectopic ureters may enter the bladder in the normal position; thus, a cystotomy may be required to determine if the ureteral openings are in their normal position in the bladder. Saline can be injected into the ureteral lumen to see if the bladder is bypassed. Alternatively, a small incision can be made in the ureter, and monofilament nylon or a small catheter inserted into the lumen. If the ureter is ectopic, the nylon or catheter should pass through from the vulva or penis.

Treatment

The treatment for urinary incontinence caused by ureteral ectopia is surgical. Surgical correction of an ectopic ureter is well documented (Owen, 1973b; Archibald and Owen, 1974; Robins and Presnell, 1974; Dingwall et al., 1976; Chiari et al., 1977).

Techniques include nephrectomy and ureterectomy in the unilateral condition and implantation of the ureter into the bladder for the bilateral condition. The combined intra- and extravesical technique of ureterovesical anastomosis (Dingwall et al., 1976) is now the method of choice. This technique takes advantage of the fact that the ectopic ureter is usually already attached to the bladder. A routine cystotomy is performed, a uretero-vesical opening created, and the ureteral mucosa sutured to the bladder mucosa. The ureter distal to this opening is ligated. A catheter is placed into the ureter via the opening and then passed through the urethra to the outside and sutured to the skin for four to five days. The catheter ensures postsurgical patency of the ureter. Extravesically, a submucosal tunnel (one and one half to three centimeters long) is created for the ureter to prevent reflux of urine as the bladder fills and empties.

The advantages of this technique are that the ureter is not severed, the ureteral blood supply is preserved, interference with outflow of urine from the ureter is minimal, and postsurgical vesicoureteral reflux should be prevented. Before surgery is attempted in the dog with ureteral ectopia, it is important to know the side(s) affected, the site or sites of termination of the ectopic ureters, and the functional capacity of the associated and the contralateral kidneys. Nephrectomy and ureterectomy are the treatments of choice when the kidney attached to the ectopic ureter shows damage due to chronic bacterial infection.

Transplantation of the ureter into the bladder is the procedure of choice if both kidneys show reduced function, if both ureters terminate outside the bladder, or if the kidney and ureter are normal in unilateral ureteral ectopia. In the case of vaginal termination, the ureter should be sectioned as close as possible to its site of termination, because infection of the distal segment may require further surgery (Pearson et al., 1965). Care is necessary to avoid damage to the vesicoureteral sphincter during dissection of ureters within the bladder wall close to the sphincter.

Vesicoureteral reflux may occur after vesicoureteral transplantation even though surgical techniques attempt to eliminate this sequela (Archibald and Owen, 1974; Dingwall et al., 1976). Reflux is more likely to occur when the ureters are grossly dilated. Even gross megaureter is reversible after successful implantation, but excessive thickening of the ureteral wall makes the procedure technically difficult (Van Den Brom et al., 1978).

Infection of the urinary system should be controlled with appropriate antibacterial therapy, preferably commenced prior to surgery.

Prognosis

Without surgical treatment, urinary incontinence will continue. However, a progressive decrease in severity of incontinence has been observed in some dogs that had concurrent chronic pyelonephritis in the associated kidney. The progressive deterioration of renal function resulted in a reduction in the rate and amount of urine produced by the diseased kidney (Osborne and Oliver, 1977). If surgical correction of unilateral ectopia is attempted, a good prognosis can be given if the ureter terminates in the vagina, no matter what surgical technique is used. If the site of termination of the ureter(s) is the urethra, however, a more guarded prognosis should be given, as some dogs continue to show signs of urinary incontinence after surgical correction.

Prevention

Because a genetic etiology for ectopic ureters is likely, retrograde urethrography might be indicated in stud male dogs of suspect breeds before they are used for breeding purposes. They can have ectopic ureters without manifesting clinical signs.

MORPHOLOGIC DISORDERS

VESICOURETERAL REFLUX

Vesicoureteral reflux is defined as regurgitation or retrograde flow of urine from the lumen of the urinary bladder into the ureter or ureters.

Pathophysiology

Anatomic ureterovesical valves are not present in dogs, but since the ureters run an oblique course through the bladder wall, retrograde flow of urine from the bladder into the ureters is prevented. Detrusor muscle tone is an important defense against reflux, in addition to the oblique course of the ureter through the bladder wall. The thin-walled intravesical portion of the ureter collapses against the bladder wall as pressure within the bladder increases (Christie, 1973b). There are a number of factors, the presence of one or more of which predispose to reflux: anatomic changes at the vesicoureteral junction, increased intravesical pressure, and diminished peristaltic power of the ureter (Goulden, 1968; Christie, 1973b; Veerecken, 1976; Schulman and Gregoir, 1977).

Vesicoureteral reflux is more likely to occur in dogs in which intravesical portion of the ureter is short. This is significant, because during development the submucosal portion of the ureter increases in diameter before it increases in length. Thus, vesicoureteral reflux occurs; as growth proceeds, however, the submucosal portion elongates, restoring a favorable length:diameter ratio to the flap valve and thus bringing about a regression of the reflux (Christie, 1971b; 1973a,b). These changes in growth of the submucosal ureter are thought to explain the high incidence of primary self-limiting vesicoureteral reflux observed in young puppies between 7 and 12 weeks of age with normal urinary systems.

Reflux can be categorized as primary or secondary on the basis of pathogenesis. Primary reflux represents a structural change related to growth and maturation of the intravesical ureter (Christie, 1973a). Secondary reflux is a sequel to cystitis, lower tract obstruction, urolithiasis, or neurogenic bladder disease (Goulden, 1968; Veerecken, 1976). Secondary vesicoureteral reflux is rare in the cat, but it has been described (Goulden, 1969; Kipnis, 1975).

Significance

There is little question that vesicoureteral reflux is responsible for the perpetuation of bacterial cystitis and that bacterial pyelonephritis results from vesicoureteral reflux (Belman, 1976). Mechanical emptying of the bladder eliminates bacteria from the bladder. If vesicoureteral reflux is present as well as cystitis, however, then the bladder will be recontaminated with infected re-

fluxed urine from the ureter. Furthermore, in addition to perpetuating cystitis, vesicoureteral reflux predisposes an animal to pyelonephritis because it permits bacteria to reach the normally sterile kidney. Still, a bladder infection does not necessarily lead to renal infection in all cases (Newman et al., 1974).

Diagnosis

The diagnosis of vesicoureteral reflux is made radiographically. Voiding cystourethrography (voiding cystogram) or voiding cinecystography are the most satisfactory methods for demonstrating this phenomenon (Goulden, 1968; Christie, 1971b). The former can be performed simply in most veterinary practices without sophisticated radiologic equipment and enables most cases of reflux to be detected (Goulden, 1968; Christie, 1973b). The dog or cat is anesthetized (without premedication) to approximately the depth required for tracheal intubation. With the animal in lateral recumbency the bladder is catheterized, the urine drained, and the bladder distended by gravity flow with a suitable nonirritating contrast agent at a pressure of 30 to 40 cm of water, using the pubic symphysis as the zero reference point. The contrast agent should be instilled slowly so that the intravesical pressure remains low; when enough has been added to stimulate receptors in the bladder wall, contraction of the detrusor muscle occurs, causing urine to be expelled around the catheter. Alternatively, with the bladder distended, the catheter is withdrawn before voiding and the depth of anesthesia lightened. Radiographs should be taken during filling, during micturition, and immediately after urination (Goulden, 1968). Lateral recumbency is preferred, since this position is said to favor reflux (Cass and Lenaghan, 1965). In some animals, especially those with abnormalities of the urinary tract that result in gross distension, micturition may not occur. In these animals, gentle digital pressure can be applied to the bladder through the abdominal wall to initiate the micturition reflex. In more than 90 per cent of cases with reflux, contrast material is observed radiographically to reach to the renal pelvis (Fig. 75–3) (Christie, 1973b).

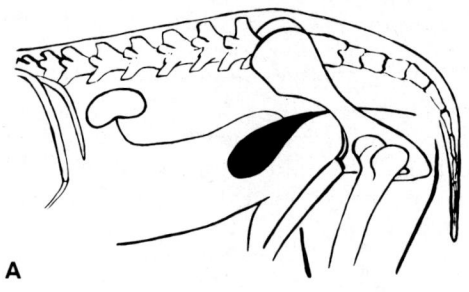

A

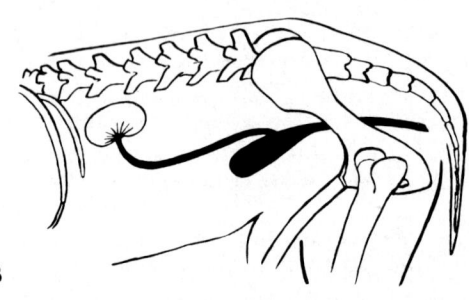

B

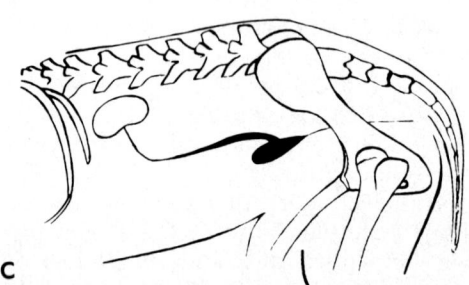

C

Figure 75–3. Diagram illustrating vesicoureteral reflux in dogs. *A*, Before micturition. *B*, During micturition. Shows regurgitation of vesical contents into the ureter and kidney pelvis. *C*, Immediately after micturition. Shows urinary retention resulting from the return of the regurgitated vesical contents into the bladder.

Treatment

Primary vesicoureteral reflux of young dogs is self limiting in most cases and therefore of little importance in the pathogenesis of renal defects or pyelonephritis. No treatment is required. Secondary vesicoureteral reflux may predispose the animal to pyelonephritis, therefore removal of the predis-

posing causes is mandatory. Treatment of bacterial cystitis, removal of calculi, and relief of lower urinary tract obstruction is essential if reflux of infected urine is to be prevented; otherwise, pyelonephritis is inevitable.

URETEROVAGINAL FISTULA

Urinary incontinence that occurs in bitches or queens soon after hysterectomy may be due to the formation of a utererovaginal fistula. Pearson and Gibbs (1980) described three bitches in which the onset of urinary incontinence occurred within two to three weeks of spaying, and Allen and Webbon (1980) described a similar condition in two cats. Excretory urography is the most useful diagnostic aid to confirm this diagnosis. The renal pelvis and affected ureter may be dilated, and in lateral radiographs the dilated ureter may be shown to terminate in the pelvic area at a site dorsal to the bladder neck. Cineradiography after injection of water soluble contrast agent into the vagina via an inflated Foley catheter may be required to demonstrate conclusively that a communication between the ureter and vagina exists. If the ureter communicates with the vagina, the contrast medium will be seen in the affected ureter.

Treatment

Exploratory laparotomy is necessary to locate the adhesion between the ureter and the vaginal stump. The affected ureter can be sectioned above the adhesion and reimplanted into the bladder by one of the submucosal tunneling techniques. The vaginal stump should also be shortened (Pearson and Gibbs, 1980). If the ureter is grossly dilated and thickened, then reimplantation may not be practicable and unilateral ureteronephrectomy is the treatment of choice. Pearson and Gibbs (1980) suggested that this uncommon accident can be prevented during surgery by careful cutting (rather than tearing) of the broad ligament down to the cervix, and by amputating as low as possible on the vagina. Despite the fact that this condition may occur after hysterectomy, it should not be forgotten that bitches with a previously ectopic ureter may become incontinent after ovariohysterectomy. Greene et al. (1978) reported a case such as this, wherein the ureter entered the bladder in the normal position and ran within the bladder wall to terminate in the urethra. The bitch urinated normally prior to surgery but became incontinent three weeks after surgery.

NEOPLASIA

Tumors of the canine and feline urinary system are uncommon, and primary benign and malignant neoplasms of the ureter are· rare. Neoplasms originating in abdominal organs of the bladder trigone may involve the ureter. In the last ten years there have been two reports in dogs of primary tumors arising from the ureter.

Liska and Patnaik (1977) described a leiomyoma of the ureter that obstructed the distal ureter, causing hydroureter; Berzon (1979) described a leiomyosarcoma of the ureter. In each of these cases the presenting clinical signs were not suggestive of urinary tract involvement. If the tumor mass is large it may be palpated or be seen in plain radiographs of the abdomen. Excretory urography is the best method of demonstrating whether a ureter is involved and obstructed by the tumor. Nevertheless, exploratory surgery may be necessary to confirm the presence of a tumor of the ureter. Removal of the tumor by ureteronephrectomy is the treatment of choice, provided that the other kidney and ureter are functional and metastasis has not occurred.

MEGAURETER (URETERECTASIS)

Dilation of the ureteral lumen and abnormal peristalsis is a common finding in diseases of the ureter. Varying degrees of megaureter are seen in cases of ectopic ureter in the dog (Owen, 1973b), in ureteral obstruction, in ureteral neoplasia (Liska and Patnaik, 1977), and in ureteral duplication (O'Handley et al., 1979), and may be present with urinary tract infection (Grana et al., 1968). Urinary incontinence associated with megaureter has been reported in the absence of other urinary tract lesions in dogs (Pollock and Schoen, 1971) and in a cat (North, 1978). In some animals the cause of the megaureter cannot be established. There is, presumably, impaired peristalsis that results in a functional ureteral obstruction and consequent ureteral dilation.

Ureterectomy and nephrectomy constitute the treatment of choice in some cases, but treatment of the primary condition— e.g., relief of obstruction, transplantation of an ectopic ureter, or treatment of urinary tract infection—can result in complete resolution (Rose et al., 1975). Ureteral plication has been used successfully to reduce the ureteral caliber and restore normal peristalsis in dogs with experimental megaureter (Starr, 1979).

UROLITHIASIS

Ureteral calculi are uncommon in the dog and cat, although they have been reported (Brown et al., 1977; Wolf et al., 1979). Calculi arise in the renal pelvis and pass from there into the ureter, where they cause partial or complete obstruction of the ureter. Clinical signs associated with ureteral calculi may be severe abdominal pain, ureteral dilation, and hydronephrosis. Plain radiography or excretory urography are the most suitable means by which a diagnosis of ureteral urolithiasis can be confirmed.

Treatment should consist of surgical removal of all calculi from the obstructed ureter and kidney and treatment of bacterial infection, if present. The calculi should be analyzed, so that specific therapy can be administered to prevent recurrence of uroliths.

URETERITIS

Ureteritis occurs in association with infection of other parts of the urinary tract. Infection may ascend from the bladder or descend from the kidney. Pyelonephritis and/or cystitis associated with vesicoureteral reflux provide a continuous source of bacteria and allow ureteritis to persist. Ureteritis may result in functional or mechanical obstruction to urine flow. Infection with some species of bacteria (Escherichia coli) has been shown to stop or slow ureteral peristalsis (Rose and Gillenwater, 1978). Treatment of ureteritis is identical to that of other urinary tract infections.

URETERAL TRAUMA

Injury to, or rupture of the ureter may occur as a result of trauma to the abdomen lumbar region or it may be iatrogenic to surgery, especially ovariohysterectomy and prostatic surgery. Rupture of the ureter that occurs as a result of trauma usually occurs near the kidney or close to the bladder trigone. Urine leaking from a damaged ureter will cause peritonitis, but renal failure should not develop if only one ureter is damaged. Nevertheless, the BUN level can rise quickly after injury, in some cases. If the ureter is obstructed, hydronephrosis of the kidney will result.

Clinical Signs

A history of recent abdominal trauma, pain in the sublumbar area or posterior abdomen, and the presence of a palpable abdominal mass near the kidney or bladder provide evidence for possible ureteral damage. Urine may be aspirated from the abdomen if large quantities of urine accumulate when the ureteral defect is not sealed off.

Plain radiographs of the abdomen may demonstrate the presence of free fluid within the abdomen or soft tissue densities in the region of the kidney or bladder trigone, and when sublumbar leakage occurs tissue fascial planes are readily recognizable. Excretory urography should demonstrate ureteral rupture; escape of contrast agent from the ureter into the peritoneal cavity or retroperitoneal tissues will confirm ureteral rupture. Exploratory laparotomy may be necessary to identify the actual site of rupture.

Treatment

Treatment of ureteral rupture or obstruction resulting from trauma is surgical. If the ureteral lesion is unilateral and the opposite kidney functions adequately, then unilateral nephrectomy and ureterectomy should be attempted. In some dogs ureteral anastomosis may be possible after resection of the damaged portion of the ureter.

URETERAL OBSTRUCTION

Ureteral obstruction can be caused by obstruction within the lumen of the ureter or pressure from external lesions. Uroliths, primary ureteral neoplasms, ureteritis, or stricture are causes of internal ureteral obstruction. Causes of external obstruction of the ureter include abdominal neoplasms,

ureteral ligation during surgery, abnormal displacement of the bladder, and space-occupying abdominal masses.

Obstruction is most often unilateral, although bilateral ureteral obstruction may occur, with lesions involving the bladder trigone. Complete unilateral ureteral obstruction will cause hydronephrosis of that kidney, but renal failure should not result if the other kidney has normal function. However, BUN levels may be significantly elevated in some dogs with unilateral obstruction. Sudden complete bilateral ureteral obstruction will result in death of the dog in three to six days from fluid, electrolyte, and acid-base imbalance. Metabolic acidosis and hyperkalemia are the most critical and significant changes. If bilateral ureteral obstruction occurs more slowly, with each ureter being obstructed sequentially (as might occur with a neoplasm in the region of the bladder trigone), renal failure will develop more slowly. The clinical course is longer, but bilateral hydronephrosis will occur eventually.

Chronic upper urinary tract obstruction complicated by infection is serious, as the presence of infection will augment the existing obstruction by impairing ureteral peristalsis leading to stasis (Rose and Gillenwater, 1978).

Clinical Signs

As with the other conditions of the ureters, the clinical signs are usually associated with the underlying cause. If the obstruction is caused by an abdominal mass, the lesion and enlarged hydronephrotic kidney(s) may be palpated. If bilateral obstruction is present, signs of renal failure will be present. Plain radiographs of the abdomen may show the lesion causing the obstruction and enlarged kidneys. Excretory urography should demonstrate obstruction of urine outflow.

Treatment

Once a diagnosis of ureteral obstruction has been made the primary cause of obstruction should be removed before irreversible renal changes develop. The effects of urinary tract obstruction on renal function have been defined and are obviously dependent on the severity and duration of the obstruction (Wilson, 1977). In experimental dogs, if obstruction was allowed to persist for two weeks before being relieved, the affected kidney regained only 50 to 60 per cent of its preobstruction function. Four weeks is considered to be the maximum time for complete obstruction to be present with any likelihood of return of significant renal function after surgical correction (Pridgin et al., 1961). If an early diagnosis of unilateral obstruction has been made, it may be possible to perform a ureterectomy and ureteral anastomosis.

Impairment of ureteral function that results from chronic obstruction even in the presence of infection can be reversed after surgical correction of the obstruction in conjunction with appropriate antibiotic treatment (Rose et al., 1975).

In most cases nephrectomy and ureterectomy is the surgical treatment of choice, especially in dogs with advanced unilateral hydronephrosis. The function of the contralateral kidney should always be assessed before considering nephrectomy. There is no treatment for chronic bilateral ureteral obstruction and hydronephrosis, because renal damage is irreversible; the animal will show signs of chronic renal failure after the obstruction is relieved.

Prognosis

In unilateral obstruction and bilateral obstruction, if diagnosed early before permanent structural damage is done to the kidney, a good to guarded prognosis can be given provided that the obstruction can be relieved and the primary cause removed. The prognosis will depend on the nature of the lesion causing the obstruction (a neoplasm, inflammation, urolith).

REFERENCES

Allen, W. E., and Webbon, P.: Two cases of urinary incontinence in cats associated with acquired vaginoureteral fistula. J. Small Anim. Pract. *21*:367, 1980.

Archibald, J., and Owen, R. R.: Urinary System. *In* Canine Surgery. 2nd ed. American Veterinary Publication Inc., Santa Barbara, California, 1974.

Bannigan, J.: The structure and function of the ureter in the dog. Irish J. Med. Sci., *144*:426, 1975.

Bebco, R. L., Prier, J. E., and Biery, D. N.: Ectopic ureters in a male cat. J.A.V.M.A. *171*:738, 1977.

Belman, A. B.: The clinical significance of vesicoureteral reflux. Pediatr. Clin. North Am. *23*:707, 1976.

Berzon, J. L.: Primary leiomyosarcoma of the ureter in a dog. J.A.V.M.A. *175*:374, 1979.

Biewenga, W. J., Rothuizen, J., and Voorhout, G.: Ectopic ureters in the cat — a report of two cases. J. Small Anim. Pract. *19*:531, 1978.

Brown, N. O., Parks, J. L., and Greene, R. W.: Canine urolithiasis: retrospective analysis of 438 cases. J.A.V.M.A. *170*:419, 1977.

Cass, A. S., and Lenaghan, D.: The influence of posture on the occurrence of vesicoureteral reflux. Invest. Urol. *2*:523, 1965.

Chiari, R., Harzmann, R., and Gilch, W.: Ureteroneocystotomy without dissection of the submucosal tunnel. Int. Urol. Nephrol. *9*:99, 1977.

Christie, B. A.: The ureterovesical junction in dogs. Invest. Urol. *9*:10, 1971a.

Christie, B. A.: Incidence and etiology of vesicoureteral reflux in apparently normal dogs. Invest. Urol. *9*:184, 1971b.

Christie, B. A.: The occurrence of vesicoureteral reflux and pyelonephritis in apparently normal dogs. Invest. Urol. *10*:359, 1973a.

Christie, B. A.: Vesicoureteral reflux in dogs. J.A.V.M.A. *162*:771, 1973b.

Dingwall, J. S., Eger, C. E., and Owen, R. R.: Clinical experiences with the combined techniques of ureterovesical anastomosis for treatment of ectopic ureters. J.A.A.H.A. *12*:406, 1976.

Feeney, D. A., Thrall, D. E., Barver, D. L., Culver, D. H., and Lewis, R. E.: Normal canine excretory urogram. Effects on dose, time and individual dog variation. Am. J. Vet. Res. *40*:1596, 1979.

Goulden, B. E.: Vesicoureteral reflux in the dog. N.Z. Vet. J. *16*:167, 1968.

Goulden, B. E.: Vesicoureteral reflux in the dog (letter). N.Z. Vet. J. *17*:211, 1969.

Grana, L., Donellan, W. L., and Swenson, O.: Effects of gram negative bacteria on ureteral structure and function. J. Urol. *99*:539, 1968.

Greene, J. A., Thornhill, J. A., and Blevins, W. E.: Hydronephrosis and hydroureter associated with a unilateral ectopic ureter in a spayed bitch. J.A.A.H.A. *14*:708, 1978.

Hayes, H. M.: Ectopic ureters in dogs: Epidemiologic features. Teratology *10*:129, 1974.

Johnston, G. R., Jessen, C. R., and Osborne, C. A.: Retrograde Contrast Urethrography. *In* Kirk, R. W. (ed.): Current Veterinary Therapy VI, W. B. Saunders Co., Philadelphia, 1977, p. 1189.

Jones, B. R.: Ureteral ectopia in the golden retriever. Breeding experiments. Unpublished data, 1980a.

Jones, B. R.: Clinical investigations of ureteral ectopia in dogs. Unpublished data, 1980b.

Kipnis, R. M.: Vesicoureteral reflux in a cat. J.A.V.M.A. *167*:288, 1975.

Lennox, J. S.: A case report of unilateral ectopic ureter in a male Siberian husky. J.A.A.H.A. *14*:331, 1978.

Liska, W. D., and Patnaik, A. K.: Leiomyoma of the ureter of a dog. J.A.A.H.A. *13*:83, 1977.

Newman, L., Bucy, J. G., and McAlister, W. H.: Experimental production of reflux in the presence and absence of infected urine. Radiology *111*:591, 1974.

North, D. C.: Hydronephrosis and hydroureter in a kitten — a case report. J. Small. Anim. Pract. *19*:237, 1978.

O'Handley, P., Carrig, C. B., and Walshaw, R.: Renal and ureteral duplication in a dog. J.A.V.M.A. *174*:484, 1979.

Orr, C.: Ectopic ureters in a cat. Bull. Feline Adv. Bureau *17*:7, 1979.

Osborne, C. A., Low, D. G., and Finco, D. R.: Canine and Feline Urology, W. B. Saunders Co., Philadelphia, 1972.

Osborne, C. A., and Oliver, J. E.: Non-neurogenic Urinary Incontinence. *In* Kirk, R. W. (ed.): Current Veterinary Therapy VI. W. B. Saunders Co., Philadelphia, 1977, p. 1165.

Owen, R. R.: Canine ureteral ectopia — a review. J. Small Anim. Pract. *14*:407, 1973a.

Owen, R. R.: Canine ureteral ectopia — a review. Incidence, diagnosis and treatment. J. Small Anim. Pract. *14*:419, 1973b.

Pearson, H., and Gibbs, C.: Urinary incontinence of the dog due to accidental vaginal-uretero fistulation during hysterectomy. J. Small Anim. Pract. *21*:287, 1980.

Pearson, H., Gibbs, C., and Hillson, J. M.: Abnormalities of the canine urinary tract. Vet. Rec. *77*:775, 1965.

Pollock, S., and Schoen, S. S.: Urinary incontinence associated with congenital ureteral values in a bitch. J.A.V.M.A. *159*:332, 1971.

Pridgin, W. P., Woodhead, D. M., and Younger, R. K.: Alterations in renal function produced by ureteral obstruction. Determination of critical obstruction time in terms of renal survival. J.A.V.M.A. *78*:563, 1961.

Robins, G. M., and Presnell, K. R.: Ureteroneocystotomy in the dog. J. Small Anim. Pract. *15*:185, 1974.

Rose, J. G., and Gillenwater, J. Y.: Effect of chronic ureteral obstruction and infection upon ureteral function. Invest. Urol. *11*:471, 1974.

Rose, J. G., Gillenwater, J. Y., and Wyker, A. T.: The recovery of function of chronically obstructed and infected ureters. Invest. Urol. *13*:125, 1975.

Rose, J. G., and Gillenwater, J. Y.: Effects of obstruction on ureteral function. Urology *12*:139, 1978.

Schulman, C. C., and Gregoir, W.: Die Physiopathologie des primären vesikoureteralen Refluxes. Urologie [A] *16*:118, 1977.

Starr, A.: Ureteral plication. A new concept in ureteral tailoring for megaureter. Invest. Urol. *17*:153, 1979.

Van Den Brom, W. E., Biewenga, W. J., Rothuizen, J., and Voorhout, G.: Ectopic megaureter in the dog. Proc. Voorjaarsdagen *9*:61, 1978.

Vereecken, R. L.: Physiology and pathophysiology of the Ureter. Eur. Urol. *2*:4, 1976.

Wilson, D. R.: Renal function during and following obstruction. Ann. Rev. Med. *28*:329, 1977.

Wolf, A. M., Leighton, R. L., and Watrous, B. J.: Uric acid ureteral calculus and pararenal cyst in a cat. J.A.A.H.A. *15*:767, 1979.

CHAPTER **76**

Diseases of the Bladder and Urethra*

RICHARD W. GREENE
and RICHARD C. SCOTT

ANATOMY

In the dog, the urinary bladder is located just anterior to the brim of the pelvis. When empty, the bladder lies almost entirely within the pelvic canal, but as urine distends the bladder, it extends over the brim of the pelvis into the posterior abdomen. In the cat, the bladder is located within the posterior abdominal cavity at all times. In both species the bladder is divided into three segments: the blind-ending dome or fundus, the middle segment or body, and the posteriorly located bladder neck, which continues as the urethra. In the cat the

*The authors acknowledge the Berkeley Veterinary Research Foundation for assistance in the preparation of this paper.

bladder neck is longer than that in the dog (Crouch, 1969).

In the cat and dog, the trigone of the bladder is a triangular bundle of thin muscles that extends from the two points where the ureters enter the bladder to the urethral orifice in the bladder neck. The muscle bundles in the trigone are thought to be extensions of the intravesical ureters. After each ureter enters the trigone, it courses through the bladder musculature as the intramural segment, then passes obliquely toward the bladder neck beneath the bladder mucosa as the submucosal segment, and ends at the ureteric orifice. It is currently believed that vesicoureteral reflux is prevented by detrusor muscle tone, and provided by detrusor muscle fascicles surrounding the submucosal segment of the ureter (Christie, 1971).

The bladder is fixed in its location by three ligaments, which are actually double layers of peritoneum. The two lateral ligaments extend from the lateral bladder walls to the pelvic canal, while the larger middle umbilical ligament extends from the ventral surface of the bladder to the pelvic symphysis and ventral abdominal wall (Christensen, 1968; Gordon, 1960).

The blood supply of the anterior bladder is derived from the umbilical arteries, which course to the bladder in the lateral umbilical ligaments. After reaching the bladder, they give rise to the cranial vesical arteries. The posterior bladder and bladder neck are supplied by the caudal vesical arteries, which arise from the urogenital arteries. They are located in the fat near the bladder neck and prostate gland (in the male) (Christensen, 1968; Gordon, 1960).

Motor innervation of the bladder is provided by both autonomic and somatic fibers. The sympathetic supply is from the hypogastric nerve, which is ultimately derived from the caudal mesenteric ganglia (Christensen, 1968; Gans, 1970; Gordon, 1968). The pelvic nerve supplies parasympathetic innervation to the bladder. It is derived from the preganglionic fibers in the intermediolateral column of sacral gray matter (Bradley and Timm, 1974). These fibers pass within the ventral sacral roots to the pelvic plexus and vesical plexus near the wall of the rectum (Christensen, 1968; Gans, 1970; Gordon, 1968). After synapse, postganglionic fibers course to the bladder within the pelvic nerve to synapse on detrusor muscle fibers. The pelvic and hypogastric nerves pass to the bladder in the lateral ligaments near the caudal vesical arteries. Somatic innervation is derived from the pudendal nucleus located in the ventral gray matter of segments-S-1, S-2, and S-3 (Bradley and Timm, 1974) which become the pudendal nerve. This supplies the external bladder sphincter and urethra, and courses to the bladder along the ventral surface of the urethra. Sensory fibers pass from the sphincters to the spinal cord on all three motor nerves (Christensen, 1968; Gans, 1970; Gordon, 1960).

There are synaptic connections between the pudendal and detrusor nuclei through interneurons. The detrusor nucleus synapses with higher centers in the pontine mesencephalic reticular formation and the frontal cortex. Complicated interrelationships between these centers are responsible for modulation of the micturition reflex, which will be discussed later (Bradley and Timm, 1974).

In the male dog, the urethra is divided into the prostatic portion, located within the prostate gland, the membranous urethra, located between the caudal end of the prostate gland and the urethral bulb of the penis, and the cavernous portion, located between the urethral bulb of the penis and the urethral meatus. The male urethra extends from the bladder neck through the pelvic canal and then curves around the pubis. In the female, the urethra courses directly from the bladder neck in a caudodorsal direction to the floor of the vagina, where it exits through the urethral orifice. The blood supply of the male urethra comes from the prostatic branch of the urogenital artery, which arises distally from the urethral artery. The artery of the urethral bulb also supplies the cavernous urethra. Innervation of the urethra is from the pudendal nerve, and fibers are derived from the pelvic plexus. In the female dog, the urethral blood supply is from the caudal vesical artery and the external and internal pudendal arteries (Christensen, 1968).

In the male cat, the anatomy of the urethra is more complex. The membranous urethra extends from the bladder neck to the bulbourethral glands and is located within the pelvic canal. The portion of the membranous urethra that passes through the prostate gland is termed the prostatic urethra, and the portion passing through the bulbourethral glands is called the bulbous urethra. The prostate gland and prostatic urethra are midway between the anterior and posterior brims of the pelvis. The bulbourethral glands are located just caudal to the pelvis and are partially surrounded by the ischiocavernous muscles. From this point, the penile urethra passes distally to the urethral meatus. The urethra of the female cat is similar to that of the female dog. The blood supply of the urethra is derived from the urogenital artery in the male and female of both species, and also from the prostatic and dorsal arteries of the penis of both species (Crouch, 1969).

PHYSIOLOGY

The micturition reflex in the cat and dog is controlled primarily by reflex arcs in spinal cord segments, but these are influenced by higher centers in the brain (Bradley and Timm, 1974).

Filling of the bladder is controlled in part by nerve impulses and medial reticular formation. These fibers inhibit motor neurons to the bladder (Gans, 1970). At the same time, the striated urethral sphincter contracts and remains closed (Bradley and Timm, 1974; Gans, 1970). This is a result of tonic impulses arising from receptors in the sphincter that pass in pudendal sensory fibers to the spinal cord. They tonically stimulate the motor unit of the pudendal nerve to maintain closure of the sphincter (Bradley and Timm, 1974).

When bladder pressure reaches a certain point, new sensory impulses come from the pelvic nerve as a consequence of detrusor muscle stretching and pass to the sacral spinal cord segments. Afferent connections with the reticular formation occur through the spinoreticular pathways; after reflex integration occurs, efferent impulses return and stimulate the detrusor nucleus and, ultimately, the pudendal nucleus (Bradley and Timm, 1974; Oliver and Osborne, 1980). Motor impulses are then transmitted in the pelvic nerve to detrusor muscle pacemaker fibers, which depolarize. The impulse is spread to adjoining muscle fibers until the detrusor muscle contracts. This opens the bladder neck (Oliver and Osborne, 1980). At the same time, new sensory

impulses arise and pass in the pelvic nerve to the spinal cord and the pudendal nucleus. These impulses inhibit the tonic activity of the pudendal nerve and allow relaxation of the striated muscle of the sphincter (Bradley and Timm, 1974). Bladder emptying can now occur as the impulse from the detrusor muscle passes from muscle fiber to muscle fiber, and the bladder contracts and empties. Continued detrusor contraction is enhanced by sensory impulses arising from receptors in the bladder wall and urethra (Gans, 1970). Bladder tone diminishes after voiding, and all afferent impulses cease. The striated urethral sphincter closes and the reflex is ended.

The sympathetic innervation of the bladder has a questionable influence on the micturition reflex (Bradley and Timm, 1974; Oliver and Osborne, 1980). Ablation of sympathetic nerves does not alter micturition (Oliver and Osborne, 1980). The role played by the sympathetic system in micturition may be to dilate smooth muscle of the proximal urethra and to modulate motor impulses to the detrusor muscle (Bradley and Timm, 1974).

ANOMALIES OF THE BLADDER

Considering the complex embryologic events that lead to the development of the bladder and urethra, it is surprising that congenital anomalies of the bladder are not seen more frequently. Agenesis, hypoplasia, reduplication, diverticulum, contracture of the bladder outlet, absence of the urinary sphincter, exstrophy, urachal cyst, urachal fistula, trigonal folds, and cloacal formation have all been reported in man as anomalies of the bladder (Campbell and Harrison, 1970), but are most unusual in the dog and cat (Bloom, 1954; Osborne et al., 1966; Greene and Bohning, 1971). Urachal cysts, urachal fistula, and bladder diverticulum are the only anomalies frequently seen in veterinary clinical practice (Bloom, 1954; Osborne et al., 1966). Exstrophy of the bladder in a dog has been reported (Hobson and Ader, 1979).

URACHAL ANOMALIES

In the fetus, the urachus or allantoic stalk is a tubular structure that connects the lumen of the bladder with the allantois. At birth, or shortly thereafter, the urachus closes and forms a cicatrix at the apex of the bladder in most animals, and the urethra takes over its function (Bloom, 1954; Jamdar, 1956). In man, the urachus persists as the medial or middle umbilical ligament (Jamdar, 1956), whereas in lower animals the middle umbilical ligament is a double form of peritoneum that connects the ventral wall of the bladder to the ventral abdominal wall (Miller et al., 1964).

If closure of the urachal canal is not complete, a urachal anomaly may develop; four variations have been described in man, dog, and cat (Bloom, 1954; Brodie, 1945; Jarzylo et al., 1965; Hansen, 1977). Type 1 is complete, and the urachus communicates with the bladder and umbilicus. Type 2 is a blind internal type and involves a failure to close at the bladder. Type 3 is a blind external type; a urachal sinus forms at the umbilicus, and the bladder is normal. Type 4 is a totally blind urachal cyst that can form anywhere along the urachal canal and may or may not communicate with the bladder or the umbilicus (Fig. 76–1).

In one study it was reported that some form of urachal remnant was found in 25 per cent of all cats dissected, and it was believed that the urachal remnant was a contributing or predisposing factor to feline urologic syndrome (Hansen, 1977).

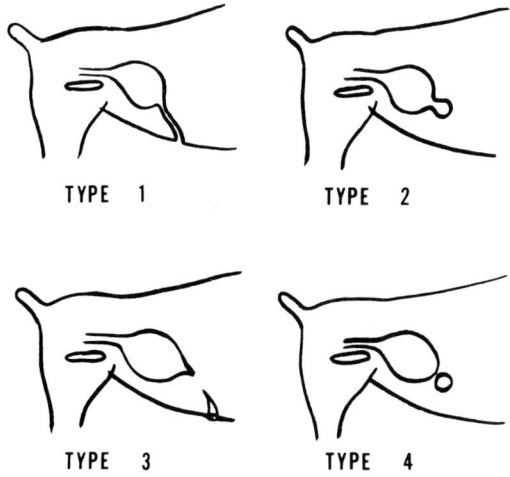

TYPE 1   TYPE 2

TYPE 3   TYPE 4

Figure 76–1. The four types of urachal anomalies. Type 1, the urachus communicates with the bladder and umbilicus. Type 2, the urachus fails to close completely at the bladder. Type 3, a urachal sinus is formed at the umbilicus. Type 4, a totally blind urachal cyst.

Type 1. Signs and treatment vary with the type of anomaly present. With the complete type, the animal is presented with urine scald of the skin at the umbilicus but is still able to urinate normally through the penile urethra. Radiographs of the abdomen may reveal an elongated urinary bladder with a pointed vertex (Park, 1978) that is displaced in a cranioventral direction, but contrast radiography, either an intravenous pyelogram or retrograde cystogram through the urethra or umbilical opening, is necessary to demonstrate the opening from the apex of the bladder to the umbilicus. Urinalysis reveals mild cystitis. Surgical removal of the fistula is the only treatment. An elliptic incision is made around the umbilical opening, and the fistula traced in the abdomen to the apex of the bladder; the fistula is excised and the bladder wall is closed in routine fashion.

Type 2. The blind internal type is the most common urachal anomaly seen in the dog and cat. It may persist unrecognized as a potential tract for many years. When it is associated with a lower urinary tract obstruction such as an enlarged prostate, urinary calculi, or urolithiasis in the cat, it may fistulate at the umbilicus or result in a diverticulum at the apex of the bladder. This tract can also be found during routine ovariohysterectomy as a fine to thick band running from the apex of the bladder to the umbilicus. These tracts should be removed, because they may potentially induce the clinical signs described below (Fig. 76–2, *A*, *B*).

Signs vary with the extent of the anomaly, from soiling at the umbilicus following urinary obstruction to signs of chronic unresponsive cystitis, the latter being more common. A dog at any age with chronic unresponsive cystitis should routinely undergo contrast radiographic studies of the bladder to rule out a diverticulum. Stasis of urine in the diverticulum may eventually lead to persistent infection, especially that caused by *Proteus, Klebsiella,* and *Pseudomonas spp.,* or to calculi formation. Urinalysis usually indicates severe infection. Treatment consists of surgically removing the diverticulum or tract from the apex to avoid urine stasis, culturing the bladder mucosa, and administering the approximate urinary antibiotics and acidifiers (Wilson et al., 1979). Visualization of the diverticulum at

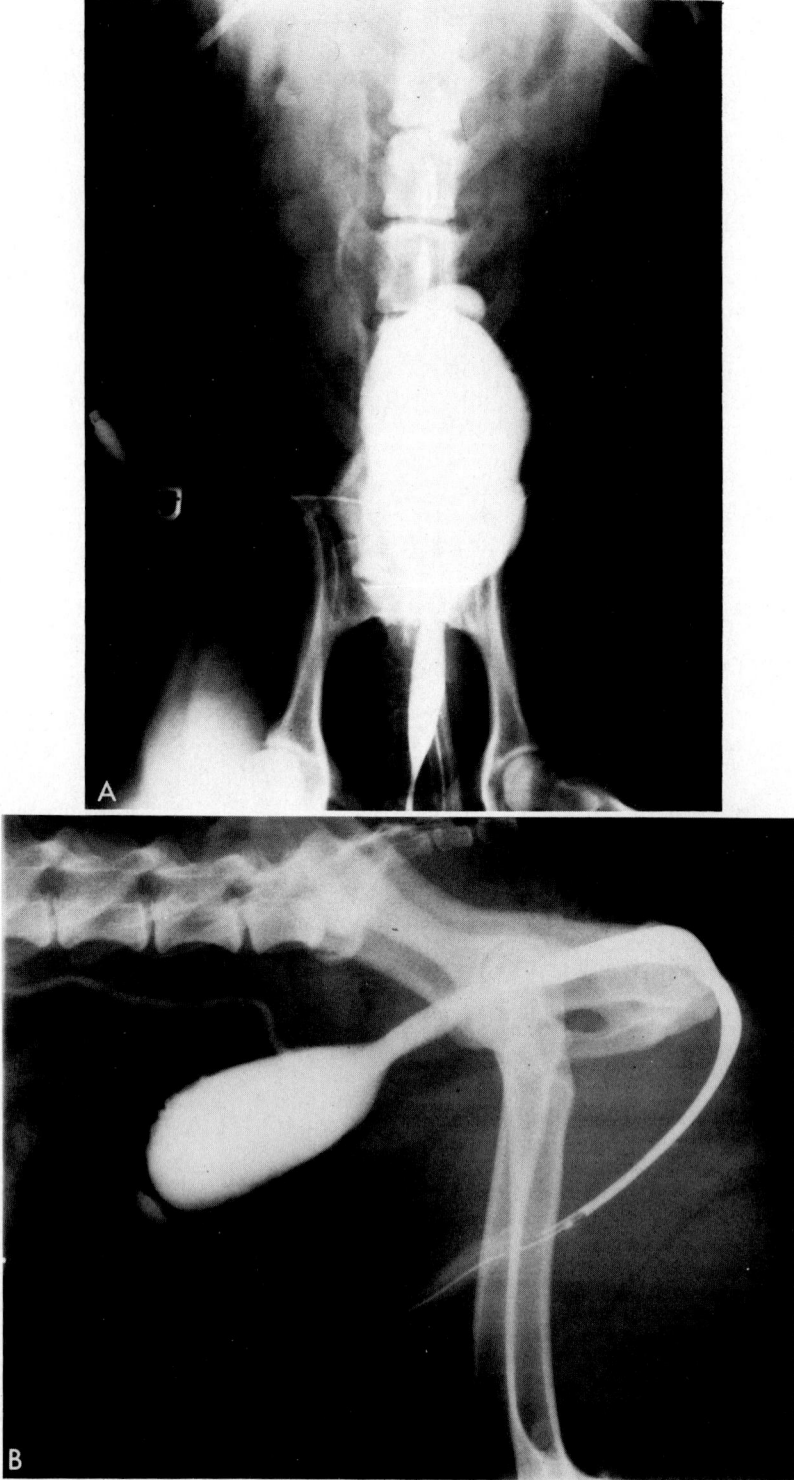

Figure 76–2. A "blind internal type" diverticulum at the apex of the bladder. *A,* Ventrodorsal and *B,* lateral views of the abdomen with a positive contrast cystogram. Note the vesicoureteral reflux of the contrast material.

surgery can be improved by placing pressure on a full bladder so that the urine distends the diverticulum.

Type 3. A urachal sinus, formed when the urachus opens only at the umbilicus, causes omphalitis. It is characterized by a persistent infection and swellings at the umbilicus in young animals and usually responds to hot packs, drainage, and antibiotics. Surgical debridement may be necessary in some cases.

Type 4. A urachal cyst can be found anywhere along the route of the urachal remnant. They vary tremendously in size and are filled with exudate from the epithelial lining. The fluid may be sterile but can become infected, possibly through hematogenous or lymphogenous routes or through ascent from the bladder itself. Noninfected cysts usually go unnoticed unless the abdomen becomes distended, or they are found incidentally during surgery or on radiography. Infected cysts can cause systemic effects, and if ruptured, they can cause peritonitis. These cysts, whether infected or not, should be surgically excised.

BACTERIAL CYSTITIS

Etiology. Various bacterial organisms have been incriminated for causing cystitis. Recent literature suggests that *E. coli* is the most common isolate (Hirsh, 1973; Kiristo et al., 1977; Osborne et al., 1972; Wooley and Blue, 1976). However, *Proteus mirabilis*, *Staphylococcus aureus*, enteric *Streptococcus spp.*, and *Klebsiella spp.* are also found frequently (Hirsh, 1973; Kiristo et al., 1977; Ling, 1979; Osborne et al., 1972; Wooley and Blue, 1976). Less common but important organisms include *Pseudomonas aeruginosa*, *Enterobacter spp.*, *Proteus vulgaris*, *Proteus rettgeri*, and *beta-hemolytic Streptococci* (Ling, 1979), and *Clostridium spp.*, (Middleton and Lomas, 1979; Sherding and Chew, 1979).

Cystitis is usually the result of an infection ascending from the lower urinary tract (Carroll, 1970; Osborne et al., 1972). Rarely, disseminated or local bacterial infections spread to the bladder via the hematogenous route (Carroll, 1970; Osborne et al., 1972). Infection in the upper urinary tract may serve as a continuing source of recurrent infection of the bladder (Campbell, 1970; Osborne et al., 1972). In the male, chronic infection of the prostate gland can also be a source of bacteria and infection (Carroll, 1970).

Factors that predispose the bladder to infection include urinary stasis, trauma, abnormal urine composition, and calculi. Urine stasis is the most important predisposing factor to infection; stasis allows bacteria present in the bladder to multiply by decreasing effective mixing of urine formed by the kidney with urine already present in the bladder (Hinman, 1968) and by decreasing bacterial elimination from the urinary tract (Osborne et al., 1979). Urine retention can be caused by any physical factors, acquired or congenital, that produce extra- or intraluminal stenosis of the urinary outflow tract. Local stasis of urine can be caused by small or large diverticula located anywhere in the lower urinary tract, but are most commonly found in the bladder (Osborne et al., 1972). Abnormalities in normal bladder innervation at any level of neurologic organization can be associated with urine retention by preventing the normal micturition reflex (Oliver and Selcer, 1974).

Trauma predisposes the bladder to infection under some circumstances by causing stenosis and urine retention. Trauma also devitalizes the mucosal lining of the urinary tract, which can disrupt normal mucosal antibacterial defenses (Norden et al., 1968) and decrease the formation of the mucoprotein lining. This may promote bacterial colonization in the urinary tract (Hutch, 1970; Parsons et al., 1977; Shrom et al., 1977) and decrease normal immunoglobulin defenses against bacterial infection (Williams and Gibbons, 1972). This subject has been reviewed (Osborne et al., 1979; Petersdorf and Turck, 1970). Regardless of the exact pathogenesis, bacteria are permitted to colonize and then multiply with increased efficacy following trauma to the mucosal lining, thereby predisposing the urinary tract to infection. Trauma may also disrupt the normal blood supply of the urinary tract, which diminishes the delivery of normal host defense mechanisms such as oxygen, immunoglobulins, and leukocytes.

The antibacterial properties of urine have been reviewed (Lees and Osborne, 1979) and include alkaline and acid pH extremes as well as urine osmolality. Changes in the composition of urine that decrease osmolality without significantly increasing urine volume and elimination of bacteria may predispose to infection. An example is oliguric renal failure, which causes impairment of the ability of the kidney to concentrate urine. Dilution of the antibacterial properties of urine may predispose to infection even when urine volume is increased (Lees et al., 1979). Likewise, decreasing urine volume without urine osmolality may also diminish delivery of antibacterial properties and enhance infection. Glycosuria due to diabetes mellitus or any other cause has been associated with increased urinary tract infections. Glycosuria allows for optimal growth of bacterial organisms that utilize glucose for their metabolism (Bailey, 1961; Finby and Begg, 1969; Teuscher, 1968).

Calculi can cause obstruction of the urine outflow tract and subsequently predispose to infection. In addition, calculi serve as a source of irritation and trauma to the urinary tract, which can predispose to infection as previously discussed. Calculi also harbor bacterial organisms that may later be a source of continuing infection (Goulden, 1968).

Physical Findings and Laboratory Findings. Patients with cystitis are examined because of variable degrees of stranguria and pollakiuria (frequency of urination). The owner often reports that the animal makes frequent attempts to urinate but produces only small amounts of urine on each occasion. Cloudy urine or hematuria may occur at any time during the course of cystitis but is often encountered early. It may become painful for the animal to urinate if the disorder goes untreated. The presence of urethral calculi may cause blockage, preventing the animal from passing urine at all. If the upper urinary tract has been involved by obstruction or infection, the patient may exhibit variable degrees of lethargy, anorexia, vomition, and dehydration caused by uremia.

Physical examination of patients with cystitis unassociated with renal involvement is usually unremarkable. Occasionally, abdominal palpation reveals a thickened bladder, or calculi may be palpated. Urethral obstruction causes bladder enlargement. Infection with bacteria causing suppuration (pyocystitis) results in hyperthermia. Pneumaturia may occur if emphysematous cystitis is present. Rarely, crepitation of the bladder caused by the presence of gas in the lumen and/or wall can be palpated.

Results of urinalysis vary with the method of collection. The preferred method is cystocentesis, since this allows for minimal contamination of the sample by bacteria and cells from the lower urinary tract. When this method of collection is used, microscopic hematuria (greater than five RBC per hpf), white blood cells (greater than four WBC per hpf), and bacteriuria indicate infection. Transitional cells, which may appear reactive, can also be seen when infection is present. The presence of granular casts and white blood cell casts suggests renal involvement (Leader and Carlton, 1970). The specific gravity varies depending on the presence of renal failure; the urine pH also varies. The presence of an alkaline pH is sometimes associated with infections caused by urea-splitting organisms. Albumin will be present in variable concentrations, depending on the degree of hemorrhage into the urine and the concentration of the sample at the time of collection. It is unusual, but theoretically possible, to see concentrations as high as 1000 mg per 100 ml. Occult blood will be present if there is sufficient hemoglobin in the sample as a result of red blood cell lysis.

When other methods of collection are used, the presence of microscopic hematuria, pyuria, and bacteriuria should be interpreted with caution, since these can be the result of contamination from the lower urinary tract.

Results of biochemical and hematologic testing may reveal high urea nitrogen and creatinine concentrations with nonregenerative anemia if there is renal involvement, or leukocytosis if pyocystitis is present. In cases of cystitis, however, results of hematologic and biochemical evaluation are usually normal.

The techniques employed for bacterial culture of the urine following proper collection have been reviewed (Barsanti and Finco, 1979; Ling and Biberstein, 1979). Quantitative culture is the most accurate method of sorting out significant bacterial growth; greater than 10^5 organisms indicate infection in voided or catheterized samples (Ling and Biberstein, 1979). When cystocentesis is the method of collection, any growth of bacteria is suspicious (Ling and Biberstein, 1979).

Treatment. The clinician should seek to diagnose and eliminate any factors predisposing to infection. Cystitis occurring for the first time in a female patient over one year of age, in the absence of predisposing factors as assessed by the history and physical examination, may be treated without investigation of the urinary tract. If, however, the patient is under one year of age, a male, or a female having had two or more episodes of cystitis, such investigation is necessary and should include plain radiography of the bladder and a urethrogram and double contrast cystogram. An intravenous pyelogram should be performed if renal involvement is suspected on the basis of results of laboratory tests.

Specific treatment is aimed at establishing sufficient blood concentrations of urinary tract antibiotics to eliminate infection. Bacterial culture of the urine and sensitivity testing are helpful in determining the drugs of choice. The various methods of sensitivity testing have been reviewed (Barsanti and Finco, 1979; Ling and Biberstein, 1979). Single-disc sensitivity testing estimates the serum concentration of various antibiotics. However, renal excretion of many antibiotics increases their concentration to levels well above these estimates (Ling, 1979; Ling and Gilmore, 1977; Ling and Ruby, 1979; Stamey et al., 1974); therefore, interpretation of single-disc sensitivity test results must be done cautiously. Other methods of sensitivity testing estimate the minimum inhibitory concentration of an antibiotic (Barsanti and Finco, 1979; Ling, 1979; Ling and Biberstein, 1979). These methods estimate the least amount of antibiotic that will result in complete inhibition of bacterial growth, and therefore, they are more accurate determinants of potential antibiotic efficacy (Ling, 1979). The cost and technical difficulties involved with these methods have prevented their gaining wide acceptance in veterinary clinical practice to date. In order to be effective, the concentration of a given antibiotic that can be achieved in the urine must also be known, and this has been determined in dogs for a small number of drugs only (Ling and Gilmore, 1977; Ling and Ruby, 1978; Ling and Ruby, 1979).

First episodes of urinary tract infections should be treated with broad spectrum antibiotics for a minimum of three weeks. One method for selecting the antibiotic to be used has been presented by Ling (1979). Alternatively, the authors have selected one of the following for initial therapy: trimethoprim-sulfa, 30 mg/kg/day;

chloramphenicol, 20 to 50 mg/kg three times per day; or cephalexin, 11 to 17.6 mg/kg three times per day. If the results of culture and sensitivity testing indicate the need for a change in the antibiotic, then a new one should be substituted. Otherwise, administration of the initial antibiotic should be continued.

Repeat urine culture and sensitivity testing is the most accurate way of determining efficacy of treatment. However, this can be expensive and time consuming. Ideally, cultures should be taken three to five days after administration of antibiotics determined to be the most efficacious by initial culture and sensitivity testing. If the culture is positive, the antibiotic should be changed and the new antibiotic used for three weeks. If a negative culture is obtained, the original antibiotic should be administered for three more weeks. If expense precludes culturing following initial therapy, the presence or absence of clinical signs and results of urinalysis can be used to determined the need for change of therapy.

Reculture and sensitivity testing should be performed 7 to 14 days after termination of treatment. If this culture is negative, treatment can be discontinued. If positive, predisposing factors for cystitis, if not already investigated, should be found and eliminated. Treatment with a new antibiotic selected on the basis of sensitivity test results should be initiated. As finances permit, reculture and sensitivity testing should be done in three to five days, and adjustments in antibiotic therapy made accordingly. The second course of antibiotic therapy should last six to eight weeks, and reculture performed 7 to 14 days after termination. If positive, antibiotic suppression therapy should be considered; if negative, antibiotics can be discontinued and reculture performed every six months, or as determined by recurrent signs.

Antibiotic suppression is a method of treatment that attempts to keep bacterial numbers low so as to prevent continuing complications from urinary tract infection, or to eradicate infection by means of a long course of treatment. A method for antibiotic suppression that has been described by Ling (1979) advocates the use of one of three agents (nitrofurantoin, trimethoprim-sulfa, or ampicillin/penicillin G) taken at one quarter the total daily dose after the last voiding of the day (Table 76–1). By admin-

Table 76–1. In Vivo Susceptibility of Common Canine Urinary Tract Bacterial Pathogens to Certain Oral Antimicrobial Agents

Predictable		Unpredictable
Approaching 100% Confidence	*About 80% Confidence*	
Staphylococcus spp (Penicillin)*	*E. coli* (Trimethoprim/Sulfa)†	*Klebsiella spp*
Streptococcus spp (Penicillin)	*Proteus mirabilis* (Penicillin)	
	Pseudomonas spp (Tetracycline)‡	

*Penicillin G: given orally at the rate of 110,000 units per kg (50,000 units per lb) of body weight in three divided doses daily, or Ampicillin: given orally at the rate of 77 mg per kg (35 mg per lb) of body weight in three divided doses daily.

†Tribrissen or Septra — given orally at the rate of 26.4 mg per kg (12 mg per kg (12 mg per lb) of body weight in two divided doses daily.

‡Tetracycline — given orally at the rate of 55 mg per kg (25 mg per lb) of body weight in three divided doses daily.

istering the drug at that time, blood concentrations remain sufficiently high for eight to ten hours to suppress or kill pathogenic bacteria (Ling, 1979). While reportedly efficacious, it requires that voiding of urine not occur during the night, and therefore the method is probably not practical in animals with polyuria or pollakiuria. Alternatively, antibacterial agents can be administered at therapeutic dosages for long periods of time. The agents that the authors have used include trimethoprim-sulfa, cephalexin, and gantrisin (0.5 gm/40 lbs, three to four times daily). Nitrofurantoin (4 mg/kg, three times per day) can also be used, unless vomition prevents chronic administration.

In either method of suppression, monthly urine cultures are recommended. Negative cultures on six occasions justify cessation of therapy. Positive cultures at any time necessitate a 14- to 20-day course of therapy with an antibiotic that is sensitive to the pathogen, followed by therapy after the last voiding as described (Ling, 1979); otherwise, a change of antibiotic, as determined by sensitivity test results, is administered for long periods of time.

Extremely resistant infections are sometimes encountered and are frequently caused by *Pseudomonas spp., Proteus spp.,* and resistant *E. coli*. Occasionally, resistant *Streptococcus faecalis* can also cause such infections. These can be treated with administrations of gentamycin, amikacin, or tobramycin at therapeutic dosages for seven to ten days, as determined by urine culture and sensitivity testing; oral antibiotic for seven days, as determined by urine culture and sensitivity testing; a second course of gentamycin, amikacin, or tobramycin (if

BUN and creatinine concentrations are normal); a second course of oral antibiotics for six to eight weeks; repeat culture in 7 to 14 days after therapy is ended; antibiotic suppression, if culture is positive. Testing for BUN or creatinine concentrations should be done prior to the second course of aminoglycoside therapy. If abnormal, the second course should not be administered.

Potentially nephrotoxic antibiotics should be avoided when preexisting renal failure is present, or a dosage adjustment should be made to account for renal failure (Kovant et al., 1973).

Urinary acidifiers may be used when the optimum pH of the pathogen is in the alkaline range (urea-splitting bacteria), or when the efficacy of a sensitive antibiotic is improved by an acid pH (penicillin, tetracycline, nitrofurantoin, and carbenicillin). Many acidifiers are available, including DL-methionine, ascorbic acid, and ammonium chloride. The client should be instructed to test the urine with hydrazine paper three times daily before meals to assure that the acidifier is working (Lewis, 1978). In the event of failure to acidify the urine, either dosage or the drug should be changed. Chronic acidification to prevent cystitis after infection has been eradicated is of questionable value.

CANINE CALCULI

Urolithiasis occurs frequently in the dog, the rate of reported occurrence being 0.4 to 2.8 per cent of cases in veterinary institutions in Europe and the United States (Finco et al., 1970; White, 1966; Weaver, 1970; Krabbe, 1949; Finco, 1970; Brown et al.,

1977). Calculi have been found throughout the urinary tract and, in one case, free in the abdominal cavity (Belkin, 1970); clinically, the majority of calculi are found in the bladder of the female and in the bladder and urethra of the male (Finco et al., 1970; White, 1966; Weaver, 1970; Finco, 1970; Brown et al., 1977; Clark, 1974). They are usually seen in dogs between three and seven years of age but have been reported in pups a few weeks old (Fig. 76–3) and in dogs over 15 years old (Hardy et al., 1972; Brodey, 1955; Finco et al., 1970; Weaver, 1970; Finco, 1970; White, 1966; White et al.,

1961; Brown et al., 1977). The mean age has been reported to be 5.5 years for all types of calculi, while the dogs with cystine calculi were younger and the dogs with oxalate calculi were older (Brown et al., 1977).

There are four different types of calculi, based on composition: phosphate, urate, cystine, and oxalate (Finco, 1970). Xanthine, sulfanilamide, carbonate, tetracycline, and silica calculi also occur rarely, although there seems to be an increase in the occurrence of silica uroliths (Kidder and Chivers, 1968; Finco, 1970; Treacher, 1966;

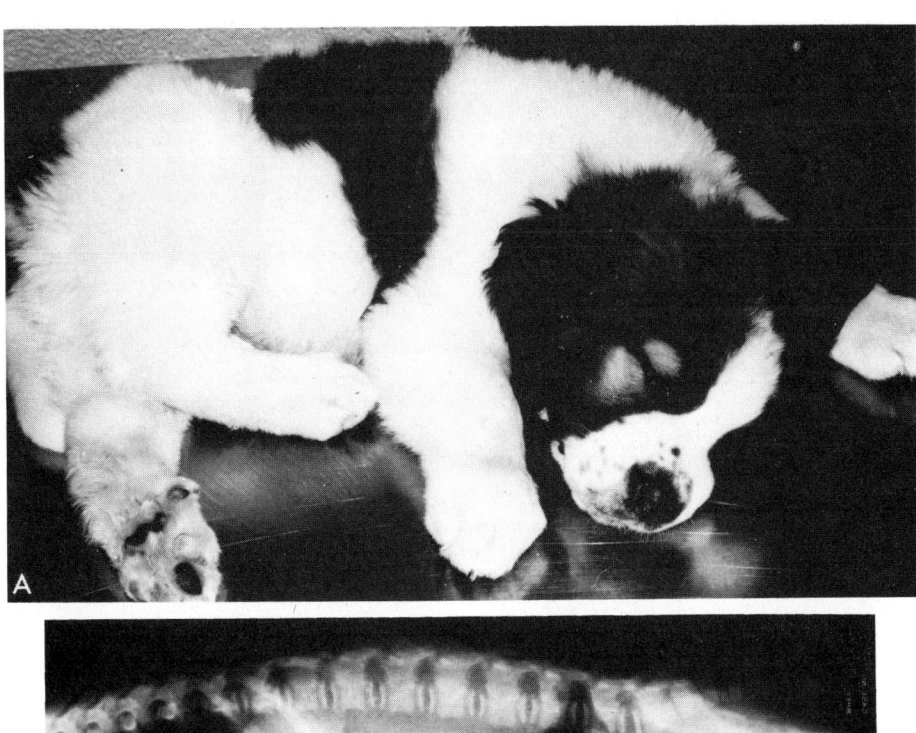

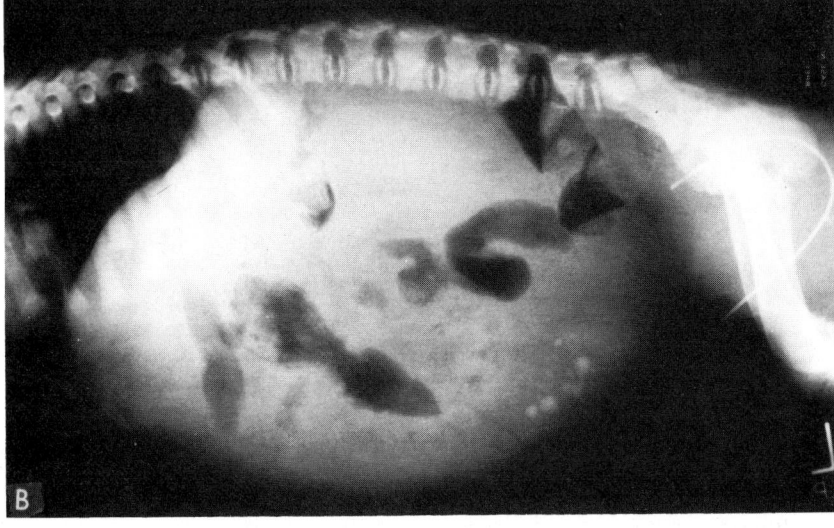

Figure 76–3. A ten-week-old St. Bernard with stranguria. *A*, Appearance at examination. *B*, Lateral radiographic view of abdomen, showing multiple phosphate cystic calculi.

Osborne and Klausner, 1978). Phosphate stones are seen most frequently, followed by cystine or urate stones (depending on the breed of dog and the geographic location), and then by oxalates (Finco, 1970; Finco et al., 1970; Weaver, 1970; Brown et al., 1977; White et al., 1961).

Breeds having the highest incidence of urolithiasis are the dachshund, Pekingese, Welsh corgi, Dalmatian, cocker spaniel, Scottish terrier, miniature schnauzer, poodle, pug, bulldog, beagle, bassett hound, and dogs of mixed breeding (Finco, 1970; Krabbe, 1949; Finco et al., 1970; Brown et al., 1977; Weaver, 1970; Brodey, 1955; White et al., 1961). The German shepherd dog has a significantly lower occurrence than other breeds (Brown et al., 1977).

The male to female sex ratio depends on the type of calculi. With phosphate (struvite) calculi affecting adults, the female is affected more often than the male (Finco, et al., 1970; Brodey, 1955; Brown et al., 1977). In dogs under one year of age, there is a higher incidence of phosphate calculi in the male (Hardy et al., 1972). Urate calculi are usually seen more often in the male than female (Brown et al., 1977). Although cystine calculi are generally thought to occur only in males, one case has been reported in a female (Brown et al., 1978) and cystinuria has been reported in a female (Bovee et al., 1977). Oxalate calculi have been reported more frequently in the male.

Signs. Most dogs with cystic calculi are examined because of some change in urinary habits, whether it be increased frequency, decreased amount, straining, or passing blood in the urine (Clark, 1966). Others show no signs at all. A history of unresponsive cystitis often accompanies the case.

The clinical signs vary with the sex of the animal and the anatomic location of the urolith within the urinary tract (Finco, 1970). A female with a short, wide urethra is rarely obstructed, as compared with a male with a long, narrow urethra; however, not all males have stones in the urethra.

A female or male dog with vesicular calculi is often in good health but exhibits signs similar to those found in dogs with cystitis (frequent urination, tenesmus, hematuria, and at times, incontinence). Abdominal palpation will often reveal the calculi in the bladder if the animal is not too fat and the bladder is empty. Females may void small calculi during urination.

In the male, calculi that are formed in the bladder may pass into the urethra, causing varying degrees of occlusion or obstruction. These calculi may lodge at any point along the urethra, but they most frequently lodge at the caudal end of the os penis, where the urethra passes through the bony groove. Early in the course, the signs are similar to those found in cystitis. When obstruction, dysuria or anuria occurs, severe tenesmus, depression, and signs of uremia develop. A distended bladder can be palpated abdominally, and the obstructing calculi may at times be palpated in the urethra, usually just posterior to the os penis. A catheter passed retrograde up the urethra will reveal the obstruction.

Evaluation. The general condition of the animal should be evaluated. Results of hematologic testing may reveal elevation in the white blood count, but it is usually not significant. Determining BUN and creatinine concentrations will aid in evaluating the degree of urinary obstruction and renal damage. Results of urinalysis may be consistent with inflammation. Bacteriologic culture and sensitivity testing or minimum inhibitory concentration testing of the urine should be done; if surgery is to be performed, however, a direct swab of the bladder wall or from the center of the calculi (Klausner and Osborne, 1979, 1980) is more effective in recovering any bacteria present.

A thorough radiographic examination of the urinary tract, including the kidneys and ureter, should be performed on all dogs with calculi. In one report, it was concluded that uroliths of the bladder were usually diagnosed antemortem, whereas uroliths of the kidney were usually diagnosed post mortem (Finco et al., 1970).

Most uroliths are radiopaque and easy to diagnose on plain films, but some are radiolucent and more difficult to diagnose. In one report, 17 of 557 calculi were radiolucent (Brown et al., 1977). Phosphate and oxalate calculi are usually radiopaque, while cystine and urate calculi vary in radiopacity (Figs. 76–4, 76–5). Cystine calculi are more often radiopaque than radiolucent, while urate calculi are more often radiolucent (Clark, 1966; Brown et al., 1977). When radiolucent calculi are suspected, especially

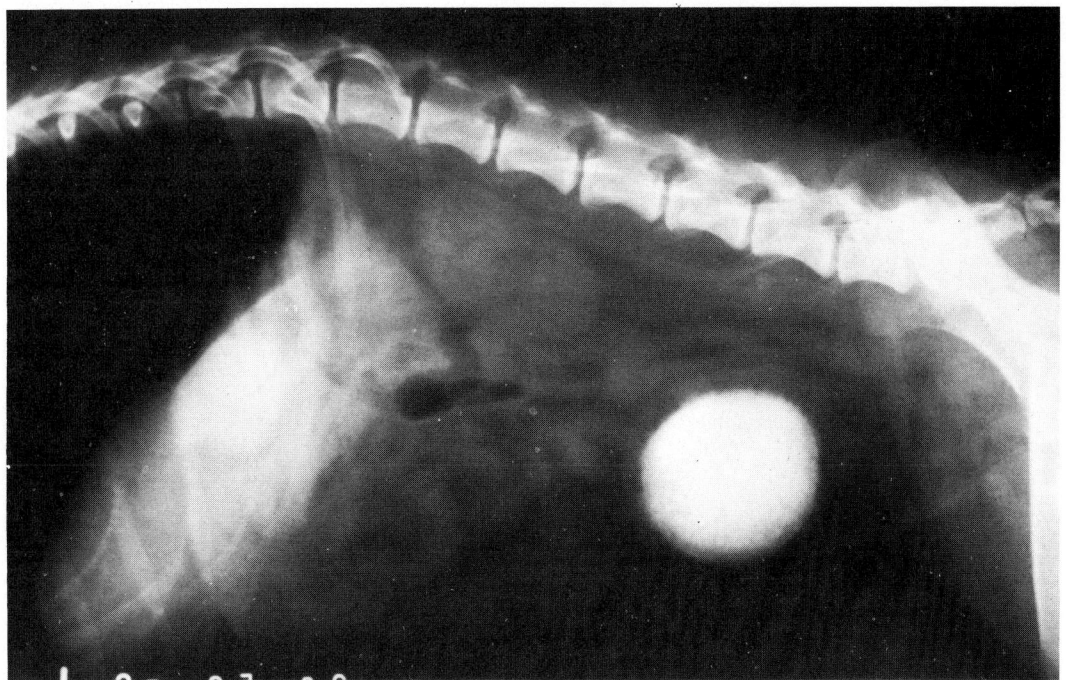

Figure 76–4. Lateral view of the abdomen of a six-year-old dog. A large, dense radiopaque (phosphate) cystic calculus can be seen.

in cases of chronic cystitis, both contrast and double contrast studies may be necessary for diagnosis. Contrast radiography should be used to identify very small calculi or anatomic abnormalities that might predispose to calculi formation.

To radiograph the perineal part of the urethra, the hind legs are pulled forward; to radiograph the penile portion, the legs are pulled back (Clark, 1966). If an obstruction is encountered with the catheter and the plain films show no calculi, contrast studies of the urethra must be performed.

With a history of change in urinary habits, palpation of hard masses in the bladder or urethra, blockage or resistance to a catheter passed retrograde up the urethra, and radiographic evidence of calculi, a diagnosis of cystic and urethral calculi is highly likely.

Treatment. An animal examined because of an obstructed urinary tract should be treated as an emergency — postrenal uremia may be present if the obstruction has been present for any length of time. Before catheterizing a dog, complete relaxation and relief from the spasm associated with urethral calculi need to be achieved; therefore, a smooth muscle relaxant may first be administered. A topical anesthetic

may also be flushed into the urethra prior to catheterization. Following sedation or general anesthesia, which is required in most cases, nonsurgical removal of the obstruction should be attempted.

There are several nonsurgical methods of relieving urethral blockage. All involve catheterization, and it is important that this procedure not be performed without flushing a lubricant or fluid through the catheter. One can attempt to forcefully push the calculi into the bladder with a well-lubricated catheter; however, this method is not recommended because of possible damage to the urethral wall.

Another technique is to flush saline solution through a well-lubricated catheter while applying gentle pressure around the catheter and distal end of the penis at the external urethral orifice. The catheter may be pushed up to the obstruction and pulled back while flushing with saline. If the pressure becomes too great within the urethra, the pressure applied at the external urethral orifice should be decreased. This should be attempted several times. The flushing will dilate the urethra over the calculi and also lubricate the urethra, decreasing the chance of injury.

A third method (Piermattei and Osborne,

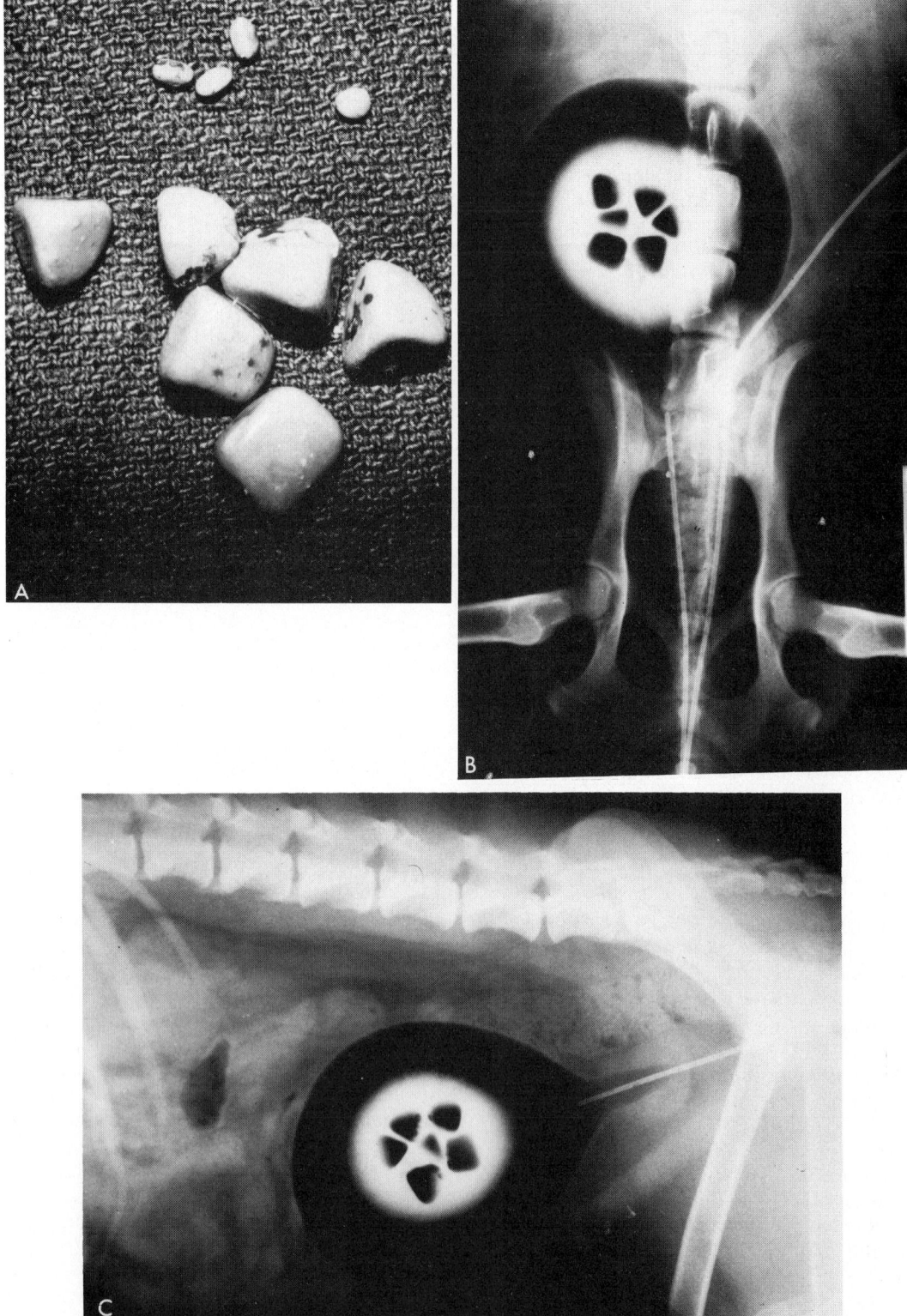

Figure 76–5. Urate cystic calculi. *A,* Gross appearance. The calculi could be demonstrated only by using double-contrast radiography. *B,* Ventrodorsal view. *C,* Lateral view.

1971) involves dilating the urethra with fluid under pressure. With sudden relief of the pressure, the calculi may be freed. This technique is performed by injecting a sterile lubricant into the urethra and inserting a teat cannula attached to a syringe full of saline into the external urethral orifice. An assistant occludes the pelvic urethra with digital pressure from the rectum, and the external urethral orifice is occluded by applying pressure around the teat cannula while the syringe of saline is injected. The urethra can be felt dilating rectally. The teat cannula and pressure to the urethral orifice should be released suddenly, allowing for a sudden release of saline from the urethral orifice. If the occlusion is due to small calculi, they will be carried out through the penile urethra with the saline. This procedure should be attempted several times. If the calculi are too large to pass through the os penis, pressure should be maintained at the external urethral orifice, and the pressure on the pelvic urethra applied from the rectum should be released suddenly, forcing the saline and calculi into the bladder. This method may be repeated several times.

Once the obstruction is relieved, the initial emergency is over. If the animal is uremic or if surgery is to be postponed until a more opportune time, a catheter can be sutured into place at the prepuce while intravenous fluids are administered. If nonsurgical methods fail to relieve the obstruction, a urethrostomy or cystotomy should be performed. Nonsurgical methods of relieving the obstruction should always be attempted prior to surgery; however, surgery is the preferred treatment for most cases of urolithiasis.

Three types of urethrostomy are recommended: the prepubic, scrotal, and perineal (Greene and Greiner, 1971; Archibald, 1965; Brown and Greiner, 1975). A urethrostomy may be temporary (the urethra is incised and no sutures are placed in the mucosa), or permanent (the mucosa is sutured to the skin to make a permanent fistula).

The prepubic urethrostomy is performed on the midline, midway between the distal end of the os penis and the scrotum. The scrotal urethrostomy involves castration and amputation of the scrotum, and suturing of the urethral mucosa to the skin in the area of the amputated scrotum. The perineal urethrostomy is performed on the midline of the perineum over the ischium midway between the ischial arch and the scrotum. The prepubic and perineal urethrostomies may be temporary or permanent; the scrotal urethrostomy is permanent. Permanent urethrostomy is preferred, inasmuch as it prevents stricture and narrowing of the urethra when the urethrostomy site heals. A permanent opening may also prevent further obstruction should calculi recur.

In cases of calculi in the bladder, a cystotomy should be performed. In the male, the urethral obstruction should first be relieved, and a catheter should remain in place to prevent further obstruction. At surgery, the bladder and urethra should be flushed many times and catheters passed to make sure no calculi remain. In cases in which there are multiple calculi, radiographs should be taken postoperatively to make sure all the calculi were removed. A direct sterile swab of the bladder or of the inside of one of the calculi should be taken for bacterial culture, and the calculi saved and analyzed. A commercial kit may be used for qualitative analysis of the calculi, but these kits are not designed to detect less common calculi, such as xanthine and silica. Quantitative analysis of calculi may be performed by a commercial laboratory and is advised, especially in recurring cases of calculi (Osborne and Klausner, 1978). Some of the calculi have typical gross appearances (Kirk et al., 1968), but this should not be relied on for identification. If the animal is not uremic, a urethrostomy and cystotomy may be performed at the same time. If the animal is uremic, the urethrostomy should first be performed to relieve the urethral obstruction, and a cystotomy performed after the proper intravenous fluid therapy has returned the dog to normal health.

Postoperatively, urinary antibiotics should be administered, using a method similar to the one described for the treatment of cystitis. Urinary acidifiers should not be used until the chemical makeup of the stones is known. At the time of suture removal or when the results of the calculi analysis and bacterial cultures are complete, treatment should be initiated to prevent recurrences of the calculi.

Prevention. The most difficult aspect of treating urolithiasis in the dog is the prevention of recurrence. This may be due in part to the fact that the exact etiopathogenesis of calculi has not been fully established (Thornton, 1968; Osborne and Klausner, 1978), but owner compliance is another important aspect. The rate of recurrence is reportedly high without the proper treatment (Bovee, 1973; Thornton, 1968; Finco, 1971; Weaver, 1970; Brodey, 1955). In a study of 438 dogs with urolithiasis, 25 per cent had known recurrences. Recurrence was observed in 17 per cent of the dogs with phosphate calculi, 33 per cent of the dogs with urate calculi, 47 per cent of the dogs with cystine calculi, and 25 per cent of the dogs with oxalate calculi (Brown et al., 1977).

The importance of stone analysis, bacterial culture, and sensitivity testing cannot be overstressed as a starting point for the prevention of recurrent urinary calculi. If treatment for one type of calculi is incorrect, it may precipitate another type.

The four basic types of calculi may be divided into primary and secondary groups. Primary calculi (cystine, urate, and oxalate) are metabolic in origin and form in acid urine. Infection may be present, usually caused by urease-negative bacteria, but it is believed that infection has no influence on primary formation (Brown et al., 1977). There may be exceptions to this, especially with oxalate calculi, which do not seem to be influenced by urine pH, but it can be followed as a general rule. Secondary calculi, the most common type, form in the presence of urea-splitting organisms, such as *Staphylococcus* or *Proteus spp.*, which cause the urine to be alkaline. This type includes magnesium ammonium phosphate (struvite) and mixed calculi. Mixed calculi are composed of primary and secondary types.

Magnesium Ammonium Phosphate Calculi

Infection plays an important role in phosphate calculi formation, since a significant clinical relationship has been shown to exist between phosphate calculi and *Staphylococcus* infection, which is rarely seen with calculi of other types (Brodey, 1955; Goulden, 1968; Weaver, 1975; Finco, 1970; Brown et al., 1980). Both *Staphylococcus* and *Proteus spp.* are common urinary bacteria associated with calculi. They are both potent urease producers that create an alkaline urine by splitting urea into ammonia and carbon dioxide. *E. coli, Klebsiella spp*, and *Pseudomonas spp.*, usually urease-negative (Klausner and Osborne, 1979). are associated with urinary tract infections but not calculi formation (Brown et al., 1977).

The exact mechanism of phosphate calculi formation is unknown, but it is believed that supersaturation of urine with magnesium ammonium phosphate crystals as a result of persistently alkaline urine is an important factor, since struvite concentration is markedly increased in alkaline urine (Klausner and Osborne, 1979; Nemoy and Stamey, 1971; Elliot et al., 1959a,b; Griffith et al., 1975). It is thought that other factors may play a role in phosphate calculi formation, since sterile urine and stone bacterial cultures have been reported in cases of phosphate calculi (Weaver, 1975; Osborne and Klausner, 1978). Genetic factors have also been investigated (Klausner et al., 1980).

Urine is usually sterile until it reaches the neck of the bladder. It may become infected via hematogenous or lymphatic routes, directly from contact with infected tissue or via infection ascending from the urinary tract. The ascending infection route is the most important (Kirk, 1972). It is necessary to first eliminate all predisposing sources of infection, and then to treat with specific urinary antibiotics as determined by the results of bacterial culture and sensitivity tests. These antibiotics should be used for a minimum of three weeks, with cultures taken within five to seven days following antibiotic therapy, and repeated at monthly intervals in cases of recurrence. The postoperative antibiotic therapy for chronic cystitis was previously described in the section on cystitis. Radiography should be repeated in cases of persistent or rapidly recurring infection; it may be necessary to provide continuous antibiotic therapy in these patients. The use of trimethoprim-sulfa, nitrofurantoin, or penicillin at one fourth the total daily dose given at bedtime has been reported (Ling, 1979) and is discussed in detail under cystitis.

As infection is controlled, urinary pH usually returns to normal (Thornton, 1968). The judicious administration of urinary acidifiers will aid in accomplishing this goal. Urinary acidifiers inhibit bacterial growth within the lower urinary tract; furthermore, the urinary salts of magnesium ammonium phosphate are more soluble at an acid pH, which reduces the chances of calculi formation (Hardy and Osborne, 1973; Thornton, 1968). Urinary acidifiers should not be used in uremic patients, but as a general rule they are nontoxic and can be used for prolonged periods of time without ill effects. Those commonly used in dogs are ascorbic acid (vitamin C), ammonium chloride, and DL-methionine (Osborne et al., 1980).

The dosage necessary to acidify urine is highly variable; it can be adjusted by the client with the use of pH paper. To be effective, urinary acidifiers must be administered three to four times daily, and the pH should be determined at the first urination of the morning (Hardy and Osborne, 1973; Osborne et al., 1980).

Sodium chloride should be used as a dietary supplement to induce polydipsia and polyuria, thus diluting the mineral components of the urine. The dosage, 1 to 10 gm/day in divided doses (Osborne, 1972), is variable, and the client can adjust it for his pet. In addition to inducing polyuria and polydipsia, frequent voiding helps to avoid stasis (Treacher, 1966). The longer the urine is retained, the greater is the chance for precipitation of foci.

Evidence incriminating diet as a cause of urolithiasis in the dog has been largely unconvincing (Jolly and Worden, 1966; Klausner and Osborne, 1980), and therefore specific diets for postoperative cystic calculi patients cannot be prescribed. Vegetable diets or any foods producing an alkaline urine should be avoided.

Spontaneous dissolution of phosphate calculi in dogs has been reported (Osborne and Klausner, 1978). Dissolution in those dogs in which surgery is impossible should be attempted by sterilizing and acidifying the urine (Klausner and Osborne, 1980). A urease inhibitor (acetohydroxamic acid) that dissolves phosphate calculi in combination with antibiotics and urinary acidifiers has been reported in humans (Griffiths et al., 1976), but this has not been reported in dogs.

Cystine Calculi

Cystinuria is an "inborn error of metabolism" in which high levels of the sulfa-containing amino acid cystine are excreted in the urine because of the abnormal transport of this and other amino acids by the proximal renal tubules. The exact mechanism of this abnormal renal transport is unknown (Osborne and Klausner, 1978). Dogs that form cystine calculi should not be used for breeding, since it has been suggested that cystinuria is transmitted by a sex-linked mode of inheritance (Medway, 1968; Tsan et al., 1972).

The only serious clinical consequence of cystinuria in the dog is precipitation of calculi; otherwise, the dog is normal in all respects (Treacher, 1966). The stones that form are usually pure cystine (Treacher, 1966; Bovee, 1973). The exact mechanism of crystallization and stone formation is unknown, but cystine is only slightly soluble at an acid pH of 6 or 7, and precipitation occurs easily at the normal urinary pH (Treacher, 1966). Not all dogs that are cystinuric form stones, but once a cystinuric dog does form calculi, it usually continues to do so every 6 to 18 months unless treatment is initiated (Bovee, 1973; Cornelius et al., 1967; Brown et al., 1977b). The age of onset of calculi in cystinuric dogs is not known, but dogs examined because of obstruction are usually between one and one half and four years of age (Bovee, 1973; Treacher, 1966).

The best method of diagnosing cystinuria is by chemical analysis of the calculi. Microscopically, it is possible to identify the flat hexagonal crystals in the urine of dogs with cystine calculi. In a crude test that can be quickly performed as a screening procedure, a drop of urine or suspension of macerated calculus is placed on a nitroprusside tablet. A drop of a ten per cent solution of potassium cyanide in normal sodium hydroxide is then added, and the appearance of a red color indicates cystine. The accuracy of the test has not been determined (Frimpter et al., 1967; Finco, 1971). Other methods of determining a cystinuric condition have been described but are not practical (Frimpter et al., 1967).

The treatment of cystine calculi is difficult and, once begun, must be continued or the calculi will recur. It is important to explain to the client that the animal is never "cured," since the renal tubular defect cannot be corrected. The aims of treatment are to decrease the amount and/or increase the solubility of the cystine produced.

Inasmuch as cystine is a nonessential amino acid, attempts have been made to decrease the amount of cystine excreted by the kidney; however, these have been ineffective (Treacher, 1966). An effort should be made to feed a diet low in animal protein and especially low in methionine (a cystine precursor) (Bovee, 1971; Finco, 1971), although in most cases this would be difficult. Raising the pH value to about 7.8 with sodium bicarbonate doubles the solubility of cystine in the urine (Treacher, 1966). In the dog, sodium bicarbonate can be administered at 1 gm/5 kg three times per day in order to maintain a pH in excess of 7.5 (Treacher, 1966). Either tablets or baking soda can be used, but baking soda mixed in the diet is more palatable. The dosage of the sodium bicarbonate necessary to alkalize the urine varies; pH paper should be used by the client to check the urine and regulate the dosage to keep the pH at 7.5 to 8. Urine is most likely to become supersaturated with cystine at night, and therefore the night dosage is important (Crawhall and Watts, 1968).

Treatment stressing dietary control, alkalization of the urine, and increased water intake alone is ineffective in most cases. The administration of D-penicillamine (Cuprimine) has been used with more success (Bovee, 1972); this drug is a chelating agent that interacts with cystine to form a penicillamine-cysteine mixed disulfide that is more soluble than free cystine in the urine. Free cystine excretion is reduced, and the likelihood of calculi formation is diminished. D-Penicillamine may be used alone with the induction of increased water consumption, or in addition to the treatment described earlier (Bovee, 1971; Greene and Greiner, 1972).

The drug is supplied in 125 to 250 mg capsules. The recommended dosage for dogs is 30 mg/kg per day divided into two doses (Bovee, 1977; Frimpter et al., 1967). The drug is bitter and cannot be mixed freely in the diet without being encapsulated; it can be given with food. Vomiting is a common sequel to the administration of this medication, especially on initiation of treatment. Antiemetics can be used to avoid vomiting, but a gradual build-up to the total dosage of D-penicillamine over a three- to four-week period is usually the best method of therapy. If vomiting is a problem, it has been recommended that the drug be administered in the evening at a dosage of 10 mg/kg in combination with increased water intake via food (Lage, 1980). B-complex vitamins should also be given, since D-penicillamine increases the requirement for pyridoxine in humans (Crawhall and Watts, 1968; Medway, 1968).

In humans undergoing therapy with D-penicillamine, toxic signs of the acute hypersensitivity syndrome have been reported in the treatment regimen, characterized by a rash, proteinuria that may progress to complete nephrotic syndrome, and bone marrow depression (Crawhall and Watts, 1968). Other than vomiting, none of these reactions have been reported in the dog, to date. Clinicians should read the drug insert before initiating treatment to become familiar with potential problems. It is also advisable to perform urinalysis and hematologic and biochemical testing every six to eight weeks to identify the occurrence of adverse reactions. Radiographs should be taken at 6- to 12-month intervals to check for recurrence.

D-Penicillamine should not be administered until all evidence of postoperative infection is gone. It has been reported (Morris et al., 1969) that D-penicillamine decreases the strength of skin wound closure by its action on collagen and, therefore, it should not be administered until after the surgical wound is completely healed. The drug is presently the most effective means of controlling cystine calculi formation (Bovee, 1971; Frimpter et al., 1967; Bovee, 1973).

Since concurrent infection may be present with cystine as with other types of calculi, the administration of urinary antibiotics is recommended for two weeks postoperatively. These infections are usually caused by *E. coli* (Brown et al., 1977). Increased fluid intake, especially at night, has been recommended as part of the therapy. This is accomplished by the gradual addition of four to six ounces of water per 30 pounds of body weight to food that already contains 70 per cent water, at each feeding (Lage, 1980).

The drug α-mercaptopropionylglycine (MPG), has been reported to be more effective than D-penicillamine in the treatment of cystine calculi in humans, with fewer side effects, but its use has not been reported in dogs (Hautmann et al., 1977).

Urate Calculi

Urate calculi are found predominantly in the Dalmatian but may be seen in other breeds (Finco, 1971; Osbaldiston and Lowrey, 1971). In any breed other than those Dalmatians in which ammonium urate calculi are diagnosed, those animals that exhibit neurologic signs or prolonged anesthetic recovery following cystotomy, portosystemic shunts should be suspected (Marretta et al., 1981). In the Dalmatian, the high rate of occurrence is caused by an inherited metabolic defect in purine metabolism; this allows high levels of uric acid to be excreted directly in the urine, whereas uric acid is converted and excreted as allantoin in other breeds (Osbaldiston and Lowrey, 1971; Benedict, 1915). The major site of this abnormality in the Dalmatian seems to be the liver, with the kidney playing only a minor role (Kuster et al., 1972).

High uric acid levels are only a predisposing factor and not the primary cause of urolithiasis. Ammonium and hydrogen ions have also been found to be powerful precipitators of urate calculi formation (Treacher, 1966; Porter, 1964). The aim of treatment is to decrease the amount of uric acid and ammonium and hydrogen ions in the urine.

Use of the drug allopurinol has been reported as the most successful method of lowering urinary uric acid levels (Bovee, 1973; Finco, 1971; Osbaldiston and Lowery, 1971). The drug acts by inhibiting the enzyme xanthine oxidase, which in turn inhibits the conversion of hypoxanthine to xanthine and of xanthine to uric acid. The net results are a decrease in uric acid and an increase in the amount of xanthine and hypoxanthine excreted in the urine. Allopurinol is supplied in 100 mg or 300 mg tablets. The recommended oral dosage of allopurinol for dogs is 30 mg/kg/day divided two or three times per day for one month. The dosage is then reduced to 10 mg/kg/day, divided two or three times per day for the life of the dog (Finco, 1977; Osborne and Klausner, 1978; Osbaldiston and Lowrey, 1971). This dosage should be reduced if the patient has renal failure. No undesirable effects have been reported in the dog, but skin rash, fever, diarrhea, and formation of xanthine calculi have been reported in man (Finco, 1971).

Alteration of diet is of questionable value in treating dogs with uric acid stones or in preventing their formation. Low purine diets, especially a diet low in meat and high in vegetables, have been advocated by some researchers (Osbaldiston and Lowrey, 1971; Dalmatian Research Foundation, 1972; Osborne and Klausner, 1978), but have not been advised by others as an effective means of lowering urinary uric acid levels (Benedict, 1915; Bovee, 1973; Osborne et al., 1972; Boulden, 1966). A low quality, dry dog food high in vegetable sources of protein is recommended (Finco, 1977), but it has been advised to use dietary control in conjunction with regulation of urine pH, the ideal pH being 6.5 (Finco, 1971; Porter, 1964). The use of sodium bicarbonate or potassium citrate in the diet has been shown to increase pH and decrease ammonium ion concentration (Porter, 1964). The value of altering the urinary pH as a preventative of the formation of uric acid stones is also questionable; if attempted, it should be done in conjunction with allopurinol therapy. Sodium bicarbonate should be administered as tablets or as powder (½ tsp baking soda equals approximately 2 gm) (Finco, 1977).

Polyuria produced by the addition of salt (NaCl) to the diet has been advocated as part of the treatment protocol. By increasing urine volume, the concentration of urates is diluted, decreasing the chance of flocculation. Sodium chloride should be given orally at a dosage of .5 to 10 gm daily to maintain a specific gravity of urine less than 1.030 (Finco and Cornelius, 1977). Table salt (½ tsp equals approximately 3½ gm NaCl) can be mixed with food or given as tablets.

Cystitis often accompanies urate calculi, and, therefore, routine urinary antibiotics should be administered.

Oxalate Calculi

Oxalate calculi, which occur frequently in man, are rarely seen in the dog in the United States. Oxalate is a metabolic end product of glyoxalate and ascorbate. As it is excreted in the urine, oxalate combines with calcium, forming an insoluble complex of calcium oxalate. Calcium oxalate calculi usually form in an acid urine. Excretion patterns were unaffected in dogs with a pH range of 5.9 to 8: the conditions favoring crystallization are unknown, making treatment very difficult (Cattell et al., 1962). Infection does not seem to play a role in the etiopathogenesis; the inflammation and hemorrhage that accompany the calculi are caused by their spiny surfaces.

There is no definitive treatment for calcium oxalate calculi in the dog, although a review of therapy in man has been reported (Osborne and Klausner, 1978). Surgical removal and polyuria induced by the addition of sodium chloride to the diet is the treatment of choice. Urinary antibiotics should be administered postoperatively to eliminate urinary tract infection. Urinary acidifiers should be avoided, especially vitamin C, which seems to influence the formation of oxalate calculi.

Silica Calculi

Silica calculi seem to be a "new type" of calculi, reported for the first time in the dog in 1976 (Legendre, 1976). Forty-eight cases of silica calculi were reported from all over the United States (Osborne et al., 1980). The German shepherd dog was the most common breed affected, while the mean age was 6.4 years. Virtually all of the calculi (47 out of 48) were found in males.

Most of the silica calculi have a characteristic "jackstone" appearance grossly. They cannot be detected by the commercial kit already mentioned and therefore must be analyzed by a commercial laboratory. Silica calculi are, however, radiodense. These calculi have been induced in experimental dogs fed diets high in silicic acid (McCullagh and Ehrhart, 1974) and have occurred naturally in Kenyan dogs, in which it was speculated that their vegetable diet may play a role in the etiopathogenesis (Brodey, 1977).

Since the exact etiology of silica calculi is unknown, only nonspecific treatment can be recommended (Osborne et al., 1980), including induced polyuria by adding sodium chloride to the diet and other dietary changes.

Mixed Calculi

Most mixed calculi are composed of a primary calculus nucleus with a secondary calculus covering. This mixture occurs because the stone irritates the bladder mucosa, initiating cystitis. The pH is altered, and the urinary phosphates further coat the primary stone. Because of the possibility that the center and shell of a calculus may differ, all such calculi analyzed should be cracked in half.

In treating mixed calculi, the cystitis should first be controlled and then specific treatment initiated for the primary type stone.

TUMORS OF THE BLADDER

It has been estimated that neoplasms of the urinary bladder account for less than 0.5 per cent of all tumors found in the dog (Catchin, 1951), and that they are seen even less frequently in the cat (Osborne et al., 1968; Dill et al., 1972; Pamukcu, 1974). The variation in occurrence is thought to be the result of a difference in the metabolic pathways of tryptophan, an essential aromatic amino acid in the dog and cat (Osborne et al., 1968; Brown and Price, 1956). Tryptophan has been incriminated as a possible cause of bladder carcinoma in dogs (Osborne et al., 1968; Radamski et al., 1971) as have other agents (Oyasu and Hopp, 1974). It has also been reported that the urine is the medium through which carcinogens come in contact with the bladder, causing tumor genesis (Hayes, 1976; McDonald and Lund, 1954), and that storage of urine in the bladder allows longer contact between carcinogens and the bladder mucosa (Staufuss and Dean, 1975).

Vesicular neoplasms are usually seen in older animals of both species, but they may also be seen on rare occasions in very young dogs. In one study of 130 bladder tumors (Osborne et al., 1968), the mean age of occurrence in the dog was 9.1 years. In the same study, the average age of nine cats with bladder tumors was 9.2 years. No breed or sex predilection was found in either species. In another study of 114 cases in the dog, there was an almost four to one greater occurrence of bladder tumors in females, and a greater than expected risk in four breeds of dogs — Scottish terrier, Shetland sheepdog, beagle, and collie (Hayes, 1976).

PRIMARY TUMORS

Primary malignant neoplasms are seen more frequently than benign or secondary tumors (tumors that have a primary origin in another organ or outside the bladder) (Jubb and Kennedy, 1970; Bloom, 1954). The papilloma and leiomyoma are commonly encountered benign epithelial and benign mesenchymal tumors, respectively. Fibroma, neurofibroma, rhabdomyoma, angioma, myxoma, and combinations of these also occur, but less frequently (Osborne et al., 1968; Jubb and Kennedy, 1970; Bloom, 1954).

The transitional cell carcinoma is the most common malignant tumor of epithelial origin, but squamous cell carcinoma and adenocarcinoma have also been found. Malignant tumors of mesenchymal tissue include fibrosarcoma, leiomyosarcoma, rhabdomyosarcoma, hemangiosarcoma, osteosarcoma, myosarcoma, or any combination of these (Osborne et al., 1968; Jubb and Kennedy, 1970; Bloom, 1954; Staufuss, 1975; Hayes, 1976). The terms "botryoid sarcoma," "botryoid rhabdomyosarcoma," and "embryonal rhabdomyosarcoma" refer to the malignant mesenchymal tumor seen in young dogs (Roszel, 1972) (Fig. 76–6).

SECONDARY TUMORS

Secondary tumors of the bladder are rare in the dog and cat. It is possible for malignant tumors to spread to the bladder by direct extension from the prostate, rectum, or uterus; by implantation from tumors of the kidneys or ureter; or via the lymph and blood.

Benign tumors are usually noninfiltrative and noninvasive, while malignant tumors are extremely invasive and infiltrative and may extend into the urethra, causing obstructive lesions. The rate of metastasis of primary transitional cell carcinoma has been reported as high as 50 per cent, with the regional nodes and lungs the most common sites of metastasis in the dog (Osborne et al., 1968). It has been reported that squamous cell carcinoma metastasizes more frequently than does transitional cell carcinoma in the dog (Bloom, 1954). Fibrosarcoma is considered highly malignant and metastasizes readily, while leiomyosarcoma metastasizes less readily (Osborne et al., 1968; Seely et al., 1978). With botryoid sarcoma, metastasis may occur but local invasion is the rule (Roszel, 1972; Robbins, 1967).

In the cat, two out of four cases of transitional carcinoma in the bladder showed metastatic lesions (Osborne et al., 1968; Dill et al., 1972), while in another study, five out of 17 cats had metastatic lesions (Wimberly and Lewis, 1979). In a report on squamous cell carcinoma of the bladder, the tumor was infiltrative and metastatic to the regional lymph nodes (Dorn, 1978). An intravenous leiomyoma was surgically removed from the bladder of a cat, and the animal remained clinically normal during a 25-month follow-up period (Patnaik and Greene, 1979).

Clinical Signs. The most common sign of an animal with neoplasia of the bladder is hematuria. Either the treatment is totally without response, or there is an initial response that decreases with time. Hematuria usually begins intermittently but progresses to constant hematuria. Other clinical findings may include frequent urination, incontinence, and tenesmus (Osborne et al., 1968). Dysuria may occur if the tumor causes total or partial obstruction of the urethra at the trigone. Generally, the signs are similar to those of chronic cystitis.

On physical examination, the mucous membranes may be pale if excessive hematuria has occurred, and abdominal palpation may reveal a thickened bladder wall; sometimes the mass can be palpated. The bladder may be full if the urethra is obstructed, and the kidney may be enlarged if hydronephrosis has developed. Enlarged abdominal lymph nodes may be palpated if metastasis has occurred. A rectal examination and palpation of the urethra and vagina will often reveal extension of the tumor to the urethra.

Hypertrophic pulmonary osteoarthropathy has been reported in association with primary carcinoma of the bladder, with metastasis to the lungs, liver, kidneys, rib, adrenal glands, and vertebrae (Brodey et al., 1973) (Fig. 76–7). Botryoid rhabdomyosarcoma and neurofibrosarcoma of the bladder have also been reported to cause hypertrophic osteoarthropathy (Halliwell and Ackerman, 1974; Theilen and Madewell, 1979).

Laboratory Examination. The urinalysis

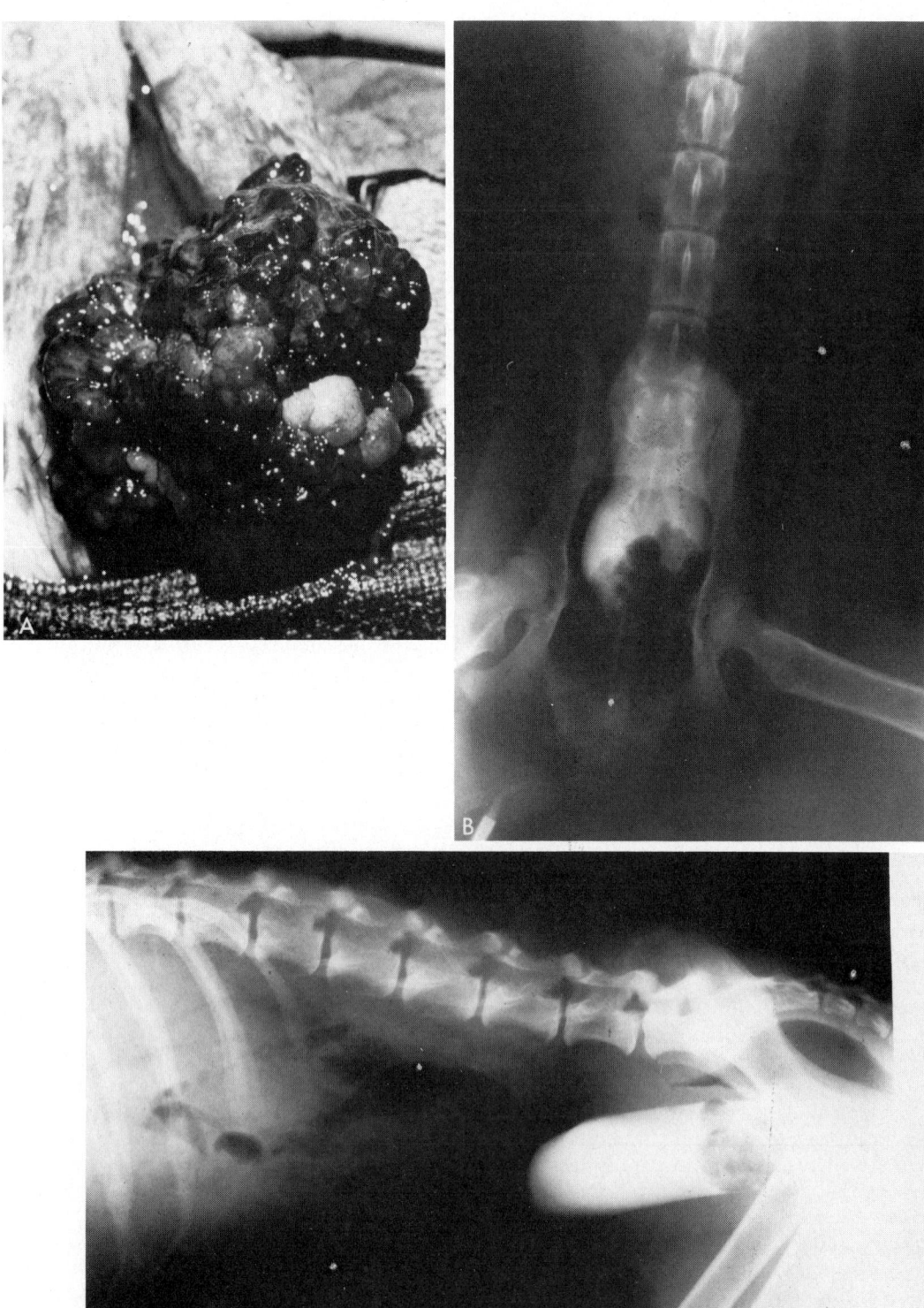

Figure 76–6. Malignant tumor of the bladder. *A*, Botryoid sarcoma of the urinary bladder in a nine-month-old Doberman pinscher. *B*, Ventrodorsal and *C*, lateral views, using positive-contrast radiography and showing the mass in the trigone area.

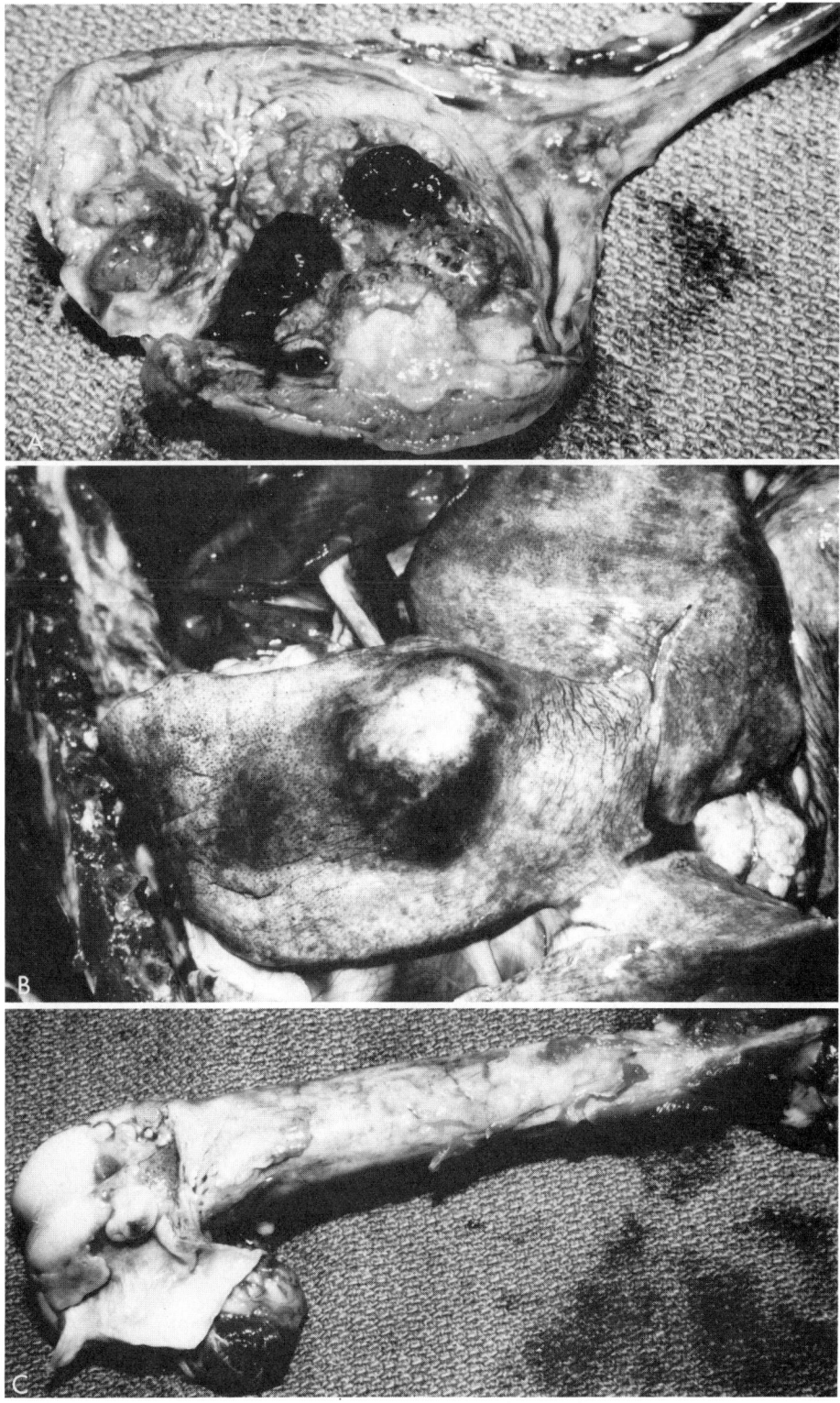

Figure 76–7. Transitional cell carcinoma. *A,* The disease originated in the bladder. *B,* Metastasis to the lungs. *C,* Result of metastasis was hypertrophic pulmonary osteoarthropathy.

is usually consistent with cystitis, but careful microscopic examination of the urinary sediment may reveal some atypical, exfoliated tumor cells among the predominantly inflammatory elements, especially in association with transitional cell carcinomas (Theilen and Madewell, 1979). This is not a constant finding, and many urine samples require special examinations before these atypical neoplastic cells can be found. The results of exfoliative cytology in the diagnosis of bladder tumors in man has been disappointing (Wiggishoff and McDonald, 1972). If hematuria has been a problem, the hemogram may show evidence of anemia. The BUN may be elevated if there is bladder or urethral obstruction.

Radiographic Examination. Plain radiographs may reveal an enlarged kidney and distended bladder if hydronephrosis and obstruction have occurred. A thickened bladder wall and, possibly, displaced organs due to lymph node metastasis may also be seen. Calcification of the tumor may occur and cause it to be confused with cystic calculi. Radiographs of the chest and lumbar vertebrae should be examined for possible metastasis.

Contrast radiography is usually necessary to demonstrate tumors of the bladder. Air or radiopaque dyes, or both, can be used as contrast mediums to aid in demonstrating neoplasia of the bladder. Space-occupying lesions that protrude into the lumen of the bladder are more readily diagnosed radiographically than the diffuse infiltrating-type tumors that cause thickening and irregularity of the bladder wall. When pneumocystography is performed in the cat, care should be taken to avoid the induction of a venous air embolism (Thayer et al., 1980; Zontine and Andrews, 1978).

Exploratory Surgery. It is sometimes difficult to differentiate between neoplasia and chronic cystitis, even after a good history has been taken and physical examination, laboratory testing, and radiographs have been completed. Exploratory surgery and biopsy of the bladder and associated lymph nodes may be necessary to make a definitive diagnosis.

Treatment. Treatment of bladder neoplasms depends upon whether the tumor is primary or secondary, benign or malignant, and whether it is metastatic. Most malignant lesions are inoperable when detected be-

cause the diagnosis is not made until late in the course of the disease.

BENIGN TUMORS. Benign tumors can usually be removed by excising the neoplasm and a rim of normal bladder tissue around it; this depends on the location of the tumor, however. A biopsy specimen of the mass should be examined histologically. A tumor at the apex of the bladder can be removed more easily than one at the trigone because of the lack of ureteral involvement. In some cases, a nephrectomy or ureteric reimplantation may be necessary. As a general rule, benign tumors respond well to surgical excision as long as they have not become so enlarged that they cause anatomic or physiologic damage to the bladder or block the ureters and urethra, causing irreversible kidney damage (Osborne et al., 1968). A benign papilloma may recur, however, and undergo malignant changes (Bloom, 1954).

MALIGNANT TUMORS. Malignant tumors of the bladder may be treated by surgical excision, but the results are often discouraging. Stay sutures should be placed in the bladder for control, and moist laparotomy pads may be used to prevent the rest of the abdomen from becoming seeded with malignant tumor cells. The surgeon should also take care to prevent iatrogenic spread. All abdominal organs should be examined for metastasis, and biopsy should be performed on the regional sublumbar lymph nodes. The tumor should be removed by wide radical excision because of the invasiveness of most malignant bladder tumors. In all cases, biopsy of the mass should be performed. Depending on the position of tumor, more radical surgery may be indicated; however, justification for this is questionable, since normal urinary function is rarely retained in such circumstances (Theilen and Madewell, 1979; Bovee et al., 1979). In cases of widely metastatic tumors or highly invasive tumors that are inoperable, the animal should be euthanatized.

Chemotherapy and radiation therapy have been used, but with poor results (Osborne et al., 1968). They may be indicated in some cases, in combination with surgical excision (Theilen and Madewell, 1979).

In general, surgery for the removal of malignant tumors has been unrewarding, and hematuria and regrowth of tumor usually occur within months. However, surgery is often the one chance the animal has for recovery and is generally necessary for a definitive diagnosis after prolonged medical treatment. In all postoperative surgical cases, routine treatment for cystitis should be administered and radiographs taken at five- to six-month intervals to check for recurrence.

TRAUMA TO BLADDER

Common Causes. Trauma to the urinary bladder may result from penetrating or nonpenetrating wounds, excessive straining at parturition, or unsuccessful attempts at urination due to lower urinary tract obstruction by tumors or calculi (Archibald, 1965).

In a study of motor vehicle accidents (which are the leading cause of trauma), 29 per cent of the dogs with confirmed intra-abdominal injuries had ruptured bladders (Kolata and Johnston, 1975). Of 281 cases of urinary tract trauma diagnosed radiographically, 175 cases (62 per cent) suffered a ruptured bladder, especially as the result of an automobile accident (Kleine and Thornton, 1971). Many of these cases also have pelvic fractures, which accompanied bladder trauma in 46.2 per cent of the cases (Burrows and Bovee, 1974).

Other causes of nonpenetrating trauma include falls from great heights and blows to the abdomen. Penetrating lesions include bullet wounds, knife wounds, or wounds made by any other sharp object that enters the abdomen directly and penetrates the bladder. Bladder tumors or ulcerative cystitis rarely penetrate the serosal wall of the bladder. Cystic calculi frequently cause trauma to the mucosa with resulting hematuria, but spontaneous rupture is rarely seen (Archibald, 1965). Often, more trauma is inflicted by the examining clinician during palpation of the bladder than by the calculi themselves. The bladder may accidentally be ruptured by the clinician in his attempt to relieve lower urinary tract obstruction by retrograde transurethral flushing with saline or by expressing a full bladder with urethral obstruction. Rupture of the bladder secondary to urethral obstruction is more common in the cat than in the dog, while traumatic rupture by automobile accident is more common in the dog.

Ruptured bladders occur more frequently in male dogs because of the length and diameter of the urethra (Rawlings, 1969; Maynard, 1961). This, however, may be due to the fact that a higher incidence of trauma, generally speaking, is reported in males (Burrows and Bovee, 1974; Kolata and Johnston, 1975).

Clinical Signs. A history of recent trauma, external evidence of trauma, or sudden onset of signs such as oliguria with hematuria or blood at the end of the prepuce or vulva aid in diagnosing trauma to urinary bladder. However, signs vary with the degree of damage.

The most common lesion of the bladder following trauma is simple contusion with resulting mild to severe hematuria (Archibald, 1965). In cases of automobile accidents, the presenting signs of shock, collapse, dyspnea, and other injuries to the skeletal system overshadow a possible ruptured bladder. The animal may initially respond to the treatment for shock and then steadily deteriorate on the second or third day. In experimental studies, the average time for death following untreated, induced bladder rupture was 65 hours. In naturally occurring cases, the mortality rate was 42.3 per cent (Burrows and Bovee, 1974).

Other signs seen on examination may include a stiff gait, a tucked up abdomen, and reluctance to walk caused by pain, anorexia, and progressive central nervous system depression. Temperatures vary, but vomiting associated with ileus and peritonitis is a consistent finding. Dehydration is usually present and progressive.

In many cases of bladder rupture, a small amount of bloody urine is passed; consequently, lack of urination is not always a cardinal sign of a ruptured bladder. Straining to urinate may also be seen. A catheter inserted into the urethra may pass through the rent in the bladder and free, extravasated urine will be removed from the abdominal cavity, giving the false impression that the bladder is intact.

Physical Examination. A routine, systematic physical examination should be performed on all traumatized patients, either on presentation or when the patient has been stabilized. This should specifically include abdominal palpation, percussion, and a rectal examination. With urethral obstruction, the animal is usually examined because of stranguria or for passing small amounts of bloody urine. If the obstruction is of long duration, signs of uremia may be present. In cases of iatrogenic rupture caused by palpation of a distended bladder with urethral obstruction, the bladder may be distended one moment and small the next, with no urine passing out the urethra. Signs of shock usually develop rapidly. While a dog with a traumatic rupture of the bladder may be overlooked for 24 hours, a ruptured bladder following urethral obstruction is an emergency because of more rapid deterioration that follows. With traumatic rupture the urine is sterile and the animal is healthy prior to trauma; with urethral obstruction, however, the animal frequently has preexisting disease. Urea nitrogen and creatinine concentrations of the abdominal fluid should be determined and, when compared to that of serum concentrations of each, should contain similar concentrations of urea nitrogen but higher concentrations of creatinine. Detection of this difference is a useful aid in the diagnosis of free urine in the abdomen (Burrows and Bovee, 1974).

In cases in which a small contracted bladder is palpated and free fluid is suspected on percussion, sterile abdominal paracentesis should be performed in two or more places and the fluid examined for odor, color, specific gravity, protein content, and cellular composition to determine whether the fluid is a transudate, an exudate, blood, or urine.

Laboratory Examination. Routine blood analysis provides useful guidelines for the evaluation of the general condition of the patient and may indicate other abnormal conditions. In most cases of ruptured bladder, the clinician can expect leukocytosis with rising neutrophilia and a rapidly rising packed cell volume. The serum concentrations of creatinine, potassium, inorganic phosphorus, and BUN become elevated, while serum sodium and chloride concentrations decrease. Acidosis might be expected in some animals; however, in cases of induced disease it has been reported that the mean acid-base values remain normal, decreasing only terminally (Burrows and Bovee, 1974).

Radiographic Examination. On radiography of the abdomen, a ruptured bladder may be suspected if there is loss of bladder detail or if the bladder is small and contracted, and if there is evidence of peritonitis and intestinal ileus. Contrast cystograms using aqueous organic iodide solution dilated to 50 per cent with sterile water or saline material have been shown to be a more accurate aid in the diagnosis of a ruptured bladder than pneumocystograms (Burrows and Bovee, 1974). The dose is variable but should be about 50 to 100 ml. Extravasation of the radiopaque dye into the peritoneum is seen more readily than is free air when pneumocystography is performed. Sometimes a tentative diagnosis may be made during administration of the contrast by the sound of it passing freely into the abdominal cavity, if resistance is not felt from the bladder (Kleine and Thornton, 1971). Contrast retrograde cystograms using air, carbon dioxide, or radiopaque dye may be necessary to confirm the diagnosis. Air or carbon dioxide usually is the best contrast medium, but any of the radiopaque dyes that are not irritating to the peritoneum may be used. The bladder should be empty and free of blood clots before a cystogram is performed. Contrast radiography demonstrates the escape of free contrast medium into the peritoneal cavity, and the dye may outline the intestine.

Radiography should also be used to evaluate other soft tissue and abdominal injuries as well as skeletal injury, especially to the pelvis. It may be necessary to perform an intravenous pyelogram or urethrogram to evaluate the status of the kidney, ureter, and urethra. Contrast radiography may reveal large blood clots in the bladder or a diverticulum, indicating trauma to the bladder less severe than a rupture.

Treatment. Contusions and injury to the bladder without evidence of rupture but with hematuria should be treated with urinary antibiotics and acidifiers. If the hematuria is excessive, an indwelling, retrograde urethral catheter should be used to infuse cold saline solution combined with antibiotics into the urinary bladder to reduce the hemorrhage and to remove any blood clots that may obstruct urine flow or act as a nidus for infection. Good urine flow is important, and if large volumes of oral fluid cannot be consumed, intravenous fluid therapy should be administered.

A diverticulum of the bladder may predispose to chronic cystitis and may have to be surgically excised if problems occur. Once the diagnosis of a ruptured bladder has been established, it is important to stabilize the patient's metabolic, fluid, and electrolyte imbalances prior to surgery. If the rupture is diagnosed within 12 hours and the patient is stable, surgery can be performed; otherwise, efforts should be made to stabilize the patient first.

Physiologic saline solution should be administered to replace the depleted sodium, chloride, and fluid deficit. An indwelling urethral catheter can be used to drain the urine from the bladder and possibly the peritoneal cavity. Abdominal drainage may be necessary if a good flow is not established from the catheter. Broad spectrum antibiotics should be administered (Burrows and Bovee, 1974).

As the animal improves clinically, usually in 6 to 12 hours, its serum biochemical concentrations should be rechecked to see if the patient is metabolically stable and surgery can be performed. The fluid should be switched to lactated Ringer's solution, and anesthesia administered. A midline incision is made from the umbilicus to the brim of the pelvis. Suction should be available to remove the extravasated urine from the abdomen, and the bladder exteriorized and packed off with moist laparotomy pads. After the tear is located, the ureters and blood supply to the bladder are examined to ensure that they are intact, and the abdominal contents are carefully examined for other evidence of trauma. In some cases, resection of a large portion of the bladder

may be required. The edges of the bladder wall are debrided to areas of healthy tissue, and the tear is closed with a double layer of 3-0 absorbable suture in a continuous inverting pattern. Care should be taken so that the ureterovesicular junction is not occluded. At times, it may be necessary to reimplant the ureter. If the rupture is iatrogenic or caused by calculi, the bladder and urethra should be flushed to remove the obstruction, and the abdominal fluid should be cultured for bacteria. The abdomen is then lavaged with large quantities of warm saline or lactated Ringer's solution.

A second operation may be required to repair a fractured pelvis if the fracture cannot be reduced during initial surgery. The postoperative recovery period and prognosis are usually satisfactory in all cases of rupture caused by trauma or associated with calculi, if the animal is stabilized metabolically before surgery.

Foreign Bodies

Most foreign bodies found in the bladder or urethra occur as a result of a gunshot or air pellet wound (Denny, 1972; Andre and Jackson, 1972); however, an encrusted grass seed comprising three awns of wild barley was removed from a canine urethra and was speculated to have gained entrance via the urethral orifice (Schneck, 1974). Clinical signs of foreign bodies are similar to those of cystitis or cystic calculi. Surgical removal

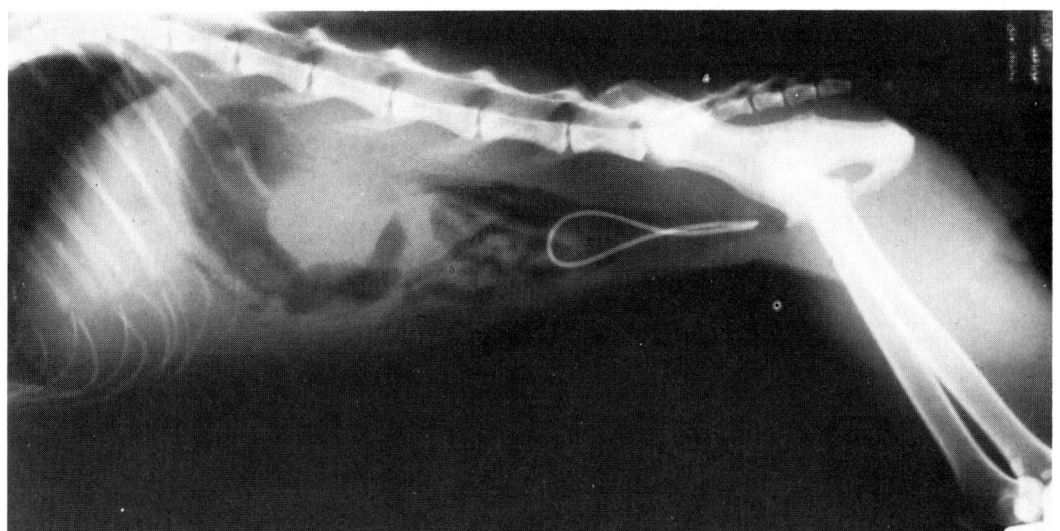

Figure 76–8. Foreign body in the bladder. Lateral view of the abdomen, illustrating a urethral catheter in the bladder.

followed by treatment with urinary antibiotics is desirable because calculi formation, chronic cystitis, or urethral obstruction may occur (Fig. 76–8).

INCONTINENCE: ATONY

Urinary incontinence is the involuntary loss of urine from the bladder, resulting in the constant or intermittent dribbling of urine. In general, this disorder is more frequent in the female than in the male, and is more common in dogs than in cats. Incontinence may be grouped by etiology into several broad categories: congenital anomalies of the urinary tract, trauma or diseases of the urinary tract, neurogenic abnormalities, and endocrine abnormalities.

CONGENITAL ANOMALIES

Ectopic ureters are the most common of the congenital anomalies of the urinary tract and have been reported as a cause of incontinence in both the male and female (Hayes, 1974; Osborne, 1967; Osborne et al., 1975a). Urine formed by the kidneys is transported directly to a point beyond the bladder sphincter, causing involuntary loss of urine. Ectopic ureters that empty proximal to the sphincter do not usually cause incontinence (Osborne et al., 1975a). Anomalies that predispose the urinary tract to infection or irritation, such as ureteroceles (Scott, 1974), can cause incontinence by rendering the external sphincter incompetent. Ureteroceles may also cause partial obstruction and inflammation of the bladder neck (Scott, 1973). Any anomalous development of the bladder, urethra, or genital tract that causes urine stasis can predispose to infection. The severity of incontinence under these circumstances varies with the degree of damage to the external sphincter. Persistent urachus causes a form of incontinence wherein urine dribbles out involuntarily through an opening other than the urethra. Other anomalies create fistulas that connect with the urinary tract (Osborne et al., 1975b). Incontinence results from dribbling of urine from these abnormal regions following urination.

TRAUMA OR DISEASE

Trauma and irritation to the external sphincter and proximal urethra may cause incontinence. Fracture of the pelvis, ovariohysterectomy, parturition accompanied by dystocia with or without surgical manipulations, and iatrogenic trauma resulting from surgical procedures on the bladder and distal urinary tract are occasionally causes of incontinence (Everett and Williams, 1970). As previously discussed, any factors that predispose the urinary tract to infection or irritation (anomalies, stones, trauma) can render the external sphincter incompetent, causing intermittent constant incontinence. In rare instances, a disease or abnormality that causes long-term obstruction can produce overflow incontinence. Pressure builds in the bladder and eventually reaches a point that overcomes the resistance to outflow. Under these circumstances, a constant dribbling of urine occurs, or a sudden release of urine may take place following coughing, sudden movement, or even simply lying down. There is usually a history of stranguria and difficulty in initiating urine flow.

NEUROGENIC ABNORMALITIES

Neurogenic abnormalities cause incontinence by disrupting motor impulses that control micturition, by disrupting sensory impulses that signal the need for micturition, or, more commonly, by both (Lapides, 1970; Oliver, 1974; Oliver and Osborne, 1980). Numerous spinal cord disorders that involve the cord segments in micturition reflex produce overflow incontinence; however, in this condition, the cause of bladder distention differs from that in long-term obstruction. Under these circumstances, the paralyzed bladder expands until pressure causes expulsion of urine through a weakened or spastic sphincter (Lapides, 1970; Oliver, 1974). In addition, lesions in the brainstem, cerebellum, and cortex can also cause incontinence on the same basis (Oliver, 1974). Diseases that affect the pelvic nerve peripherally can cause overflow incontinence, while lesions affecting the pudendal nerve can cause either overflow incontinence or incompetent striated sphincter function (Bradley and Timm, 1974).

ENDOCRINE ABNORMALITIES

Endocrine abnormalities may cause incontinence in the dog. This may occur following ovariohysterectomy and occasionally is seen in old, intact male and female dogs. The exact pathogenesis of this abnormality remains unclear. Estrogens may influence the response of the urethra and urinary bladder to alpha-adrenergic stimulation; estrogen deficiency decreases the alpha-adrenergic response in the urethra and bladder (Hodgson et al., 1978; Osborne et al., 1980c).

Treatment of Incontinence. Treatment of urinary incontinence depends on accurate diagnosis of the cause. Urinary tract anomalies can be diagnosed by contrast radiography, including intravenous pyelography and cystography. After the anomaly has been characterized, surgical intervention is indicated to reconstruct the urinary tract and correct the cause or predisposing factor. Such procedures have been described in detail (Everett and Williams, 1970).

Estrogens may influence the response of the urethra and urinary bladder to alpha-adrenergic stimulation; estrogen deficiency decreases the alpha-adrenergic response in the urethra and bladder (Hodgson et al., 1978; Osborne et al., 1980c).

Incontinence caused by weakening of the external sphincter or chronic bladder distention may be treated conservatively with bethanechol chloride (Urecholine). The initial dosage is 5 to 10 mg three times daily, which may be altered according to the response obtained. Therapy should be continued for three to five days, then discontinued. Prolonged therapy with Urecholine is not indicated, regardless of whether initial therapy fails or succeeds. Infection that causes incontinence or accompanies incontinence due to other causes should be treated with appropriate urinary tract antibiotics, as determined by bacterial culture and sensitivity testing (see Bacterial Cystitis). Other management includes periodic evacuation of the distended bladder by manual expression or by catheterization, and surgical correction of the underlying etiologic factor when this is possible.

Hormonal abnormalities may respond to replacement therapy with stilbestrol (equivalent to 0.05 mg of Estinyl), given orally at a dosage of one mg every third day. The dosage should be adjusted according to clinical response and recurrence of incontinence. Thus, the dosage can be tapered to every four days, then every five days, then

every six days at weekly intervals consecutively. If incontinence does not recur with a dosage of one mg every seven days, the drug should be discontinued. Recurrence of incontinence can be treated in the same way, starting at one mg every three days. When estrogens are used, a platelet count and a CBC should be determined monthly in order to detect abnormalities resulting from therapy. If thrombocytopenia or hemorrhagic diathesis develops, therapy must be discontinued. Nonregenerative anemia is rare when the dosages given are followed, but if this should occur, therapy should be discontinued.

CONGENITAL ABNORMALITIES OF THE URETHRA

Congenital anomalies of the urethra occur infrequently in the dog and cat and are seen more often in the male than in the female (Archibald, 1965). Anomalies that have been reported include absence of the urethra associated with absence of the penis, urethral duplication, hypospadias and epispadias, diverticulum, and accessory meatus (Osborne et al., 1972; Bloom, 1954). Other anomalies may occur with hermaphroditism and pseudohermaphroditism.

BACTERIAL URETHRITIS AND GRANULOMATOUS URETHRITIS

Etiology. Bacterial urethritis is usually associated with infection of the urinary bladder. The etiologic agents and predisposing factors are the same as in cystitis. Trauma is particularly important. Granulomatous urethritis is a disease of unknown etiology that occurs only in female dogs, or is only symptomatic in females. Bacterial infection can complicate this disease.

Clinical Signs and Laboratory Findings. The clinical signs associated with bacterial urethritis include stranguria and pollakiuria. Blood is usually passed initially, followed by a stream of clear urine, unless there is concomitant bacterial cystitis. Dribbling of blood unassociated with micturition may also occur. Brisk hemorrhage from the penis can occur. When inflammation is severe and the urethral lumen becomes partially or completely occluded, signs progress to severe stranguria with small amounts of urine, or no urine passed on each attempt to urinate. Urethritis associated with feline urolithiasis is discussed later in the chapter (see p. 1923). Laboratory findings are the same as those for bacterial cystitis.

A dog with granulomatous urethritis is frequently examined because of partial urethral obstruction associated with moderate to severe stranguria. Hematuria can occur when bacterial infection arises concomitantly. Results of laboratory testing include microscopic hematuria initially; however, bacterial cystitis frequently occurs simultaneously. Thus, in most cases, the laboratory findings are the same as those seen in cystitis (see Bacterial Cystitis).

Treatment. When obstruction is severe enough to cause urine retention, the clinician must pass a catheter so that the animal can urinate while medical therapy is administered. The catheter should be removed as soon as possible (usually three to five days after instituting specific therapy). Urinary tract antibiotics should be administered as in the treatment of bacterial cystitis according to results of urine culture and sensitivity testing.

Therapy for granulomatous urethritis includes treatment with corticosteroids (prednisone) and antibiotics (see Bacterial Cystitis). Corticosteroids are administered at a dosage of 1 mg per lb, divided into two daily doses. This level is continued for 7 to 14 days, and then tapered by 50 per cent every seven days until the dosage reaches .0625 mg per lb. Corticosteroids are then discontinued. Recurrence of obstruction with stranguria should be treated by re-initiating corticosteroid therapy at the highest dosage and tapering every 14 days. Antibiotics are administered along with corticosteroids and are continued for three weeks beyond cessation of corticosteroid therapy. Rarely, urethral bypass surgery is necessary if medical therapy fails to control the signs of granulomatous urethritis.

URETHRAL TUMORS

Urethral tumors in the dog and cat are rare. In a study of 20 cases of primary urethral tumors in the dog, the average age was 10.4 years. While there was no breed predisposition, the tumors occurred more frequently in the female (Tarvin et al., 1978). One case of urethral tumor in a six-year-old intact male cat has also been reported (Barnett and Nobel, 1975).

The most common signs on examination are hematuria and stranguria, progressing over several weeks, to almost total urinary retention (Pearson and Gibbs, 1971; Pollock, 1968; Tarvin et al., 1978). Severe tenesmus and incontinence may also be present. Diagnosis of urethral tumors is difficult and is often considered only after the elimination of other more common lesions of the lower urinary tract. In the study cited, physical examination was helpful in diagnosing 50 per cent of the cases; rectal and vaginal examination, abdominal palpation, and difficulty in passing a urinary catheter were all helpful in localizing the disease to the urethra (Tarvin et al., 1978).

Results of hematologic and biochemical testing are normal in most cases. Urinalysis may reveal anaplastic tumor cells. Urinary catheterization may be used as a simple method of obtaining a biopsy specimen of the urethra (Mehlhoff and Osborne, 1977). The most useful diagnostic procedure for localizing the lesion to the urethra and determining its extent is contrast radiography (voiding cystography-urethrography). Plain thoracic radiographs are helpful in locating pulmonary metastases, enlarged sublumbar lymph nodes, vertebral metastases, and caudal abdominal masses (Tarvin et al., 1978).

Squamous cell carcinoma was the most common tumor type encountered in one study (Tarvin et al., 1978), while transitional cell carcinoma was the most common in another (Wilson et al., 1979) (Fig. 76–9). Metastasis was seen in 6 of 20 cases, with regional lymph nodes being the most common site (Tarvin et al., 1978).

While biopsy and resection via episiotomy may be performed, an exploratory laparotomy and biopsy is the only means of confirming the diagnosis. Surgical excision is the treatment of choice, but in most cases it is difficult, since the entire urethra is involved. Chemotherapy, radiation hyperthermia, and immunotherapy may be considered as adjuncts to surgical excision. The prognosis is usually poor because of the extent and obstructing nature of the tumor.

URETHRAL TRAUMA

Trauma to the urethra in the dog and cat may be seen in association with pelvic frac-

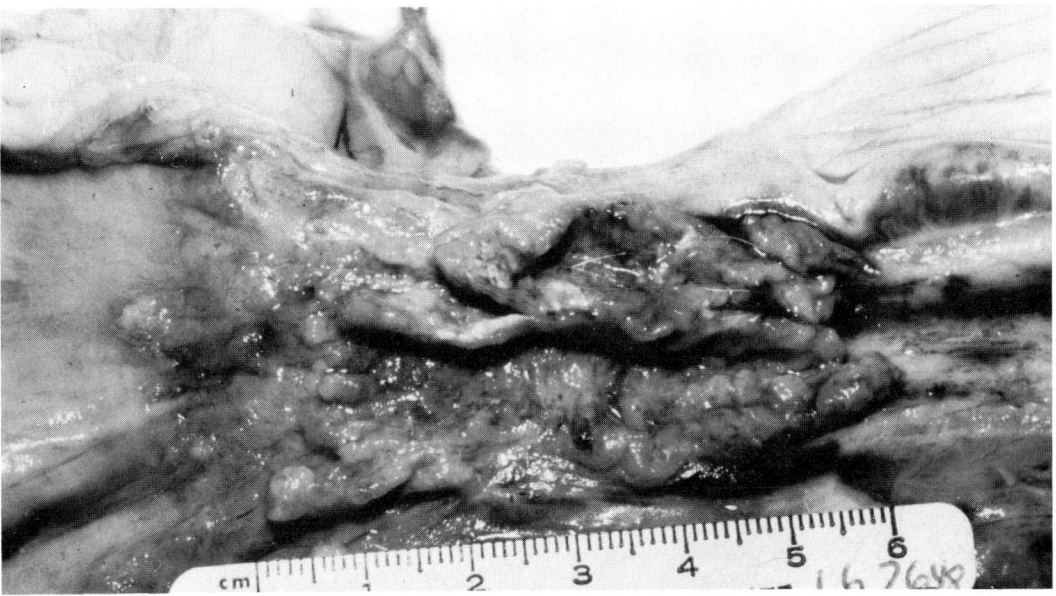

Figure 76–9. Transitional cell carcinoma of the female urethra.

tures, or fractures of the os penis in the dog resulting from automobile accidents. It occurs more commonly as a result of urethral catheterization or in conjunction with urethral blockage caused by calculi. Bite wounds of the urethra damage tissue more extensively than do sharp lacerations and increase the potential for infection. Foreign objects occasionally injure the urethra (Fig. 76–10).

The extent of the trauma may vary from mild urethritis to a more serious perforation or complete severance. The management of urethritis, urethral calculi, and urethral obstruction is discussed elsewhere in this chapter.

Clinical Signs. Clinical signs depend on the location of the rupture and whether or not there is obstruction of urine outflow. The signs of urethral rupture may be identical to those already described for rupture of the bladder, if the rupture is in the pelvic urethra. Other ruptures are usually manifested by swelling, pain, cellulitis, and tenderness caused by extravasation of urine into the surrounding tissue, with necrosis and sloughing of the tissue if the rupture site is not determined early. Urine extravasated into the abdomen may cause peritonitis. Hematuria, oliguria, or anuria maybe present (Putnam and Pennock, 1969).

Radiographic Examination. Positive contrast retrograde urethrography usually reveals contrast medium in the periurethral tissue if a withdrawal rupture exists. Small tears may be very difficult to see on a radiograph but may show up as filling defects on a urethrogram. Retrograde urethrograms are indicated in all patients sustaining pelvic fractures because of the associated frequency of urethral trauma (Fig. 76–11).

Treatment. Repair of a ruptured urethra depends on the severity and location of the tear. Small tears may heal spontaneously if resection is not complete, and if an indwelling Foley catheter is placed in the urethra and sutured at the prepuce (Weaver and Schulte, 1962). An Elizabethan collar should be used to prevent the animal from removing the catheter, and the catheter should be left in place for seven to ten days (Weaver and Schulte, 1962). A prescrotal or perineal urethrostomy in the dog, or perineal urethrostomy in the cat, may be necessary to introduce the Foley catheter.

In cats with ruptured urethras, a urethrostomy may have to be performed. In male cats with ruptured urethras caused by attempts to catheterize to relieve urethral blockage, a perineal urethrostomy can be performed, since most of the ruptures occur in the penile urethra. In cats with ruptures of the pelvic or abdominal urethra, an antepubic urethrostomy can be performed if other measures fail.

If a laceration occurs in the distal urethra

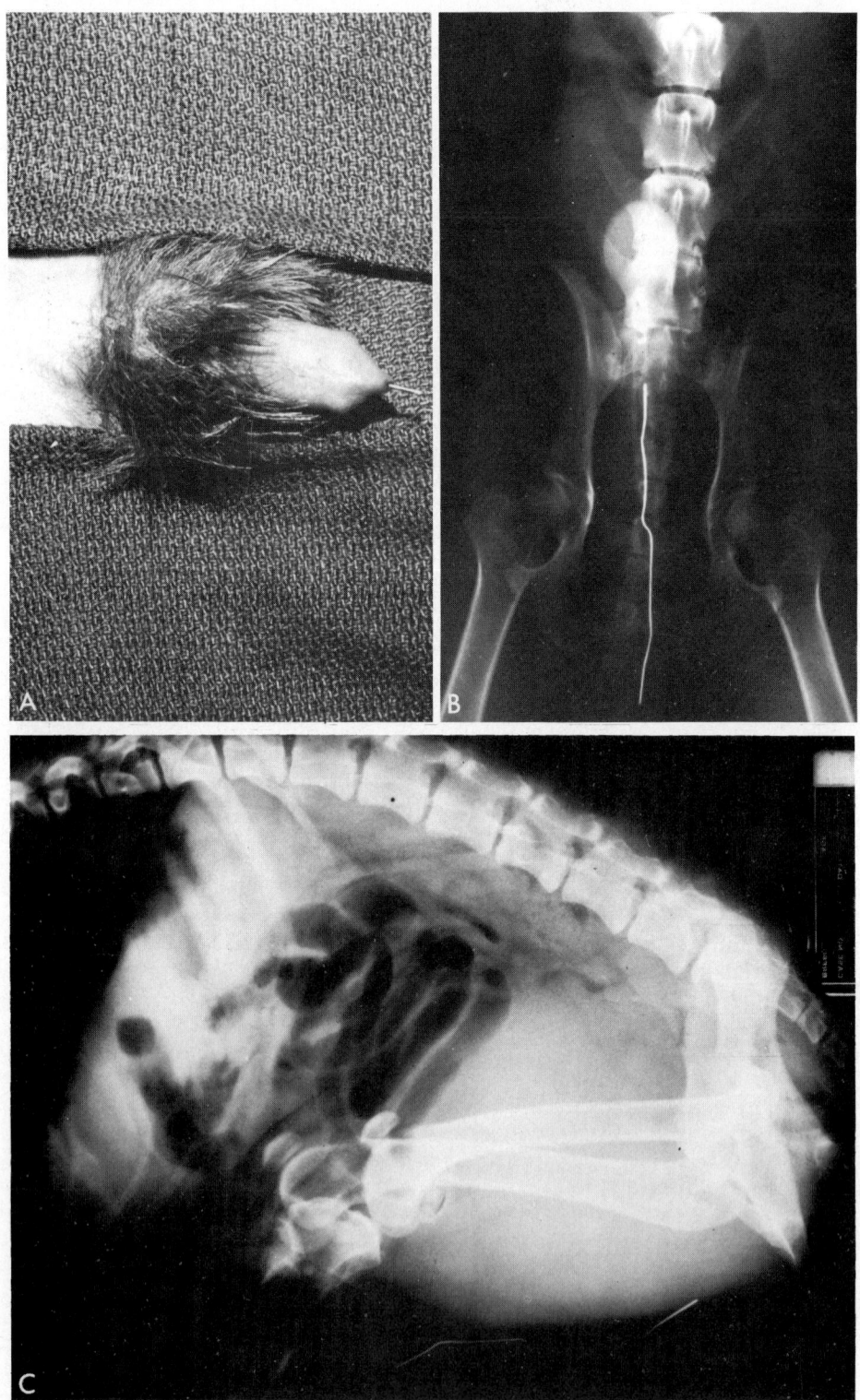

Figure 76–10. Urethral foreign body (paper clip) causing trauma in a dog. *A*, Gross appearance. *B*, Ventrodorsal view. *C*, Lateral view.

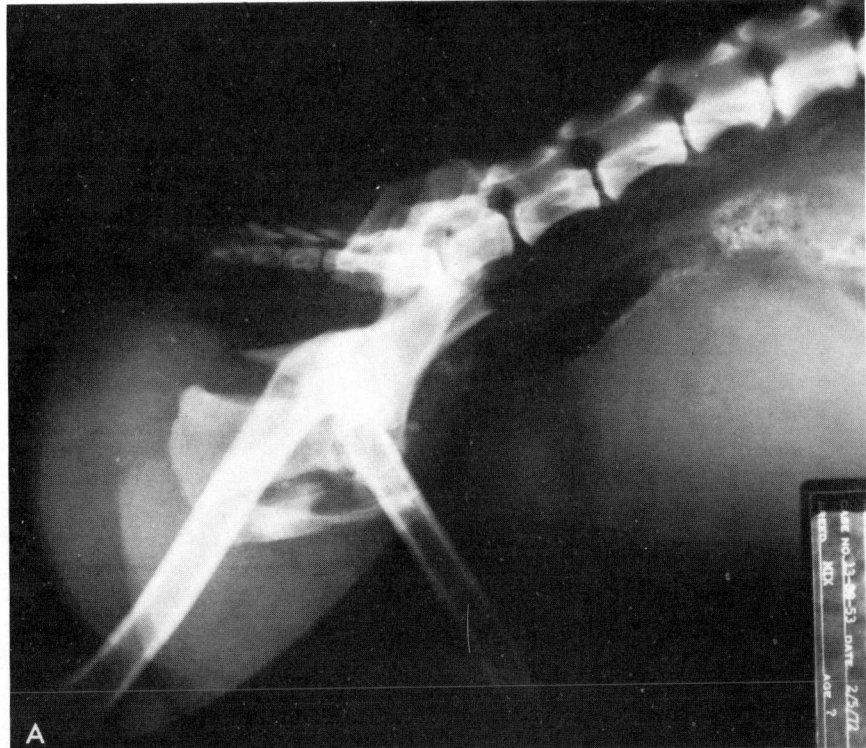

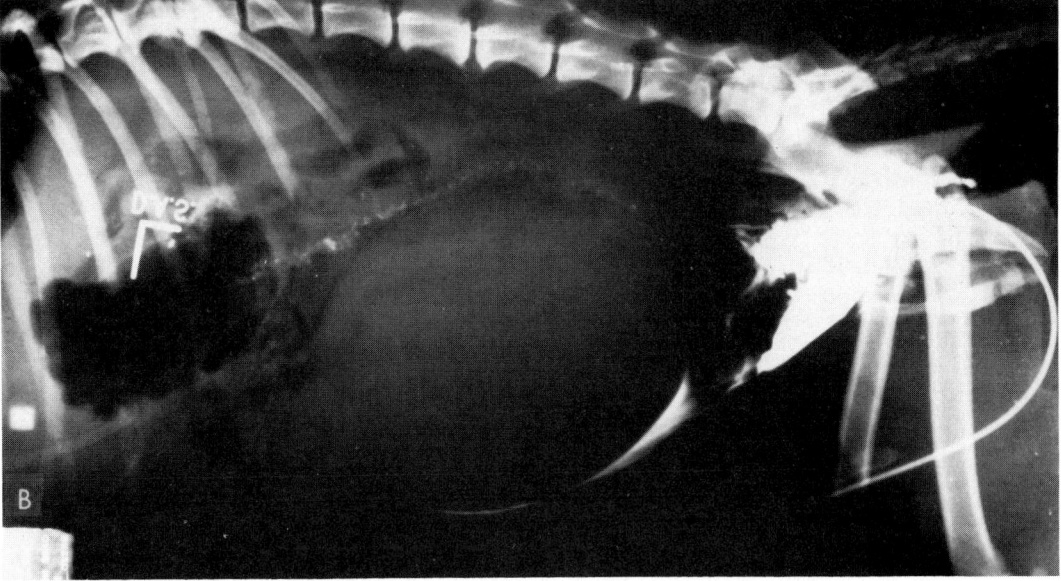

Figure 76–11. Ruptured urethra resulting from a pelvic fracture caused by an automobile accident. *A,* Lateral projection demonstrating the fractured pelvis. *B,* Retrograde urethrogram illustrating extravasation of contrast material into the abdominal and periurethral tissue.

of a male dog, a prepubic, scrotal, or perineal urethrostomy can be performed proximal to the rent. If the rent can be identified, it can be sutured closed over an indwelling Foley catheter with interrupted catgut sutures (Greiner and Brown, 1975). If the laceration is in the pelvic urethra and there is extravasation of urine into the periurethral tissue or abdominal cavity, a Foley catheter should be placed retrograde into the bladder as a urinary diversion measure, so that the dog can be stabilized metabolically before surgery. If the catheter cannot be passed into the bladder, a temporary tube cystostomy using a Foley catheter can be performed using local anesthesia. The animal can then be stabilized (see Trauma to Bladder) and the periurethral tissues have a chance to return to normal before primary repair is attempted. By using a tube cystostomy, surgery can be delayed for three to five days, which ensures that the patient is a better surgical candidate.

If the laceration is in the pelvic urethra, a laparotomy and symphysiotomy may be necessary to expose the urethra (Putnam and Pennock, 1969). A small laceration can be sutured with 3–0 chromic catgut in an interrupted pattern over an indwelling Foley catheter. The catheter should be left in place for seven to ten days. It is possible to anastomose the external pelvic urethra to the neck of the bladder, in front of the ischium, in cases in which the ends of the urethra have distracted, or when granulation tissue invades the rupture site (Knecht and Slusher, 1970).

Following surgical intervention, the administration of appropriate fluid and antibiotic therapy is extremely important, and drainage at the site of the laceration is mandatory to remove collected urine. If the rupture is in the external urethra, hot compresses should be applied to the area; indwelling catheters should be removed in seven to ten days. The most serious postoperative complication is urethral stricture.

PROLAPSE OF THE MALE URETHRA

Prolapse of the penile urethra is rare in the dog; it occurs most often in the brachiocephalic breeds. Clinical signs are usually excessive licking of the prepuce and hemorrhage from the preputial orifice. Examination of the penis reveals that the mucosa protrudes from the urethral orifice. The protruding portion varies in length, and in color varies from bright red to purple. Prolapse of the penile urethra results most frequently from excessive sexual excitement or masturbation. Excessive straining when urinating due to genitourinary infection or urethral calculi may also be causative.

Treatment. A prolapsed penile urethra should be reduced as soon as possible before irreversible damage and edema occur; therapy should then be directed toward the cause of the prolapse. The prolapsed portion may reduce itself spontaneously; in most cases it will recur, however, and a permanent cure is unlikely.

Two types of surgical procedures have been used to treat the prolapsed portion of the urethra. One method involves placing the dog under general anesthesia and manually reducing the prolapse with a male urinary catheter. While the catheter is held in place, a purse-string suture of nonabsorbable material is placed at the penile orifice. The catheter is then removed and the suture is left in place for five days (Firestone, 1941).

The second method of surgical correction is amputation of the prolapsed portion of the urethra, again while the animal is under anesthesia. The mucosa is resutured to the penile tissue with fine chromic catgut. This can be done either by placing stay sutures in the mucosa or by placing two straight intestinal needles perpendicular to one another through the penile tissue to prevent retraction of the mucosa distally (Sinibaldi and Greene, 1973; Hobson and Heller, 1971). If any calculi, foreign bodies, or congenital defects are present, correction should be made at the time of surgery. Balanoposthitis, if present, should also be treated at this time.

Whichever surgical technique is used, careful postoperative treatment is imperative to success of the operation. Failures are usually due to poor postoperative management.

If urethritis is present, either as a cause or result of the prolapse, urinary antibiotics should be administered at the recommended dosage for a minimum of seven to ten days. Antispasmodics and antiinflammatory agents are helpful in relieving the spasms, inflammation, and straining that occur as a result of urethritis. They should be continued for two to three days postoperatively.

Elizabethan collars or tranquilizers must be used to prevent self-multilation. Estradiol cypionate (1 mg intramuscularly) or diethylstilbestrol (1 mg daily) for three to five days can be administered to prevent excessive sexual excitement and bleeding from the surgical site. In many cases, castration may be necessary, especially if masturbation was the initiating cause of the prolapse. The dog's cage should be covered and darkened to prevent his becoming excited and cleared of any material that will allow masturbation. Ointments can be infused into the prepuce to reduce inflammation or infection of the prepuce or penis.

The dog may be released from the hospital on the fourth postoperative day on urinary antibiotics and tranquilizers and/or with an Elizabethan collar. The client should be instructed to infuse the prepuce twice daily with an antibiotic and anti-inflammatory ointment. The animal should be reexamined in seven to ten days.

FELINE UROLITHIASIS SYNDROME (FUS)

Incidence. Urolithiasis accounts for up to ten per cent of the total male cat population seen in veterinary practice (Foster, 1967). Although the syndrome is more severe in male cats, owing to the occurrences of urinary obstruction, it also occurs in female cats (Bohonowych et al., 1978; Engle, 1977). The incidence of FUS in the total population of male and female cats is between .6 and 9.8 per cent (Engle, 1977; Tomey and Follis, 1978; Walker et al., 1977). Overall recurrence rates of 32 to 50 per cent have been reported in cats that were hospitalized because of obstruction (Bovee et al., 1979b; Foster, 1967; Walker et al., 1977). Some studies have associated obesity (Walker et al., 1977; Willeberg and Priester, 1976) and decreased activity (Reif et al., 1977) with occurrence of FUS. A seasonal incidence of late autumn and winter has been reported by some investigators (Walker et al., 1977; Willeberg, 1975; Willeberg and Priester, 1976), although the syndrome can occur at any time of the year. Animals one to six years of age are generally affected (Willeberg and Priester, 1976). FUS is infrequently encountered in cats less than one year of age (Bohonowych et al., 1978; Reif et al., 1977). It is generally agreed that there is no breed predilection; however, one investigator reported an increase risk in Persian cats and a decreased risk in Siamese cats (Willeberg and Priester, 1976). Mortality rates have been reported to be 1.2 per cent (Engle, 1977) and 22 per cent (Walker et al., 1977).

Etiology. In spite of extensive clinical and research studies, the etiology of FUS remains poorly understood, although a number of predisposing factors have been implicated. The theories that have been advanced can be grouped into four major categories: (1) viral etiologies, including Manx calicivirus, (formerly picornavirus), feline cell-associated herpes virus, and feline syncytium-forming virus (paramyxovirus); (2) struvite crystalluria, a unique urinary protein, influence of pH, and influence of diet; (3) anatomic factors, including effect of the penile urethra, effect of castration; and (4) other factors, including urinary tract infection, urine stasis.

Viral etiologic agents have been implicated as causative, and there is experimental evidence to support this hypothesis. Manx calcivirus induces FUS when directly infused into the bladder or passed by aerosol transmission (Rich and Fabricant, 1969; Fabricant and Rich, 1971; Rich et al., 1971); associated with this virus is the feline syncytium-forming virus, which is either a passenger virus or a second virus that acts synergistically with Manx calicivirus to produce the syndrome (Fabricant, 1973.)

The herpes virus subsequently designated feline cell-associated herpes virus (Fabricant, 1979) was first isolated from the kidneys and bladders of two littermate kittens with respiratory disease (Fabricant and Rich, 1971). The role that this virus plays in association with the Manx calicivirus in inducing urolithiasis was demonstrated in specific pathogen-free cats (Fabricant, 1977). The feline cell-associated herpesvirus alone was capable of inducing urolithiasis, but when both Manx calicivirus and the herpesvirus were inoculated together, urolithiasis developed earlier and in more cats (Fabricant, 1977). Thus, it appears that in natural disease the Manx calicivirus may stimulate latent viruses in the bladder, such as a feline cell-associated herpes virus, which together produce urolithiasis (Fabricant, 1979). Further studies are needed to clarify the exact role of viruses in the etiology of FUS.

Struvite Crystalluria. Struvite crystalluria (magnesium ammonium phosphate hexahydrate) is common to all cats, both normal ones and those affected by FUS (Carbone, 1965; Rich and Kirk, 1969). Several factors influence formation of struvite crystals in the urine. A unique protein has been isolated from the urine and urethral plugs of cats with FUS, and this may bear some relationship to the growth of crystals that subsequently cause obstruction (Rich and Norcross, 1969). However, the exact role that this unique protein plays in etiology of urolithiasis remains unknown. The source of this protein has not been established, but it is not the result of tissue breakdown or other processes occurring after obstruction. Urine pH above 6.8 is also associated with increased occurrence of struvite crystals (Rich and Kirk, 1968).

Mineral composition of the diet may play an important role in struvite crystal and calculus formation and in the production of urolithiasis experimentally (Lewis et al., 1978). Diets containing high magnesium (0.75 per cent dry matter) caused obstruction when combined with low calcium intake, whether the phosphorus content was high or low (Lewis et al., 1978). Increasing the calcium content of the diets had a variable effect on calculus formation, depending on the concentrations of magnesium and phosphorus (Lewis et al., 1978). When both of these minerals were high, there was increased calculus formation; when both were low, there was decreased calculus formation. Diets containing low magnesium (less than 0.1 per cent dry matter) did not produce obstruction of the urinary tract, regardless of the phosphorus or calcium content of the diet (Lewis et al., 1978); calculi composed of calcium phosphate were found in a small percentage (4 of 43) of these cats with a magnesium deficiency produced by the diet (Lewis et al., 1978). Most commercial cat foods have a lower magnesium level than that found in experimental, calculogenic diets, and feeding such diets may reduce recurrence of urolithiasis (Feldmann, et al., 1977). Only a few diets contain less than 0.1 per cent magnesium and 0.8 per cent phosphorus, which was found to be the least calculogenic, provided that dietary calcium was high or adequate (Lewis et al., 1979). They are C/D (Hill) and Beef and Liver Buffet by Friskies (Lewis, 1981).

The exact role played by struvite crystals in the etiology of urolithiasis and the factors that influence their formation, including diet, are being studied. Since struvite crystals are always found in sabulous plugs

(Carbone, 1965; Rich and Kirk, 1968; Jackson, 1971), and because infusion of massive doses of struvite crystals into the bladder has produced urolithiasis experimentally (Rich and Kirk, 1968), it is thought that together with other factors, they do play some role in the etiology of urolithiasis.

Anatomic Factors. The predominant occurrence of urolithiasis in male cats has been associated with the narrowness of the urethral lumen in comparison to that of the female (Foster, 1967). The exact region of the penile urethra where uroliths first lodge is not known; however, the narrowest distal portions are considered the most likely areas. Early castration was thought to predispose to obstruction by inducing a smaller, narrower urethra, but subsequent investigations have failed to substantiate this hypothesis (Herron, 1972). The effect of later castration has also been shown not to increase the risk of developing FUS (Bohonowych et al., 1978; Bovee et al., 1979b; Jackson, 1971; Reif et al., 1977), although some investigators report a higher incidence in castrated and spayed cats (Engle, 1977; Willeberg and Priester, 1976).

Other Factors. Urinary bacterial infection is now thought to occur after the formation of sabulous plugs, and as such it is a complication, rather than a cause, of urolithiasis (Schechter, 1970). The fact that continued urinary tract infection contributes to recurrence of obstruction cannot be doubted. Infection and urethral trauma cause swelling and devitalization of the lining of the urinary tract, which then predisposes to stenosis and reobstruction caused by crystals and sabulous plugs consisting of crystals, mucus, and degenerative cellular debris. Infection can also enhance struvite crystalluria and calculus genesis, especially if the infection is caused by urease-producing bacteria. Finally, infection can have a deleterious effect on renal function if it ascends to the kidneys.

Obstruction and subsequent urine stasis caused by sabulous plugs, swelling, and infection of the urethral lining predispose to infection of the bladder by allowing bacteria to multiply (Hinman, 1968). In addition, urine stasis allows the precipitation of struvite microcrystals that ordinarily would be passed, thereby generating further obstruction and further complicating urine stasis.

Cats that are obese and lazy and do not

use the litter pan or go outside as often as other cats may be predisposed to FUS because of urine stasis (Reif et al., 1977; Walker et al., 1977; Willeberg and Priester, 1976), as may be cats that are confined indoors, especially during the winter months (Walker et al., 1977; Willeberg, 1975; Willeberg and Priester, 1976).

In summary, various etiologic factors are probably involved in the etiology of FUS. The importance of each factor remains the subject of ongoing investigations.

Clinical Signs and Laboratory Findings. Initially, there are frequent attempts to urinate, with straining over the litter pan or other, unusual places. Between these episodes, the cat usually licks the penis. The observant client may eventually report that small amounts of urine, which may contain blood, are passed on each occasion.

As the syndrome progresses, the cat does more straining at the litter pan, and eventually little or no urine is passed because of complete or nearly complete obstruction. After 48 hours, the signs of anorexia and vomition, progressive depression and lethargy, and dehydration develop (Burrows and Bovee, 1978). In female cats, urethral obstruction is encountered less frequently, and thus, the predominant signs include pollakiuria, stranguria, and hematuria.

The BUN and creatinine concentrations are variably elevated according to the duration of obstruction (Burrows and Bovee, 1978; Finco and Cornelius, 1977). Serum sodium concentration is usually normal (Burrows and Bovee, 1978) but it can be low (Finco and Cornelius, 1977). Serum chloride is usually normal (Burrows and Bovee, 1978). There is variable hyperkalemia (Burrows and Bovee, 1978; Finco and Cornelius, 1977), depending on the duration of obstruction. Hyperphosphatemia and metabolic acidosis are common (Burrows and Bovee, 1978; Finco and Cornelius, 1977). Other possible laboratory findings include hypocalcemia, hyperglycemia, and hyperproteinemia (Finco and Cornelius, 1977). Urinalysis shows a wide range of pH and specific gravity, and numerous red blood cells in the urine sediment; white blood cells and bacteria are seen if there is bacterial infection, and struvite crystals are usually seen.

Patient Management. The status and management of the patient depends on the severity of fluid and electrolyte disturbances (or uremia), the duration and severity of obstruction, and the association of gross hematuria and urinary tract infection. If the patient is examined early in the course of urolithiasis, the bladder may be small, and any urine that is present is usually expressed easily by manual pressure on the bladder. The animal may void clear urine, or there will be variable degrees of hematuria. At this stage, a broad-spectrum urinary tract antibiotic and urine acidifiers should be administered for a minimum of 21 days. A wide variety of agents are available (see p. 360). Urine culture and sensitivity testing are usually not necessary at this time, unless there is gross hematuria, which suggests bacterial infection. In such cases, the urinary tract antibiotic that was initially chosen should be changed if indicated by culture and sensitivity testing.

Clients should be thoroughly educated regarding the signs of recurrent obstruction and uremia. They should be advised to watch closely for continued passage of urine, and in the event of obstruction or continued gross hematuria, they should be instructed to return the cat to the clinic immediately. If the history includes the feeding of dry cat food or fish, the diet should be changed to canned cat food other than fish. The role that dry cat food plays in influencing FUS remains controversial (see previous discussion). Increased risk of FUS and urinary tract obstruction with the feeding of dry cat foods has been reported (Reif et al., 1977; Willeberg, 1975). The incidence of recurrence of FUS, however, could not be associated with dry cat food feeding (Bovee, 1979b). Ideally, the recommended diet should be low in magnesium and phosphorus (Lewis et al., 1978), as described previously (see Etiology). Water should be made readily available to the cat, and the diet might even be salted to encourage water consumption.

A cat is admitted to the hospital when obstruction is present and there is a history of vomition, depression, dehydration, and lethargy. From this point, management of urolithiasis can be placed into the following categories: initial therapy, which consists of relief of obstruction, management of dehydration, management of acidosis, and management of hyperkalemia; diuresis, which involves management of fluid balance, management of electrolyte abnormalities, tapering fluids in diuresis, and management of "high output" renal failure; antibiotic therapy; care of the urinary catheter; and surgical management.

The first aim of treatment is to establish a patent urethra. The patient may require chemical restraint in order to accomplish this, and a wide variety of drugs are available. The choice of agent depends on the severity of uremia and dehydration as evaluated clinically. A safe combination is an ultra-short barbiturate anesthetic (sodium thiamylal, sodium thiopental, or sodium methohexital) and atropine. These agents provide short-acting anesthesia. Since they are metabolized by the liver, they do not accumulate in toxic concentrations as a result of renal failure (Sharpless, 1971). Care should be taken to avoid anesthetic agents which are excreted by the kidney. In severely depressed cats that are dehydrated, nitrous oxide and halothane can be administered by face mask. More often, restraint can be accomplished under these circumstances by rolling the cat in a blanket. An assistant can then hold the two hindlegs pulled forward to support the patient in dorsal recumbency for catheterization.

The urethral plug occasionally can be removed from the urethra by gently rolling the penis between the thumb and forefinger. If this is not immediately successful, however, further attempts should not be made because urethral trauma may ensue, complicating the urethral obstruction. At this point, backflushing the urethral plugs with sterile saline or other suitable antiseptic solutions should be performed. The silver abscess cannula (or any reasonable facsimile) is excellent for this purpose, since it is nontraumatic and provides an opening at the end of the cannula for maximum efficiency in backflushing. With the cat adequately restrained in dorsal recumbency, the prepuce is grasped gently to hold the penis. The cannula is carefully inserted into the distal tip of the penile urethra. After lifting dorsally on the prepuce to straighten the urethra, the sterile solution is gently flushed into the urethra. If the plug is not immediately dislodged, several attempts should be made, as continued flushing will eventually loosen the plug in the majority of cases. Following this, a polyethylene tomcat catheter is inserted into the urethra to the bladder.

Cats that are depressed and dehydrated usually require prolonged catheterization, in which cases the tomcat catheter should be sutured in place. An adhesive tape tag is attached to the flanged end of the catheter and sutured to the prepuce, making certain that the penis is avoided. The bladder is then flushed with sterile saline solution containing urinary tract antiseptics. The solution may be chilled if there is gross hematuria. The procedure is to infuse 7 to 15 ml of solution into the bladder, retrieve this, and repeat infusions until the return solution is reasonably clear and absent of crystals and debris. The usual total volume required is 50 to 100 ml. Sterile tubing (a sterile administration set may be used) is then attached to the catheter and allowed to run to a bottle for continued collection of urine. An Elizabethan collar is occasionally necessary to prevent the cat from licking the catheter and penis. With this system, urine output can be easily monitored with reasonable asepsis. Such monitoring of urine output is extremely important in early parenteral fluid therapy. If the cat is not depressed and dehydrated and a full stream of urine is elicited by urethral backflushing, it may not be necessary to suture the catheter in place. Under these circumstances, bladder size and urethral patency should be checked frequently. If obstruction occurs later, the cat should be catheterized as described.

Parenteral fluid therapy should initially aim to replace fluid and electrolyte losses, as well as provide daily maintenance of insensible fluid losses and urine output. The fluid given should be isotonic and provide a balanced solution of electrolytes (e.g., lactated Ringer's solution). Rehydration fluid volumes may be calculated by estimating clinical dehydration and applying this to the following formula: percentage of dehydration (decimal figure) $\times$ weight (lb) $\times$ 500 = ml fluid replacement.

Empirically, maintenance of insensible water loss is 10 ml per lb of body weight daily and should be added to the rehydration volume. Finally, daily urine output can be estimated by continuously monitoring it over a certain period of time (two to four hours) and then converting this to an average hourly output figure. This figure, multiplied by 24 hours, roughly estimates daily urine volume, which should be added to make a total 24-hour parenteral fluid volume.

Electrolyte abnormalities are common after prolonged obstruction. Initially, acidosis and hyperkalemia are the most significant, clinically. Acidosis is manifested by variable degrees of lethargy and deep respiration. This can be treated by adding sodium bicarbonate to the parenteral fluids. The requirement can be empirically replaced by adding 10 to 15 mEq sodium bicarbonate per 250 ml of fluid, or more accurately determined by laboratory testing with subsequent administration of the base deficit over 24 hours as follows: normal bicarbonate − measured bicarbonate × .6 × weight (kg).

Hyperkalemia occurs after prolonged obstruction as a consequence of impaired potassium excretion by the damaged kidney (Burrows and Bovee, 1978; Finco and Cornelius, 1977). It is manifested clinically as variable lethargy progressing to profound depression and coma as serum concentrations approach 9 to 10 mEq per liter. When hyperkalemia is suspected, an electrocardiogram (ECG) should be taken and serum-electrolyte studies made. The electrocardiographic criteria for establishing hyperkalemia have been discussed (see Chapter 49). Life-threatening hyperkalemia appears clinically as coma or depression bordering on coma. There is usually simultaneous hypothermia and severe dehydration. The ECG is abnormal in all such cases. It may be treated vigorously by infusing sodium bicarbonate intravenously (10 to 25 mEq) for 30 minutes. Alternately, insulin may be given at 0.35 unit per lb of body weight intravenously, immediately followed by dextrose given intravenously; the dosage of dextrose should be two gm of dextrose per one unit of insulin. This is provided by giving one gm per unit STAT, and the remainder as a 2.5 per cent dextrose solution. Continued dextrose administration is usually not necessary after the effects of insulin have abated (six to eight hours). The salutary effects of insulin on hyperkalemia can be documented by monitoring the ECG, which should become normal. After relief of the urethral obstruction, continued therapy with insulin and dextrose is rarely required. The serum-potassium concentration should be monitored daily in order to determine the need for further therapy.

There is usually moderate to massive diuresis following relief of obstruction (Witte et al., 1964; Brucker, 1957; Jaenike, 1972; Falls and Stacy, 1973). The magnitude of diuresis and renal impairment correlates with duration of obstruction. Diuresis is believed to result from a proximal tubular defect in the resorption of solutes, mainly sodium, and from a solute diuresis resulting from metabolites retained during obstruction (Bricker, 1957; Witte et al., 1964; Jaenike, 1972; Falls and Stacy, 1973). Diuresis in the first 24 to 36 hours following relief of obstruction must be diagnosed by monitoring urine output, since it poses problems for both fluid and electrolyte management.

While hyperkalemia may occur initially, hypokalemia and hyponatremia may ensue, as urine that is rich in sodium and potassium is excreted in massive volumes. By monitoring urine output, the clinician can detect significant changes in urine volume, so that the total daily fluid volume can be adjusted to prevent dehydration.

The choice of fluid to be administered is determined by daily monitoring of serum sodium and potassium concentrations. In addition, renal function should be monitored by determining BUN or creatinine concentrations. As mentioned previously, the fluid used initially may be lactated Ringer's solution, or similarly balanced isotonic fluid. Should there be a decline in the serum of either sodium or potassium, the clinician must supplement therapy with additional electrolytes. If the patient can tolerate oral therapy, hyponatremia can be treated with enteric-coated salt tablets. The dosage varies with the severity of hyponatremia, but in general, a dosage of 1 gm three times daily is adequate initially. This can be raised to 4 gm daily if necessary, as determined by continued monitoring of serum sodium. Hypokalemia can be treated with oral potassium elixirs or wax matrix potassium chloride tablets, if oral therapy is feasible. The latter has been found superior, since they are nonirritating, palatable, and do not cause vomiting. The latter should be dosed at one-half to one tablet twice daily, but the actual dosage must be adjusted to the individual requirements of the patient. The elixirs should be diluted with tap water prior to administration in order to avoid vomition. A starting dosage is one-half teaspoon (2.5 ml) three times daily; however, with massive hypokalemia (less than 2.5 mEq per liter) and kaliuresis, the starting dosage should be as high as one teaspoon three times per day. As with hyponatremia, the initial dose of the potassium supplement may be raised by one-half to one teaspoon three times per day, as determined by monitoring the serum potassium daily. If a further decline in the serum concentration is encountered, the dosage can be raised to as much as two to three teaspoons three times daily. Supplementation of parenteral fluids with potassium salts may eventually become necessary if hypokelemia continues.

If the patient is unable to tolerate oral therapy, intravenous therapy is an alternative. Hyponatremia may be treated by changing the fluid to normal saline if the patient was previously on lactated Ringer's solution, or by adding sodium salts to the parenteral fluids. It is rarely necessary to add more sodium than is present in normal saline. Hypokalemia can be corrected by adding potassium salts to parenteral fluids. The amount added depends on the degree of hypokalemia. The authors add potassium according to the serum concentration of the electrolyte as in Table 76–2.

If the patient has kaliuresis, it may be necessary to administer large amounts of potassium intravenously. It is unsafe to administer more than 20 mEq of potassium supplement within one hour, since life-threatening cardiac arrhythmias or cardiac arrest can occur. In rare situations, with massive kaliuresis, this rate of potassium administration may need to be exceeded. The dosage of the potassium added to the fluids may be altered according to clinical response. If the serum potassium moves into the normal range after a day of treatment, the dosage of potassium supplement per 250 ml of fluid should be maintained at the same level. If the serum concentration rises only slightly or declines, the dosage must be raised to the next level. Rarely do patients require more than 20 mEq per 250 ml. If the serum potassium elevates over 5.5 mEq per liter, the dosage should be decreased to the next lower level. If it is more than 7 mEq per liter, potassium supplements may be discontinued. Whenever potassium salts are administered intravenously, it is essential to monitor the ECG for signs of S-T and T wave changes, as well as arrhythmias.

Continued treatment of acidosis during diuresis is rarely necessary. For this reason, unless the patient shows symptomatic acidosis, sodium bicarbonate should not be routinely added to parenteral fluids once acidosis is initially corrected and once the diuresis phase begins.

As renal function improves, the diuresis phase of postrenal azotemia will decline. The dilemma facing the clinician is whether parenteral fluid therapy is potentiating the diuresis phase. The average duration of diuresis is two to five days after correction of urethral obstruction; longer periods can occur as a result of additional renal damage, however. During therapy, renal function should be monitored by determining BUN or creatinine concentrations. The clinician can attempt reduction of the total daily fluid volume when blood concentrations are stable or in the normal range. The urine output is monitored as before, but only 50 to 75 per cent of the estimated daily urine volume is provided. Renal function of the patient should be followed closely, as well as state of hydration. If moderate dehydration develops, or if renal function deteriorates, the clinician should reinstitute fluid therapy at the higher volume originally determined for one to two days. At this point, a second tapering-off procedure can be attempted. If the patient remains hydrated or becomes minimally hydrated and renal function does not deteriorate dramatically, fluid therapy may be tapered off again. Eventually, the volume of fluids given will provide only normal daily maintenance (10 ml per lb insensible loss and 0.5 to 1 ml per lb per hour of urine output), at which time parenteral

Table 76–2. **Addition of Potassium Salts to Parenteral Fluids for Correction of Hypokalemia**

Serum Potassium (mEq per liter)	mEq per 250 ml of Fluid
Below 2.0	20
2.0 to 2.5	15
2.6 to 3.0	10
3.1 to 3.5	7

DISEASES OF THE BLADDER AND URETHRA / **1929**

fluids may be discontinued and the patient provided with adequate drinking water. Electrolyte therapy during this tapering-off procedure may also require adjustment. This is determined by continued daily monitoring of the serum sodium and potassium in order to detect significant changes. When parenteral fluids are stopped, continued oral electrolyte therapy may occasionally be necessary should there be a continued defect in electrolye excretion resulting from renal damage, as shown by severe potassium alterations.

Occasionally, a patient's hospital course is characterized by relief of obstruction followed by diuresis that does not lower the BUN or creatinine concentrations. Electrolyte abnormalities may develop as a result of solute diuresis. This is termed *high output renal failure*. Under these circumstances, the clinician may use mannitol, in spite of the presence of diuresis, to improve renal function. Mannitol is an osmotic agent that has been shown to increase renal blood flow during hypotension and hypoperfusion (Gagnon et al., 1963; Dragon and Deutsch, 1971; Morris et al., 1972). Regardless of the exact mechanism of action, mannitol can be given at a dosage of 0.5 gm per kg and is dripped intravenously over a 15- to 30-minute period. In some cases of high output renal failure, significant improvement in renal function follows. Diuresis is enhanced, which necessitates accurate monitoring of urine output as well as of the fluid and electrolyte disturbances that may ensue. Management of the patient after administration of mannitol is the same as that described previously.

In-patient therapy should include urinary tract antibiotics, both to prevent infection from the catheter and to treat preexisting infection. Broad-spectrum antibiotics that are not nephrotoxic (see Chapter 29) should be used initially. Urine culture and sensitivity testing may be performed after catheterization, and the antibiotics altered as indicated. After renal function has become normal even the more nephrotoxic antibiotics can be used if they are needed, as shown by culture and sensitivity testing. Urine acidifiers should be avoided early in the course of therapy, since acidosis is common and therapy can be complicated by the use of acidifiers. Later, however, when renal function is normal and acidosis is corrected,

urine acidifiers may be added to the regimen.

Other supportive therapy that can be given during hospitalization includes force-feeding a high-quality diet and providing water as soon as the patient can tolerate alimentation.

The clinician must determine when to remove the urinary catheter. This varies with the patient's status on admission and the rapidity of recovery of renal function. When renal function and electrolyte disturbances are stable and when diuresis has ended, the catheter can be removed. Prior to removal, the bladder should be flushed. The clinician should frequently monitor the flow of the urine through the urethra, as well as the bladder size, in order to diagnose recurrence of the urethral obstruction. In the event of recurrence, the clinician must determine whether recatheterization and extensive flushing of the bladder or surgical intervention with perineal urethrostomy is preferable. The latter is the procedure the authors use in most cases.

Aftercare. Moderate output can be maintained by allowing an adequate supply of water. By salting the diet, water consumption by the patient is encouraged. Salt tablets can be used in the occasional patient for which salting the diet causes anorexia. Increased urine output tends to diminish the opportunity for sabulous plug formation in the urethra and may diminish hematuria in cats fed calculogenic diets (Lewis et al., 1978).

Recurrent urinary tract infection may become a serious problem following an episode of urethral obstruction. If infection goes unattended, obstruction may recur, and for this reason clients should be thoroughly educated regarding the clinical signs of urinary tract infection. Antibiotics for the urinary tract should be used for at least four weeks after hospitalization, as determined by initial urine culture and sensitivity testing. During this time, and thereafter in patients with recurrent infection, periodic culture and sensitivity testing should be done by the clinician to determine the need for continued antibiotics and to determine the proper antibiotic if one is required. Long-term therapy occasionally is indicated to prevent or control infection and, subsequently, urethral obstruction (see Bacterial Cystitis).

Acidifiers theoretically diminish the solubility of struvite crystals, which are a component of the sabulous plugs found in FUS. Although the use of acidifers has not been proven to reduce the incidence of FUS, their use seems justified on the basis of the effect that urine pH has on struvite solubility. Chlorethamine has a questionable effect on urine pH in the cat (Bovee, 1979b). DL-Methionine and ascorbic acid have little or no effect on urine pH (Chow et al., 1978). Ammonium chloride, however, was found to be effective as an acidifier for longer periods when given once daily (Chow et al., 1978). A dosage of one gm per day has been recommended (Lewis et al., 1978). DL-Methionine is not a potent urine acidifier, but it has been shown to delay urethral obstruction in cats fed a calculogenic diet when given at a rate of one gm per day (Chow et al., 1976; Lewis et. al., 1981).

A noncalculogenic diet as described is recommended after urethral obstruction has been resolved (Lewis et al., 1978); whether or not dietary measures will have any effect on the incidence of reobstruction, however, is debatable (Bovee, 1979b; Feldmann et al., 1977).

Finally, clients should be thoroughly advised of the clinical signs associated with recurrent urethral obstruction and urinary tract infection. Early diagnosis and treatment of obstruction is beneficial to the patient; otherwise, uremia and postobstructive diuresis may complicate therapy. The client should allow the cat free and unlimited access to water and a clean litter pan, or free access to the outside environment. The importance of properly medicating the cat for the total duration of therapy must also be emphasized.

Surgical Treatment of Urolithiasis. Surgical correction to date has been the most effective means of managing chronic cases of urolithiasis. Surgical intervention should be considered when a cat has had two or three recurrences of obstruction and the clinician feels that the recurrences will continue. The length of time between each occurrence is also an important consideration. Each clinician must determine when the medical treatment has failed and surgery must be performed. In cases in which the obstruction can only be partially relieved, owing to either a stricture from pre-

vious catheterizations or calculi "plugs," surgery must be performed. If the urethra is damaged during the catheterization process, surgery must be performed immediately. In cases in which urethral obstruction can not be relieved, immediate surgical relief is necessary. The authors believe that abdominal paracentesis should not be performed because of the poor prognosis following this procedure. The risk is high in these cases with any procedure, and the owners must be prepared for the worst, but the overall chance for a normal animal is better with surgery than with other techniques.

Many surgical procedures have been described for the treatment of FUS (Carbone, 1963, 1967; Manziano and Manziano, 1966; Blake, 1968; Ford, 1968; Mendham, 1970; Wilson and Harrison, 1971; Richards et al., 1972; Johnston, 1974; Biewenga, 1975). Their aim is to eliminate or bypass the penile urethra with its narrow lumen, where most of the blockage occurs. In its place, surgeons make a new opening using the pelvic urethra or prostatic urethra with its larger lumen. Perineal urethrostomy and preputial urethrostomy use the pelvic urethra just posterior to the bulbourethral glands, while antepubic urethrostomy uses the abdominal urethra, just anterior to the prostate, for the opening.

It is beyond the scope of this chapter to describe the various surgical techniques. One of the authors (Greene) has performed many urethrostomies using the perineal urethrostomy technique described by Wilson and Harrison (1971) and the antepubic technique described by Ford (1968) with a high rate of success. Specific information relative to these surgical procedures is thoroughly discussed in the original articles.

A perineal urethrostomy should be attempted first, but if the urethra is ruptured anterior to the bulbourethral glands or if problems are encountered with the surgery, an antepubic urethrostomy should be performed. If any strictures have occurred from previous perineal urethrostomies, surgery may be redone, using the technique described by Wilson and Harrison (1971). Postoperative stricture formation occurred in 11.5 per cent of the cases in which the technique described by Wilson and Harrison was used (1971), and postoperative cystitis occurred in 25 per cent of the cases reported by Smith and Schiller, 1978.

For good surgical results, it is important for (1) the surgeon to have a thorough understanding of the normal anatomy of the perineal area, (2) the cat to be treated medically (as already described) whenever possible, and (3) the bladder to be empty at the time of surgery. A cystotomy may have to be performed in the male or female if there are large calculi in the bladder.

The surgical procedure only provides a larger opening for the urine and crystals to pass through. It is still necessary to administer antibiotics and long-term urinary acidifiers and to add salt to the diet. The chance of urethral blockages decreases with surgery, but cystitis can occur and needs frequent medication. If chronic cystitis occurs, radiographic evaluation of the bladder is indicated in order to differentiate this malady from that due to cystic calculi.

CYSTIC CALCULI IN THE CAT

Although cystic calculi in the cat have been described, they appear to be relatively rare (Ryan and Wolfer, 1978; Kirkpatrick, 1977; Davidson, 1975; Bohonowych et al., 1978). In one report the mean annual rate of occurrence of cystic calculi in the cat was approximately 0.08 per cent. The mean age for all first occurrences was 4.9 years. Calculi were found in spayed and intact females and in castrated and intact males, but there was a higher incidence of calculi in spayed females (Bohonowych et al., 1978).

The etiology of cystic calculi in cats is unknown but is probably multifactoral. A virus was isolated from a female cat with a cystic calculus, but the significance of the virus is not known (Fabricant, 1971b). More research on etiology is necessary for this disease as well as for FUS. In fact, cystic calculi in the cat may be a part of this syndrome.

Cats with cystic calculi usually develop signs similar to those associated with cystitis (i.e., hematuria, stranguria, and pollakiuria). Some cats may have history of little or no response to previous antibiotic therapy. Since the bladder is usually thickened, the calculi may be difficult to palpate. Radiography is the best method of confirming the diagnosis. Ninety-six per cent of the calculi were radiopaque in one study (Bohonowych et al., 1978). Contrast radiography or exploratory cystotomy should be used to confirm the existence of radiolucent calculi (Bohonowych et al., 1978; Kirkpatrick, 1977). Radiodense and radiolucent calculi are both large and small, single and multiple (Bohonowych et al., 1978; Ryan and Wolfer, 1978).

Surgical removal of the calculi, followed by proper medical therapy, is the recommended treatment. The mineral composition of the calculi should be analyzed to aid in formulating prophylactic therapy. Bacterial culture and sensitivity testing should be performed with swabs taken directly from the bladder wall and calculi. In one report, 96.8 per cent of the calculi were phosphate, and 1.6 per cent of the cultures were positive for bacteria, with *Staphylococcus spp.* the most common organism isolated. *In vitro* sensitivity test results showed that gentamicin, cephalothin, and chloramphenicol were the most effective antibiotics (Bohonowych, 1978). Antibiotics selected on the basis of culture should be used postoperatively for 14 to 21 days, and the clinician should be aware of the side effects of various antibiotics in cats. Other medications already described in this chapter for the treatment of FUS should also be prescribed for the prevention of recurrence.

REFERENCES

Andre, P. G., and Jackson, O. F.: Lead foreign body in a cat's bladder. J. Small Anim. Pract. *13*:101, 1972.

Archibald, J.: Urinary System. *In* Archibald, J. (ed.): Canine Surgery. American Veterinary Publications, Inc., Santa Barbara, Calif., 1965.

Bailey, H.: Cystitis emphysematosa. Am. J. Roentgenol. *86*:850, 1961.

Barrett, R., and Nobel, T.: Transitional cell carcinoma of the urethra in a cat. Cornell Vet. *66*:14, 1976.

Barsanti, J. A., and Finco, D. R.: Laboratory findings in urinary tract infections. Vet. Clin. North Am. *9*:729, 1979.

Belkin, P. V.: Clinical briefs: Intra-abdominal vesicular calculus in a dog. Modern. Vet. Pract. *51*:63, 1970.

Benedict, S. R.: Uric acid in its relations to metabolism. Harvey Lectures II:346, 1915.

Biewenga, W. J.: Preputial urethroplasty for relief of urethral obstruction in the male cat. J.A.V.M.A. *166*:460, 1975.

Blake, J. A.: Perineal urethrostomy in cats. J.A.V.M.A. *152*:1499, 1962.

Bloom, F.: Pathology of the Dog and Cat. American Veterinary Publications, Inc., Evanston, Ill., 1954.

Bohonowych, R. O., Parks, J. L., and Greene, R. W.: Features of cystic calculi cats in a hospital population. J.A.V.M.A. *173*:301, 1978.

Bovee, K. C.: Cystine urolithiasis. *In* Kirk, R. W. (ed.): Current Veterinary Therapy VII. W. B. Saunders Co., Philadelphia, 1980.

Bovee, K. C.: Cystinuria and Cystine Calculi. *In* Kirk, R. W. (ed.): Current Veterinary Therapy IV. W. B. Saunders Co., Philadelphia, 1971.

Bovee, K. C.: Urolithiasis in the dog. Proceedings, 40th Annual American Animal Hospital Association Meeting, 1973.

Bovee, K. C.: Canine cystinuria and cystine calculi. Gaines Progress. Winter, 1972.

Bovee, K. C., Pass, M. A., Wardley, R., et al.: Trigonal-colonic anastomosis: A urinary diversion procedure in dogs. J.A.V.M.A. *174*:184, 1979a.

Bovee, K. C., Reif, J. S., Maguire, T. G., et al.: Recurrence of feline urethral obstruction. J.A.V.M.A. *174*:93, 1979b.

Bovee, K. C., Thier, S. O., Rea, C., et al.: Renal clearance of amino acids in canine cystinuria. Metabolism *23*:51, 1974.

Bradley, W. E., and Timm, G. W.: Physiology of micturition. Vet. Clin. North Am. *4*:487, 1974.

Bricker, N. S., Shawyri, E. D., Reardan, J. B., et al.: An abnormality in renal function resulting from urinary tract obstruction. Am. J. Med. *23*:554, 1957.

Brodey, R. S.: Silicate renal calculi in Kenyan dogs. J. Small Anim. Pract. *18*:523, 1977.

Brodey, R. S.: Canine urolithiasis. J.A.V.M.A. *126*:1, 1955.

Brodie, N.: Infected urachal cysts. Am. J. Surg. *69*:243, 1945.

Brodey, R. S., Riser, W. H., and Allen, H.: Hypertrophic pulmonary osteoarthropathy in a dog with carcinoma of the urinary bladder. J. Am. Vet. Med. Assoc. *162*:474, 1973.

Brown, N. O., Parks, J. L., and Greene, R. W.: Canine urolithiasis: Retrospective analysis of 438 cases. J.A.V.M.A. *170*:414, 1977a.

Brown, N. O., Parks, J. L., and Greene, R. W.: Recurrence of canine urolithiasis. J.A.V.M.A. *157*:419, 1977b.

Brown, R. R., and Price, J. M.: Quantitative studies on metabolites of tryptophan in the urine of the dog, cat, rat, and man. J. Biol. Chem. *219*:985, 1956.

Brown, S. G., and Greiner, T. P.: Surgery of the Urethra. *In* Bojrab, M. J. (ed.): Current Techniques in Small Animal Surgery. Lea & Febiger, Philadelphia, 1975.

Burrows, C. F., and Bovee, K. C.: Characterization and treatment of acid-base and renal defects due to urethral obstruction in cats. J.A.V.M.A. *172*:801, 1978.

Burrows, C. F., and Bovee, K. C.: Metabolic changes due to experimentally induced rupture of the canine urinary bladder. Am. J. Vet. Res. *35*:1083, 1974.

Campbell, M. F.: Urinary Infections. *In* Campbell, M. F., and Harrison, J. H. (eds.): Urology 2. W. B. Saunders Co., Philadelphia, 1970.

Carbone, M. G.: Urethal surgery in the cat. Vet. Clin. North Am. *1*:281, 1971.

Carbone, M. G.: A modified technique for perineal urethrostomy in the male cat. J.A.V.M.A. *151*:301, 1967.

Carbone, M. G.: Phosphocrystalluria and urethral obstruction in the cat. J.A.V.M.A. *147*:1195, 1965.

Carbone, M. G.: Perineal urethrostomy to relieve urethral obstruction in the male cat. J.A.V.M.A. *143*:34, 1963.

Carroll, G.: Nontuberculous Infections of the Urinary Tract. *In* Campbell, M. F., and Harrison, J. H. (eds.): Urology 1. W. B. Saunders Co. Philadelphia, 1970.

Catchin, E.: Neoplasms in small animals. Vet. Rec. *63*:67, 1951.

Cattell, W. R., Spencer, A. G., Taylor, G. W., and Watts, R. W.: The mechanism of the renal excretion of oxalate in the dog. Clin. Sci. *22*:43, 1962.

Chow, F. H. C., Taton, G. F., Lewis, L. D., and Hamar, D. W.: Effect of dietary ammonium chloride, DL-methionine, sodium phosphate and ascorbic acid on urinary pH and electrolyte concentrations of male cats. Feline Pract. *8*:29, 1978.

Chow, F. H. C., Dysart, M. I., Hamar, D. W., et al.: Effect of dietary additives on experimentally produced feline urolithiasis. Feline Pract. *6*:51, 1976.

Christensen, G. C.: The Urogenial System and Mammary Glands. *In* Miller, M. E. (ed.): Anatomy of the Dog. W. B. Saunders Co., Philadelphia, 1968.

Christie, B. A.: The ureterovesical junction in dogs. Invest. Urol. *9*:10, 1971.

Clark, W. T.: Staphylococcal infection of the urinary tract and its relation to urolithiasis in the dog. Vet. Rec. *95*:204, 1974.

Clark, W. T.: Urolithiasis in the dog. IV. Diagnosis. J. Small Anim. Pract. *7*:553, 1966.

Cornelius, C. E., Bishop, J. A., and Schaffer, M. H.: A quantitative study of amino aciduria in dachshunds with a history of cystine urolithiasis. Cornell Vet. *57*:177, 1967.

Crawhall, J. C., and Watts, R. W. E.: Cystinuria. Am. J. Med. *45*:736, 1968.

Crouch, J. E.: Text-Atlas of Cat Anatomy. Lea & Febiger, Philadelphia, 1969.

Dalmatian Research Foundation: Low Protein, Low Purine Diet for Dalmatians with Skin or Kidney Problems. Dalmation Research Foundation, York, Pennsylvania, 1972.

Davidson, S.: A large urinary calculus in a cat. Feline Pract. *5*:45, 1975.

Denny, H. R.: An unusual cause of urethral obstruction in the dog. J. Small Anim. Pract. *13*:339, 1972.

Dill, G. S., McElvea, R., and Stookey, J. L.: Transitional cell carcinoma of the urinary bladder in a cat. J.A.V.M.A. *160*:743, 1972.

Dorn, A. S.: Squamous cell carcinoma of the urinary bladder in a cat. Feline Pract. *8*:14, 1978.

Dragon, P., and Deutsch, G.: The effect of intravenous fluids on renal medullary flow after hemorrhage. Invest. Urol. *8*:695, 1971.

Elliot, J. S., Sharp, R. F., and Lewis, L.: The solubility of struvite in urine. J. Urol. *81*:365, 1959a.

Elliot, J. S., Sharp, R. F., and Lewis, L.: Urinary pH. J. Urol. *81*:339, 1959b.

Engle, C. G.: A clinical report on 250 cases of feline urological syndrome. Feline Pract. *7*:24, 1977.

Everett, H. S., and Williams, T. J.: Urology in the Female. *In* Campbell, M. F., and Harrison, J. H. (eds.): Urology 3. W. B. Saunders Co., Philadelphia, 1970.

Fabricant, C. G.: Herpesvirus-induced feline urolithiasis. A review. J. Comp. Microbiol. Immunol. Infect. Dis. *1*:121, 1979.

Fabricant, C. G.: Herpesvirus-induced urolithiasis in specific pathogen-free male cats. Am. J. Vet. Res. *38*:1837, 1977.

Fabricant, C. G.: Urolithiasis: A review with recent viral studies. Feline Pract. *3*:22, 1973.

Fabricant, C. G., and Rich, L. J.: Microbial studies of feline urolithiasis. J.A.V.M.A. *158*:976, 1971.

Fabricant, C. G., Gillespie, J. H., and Krook, L.: Intracellular and extracellular mineral formation induced by viral infection of cell cultures. Infect. Immun. *3*:416, 1971a.

Fabricant, C. G., King, J. M., Gaskin, J. M., et al.: Isolation of a virus from a female cat with urolithiasis. J.A.V.M.A. *158*:200, 1971b.

Falls, W. F., and Stacy, W. K.: Postobstructive diuresis. Am. J. Med. *54*:404, 1973.

Feldmann, M. B., Kennedy, B. M., and Schelstraete, B. S.: Dietary minerals and the feline urological syndrome. Feline Pract. 7:39, 1977.

Finby, N., and Begg, C. F.: Correlation conferences in radiology and pathology. Diabetes mellitus and cystitis emphysematosa. N.Y. J. Med. *69*:1315, 1969.

Finco, D. R.: Urate Urolithiasis. *In* Kirk, R. W. (ed.): Current Veterinary Therapy VI. W. B. Saunders Co., Philadelphia, 1977.

Finco, D. R.: Current status of canine urolithiasis. J.A.V.M.A. *157*:327, 1970.

Finco, D. R., and Cornelius, L. M.: Characterization and treatment of water, electrolyte, and acid-base imbalances of induced urethral obstruction in the cat. Am. J. Vet. Res. *28*:823, 1977.

Finco, D. R., Rosen, E., and Johnson, K. H.: Canine urolithiasis: A review of 133 clinical and 23 necropsy cases. J.A.V.M.A. *157*:1225, 1970.

Firestone, W. M.: Prolapse of the male urethra. J.A.V.M.A. *99*:135, 1941.

Ford, D. C.: Antepubic urethrostomy in the cat. J. Am. Anim. Assoc. *4*:145, 1968.

Foster, S. J.: The "urolithiasis" syndrome in male cats; a statistical analysis of the problems with clinical observations. J. Small Anim. Pract. *8*:207, 1967.

Frimpter, G. W., Thouin, P., and Ewalds, B. H.: Penicillamine in canine cystinuria. J.A.V.M.A. *151*:1084, 1967.

Gagnon, J. A., Murphy, G. D., and Teschan, P. E.: Renal hemodynamic effects of hypertonic mannitol in the dog. Fed. Proc. *22*:173, 1963.

Gans, J. H.: The Kidneys. *In* Swenson, M. (ed.): Dukes' Physiology of Domestic Animals. 8th ed. Comstock Publishing Associates, Ithaca, N.Y., 1970.

Gordon, N.: Surgical anatomy of the bladder, prostate gland, and urethra. J.A.V.M.A. *136*:215, 1960.

Goulden, B. E.: Clinical observations on the role of urinary infection in the aetiology of canine urolithiasis. Vet. Rec. *83*:509, 1968.

Goulden, B. E.: Urolithiasis in the dog — treatment and prophylaxis. J. Small Anim. Pract. 7:557, 1966.

Greene, R. W., and Bohning, R.: Patent persistent urachus associated with urolithiasis in a cat. J.A.V.M.A. *158*:489, 1971.

Greene, R. W., and Greiner, T. P.: Surgery of the urogenital tract. Proceedings, 39th Annual American Animal Hospital Association Meeting, 1972.

Greene, R. W., and Greiner, T. P.: Scrotal urethrostomy for relief of urethral blockage in the dog. J.A.V.M.A. *158*:1864, 1971.

Griffith, D. P., Borgin, S., and Musher, D. M.: Dissolution of struvite urinary stones. Invest. Urol. *13*:351, 1976.

Griffith, D. P., Musher, D. M., and Itin, C.: Urease: The primary cause of infection induced urinary stones. Invest. Urol. *13*:346, 1976.

Halliwell, W. H., and Ackerman, N.: Botryoid rhabdomyosarcoma of the urinary bladder and hypertrophic osteoarthropathy in a young dog. J.A.V.M.A. *165*:911, 1974.

Hamar, O., Chow, F. C. H., Dysart, M. I., and Rich, L. J.: Effect of sodium chloride in prevention of experimentally produced urolithiasis in male cats. J.A.A.H.A. *12*:514, 1976.

Hansen, J. S.: Urachal remnant in the cat: Occurrence and relationship to the feline urological syndrome. Vet. Med. Small Anim. Clin. *72*:1735, 1977.

Hardy, R. M., and Osborne, C.: The use and misuse of urinary acidifiers. Proceedings, 40th Annual American Animal Hospital Association Meeting, 1973.

Hardy, R. M., Osborne, C. A., Cassidy, F. C., and Jackson, K. H.: Urolithiasis in immature dogs. Vet. Med. Small Anim. Clin. *67*:1205, 1972.

Hautmann, R., Terhost, B., Stuklsatz, H. W., and Lulzezer, W.: Mercaptopropionylglycine: A progress in cystine stone therapy. J. Urol. *117*:628, 1977.

Hayes, H. M., Jr.: Canine bladder cancer: Epidemiologic features. Am. J. Epidemiol. *104*:673, 1976.

Hayes, H. M., Jr.: Ectopic ureter in dogs. Epidemiologic features. Teratology *10*:129, 1974.

Herron, M. A.: The effect of prepubertal castration on the penile urethra of the cat. J.A.V.M.A. *160*:208, 1972.

Hinman, F., Jr.: Bacterial elimination. J. Urol. *99*:811, 1968.

Hirsh, D. C.: Multiple antimicrobial resistance in *Escherichia coli* isolated from the urine of dogs and cats with cystitis. J.A.V.M.A. *162*:885, 1973.

Hobson, H. P., and Ader, P. L.: Exstrophy of the bladder in a dog. J.A.A.H.A. *15*:103, 1979.

Hobson, H. P., and Heller, R. A.: Surgical correction or prolapse of the male urethra. Vet. Med. Small Anim. Clin. *66*:1177, 1971.

Hodgson, B. J., Samas, S., Bolling, D. R., and Heesch, C. M.: Effect of estrogen on sensitivity of rabbit bladder and urethra to phenylephrine. Invest. Urol. *16*:67, 1978.

Hutch, J. A.: The role of urethral mucus in the bladder defense mechanism. J. Urol. *103*:165, 1970.

Jackson, D. A., Osborne, C. A., Brasmer, T. H., and Jessen, C. R.: Nonneurogenic urinary incontinence in a canine female pseudohermaphrodite. J.A.V.M.A. *172*:926, 1978.

Jackson, D. F.: The treatment and subsequent prevention of struvite urolithiasis in cats. J. Small Anim. Pract. *12*:555, 1971.

Jaenike, J. R.: The renal functional defect of postobstructive nephropathy. J. Clin. Invest. *51*:2999, 1972.

Jamdar, M. N.: Urachal remnant of domestic animals as compared to that of man and two cases of partially involuted urachus in equines. Indian Vet. J. *33*:143, 1956.

Jarzylo, S., Challis, T., and Bruce, A.: Urachal abnormalities. J. Canad. Assoc. Radiol. *16*:175, 1965.

Johnston, D. E.: Feline urethrostomy — a critique and a new method. J. Small Anim. Pract. *15*:421, 1974.

Jolly, D. W., and Worden, A. N.: Urolithiasis in the dog. III. Nutritional aspects. J. Small Anim. Pract. 7:549, 1966.

Jubb, K. V. F., and Kennedy, P. C.: Pathology of

Domestic Animals, Vol. 2, 2nd ed. Academic Press, New York, 1970.

Kidder, D. E., and Chivers, R. P.: Xanthine calculi in a dog. Vet. Rec. *83*:228, 1968.

Kiristo, A. K., Vasenius, H., and Sandholm, M.: Canine bacteriuria. J. Small Anim. Pract. *18*:707, 1977.

Kirk, R. W.: Antimicrobial therapy. Proceedings, 39th Annual American Animal Hospital Association Meeting, 1972.

Kirk, R. W.: Treatment of urinary tract infections. Proceedings, 39th Annual American Animal Hospital Association Meeting, 1972.

Kirk, R. W., McEntee, K., and Bentinck-Smith, J.: Diseases of the Urogenital System. *In* Catcott, E. J. (ed.): Canine Medicine. American Veterinary Publications, Santa Barbara, Calif., 1968.

Kirkpatrick, R. M.: Urate calculus in a male cat. Vet. Med. Small Anim. Clin. *72*:1171, 1977.

Klausner, J. S., and Osborne, C. A.: Struvite urolithiasis. *In* Kirk, R. W. (ed.): Current Veterinary Therapy VII. W. B. Saunders Co., Philadelphia, 1980.

Klausner, J. S., and Osborne, C. A.: Urinary tract infection and urolithiasis. Vet. Clin. North Am. *9*:701, 1979.

Klausner, J. S., Osborne, C. A., O'Leary, T. P., et al.: Experimental induction of struvite uroliths in miniature schnauzer and beagle dogs. Invest. Urol. *18*:127, 1980.

Klausner, J. S., Osborne, C. A., O'Leary, T. P., et al.: Struvite urolithiasis in a litter of miniature schnauzer dogs. Am. J. Vet. Res. *41*:712, 1980.

Kleine, L. J., and Thornton, G. W.: Radiographic diagnosis of urinary tract trauma. J.A.A.H.A. 7:318, 1971.

Knecht, C. D., and Slusher, R.: Extra-pelvic anastomosis of the bladder and penile urethra in a dog. J.A.A.H.A. *6*:247, 1970.

Kolata, R. J., and Johnson, D. E.: Motor vehicle accidents in urban dogs: A study of 600 cases. J.A.V.M.A. *167*:938, 1975.

Kovant, P., Labovitz, E., and Levinson, S. P.: Antibiotics and the kidney. Med. Clin. North Am. 57:1045, 1973.

Krabbe, A.: Urolithiasis in dogs and cats. Vet. Rec. *61*:751, 1949.

Kuster, G., Shorter, R. G., Dawson, B., and Hallenbeck, G. A.: Uric acid metabolism in Dalmatians and other dogs. Arch. Intern. Med. *129*:492, 1972.

Lage, A. L.: Cystinuria and cystine urolithiasis. *In* Kirk, R. W. (ed.): Current Veterinary Therapy VII. W. B. Saunders Co., Philadelphia, 1980.

Lapides, J.: Neuromuscular Vesical and Ureteral Dysfunction. *In* Campbell, M. F., and Harrison, J. H. (eds.): Urology 2. W. B. Saunders Co., Philadelphia, 1970.

Leader, A. J., and Carlton, C. E., Jr.: Urologic Diagnosis and the Urologic Examination. *In* Campbell, M. F., and Harrison, J. H. (eds.): Urology 1. W. B. Saunders Co., Philadelphia, 1970.

Lees, G. E., and Osborne, C. A.: Antibacterial properties of urine: A comparative review. J.A.A.H.A. *15*:125, 1979.

Lees, G. E., Osborne, C. A., and Steven, J. B.: Urine: A medium for bacterial growth. Vet. Clin. North Am. *9*:611, 1979.

Legendre, A. M.: Silica urolithiasis in a dog. J.A.V.M.A. *168*:418, 1976.

Lewis, L. D., Chow, F. H. C., Taton, G. F., and Hamar, D.: Effect of various dietary mineral concentrations on the occurrence of feline urolithiasis. J.A.V.M.A. *172*:559, 1978.

Ling, G. V.: Treatment of urinary tract infections. Vet. Clin. North Am. *9*:795, 1979.

Ling, G. V., and Gilmore, C. J.: Penicillin G or ampicillin for oral treatment of canine urinary tract infections. J.A.V.M.A. *171*:358, 1977.

Ling, G. V., and Ruby, A. L.: Trimethoprin in combination with sulfonamide for oral treatment of canine urinary tract infections. J.A.V.M.A. *174*:1003, 1979.

Ling, G. V., and Ruby, A. L.: Chloramphenicol for oral treatment of canine urinary tract infections. J.A.V.M.A. *172*:914, 1978.

Ling, G. V., Biberstein, E. L., and Hirsh, D. C.: Bacterial pathogens in urinary tract infections. Vet. Clin. North Am. *9*:617, 1979.

McCullagh, K. G., Ehrhart, L. A.: Silica urolithiasis in laboratory dogs fed semisynthetic diets. J.A.V.M.A. *164*:712, 1974.

McDonald, D. F., and Lund, R. R.: The role of the urine in vesical neoplasms. J. Urol. *71*:560, 1954.

Mandel, M.: Hypertrophic osteoarthropathy secondary to neurofibrosarcoma of the urinary bladder in a cocker spaniel. Vet. Med. Small Anim. Clin. *70*:1307, 1975.

Manziano, C. F., and Manziano, T. R.: Perineal urethrostomy for relief of urethral blockage in the male cat. J.A.V.M.A. *149*:1312, 1966.

Marretta, S. M., Pask, A. J., Greene, R. W., and Liu, S. K.: Urinary calculi associated with portosystemic shunts in six dogs. J.A.V.M.A. *178*:133, 1981.

Maynard, J. A.: Traumatic rupture of the bladder in the dog — a clinical study of nine cases. J. Small Anim. Pract. *2*:131, 1961.

Medway, W.: Cystinuria and Cystine Calculi. *In* Kirk, R. W. (ed.): Current Veterinary Therapy III. W. B. Saunders Co., Philadelphia, 1968.

Mehlhoff, T., and Osborne, C. A.: Catheter biopsy of the urethra, urinary bladder and prostate gland. *In* Kirk, R. W. (ed.): Current Veterinary Therapy VI. W. B. Saunders Co., Philadelphia, 1977.

Mendham, J. H.: A description and evaluation of antepubic urethrostomy in the male cat. J. Small Anim. Pract. *11*:709, 1970.

Middleton, D. J., and Lomas, G. R.: Emphysematous cystitis due to *Clostridium perfringens* in a non-diabetic dog. J. Small Anim. Pract. *20*:433, 1979.

Miller, M. E., Christensen, G. C., and Evans, H. E.: Anatomy of the Dog. W. B. Saunders Co., Philadelphia, 1964.

Morris, C. R., Alexander, E. A., Bruns, F. J., and Levinsky, N. G.: Restoration and maintenance of glomerular filtration by mannitol during hypoperfusion of the kidney. J. Clin. Invest. *51*:1555, 1972.

Morris, J. J., Seifter, E., Tettura, G., et al.: Effect of penicillamine upon healing wounds. J. Surg. Res. *9*:143, 1969.

Nemoy, N. T., Stamey, R. A.: Surgical, bacteriological and biochemical management of infection stones. J.A.M.A. *215*:1470, 1971.

Norden, C. W., Green, C. H., and Kass, E. H.: Antibacterial mechanisms of the urinary bladder. J. Clin. Invest. *47*:2689, 1968.

Oliver, J. E., Jr., and Osborne, C. A.: Neurogenic Urinary Incontinence. *In* Kirk, R. W. (ed.): Current Veterinary Therapy VII. W. B. Saunders Co., Philadelphia, 1980.

Oliver, J. E., Jr., and Selcer, R. R.: Neurogenic causes of

abnormal micturition in the dog and cat. Vet. Clin. North Am. *4*:517, 1974.

Oliver, J. E., Jr.: Neurology of visceral function. Vet. Clin. North Am. *4*:517, 1974.

Osbaldiston, G. W., and Lowrey, J. L.: Allopurinal in the prevention of hyperuricemia in Dalmatian dogs. Vet. Med. Small Anim. Clin. *66*:711, 1971.

Osborne, C. A., and Hanlon, G. F.: Canine congenital ureteral ectopia: A case report and. review of the literature. J.A.A.H.A. *3*:111, 1967.

Osborne, C. A., and Klausner, J. S.: War on canine urolithiasis: Problems and solutions. Proceedings, 45th Annual American Animal Hospital Association Meeting, 1978.

Osborne, C. A., Dieterich, H. F., Hanlon, G. F., and Anderson, L. D.: Urinary incontinence due to ectopic ureter in a male dog. J.A.V.M.A. *166*:911, 1975a.

Osborne, C. A., Engen, M. H., Yaro, B. L., et al.: Congenital urethrorectal fistula in two dogs. J.A.V.M.A. *166*:999, 1975b.

Osborne, C. A., Hammer, R. F., and Klausner, J.S.: Canine Silica Urolithiasis. In Kirk, R.W. (ed.): Current Veterinary Therapy VII. W. B. Saunders Co., Philadelphia, 1980a.

Osborne, C. A., Klausner, J. S., Hardy, R. M., and Lees, G. E.: Ancillary Treatment of Urinary Tract Infections. In Kirk, R. W. (ed.): Current Veterinary Therapy VII. W. B. Saunders Co., Philadelphia, 1980b.

Osborne, C. A., Oliver, J. E., and Polzin, D. W.: Non-neurogenic Urinary Incontinence. In Kirk, R. W. (ed.): Current Veterinary Therapy VII. W. B. Saunders Co., Philadelphia, 1980c.

Osborne, C. A., Klausner, J. S., and Lees, G. E.: Urinary tract infections: Normal and abnormal host defense mechanisms. Vet. Clin. North Am. *9*:587, 1979.

Osborne, C. A., Low, D. G., and Finco, D. R.: Canine and Feline Urology. W. B. Saunders Co., Philadelphia, 1972.

Osborne, C. A., Low, D. G., and Perman, V.: Neoplasms of the canine and feline urinary bladder: Clinical findings, diagnosis, and treatment. J.A.V.M.A. *152*:247, 1968a.

Osborne, C. A., Low, D. G., and Perman, V.: Neoplasms of the canine and feline urinary bladder: Incidence, etiology, occurrence, and pathology. Am. J. Vet. Res. *29*:2041, 1968b.

Osborne, C., Rhoades, J., and Hanlan, G.: Patent urachus in the dog. J.A.A.H.A. *2*:245, 1966.

Oyasu, R., and Hopp, M. L.: Collective review: The etiology of cancer of the bladder. Surg. Gynecol. Obstet. *138*:97, 1974.

Pamukcu, A. M.: Tumors of the urinary bladder. Bull. WHO *50*:43, 1974.

Park, R. D.: Radiology of the urinary bladder and urethra. In O'Brien, T. R. (ed.): Radiologic Diagnosis of Abdominal Disorders in the Dog and Cat. W. B. Saunders Co., Philadelphia, 1978, pp. 543–614.

Parsons, C. L., Greenspan, C., Moore, S. W., et al.: Role of surface mucin in primary antibacterial defense of the bladder. Urology *9*:48, 1977.

Patnaik, A. K., and Greene, R. W.: Intravenous leiomyoma of the bladder in a cat. J.A.V.M.A. *175*:381, 1979.

Pearson, H., and Gibbs, C.: Urinary tract abnormalities in the dog. J. Small Anim. Pract. *12*:67, 1971.

Petersdorf, R. G., and Turck, M.: Some current concepts of urinary tract infections. Disease-A-Month, December, 1970, p. 9.

Piermattei, D. L., and Osborne, C. A.: Non-surgical

removal of calculi from the urethra of a male dog. J.A.V.M.A. *159*:1755, 1971.

Pollock, S.: Urethral carcinoma in the dog: A case report. J. Am. Vet. Rad. Soc. *9*:95, 1968.

Porter, P. J.: Comparative study of the macromolecular components excreted in the urine of dog and man. J. Comp. Pathol. *74*:108, 1964.

Putnam, R. W., and Pennock, P. W.: Emergency surgery following urogenital trauma. Mod. Vet. Pract. *50*:34, 1969.

Radamski, J. L., Glass, E. M., and Deichman, W. B.: Transitional cell hyperplasia in the bladders of dogs fed DL-tryptophan. Cancer Res. *31*:1690, 1971.

Rawlings, C. A.: Extraperitoneal urinary bladder rupture and urinary fistula in a dog. J.A.V.M.A. *155*:123, 1969.

Reif, J. S., Bovee, K. C., Gaskell, C. J., et al.: Feline urethral obstruction. A case-control study. J.A.V.M.A. *170*:1320, 1977.

Rich, L. J., and Fabricant, C. G.: Urethral obstruction in male cats: Transmission studies. Can. J. Comp. Med. *33*:164, 1969.

Rich, L. J., and Kirk, R. W.: The relationship of struvite crystals to urethral obstruction in cats. J.A.V.M.A. *154*:153, 1969.

Rich, L. J., and Kirk, R. W.: Feline urethral obstruction: Mineral aspects. Am. J. Vet. Res. *29*:2149, 1968.

Rich, L. J., and Norcross, N. L.: Feline urethral obstruction: Immunologic identification of a unique urinary protein. Am. J. Vet. Res. *30*:1001, 1969.

Rich, L. J., Fabricant, C. G., and Gillespie, J. H.: Virus induced urolithiasis in male cats. Cornell Vet. *61*:542, 1971.

Richards, D. A., Hinko, P. J., and Morse, E. M.: Feline perineal urethrostomy — a new technique for an old problem. J.A.A.H.A. *8*:66, 1972.

Robbins, S. L.: Pathology. 3rd ed. W. B. Saunders Co., Philadelphia, 1967.

Roszel, J. F.: Cytology of urine from dogs with botryoid sarcoma of the bladder. Acta Cytol. *16*:443, 1972.

Ryan, C. P., and Wolfer, J. J.: Cystic calculi in four cats. Vet. Med. Small Anim. Clin. *73*:1414, 1978.

Schechter, R. D.: The significance of bacteria in feline cystitis and urolithiasis. J.A.V.M.A. *156*:1567, 1970.

Schneck, G. W.: Grass-seed urinary calculus. Vet. Rec. *94*:431, 1974.

Scott, R., Greene, R., and Patnaik, A.: Unilateral ureterocele associated with hydronephrosis in a dog. J.A.A.H.A. *10*:126, 1974.

Seely, J. C., Cosenzy, S. F., Montgomery, C. A.: Leiomyosarcoma of the canine urinary bladder, with metastasis. J.A.V.M.A. *172*:1427, 1978.

Sharpless, S. K.: Hypnotics and Sedatives. In Goodman, L. S., and Gilman, A. (eds.): The Pharmacological Basis of Therapeutics. 4th ed. The Macmillan Company, Toronto, 1971.

Sherding, R. G. and Chew, D. J.: Non-diabetic emphysematous cystitis in two dogs. J.A.V.M.A. *174*:1105, 1979.

Shrom, S. H., Parson, C. L., and Mulholland, S. G.: Role of urothelial surface mucoprotein in intrinsic bladder defense. Urology *9*:526, 1977.

Sinibaldi, K. R., and Greene, R. W.: Surgical correction of prolapse of the male urethra in three English bulldogs. J.A.A.H.A. *9*:450, 1973.

Smith, C. W., and Schiller, A. G.: Perineal urethrostomy in the cat: A retrospective study of complications. J.A.A.H.A. *14*:225, 1978.

Stamey, T. A., Fair, W. R., Timothy, M. M., et al.: Serum vs. urinary antimicrobial concentrations in cure of urinary tract infections. N. Engl. J. Med. *291*:1159, 1974.

Staufuss, A. C., and Dean, B. A.: Neoplasms of the canine urinary bladder. J.A.V.M.A. *166*:1161, 1975.

Tarvin, G., Patnaik, A., and Greene, R. W.: Primary urethral tumors in dogs. J.A.V.M.A. *172*:931, 1978.

Teuscher, A.: Urinary tract infections in diabetes. Schweiz. Med. Wochenschr. *97*:1161, 1968.

Thayer, G. W., Carrig, C. B., and Evans, A. T.: Fatal venous air embolism associated with pneumocystography in a cat. J.A.V.M.A. *176*:654, 1980.

Theilen, G. H., and Madewell, B. R.: Tumors of the Urogenital Tract. *In* Theilen, G. H., and Madewell, B. R. (eds.): Veterinary Cancer Medicine. Lea & Febiger, Philadelphia, 1979.

Thornton, G. W.: Urinary calculi in the Dog. *In* Kirk, R. W. (ed.): Current Veterinary Therapy III. W. B. Saunders Co., Philadelphia, 1968.

Tomey, S. L., and Follis, T. B.: Incidence rates of feline urological syndrome in the United States. Feline Pract. *8*:39, 1978.

Treacher, R. J.: Urolithiasis in the dog. II. Biochemical aspects. J. Small Anim. Pract. *7*:537, 1966.

Tsan, M. F., Jones, T. C., Thornton, G. W., et al.: Canine cystinuria: Its urinary amino acid pattern and genetic analysis. Am. J. Vet. Res. *33*:2455, 1972.

Walker, A. D., Weaver, A. D., Anderson, R. S., and Crighton, D. W.: An epidemiological study of the feline urological syndrome. J. Small Anim. Pract. *18*:283, 1977.

Weaver, A. D.: Relationship of bacterial infection in urine and calculi to canine urolithiasis. Vet. Rec. *97*:48, 1975.

Weaver, A. D.: Canine urolithiasis: Incidence, chemical composition and outcome of 100 cases. J. Small Anim. Pract. *11*:93, 1970.

Weaver, R. G., and Schulte, J. W.: Experimental and clinical studies of urethral regeneration. Surg. Gynecol. Obstet. *115*:729, 1972.

White, E. G.: Synposium on urolithiasis in the dog. Introduction and Incidence. J. Small Anim. Pract. *7*:529, 1966.

White, E. G., Treacher, R. F., and Porter, P.: Urinary calculin in the dog. I. Incidence and chemical composition. J. Comp. Pathol. *7*:201, 1961.

Wiggishoff, C. C., and McDonald, J. H.: Urinary exfoliative cytology in the diagnosis of bladder tumor. ACTA Cytol. *16*:139, 1972.

Willeberg, P. A.: A case-control study of some fundamental determinants in the epidemiology of the feline urological syndrome. Nord. Vet. Med. *27*:1, 1975.

Willeberg, P., and Priester, W. A.: Feline urological syndrome: Association with some time, space, and individual patient factors. Am. J. Vet. Res. *37*:975, 1976.

Williams, R. C., and Gibbons, R. J.: Inhibition of bacterial adherence by secretory immunoglobin A: a mechanism of antigen disposal. Science *177*:697, 1972.

Wilson, G. P., and Harrison, J. W.: Perineal urethrostomy in cats. J.A.V.M.A. *159*:1789, 1971.

Wilson, G. P., Hayes, H. M., and Casey, W. C.: Canine urethral cancer. J.A.A.H.A. *15*:741, 1979.

Wilson, W. W., Klausner, J. S., Stevens, J. B., and Osborne, C. A.: Vet. Surg. *8*:63, 1979.

Wimberly, H. C., and Lewis, R. M.: Transitional cell carcinoma in the domestic cat. Vet. Pathol. *16*:223, 1979.

Witte, M. H., Short, F. A., and Hollander, W., Jr.: Massive polyuria and naturesis following relief of urinary tract obstruction. Am. J. Med. *37*:320, 1964.

Wooley, R. E., and Blue, J. L.: Quantitative and bacteriological studies of urine specimens from canine and feline urinary tract infections. J. Clin. Microbiol. *4*:326, 1976.

Zontine, W. J., and Andrews, L. K.: Fatal air embolism as a complication of pneumocystography in two cats. J. Am. Vet. Radiol. Soc. *19*:8, 1978.

Diseases of the Blood Cells, Lymph Nodes, and Spleen

CHAPTER 77

Diseases of the Red Blood Cells

VICTOR PERMAN
and WILLIAM D. SCHALL

Knowledge of canine and feline red cell disorders has expanded greatly. The concept of the minimal data base to include hematologic data has uncovered the mild to moderately anemic patient in greater numbers. The general availability of more precise measurement of erythrocyte parameters has generated data that require a deeper insight into erythropoiesis. Simple description of a disease in morphologic terms is no longer adequate for meeting accepted diagnostic and therapeutic standards. Therefore, much of this chapter is concerned with the biochemical and physiologic concepts pertinent to present-day hematology.

PHYSIOLOGY OF THE ERYTHRON

A logical approach to the solution of problems involving red blood cells is possible only if the veterinarian applies known physiologic principles. Basic information regarding the functional state of the erythron at the biochemical, cellular, and tissue or organ level is necessary.

HEMOGLOBIN BIOSYNTHESIS

Immature red cells synthesize hemoglobin in the bone marrow. In the normal cat or dog, immature red cells perform this function at a rate commensurate with the needs of the animal. The production of heme begins with the interaction of the amino acid, glycine, and succinate, an intermediate of the tricarboxylic acid (Kreb's) cycle. Seven successive steps follow, the last of which involves the incorporation of ferrous iron into a protoporphyrin IX molecule to form heme. In the process of heme synthesis, three porphyrin precursor compounds are formed. Specific examples of abnormalities in heme synthesis include feline porphyria, lead poisoning, and chloramphenicol toxicity.

Four heme molecules combine with a globin molecule to form hemoglobin. The hemoglobin molecule is symmetric. Each half-molecule is composed of two polypeptide chains arbitrarily designated α and β chains in the adult. Like heme, globin and hemoglobin are formed within the developing red blood cell.

In contrast to heme, which is identical for all hemoglobin molecules, regardless of stage of maturity or species, the globin portion exhibits structural differences. Both inter- and intraspecies variations exist. The cat and dog have embryonic and adult hemoglobin but no fetal hemoglobin (Kitchen, 1969). Embryonic hemoglobin is composed of two α and ϵ chains (Fantoni et al., 1981). Feline and canine embryonic hemoglobin disappears during the third week of gestation and is replaced by adult hemoglobin.

The adult cat has two types of hemoglobin, whereas the adult dog has only one. The two feline hemoglobins occur because of two different β chain structures. Because the two hemoglobins differ in oxygen affinity and because their proportions vary among cats, individual cats may have differences in oxygen affinity.

Although several abnormal hemoglobins linked to deleterious side effects are known in man, none has been clearly demonstrated in cats or dogs. The existence of hemoglobin C in the cat has been suggested (Altman et al., 1972).

Feline Hemoglobin. Feline hemoglobin differs significantly from that of the dog and man. The heterogeneity of feline hemoglobin is variable. The two different β chains form two different hemoglobins designated hemoglobin A (HbA) and hemoglobin B (HbB). Ten to 50 per cent of the total hemoglobin present in cats is HbB (Taketa et al., 1972). It differs from HbA in its relative insensitivity to the modulating effects of 2,3-diphosphoglycerate (2,3-DPG) (Bunn, 1971). For this reason, there is probably variation among individual cats in their ability to adapt and tolerate a given degree of anemia. Cats have a red cell 2,3-DPG concentration much lower than that of dogs, but increases in the anemic state are of a greater magnitude than those reported for other species (Searcy, 1972a; Mauk et al., 1974). Feline hemoglobin also differs in that its heme-heme interaction is pH dependent (Hamilton and Edelstein, 1972). In acidosis, heme-heme interaction is suppressed.

TRANSPORT OF OXYGEN TO TISSUES

The uptake and transport of oxygen by hemoglobin is complicated by the presence of four heme groups per hemoglobin molecule. Each ferrous hemoglobin molecule may bind none, one, two, three, or four oxygen molecules.

Oxyhemoglobin Dissociation. When the percentage of hemoglobin saturated with oxygen is determined with respect to the partial pressure of oxygen, a sigmoidal curve is obtained (Fig. 77–1). This curve is called the *oxygen dissociation curve of hemoglobin* or the *oxyhemoglobin dissociation curve.* At low oxygen tensions (concave portion of the sigmoidal curve) oxygenation of only one heme group occurs. This initial oxygenation causes an intramolecular alteration that facilitates more rapid oxygenation of second

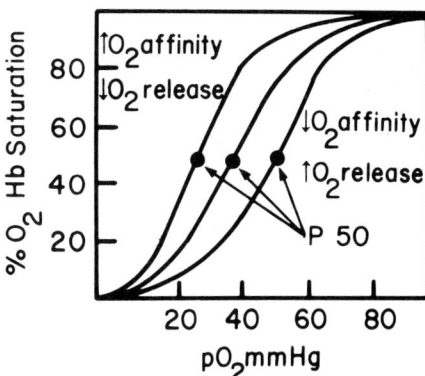

Figure 77–2. Shifts in the oxyhemoglobin dissociation curve. If the curve shifts to the right, there is decreased oxygen affinity and greater release of oxygen to tissues. As the curve shifts to the left there is increased oxygen affinity and less release of oxygen to tissues. The P_{50} value is the partial pressure of oxygen at which hemoglobin is 50 per cent saturated. (Adapted from Williams, W. J. et al. McGraw-Hill, Inc., 1972.)

and third heme groups within the molecule (straight portion of the curve). This alteration in oxygen affinity is usually called *heme-heme interaction* (Roughten et al., 1955; Harris and Kellermeyer, 1970). The straight part of the curve falls in the region of usual partial pressures of oxygen, and in this region, minor changes in the partial pressure bring about the dissociation or association of large amounts of oxygen.

FACTORS THAT AFFECT OXYHEMOGLOBIN DISSOCIATION. The position and shape of the oxygen dissociation curve can be altered by factors such as changes in pH, temperature, and organic phosphate concentrations. Thus, the affinity of hemoglobin for oxygen can be altered so that there is a decreased affinity and more oxygen released to the tissues (shift of the oxyhemoglobin curve to the right), or an increased affinity and less oxygen released to the tissues (shift of the oxyhemoglobin dissociation curve to the left). As illustrated in Figure 77–2, a shift of the oxyhemoglobin dissociation curve to the right results in less oxygen saturation at a given partial pressure of oxygen. The partial pressure of oxygen at which 50 per cent of the hemoglobin is saturated (P_{50}) is often used to compare oxyhemoglobin dissociation curves.

pH. Decrease in pH has both an immediate and a delayed effect on the affinity of hemoglobin for oxygen. The immediate effect of decreased pH is decreased affinity or a shift of the oxyhemoglobin dissociation

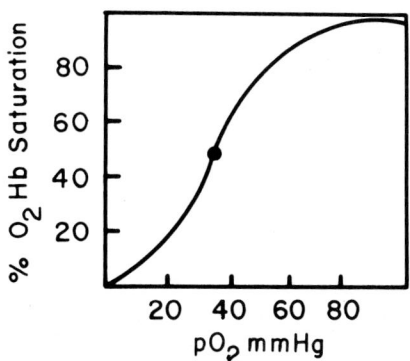

Figure 77–1. The oxyhemoglobin dissociation curve. As the partial pressure of oxygen (P_{O_2}) increases, the per cent of hemoglobin saturated with oxygen increases. In the straight part of the curve, a small increase in the P_{O_2} results in a large increase in the per cent of hemoglobin saturated with oxygen.

curve to the right. Within hours, however, the delayed effect of decreased pH results in diminished amounts of red cell 2,3-DPG and shifts the oxyhemoglobin dissociation curve back to the original position (Rorth, 1971).

Temperature. Hypothermia leads to increased oxygen affinity and a shift of the oxyhemoglobin curve to the left. The mechanism of this temperature effect is unknown.

2,3-Diphosphoglycerate. Increased erythrocyte organic phosphate concentrations result in decreased oxygen affinity and shift the oxyhemoglobin dissociation curve to the right. Quantitatively, the most important of the organic phosphates in modulating hemoglobin-oxygen affinity is 2,3-diphosphoglycerate (2,3-DPG). Of lesser significance is adenosine triphosphate (ATP). Other organic phosphates are of negligible importance. Several clinical conditions in man (Table 77–1) are associated with changes in 2,3-DPG concentrations (Oski and Delivoria-Papadopoulos, 1970). Canine hemoglobin is known to be 2,3-DPG responsive, and canine erythrocytes contain quantities of 2,3-DPG comparable to that found in human erythrocytes (Bunn, 1971; Searcy, 1972). Consequently, data from studies of 2,3-DPG in man are likely to be applicable to the dog.

Table 77–1. Clinical Conditions Known to Be Associated with 2,3-DPG-Mediated Changes in the Oxygen Affinity of Blood in Man or Dog or Both

Increased red cell 2,3-DPG, decreased oxygen affinity
Hypoxemia
    High altitude adaptation
    Chronic pulmonary disease
    Chronic cyanotic heart disease
Anemia
    Iron deficiency
    Red cell pyruvate kinase deficiency
    Aplastic and hypoplastic anemias
        (decreased red cell mass)
    Chronic liver disease
Hyperphosphatemia
    Chronic renal failure
    Physiological anemia of the young

Decreased red cell 2,3-DPG, increased oxygen affinity
Prolonged Acidosis
Following Massive Transfusions of Stored Blood

Factors known to affect red cell 2,3-DPG concentration include pH, the partial pressure of oxygen, and inorganic phosphate concentration. Hypoxemia resulting from conditions such as high altitude and congestive heart failure leads to increased 2,3-DPG concentration and shift of the oxyhemoglobin dissociation curve to the right. Children with slowly evolving iron-deficiency anemia have developed elevated 2,3-DPG values and right-shifted P_{50} values. A hemoglobin of 7.0 gm/dl and a P_{50} value shifted to the right by ten mm Hg would have oxygen delivery equivalent to that of a Hg level of 12 gm/dl (Lovric et al., 1975). 2,3-DPG is important when stored blood is used for transfusion, since the decreased level of erythrocyte inorganic phosphate concentration results in a left-shift oxygen dissociation curve and may not correct the tissue anoxia.

Inorganic Phosphate. Increased erythrocyte 2,3-DPG concentrations result from rather minor increases of inorganic phosphate concentration. This effect is important *in vivo* and *in vitro.* Card and Brain (1973) have provided evidence that the anemia of childhood is a physiologic response to hyperphosphatemia. The normal hyperphosphatemia of children results in increased erythrocyte, 2,3-DPG concentration and shifts the oxyhemoglobin dissociation curve to the right. As a result, oxygen delivery to the tissues is normal in children in spite of packed-cell volumes (PCV) and hemoglobin concentrations that are significantly lower than those found in adults. Hyperphosphatemia and associated physiologic anemia is also present in puppies (Huggins et al., 1971; Ewing et al., 1972; Fletch and Smart, 1972).

The hyperphosphatemia of renal failure is also associated with increased red cell 2,3-DPG and shift of the oxyhemoglobin dissociation curve to the right (Lichtman and Miller, 1970). The adaptive sequence partly compensates for anemia caused by decreased production of the renal erythropoietic factor.

Inorganic phosphate concentration and associated concentration of red cell 2,3-DPG is also important *in vitro.* Eisenbrandt and Smith (1973) have shown that 2,3-DPG concentration in canine erythrocytes is maintained better by citrate phosphate dextrose (CPD) solutions than by acid citrate dextrose (ACD) solutions.

THE ERYTHRON AND NORMAL RED CELL PRODUCTION

The main functions of the cells in the erythroid series are production, transportation, and protection of hemoglobin.

Site of Production. The process of erythropoiesis normally takes place within the bone marrow stroma (Alsaker, 1977). The stroma is both extravascular and extrasinusoidal. Normoblasts usually develop near the sinus wall and cluster about reticulum cells. The reticulum cell and its associated normoblasts constitute the "erythrocytic islet" (Bessis, 1967; Bessis, 1973b). In chronic stimulatory steady states, extramedullary erythropoiesis of the spleen, liver, and other tissues may occur.

Stem Cells. Rapid accumulation of information on hematopoiesis has required reevaluation of traditional concepts of blood cell production (Fig. 77–3). A pluripotent stem cell gives rises to all cell lines in discrete and separate colonies called *colony forming units–spleen* (CFU-S) (Till and McCulloch, 1961). Stem cells to cell lines have been grown *in vitro* and provide new insight into the control of blood cell production (Bradley and Metcalf, 1966; Pluznik and Sachs, 1965). The cultivation of erythroid cells in culture has revealed a *burst forming unit–erythroid,* (BFU-E) (Axelrod et al., 1973) amid a *colony forming unit–erythroid* (CFU-E) (Stephenson et al., 1971). The BFU-E cells are of low sensitivity to erythropoietin, and their progeny give rise to the CFU-E, which interacts with erythropoietin and in turn gives rise to morphologically identifiable erythroid cells. Erythropoiesis is also stimulated by nonhemopoietic hormones such as thyroid, steroids, and growth hormones (Singer and Adamson, 1976; Golde et al., 1976). Stem cells are found in fetal liver, bone marrow, and peripheral blood, since cell concentrates from these tissues will effect engraftment of bone marrow. Self-renewal of the committed cell compartments takes place in the stem cells. The significance of stem cells to clinical disease has been reviewed (Cline and Golde, 1978; Cline and Golde, 1979).

The Maturation Sequence. The continuum of maturation from stem cell to mature erythrocyte has several morphologically identifiable stages. Different names have been assigned to identical cells (Table 77–2). The most immature cell that can be identified as belonging to the erythrocytic series is the pronormoblast. Through multiplication and irreversible processes of maturation, the pronormoblast produces red blood cells. Because the cells that can be identified as stages of the erythrocytic series all divide and differentiate into nondividing cells that are released into peripheral blood, they are not capable of self-maintenance. Some of the stem cells contribute to self-renewal, while others differentiate into the erythrocytic, granulocytic, or megakaryocytic series.

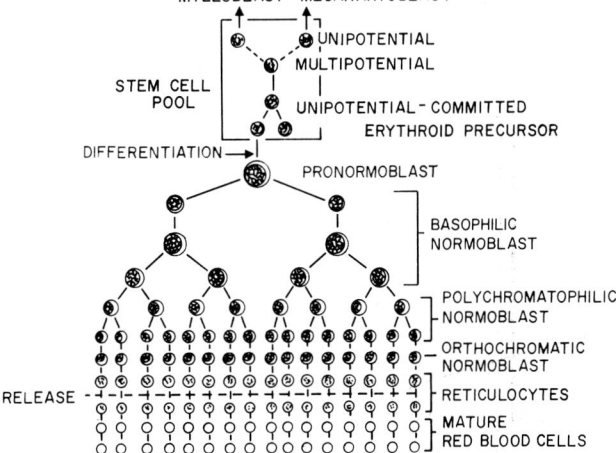

Figure 77–3. Model of the stem-cell pool and erythrocyte-maturation sequence. (Adapted from Williams, W. J., et al., Hematology, McGraw-Hill, Inc, 1972.)

Table 77–2. Erythrocyte Precursor Nomenclature*

1	2	3
Rubriblast	Proerythroblast	Pronormoblast
Prorubricyte	Early erythroblast	Basophilic normoblast
Rubricyte	Late erythroblast	Polychromatophilic normoblast
Metarubricyte	Normoblast	Orthochromatic normoblast
Reticulocyte	Reticulocyte	Reticulocyte
Erythrocyte	Erythrocyte	Erythrocyte

*Nomenclature from Column 3 is used throughout this chapter.
1. From Schalm, O. W.: Veterinary Hematology, 2nd ed. Lea & Febiger, Philadelphia, 1965.
2. From Harris, J. W., and Kellermeyer, R. W.: The Red Cell, revised ed. Harvard University Press, Cambridge, 1970.
3. From Williams, W. J., Beutler, E., Erslev, A. J., and Rundles, R. W.: Hematology. McGraw-Hill Book Co., Inc., New York, 1972. Used with permission of McGraw-Hill Book Company.

The maturation of the canine pronormoblast into the mature red cell takes about three to four days (Stohlman, 1960). Peak reticulocytosis is detected at five days in the dog. Maturation time in the cat is slightly shorter, with peak reticulocytosis occurring on the fourth day (Alsaker et al., 1977).

During the first part of the maturation process, usually four mitotic divisions take place, so that each pronormoblast gives rise to 16 mature red cells. At the late polychromatophilic normoblast stage, the nucleus becomes pyknotic; the cell is incapable of DNA synthesis and, hence, is incapable of further division. The nucleus is then extruded from the cell; the cell usually retains some of its RNA. Denucleation of the normoblasts is incompletely understood. A recent study on rabbit bone marrow demonstrated that nuclear extrusion occurs as normoblasts traverse small openings in the sinus wall (Fig. 77–4) (Tavassoli and Crosby, 1973). If this mechanism is predominate, one would expect that reticulocytes would not be present in extravascular hematopoietic space, while they indeed are present in numbers about equal to normoblasts in the normal marrow (Reiff et al., 1958). Based on *in vitro* studies, alternate mechanisms have been proposed and were reviewed by Alsaker (1977). The nucleus and other particulates appear to separate from the emerging reticulocytes by a process likened to reverse pinocytosis and in part are removed from the cell (Figs. 77–5 and 77–6). Thus, the cell exhibits polychromatophilic properties when stained with Wright stain and reticulated characteristics when stained with new methylene blue. The number of polychromatophilic cells approximates the number of reticulocytes in the dog and in

the cat, provided aggregate reticulocytes are counted (Laber et al., 1974). The cat has more than one form of reticulocyte when stained by supravital methods (Schalm et al.,

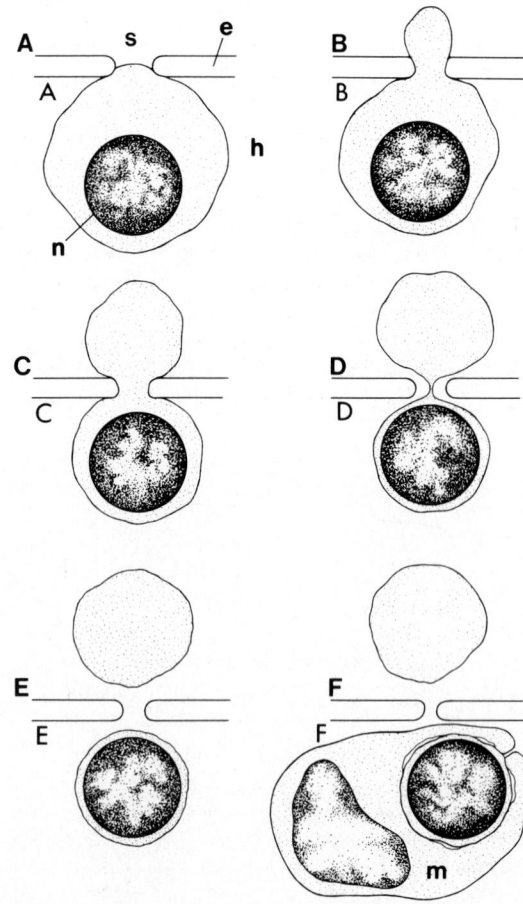

Figure 77–4. Schematic representation of the formation of a reticulocyte from a normoblast during progressive passage through an endothelial cell aperture (A–F). Endothelial cell (e); normoblast nucleus (n); macrophage with engulfed nucleus (m); sinus lumen (s); hematopoietic compartment (h).

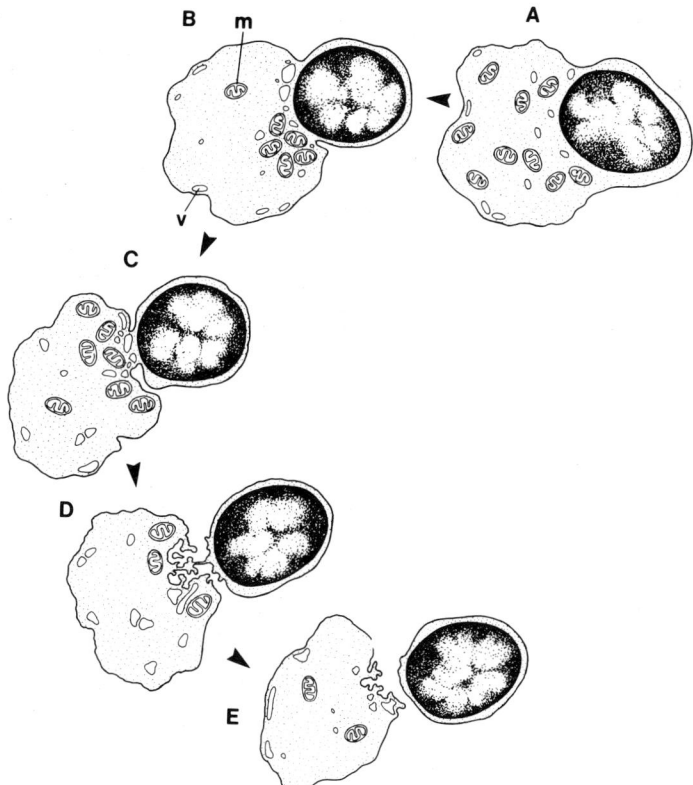

Figure 77–5. The process of normoblast denucleation as proposed by Simpson and Kling (1967). Nucleus becomes eccentric; vesicles coalesce between nucleus and mitochondria; with further coalescence, tenuous connection is finally broken. Mitochondrion (m); vesicle (v). (From Alsaker, R. D.: Vet. Clin. Pathol. *6*:7, 1977. Used with permission of author and publisher.)

1975). Schalm and coworkers (1975) divided the cat reticulocytes into Type I, containing faint blue stippling; Type II, containing large dark granules; and Type III, containing a heavy dark granular network. Cramer and Lewis (1971) divided the reticulocytes into two types, punctate and aggregate.

Maturation of the reticulocyte is thought to take place by extrusion of ribosomal aggregates at the time of nuclear extrusion. Thereafter, loss of polyribosomes occurs through degradation of purines, the products of which are metabolically utilized, pyrimidines that are diffused through the cell membrane (Bertles and Beck, 1962), and through a method suggested by electron microscopic studies, in which clusters of ribosomes appear to be discharged by exocytosis (Campbell, 1972).

Fan et al. (1978) indicate that maturation time of the Type II and III reticulocytes was about 12 hours both *in vivo* and *in vitro*, while the maturation time of the Type I reticulocyte was about three days. There appears to be no difference in response to acute blood loss between the Type II and Type III reticulocyte of the cat. The Type I

reticulocyte more nearly paralleled the return to normal of the packed cell volume (PCV) than did the Type II and III reticulocytes. Fan et al. (1977) suggest that both heavy and light reticulocyte types be counted independently for the cat.

The Erythron. *Erythron* (Boycott, 1929) is a term used to designate the combined mass of immature and mature red cells, whether extravascular or intravascular, fixed or circulating. The erythron, in other words, is composed primarily of the erythroid marrow and the circulating erythrocytes. This concept emphasizes the functional unity of the red cells and their precursors and implies that evaluation of both is necessary for an understanding of the true functional state.

The erythron is normally maintained in a steady state, in which the rate of red cell production precisely balances the rate of destruction. This steady state is maintained by modulation in the rate of red cell production through control of the number of stem cells that differentiate into committed erythrocyte precursors. Although it is conceivable that the rate of red cell production

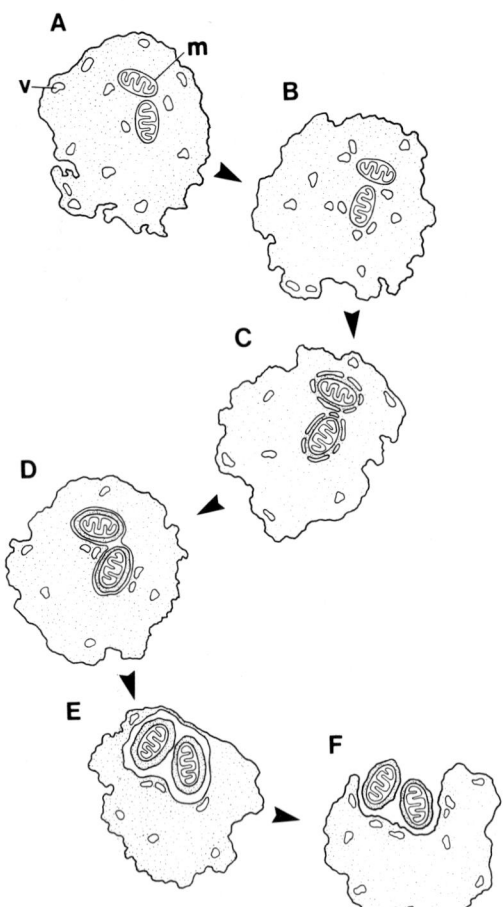

Figure 77–6. Mechanism of mitochondrial extrusion from the reticulocyte as proposed by Simpson and Kling (1968). Mitochondria are progressively surrounded by vesicles, which fuse end to end, leaving mitochondria rimmed by double-layered membrane. Outer membrane of mitochondrial vacuole fuses with cell membrane, resulting in extrusion of mitochondria surrounded by a single membrane. (From Alsaker, R. D.: Vet. Clin. Pathol. 6:7, 1977. Used with permission of author and publisher.)

could be controlled by altering the rate of mitosis and maturation, no evidence has been gathered to support this notion.

The mechanism of erythropoiesis control is now well established as a sensitive feedback system. The fundamental stimulus for erythropoiesis, and hence for increase in the size of the erythron, is tissue hypoxia. The rate of red cell production determines the size of the hemoglobin mass, which determines the circulating hemoglobin concentration. The hemoglobin concentration is the major determinant of the degree of tissue oxygenation, which determines the rate of red cell production (Harris and Kellermeyer, 1970). Several other factors influence the amount of oxygen delivered to tissues, however. Among these are oxygen tension of inspired air, pulmonary function, cardiac output, shifts in the oxyhemoglobin dissociation curve (changes in the affinity of hemoglobin for oxygen), and the distribution of blood to different tissues.

Erythropoietin. Tissue hypoxia does not directly control or stimulate red cell production. Instead, a circulating factor produced in response to hypoxia and referred to as *erythropoietic stimulating factor* (ESF) or *erythropoietin* has been identified as the mediator of erythropoiesis. It is now generally agreed that erythropoietin is a hormone that is characterized as a nondialyzable, relatively thermostable α globulin. Estimates of its molecular weight range from 39,000 to 70,000.

The primary site of erythropoietin production in those species studied is the kidney. Experimental evidence indicates that in the dog, the *only* site of erythropoietin production is the kidney (Harris and Kellermeyer, 1970), and canine end-stage kidney disease is reliably associated with nonregenerative anemia.

The action of erythropoietin is complicated (Fig. 77–7). In response to hypoxia, renal tissue elaborates renal erythropoietic factor (REF), which activates inactive erythropoietin (erythropoietinogen) of hepatic origin to active erythropoietin (ESF).

Clinical conditions that may be associated with decreased production of erythropoietin include end-stage kidney disease and aplastic anemias. In contrast, canine renal carcinoma accompanied by polycythemia is thought to entail excess production of erythropoietin (Scott and Patnaik, 1972).

Ineffective Erythropoiesis. Total erythropoiesis is the total production of red cells, regardless of entrance to the circulating blood. That portion of the red cell mass that

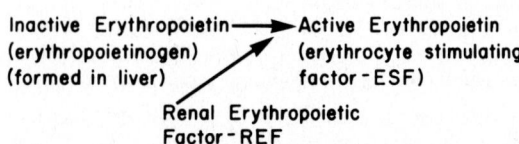

Figure 77–7. The erythropoietin system. In the dog, REF has no extrarenal production site. End-stage canine kidney disease, therefore, is reliably associated with nonregenerative anemia.

enters, into the circulation and remains there long enough to be detected or to contribute to the steady state is referred to as *effective erythropoiesis. Ineffective erythropoiesis* refers to that portion of the red cell mass not appearing in the circulation or not remaining in the circulation long enough to be detected. In some diseases such as erythemic myelosis, the bone marrow processes hemoglobin and produces immature red cells but does not deliver mature erythrocytes to the circulation. In normal dogs, only a small portion of the total erythropoietic activity is ineffective (Odartchenko et al., 1971).

Erythrokinetic studies that include the bone marrow ratio of erythrocytic to myelocytic cells, plasma-iron turnover, red cell utilization of iron, the reticulocyte count, red cell life span, fecal urobilinogen determinations, and autoradiographic cytokinetic analysis provide the most accurate assessment of effective erythropoiesis. The reticulocyte count provides the most practical means of evaluating erythropoiesis in terms of bone marrow response to stimulation and delivery of red cells to peripheral blood.

Definition of Anemia. Anemia is traditionally defined in terms of the concentration of hemoglobin in peripheral blood or in terms of a reasonable equivalent such as the packed-cell volume (PCV). This definition has merit because the major determinant of tissue oxygen supply is the circulating hemoglobin concentration, which is relatively easy to determine. However, a definition of anemia based on hemoglobin concentration does not take into account other factors that influence the delivery of oxygen to the tissues, such as the rate of circulation, the position of the oxyhemoglobin dissociation curve, the rate of dissociation of oxygen from hemoglobin, and the functional adequacy of circulatory beds. Because of the difficulty in assessing all the variables that influence the delivery of oxygen to the tissues, it is best to define anemia in terms of the deviation from accepted normal hemoglobin concentration or PCV for the species, age, and sex.

Control and Effectiveness of the Erythron. From a pool of stem cells in the bone marrow, immature red cells are produced and pass through successive morphologic stages of maturation. Nearly mature red cells are released to the peripheral blood as reticulocytes, a practical indicator of bone marrow response.

The stimulus for increased erythropoiesis is tissue hypoxia, which causes increased production of erythropoietin. The erythropoietin produced primarily by the kidney stimulates bone marrow stem cells to differentiate erythrocyte precursors. The process of erythropoiesis may not be effective if red cells are not released or are prematurely destroyed.

The ability of erythrocytic hemoglobin to oxygenate tissues varies and can be affected by factors such as environmental oxygen tension and cardiac function. The effectiveness of erythrocytic hemoglobin oxygen delivery can be increased if red cell 2,3-DPG concentrations are increased by factors such as hypoxia and inorganic phosphate concentrations. These modulations in the effectiveness of hemoglobin in oxygen delivery to tissues are physiologically and pathophysiologically significant.

Endocrine Function and the Erythron. The endocrine glands regulate normal erythropoiesis indirectly through their effects on metabolism and oxygen requirements and not through a direct effect on the bone marrow or direct modification of the fundamental stimulus of hypoxia. Some endocrine disorders, however, are often associated with hematologic alterations.

Hypothyroidism is associated with decreased red cell production due to decreased size of the erythron as an adaptation to the diminished needs of tissue for oxygen (Harris and Kellermeyer, 1970). The anemia is normocytic and normochromic (Schalm et al., 1975); the bone marrow is hypocellular. The anemia responds slowly to thyroid replacement (Hollander et al., 1967).

In man, hyperthyroidism is associated with increased red cell 2,3-DPG concentrations and a right shift of the oxyhemoglobin dissociation curve. Erythrocyte-survival time is slightly shortened, but erythropoiesis is increased. Hypofunction of the anterior pituitary in man is associated with moderate normocytic, normochromic anemia.

Normocytic, normochromic anemia accompanies human Addison's disease, but the PCV and hemoglobin concentration may not be decreased because of the significant decrease in plasma volume and hemoconcentration. Data from dogs with hypoadrenocorticism suggest that the situation is similar in this species (Mulnix, 1971; Keeton et al., 1972).

That men have a higher PCV than women is attributed to differences in androgen activity. This sex difference does not exist in cats or dogs except in the postestrus non-pregnant and the pregnant bitch (Tietz et al., 1967; Anderson and Schalm, 1970; Concannon et al., 1977). Pharmacologic doses of anabolic androgenic steroids do increase the size of the erythron, and are used therapeutically (Shahidi, 1973).

Pharmacologic doses of estrogens, including diethylstilbestrol, are known to cause bone marrow suppression and aplastic anemia in the dog (Crafts, 1948; Chiu, 1974). Sertoli-cell tumor in the dog has been associated with aplastic anemia that has been attributed to excess production of estrogens (Mulkey and Schall, 1972).

Red Cell Sodium and Potassium. In contrast to man and some other mammals, the dog and cat have normal red cell sodium and potassium concentrations that approach the levels of plasma concentrations. Cat and dog erythrocytes are high in sodium and low in potassium; for human erythrocytes the reverse is true (Romualdez et al., 1972). In addition, it is known that the red cells of newborn puppies (Miles and Lee, 1972) and reticulocytes of mature dogs (Parker, 1973) have relatively high concentrations of potassium. Puppy red cells gradually acquire adult concentrations of sodium and potassium over a period of weeks.

These observations are clinically significant from at least two standpoints. Serum-potassium determinations conducted on either hemolyzed or long-standing canine and feline blood samples are less likely to yield fallaciously high determinations than are similar human samples, and hyperkalemia is less likely to result from the transfusion of stored feline or canine blood (Coulter and Small, 1971).

Iron Metabolism. The precise regulatory mechanism for iron absorption is still not known despite extensive studies and reviews. Dietary iron is principally in the Fe^{3+} form as bound iron. Iron bound to phytates and phosphates is unavailable for absorption. Other dietary iron is acted on in the stomach, where the acidity releases the iron

from proteins and maintains both Fe^{3+} and Fe^{2+} in solution. The alkaline environment of the small intestine contains reducing substances that favor reducing Fe^{3+} to Fe^{2+}, which is the more absorbable form.

Heme iron is readily absorbed, whereas iron in foods bound to oxalates, phytates, and phosphates is less readily available (Kaneko, 1980a). Normally, only ten to 15 per cent of dietary iron is absorbed to maintain body iron in the dog (Stewart and Gambino, 1961).

Iron in the Fe^{2+} form is absorbed by the intestinal mucosa and bound to apoferritin to form ferritin. Transfer of ferritin to the plasma takes place mainly in the duodenum.

Body iron is regulated by intestinal absorption rather than by excretion. If dietary intake is increased, the amount of iron absorbed is increased but the percentage absorbed decreases. Iron absorption is increased in blood-loss anemia, in iron-deficient states, and to a lesser degree, in hemolytic anemias (Koepke et al., 1970).

Plasma transport of iron is by a specific iron-binding protein called transferrin. Normally, two thirds of the transferrin is unbound and the other third is bound to Fe^{3+}. The total iron-binding capacity of plasma is the serum iron level and the unbound iron-binding capacity (UIBC). Transferrin transports iron to and from iron compartments and acceptor sites on cell membranes. The readily available pool of iron is termed the "labile iron pool" and in part has been shown by Pollycove and Mortimer (1961) to exist on cell membranes of developing normoblasts.

In the normal steady state, about two thirds of the body iron is distributed throughout the erythron as hemoglobin iron. Approximately one fourth of the iron is stored as ferritin or hemosiderin in macrophages of the spleen, liver, and bone marrow. The remaining body iron is incorporated in myoglobin, is present in a labile pool, and exists as other tissue iron or as transport iron. The transport iron is less than 0.1 per cent of the total body iron (Beutler et al., 1963).

Iron excretion is minimal through the major excretory routes and from exfoliated cells and tissues. When normal canine and feline red cells become senescent, they are trapped by the macrophage system, phagocytized, and metabolically degraded. The

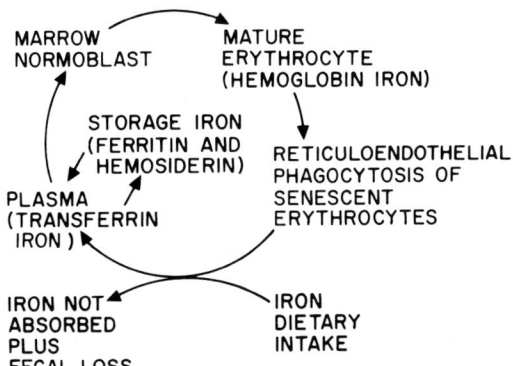

Figure 77–8. Internal and external iron cycle. Most body iron cycles exist in a virtually closed internal system. The small quantity of iron lost daily is replaced by absorption from the amount ingested.

released iron is stored in the macrophage system or enters circulation pathways. Thus, the body iron of mammals is conserved and recycled in an efficient manner (Fig. 77–8).

Physiologic Changes. Detailed information regarding physiologic changes in the erythron is available for the dog and to a lesser extent for the cat. With few exceptions (Smith et al., 1972), data are restricted to examinations of venous blood.

AGE. From birth to about three days of age, the puppy PCV is greater than or equal to that of the adult (Huggins et al., 1971). Thereafter, the PCV progressively declines until about six weeks of age, at which time the PCV may be less than 25 per cent but is usually between 25 and 30 per cent (Anderson and Schalm, 1970; Huggins et al., 1971; Ewing et al., 1972). From six weeks to six months of age, the PCV gradually increases until normal adult values are attained. The PCV of cats undergoes similar changes, but the lowest feline PCV is present at four weeks of age and the adult values are attained at five months of age (Windle et al., 1940). The lower PCV of puppies is accompanied by hyperphosphatemia and is probably associated with a shift of the oxyhemoglobin dissociation curve to the right due to increased red cell 2,3-DPG concentrations.

SEX. In contrast to humans, the bitch does not usually have a PCV less than that of the male dog. The canine female has a PCV either equal to or greater than that of the canine male (Tietz et al., 1967; Porter and Canaday, 1971; Anderson and Schalm, 1970; Concannon et al., 1977), except during estrus and pregnancy. The PCV of adult queens and toms is not significantly different (Windle et al., 1940).

ESTRUS AND PREGNANCY. Tietz et al. (1967) determined that normally there is a 20 per cent decrease in a bitch's PCV following estrus. The lowest postestrus PCV is reached during the seventh week after the onset of estrus. Pregnant bitches have a similar decrease in PCV, but the magnitude of the decrease is greater (33 per cent) and occurs later (during the eighth week after the onset of estrus) (Doxey, 1966; Tietz et al., 1967; Concannon et al., 1977). The PCV of the queen progressively decreases during pregnancy (Berman, 1974). A 20 per cent decrease is reached just before parturition and is accompanied by reticulocytosis. The PCV approaches normal 100 days after parturition.

SEASON. The PCV in the male dog is greater during the winter (Thomas and Kittrell, 1966; Tietz et al., 1967). The magnitude of the seasonal increase is less than ten per cent.

ALTITUDE. Thomas and Kittrell (1966) have determined that dogs moved from sea level to altitudes between 6000 and 10,000 feet above sea level have PCV increases between 15 and 20 per cent.

EXERCISE. Although, theoretically, chronic strenuous exercise should cause an increase in the PCV, no convincing data support this hypothesis. The PCV of racing greyhounds was greater than generally accepted normal values for dogs but was not compared with the PCV of greyhounds not conditioned by training (Porter and Canaday, 1971).

BREED. Few specific breeds of dogs have been studied in detail (Schalm, 1965; Huggins et al., 1971; Porter and Canaday, 1971; Ewing et al., 1972). Insufficient data are currently available for definitive generalizations, although Schalm (1965) has suggested that poodles, German shepherds, boxers, beagles, dachshunds, and Chihuahuas often have hemoglobin concentrations greater than 18 gm per 100 ml.

ENVIRONMENT. The PCV of dogs is influenced by inapparent or subclinical disease or accepted degrees of health. In the more temperate and tropical zones, where the incidence of parasitic disease is greater, accepted values for "normal dogs" tend to be lower than values for "healthy" dogs.

EVALUATION OF THE ERYTHRON

Laboratory evaluation of the erythron requires an orderly clinical approach. Anemia or polycythemia may be apparent from examination of the patient, packed-cell volume, or hemoglobin determination. Definition of the problem requires systematic evaluation of red cell morphology, bone-marrow production, red cell destruction, and even blood-volume measurements.

A simple classification of polycythemia and anemia is given in Table 77–3. The characteristics of response to increased red blood cell production provide a basis for logical evaluation of the anemia patient. Understanding the differences in response between the dog and cat, the limitations of laboratory methods, and the variations in normal values is fundamental to accurate interpretation of laboratory data.

BLOOD VOLUME

Blood-volume determinations have limited clinical usefulness. The differential diagnosis of shock and states of rapidly changing fluid balance, blood-volume loss or replacement, and the polycythemias is, in part, based on blood-volume measurements.

Blood-Volume Measurement. Measurement of plasma volume can be made by dilution techniques employing the dye Evans' blue, T1824, or vital red, or albumin tagged with ^{131}I.

$$\text{Volume of plasma in ml} = \frac{\text{mg dye injected}}{\text{mg/ml in plasma of venous blood}}$$

$$\text{Blood volume in ml} = \frac{\text{plasma volume}}{100 - \text{venous hematocrit}}$$

Correction factors have been applied in the packed-cell measurement to determine total blood volume. In the dog, measurements made by Gregerson and Schiro

Table 77–3. Classification of Polycythemia and Anemia

Polycythemia
  Primary
  Secondary
Anemia
  Regenerative (increased red cell production)
  Nonregenerative (decreased red cell production)

(1938) with vital red or T1824 indicate 4.0 per cent of the dye is trapped in the venous hematocrit. The correction factor is introduced in blood-volume calculation as follows:

$$\text{Blood volume in ml} = \frac{\text{plasma volume in ml}}{100 - (\text{venous hematocrit} \times 0.96)} \times 100$$

The blood cell volume may be measured with dilution techniques by tagging erythrocytes with ^{51}Cr, ^{32}p, ^{55}Fe, or ^{59}Fe. The red cell mass is obtained from the formula:

$$\frac{\text{Total counts injected}}{\text{Counts/ml whole blood}}$$

$$\times \text{ hematocrit} = \text{red cell mass (ml)}$$

$$\text{Total blood volume} = \frac{\text{red cell mass}}{\text{hematocrit} \times 0.91}$$

The correction factor (0.91) is used for man to make the observed venous hematocrit match the true body hematocrit. The venous hematocrit is higher than arterial and capillary hematocrits because of protein and fluid distribution in the capillary bed. Simultaneous red-cell-volume measurement with ^{51}Cr and plasma-volume measurement with ^{131}I-labeled serum albumin or T1824 is required for accurate blood-volume determination.

Woodward et al. (1968) questioned whether correction factors should be used in blood- or plasma-volume measurements for the dog, since blood-volume determinations are relative. The early observations of Barcroft and Stephens (1927) demonstrated that the spleen of the dog may contain one fifth of the total red blood cells. Reece and Wahlstrom (1970), in studies of normal beagles, indicated an 11.4 per cent rise in mean venous hematocrit, associated with excitement, and a drop of 8.8 ml per kg in mean plasma volume, associated with feeding. In dogs placed under barbiturate anesthesia, Usenik and Cronkite (1965) observed a drop of 8.0 per cent in venous hematocrit within 30 minutes. A similar drop was seen following administration of acetyl promazine to dogs. The fall in erythrocyte parameters was 23 per cent, with a nadir of 60 minutes (Lang et al., 1979). Because the status of the spleen of diseased dogs may be uncertain, the application of correction factors to total body packed-cell volume or trapped plasma is questionable.

Schalm (1965) indicates that for practical application to the dog and cat, the blood volume may be estimated on the basis of millimeters per pound of body weight or stated as a percentage of body weight. Thus, the canine blood volume is 35 to 40 ml per pound (eight to nine per cent of body weight) and the feline 28 to 30 ml per pound (six to seven per cent of body weight).

Alterations in Blood Volume. Erythrocytes in normal states compose slightly less than half the blood volume in dogs and a lesser portion in cats. Regulation of the blood volume is influenced by factors that control erythropoiesis and the plasma fraction.

The cellular compartment may be decreased by several mechanisms and may be associated with concurrent change in the plasma compartment. The spleen serves as a major reserve store of erythrocytes and may sequester or release large numbers of erythrocytes with no changes in plasma constituents.

The plasma volume is influenced by changes in blood pressure, water intake and elimination, and the action of antidiuretic hormone and aldosterone. Empirical attempts at fluid balance in clinical situations may result in major changes in plasma volume.

ERYTHROCYTES

Evaluation of erythrocyte alterations and changes in function requires diverse laboratory tests. Quantitative, morphologic, functional, and immunologic tests are used.

Quantitation

Erythrocyte measurements and indices are used to find specific red blood cell changes associated with various pathologic processes.

Packed-Cell Volume (PCV). The packed red cell volume is best determined by the microhematocrit method. The macro method of Wintrobe is seldom used because of problems inherent in centrifugation and the inaccuracy caused by inadequate packing. Measurement of the red cell mass per unit volume of blood by the Coulter Model S and ZBI particle counters are based on measurement of the mean cell volume and erythrocyte number. The product is referred to as hematocrit (Hct) to distinguish it from the PCV by the centrifuge method (Harvey, 1981). Fairbanks (1978) has shown nonequivalence of automated Hct and manual PCV. The automated erythrocyte count is a linear function of hemoglobin concentration in serially diluted specimens. The MCV as measured by the Coulter S and ZBI is nearly a constant across serially diluted specimens. However, the relationship between the centrifuged PCV and the erythrocyte count is curvilinear; i.e., the PCV was disproportionately higher when the erythrocyte count was high and disproportionately lower when the erythrocyte count was low. There is good agreement between the Coulter S Hct and the centrifuged PCV from about PCV 25 to 50. The Coulter Hct is calibrated to centrifuged hematocrit values obtained with normal blood. The nonequivalence of the Hct and the microhematocrit (PCV) is attributed in part to variable amounts of trapped plasma and to erythrocyte shapes. When properly conducted, these two methods result in reliable measurements of the blood portion of the erythron. The PCV calculated by measurements made with the Coulter Model S particle size counter does not change with anticoagulant type or quantity of blood (Duben and Syopniewski-Radovsky, 1973). With proper techniques, the microhematocrit method is accurate to ±0.5 per cent.

The PCV of human venous blood may be increased by prolonged occlusion of veins during sampling. Attention to venous stasis is also necessary during canine and feline sampling.

The influence of using a large bore needle for sampling to avoid hemolysis has been perpetuated as an old wives' tale (Moss and Staunton, 1970). Hemolysis is due to the velocity of blood and the nature of the entrance and existing openings. Small bore needles have lower potential blood velocity. Under usual sampling conditions, aspiration through 20-gauge, 22-gauge and 25-gauge needles should not be associated with hemolysis. Short needle lengths and large bores increase the velocity of flow, hence the potential for hemolysis (Forstrom and Blackshear, 1970).

Penny et al. (1970) indicated that up to a 37 per cent reduction in PCV occurs with the use of excessive amounts of the anticoagulant ethylenediamine-tetraacetic acid (EDTA). Commercially prepared sample tubes contain approximately 1.5 mg of EDTA for each milliliter of blood to be preserved. A canine blood sample containing ten mg per ml EDTA would have a PCV 90 per cent of the normal value if determined within one hour after sampling. When EDTA affects the PCV measurement, greater reliance should be placed on the hemoglobin value in interpretation.

Excitement of the animal at the time of sampling causes epinephrine release and splenic contraction, resulting in a 10 to 15 per cent increase in PCV due to release of red blood cells. The PCV of venous blood of the spleen approximates 80 per cent.

The range for PCV values of the dog and cat is determined by several factors, such as age, breed, hormonal influence, environment, physical condition, and laboratory measurement. The "normal" PCV for the dog and cat falls within a narrower range when physiologic variables are considered in the clinical evaluation of the patient.

Since the clinical diagnosis is greatly dependent upon the PCV measurement, physiologic and sampling variables must be considered in data interpretation. Furthermore, body fluid balance and changes in blood volume may drastically alter the PCV and mask an underlying anemia.

Hemoglobin. Hemoglobin (Hb) may be determined by several spectrophotometric methods. The cyanmethemoglobin method is most commonly used and gives slightly higher values than acid or alkaline hematin methods. Although hemoglobin determination alone is less useful than the PCV determination, when used in conjunction with the PCV, it provides a reliable index of hemoglobin concentration in red blood cells.

Red Blood Cell Count. The hemocytometer red blood cell (RBC) count is subject to greater laboratory error than are the PCV or Hb determinations. Red cell counts obtained by electronic particle counters are more accurate than those obtained by hemocytometer methods. Indices calculated from accurate RBC counts provide useful information about RBC size and Hb content (i.e., normocytic, microcytic, macrocytic, normochromic, and hypochromic states). Comparable information may be obtained from morphologic evaluation of Wright-stained smears. The indices and RBC values

obtained with particle counters are useful when samples are properly collected, preserved, measured, and interpreted.

RBC Indices. The red blood cell indices or mean cell constants, based on the method used for man (Wintrobe, 1967), provide useful clinical information only when the limitations of the method and the normal values are understood. The mean corpuscular volume (MCV), mean corpuscular hemoglobin (MCH), and mean corpuscular hemoglobin concentration (MCHC) may be calculated in the following manner:

$$\text{MCV (femtoliters)} = \frac{\text{PCV} \times 10}{\text{RBC count in millions}}$$

EXAMPLE: PCV = 48; RBC = 7.0 million.

$$\text{MCV} = \frac{48 \times 10}{7} = 68.8 \text{ fl}$$

$$\text{MCH (picograms)} = \frac{\text{Hb} \times 10}{\text{RBC count in millions}}$$

EXAMPLE: Hb = 16.0; RBC = 7.0 million.

$$\text{MCH} = \frac{16.0}{7} \times 10 = 22.9 \text{ pg}$$

$$\text{MCHC (g/dl)} = \frac{\text{Hb}}{\text{PCV}} \times 100$$

EXAMPLE: Hb = 16.0; PCV = 48.0

$$\text{MCHC} = \frac{16.0}{48} \times 100 = 33 \text{ gm/dl}$$

Recent insight into nonequivalence of the Coulter Hct and the microhematocrit PCV must be considered in interpretation of the red blood indices (Fairbanks, 1980; Harvey, 1981). The MCH is not influenced by instrumentation, since automated erythrocyte counts and cyanmethemoglobin determinations yield constant MCH values across all serial dilutions. The MCV as determined by instrument measurement of the erythrocyte volumes (Coulter S and ZBI) is essentially constant across serial dilutions of blood. The MCV as determined by the microhematocrit is not linear, since the relationship between the centrifuged PCV and the erythrocyte count was curvilinear; i.e., the PCV was disproportionately higher when the erythrocyte count was high and disproportionately lower when the erythrocyte count was low (Fairbanks, 1980). Thus, the MCV based on the centrifuged PCV is more inconsistent and was normal in about one third of the specimens of microcytic anemia of people in that study. Similar findings in microcytic anemias of dogs have been mentioned (Harvey, 1981). In contrast to the MCV discrepancy, the MCHC is usually decreased in microcytic hypochromic anemia of dogs when the microhematocrit is used in calculation of the PCV; however, when the MCHC is determined by the Hct based on a calculated value, the value is within normal limits when slight to moderate microcytic hypochromic anemias are evaluated (Harvey, 1981). Thus, it becomes important to reference the method of study and to carefully interpret erythrocyte indices when evaluating the anemic patient.

Fairbanks (1980) concludes that when the MCV and MCH are obtained from the calculated Hct and automated erythrocyte counts, recognition and discrimination of anemias may be possible with greater sensitivity and reliability. The MCHC determined by these methods may be less sensitive.

Schalm (1974) outlined a morphologic classification of the anemias based on the red cell indices (Table 77–4). This classification is not all-inclusive but does provide an approach to more precise evaluation of the anemic patient.

The MCV and MCH increase proportionately in responsive anemia, with premature release of macroerythrocytes into the circulation. These "shift" reticulocytes appear in the circulation two to four days after stimulation and spend an increased time in the peripheral blood as reticulocytes. Since these reticulocytes remain enlarged, the MCV and MCH are elevated, but the MCHC is decreased. Thus, normal red cell indices can only be interpreted correctly in relation to the degree of marrow stimulation. For example, with marked stimulation of erythropoiesis in the dog, the MCV increases to 85 or 95 and the MCH to 26 or 30. The MCHC may decrease to 24.

Polychromatophilic macrocytes produced in response to marked erythropoietin stimulation have a survival time less than half of erythrocytes produced in near steady states. Card et al. (1969) suggest that the accelerated destruction of macrocytes in vivo may be related to glucose deprivation in tissues where they are sequestered because of their large size.

Macrocytosis not associated with responsive erythropoiesis reflects nuclear matura-

Table 77–4. Morphologic Classification of the Anemia

I. Macrocytic normochromic
   A. Pernicious anemia in man and primates
   B. Vitamin B_{12} and folate deficiencies
   C. Cobalt deficiency in ruminants
   D. Erythremic myelosis: a myeloproliferative disorder in cats
   E. Macrocytosis of poodles

II. Macrocytic hypochromic
   A. During recovery from massive erythrocyte loss
      1. Hemorrhage
         a. Injury
         b. Neoplasms
         c. Thrombocytopenia
         d. Blood clotting disorders
      2. Hemolytic destruction of erythrocytes
         a. Hemoparasites (anaplasmosis, haemobartonellosis)
         b. Autoimmune hemolytic anemia
         c. Heinz body anemia from drug toxicity
         d. Erythrocyte pyruvate kinase deficiency in basenji dogs

III. Normocytic normochromic
   A. Chronic diseases leading to depression of erythrogenesis as in hypoplastic and aplastic bone marrow
      1. Chronic infection, particularly suppurative and granulomatous
      2. Nephritis with uremia
      3. Malignancies
      4. Hormone deficiency (hypothyroidism, hypoadrenocorticism)

IV. Microcytic hypochromic
   A. Iron deficiency (also copper deficiency)
   B. Vitamin B_6 (pyridoxine) deficiency
   C. Chronic blood loss (ulcer, leiomyoma of duodenum, blood sucking parasites)

From Schalm, O. W.: Morphological classification of the anemia. Calif. Vet. October 30, 1974, p. 28. Used with permission.

tion defects. Such changes are associated with folic acid and vitamin B_{12} deficiency, some forms of hepatic disease, and some myeloproliferative disorders. Schalm (1976) described erythrocyte macrocytosis in miniature poodles not accompanied by anemia. Megaloblastoid changes and nuclear abnormalities were reported.

Microcytosis reflects cytoplasmic maturation defects. Some nutritional factors, absent or inhibited, may cause extra cell divisions in proliferative compartments, resulting in smaller erythrocytes. The most common cause of microcytosis is iron deficiency, which also results in hypochromic cells.

Normocytic erythrocytes occur when there is selective depression of erythropoiesis, as seen in chronic infections, malignancies, chronic renal failure, and hypoplastic disorders. The hemoglobin content of these cells is normal.

The MCHC is relatively constant for all mammals and ranges from 32 to 36, with accurate measurements of Hb and PCV. A decrease in MCHC indicates a decrease in mean hemoglobin content, which is indicative of hypochromic red blood cells and usually equated with iron deficiency. In the absence of a significant reticulocytosis, a low MCHC of 25 to 30 indicates hypochromic anemia. In the presence of a significant reticulocytosis, such as that which characterizes markedly responsive anemia, the MCHC will also be decreased because polychromatophilic macrocytes do not have a full complement of hemoglobin relative to cell size.

Morphology

Accurate red blood cell indices are helpful in the initial classification of an anemia. The indices should be interpreted in light of morphologic changes observed on careful inspection of Romanowsky-stained blood smears. Erythrocyte size and color saturation can not be determined as accurately from morphology as from measured erythrocyte indices. However, the size, color, shape changes, and erythrocyte inclusions need to be evaluated on the blood of anemic patients for completeness.

Blood Smears. Red blood cell morphology is easily defined on well-stained, properly made blood smears. The smears should be prepared from fresh blood, rapidly air dried, and stained with a Wright-type stain. Areas to be examined should have a uniform distribution of evenly spaced and separated red blood cells, free of precipitate artifact. Overly thin areas and areas of overlapping red blood cells should be avoided. The area between is appropriately termed the "red cell area" of the smear, and shape changes are more apparent. In thin areas, the cells are overly spread and central pallor is lacking. Misshapen cells appear round owing to reduced surface tension effects. Further, in areas that are too thick, noted by beginning rouleau formation, the erythrocytes contain punched-out centers. The stomatocytes induced in these thick areas are common artifacts of dog blood. Red blood cells in smears made from blood preserved with anticoagulants will have time- and anticoagulant-induced morphologic changes. In blood collection systems (Vacutainer, Becton-Dickinson), blood is drawn into tubes containing anticoagulant (EDTA). Smears made immediately following collection will be satisfactory.

SLIDE METHOD. Cell distribution is dependent upon proper preparation of blood smears. A small drop of fresh blood is placed near the end of a clean glass slide. The edge of a second slide is drawn over the drop with a smooth, even motion. The thickness of the smear may be adjusted by varying the speed and angle of the pusher slide.

The drop of blood may be varied in size to compensate for changes in blood viscosity. High-PCV blood is more viscous and results in short, thick smears, while low-PCV blood results in long, thin smears when the drop size and speed of the pusher slide are constant. The ultimate objective is a feathered edge of the smear located on the middle two thirds of the slide, even distribution of white blood cells, and an area of evenly spread red cells.

Smears made too slowly will result in large-sized, low-density cells (such as polychromatophiles) being drawn to the feathered edge in greater than normal numbers.

COVERSLIP SMEARS. Properly made coverslip smears result in even distribution of cells with minimal distortion artifacts. Number 1, 22-mm-square coverslips are used. A small drop of fresh blood is placed on the center of a clean coverslip. A second coverslip is placed over the drop to create an even, circular spreading of the blood. The coverslips are pulled apart with even motion and the films dried.

BLOOD-SMEAR STAINING. Blood smears may be stained with Wright or similar Romanowsky stains. The staining procedure is usually divided into three parts (1) fixations, two to five minutes; (2) buffering, five to 20 minutes; and (3) washing. The stain, buffer, staining time (buffering time), and washing are extremely important. The optimal time for buffering and the proper pH of the buffer are determined by trial and examination. In general, precipitated stain is the result of inadequate washing. Periodically, stained smears should be reviewed by qualified technologists or clinical pathologists to assure quality of preparation.

Morphologic Features. The stained blood smear provides a suitable means of verifying the cellular indices and detecting changes in morphology. The color change of polychromasia may be used like the reticulocyte count as a function test of effective erythropoiesis. Various morphologic features, especially of canine red blood cells, yield useful diagnostic or prognostic information. The following morphologic features should be considered:

Size — Normo-, micro-, and macrocytes.

Shape — Normal, spherocytes, crystallized hemoglobin, various poikilocytes.

Color — Normo-, hypochromic. Hyperchromasia is an artifact of the shape change, spherocyte. Polychromasia is the presence of ribonucleic acid (RNA) in young red cells.

Inclusions — Howell-Jolly bodies (nuclear fragments), precipitated hemoglobin, iron granules (siderocytes), basophilic stippling, and blood parasites.

MATURE ERYTHROCYTES. The normal red blood cell of the dog from birth until three to four weeks of age is a biconcave disk approximately 8.0 μ in diameter. Thereafter the mature erythrocyte of the dog approximates 7.0 μ in diameter. The average red blood cell of the cat is 5.8 μ in diameter. The hemoglobin is evenly distributed in red cells devoid of artifacts. The central pale depressed area of the canine red cell is prominent in contrast to the small central area of the feline red cell (Figs. 77–9 and 77–10). In areas of the blood smears where the cells are spread thinly, the central area may be less apparent.

POLYCHROMATOPHILS. Polychromasia is the presence of pale bluish red erythrocytes on a Wright-stained smear (Fig. 77–15). The blue color is due to the presence of RNA in immature erythrocytes. In man, these cells are termed marrow reticulocytes that have "shifted" out of the marrow prematurely in response to high erythropoietin stimulation.

In diseases of the bone marrow stroma,

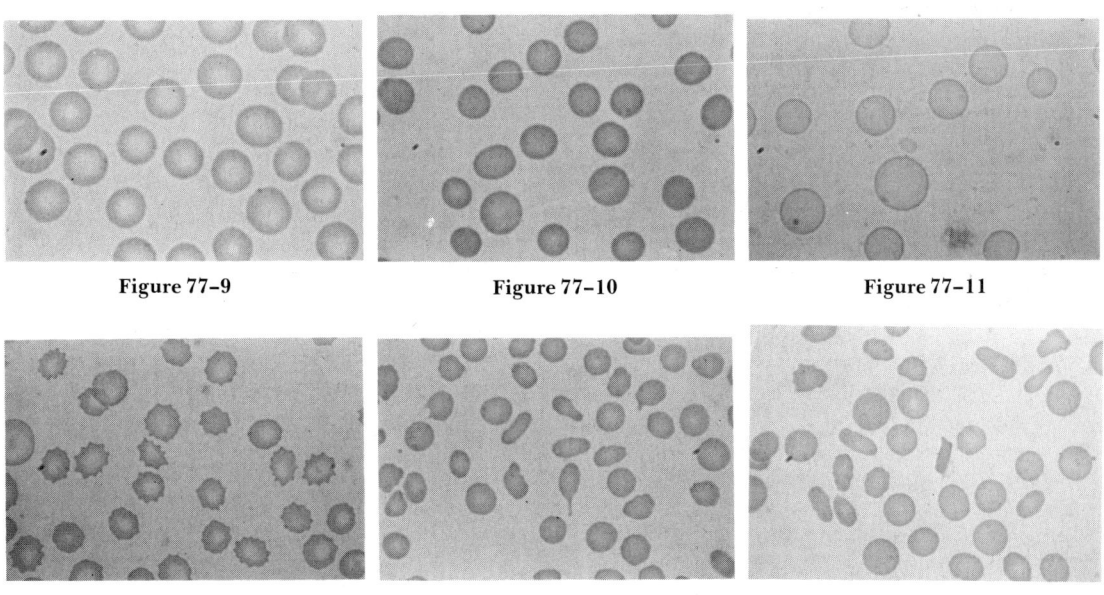

Figure 77–9   **Figure 77–10**   **Figure 77–11**

Figure 77–12   **Figure 77–13**   **Figure 77–14**

Figure 77–9. Normal dog erythrocytes. Central pallor and uniform size are characteristic features. Wright's stain. ×1250.

Figure 77–10. Normal cat erythrocytes. Minimal central pallor and variation in size are characteristic features. Wright's stain. × 1600.

Figure 77–11. Erythemic myelosis. Note macrocytic erythrocytes. Wright's stain. × 1600.

Figure 77–12. Cremation artifact of dog erythrocytes. Smear made from blood preserved with ethylenediaminetetraacetic acid. Wright's stain. × 1250.

Figure 77–13. Keratocytes in a cat with microangiopathy associated with disseminated intravascular coagulopathy. Wright's stain. ×1250.

Figure 77–14. Crystallized hemoglobin in a cat erythrocyte.

there is a disproportionate increase in polychromatophilic erythrocytes in relation to the degree of anemia present. In man, anemia not associated with a rise in erythropoietin is characterized by the absence of the polychromatophil (Perotta and Finch, 1971).

The number of reticulocytes that are recognized as polychromatophilic erythrocytes in the dog and cat has been defined. Based on observations in the authors' laboratory, the polychromatophilic erythrocyte count and the aggregate reticulocyte count are the same for the dog and cat (Laber et al., 1974). In these studies, the finely reticulated erythrocytes of the cat described by Cramer and Lewis (1972) were not counted.

In man, both reticulocytes and polychromatophilic erythrocytes reflect changes in the rate of erythropoiesis or alterations in release mechanisms. Minor increases in polychromatophilic erythrocytes in nonanemic animals do not necessarily reflect increased erythropoiesis or changes in the bone marrow microenvironment. This may be explained in part by the release of sequestered polychromatophilic erythrocytes from capillary beds and sinus areas of the spleen at the time of sampling. The large-sized polychromatophilic erythrocytes are selectively trapped in capillaries and spleen. Release may occur from splenic contraction or increased blood flow resulting from muscular contraction associated with excitement at the time of sampling.

MACROCYTES. Abnormally large erythrocytes are macrocytes. Macrocytes produced in response to the erythropoietin stimulation are reported by Card et al. (1969) to have a shorter life span than that of erythrocytes produced during normal steady-state erythropoiesis. Macrocytes not associated with erythropoietin stimulation are diagnostically important (Fig. 77–11). Vitamin B_{12} and folic acid deficiency induce maturation changes characterized by macrocytosis. Macrocytosis may also occur with production defects resulting from or associated with myeloproliferative diseases. A hereditary macrocytosis of miniature poodles has been described (Schalm, 1976). Maturation defects and macrocytosis were prominent features in nonanemic dogs.

MICROCYTES. Microcytes are smaller than the normal erythrocytes produced during erythropoiesis. Microcytes are most frequently caused by iron deficiency (Fig. 77–16). The smaller erythrocytes produced are hypochromic and are predisposed to shape changes.

Microcytic anemia in man and animals may be associated with chronic infection, lead poisoning, copper deficiency, protein abnormality, and other conditions characterized by ineffective erythropoiesis.

Erythrocytes produced as a result of erythropoietin stimulation are normocytic or may be macrocytic. There is an erythrocytosis-stimulating factor that differs from erythropoietin and is derived from the plasma of animals made anemic by a variety of means. This factor has been identified by Linman et al. (1958) as a lipid and may be identical or closely related to batyl alcohol. This factor and batyl alcohol produce erythrocytosis characterized by microcytes but without commensurate increases in hemoglobin. The role of this erythrocytosis-stimulating factor in disease has not been defined.

HYPOCHROMIC CELLS. Hypochromic cells have increased areas of central pallor (Fig. 77–17) and are usually microcytic. Calculations of red cell indices reveal a decreased MCV, MCH, and MCHC. The MCHC may be in the range of 24 to 30. Hypochromic microcytic anemia is ineffective erythrogenesis and nonresponsive, with a diminished or absent reticulocyte response. The hypochromic cells formed are easily distorted, and shape changes occur. Hypochromic cells represent a late change in iron-deficiency anemia.

Lack of available iron during hemoglobin synthesis results in hemoglobin-deficient erythrocytes. The most frequent cause of iron deficiency is chronic blood loss. However, in dogs and cats, inadequate dietary intake and absorption are significant factors, particularly in young growing animals with rapidly increasing blood volumes, since available stored iron in young animals may be negligible.

NUCLEATED RED BLOOD CELLS. The release of nucleated red blood cells into the general circulation is a poorly understood phenomenon. In general, the more severe the anemia, the greater the likelihood of nucleated cell release, particularly in the cat, regardless of the degree of bone marrow activity. Nucleated red cells in the peripheral blood should not be equated to increased

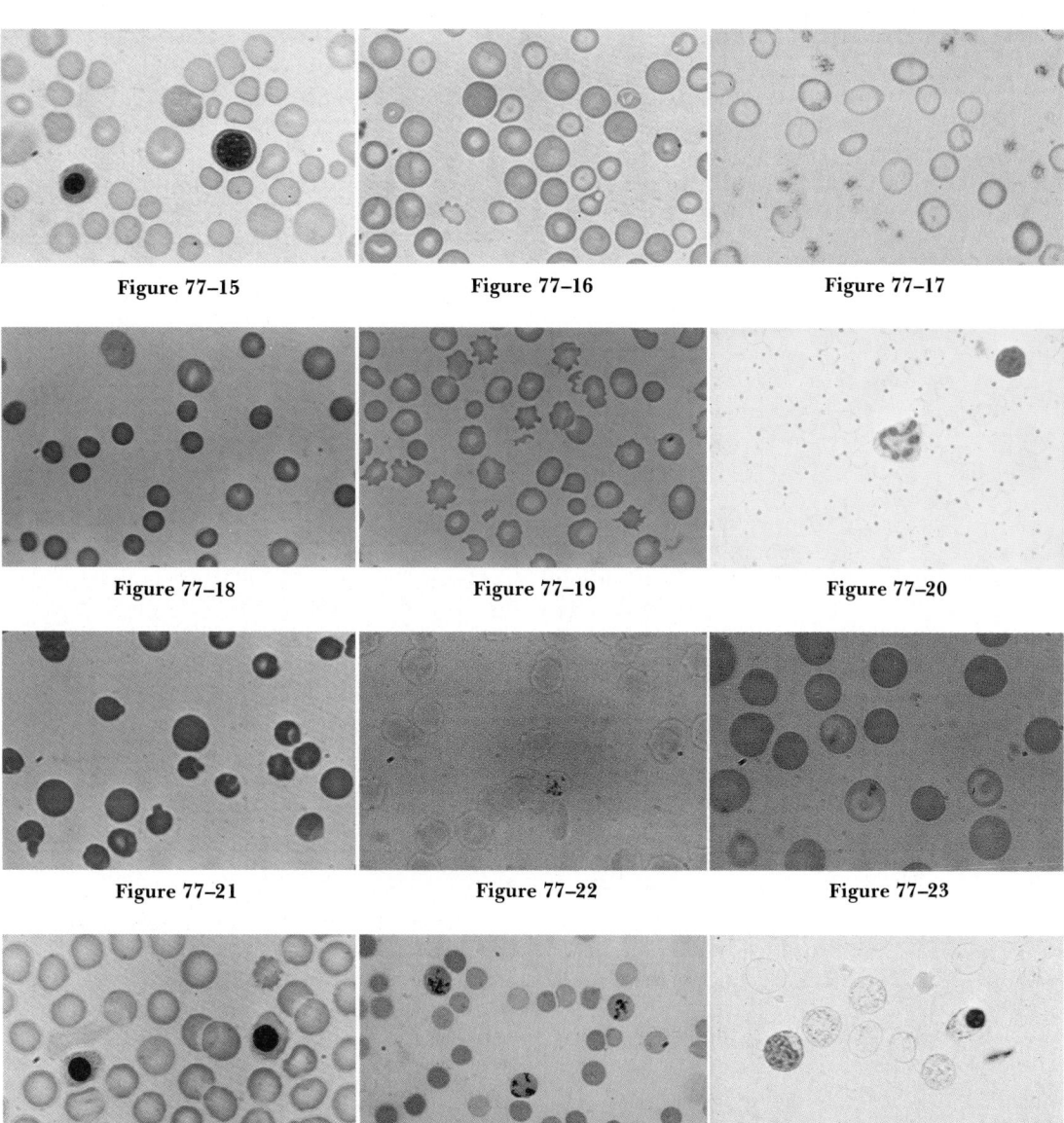

Figure 77–15.

Figure 77–16.

Figure 77–17.

Figure 77–18.

Figure 77–19.

Figure 77–20.

Figure 77–21.

Figure 77–22.

Figure 77–23.

Figure 77–24.

Figure 77–25.

Figure 77–26.

Figure 77–15. Feline autoimmune hemolytic anemia. The regenerative response is characterized by polychromasia, anisocytosis, nucleated erythrocytes, and a Howell-Jolly body. Wright stain. ×1250.

Figure 77–16. Hypochromic anemia in a dog. Note hypochromasia, microcytes, and codocytes (target cells). Wright stain. ×1250.

Figure 77–17. Hypochromic anemia in a dog. Marked hypochromasia and microcytosis in severe blood loss caused by hookworms. Wright stain. ×1250.

Figure 77–18. Canine autoimmune hemolytic anemia. Small intensely stained erythrocytes are spherocytes. Wright stain. ×1250.

Figure 77–19. Poikilocytosis and spherocytes in a dog with microangiopathy associated with disseminated intravascular coagulopathy. Wright stain. ×1250.

Figure 77–20. Heinz bodies (erythrocyte refractile bodies) in cat erythrocytes. Air-dried blood film stained with new methylene blue. ×1250.

Figure 77–21. Methylene-blue-induced hemolytic anemia in a cat. Note Heinz bodies on smaller erythrocytes. Wright stain. ×1250.

Figure 77–22. Siderocyte in dog blood stained by Prussian blue to demonstrate iron. ×1250.

Figure 77–23. Pappenheimer body in a dog erythrocyte. The blue-black aggregate is seen in a codocyte. Wright stain. ×1250.

Figure 77–24. Sideroblast in dog blood. The fine stippling of the cytoplasm of the nucleated erythrocyte resembles basophilic stippling. Wright stain. ×1250.

Figure 77–25. Reticulocytes in dog blood stained vitally with new methylene blue and counterstained with Wright's stain. Three aggregate forms present. ×1250.

Figure 77–26. Reticulocytes in dog blood stained with new methylene blue by the method of Schalm. ×1250.

erythropoiesis, but rather to damage to the restraining barrier that keeps the cells confined to production sites. Clinical conditions associated with the release of nucleated red blood cells are varied, namely endotoxemia, neoplasia of the bone marrow, myelofibrosis, hemorrhage in the marrow, extramedullary erythropoiesis, lead poisoning, and anemia (regardless of type). The highest numbers have been seen in erythroleukemia and severe nonregenerative anemias of cats. On occasion, nucleated red blood cells and immature leukocytes are released from the bone marrow, the so-called "leukoerythroblastic reaction."

The appearance of nucleated blood cells disassociated from a reticulocyte response should focus attention on a serious problem that may not involve erythropoiesis but rather may reflect damage to the normal restraining barrier between the extravascular bone marrow space and blood.

HOWELL-JOLLY BODIES. Howell-Jolly bodies are one to two μ nuclear fragments, usually single but occasionally multiple, which are located in non-nucleated erythrocytes (Fig. 77–15). The Howell-Jolly body is removed by the pitting action of splenic sinus endothelium (Jandl, 1965). Postsplenectomy and functional disease states of the spleen are associated with increased numbers of Howell-Jolly bodies in blood erythrocytes.

The removal of Howell-Jolly bodies from the erythrocytes of normal dogs is relatively complete; however, Howell-Jolly bodies are frequently found in erythrocytes of clinically normal cats. Perhaps splenic contraction at the time of sampling forces Howell-Jolly body–containing erythrocytes from sludged areas and sites of extramedullary erythropoiesis into the general circulation.

POIKILOCYTES. Variation in red blood shape is termed poikilocytosis. The cells may be round, oval, pear-shaped, crenated, spiculed, and many other shapes. Care must be taken to recognize artifacts due to smear preparation. The "red cell area" of the smear must be selected carefully. Areas of the smear that are too thin cause decreased surface tension and deformed cells that round up, abolishing significant findings. In areas too thick, drying artifacts may cause unusual punched-out or spiculed cells. The glass slide itself may influence red cell shape.

When the deformity is questionable, examination with the phase microscope can usually separate whether the deformities existed previously or were induced in smear preparation.

Considerable variation in terminology exists for the various poikilocytes. The terminology used in this chapter is that of Bessis (1973a; 1977) developed for man and applicable to blood of other mammals (Table 77–5).

Poikilocytes are commonly found in some diseases of the dog and provide useful clues as to the disease. Poikilocytes do not commonly occur in cats. This may reflect physical features of the smaller erythrocytes rather than disease conditions.

SPHEROCYTES. In dogs, the spherical nature of the erythrocytes is caused by increased intracellular fluid or by loss of cell membrane without significant loss of internal cellular substance. The spherocyte is recognized as a smaller than normal erythrocyte. Its hyperchromic appearance reflects increased central thickness (Fig. 77–18). Spherocytes are readily distinguished in canine blood; however, because of the small size of feline erythrocytes, this shape change may not be recognized in cats.

A discussion of the mechanism of sphering is beyond the scope of this chapter. In man, hereditary spherocytosis is associated with membrane alterations resulting in sodium retention and subsequent swelling. There is no documentation of hereditary spherocytosis in the dog and cat. Acquired spherocytosis, induced by immune-mediated factors or red cell aging, occurs in the dog. Acquired spherocytosis is commonly seen in systemic lupus erythematosus of the dog as described by Lewis et al. (1963; 1965a,b). Frequently, the spherocytic anemia is Coombs-positive; however, immune-mediated spherocytic anemia need not be Coombs-positive (Avolt et al., 1973).

Aged red blood cells tend to sphere. The clinician should be aware of this fact when examining the blood of dogs receiving several large transfusions of stored blood.

Spherocytosis has been described in feline immune-mediated anemia (Scott et al., 1973). However, the small size of the feline red blood cells makes detection difficult (Fig. 77–15).

Spherocytes are seen in fragmentation anemias regardless of cause as the result of

Table 77–5. Nomenclature of Abnormally Shaped Erythrocytes

Term	Meaning in Greek	Description	Conditions Observed in
Discocyte	Disc	Normal biconcave erythrocyte	Health
Echinocyte	Sea urchin	Different stages of crenation, 10 to 30 spicules; regular distribution on surface	Mainly *in vitro* but can be seen *in vivo*
Stomatocyte	Mouth	Different stages of cup shape	Artifact in thick portions; hereditary
Acanthocyte	Spike	Spheroidal cells with 2 to 20 spicules irregularly distributed	and acquired syndrome
Codocyte	Bell, Hat	Thin bell-shaped erythrocyte (target cell = codocyte flattened on a surface)	Retention icterus hepatic insufficiency
Dacrocyte	Teardrop	A single spicule in teardrop shape	Fragmentation anemias
Drepanocyte	Sickle	Sickle shape, rigid spicules	S Hemoglobin
Elliptocyte	Oval	Oval shape	Congenital or acquired
Keratocyte	Horn	1 to 6 spicules	Fragmentation anemia, DIC, myelofibrosis
Knizocyte	Pinch	Triconcave erythrocyte	Hemolytic anemia
Leptocyte	Thin	Flattened cell	Hypochromic cells
Megalocyte	Giant	Oval macrocyte	Maturation defect
Schizocyte	Cut	Fragment of discocyte, 2 to 4 angular projections	Smear keratocyte
Spherocyte	Sphere	Spherical shape; macro = swollen sphere; micro = reduced volume	Immune-mediated fragmentation anemia

Modified and adpated from Bessis, M.: Living blood cells and their ultrastructure. Springer-Verlag, New York, 1973. Bessis, M.: Blood Smear Reinterpreted. Springer-International, Berlin, 1977.

erythrocyte damage. The percentage of cells as spherocytes may be quite high and easily confused with autoimmune hemolytic anemia (AIHA).

The final outcome of the spherocyte is removal from the circulation and destruction, usually within macrophages. The spherocytes do have restricted deformability, and entrapment by the microcirculation of spleen leads to destruction.

In clinical evaluation of the AIHA spherocytic anemia patient, the percentage of cells with spherocytic change should be determined. In general, the more spherocytes, the lesser the reticulocyte response and the longer before remission is achieved. The spherocyte cells must be replaced by normal cells.

ACANTHOCYTES. Acanthocytes are red cells with 2 to 20 rounded projections, irregularly distributed. In man, they result from plasma abnormalities such as decreased cholesterol, phospholipids, depressed triglycerides, free fatty acids, and specifically, abetalipoproteinemia. Membrane studies reveal decreased lecithin and linoleic acid, and increased cholesterol and sphingomyelin. Evidence indicates that acanthocytes contain excessive membrane cholesterol, resulting in their destruction while traversing the small orifices of the spleen. The presence of acanthocytes indicates an underlying metabolic defect and may be seen in forms of hepatic disease, uremia, hemolytic uremic syndrome, and hereditary abetalipoproteinemia. Acanthocytes have been found in hepatic diseases of dogs. The spur cell anemia of the dog described by Schull et al. (1978) would be termed acanthocytic by these criteria. Crenation changes resemble acanthocytes but occur in erythrocytes exposed to anticoagulants (Fig. 77–12). Acanthocytes can only be defined on properly stained fresh blood smears.

CODOCYTES AND LEPTOCYTES. Codocytes (target cells) are large thin red cells with a peripheral rim and a central mass of hemoglobin. Codocytes result from cholesterol loading of the red cell membrane, caused by a plasma-transesterase deficiency. Codocytes are seen in some forms of chronic hepatic disease and some splenic disorders. Review of the University of Minnesota Veterinary Hospital files on portal-caval shunts of dogs revealed that 80 per cent of hemograms contained the report of target cells (Toombs, 1980). The distinction between codocytes and leptocytes in dogs remains to be made. Hypochromic and polychromatophilic cells are frequently shaped as codocytes or leptocytes (Fig. 77–16). Schalm (1965) states, "The appearance of target cells or other forms of leptocytes in the absence of frank evidence of active erythrogenesis may be interpreted as an expression of a chronic disease process."

SCHIZOCYTES. A red cell fragment occurring as the result of a complete cut is a schizocyte (Fig. 77–19). Schizocytes are found in low numbers in diseases with alteration of the microcirculation and some forms of hemolytic anemias. Microangiopathy due to intravascular coagulation results in injury to normal red cells.

KERATOCYTES AND DACROCYTES. Red cells entrapped in fibrin meshwork of intravascular coagulation events and in microangiopathy may develop several (one to six) blunt, rounded, irregularly spaced projections of the surface membrane. Keratocytes associated with schizocytes and fragmentation-induced spherocytes are indicative of fragmentation anemia (Fig. 77–19).

KNIZOCYTES. Pinched erythrocytes with a triconcave appearance are indicative of hemolytic anemia. Such cells are seen in Heinz body-induced anemias of dogs.

STOMATOCYTES. The "pinched out" appearance of erythrocytes with round or elongated openings are artifacts when encountered in dogs. The cells are found in the smear in the thicker reaches of the area of red cells and reflect smear thickness. A hereditary spherocytosis of the Alaskan malamute has been reported (Fletch and Pinkerton, 1972).

INTRAERYTHROCYTIC CRYSTALLOID BODY. Rectangular crystalloid bodies within erythrocytes have been described by Altman et al. (1972) and reported to be similar to crystals seen in red cells of man with hemoglobin C disease. Similar crystals (Fig. 77–14) are found in red cells of anemic cats and following therapy for leukemia with different chemotherapeutic agents.

HEINZ BODIES (SCHMAUCH OR ERYTHROCYTE REFRACTILE BODIES). Intracellular erythrocyte aggregates demonstrated with (1) wet unstained preparations, (2) supravital stains, and (3) phase-contrast microscopy are termed Heinz bodies (1890) (Fig. 77–20). Schmauch, as cited by Beritic (1964), first described the appearance of these bodies in erythrocytes of normal cats. Schalm and Smith (1963) later called the bodies, when stained with new methylene blue, "erythrocyte refractile bodies." Heinz-body formation causes red cell destruction in most animals by the pitting action of the spleen. Cats normally have Heinz bodies, and only some large forms are associated with hemolysis.

Several chemical oxidants, such as phenylhydrazine and methylene blue, serve as models for the study of Heinz-body formation. Methylene blue has induced hemolytic anemia in the cat (Schechter et al., 1972). Techniques for the detection of Heinz bodies in erythrocytes have been reviewed by Jain (1973). Heinz bodies in the blood of normal cats are usually not demonstrable with Romanowsky stains; however, when observed, these bodies have been exceptionally large and associated with hemolysis (Fig. 77–21).

The interaction between oxidant drugs and erythrocytes is not completely understood. Several effects are noted, including Heinz body formation, hemolysis, and methemoglobin formation. Oxidant drugs react with hemoglobin, generating the superoxide free radical. The protective enzyme superoxide dismutase catalyzes the dismutation of superoxide radicals to hydrogen peroxide. Erythrocytes contain catalase and glutathione peroxidase, which degrade the hydrogen peroxide, thus protecting the cell from damage. Glutathione peroxidase also reacts with lipid peroxides. Hemoglobin is therefore dependent for its functional integrity on the hexomonophosphate shunt pathway to drive these reactions (Kaneko, 1980). This auxiliary energy-generating mechanism couples oxidative glycolysis with tripuridine nucleotide and glutathione reduction to protect hemoglobin against dematuration. Oxidative dematuration results in globin precipitates that attach themselves as large aggregates (Heinz bodies) to the inner cell membrane.

Oxidant drugs in toxic doses vary in their production of methemoglobinemia, which may obscure the underlying Heinz body anemia (Harvey and Kornick, 1976).

BASOPHILIC STIPPLING. The appearance of fine to coarse basophilic granulation in erythrocytes stained with Romanowsky stains is called basophilic stippling. Basophilic stippling is frequently observed in conditions of ineffective erythropoiesis, such as lead poisoning (Zook et al., 1969). Basophilic stippling occurs in young erythrocytes that contain ribosomes. In stippled cells, the ribosomes aggregate during drying of the smear before staining with Wright-type stains (George and Duncan, 1979). Zook et al. (1970) have reported that the anticoagulants sodium versenate and potassium oxalate decrease the number of stippled cells that can be found in blood. Rapid drying of film apparently does not alter the occurrence of stippling, but alcohol-fixed smears or stains that are overly acidic owing to the pH of the buffer result in fewer detectable stippled erythrocytes.

SIDEROCYTES AND SIDEROBLASTS. A siderocyte is a non-nucleated red cell in which iron-containing granules are distributed at random throughout the cytoplasm and can be demonstrated by the Prussian blue reaction (Fig. 77–22). In normal animals, a rare siderocyte may be found in peripheral blood and a small percentage of marrow reticulocytes.

Deiss et al. (1966) have defined two types of siderocytes in animals that are separable on the basis of pathogenic mechanism, behavior of cells, and siderotic granules. One type of siderocyte is not demonstrated by Romanowsky stains; a second type, Pappenheimer bodies, includes siderotic granules that are associated with mitochondria and appear as blue-black aggregates with Wright's stain (Fig. 77–23). The Pappenheimer body may be confused with basophilic stippling.

A sideroblast is a nucleated red cell in which siderotic granules may be demonstrated in the cytoplasm (Fig. 77–24). In man, 30 to 90 per cent of developing nucleated red cells in bone marrow contain a few small, randomly dispersed siderotic granules. Abnormal siderotic granules are large and more numerous, assuming a perinuclear ring or collar around at least three fourths of the nucleus (an abnormally ringed sideroblast). In these situations, a population of normochromic red cells appear in the peripheral blood. The association of abnormal nucleated sideroblasts in the marrow and the dimorphic peripheral blood combination of hypochromic and normochromic erythrocytes indicates a sideroachrestic anemia (Bjorkman, 1956).

Sideroblasts in man are both hereditary and acquired. The acquired sideroblastic anemias have been classified as primary and secondary. The latter type of anemia is seen in association with a large range of disorders and drug toxicities of man (Harris and Kellermeyer, 1970).

Function Tests

Quantitative measurement of erythropoiesis requires the simultaneous measurement of red cell total volume, rate of production, and life span. In clinical veterinary medicine, precise measurements are usually neither practical nor necessary to patient management. Analysis of bone marrow function is, however, essential in anemia diagnosis and evaluation.

The first step in anemia assessment is an evaluation of erythroid marrow production and red blood cell destruction characteristics. The anemia caused by decreased bone marrow production can be separated from that associated with increased bone marrow production. In cases of erythroid hyperplasia of bone marrow, effective erythropoiesis must be differentiated from ineffective erythropoiesis.

Production Measurements. In the majority of clinical conditions of the dog and cat, the reticulocyte or polychromatophile count and the bone marrow may be used to define production and destruction patterns.

Table 77–6. Reticulocyte Maturation Correction Figures

Packed Cell Volume (Percentage)	Maturation Time in Days
45	1.0
35	1.5
25	2.0
15	2.5

Adapted from Finch, C. A., "The Red Cell Manual." University of Washington, Seattle, 1969.

Studies of plasma iron turnover, percentage of utilization, and iron storage provide additional valuable data.

RETICULOCYTE COUNT. The reticulocyte is a young erythrocyte with demonstrable RNA precipitated on red cell stroma by use of vital stains (Figs. 77–25 and 77–26).

Brecher's (1949) procedure for reticulocyte counts is to mix EDTA anticoagulated blood with a 0.5 per cent saline solution of new methylene blue (color index No. 52030) in equal amounts in a test tube or pipette. After 10 to 15 minutes of incubation, the mixture is shaken and coverslip or conventional smears are made. The smears are counterstained with Wright's stain after ten minutes of air drying. Coverslip smears are superior to conventional glass slide films, because reticulocytes tend to be pulled to the feathered edge on the latter.

Cramer and Lewis (1972) studied the reticulocyte response in cats and described a finely reticulated punctate form of reticulocyte and a heavily reticulated aggregate form. The aggregate form of reticulocyte composes a small portion (0 to 0.4 per cent) of the circulating erythrocyte, while the punctate form predominates (total reticulocyte count 1.4 to 10.8 per cent of erythrocytes).

Reticulocyte preparations stained with new methylene blue applied directly to air-dried blood films and polychromatophilia of Wright-stained smears demonstrate the equivalent of the aggregate form of reticulocyte by the criteria of Cramer and Lewis (1972). The aggregate form gives an accurate assessment of increased erythropoiesis when interpreted in light of relevant factors.

Marked erythropoietin stimulation of the bone marrow, resulting in increased effective erythropoiesis, is associated with a proportionate increase in reticulocytes in the circulation. Heavily reticulated macrocytic erythrocytes released into the circulation one to three days before their maturation under conditions of marked erythropoietin stimulation are called *shift reticulocytes*. A correction for this phenomenon of marrow reticulocyte "shift" is made for man. Corresponding factual data are not available for the dog and cat, although subjective correction is frequently made.

DOG RETICULOCYTE RESPONSE. The polychromatophilic erythrocyte of Wright-stained smears is comparable to the aggregate form of reticulocyte in the dog and cat (Laber et al., 1974). The erythrocyte-production index based on the polychromatophilic erythrocyte for the dog is the same as that based on reticulocytes (Tables 77–6 and 77–7). Following significant blood loss by phlebotomy, a mean reticulocytosis of 4.0 per cent (SD ± 3.4 per cent) was found (Fig. 77–27). Thus, considerable variation between dogs is possible and significant anemia (PCV 30) may not effect significant reticulocytosis in all dogs.

CAT RETICULOCYTE RESPONSE. The morphology of cat reticulocytes has been described. The aggregate reticulocyte of the cat (Fig. 77–28) has been shown to correspond in number to polychromasia or to reticulocytes (Alsaker et al., 1977). The punctate reticulocyte response was similar to that observed by Cramer and Lewis (1972).

Recently, Fan et al. (1978) further characterized the reticulocyte response of the cat following experimental acute blood loss.

Table 77–7. Erythrocyte Production Level Scored on the Basis of Reticulocyte or Polychromatophil Erythrocyte Percentage for Anemic Dogs and Cats

Percentage of Reticulocytes	Degree of Stimulation			
	Normal	*Slight*	*Moderate*	*Marked*
Dog	1	1–4	5–20	21–50
Cat	0–0.4	0.5–2	3–4	5.0

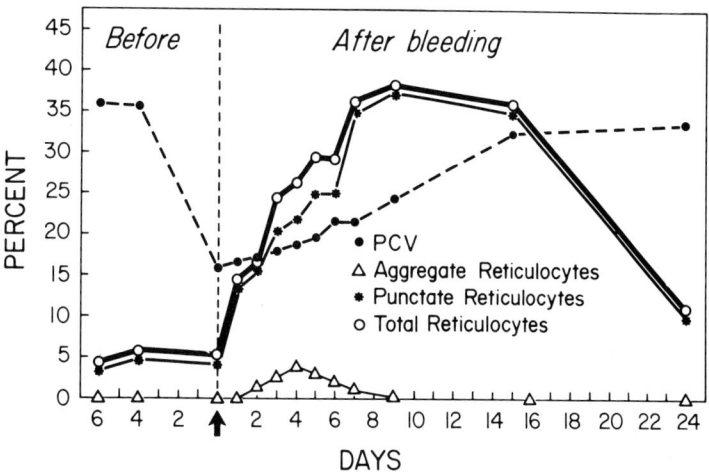

Figure 77–27. Comparison of aggregate reticulocyte count (including 1 standard deviation) to both the polychromatophilic cell count on Wright's-stained smears and the reticulocyte count, using new methylene blue, as described by Schalm (1965). Arrow indicates day of phlebotomy. (From Alsaker, R. D., et al.: J.A.V.M.A. *170*:39, 1977. Used with permission of author and publisher.)

The heavily reticulated erythrocyte response was detectable when 30 per cent or 45 per cent of the blood volume was removed. Aggregate reticulocytes were not increased to clinically significant levels when 15 per cent of the blood volume was removed. It was concluded that the punctate reticulocyte is not a manifestation of prolonged maturation as previously suggested (Cramer and Lewis, 1972) but is a true indicator of bone marrow response.

Fán et al. (1978) studied the effect of epinephrine stimulation on reticulocyte numbers and erythrocyte parameters. The PCV increased 26 per cent and the total reticulocytes 66 per cent with comparable increases in the subtypes.

The reporting of reticulocytes in absolute values is useful and proper. However, in order to report absolute values, total erythrocyte counts are necessary. Expression of reticulocyte values as a percentage is valid and must be interpreted in light of the PCV, state of hydration, and sampling conditions.

THE REGENERATIVE RESPONSE. The reticulocyte or polychromatophilic erythrocyte response is the best single test for evaluation of the level of increased erythrocyte production. The introduction of the larger young erythrocyte results in anisocytosis of a degree comparable to the production level. Nucleated red blood cells and Howell-Jolly bodies occur in similar relative proportions.

The presence of anisocytosis, nucleated red cells, or Howell-Jolly bodies in the circulation in the absence of proportionate

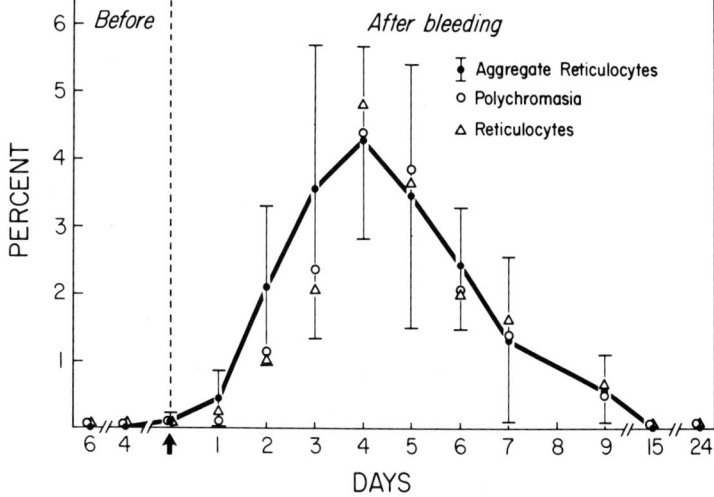

Figure 77–28. Changes in the mean PCV (5 cats) and the aggregate and punctate reticulocyte counts in blood smears stained by Brecher's (1949) method. Arrow indicates day of phlebotomy.

numbers of reticulocytes or polychromatophilic erythrocytes does not indicate accelerated erythropoiesis. Anisocytosis may accompany, for example, macrocytic anemia, spherocytic anemia, iron-deficiency anemia, and myeloproliferative disorders. The presence of nucleated red blood cells and Howell-Jolly bodies also reflects the degree of integrity of the microcirculation and the presence of extramedullary erythropoiesis. For these reasons, the regenerative signs (signs of increased erythrocyte production) are interpretable when viewed collectively and may lead to misdiagnosis when viewed singularly.

BONE MARROW. Biopsy of bone marrow from sites of active erythropoiesis is accomplished by aspiration or core biopsy. Techniques of bone marrow biopsy have been reviewed (Perman et al., 1974). Aspiration biopsy allows a practical clinical approach to evaluation of erythrocyte production. The sites of biopsy (ileum, femur, rib, or sternebrae) are selected for known activity in the normal animal.

Quantitation on aspiration biopsy is limited to subjective evaluation of cell density and inspection of unit particles of bone marrow. The marrow aspirate is evaluated for megakaryocyte number, abnormal cells, maturation patterns of red and white blood cells, and the ratio of erythroid to myeloid cells. Erythroid hyperplasia with a commensurate reticulocyte response indicates effective erythropoiesis. On the other hand, erythroid hyperplasia without a commensurate reticulocytosis indicates ineffective erythropoiesis.

Erythroid hypoplasia on marrow aspirate requires careful evaluation of unit particles for assessment of overall cellularity. A decrease in fat spaces indicates a hyperplastic bone marrow, while unit particles composed mainly of fat spaces indicate bone marrow hypoplasia. The erythroid to myeloid ratio estimate or count determines the final assessment. More definitive bone marrow evaluation is obtained by tissue biopsy using the Jamshidi (Jamshidi and Swaim, 1971), Conrad-Crosby (Conrad and Crosby, 1961), or Westerman-Jensen biopsy needles (Ellis et al., 1964). The tissue biopsy specimens are processed for histopathologic examination. Tissue biopsy should be done on all low cellularity bone marrow as judged from aspirate biopsy. The most hypercellular bone marrows at times yield low cellularity aspirates or "dry" taps.

Tests of Iron Metabolism

Serum Iron (SI). Limited studies on serum iron have been done on dogs and cats. Kaneko (1980) finds the serum iron level for dogs to range from 94 to 122 $\mu g/dl$ (mean 108) and from 68 to 215 (140) $\mu g/dl$ for cats. Lombardi used mongrel dogs with low mean PCV (36 per cent ± five per cent) in his study and found the SI for dogs to be 161 ± 44 $\mu g/dl$. Harvey (1981) gives SI values of 149 (84 to 233) $\mu g/dl$.

Unbound Iron Binding Capacity (UIBC). The UIBC is measured by the amount of iron that plasma can bind and is expressed as $\mu g/dl$. Kaneko (1981) gives UIBC values of 170 to 222 (200) $\mu g/dl$ for dogs and 105 to 205 (150) $\mu g/dl$ for cats. Harvey (1981) gives slightly high UIBC values for dogs: 243 (142 to 393) $\mu g/dl$.

Total Iron Binding Capacity (TIBC). Serum iron represents the portion of tranfusion that is bound to iron, and UIBC represents the unbound plasma transferrin that can combine. The sum equals the TIBC. Harvey (1981) gives 391 (284 to 572) $\mu g/dl$ as the TIBC for dogs. The per cent saturation of transferrin can then be calculated as 39.3 (19.6 to 59.3).

Bone Marrow Iron. About one-half of the total body iron is in the form of hemosiderin. Prussian blue stain of the bone marrow demonstrates this iron storage compartment. Kaneko (1980) indicates the normal amount to be 1+ to 2+ on a 0 to 4+ scale.

Serum Ferritin. Ferritin is, next to hemoglobin, the most abundant iron-containing protein and is the principal labile iron storage form. Measurement of serum ferritin gives an accurate and convenient appraisal of storage iron and thus provides a means of distinguishing iron deficiency anemia from other anemias with low serum iron and increased storage iron pools. Serum ferritin values have been reviewed by Kaneko (1980). Pollack et al. (1977) reported mean values of 24 ng/ml (7.05 to 7.5 ng/ml), about one-third the normal human value. In recent studies of humans, Krause and Stole (1980) found that serum ferritin was useful in distinguishing the iron-deficient state from other disorders associated with low serum iron and low saturation of transferrin. However, a low number of iron-deficient patients had normal ferritin levels. These individuals had liver disease or neoplasms of hemic tissue.

Ferrokinetics. The mean ^{59}Fe clearance half-time in the dog, determined by Kaneko and Cornelius (1970) to be 56 minutes (range, 39 to 63), is intermediate between values found by Lombordi (1973) and by Naets and Heuse (1964). The value determined by Quaife and Odland (1967) was much higher (85 ± 14 minutes). Plasma-iron turnover rate in the dog was determined to be 2.64 ± 0.99 mg per 100 ml per day by Lombardi and 1.96 mg per 100 ml per day (range 1.71 to 2.22) by Kaneko and Cornelius.

Destruction Measurements. Measurement of red cell destruction is more difficult than are production measurements. Accurate assessment of blood volume and changes in packed red cell volume over a period of time gives an estimate of the destruction index. For example, if production is increased, based on assessment of the regenerative response, and the packed-cell volume is falling over several days, the destruction index is greater than the production rate.

The rate of destruction considers the life span of red blood cells. Shorter red cell life span leads to increased red blood production. Measurement of the life span of red blood cells is of value in chronic hemolytic anemia and in hemolytic crisis, when the packed-cell volume is changing.

RED CELL LIFE SPAN. Red cell life span measurement may be accomplished by *in vitro* labeling of a red cell cohort with ^{51}Cr or [32]p isotope and observing the disappearance curve after infusion (Cline and Berlin, 1962). The ^{51}Cr technique is most commonly used but does not give true life span measurements because elution of label prior to cell death necessitates the application of correction factors (Mollison and Veall, 1955).

Destruction of red blood cells may be intravascular or extravascular. In extravascular red blood cell destruction, the products of hemolysis in reticuloendothelial cells may be measured by the icterus index, indirect bilirubin, and fecal urobilinogen levels. Fecal urobilinogen determination is sel-

dom done, and the more commonly done urine urobilinogen provides little additional information over indirect bilirubin measurement. Intravascular hemolysis may be determined by measuring plasma hemoglobin, urine hemoglobin, urine hemosiderin, blood heptoglobin, and blood methemalbumin. In many clinical cases, gross observation will separate intravascular hemolysis from extravascular hemolysis. Frequently, examination of bone marrow phagocytic cells for erythrophagia will distinguish the method of destruction.

Red Blood Cell Metabolism Defects. Disturbances in red blood cell metabolism may be classified according to the mechanism and site of action, i.e., metabolic defects, membrane defects, or extravascular abnormality.

Metabolic Enzyme Abnormalities. The principal metabolic abnormality of red cell metabolism is hereditary pyruvate kinase deficiency of the basenji (Ewing, 1969b; Tasker et al., 1969; Searcy et al., 1971) and the beagle (Prasse et al., 1974). Enzymatic defects require sophisticated research techniques for assay and characterization of the deficiency. Several other enzyme deficiencies have been described in man.

Immunologic Tests

Membrane Abnormalities. A hereditary spherocytosis of man is the result of an imperfect red cell membrane (Dacie, 1962). The occurrence of hereditary spherocytosis of the dog is probable, considering the frequency of spherocytic anemia. Differential diagnosis of hereditary and acquired spherocytic hemolytic anemia is based on differences in osmotic fragility of red blood cells, autohemolysis, and immunologic demonstration of membrane antigen or extracellular antibody.

Autoimmune Defects. The interaction of a membrane antigen and extracellular antibody can result in cell lysis, phagocytosis, or intravascular agglutination of red cells. Antibodies directed against RBC belong to either the IgG (warm reacting antibody) or IgM (cold reacting antibody). The incomplete nonagglutinating antibodies (IgG) and complement cause injury to red blood membranes, including the sphering phenomena (Avolt et al., 1973; Halliwell, 1978). The spherocytes are selectively sequestered by the microcirculation of the spleen and phagocytized by reticuloendothelial lining cells (Costea, 1972).

PRINCIPLES OF THERAPY

The goal of diagnostic efforts in the anemic patient is to establish cause so that specific therapy can be instituted. In those instances in which a definitive diagnosis is not established, the information obtained still enables a logical therapeutic approach. In this section, therapy that can be employed for anemias of various causes will be reviewed. Fixed-dose combination hematinics marketed for use in anemic cats and dogs, which are sometimes indiscriminately used, will not be considered.

TRANSFUSION

The objectives of transfusion for anemia are to sustain life when threatened by reduction in the red cell mass, and to maintain circulating hemoglobin levels that ameliorate most clinical signs. Patients with chronic nonregenerative, nonhemolytic anemia are likely to derive substantial benefit from a single therapeutic transfusion for little more than three weeks, even if the transfused red cells are relatively fresh and all other influencing factors such as anticoagulant, storage, and mechanical handling are optimal.

Indications. Replacement of red cell mass deficit is indicated when the magnitude of the deficit approaches that associated with clinical signs. Arbitrarily, when the PCV of the dog is 15 per cent or less (hemoglobin 5 gm per 100 ml), transfusion is indicated. Cats appear to tolerate a greater red cell deficit than dogs and may not require transfusion until the PCV is 12 per cent or less (hemoglobin, 4 gm per 100 ml).

Contraindication. The transfusion of incompatible blood to an anemic patient is contraindicated. Incompatible blood, however, may be lifesaving in instances of acute hemorrhage when the emergency precludes the determination of compatibility. Intraspecies transfusion is always contraindicated because of reactions and failure of erythrocyte survival.

Transfusions are to be avoided in cats and dogs with autoimmune hemolytic anemia, because transfused red cells are likely to be rapidly hemolyzed and add to the existing burden. Only when the degree of anemia is apt to cause death should patients with autoimmune hemolytic anemia be transfused.

The degree to which transfusions further suppress erythropoiesis in anemic patients is not exactly known. Unless replacement therapy maintains hemoglobin levels near normal, however, the stimulus for erythropoiesis (tissue hypoxia) is present. Deliberate attempts at suppression of erythropoiesis by transfusion in human thalassemia patients require maintenance of hemoglobin above 10 gm per 100 ml (Beard et al., 1969). Transfusion is usually used to maintain anemic cats and dogs; therefore, it is not likely to significantly suppress erythropoiesis.

Collection and Storage of Blood. Three anticoagulants are most commonly used for the collection of donor blood: acid citrate dextrose (ACD), citrate phosphate dextrose (CPD), and heparin. The latter is most commonly used for feline blood.

Blood collected in commercial glass or plastic containers with predetermined amounts of either ACD or CPD anticoagulant should be filled to the appropriate level so that excess anticoagulant is not present. The dextrose present in these two anticoagulants has a red cell preservative effect. Canine whole blood collected in these solutions should be maintained at a temperature between 1°C and 6°C (32°F and 43°F). If properly collected and stored, blood can be used at any time within 21 days. After 21 days of storage, at least 70 per cent of transfused canine erythrocytes survive 24 hours after administration (Eisenbrandt and Smith, 1973).

Although the dextrose present in either ACD or CPD anticoagulant helps maintain the viability of stored erythrocytes, canine red cell 2,3-DPG concentration decreases during storage to less than half normal values at 21 days after collection. The decreased erythrocyte 2,3-DPG concentration results in a shift of the oxyhemoglobin dissociation curve to the left and decreased oxygen delivery to tissues. Within three to four hours after transfusion, the 2,3-DPG concentration returns to normal. Transfusion of massive amounts of stored blood, however, may be temporarily associated with inadequate tissue oxygenation because of the high oxygen affinity of the transfused hemoglobin. Eisenbrandt and Smith (1973) have shown that CPD anticoagulant maintains canine erythrocyte 2,3-DPG concentration better than ACD, but the difference is quantitatively small.

Because of the small volumes, feline blood is seldom stored in standard ACD or CPD containers. Instead, a small quantity of heparin is usually drawn into a 35- to 100-ml syringe; blood is withdrawn from the donor cat and immediately administered to the recipient. The amount of heparin used often exceeds that needed and may result in heparinization of the recipient. Heparin, 450 units in six ml of saline, is recommended for the anticoagulation of 100 ml of human blood. Thus, no more than 0.25 ml of standard sodium heparin (1000 USP units per ml) is needed as the anticoagulant for 50 ml of blood. This amount of heparin may be more effective if diluted with three ml of saline for infusion.

Heparin anticoagulant solution lacks dextrose and therefore has no erythrocyte preservative effect. Moreover, its anticoagulant effect is eventually neutralized by thromboplastic and antiheparin materials liberated by cellular elements of the blood. For these reasons, heparinized blood must be used immediately or stored at 1°C to 6°C and used within 48 hours of collection.

Blood Groups and Blood Compatibility. The currently recognized canine erythrocyte antigens (DEA) consist of eight types that have been identified with the use of monospecific sera produced by deliberate isoimmunization. Revisions in nomenclature are outlined in Table 77–8 (Vriesendorp et al., 1973). Of these eight erythrocyte antigens, DEA-1 (old A_1) and DEA-2 (old A_2) are the most reactive. Severe hemolytic reactions are reliably produced when DEA-1 or DEA-2 erythrocytes are transfused to dogs that are normally without these antigens but that have been previously sensitized by transfusion. Because of prior sensitization, recipient dogs will have produced anti-DEA-1 or anti-DEA-1,2 isoantibodies. Naturally occurring anti-DEA-1 and anti-DEA-1,2 isoantibodies (in dogs not previously sensitized by transfusion) have not been detected.

The remaining canine erythrocyte antigens are more weakly reactive in previously

Table 77–8. Nomenclature of Canine Erythrocyte Antigens

New	Old	Population Incidence
DEA-1	A_1	40%
DEA-2	A_2	20%
DEA-3	B	5%
DEA-4	C	98%
DEA-5	D	25%
DEA-6	F	98%
DEA-7	Tr	45%
DEA-8	He	40%

From Ball, R. W.: New knowledge about blood groups in dogs. Proc. Gaines Veterinary Symposium, 1973.

sensitized dogs. Naturally occurring antibodies to some of these erythrocyte antigens do exist, however. Increased rate of destruction of the tranfused erythrocytes rather than transfusion reaction can result from inappropriate transfusion (Swisher and Young, 1961).

Based on current knowledge of canine erythrocyte antigen systems, some recommendations regarding the transfusion of erythrocytes are possible. Random transfusions should be avoided, primarily because of the risk of sensitizations and subsequent severe transfusion reaction, and also because transfused red cells may have a shortened life span. Donor dogs should be blood typed to assure that they do not have DEA-1 and DEA-2. Unfortunately, specific antisera for typing are difficult to obtain. Canine blood typing or use of a DEA-1 and DEA-2 negative donor does not ensure compatibility (Swisher and Young, 1961). Accordingly, cross-matching by standard techniques should be done whenever possible (Swisher and Young, 1961).

Information regarding blood compatibility of cats is not complete. At least three blood groups have been identified and the presence of isoagglutinins has been documented (Holmes, 1953). Until more data are accumulated, cat blood should be cross-matched prior to transfusion when possible.

Products for Transfusion. When blood is tranfused for its temporary therapeutic benefit to the anemic patient (as compared with the patient with acute blood loss or hemorrhagic shock), the need is for the oxygen-carrying capacity of hemoglobin

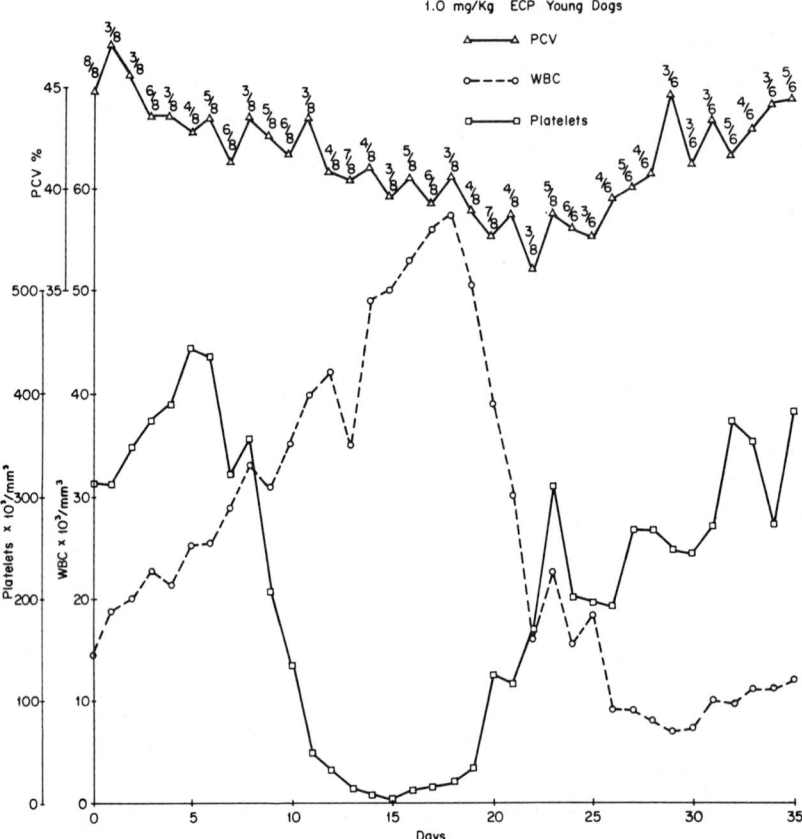

Figure 77–29. Mean PCV, WBC, and platelet counts on young dogs (<2 years of age) receiving an intramuscular injection of 1.0 mg/kg of β-estradiol cypionate.

rather than blood-volume expansion provided by the use of whole blood. Anemia, defined as deficit of red cell mass only, is not an indication for the transfusion of whole blood. The transfusion of plasma present in whole blood may be contraindicated, as well as unnecessary. Further, the transfused cells appear as spherocytes in the recipient's blood and may lead to diagnostic confusion.

Since patients with chronic anemia are deficient in erythrocytes, packed or sedimented red cells are the replacement products of choice. Packed red cells are separated from whole blood by centrifugation, whereas sedimented red cells are separated by gravity. Centrifugation of stored whole blood requires equipment not usually available in veterinary practice, but sedimented red cells can be obtained by aspiration of plasma with needle and syringe. First, whole blood is allowed to remain undisturbed for at least 24 hours. A three-inch 20-gauge needle with attached 50- to 100-ml syringe is then used to withdraw the plasma. Erythrocytes can be separated by sedimentation and aspiration up to 21 days after collection. Another means of obtaining sedimented red cells is to store blood containers upside down. The transfusion can then be stopped when the sedimented red cells have been administered, leaving the plasma in the container. The hematocrit of sedimented red cells approaches 70 per cent. Sedimented red cells are administered according to the method used for whole blood.

Dose of Blood. The dose of blood is often arbitrarily stated to be 10 to 20 ml per kg of body weight. This arbitrary dose is illogical, because hemoglobin concentration may not be increased to the desired level. Bild (1959) has suggested that the dose of blood to be administered should be estimated by calculating the patient's hemoglobin deficit. His method of estimation can be easily modified to calculate the mass of hemoglobin necessary to increase the patient's hemoglobin concentration to 7 gm per 100 ml. The volume of transfused plasma is ignored in these estimations and can be minimized by the administration of sedimented red cells rather than whole blood.

Administration of Blood. Whole blood and sedimented red cells are usually administered intravenously. The cephalic, recurrent tarsal, and jugular veins are most often used. The rate of intravenous administration of blood to an anemic patient is usually less than ten ml per kg per hour. The first portion of the transfusion is usually administered more slowly, and the procedure is stopped if urticaria develops. Blood need not be warmed unless it is to be administered more rapidly than 50 ml per kg per hour.

The rate of administration of blood of plasma relates to the time sequence of the development of the deficit. Following rapid blood loss, blood transfusions need to be rapid. Conversely, a prolonged severe anemia is associated with marked systemic effects on the cardiovascular system. In such cases, the blood tranfusion should proceed by small increments to prevent cardiac overload. In the classic hookworm puppy, Bild (1959) recommends that fluid administration precede the blood transfusion or be given simultaneously.

In small puppies and kittens, blood is often administered in the medullary canal of a femur. A 20-gauge, 1- to 1.5-inch needle with stylet is preferred. The stylet prevents a core of bone from occluding the needle lumen. If a needle with stylet is not available, standard disposable 20- or 18-gauge needles usually can be used successfully because of the softness of puppy and kitten bone (although occasionally bone will plug the needle). The needle should be directed into the trochanteric fossa of the femur and passed through the cortical and trabecular bone into the medullary cavity. Whole blood or sedimented red cells can then be gravity dripped or injected by syringe. If the infusion is made with a syringe, care must be taken to inject slowly to minimize endosteal pain. The intraosseous administration of blood should be restricted to those small puppies and kittens in which venipunctures cannot be made or maintained because the route has the following disadvantages: slow infusion rate, associated pain, and the possibility of inducing osteomyelitis.

Intraperitoneal transfusions have also been used in puppies and kittens. The fate of erythrocytes transfused by this route into normal dogs has been established (Clark and Woodley, 1959) and suggests that the intraperitoneal route is not useful. In acutely anemic puppies and kittens, however, this route of transfusion has been satisfactory (Thornton, 1974).

Plasma Transfusion and Reactions. Nonautologous (homologous) canine plasma is often incompatible (Bliss et al., 1959; Huggin et al., 1965; Jahn, 1967). As a plasma extender, Bliss and coworkers (1959) found nonautologous canine plasma proteins to be rejected 50 per cent of the time. Intradermal injections of small amounts of test plasma produced a well-marked wheal within minutes. Systemic reaction to incompatible plasma and whole blood may reach severity sufficient to cause death. The reaction is blocked or controlled by antihistamine or corticosteroid administration.

Transfusions for Other Blood Elements. Generalizations regarding the administration and storage of blood to be transfused for increasing the red cell mass do not all hold true for other uses of blood. Platelets do not store well, and for this reason, fresh whole blood is usually transfused to thrombocytopenic dogs and cats. Platelet concentrates used in man are not generally used in animals. Platelet compatibility in dogs is probably linked to tissue antigen (DL-A) rather than to blood groups (Vriesendorp et al., 1973) but is usually ignored. The compatibility of leukocytes is also a function of histocompatibility, but the effectiveness of leukocyte transfusion is equivocal (Boggs, 1974). Transfusion for replacement of deficient coagulation factors must be fresh but need not contain the formed blood elements.

Blood Substitutes. Recent developments in the use of perfluocarbon-polyols indicate the potential for a blood substitute (Zucali et al., 1979). The applicability to the dog and cat on a clinical basis is not known.

SPLENECTOMY

Splenectomy occasionally has been advocated for the therapy of chronic anemia in the cat and dog. In many instances, the term

Table 77–9. Androgenic Anabolic Steroids Used for the Treatment of Aplastic and Other Nongenerative Anemias*

Type of Androgen	Chemical Name (Trivial Name)	Trade Name	Dosage and Route of Administration
17 α-Alkylated androgens	17 α-Methyl-11 β, 17 β-dihydroxy-9 α-fluoro-androst-4-en-3-one (fluoxymesterone)	Halotestin, Ultandren	0.25 to 1 mg/kg/day orally
	17 α-Methyl-17 β-hydroxy-2-hydroxymethylene-5 α-androstan-3-one (oxymetholone)	Ora-Testryl, Adroyd, Anapolon, Anadrol-50	0.25 to 4 mg/kg/day orally
	17 α-Methyl-17 β-hydroxy-5 α-androstane-(3, 2-c)-pyrazole (stanazolol)	Wistrol-V	0.25 to 3 mg/kg/day orally
	17 α-Methyl-17 β-hydroxy-androsta-1, 4-dien-3-one (methandrostenolone)	Dianabol	2 to 10 mg/kg/week intramuscularly 0.25 to 3 mg/kg/day orally
	17 α-Ethyl-17 β-hydroxy-19-norandrost-4-en-3-one (norethandrolone)	Nilevar	0.25 to 3 mg/kg/day orally
Testosterone esters	Testosterone heptanoate (testosterone enanthate)	Delatestryl	4 to 7 mg/kg/week intramuscularly
	Testosterone cyclopentylpropionate (testosterone cypionate)	Depotestosterone	4 to 7 mg/kg/week intramuscularly
	Testosterone ester mixture (phenylpropionate, isocaproate, propionate, decanoate)	Sustanon 250	4 to 7 mg/kg/week intramuscularly
Other non-17 α-alkylated androgens	19-Nortestosterone phenylpropionate (nandrolone phenylpropionate)	Durabolin	1 mg/kg biweekly intramuscularly
	19-Nortestosterone decanoate (nandrolone decanoate)	Deca-Durabolin	1 to 1.5 mg/kg/week intramuscularly
	1-Methyl-17 β-hydroxy-5 α-androst-1-en-3-one acetate (methenolone acetate)	Primobolan	0.25 to 3 mg/kg/day orally

*From Shahidi, N. T.: Androgens and erythropoiesis. N. Engl. J. Med., 289:72, 1973.

hypersplenism has been loosely used by veterinary surgeons to justify splenectomy. Unequivocal indications for splenectomy in the dog or cat are rarely encountered.

Although documentation in cats and dogs is lacking, splenectomy in man may result in substantial improvement and may lessen the transfusion requirements in some chronic hemolytic anemias. One such anemia known to exist in dogs is pyruvate kinase deficiency.

Usually, splenectomy should not be considered for, nor should the diagnosis of hypersplenism be applied to, immune-mediated hemolytic anemia documented by Coombs' test or other immunologic techniques (Jacob, 1972). In these diseases, destruction of antibody-coated erythrocytes is a generalized response of the reticuloendothelial system in which the spleen participates in a nonspecific way. Therapy in these instances should be directed against the inappropriate production of autoantibodies rather than against splenic function.

ANABOLIC ANDROGENIC STEROIDS

The anabolic androgenic steroids are currently regarded as the most useful nonspecific stimulants of erythropoiesis. A clear distinction should be made between their use and the use of glucocorticoids, which have not been shown to have a definite erythropoietic effect. Because of extreme toxicity and ineffectiveness, the use of other chemicals such as cobalt and batyl alcohol has been abandoned.

Most of the anabolic androgenic steroids presently in use are listed in Table 77–9. Of these, stanozolol has been approved for use in cats and dogs; others, especially oxymetholone and testosterone enanthate, are commonly used in these species. The number of available compounds reflects efforts to discover steroids with substantial protein anabolism but without androgenic properties. None is completely devoid of virilizing effect when used in man, but this side effect is not objectionable or obvious in cats and dogs.

Although the erythropoietic activity of the anabolic androgenic steroids is well established, the exact mechanisms of action have not been clarified. Experimental evidence strongly indicates, however, that the administration of these compounds results in an increased production of renal erythropoietic factor and an increase in the pool of erythropoietin-responsive stem cells (Shahidi, 1973). Parker et al. (1972) have reported androgen-induced increase in red cell 2,3-DPG in human patients with chronic renal failure. The magnitude of the increase was such that the unloading of oxygen to the tissues would be greatly enhanced.

The androgenic anabolic steroids are used in disorders such as acquired aplastic anemia, myeloproliferative disorders, and lymphoma with associated nonregenerative anemia in cats and dogs. Although adequate data are lacking, it appears that about one third of canine and feline patients show erythropoietic response to these compounds. This response route is comparable to that documented in man (Sanchez-Medal et al., 1969; Shahidi, 1973).

Data from dogs with the anemia of renal failure are inconclusive, but because of the lack of extrarenal production of erythropoietin, dogs are less likely to respond erythropoietically. However, androgenic anabolic steroids increase erythrocyte 2,3-DPG concentration in humans with anemia of renal failure (Parker et al., 1972), and their use is justified in anemic cats and dogs with renal failure.

Nutrition. It has long been established that common dietary factors influence hemoglobin production in dogs (Hahn and Whipple, 1939; Robscheit-Robbins et al., 1940). These studies were conducted in dogs made anemic by bleeding. Meat diets were more effective than plant and animal products low in iron. The quality and completeness of the diet for the anemic patient is of greatest importance.

Vitamins. The essential vitamins for hemoglobin synthesis are pyridoxine, riboflavin, and niacin. These vitamins have a metabolic role as coenzymes in the synthesis of the hemoglobin molecule. Vitamin B_{12} and folic acid are necessary to the synthesis of purine and pyrimidine bases, constituents of DNA and RNA.

Minerals. The dog and cat require iron and copper for hemoglobin synthesis. (Copper is a cofactor for the enzyme delta-aminolevulinic acid dehydrase necessary to heme synthesis.)

Mineral-Vitamin Therapy. Combination drug therapy does not have a place in the management of the anemic patient unless a need is established. Some water soluble vitamins have a fast turnover, i.e., riboflavin, niacin, and pyridoxine. Vitamin B_{12} is stored for long periods and folic acid for shorter periods. Except for iron deficiency anemia, iron therapy is not indicated.

DISORDERS OF THE ERYTHRON

POLYCYTHEMIA

Increased numbers of circulating red blood cells is termed polycythemia. It may be relative, in which case the condition is due to a decrease in quantity of blood plasma, or it may be absolute, in which case there is an actual increase in the number of red cells (Table 77–10). Although this approach to classification is convenient, it does not consider the concept of *total red cell volume*, which is necessary to differential diagnosis.

Relative Polycythemia (Hemoconcentration)

The loss of plasma results in hemoconcentration of red blood cells and may occur as the result of diverse mechanisms. Packed red cell volumes of 70 per cent and over are recorded. The degree of polycythemia is based on the increase of PCV above normal. For young dogs and cats, and obese animals with normally low PCV, polycythemia may occur secondary to fluid loss of plasma shift. In dehydration, the rapid loss of plasma results in a relative increase in PCV and total plasma protein (TPP). Normal values for the patient in question or animals of comparable breed, age, and sex must form the basis for interpretation. Disproportionate increases in erythrocytes and plasma proteins may lead to erroneous conclusions.

Decreased plasma volume may be the

Table 77–10. Classification of Polycythemia

Relative Polycythemia (Hemoconcentration)
  Secondary to fluid or plasma shift
  Secondary to splenic contraction
Absolute Polycythemia
  Primary
    Polycythemia vera
  Secondary
    Caused by hypoxemia
    Caused by hormones or chemicals

result of total body salt deficit or a fluid shift from intravascular to extravascular spaces. Increased hydrostatic pressure in veins and capillaries or increased vascular permeability, as with anoxia or anaphylaxis, may cause a shift of fluid to the extravascular space.

In hyperadrenocorticism, a decrease in plasma volume with a normal red cell mass may give rise to increased packed-cell volumes. In hypoadrenocorticism, a relative polycythemia may be present owing to shift in extracellular water and dehydration. Correction of the dehydration may uncover a mild to marked anemia (Keeton et al., 1972). Polycythemia may also occur secondary to splenic contraction. The occurrence of splenic contraction at the time of blood sampling for hematologic examination may result in a 10 to 15 per cent rise in PCV. This phenomenon is less noticeable in the cat than in the dog. In the patient that is visibly excited at the time of sampling, splenic contraction should be considered in the interpretation of the hemogram. The addition of sequestered red cells from the spleen is not accompanied by an increase in plasma proteins.

Splenic contraction may result in PCV as high as 55 to 60 per cent in healthy, active, adult dogs. This is particularly true for the small and toy breeds of dogs that tend to have PCV values in the high-normal range. Splenic contraction also may cause the release of sequestered reticulocytes, so that a mild reticulocytosis (one to two per cent) occurs.

Absolute Polycythemia

An increase in total hemoglobin–red cell mass with a plasma volume near normal is absolute polycythemia (Harris and Kellermeyer, 1970). Absolute polycythemia may be classified as primary or secondary.

Polycythemia vera is a primary polycythemia of unknown cause that is a chronic hematologic disease of erythropoietic tissue classified as a myeloproliferative disorder. The disease is rare in cats and dogs. McGrath (1974) reported three canine cases and reviewed five previously reported cases (Cole, 1954; Donovan and Loeb, 1959; Miller, 1968; Carb, 1969; Bush and Frankhauser, 1972). Reed et al. (1970) reported the occurrence of polycythemia vera in a cat.

There are insufficient data for substantial

conclusions regarding breed, age, and sex predisposition of this disease in cats and dogs. The age of affected dogs ranges from one to nine years.

Erythema of the mucous membranes was present in all eight of the reported dogs with polycythemia vera. Other common clinical signs are polydipsia and polyuria, hemorrhage, and signs referable to neurologic or neuromuscular disorders. In contrast to the clinical features of the disease in man, splenomegaly and thrombosis have not been commonly detected in dogs, whereas polydipsia and polyuria are not reported in man. The relationship between the observed clinical signs and the absolute increase in red cell mass of polycythemia vera has not been clearly established but is generally thought to be linked to increased blood viscosity.

The PCV of affected dogs and cats ranges from 70 to 80 per cent. The total RBC mass was increased to an average of twice normal in the five dogs (McGrath, 1974) and one cat (Reed et al., 1970) in which it was determined. The blood volume was also increased but to a lesser extent. RBC ^{51}Cr survival times in one affected cat and one affected dog were normal, but RBC ^{58}Fe incorporation studies indicated accelerated erythropoiesis. Plasma protein and platelet concentrations are usually normal, but a leukocytosis is often present.

Therapy for polycythemia vera is usually initiated by the withdrawal of 20 to 30 ml per kg of body weight of blood at two- to four-day intervals until the PCV is within normal limits. Based on the few reports of therapeutic trials, repeat phlebotomy is usually necessary at two- to three-month intervals. In addition, myelosuppression with ^{32}p is used in man, but reports of ^{32}p use in dogs are meager (McGrath, 1974). Busulfan and other chemical myelosuppressive agents have also been employed in man and dog.

Secondary polycythemia can occur as a result of hypoxemia or as the result of excessive endogenous production of compounds with erythropoietin-like activity. Secondary polycythemia can also be experimentally produced by the administration of certain chemicals.

The secondary polycythemia caused by hypoxemia is mediated by increased release of erythropoietin by the kidney. The hypox-

emia may be generalized or renal, but it must be sustained to stimulate polycythemia. The principal forms of hypoxia (anoxia) producing polycythemia are hypoxic (anoxic), stagnant, and histotoxic.

Hypoxic hypoxia may result from environmental or *in vivo* factors. Reduced oxygen tension of high altitude causes mild polycythemia with increases in PCV of 15 to 20 per cent in dogs (Thomas and Kittrell, 1966). Definitive data are lacking for the cat.

Another cause of hypoxic hypoxia is interference with oxygenation because of obstructive changes in major air passages, or parenchymatous damage at the alveolus, or both. The secondary polycythemia that occurs as the result of severe pulmonary disease is usually mild, and the PCV returns to normal if the primary cause is corrected.

Congenital heart disease characterized by right-to-left shunting of blood and consequent hypoxemia result in secondary polycythemia (Ettinger and Suter, 1970). The polycythemia may be profound (Legendre et al., 1974).

Stagnant hypoxia due to circulatory insufficiencies, such as congestive heart failure or heartworm disease, can cause secondary polycythemia. The increase in PCV is usually slight but is often accompanied by mild reticulocytosis and the appearance of orthochromatophilic normoblasts in peripheral blood. In the late stages of uncompensated cardiac disease, the PCV is variable. Polycythemia should not be considered a reliable sign of cardiac insufficiency.

Histotoxic hypoxia can occur as the result of methemoglobin formation. This compound is incapable of carrying oxygen. Brownish blood and cyanosis rather than polycythemia, however, are the most prominent clinical features. Normally, hemoglobin iron is maintained in the ferrous (reduced) state. Methemoglobinemia occurs when hemoglobin iron is in the ferric (oxidized) state and may result from oxidant compounds such as nitrites and certain analgesics and sulfonamides or from deficiency of enzymes necessary to maintain hemoglobin in the reduced state. Harvey et al. (1974) reported methemoglobin reductase deficiency. Approximately 30 per cent of the dog's total hemoglobin was methemoglobin. The only clinical signs were brownish mucous membranes and blood. Methemo-globinemia and cyanosis have been observed in cats to which acetaminophen was administered (Finco et al., 1974), and it has been observed with other oxidant drugs. Heinz-body anemia also resulted.

Secondary polycythemia as the result of excess production of erythropoietin or substances with erythropoietin-like activity occurs in man. Conditions associated with secondary polycythemia in man and thought to be mediated by such substances include renal cysts, hydronephrosis, polycystic kidneys, and neoplasms of the kidney, ovary, adrenals, cerebellum, and liver (Seim, 1970). Scott and Patnaik (1972) reported polycythemia secondary to renal carcinoma in two dogs. The polycythemia disappeared after excision of the neoplastic kidney.

Polycythemia secondary to the administration of testosterone or to the androgenic anabolic steroids is theoretically possible but not of practical concern. The administration of cobalt is known to cause secondary polycythemia by interfering with certain enzymes necessary for oxygen transport and utilization (Levy et al., 1950).

ANEMIA

Anemia is a decrease in PCV or hemoglobin resulting in decreased oxygen-carrying capacity of the blood. Classifications of the types of anemia have been based on red cell morphology, etiology, or mechanism of altered red cell production.

Anemia is a clinical sign of disease, not a disease per se. A logical approach to evaluation uses all clinical and laboratory data available. The broad classification in Table 77–11 combines morphology and pathophysiology to form a basis for discussing disorders of erythropoiesis characterized by anemia. It is obvious that categorically not all blood-loss anemias are regenerative.

Table 77–11. Classification of Anemia

Regenerative Anemia: Anemia associated with increased red cell production
  Blood loss
  Blood destruction
Nongenerative Anemia: Anemia associated with decreased red cell production
  Nutritional
  Hypoplastic and aplastic

Consideration must be given to time sequence, nutritional considerations, and biological variations.

Since several chapters deal with diseases in which anemia occurs, discussion of these disorders will be brief in this chapter.

Effects of Anemia. The pathophysiologic basis for clinical signs of anemia exists regardless of the causative disorder. The development of these signs depends upon the following factors: (1) the degree of anemia, (2) the rapidity of development, (3) changes in blood volume, (4) cardiopulmonary functions, (5) the age of the animal, (6) the activity of the patient, and (7) the causative disorder.

In general, all of these effects relate to the ability of blood to transport oxygen to the tissues. The supply of oxygen to the tissues depends on several factors, including oxygenation of hemoglobin, transport, and tissue utilization. Hemoglobin carries 1.36 ml of oxygen per gram at complete saturation. Assuming complete saturation of hemoglobin with oxygen, arteriovenous blood-oxygen differences reflect tissue removal of oxygen. For man, six ml of oxygen per 100 ml of blood is removed by the tissues. Thus, five gm of hemoglobin per deciliter would be necessary to supply tissue oxygen needs, provided hemoglobin was the sole factor in oxygen delivery.

Clinical experience indicates that in the dog and cat with chronic uncomplicated anemia, four to five gm of hemoglobin per deciliter provides sufficient oxygen-carrying capacity for tissues in animals at rest. Compensatory changes allow for survival of cats with hemoglobin concentrations as low as two gm per 100 deciliter. In uncomplicated chronic anemia with mild hemoglobin deficit, clinical signs of anemia may be evident upon exercise. Lack of endurance may be observed in working dogs, but in less active animals, clinical signs may not become apparent until anemia is marked. Moderately anemic animals may exhibit difficulties when exercised or engaged in play. Tiring and collapse are frequent complaints. A frequent complaint is seizure, a mistaken interpretation of cerebral hypoxia. Severely anemic animals, on the other hand, may be presented with no obvious outward sign to the owner that a serious problem exists. The clinical signs most frequently encountered in anemia regardless of cause are outlined in Table 77–12.

Table 77–12. Clinical Signs of Anemia

Digestive
  Anorexia, diarrhea or constipation
Neuromuscular
  Weakness, fainting, reduced performance
  Listlessness, depression
  Sensitivity to cold
  Lesions in optic fundus
Cardiopulmonary
  Increased rate and depth of respiration
  Dyspnea on exercise
  Tachycardia
  Increased arterial pulsation
  Systolic (anemic) murmur
  Cardiac enlargement
Integumentary
  Pale mucous membranes
  Lack of care to hair coat in cats

Anemias Associated with Increased Red Cell Production

The regenerative anemias are characterized by the appearance in the circulation of reticulocyte-polychromatophilic cells in numbers commensurate with the degree of anemia and the stage of the disease.

Blood-Loss (Posthemorrhagic) Anemia. Blood-loss anemia differs in affected animals principally according to the disease process, the rapidity of loss (peracute, acute, or chronic), and the location of the hemorrhage (body exterior, cavities, or tissues).

PERACUTE BLOOD LOSS. Very rapid blood loss to the body exterior is manifested as hypovolemia, and not hemorrhagic anemia. It is only after restoration of plasma volume that decreases in PCV may be observed. Blood-volume restoration, however, begins immediately after significant hemorrhage. In dogs, one fifth of the blood volume with a PCV of approximately 80 per cent is added to the circulation with splenic contraction. Fluid shifts from extravascular spaces contribute to plasma restoration. With adequate fluid intake and cessation of the hemorrhage, apparent blood-volume restoration and appropriate decrease in PCV are observed within 12 to 24 hours. Figures 77–30 and 77–31 illustrate the sequence of cellular responses to controlled phlebotomy. The amount of blood withdrawn on three successive days was 20 per cent of the blood volume based on 88 ml per kg of body weight. Assuming that there was no splenic reserve and minimal contribution from new red cell production, a calculated drop in PCV of 50 per cent was expected. The contribution of splenic blood is apparent, since the low mean PCV was greater than 60 per cent of base-line values.

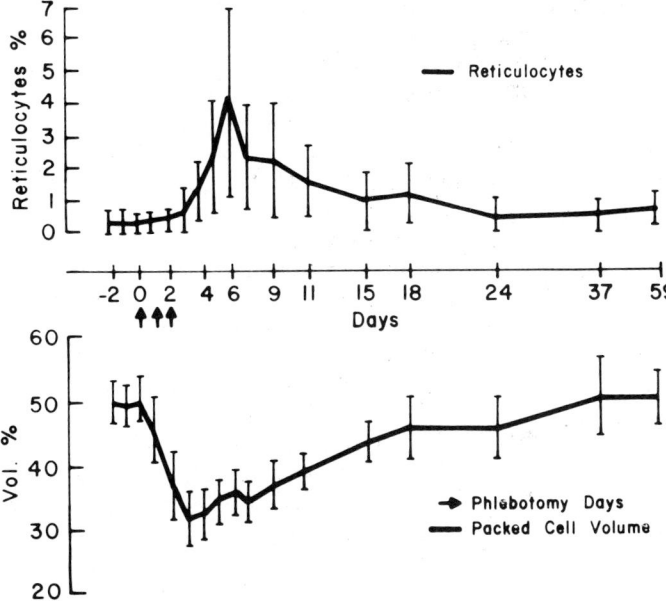

Red Blood Cell Response to Controlled Bleeding in Dogs

Figure 77–30. Changes in the PCV and reticulocyte numbers in response to acute hemorrhage of the dog.

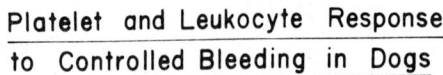

Platelet and Leukocyte Response to Controlled Bleeding in Dogs

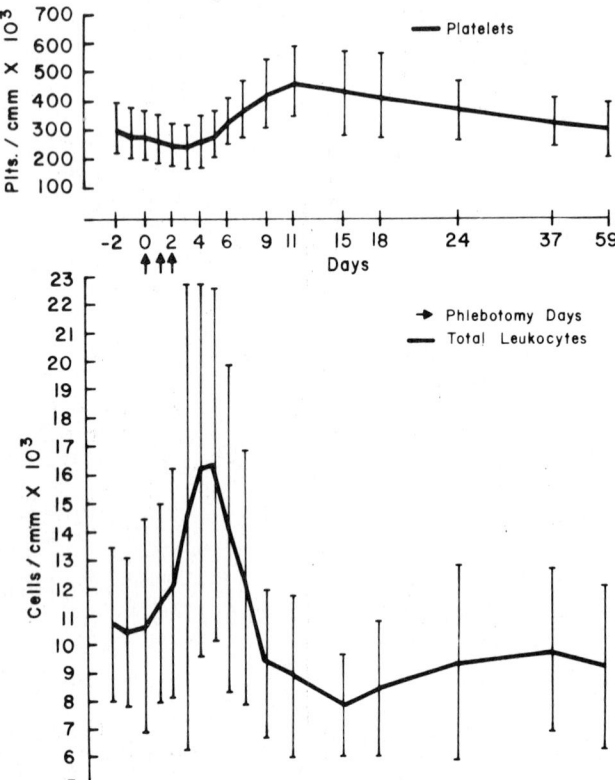

Figure 77–31. Changes in the total WBC and platelet numbers in response to acute blood loss in the dog.

Bone marrow red cell production is manifested as reticulocyte increases within 72 hours after the hemorrhagic stimulus. A peak response is achieved by the fifth day after a single hemorrhagic episode. Restoration of red cell mass by new production is essentially complete in four weeks.

Peracute blood loss in the peritoneal cavity or pleural space may be greatly affected by autotransfusion of red blood cells via lymphatic circulation (Clark and Woodley, 1959). Splenic rupture in dogs, leading to circulatory collapse caused by internal bleeding, may be followed by restoration of blood volume through recirculation. Bleeding into either the pleural space or the peritoneal cavity is associated with recirculation of 80 to 90 per cent of the extravasated red cell mass (Clark and Woodley, 1959).

Peracute blood loss into tissues differs from loss to the exterior and body cavities in that the majority of extravasated red cells are destroyed at the site of hemorrhage. Recirculation is insignificant.

In contrast to blood loss to the exterior, blood loss into body cavities and body tissues is essentially through blood destruction mechanisms. Erythrocytes that do not reenter the circulation are broken down *in situ*. Sufficient erythrocyte destruction may lead to jaundice, and the process is in essence a hemolytic event.

After restoration of blood volume following peracute hemorrhage, the PCV, Hb, and RBC values are all proportionately decreased — commensurate with the degree of blood loss — and modified by recirculation of red cells into body cavities in the case of hemorrhage. The erythrocytes are normochromic and normocytic. Another laboratory finding is a proportionate decrease in total plasma-protein concentration. Stress leukocytosis is usually evident within hours after significant hemorrhagic stimulus and rapidly returns to normal after cessation and correction of the hemorrhagic episodes (Fig. 77–30). Platelet numbers usually remain normal, but after massive blood loss, both a decrease in platelet number (consumption) and an increase in platelet size (release of newly formed platelets) may occur. Thrombocytosis is evident by the third posthemorrhagic day, and persistently high levels of platelets are found during the regenerative period. Careful examination of the serum, urine, and tissue for blood destruction pigments is helpful to distinguish blood loss from blood destruction.

The immediate therapeutic efforts for acute blood loss are directed at cessation of hemorrhage and restoration of circulating blood volume as indicated by the severity and location of hemorrhage. After the crisis, adequate dietary intake, provided by balanced commercial rations, is sufficient to replenish losses and provide the basis for regeneration. In the case of young animals, iron supplementation may be indicated, but combination hematinics are seldom indicated in young or old cats or dogs.

ACUTE BLOOD LOSS. Acute blood loss is the loss of significant quantities of blood over a short period of time (usually days), accompanied by plasma restoration sufficient to maintain adequate blood volume. Hypovolemia is not a significant problem, but loss of red cell mass (anemia) is. In many instances, acute blood loss is of sufficient duration that demonstrable stimulation of red blood cell production is evidenced by a significant reticulocyte response. The response to acute blood loss is modified by the location of bleeding, as previously described. Therapeutic considerations of acute blood loss are similar to those of peracute blood loss, except that additions to the red cell mass are more often indicated. Acute blood loss and chronic blood loss are clinically distinguished by availability of adequate quantities of iron.

CHRONIC BLOOD LOSS. Chronic blood loss is the continued loss of blood to the exterior over sufficiently long periods of time so that a deficiency of iron exists. The iron deficiency results from exhausted iron storage and inadequate iron intake or absorption. The onset of microcytic and hypochromic red cells in the circulation is a late effect of iron deficiency (Harris and Kellermeyer, 1970).

This arbitrary distinction between acute and chronic blood loss involves differences in time intervals and differences in volume considerations when applied to the young puppy with inadequate iron storage versus the adult dog. For example, hookworm disease in young puppies leads to iron-deficiency anemia over a relatively short period of time because of inadequate iron stores. A proportionate hookworm burden in the adult dog will take much longer to produce iron deficiency.

The laboratory evaluation of peripheral blood and bone marrow from patients with chronic blood-loss anemia varies with the progression of the disease. Generally, the anemia is severe. Although both plasma and red cells are lost, circulating volume is maintained.

Early in the course of chronic blood loss, the reticulocyte response usually reflects the degree of anemia, and the bone marrow is proportionately hyperplastic. Often, there is modest decrease in the MCH, MCV, and MCHC. The MCHC must be carefully interpreted, because reticulocytosis may be present.

Later in the course of anemia caused by chronic blood loss, microcytic and hypochromic red cells are present in significant numbers as the severely iron-deficient state is reached. Poikilocytosis is often present. Erythrocytes tend not to be uniform in size (anisocytosis), depending on the rate of blood loss. The reticulocyte response diminishes. The bone marrow remains hyperplastic, but pronormoblasts and basophilic normoblasts predominate because of the lack of iron for incorporation into polychromatophilic staining normoblasts.

Still later in the course of the anemia, red cells tend to be uniformly microcytic and hypochromic (Figs. 77–16 and 77–17). The reticulocyte response becomes nil and the bone marrow, hypoplastic. There is a decrease in MCH and MCHC. The erythrocytes are microcytic (MCV < 60 fl) and a low serum iron concentration (< 84 μg/dl) has been found (Harvey, 1981). Further, the MCHC may be normal in one third of the cases when the determination is made by calculation from the Hct. MCHC calculated from centrifuge-determined PCV would tend to be decreased. The MCH is decreased, depending on the severity of the anemia. The Japanese Akita normally has microcytic erythrocytes (Schalm, 1980).

Considerable attention has been given to canine hookworm disease, one cause of iron-deficiency anemia in the dog (Clark et al., 1961; Beaver et al., 1964; Georgi et al., 1969). It is conceivable that iron-deficiency anemia could result from decreased dietary intake, but unlikely, particularly if dogs are fed commercial rations. It is also conceivable that chronic intestinal malabsorption could result in iron deficiency. However, because of the large quantity of iron stored in the normal adult animal, failure of iron absorption or lack of dietary intake will result in iron-deficiency anemia only after many years.

Acute blood loss does not cause iron-deficiency anemia, because exsanguination precedes depletion of iron stores. The most likely and most commonly documented cause is chronic blood loss, usually through the intestine. In old cats and dogs, neoplasia may be the cause of chronic intestinal blood loss; in puppies, however, the most common cause is *Ancylostoma caninum* infestation (see Chapter 58).

The therapy for chronic blood-loss anemia leading to iron deficiency involves transfusion (see p. 1967), adequate diet, and iron replacement. The importance of adequate diet has long been established (Hahn and Whipple, 1939; Miller et al., 1947), and quality commercial balanced rations are sufficient to support regeneration of the erythron.

Data regarding iron-replacement therapy in the cat and dog are incomplete. Traditionally, veterinarians have used parenteral iron dextran replacement. This route of administration is convenient and eliminates the variable of intestinal iron absorption that has been documented to be reduced in man (Kimber and Weintraub, 1968). Parenteral iron is painful and requires multiple injections. The oral administration of iron is favored in man and should be for dogs. The oral administration of various uncoated ferrous salts is favored in man. Hathway (1974) recommends oral iron at a daily dose of three mg per kg per dog for an unspecified duration. Recently, Dodds and Ward (1980) recommended 100 to 300 mg ferrous sulfate per day. Based on studies in chicks, rats, and swine (Miller, 1977), good bioavailability of iron is provided by the salts of ferrous sulfate (1, 2, or 7) hydrated, ferrous ammonium sulfate, ferrous chloride, ferrous fumarate, ferrous gluconate, ferric ammonium citrate, ferric-choline citrate, ferric glycerophosphate, ferric chloride, and ferric sulfate. Other salts were poorly available, namely, ferrous carbonate, reduced iron, ferric pyrophosphate, ferric orthophosphate, and ferric oxide. Harvey (1981) observed serum iron values to normalize following therapy with oral iron; however, the MCV was delayed in returning to normal levels. Formulae for the calculation of total iron replacement are available for use in man (Goodman and Gilman, 1970), but it is not known if they are applicable to the cat or dog. Iron deficiency anemia does occur infrequently in cats. Like the dog, the majority of cases relate to infections caused by blood-sucking internal and external parasites, usually in young animals.

Hemolytic Anemia. Hemolytic anemia is characterized by decreased red blood cell survival time. In most instances, hemolytic anemia is detected by demonstrating hemoglobin degradation products and increased red cell production. Red cell survival studies allow more precise characterization of hemolytic disease but are not routinely used at present. Red cell survival approximates 100 to 110 days in the dog and 66 to 78 days in the cat (Schalm, 1965; Kaneko et al., 1966).

The site, rate, and manner of red blood cell destruction alter the clinical and laboratory manifestations of hemolytic disease. Red cell destruction may occur intravascularly or extravascularly within phagocytic cells. In some hemolytic diseases, increased red cell destruction occurs both intravascularly and extravascularly. Extravascular hemolysis is more common in the cat and dog.

Hemolytic disease may have different chemical manifestations, depending on the rapidity and amount of red cell destruction. Sudden onset of significant hemolysis occurs in diverse conditions, such as isoimmune and autoimmune hemolytic disease, Heinz-body anemia, babesiasis, and the caval syndrome in dirofilariasis. The clinical manifestations of anorexia, fever, anemia, and hemoglobinuria characterize acute hemolytic crises. Other signs may be present, depending on the mechanism or primary disease process.

Multisystemic effects of acute hemolytic anemia occur. The effects of anemia per se have been discussed. Pigment metabolism or excretion may have significant hepatorenal effect when combined with hypoxemia of severe anemia. The sudden release of hemoglobin and erythrocyte products may cause consumption of coagulation factors, resulting in disseminated intravascular coagulation (DIC). This is well documented in fulminant babesiasis (Moore, 1979; Moore and Williams, 1979).

Hemoglobin degradation products are not always obvious in hemolytic disease, and animals are not necessarily icteric, in spite of profound disease. The determinant is the rate of hemolysis and degree of hepatic function in metabolic degradation of pigment.

The regenerative response of eyrthropoietic tissue is usually consistent with the degree of anemia and the time sequence of the disease process, but the reticulocyte response is comparably greater in hemolysis than in blood loss. This effect may be due to hemolysates (Sanchez-Medal et al., 1963) or the ready availability of iron. The reticulocyte response may be as high as 30 to 50 per cent in chronic hemolytic disease of the dog, but peripheral evidence of bone marrow response in the cat is usually substantially less (three to eight per cent) if the aggregate form reticulocytes are counted.

Intravascular hemolysis is characterized by the release of free hemoglobin. If the intravascular hemolysis is sufficiently rapid, the hemolysis will be grossly evident in centrifuged blood. Free hemoglobin released into plasma is bound to haptoglobin. The size of the resultant complex precludes passage into the glomerular filtrate. If the rate of hemolysis is rapid, haptoglobin may become saturated, in which case free hemoglobin may (1) dissociate into globin and heme (if in the form of methemoglobin), (2) be removed by the liver, or (3) be excreted by the kidney. Free hemoglobin passing into the glomerular filtrate may exceed the resorptive capacity of proximal tubules, in which case hemoglobinuria results. Because of desquamation and disruption of tubular cells containing hemosiderin, chronic intravascular hemolysis is often characterized by hemosiderinuria.

Extravascular hemolysis ordinarily takes place within the reticuloendothelial system of the spleen, liver, and bone marrow. In a sequence of events not fully understood, hemoglobin is catabolized and the heme is ultimately converted to free (unconjugated) bilirubin. If extravascular hemolysis occurs

rapidly, icterus results, owing to increased free (unconjugated or indirect reading) bilirubin. Since free bilirubin is virtually insoluble in water, it does not appear in the urine. Instead, it is transported to the liver bound to albumin. Within the liver, the free bilirubin is conjugated primarily to bilirubin diglucuronide, which is then excreted into bile. In the gut, the bilirubin is progressively reduced by bacteria to the urobilinogens, an excess of which may result in orange feces. Since a portion of the urobilinogens is absorbed and appears in the urine, rapid extravascular hemolysis is characterized by increased concentration of urobilinogen in urine.

Extravascular hemolysis is sometimes accompanied by hepatic damage, in which case conjugated (direct reading) bilirubin may contribute to icterus.

Aplastic crisis is a reasonably well-defined phenomenon in man (Harris and Kellermeyer, 1970) that probably occurs in cats and dogs. Aplastic crisis is characterized by temporary bone marrow failure in association with inflammatory, neoplastic, toxic, or allergic disease in patients with steady-state chronic hemolytic disease. Temporary cessation of bone marrow response in such patients can result in a fall of PCV from a functionally borderline level of 18 per cent to a critical nine per cent in a 48-hour interval. Rigorous laboratory monitoring may allow detection of aplastic crisis in sufficient time for successful replacement therapy.

Classification of hemolytic disease can be based on whether abnormalities are intracorpuscular or extracorpuscular. This is useful to the clinician interested in precise definition of the hemolytic disease. A classification based on intravascular or extravascular destruction with subclassification as to rapidity of red cell destruction appears to be useful in cliniical assessment of the hemolytic process. Additional classification may be based on etiologic cause. Because of the complexity of hemolytic disorders, the logical approach of Harris and Kellermeyer (1970) will be followed (Table 77–13).

Intracorpuscular Abnormalities. Hereditary abnormalities of the red blood cell membrane, metabolic pathways, and hemoglobin account for a wide variety of hemolytic disorders in man. Hemoglobinopathies leading to decreased red cell survival have

Table 77–13. Classification of Hemolytic Diseases

Intracorpuscular Abnormalities
Hereditary Defects of Red Blood Cells
  Stomatocytosis (hemolytic anemia of the chondrodysplastic malamute)
  Hereditary nonspherocytic disease (pyruvate kinase deficiency of the basenji)
  Congenital feline porphyria
Interaction of Intra- and Extracorpuscular Abnormalities
Acquired Defects (Lead Poisoning)
Extracorpuscular Abnormalities
Acquired Defects Associated with Demonstrable Antibody
  Isoimmune diseases
  Autoimmune diseases
Acquired Defects Nonassociated with Demonstrable Antibody
  Disorders caused by chemicals toxic to red blood cells (Heinz body anemia)
  Disorders caused by infectious agents
  Miscellaneous disorders associated with hemolytic disease

not been documented in the cat or dog. An abnormal hemoglobin was found in a nonanemic dog associated with reduced exercise tolerance (Jones and Hinton, 1978). The anemia of the basenji is the first enzymatic deficiency of red cell metabolism recognized in the dog. The macrocytic anemia of the Alaskan malamute may represent a red cell membrane disorder. As the anemias of animals are more intensely studied, additional hereditary problems are likely to be identified.

HEMOLYTIC ANEMIA OF THE CHONDRODYS-PLASTIC MALAMUTE. Hereditary chondrodysplasia of the Alaskan malamute has been recognized by breeders for some time. Recent investigations of altered bone formation in malamutes revealed a mild hemolytic anemia and splenomegaly (Fletch and Pinkerton, 1972). Although the PCV is normal in affected animals, the hemoglobin content is reduced, resulting in altered red blood cell indices. The MCHC is consistently below 30 per cent, and the MCV is over 80 cu μ. In adult dwarf malamutes, there is mild reticulocytosis. Blood smears show macrocytosis and variable numbers of stomatocytes (Fletch and Pinkerton, 1972).

The gene symbol "dan" has been adopted for the syndrome. Affected animals are designated dan/dan, carriers dan/+, and normal dogs +/+ (Fletch and Pinkerton, 1972).

FAMILIAL BASENJI ANEMIA. Familial nonspherocytic hemolytic anemia in basenji dogs (Ewing, 1969b; Tasker et al., 1969) has been identified as erythrocyte pyruvate kinase (PK) deficiency (Searcy, 1970; Searcy et al., 1971). PK deficiency has been identified in beagles (Praase et al., 1975). The enzyme is necessary in the Embden-Meyerhof glycolytic pathway essential for red cell metabolism. The mode of inheritance appears to be mendelian recessive.

Anemia is severe, with hemoglobin levels ranging from four to nine gm per 100 ml. Hyperbilirubinuria, urobilinogenuria, pigmented feces, and erythroid hyperplasia of the bone marrow are found. All affected animals show marked reticulocytosis-polychromasia, macrocytosis, and normoblasts in the peripheral blood. The MCV is raised as the result of the macrocytic reticulocytes, which may be in the 30 to 50 per cent range. The MCHC is reduced to between 24 and 29 per cent as a result of macrocytic reticulocytes that have not completed iron incorporation into hemoglobin.

The hemolytic disease is a disorder of young basenjis. Animals surviving to two to three years of age are affected with myelofibrosis and osteosclerosis (Searcy, 1972b). Increased density of trabecular bone can be demonstrated radiographically. The bone marrow cavity is replaced with fibrous tissue. The myelofibrosis and osteosclerosis impair erythropoiesis and eventually lead to death from anemia (Search, 1970, 1972b).

Carrier animals can be identified by pyruvate kinase assay. As pointed out by Searcy (1970) and Searcy et al. (1971), correction for high levels of enzyme in reti̶c̶y̶t̶e̶s̶ and leukocytes must be made in order to detect deficiency in the carrier animals. Incomplete leukocyte removal may result in failure of carrier animal detection. That PK deficiency is a stem cell disorder has been proved by bone marrow transplantation studies (Weiden et al., 1976). Three severely anemic PK dogs were engrafted with bone marrow from histocompatible littermates. The recipients all recovered from the anemic state and short erythrocyte life span. The dogs were followed for 5.5 years. Long-term survival with complete reversal of iron overload and without cirrhosis and osteosclerosis was recently reported (Weiden et al., 1981). These investigators effected correction by bone marrow transplantation and determined the stem cell nature of the disease (Weiden et al., 1974).

FELINE PORPHYRIA. Porphyria of domestic cats is characterized by biochemical changes that overlap erythropoietic and nonerythropoietic forms of the disease in man. The clinical features of feline porphyria appear to be similar to those recorded for congenital erythropoietic porphyria (Glenn et al., 1968). The first case of feline porphyria was recorded by Tobias (1964).

The excessive accumulation of brownish pigment in bones and teeth, which fluoresces under ultraviolet light, is caused by overproduction of uroporphyrins and coproporphyrins. These porphyrins are predominantly of the type I isomer, which cannot be utilized in the heme-biosynthesis pathway. It is presumed that the deficiency in feline porphyria is a deficiency of uroporphyrinogen II cosynthetase activity, allowing excessive accumulations of uroporphyrin I, coproporphyrin I, and protoporphyrinase in erythrocytes, urine, feces, and tissues. Affected cats have photosensitivity, severe anemia, and severe renal disease (Giddens et al., 1975).

Hereditary porphyria is inherited as an autosomal dominant trait (Glenn et al., 1968).

Interaction of Intra- and Extracorpuscular Abnormalities. Hemolytic anemia resulting from extracorpuscular chemical interference of normal erythrocytes or enzyme-deficient erythrocytes produces several serious hemolytic diseases in man. One example in the dog and cat is lead poisoning, in which lead interferes with erythrocyte function, resulting in a shortened survival time.

LEAD POISONING. The ingestion of lead-containing substances such as paint and linoleum can result in lead poisoning (Zook et al., 1969, 1970, 1972a, b). The disease is characterized by gastrointestinal, central nervous system, and hematologic disorders. Zook et al. (1972a) reported 214 cases of lead-poisoned dogs; 97 per cent had normoblastosis and 95 per cent had basophilic stippling. The presence of 15 or more stippled RBC per 10,000 RBC should be considered suggestive of, and 40 or more diagnostic of, lead poisoning in dogs with signs typical of the disease. Dogs with lead poisoning may be anemic. The anemia is normocytic and slightly hypochromic and tends to

occur only in poisonings of long duration. The hematology of lead poisoning in man and animals has been reviewed by George and Duncan (1979). Lead inhibits a number of enzymes in heme synthesis and results in the production of increased quantities of heme precursors. The detection of these precursors in urine can be used as a screening test for lead poisoning. The enzymes most sensitive to inhibition by lead are delta amino levulinic acid dehydratase (ALAD) and ferrochelatase (Bottomley, 1977). The substrate for ALAD, amino levulinic acid urine levels are insensitive for the diagnosis of lead poisoning at present (McSherry et al., 1971).

In addition to the inhibition of erythropoiesis caused by suppression of heme synthesis, there is evidence that lead partially inhibits globin synthesis and has direct effect on erythrocytes, resulting in significantly decreased red cell half-life (Griggs and Harris, 1958). The definitive diagnosis of lead poisoning is based on direct measurement of lead in blood, body fluids, or tissues (see Chapter 23).

Mitema et al. (1980) investigated the effect of chronic lead exposure on canine bone marrow and found that increased myeloid-erythroid ratios in dogs give 2 mg/kg and 5 mg/kg daily of lead acetate. Only one dog of four given five mg/kg for six weeks developed clinical signs. Blood lead levels significantly above 60 μg/dl did not produce clinical signs of disease. Zook and Carpenter (1977) considered blood lead levels of 40 to 50 μg/dl indicative of disease in the presence of clinical signs and > 60 μg/dl as being diagnostic.

Extracorpuscular Abnormalities. Acquired defects of red cell production or life span induced by extracorpuscular factors may be separated into immunologic and nonimmunologic categories. In general, these disorders are difficult to diagnose definitively in clinical practice.

ACQUIRED DEFECTS WITH DEMONSTRABLE ANTIBODY

Isoimmune Disease. Significant naturally occurring demonstrable antibody is lacking in the dog and cat. Newborn puppies of the blood group CEA-1 (A system) born of immunized CEA-1 negative bitches, if permitted to nurse on the first day of life, may receive large amounts of CEA-1 antibody (Swisher and Young, 1961). A hemolytic crisis is produced in CEA-1 negative pups and may be fatal during the first two to three days of life. Pups of blood type CEA-2 are generally mildly affected and exhibit positive direct antiglobin tests of their red cells. Isoantibodies to other blood-group types have not been implicated in diseases of newborn pups; however, isoimmunization to CEA-7 (Tr antigen) is possible. Natural or transplacental immunization of the bitch does not occur during pregnancy; hence, previous blood transfusion (sensitization) with red cell antigens is necessary for the disease.

Isoimmune disease of newborn kittens has been recorded by Majka (1974). The mechanism has not been determined.

AUTOIMMUNE HEMOLYTIC ANEMIA. Autoimmune hemolytic anemia occurs in both the dog (Miller et al., 1954; Lewis et al., 1963) and the cat (Sodikoff and Custer, 1965; Scott et al., 1973).

The disease in dogs and cats is associated with a variety of disorders and classified on the basis of autoantibody type and to some extent the prognosis for patients with autoimmune hemolytic anemia (AIHA) (Halliwell, 1978; Halliwell and Werner, 1979). This classification is based on a limited number of cases.

Class I, or In-Saline-Acting Autoagglutinins. These animals develop agglutinating autoantibody, which results in direct or intravascular hemagglutination. Agglutination can be seen immediately on withdrawal of blood into syringe or tube or when blood is placed on a glass slide. Agglutination can be distinguished from rouleau formation by one-half dilution of blood with saline; rouleau formation will disperse and agglutination persists. The demonstration of a saline-acting autoagglutinin is diagnostic for AIHA, and a Coombs' test is not necessary. This form of AIHA is the most difficult to treat. In addition to the anemia, the liver is overloaded with damaged cells and pigment. Specific therapy includes high-dose steroids and immunosuppressive drugs.

Class II, In Vivo Hemolysins. There is massive destruction of erythrocytes in the circulation. Hemoglobinemia and hemoglobinuria both are seen. There is usually profound reticulocytosis and spherocytic change. Antibody types are IgG and IgM, with complement fixation.

Class III, Incomplete Antibody Type. This appears to the commonest form of AIHA. There is seldom evidence for rapid erythrocyte destruction as in hemoglobinuria. Reticulocytosis is variable, as is spherocytosis. The antibody type is usually IgG.

Class IV, Cold Hemagglutinin Disease. The autoantibody is not fully active at body temperature 37° C. Optimal activity is at colder temperatures, thus intravascular agglutination occurs in the small blood vessels of the extremities (Slappendel et al., 1975; Greene et al., 1977). The disease is characterized in the dog by cyanosis and necrosis of the extremities.

Class V, Cold Autoimmune Anemia — Nonagglutinating Type. The autoantibodies are cold reactive but not agglutinating. Acrocyanosis and necrosis of extremities are not seen. The course of the disease is characterized by episodes of hemolysis that exacerbate in cold weather. The diagnosis is made by a positive Coombs' test performed at +4° C.

The Class I, IV, and V type AIHA persist clinically, with signs that are distinct for each mechanism of antibody injury. The Class II and III AIHA cases do not have clear definition. Morphologic changes of erythrocytes are important to diagnosis. Spherocytes are a prominent feature of these cases (Figure 77–18).

Since the spherocytes are deformed cells destined to be removed from the circulation, the degree of reticulocytosis and spherocytosis should be assessed for determining response to therapy and prognosis. The high reticulocyte count, low spherocyte count patient goes into remission more readily than does the low reticulocyte count, high spherocyte count patient. The bone marrow in AIHA with nearly all spherocytes is essentially aplastic with regard to erythroid elements. Morphologically, the blood smear has the appearance of feline blood because of the uniformly small sized cells.

Mechanisms of Autoimmune Hemolytic Anemia (AIHA)

The pathogenesis of Coombs-positive anemias in dogs and cats is multiple (Werner, 1980). Drugs have been shown to act as haptens, or injure erythrocytes to expose sequestered antigenic sites. Although the list of drugs capable of inducing hemolytic anemias in man is large, documentation in animals is scanty. Atwell et al. (1978) demonstrated Coombs-positive, steroid-responsive hemolytic anemia in two dogs suspected to have been induced by levamisole. Appropriate confirmatory studies were not made. Of greater frequency are microorganisms that alter antigenic determinants of erythrocytes. *Hemobartonella felis* produces a Coombs-positive anemia (Maede and Hata, 1975) that is responsive to steroid therapy (Harvey and Gaskin, 1978). Perman (1978) found three of six cases of ehrlichiosis to be Coombs positive. Werner (1980) summarizes diseases that have been associated with Coombs-positive anemia (Table 77–14). It is apparent that the erythrocyte is an "innocent bystander" and bears the brunt of the punishment (Werner, 1980).

AIHA often occurs in systemic lupus erythematosus (SLE) of the dog (Lewis et al., 1963, 1965a, b; Lewis and Schwartz, 1971). AIHA is an occasional complication of malignant disease of lymphoreticular tissue and has been reported with myeloproliferative disease and hemangiosarcoma (Werner, 1980).

Table 77–14. Diseases That Have Been Associated with Coombs-Positive Anemias in Dogs and Cats*

Neoplastic
  Lymphoid
  Myeloid
  Hemangiosarcoma
Infectious
  Bronchopneumonia
  FeLv infection
  Rickettsial
    Hemobartonellosis
    Ehrlichiosis
Parasitic
  Dirofilariasis
  Piroplasmosis
  Leishmaniasis
Autoimmune
  Systemic lupus erythematosus
  *Immune-mediated thrombocytopenia
Miscellaneous
  Granulomatous disease
  Glomerulonephritis

*Some patients had significant hemolytic anemia, while many did not.

From Werner, L. L.: Coombs-positive anemias in the dog and cat. Comp. Cont. Ed. 2:96, 1980. Used with permission.

Autoimmune Hemolytic Anemia in the Cat

Autoimmune hemolytic anemia in the cat is characterized by anemia, a positive direct antiglobulin reaction, and reticulocytosis (Scott et al., 1973). Clinical findings of red cell destruction are similar to those of hemolytic anemia due to other causes. Autoimmune hemolytic anemia of the cat is not characterized by detectable spherocytosis, because the small size of normal feline erythrocytes does not allow for perceptible, morphologic differentiation. Diagnosis is based on a regenerative, Coombs-positive anemia, responsive to steroid therapy and elimination of other possible causes. Serum haptoglobin may be normal, owing to rapid synthesis of haptoglobin (Harvey and Gaskin, 1978).

Since hemobartonellosis frequently presents as a Coombs-positive steroid-responsive anemia, it is not possible to distinguish the disease from that described by Scott et al. (1973).

Coombs-Negative, Spherocytic, Steroid-Responsive Anemia

Not all spherocytic steroid-responsive anemias are Coombs positive. Recognition of the type anemia is not based solely on the presence of spherocytes, since other causes of spherocytes such as fragmentation anemia and transfused stored blood are recognized.

Immune-Mediated Stem Cell Disorders

Recent reports indicate that immune injury to hematopoietic stem cells may involve either humoral antibody or cell-mediated cytotoxic mechanisms. Injury may affect a single cell series or involve several cell lines, including the pluripotent stem cell (Cline and Golde, 1978). In humans, immune suppression of hematopoiesis has been described for pure red cell aplasia, systemic lupus erythematosus, immune panleukopenia, and some cases of aplastic anemia.

Pure Red Cell Aplasia

Little is known about the antigenic constitution of erythrocyte precursor cells. Kim et al. (1976) showed that heterologous antierythrocyte antibody causes complement-mediated lysis of hemoglobinized human erythroblasts, reticulocytes, and mature red cells but does not destroy erythropoietin-responsive precursors. Whether this mechanism is operative in canine pure red cell aplasia is speculative (Lund and Avolt, 1972). Both spherocytic and nonspherocytic pure red cell aplasia have been seen in the dog. The anemias are steroid responsive. Whether the mechanism is immune-mediated or an aplastic crisis due to other causes remains to be shown (Perman, 1978). The condition has been seen in lupus erythematosus (LE)-positive patients with multisystemic signs of disease and in LE-negative patients. The impaired erythropoiesis dog described by Fletch et al. (1975) appears to be similar.

Prognosis and Therapy of AIHA

The prognosis of autoimmune hemolytic anemia is guarded and based on the associated underlying disease if demonstrable. The rationale for therapy is to manage the anemic crisis, inhibit immune destruction of erythrocytes, and treat the underlying associated disease if present.

The anemic crisis seldom necessitates blood transfusion of the patient. There needs to be evidence for hypoxia. A low PCV is not necessary, nor is it an indication for blood transfusion. Furthermore, the transfused cells may add to the burden of erythrocyte destruction. The use of cold stored blood must be avoided in cold hemagglutin disease (Rosenfield and Jagathambal, 1976).

The mechanism of erythrocyte injury is of importance to steroid therapy. Frank et al. (1977) summarize *in vivo* and *in vitro* studies on the pathophysiology of immune hemolytic anemia of humans and guinea pigs. These findings are of importance to the management and therapy.

Regarding immune-mediated erythrocyte destruction, IgG-coated cells are destroyed principally in the spleen. Large numbers of IgG molecules may change the primary site of sequestration from spleen to liver. Complement-fixing IgG antibodies have augmented clearance of erythrocyte by both spleen and liver. Synergism between the binding sites on the IgG and complement

molecules for receptors on macrophages has been postulated. IgM antibody fixes complement, and these coated erythrocytes are cleared primarily by the liver. Thus, the variable results of splenectomy as a modality for therapy are in part explained. The spleen is a major source of IgG antibody production, which also contributes to the beneficial effect of splenectomy in some cases. Splenectomy for AIHA should be avoided and considered as a last resort (Bowdler, 1976). Newer developments in nuclear medicine allow for precise location of destruction sites of erythrocytes in AIHA (McIntyre, 1977).

Corticosteroids are most commonly used to induce remission in AIHA. The mechanism is not completely elucidated. Frank et al. (1978) suggest that the principal mechanism of steroid action is to inhibit clearance of antibody-coated erythrocytes by the fixed macrophages of the spleen and liver. There is little effect on circulating antibody level or antibodies on erythrocytes. Moreover, their studies have shown that glucocorticoids were most effective in reducing clearance of IgG-coated cells, moderately effective in reducing clearance of IgG plus complement-coated cells, and least effective in reducing clearance of IgM and complement-coated cells. As clearance rates were reduced, depending on antibody coating, increasingly higher steroid levels were necessary. Thus, high steroid concentrations were necessary to effect any improvement in IgM cold agglutinin syndromes. When steroids were ineffective in controlling clearance of erythrocytes, cyclophosphamide and azathioprine improved survival by interfering with antibody production rather than by altering macrophage function.

The duration of corticosteroid therapy may be long. Stabilization of the PCV may take several days. The degree of reticulocytosis and numbers of spherocytes may be used to indicate recovery periods. A low reticulocyte count and high spherocyte numbers (>95 per cent) will require several weeks before remission is complete. In the pure red cell anemias, response to steroids was of the order of two to three weeks before reticulocytes was demonstrable and two to three months before complete remission. See Chapter 83 for additional remarks concerning therapy.

Nonautoimmune Coombs-Positive Anemias

Several diseases (Table 77–14) have an immune component to the pathogenesis of anemia. The infectious anemias caused by *Rickettsia* and parasitic agents have been shown recently to be frequently Coombs positive and will be discussed separately.

Feline Hemobartonellosis. Feline infectious anemia is caused by *Hemobartonella felis*, a rickettsial organism. Recent studies (Maede and Hata, 1975; Maede and Sonoda, 1975; Maede, 1975; Maede, 1978; Maede and Murata, 1978; Maede, 1979; Harvey and Gaskin, 1977, 1978a, b; and Harvey, 1980) have led to a better understanding of the pathogenesis of this disease.

The natural transmission may be by bloodsucking arthropods, from queen to offspring, and iatrogenically from blood transfusions. The clinical signs are weakness, depression, weight loss, and pale mucous membranes. Fever, jaundice, and splenomegaly are variable. Experimentally, Harvey and Gaskin (1977) have shown the disease to be characterized by episodes of hemolysis. A chronic carrier state is seen in surviving animals. Harvey and Gaskin (1977) also report that over 50 per cent of the time rare or no organisms could be demonstrated on erythrocytes. Maede and Hato (1975) found marked increase in osmotic fragility of erythrocyte following the appearance of organisms. The direct Coombs' test was positive for an average of 15 days after *H. felis* was demonstrated. [51]Cr life span studies showed erythrocyte half-lives of 8.8 days for noninfected cats and 4.3 days for infected cats (Maede, 1975). Ultrastructural observations on the removal of organisms in the spleen demonstrate the role of macrophages in removal of organisms from the surface of erythrocytes (Maede and Murata, 1978; Maede, 1978). Erythrocyte destruction was by erythrophagocytosis. Macrophage-laden erythrocytes are demonstrable in spleen, liver, bone marrow, and blood. Clearance of organisms from the erythrocytes may occur within hours (Harvey, 1978). Jaundice occurs with initial hemolytic crisis; however, after repeat episodes, jaundice may be absent. The liver's ability to clear pigment may be a factor.

The disease is frequently associated with FeLV infection or other disease conditions. That hemobartonellosis is a secondary disease precipitated by stress has not been shown. Harvey and Gaskin (1975) failed to induce relapses with corticosteroids. The beneficial effects of corticosteroids on recovery from the anemia in the presence of parasitemia was demonstrated. These observations and the Coombs-positive result following parasitemia have led to the use of corticosteroids in therapy.

DIAGNOSIS. The diagnosis of *H. felis* may be difficult. The only consistent finding is anemia, which may be mild in the carrier state. Since organisms are absent or in low number over 50 per cent of the time, demonstration of parasitemia is not always possible. The coccoid and ring forms of the organisms are demonstrated on Wright-stained smears. Observation of erythrocytes at the feathered end or thin areas shows organisms at the periphery of the erythrocyte. These areas are usually free of precipitated stain. Small and Ristic (1967) recommend acridine orange for demonstrating the organisms.

The anemia is usually regenerative. However, with concurrent diseases causing suppression of the bone marrow, nonregenerative anemias are found and bone marrow examination is necessary. The bone marrow may show intense erythropoiesis, with the PCV in the 15 to 20 range in the cat.

Leukocyte responses are variable. Erythrophagocytosis, monocytosis, and reactive lymphocytes are indicative of immune-mediated red cell destruction. Differentiation from autoimmune hemolytic anemia is not possible, since both are Coombs positive and may respond to steroid therapy.

THERAPY. The initial objective should be to correct fluid deficits in dehydrated animals. Blood transfusion may be required when the PCV is less than 15 in hydrated patients. However, many cats having PCV as low as six to nine may recover without transfusion. Indication of glucocorticoids (prednisone or prednisolone, one to two mg/kg of body weight twice daily) is based on the mechanism of the anemia (Harvey, 1980). The tetracyclines, 20 mg/kg body weight three times per day, are the treatment of choice (Ristic, 1969; Harvey, 1980). Thiacetarsamide sodium, one per cent (1 mg/kg is repeated 48 hours apart) has been recommended by Fishler and Birzele (1974).

Since hemobartonellosis is frequently associated with other concurrent diseases, response to therapy may be transient or not at all.

Canine Hemobartonellosis. *Haemobartonella* rarely causes hemolytic disease in dogs that have not been splenectomized. In affected dogs, the organisms are present in variable numbers on individual red cells. The number of red cells affected with organisms is relatively low, and many microscopic fields must be searched to identify the agent. The anemia is regenerative. In splenectomized dogs, target cells, Howell-Jolly bodies, and poikilocytes commonly associated with splectomy are observed. Bundza et al. (1976) report hemobartonellosis in a dog in association with Coombs-positive anemia. Since Coombs positivity in the cat with hemobartonellosis occurs during parasitemia, the same must be true in the dog. *Haemobartonella canis* may be seen in nonsplenectomized dogs (Pryor and Bradbury, 1975; Sonada et al., 1978).

Cytauxzoonosis-like Disease of Cats. A cytauxzoon-like organism has been reported to cause fatal disease in cats in Missouri (Wagner, 1976; Bendele et al., 1976a,b). The protozoan is morphologically similar to *Cytauxzoon* and is classified in the family Therileriidae. Clinical signs include lethargy, pale icteric mucous membranes, fever, and depression. The Missouri cats were from heavily wooded areas. The disease is thought to occur througout the entire southeastern United States where significant populations of ixodes ticks are found.

Clinically, the disease may be confused with hemobartonellosis. The piroplasm or ring forms may be found in erythrocytes on Wright-stained smears or at necropsy when large numbers of schizonts are found in liver, lung, spleen, and lymph nodes. The disease, when recognized, has been invariably fatal, and treatment is not known.

Canine Ehrlichiosis (see Chapter 27). Canine ehrlichiosis is a tick-borne disease of dogs caused by the rickettsial organism *Ehrlichia canis* (Ewing, 1969; Huxsoll et al., 1972; Buhles et al., 1975; Huxsoll, 1975; Pierce et al., 1977; Reardon and Pierce, 1981a,b). The disease varies from an acute febrile syndrome to a severe, chronic, and often fatal disease. The anemia that is frequently associated is mild to moderate. The bone marrow may be hyperplastic to severely hypoplastic. The genesis of the anemia may be of different causes, e.g., blood loss, chronic inflammation, bone marrow hypoplasia, and immunologically mediated, since it is frequently Coombs positive (Perman, 1978; Werner, 1980).

DIAGNOSIS. Canine ehrlichiosis is most often reported in tropical and subtropical climates where the tick vector populations are high. The temperate climates where the *Rhipicephalus sanguineus* tick is distributed may be endemic areas. The infection of *E. canis* is often complicated by current hemotropic agents such as *Babesia, Hepatozoon,* and *Haemobartonella.* In nonendemic areas, the demonstration of *Babesia canis* in erythrocytes is suggestive that the disease is probably ehrlichiosis.

Demonstration of the organism within monocytes, lymphocytes, and neutrophils is facilitated by appropriate sampling techniques. The shallow ear prick and squeezing of the capillary bed yields higher numbers of appropriate cells. Since the lung, lymph node, and bone marrow are involved, aspirate biopsies of these tissues may yield diagnostic specimens. An IFA test for canine ehrlichiosis is available (Lewis and Huxsoll, 1977).

Canine Babesiosis (See Chapter 27). Canine babesiosis (*Babesia canis* and *B. gibsoni*) occurs as an acute hemolytic anemia with variable complications (Malherbe, 1956; Groves and Yap, 1968; and Moore, 1978). The acute stage may last for hours to days, during which time the organism can be seen on blood smears. Ear prick smears are best. The carrier or latent state is common and parasites may be difficult to find. Serology has proved useful to diagnosis (Ristic et al., 1971; Anderson et al., 1980). The disease is frequently complicated by concurrent infections with other hematropic agents such as *Ehrlichia canis, Haemobartonella,* and *Hepatozoon.*

The progressive anemia may be regenerative and Coombs positive. Complications with *E. canis* suggest that many atypical manifestations may relate to concurrent infection. Recently, Moore (1977) and Moore and Williams (1979) described disseminated intravascular coagulation (DIC) as a complication to *B. canis* infection in the dog. In acute fulminant disease, DIC should be suspected and evaluated (Moore, 1979a,b).

Feline Babesiosis. Feline babesiosis has received scant attention on a world-wide basis. The parasite is recognized from blood smear examination, and endemic areas are known (Futter and Belonji, 1980).

Canine Hepatozoonosis Trypanosomiasis, Leishmaniasis, and Histoplasmosis. These organs cause disease manifested by a variety of clinical signs, including anemia. The anemia is generally nonregenerative, but since the monocyte-macrophage system is usually involved, increased rate of red cell destruction associated with splenomegaly may contribute to anemia (Williams et al., 1977; Craig et al., 1978).

ACQUIRED DEFECTS WITHOUT DEMONSTRABLE ANTIBODY

Acquired hemolytic anemias of nonimmune type are of diverse etiology. A frequent manner of erythrocyte destruction is through fragmentation mechanisms. The fragmentation disorders were recently reviewed by Rebar et al. (1981). The nomenclature (Table 77–5) of Bessis (1977) will be followed.

Disorders Caused by Toxic Chemicals (Heinz Body Anemia). Heinz bodies (erythrocyte refractile bodies) are denatured hemoglobin produced in red blood cells when oxidants cause globin precipitation in glucose-6-phosphate dehydrogenase (G-6-PD) deficient cells. Naturally occurring G-6-PD deficiency occurs in man but has not been described in animals. Older red cells are known to contain reduced amounts of G-6-PD, rendering these cells more sensitive to Heinz body formation. The cat appears to be predisposed to Heinz body formation, since these structures are found in red blood cells of normal cats (Beritic, 1964; Schalm and Smith, 1963).

Cats treated with urinary antiseptics containing methylene blue form large Heinz bodies in many red blood cells. The cells may be destroyed by passage through the spleen, resulting in a hemolytic crisis. The anemia varies in severity (Schechter et al., 1973). Hemolytic crisis may be followed by a period of red cell refractoriness to Heinz body formation. Variability in absorption of enteric-coated tablets containing methylene blue (Schechter et al., 1973) and the refrac-

toriness of young cells or cells following a hemolytic episode tend to explain long-term use of these drugs in cats that do not acquire Heinz body hemolytic anemia in cats. Methemoglobinemia was a profound feature of affected cats in the reports of Schechter et al.

The combination urinary tract compound frequently contains an analgesic, phenazopyridine (Harvey and Kornick, 1976), which produces both Heinz body anemia and methemoglobinemia at high doses.

The analgesic acetaminophen produces methemoglobinuria (Leyland, 1974) and Heinz body anemia (Finco et al., 1975). Schalm (1980) describes Heinz body anemia in a cat resulting from autointoxication. The oxidant principle was not determined. Whether reduced levels of vitamin E and/or selenium effect the pentose phosphate pathway, rendering the cells more susceptible to oxidative stress in cats, has not been shown. The additive effect of oxidative stress may be a factor, since Heinz body anemia has been seen by the authors in cats receiving low dose phenazopyridine (10 mg/kg/day). Ingestion by cats of oxidative compounds and foods with Heinz body potential in other species should be avoided.

Heinz body anemia in dogs is probably more common than previously recorded. Farkas and Farkas (1974) described hemolytic anemia due to ingestion of onions in a dog. Sebrell (1930) produced anemia in dogs by feeding subjects whole onions; later, Grukzit (1931a,b) showed that the toxic principle resided in the oil of onion. The main constituent of onion oil is allylpropyl disulfide and the synthesized compound *N*-propyl disulfide (Grukzit, 1931a; Williams et al., 1941) is probably the toxic principle. The mechanism of the anemia as caused by Heinz bodies was not shown at that time. Onion-induced Heinz body anemia in cattle, sheep, and horses is well documented (Schalm et al., 1975). Recently, Lees et al. (1979) and Rebar and Lewis (1979) report Heinz body anemia in dogs associated with onion ingestion. Other causes are postulated. The feeding of human cuisine to dogs accounts for the higher frequency of onion poisoning in some geographic areas. Plants belonging to the family Brassicaceae, including cabbage, brussels sprouts, kale, rape, watercress, broccoli, and kohlrabi, induce Heinz body anemia in cattle. The potential for ingested plants of the family Brassicaceae to induce Heinz body anemia in dogs remains to be shown.

The simultaneous occurrence of methemoglobinemia and Heinz body anemia may lead to missed diagnosis and errors in treatment. Although hereditary and acquired methemoglobinemia occurs (Letchworth et al., 1977), all dogs and cats exhibiting cyanosis and chocolate-brown blood should have blood smears stained with new methylene blue to demonstrate the presence or absence of Heinz bodies as a concurrent problem. Benzocaine induces methemoglobinemia and a mild Heinz body anemia when applied topically (Harvey et al., 1979). Benzocaine applied as an aerosol spray to the buccal mucosa produced methemoglobinemia. A presumptive test for methemoglobin is the spot filter test. A drop of blood with significant methemoglobin will turn brown on filter paper. Oxyhemoglobin will remain red. Approximately ten per cent methemoglobin is required before browning in EDTA tubes (Harvey, 1981) and 40 to 80 per cent methemoglobinemia before clinical signs are manifest. The 30 per cent methemoglobinemia associated with hereditary enzyme deficiency in the dog is usually not sufficient to induce clinical signs.

The anemia of Heinz body red cell destruction may be mild to severe. It is usually markedly regenerative. Hemoglobinemia, hemoglobinuria, and jaundice may be present. If the oxidant is methylene blue, bluish-green discoloration of the urine is often seen.

Heinz bodies (Fig. 77–21) may be seen in many red blood cells and are usually recognized on Wright-stained smears. New methylene blue stain should be used to demonstrate the precise nature of the cells. Fragmenting erythrocytes and low numbers of spherocytes are seen in dogs but not cats.

THERAPY OF HEINZ BODY ANEMIA AND METHEMOGLOBINEMIA. The initial approach to therapy is accurate diagnosis and assessment of the clinical status. When methemoglobinemia is significant, administration of one to two mg/kg of body weight of a one per cent solution of methylene blue in a single intravenous injection is advised for man and repeated if necessary. Harvey (1979) states that the dose of 8.8 mg/kg IV for the dog, which has been recommended

in one veterinary reference text, is in the toxic range for Heinz body anemia. Whole blood transfusion or even exchange blood transfusion may be indicated. Oxygen therapy is advised.

In Heinz body anemia, uncomplicated by methemoglobinemia, recovery is usually associated with removal of the toxic principle. In idiopathic cases, a change in diet and environment may be all that is required. Blood transfusion may be necessary when the anemic state is marked.

Acetaminophen Toxicosis. In man, the severity of the toxic signs of acetaminophen toxicosis results in renal and hepatic necrosis. Acetylcysteine, a precursor of glutathione, has been reported to reduce the severity of the toxicosis (St. Omer and McKnight, 1980). The antidote is given at a rate of 1.4 ml/kg of body weight for the ten per cent solution.

Erythrocyte Fragmentation Associated with Systemic Diseases. A variety of diseases have been associated with fragmentation and morphologic alterations of erythrocytes. The terminology of Bessis (Table 77–5) for human erythrocytes is followed. It appears to be applicable to the dog and cat.

Fragmentation anemia has been recently reviewed by Rebar et al. (1981). The spherocytic and Heinz body anemias are forms of fragmentation anemia. Fragmentation anemia may be synonymous with the microangiopathic hemolytic anemia described by Brain et al. (1962).

Disseminated Intravascular Coagulation (DIC). DIC in its chronic form is associated with intravascular fibrin formation distributed in small blood vessels, or focally, as it might appear in hemangiosarcoma of the spleen (Rebar et al., 1980). Erythrocytes entrapped in fibrin are literally torn apart. Bessis (1977) describes the phenomenon as a red cell draped over a fibrin strand — like two saddle bags. The opposing membranes adhere. As the cell is freed, the fused portion, which appears as a pseudovacuole, ruptures, leaving a notch in the cell with its bordering spicules or horns, the keratocyte (Fig. 77–19). The cell is seen when Heinz bodies of the dog are pitted, resulting in the so-called bite or helmet cells (Lees et al., 1979). The keratocytes have from one to six spicules and are associated with schizocytes and spherocytes, further evidence for fragmentation anemia. Usually, the anemia is mild, the reticulocytosis slight, and the thrombocytopenia apparent. This form of fragmentation anemia is present in chronic DIC, which may terminate into fulminating DIC, such as that seen in caval syndrome of dogs with dirofilariasis. Fragmentation anemia is not restricted to chronic DIC, since microangiopathy associated with glomerulonephritis and myelofibrosis predisposes to fragmentation events.

The acanthocyte forms blunted spicules on its surface. It differs from the keratocyte in that it has lost its normal discoid shape and appears spherocytic. The spicules (3 to 12) are irregularly distributed over the surface of the cells and have blunt, club-like tips. Rebar et al. (1981) do not distinguish between acanthocytes and keratocytes and call the cells acanthocytes, thus associating these cells with fragmentation events.

Some acanthocyte forms are called spur (Schull et al., 1978) and burr cells (Schwartz and Motto, 1949). The terminology is confusing to the translator, although it is descriptive of the appearance of the cells. Acanthocytes are associated with hepatic disease. Reduced levels of lecithyl cholesterol acyl transferase alter transfer of fatty acid from lecithin to cholesterol, resulting in accumulation of free cholesterol and lecithin within red cell membranes. The cells affected may appear as leptocytes or acanthocytes.

Regardless of the terminology and distinction between acanthocytes and keratocytes, when evidence for fragmentation — i.e., schizocytes, spherocytes, or hemolysis — is demonstrated, fragmentation anemia is present. Feldman et al. (1981) state that examination of blood smears reveals fragmentation of erythrocytes in 71 per cent of DIC dogs examined.

THERAPY. Fragmentation anemia is secondary to a variety of diseases of diverse etiology. Definition of the predisposing primary disease is necessary. When the primary disease is reversible, the fragmentation anemia regresses spontaneously.

Hypophosphatemia. Severe hemolysis of canine red blood cells has been produced experimentally by hyperalimentation, resulting in marked hypophosphatemia (less than 1.0 mg/dl) (Jacob and Amsden, 1971; Yawata et al., 1974; and Fleming et al., 1976). Perman (1974) documented severe

hemolysis in a hypophosphatemic (less than 1.0 mg/dl) dog with diabetes mellitus. Anemia, hemoglobinemia, and hemoglobinuria were present. Knochel (1977) noted that serum phosphorus levels may be normal or slightly elevated in patients with untreated diabetic ketoacidosis. Usually, large quantities of phosphorus have been eliminated in the urine. With insulin and fluid therapy and correction of the ketoacidosis, severe hypophosphatemia occurred. Under these circumstances, erythrocyte hemolysis is possible.

Hypersplenism. In virtually every disease of man that profoundly affects metabolism, shorter erythrocyte life span has been documented. Somes investigators think that splenomegaly is associated with increased erythrophagocytic activity (Weiss and Tavossoli, 1970), and the occurrence of hypersplenism has been cited (Jandl and Aster, 1967). Splenectomy of cats and dogs has often been performed when data have been insufficient to warrant the diagnosis of hypersplenism, but significant improvement has occasionally been reported to follow splenectomy in chronic hemolytic disease (Schalm, 1965).

The immunologic nature of the preneoplastic, hyperactive spleen is difficult to demonstrate. Splenectomy should be a last resort in these forms of chronic hemolytic disease.

Bedlington Chronic Progressive Hepatitis. A genetically transmitted hepatocellular disease of Bedlington terriers (Hardy et al., 1975; Twedt et al., 1979) is associated with hemolytic episodes due to copper toxicosis. The hemolytic events are similar to copper poisoning in sheep. The nature of the hemolysis in human Wilson's disease with copper toxicosis is the effect of copper through its oxidant action on membrane phospholipids rather than inhibitory effects on intracellular enzymes (Forman et al., 1980).

Anemia Associated with Decreased Red Cell Production. The nonregenerative anemias are characterized by reduced or absent reticulocyte response. The bone marrow is usually hypoplastic, although ineffective erythropoiesis with normal bone marrow cellularity is rarely encountered. The nonregenerative anemias can be divided into nutritional and hypoplastic (aplastic) types (Table 77–15).

Table 77–15.   Anemias Associated with Decreased Red Cell Production

Nutritional Anemias
   Mineral
   Vitamin
   Protein
Hypoplastic and Aplastic Anemia
   Spontaneous
   Drug-induced
   Infectious
Anemia Associated with Feline Leukemia Virus
Anemia of Chronic Renal Disease
Anemia of Chronic Inflammatory Disease
and Malignancy

Nutritional Anemias. Nutritional anemias of the cat and dog are rare, except iron-deficiency anemia, which is usually the result of chronic blood loss. The microcytic hypochromic nonregenerative anemia associated with iron loss is a late manifestion of the disease and reflects severe iron deficiency. (See Chronic Blood Loss.)

Deficiency anemias other than that caused by lack of iron have been produced experimentally. Microcytic hypochromic anemia results from experimental copper deficiency in dogs (Van Wyk et al., 1953), but naturally occurring disease has not been documented.

Megalobastic Anemia. Pernicious anemia is an important disease of man that has not been documented in the dog or cat. This macrocytic (megaloblastic) anemia is due to vitamin B_{12} (cyanocobalamin) deficiency, which is the result of genetically determined failure of the stomach to secrete intrinsic factor in amounts adequate for the physiologic absorption of vitamin B_{12}. Yamaguchi et al. (1967) have shown that intrinsic factor is not necessary for vitamin B_{12} absorption in the dog. Megaloblastic anemia in the dog has been reported by Schalm (1965) and in the cat by Schalm et al., 1975.

The megaloblastic changes in erythrocytes reflect asynchronism in maturation between cytoplasm and nucleus. Macrocytic normochromic erythrocytes are released into the circulation. The nucleus of abnormally nucleated red cells has a lacy, moth-eaten appearance. Abnormal mitotic figures are seen. Hypersegmentation of granulocyte nuclei is another morphologic feature of deficiency in this species and is related to the folic acid requirement for nucleotide synthesis (Thenen and Rasmussen, 1978). Because of the relatively short biological half-life of folic acid, animals may be predisposed to deficiency of this vitamin. Theoretically, deficiency can occur as the result of inadequate intake, poor absorption, excessive utilization, or the administration of folic acid antagonists. Folate antagonists include antineoplastic drugs, such as methotrexate and anticonvulsive agents such as phenytoin (Waxman, 1973). Folic acid–responsive, macrocytic anemia has been documented in a dog to which phenytoin was administered (Perman and Hall, 1973). Malabsorption syndromes in the dog have been associated with macrocytic anemia that was folic acid responsive (Schalm, 1965). Many cases of canine malabsorption have not been associated with macrocytic anemia (Finco et al., 1973). Sims (1979) reports megaloblastic anemia in dogs with chronic diarrhea of several weeks' or months' duration.

The role of vitamin B_{12} and folic acid in hemato- and other cell-poiesis has been reviewed (Herbert and Das, 1976). Problems in diagnosis of megaloblastic anemia exist, in that false-positive and false-negative results may occur in a spectrum of laboratory tests, including complete blood count, serum and erythrocyte folate assays, serum B_{12} assays, and tests of vitamin B_{12} absorption (Shojania, 1980). Demonstration of megaloblastic changes from careful examination of stained blood smears is probably the diagnostic method of choice.

Erythrocyte Macrocytosis in Miniature Poodles. Schalm (1976) described an erythrocyte macrocytosis in 24 miniature poodles. The erythrocyte macrocytosis (MCV 92.6 ± 6.9 fl) was not accompanied by anemia (PCV 45.5 ± 4.9) although the RBC was $4.93 \pm 0.66 \times 10^6$. Neutrophil hypersegmentation was recorded. The abnormalities persisted and were not altered by B_{12} administration.

Vitamin B_{12}, Folic Acid, and Erythroleukemia. Megaloblastic change in erythroleukemia in the cat has been described (Schalm et al., 1975) and in vitamin B_{12} and folic acid deficiency (Schalm, 1980). Similar changes were described by Lewis and Rebar (1979) in a cat. The megaloblastic changes responded to folic acid therapy only to have the patient develop erythroleukemia four months later.

Pyridoxine Deficiency. Pyridoxine (vitamin B_6) deficiency has been produced experimentally in dogs. The anemia is microcytic hypochromic (Schalm, 1965). Scott (1964) suggests that pyridoxine-deficiency anemia occurs in cats.

The occurrence of nonregenerative anemia characterized by siderocytes and sideroblasts has been reported in man in association with a variety of disorders, including pyridoxine and folic acid deficiencies (Harris and Kellermeyer, 1970). Since siderocytes (Fig. 77–22) and sideroblasts (Fig. 77–24) occur in the dog, consideration should be given to conditions associated with these cells in man whenever they are encountered in dogs.

The documentation of naturally occurring vitamin-deficiency anemias in cats and dogs is in its infancy and will remain at this level until more sophisticated methodology, including vitamin assay, is applied in veterinary medicine. Until existing technology is applied to the cat and dog, crude diagnostic inferences and therapeutic efforts will prevail.

Protein Deficiency. The importance of protein for hemoglobin production in dogs has long been known (Hahn and Whipple, 1939; Miller et al., 1947). The widespread use of balanced commercial rations has minimized anemia associated with inadequate protein intake, but the condition is still occasionally encountered in dogs owned by the uninformed or impoverished.

MINERAL AND VITAMIN THERAPY. The beneficial results of specific replacement mineral and vitamin therapy is well documented. The use of combination vitamin preparations in all anemic patients is unnecessary. Consideration should be given to dietary and alimentary status and excretion pathways. The water-soluble vitamins pyridoxine, niacin, and riboflavin are rather quickly eliminated from the body. Dietary folic acid requirements are known for the cat. Vitamin B_{12} usually has a long-lasting body storage pool. Iron therapy is only beneficial in iron deficiency. Attention should be given to providing a balanced ration.

Hypoplastic and Aplastic Anemia

The term *aplastic anemia* generally denotes pancytopenia caused by generalized bone marrow suppression. It is characterized by granulocytopenia and thrombocytopenia as well as anemia. The clinical manifestations of pancytopenia are dependent upon the predominate circulating cellular deficit. The animal may be presented for examination because of a bleeding tendency associated with thrombocytopenia, because of signs of infection referable to leukopenia, or because of signs of anemia. Owing to differences in cellular half-life, acute stem-cell aplasia is more likely to be associated with signs referable to thrombocytopenia or leukopenia, whereas more chronic hypoplastic bone-marrow disease is likely to be associated with anemia.

Aplastic anemia may be idiopathic or may be associated with various diseases and conditions such as malignancy, chronic bacterial or viral infection, ionizing radiation, and myelophthisis. Drug-induced aplastic anemias occur. Regardless of cause, aplastic anemias are usually normocytic and normochromic and, by definition, lack peripheral signs of regeneration.

Congenital Bone Marrow Hypoplasia. Severe nonregenerative anemia associated with osteopetrosis in the dog has been described (Lees and Sautter, 1979). The entity (Riser and Frankhauser, 1970) appears to be similar to osteopetrosis of humans, cattle, mice, and rats. The gradual development of sclerotic bone obliterates the marrow space, resulting in a myelophthisic type anemia. Because of the gradual onset, anemia is the prominent feature. Leukocyte counts tend to be normal to decreased. A variable degree of thrombocytopenia may be present. The condition is thought to be an osteoclast defect and has been corrected by bone marrow transplantation in humans and rats.

Drug-Induced Hypoplastic and Aplastic Anemia. The toxicity of chemotherapeutic agents for neoplastic and immunologic disorders is well documented (Cadman, 1977). With the exception of the plant alkaloids vinblastine and vincristine, and the antibiotic bleomycin, all are marrow suppressive. In general, the neoplastic and immunosuppressive chemotherapeutic agents are dose dependent and at the stem cell level. Variability does exist in effect on cell lines and when the nadir counts occur. Unless overdosed, complete recovery of the bone marrow is expected.

Estrogen-Induced Aplastic Anemia of Dogs. Estrogens, including synthetics such as diethylstilbestrol, exert a depressive effect on canine bone marrow that can result in aplastic anemia (Arnold et al., 1973; Crafts, 1948; Steinberg, 1970; Lowenstine et al., 1972). Chiu (1974) has characterized more fully the toxic manifestations of estrogen administration in the dog (Fig. 77–31). The initial response to excess estrogen is thrombocytosis followed by thrombocytopenia 12 to 14 days after administration. The leukocyte count progressively increases for 17 to 22 days but is followed by an abrupt fall to normal or leukopenic levels. The more gradual fall in the PCV is caused primarily by red cell senescence and failure of normal replacement but may be complicated by hemorrhage. Peripheral blood changes reflect bone marrow alterations. The initial effects are depression of erythroid and megakaryocytic cells, accompanied by marked myeloid hypoplasia. Bone marrow recovery may be complete if sublethal doses of estrogens are administered, but chronic aplastic anemia or acute fulminating aplastic anemia may result, depending on the dose and the individual dog. It is not known whether the bone marrow of cats is as sensitive to estrogens as the bone marrow of dogs.

The best therapy for estrogen-induced aplastic anemia of dogs is prevention. The dose of diethylstilbestrol administered to dogs should rarely exceed 0.75 mg per pound and never exceed 1.0 mg per pound or a total dose of 20 mg for any purpose. Doses as high as these should not be repeated for two months. Estradiol is generally considered to be a minimum of ten times as potent as diethylstilbestrol and should be administered at a proportionately reduced dose. If inadvertently high or repeat doses of estrogens are administered, platelet and red cell replacement, as well as antibiotic administration, should be instituted when indicated by peripheral blood changes. All therapeutic efforts are likely to be futile if thrombocytopenia persists for two weeks or more (Chiu, 1974).

Endogenous estrogen depression of the bone marrow occurs with estrogen-secreting neoplasms, as in some Sertoli cell tumors. Aplastic anemia in ferrets has been attributed to prolonged estrogenic exposure during protracted estrus (Kociba and Caputo, 1981).

Estrogen toxicity has not been reported in cats. The authors' observations are that cats differ from the dog in that doses five times greater than those inducing aplastic anemia in dogs are associated with only mild stem cell depression.

Chloramphenicol-Induced Anemia. Chloramphenicol administered orally or parenterally at therapeutic doses results in mild nonregenerative anemia that reverses when drug administration is stopped (Penny et al., 1970b; Manyan et al., 1972). The resultant anemia is induced by chloramphenicol inhibition of ferrochelatase, an enzyme necessary for the incorporation of ferrous iron into protoporphyrin IX. This side effect of chloramphenicol is also recognized in man and is considered to be distinct from severe bone marrow aplasia (Petitpierre-Gabathuler and Beck, 1972). The latter toxicity has not been documented in cats or dogs.

High doses of chloramphenicol administered to the cat may result in inappetence and depression, which may lead to death in the second or third week of continuous administration (Penny et al., 1970b). Chloramphenicol is also known to cause vacuolization of pronormoblasts and immature myeloid cells in man, cat, and dog (Schober et al., 1972; Perman, 1974). In more recent studies (Watson and Middleton, 1978), the oral administration of 120 mg/kg/day in three divided doses causes severe toxic effects of reduced food intake, dehydration, CNS depression, vomiting, diarrhea, and bone marrow changes. Toxic changes were observed at the 60 mg/kg/day level.

Chloramphenicol toxicity in dogs dosed at 175, 225, and 275 mg/kg/day was manifest by reduced appetite and weight loss (Watson, 1977). Bone marrow suppression occurred in four of nine dogs dosed at 225 or 275 mg/kg/day.

Chloramphenicol should not be administered to cats or dogs with nonregenerative anemia if another antibiotic is likely to be equally effective. Administration of the antibiotic should cease if toxic effects such as inappetence are detected in any patient to which it is administered.

Phenylbutazone-Induced Bone Marrow Suppression. Phenylbutazone-induced blood dyscrasias have been reported in dogs (Watson et al., 1980; Schalm, 1980). The marrow suppression is variable. Thrombocytopenia and leukopenia are early manifestations followed by nonregenerative anemia, which may be severe when accompanied by blood loss. This type of reaction differs from the usual response to cytotoxic drugs in that it is not dose dependent and is unpredictable. The mechanism of injury is not known. Speculation from our observations during therapy suggests immunologic mediated injury. The fatal aspects of the side reaction to this drug need to be considered when its use is anticipated.

Infectious Hypoplastic or Aplastic Anemia

Ehrlichiosis (Tropical Canine Pancytopenia). A fatal infectious disease of dogs characterized by hemorrhage, pancytopenia, and emaciation, ehrlichiosis is caused by infection with *Ehrlichia canis* (Ewing, 1969; Huxsoll et al., 1972; Seamer and Snape, 1972). In the chronic form, the disease is manifested by anemia, leukopenia, and variable degrees of thrombocytopenia. Diagnosis is based on the recognition of intracytoplasmic inclusions in lymphocytes, monocytes, or neutrophils. Affected dogs may be Coombs positive (Perman, 1974).

Pure Red Cell Aplasia Anemia. Since the term *aplastic anemia* generally indicates generalized bone marrow hypoplasia and associated peripheral consequences, pure red cell aplasia (anemia) is used to denote selective erythroid bone marrow depression and associated anemia (Lund and Avolt, 1972). In most instances, pure red cell aplasia is idiopathic. It is seen in SLE of humans and dogs. Immunologic injury to the committed stem cell as a mechanism of this entity is discussed by Cline and Golde (1978). A report by Stockham et al. (1980) describes such a case in the dog. Fletch et al. (1975) describe impaired erythropoiesis in two dogs. Similar descriptions have been made in which androgen therapy for stimulation of the bone marrow has been suggested to be beneficial (Eldor et al., 1978) while the dog was simultaneously receiving prednisone. The appropriate definition studies are lacking and the choice remains to use corticosteroids, based on the hypothesis that immune-mediated disease is the cause or that androgens act as a marrow stimulant, or both. In either case, blood transfusions are frequently necessary, along with chemotherapy for several weeks before a response is to be expected.

Anemia Associated with Feline Leukemia Virus. Both aplastic anemia (pancytopenia) and pure red cell aplasia of the cat are often associated with positive fluorescent antibody test for feline leukemia virus (Hardy, 1974). Affected cats do not have lymphoma or leukemia but may develop either if survival is of sufficient duration.

The anemia induced by feline leukemia virus is normocytic and normochromic and void of significant reticulocyte response (Hoover et al., 1974). Hardy (1974) has described features of pancytopenia associated with positive fluorescent antibody tests that distinguish the syndrome from feline panleukopenia (feline enteritis). Feline pancytopenia associated with leukemia virus infection tends to occur more often in adult cats, has a more chronic course, and is characterized by less severe leukopenia (1500 to 4000 WBC per cu mm). Thrombocytopenia may be present, in contrast to feline panleukopenia (enteritis), which is rarely characterized by thrombocytopenia. Feline panleukopenia (enteritis) occurs more frequently in young (often unvaccinated) cats and is characterized by less severe anemia but more profound leukopenia.

Pedersen (1981) states that the anemia is a common long-term sequela to FeLV, appearing from six months to three years after the initial infection. It is often associated with deficiency of white blood cells and blood platelets. A similar self-limiting anemia is seen in the primary phase of the infection. The anemia of the secondary stage is often progressive and fatal.

The anemia associated with FeLV infection was studied clinically in 100 FeLV virus-positive cats by Cotter (1979). The median survival was four months in the treated group of 29 cats (range two weeks to seven years). Eight cats had return of normal counts, and one cat converted from FeLV-positive to FeLV-negative.

Cotter (1979) stresses the need for bone marrow examination to aid in differential diagnosis. Inasmuch as remissions are possible, supportive therapy is necessary. Blood transfusions are most beneficial.

Erythropoietin Deficiency. Chronic renal disease leading to end-stage kidneys is reliably associated with nonregenerative anemia caused by lack of erythropoietin production (Osborne et al., 1972). The anemia is normochromic and normocytic and is not accompanied by reticulocytosis. The anemia may be mild or marked. Young dogs with chronic progressive renal disease frequently have signs referable to anemia rather than uremia because the expanding blood volume associated with growth aggravates the erythropoietin deficiency. Adult animals are usually examined because of signs referable to renal insufficiency or uremia rather than anemia.

Therapy of the anemia associated with chronic renal failure is restricted to the administration of androgenic anabolic steroids and the short-term benefits of red cell replacement. If histocompatibility testing gains more widespread use, renal transplantation may have more practical application in the future, as may the use of dialysis techniques. Dialysis techniques may alleviate uremia, but anemia persists because erythropoietin is not replaced.

Therapy of Hypoplasia and Aplastic Anemia. The therapy of severe aplastic anemia is dependent on the etiology and the hematologic alterations present. When the inciting cause is known, dose response data may prove useful in prognosis. The disease needs to be characterized by clinical, blood, and bone marrow findings.

Acute Aplastic Anemia. The principal clinical features relate to thrombocytopenia and severe leukopenia. Perman et al. (1962) studied the regenerative ability of hemopoietic tissue following lethal x-irradiation in dogs. The principles of therapy were replacement of blood elements, antibiotics, and supportive care. Fresh whole blood, platelet-rich plasma, or platelet concentrates are necessary to control hemorrhage. Post-transfusion platelet counts of 25,000 to 75,000 should be achieved. Without augmented use or destruction, a single blood or platelet concentrate transfusion will maintain > 5000 platelets for three to five days. Repeat transfusions are necessary.

Severe leukopenia, and neutropenia specifically (< 200 neutrophil/dl), is invariably associated with high fever caused by opportunistic organisms. High-dose single broad-spectrum antibiotic therapy is usually effective for five to seven days, after which time fever returns, indicating resistant organisms. The second antibiotic is usually less effective and may control fever for up to five days. The third antibiotic is still less effective in the neutropenic dog or cat.

In general, appropriate platelet and red cell replacement, antibiotic therapy, and general supportive care will keep the patient alive for at least two weeks, a period usually of sufficient length to allow bone marrow recovery if regeneration is possble.

Chronic Aplastic Anemia. The chronic form of stem cell injury results in severe nonregenerative anemia. Erythrocyte production is of low order for a long time. Leukocyte and platelet deficiency is of variable degree, although fatal. Thus, anemia develops over an extended period.

The therapy of this form of anemia requires repeat blood transfusion to replace red cell deficits. A gradual return of hemopoiesis is all that can be expected. Androgen stimulation of the bone marrow may be attempted.

Bone Marrow Transplantation. Extensive studies on canine bone marrow transplantation have been reported from several laboratories (Storb et al., 1976). Successful treatment of PK deficiency anemia and cyclic neutropenia have been described (Weiden et al., 1974; Weiden et al., 1976). Autologous transplants have been used in therapeutic modalities for hemopoietic neoplasms. Long-term preservation of bone marrow and stem cell pools in dogs is possible (Gorin et al., 1978; Northdurft et al., 1977).

The application of bone marrow transplantation to hypoplastic and aplastic anemia is restricted by the availability of compatible and matched donors. The technology and expertise are available.

Anemia of Infection and Malignancy. Both malignancy and chronic infection are often accompanied by normocytic, normochromic nonregenerative anemia. The mechanism of the associated anemia is obscure (Kurnick et al., 1972). The anemia of chronic infection is often characterized by rouleau formation, hyperglobulinemia, and leukocytosis. An anemia associated with malignancy often occurs and cannot be attributed to blood loss, hemolysis, anorexia, or myelophthisis. The anemia of malignancy occurs prior to the administration of myelosuppressive or immunosuppressive drugs. Cancer chemotherapy, however, may be accompanied by iatrogenic anemia caused by inhibition of DNA or RNA synthesis, suppression of mitosis, or direct cytotoxic properties of the chemotherapeutic agents (Pisciotta, 1971).

Recent studies have yielded additional information on the pathogenesis of the anemia of inflammatory disease in the dog (Feldman, 1979; Feldman et al., 1981a,b,c,d) and in the cat (Weiss, 1981).

The anemia is normocytic and normochromic. There is shortened red cell survival (Weiss, 1981). The bone marrow is less responsive and somewhat hypoplastic. There is no significant reticulocyte response. Iron metabolism is altered, in that serum iron and iron binding capacity de-

creases. Transferrin saturation decreases and free red cell protophyrin increases (Feldman et al., 1981). The monocyte-macrophage iron storage compartment increases. This is in contrast to iron deficiency anemia, which is differentiated by the reduced iron storage compartment or serum ferritin levels. The anemia is insidious in development and mild in the dog. In contrast, the shorter life span and the decreased survival time of erythrocytes may lead to rapid and profound anemia in the cat (Weiss, 1981).

The anemia is unresponsive to hematinics. It regresses with recovery from the underlying inflammatory or neoplastic process. Therapy is therefore directed toward the primary disease.

REFERENCES

Alsaker, R. D.: The formation, emergence, and maturation of the reticulocyte: A review. Vet. Clin. Pathol. *6*:7, 1977.

Alsaker, R. D., Laber, J., Stevens, J., and Perman, V.: A comparison of polychromasia and reticulocyte counts in assessing erythrocytic regenerative response in the cat. J.A.V.M.A. *170*:39, 1977.

Altman, N. H., Melby, E. C., and Squire, R. A.: Intraerythrocytic crystalloid bodies in cats. Blood *39*:901, 1972.

Anderson, A. C., and Schalm, O. W.: Hematology. *In* Anderson, A. C. (ed.): The Beagle as an Experimental Animal. Ames, Iowa, Iowa State Univ. Press, 1970.

Anderson, J. F., Magnarelli, L. A., and Sulzer, A. J.: Canine babesiosis: Indirect fluorescent antibody test for a North American isolate of *Babesia gibsoni*. J.A.V.M.A. *41*:2102, 1980.

Arnold, O., Holtz, F., and Marx, H.: Ueber die Wirkung Des Follikelhormons auf Knochenmark und Blut bei Hunden. Arch. Exp. Pathol. Pharmacol. *186*:1, 1973.

Atwell, R. B., Johnstone, I., Read, R., Reilly, S., and Wilkins, S.: Haemolytic anemia in two dogs suspected to have been induced by levamisole. Aust. Vet. Jour. *55*:292, 1979.

Avolt, M. D., Lund, J. E., and Pickett, J. C.: Autoimmune hemolytic anemia in a dog. J.A.V.M.A. *162*:45, 1973.

Axelrod, A. A., McLeod, O. L., Shreeve, M. M., and Heath, D. S.: Properties of cells that produce erythrocytic colonies *in vitro*. *In* Robinson, W. A. (ed.): Proceedings of the Second International Workshop on Hemopoiesis in Culture. Airlie House, Va., Grune & Stratton, New York, 1973.

Baran, D. T., Griner, P. F., and Klemperer, M. R.: Recovery from aplastic anemia after treatment with cylcophosphamide. N. Eng. J. Med. *295*:1522, 1976.

Barcroft, J., and Stephens, J. G.: Observations upon the size of the spleen. J. Physiol. *64*:1, 1927.

Beard, M. E. J., Necheles, T. F., and Allen, D. M.:

Clinical experience with intensive transfusion therapy in Cooley's anemia. Ann. N.Y. Acad. Sci. *165*:415, 1969.

Beaver, P. C., Yoshida, Y., and Ash, L. R.: Mating of *Ancylostoma caninum* in relationship to blood loss in the host. J. Parasitol. *50*:286, 1964.

Bendele, R. A., Schwartz, W. L., and Jones, L. P.: Cytauxzoonosis-like diseases in Texas cats. Friskies Research Digest *12*:10, 1976a.

Bendele, R. A., Schwartz, W. L., and Jones, L. P.: Cytauxzoonosis-like diseases in Texas cats. Southwest. Vet. *29*:244, 1976b.

Beritic, T.: Studies on Schmauch bodies. I. The incidence in normal cats and the relationship to Heinz bodies. Blood *25*:999, 1964.

Berman, E.: Hemogram of the cat during pregnancy and lactation and after lactation. Am. J. Vet Res. *35*:457, 1974.

Bertles, J., and Beck, W.: Biochemical aspects of reticulocyte maturation. J. Biol. Chem. *237*:3770, 1962.

Bessis, M.: Blood Smear Reinterpreted. Springer-International, Berlin, 1977.

Bessis, M.: Red cell shapes. An illustrated classification and its rationale. *In* Bessis, M., Wood, R. I., and Lebland, P. F. (eds.): Red Cell Shape. Springer-Verlag, New York, 1973a.

Bessis, M.: Living Blood Cells and their Ultrastructure. Springer-Verlag, New York, 1973b.

Bessis, M.: Morphology of the different stages of maturation of the cells of the erythrocytic series in mammals. Exp. Biol. Med. *1*:220, 1967.

Beutler, E., Fairbanks, V. F., and Fahey, J. L.: Clinical Disorders of Iron Metabolism. Grune & Stratton, New York, 1963.

Bild, C. E.: Clinical aspects of canine blood transfusion. Vet. Med. *54*:459, 1959.

Bjorkman, S. E.: Chronic refractory anemia with sideroblastic bone marrow. Study of 4 cases. Blood *11*:250, 1956.

Bliss, J. Q., Johns, D. G., and Burgen, A. S. V.: Transfusion reactions due to plasma incompatibility in dogs. Circ. Res. 7:79, 1959.

Boggs, D. R.: Transfusion of neutrophils as prevention or treatment of infection in patients with neutropenia. N. Eng. J. Med. *290*:1055, 1974.

Bottomley, S. S.: Porphyrin and iron metabolism in sideroblastic anemia. Semin. Hematol. *14*:169, 1977.

Bowdler, A. J.: The role of the spleen and splenectomy in autoimmune hemolytic disease. Semin. Hematol. *13*(4):335, 1976.

Boycott, A. E.: The blood as a tissue: Hypertrophy and atrophy of the red corpuscles. Proc. Roy. Soc. Med. *23*:15, 1929.

Bradley, T. R., and Metcalf, D.: The growth of mouse bone marrow cells in vitro. Aust. J. Exp. Biol. Med. Sci. *44*:287, 1966.

Brain, M. C., Dacie, J. V., and Hourihene, D. O. B.: Microangiopathic hemolytic anemia: The possible role of vascular lesions in pathogenesis. Br. J. Haematol. *8*:358, 1962.

Brecher, G.: New methylene blue as a reticulocyte stain. Am. J. Clin. Pathol. *19*:895, 1949.

Buhles, W. C., Huxsoll, D. L., and Hildebrant, P. K.: Tropical canine pancytopenia: Role of aplastic anemia in the pathogenesis of severe disease. J. Comp. Pathol. *85*:511, 1975.

Bull, R. W.: New knowledge about blood groups in dogs. Proc. Gaines Vet. Symp., 1972.

Bundza, A., Lumsden, J. H., McSherry, B. J., Valli, V. E. O., and Janzen, E. A.: Haemobartonellosis in a dog in association with Coombs positive anemia. Can. Vet. J. *17*:267, 1976.

Bunn, H. F.: Differences in the interaction of 2,3-diphosphoglycerate with certain mammalian hemoglobins. Science *172*:1049, 1971.

Bush, B. M., and Frankhauser, R.: Polycythemia vera in a bitch. J. Small Anim. Pract. *13*:75, 1972.

Cadman, E.: Toxicity of chemotherapeutic agents. *In* Becker, F. F. (ed.): Cancer, A Comprehensive Treatise. Vol. 5, Plenum Press, New York, 1977.

Campbell, F. R.: Electron microscopic studies on fate of erythroblast ribosomes. Anat. Res. *174*:513, 1972.

Carb, A. V.: Polycythemia vera in a dog. J.A.V.M.A. *154*:289, 1969.

Card, R. T., and Brain, M. C.: The "anemia" of childhood: Evidence for a physiological response to hyperphosphatemia. N Engl. J. Med. *288*:388, 1973.

Card, R. T., McGrath, M. J., Paulson, E. J., and Valberg, L. S.: Life-span and autohemolysis of macrocytic erythrocytes produced in response to hemorrhage. Am. J. Physiol. *216*:974, 1969.

Chiu, T.: Studies on estrogen-induced proliferative disorders of hemopoietic tissue in the dog. Thesis, University of Minnesota, 1974.

Clark, C. H., and Woodley, C. H.: The absorption of red blood cells after parenteral injection at various sites. Am. J. Vet. Res. *20*:1062, 1959.

Clark, C. H., Kling, J. M., Woodley, C. H., and Sharp, N.: A quantitative measurement of the blood loss caused by ancylostomiasis in dogs. Am. J. Vet. Res. *22*:370, 1961.

Cline, M. J., and Berlin, N. I.: Red blood cell lifespan using DFP[32] as a cohort label. Blood *19*:715, 1962.

Cline, M. J., and Golde, D. W.: Controlling the production of blood cells. Blood *53*:157, 1979.

Cline, M. J., and Golde, D. W.: Immune suppression of hematopoiesis. Am. J. Med. *301*, 1978.

Cole, N.: Polycythemia in a dog. N. Am. Vet. *35*:601, 1954.

Concannon, P. W., Powers, M. E., Holder, W., and Hansel, W.: Pregnancy and parturition in the bitch. Biol. Reprod. *16*:517, 1977.

Conrad, M. E., and Crosby, W. H.: Bone marrow biopsy modification of the Vim-Silverman needle. J. Lab. Clin. Med. *57*:642, 1961.

Costea, N.: The differential diagnosis of hemolytic anemia. Med. Clin. North Am. *57*:289, 1972.

Cotter, S. M.: Anemia associated with feline leukemia virus infection. J.A.V.M.A. *175*:1191, 1979.

Coulter, D. B., and Small, L. L.: Effects of hemolysis on plasma electrolyte concentrations of canine and porcine blood. Cornell Vet. *61*:660, 1971.

Crafts, R. C.: The effects of estrogen on the bone marrow of adult female dogs. Blood *3*:276, 1948.

Craig, T. M., Smallwood, J. E., Knauer, K. W., and McGrath, J. P.: *Hepatozoan canis* infections in dogs: Clinical radiographic, and hematologic findings. J.A.V.M.A. *173*:967, 1978.

Cramer, D. V., and Lewis, R. M.: Reticulocyte response in the cat. J.A.V.M.A. *160*:61, 1972.

Dacie, J. V.: The Hemolytic Anemias — Congenital and Acquired. *In*: The Autoimmune Hemolytic Anemias, 2nd ed., Grune & Stratton, New York, 1962.

Davies, M., Muckle, T. J., Cassells-Smith, A., Webster, D., and Kerr, D. N. S.: Oxymetholone in the treatment of anaemia in chronic renal failure. Br. J. Urol. *44*:387, 1972.

Deiss, A., Kurth, D., Cartwright, G. E., and Wintrobe, M. M.: Experimental production of siderocytes. J. Clin. Invest. *45*:353, 1966.

Dodds, W. J., and Ward, M. O.: Iron supplementation in dogs and cats. Mod. Vet. Pract. *61*:496, 1980.

Donovan, E. F., and Loeb, W. F.: Polycythemia rubra vera in the dog. J.A.V.M.A. *134*:36, 1959.

Doxey, D. L.: Some conditions associated with variations in circulating oestrogens — Blood picture alterations. J. Small Anim. Pract. *7*:375, 1966.

Dubin, S., and Syopniewski-Radovsky, A.: Variations of hematocrit values with choice of anticoagulant and choice of measurement method. Bull. Am. Soc. Vet. Clin. Pathol. *2*:25, 1973.

Eisenbrandt, D. L., and Smith, J. E.: Evaluation of preservatives and containers for storage of canine blood. J.A.V.M.A. *163*:989, 1973.

Eisenbrandt, D. L., and Smith, J. E.: Use of biochemical measures to estimate viability of red blood cells in canine blood stored in acid citrate dextrose solution, with and without ascorbic acid. J.A.V.M.A. *163*:984, 1973.

Eldor, A., Hershko, C., and Bruchina, A.: Androgen responsive aplastic anemia in a dog. J.A.V.M.A. *173*:304, 1978.

Ellis, L. D., Jensen, W. M., and Westerman, M. P.: Needle biopsy of bone and marrow. Arch. Intern. Med. *114*:213, 1964.

Ettinger, S. J., and Suter, P. F.: Canine Cardiology. W. B. Saunders Co., Philadelphia, 1970.

Ewing, G. O.: Familial nonspherocytic hemolytic anemia of Basenji dogs. J.A.V.M.A. *154*:503, 1969b.

Ewing, G. O., Schalm, O. W., and Smith, R. S.: Hematologic values of normal basenji dogs. J.A.V.M.A. *161*:1661, 1972.

Ewing, S. A.: Canine ehrlichiosis. Adv. Vet. Sci. Comp. Med. *13*:331, 1969a.

Fairbanks, V. F.: Nonequivalence of automated and manual hematocrit and erythrocyte indices. Am. J. Clin. Pathol. *73*:55, 1980.

Fan, L. C., Dorner, J. L., and Hoffmann, W. E.:

Reticulocyte response and maturation in experimental acute blood loss anemia in the cat. J.A.A.H.A. *14*:219, 1978.

Fantoni, A., Farace, M. G., and Gambari, R.: Embryonic hemoglobins in man and other mammals. Blood *57*:623, 1981.

Farkas, M. C., and Farkas, J. N.: Hemolytic anemia due to ingestion of onions in a dog. J.A.A.H.A. *10*:65, 1974.

Feldman, B. F.: The anemia of inflammatory disease in the dog. Vet. Clin. Pathol. *9*:44, 1980.

Feldman, B. F., Kaneko, J. J., and Farver, T. B.: Anemia of inflammatory disease in the dog: Ferrokinetics of adjuvant-induced anemia. Am. J. Vet. Res. *42*:583, 1981a.

Feldman, B. F., Kaneko, J. J., and Farver, T. B.: Anemia of inflammatory disease in the dog: Availability of storage iron in inflammatory disease. Am. J. Vet. Res. *42*:586, 1981b.

Feldman, B. F., Kaneko, J. J., and Farver, T. B.: Anemia of inflammatory disease in the dog. Clinical characterization. Am. J. Vet. Res. *42*:1109, 1981c.

Feldman, B. F., Keen, C. L., Kaneko, J. J., and Farvar, T. B.: Anemia of inflammatory disease in the dog: Measurement of hepatic superoxide dismutase, hepatic nonheme iron, copper, zinc, and ceruloplasmin and serum iron, copper, and zinc. Am. J. Vet. Res. *42*:1118, 1981.

Feldman, B. F., Madewell, B. R., and O'Neill, S.: Disseminated intravascular coagulation: Antithrombin, plasminogen, and coagulation abnormalities in 41 dogs. J.A.V.M.A. *179*:151, 1981.

Finco, D. R., Duncan, J. R., Schall, W. D., Hooper, B. E., Chandler, F. W., and Keating, K. A.: Chronic enteric disease and hypoproteinemia in 9 dogs. J.A.V.M.A. *163*:262, 1973.

Finco, D. R., Duncan, J. R., Schall, W. D., and Prasse, K. W.: Acetaminophen toxicity in the cat. J.A.V.M.A. *166*:469, 1975.

Fisher, J. W.: Erythropoietin: Pharmacology, biogenesis and control of production. Pharmacol. Rev. *24*:459, 1972.

Fishler, J. J., and Birzele, F. D.: Feline infectious anemia. *In* Kirk, R. W. (ed.): Current Veterinary Therapy V. W. B. Saunders Company, Philadelphia, 1974.

Fleming, C. R., McGill, D. B., Hoffman, H. N. II, and Nelson, R. A.: Subject review: Total parenteral nutrition. Mayo Clin. Prac. *51*:187, 1976.

Fletch, S. M., and Pinkerton, P. H.: An inherited anemia associated with hereditary chondrodysplasia in the Alaskan malamute. Can. Vet. J. *13*:270, 1972.

Fletch, S. M., and Smart, M.: Normal biochemical and hematologic parameters in the growing canine. Bull. Am. Soc. Vet. Clin. Pathol. *1*:11, 1972.

Fletch, S. M., DeGeer, T. F., and Catherwood, J.: Impaired erythropoiesis in two dogs. Bull. Am. Soc. Vet. Clin. Pathol. *4*:31, 1975.

Forman, S. J., Kumar, K. S., Redeker, A. G., and Hochstein, P.: Hemolytic anemia in Wilson disease: Clinical findings and biochemical mechanisms. Am. J. Hematol. *9*:269, 1980.

Forstrom, R. J., and Blackshear, P. I.: Needles and hemolysis. N. Engl. J. Med. *282*:967, 1970.

Frank, M. M., Schreiber, A. D., Atkinson, M. D., and Joffe, C. J.: Pathophysiology of Immune Hemolytic Anemia. Ann. Int. Med. *37*:210, 1977.

Futter, G. J., and Belonji, P. C.: Studies on feline babesiosis. I. Historical review. J. S. Afr. Vet Assoc. *50*:105, 1980.

George, J. W., and Duncan, J. R.: The hematology of lead poisoning in man and animals. Vet. Clin. Pathol. *8*:23, 1979.

Georgi, J. R., LeJambre, L. F., and Ratcliffe, L. H.: *Ancylostoma caninum* burden in relationship to erythrocyte loss in dogs. J. Parasitol. *55*:1205, 1969.

Giddens, W. E., Jr., Labbe, R. F., Swango, L. J., and Padgett, G. A.: Feline congenital erythropoietic porphyria associated with severe anemia and renal disease. Am. J. Pathol. *80*:367, 1975.

Glenn, B. L., Glenn, H. G., and Omtvedt, I. T.: Congenital porphyria in the domestic cat *(Felis catus)*: Preliminary investigations on inheritance pattern. Am. J. Vet. Res. *29*:1653, 1968.

Golde, D. W., Bersch, N., and Li, C. H.: Growth hormone: Species specific stimulation of erythropoieses *in vitro*. Science *196*:1112, 1977.

Goodman, L. S., and Gilman, A.: The Pharmacological Basis of Therapeutics, 4th ed. The Macmillan Co., London, 1970.

Gorin, N. C., Herzig, G., Bull, M. I., and Graw, R. G.: Long-term preservation of bone marrow and stem cells in dogs. Blood *51*:257, 1978.

Greene, C. E., Kristensen, F., Hoff, E. J., and Wiggins, M. D.: Cold hemagglutinin disease in a dog. J.A.V.M.A. *170*:505, 1977.

Gregerson, M. L., and Schiro, H.: The behavior of the dye T-1829 with respect to its absorption by red blood cells and its fate in blood undergoing coagulation. Am. J. Physiol. *121*:284, 1938.

Griggs, R. D., and Harris, J. W.: Erythrocyte survival and heme synthesis in lead poisoning. Clin. Res. *6*:188, 1958.

Groves, M. G., and Yap, L. F.: *Babesia gibsoni* in a dog. J.A.V.M.A. *153*:689, 1968.

Grukzit, O. M.: I. Anemia of dogs produced by feeding the whole onions and of onion fraction. Am. J. Med. Sci. *181*:812, 1931a.

Grukzit, O. M.: II. Anemia in dogs produced by feeding disulphide compounds. Am. J. Med. Sci. *181*:815, 1931b.

Hahn, P. F., and Whipple, G. H.: Hemoglobin production in anemia limited by low protein intake. Influence of iron intake, protein supplements and fasting. J. Exp. Med. *69*:315, 1939.

Halliwell, R. E. W.: Autoimmune disease in the dog. Adv. Vet. Sci. Comp. Med. *22*:221, 1978.

Halliwell, R. E. W., and Werner, L. L.: Autoimmune Disease. *In* Chandler, E. A., et al. (eds.): Canine Medicine and Therapeutics. Blackwell Scientific Publications, Oxford, 1979.

Hamilton, M. N., and Edelstein, S. J.: Cat hemoglobin: pH dependent cooperativity of oxygen binding. Science *178*:1104, 1972.

Hardy, R. M., Stevens, J. B., and Stowe, C. M.: Chronic progressive hepatitis in Bedlington terriers associated with elevated liver copper concentrations. Minn. Vet. *15*:13, 1975.

Hardy, W. D., Jr.: Feline leukemia virus-related diseases. Proc. Am. Anim. Hosp. Assoc., South Bend, 1974.

Harris, J. W., and Kellermeyer, R. W.: The Red Cell. Text Ed. Harvard University Press, Cambridge, 1970.

Harvey, J. W.: College of Veterinary Medicine, University of Florida, Gainesville, Fl., 1981. Personal communication.

Harvey, J. W.: Feline hemobartonellosis. *In* Kirk, R. W. (ed.): Current Veterinary Therapy VII. W. B. Saunders Company, Philadelphia, 1980.

Harvey, J. W., and Gaskin, J. M.: Feline haptoglobin. Am. J. Vet. Res. *39*:549, 1978a.

Harvey, J. W., and Gaskin, J. M.: Feline haemobartonellosis. Proc. Am. Anim. Hosp. Assoc., South Bend, *45*:117, 1978b.

Harvey, J. W., and Gaskin, J. M.: Feline hemobartonellosis: attempts to induce relapses of clinical disease in chronically infected cats. J.A.A.H.A. *14*:453, 1978c.

Harvey, J. W., and Gaskin, J. M.: Experimental feline haemobartonellosis. J.A.A.H.A. *13*:28, 1977.

Harvey, J. W., and Kornick, H. P.: Phenazopyridine toxicosis in the cat. J.A.V.M.A. *169*:327, 1976.

Harvey, J. W., Ling, G. V., and Kaneko, J. J.: Methemoglobin reductase deficiency in a dog. J.A.V.M.A. *164*:1030, 1974.

Harvey, J. W., Sameck, J. H., and Burgard, F. J.: Benzocaine-induced methemoglobinemia in dogs. J.A.V.M.A. *175*:1171, 1979.

Hathaway, J. E.: Anemia in the dog. *In* Kirk, R. W. (ed.): Current Veterinary Therapy V. W. B. Saunders Co., Philadelphia, 1974.

Heinz, R.: Morphologische Veranderungen der rothen Blutkorperchen durch Sifte. Virchows Arch. (Pathol. Anat.) *122*:122, 1890.

Herbert, V., and Das, K. C.: The role of vitamin B_{12} and folic acid in hemato- and other cell-poiesis. Vitam. Horm. *34*:1, 1976.

Hillman, R. S.: Hematology Laboratory Manual. University of Washington Press, Seattle, 1970.

Hollander, C. S., Thompson, R. H., Barrett, P. V. D., and Berlin, N. I.: Repair of the anemia and hyperlipidemia of the hypothyroid dog. Endocrinology *81*:1007, 1967.

Holmes, R.: The occurrence of blood groups in cats. J. Exp. Biol. *30*:350, 1953.

Hoover, E. A., Kociba, G. J., Hardy, W. D., Jr., and Yohn, D. S.: Erythroid hypoplasia in cats inoculated with feline leukemia virus. J. Natl. Cancer Inst. *53*:1271, 1974.

Huggins, R. A., Deavers, S., and Smith, E. L.: Growth in beagles: Changes in body weight, plasma volume, and venous hematocrit. Pediatr. Res. *5*:193, 1971.

Huggins, R. A., Smith, E. L., and Deavers, S.: Some effects of autologous and homologous blood or plasma over transfusions in the dog. Am. J. Physiol. *209*:673, 1965.

Huxsoll, D. L.: Canine ehrlichiosis (tropical canine pancytopenia): A review. Vet. Parasitol. *2*:49, 1976.

Huxsoll, D. L., Amyx, H. L., Hemelt, I. E., Hildebrandt, P. K., Nims, R. M., and Gochenour, W. S., Jr.: Laboratory studies on tropical canine pancytopenia. Exp. Parasitol. *31*:53, 1972.

Jacob, H. S.: Hypersplenism. *In* Williams, W. J., Beutler, E., Erslev, A. J., and Rundles, R. W. (eds.): Hematology, McGraw-Hill Book Co., Inc., New York, 1972.

Jacob, H. S., and Amsden, T.: Acute hemolytic anemia with rigid red cells in hypophosphatemia. N. Engl. J. Med. *285*:1446, 1971.

Jahn, H.: Vertraglichkeitsuntersuchungen vor Blutund Plasmatransfusion en beium Hung. Inaugural-Dissertation, Universitat München, 1967.

Jain, N. C.: Demonstration of Heinz bodies in erythrocytes in the cat. Bull. Am. Soc. Vet. Clin. Pathol. *2*:13, 1973.

Jamshidi, K., and Swain, W. R.: Bone-marrow biopsy with unaltered architecture: a new biopsy device. J. Lab. Clin. Med. *77*:335, 1971.

Jandl, J. H.: Mechanisms of antibody-induced red cell destruction. Series Haematol. *9*:35, 1965.

Jandl, J. H., and Aster, R. H.: Increased splenic pooling and the pathogenesis of hypersplenism. Am. J. Med. Sci. *253*:383, 1967.

Jensen, W. M., Moreno, G. D., and Bessis, M. C.: An electron microscope description of basophilic stippling in red cells. Blood *25*:933, 1965.

Jones, D. R. E., and Hinton, M.: Reduced exercise tolerance in a dog associated with an abnormal haemoglobin. Vet. Rec. *102*:105, 1978.

Kaneko, J. J.: Iron Metabolism. *In* Kaneko, J. J. (ed.): Clinical Biochemistry of Domestic Animals. 3rd ed. Academic Press, New York, 1980a.

Kaneko, J. J.: Porphyrin, Heme and Erythrocyte Metabolism. *In* Kaneko, J. J. (ed.): Clinical Biochemistry of Domestic Animals. 3rd ed. Academic Press, New York, 1980b.

Kaneko, J. J., and Cornelius, C. E.: Clinical Biochemistry of Domestic Animals. 2nd ed. Vol. I. Academic Press, New York, 1970.

Kaneko, J. J., Green, R. A., and Mia, A. S.: Erythrocyte survival in the cat as determined by glycine-2-C^{14}. Proc. Soc. Exp. Biol. Med. *123*:784, 1966.

Keeton, K. S., Schechter, R. D., and Schalm, O. W.: Adrenocortical insufficiency in dogs. Calif. Vet. *26*:12, 1972.

Kimber, C., and Weintraub, L. R.: Malabsorption of iron secondary to iron deficiency. New Engl. J. Med. *279*:453, 1968.

Kitchen, H.: Heterogeneity of animal hemoglobins. Adv. Vet. Sci. Comp. Med. *13*:247, 1969.

Knockel, J. P.: The pathophysiology and clinical characteristics of severe hypophosphatemia. Arch. Intern. Med. *137*:203, 1977.

Kociba, G. J., and Caputo, C. A.: Aplastic anemia associated with extrus in pet ferrets. J.A.V.M.A. *178*:1293, 1981.

Koepke, J. A., Sankaran, S., Rose, S. D., and Stewart, W. B.: Multicompartmental analysis or iron kinetics in anemic dogs. Indian J. Med. Res. *58*:39, 1970.

Krause, J. R., and Stole, V.: Serum ferritin and bone marrow biopsy iron stores. II. Correlation with low serum iron and Fe/TIBC ratio less than 15%. Am. J. Clin. Pathol. *74*:461, 1980.

Kurnick, J. E., Ward, H. P., and Pickett, J. C.: Mechanism of anemia of chronic disorders. Arch. Intern. Med. *130*:323, 1972.

Kurth, D., Deiss, A., and Cartwright, G. E.: Circulatory siderocytes in human subjects. Blood *34*:754, 1969.

Laber, J., Perman, V., and Stevens, J. B.: Polychromasia or Reticulocytes—An Assessment of the Dog. J.A.A.H.A. *10*:399, 1974.

Lang, S. M., Eglen, R. M., and Henry, A. C.: Acetylpromazine administration: its effect on canine hematology. Vet. Rec. *105*:397, 1979.

Lees, G. E.: Heinz body hemolytic anemia and methemoglobinemia. *In* Kirk, R. W. (ed.): Current Veterinary Therapy VII. W. B. Saunders Co., Philadelphia, 1980.

Lees, G. E., and Sautter, J. H.: Anemia and osteopetrosis in a dog. J.A.V.M.A. *175*:820, 1979.

Lees, G. E., Polzin, D. J., Perman, V., Hammer, R. F., and Smith, J. A.: Idiopathic Heinz body hemolytic anemia in three dogs. J.A.V.M.A *15*:143, 1979.

Legendre, A. M., Appleford, M. D., Eyster, G. E., and

Dade, A. W.: Secondary polycythemia and seizures due to right and left shunting patent ductus arteriosus in a dog. J.A.V.M.A. *164*:1198, 1974.

Letchworth, G. J., Bentinck-Smith, J., Bolton, G. R., Wootlon, J. F., and Family, L.: Cyanosis and methemoglobinemia in two dogs due to NADH methemoglobin reductose deficiency. J.A.A.H.A. *13*:75, 1977.

Levy, H., Leveson, V., and Schode, A. L.: Effect of cobalt on the activity of certain enzymes in homogenates of rat tissue. Arch. Biochem. *27*:34, 1950.

Lewis, H. B., and Rebar, A. H.: Bone Marrow Evaluation in Veterinary Practice. Ralston Purina Co., St. Louis, 1979.

Lewis, R. M., and Schwartz, R. S.: Canine systemic lupus erythematosus. Genetic analysis of an established breeding colony. J. Exp. Med. *134*:417, 1971.

Lewis, R. M., Henry, W. B., Thornton, G. W., and Gilmore, C. E.: A syndrome of autoimmune hemolytic anemia and thrombocytopenia in dogs. J.A.V.M.A *1*:140, 1963.

Lewis, R. M., Schwartz, R. S., and Gilmore, C. E.: Autoimmune diseases in domestic animals. Ann. N.Y. Acad. Sci. *124*:718, 1965a.

Lewis, R. M., Schwartz, R. S., and Hendry, W. B.: Canine systemic lupus erythematosus. Blood *25*:143, 1965b.

Leyland, A.: Probable paracetamol toxicity in a cat. Vet. Rec. *94*:104, 1974.

Lichtman, M. A., and Miller, D. R.: Erythrocyte glycolysis, 2,3-diphosphoglycerate and adenosine triphosphate concentration in uremic subjects: Relationship to extracellular phosphate concentration. J. Lab. Clin. Med. *65*:267, 1970.

Linman, J. W., Bethell, F. H., and Long, M. J.: Studies on the nature of the plasma erythropoietic factor(s). J. Lab. Clin. Med. *51*:8, 1958.

Lombardi, M. H.: Plasma iron-59 clearance and plasma iron turnover rate in dogs. Am. J. Vet. Res. *34*:1437, 1973.

Lovric, V. A., Beal, P. J., and Lamini, A. T.: Iron-deficiency anemia: Evaluation of compensatory changes. J. Pediatr. *86*:198, 1975.

Lowenstine, L. J., Ling, G. V., and Schalm, O. W.: Exogenous estrogen toxicity in the dog. Calif. Vet. *26*:14, 1972.

Lund, J. E., and Avolt, M. D. L.: Erythrocyte aplasia in a dog. J.A.V.M.A. *16*:1500, 1972.

Maede, Y.: Studies on feline haemobartonellosis. IV. Life span of erythrocytes of cats infected with *Hemobartonella felis*. Jap. J. Vet. Sci. *37*:269, 1975.

Maede, Y.; Studies on feline haemobartonellosis. V. Role of the spleen in cats infected with *Haemobartonella felis*. Jap. J. Vet. Sci. *40*:141, 1978.

Maede, Y.: Sequestration and phagocytosis of *Hemobartonella felis* in the spleen. Am. J. Vet. Res. *40*:691, 1979.

Maede, Y., and Hata, R.: Studies on feline hemobartonellosis. II. Mechanism of anemia produced by infection with *Haemobartonella felis*. Jap. J. Vet. Sci. *37*:49, 1975.

Maede, Y., and Murata, H.: Ultrastructural observations on the removal of *Hemobartonella felis* from erythrocytes in the spleen of a cat. Jap. J. Vet. Sci. *40*:203, 1978.

Maede, Y., and Sonoda, M.: Studies on feline hemobartonellosis. III. Scanning electron microscopy of *Hemobartonella felis*. Jap. J. Vet. Sci. *37*:290, 1975.

Majka, J.: Personal communication, 1974.

Malherbe, W. P.: The manifestations and diagnosis of *Babesia* infections. Ann. N. Y. Acad. Sci. *69*:128, 1956.

Manyan, D. R., Arimura, G. K., and Yunis, A. A.: Chloramphenicol-induced erythroid suppression and bone marrow ferrochelatase activity in dogs. J. Lab. Clin. Med. *79*:137, 1972.

Mauk, A. G., Whelan, H. T., Putz, G. R., and Taketa, F.: Anemia in domestic cats: Effect on hemoglobin components and whole blood oxygenation. Science *185*:447, 1974.

McCredie, K. B.: Oxymetholone in refractory anaemia. Br. J. Haematol. *17*:265, 1969.

McGrath, C. J.: Polycythemia vera in dogs. J.A.V.M.A. *164*:1117, 1974.

McIntyre, P. A.: Newer developments in nuclear medicine applicable to hematology. *In* Brown, E. B. (ed.): Progress in Hematology X. Grune & Stratton, New York, 1977.

McSherry, B. J., Willoughby, R. A., and Thomson, R. G.: Urinary delta amino levulinic acid (ALA) in the cow, dog, and cat. Can. J. Comp. Med. *35*:136, 1971.

Miles, P. R., and Lee, P.: Sodium and potassium content and membrane transport properties in red blood cells from newborn puppies. J. Cell Physiol. *79*:367, 1972.

Miller, E. R.: Iron for pigs. Animal Nutrition and Health, March, 1977.

Miller, G., Swisher, S. N., and Young, L. E.: A case of autoimmune hemolytic disease in the dog. Clin. Res. Proc. *2*:60, 1954.

Miller, L. L., Robscheit-Robbins, F. S., and Whipple, G. H.: Anemia and hypoproteinemia. J. Exp. Med. *85*:267, 1947.

Miller, R. M.: Polycythemia vera in a dog. Vet. Med. Small Anim. Clin. *63*:222, 1968.

Mitema, E. S., Achme, F. W., Penumarthy, L., and Moore, W. E.: Effects of chronic lead exposure on the canine bone marrow. Am. J. Vet. Res. *41*:682, 1980.

Mollison, P. L., and Veall, N.: The use of the isotope 51^{Cr} as a label for red cells. Br. J. Haematol. *1*:62, 1955.

Moore, D. J.: Disseminated intravascular coagulopathy: A complication of *Babesia canis* infection in the dog. Dissertation (M. Med. Vet. (Med.)), University of Pretoria, Pretoria, 1978.

Moore, D. J.: Disseminated intravascular coagulation: A review of its pathogenesis, manifestations and treatment. J. S. Afr. Vet. Med. Assoc. *50*:259, 1979a.

Moore, D. J.: Therapeutic implications of *Babesia canis* infections in dogs. J. S. Afr. Vet. Med. Asso. *50*:346, 1979b.

Moore, D. J., and Williams, M. C.: Disseminated intravascular coagulation: A complication of *Babesia canis* infection in the dog. J. S. Afr. Vet. Med. Assoc. *50*:265, 1979.

Moss, G., and Staunton, C.: Blood flow, needle size and hemolysis — examining an old wives tale. N. Engl. J. Med. *282*:967, 1970.

Mulkey, O. C., Jr., and Schall, W. D.: Unpublished data, 1972.

Mulnix, J. A.: Hypoadrenocorticism in the dog. J.A.A.H.A. *7*:220, 1971.

Naets, J. P., and Heuse, A.: Effect of anemic hypoxia on erythropoiesis of normal and uremic dogs with or without kidneys. J. Nucl. Med. *5*:471, 1964.

Najean, Y., Pecking, A., and Le Danvic, M. (Secretaries). Androgen therapy of aplastic anemia. A prospective study of 352 cases. Scand. J. Hematol. 22:343, 1979.

Northdurft, W., Bruch, C., Fleidner, T. M., and Rüber, E.: Studies on the regeneration of the CFU-C population in blood and bone marrow of lethally irradiated dogs after autologous transfusion of cryopreserved mononuclear blood cells. Scand. J. Hematol. 19:470, 1977.

Odartchenko, N., Cottier, H., and Bond, V. P.: A study on ineffective erythropoiesis in the dog. Cell Tissue Kinet, 4:107, 1971.

Osbone, C. A., Low, D. G., and Finco, D. R.: Canine and Feline Urology. W. B. Saunders Co., Philadelphia, 1972.

Oski, F. A., and Delivoria-Papadopoulos, M.: The red cell 2,3-diphosphoglycerate and tissue oxygen release. J. Pediatr. 77:941, 1970.

Parker, J. C.: Dog red blood cells — adjustment in density *in vivo.* J. Gen. Physiol. 61:146, 1973.

Parker, J. P., Beirne, G. J., Desai, J. N., Raich, P. C., and Shahidi, N. T.: Androgen-induced increase in red cell 2,3-diphosphoglycerate. N. Engl. J. Med. 287:381, 1972.

Pedersen, N. C.: Immunosuppressive drugs and their role in the treatment of immunologic diseases of the dog. In Proc., 28th Gaines Veterinary Therapy, Tuskegee Institute, Alabama, 1978.

Pedersen, N. C.: Feline infectious disease. Proc. 48th Annual Meeting Am. An. Hosp. Assoc., Atlanta, 1981.

Penny, R. H. C., Carlisle, C. H., Davidson, H. A., and Gray, E. M.: Some observations on the effect of the concentration of etyhlenediamine tetraacetic acid (EDTA) on the packed cell volume of domesticated animals. Br. Vet. J. 126:383, 1970a.

Penny, R. H. C., Carlisle, C. H., Prescott, C. W., and Davidson, H. A.: Further observations on the effect of chloramphenicol on the haemopoietic system of the cat. Br. Vet. J. 126:453, 1970b.

Perman, V.: The anemic dog. Proc. Am. Anim. Hosp. Assn. South Bend, Ind., 1978.

Perman, V.: Unpublished data, 1974.

Perman, V., and Hall, M.: Unpublished observations, 1973.

Perman, V., Cronkite, E. P., Bond, V. P., and Sorensen, D. K.: The regenerative ability of hematopoietic tissue following lethal x-irradiation in dogs. Blood 19:724, 1962.

Perman, V., Cronkite, E. P., Bond, V. P., and Sorensen, D. K.: Hemopoietic regeneration in control and recovered heavily irradiated dogs following severe hemorrhage. Blood 19:738, 1962.

Perman, V., Osborne, C. A., and Stevens, J. B.: Bone marrow biopsy. Vet. Clin. North Am. 4:293, 1974.

Perrotta, D. O., and Finch, C. A.: The polychromatophilic erythrocyte. Am. J. Clin. Pathol. 57:57, 1971.

Petitpierre-Gabathuler, M. P. I., and Beck, E. A.: Effects of chloramphenicol on heme synthesis. Acta Haematol. 47:257, 1972.

Pierce, K. R., Marrs, G. E., and Hightower, D.: Acute canine ehrlichiosis: Platelet survival and factor 3 assay. Am. J. Vet. Res. 38:1821, 1977.

Pisciotta, A. V.: Drug-induced leukopenia and aplastic anemia. Clin. Pharmacol. Ther. 12:13, 1971.

Pluznik, D. H., and Sachs, L.: The cloning of normal "mast" cells in tissue culture. J. Cell Physiol. 66:319, 1965.

Pollack, A. S., Lipschitz, D. A., and Cook, J. P.: The kinetics of serum ferritin. Proc. Soc. Exp. Biol. Med. 157:481, 1978.

Pollycove, A., and Mortimer, A.: The quantitative determination of iron kinetics and hemoglobin synthesis in human subjects. J. Clin. Invest. 40:753, 1961.

Porter, J. A., Jr., and Canday, W. R.: Hematologic values in mongrel and greyhound dogs being screened for research use. J.A.V.M.A. 159:1630, 1971.

Prasse, K. W., Crouser, D. R., Beutler, E., Walker, M., and Schall, W. D.: Pyruvate kinase deficiency anemia with terminal myelofibrosis and osteosclerosis in a beagle. J.A.V.M.A 166:1170, 1975.

Pryor, W. H., and Bradbury, R. P.: *Haemobartonella canis* infection in research dogs. Lab. Anim. Sci. 25:266, 1975.

Quaife, M. A., and Odland, L. T.: The variation of plasma iron-59 clearance T1/2 with plasma iron concentration. J. Nucl. Med. 8:297, 1967.

Reardon, M. J., and Pierce, K. R.: Acute experimental canine ehrlichiosis. Vet. Pathol. 18:48, 1981a.

Reardon, M. J., and Pierce, K. R.: Acute experimental canine ehrlichiosis. II. Sequential reaction of the hemic and lymphoreticular system of selectively immunosuppressed dogs. Vet. Pathol. 18:384, 1981b.

Rebar, A. H., and Lewis, H. B.: Blood cells in disease. In Catcott, E. J. (ed.): Canine Medicine, Vol. 2, Santa Barbara, American Veterinary Publications, 1979.

Rebar, A. H., Hahn, F. F., Halliwell, W. H., De Nicola, D. B., and Benjamin, S. A.: Microangiopathic hemolytic anemia associated with radiation-induced hemangiosarcomas. Vet. Pathol. 17:443, 1980.

Rebar, A. H., Lewis, H. B., De Nicola, D. B., Halliwell, W. H., and Boon, G. D.: Red cell fragmentation in the dog: An editorial review. Vet. Pathol. 18:415, 1981.

Reece, W. O., and Wahlstrom, J. D.: Effect of feeding and excitement on the packed cell volume of dogs. Lab. Anim. Care 20:1114, 1970.

Reed, C., Ling, G. V., Gould, D., and Kaneko, J. J.: Polycythemia vera in a cat. J.A.V.M.A. 157:85, 1970.

Reiff, R. H., Nutter, J. Y., Donohue, D. M., and Finch, C. A.: The relative number of marrow reticulocytes. Am. J. Clin. Pathol. 30:199, 1958.

Richardson, J. R., Jr., and Weinstein, M. B.: Erythropoietic response of dialyzed patients to testosterone administration. Ann. Intern. Med. 73:403, 1970.

Riser, W. H., and Frankhauser, R.: Osteopetrosis in the dog: A report of three cases. J. Am. Vet. Radiol. Soc. 11:29, 1970.

Ristic, M.: Infectious blood disease of dogs. Ill. Vet. 12:6, 1969.

Ristic, M., Lykens, J. D., Smith, A. P.: *Babesia canis* and *Babesia gibsoni.* Soluble and corpuscular antigens isolated from blood of dogs. Exp. Parasitol. 30:385, 1971.

Robscheit-Robbins, F. S., Madden, S. C., Rowe, A. D., Turner, A. P., and Whipple, G. H.: Hemoglobin and plasma protein. J. Exp. Med. 72:479, 1940.

Romualdez, A., Sha'afi, R. I., Lange, Y., and Solomon, A. K.: Cation transport in dog red cells. J. Gen. Physiol. 60:46, 1972.

Rorth, M.: Effect of acid-base disturbances on the oxygen transport of the human red cell. Acta Anaesthesiol. Scand. 45 (Suppl.):49, 1971.

Rosenfield, R. E., and Jagathambal: Transfusion therapy for autoimmune hemolytic anemia. Semin. Hematol. 13:(4)311, 1976.

Roughton, J. F. W., Otis, A. B., and Lyster, R. L. J.: The determination of the individual equilibrium constants of the four intermediate reactions between oxygen and sheep haemoglobin. Proc. Roy. Soc. Lond. (Biol.) *144*:29, 1955.

St. Omer, U. V., and McKnight, E. B.: Acetylcysteine for treatment of acetaminophen toxicosis in the cat. J.A.V.M.A. *176*:911, 1980.

Sanchez-Medal, L., Bomez-Leal, A., Duarte, L., and Rico, M. G.: Anabolic androgenic steroids in the treatment of acquired aplastic anemia. Blood *34*:283, 1969.

Sanchez-Medal, L., Labardin, J., and Lorin, A.: Hemolysis and erythropoiesis. I. Influence of intraperitoneal administration of whole hemolysates on the recovery of bled dogs, as measured by changes in the total erythrocytic volume. Blood *21*:586, 1963.

Schalm, O. W.: Phenybutazone toxicity in two dogs. *In* Schalm, O. W.: Manual of Feline and Canine Hematology. Veterinary Practice Publishing Company, Santa Barbara, 1980a.

Schalm, O. W.: Clinical significance of the morphologic classification of erythrocyte population. Canine Pract. 7:59, 1980b.

Schalm, O. W.: Methylene blue induced Heinz body hemolytic anemia in a dog. Canine Pract. 5:20, 1978.

Schalm, O. W.: Erythrocyte macrocytosis in miniature poodles. Calif. Vet. April 29, 1976.

Schalm, O. W.: Morphological classification of the anemia. Calif. Vet. Oct. 30, 1974, p. 28.

Schalm, O. W.: Veterinary Hematology, 2nd ed. Lea & Febiger, Philadelphia, 1965.

Schalm, O. W., and Smith, R.: Some unique aspects of feline hematology in disease. Small Anim. Clin. *3*:311, 1963.

Schalm, O. W., Jain, N. C., and Carroll, E. J.: Veterinary Hematology, 3rd ed., Lea and Febiger, Philadelphia, 1975.

Schechter, R. D., Schalm, O. W., and Kaneko, J. J.: Heinz body hemolytic anemia associated with the use of urinary antiseptics containing methylene blue in the cat. J.A.V.M.A. *162*:37, 1973.

Schober, R., Kosek, J. C., and Wolf, P. L.: Chloramphenicol-induced vacuoles. Arch. Pathol. *94*:298, 1972.

Schull, B. M., Bunch, S. E., Maribei, J., and Spaulding, G. L.: J.A.V.M.A. *173*:978, 1978.

Schwartz, S. E., and Motto, S. A.: The diagnostic significance of burr red blood cells. Am. J. Med. Sci. *218*:563, 1949.

Scott, D. W., Schultz, R. D., Post, J. E., Bolton, G. R., and Baldwin, C. A.: Autoimmune hemolytic anemia in the cat. J.A.A.H.A. *9*:530, 1973.

Scott, P. O.: Nutritional requirements and deficiencies. *In* Catcott, E. J. (ed.): Feline Medicine and Surgery. American Veterinary Publications, Inc., Wheaton, Ill., 1964.

Scott, R. C., and Patnaik, A. K.: Renal carcinoma with secondary polycythemia in the dog. J.A.A.H.A. *8*:275, 1972.

Seamer, J., and Snape, T.: *Ehrlichia canis* and tropical canine pancytopenia. Res. Vet. Sci. *13*:307, 1972.

Searcy, G. P.: Bone marrow failure in the dog and cat. *In* Kirk, R. W. (ed.): Current Therapy VII. W. B. Saunders Co., Philadelphia, 1980.

Searcy, G. P.: Significance of oxygen hemoglobin dissociation in anemia. Bull. Am. Soc. Vet. Clin. Pathol. *1*:10, 1972a.

Searcy, G. P.: Myelofibrosis and osteosclerosis as sequelae to congenital hemolytic anemia in the Basenji dog. Proc. Am. Soc. Vet. Clin. Pathol., New Orleans, 1972b.

Searcy, G. P.: Congenital hemolytic anemia in the basenji dog due to erythrocyte pyruvate kinase deficiency. Ph.D. thesis. Cornell University, 1970.

Searcy, G. P., Miller, D. R., and Tasker, J. B.: Congenital hemolytic anemia in the Basenji dog due to erythrocyte pyruvate kinase deficiency. Can J. Comp. Med. *35*:67, 1971.

Sebrell, W. H.: An anemia of dogs produced by feeding onions. Pub. Health Rep. *45*:175, 1930.

Seim, H.: Polycythemias. Differential diagnosis and treatment. Minn. Med. *53*:557, 1970.

Shahidi, N. T.: Androgens and erythropoiesis. N. Engl. J. Med. *289*:72, 1973.

Shaldon, S., Koch, K. M., Oppermann, F., Wolf, D. P., and Schoeppe, W.: Testosterone therapy for anaemia in maintenance dialysis. Br. Med. J. *3*:212, 1971.

Shojania, A. M.: Problems in the diagnosis and investigation of megaloblastic anemia. C.M.A. Jour. *122*:999, 1980.

Simpson, C. F., and Kling, J. M.: The mechanism of mitochondrial extrusion from phenylhydrazine-induced reticulocytes in the circulating blood. J. Cell. Biol. *36*:103, 9168.

Simpson, C. F., and Kling, J. M.: The mechanism of denucleation in circulating erythroblasts. J. Cell. Biol. *35*:237, 1967.

Sims, M. A.: Megaloblastosis in the dog. Vet. Res. *105*:359, 1979.

Singer, J. W., and Adamson, J. W.: Steroids and hematopoiesis. III. The response of granulocytic and erythroid colony-forming cells to steroids of different classes. Blood *48*:855, 1976.

Slappendel, R. J., Van Erp, C.L.G.M., Goudswaard, J., and Bethlehem, M.: Cold hemagglutinin disease in a toy pinscher dog. Tijdschr. Diergeneeskd. *100*:445, 1975.

Small, E., and Ristic, M.: Morphological features of *Haemobartonella felis*. Am. J. Vet. Res. *28*:845, 1967.

Smith, E. L., Deavers, S., and Huggins, R. A.: Absolute and relative residual organ blood volumes and organ haematocrits in growing beagles. Proc. Soc. Exp. Biol. Med. *140*:285, 1972.

Sodikoff, C. H., and Custer, M. A.: Autoimmune hemolytic anemia in a cat. J.A.A.H.A. *1*:261, 1965.

Sonoda, M., Takahaski, K., Tamura, T., and Koiwa, M.: Studies on canine haemobartonellosis. I. *Haemobartonella canis* detected in the blood of dogs inoculated with *Babesia gibsoni*. Jap. J. Vet. Sci. *40*:335, 1978.

Steinberg, S.: Aplastic anemia in a dog. J.A.V.M.A. *157*:966, 1970.

Stephenson, J. R., Axebrad, A. A., McLeod, D. L., Shreeve, M. M.: Induction of colonies of hemoglobin-synthesizing cells by erythropoietin *in vitro*. Proc. Natl. Acad. Sci. USA *68*:1542, 1971.

Stewart, W. B., and Gambino, S. F.: Kinetics of iron absorption in normal dogs. Am. J. Physiol. *201*:67, 1961.

Stockham, S. L., Ford, R. B., and Weiss, D. J.: Canine autoimmune hemolytic disease with a delayed erythroid regeneration. J.A.A.H.A. *16*:929, 1980.

Stohlman, F., Jr.: Observations on the changes in the kinetics of red cell proliferation following irradiation and hypertransfusion. Blood *16*:177, 1960.

Storb, R., Weiden, P. L., Graham, T. C., and Thomas, E. D.: Studies of marrow transplantation in dogs. Transplant. Proc. *8*:545, 1976.

Swisher, S. N., and Young, L. E.: The blood grouping systems of dogs. Physiol. Rev. *41*:495, 1961.

Taketa, F., Attermeier, M. H., and Mauk, A. G.: Acetylated hemoglobins in feline blood. J. Biol. Chem. 247:33, 1972.

Tasker, J. B., Severin, G. A., Young, S., and Gillette, E. L.: Familial anemia in the basenji dog. J.A.V.M.A. 154:158, 1969.

Tavassoli, M., and Crosby, W. H.: Fate of the nucleus of the marrow erythroblast. Science 1979:912, 1973.

Thenen, S. W., and Rasmussen, K. M.: Megaloblastic erythropoiesis and tissue depletion of folic acid in the cat. Am. J. Vet. Res. 39:1205, 1978.

Thomas, R. E., and Kittrell, J. E.: Effect of altitude and season on the canine hemogram. J.A.V.M.A. 148:1163, 1966.

Thornton, G. W.: Blood transfusion. In Kirk, R. W. (ed.): Current Veterinary Therapy V. W. B. Saunders Co., Philadelphia, 1974.

Tietz, W. J., Jr., Benjamin, M. M., and Angleton, G. M.: Anemia and cholesterolemia during estrus and pregnancy in the beagle. Am. J. Physiol. 2(2):693, 1967.

Till, J. E., and McCulloch, E. A.: A direct measurement of the radiation sensitivity of normal mouse bone marrow cells. Radiat. Res. 14:213, 1961.

Tobias, G.: Congenital porphyria in a cat. J.A.V.M.A. 145:462, 1964.

Toombs, J.: Personal communication, 1980.

Twedt, D. C., Sternlieb, I., and Gilbertson, S. R.: Clinical, morphologic, and chemical studies on copper toxicosis of Bedlington terriers. J.A.V.M.A. 175:269, 1979.

Usenik, E. A., and Cronkite, E. P.: Effects of barbiturate anesthetic on leukocytes in normal and splenectomized dogs. Anesth. Analg. (Cleve.) 44:167, 1965.

Van Wyk, J. J., Baxter, J. H., Aberoyd, J. H., and Motulsky, A. G.: The anemia of copper deficiency in dogs compared with that produced by iron deficiency. Bull. Johns Hopkins Hosp. 93:41, 1953.

Vriesendorp, H. M., et al.: Joint report of First International Workup on Canine Immunogenetics. Tissue Antigens 3:145, 1973.

Wagner, J. E.: A fatal cytauxzoonosis-like disease in cats. J.A.V.M.A. 168:585, 1976.

Watson, A. D. J.: Chloramphenicol toxicity in dogs. Res. Vet. Sci. 23:66, 1977.

Watson, A. D. J., and Middleton, D. J.: Chloramphenicol toxicosis in cats. Am. J. Vet. Res. 39:1199, 1978.

Watson, A. D. S., Wilson, J. T., and Turner, D. M.: Phenylbutazone-induced blood dyscrasias suspected in three dogs. Vet. Rec. 107:239, 1980.

Waxman, S.: Metabolic approach to the diagnosis of megaloblastic anemias. Med. Clin. North Am. 57:315, 1973.

Weber, P. M., Pollycove, M., Bacaner, M. B., and Lawrence, J. H.: Cardiac output in polycythemia vera. J. Lab. Clin. Med. 73:753, 1969.

Weiden, P. L., Hackman, R. C., Deeg, H. J., Graham, T. C., Thomas, E. D., and Storb, R.: Long-term survival and reversal of iron overload after marrow transplantation in dogs with congenital hemolytic anemia. Blood 57:66, 1981.

Weiden, P. L., Ribinett, B., Graham, T. C., Adamson, J., and Storb, R.: Canine cyclic neutropenia. A stem cell defect. J. Clin. Invest. 53:950, 1974.

Weiden, P. L., Storb, R., Graham, T. C., and

Schroeder, M.: Severe hereditary haemolytic anemia in dogs treated by marrow transplantation. Br. J. Haematol. 33:357, 1976.

Weiss, D. J.: The role of serum iron, erythropoietin and erythrocyte survival in anemia of inflammatory disease. A Ph.D. dissertation, Michigan State University, E. Lansing Mich. 1981.

Weiss, L., and Tavossoli, M.: Anatomical hazards to the passage of erythrocytes through the spleen. Semin. Hematol. 7:372, 1970.

Weiss, R. C., Dodds, W. J., and Scott, F. W.: Disseminated intravascular coagulation in experimentally induced feline infectious peritonitis. Am. J. Vet. Res. 40:663, 1980.

Werner, L. L.: Coombs-positive anemias in the dog and cat. Comp. Cont. Ed. 2:96, 1980.

Williams, G. D., Adams, L. G., Yaeger, R. G., McGrath, R. R., Read, W. K., and Bilderback, W. R.: Naturally occurring trypanosomiasis (Chagas' Disease) in dogs. J.A.V.M.A. 171:171, 1977.

Williams, H. H., Erickson, B. N., Beach, E. F., and Macy I. G.: Biochemical studies of the blood of dogs with N-propyl disufide anemia. J. Lab. Clin. Med. 26:996, 1941.

Williams, W. J., Beutler, E., Erslev, A. J., and Rundles, R. W.: Hematology. McGraw-Hill Book Co., Inc., New York, 1972.

Windle, W. F., Sweet, M., and Whitehead, W. H.: Some aspects of prenatal postnatal development of the blood of the cat. Ant. Rec. 78:321, 1940.

Wintrobe, M. M.: Clinical Hematology. Lea & Febiger, Philadelphia, 1967.

Woodward, K. T., Berman, A. R., Michaelson, S. M., and Odland, L. T.: Plasma erythrocyte, and whole blood volume in the normal beagle. Am. J. Vet. Res. 29:1935, 1968.

Yamaguchi, N., Weisberg, H., and Glass, G. B. J.: Intestinal vitamin B-12 absorption in the dog. Evidence against an intrinsic factor mechanism. Gastroenterology 52:1145, 1967.

Yawata, Y., Hebbel, R. P., Silvis, S., Howe, R., and Jacob, H.: Blood cell abnormalities complicating the hypophosphatemia of hyperalimentation: erythrocyte and platelet ATP deficiency associated with hemolytic anemia and bleeding in hyperalimented dogs. J. Lab. Clin. Med. 84:643, 1974.

Zook, B. C., and Carpenter, J. L.: Lead Poisoning. In Kirk, R. W. (ed.): Current Veterinary Therapy. VI. W. B. Saunders Co., Philadelphia, 1977.

Zook, B. C., Carpenter, J. L., and Leeds, E. B.: Lead poisoning in dogs. J.A.V.M.A. 155:1329, 1969.

Zook, B. C., Carpenter, J. L., and Roberts, R. M.: Lead poisoning in dogs: Occurrence, source, clinical pathology and electroencephalography. Am. J. Vet. Res. 33:892, 1972.

Zook, B. C., Kopito, L., Carpenter, J. L., Cramer, D. V., and Schwachman, H.: Lead poisoning in dogs: Analysis of blood, urine, hair, and liver for lead. Am. J. Vet. Res. 33:903, 1972.

Zook, B. C., McConnell, G., and Gilmore, C. E.: Basophilic stippling of erythrocytes in dogs with special references to lead poisoning. J.A.V.M.A. 157:2092, 1970.

Zucali, J. R., Mirand, E. A., and Gordon, A. S.: Erythropoiesis and artificial blood substitution with a perfluocarbon-polyol. J. Lab. Clin. Med. 94:742, 1979.

CHAPTER 78

KEITH W. PRASSE

White Blood Cell Disorders

The term *leukocyte* refers to all nucleated blood cells and their precursors, excluding nucleated cells of the erythrocytic series. Clinical evaluation of disorders of the leukocytes is routine, employing both quantitative, total, and differential leukocyte counts, and qualitative observations of leukocyte morphology. Occasionally, cytologic examination of bone marrow, lymph node, other solid tissues, and exudates or fluids facilitates the blood examination. Change in blood leukocyte number and morphology occurs in a wide variety of diseases and may be referred to as the *leukocyte response*. The leukocyte response is seldom diagnostic, if viewed by itself, but it is an important adjunct to information obtained from the case history, observation of clinical signs, and findings from the physical examination.

A therapeutically useful interpretation of leukocyte response requires knowledge of the following: leukocyte function, leukocyte production, distribution and fate, normal leukocyte number and morphology, and physiopathologic mechanisms that result in change in number or morphology of leukocytes. In addition to general leukocyte responses, certain non-neoplastic diseases affecting principally leukocytes and hematopoietic neoplasms will be described. (Lymphosarcoma and feline mastocytosis are described in detail in Chapter 30.)

DESCRIPTION OF THE LEUKON

QUANTITATIVE AND QUALITATIVE ASSESSMENT OF LEUKOCYTES

The leukogram comprises total (WBC) and differential leukocyte counts and morphologic assessment of cells on blood smears. The leukogram should be obtained with other laboratory data as part of the minimum data base used in assessment of the patient. Various methods for obtaining the total WBC count and staining blood smears are described by Benjamin (1978), Bentinck-Smith (1969), Coles (1974), and Schalm et al. (1975). Normal values must be known in order to properly interpret leukocyte responses to disease. Although interpretations are based on changes from the expected norm, it must be understood that there is an error factor inherent in the means of data collection. Standard error in total leukocyte (WBC) counts for experienced technicians using manual methods may be ± 20 per cent (Biggs and MacMillan, 1948). Electronic counters and automated diluting techniques reduce the error to less than five per cent, but more error occurs with very low and very high counts. Any error in the total count is extended to the absolute differential count, in which further error may be introduced by cell-identification problems on the stained blood film. The greatest identification error involves segmenter versus band neutrophil counts made by technicians experienced with human blood, but not with canine and feline blood. The common error is to identify too many band neutrophils. Error on the differential count can be minimized by counting more cells (Koepke, 1977).

Examination of bone marrow is an important adjunct to blood evaluation in certain anemias, pancytopenias, neutropenias, thrombocytopenias, and suspected hyperproliferative or neoplastic disorders. A detailed and illustrated approach to collection and interpretation of bone marrow is available (Lewis and Rebar, 1979). Once the skills of collection and cell identification are attained, evaluation of the bone marrow aspiration smear can become a routine, practical, clinical procedure. Cellularity of marrow can be estimated from particle smears, and the myeloid (granulocytic):

erythroid ratio (M:E ratio) can be determined by counting cells in the respective series on several fields of view. The time required to perform a differential count of all maturation stages in each series may not be worthwhile, but while deriving the M:E ratio, an impression of the relative distribution of these various stages should be obtained; in general, rubricytes and metarubricytes comprise 90 per cent of the erythroid cells, and metamyelocytes, bands, and segmenters make up about 80 per cent of the granulocytic cells in canine and feline bone marrow (Duncan and Prasse, 1976). Hyperplasia of either the granulocytic or erythroid series is characterized by an increase in the relative percentage of more immature stages, and the converse characterizes hypoplasia. An increased M:E ratio indicates myeloid hyperplasia, erythroid hypoplasia, or both, whereas a low M:E ratio indicates the reverse.

Other important adjuncts to blood counts for evaluation of the leukon are cytologic examination of extramarrow hemic tissues such as lymph nodes, spleen, and liver, and cytologic examination of exudates and effusions. The extension of standard hematologic techniques to study the cells of these fluids and solid tissues is described and illustrated by Perman et al. (1979). Enlarged lymph nodes reacting to antigenic stimulation, inflammation, or neoplasia usually can be differentiated. Likewise, cytologic examination of exudates or other bodily fluids may provide a more direct assessment of disease than blood examination alone.

To date, the clinical assessment of the functional status of leukocytes in dogs and cats is still in developmental stages. Some of the procedures being used include *in vitro* lymphocyte responses to mitogens (blast transformation) (Cockerell et al., 1975; Kelly et al., 1977; Taylor and Siddique, 1977; Angus and Yang, 1978; Angus et al., 1978; Dutta et al., 1978), culture of granulocytic stem cells from bone marrow (Rudolph and Kaneko, 1980), and neutrophilic chemotactic responsiveness (Latimer et al., 1981). The nitroblue tetrazolium test (NBT) measures oxidative metabolism of neutrophils, and it has been studied as a clinical aid for detecting infection in the dog and cat. Infected animals have higher percentages of reactive cells than uninfected ones (Poli et al., 1973; Poli and Faravelli, 1974).

Cytochemical characteristics of leukocytes can be studied with the use of histochemical staining techniques; included are stains for alkaline phosphatase, acid phosphatase, peroxidase, lipid, nonspecific esterase, and glycogen (Jain, 1970; Schalm et al., 1975). Clinically, the staining reactions are being developed to aid differentiation of cell types in certain leukemias of dogs and cats. In human beings, neoplastic cells of acute lymphoblastic, myeloblastic, and monocytic leukemias are differentiated by these techniques (Yam et al., 1971; Hayhoe and Cawley, 1972; Li et al., 1973; Glick and Horn, 1974).

Normal Values for the Dog. Normal blood and bone marrow values for canine leukocytes are listed in Table 78–1. Available data indicate that the effect of breed differences on normal blood-leukocyte values is slight. Beagles and basenjis have slightly higher mean total WBC counts than those listed in Table 78–1, with increases due to higher neutrophil and lymphocyte numbers (Michaelson and Scheer, 1966; Ewing et al., 1972). Porter and Canaday (1971) report lower eosinophil counts in greyhounds. It should be noted that eosinophils of adult greyhounds contain few granules and many vacuoles, which may cause problems in identification of the cell (Jones and Paris, 1963).

The principal effect of age on blood-leukocyte counts involves the number of lymphocytes. In general, lymphocytes may exceed 30 per cent of the total count in dogs under six months of age (Schalm et al., 1975). Ewing et al., (1972) observed that basenji lymphocyte counts increase with age, from 3157 per microliter at less than 35 days of age to 5564 per microliter at 85 to 120 days of age (mean values), and then decline to values approximating those listed in Table 78–1.

Of the few studies that indicate differences in leukocyte numbers between male and female dogs, one reports lymphocyte counts in the female beagle to be slightly higher, and monocyte counts to be lower, than those in the male. In addition, the age regression for lymphocytes, which is found in the female beagle, is not present in the male (Michaelson and Scheer, 1966).

Normal Values for the Cat. Normal blood and bone marrow leukocyte values for kittens and adult cats are listed in Table 78–2. As indicated, age does influence normal values. Neutrophils, lymphocytes, and

Table 78–1. Normal Blood and Bone Marrow Values in the Dog *

Blood

Total WBC count per microliter	6,000–17,000	
	Per Microliter	*Percentage*
Segmented neutrophil	3,000–11,500	60–77
Band neutrophil	0– 300	0– 3
Lymphocyte	1,000– 4,800	12–30
Eosinophil	100– 1,250	2–10
Basophil	Rare	Rare
Monocyte	150– 1,350	3–10

Bone Marrow (Iliac Crest)

Myeloid:erythroid ratio	1 to 2:1	
	Percentage	*Percentage of Myeloid Cells*
Rubriblasts, prorubricytes	4.1	8.8
Rubricytes, metarubricytes	42.3	91.2
Total erythroid cells	46.4	100
		Percentage of Myeloid Cells
Myeloblasts, promyelocytes, myelocytes	10.3	19.3
Metamyelocytes, bands, segmenters	43.1	80.7
Total myeloid cells	53.4	100
Lymphoid cells	0.2	

*From Schalm, O. W. et al.: Veterinary Hematology. 3rd ed. Lea & Febiger, Philadelphia, 1975.

Table 78–2. Normal Blood and Bone Marrow Values in the Cat

Blood	**Adult** *		**Kitten** †	
Total WBC count per microliter	5,500–19,500		600–40,900	
	Per Microliter	*Percentage*	*Per Microliter*	*Percentage*
Segmented neutrophil	2,500–12,500	35–75	4,200–29,200	25–87
Band neutrophil	0– 300	0– 3	0– 2,300	0– 7.5
Lymphocyte	1,500– 7,000	20–55	2,400– 7,100	8–68
Eosinophil	0– 1,500	2–12	0– 5,900	0–26.5
Basophil	Rare		Rare	
Monocyte	0– 850	1– 4	Rare	

Bone Marrow (Femur)‡

Myeloid:erythroid ratio	0.6 to 3.9:1	
	Percentage	*Percentage of Erythroid Cells*
Rubriblasts	1.2	3.1
Prorubricytes, rubricytes	18.9	49.5
Metarubricytes	18.2	47.4
Total erythroid cells	38.3	100
		Percentage of Myeloid Cells
Myeloblasts, promyelocytes, myelocytes	10.1	18.2
Metamyelocytes, bands, segmenters	45.5	81.8
Total myeloid cells	55.6	100
Lymphoid cells	5.6	

*Ear vein in cats over one year old (Schalm and Smith, 1963).
†Jugular vein in kittens eight to 30 weeks old (Johnson and Perman, 1968).
‡Gilmore et al., 1964a.

eosinophils have higher values in kittens. Johnson and Perman (1968) found that kittens 8 to 12 weeks old have higher and more variable WBC counts than 14- to 26-week-old kittens. The possible influence of breed and sex on leukocyte values in cats has not been reported.

The frequent occurrence of physiologic leukocytosis, characterized by increased neutrophil and lymphocyte counts, is common in cats, especially in those under one year of age (Schalm and Smith, 1963). Normally, this condition may be induced by fear or excitement. In clinically ill cats, the effect of such a stimulus is probably minimal.

MORPHOLOGY OF LEUKOCYTES IN DOGS AND CATS

Canine and feline leukocytes have been described and illustrated by several authors (Gilmore et al., 1964a; Schalm, 1964; Bentinck-Smith, 1969; Schalm et al., 1975). These descriptions are briefly outlined below. They are based on observations of Romanowsky-stained (Wright stain, Wright-Leishman stain, and Giemsa stain) blood films. Differences observed using new-methylene-blue (NMB) stain, which gives more easily reproducible results, are noted when appropriate. For descriptions of cy-

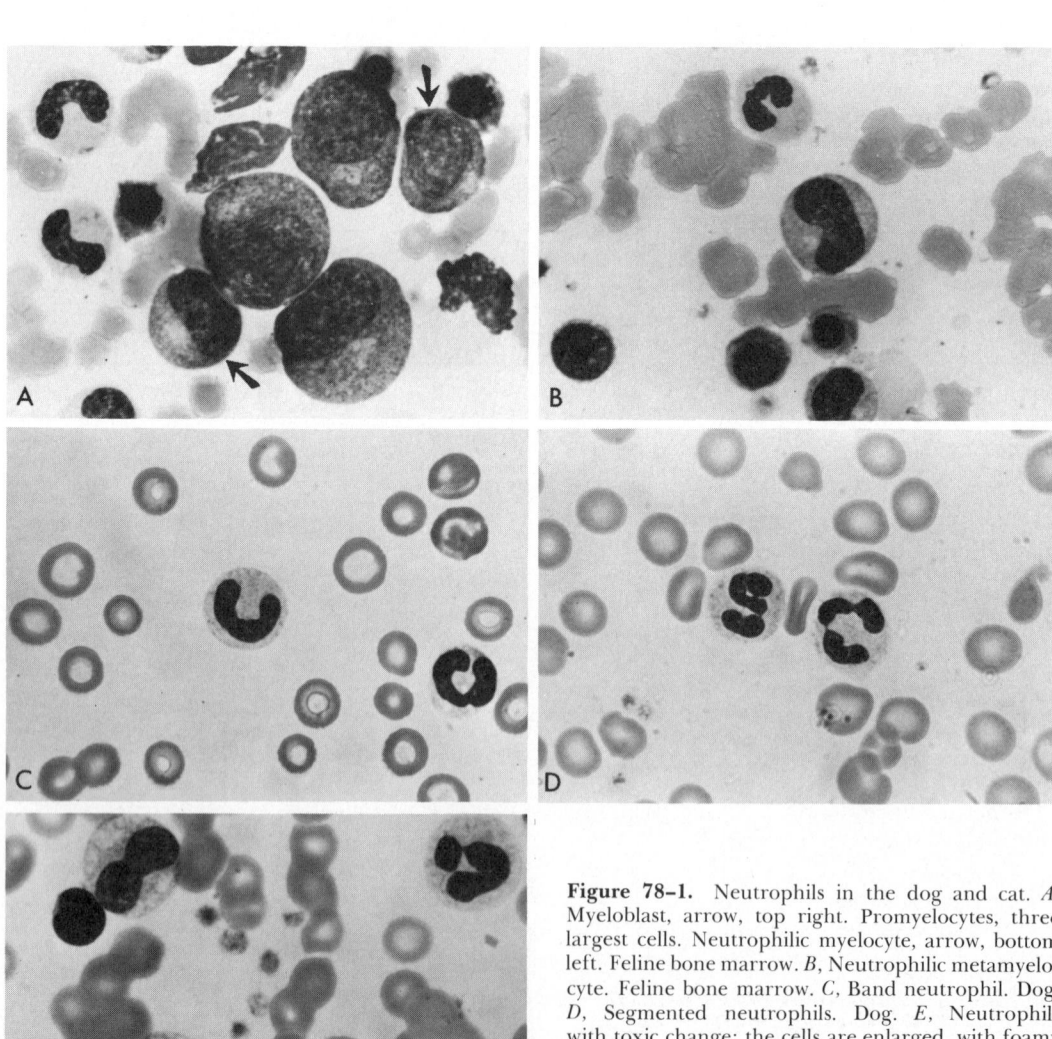

Figure 78–1. Neutrophils in the dog and cat. *A,* Myeloblast, arrow, top right. Promyelocytes, three largest cells. Neutrophilic myelocyte, arrow, bottom left. Feline bone marrow. *B,* Neutrophilic metamyelocyte. Feline bone marrow. *C,* Band neutrophil. Dog. *D,* Segmented neutrophils. Dog. *E,* Neutrophils with toxic change; the cells are enlarged, with foamy basophilic cytoplasm. Small lymphocyte, upper left. Monocyte, lower right. Platelets, center. Dog.

Illustration continued on opposite page

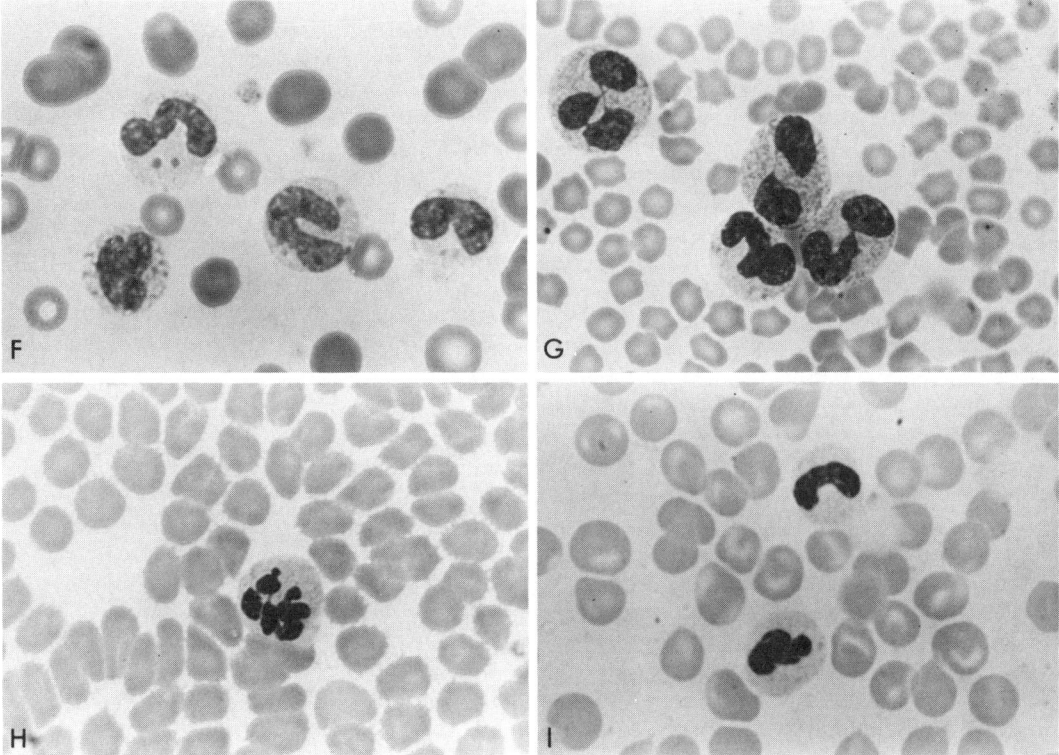

Figure 78–1 *Continued.* F, Neutrophils with toxic change; the cells are enlarged, with foamy basophilic cytoplasm and cytoplasmic Döhle bodies. Dog. G, Neutrophils with toxic change; the cells are enlarged, with foamy basophilic cytoplasm; the cells also have asynchronous nuclear maturation characterized by premature nuclear segmentation. Cat. H, Hypersegmented neutrophil. Dog with chronic suppurative disease. I, Mature neutrophils with hyposegmentation of nuclei and aggregated nuclear chromatin; pseudo–Pelger-Huët anomaly. Dog with hyperadrenocorticism.

Wright or Wright-Leishman stains. Magnification is the same on all cells in the composite. (Photomicrographs *D* and *E*, courtesy of Dr. J. R. Duncan, University of Georgia, Athens, GA.)

tochemistry of canine and feline leukocytes, the reader is referred to other sources (Atwal and McFarland, 1967; Jain, 1970; Rausch and Moore, 1975; Schalm et al., 1975).

Myeloblast (Fig. 78–1,*A*). This cell is round, measures 15 to 20 μ in diameter, and contains a round to oval nucleus. The chromatin stains purple, is evenly dispersed, and reveals one to two nucleoli.

Promyelocyte (Fig. 78–1,*A*). This cell is about the same size or slightly larger than the myeloblast, and its nucleus has slight clumping of chromatin, with nucleoli less readily visible. The abundant cytoplasm contains variable numbers of azurophilic granules.

Neutrophilic Myelocyte (Figs. 78–1,*A*, 78–3,*G*). This cell is slightly smaller than the myeloblast and the promyelocyte, and its nucleus is usually oval and often eccentri-

cally positioned. The nuclear chromatin is more condensed than that of the promyelocyte, and nucleoli are absent. With maturation and division the azurophilic granules become fewer and nearly invisible, and the specific granules may be difficult to discern in the pale blue cytoplasm.

Neutrophilic Metamyelocyte (Figs. 78–1,*B*, 78–3,*G*). This cell is variable in size but tends to be smaller than the myelocyte. The nucleus is almost bean-shaped, and later, as maturation proceeds, the nucleus becomes thinner and more elongated. The nuclear chromatin is condensed into evenly dispersed clumps. The cytoplasm is grayer than that of the myelocyte, and, as in myelocytes, the specific neutrophilic granules may be difficult to discern.

Band Neutrophil (Figs. 78–1,*C*, 78–3,*G*). This cell is smaller than the metamyelocyte and has a gently curved, elongated nucleus with smooth parallel sides. The nucleus may form a U or S shape. The cytoplasm is pale gray, with pale-staining neutrophilic granules dispersed throughout the cell.

In order to achieve interlaboratory uniformity of differential leukocyte counts and the assessment of severity of the left shift in diseased dogs and cats, strict attention to the differentiation between band neutrophils and segmented neutrophils is required. According to Schalm et al. (1975), "irregularity of the nuclear membrane or beginning indentation are features indicating that maturity has been attained, requiring classifications as a segmenter and not a band form."

Segmented Neutrophil (Figs. 78–1,*D*, 78–3,*D*, 78–3,*G*). This cell is six to nine μ in diameter, with cytoplasm similar in color to that of band cells. It is classified as segmented if the nuclear membrane has irregularities or constrictions beginning to form at least two lobes, but most circulating neutrophils have two or three nuclear lobes or segments. The nuclear membrane is irregular, and the chromatin consists of dark clumps and strands. The sex chromatin (an appendage of chromatin) may be found on the neutrophil nucleus in the female dog and cat.

Nonspecific Morphologic Abnormalities of Neutrophils. Circulating neutrophils frequently manifest changes induced by systemic toxemia or other consequences of severe illness. The changes are most common with endotoxin-producing bacterial infections, but they are not specific for bacterial infection. Toxic changes usually warrant a guarded prognosis. The most common toxic manifestation in canine and feline neutrophils is enlargement of the cells with a faintly basophilic, foamy, vacuolated cytoplasm (Figs. 78–1,*E–G*, 78–3,*A,B*) (Schalm et al., 1975). Another toxic change, less common in dogs and cats, is referred to as toxic granulation; the "toxic granules" have been shown to be primary granules of the neutrophil, which stain more intensely than normal (Fig. 78–3,*C*) (McCall et al., 1969). A third manifestation of toxic change is the presence of Dohle bodies, more common in cats than in dogs. Dohle bodies are angular, bluish cytoplasmic aggregates in Romanowsky-stained neutrophils and represent aggregation of residual rough endoplasmic reticulum normally removed

during maturation of the cell (Fig. 78–1,*F*) (Schalm et al., 1975). Occasionally all three types of toxic changes — foamy basophilic cytoplasm, intensely stained granules, and Dohle bodies — can be found at the same time.

Neutrophils characterized by asynchronous nuclear and cytoplasmic maturation, and occasionally giant size, represent another of the nonspecific abnormalities (Schalm et al., 1975). Asynchronous maturation is seen most often during conditions of intense granulopoietic effort marked by neutrophilic leukocytosis and many immature neutrophils in the blood (left shift). The change is recognized by the appearance of nuclear segmentation in a large cell with only moderately condensed chromatin, more like that of the neutrophilic myelocyte or metamyelocyte (Fig. 78–1, *G*).

Cells of normal size with hypersegmented nuclei may be seen in low numbers, when the average circulating transit time is prolonged (Fig. 78–1, *H*). Examples of such circumstances are hyperadrenocorticism and late stages of chronic suppurative disease. This nonspecific change may be seen with the simultaneous appearance of immature neutrophils in the same blood sample.

Cells of normal size with hyposegmented nuclei, mature, densely aggregated chromatin, and mature cytoplasm are an acquired abnormality of rare occurrence in the dog (Fig. 78–1, *I*). This change is referred to as pseudo–Pelger-Huët anomaly, and in fact, the true Pelger-Huët anomaly must be differentiated (see discussion on Canine Pelger-Huët Anomaly). The transient, acquired hyposegmentation must be differentiated from that of the left shift, i.e., the appearance of band or metamyelocyte neutrophils in blood. The chromatin and cytoplasm of the cells are mature in this condition of acquired hyposegmentation. Pseudo–Pelger-Huët anomaly has been described in the dog (Shull and Powell, 1978) and in man (Dorr and Moloney, 1959; Kaplan and Barrett, 1967).

Monocyte (Figs. 78–2,*A–C*, 78–3,*A*). Monocytes are the largest cells in the blood of healthy dogs and cats, but they are usually smaller than neutrophilic metamyelocytes and myelocytes. The cell is frequently vacuolated, especially if blood is allowed to remain in an anticoagulated tube for a while before smears are made. The monocyte nucleus varies in shape; it may be oval, trilobate, or otherwise irregular. The cytoplasm is gray-blue and always darker than that of cells in the neutrophilic series. Fine, dustlike azurophilic granulation may be seen, and fine, hairlike projections or pseudopodia often occur on the plasma membrane.

Eosinophil (Figs. 78–2,*D,E*, 78–3,*D,F*). The eosinophil, in all its stages of matura-

tion from the myelocyte to segmented cell, is readily identified by its large granules. These granules stain orange in Romanowsky-stained preparations but remain unstained in NMB-stained films. In the latter, the eosinophil may be differentiated by the brilliance of the cytoplasm, caused by sharply refracted light from the granules. Canine eosinophilic granules are round, vary widely in size, and do not com-

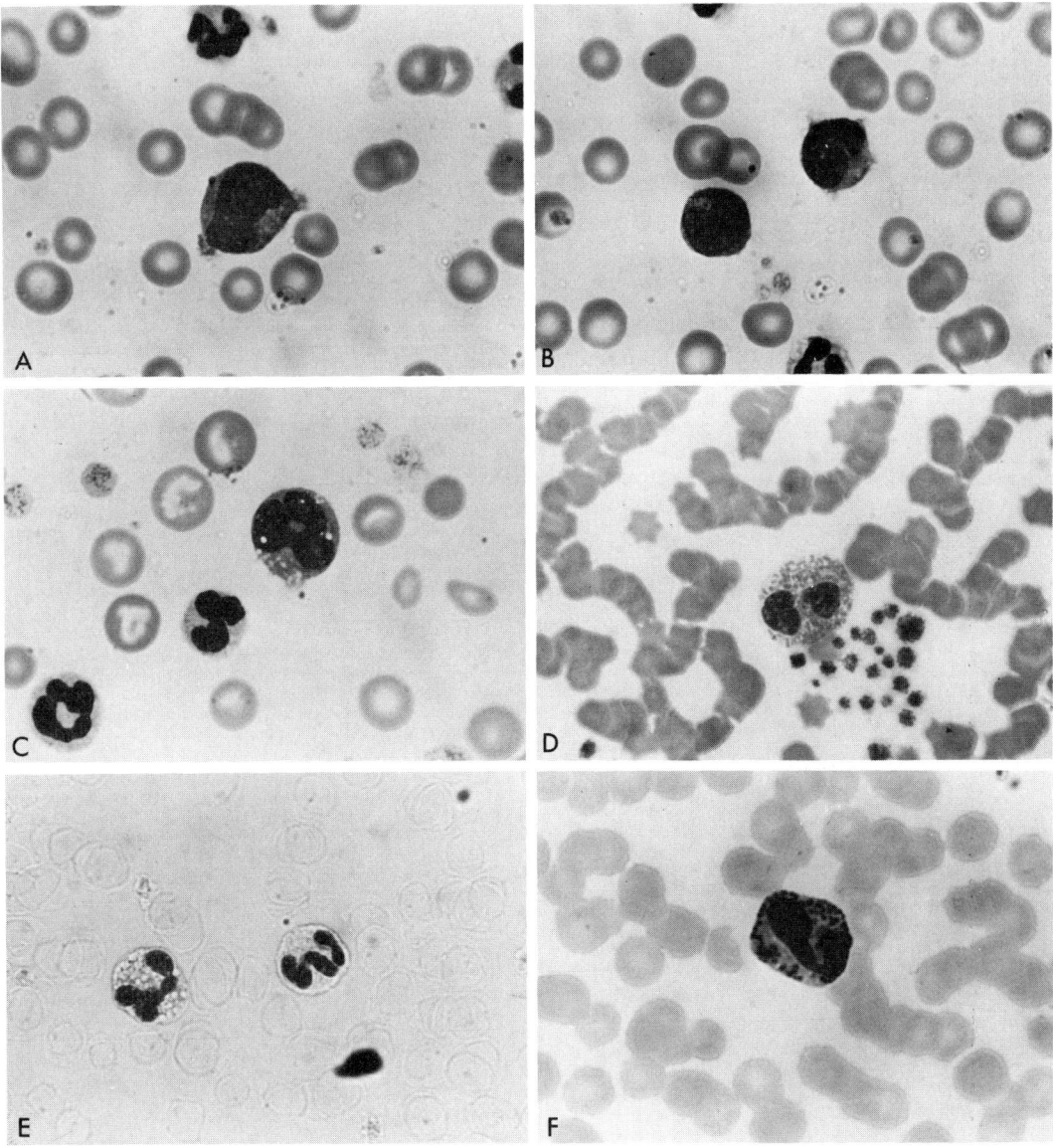

Figure 78–2. Monocytes, eosinophils, basophils, and lymphocytes in dog and cat. *A*, Monocyte with blue-gray cytoplasm, irregular nucleus and pseudopodia. Dog. *B*, Monocytes with blue-gray cytoplasm, fine pseudopodia and irregular nuclei. Dog. *C*, Monocytes with neutrophilic features and segmented neutrophils, lower left. Dog. *D*, Eosinophil. Platelets. Cat. *E*, Eosinophil, left. Neutrophil, right. New methylene blue stain, wet preparation. Dog. *F*, Basophil with sparse basophilic (purple) granules. Dog.

Illustration continued on following page

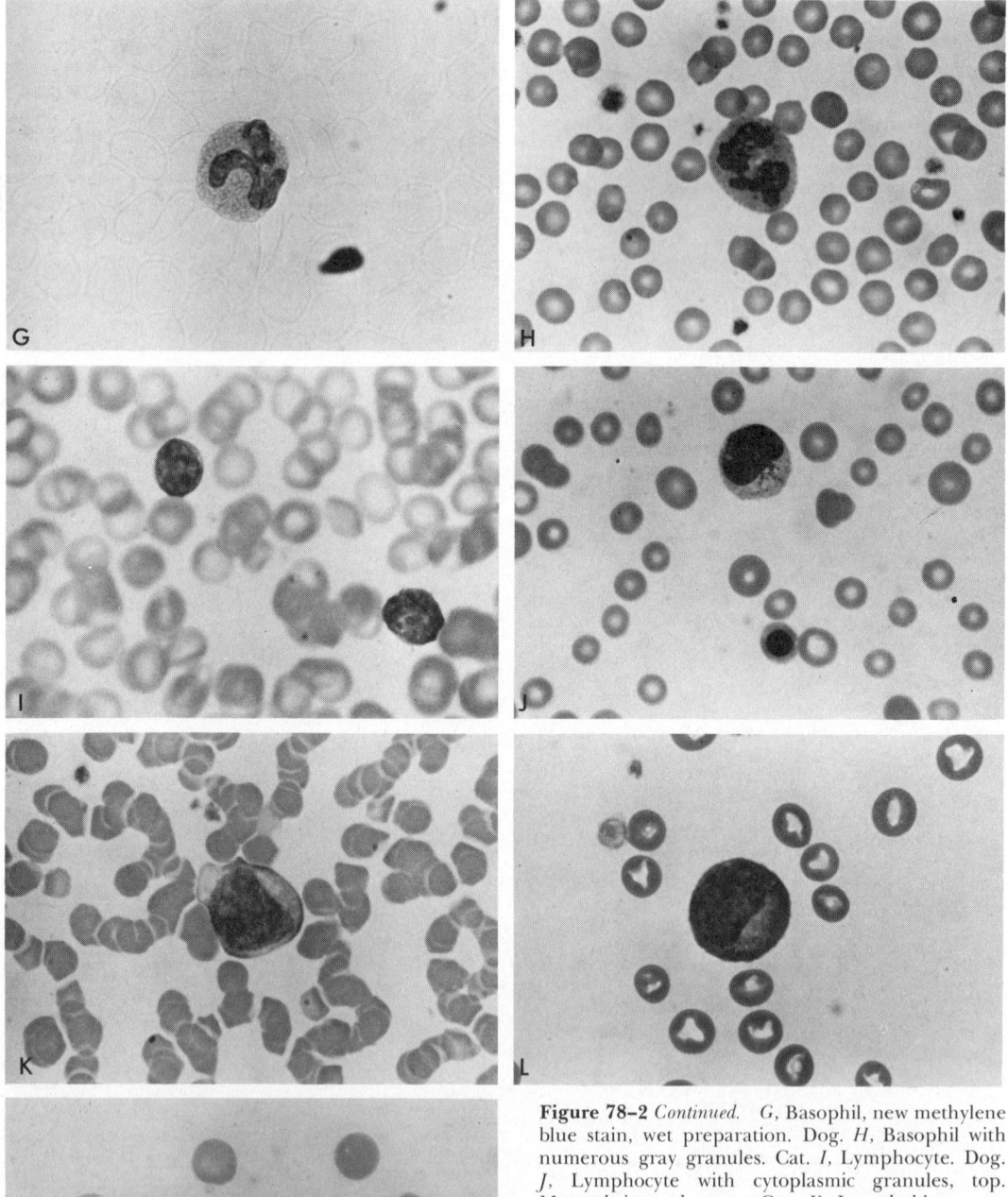

Figure 78–2 *Continued.* *G*, Basophil, new methylene blue stain, wet preparation. Dog. *H*, Basophil with numerous gray granules. Cat. *I*, Lymphocyte. Dog. *J*, Lymphocyte with cytoplasmic granules, top. Metarubricyte, bottom. Cat. *K*, Lymphoblast, very rare in blood. Cat. *L*, Immunocyte, an antigenically stimulated lymphocyte with intensely basophilic cytoplasm and densely aggregated chromatin. Dog. *M*, Plasma cell, very rare in blood. Segmented neutrophil. Dog.

Wright or Wright-Leishman stain unless otherwise noted. Magnification is the same on all cells in the composite. (Photomicrographs *A*, *B*, and *C*, courtesy of Dr. J. R. Duncan, University of Georgia, Athens, GA.)

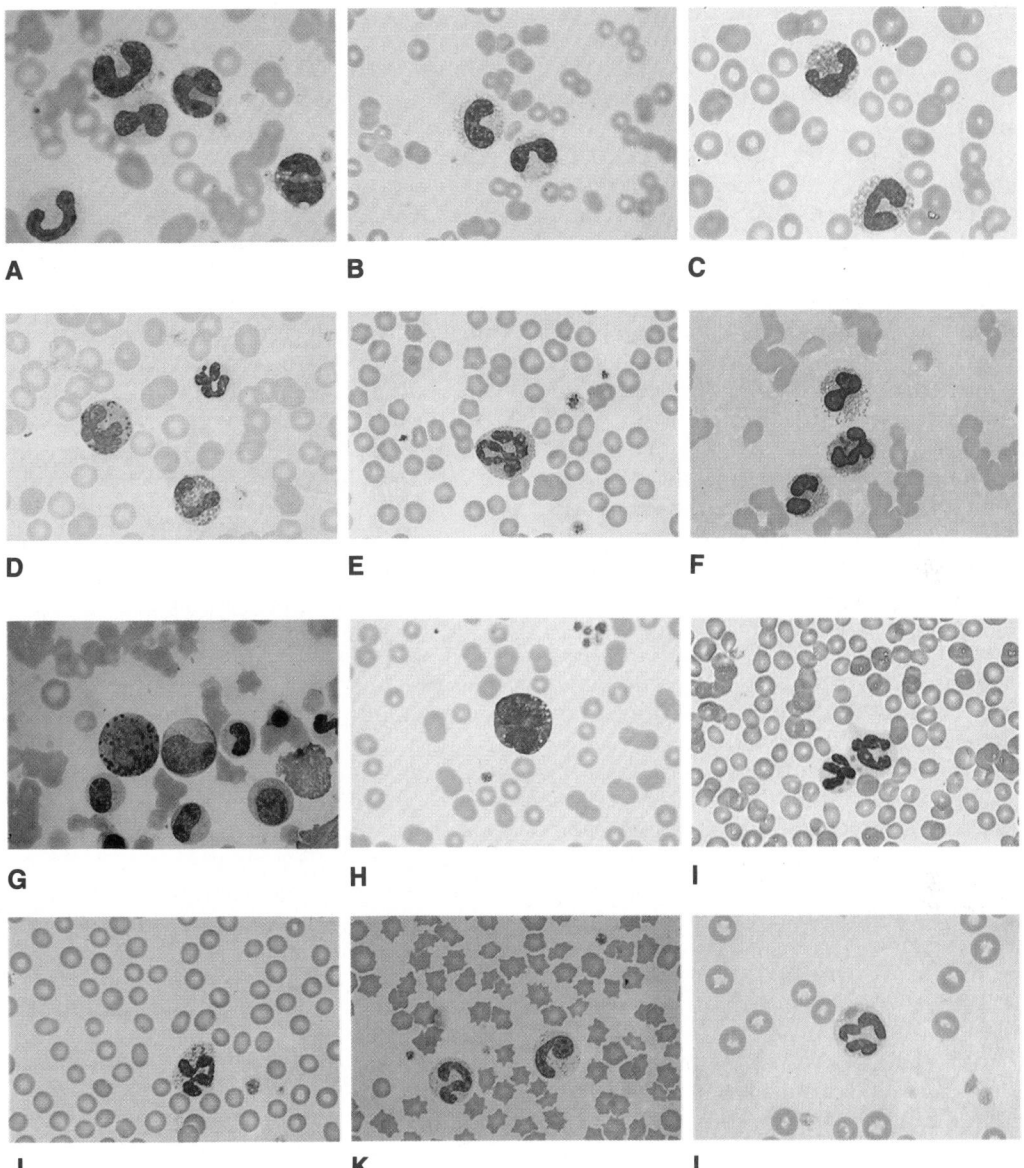

Figure 78–3. *A,* Band neutrophils with basophilic, foamy toxic cytoplasm, three cells on left. Monocytes, two cells on right. Dog. *B,* Band neutrophils with basophilic, foamy toxic cytoplasm. Cat. *C,* Band neutrophils with intensely stained, toxic granules. Dog. *D,* Normal segmented neutrophil, top right, eosinophil, bottom and basophil, left. Dog. *E,* Basophil. Cat. *F,* Eosinophils and basophil, center cell, in lipemic blood (notice the lipid-proteinic background). Cat. *G,* Basophilic myelocyte, neutrophilic myelocyte, band neutrophil, rubricyte, segmented neutrophil, smudged cell, neutrophilic myelocyte, neutrophilic metamyelocyte, and neutrophilic metamyelocyte, from top left, clockwise. Feline bone marrow. (Photomicrograph courtesy of Dr. J. R. Duncan, University of Georgia, Athens, GA.) *H,* Antigenically activated lymphocyte, immunocyte. Cat. *I,* Segmented neutrophils with giant cytoplasmic granules in a Persian cat with Chediak-Higashi syndrome. (Blood smear provided courtesy of Dr. John W. Kramer, Washington State University, Pullman, Washington.) *J,* Segmented neutrophil with large purple cytoplasmic granules from a Siamese cat with mucopolysaccharidosis. (Blood smear provided courtesy of Dr. John W. Kramer, Washington State University, Pullman, Washington.) *K,* Segmented neutrophils with large purple cytoplasmic granules from a Siamese cat with sphingolipidosis. *L,* Segmented neutrophil with an eosinophilic cytoplasmic inclusion of canine distemper. Dog.

Wright or Wright-Leishman stain. Magnification is the same on all cells in the composite.

pletely fill the cytoplasm, which appears pale gray between granules. Feline eosinophilic granules are elliptic, smaller and brighter orange than those of the dog, and uniform in size.

Basophil (Figs. 78–2,F–H, 78–3,D–G). The basophil and its precursors (back to the myelocyte stage) may be identified by intensely purple (metachromasia) cytoplasmic granules in a gray cytoplasm. These granules are water soluble and may not be observed in NMB-stained preparations. In the cat, as the basophilic granules mature, the metachromatic staining quality of the granules disappears. In Romanowsky stains, feline basophil granules are gray, elliptic, and numerous. Feline basophils are larger than neutrophils, and a trained microscopist can identify the cells with ease. Occasionally a feline basophil retains metachromasia in a few granules, which facilitates identification.

Lymphocyte (Fig. 78–2,I,J). The functional types of lymphocytes, T cells and B cells, are morphologically indistinct. Although small, medium, and large lymphocytes can be seen, the size is more continuous than trimodal and relates to metabolic status and degree of flattening on smears rather than any specific classification. Lymphocytes are usually 7 to 9 μ but range from 4 to 12 μ in diameter. The nucleus often nearly fills the cell, leaving visible only a narrow rim of pale blue cytoplasm. The chromatin is coarsely granular, and the nucleolus is obscure in Romanowsky-stained cells but may be visible in NMB-stained preparations. Occasionally, a few purple granules can be seen in the cytoplasm of Romanowsky-stained cells.

Lymphoblast (Fig. 78–2,K). Cells referred to as lymphoblasts (not to be considered a precursor cell, but rather a stage in the life cycle of a lymphocyte) are very rare in blood in health or disease. They are larger, more basophilic, and have finer chromatin than lymphocytes. Their nucleoli are usually visible in Romanowsky-stained cells.

Immunocyte and Plasma Cell (Figs. 78–2,L,M, 78–3,H). Metabolically activated lymphocytes, called immunocytes (Greaves et al., 1973), are seen occasionally in blood of healthy dogs and cats and more frequently during infections or other causes of antigenic challenge (Wood and Frenkel,

1967; Wilkins, 1974). Immunocytes have intensely basophilic cytoplasm on Romanowsky-stained smears, and the cells vary from 7 to 15 μ in diamter. Unlike lymphoblasts, the chromatin is densely aggregated, nucleoli are usually invisible, and the nuclear outline may be irregular. These cells are variously referred to as atypical lymphocytes, immunocytes, plasmacytoid lymphocytes, or virocytes.

Plasma cells are a specific type of immunocyte. Nuclear and staining characteristics are the same as in other immunocytes, but the cell is identifiable by an eccentrically placed nucleus and a pale perinuclear zone in the cytoplasm. Plasma cells are immunocytes that occur in lymph nodes and bone marrow and only rarely in blood.

FUNCTION, PRODUCTION, AND KINETICS OF LEUKOCYTES

Neutrophil. The function of neutrophils is to phagocytize and kill microbes. Constituents in cytoplasmic granules include microbiocidal systems, equally toxic to bacteria, fungi, and viruses, and digestive acid hydrolases and other proteases. The principal microbiocidal systems include myeloperoxidase, which works with H_2O_2 and superoxide ion generated by the cell during phagocytosis, lysozyme, lactoferrin, and cationic proteins (Baggiolini, 1980). Microbes are internalized by neutrophils into a phagocytic vacuole. The cytoplasmic granules fuse with the vacuole, and the microbiocidal and digestive contents are exposed to the microbe. This important defense mechanism may be used anywhere, but the function is primarily conducted in tissues and not in blood. Certain of the neutrophilic enzymes have substrate specificities that suggest an extracellular digestive function for the cell. For example, neutrophil elastase digests fibrinogen, components of complement, and other extracellular substrates (Baggiolini, 1980); other neutrophil products stimulate the generation of mediators of inflammation (Weismann et al., 1980).

Granule and cytoplasmic contents also provide a basis for histochemical differentiation of precursor neutrophils from other types of primitive cells that may be encountered in leukemia. Species differences for neutrophilic granule contents are described; specifically, canine and feline neutrophils lack alkaline phosphatase (Atwal and McFarland, 1967; Rausch and Moore, 1975).

Neutrophils respond to chemotactic stimuli. Chemotaxis is the directional migration of cells toward the greatest concentration of chemotactic agents. Bacterial products released during the growth phase have been shown to be chemotactic (Ward et al., 1968). Injured tissue, in the absence of bacteria, also provides chemotactic stimuli to neutrophils (Hurley, 1964). In certain instances, complement components seem to play a significant role in the attraction of neutrophils to affected tissues (Boyden, 1962; Ward et al., 1965).

While neutrophils are among the most important of the body's defense mechanisms, they can also exert pathologic effects. Neutrophils produce the Arthus reaction, an inflammation and necrosis of tissue that follows an antigen-antibody reaction in blood-vessel walls (Cochrane et al., 1959). Pathologic effects of neutrophilic contents have been demonstrated experimentally in dogs with urate-induced gouty arthritis (Phelps and McCarty, 1966). Certain granule proteins of neutrophils are pyrogenic (Herion et al., 1966), and neutrophilic lysosomal contents can produce reduction in blood pressure, cardiac output, and peripheral vascular resistance during endotoxemia in dogs (Jolley et al., 1970).

Neutrophils compose a population of cells that are continuously being destroyed and replaced by both the healthy and the diseased body. They are produced in the bone marrow and released into the blood, in which their presence is transitory, and their number is subject to the influence of infectious and noninfectious physiopathologic changes. After a brief sojourn in the blood, they migrate to tissues and remain there. The principal sites of neutrophil loss in healthy animals are the mucous membranes of the respiratory and gastrointestinal tracts (Fliedner et al., 1964), and recently the monocyte-macrophage population in the bone marrow, liver, and spleen has been suggested to be responsible for normal neutrophil death (Cronkite, 1979). In disease, the cells are lost in those tissues in which their functional potential has been utilized.

Neutrophil production in the bone marrow is an orderly maturing process that occurs in sequential stages through the following catenated cytologic compartments: myeloblast, promyelocyte (progranulocyte), neutrophilic myelocyte, neutrophilic metamyelocyte (juvenile), band neutrophil, and segmented neutrophil (Fig. 78–4). Myeloblasts are genetically committed to a specific granulocytic cell line, but the specific type cannot be visually identified. Once the myelocyte stage of maturation is reached, granulocytes may be identified by the presence of specific granules. Myeloblasts and promyelocytes are believed to divide once, with daughter cells becoming members of the next compartment in sequence. Myelocytes are believed to divide about three times before daughter cells of the third generation become metamyelocytes. The occurrence of additional myelocyte divisions before the metamyelocyte stage, at which division stops, would account for a doubling of neutrophil output with each additional division (Cronkite and Vincent, 1970; Prasse et al., 1973b). In dogs, however, there is evidence to suggest that myelocyte overproduction and cell attrition normally occur in the bone marrow (Patt and Malo-

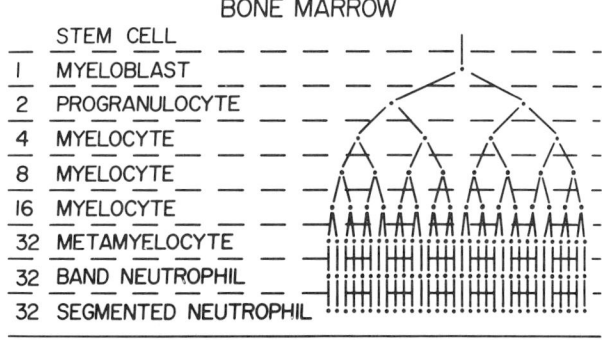

Figure 78–4. Schema of granulopoiesis. Granulopoiesis is an orderly maturation through catenated cytologic compartments. Cell division stops at the metamyelocyte compartment. Mechanisms for increased neutrophil production with times for effects to be manifested in the blood are increased stem-cell input, approximately 120 hours, and increased number of divisions or reduction in cell attrition in the myelocyte compartment, approximately 72 to 96 hours. Increased rate of release of mature neutrophils into the blood may occur rapidly, with appropriate stimuli.

BONE MARROW

	STEM CELL
I	MYELOBLAST
2	PROGRANULOCYTE
4	MYELOCYTE
8	MYELOCYTE
16	MYELOCYTE
32	METAMYELOCYTE
32	BAND NEUTROPHIL
32	SEGMENTED NEUTROPHIL

BLOOD

ney, 1964; Maloney et al., 1971; Smith et al., 1972b). This finding indicates that increased neutrophil production would occur by reduction in cell attrition. Intramarrow death of granulocytes, referred to as ineffective granulopoiesis, has been estimated at 15 to 20 per cent of the cells at the myelocyte level in dogs (Deubelbeiss et al., 1975).

Neutrophilic metamyelocyte and band and segmented neutrophils do not divide but constitute the final maturation stages and reserve or storage pool of neutrophils in the bone marrow. The postmitotic cells comprise about 80 per cent of the granulocytes in bone marrow of healthy dogs and cats.

Increased movement of neutrophils from the bone marrow to the blood is accomplished in several ways: release of the more mature cells from the storage pool occurs in a few hours; amplification of production or regulation by reduced attrition at the myelocyte level requires about 72 to 96 hours for the effect to be manifested in blood; and increased stem-cell input to the myeloblast stage requires about 120 hours for the production of mature cells (Patt and Maloney, 1964; Cronkite and Vincent, 1970; Prasse et al., 1973b). This enhancement of cell production is believed to be effected by colony stimulating factor, the putative regulator of granulopoiesis (Hays and Craddock, 1978). Colony stimulating factor is a term applied to a group of glycoproteins absolutely required for *in vitro* production of granulocytes and isolated from many different tissues. Monocytes and macrophages throughout the body are the richest source of glycoproteins, and bone marrow mac-

rophages are considered to be the principal source (Cronkite, 1979). As the storage pool of neutrophils depletes, colony stimulating factor synthesis by marrow macrophages increases, followed by increased stem cell input and increased mitotic activity among the early granulocytes. Replenishment of the storage pool would diminish the stimulation.

Neutrophils are released from the bone marrow into the blood in an orderly fashion, according to the age of cells (Maloney and Patt, 1968). In other words, the blood is supplied with mature segmented neutrophils, and as a peripheral demand for cells develops, segmented neutrophils are called from the storage pool at a greater rate. As the demand intensifies and the reserve of mature cells diminishes, band neutrophils appear in the blood. This may be followed by the appearance of neutrophilic metamyelocytes, or even more immature cells in severe situations.

Neutrophils are unevenly distributed in the blood of the dog and cat. The cells move through capillaries and postcapillary venules at a slower pace than other cellular elements of the blood. The cells move slowly, marginating along the vessel walls. In healthy dogs, the marginal pool of neutrophils is about 50 per cent larger than the circulating pool of cells in the freely flowing blood of macroscopic vessels (Raab et al., 1964). In healthy cats, the marginal pool is about 70 per cent larger than the circulating pool (Prasse et al., 1973a). Neutrophils in the circulating pool are those encountered on routine, total, and differential leukocyte counts (Fig. 78–5). Differing physiopathologic states induce numeric changes in neu-

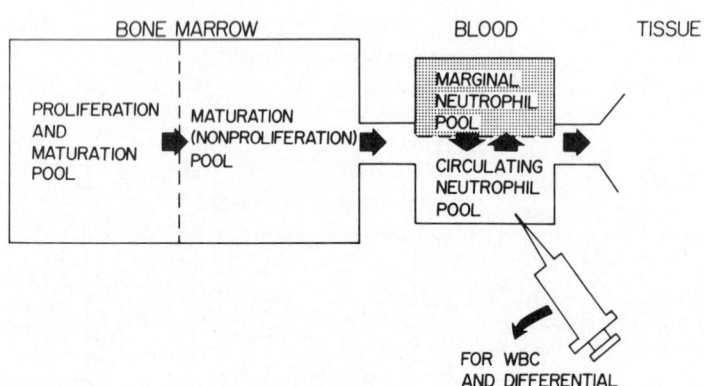

Figure 78–5. Schema of neutrophil kinetics. Release of neutrophils from the bone marrow into the blood is ordered according to the age of the cells. Neutrophils are unevenly distributed in the blood and form two dynamic neutrophil pools: the marginal pool in small blood vessels and the circulating pool in large blood vessels. The total blood-neutrophil pool is about 50 per cent greater in healthy dogs and 70 per cent greater in healthy cats than the product of blood volume × WBC count × percentage of neutrophils in the circulating pool. Neutrophils randomly enter tissues after an average blood sojourn of five to eight hours.

trophil distribution in the marginal and circulating pools. These changes (which will be described later in this chapter) influence the interpretation of neutrophil responses in disease.

Since the biological half-life of neutrophils in the blood is about 5.7 hours in healthy dogs (Raab et al., 1964) and 7.4 hours in cats (Prasse et al., 1973a), the average transit time (half-life divided by natural log of 2) for a neutrophil in blood is about ten hours, and the entire population of neutrophils in the blood is replaced about two and one-half times each day. Cells leave the blood in health and disease in random fashion unrelated to the age or maturation state. Physiopathologic factors may influence the rate at which neutrophils leave the blood.

Monocyte. Monocytes are members of the population of cells that constitute the mononuclear phagocyte system. They are produced in the bone marrow and migrate into blood and finally into tissues, where they mature into macrophages. In addition to wandering macrophages of interstitial tissues, fixed macrophage populations such as hepatic Kupffer cells and alveolar macrophages have been shown to be bone marrow–monocyte derived (Diesselhoff-Den Dulk et al., 1979; Johnson et al., 1980). Macrophages function in remodeling of tissues, removal of dead or effete cells, and phagocytosis of foreign particulate material. They participate in all types of inflammation. In addition to the phagocytic activities, macrophages are secretory cells, and the extensive array of secretory products place macrophages directly into a complex role in immunologic and inflammatory humoral mechanisms (Dannenberg, 1975; Nathan et al., 1980).

Secretory products of macrophages include protease, which activate components of the fibrinolytic, complement, and kinin systems; inhibitors of the same systems; complement components; carrier proteins, such as transferrin; several prostaglandins with a variety of biological activities; mitogens for lymphocytes, erythroid cells, and granulocytes (colony stimulating factor); interferon; endogenous pyrogen, for which macrophages may be the main source that affects temperature regulation and causes fever; and still other substances.

Although they are responsive to infection, macrophages are less responsive than neutrophils in the defense of blood-borne pyogenic bacteria (Cohen, 1968). Macrophages possess microbiocidal systems like that of neutrophils, but certain organisms may be destroyed by the cell or may successfully parasitize the cell, depending on the activity-status of the macrophage. Such organisms include *Listeria, Salmonella, Brucella, Mycobacteria, Chlamydia, Rickettsia, Leishmania, Toxoplasma,* and *Trypanosoma* (Nathan et al., 1980).

Monocyte production in bone marrow is closely related to that of neutrophils; the two phagocytes have the same or closely related stem cells (Cronkite, 1979). Only subtle structural differences such as microfilaments in monocytic cells allow electron microscopic differentiation of promonocytes from promyelocytes (Nichols and Bainton, 1973). The next maturation stage — monocyte — is released to the blood, unlike neutrophils, which mature and are stored in bone marrow. Kinetic studies in man reveal that the distribution of monocytes in the blood is similar to neutrophil distribution (Meuret and Hoffman, 1973). The cells are unevenly distributed, with the number of monocytes in the marginal pool being nearly five times larger than the number of cells in the large vessels of the circulating pool. Monocytes are lost randomly from the blood, with a circulating half-life of 8.4 hours in human beings. Similar studies have not been done in the dog or cat.

Eosinophil. The functions of eosinophils relate primarily to defense against metazoan parasites and to an anti-inflammatory or moderating role in immediate or delayed hypersensitivity inflammatory reactions (Beeson and Bass, 1977). The cells possess many metabolic and granular components that are identical to those of neutrophils, but eosinophils are not protective against bacterial infection. Eosinophils isolated from mice infected with *Trichinella spiralis* or *Schistosoma mansoni* damage or kill migratory stages of these parasites by antibody-dependent, complement-independent mechanisms (Butterworth et al., 1977; Kazura and Grove, 1978). The anti-inflammatory or moderating role of eosinophils in hypersensitivity reactions is mediated by secretions from stimulated cells. The cells are chemotactically attracted to the inflammatory site by factors derived from degranulating mast cells or basophils. The attracted eosinophils secrete substances that suppress further mast cell or basophil degranulation, inactivate histamine and other mediators of inflammation, and prevent mast cells from resynthesizing more of the inflammatory mediators (Beeson and Bass, 1977).

The bone marrow production of eosinophils closely parallels that of neutrophils, but they are derived from different stem cells (Dao et al., 1977). The precursors of eosinophils are identifiable microscopically at the myelocyte stage when the specific granules appear, and maturation proceeds through metamyelocyte, band, and segmented stages. Eosinophilopoiesis is subject to immunologic control. Poietic factors for eosinophils have been derived from antigenically stimulated T lymphocytes, and further, eosinophils so produced have been shown to possess surface receptors specific for the antigen used to stimulate the lymphocytes (Basten and Beeson, 1970; Weller and Goetzl, 1980).

Little is known about blood-eosinophil kinetics in animals. In human beings, eosinophils move randomly from blood into tissues with a half-life of two hours, but kinetics is more complicated during eosinophilia (Weller and Goetzl, 1980). Eosinophils are more numerous in tissues than in blood, and they are found principally below epithelial surfaces exposed to the external environment.

Basophil. Basophils and mast cells are functionally similar cells with large metachromatic granules when stained with Romanowsky stains. Their nuclear and granular fine structure are dissimilar, however, and they are believed to be distinct cell lines (Bainton, 1980). Basophils originate in bone marrow, and the cell line is visually identified when specific granules appear in the myelocyte stage of development. The origin of mast cells remains controversial. In general, animals that have few blood basophils, such as cats, have numerous mast cells in interstitial tissues, whereas animals with numerous basophils, e.g., rabbits, have fewer tissue mast cells (Michels, 1938).

Granules of basophils and mast cells contain mediators of inflammation, including histamine, eosinophil chemotactic factor of anaphylaxis, heparin, slow reactive substance of anaphylaxis, platelet activating factor, and other substances (Dvorak and Dvorak, 1979; Bainton, 1980). Interaction of the cell membrane with anaphylatoxin (C3a and C5a components of complement), or with allergen and specific immunoglobulin E, which may coat the cell, results in degranulation and release of the mediators. The various effects include smooth muscle and endothelial cell contraction, edema formation, attraction of eosinophils, platelet activation, activation or inhibition of coagulation, and promotion of fibrinolysis (Dvorak and Dvorak, 1979). Consequently, basophils and mast cells promote inflammation, whereas eosinophils (described previously) are primarily anti-inflammatory. The inflammatory reactions mediated by basophil or mast cell degranulation include immediate and delayed hypersensitivity responses (Dvorak and Dvorak, 1979).

Lymphocyte. Lymphocyte production, distribution, and fate have been studied primarily in birds and small rodents (Greaves et al., 1973), but the details are largely accepted for all species. Lymphocytes are distributed in lymph nodes, spleen, thymus, tonsils, gastrointestinal lymphoid tissues, bone marrow, and blood. Differentiation of lymphocyte types is marked by the acquisition of surface receptors and markers rather than by dramatic morphologic changes. The life span of lymphocytes is defined by either the time interval between cell divisions or the interval between the last division and cell death. The interval between cell divisions is variable, but in general, some cells are believed to be short-lived (about two weeks), and others are long-lived, with intermitotic intervals of weeks, months, or years. Most lymphocytes are morphologically indistinct. Although morphologically defined, lymphoblasts are not to be considered precursor or poorly differentiated cells; instead, they are a morphologic manifestation to antigenic or mitogenic stimulation representing some stage in the cell cycle of an individual lymphocyte. Other morphologically distinct lymphocytes are immunocytes, one of which is the plasma cell line. Plasma cells are secretory lymphocytes, but not all secreting or otherwise functional lymphocytes have morphologic identity.

Immune function can be assessed by measuring humoral antibody levels, *in vivo* manifestations of delayed hypersensitivity such as skin graft rejection, and *in vitro* lymphocyte blast transformation to mitogenic stimulation. Screening for general immunocompetence by lymphoblast transformation induced by mitogens is described for dogs and cats (Cockerell et al., 1975; Taylor and Siddique, 1977; Angus and Yang, 1978).

Change in blood lymphocyte number correlates poorly with the functional status of the lymphocyte population, but the blood number is affected by a variety of pathophysiologic processes. Among the leukocytes, lymphocytes are unique because they recirculate. The majority of T cells recirculate, whereas most of the B cells found in blood are thought to be transient members of the recirculating population; the majority of B cells do not recirculate (Greaves et al., 1973). Estimates based on surface marker analyses of the proportions of T and B cells in the blood of dogs and cats are widely varied (Mackey, 1977; Miller et al., 1978). The primary route of recirculating lymphocytes is from the efferent ducts of lymph nodes, through thoracic duct and right lymphatic duct and into the bloodstream; the lymphocytes then emigrate from the blood through venules of the cortex of lymph nodes and eventually return to the efferent lymph again. The recirculation of lymphocytes in the spleen is different, and another, more direct lymph node to blood to lymph node route is described also (Schunda, 1978). Pathophysiologic processes that affect the recirculation of lymphocytes form the basis for interpretation of blood lymphocyte counts.

PHYSIOLOGIC LEUKOCYTOSIS

Physiologic events in *healthy* cats and dogs can cause mild leukocytosis. The changes are slight neutrophilia (5000 to 15,000 neutrophils per microliter) and marked lymphocytosis (3000 to 15,000 lymphocytes per microliter) accompanied by normal monocyte and eosinophil counts, although eosinopenia may occur in some cases (Schalm and Smith, 1963; Schalm et al., 1975; Kleinsorgen et al., 1976; Niepage, 1978). The changes are immediately apparent in healthy animals excited by strange surroundings or forcibly restrained for sample collection. After a few hours of acclimation to the surroundings or after the animal is accustomed to the routine of

bleeding, the leukocyte changes may not be seen. Physiologic leukocytosis is seen more often in cats than in dogs because of their more excitable nature, and because values more often exceed normal limits in cats.

Physiologic leukocytosis is believed to be mediated by epinephrine released because of fear, excitement, or sudden strenuous physical activity. Increased muscular activity, heart rate, and blood pressure are associated with the neutrophilia. Neutrophils that are slowly traversing along the walls of small blood vessels (the marginal pool) are mobilized, resulting in a larger number of neutrophils in the circulating pool. Experimentally, this redistribution of neutrophils has been induced by exogenous epinephrine (Fig. 78–6) (Athens et al., 1961a, 1961b). These studies have further shown that the total number of neutrophils in the blood (marginal pool plus circulating pool) does not change, and that the neutrophil transit time remains normal. The neutrophil response is less in dogs because the marginal pool in dogs is smaller than that in cats (Raab et al., 1964; Prasse et al., 1973a). These findings indicate that increased movement from blood to tissue, and from bone marrow to blood, does not occur in physiologic neutrophilia.

Compared with neutrophilia, physiologic lymphocytosis is more dramatic, but the mechanism is unexplained. Epinephrine may interfere with cell receptors in the lymph nodes, preventing egress of recirculating lymphocytes from blood, or the arrival of recirculating lymphocytes into blood from the thoracic duct may be facilitated by the effects of muscular activity on efferent lymph flow. Since the estimated average blood transit time for lymphocytes is about 20 minutes (Pattengale et al., 1972; Greaves et al., 1973), either impaired egress or facilitated reentry of cells would have an immediate, dramatic effect on the blood lymphocyte number, as seen in physiologic leukocytosis.

LEUKOCYTE RESPONSE TO CORTICOSTEROIDS

Corticosteroids cause predictable changes in blood leukocyte numbers in dogs and cats. The peak of the response is characterized by neutrophilia, lymphopenia, monocy-

NEUTROPHIL KINETICS IN HEALTH

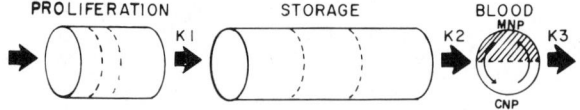

EPINEPHRINE RESPONSE

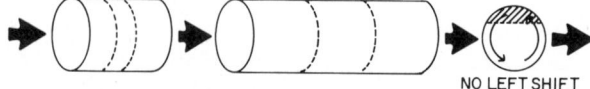

CORTICOSTEROID RESPONSE

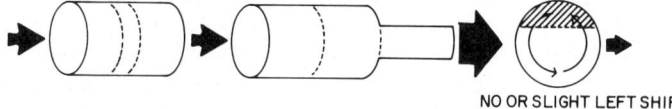

ACUTE PURULENT INFLAMMATION

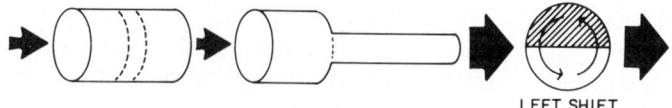

Figure 78–6. Mechanisms of neutrophilia. Size of arrows represent rates of movement of cells through the compartments of granulopoiesis, marrow storage, and blood. The size of the tubes, circle, and shaded area represent bone marrow proliferation and storage pools, blood total neutrophil pool, and blood marginal neutrophil pool, respectively.

ESTABLISHED PURULENT INFLAMMATION

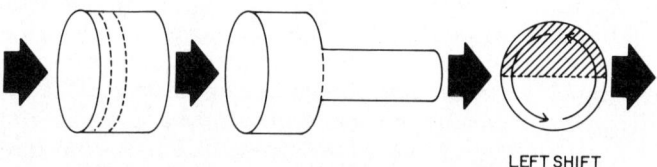

CHRONIC SUPPURATIVE DISEASE

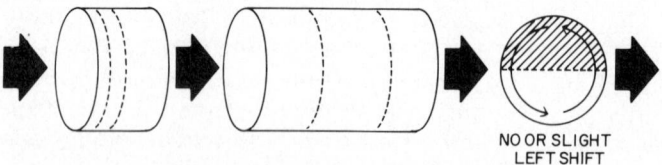

tosis, and eosinopenia. A minimal left shift may be seen, depending upon the adequacy of the bone marrow storage pool of neutrophils at the onset of the response. Monocytosis is the least consistent change in the characteristic response. Total WBC counts may range from normal to about 30,000 per

microliter in cats and to about 40,000 per microliter in dogs.

Experimentation with corticosteroids and ACTH has helped to explain the mechanism for the leukocyte response. These drugs cause mobilization of marginal neutrophils from the small blood vessels, with an increase in the number of cells in the circulating pool, impaired emigration of neutrophils into the tissue through vessel walls, and consequently, prolongation of the blood neutrophil transit time and increase in the number of neutrophils in the blood with time. An increased rate of release of the cells from the bone marrow to the blood also occurs (Athens et al., 1961a; Bishop et al., 1968). The net effect of these changes is a one- to fivefold increase in the blood neutrophil count, which may be accompanied by a slight left shift (Fig. 78–6).

The finding of Meuret and Hoffman (1973) that a large marginal monocyte pool may exist in the vascular bed of human beings (i.e., the monocytes are unequally distributed in the blood) provides speculative evidence for the occurrence of a large, marginal, monocyte pool in other species. As with blood neutrophils, the action of corticosteroids may result in mobilization of marginal cells, and monocytosis ensues.

The mechanism whereby corticosteroid causes lymphopenia is poorly understood. Lymphocytes in the cortex of the thymus and uncommitted T and B cells of the lymph nodes are susceptible to lysis by corticosteroids. In contrast, lymphocytes in the thymic medulla and bone marrow and committed effector T and B lymphocytes and plasma cells are resistant to corticosteroid-induced lysis (Craddock, 1978). The principal effect on the recirculating lymphocytes, however, is an immediate redistribution, so that the blood lymphocyte number is diminished. Experiments in rodents have shown that recirculating lymphocytes remain transiently sequestered in lymph nodes or in the blood vasculature of bone marrow following injection of corticosteroid (Greaves et al., 1973; Yu et al., 1974; Fauci and Dale, 1975; Fauci et al., 1976).

Although the actual mechanisms are not understood, research findings from dogs and other species on the eosinopenic effects of corticosteriods are summarized by Beeson and Bass (1977) as follows.

There is a rapid, reversible peripheral sequestration of eosinophils; the site is unknown, but it is at least immediately accessible to the circulation. This probably involves margination of the cells within the vascular compartments. Egress of the mature cells from the marrow into the blood is inhibited. Marrow production continues for at least 36 hours in most species, and there is an increase in total marrow eosinophils during this time. With prolonged steroid action there is eventually a depression of marrow production and in numbers of marrow eosinophils.

Following a single dose of ten units of ACTH or 20 mg of prednisolone in dogs and 5 mg of prednisolone in cats, peak neutrophilia, greater than a 50 per cent decrease in lymphocyte count, eosinopenia, and monocytosis occur by four to six hours after administration. Baseline values return by 24 hours after treatment (Jasper and Jain, 1965; Jain and Schalm, 1966; Schalm et al., 1975). Prolonged administration of the drug produces continual change, and a longer period is necessary to reach baseline values after cessation of treatment. But the magnitude of leukocytosis (which is dose dependent) tends to diminish as daily treatment continues (Jasper and Jain, 1965; Jain and Schalm, 1966). In cats given weekly injections of repositol corticosteroid, the leukocyte response was inconsistently observed (Scott et al., 1978), and alternate day therapy with short-acting corticosteroids may obviate the effects.

The endogenous release of corticosteroids following stimulation of the pituitary-adrenal axis is a common response in clinical diseases resulting in the corticosteroid-induced leukogram. This response, often referred to as systemic stress, is stimulated by pain and extremes in heat or cold exposure. Hyperadrenocorticism in dogs is characterized also by neutrophilia, lymphopenia, eosinopenia, and monocytosis, but as the disease progresses, neutrophilia disappears and total WBC counts may be within normal limits (Schalm et al., 1975). In a retrospective study of 760 canine and 225 feline leukograms, the stress leukogram was observed at the time of admission to the hospital in dogs with the following conditions: accidental trauma, fracture, shock, biliary obstruction, dystocia, epileptiform seizure, gastrointestinal obstruction, intervertebral disc syndrome, organophosphate poisoning, and pylorospasm. In cats, it was seen in accidental trauma, fractures, intestinal obstruction, urethral obstruction, and oxalate poisoning (Prasse, 1975).

It should be noted that stimulation of the pituitary release of ACTH followed by adrenocortical release of steroids is the cause of the "stress leukogram," and that the "fight or flight" response of the sympathetic nervous system with epinephrine release is the cause in healthy animals of "physiologic leukocytosis," a considerably different leukogram (described earlier). Systemic stress may accompany diseases in which other stimuli of neutrophilia coexist with the endogenous corticosteroid stimulation; lymphopenia and eosinopenia may be the only indicators of the stressful component. Stress may also accompany diseases usually characterized by eosinophilia; the eosinophil response may be absent or tempered by the corticosteroid stimulation (Beeson and Bass, 1977).

NEUTROPHIL RESPONSES IN INFLAMMATION

Inflammation is a complex humoral and cellular response to tissue injury. Its detection is a primary reason for the routine examination of blood leukocytes, and once detected, its clinical course can be monitored by repeated blood-leukocyte evaluation. With respect to hematology, inflammation represents a local or generalized tissue demand for neutrophils. Neutrophils respond to chemotactic stimuli in the affected tissue and become an integral part of the inflammatory reaction itself. In addition to bacteria, virus, fungi, or other infectious agents, chemical, thermal, and other noninfectious agents may induce the inflammation that stimulates the neutrophil response. Immune-mediated diseases such as polymyositis, autoimmune hemolytic anemia, and lupus erythematosis elicit marked neutrophilic leukocytosis. In general, local inflammation (such as pyometra or abscess) produces neutrophilia of greater magnitude than that produced by generalized inflammatory diseases, and pyogenic bacteria produce more intense neutrophilia than other etiologic agents.

As the tissue demand for neutrophils develops, increased rate of release from bone marrow into blood and granulopoiesis (neutrophil production) are stimulated. The mode of stimulation for increased neutrophil production has not been clearly identified, but by analogy to the action of erythropoietin (the stimulus for erythropoiesis), it is surmised that a granulopoietin (colony stimulating factor) also exists (Bierman, 1964; Metcalf and Moore, 1971). As release to blood depletes the marrow granulocyte storage pool of mature neutrophils, bone marrow macrophages secrete the factor, which stimulates cellular proliferation. Rytöma (1968, 1973) demonstrated the existence of a negative-feedback, chalone mechanism, whereby after a sudden loss of neutrophils (and thereby loss of granulocyte chalone) in an inflamed tissue, the resulting fall in granulocyte chalone permits a higher mitotic rate among granulocytic precursors.

The number of neutrophils ultimately encountered in the blood during inflammatory disease represents the balance between the tissue demand for cells and the rate of bone-marrow release of new cells. This balance, including the factors that influence it, has been examined in leukokinetic studies of experimentally induced inflammatory disease. As acute inflammation develops, the marginal pool increases, followed shortly by an increase in the circulating pool (Marsh et al., 1967; Athens et al., 1965; Gailbraith et al., 1965) (Fig. 78–6). The rates of bone marrow granulopoiesis and release of cells into the blood are stimulated. If production and release of cells by the bone marrow sufficiently exceed the tissue demand, a neutrophilic leukocytosis with a regenerative left shift will be found. The converse condition, in which tissue demand exceeds the bone marrow production and release of cells, results in a degenerative left shift, and in severe instances, neutropenia is observed. During the peak of inflammation, neutrophil transit time is nearly normal, and the WBC count stabilizes, although it may fluctuate slightly. At this time, tissue demand and bone marrow production and release are nearly balanced.

The magnitude of neutrophilic leukocytosis is roughly parallel to the magnitude of inflammation. Schalm (1962, 1963) summarized findings in canine patients with neutrophilic leukocytosis as follows: WBC counts of 20,000 to 30,000 per microliter were common, with typical diseases being nephritis, neoplasia, and distemper with secondary bacterial infection. Of 683 canine patients, seven per cent had WBC counts between 30,000 and 50,000 per microliter, and three per cent had counts exceeding 50,000 per microliter, common diseases being pyometra, pyogenic infections (abscesses, suppurative pleuritis, pneumonia, and pyelonephritis), malignancies, endocarditis, and leptospirosis. On rare occasions, suppurative diseases may result in WBC counts exceeding 100,000 per microliter in the dog. The majority of feline patients with suppurative infectious diseases have WBC counts from 19,500 to 30,000 per microliter, and extreme counts in the cat begin at 30,000 per microliter and range to 75,000 per microliter (Schalm and Smith, 1963).

The magnitude of the left shift is an index of the intensity of inflammation or the nature of the particular inflammatory exudate. Mild left shift, about 300 to 1000 immature neutrophils per microliter, is a typical finding in canine and feline diseases in which the neutrophil is a minimal component of the exudate. Examples are hemorrhagic cystitis, seborrheic dermatitis, tracheobronchitis, catarrhal or hemorrhagic enteritis, and certain nonsuppurative granulomatous diseases. This neutrophil response may be difficult to differentiate from corticosteroid-induced neutrophilia without knowledge of the nature of the disease at hand. Immature neutrophils in excess of 1000 per microliter or in excess of ten per cent of the total neutrophil count in dogs or cats usually indicates more intensity, a purulent exudative process. Purulent diseases may cause the total WBC count to be low, within normal limits, or high, depending on the balance between the rate of tissue utilization and the rate of neutrophil release from bone marrow. In any case, since the rate of utilization and release are high, bone marrow storage depletes faster than production replenishes it, and immature neutrophils mark the differential leukocyte counts in these diseases.

Figure 78–7 schematically illustrates the course of neutrophilic leukocytosis in those suppurative disorders that become chronic. When the number of immature neutrophils approaches, equals, or exceeds the number of segmented neutrophils, the presence of an intense suppurative disease is indicated. After a period of time, the magnitude of the left shift begins to diminish, and eventually a right shift with hypersegmented neutrophils is observed in the blood. Although a significant neutrophilic leukocytosis continues, a declining or minimal left shift (in the face of continued clinical illness), with the appearance of hypersegmented neutrophils, denotes a chronic suppurative disease in which granulopoiesis simultaneously has maintained the supply for tissue utilization and replenished the bone marrow storage pool of neutrophils (Fig. 78–6).

Occasionally when neutrophilic leukocytosis and marked left shift are observed, the location of tissue utilization of neutrophils remains totally obscure in clinical or even gross necropsy inspection. Examples of such conditions include purulent enteritis and purulent dermatitis. In these circumstances neutrophils emigrate to the gut lumen or body surface and are immediately lost without visible accumulation; histologic examination usually reveals the neutrophilic exudation in the mucous membrane or skin. These tissues represent "local" sites of inflammation, and the neutrophilia may be very dramatic compared with the unimpressive tissue reaction. Other diseases in which the site of neutrophil loss remains obscure include hemolytic anemias, particularly autoimmune hemolytic anemia. Surgical extirpation of a localized area of suppuration such as pyometra is often followed by inten-

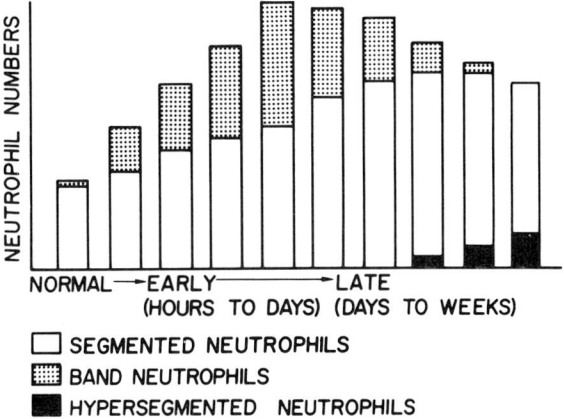

Figure 78–7. Course of blood-neutrophil response in chronic suppurative disorders. Intense suppuration may be indicated when the number of immature neutrophils nearly equals or exceeds the number of mature neutrophils. Repetitive examination is necessary to establish if the left shift is increasing or decreasing during continued suppuration. The occurrence of hypersegmented neutrophils may reflect the existence of a long-standing suppuration.

sification of the neutrophilia for a few days; this should not be confused with complications from the surgery itself.

NEUTROPENIA

Neutropenia, which is almost always concomitant with leukopenia in the dog and cat, is an important finding, frequently associated with grave consequences. The seriousness of neutropenia stems not only from the added risk of bacterial infection but also from the general nature of the clinical disorders with which it is associated. Neutropenias may be categorized as reduced survival of mature cells, reduced production by the bone marrow, and increased ineffective granulopoiesis (Finch, 1977). These types of neutropenia are shown schematically in Figure 78–8.

In reduced survival neutropenia, the destruction of mature neutrophils or the tissue utilization of the cells is massive, blood transit time is decreased, and the rate of cell loss exceeds the rate of replenishment from bone marrow (Greenberg et al., 1967). If the process persists for one or two days, the bone marrow exhibits granulopoietic hyperplasia (Fig. 78–9,A). In reduced production neutropenia, the principal effect occurs at the stem cell level, the development of neutropenia is often insidious, and the clinical course may be more prolonged. The diseases are characterized often by pancytopenia, i.e., anemia, neutropenia, and thrombocytopenia. The bone marrow exhibits granulopoietic hypoplasia and often hematopoietic hypoplasia (Fig. 78–9,B). Neutropenia that results from increased ineffective granulopoiesis is characterized by neutropenia and granulopoietic hyperplasia in the bone marrow and is essentially indistinguishable from reduced survival neutropenia except by clinical course or outcome. Ineffective granulopoiesis is due to arrested maturation, usually at the myelocyte level; intramedullary death of granulocytes; or failure to release mature cells into the blood. Use of the term "maturation arrest" should be applied only when true arrest of maturation is proven; application of the term to describe the granulopoietic

NEUTROPHIL KINETICS IN HEALTH

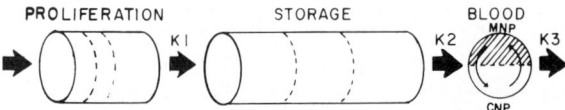

REDUCED SURVIVAL NEUTROPENIA

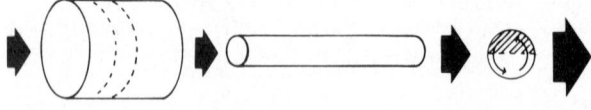

Figure 78–8. Mechanisms of neutropenia. Size of arrows represent rates of movement of cells through the compartments of granulopoiesis, marrow storage, and blood. The size of the tubes, circle, and shaded area represent bone marrow proliferation and storage pools, blood total neutrophil pool, and blood marginal neutrophil pool, respectively.

REDUCED GRANULOPOIESIS

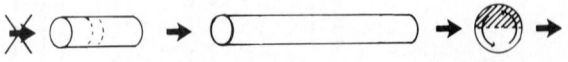

INCREASED INEFFECTIVE GRANULOPOIESIS

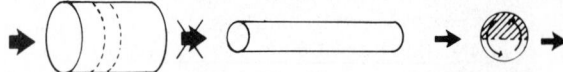

hyperplasia that accompanies reduced survival neutropenia is incorrect.

The various neutropenic disorders of dogs and cats will be briefly described; many of the diseases mentioned are discussed in greater detail elsewhere in this text. It should be noted that the listing of a particular neutropenic disease by mechanism of neutropenia is presumptive, and future research findings may impose reclassification.

Reduced Survival Neutropenia. Neutropenia caused by sudden, massive utilization of cells is associated with certain localized acute bacterial infections (Schalm, 1963). The purulent exudative diseases are located particularly in the lung, thorax, peritoneal cavity, or uterus in dogs and cats. The associated syndromes are inhalation pneumonia, intestinal rupture, intussusception with necrosis, acute metritis, or ruptured internal abscess. Gram-negative bacteria are common causes. A similar response may be seen in feline (Timoney et al., 1978) and canine salmonellosis. In these diseases the neutropenia is characterized by toxic, immature cells in the blood and, in the bone marrow, decreased proportion of metamyelocytes, bands, and segmenters with increased proportion of early granulocytic precursors. If the animal survives, neutrophilic leukocytosis is hopefully observed over the following 72 to 96 hours.

Antibody-mediated, immune neutrope-

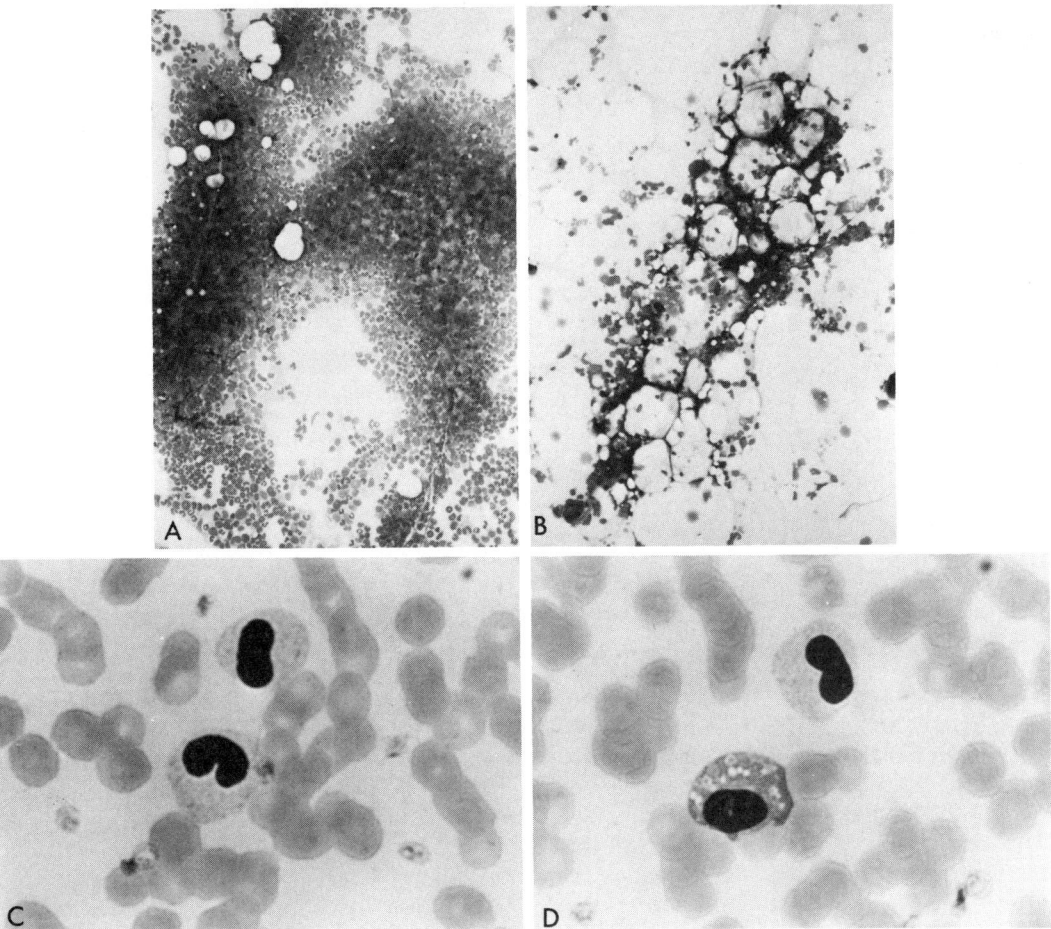

Figure 78–9. *A,* Bone marrow particle smear. Particle exhibits many cells and little fat, a hypercellular bone marrow. Cat. (Low magnification.) *B,* Bone marrow particle smear. Particle exhibits few cells and much fat, a hypocellular bone marrow. Cat. (Low magnification.) *C,* Mature neutrophils with hyposegmented nuclei and dense nuclear chromatin from a dog with Pelger-Huët anomaly. (Blood smear provided courtesy of Dr. O. W. Schalm, University of California, Davis, California.) *D,* Neutrophil and eosinophil, bottom, from a dog with Pelger-Huët anomaly. (same dog as *C*).

Illustration continued on following page

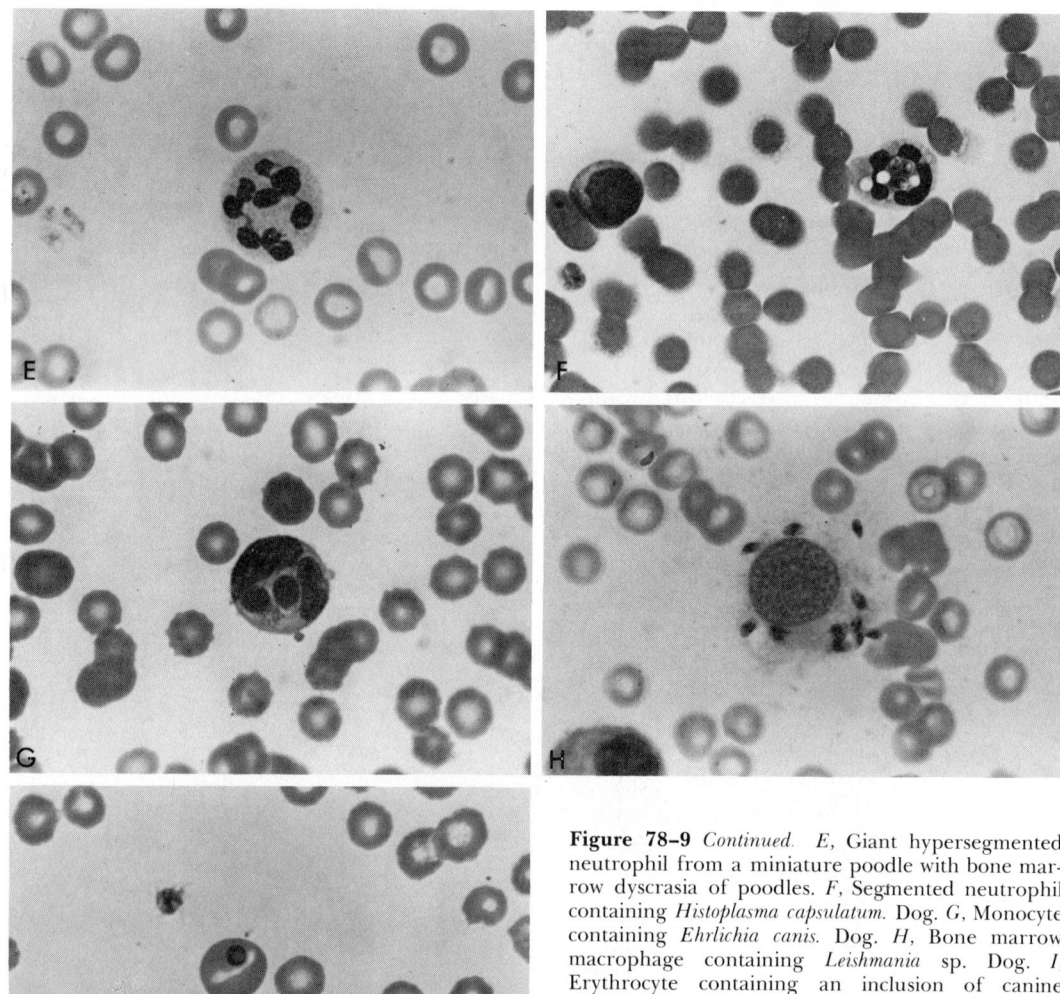

Figure 78–9 *Continued.* *E,* Giant hypersegmented neutrophil from a miniature poodle with bone marrow dyscrasia of poodles. *F,* Segmented neutrophil containing *Histoplasma capsulatum.* Dog. *G,* Monocyte containing *Ehrlichia canis.* Dog. *H,* Bone marrow macrophage containing *Leishmania* sp. Dog. *I,* Erythrocyte containing an inclusion of canine distemper. Dog.

Wright or Wright-Leishman stain. Magnification on cells in *C* through *I* is the same. (Photomicrographs *A, B, F,* and *G* provided courtesy of Dr. J. R. Duncan, University of Georgia, Athens, GA.)

nia is classified also as reduced survival neutropenia. Certain neutropenic animals, sometimes with episodic or cyclic neutropenia in which immune neutropenia was suspected, have been successfully managed with corticosteroid treatment, but immune-mediated neutropenia is an equivocal diagnosis unless antineutrophil antibody is demonstrated in the serum or on the cells of the patient.

Reduced Production Neutropenia. Neutropenia caused by diminished bone marrow production may occur in acute diseases, or the onset may be insidious, depending on the cause. Certain neutropenic viral diseases may present with febrile illness of acute onset, whereas some pancytopenic diseases progress more slowly, and hemorrhages due to thrombocytopenia may be the early clinical findings.

Feline panleukopenia virus (see Chapter 27) causes profound neutropenia, and the mechanism appears to be that of reduced production. During the course of illness, neutropenia persists with few immature neutrophils appearing in the blood (Schalm et al., 1975). Neutropenia and lymphopenia with total WBC counts ranging from less than 100 to 2000 per microliter occur in dogs with parvovirus infection (see Chapter 27); leukopenia accompanies the clinical signs of illness (Appel et al., 1978a, 1979b).

Reduced production is the mechanism of neutropenia in dogs with estrogen toxicity (Chiu, 1974; Bland-van den Berg et al., 1978; Schalm, 1978) and in dogs with testicular neoplasia (Kasbohm and Saar, 1975). In estrogen toxicity the following hematologic changes take place; platelet number increases within five to seven days after the overdosage and is followed by thrombocytopenia by day 13; on day 5, the bone marrow exhibits erythroid hypoplasia, decreased megakaryocytes, and myeloid hyperplasia; marked neutrophilic leukocytosis peaks by days 17 to 23 and is followed by decreasing counts progressing to neutropenia; anemia progresses, and by day 10 the bone marrow is hypocellular and depleted of all hematopoietic elements (Chiu, 1974). The magnitude of changes in cell numbers and potential for recovery apparently depend on the dose of estrogen. In 3 of 138 dogs with testicular tumors, both Sertoli cell and interstitial cell tumors were associated with the syndrome (Kasbohn and Saar, 1975). The affected dogs had nonregenerative anemia, neutropenia, and thrombocytopenia.

Other cases of reduced production neutropenia include cyclic hematopoiesis of collies, and canine ehrlichiosis (a pancytopenic disease) (see Chapter 27). The thrombocytopenia of ehrlichiosis is believed to be due to increased destruction rather than reduced production (Lovering et al., 1980), but granulopoiesis is decreased (Schalm and Strombeck, 1974). Cytotoxic agents used for cancer treatment may also cause reduced production neutropenia.

Feline leukovirus–infected, nonleukemic cats present with a broad spectrum of clinical illnesses, but typically they exhibit anorexia, depression, pyrexia, and nonregenerative anemia. In a review of case records at The University of Georgia Veterinary Teaching Hospital, about 50 per cent of the infected, nonleukemic cats had neutropenia. Bone marrow in these cats is found to have either granulopoietic hypoplasia (hence, reduced production neutropenia), or, surprisingly, marked granulopoietic hyperplasia. The latter cases are believed to represent an example of ineffective granulopoiesis. In the cases with granulopoietic hypoplasia, other clinical findings may mimic infectious panleukopenia (Hardy et al., 1976).

Increased Ineffective Granulopoiesis. Neutropenia caused by increased ineffective granulopoiesis may be difficult to clinically distinguish from reduced survival neutropenia, because both types are accompanied by granulopoietic hyperplasia in the bone marrow.

Certain feline leukovirus–infected, nonleukemic, neutropenic cats are found to have marked granulopoietic hyperplasia on bone marrow examination. Myeloblasts, promyelocytes, and myelocytes predominate, and more mature neutrophils are nearly absent in bone marrow. Placement of this syndrome as an example of ineffective granulopoiesis is presumptive, but if the cats survive, the hematologic pattern may persist unchanged for days or even weeks. Cats originally described as having "subleukemic granulocytic leukemia" (Schalm, 1972; Duncan and Prasse, 1976) may be representative of this syndrome. Affected cats may either die from secondary infection, eventually recover clinically and hematologically, or in rare instances, progress into neoplasia, i.e., granulocytic leukemia. In this regard, the feline syndrome is remarkably similar to human "preleukemic syndrome" (Madewell et al., 1979).

Another example of ineffective granulopoiesis is myelofibrosis, a lesion associated with feline leukovirus infection (Hoover and Kociba, 1974; Flecknell et al., 1978; Zenoble and Rowland, 1979). It is characterized by hematopoietic hyperplasia with impaired marrow release of cells and progressive neutropenia and anemia. In the developing stages, the blood neutrophil number is persistently low in spite of numerous mature and immature precursors seen in bone marrow aspiration smears.

Diphenylhydantoin, phenylbutazone, and other drugs may cause maturation arrest and neutropenia in human beings (Taetle et al., 1979). Diphenylhydantoin has been shown to inhibit granulocyte proliferation in concert with the presence of serum from the neutropenic patient, a true measure of ineffective granulopoiesis. Dogs treated with diphenylhydantoin may develop neutropenia that is reversible after cessation of therapy. Phenylbutazone may induce neutropenia in dogs (Schalm, 1979) by a similar mechanism, but hapten-induced antibody mediated neutropenia (reduced survival) is attributed also to this drug in humans (Finch, 1977).

NEUTROPHIL RESPONSES IN VIRAL INFECTIONS

The feline infectious panleukopenia virus, canine parvovirus, and feline leukovirus were discussed with the mechanisms of neutropenia. In each of these infections, neutropenia predictably occurs during the stages of clinical illness, and the mechanisms leading to neutropenia are presumed to be reduced production based on the hematologic patterns observed. In most other viral infections neutropenia is less remarkable, if it occurs at all, and in some diseases neutrophilia may be seen.

Canine coronavirus infection may cause lymphopenia, but neutropenia does not occur, which serves as a useful means for differentiating it from canine parvovirus infection (Appel et al., 1979a, 1979b). Canine distemper and infectious hepatitis viruses cause low normal neutrophil counts, or high normal counts, or neutrophilic leukocytosis if secondary bacterial infections accompany the diseases (Schalm, 1963).

Upper respiratory virus infections in cats usually have normal neutrophil counts (Report, 1970). Feline infectious peritonitis is found often with neutrophilic leukocytosis (Ward and Pederson, 1969).

MONOCYTE RESPONSES

Absolute monocytosis, defined as counts exceeding 1350 per microliter in the dog and 850 per microliter in the cat, occurs quite frequently. Its occurrence is related to disorders characterized by suppuration, necrosis, malignancy, hemolysis, hemorrhage (Schalm, 1962, 1963), and immune-mediated diseases and certain pyogranulomatous conditions. Monocytosis in response to endogenous or exogenous corticosteroids was described earlier in the chapter. In a consecutive series of approximately 760 cases involving dogs that had been hospitalized and examined hematologically, 232 cases (30.6 per cent) had monocytosis. One hundred thirty-five cases were chronic disorders, and 97 were acute, stressful disorders (Prasse, 1975). In the same study, 225 feline cases were examined hematologically, and 27 (11.1 per cent) had monocytosis. Sixteen cases were chronic disorders and 11 were acute, stressful disorders. Most of the acute cases with monocytosis were accidental trauma.

It is generally accepted that monocytes transform into active phagocytic cells, or macrophages, within tissues. On rare occasions, this phagocytic tendency may be observed on a blood film, and monocytes bearing erythrocytes within the cytoplasm may be seen in autoimmune hemolytic anemia. Although monocytes apparently leave the blood and enter an affected tissue at the same time as neutrophilic leukocytes, they appear in much lower numbers than the neutrophils, and the latter predominate in early inflammatory exudates. Apparently, monocytes have a longer tissue life span (as transformed macrophages), and their numbers steadily increase in the exudate as the condition becomes chronic. During these later stages of the disorder, monocytosis may be observed. In general, monocytosis is expected any time neutrophilia occurs, and it only rarely represents the sole change from normal in a leukogram.

EOSINOPHIL RESPONSES

Eosinophilia and eosinopenia are common findings in dogs and cats. In general, eosinophilia is associated with parasitism and hypersensitivity states, whereas eosinopenia occurs with acute infections that cause inflammation and with the endogenous or exogenous corticosteroid response (see Leukocyte Response to Corticosteroids). It should be kept in mind that eosinophils are present in low numbers in blood. Therefore, differential counts have more inherent error in eosinophil counts than in counts for neutrophils or lymphocytes; variation in observing plus or minus two or three eosinophils, which is entirely within biological limits of variation, may definitely influence the interpretation of the leukogram. No eosinophils may be observed in the blood of clinically normal animals; in contrast, animals with eosinophilic disorders may have a response tempered by the corticosteroid-eosinophilic effect, if they are severely stressed. Another observation that seems paradoxical is the occurrence of local lesions that contain significant numbers of eosinophils in the exudate but without concomitant circulating eosinophilia. Eosinophilic and eosinopenic conditions, however, have rather predictable patterns of occurrence.

Eosinophilia. Eosinophilia occurs in disorders characterized by immediate hypersensitivity reaction. These conditions are IgE-producing disorders, and the IgE is surface-bound to mast cells and basophils. Interaction of antigen with specific IgE causes the mast cells and basophils to secrete their granule contents. Histamine, slow reactive substance of anaphylaxis, and chemotactic factors for eosinophils and neutrophils are released. Another feature of eosinophilic disorders is T lymphocyte sensitization, which apparently is necessary to stimulate eosinophilopoiesis and to produce and sustain eosinophilia (Basten and Beeson, 1970; Beeson and Bass, 1977). The tissues usually affected in eosinophilic disorders are skin, lung, gastrointestinal tract, and reproductive tract (Schalm, 1966a, 1966b). These tissues are constantly in contact with external, foreign material, and the subepithelial tissues of these organs are rich in mast cells. The response is a matter of degree. Many local inflammatory reactions may be found on histologic examination to have numerous eosinophils among the cells in the exudate, yet no circulating eosinophilia is observed.

In a survey of 760 sequentially hospitalized dogs examined hematologically, 184 dogs (24 per cent) presented with eosinophilia. One hundred seventeen of the 184 dogs were parasitized, and of these, parasitism was the primary clinical problem in 60 dogs (the population had a geographic bias for a high incidence of dirofilariasis) (Prasse, 1975). In the same study, 43 of 225 cats (8.8 per cent) presented with eosinophilia; none of the eosinophilic cats were kittens.

Usually an examination for parasites follows observation of eosinophilia in an animal. Only those parasites that are migratory and invasive produce eosinophilia. Those that cause only a slight focal lesion generally do not cause eosinophilia (Beeson and Bass, 1977). Dirofilariasis consistently produces eosinophilia in dogs, and increased basophil counts frequently accompany the eosinophilia, especially in microfilaria-negative

dogs. Other parasitisms of dogs that quite consistently induce eosinophilia are ancylostomiasis, infestation with *Spirocerca lupi*, *Strongyloides stercoralis* (Soulsby, 1965), and *Filaroides osleri* (Soulsby, 1965), and flea-allergy dermatitis. Occasionally, whipworms are associated with circulating eosinophilia in dogs. Parasites such as ascarids, tapeworms, and *Coccidia* rarely induce a sustained eosinophilia, but in a survey of dogs with gastrointestinal parasitism, mean circulating eosinophil counts were higher than in uninfected dogs (Saror et al., 1979). Eosinophil counts were normal in 20 dogs with microfilaremia of *Dipetalonema sp.* (Wittmer et al., 1979).

No difference in eosinophil counts between 30 noninfected cats and 35 cats infected with *Taenia taeniaformis, T. pisiformis, T. hydatigena, Hymenolepis nana, Toxocara cati, T. canis, Toxascaris leonina, Uncinaria stenocephala,* or *Ancylostoma caninum* was seen (Roth and Schneider, 1971). In contrast, aelurostrongylosis (Scott, 1973), paragonimiasis (Hoover and Dubey, 1978), trichinosis (Holzworth and Georgi, 1974), and flea infestation (particularly flea-allergy dermatitis) are parasitisms accompanied by eosinophilia in cats.

A wide variety of nonparasitic disorders cause eosinophilia, including atopic hypersensitivity conditions such as staphylococcal hypersensitivity dermatitis in dogs, eosinophilic pneumonitis in dogs and cats, oral eosinophilic granuloma of Siberian huskies (Potter et al., 1980), and eosinophilic granuloma complex of cats. In some diseases, local eosinophil infiltration may be marked, but circulating eosinophilia is uncommon. An example is canine eosinophilic myositis and atrophy of head muscles; only 3 of 20 dogs (two of the three were Alsatian) with myositis and atrophy of head muscles had eosinophilia (Irfan, 1971). Dogs with panosteitis (it has been called eosinophilic panosteitis) inconsistently have eosinophilia (Bone, 1980). Whereas hyperadrenocorticism causes eosinopenia, the converse is not true; adrenal insufficiency does not usually cause eosinophilia.

In human beings, eosinophilic leukemoid reaction may accompany certain types of lymphoblastic leukemia (Spitzer and Garson, 1973). The author has observed two cats with eosinophilia in excess of 60,000 cells per microliter. They were initially diagnosed as having eosinophilic leukemia because the change persisted, but both cats had alimentary lymphosarcoma at necropsy.

BASOPHIL RESPONSES

Basocytophilia (basophilia) is seldom numerically dramatic, but observing even a few cells usually attracts attention to this leukogram change. The response is infrequent in dogs and cats. Recognition of basophilia in cats depends on the ability of the microscopist to identify the cell. Cat basophil granules lack the usual metachromatic staining quality, but the cell can be readily identified (see discussion on morphology earlier in the chapter).

Basophilia is encountered usually in conditions that stimulate IgE production. Such basophilias are almost always concomitant with eosinophilia. Basophilia, usually without concomitant eosinophilia, also occurs during persistent hyperlipoproteinemias. These conditions include hyperadrenocorticism (Schalm et al., 1975), chronic liver disease, nephrotic syndrome, and diabetes mellitus.

LYMPHOCYTE RESPONSES

Lymphopenia is a frequent abnormality in the canine and feline leukogram, but it is almost never the sole cause of leukopenia. Lymphocytosis is uncommon, and when observed, it accounts for only mild leukocytosis. The recirculating lymphocytes, which comprise the population of cells found in blood, account for only part of the total lymphocyte population. Tremendous lymphoid hyperplasia may cause enlargement of lymph nodes, yet a normal blood lymphocyte number or even lymphopenia may be observed simultaneously. Certain specific interpretations can be applied to changes in the blood lymphocyte number, but the correlation between the functional status of the immune system and blood lymphocyte number is poor.

Lymphocytosis. An absolute lymphocytosis is defined as an increase in the lymphocyte count above 4800 per microliter in the dog and 7000 per microliter in the cat. Relative lymphocytosis (i.e., elevation of the count with the value remaining in the normal range) may be more common, but it is difficult to detect, since baseline data are seldom available for the patient in question. Therefore, interpretative logic applied to lymphocyte increases tends to be appropriate only when the rise in the lymphocyte count is absolute, or when a decline has been anticipated. Care must also be taken to avoid mistaking high percentage lymphocyte counts as lymphocytosis. Although the percentage will be high in conjunction with neutropenia, the absolute lymphocyte number may be within, or even below, the normal range of values. In contrast, a low percentage lymphocyte count in conjunction with neutrophilia may belie the actual presence of a normal or elevated absolute lymphocyte count. Therefore, reliance on the absolute lymphocyte number for interpretative purposes cannot be overemphasized.

When absolute lymphocytosis is observed, the first consideration should be given to physiologic causes. It should be noted that lymphocyte values in kittens and puppies may be higher than those in adults. In cats alone, the occurrence of lymphocytosis may be observed in conjunction with fear or excitement (i.e., physiologic leukocytosis), although this response tends not to occur in clinically ill cats (Schalm and Smith, 1963).

Pathologic causes of absolute lymphocytosis are few but include lymphocytic leukemia, adrenal insufficiency (Schalm et al., 1975), and illnesses characterized by prolonged antigenic stimulation (such as chronic infection, hypersensitivity diseases, and autoimmune diseases). It should be noted that the patient having an illness with obvious, severe systemic disease would be expected to have lymphopenia. Finding a high-normal lymphocyte count or absolute lymphocytosis in this patient warrants consideration of the above disorders.

The occurrence of antigenic stimulation may be substantiated by finding a small number of lymphocytes to be larger and more basophilic than normal (see morphologic description of immunocytes earlier in the chapter).

Lymphoid neoplasia may be accompanied by lymphocytic leukemia in the dog and cat (see Chapter 79). This should also be included in the differential diagnosis, when high-normal or moderate absolute lymphocytosis is detected in patients with undiagnosed clinical illness. Occasionally, lymphocytic leukemia is manifested by significant lymphocytic leukocytosis (50,000 per microliter or greater) in which a high proportion of the lymphocytes are atypical.

Lymphopenia. Lymphopenia is a common abnormality. In a series of 760 dogs sequentially hospitalized and examined hematologically, 198 (26 per cent) had lymphopenia, less than 1000 cells per microliter. Of the 198 dogs, 68 died, were euthanatized, or did not recover by the time of dismissal from the hospital (Prasse, 1975). In the same study, 66 of 225 cats (29 per cent) had lymphopenia, less than 1500 per microliter, and 35 died, were euthanatized, or did not recover by the time of dismissal.

The general causes of lymphopenia include exogenous or endogenous corticosteroids (see Leukocyte Response to Corticosteroids), acute infection, loss of efferent lymph, and replacement or hypoplasia of the recirculating population of lymphocytes. When lymphopenia is observed on a leukogram, these general causes may be difficult to differentiate. Lymphopenia of stress may be particularly hard to differentiate from lymphopenia of acute infection.

The mechanism of lymphopenia in acute infection can be only surmised from assessment of certain research findings. Immunization by intravenous route causes uncommitted circulating lymphocytes to be transiently entrapped in the spleen of mice, and subcutaneous immunization causes transient entrapment of uncommitted lymphocytes in the regional lymph node (Zatz and Lance, 1971). Hall and Morris (1965) observed a transient arrest of drainage of efferent lymph from specific lymph nodes injected with antigen in sheep. In addition to transient entrapment of uncommitted lymphocytes, committed lymphocytes (perhaps the memory cells) are entrapped in lymph nodes for one to two days after antigenic challenge in a sensitized host (Graves et al., 1973). These findings suggest that lymphopenia may be a consequence of acute stages of infection as a natural mechanism for antigen assessment or management in the lymphoid tissues. An alternative explanation is lymphocyte death by direct injury from the infectious agent.

Examples of infections that are characterized by lymphopenia in the acute stages of clinical illness in dogs are infectious hepatitis, distemper, salmon poisoning, ehrlichio-

sis, parvovirus gastroenteritis, and coronavirus enteritis (Schalm and Strombeck, 1974; McCullough et al., 1974; Schalm et al., 1975; Appel et al., 1979). In cats, feline leukovirus infection and infectious panleukopenia virus cause lymphopenia (Rohovsky and Fowler, 1971; Cotter et al., 1979). Bacterial infection is less consistently associated with lymphopenia.

Lymphopenia secondary to loss of efferent lymph occurs with ruptured thoracic duct and chylothorax in dogs and cats. It also occurs as a consequence of feline cardiomyopathies accompanied by chylous thoracic effusion, and by loss of enteric lymphocyte-rich lymph into the gut lumen during certain chronic enteric diseases in dogs (Finco et al., 1973). Lymphopenia can occur as a consequence of loss of lymph node architecture in diseases that destroy the route of recirculating lymphocytes. Such diseases include generalized lymphosarcoma and diffuse granulomatous inflammatory diseases. Hypoplasia of the T cell system, the principal cell type in the recirculating lymphocyte population, causes lymphopenia. It occurs as a consequence of feline leukovirus–induced thymic atrophy in kittens (Anderson et al., 1971).

PROGNOSIS AND LEUKOCYTE RESPONSES

If a leukogram contains abnormalities and sequential studies show a return toward normal values, the change obviously reflects a favorable prognosis, if it is accompanied by convalescence in the animal in question. Nevertheless, certain patterns in neutrophil changes can be used as signalment of a particularly severe disease process, and some changes in eosinophil and lymphocyte numbers may signal significant change in health status before the change is manifested by physical findings in the animal.

Neutropenia, regardless of the mechanism or cause, should signal an unfavorable clinical circumstance. Affected animals have an added risk of infection, and the neutropenic disease itself is often life threatening or difficult to manage. Other neutrophil patterns that clearly denote a serious illness include left shifts in which immature neutrophils exceed the segmented neutrophil number in blood. This implies an intensive tissue demand for cells, which at the moment is progressing more rapidly than the granulopoietic effort. Any neutrophil response that prompts the observer to consider granulocytic leukemia in the differential diagnosis, i.e., a leukemoid response, is generally associated with a severe, purulent disease, a circumstance warranting careful clinical management. One exception is neutrophilic leukocytosis accompanied by very immature neutrophils, a few myelocytes, and promyelocytes; this may occur during clinical recovery from previous granulopoietic hypoplasia — a favorable finding, for example, during recovery from infectious panleukopenia.

In animals being monitored for health status by hematology on a daily or near daily basis, a sudden fall in lymphocyte number signals impending clinical illness, either the onset of acute infection or severe system stress. In contrast, lymphopenic animals being managed for a severe illness and monitored hematologically may have impending clinical remission if the lymphocyte number is found to return to normal limits. A reappearance of eosinophils in an ill, eosinopenic animal also denotes impending remission of illness.

SPECIFIC, NON-NEOPLASTIC DISEASES OF LEUKOCYTES

CANINE CYCLIC HEMATOPOIESIS (GRAY COLLIE SYNDROME)

Cyclic hematopoiesis (formerly called cyclic neutropenia) is a noninfectious disease reported only in the collie. This cyclic disease is believed to be inherited as a simple, autosomal recessive trait. In an experimental colony of collies and collie-beagle crosses, matings of heterozygotes yielded 110 pups; 28 pups (15 female and 13 male) were affected with cyclic hematopoiesis (Jones et al., 1975a). All affected collies have a specific dilution of their hair color, being silver-gray in character. Whether the blood dyscrasia and the dilution of hair color are closely linked traits or are caused by the same genetic defect is unknown (Cheville, 1968; Ford, 1969; Lund, 1973). Gray collies having cyclic hematopoiesis may coincidentally be affected by various features of the collie ocular ectasia syndrome, a congenital disease common to the breed.

Cyclic neutropenic episodes occur at 11- to 12-day intervals (Fig. 78–10). Neutropenia (defined by a low count of 0 to 400 per microliter) lasts an average of three days, followed by normal to slightly increased neutrophil counts lasting six to seven days. A single minor dip and peak of blood-neutrophil number usually antecedes the recurrence of neutropenia (Dale et al., 1972). During the neutropenic stage, a large proportion of the circulating neutrophil population is immature. Ultrastructural lesions have been observed in granulocyte precursors, coincident with interruption of further differentiation of the cells in the bone marrow. This precedes the development of peripheral neutropenia by two to three days (Scott et al., 1973). Recovery from neutropenia occurs in a single wave of granulopoietic activity.

The blood numbers of reticulocytes, platelets, and monocytes also cycle in affected collies (Patt et al., 1973; Weiden et al., 1974; Jones et al., 1975b). These observations, plus the finding of in vitro cyclic cyto-

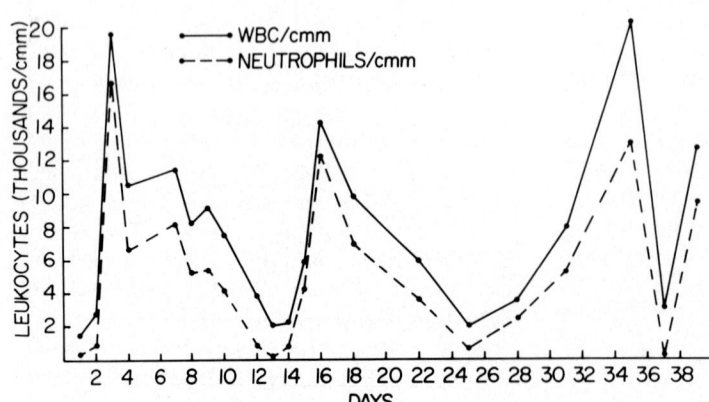

Figure 78–10. Leukocyte response in cyclic hematopoiesis. This 38-day leukocyte response from a gray collie with cyclic hematopoiesis illustrates the 11- to 12-day interval between neutropenic stages.

poietic potential of marrow from affected dogs, implies that the principal defect in cyclic hematopoiesis is at the multipotential hematopoietic stem cell level (Dunn et al., 1978). In addition to the stem cell defect, neutrophils isolated from affected dogs have been shown to have metabolic and functional abnormalities characterized by decreased bactericidal potential (Chusid et al., 1975).

Bone marrow from unaffected littermates has been transplanted into supralethally irradiated affected collies, and the cyclic changes in blood cells have disappeared in the recipients. Conversely, marrow from affected dogs transplanted into normal recipients has resulted in the appearance of cyclic changes in blood cells of the recipients (Dale and Graw, 1974; Weiden et al., 1974; Jones et al., 1975b; 1975c). In gray collies in which cyclic hematopoiesis had been eliminated by supralethal irradiation and transplantation with marrow from normal littermates two years earlier, normal Collie coloration of hair showed on their tails and other areas (Yang, 1978).

Clinical Findings. Collies affected by cyclic hematopoiesis will usually become ill within the first six months of life. The cyclic changes in blood cells may be observed as early as the eighth day of life, and PCV and hemoglobin values are lower and increase more slowly than those in unaffected littermates (Jones et al., 1974). Case histories may include such information as weakness during the postnatal period, early death of littermates, slow healing of minor wounds, and slow or retarded growth compared with that of unaffected littermates. Hair on affected dogs is characteristically silver-gray but may vary from a pale collie tricolor to dark charcoal gray. Gradual pigmentary change from brown to gray may also be noted (Lund et al., 1967; Cheville, 1968).

Presenting clinical signs that are commonly reported in varying combinations include anorexia, lethargy, arthralgia, diarrhea, epistaxis, and gingivitis or gingival hemorrhages. Rectal temperature is usually increased. Signs parallel the neutropenic phase, and recovery from neutropenia is followed by remission of the signs. Repeated neutropenic episodes are accompanied by recurrent and often intensified illness, such as septicemia, pneumonia, hemorrhagic enteritis, or other pyogenic infections. Increas-ing dependency on antibiotic therapy is necessary for survival. Profuse hemorrhage occurs in some cases, and prolonged clotting times are reported (Cheville, 1968); this may be a manifestation of disseminated intravascular coagulation. Anemia may be found in late stages of the disease. Amyloidosis may be found in those dogs that survive multiple episodes of infection (Cheville, 1968; Machado et al., 1978).

Diagnosis is made by demonstration of the cyclic change in blood neutrophil, platelet, and reticulocyte numbers. Experimentally, daily injection of affected collies with endotoxin sufficiently stimulates the flux of cells in the proliferation compartment of granulopoiesis to obviate the cyclic changes (Hammond et al., 1979). Similarly, the cyclic change in neutrophils may be less obvious during prolonged episodes of bacterial infection.

CANINE GRANULOCYTOPATHY SYNDROME

Renshaw et al. (1975, 1977, 1979) have described a disease originally diagnosed in an Irish setter and characterized by reduced bactericidal function of neutrophils. The disease is inherited as an autosomal recessive trait. From puppyhood, life-threatening recurrent infections are associated with neutrophilic leukocytosis and pyrexia. The neutrophils have defective hexose monophosphate shunt activity (although, paradoxically, ability to reduce nitroblue tetrazolium is increased). The cells have a decreased ability to kill catalase-positive and catalase-negative bacteria.

PELGER-HUËT ANOMALY

Dogs. Pelger-Huët anomaly is a condition characterized by hyposegmentation of nuclei of neutrophils and eosinophils. The nuclei remain round, oval, or bean-shaped; the nuclear chromatin appears condensed; the cell size is normal; and the cytoplasm appears mature (Fig. 78–9,*C,D*). The anomaly is uncommon in dogs, but has been reported in the redbone hound (Schalm et al., 1975), cocker spaniel (Feldman and Romans, 1976), black and tan coonhound (Pace, 1977), and foxhound (Bowles et al., 1979). Case files at the University of Georgia Veterinary Teaching Hospital list Pelger-

Huët anomaly in a Basenji, a Boston terrier, and a mixed-breed dog. Other clinical pathologists in the United States and elsewhere (Kiss and Komar, 1967) have seen the anomaly in leukocytes of dogs. The inheritance mode in dogs is not determined, but in the foxhound study (Bowles et al., 1979), non–sex-linked dominant transmittance was suggested.

The anomaly is usually encountered as an incidental finding unrelated to abnormal health. When a persistent left shift concomitant with a normal WBC count cannot be equated with the health status of the dog in question, Pelger-Huët anomaly should be considered. Nearly all of the neutrophils and eosinophils have the round, oval, or bean-shaped nuclei; two-lobed or three-lobed segmenters are rare in the blood. Bone marrow precursors exhibit normal nuclear maturation in the early granulocyte precursors and normal cytoplasmic maturation throughout the series. A very similar problem confronts the diagnostician in animals with acquired hyposegmentation, pseudo–Pelger-Huët anomaly (see p. 2006).

In the foxhounds (Bowles et al., 1979) with Pelger-Huët anomaly, blast transformation studies indicated a factor or factors in the affected dogs' plasma that inhibited B lymphocyte reactivity. Neutrophil mobility into skin abrasion sites was impaired also. And affected females had a lower percentage of pups weaned than did unaffected females.

Cats. Pelger-Huët anomaly was diagnosed in two ten-year-old castrated male feline littermates (Weber et al., 1981). The classical nuclear changes were in neutrophils and eosinophils.

BONE MARROW DYSCRASIA IN POODLES

Poodles, particularly miniature and toy breeds, are affected by a bone marrow dyscrasia that results in asymptomatic abnormalities of erythrocytes and neutrophils (Schalm et al., 1975; Schalm, 1976b). Macrocytic normochromic erythrocytes and hypersegmented neutrophils, sometimes of giant size (Fig. 78–9,*E*), characterize the dyscrasia. The changes are discovered during hematologic examination when the patient has been presented for complaints unrelated to the hematologic abnormality.

Affected dogs go unnoticed unless MCV is calculated, or unless the hypersegmented neutrophils are noticed during routine differential counting. The MCV is typically 85 to 96 femtoliters, and the dogs are not anemic.

FELINE CHEDIAK-HIGASHI SYNDROME

Kramer et al. (1975, 1977) have described Chediak-Higashi syndrome in a line of Persian cats being bred to develop the blue-smoke hair. As reviewed by Kramer et al. (1977), Chediak-Higashi syndrome has been described in human beings, mink, cattle, mice, and a killer whale. The disease is manifested by partial oculocutaneous albinism, an increased susceptibility to infection, enlarged granules in leukocytes and melanocytes, and a bleeding tendency. As in other animals, the disease in cats is inherited as an autosomal recessive trait (Kramer et al., 1977).

The affected Persian cat's blue-smoke hair was lighter colored than unaffected blue-smoke–colored cats. The hair color was always seen in conjunction with yellow-green irises, compared with copper-colored irises in normal Persians. Fundic pigmentation was decreased. The fundus reflected red on ophthalmoscopic examination. Photophobia was obvious, and affected cats tended to develop cataracts at an early age (Prieur et al., 1979). No increased tendency for infection has been seen in affected cats (Kramer et al., 1977; Prieur et al., 1979).

Abnormally large, peroxidase-positive, sudanophilic granules are found in neutrophils (Fig. 78–3, *I*). Eosinophil and basophil granules are enlarged, and melanin granules in skin and hair are enlarged (Kramer et al., 1977).

The affected cats have a tendency to bleed following minor surgery and to form hematomas at venapuncture sites (Prieur et al., 1979). Clotting times and platelet counts are normal, but platelet function is abnormal (Meyers, 1980).

CYTOPLASMIC INCLUSIONS IN LEUKOCYTES OF DOGS AND CATS

Mucopolysaccharidosis. Cytoplasmic mucopolysaccharide granules in leukocytes associated with certain heritable disorders characterized by skeletal deformities, functional deficits of the central nervous system, and other signs attributed to enzyme deficiency in the catabolism of mucopolysaccharides have been described in Siamese cats (Crowell et al., 1976; Jezyk et al., 1977; Langweiler et al., 1978) and dachshunds (Schalm, 1977). The specific deficient enzyme was not identified in the canine report, but the cats were deficient in arylsulfatase B (Jezyk et al., 1977; Langweiler et al., 1978).

The granules in feline neutrophils stain purple (metachromatic) on Romanowsky-stained smears (Fig. 78–3,*J*), and the metachromasia can be confirmed by positive staining with toluidine blue. Diagnosis may be aided by finding the cytoplasmic inclusions in leukocytes, but it also depends on demonstration of the skeletal defects and glycosaminoglycans excreted in urine (Langweiler et al., 1978). Purple granules can be found in the leukocytes in other, so-called storage diseases; a cat with sphingolipidosis had numerous large granules in neutrophils (Fig. 78–3, *K*).

Schalm (1977) suggested that "the mucopolysaccharide granules can be distinguished from so-called 'toxic' granules by the fact that the cytoplasm takes a normal stain rather than the bluish staining of the cytoplasm of 'toxic' neutrophils. Furthermore, 'toxic' granulation is not of common occurrence in the dog or cat."

Inclusions in Infections. Viral inclusions of canine distemper may be found infrequently in erythrocytes or any of the various leukocytes (Schalm, 1974). The inclusions stain light red in leukocyte cytoplasm and a different shade of red than hemoglobin in erythrocytes (Figs. 78–3,*L*, 78–9,*I*). The inclusions tend to disappear in anticoagulated blood left standing for some time before smears are made. The author has seen these inclusions quite often in young dogs just vaccinated in the previous days or weeks; the question of whether or not the inclusions are infectious or vaccine virus remains unanswered. These dogs have not always had typical canine distemper hemograms (see earlier discussion) or clinical findings.

Other infectious agents can be found in the cytoplasm of blood and bone marrow leukocytes. Included are *Histoplasma capsulatum*, *Ehrlichia canis*, and *Leishmania sp.* (Fig. 78–9,*F–H*).

NEOPLASTIC DISEASES OF LEUKOCYTES

HEMATOPOIETIC NEOPLASIA

Terminology and Classification. Malignant proliferation of hematopoietic cells is the most common form of neoplasia in the cat and among the most common in the dog. A characteristic of many components of the hematopoietic system is entry into the blood. When neoplastic proliferation of any of these hematopoietic components gives rise to the presence of detectable numbers of malignant cells in the blood, a leukemic state ensues. For this reason hematopoietic neoplasms may be subdivided on the basis of obvious blood involvement (leukemia) or no obvious involvement (aleukemia). As an example, a lymphoid neoplasm may have no blood abnormality, or it may be accompanied by malignant cells in the blood (e.g., lymphocytic leukemia). This subdivision may not reflect any pathogenic difference but is useful for clinical differentiation.

Hematopoietic neoplasms may be further classified as either lymphoproliferative or myeloproliferative. This classification has clinical significance. Lymphoproliferative neoplasia is nearly always manifested by tumor formation in affected organs. Possible exceptions are lymphocytic leukemia involving only bone marrow and the diffuse or soft tissue form of plasma-cell myeloma. In contrast, myeloproliferative neoplasia is rarely associated with tumor formation. The major exception is mast cell leukemia, which should probably not be included with hematopoietic neoplasia. In domestic animals, the ratio of incidence of lymphoproliferative to myeloproliferative disorders is reported to be ten to one (Nielsen, 1970).

As advances in research are made on the etiology, epidemiology, and therapy of hematopoietic neoplasms, the clinical differentiation of the various types becomes more important. Several authoritative reviews of hematopoietic neoplasia occur in the recent literature (Anderson et al., 1969; Nielsen, 1969, 1970; Gilmore and Holzworth, 1971; Schalm et al., 1975). (Lymphosarcoma and feline mastocytosis are described in detail in Chapter 30. Fig. 78–11,*H,I* illustrates lymphosarcoma for comparison with other leukemias here.) The remaining portion of this chapter will be devoted to a general discussion of clinical and hematologic manifestations of leukemias, followed by descriptions

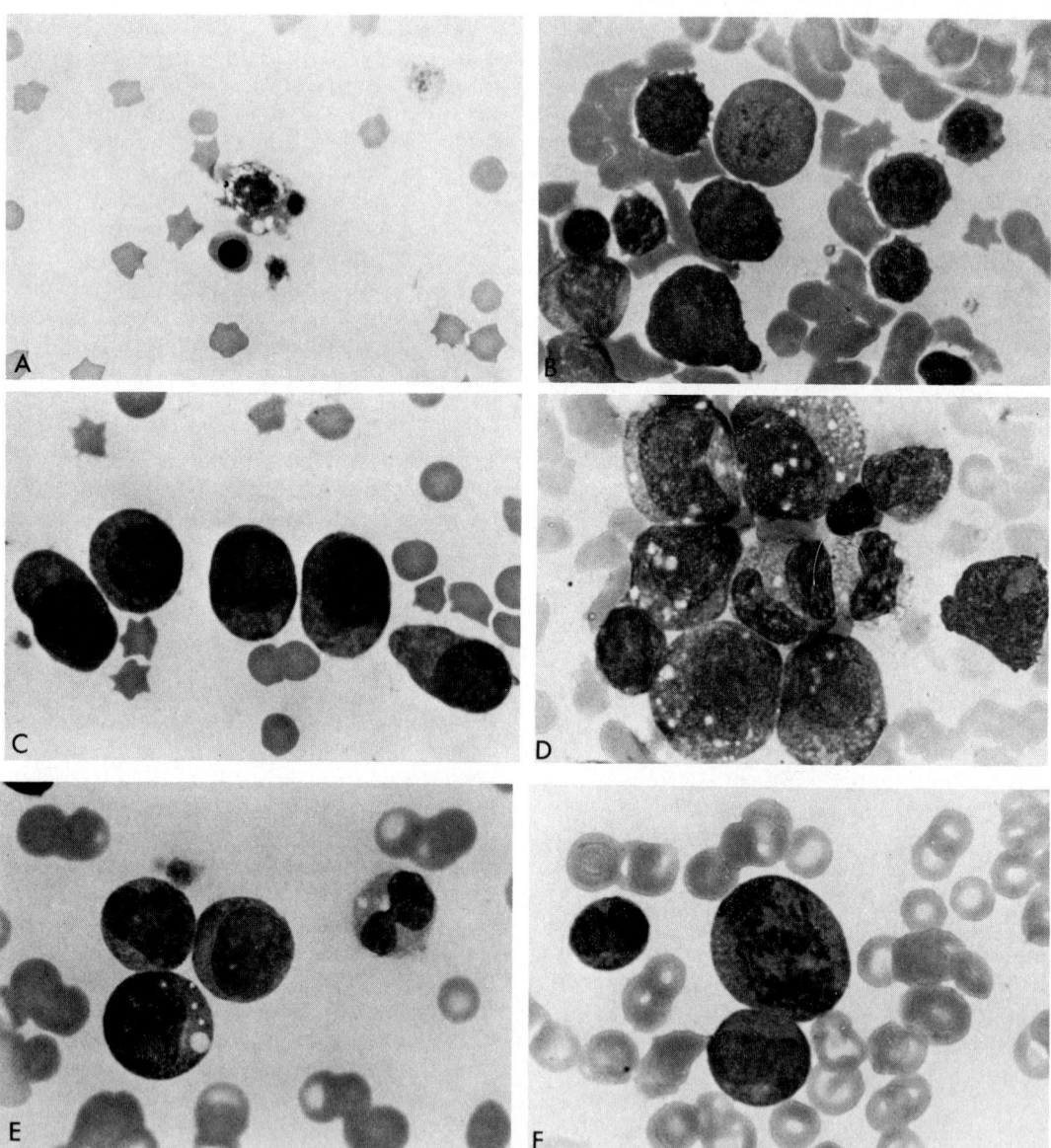

Figure 78–11. *A,* Giant bizarre platelet (top) in the blood of a cat with myeloproliferative disease. *B,* Erythremic myelosis in a cat. Several rubricytes, a rubriblast, bottom left, and a bizarre megalobastic rubricyte, top center. Feline bone marrow. *C,* Blast-form of erythremic myelosis (reticuloendotheliosis) in a cat. Large undifferentiated erythroid cells with eccentric nuclei, nucleoli, and broad pseudopodia. Feline bone marrow. *D,* Granulocytic leukemia in a cat. Undifferentiated granulocyte precursors with faintly granular and vacuolated cytoplasm and a neutrophilic metamyelocyte with abnormal nuclear segmentation. Feline bone marrow. *E,* Granulocytic leukemia in a dog. Undifferentiated granulocyte precursors with faintly granular basophilic cytoplasm, vacuoles and nucleoli. A differentiated cell with abnormal nuclear segmentation, right. Canine blood. *F,* Granulocytic leukemia in a dog. Abnormal mitotic figure and a smaller blast cell. Canine blood.

Illustration continued on opposite page

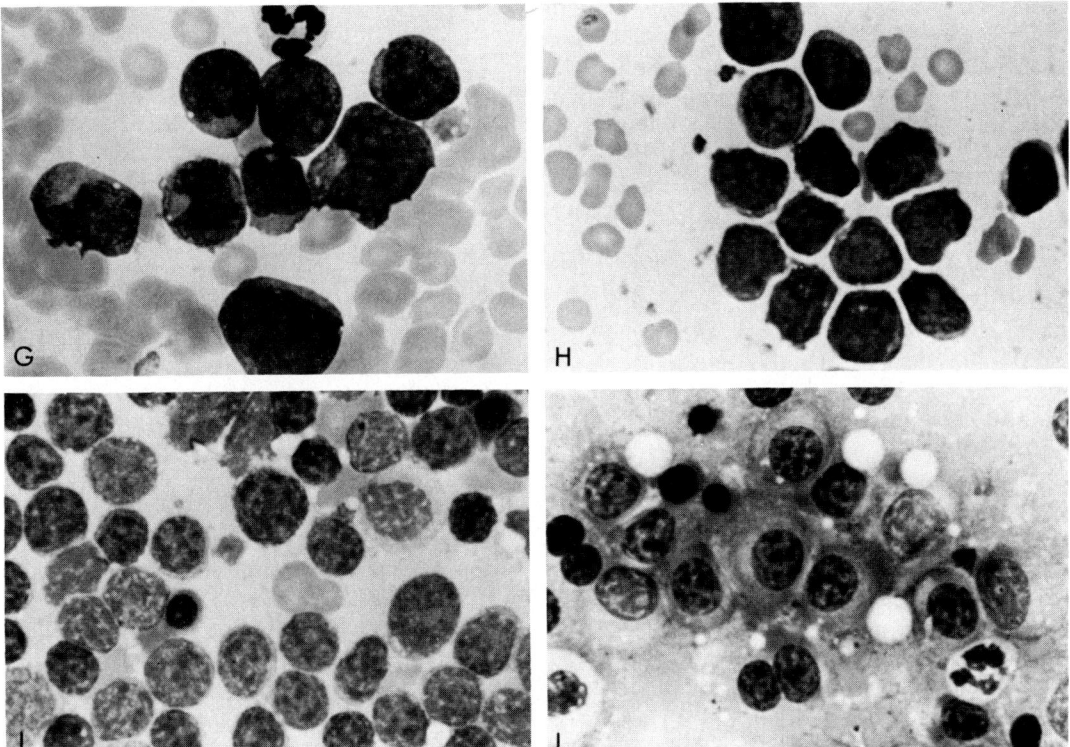

Figure 78–11 *Continued*   *G,* Myelomonocytic leukemia in a dog. Several blasts and undifferentiated cells with faintly granular cytoplasm and irregular nuclei. Canine blood. *H,* Lymphosarcoma in a cat. Numerous lymphoblasts. Feline bone marrow. *I,* Lymphosarcoma in a dog. Numerous lymphoblasts. Canine bone marrow. *J,* Plasma cell myeloma in a dog. Several plasma cells with normal appearance and one binucleated cell, center-bottom. Canine bone marrow.

Wright or Wright-Leishman stain. Magnification is the same for all cells in the composite. (Photomicrographs *B* and *C* provided courtesy of Dr. J. R. Duncan, University of Georgia, Athens, GA.)

of the myeloproliferative disorders and plasma cell myeloma as they occur in the dog and cat.

Leukemia — General Comments. The clinical detection of hematopoietic neoplasia in the dog or cat frequently offers considerable challenge to the clinician, hematologist, and pathologist. Perhaps more than any other group of diseases, the definitive diagnosis depends on cytology. Certainly, a dog or cat having greatly enlarged peripheral lymph nodes may be easily diagnosed as having lymphosarcoma by cytologic or histopathologic examination. Likewise, a dog having a WBC count exceeding 200,000 per microliter and a predominance of immature granulocytes, with numerous mitotic figures, would be highly suspicious for granulocytic leukemia. However, many cases are more subtle with respect to initial manifestations, and even more careful inspection is necessary to include hematopoietic neoplasia in the differential diagnosis. This is particularly true in the myeloproliferative disorders in which the formation of sarcomatous masses is not characteristic. The following discussion is an attempt to

place in perspective the various subtleties and clues that may lead eventually to definitive diagnosis of the various hematopoietic neoplasms.

The clinical signs common to all hematopoietic neoplasms are weight loss, pallor, and fever. Other signs that also are common but are more variable in occurrence include anorexia, splenomegaly, hepatomegaly, and enlargement of lymph nodes (Gilmore and Holzworth, 1971). Any or all of these signs may be caused by a variety of infectious and noninfectious diseases. But when routine diagnostic procedures fail to yield a diagnosis and routine supportive therapy seems of no avail, the persistence of these signs should lead to inclusion of hematopoietic neoplasia in the differential diagnosis. Other, equally nonspecific clinical signs may be more acute in nature and pertain to the various organ systems affected by neoplasia. These signs include dyspnea, signs of uremia, lameness, vomiting, diarrhea, and hemorrhage.

Anemia is perhaps the most consistent hematologic feature of hematopoietic neoplasia. Generally, it is more severe with myeloproliferative than with lymphoproliferative disorders. The pathogenesis of the anemia influences the morphologic features found in blood erythrocytes (i.e., the anemia may appear to be regenerative or nonregenerative). Pathogenic mechanisms may include simple depression of erythropoiesis associated with the cachectic disease (anemia of lesser severity than others), myelophthisic anemia, hemorrhage associated with myelophthisic thrombocytopenia (Medway and Rapp, 1962; Skelly, 1963), or possibly, immune-mediated hemolysis. With these and perhaps other pathogenic mechanisms in play, the morphology of blood erythrocytes will be variable. In some cases, certain patterns of erythrocyte morphology may even indicate leukemia. Myeloproliferative disease in cats is frequently characterized by the presence of nucleated erythrocytes in the blood, with concomitant absence of polychromasia and reticulocytosis (Schalm, 1971). These cells may also be morphologically abnormal or present in vast numbers, which would suggest the presence of erythroleukemia or erythremic myelosis, variant forms of feline myeloproliferative disease (Gilmore and Holzworth, 1971; Schalm, 1971). Schalm (1971) cautions, however, that large numbers of nucleated erythrocytes may be encountered in cats with regenerative anemias that are unrelated to hematopoietic neoplasia.

The single most valuable (and sometimes the only) way to make a definitive diagnosis of leukemia is through examination of well-stained blood or bone marrow films. Leukemic cells may be observed in low or high numbers among the leukocytes in the blood. In some cases, only a few atypical cells may be observed along the edges or feathered tip of the film. Examination of bone marrow films may reveal a few cells that are difficult to differentiate from the normal population of immature hematopoietic cells, or one may find large numbers of anaplastic cells. Although such changes may not be sufficient for diagnosis, they suggest the need for further observation and examination.

Other blood leukocyte changes may be even more subtle but offer additional indications of leukemia. Large numbers of atypical lymphocytes, or a normal to high-normal lymphocyte count concomitant with severe systemic stress, may strongly indicate lymphocytic leukemia. An uneven left shift of neutrophils (e.g., 41 per cent segmented,

5 per cent band, 15 per cent metamyelocyte, 1 per cent myelocyte, and 10 per cent promyelocyte) may denote granulocytic leukemia (Skelley, 1963). (It must be remembered, however, that an uneven left shift may also be observed during resurgence from neutropenia by depression of granulopoiesis.)

In human beings, a recognized state of hematologic abnormality, referred to as preleukemia, is characterized by chronic anemia, neutropenia, thrombocytopenia, and hyperplastic bone marrow (Dreyfus, 1976). This preleukemic state may disappear, remain stable almost indefinitely, or progress slowly or explosively to overt myeloid or myelomonocytic leukemia. A similar phenomenon is seen in certain feline leukovirus-infected cats (Madewell et al., 1979). The cats present with anorexia, depression, pyrexia, and various other signs, and they have anemia, severe neutropenia, and concomitant granulocytic hyperplasia in the bone marrow. The disease syndrome in these cats, originally called subleukemic granulocytic leukemia (Schalm, 1972; Duncan and Prasse, 1976), leads either to death from secondary infection, to an unchanging state of chronic debilitation, or in some cases, to classic granulocytic leukemia.

MYELOPROLIFERATIVE DISEASE IN CATS

Myeloproliferative disease in cats is a progressive, fatal leukemic disorder characterized by abnormal proliferation of erythrocytic, granulocytic, or megakaryocytic cells. Feline leukovirus has been associated with the clinical disease (Herz et al., 1979; Schalm and Theilen, 1970; Cotter et al., 1975). Jarrett et al. (1971) experimentally infected a cat with virus isolated from a feline lymphoma, and the recipient developed myeloid leukemia, one of the forms of myeloproliferative disease. It remains uncertain, however, if all types of myeloproliferative disease are caused by the feline leukemia virus. The cellular proliferation occurs in bone marrow and other organs of the monocyte-macrophage system (reticuloendothelial system). Sarcomatous masses do not occur, but diffuse enlargement of liver and spleen and mild enlargement of lymph nodes occur as these organs become affected by the disease.

The disease occurs frequently, although

lymphosarcoma is more common. Over the course of approximately 15 months at The University of Georgia Veterinary Teaching Hospital, 95 feline leukovirus positive cats were seen. Seventy-seven of these cats were nonleukemic, and 18 were leukemic. Of the leukemic cats, ten had lymphosarcoma and eight had myeloproliferative disease. Any age cat is susceptible, but the disease is rare in cats less than one year old.

The clinical signs of myeloproliferative disease are rather constant (Gilmore et al., 1964b; Ward et al., 1969; Schalm and Theilen, 1970; Schalm et al., 1975). Weight loss, listlessness, anorexia, pallor, and fever are most common. Temperatures range from 103 to 106° F. Other signs, which are more inconsistent among cases but are frequently observed, include splenomegaly, hepatomegaly, and, less frequently, slightly enlarged lymph nodes. Icterus tends to occur in those cats with severe liver involvement. Hemobartonellosis is probably most often misdiagnosed on the basis of the clinical signs and the severe anemia. Concomitant hemobartonellosis, toxoplasmosis, and lymphosarcoma have been observed with myeloproliferative disease (Ward et al., 1969).

Myeloproliferative disease is progressive, with a fatal outcome usually within one week to several months. Temporary remission of clinical signs can be achieved with supportive therapy, which includes periodic blood transfusion. One patient that underwent apparent remission of clinical signs suffered a relapse and died two years later (Schalm, 1973). Attempts to treat the disease with cancer chemotherapeutic drugs usually have not altered the fatal course (Crow et al., 1977; Madewell et al., 1979).

The hematologic findings provide the means for diagnosis in all cats with myeloproliferative disease. Anemia is constant. Packed cell volumes range from 6 to 20 per cent. White blood cell counts are variable, ranging from leukopenia to marked leukocytosis. Platelet numbers may be decreased in some cases, but more importantly, large and bizarre platelets are common in these cats (Fig. 78–11, *A*). The cytologic characteristics in the blood and bone marrow vary with the type of myeloproliferative disease. On the basis of hematologic cytology, myeloproliferative disease is separated into the following types: erythremic myelosis, a blast form of erythremic myelosis (reticuloen-

dotheliosis), myeloid or granulocytic leukemia, monocytic leukemia, myelomonocytic leukemia, eosinophilic leukemia, and megakaryocytic myelosis.

Erythremic Myelosis. In this type of myeloproliferative disease, the abnormally proliferating cells are erythrocytic (Schalm and Theilen, 1970; Schalm, 1975a; Schalm et al., 1975). Erythremic myelosis may be suspected when the blood smear from a severely anemic cat exhibits erythrocytic anisocytosis, a variable number of nucleated erythrocytes, and an absence of polychromasia or reticulocytosis. The bone marrow contains a preponderance of rather normal-appearing erythrocytic precursors in all stages of maturation. A few bizarre forms of erythrocytic precursors are scattered among the excessive number of rubricytes. The bizarre cells are megaloblastoid rubricytes (Fig. 78–11, *B*). Occasionally binucleated rubricytes or metarubricytes may be seen.

Erythremic myelosis may change with time in certain cats. Some cats develop abnormal granulocyte proliferation simultaneously with erythremic myelosis, and these types of myeloproliferative disease may be called erythroleukemia. Such a progression is analogous to the Di Guglielmo syndrome in human beings (Zawidzka et al., 1964). In rare instances, erythroleukemia may progress to granulocytic leukemia with little evidence of continued abnormal erythrocytic proliferation (Schalm, 1975b). Erythremic myelosis has been seen to progress into reticuloendotheliosis, a blast form of the disease (Harvey et al., 1978).

Blast Form of Erythremic Myelosis (Reticuloendotheliosis). In one of the earliest reports on the subject, myeloproliferative disease in cats was called reticuloendotheliosis (Gilmore et al., 1964b). The primitive cells that characterize the disease were believed to be early erythroid cells on the basis of electron microscopic examination (Hurvitz, 1970). Erythremic myelosis of primitive or blast erythroid cell type is now considered more descriptive than the term reticuloendotheliosis (Harvey et al., 1978).

The primitive cells in this type of myeloproliferative disease are very distinctive (Schalm, 1975c; Schalm et al., 1975; Giles et al., 1974; Crow et al., 1977). In severely anemic cats the cells predominate in bone marrow and may be found in variable numbers in blood. The cells (Fig. 78–11, *C*) have round nuclei with coarse granular chromatin and distinct nucleoli. The nucleus is eccentrically placed in many of the cells. The cytoplasm is dark blue with occasional purple granules and a lighter blue Golgi zone adjacent to the nucleus. The cells vary in size, and sometimes large, broad pseudopodia may be seen. In some cases these primitive cells are seen simultaneously with differentiated erythrocytic precursors and megaloblastoid rubricytes, as described for erythremic myelosis.

Myeloid or Granulocytic Leukemia. Granulocytic leukemia usually refers to abnormal proliferation of neutrophils, unless otherwise specified. Cats with this form of myeloproliferative disease have severe nonresponsive anemia and variable WBC counts, from leukopenia to greater than 300,000 per microliter (Fraser et al., 1974; Sutton et al., 1978; Madewell et al., 1979). Primitive myeloblasts, promyelocytes, and myelocytes predominate in bone marrow and may be seen in variable numbers in blood (Fig. 78–11, *D*).

Cells may be differentiated sufficiently to be identified as granulocytic precursors, but in some cases differentiation from monocytes may be very difficult on Romanowsky-stained smears. Furthermore, some cases have abnormal proliferation of granulocytes and monocytes, or features of both cell types; these may be called myelomonocytic leukemia. Special stains may facilitate differentiation of these cell types. Granulocytic precursors stain positive for peroxidase and naphthol-AS-D-chloroacetate esterase. Monocytic precursors stain positive for peroxidase, lipase, and alpha-naphthol-acetate esterase (Yam et al., 1971; Hayhoe and Cawley, 1972; Li et al., 1973; Glick and Horn, 1974).

The greatest difficulty in diagnosing granulocytic leukemia is differentiation from nonhematopoietic diseases that cause marked proliferation of neutrophils. Acute localized purulent diseases may mimic granulocytic leukemia clinically and hematologically. Disease progression may be the only means of differentiation in some cases.

Erythroleukemia. Erythroleukemia is a term used to identify myeloproliferative disease in which hematologic features of erythremic myelosis and granulocytic leukemia are concomitant. Progression from erythremic myelosis to erythro-

leukemia and to granulocytic leukemia has been observed in cats (Zawidzka et al., 1964; Schalm, 1975b).

Monocytic Leukemia. Cats affected with monocytic leukemia have less severe anemia than cats with the other forms of myeloproliferative disease. Packed cell volumes have been reported at about 20 per cent, and WBC counts were near or greater than 300,000 per microliter (Holzworth, 1960; Schalm, 1976d; Henness et al., 1977). Monocytoid cells predominated in bone marrow and comprised about 90 per cent of blood leukocytes. Monocytoid cells have convoluted nuclear membranes, and sometimes pseudopodia. Special stains can be used to differentiate these cells with neutrophilic precursors (see discussion of Granulocytic Leukemia).

Myelomonocytic Leukemia. Cats with myelomonocytic leukemia have hematologic features of both granulocytic and monocytic leukemia. Several cases have been described (Loeb et al., 1975; Schalm, 1976; Stann, 1979). A noteworthy feature of the descriptions was the wide tissue distribution of tumor cells observed at necropsy. In addition to tissues usually affected in granulocytic leukemia (bone marrow, spleen, liver, and lymph nodes), monocytic and myelomonocytic leukemias infiltrate virtually every other organ. Monocytoid cells were seen in brain, heart, lung, diaphragm, eye, gallbladder, kidney, and other organs. And some infiltrations caused raised nodules, contrary to the general premise that sarcomatous masses usually do not occur in myeloproliferative diseases.

Megakaryocytic Myelosis. A cat with thrombocytosis, undifferentiated blast cells in blood, bizarre forms of platelets in blood, and marked megakaryocytic proliferation in bone marrow, liver, and spleen was diagnosed as having megakaryocytic myelosis (Michel et al., 1976).

Eosinophilic Leukemia. Eosinophilic leukemia is characterized by marked eosinophilic leukocytosis. Counts have been reported to exceed 200,000 per microliter (Holzworth, 1960; Simon and Holzworth, 1967; Silverman, 1971; Schalm, 1976b). The bone marrow, spleen, liver, and lymph nodes are infiltrated by eosinophils in various stages of maturation. This author has seen eosinophil counts in excess of 60,000 per microliter in two cats that subsequently died and were found to have alimentary lymphosarcoma. In retrospect, the eosinophilia was believed to be an eosinophilic leukemoid response similar to that described in certain types of human lymphoblastic leukemia (Spitzer and Garson, 1973).

CANINE MYELOGENOUS LEUKEMIAS

Myelogenous leukemia is not common in dogs. Affected dogs have progressive disease, although acute crises can occur. Dogs of any age from less than one year to more than 15 years old may be affected. Consistent clinical signs are protracted, with progressive weakness, weight loss, fever, slight to moderate lymph node enlargement, splenomegaly, sometimes hepatomegaly, and pallor (Schalm et al., 1975). Unusual signs may develop as a result of neoplastic proliferation in a variety of tissues. Canine myelogenous leukemia comprises granulocytic (neutrophilic cell line) leukemia, monocytic leukemia, myelomonocytic leukemia, basophilic leukemia, and megakaryocytic leukemia. These types of myelogenous leukemia may be difficult to differentiate on Romanowsky-stained smears. Special staining reactions are useful for differentiation: Sudan black stains granules in myeloblasts and monoblasts; lipase and alpha-naphthol acetate esterase are positive in monoblasts; naphthol-AS-D-chloroacetate esterase is positive in myeloblasts; and lymphoblasts are negative in each of these stains (Yam et al., 1971; Hayhoe and Cawley, 1972; Li et al., 1973; Glick and Horn, 1974). Canine eosinophilic leukemia has been diagnosed only histopathologically in dogs (Christoph and Pollaske, 1952).

Granulocytic Leukemia. Descriptions of naturally occurring canine granulocytic leukemia are quite numerous and often well illustrated (Meier, 1957; Medway and Rapp, 1962; Lucke and Sumner-Smith, 1963; Skelly, 1963; Cameron et al., 1969; Schalm et al., 1975; Cooper and Watson, 1975; Schalm, 1976; Pollet et al., 1978), although the disease is rare. The neoplastic proliferation is limited to the neutrophilic cell line. Usually, neoplastic cells are in the blood and WBC counts are very high, some in excess of 300,000 per microliter. Myeloblasts, promyelocytes, and myelocytes predominate in bone marrow and are seen in blood (Fig. 78–11,*E,F*).

Differentiation of granulocytic leukemia from other blast form leukemias, lymphosarcoma, and nonleukemic pyogenic diseases may be difficult. Bone marrow examination may be nondiagnostic if the cells are well differentiated. Localized purulent or necrotic lesions or nonhematopoietic malignancy can induce a leukemoid response remarkably similar to granulocytic leukemia. Disorderly release of immature neutrophils from the bone marrow is suggestive of leukemia, and abnormal maturation with the appearance of nucleoli in maturing neutrophils denotes neoplasia.

Bone marrow, spleen, liver, and lymph nodes are the usual tissues affected. Occasionally greenish nodules may be seen in parenchymal organs (Schalm, 1976c). A very rare form of the disease is called myelosarcoma, in which the principal organ affected is the spleen (Smith et al., 1972a). Splenectomy may be followed by reduction in WBC count and remission of clinical signs for some time. Chemotherapy of granulocytic leukemia is not very rewarding (MacEwen et al., 1977).

Monocytic Leukemia. Dogs with monocytic leukemia have milder anemia, and neoplastic infiltration often affects more tissues than granulocytic leukemia; clinical findings are very similar in the two diseases, however. The monocytic neoplastic cells cause marked leukocytosis and have convoluted nuclei and sometimes cytoplasmic pseudopodia. Microfilaments can be seen in cells by electron microscopy. Several canine cases are described (Meier, 1957; Loeb et al., 1970; Mackey et al., 1975; Schalm, 1976a).

Myelomonocytic Leukemia. Myelomonocytic leukemia in dogs was reviewed by Linnabary et al. (1978). In this disease the neoplastic cells have features of both myeloblasts and monocytes. The disease is rare, but several cases have been reported (Barthel, 1974; Ragan et al., 1976; Green and Barton, 1977; Linnabary et al., 1978). Anemia is mild, but other signs are similar to granulocytic leukemia. The undifferentiated cells predominate in bone marrow and cause marked leukocytosis (Fig. 78–11,*G*). Neoplastic cells infiltrate lymph nodes, spleen, liver, bone marrow, tonsils, lung, intestine, kidney, and other tissues.

Megakaryocytic Leukemia. Holscher et al. (1978) diagnosed megakaryocytic leukemia in a dog at necropsy. Although the

WBC count had been low, blast cells had been seen in blood smears, and the dog was anemic and thrombocytopenic. Bone marrow, spleen, liver, lung, kidney, and lymph nodes contained numerous megakaryocytic cells. The cells stained positive with alpha-naphthal acetate esterase and negative with naphthol-AS-D-chloroacetate esterase, the staining pattern expected for normal megakaryocytes.

Basophilic Leukemia. Dogs with signs similar to those for granulocytic leukemia have been seen in which basophils predominate in bone marrow and blood (Rampichini and Coluzzi, 1962; Romanelli, 1962; Kammermann-Leuscher, 1966; Alroy, 1972; MacEwen et al., 1975). MacEwen et al. (1975) produced clinical remission after two months on therapy with hydroxyurea, and the dog remained in remission for eight months, the limit of the report.

PLASMA CELL MYELOMA

Neoplasms of plasma cells (or plasma cell precursors) are referred to synonymously as plasma cell myeloma, multiple myeloma, or myelomatosis. A macroglobulinemia syndrome may be a closely related disorder. Plasma cell myeloma is characterized by tumors of bone marrow that occur in solitary or multiple sites. Soft tissue dissemination is common, especially in the spleen, liver, and kidney. Plasma cells produce immunoglobulins, and neoplasia of plasma cells is frequently characterized by production of a homogenous, monoclonal immunoglobulin. These immunoglobulins, also referred to as M components or myeloma paraproteins, are a single protein produced by a clone of cells. (See Chapter 81.)

Osborne et al. (1968) thoroughly reviewed 20 canine cases reported in earlier literature (including one case mentioned above) and described two additional cases. More recent cases have also been described (Oduye and Losos, 1972; Walton and Gopinath, 1972; Braund et al., 1979). Affected dogs have ranged in age from 8 months to 16 years, with most of them being 8 to 10 years old. Plasma cell myeloma has been reported in cats (Farrow and Penny, 1971; Hay, 1978).

Clinical Findings. In dogs, plasma cell myeloma usually occurs in the bone marrow. Clinical signs are most frequently referable to some musculoskeletal disorder, such as lameness, pathologic fracture, joint swelling, arthralgia, pain on palpation of bones, and occasionally paraplegia (Osborne et al., 1968). Lesions within bone marrow can be demonstrated radiographically (Fig. 78–12). They are characterized by "punched-out" areas of osteolysis occurring in single or multiple sites within various flat bones or at the ends of long bones. The review of cases by Osborne et al. (1968), however, shows that this finding is not a constant feature of plasma cell myeloma. In addition, the bone marrow lesion cannot be considered pathognomonic, since various other diseases may cause osteolysis.

Plasma cell myeloma commonly has soft tissue distribution. Multiple nodules or diffuse infiltrations may be found in the liver, spleen, kidney, or lymph nodes (Osborne et al., 1968); recently, a case with extensive skin lesions was described (Walton and Gopinath, 1972).

Anemia, abnormal bleeding tendencies, weight loss, and palpable tumors are inconsistently but frequently reported signs.

Laboratory Findings. Electrophoresis of serum or urine that has been concentrated may reveal a sharply defined protein band migrating in the β- or γ-globulin zone (see Chapter 83). This may represent the myeloma paraprotein. Such a finding in serum must be interpreted carefully, however, since similar (although usually wider) bands may occur in inflammatory or other neoplastic diseases. Likewise, globulin may be found in urine during inflammatory disorders of the urogenital tract, although in these instances, albumin and other globulins should be expected findings. The commonly used urine-albumin tests will not detect paraproteins, and the heat test is also considered unreliable (Hurvitz et al., 1971).

Aspiration biopsy of suspected bone lesions or imprints of soft tissue tumors may reveal pleomorphic plasma cells (Fig. 78–11,*J*), which may be quite large (15 to 30 μ in diameter), with moderately basophilic and vacuolated cytoplasm. Occasional binucleated or trinucleated cells may be seen, but mitotic figures are rare. A gradation from well-differentiated plasma cells to undifferentiated, primitive cells may be observed (Osborne et al., 1968; Hurvitz et al., 1971).

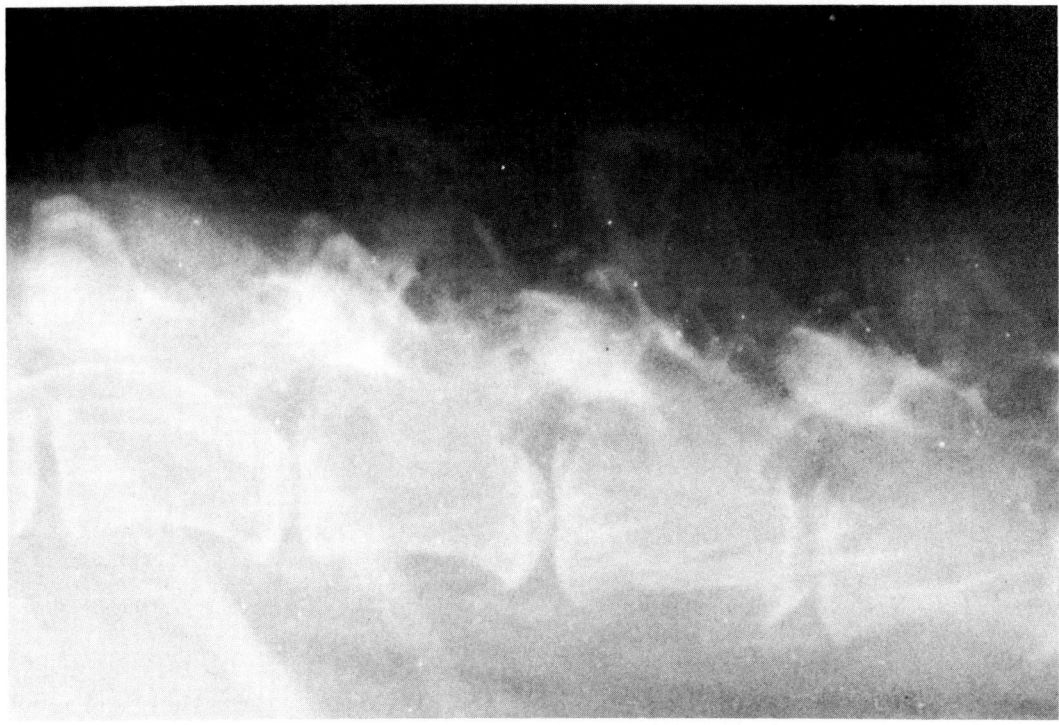

Figure 78–12. Canine plasma-cell myeloma. Lateral radiograph of lumbar spine of a 12-year-old female cocker spaniel that had developed pain of the lumbar area with hindleg paralysis. There are demineralized areas in the dorsal spines and dorsal laminae. There is no sclerosis around the margins of demineralized areas. (Photograph provided courtesy of Dr. R. E. Lewis, Athens, GA.)

Affected dogs presenting with intermittent or persistent hemorrhage episodes are found to have prolonged bleeding times but normal clotting tests (Hurvitz et al., 1970; Shepard et al., 1972). The mechanism producing this change in myeloma is unclear but may involve thrombocytopenia, abnormal platelet function, or acquired vessel wall damage. The bleeding tendency has been observed to parallel periods of increased plasma protein concentration (Shepard et al., 1972).

Therapy. Specific therapy in a dog with γ-A myeloma has been successful, with apparent clinical recovery (Shepard et al., 1972). Dogs may be treated with control of secondary infection and with plasmapheresis to relieve the hyperviscosity that accompanies some cases of paraproteinemia, and for depression of neoplastic plasma cells.

REFERENCES

Alroy, J.: Basophilic leukemia in a dog. Vet. Pathol. *9*:90, 1972.

Anderson, L. J., Jarrett, W. F. H., and Crighton, G. W.: A classification of lymphoid neoplasms of domestic mammals. Natl. Cancer Inst. Monogr. *32*:343, 1969.

Anderson, L. J., Jarrett, W. F. H., Jarrett, O., and Laird, H. M.: Feline leukemia-virus infection of kittens: mortality associated with atrophy of the thymus and lymphoid depletion. J. Natl. Cancer Inst. *47*:807, 1971.

Angus, K., Wyand, D. S., and Yang, T. J.: Impaired lymphocyte response to phytohemagglutinin in dogs affected with cyclic neutropenia. Clin. Immunol. Immunopathol. *11*:39, 1978.

Angus, K., and Yang, T. J.: Lymphocyte response to phytohemagglutinin: temporal variation in normal dogs. J. Immunol. Methods *21*:261, 1978.

Appel, M. J. G., Cooper, B. J., Greisen, H., Scott, F., and Carmichael, L. E.: Canine viral enteritis. I Status report on corona- and parvo-like viral enteritides. Cornell Vet. *69*:123, 1979a.

Appel, M. J. G., Meunier, P., Greisen, H., Carmichael, L. E., and Glickman, L.: Enteric viral infections of dogs. Gainesville, 29th Gaines Veterinary Symposium, October 17, 1979b.

Athens, J. W., Haab, O. P., Raab, S. O., Boggs, D. R., Ashenbrucker, H., Cartwright, G. E., and Wintrobe, M. M.: Leukokinetic studies. IV. The total blood, circulating and marginal granulocyte pools and the granulocyte turnover rate in normal subjects. J. Clin. Invest. 40:989, 1961a.

Athens, J. W., Haab, O. P., Raab, S. O., Boggs, D. R., Ashenbrucker, H., Cartwright, G. E., and Wintrobe, M. M.: Leukokinetic studies. XI. Blood granulocyte kinetics in polycythemia vera, infection and myelofibrosis. J. Clin. Invest. 44:778, 1965.

Athens, J. W., Raab, S. O., Haab, O. P., Mauer, A. M., Ashenbrucker, H., Cartwright, G. E., and Wintrobe, M. M.: Leukokinetic studies. III. The distribution of granulocytes in the blood of normal subjects. J. Clin. Invest. 40:159, 1961b.

Atwal, O. S., and McFarland, L. Z.: Histochemical study of the distribution of alkaline phosphatase in leukocytes of the horse, cow, sheep, dog and cat. Am. J. Vet. Res. 28:971, 1967.

Baggiolini, M.: The Neutrophil. In Glynn, L. E., Houck, J. C., and Weissmann, G. (eds.): Handbook of Inflammation. Vol. 2. The Cell Biology of Inflammation, Elsevier/North Holland Biomedical Press, New York, 1980.

Bainton, D. F.: The Cells of Inflammation: A General Review. In Glynn, L. E., Houck, J. C., Weissman, G. (eds): Handbook of Inflammation. Vol. 2. The Cell Biology of Inflammation, Elsevier/North Holland Biomedical Press, New York, 1980.

Barthel, C. H.: Acute myelomonocytic leukemia in a dog. Vet. Pathol. 11:79, 1974.

Basten, A., and Beeson, P. B.: Mechanism of eosinophilia: II. Role of the lymphocyte. J. Exp. Med. 131:1288, 1970.

Beeson, P. B., and Bass, D. A.: The Eosinophil. W. B. Saunders Co., Philadelphia, 1977.

Benjamin, M. M.: Outline of Veterinary Clinical Pathology. 3rd ed. The Iowa State University Press, Ames, Iowa, 1978.

Bentinck-Smith, J.: Hematology. In Medway, W., Prier, J. E., and Wilkinson, J. S. (eds.): Textbook of Veterinary Clinical Pathology. The Williams and Wilkins Co., Baltimore, 1969.

Bierman, J. R.: Characteristics of leukopoietin G in animals and man. Ann. N.Y. Acad. Sci. 113:753, 1964.

Biggs, R., and MacMillan, R. L.: The errors of some hematological methods as they are used in a routine laboratory. J. Clin. Pathol. 1:269, 1948.

Bishop, C. R., Athens, J. W., Boggs, D. R., Warner, H. R., Cartwright, G. E., and Wintrobe, M. M.: Leukokinetic studies. XIII. A nonsteady state kinetic evaluation of the mechanism of cortisone-induced granulocytosis. J. Clin. Invest. 47:249, 1968.

Bland-van den Berg, P., Bomzon, L., and Lurie, A.: Oestrogen-induced bone marrow aplasia in a dog. J. S. Afr. Vet. Med. Assoc. 49:363, 1978.

Bone, D. L.: Canine panosteitis: a review. Canine Pract. 7(4):61, 1980.

Bowles, C. A., Alsaker, R. D., and Wolfle, T. L.: Studies of the Pelger-Huët anomaly in foxhounds. Am. J. Pathol. 96:237, 1979.

Boyden, S.: The chemotactic effect of mixtures of antibody and antigen on polymorphonuclear leukocytes. J. Exp. Med. 115:453, 1962.

Braund, K. G., Everett, R. M., Bartels, J. E., and DeBuysscher, E.: Neurologic complications of IgA multiple myeloma associated with cryoglobulinemia in a dog. J.A.V.M.A. 174:1321, 1979.

Butterworth, A. E., David, J. R., Franks, D., et al.: Antibody-dependent eosinophil-mediated damage to ^{51}Cr-labeled schistosomula of Schistosoma mansoni: damage by purified eosinophils. J. Exp. Med. 145:136, 1977.

Cameron, T. P., Kinard, R., and Johnson, R.: Irradiation of a dog with myelogenous leukemia. J.A.V.M.A. 154:279, 1969.

Cheville, N. F.: The grey collie syndrome. J.A.V.M.A. 152:620, 1968.

Chiu, T.: Studies on estrogen-induced proliferative disorders of hemopoietic tissue in dogs. Thesis, University of Minnesota, Minneapolis, 1974.

Christoph, H. J., and Pollaske, G.: Beitrag zur Leukose des Hundes. Monatsschr. Vet. 7:1, 1952.

Chusid, M. J., Bujal, J. S., and Dale, D. C.: Defective polymorphonuclear leukocyte metabolism and function in canine cyclic neutropenia. Blood 46:921, 1975.

Cochrane, C. G., Weigle, W. O., and Dixon, F. J.: The role of the polymorphonuclear leukocytes in the initiation and cessation of the Arthus vasculitis. J. Exp. Med. 110:481, 1959.

Cockerell, G. L., Hoover, E. A., LoBuglio, A. F., and Yohn, D. S.: Phytomitogen- and antigen-induced blast transformation of feline lymphocytes. Am. J. Vet. Res. 36:1489, 1975.

Cohen, Z. A.: The structure and function of monocytes and macrophages. Adv. Immunol. 9:163, 1968.

Coles, E. M.; Veterinary Clinical Pathology. 2nd ed. W. B. Saunders Co., Philadelphia, 1974.

Cooper, B. J., and Watson, A. D. J.: Myeloid neoplasia in a dog. Austr. Vet. J. 51:150, 1975.

Cotter, S. M.: Anemia associated with feline leukemia virus infection. J.A.V.M.A. 175:1191, 1979.

Cotter, S. M.; Hardy, W. D., and Essex, M.: Association of feline leukemia virus with lymphosarcoma and other disorders in the cat. J.A.V.M.A. 166:449, 1975.

Cowell, K. R., Jezyk, P. F., Haskins, M. E., and Patterson, D. F.: Mucopolysaccharidosis in a cat. J.A.V.M.A. 169:334, 1976.

Craddock, C. G.: Corticosteroid-induced lymphopenia, immunosuppression, and body defense. Ann. Intern. Med. 88:564, 1978.

Cronkite, E. P.: Kinetics of granulopoiesis. Clin. Haematol. 8:351, 1979.

Cronkite, E. P., and Vincent, P. C.: Granulocytopoiesis. In Proceedings of the 8th Annual Hanford Biology Symposium, Richland, Washington, 1968: Myeloproliferative disorders of animals and man. U.S.A.E.C. Conference 680529, 1970.

Crow, S. E., Madewell, B. R., and Henness, A. M.: Feline reticuloendotheliosis: a report of four cases. J.A.V.M.A. 170:1329, 1977.

Dale, D. C., and Graw, R. G.: Transplantation of allogeneic bone marrow in canine cyclic neutropenia. Science 183 (No. 4120):83, 1974.

Dale, D. C., Wards, S. B., Kimball, H. R., and Wolff, S. M.: Studies of neutrophil production and turnover in grey collie dogs with cyclic neutropenia. J. Clin. Invest. 51:2190, 1972.

Dannenberg, A. M.: Macrophages in inflammation and infection. New Eng. J. Med. 293:489, 1975.

Dao, C., Metcalf, D., and Bilski-Pasquier, G.: Eosinophil and neutrophil colony-forming cells in culture. Blood 50:833, 1977.

Deubelbeiss, K. A., Dancey, J. T., Harker, L. A., and Finch, C. A.: Neutrophil kinetics in the dog. J. Clin. Invest. 55:833, 1975.

Diesselhoff-Den Dulk, M. M. C., Crofton, R. W., and Van Furth, R.: Origin and kinetics of Kupffer cells during an acute inflammatory response. Immunology 37:7, 1979.

Dorr, A. D., Moloney, W. C.: Acquired pseudo-Pelger anomaly of granulocytic leukocytes. N. Engl. J. Med. 261:742, 1959.

Duncan, J. R., and Prasse, K. W.: Clinical examination of bone marrow. Vet. Clinics North Am. 6(4):597, 1976.

Dunn, C. D. R., Jones, J. B., Jolly, J. O., and Lange, R. D.: Cell proliferation of canine cyclic hematopoietic marrow in diffusion chambers. Proc. Soc. Exp. Biol. Med. 158:50, 1978.

Dutta, S. K., Novilla, M. N., Bumgardner, M. K., and Ingling, A.: Lymphocyte responsiveness to mitogens and quantitation of T and B lymphocytes in canine malignant lymphoma. Am. J. Vet. Res. 39:455, 1978.

Dvorak, A. M., and Dvorak, H. F.: The basophil. Its morphology, biochemistry, motility, release reactions, recovery, and role in the inflammatory responses of IgE-mediated and cell-mediated origin. Arch. Pathol. Lab. Med. 103:551, 1979.

Ewing, G. O., Schalm, O. W., and Smith, R. S.: Hematologic values of normal basenji dogs. J.A.V.M.A. 151:1661, 1972.

Fauci, A. S., and Dale, D. C.: The effect of hydrocortisone on the kinetics of normal human lymphocytes. Blood 46:235, 1975.

Fauci, A. S., Dale, D. C., and Balow, J. E.: Glucocorticosteroid therapy: mechanisms of action and clinical considerations. Ann. Intern. Med. 84:304, 1976.

Feldman, B. F., and Romans, A. U.: The Pelger-Huët anomaly of granulocytic leukocytes in the dog. Canine Pract. 3(5):22, 1976.

Finch, S. C.: Granulocytopenia. In Williams, W. J., Beutler, E., Erslev, A. J., and Rundles, R. W. (eds.): Hematology. 2nd ed. McGraw-Hill Book Company, New York, 1977.

Finco, D. R., Duncan, J. R., Schall, W. D., Hooper, B. E., Chandler, F. W., and Keating, K. A.: Chronic enteric disease and hypoproteinemia in 9 dogs. J.A.V.M.A. 163:262, 1973.

Flecknell, P. A., Gibbs, C., and Kelly, D. F.: Myelosclerosis in a cat. J. Comp. Pathol. 88:627, 1978.

Fliedner, T. M., Cronkite, E. P., and Robertson, J. S.: Granulopoiesis. I. Senescence and random loss of neutrophilic granulocytes in human beings. Blood 24:402, 1964.

Ford, L.: Hereditary aspects of human and canine cyclic neutropenia. J. Hered. 60:293, 1969.

Fraser, C. J., Joiner, G. N., Jardine, J. H., and Gleiser, C. A.: Acute granulocytic leukemia in cats. J.A.V.M.A. 165:355, 1974.

Gailbraith, P. R., Valberg, L. S., and Brown, M.: Patterns of granulocyte kinetics in health, infection and carcinoma. Blood 25:683, 1965.

Giles, R. C., Buhles, W. C., and Montgomery, C. A.: Myeloproliferative disorder in a cat. J.A.V.M.A. 165:456, 1974.

Gilmore, C. E., Gilmore, V. H., and Jones, T. C.: Bone marrow and peripheral blood of cats: Technique and normal values. Pathol. Vet. 1:18, 1964a.

Gilmore, C. E., Gilmore, V. H., and Jones, T. C.: Reticuloendotheliosis, a myeloproliferative disorder of cats: A comparison with lymphocytic leukemia. Pathol. Vet. 1:161, 1964b.

Gilmore, C. E., and Holzworth, J.: Naturally occurring feline leukemia: Clinical, pathologic, and differential diagnostic features. J.A.V.M.A. 158:1013, 1971.

Glick, A. D., and Horn, R. G.: Identification of promonocytes and monocytoid precursors in acute leukemia of adults: Ultrastructural and cytochemical observations. Br. J. Haematol. 26:395, 1974.

Greaves, M. F., Owen, J. J. T., and Raff, M. C.: T and B Lymphocytes. Origins, Properties and Roles in Immune Responses. American Elsevier Publishing Company, New York, 1973.

Green, R. A., and Barton, C. L.: Acute myelomonocytic leukemia in a dog. J.A.A.H.A. 13:708, 1977.

Greenberg, M. S., Zanger, B., and Wong, H.: Studies in granulocytopenic subjects. Blood 30:891, 1967.

Hall, J. G., and Morris, B.: The immediate effect of antigens on the cell output of a lymph node. Br. J. Exp. Pathol. 46:450, 1965.

Hammond, W. P., Engelking, E. R., and Dale, D. C.: Cyclic hematopoiesis. Effects of endotoxin on colony-forming cells and colony-stimulating activity in grey collie dogs. J. Clin. Invest. 63:785, 1979.

Hardy, W. D., Hess, P. W., MacEwen, E. G., McClelland, A. J., Zuckerman, E. E., Essex, M., Cotter, S. M., and Jarrett, O.: Biology of feline leukemia virus in the natural environment. Cancer Res. 36:582, 1976.

Harvey, J. W., Shields, R. P., and Gaskin, J. M.: Feline myeloproliferative disease: Changing manifestations in peripheral blood. Vet. Pathol. 15:437, 1978.

Hay, L. E.: Multiple myeloma in a cat. Aust. Vet. Pract. 8(1):45, 1978.

Hayhoe, F. G. H., and Cawley, J. C.: Acute leukemia: Cellular morphology, cytochemistry and fine structure. In Roath, S. (ed.): Clinics in Hematology: Acute Leukemia, Vol. 1:49, 1972.

Hays, E. F., and Craddock, C. G.: Colony-stimulating activity. Arch. Pathol. Lab. Med. 102:165, 1978.

Henness, A. M., Crow, S. E., and Anderson, B. C.: Monocytic leukemia in three cats. J.A.V.M.A. 170:1325, 1977.

Herion, J. C., Spitznagel, J. K., Walker, R. I., and Zeya, H. I.: Pyrogenicity of granulocyte lysosomes. Am. J. Physiol. 211:693, 1966.

Herz, A., Theilen, G. H., Schalm, O. W., and Munn, R. J.: C-type virus in bone marrow of cats with myeloproliferative disorders. J. Natl. Cancer Inst. 44:339, 1970.

Holscher, M. A., Collins, R. D., Glick, A. D., and Griffith, B. O.: Megakaryocytic leukemia in a dog. Vet. Pathol. 15:562, 1978.

Holzworth, J.: Leukemia and related neoplasms in the cat. II. Malignancies other than lymphoid. J.A.V.M.A. 136:107, 1960.

Holzworth, J., and Georgi, J. R.: Trichinosis in a cat. J.A.V.M.A. 165:165, 1974.

Hoover, E. A., and Dubey, J. P.: Pathogenesis of experimental pulmonary paragonimiasis in cats. Am. J. Vet. Res. 39:1827, 1978.

Hoover, E. A., and Kociba, G. J.: Bone lesions in cats with anemia induced by feline leukemia virus. J. Natl. Cancer Inst. 53:1277, 1974.

Hurley, J. V.: Substances promoting leukocyte emigration. Ann. N.Y. Acad. Sci. 116:918, 1964.

Hurvitz, A. I.: Fine structure of cells from a cat with myeloproliferative disorder. Am. J. Vet. Res. 31:747, 1970.

Hurvitz, A. I., Haskins, S. C., and Fischer, C. A.: Macroglobulinemia with hyperviscosity syndrome in a dog. J.A.V.M.A. 157:455, 1970.

Hurvitz, A. I., Kihoie, J. M., Capra, J. D., and Prats, R.: Bence Jones proteinemia and proteinuria in a dog. J.A.V.M.A. *159*:1112, 1971.

Irfan, M.: The peripheral blood picture in myositis and atrophy of head muscles in dogs. Ir. Vet. J. *25*(10):189, 1971.

Jain, N. C.: A comparative cytochemical study of leukocytes of some animal species. Folia Haematol. *94*:49, 1970.

Jain, N. C., and Schalm, O. W.: Influence of corticosteroids on total and differential blood leukocyte counts. Calif. Vet. *20*(6):28, 1966.

Jarrett, W. F. H., Anderson, L. J., Jarrett, O., Laird, H. M., and Stewart, M. F.: Myeloid leukemia in a cat produced experimentally by feline leukemia virus. Res. Vet. Sci. *12*:385, 1971.

Jasper, D. E., and Jain, N. C.: The influence of adrenocorticotropic hormone and prednisolone upon marrow and circulating leukocytes in the dog. Am. J. Vet. Res. *26*:844, 1965.

Jezyk, D. F., Haskins, M. E., Patterson, D. F., Mellman, W. J., and Greenstein, M.: Mucopolysaccharidosis in a cat with arylsulfatase B deficiency: a model of Maroteaux-Lamy syndrome. Science *198*:834, 1977.

Johnson, K. H., and Perman, V.: Normal values for jugular blood in the cat. VM SAC *63*:837, 1968.

Johnson, K. J., Ward, P. A., Striker, G., and Kunkel, R.: A study of the origin of pulmonary macrophages using the Chediak-Higashi marker. Am. J. Pathol. *101*:365, 1980.

Jolley, W. B., Meyers, F. J., Smith, L. L., and Brizuele, H.: The effect of leukocyte lysosomal contents on circulatory dynamics. Fed. Proc. *29*:447, 1970.

Jones, J. B., Jones, E. S., and Lange, R. D.: Early-life hematologic values of dogs affected with cyclic neutropenia. Am. J. Vet. Res. *35*:849, 1974.

Jones, J. B., Lange, R. D., and Jones, E. S.: Cyclic hematopoiesis in a colony of dogs. J.A.V.M.A. *166*:365, 1975a.

Jones, J. B., Lange, R. D., Yang, T. J., et al.: Canine cyclic neutropenia: Erythropoietin and platelet cycles after bone marrow transplantation. Blood *45*:213, 1975b.

Jones, J. B., Yang, T. J., Dale, J. B., and Lange, R. D.: Canine cyclic haematopoiesis: marrow transplantation between littermates. Br. J. Haematol. *30*:215, 1975c.

Kammermann-Leuscher, B.: Blutbasophilen-Leukose bei Hund und Gewebsbasophilen-Retikulose bei der Katze. Berl. Muench. Tieraerztl. Wochenschr. *79*:459, 1966.

Kaplan, J. M., and Barrett, O.: Reversible pseudo-Pelger anomaly related to sulfasoxazole therapy. N. Engl. J. Med. *277*:421, 1967.

Kasbohm, C., and Saar, C.: Ostrogenbedingte Knochenmarkschaden bei Huden mit Hodenneoplasien. Tierarztk Oraxus *3*:225, 1975.

Kazura, J. W., and Grove, D. E.: Stage-specific antibody-dependent eosinophil-mediated destruction of Trichinella spiralis. Nature *274*:588, 1978.

Kelly, J. D., Kenny, D. F., and Whitlock, H. V.: The response to phytohemagglutinin of peripheral blood lymphocytes from dogs infected with Ancylostoma caninum. N.Z. Vet. J. *25*:12, 1977.

Kiss, M., and Komár, G.: Pelger-Huët'sche Kernanomalie der Leukozyten bei einem Hunde. Berl. Muench. Tierrarztl. Wochenschr. *24*:474, 1967.

Kleinsorgen, A., Bradenberg, C., and Brummer, H.: Untersuchungen uber den Einfluss von Zwangsmass-nahmen auf Blutparameter bei den Hauskatze. Berl. Muench. Tierarztl. Wochenschr. *89*:358, 1976.

Koepke, J. A.: A delineation of performance criteria for the differentiation of leukocytes. Am. J. Clin. Pathol. *68*:202, 1977.

Krakowa, S., Wallace, A. L., Ringler, S. S., and Koestner, A.: Evaluation of B lymphocyte levels and functions in gnotobiotic dogs. Am. J. Vet. Res. *39*:1881, 1978.

Krammer, J. W., Davis, W. C., and Prieur, D. J.: The Chediak-Higashi syndrome of cats. Lab. Invest. *36*:554, 1977.

Kramer, J. W., Davis, W. C., Prieur, D. J., Baxter, J., and Norsworthy, G. D.: An inherited disorder of Persian cats with intracytoplasmic inclusions in neutrophils. J.A.V.M.A. *166*:1103, 1975.

Langweiler, M., Haskins, M. E., and Jezyk, P. F.: Mucopolysaccharidosis in a litter of cats. J.A.A.H.A. *14*:748, 1978.

Latimer, K. S., Crane, L. S., and Prasse, K. W.: Quantitative evaluation of neutrophilic chemotaxis in twelve beagle dogs. Am. J. Vet. Res. *42*:1254, 1981.

Lewis, H. B., and Rebar, A. H.: Bone Marrow Evaluation in Veterinary Practice. Ralston Purina Company, Saint Louis, 1979.

Li, C. Y., Lam, K. W., and Yam, L. T.: Esterases in human leukocytes. J. Histochem. Cytochem. *21*:1, 1973.

Linnabary, R. D., Holscher, M. A., Glick, A. D., Powell, H. S., and McCollum, H. M.: Acute myelomonocytic leukemia in a dog. J.A.A.H.A. *14*:71, 1978.

Loeb, W. F., Lamont, P. H., and Capen, C. C.: Monocytic leukemia in a dog. *In* Proceedings of the 8th Annual Hanford Biology Symposium, Richland, Washington, 1968: Myeloproliferative Disorders of Animals and Man. USAEC Conference 680529, 1970.

Loeb, W. F., Rininger, B., Montgomery, C. A., and Jenkins, S.: Myelomonocytic leukemia in a cat. Vet. Pathol. *12*:464, 1975.

Lovering, S. L., Pierce, K. R., and Adams, G.: Serum complement and blood platelet adhesiveness in acute canine ehrlichiosis. Am. J. Vet. Res. *41*:1266, 1980.

Lucke, V. M., and Sumner-Smith, G.: A case of myeloid leukemia in the dog. J. Small Anim. Pract. *4*:23, 1963.

Lund, J. E.: Canine cyclic neutropenia. Comp. Pathol. Bull. *5*(2):2, 1973.

Lund, J. E., Padgett, G. A., and Ott, R. L.: Cyclic neutropenia in grey collie dogs. Blood *29*:452, 1967.

MacEwen, E. G., Drazner, F. H., McClelland, A. J., and Wilkins, R. J.: Treatment of basophilic leukemia in a dog. J.A.V.M.A. *166*:376, 1975.

MacEwen, E. G., Patnaik, A. K., and Wilkins, R. J.: Diagnosis and treatment of canine hematopoietic neoplasms. Vet. Clinics North Am. *7*(1):105, 1977.

Machado, E. A., Gregory, R. S., Jones, J. B., and Lange, R. D.: The cyclic hematopoietic dog: a model for spontaneous secondary amyloidosis. A morphologic study. Am. J. Pathol. *92*:23, 1978.

Mackey, L. J.: Distribution of T and B cells in thymus, blood and lymph nodes of the cat. Res. Vet. Sci. *22*:225, 1977.

Mackey, L. J.: Monocytic leukaemia in the dog. Vet. Rec. *96*:27, 1975.

Madewell, B. R., Jain, N. C., and Weller, R. E.: Hematologic abnormalities preceding myeloid leukemia in three cats. Vet. Pathol. *16*:510, 1979.

Maloney, M. A., and Patt, H. M.: Granulocyte transit from bone marrow to blood. Blood 31:195, 1968.

Maloney, M. A., Patt, H. M., and Lund, J. E.: Granulocyte dynamics and the question of ineffective granulopoiesis. Cell Tissue Kinet. 4:201, 1971.

Marsh, J. C., Boggs, D. R., Cartwright, G. E., and Wintrobe, M. M.: Neutrophil kinetics in acute infection. J. Clin. Invest. 46:1943, 1967.

McCall, C. E., Katayama, I., Cotran, R. S., and Finland, M.: Lysosomal and ultrastructural changes in human "toxic" neutrophils during bacterial infection. J. Exp. Med. 120:267, 1969.

McCullough, B., Krakowka, S., and Koestner, A.: Experimental canine distemper virus-induced lymphoid depletion. Am. J. Pathol. 74:155, 1974.

Medway, W., and Rapp, J. P.: A case of chronic granulocytic leukemia with thrombocytopenic purpura in a dog. Cornell Vet. 52:247, 1962.

Medway, W., Weber, W. T., O'Brien, J. A., and Krawitz, L.: Multiple myeloma in a dog. J.A.V.M.A. 150:386, 1967.

Meier, H.: Neoplastic diseases of the hematopoietic system (so-called leukosis complex) in the dog. Zentralbl. Veterinaermed. 4:633, 1957.

Metcalf, D., and Moore, M. A. S.: Haematopoietic Cells. North-Holland, Amsterdam, 1971.

Meuret, G., and Hoffman, G.: Monocytic kinetic studies in normal and disease states. Br. J. Haematol. 24:275, 1973.

Meyers, K. M.: Personal communication, University of Florida, Gainesville, 1980.

Michaelson, S. M., and Scheer, K.: The blood of the normal beagle. J.A.V.M.A. 148:532, 1966.

Michel, R. L., O'Handley, P., and Dade, A. W.: Megakaryocytic myelosis in a cat. J.A.V.M.A. 168:1021, 1976.

Michels, N. A.: The mast cells. In Downey, J. (ed.): Handbook of Hematology. Hoeber, New York, 1938.

Miller, C. H., Carbonell, A. R., Peng, R., McKenzie, M. R., and Shifrine, M.: Cell surface markers on canine lymphocytes. Am. J. Vet. Res. 39:1191, 1978.

Nathan, C. F., Murray, H. W., and Cohn, Z. A.: The macrophage as an effector cell. N. Eng. J. Med. 303:622, 1980.

Nichols, B. A., and Bainton, D. F.: Differentiation of human monocytes in bone marrow and blood. Lab. Invest. 29:27, 1973.

Nielsen, S. W.: Myeloproliferative disorders in animals. In Proceedings of the 8th Annual Hanford Biology Symposium, Richland, Washington, 1968: Myeloproliferative Disorders of Animals and Man. USAEC Conference 680529, 1970.

Nielson, S. W.: Spontaneous hematopoietic neoplasms of the domestic cat. Natl. Cancer Inst. Monogr. 32:73, 1969.

Niepage, H.: Das Blutbild beim Hund unter kurzfristig wechselnden physiologischen Bedingungen. Zentralbl. Veterinaermed. 25A(7):520, 1978.

Oduye, O. O., and Losos, G. J.: Multiple myeloma in a dog. J. Small Anim. Pract. 13:257, 1972.

Osborne, C. A., Perman, V., Sautter, J. H. et al.: Multiple myeloma in the dog. J.A.V.M.A. 153:1300, 1968.

Pace, E. M.: Pelger-Huët anomaly transmission. Canine Pract. 4(3):33, 1977.

Patt, H. M., Lund, J. E., and Maloney, M. A.: A model of granulocyte kinetics. Ann. N.Y. Acad. Sci. 113:515, 1965.

Pattengale, P. K., Sahl, W. M., and Thorbecke, G. J.: Fate of autogenous canine lymphocytes after injection into an afferent lymphatic of the popliteal lymph node. Am. J. Pathol. 67:527, 1972.

Perman, V., Alsaker, R. D., and Rüs, R. C.: Cytology of the Dog and Cat. American Animal Hospital Association, South Bend, Indiana, 1979.

Phelps, P., and McCarty, J.: Crystal-induced inflammation in canine joints. II. Importance of polymorphonuclear leukocytes. J. Exp. Med. 124:155, 1966.

Poli, G., and Faravelli, G. L.: Nitroblue tetrazolium test in cats. Clin. Vet. 97:248, 1974.

Poli, G., Nicoletti, G., and Faravelli, G.: Nitroblue tetrazolium test nel cane. Foli. Vet. Lat. 3:215, 1973.

Pollet, L., van Hove, W., and Mattheeuws, D.: Blastic crisis in chronic myelogenous leukemia in a dog. J. Small Anim. Pract. 19:469, 1978.

Porter, J. A., and Canaday, W. R.: Hematologic values in mongrel and greyhound dogs being screened for research use. J. Am. Vet. Med. Res. 159:1603, 1971.

Potter, K. A., Tucker, R. D., and Carpenter, J. L.: Oral eosinophilic granuloma of Siberian huskies. J.A.A.H.A. 16:595, 1980.

Prasse, K. W.: Disorders of the leukocytes. In Ettinger, S. J. (ed.): Textbook of Veterinary Internal Medicine. W. B. Saunders Co., Philadelphia, 1975.

Prasse, K. W., Kaeberle, M. L., and Ramsey, F. K.: Blood neutrophilic granulocyte kinetics in cats. Am. J. Vet. Res. 34:1021, 1973a.

Prasse, K. W., Seagrave, R. C., Kaeberle, M. L., and Ramsey, F. K.: A model of granulopoiesis in cats. Lab. Invest. 28:292, 1973b.

Prieur, D. J., Collier, L. L., Bryan, G. M., and Meyers, K. M.: The diagnosis of feline Chediak-Higashi syndrome. Feline Pract. 9(5):26, 1979.

Raab, S. O., Athens, J. W., Haab, O. P., Boggs, M. R., Ashenbrucker, H., Cartwright, G. E., and Wintrobe, M. M.: Granulokinetics in normal dogs. Am. J. Physiol. 206:83, 1964.

Ragan, H. A., Hackett, P. L., and Dogle, G. E.: Acute myelomonocytic leukemia manifested as myelophthisic anemia in a dog. J.A.V.M.A. 169:421, 1976.

Rampichini, L., and Coluzzi, G.: Contributo allo studio della leucemia basofila negli animali domestica. Descrizione di un caso rescontrato in un cane. Atti. Soc. Ital. Sci. Vet. 16:271, 1962.

Rausch, P. G., and Moore, T. G.: Granule enzumes of polymorphonuclear neutrophils: A phylogenetic comparision. Blood 46:913, 1975.

Renshaw, H. W., Catburn, C., Bryan, G. M., Bartsch, R. C., and Davis, W. C.: Canine granulocytopathy syndrome: Neutrophil dysfunction in a dog with recurrent infections. J.A.V.M.A. 166:443, 1975.

Renshaw, H. W., and Davis, W. C.: Canine granulocytopathy syndrome. Am. J. Pathol. 95:731, 1979.

Renshaw, H. W., Davis, W. C., and Renshaw, S. J.: Canine granulocytopathy syndrome: Defective bacteriocidal capacity of neutrophils from a dog with recurrent infections. Clin. Immunol. Immunopathol. 8:385, 1977.

Report of the Panel of the Colloquium on Selected Feline Infectious Diseases. J.A.V.M.A. 157:2043, 1970.

Rohovsky, M. W., and Fowler, E. H.: Lesions of experimental panleukopenia. J.A.V.M.A. 158:872, 1971.

Romanelli, V.: Sopra la leucemia basofila leucemia del cane. Arch. Vet. Ital. 4:499, 1962.

Roth, B., and Schneider, C. C.: Untersicchungen zur Abhängigkeit des "weiken Blutbildes" bei Hauskatzen (Felis domestica) von Wurminfektionen des Darmes. Berl. Muench. Tierarztl. Wochenschr. 22:435, 1971.

Rudolph, W. G., and Kaneko, J. J.: Effect of neutropenia on colony stimulating and inhibiting activity of dog serum. Proc. Soc. Exper. Biol. Med. 163:421, 1980.

Rytöma, T.: Chalone of the granulocyte system. Chalones: Concepts and current researches. Natl. Cancer Inst. Monogr. 38:143, 1973.

Rytöma, T. and Kiviniemi, K.: Control of granulocyte production. Cell Tissue Kinet. 1:5, 1968.

Saror, D. I., Schillhorn Van Veen, T. W., and Adevabju, J. B.: The haemogram of dogs with intestinal parasites in Zaria, Nigerio. J. Small Anim. Pract. 20:243, 1979.

Schalm, O. W.: Leukocyte responses to disease in various domestic animals. J.A.V.M.A. 140:557, 1962.

Schalm, O. W.: Interpretation of leukocyte responses in the dog. J.A.V.M.A. 142:147, 1963.

Schalm, O. W.: Clinical significance of the eosinophil leukocyte. Calif. Vet. 20(3):17, 1966a.

Schalm, O. W.: Eosinophilia in canine diseases. Calif. Vet. 20(4):11, 1966b.

Schalm, O. W.: Comments on feline leukemia: Clinical and pathologic features, differential diagnosis. J.A.V.M.A. 158:1025, 1971.

Schalm, O. W.: Interpretations in feline bone marrow cytology. J.A.V.M.A. 161:1418, 1972.

Schalm, O. W.: Myeloproliferative disorder in a cat with a period of remission followed by a relapse two years later. Calif. Vet. 27(4):18, 1973.

Schalm, O. W.: Viral inclusions in blood cells and hemograms in canine distemper. Calif. Vet. 28(12):23, 1974.

Schalm, O. W.: Canine hematology. Vet. Scope 9:2, 1975a.

Schalm, O. W.: Myeloproliferative disorders in the cat: 3. Progression from erythroleukemia into granulocytic leukemia. Feline Pract. 5(6):31, 1975b.

Schalm, O. W.: Myeloproliferative disorders in the cat: 1. Reticuloendotheliosis. Feline Pract. 5(4):16, 1975c.

Schalm, O. W.: 1. Acute monocytic leukemia. 2. Reticulum cell sarcoma (Dog). Canine Pract. 3(4):19, 1976a.

Schalm, O. W.: Erythrocyte macrocytosis in miniature and toy poodles. Canine Pract. 3(6):55, 1976b.

Schalm, O. W.: Granulocytic (myelogenous) leukemia in the dog. Canine Pract. 3(3):22, 1976c.

Schalm, O. W.: The feline leukemia complex: 2. Less common forms of leukemic leukemia. Feline Pract. 6(3):36, 1976d.

Schalm, O. W.: Mucopolysaccharidosis. Canine Pract. 4(6):29, 1977.

Schalm, O. W.: Exogenous estrogen toxicity in the dog. Canine Pract. 5(5):57, 1978.

Schalm, O. W.: Phenylbutazone toxicity in two dogs. Canine Pract. 6(4):47, 1979.

Schalm, O. W., Jain, N. C., and Carroll, E. J.: Veterinary Hematology. 3rd ed. Lea & Febiger, Philadelphia, 1975.

Schalm, O. W., and Smith, R.: Some unique aspects of feline hematology in disease. J. Small Anim. Clin. 3:311, 1963.

Schalm, O. W., and Strombeck, D. R.: Pancytopenia in a dog due to Ehrlichia canis. Canine Pract. 1(4):13, 1974.

Schalm, O. W., and Theilen, G. H.: Myeloproliferative disease in the cat, associated with C-type leukovirus particles in bone marrow. J.A.V.M.A. 157:1686, 1970.

Schnuda, N. D.: Circulation and migration of small blood lymphocytes in the rat. Am. J. Pathol. 93:623, 1978.

Scott, D. W., Kirk, R. W., and Bentinck-Smith, J.: Some effects of short-term methylprednisolone therapy in normal cats. Cornell Vet. 69:104, 1978.

Scott, R. E., Dale, D. C., Rosenthal, A. S., and Wolff, S. M.: Cyclic neutropenia in grey collie dogs: Ultrastructural evidence for abnormal neutrophil granulopoiesis. Lab. Invest. 28:514, 1973.

Shepard, V. J., Dodds-Laffin, W. J., and Laffin, R. J.: Gamma A myeloma in a dog with defective hemostasis. J.A.V.M.A. 160:1121, 1972.

Shull, R. M., and Powell, D.: Acquired hyposegmentation of granulocytes. Cornell Vet. 69:241, 1979.

Silverman, J.: Eosinophilic leukemia in a cat. J.A.V.M.A. 158:199, 1971.

Simon, N., and Holzworth, J.: Eosinophilic leukemia in a cat. Cornell Vet. 57:579, 1967.

Skelly, J. F.: Clinico-pathologic conference from the School of Veterinary Medicine, University of Pennsylvania (myelogenous leukemia). J.A.V.M.A. 142:646, 1963.

Smith, H. A., Jones, T. C., and Hunt, R. D. Veterinary Pathology. 4th ed. Lea & Febiger, Philadelphia, 1972a.

Smith, V. D., Blackwell, L. H., and Overman, R. R.: Evidence for bone marrow cell attrition as a mechanism for granulocyte regulation in the canine. Fed. Proc. 31:342, 1972b.

Soulsby, E. J. L.: Textbook of Veterinary Clinical Parasitology. Vol. I. Helminths. F. A. Davis Co., Philadelphia, 1975.

Spitzer, G., and Garson, O. M.: Lymphoblastic leukemia with marked eosinophilia: a report of 2 cases. Blood 42:377, 1973.

Stann, S. E.: Myelomonocytic leukemia in a cat. J.A.V.M.A. 174:722, 1979.

Sutton, R. H., McKellow, A. M., and Bottrill, M. B.: Myeloproliferative disease in the cat: A granulocytic and megakaryocytic disorder. N.Z. Vet. J. 26:273, 1978.

Taetle, R., Lane, T. A., and Mendelsohn, J.: Drug-induced agranulocytosis and a cross-reacting lymphocyte antibody. Blood 54:501, 1979.

Taylor, D. W., and Siddique, W. A.: Responses of enriched populations of feline T and B lymphocytes to mitogen stimulation. Am. J. Vet. Res. 38:1969, 1977.

Timoney, J. F., Neibert, H. C., and Scott, F. W.: Feline salmonellosis. A nosocomial outbreak and experimental study. Cornell Vet. 68:211, 1978.

Walton, G. S., and Gopinath, C.: Multiple myeloma in a dog with some unusual features. J. Small Anim. Pract. 13:703, 1972.

Ward, B. C., and Pederson, N.: Infectious peritonitis in cats. J.A.V.M.A. 154:26, 1969.

Ward, J. M., Sodikoff, C. H., and Schalm, O. W.: Myeloproliferative disease and abnormal erythrogenesis in the cat. J.A.V.M.A. 155:879, 1969.

Ward, P. A., Cochrane, C. G., and Muller-Eberhard, H. J.: The role of serum complement in chemotaxis of leukocytes in vitro. J. Exp. Med. 122:327, 1965.

Ward, P. A., Lepow, I., and Newman, L. J.: Bacterial

factor chemotactic for polymorphonuclear leukocytes. Am. J. Pathol. *52*:725, 1968.

Weber, S. E., Evans, D. A., and Feldman, B. F.: Pelger-Huët anomaly of granulocytic leukocytes in two feline littermates. Feline Pract. *11*(1):44, 1981.

Weiden, P. L., Robinett, B., Graham, T. C., Adamson, J., and Storb, R.: Canine cyclic neutropenia: a stem cell defect. J. Clin. Invest. *53*:950, 1974.

Weissmann, G., Smolen, J. E., and Korchak, H. M.: Release of inflammatory mediators from stimulated neutrophils. N. Engl. J. Med. *303*:27, 1980.

Weller, P. F., and Goetzl, E. J.: The human eosinophil. Roles in host defense and tissue injury. Am. J. Pathol. *100*:793, 1980.

Wilkins, R. J.: Morphologic features of feline peripheral blood lymphocytes. J.A.A.H.A. *10*:362, 1974.

Wittwer, F., Bohmwald, H., Vidal, E., and Obert, C.: Valores hematologicos en perros infectados con microfilaria (Dipetalonema sp.). Zentralbl. Veterinaermed. *25*:424, 1979.

Wood, T. A., and Frenkel, E. P. The atypical lymphocyte. Am. J. Med. *42*:923, 1967.

Yam, L. T., Lu, C. Y., and Crosby, N. J.: Cytochemical identification of monocytes and granulocytes. Am. J. Clin. Pathol. *55*:283, 1971.

Yang, T. J.: Recovery of hair coat color in grey collie (cyclic neutropenia) — normal bone marrow transplant chimeras. Am. J. Pathol. *91*:149, 1978.

Yu, D. T. Y., Clements, P. J., Paulus, H. E., Peter, J. B., Levy, J., and Barnett, E. V.: Human lymphocyte subpopulations. Effect of corticosteroids. J. Clin. Invest. *53*:565, 1974.

Zatz, M. M., and Lance, E. M.: The distribution of ^{51}Cr-labelled lymphocytes into antigen-stimulated mice. Lymphocyte trapping. J. Exp. Med. *134*:224, 1971.

Zawidzka, Z. Z., Janzen, E., and Grice, H. C.: Erythremic myelosis in a cat. A case resembling Di Guglielmo's syndrome in man. Pathol. Vet. *1*:530, 1964.

Zenoble, R. D., and Rowland, G. N.: Hypercalcemia and proliferative, myelosclerotic bone reaction associated with feline leukovirus infection in a cat. J.A.V.M.A. *175*:591, 1979.

CHAPTER **79**

BERNARD F. FELDMAN
and JOSEPH G. ZINKL

Diseases of the Lymph Nodes and Spleen

Lymphocyte production and immunologic activity occur in many different settings. There is no single organ in which immune activity is concentrated; it develops from an entire class of tissue called the lymphoreticular system. This anatomically dispersed network comprises the cells, both fixed and mobile, that are actively involved in body defense. These defenses include cells with primary phagocytic function as well as immunologically active cells; granulocytes are not ordinarily included (Widmann, 1978). The immune system consists of a number of lymphoid organs, including the thymus, lymph nodes, spleen, parts of the liver, parts of the bone marrow, and elements in the lining of the alimentary and respiratory tracts (Table 79–1) (David, 1980). A variety of cells that travel between the various lymphoid organs and the rest of the body make up the immune system. The immunologically active cells of the immune system compose the various classes of lymphocytes. A number of other cells, however, including monocytes (macrophages) and polymorphonuclear leukocytes (neutrophils, eosinophils, basophils, mast cells) play important accessory roles in the immune system.

The stem cells from which lymphocytes derive arise from the yolk sac and the fetal liver; later, some stem cells originate from the bone marrow. Such cells differentiate into lymphocytes in the primary lymphoid organs, namely the thymus and the bursa

Table 79–1. Organs of the Immune System

Primary Lymphoid Organs
  Thymus
  The Bursa equivalent
    Liver?
    Gut associated lymphoid tissue?
    Bone marrow?

Secondary Lymphoid Organs
  Lymph nodes
  Spleen
  Other lymphoid tissue
    Peyer's patches
    Lymphoid accumulation in:
      Small intestine
      Epithelial tissue
      Connective tissue
      Respiratory tissue

---

equivalent. In this chapter, two of the secondary lymphoid organs, the lymph nodes and the spleen, will be considered.

THE LYMPH NODES

LYMPH NODE STRUCTURE

The structure of normal lymph nodes varies with site and age. A proposal for correlating structure with immunologic function has been put forward by Cottier et al. (1973). A normal cervical lymph node in an adult dog is bean-shaped and measures 0.5 to 1.5 cm in maximum diameter. The capsule is composed of two to three layers of fibroblasts and the collagen that they lay down. Below the capsule lies a subcapsular sinus lined peripherally by endothelial cells, and lined elsewhere by macrophages with gaps in between. Across the sinusoid run strands of collagen covered by the cytoplasm of endothelial cells. The macrophages lining the inner layer of the sinusoid lie on a layer of collagen, which contains few fibroblasts. The subcapsular sinus is continuous with radial sinusoids, which in turn join to form the efferent ducts of the node. The structure of the wall of the sinusoids is similar. Macrophages form a particularly prominent part of the wall of the medullary sinusoids.

The parenchyma of the lymph node outside the sinusoids is built on a framework of elongated fibroblasts with numerous long, spidery processes, each lying upon and surrounding a trabecula of collagen. This is often described as the reticulin framework of the node. In between there are packed lymphocytes and other lymphoreticular cells in varying proportions; the areas of the parenchyma are conveniently divided into the outer cortex, the germinal centers and lymphocytic follicles, the inner cortex or paracortex, and the medullary cords (Cottier et al., 1973). The outer cortex is composed of undifferentiated areas that contain predominantly small lymphocytes with a few plasma cells.

The germinal centers are spherical and are surrounded by small lymphocytes and blast cells. Sometimes a lighter staining superficial zone is less densely packed and may show a few plasma cells, while in a darker staining deep zone, mitosis is evident. The background framework contains dendritic reticular cells and conventional macrophages. Germinal centers vary in structure depending upon activity. It is thought, though by no means proved, that B-lymphocytes migrate into the follicle, enlarge and develop irregularly shaped nuclei, divide, and ultimately leave the follicle as immature plasma cells (Carr et al., 1977). Sometimes the center may be largely replaced by epithelioid macrophages.

The inner cortex or paracortex is composed of more loosely arranged lymphoid tissue; most of the lymphocytes in this area are thymus-derived (Parrott et al., 1966), and there is a moderate number of macrophages. These nodular aggregates do not contain plasma cells and are found in increasing numbers in reactive lesions. They are commoner in superficial glands (Ree and Fanger, 1975). During a cell-mediated immune response, this area becomes edematous owing to blockage of the sinusoids; numerous lymphocytes migrate through the wall of the post-capillary venules into the paracortex and proliferate.

The medullary cords are the areas of lymph nodes that lie between the medullary sinusoids. They are packed with plasma cells during an immune response (Carr et al., 1977). The variations in structure of lymph nodes that occur during lymph node reactions are delineated in Table 79–2.

IMMUNOCOMPETENT CELLS OF THE IMMUNE RESPONSE

The Lymphocyte

The biology of the lymphocyte has been reviewed by Henry and Goldman (1975). Lymphocytes range in size from 5μ to 10μ

Table 79–2. Lymph Node Reactions

1. Stimulation of germinal center activity
2. Plasma cell proliferation and maturation
3. Maturation and enlargement and division of sinus and interstitial macrophages
4. Increased cell traffic through the node:
   a. Increased passage of monocytes and lymphocytes in afferent lymph
   b. Increased migration and maturation of T lymphocytes
   c. Acute inflammatory reaction
   d. Increased monocyte immigration, macrophage maturation and formation of granulomata, often with epithelioid cells

and are conveniently described as small or large. The small lymphocyte has a nucleus that stains heavily in standard light microscopic preparations. The scanty cytoplasm contains a few small mitochondria, a centriole, and some ribosomes.

The large lymphocyte, according to some authors (Carr et al., 1977; David, 1980), is synonymous with the lymphoblast. This cell has a nucleus with much less dense chromatin in an open meshwork. There is much more cytoplasm than in the small lymphocyte. When cell division is stimulated in lymphoid tissue, as in an immune reaction, both thymidine uptake and mitoses are seen in large lymphocytes. In descriptions of the changes occurring in tissues during immune responses, a separate cell type is described as the "immunocyte" or "immunoblast." This term refers to the functional properties of differentiating forms of lymphocytes. The B cells differentiate into the antibody-producing plasma cells. The T cells are involved in cell-mediated reactions and also interact with B lymphocytes to regulate the production of antibody.

Thymic (T) lymphocytes derive originally from the bone marrow but are conditioned by the thymus in the early neonatal period. Their life span may be fairly long (months or years). Many lymphocytes recirculate, leaving the bloodstream through post-capillary venules to enter peripheral lymphoid organs and draining with the lymph back into the venous circulation (via the thoracic duct). The major part of the recirculating pool is composed of T lymphocytes, which are involved in the production of soluble mediators, or lymphokines. Lymphokines include *migration inhibition factor,* which inhibits *in vitro* movement of macrophages and, presumably, immobilizes

macrophages at the site of the inflammation event *in vivo; macrophage activation factor,* by which macrophages develop increased phagocytic ability, increased RNA syntheses, and increased ability to destroy ingested microbes; *chemotaxin,* which actively causes *in vitro* movement of macrophages; *lymphotoxin,* a soluble factor nonspecifically toxic for a variety of target cells; *interferon,* an inhibitor of viral growth; *bone resorption factor,* which is associated with an increase in osteoclastic activity, elevation in total and ionized calcium levels in many canine lymphomas; *lymphocyte transforming factor(s),* which permit nonsensitive lymphocytes to be stimulated by antigen *in vitro;* and *transfer factors,* which transfer delayed hypersensitivity *in vitro.* Transfer factors have been obtained by disrupting lymphocytes from sensitized animals in the absence of antigen.

Bursa-dependent or B lymphocytes appear to derive ultimately from the marrow. In birds they derive immediately from the bursa of Fabricius, a hindgut diverticulum, while in mammals their origin is less clear but is thought to be similarly related to intestinal lymphoreticular tissue. B cells have a shorter life — days or weeks rather than months — and are a less important component (in terms of numbers) of the recirculating pool. B cells interact with T lymphocytes in the induction of many humoral immune responses, though other responses are T-cell independent. B cells carry a prominent and easily recognizable surface immunoglobulin component and mature into plasma cells, producing immunoglobulin (antibody) at various stages during maturation. B cells also carry surface receptors for complement, enabling them to bind antigen-antibody complexes. Some of the characteristics of T and B lymphocytes are indicated in Table 79–3 and Figures 79–1 through 79–3.

The Plasma Cell

Under the influence of antigen, T lymphocytes, and macrophages, B cells differentiate into antibody-producing cells, the plasma cells. These are larger than lymphocytes and are characterized by an eccentric nucleus with coarse heterochromatin arranged in a "clock-face" or "cartwheel" pattern. Plasma cells have a highly basophilic cytoplasm and a well-developed endoplasmic reticulum, often organized in parallel,

Table 79–3. Characteristics of T and B Lymphocytes

	T	B
Origin		
Ultimate	Marrow	Marrow
Proximate	Thymus	Gut-associated lymphoid tissue? Marrow
Recirculation	Important	Less important
Longevity	More are long-lived	Fewer are long-lived
Site		
Lymph node	Interfollicular	Subcapsular medullary, germinal centers
Spleen	Periarteriolar	Peripheral white pulp, red pulp
Peyer's patch	Perifollicular	Follicular
Function		
Cell-mediated immunity	Important	Trivial involvement
Humoral immunity		
Induction	Important	Important
Antibody synthesis	Uninvolved	Important
Memory	Important	Important

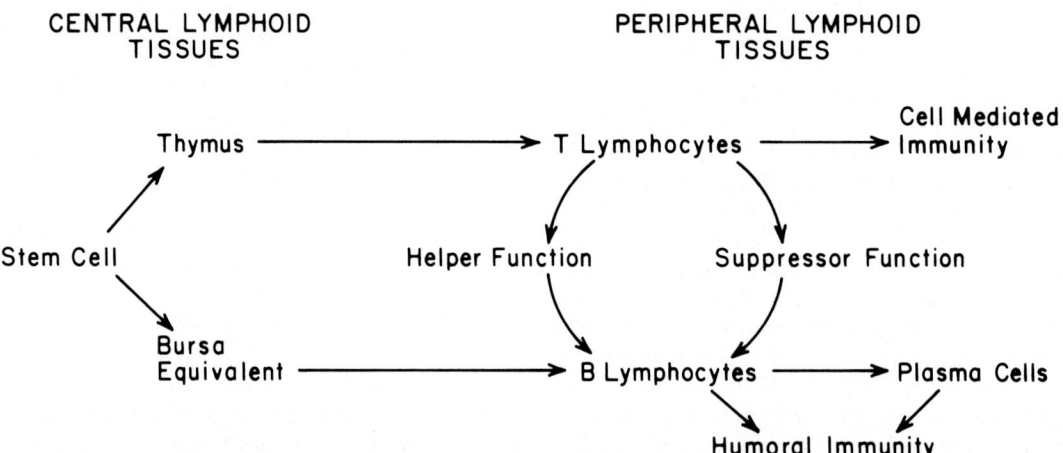

Figure 79–1. Schematic representation of development of the lymphoid system.

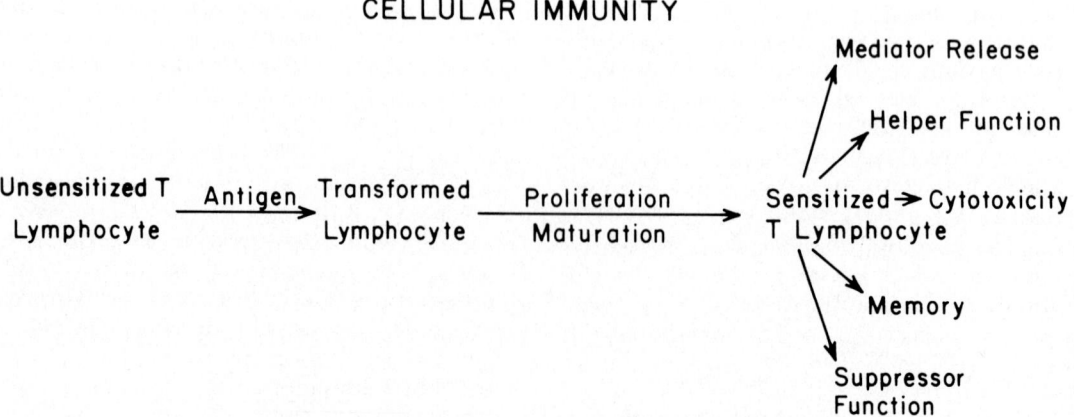

Figure 79–2. Reactions of T lymphocytes to antigens.

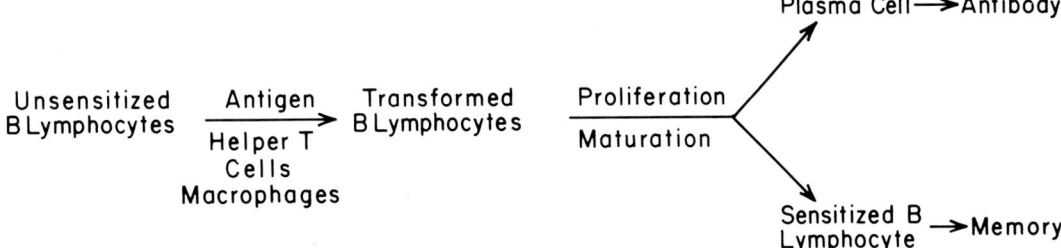

Figure 79–3. Reactions of B lymphocytes to antigens.

concentric layers. Plasma cells may be distended with granular material, which is the antibody they are producing. Sometimes one or more of the endoplasmic cisterns are distended by large inclusions, called Russell bodies. These are aggregates of incompletely formed immunoglobulin molecules. The immature precursors of plasma cells, the plasmablasts, are difficult to differentiate from lymphoblasts and large lymphocytes.

Monocytes (Macrophages)

Monocytes belong to the monocyte-macrophage system, previously called the reticuloendothelial system (RES). They are large mononuclear cells that constitute three to eight per cent of the peripheral blood leukocytes. Their cytoplasm is much more abundant than that of the lymphocytes. Their nucleus is usually eccentric and oval or kidney-shaped. Small vacuoles in the cytoplasm are the lysosomes filled with degradative enzymes. Monocytes originate from promonocytes, which divide rapidly. Precursors are difficult to identify in the bone marrow. When the mature cells enter the peripheral blood, they are called monocytes, and when they leave the blood and infiltrate tissues, they are referred to as macrophages. Macrophages play an important part in the induction of the immune response. They present antigen to the lymphocytes that bear specific receptors for the antigen. They also act as effector cells, attacking certain microorganisms and neoplastic cells. Monocytes have surface F_c receptors for immunoglobulins IgG1, IgG3 and for the complement components C3b and C3d.

Allied Immunocompetent Cells

Neutrophils, eosinophils, basophils, and mast cells are important cells in the immune

response and defense mechanisms. They are covered in detail in Chapters 78 and 81.

LYMPHOCYTES AND LYMPHOCYTE TRAFFIC

There are three types of lymphocyte circulation: (1) the seeding of stem cells from fetal liver or bone marrow to primary lymphoid organs and the subsequent differentiation and distribution of these cells to the peripheral lymphoid system; (2) the recirculation of lymphocytes from blood to lymph to blood; and (3) the distribution of effector cells to particular parts of the body.

In the first type of circulation, stem cells destined to become T lymphocytes from the bone marrow enter the thymus, where they proliferate and differentiate into immunocompetent cells within two or three days; these cells are seeded to the peripheral lymphoid organs. The B stem cells move from the bone marrow to the secondary lymphoid organs. Mature B and T lymphocytes do not reenter the primary lymphoid organs in substantial numbers.

The second pattern, the recirculation of lymphocytes from the blood through the nodes to the lymphatics and back to the blood is much more rapid and does not involve cell proliferation. Average transit times of small lymphocytes, most of which are long-lived T cells, are 0.6 hour in blood, 5 to 6 hours in the spleen, and 15 to 20 hours in the lymph nodes (Weiss, 1980; David, 1980). The transit time for B cells is longer, for example, 30 hours in lymph nodes (Weiss, 1980). Both T and B lymphocytes enter the lymph nodes via a specialized part of the post-capillary venule. T cells remain in the inner cortex, whereas B cells slowly move to the germinal centers. Presumably, B cells must have time to traverse the thymic-dependent areas and go to the medulla, because this is where most of the plasma cells (B lymphocyte-derived) are found. If lymphocytes are drained from the thoracic duct (mostly T cells) and not allowed to reenter the blood, the thymus-dependent areas of the peripheral lymphoid system are depleted of lymphocytes much more rapidly than germinal centers.

A third, not well defined traffic pattern consists of the movement of effector cells, both T and B lymphocytes, to areas where they participate in an overall inflammatory reaction. This traffic pattern is associated with cell proliferation, and examples of it include the movement of lymphocytes to the site of an invading antigen at the periphery.

CLASSIFICATION OF LYMPH NODE DISEASE

Including leukemia, lymph node disease is classified in relation to histologic appearances in biopsy. Such a biopsy may have four basic changes, hypoplasia, reactive hyperplasia, primary or secondary neoplasia, and histiocytic or plasma cell disorders.

Lymph Node Hypoplasia

Lymph node hypoplasia is a histologic classification based on appearances in a biopsy. Primary hypoplasia is rare and is found in the immune deficiency states. In small animal veterinary medicine, secondary (acquired) immunodeficiency in association with lymphoreticular disease, tumor, or immunosuppression is more common and is becoming more widespread as therapeutic regimens for many diseases become more intense.

Congenital Deficiency Syndromes. The causes of congenital immunodeficiency are unknown. No clear antecedent event like maternal illness or chemical exposure during pregnancy precedes sporadic cases. Several defects are known to have been transmitted by genes on the X chromosome in man, and a few exceedingly rare autosomal defects have been described (Webster, 1974). Combined immunodeficiency has been described in Arabian foals (Deem et al., 1979) but not in pet animals. DiGeorge's syndrome is a congenital athymic problem associated with a lack of cell-mediated im-

munity. Bruton-type agammaglobulinemia is associated with a lack of humoral immunity. Other syndromes affecting both cell-mediated and humoral immunity have been described in man.

Acquired Secondary Immunodeficiency. Defective immune function often accompanies disease of the lymphoid tissues. Lymphoma consistently depresses T cell activity (Bennett and Lichtman, 1980). Multiple myeloma (see following discussion), a neoplasm of plasma cells, causes defects in humoral responsiveness (Bernier and Lichtman, 1980). In chronic lymphocytic leukemia, a neoplasm of B lymphocytes but not of the plasma cells, circulating antibody levels are often low; autoantibodies against red cells sometimes develop late in the disease (MacEwen et al., 1977b). Prolonged illness of any kind, protein deficiency or protein loss, and general debility create a predisposition to infection even though no specific lesion of the immune mechanisms can be identified.

Immunosuppression. Probably the most common form of immunodeficiency is iatrogenic. This includes nearly all drugs used in treating cancer as well as ionizing radiation and adrenal cortical steroids, which are used to treat many diseases, including autoimmune disorders. Since the immunosuppressive effects of therapy are superimposed on the debilitating effects of the primary disease, the patient becomes extremely susceptible to each infectious agent to which he is exposed.

In immunosuppressed patients, organisms that are numerous in the environment but rarely infect normal individuals are particularly troublesome. The compromised patient cannnot repel these opportunistic invaders, and the resulting infections are difficult to eradicate. Environmental fungi are an enormous problem, especially *Aspergillus* and *Candida* species, because the drugs given to combat fungi are less effective than is antibacterial therapy and, in addition, carry a high incidence of side effects. Immunologic deficiency in leukemia and lymphoma is one of the most characteristic features of this group of diseases. It relates to direct involvement of the immune system by the malignant process and indirectly to the extent that the tumor burden is immunosuppressive. Also, the immunosuppressive effects of antitumor therapy must not be forgotten. Specific reactivity on the part of the tumor-bearing patient to his own tumor has been clearly documented in leukemias in man (Bernier and Lichtman, 1980). However, it is not known which of the several immunologic mechanisms of specific tumor immunity is actually responsible for host control of the tumor.

Lymphadenopathy (Hyperplasia)

Lymphadenopathy results from either neoplastic proliferation of a clone of lymphocytes or reactive hyperplasia of lymphocytes. Metastatic tumors commonly enlarge lymph nodes. The common causes of reactive lymphadenopathy are bacterial and viral infections, immune processes, toxoplasmosis, and less commonly, granulomatous disease. Lymphoid hyperplasia involves not only regional lymph nodes but in some cases the spleen and liver as well. Metastatic carcinoma usually enlarges a localized group of lymph nodes, which drain the primary site.

Diagnostic Evaluation of Lymphadenopathy. The logical sequence of diagnostic evaluation involves noninvasive techniques to document the underlying disease before biopsy is performed. Physical examination determines the extent of lymphadenopathy. Other diagnostic studies include

1. Radiograph of the chest to document hilar adenopathy, infections, or tumor.
2. Serologic tests for infectious agents, including tests for *Toxoplasma* or *Ehrlichia.*
3. Skin tests for coccidioidomycosis or histoplasmosis, especially if the radiographs of the chest are suggestive.
4. Cytology of the lymph node obtained by aspiration to document infection, granuloma, or tumor.
5. Biopsy of the lymph node to establish lymph node morphology and to document infection, granuloma, or tumor.
6. Bone marrow biopsy and liver biopsy; these are less helpful in benign lymphadenopathy.
7. Culture of biopsy material for bacteria and fungus. Cultures of bone marrow may be considered but are less successful than those of lymph nodes because of the limited volume of material.

Laboratory Studies for Lymphadenopathy
HEMATOLOGIC TESTS. Lymphocytosis may be transient in many diseases that cause

Table 79–4. Summary of Causes of Lymphadenopathy without Lymphocytosis

Infections
  Parasitic
    Toxoplasmosis
    Filaria
  Bacterial
  Fungal
    Coccidioidomycosis
    Histoplasmosis
  Viral
Collagen Disease
  Rheumatoid arthritis
  Systemic lupus erythematosus
Drugs
  Diphenylhydantoin
Neoplastic
  Lymphoma or leukemia
  Metastatic carcinoma
Other
  Reactive follicular hyperplasia

lymphadenopathy and, thus, absent at the time of diagnosis (Table 79–4). Therefore, hematologic findings may be minimal. Anemia and thrombocytopenia suggest lymphoproliferative malignancy but may be seen in collagen vascular disease and other conditions. Regional lymphadenopathy may suggest the port of entry of infection. Cervical lymphadenopathy suggests respiratory disease; inguinal suggests genitourinary disease; axillary or inguinal suggests pleuritis or peritonitis; and pulmonary hilus suggests neoplasia of the lung or heart. Regional lymphadenopathy draining tumors may suggest the primary site: Cervical suggests the nasopharynx, lung, or thyroid; axillary suggests the chest or anterior mammary chain; pulmonary hilus suggests lung or, rarely, upper gastrointestinal tract. Peripheral blood findings are nonspecific. Variable lymphocytosis may be seen in some infectious diseases, neutrophilia in others. Bone marrow biopsy occasionally reveals disseminated fungal disease.

OTHER USEFUL TESTS. *Serologic tests* for infectious agents may be useful. High titers for ubiquitous organisms (e.g., *Toxoplasma*) or titers of unusual organisms (as coccidioidomycosis) suggest the cause (Kaufman, 1976).

Skin tests show strongly positive results in certain fungal diseases with lymphadenopathy, including histoplasmosis and coccidioidomycosis (Kaufman, 1976). Prolonged stimulation with fungal organisms provokes a cellular immune response that is recalled when killed organisms are injected intradermally. T lymphocytes aggregate at the site of injection, releasing chemotactic factors for monocytes that then release vasoactive amines, which in turn produce redness and induration. Skin tests become positive 4 to 12 weeks after infection (Maslow et al., 1980).

Cultures document the specific organism in infectious lymphadenopathy. They are most applicable for bacterial causes. Blood cultures are usually not helpful unless obvious systemic signs of high fever and leukocytosis are present. Cultures of specific lymph nodes may be helpful. Bone marrow culture is not usually diagnostic, because limited numbers of organisms are usually present and the sample size is limited.

Radiography of the chest helps detect pulmonary hilar adenopathy. With fungal infections, diffuse fibrosis to single lesions are found.

Biopsy of the lymph node provides specific diagnosis and tissue for culture. Easily accessible lymph nodes are preferred. The presence of acute inflammatory cells in follicular necrosis suggests a reactive origin. If present, granulomas may be epithelioid or caseating. Plasma cells may be seen in reactive lesions and, when accompanied by inflammatory cells, in septic lesions (see Lymph Node Cytology). Tumors metastatic to lymph nodes from previously unsuspected malignancy may suggest the primary tumor by their histology (for example, adenocarcinoma versus squamous carcinoma versus melanoma).

LYMPH NODE NEOPLASIA
Lymph Node Cytology

Lymph node biopsy is indicated when local or generalized lymph node enlargement occurs. Enlarged nodes always suggest the possibility of a neoplastic process, either primary or metastatic. Examination of needle aspiration biopsies may reveal the cause of enlargement. Aspiration biopsy may be performed on lymph nodes of any size, provided they can be immobilized. In general, peripheral nodes are best for obtaining specimens for examination. The skin through which the needle will be introduced is surgically prepared. The node is immobi-

lized with one hand and a needle (18 to 25 gauge) of sufficient length to reach the node and attached to a syringe (3 to 6 ml) is inserted through the skin into the node. Usually no anesthetic is necessary, but local anesthesia may be desirable in some situations. Sedation of excitable patients may be necessary. Following introduction of the needle into the node, negative pressure is applied to the syringe while the needle is advanced through the node. The application of negative pressure while advancing the needle should be repeated several times in different areas of the node. Excessive trauma should be avoided, however. By following this procedure, a larger volume of the node is sampled, and contamination of the sample by blood is less than if the needle is allowed to remain in one location (Perman et al., 1974). Only a few drops of material are required for examination. Attempting to obtain a large amount of material will often result in major contamination with blood, owing to capillary hemorrhage.

Smears are prepared in a manner identical to that of blood. Either slide smears or coverslip smears can be used; however, coverslip smears are more uniform, more easily stained, and easier to examine. Impression smears from surgically excised nodes can be made by gently touching a slide or coverslip to the freshly cut surface. If the surface of the node is covered with a film of blood or fluid, lightly blot the surface with absorbent paper before making the imprint.

After rapid air drying, films can be stained in a manner similar to that used for blood films. Cellular preparations that are thick may understain. Staining with Giemsa after Wright's staining will often enhance the stain.

Interpretation of cytologic preparations requires that one be familiar with cells found in lymph nodes. There are four main categories of cells in lymph nodes: mature lymphocytes, stem or blast cells, macrophages, and other cell types (Soderstrom, 1966; Perman et al., 1979) (Figs. 79–4 through 79–6).

The primary cells of normal nodes are mature lymphocytes making up 90 to 95 per cent of the cells. They are similar to the lymphocytes of the blood, except they may have a more coarsely clumped chromatin. These cells are small (approximately 10 μ in diameter) and usually have a sparse cy-

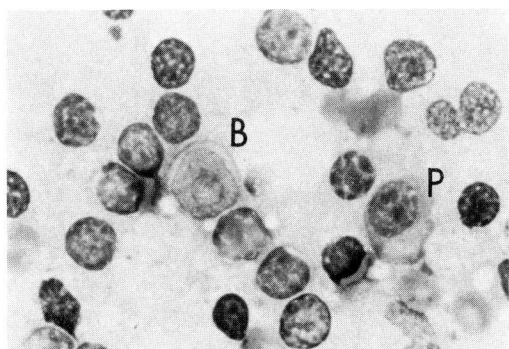

Figure 79–4. Lymph node aspirate containing a lymphoblast (B), a plasma cell (P), and several lymphocytes. The lymphoblast is a pale type, and its nucleus contains a distinct nucleolus. The abundant basophilic cytoplasm with a pale perinuclear area is typical of plasma cells. (×1400.)

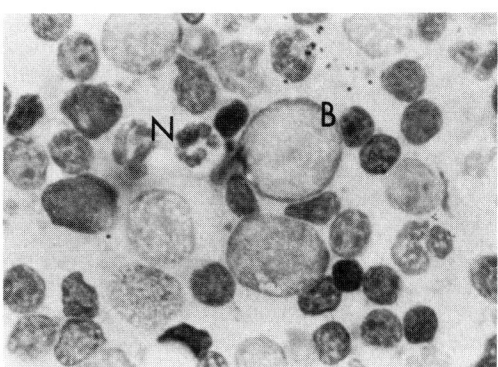

Figure 79–6. Basophilic lymphoblast (B), neutrophils (N) and lymphocytes in a reactive node. The lymphoblast nucleus contains two distinct nucleoli. (×1400.)

toplasm, which may not completely surround the nucleus. Two distinct types of lymphocytes include dark and pale types. Dark lymphocytes have small, dark-staining, compact nuclei and generally a moderately basophilic cytoplasm. Pale lymphocytes have less condensed nuclei, which stains less intensely. Their cytoplasm is usually more abundant and lighter than that of dark lymphocytes.

Lymphoblasts or stem cells are encountered much less frequently. These cells are larger (1 1/2 to 3 times) than lymphocytes, contain a fine, diffuse nuclear chromatin, and may have a distinct nucleolus. Both pale and dark types are found.

Macrophages, sometimes called tissue-bound reticulum cells, reticuloendothelial cells (RE cells), or histocytes, make up a

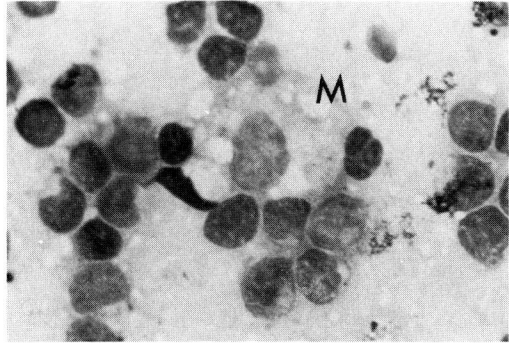

Figure 79–5. Lymph node aspirate containing a macrophage (M), a neutrophil and several lymphocytes. The macrophage (or fixed phagocyte) has a fine, netlike chromatin pattern and an indistinct cytoplasmic border. (×1400.)

small percentage of the cells of a node. Their function is to phagocytose foreign material presented to the node. They have round, oval, or oblong nuclei with a netlike or widely stippled chromatin pattern in which there may be one to two nucleoli. The cytoplasm stains pale blue or gray and is often vacuolated. The cytoplasmic borders are often indistinct.

Plasma cells are found in aspirates in varying numbers. They are related to lymphoid cells, since they are derived from antigenically stimulated B-lymphocytes after blastic transformation, division, and differentiation. They have a dark-staining, moderately condensed nucleus, which is usually eccentrically placed. The cytoplasm is very basophilic and usually has a perinuclear clear area (halo).

Other cells that may be found in lymph node aspirates are neutrophils, eosinophils, mast cells, erythrocytes, and monocytes. These cells are similar to their counterparts in blood and other tissues.

An object often found in lymph node aspirates is the lymphoglandular body. These bodies probably are cytoplasmic fragments of lymphocytes or lymphoblasts (Soderstrom, 1966). They usually stain blue-gray and vary in size from that of a small platelet to that of an erythrocyte.

Classification of Lymph Node Aspirates

In order to better interpret the cause of lymph node changes, a general classification scheme based upon the cytology is presented (Table 79–2) (Zinkl and Keeton, 1979a, 1979b, and 1981). This is a general classification and does not offer specific diagnosis. Each cytologic picture might be produced by different diseases. In some cases, however, a specific diagnosis may be reached on the basis of the cytologic examination. Most aspirates fall into the following classes: normal, reactive, purulent, mixed (reactive and purulent) and neoplastic (either primary or metastatic).

The normal node contains all of the above elements. Mature lymphocytes are the predominant cell. Blast cells of both the basophilic and pale types and fixed phagocytes make up most of the remaining cells. Inflammatory cells, plasma cells, and erythrocytes are usually present in small numbers, although trauma induced during the tap will cause blood cells to be increased artifactually. Lymphoglandular bodies are present in varying numbers but generally can be found without difficulty.

The reactive node is characterized by increased numbers of basophilic blast cells and/or plasma cells. In highly reactive nodes, mitotic figures and basophilia of cells may be prominent. Tissue-bound phagocytes or macrophages may also be increased. Some increase in other inflammatory cells such as neutrophils, eosinophils, mast cells, and basophils may also be seen (Fig. 79–7).

The reactive nature of these nodes is assumed to indicate an immunologic reaction to foreign antigen being presented to the node. The nature of the cytologic picture (i.e., basophilic blast cell proliferation or plasma cell proliferation) may represent different types of immunologic responses or different stages of the same basic reaction.

In the purulent reaction, neutrophils are

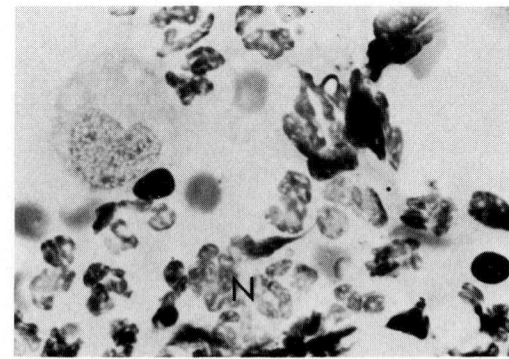

Figure 79–8. Degenerating neutrophils (N) and macrophage in a purulent node. When large numbers of neutrophils are found, or when neutrophils are degenerating, the sample should be cultured. (×1400.)

greatly increased in numbers. Macrophages may also be increased. Many of these nodes may be septic even though bacteria are difficult to identify. Neutrophils often appear to be degenerating, with pyknotic or dissolving nuclei and ruptured cytoplasm. Purulent nodes, especially with degenerating neutrophils, should be collected aseptically, and bacteriologic examination should be performed. Nodal reactions of this type probably occur when organisms gain access to the node from septic sites drained by the node (Figure 79–8).

Nodes exhibiting both reactive and purulent characteristics may be encountered. In these, increased numbers of plasma cells, basophilic blast cells, neutrophils, and macrophages are found (Fig. 79–9).

Lymphoma. When precursor lymphocytes become malignant, large numbers of pleomorphic, primitive lymphoblasts dis-

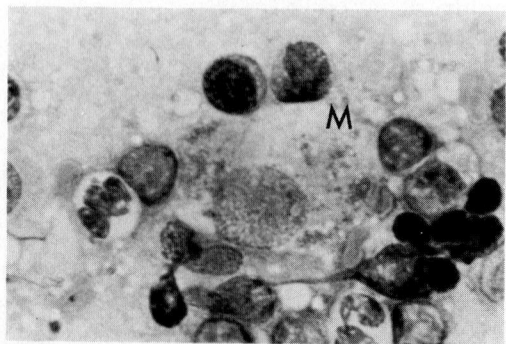

Figure 79–7. Macrophage (M) in a reactive node. The macrophage (M) contains numerous *Neorickettsia helminthoeca* elementary bodies in the cytoplasm. (×1400.)

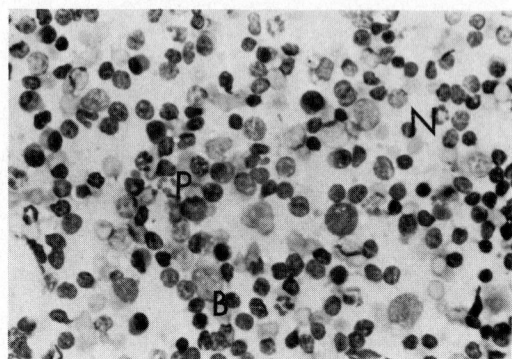

Figure 79–9. Mixed reactive-purulent reaction containing plasma cells (P), basophilic lymphoblast (B), and neutrophils (N). (×560.)

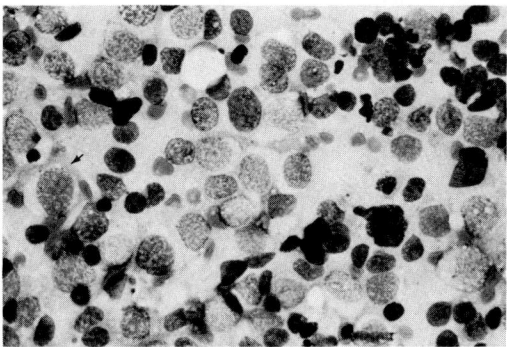

Figure 79–10. Lymph node aspirate of a histiocytic lymphoma. The cells are large with moderate amounts of foamy or vacuolated cytoplasm. The nuclei are netlike, and several contain distinct nucleoli. Only a few smaller, normal lymphocytes are present. (×560.)

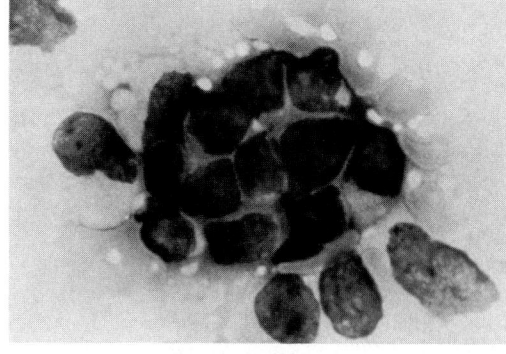

Figure 79–12. Pleomorphic lymphoblast in lymphoma. Nuclear crowding is evident by the molding of the nuclei into irregular shapes with flattened edges. Several nuclei contain nucleoli. (×1400.)

place the normal cell population of the lymph node. The major finding in cytologic preparations is large numbers of a monomorphic population of immature lymphoid cells. Few normal cells remain. These neoplastic cells vary in size, have variable sized nuclei, may have multiple or large nucleoli, and there may be increased numbers of mitotic figures present.

The morphology of malignant cells can vary markedly between cases. Some cases may have cells that are unmistakably lymphoid in nature but are primarily very immature, with many lymphoblasts and prolymphocytes being present. Other cases may have light staining cells with abundant cytoplasm, which is often vacuolated or foamy. They have irregular nuclei as well. Occasionally, extremely undifferentiated cells are found. The cells are usually difficult to

identify as being of a lymphoid nature. These cells have nuclear irregularities and a deeply basophilic cytoplasm that may contain a few distinct vacuoles. Although the morphology of the cells is quite variable in lymphoma, it is not possible to distinctly and accurately subclassify the tumors based on cytology, because gradations from one morphologic type to another occurs. Thus it is best to classify them simply as lymphoma (Figs. 79–10 through 79–13).

Myeloma. Lymph nodes may be heavily infiltrated with plasma cells in malignant myelomas. Myeloma cells are similar to normal plasma cells, having a moderate amount of deeply basophilic cytoplasm and an eccentrically placed nucleus. Malignant plasma cells usually have much less condensed nuclei than normal plasma cells. Some cells may be binucleated, and some may have distinct nucleoli. Mitotic figures may also be

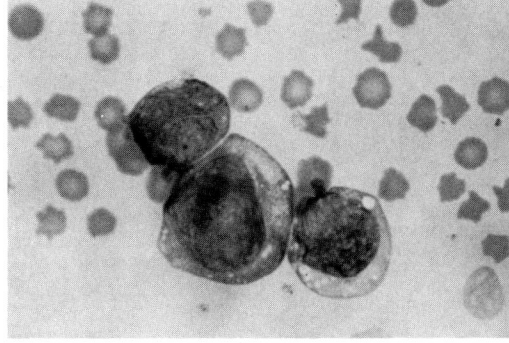

Figure 79–11. Three large lymphoblasts in an aspirate of lymphoma. The largest cell (center) has an irregular shaped nucleolus, while the smaller cells have irregular nuclei. (×1400.)

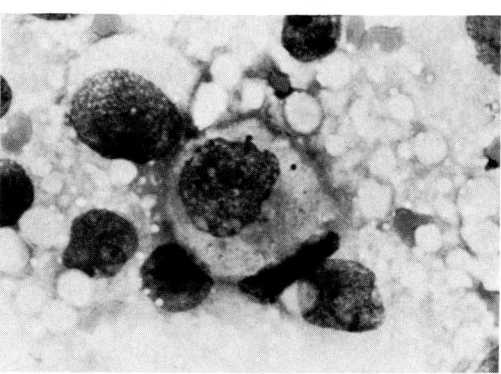

Figure 79–13. Two very large cells with macrophage characteristics in histiocytic lymphoma. (×1400.)

present. Protein electrophoresis usually reveals a monoclonal gammopathy, which is the major diagnostic feature of plasma cell myeloma (Fig. 79–14).

Metastatic Tumors. It is not uncommon to find tumor cells of various types in lymph node aspirates, since many tumors metastasize by way of lymphatics. In general, any cell that appears to be foreign to the normal cytologic makeup of a node could be a cell of a distant tumor (Zinkl and Keeton, 1981). The numbers of such cells may be very sparse or they may completely displace the nodal tissue. Therefore, a prolonged search of an aspirate may be necessary in order to rule out metastasis (Figs. 79–15 through 79–27).

Tumor cells may be differentiated enough to allow identification of the tumor. Conversely, undifferentiated cells may be present, indicating that a tumor is present, but such cells make a specific diagnosis impossible.

In addition to disclosing the presence of tumor cells, smears of nodes involved with metastatic tumors may have reactive changes. Basophilic lymphoblasts and plasma cells may be increased in numbers, perhaps in response to stimulation of the immune system by the tumor cells or cell products. Inflammatory reactions may also occur if the tumor becomes necrotic or infected and these products reach the node.

LYMPHOPROLIFERATIVE DISEASES

Lymphoproliferative responses occur in diseases and conditions that have an associated abnormal proliferation of lymphoid tissue and abnormal numbers of lymphoid elements circulating in peripheral blood. The primary lymphoid tissue proliferation is found in lymph nodes, but lymphoid tissue in spleen, liver, and even bone marrow may also participate in this process. These responses may primarily involve the tissue (lymphoma) with little, if any, peripheral blood involvement or may be manifested primarily by peripheral blood changes (leukemia) (Table 79–5; Figure 79–28).

Several concepts are particularly useful in understanding the problem of variation in the laboratory picture of lymphoproliferative responses of the malignant variety (lymphoproliferative or lymphoreticular disorder). These include appreciation of a

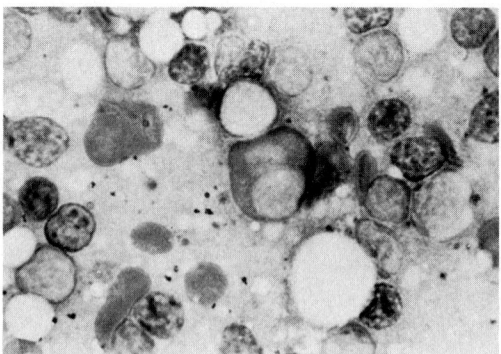

Figure 79–14. Plasma cell in lymph node of multiple myeloma. Many such cells were present in the bone marrow; there were fewer in the lymph node, but they were increased. (×1400.)

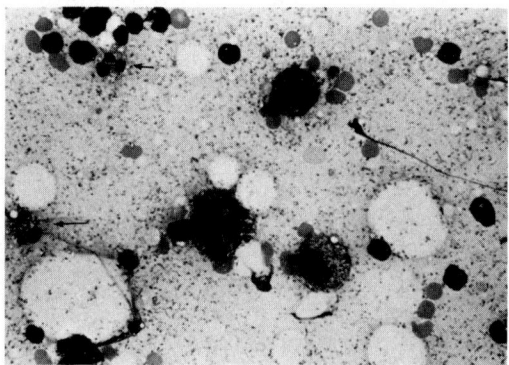

Figure 79–15. Mast cells in lymph node aspirate of mastocytosis. The cells are larger than normal mast cells. They contain variable numbers of granules. In mastocytomas there can be extreme variations in the number of granules and the size of the granules. In some mastocytomas a polarization of granules and the nucleus occurs in which the granules are found at one pole of the cell and the nucleus at the other pole. In mastocytomas, eosinophils (arrow) are usually present. (×560.)

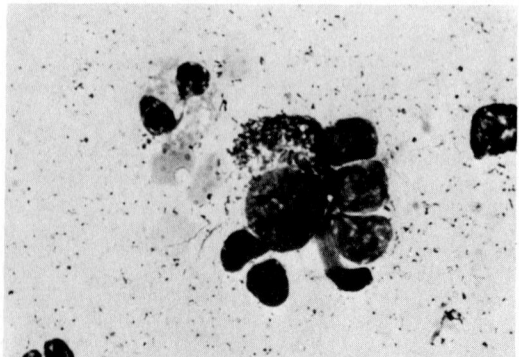

Figure 79–16. A mast cell surrounded by several lymphocytes in a mastocytoma. An eosinophil is to the left of the mast cell. Eosinophils are nearly always found in aspirates of mastocytomas. In this figure and in Figure 79–15 many mast cell granules are in the background. (×1400.)

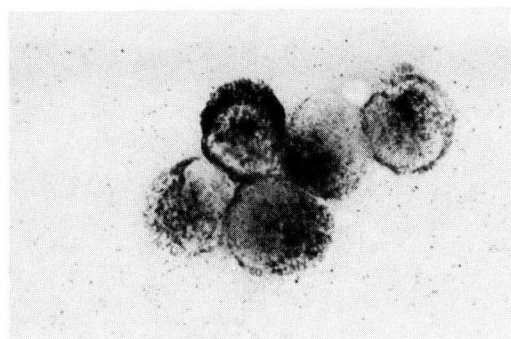

Figure 79–17. Aggregate of malignant melanocytes from a tumor that metastasized to the lymph node.

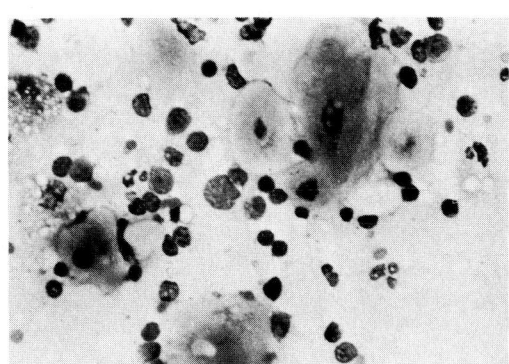

Figure 79–20. Metastasis of a squamous cell carcinoma to the lymph node. The squamous cells are very large, flat cells. In this tumor the nuclei are moderately pyknotic. (×500.)

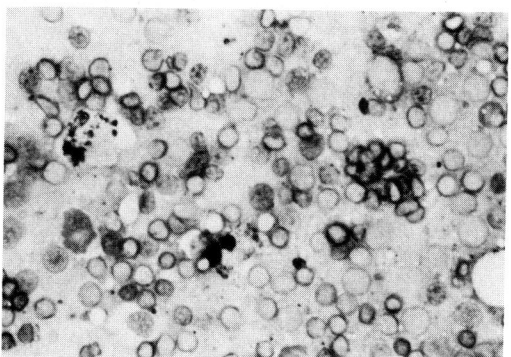

Figure 79–18. Aspirate of lymph node with macrophages containing large amounts of melanin. A search of the slide revealed a few melanocytes, which suggested malignant melanoma. Occasionally the first suggestion of the tumor type is provided by the substances found in macrophages. (×560.)

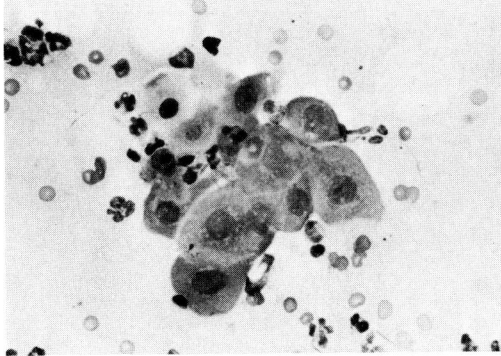

Figure 79–21. Squamous cell carcinoma cells in lymph node aspirate. The cells are less differentiated than those of Figure 79–20. Many neutrophils are often seen in aspirates of squamous cell carcinomas. Occasionally a tumor cell such as in the center of this aggregate will phagocytize a neutrophil. (×560.)

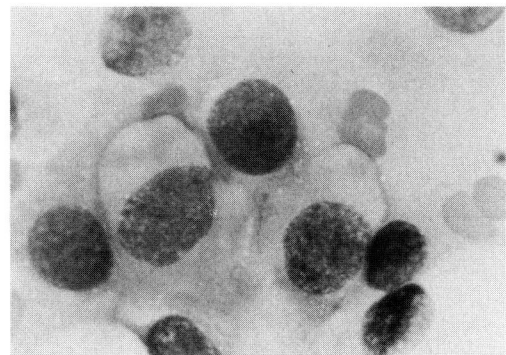

Figure 79–19. Aspirate of lymph node to which an amelanotic melanoma has metastasized. These cells are large and contain nucleoli. They nearly completely crowded out the normal lymph node cells. Most of the cells such as these contained no melanin. Prolonged searching of the slide revealed a rare cell with very fine dusting of melanin in the cytoplasm. (×1400.)

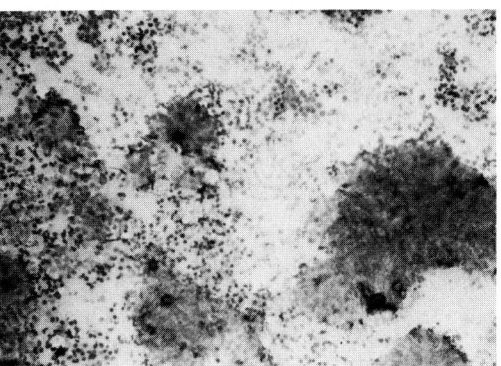

Figure 79–22. Aspirate of perianal adenocarcinoma metastasis to a lymph node. Many large aggregates of cells are present. The tumor cells completely displaced the lymph node cells. (×140.)

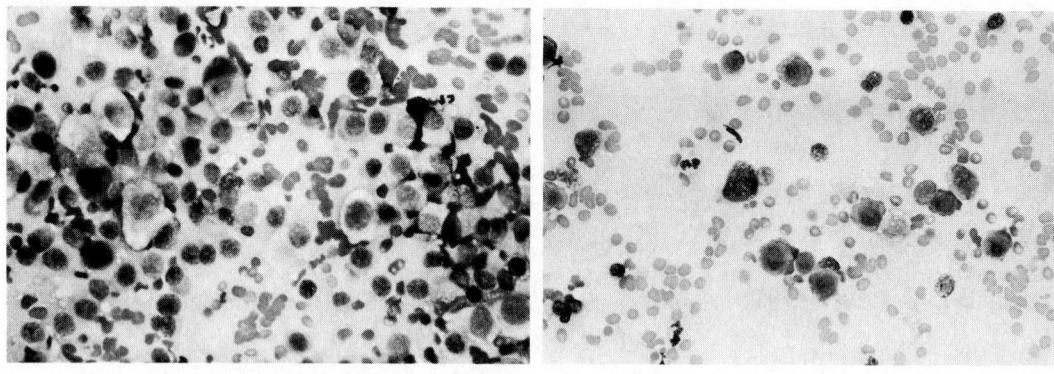

| Figure 79–23 | Figure 79–24 |

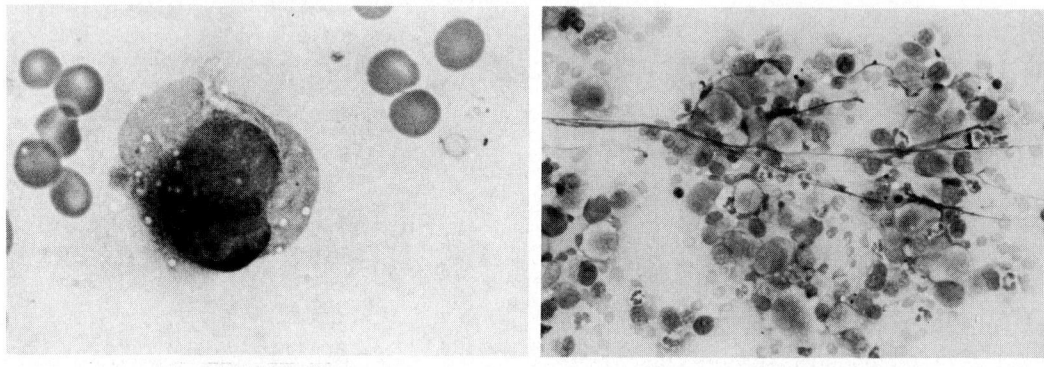

Figure 79–25

Figure 79–26

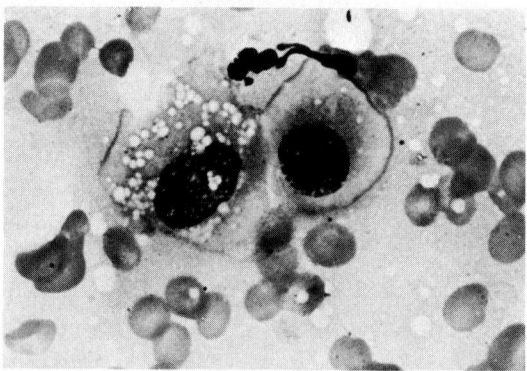

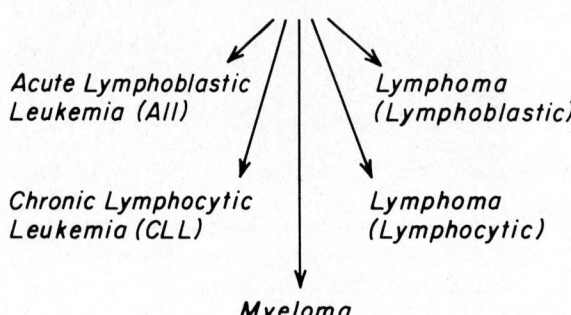

Figure 79–27

Figure 79–23 to 79–27. Many times it is not possible to determine the kind of tumor that has metastasized to the lymph node. These five figures show examples of cytologic preparations that indicated that a tumor was present but did not suggest the tumor type. Figure 79–23 shows an extremely pleomorphic cell population. The cells vary in size and have irregular nuclei and cytoplasmic borders. Some large nucleoli are present. (×560.) Figure 79–24 has a population of large cells which are somewhat pleomorphic and irregular. Although a specific diagnosis is not possible, the fact that the cells are found as individual cells rather than in aggregates suggests that the tumor is a sarcoma. (×560.) Figure 79–25 shows the irregular nucleus of one of the cells in the tumor of Figure 79–24. (×1400.) Figure 79–26 is from an unknown type tumor. There is marked variation in cell size. The cells are adhered to each other, suggesting that the tumor may be a carcinoma. (×560.) Figure 79–27 shows two large cells from an undifferentiated tumor. Many cells were similar to this and displaced the normal lymph node cells. Vacuoles as seen in the cell on the left are common in tumor cells obtained by aspiration. (×1400.)

LYMPHOPROLIFERATIVE DISORDERS

Acute Lymphoblastic Leukemia (All)

Lymphoma (Lymphoblastic)

Chronic Lymphocytic Leukemia (CLL)

Lymphoma (Lymphocytic)

Myeloma

Figure 79–28. Lymphoproliferative disorders.

Table 79–5. **Classification of Lymphoid Neoplasia**

I. Lymphocytes
   A. Lymphoma
      1. Multicentric
      2. Alimentary
      3. Anterior mediastinal
      4. Cutaneous
   B. Lymphocytic leukemia
      1. Chronic lymphocytic leukemia
      2. Acute lymphoblastic leukemia
II. Immunoglobulin secreting plasma cells
   A. Myeloma
   B. Macroglobulinemia
III. Reticulum cell
   A. Lymphoma, histiocytic type (reticulum cell sarcoma)
IV. Hodgkin's-like disease

continuum between a "pure" lymphocytic leukemia and a "pure" tissue lymphoma; all gradations in between are found. In addition, lymphomas often apparently change into leukemias. There can be an apparent change in the disease process so that primary tissue involvement may progress to a frank leukemia. In fact, this is frequently seen in clinical practice.

It may be difficult to decide from examination of the peripheral blood whether the proliferating cells are of myeloid or lymphoid origin. The blastic leukemias are examples of this problem. Studies involving special cytochemical stains are sometimes helpful; experience and expert judgment are also helpful, but in other cases the question will be answered only with time. Figure 79–28 illustrates the most important clinical entities involving the lymphoproliferative response and will serve as a general outline for the short discussions that follow.

Acute Lymphoblastic Leukemia

Acute lymphoblastic leukemia (ALL) is regarded as a proliferation of lymphoblasts originating in marrow and perhaps extramyeloid lymphatic tissue. Anemia, thrombocytopenia, and granulocytopenia in ALL result from the effects of masses of leukemic lymphoblasts on normal hematopoietic stem cells (Simone, 1978; Lichtman, 1980).

Accumulation of leukemic blast cells in peripheral tissue occasionally leads to signs referable to specific organs. Malaise and easy fatigability are nearly always present. Fever and gingival, cutaneous, or nasal bleeding are present in as many as half the patients. Lymphadenopathy, pallor, and hepatosplenomegaly may be present (Mac-Ewen et al., 1977b). As the bone marrow is replaced by leukemic lymphoblasts, normal erythroid, granulocytic, and megakaryocytic cells are greatly reduced in number.

Treatment of ALL is based on the premise that eradication of leukemic blast cells will allow regrowth and ascendancy of suppressed normal hematopoietic cells. ALL cells are sensitive to antileukemic drugs. The cytocidal drugs initially used to reduce the body burden of leukemic lymphoblasts, vincristine and glucocorticoids, are not exquisitely toxic to hematopoietic cells. Infection during remission is a serious and sometimes terminal threat. Presumably these infections are a result of the immunosuppression from intensive chemotherapy.

Chronic Lymphocytic Leukemia

Chronic lymphocytic leukemia (CLL) is a neoplastic disorder of small lymphocytes. As a result of increased proliferation and prolonged survival of lymphocytes, there is an enormous accumulation of lymphoid cells in marrow, blood, lymph nodes, liver, and spleen. The proliferative disorder may originate in the marrow but also occurs in lymph nodes and spleen. CLL is a monoclonal proliferation of B lymphocytes, and cells usually carry determinants for IgM on their surfaces (Bennett and Lichtman, 1980). Normal hematopoietic cell proliferation is thought to be impaired because of the massive lymphocytic accumulation in marrow. Varying degrees of anemia, neutropenia, and thrombocytopenia develop. Later in the disease, a generalized defect in B lymphocyte function can result in insufficient immunoglobulin synthesis. This can result in serious difficulties with antibody production against challenging microbes.

Most dogs with CLL are asymptomatic at the time of diagnosis. The disorder is discovered while the patient is being evaluated for an unrelated medical problem. In patients that are ill, signs include malaise, easy fatigability, and weight loss. Often enlarged lymph nodes are discovered and lead to the diagnosis. Splenomegaly and hepatomegaly are very common.

Red cell and platelet counts may be normal or a slight anemia may be present. When more severe anemia and thrombocytopenia are found at the time of diagnosis, prognosis is poor. An absolute lymphocytosis is always present. The white cell count usually varies between 30,000 to 50,000 per microliter, with 40 to 80 per cent being lymphocytes (MacEwen et al., 1977b). Bone marrow aspiration reveals a high percentage of lymphocytes (60 to 80 per cent), together with a few lymphoblasts. Three canine patients with this form of leukemia had a monoclonal gammopathy, which resulted in hyperviscosity syndrome (MacEwen et al., 1977b).

The alkylating agent chlorambucil, administered at two doses of 0.2 mg per kg of body weight orally for seven to ten days, has been effective. The dose is then reduced to 0.1 mg per kg orally per day. In one dog, remission was observed for at least two years after having been treated for five and one-half months (MacEwen et al., 1977b). We give 2.0 mg/m² every other day as needed.

Many patients, despite marked increase of lymphocytes in blood and in marrow, and moderate lymph node and splenic enlargement, are able to maintain comfortable lives (Harvey et al., 1981). In patients with active disease in which either anemia, thrombocytopenia, or enormous splenic or lymph node enlargement is present, an attempt to reduce the lymphocyte mass in marrow and tissues is justified.

Variants of Chronic Lymphocytic Leukemia. CLL bears a close relationship to lymphoma. The histologies of CLL and lymphocytic lymphoma are identical and this can lead to a diagnosis of lymphoma in a patient with CLL if lymph nodes are examined without giving consideration to blood counts. Studies have suggested that patients with CLL having cells morphologically similar to lymphoma cells have a shorter life span than those with typical well differentiated cells (Gunz, 1977)

Lymphoma with Leukemic Manifestations. Diffuse involvement of marrow and the presence of circulating pathologic cells may accompany any histologic type of lymphoma. This pattern is most frequently seen with poorly differentiated lymphoma. When this clinical syndrome develops in the course of a previously diagnosed lymphoma, it indicates disease progression. If lymphoma with leukemic manifestations represents the initial presentation of a lymphoproliferative disorder, it can be distinguished from classical CLL by the fact that there are fewer cells in the blood and the cells are more immature. This type of presentation is a more progressive disease and usually requires more intensive chemotherapy or local radiotherapy.

Myeloma

Myeloma is a malignant disease that results from the neoplastic proliferation of a clone of cells with features of differentiated B lymphocytes. The malignant clone has the morphologic features of plasma cells. They produce a monoclonal immunoglobulin that reflects the nature and the size of the tumor cell mass. The neoplastic plasma cells are confined largely to the bone marrow when the tumor mass is small, but as the number of malignant cells increases, lymph nodes, liver, spleen, and other organs may be infiltrated with abnormal cells. Concomitant with the malignant plasma cell growth is an impaired ability to mount a normal humoral immune response. The consequences of myeloma are related to the tumor cell mass, the immunoglobulin produced, and the associated immune deficiency (MacEwen and Hurvitz, 1977a; Bernier and Lichtman, 1980).

Cell Mass. The bulk of the plasma cell tumor involves the marrow and compromises hematopoietic cell production. Thus cytopenias, especially anemia, are nearly always associated with clinically apparent disease. Bone destruction, while rare in myelomas of small animals, is also related to the intramedullary cell mass. Bone destruction occurs when myeloma cells secrete osteoclast activating factor, which stimulates osteoclasts to induce bone resorption and leads to radiographic evidence of osteolysis.

Monoclonal Immunoglobulins. In the dog and the cat, several disease conditions have been found to be associated with monoclonal gammopathies (myeloma, macroglobulinemia, lymphoma, lymphocytic leukemia, neoplasms of cells not known to produce immunoglobulins, and benign monoclonal gammopathies). The malignant plasma cells may secrete IgG or IgA, or have light chains of immunoglobulin, which, because of their small size, are rapidly excreted in the urine and represent Bence

Jones protein. (These same light chains are chief among the proteins incriminated in *amyloidosis*) (Isobe and Osserman, 1974). When IgG or IgA is present in high concentration or has a high intrinsic viscosity, an increase in blood viscosity may occur. When immunoglobulins are cold-insoluble, cryoglobulinemia may occur. Light chains, when excreted in large quantities, have been implicated in renal dysfunction by forming casts and causing amyloidosis (Wiltshaw, 1976).

Immune Deficiency. Patients with myeloma suffer from an inability to mount an adequate humoral immune response. As a result, encapsulated organisms that require antibody attachment prior to phagocytosis are particularly virulent in myeloma patients. The humoral deficit is aggravated by diminished leucocyte production and faulty granulocytic function. The effects of treatment with cytotoxic agents further impair host defenses.

Laboratory Findings. Monoclonal gammopathy occurs in myeloma. The peak in the electropherogram may be in any of the globulin regions. Most often it is in the gamma region. Very rarely two sharp peaks are found, one of which probably is an aggregate or polymer of the other. Marked to moderate anemia is very common, and granulocytopenia or thrombocytopenia may also be present. Plasma cells or plasmacytoid lymphocytes ("plymphocytes") are not usually evident in the blood, though rarely plasma cell leukemia may occur in myeloma. Marrow examination nearly always reveals an increase in plasma cells, which may compose 10 to 90 per cent of the aspirated cells. Plasmocytosis can occur with other diseases, although the greater the percentage of plasma cells and the more cytologic atypia, the more likely they are to represent myeloma cells.

Radiography may occasionally show osteoporosis or osteolytic lesions in skull, ribs, pelvis, or vertebrae. Hypercalciuria and hypercalcemia may occur. Renal insufficiency may be present. Alkaline phosphatase levels are variable, since osteoblastic activity (the cause of elevations of the bone isozyme of alkaline phosphatase) does not increase to compensate for osteolysis. Hemorrhagic diatheses occurs as a result of coagulation activation due to stasis (hyperviscosity) or because the myeloma proteins coat platelets

Table 79–6. Clinical Staging of Canine Myeloma*

Finding	†High Tumor Mass	Low Tumor Mass
Hematocrit	< 30%	> 30%
Calcium	> 12 mg/dl	< 12 mg/dl
Lytic bone	Multiple	Solitary or None
Monoclonal IgG	> 7 gm/dl	< 5 gm/dl
Monoclonal IgA	> 5 gm/dl	< 3 gm/dl
Bence Jones proteinuria	+ or −	−

*Modified from Bernier, G. M., and Lichtman, M. A.: Myeloma. *In* Lichtman, M. A. (ed.): Hematology and Oncology. Grune and Stratton, New York, 1980.

†If one or more of the high mass findings are present the patient is regarded as having a large number of tumor cells. All of the low mass findings must be present to be regarded as low mass. Other findings are intermediate cell mass. The finding of elevated serum urea nitrogen or serum creatinine conveys a poor prognosis.

and render them nonfunctional. The diagnosis of myeloma is sometimes established following evaluation of obscure renal disease, hypercalcemia, or hemorrhage. The clinical staging of myeloma is outlined in Table 79–6.

Treatment. Increasing concentrations of serum monoclonal immunoglobulins, advancing anemia, evidence of bone destruction, granulocytopenia, and thrombocytopenia are some findings that indicate treatment of the tumor is warranted. Alkylating agents, especially melphalan or cyclophosphamide, have been very effective in the management of myeloma. Glucocorticoids used in conjunction with alkylating agents may slightly enhance the response rate. Hydration during initial cytotoxic therapy, especially with preexisting hypercalcemia, will lessen the chance of nephropathy (MacEwen and Hurvitz, 1977a). Surgical excision or radiation therapy for localized plasma cell tumors may also be used.

Lymphoma

The lymphomas are a group of diseases that, although varying widely in histologic features, natural history, and prognosis, share a common characteristic, namely a neoplastic proliferation of lymphoid cells. The lymphomas may arise in lymph nodes or in other sites of lymphoid tissue, including the spleen, gastrointestinal tract, or bone marrow. In some cases the disease may remain localized, involving one node or group of nodes or a single extranodal site, for months. In other instances multiple lymph nodes are involved at the onset, and dissemination to bone marrow, liver, lung, and other organs may occur as well. As a group, lymphomas differ from Hodgkin's-like disease in their greater tendency to involve extralymphatic tissues often at the time of clinical presentation (Rosenberg et al., 1961; Jones and Godden, 1977).

Incidence. Of 741 dogs with hemolymphatic neoplasia whose case reports were compiled from 12 veterinary schools in North America from 1967 to 1971, approximately 94 per cent were lymphoid in origin, of which 83 per cent were lymphomas and 11 per cent were reticulum cell sarcomas (lymphoma, histiocytic type) (Priester, 1972).

In 245 cats with hemolymphatic neoplasia 57 per cent were lymphomas (Holzworth, 1960). Lymphoproliferative disorders are associated with Feline Leukemia Virus (FeLV) in 70 per cent or more of the cases (Pedersen and Madewell, 1980). There is a tendency for aged cats and cats with solitary lymphoid neoplasms to be virus-negative. These neoplasms are categorized anatomically into four major forms: anterior mediastinal (thymic), alimentary, multicentric, and leukemic (in peripheral blood). Staging of lymphomas is outlined in Table 79–7.

Classification. Several classifications of lymphomas based on the histologic, cytologic, and immunologic properties of the tumor are in current use. Considerable controversy and uncertainty exist among pathologists concerning the relative utility and scientific validity of the various classification schemes, and no general agreement on nomenclature schemes has yet been reached (Jones and Godden, 1977). For the clinician the Rappaport (1966) classification is most useful. Further understanding of lymphocytic function and new methods to detect cell surface markers may require modification of the Rappaport scheme in the future.

Neoplastic tissues from 72 dogs with lymphoma were classified according to the Rappaport scheme. In seven dogs (9.7 per cent) the neoplasms were classified as nodular and in 65 dogs (90.3 per cent) they were classified as diffuse. The principal cytologic types were lymphocytic (poorly differentiated) and histiocytic, and composed 39 per cent and 56 per cent of the lymphomas, respectively; lymphocytic (well differentiated), mixed, and undifferentiated types composed six per cent. Analysis revealed no significant differences among nodular histiocytic, diffuse lymphocytic (poorly differentiated), and diffuse histiocytic groups relative to days remission as well as days survival. Hence, the Rappaport scheme cannot be used as a prognostic criterion in predicting therapeutic response, remission, or survival (Weller et al., 1980).

Signs. The most common presenting sign is painless lymphadenopathy. This may occur in any area but frequently involves the tumor-palpable node-bearing areas, the prescapular, inguinal, and popliteal. Pleural effusions may be caused by hilar (mediastinal) adenopathy or lymphomatous involvement of the pleura. Ascites may be a presenting sign secondary to extensive abdominal adenopathy. Tonsils may be enlarged. Hypercalcemia may be observed in 10 to 15 per cent of the dogs with lymphoma (MacEwen et al., 1977b).

Alimentary System. Animals with the alimentary form of the disease are usually presented with, or because of, weight loss, vomiting, and diarrhea. Involvement is more frequently diffuse, and the sites of involvement are the stomach and small intestine. Ascites may be seen as a result of mesenteric lymph node obstruction (Theilen and Madewell, 1979).

Respiratory System. Pleural involvement may be associated with pleural effusion. Pleural effusion may also arise from lymphatic destruction by intrathoracic tumor. Hypertrophic (pulmonary) osteopathy is a rare finding with intrathoracic lymphoma. In the cat, the mediastinal type involves infiltrated thymus, mediastinal lymph nodes, and rarely, other organs (Theilen and Madewell, 1979). Fifty per cent of dogs with mediastinal lymphoma in one study had hypercalcemia (MacEwen et al., 1977b).

Hemopoietic System. Normocytic, normochromic anemia can be a presenting feature of lymphoma. Often anemia is a feature of generalized disease, but it may be exacerbated by blood loss, myelosuppressive therapy, bone marrow infiltration, hypersplenism, and uremia.

A particular feature of lymphoma is the incidence of autoimmune hemolytic anemia (Werner, 1980). Both warm and cold antibodies have been incriminated and may occur even in the presence of hypogammaglobulinemia (Davie, 1967). The warm antibodies are usually IgG, while the cold antibodies are usually IgM. In both types of autoimmune hemolytic anemia the broad spectrum Coombs' antiglobulin test is positive.

Bone marrow infiltration occurs in about 15 per cent of cases of lymphoma at presentation, usually in the presence of generalized disease (MacEwen, 1980). The harder it is sought the more often it is identified. Positive identification is easier in marrow sections than in smears and is easier with more numerous and larger biopsies. The high incidence of bone marrow involvement may cause confusion with leukemia. Indeed, leukemic transformation occurs with lymphocytic lymphomas with peripheral blood involvement.

Rarely marrow infiltration may cause leukoerythroblastosis (Madewell and Feldman, 1980). Leukocytosis and thrombocytosis may occasionally be seen. Neutropenia and thrombocytopenia usually follow intensive myelosuppressive therapy or may occur with hypersplenism (Madewell and Feldman, 1980). Chronic thrombocytopenia is an occasional finding and may be caused by antiplatelet immune activity. Lymphopenia may occur with generalized disease (particularly of lymphoma, histiocytic type) and is exacerbated by cytotoxic chemotherapy.

OTHER SIGNS. Lymphomatous infiltration of the heart may obstruct inflow, cause cardiac tamponade, and restrict cardiac function. Lymphoma, histiocytic type, has a predilection for long bones. Splenomegaly is seen in one third of patients presenting with multicentric lymphoma. It is a less common finding with lymphoma, histiocytic type. Clinical size does not always correlate with pathologic involvement (MacEwen, 1980). About one third of patients with multicentric lymphoma have hepatomegaly at presentation, and in many cases this indicates hepatic involvement with lymphoma. Elevation of alkaline phosphatase is often seen in patients with lymphoma. It is often difficult to assess the isoenzyme contribution by bone and hepatic diseases. Isoenzyme studies may be of help (Moore and Feldman, 1974). Solitary malignant lympho-

ma may occur in the central nervous system. For example, malignant lymphoma infiltrated and destroyed the pituitary gland in a dog, causing diabetes insipidus (Madewell, 1975). Infiltration of renal parenchymal tissue occurs with lymphocytic lymphoma. Kidney involvement occurred in 45 per cent of cats with lymphoma (Theilen and Madewell, 1979). Cutaneous lymphomas are exceedingly rare in cats (Scott, 1980). In dogs, cutaneous involvement is infrequent and primary cutaneous lymphomas appear to be rare (Miller, 1980). The cutaneous conditions of mycosis fungoides and Sézary syndrome are discussed in the following section. Mammary, thyroid, adrenal, and pancreatic lymphomas have been described or observed. Clinical involvement is rare (Theilen and Madewell, 1979).

Diagnosis. The planned investigation of lymphoma is aimed at providing an accurate assessment of the extent of the disease. Careful staging (Table 79–7) is essential to facilitate comparison of results from different oncologic centers and, more importantly to the patient and client, to give a guide to therapy and prognosis. Most patients presented to the authors are classified in the advanced stages III, IV, and V. Criteria used to establish stages include hematologic investigation, biochemical investigation, immunologic investigation, cytology, radiography, and tissue biopsy (Theilen and Madewell, 1979). The following discussion focuses on the hematologic and biochemical investigation of lymphoma.

HEMATOLOGIC INVESTIGATION. A full peripheral blood count with examination of a blood film is mandatory. Many forms of

Table 79–7. Staging of Lymphoma*†

Stage‡	Involvement
I	Limited to a single node or lymphoid tissue in single organ (excluding bone marrow)
	Many lymph nodes in a regional area
III	Generalized lymph node
IV	Liver and/or spleen (+ stage III)
V	Manifestation in the blood; bone marrow and/or other organ systems

*Excluding myeloma
†Approved by World Health Organization, Geneva, April 1978.
‡Each stage is subclassified into: Stage A, without systemic signs and Stage B, with systemic signs.

anemia and white cell and platelet abnormalities occur with lymphoma, and tumor cells may be seen in the blood. The erythrocyte sedimentation rate may provide a guide as to disease activity and should be assessed serially.

Bone marrow aspiration and *biopsy* is also essential. The incidence of marrow lesions in lymphoma is only appreciated when thorough marrow examination is undertaken. Examination of marrow aspiration smear preparation rarely leads to the identification of lymphoma cells. When a trephine biopsy is examined (as in touch preparations and cytologic and histologic sectioning), the incidence of positive identification rises. The specimen should be slowly decalcified and serially sectioned throughout. The earliest typical foci often lie in a paratrabecular position (Han et al., 1971).

Hemolysis (particularly of an autoimmune type) may be a feature of advanced, diffuse lymphoma. If the Coombs' antiglobulin test were used more often or was more sensitive, autoimmune anemia would probably be diagnosed more frequently (Feldman and O'Neill, 1981).

BIOCHEMICAL INVESTIGATION. Blood samples should be taken for liver tests (serum bilirubin, alkaline phosphatase, liver enzymes, proteins) for urea, calcium, and electrolyte assessment (looking particularly for renal involvement). Where it is available, a multifactorial serum analysis gives a good general screen for biochemical abnormalities. Disease activity can be assessed by serial measurements of concentrations of serum iron (depressed) and serum copper (elevated) (Feldman and Kaneko, 1981a, 1981b, 1981c; Madewell and Feldman, 1980). It is often difficult to get an accurate clinical assessment of hepatic involvement. Hepatomegaly does not imply pathologic involvement, and conversely, hepatic infiltration may be seen in the presence of a clinically appearing normal liver and normal liver tests. With clinical staging evaluation criteria, hepatic involvement is strongly suggested by abnormal alkaline phosphatase and two or more other liver test abnormalities (Feldman, 1980). A hepatic biopsy is the most accurate way of assessing liver involvement when there is a high index of clinical suspicion and little laboratory corroboration.

HYPERCALCEMIA. Hypercalcemia can be one of the major problems in the management of canine lymphoma, since it can damage the kidneys. Approximately 15 per cent of dogs with lymphoma have elevated serum calcium concentrations (greater than 12 mg/dl). The usual presenting signs of hypercalcemia are polydipsia, polyuria, muscle weakness, and renal insufficiency. Hypercalcemia is caused by the production of physiologically active substances that stimulate bone resorption. Current studies (Heath et al., 1979) have shown that these substances are not parathyroid-like hormones or prostaglandin derivatives. The substances appear to be similar to osteoclast stimulating factor elaborated by myeloma cells (MacEwen, 1980).

The most critical problem associated with hypercalcemia is its effect on the kidney. Hypercalcemia can cause degeneration and necrosis of the renal tubules and the eventual development of nephrocalcinosis leading to progressive renal failure (MacEwen, 1980).

Therapy of hypercalcemia is directed at restoring hydration, maintaining urine output, inducing calcium excretion with saline diuresis and diuretics, reducing calcium intake, reducing calcium uptake with calcium chelating drugs, and administering antitumor therapy to eliminate the malignant cells that elaborate the substances causing hypercalcemia. Mithramycin ($2\mu g/kg$) may be given for one or two days in refactory cases (MacEwen, 1980).

IMMUNOLOGIC INVESTIGATION. It is not established that immune status is related to prognosis. When it occurs, however, markedly depressed immunity is nearly always a feature of disseminated disease.

In vivo investigations of cellular immunity include skin tests (recall antigens) or active sensitization with dinitrochlorobenzene (DNCB). *In vitro* tests include lymphocyte transformation, macrophage inhibition, and rosette techniques. Humoral immunity may be assessed by measuring serum immunoglobulin levels and by estimating the proportion of B cells by immunofluorescent cell surface immunoglobulin labeling techniques. Classically, when they occur, immunologic defects are of cellular immunity in Hodgkin's disease and of humoral immunity in lymphoma; in practice there may be overlap (Carr et al., 1977).

In lymphoma, monoclonal gammopathies are occasionally found. Immunoglobulin quantitation and immunoelectrophoretic examination of blood and urine should be carried out in all cases with monoclonal gammopathies.

TISSUE BIOPSY. The diagnosis of lymphoma is established by the cytologic and histologic examination of aspirated or biopsied specimens from clinically involved tissue, usually a lymph node, or occasionally an extralymphatic site (liver, lungs, bone, bone marrow). If several nodes are available for biopsy, a large node, preferably one not draining any site of overt or recent infection or inflammation, should be selected.

Treatment. After accurate staging the chemotherapeutic treatment of canine and feline lymphomas is undertaken (Table 79–7). The aim of the therapy is to control the disease process and extend the life of the animal with as few undesirable side effects as possible (treatment is discussed in Chapter 30).

CANINE LYMPHOMA. *Chemotherapy* is more effective in dogs in early clinical stages than in those with advanced disease (Crow, 1977). Dogs with multicentric type usually respond better than do those with thymic and alimentary types. All types with severe liver and kidney disease do very poorly. Dogs with hypercalcemia should be treated as emergency cases. Lymphocytic cell types are more responsive than are histiocytic cell types. Combination chemotherapy is more effective than single agent chemotherapy. Dogs that achieve complete remission survive significantly longer than those that have a partial remission. It is more beneficial to maintain a first remission than to try to

attempt a second remission (Theilen and Madewell, 1979; MacEwen, 1980). *Chemoimmunotherapy* appears to hold considerable promise for treatment of canine lymphoma (Crow, 1977; Theilen et al., 1977). *Radiotherapy* is of little benefit in canine lymphoma (Johnson, 1969). This may be partially due to the disseminated nature of the disease at presentation, which may preclude the use of this modality. Solitary lesions may be effectively treated with radiation.

FELINE LYMPHOMA. *Chemotherapy* has been established as a therapy in man and dog, and the programs used for cats have been derived from these experiences. *Radiotherapy* is successful in solitary lesions but is precluded as a treatment when lymphoma is generalized.

Hodgkin's-Like Disease

Hodgkin's disease is a lymphoproliferative disorder that is thought to represent a neoplastic proliferation of malignant cells, called Reed-Sternberg cells (Fig. 79–29). The disease may be provoked by or be a response to an underlying immune derangement or infectious process (Arseneau and Rosenthal, 1980). The diagnostic Reed-Sternberg cell is one with a deeply lobulated nucleus that gives the impression of two or more separate nuclei, or sometimes true multiple nuclei. A characteristic feature is that nucleoli are large, "inclusion-like," and acidophilic (Moulton and Dungworth, 1978; Wells, 1974). True Hodgkin's-like lesions occur rarely in the dog (Hoerni et al., 1970). The distribution of Hodgkin's-like lesions in the dog has included lymph nodes of the neck, inguinal and pelvic areas, mesentery, anterior mediastinum, and prescapular regions.

Malignant Histiocytosis

Malignant histiocytosis (formerly named histiocytic medullary reticulosis) is a disorder characterized by phagocytosis of red cells by malignant histiocytes (Scott et al., 1979; Madewell and Feldman, 1980) (Fig. 79–30). *Histiocytic leukemia* and *reticulum cell leukemia* are terms used synonymously or to indicate variants of the disorder (Rappaport, 1966). The disease is characterized by a systemic, progressive, invasive proliferation of morphologically atypical histiocytes

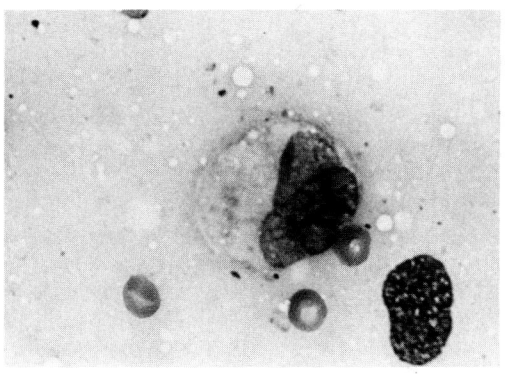

Figure 79–29. Reed-Sternberg-like cell in a lymph node aspirate. The nucleus appears to be made up of several distinct nuclei. Such cells are very large and have irregular nuclei which are often multiply lobulated. (×1400.)

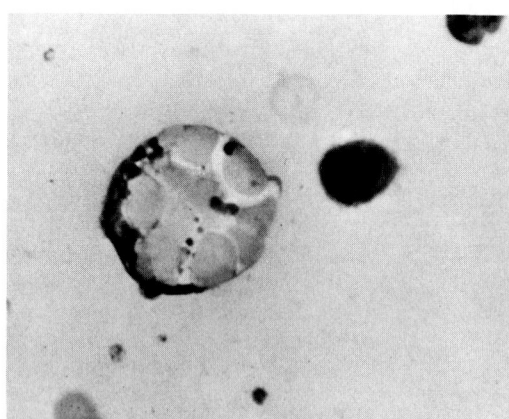

Figure 79–30. Extensive phagocytosis of erythrocytes in a histiocytic cell of malignant histiocytosis. The nucleus of the cell has been flattened against the cell membrane by the erythrocytes. (×1400.)

or their precursors. Hemogram findings include anemia, thrombocytopenia, and occasionally leukopenia. There may be poikilocytosis. Abnormal or immature histiocytes are found on bone marrow smears and occasionally on blood smears. A leukemic blood profile is rare. The histiocytes have abundant pale blue, foamy cytoplasm that is irregular in outline. The cytoplasm may be vacuolated and contain sudanophilic material. The nuclei have lacelike chromatin that is coarser than that of leukemic monocytoid cells, and a distinct nucleolus usually is present (Rappaport, 1966).

Malignant histiocytosis is characterized microscopically by multifocal proliferation of histiocytes or precursors of histiocytes in the spleen, liver, lymph nodes, and bone marrow. The neoplastic cells may contain phagocytized red cells, white cells, pyknotic material, hemosiderin, and fat. In addition to histiocytes, smaller, nonphagocytizing cells with less cytoplasm also proliferate; these cells may be prohistiocytes (Marshall, 1956). Malignant histiocytosis has been described in the dog (Schalm, 1978; Scott et al., 1979).

Mycosis Fungoides and Sézary Syndrome

Mycosis fungoides is a chronic lymphoproliferative disorder arising in the skin. The disease generally evolves in three distinct stages: the premycotic phase, early skin infiltration with plaquelike involvement, and finally the development of skin nodules

(Epstein et al., 1972; Shadduck, 1979; Ihrke, 1979; Miller, 1980; Rosenthal and Arseneau, 1980).

Sézary syndrome is a variant of mycosis fungoides. In this disorder, the skin is involved with a generalized exfoliative erythroderma and the blood contains numerous abnormal monocytoid cells identical to those involving the skin and tissues in mycosis fungoides. Sézary syndrome can be thought of as the leukemic phase of mycosis fungoides (Lutzner et al., 1975).

LYMPHANGIECTASIA

Intestinal lymphangiectasia is a nonspecific abnormality of the lymphatics that results in their obstruction (Mattheeuws et al., 1974). It may be present at birth or it may be acquired later in life. In congenital lymphangiectasia, lymph flow is in stasis because there is an insufficient number of lymphatic vessels to remove interstitial fluid. The stasis that appears in adult animals is usually caused by obstructive lesions developing throughout the lymphatics. The obstruction is usually caused by granulomatous lesions within and around the lymphatics. It has been suggested that acquired lymphangiectasia develops in dogs with lymphatics that are incompletely developed from birth (Strombeck, 1979). Lymphatic hypertension appears during digestion and absorption, when lymph flow is maximum, causing lipids to diffuse from lymph vessels. Lipids are foreign and irritating to interstitial structures. Irritation by the unphagocytized lipids stimulates granuloma formation, and clinical signs of lymphangiectasia appear when lymph flow is reduced even further. The stasis causes increased lymphatic hypertension and interstitial fluid leakage into the abdominal cavity and intestinal lumen. Hypoproteinemia develops because the lost fluids contain plasma proteins, and losses are faster than hepatic synthesis. Lymphangiectasia can be differentiated from other causes of protein loss on the basis of reduced numbers of lymphocytes in the hemogram. The lymphatic obstruction causes loss of lymphocytes into the intestine. T lymphocytes are lost into the intestinal lumen. The loss of large numbers of T lymphocytes leaves the animal with a deficiency in the cellular immune response. Thus, the animal with lymphangiectasia has lymphopenia, hypoproteinemia, and immunologic deficiency (Munro, 1974).

Clinical Findings. Diarrhea may be observed long before signs of hypoproteinemia. Nutritional deficiency is often associated with weight loss and changes in skin and haircoat. When hypoproteinemia is marked, ascites and dependent edema appear. Lymphangiectasia is often severe enough to cause ascites and edema in some of the cases when there is no clinical evidence for diarrhea or malabsorption. The absence of diarrhea does not rule out lymphangiectasia.

Laboratory Findings. Hemograms and blood chemistries identify hypoproteinemia. Edema and ascites appear variably when plasma albumin decreases below 1.5 gm/dl. Total proteins decrease (as albumin decreases so does the globulin fraction). When hepatic disease and renal disease are ruled out, intramural intestinal disease must be ruled out as the cause of the hypoproteinemia. In lymphangiectasia, fecal examination for parasites and maldigestion are negative, while fecal fat excretion is increased. Fat malabsorption is a constant feature of lymphangiectasia, since the transport of chylomicrons through lymphatics is impaired. Hypocalcemia is sometimes found, since serum calcium is partially bound to serum albumin and their levels change in parallel. Anemia due to iron deficiency caused by absorptive failure is sometimes apparent (Strombeck, 1979).

Diagnosis and Management. Protein-losing enteropathy is diagnosed when hypoproteinemia is found not to be due to renal disease, malnutrition, or chronic hepatic disease. Diagnosis is confirmed on biopsy of the gastric or small intestinal mucosa. The medical management of lymphangiectasia is considered in Chapter 58, Diseases of the Small Bowel.

SYSTEMIC MASTOCYTOSIS

Mastocytosis is considered here for the sake of completeness, though it does not fit neatly into any classification of lymphoreticular disease (Carr et al., 1977). Mastocytosis, an abnormal proliferation of tissue mast cells, involves skin, lymph nodes, viscera, bones, and the entire monocyte-macrophage system (RES). Histologically, the typi-cal cells of mastocytosis differ from normal mast cells (Gonella, 1967) in that they may contain several nuclei of bizarre shapes and the cytoplasmic granules may vary in size, number, and distribution (Figure 79–15). In addition to the many mast cells, the lesions nearly always contain numerous eosinophils.

Lymph node involvement may be regional or generalized (Havard and Scott, 1959). Hepatosplenomegaly occurs with widespread mast cell infiltration of the Monocyte-macrophage system. Skin changes may occur as successive urticarial eruptions followed by persistent pigmented lesions. Ulcers also occur and hematologic changes are common. Anemia, leukopenia, monocytosis, thrombocytopenia, bleeding, diatheses, and mast cell leukemia have all been described in the cat (Garner and Lingeman, 1970; Gilmore and Holzworth, 1971; Schalm et al., 1975). Feline cutaneous mastocytoma occurs in various regions in the body (Holzinger, 1973). These diseases may be progressive and fatal. Corticosteroid therapy may give temporary benefit, but antimitotic drugs and radiotherapy have not proven helpful.

METASTATIC TUMORS

Lymph nodes may be the site of metastasis of many tumors. The regional nodes are first involved, but generalized lymphadenopathy can occur later. Cytologic and histologic examination may be diagnostic. Excision of localized tumors should be attempted. Radiation therapy of tumors may be helpful, depending upon the sensitivity of the tumor and the extent of involvement. The cytology of a few neoplastic lesions involving the nodes is briefly described in Figures 79–17 through 79–22.

THE SPLEEN

INTRODUCTION

Existence of monocyte-macrophage (reticuloendothelial-RES) system has, for the most part, been a rather nebulous concept. One reason for this confusion is that cellular components of the monocyte-macrophage system are so widely scattered, so diverse in their structural elements, and so pleomorphic that a confusion of terms and concepts concerning their morphology and function exists. These cells include macrophages lining the sinuses of various organs, microglia, macrophages of lymphatic tissue, and specialized cells in the liver (Kupffer's cells), spleen, and bone marrow. The following functions are attributed to the monocyte-macrophage system:

1. Immune responses–antibody formation, cell and humorally mediated responses.

2. Phagocytosis (and sometimes killing) of bacteria and other microorganisms and phagocytosis of foreign particles.

3. Filtration of blood and extravascular fluids and removal of cells, damaged cells, or cells coated with antibody.

4. Hematopoiesis and replenishment of stem cell compartment.

The spleen contains macrophages (the so-called RE cells), lymphocytes, and plasma cells. Its primary functions are to filter blood, to form antibodies, and to serve as a stem cell compartment. The spleen is not essential to life. Enlargement of the spleen is usually, but not always, accompanied by signs of disease. In most instances, splenomegaly is a result of underlying disease such as leukemia, lymphoma (Fig. 79–31), or infection. Therefore it is not, in itself, a cause of disease but rather an accessory finding. Splenectomy is performed because of splenomegaly, because of an obscure hemolytic anemia or thrombocytopenia, because of splenic rupture, or because of splenic hemangiomas and hemangiosarcomas (Figs. 79–32 and 79–33).

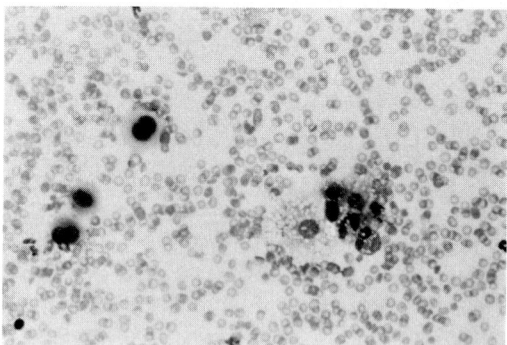

Figure 79–32

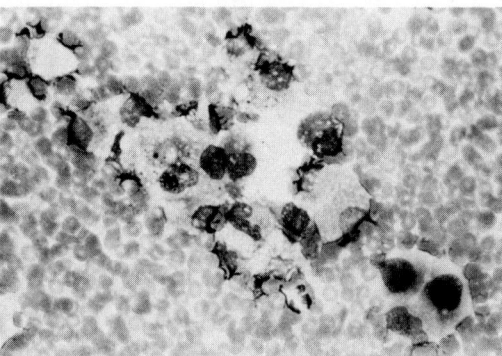

Figure 79–33

Figures 79–32 and 79–33. Aspirates from the abdomen of two dogs having splenic hemangiosarcoma showing large size and variation in morphology. Figure 79–32 shows an aggregate of large pleomorphic cells. (×350.) The vacuolated cells in Figure 79–33 are very large and some contain pigment. Cells of these types appear similar to transformed mesothelial cells or macrophages except they are larger. (×560.) Cells with multiple nuclei are occasionally seen in aspirates of hemangiosarcomas. (×1400.)

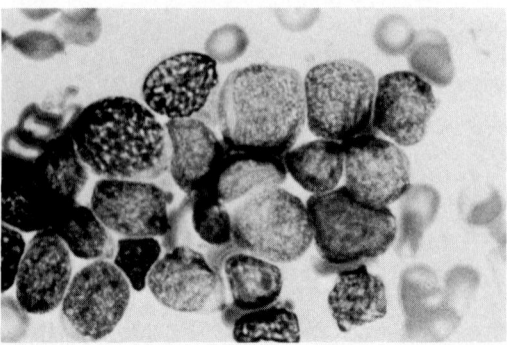

Figure 79–31. Lymphoma of the spleen showing a population of immature lymphoid cells. The cells vary in size and chromatin pattern. Molding and crowding is evident. Several cells contain indistinct nucleoli. (×1400.)

THE STRUCTURE OF THE NORMAL SPLEEN

The spleen consists of a capsule and trabeculae enclosing a pulp. The pulp is divided into four zones: the white pulp, a marginal zone, the ellipsoids, and the red pulp. The spleen of dogs and cats is relatively large, rich in trabeculae and smooth muscle, and poor in white pulp. The white pulp is immunologically competent because it sequesters lymphocytes, macrophages, and antigens and permits them to interact. The red pulp stores and tests the viability of red cells, granulocytes, and platelets (Weiss and Blue, 1980). The dog spleen has the unusual capacity to become engorged with blood during sleep or anesthesia and, in some cases, increase in weight several times greater than normal. The dog spleen also has a muscular capsule that is capable of contraction. Thus, the canine spleen can both sequester large numbers of circulating cells of all types and spill these same cells back into the bloodstream upon contraction.

A system of vascular sinuses drains into major veins in the dog. There is a very scanty sinusoidal system in the cat. Splenic cords are sometimes referred to as pulp spaces. Within the interstices of vessels are a variety of cells, including lymphocytes, macrophages, and plasma cells. Blood flows through the spleen via the splenic artery, which penetrates the splenic capsule at the hilar notch in the medial aspect of the organ. The artery then branches within the trabeculae in company with veins and with efferent lymphatics. The trabecular arteries enter the periarterial sheaths as central arteries, which empty in the cords. Virtually all the arterial blood cells then pass between lining cells and also through the basement membrane into the pulp veins or sinuses. The phagocytic function of the spleen is extremely efficient, since red blood cells can move only slowly among the interstices of the pulp and therefore come into contact with macrophages. There is a second type of blood flow in which blood passes quite rapidly through the pulp into the splenic veins. The normal circuit through the spleen is rapid. However, when the spleen is enlarged because of an accumulation of cells in the splenic cords, pooling of blood and subsequent slow passage occurs through the spleen. This leads to "conditioning" of the cells, causing membrane changes that may lead to premature cell death.

Relation of the Spleen to Erythrocytes

Sequestration Without Erythrocyte Destruction. More than ten per cent of the total red cell mass of a dog or cat can be held in the red pulp spaces of a relaxed spleen, to be injected into the circulation as a concentrated mass by contractions of the muscular capsule (Barcroft and Florey, 1928) and trabeculae, in response to adrenergic stimulation.

Reticulocytes are selectively trapped and held in the normal spleen, where they com-plete their maturation following release from the bone marrow. Certain maturational events are dependent on a normally functioning spleen. One such event is surface remodeling, during which reticulocytes lose surface area without a concurrent decrease in volume. Since the number of target cells and cells bearing Howell-Jolly bodies increases in peripheral blood after splenectomy, it is likely that the spleen removes such cells and cell structures.

Sequestration With Erythrocyte Destruction. Splenic arterioles have a few direct branches leading to the venous system, but most terminal arterioles open into the splenic cords. Blood cells pass from the cords to the pulp through slits in the sinus or endothelial walls. Blood cells must squeeze between the spaces, which are lined with reticular fibers, and between adventitial cells found outside the spaces. Macrophages are found in large numbers in these areas. There is repeated intimate contact of blood cells with these macrophages.

Blood flow in the congested spleen is slow. The pH and Po_2 fall, glucose is consumed, and metabolism is impaired. The intrasplenic hematocrit may increase, producing increased viscosity and resistance to flow. The net result is metabolic and mechanical stress to the blood cells in the presence of macrophages and other leukocytes that have the capacity to recognize membrane damage. Phagocytes remove defective areas on the cells' surface, transforming the biconcave erythrocytes into rigid spherocytes or red cell fragments, which are trapped and removed by other phagocytes.

In certain diseases affecting either the red cells or the spleen, large numbers of red cells as well as platelets and leukocytes are trapped within the red pulp. Red cells with abnormalities resulting in loss of deformability (spherocytes, Heinz bodies, *Hemobartonella*, antibody coating) will be pooled in a normal spleen and normal red cells may be trapped in abnormal spleens. Trapped red cells undergo prolonged exposure to conditions attending stasis, resulting in shortened red cell survival (Weiss and Blue, 1980).

In summary, red cells encounter their first obstacle in the terminal arterioles. Abnormal cells such as spherocytes or even normal but aged cells, are mechanically fragile and tend to fragment. Exposure to macrophages with concurrent hyperviscosity and low oxygen tension makes the cells less fluid, less deformable. Increased osmotic fragility results from decreased adenosine triphosphate production (from lack of glucose) and increased lactic acid accumulation (dropping pH). Phagocytes have, in addition, receptors for portions of immunoglobulin molecules, which, if attached to red cells, increase the chance of cell phagocytosis (Schrier, 1980).

Relation of the Spleen to Platelets

Sequestration Without Premature Destruction. Platelet concentration in the circulation is due to an equilibrium between the production of platelets in the bone marrow and the destruction of platelets caused by aging somewhere in the periphery of the body. Decreases in platelet numbers can occur as the result of decreased bone marrow production, increased peripheral destruction, or splenic sequestration. The process of sequestration can be accelerated beyond the marrow's capacity to compensate when there is increased blood flow to the spleen, such as that which occurs in diffuse hepatic disease, or congestion due to cardiac disease. Splenic pooling causes an increased proportion of platelets to be sequestered in the spleen. This may result in the decreased concentration of platelets in the general circulation. In many conditions associated with increased splenic pooling there is some reduction in platelet survival and also some impairment in platelet production, both of which contribute to thrombocytopenia.

Sequestration With Increased Platelet Destruction. The spleen may play a major role in destroying platelets in certain diseases. The most common and best studied entity in this category is immune thrombocytopenia. Three forms of immune thrombocytopenia are recognized clinically. The first is chronic immune thrombocytopenia, the second is acute thrombocytopenia, and the third is drug-induced immune thrombocytopenia.

Chronic immune thrombocytopenia is usually unaccompanied by other disease but is also seen in association with systemic lupus erythematosus and chronic lymphocytic leukemia. In this disorder the platelets are sensitized by platelet antibodies. These antibodies are autoantibodies. They coat the platelets and sensitize them so that they are destroyed by the monocyte-macrophage system. Lightly sensitized platelets are destroyed mainly in the spleen, while very heavily sensitized platelets are destroyed in the liver and in other phagocytic tissues throughout the body.

The treatment of chronic immune thrombocytopenia is aimed at reducing the rate of destruction of the sensitized platelets by the spleen and the remainder of the monocyte-macrophage system. Immunosuppressive drug therapy such as cyclophosphamide or corticosteroids acts by decreasing the titer of circulating autoantibody. This effect may be due, in part, to inhibition of immunoglobulin synthesis or increased immunoglobulin catabolism. Splenectomy relieves thrombocytopenia by removing the principal site of destruction of sensitized platelets. Corticosteroids also decrease the speed of removal of sensitized platelets by the spleen (Hirsh and Brain, 1979).

Acute thrombocytopenia is usually self-limiting (Hirsh and Brain, 1979). This mechanism of thrombocytopenia is less well understood than the chronic immune thrombocytopenic states. In a number of cases there is a preceding infection, and it may well be that the thrombocytopenia represents an immune reaction to the infection. Alternatively, it is possible that platelets are destroyed as a result of interaction with the antigen/antibody complex that forms about seven to ten days after any acute viral or bacterial infection (Champion, 1980).

An immune reaction with destruction of platelets in the peripheral blood is occasionally seen after the ingestion of certain drugs. It is likely that in most cases the drug combines with a plasma protein to form an antigen, which results in antibody formation. When the drug is readministered, the antibody combines with the antigen to form an immune complex that is adsorbed on to the platelet surface. This platelet-hapten-antibody complex is destroyed in the spleen.

Relation of the Spleen to Granulocytes

In dogs, the circulating granulocyte count is dramatically increased and sometimes doubled following injection of epinephrine (Raab, 1974). This is because of the contractile nature of the canine spleen and the fact that it is a portion of the marginal granulocyte pool that is affected by exercise or epinephrine.

The role of the spleen in leukopenia has not been clearly defined. Some patients with splenomegaly exhibit an increased rate of disappearance of granulocytes from circulation when they are measured with a radioactive label (Raab, 1964). Recent evidence suggests that the spleen is the major site of removal of neutrophils that have not migrated into tissues (Henry and Goldman, 1975).

SPLENIC CYTOLOGY

Biopsy of the spleen is indicated to determine the cause of clinically significant splenomegaly that *cannot* be determined by clinical examination, radiography, or laboratory procedures. Diseases most commonly diagnosed with the aid of spleen biopsy are extranodal lymphomas, myelogenous leukemias, and leiomyosarcomas. The suspected presence of splenic hemangiosarcoma is an absolute contraindication for splenic biopsy, owing to predisposition of this tumor to metastasize. Other contraindications are the tendency for the spleen to hemorrhage or the inability to localize the spleen by palpation or radiography (Osborne et al., 1974).

The Standard Cytologic Picture. Splenic aspirates are always rich in blood and may appear like ordinary blood smears to the naked eye. The tissue found in the smears consists of two main components: lymphoid cells and cells from the red pulp. The lymphoid cells are usually concentrated in dense aggregates that spread patchily over the smear. These cells can represent normal or abnormal types of lymphoid tissue described in the section on lymph node cytology. Typically in spleen aspirates, lymphoid cells are less dominant and tissue-bound phagocytes or macrophages more prominent than in material from lymph nodes (Soderstrom, 1966).

The red pulp is the source of the greater part of the biopsy material. Its contribution to the biopsy material embraces all types of peripheral blood cells, endothelial cells, tissue-bound phagocytes, and monocytoid cells.

Extremely large and dense platelet aggregates are usually seen at the periphery of smears. Their presence is strongly suggestive of a splenic aspirate. Splenic sinus endothelial cells are called "stave cells" by Soderstrom (1966) because of the two long, ribbon-shaped projections that continue the cytoplasm in opposite directions. Stave cells are specific to spleen aspirates.

Active phagocytes may be scarce in spleen aspirates though tissue bound phagocytes may be conspicuous in some cases. Single biopsies if inconclusive, should be repeated. Cytologically, diagnostic findings are by no means expected in all cases of splenomegaly.

Stem Cell Reactions. Basophilic stem cell reactions, often with conspicuous plasmacytosis, are especially common in splenic lupus erythematosus, in chronic hepatitis, and in hemolytic conditions.

Infectious Reactions. Reactions to infections are rarely noted in splenic aspirates and are often associated with granulomatous diseases. Increased numbers of monocytoid cells in combination with numerous neutrophilic leukocytes is a nonspecific reaction. It may be seen in infections as well as in a potpourri of other conditions.

Lymphomas. The spleen is rarely the primary site of lymphoma but is often a secondary site. In untreated terminal lymphoma the spleen may be very large and show nodular or diffuse infiltration. Lymphomas may be found in splenic aspirates (Fig. 79–31). Mature lymphoid cells all over the smear is more typical of lymphatic leukemia and is striking in the extreme monotony of the type of cells. When the lymphoid cell type shifts to a high percentage of lymphoblasts, lymphoma is the most probable diagnosis. Lymphoma, histiocytic type may be diagnosed from splenic aspirates.

Myeloid Metaplasia (Extramedullary Hematopoieses). A few myelocytes, erythroid precursors, and megakaryocytes may be found in many types of splenic reactions. Massive myeloid metaplasia (in which ordinary spleen cells are difficult to find among the bone marrow–like cells) is the typical finding in chronic myelogenous leukemia and in myelosclerosis. Soderstrom (1966) regards the scarcity of megakaryocytes in splenic aspirates in leukemia and the rich occurrence of these cells in myelosclerosis as a diagnostic clue. The liver may also be involved in massive myeloid metaplasia.

Hemolytic Anemias. Spleen aspirates may be nearly normal or present different degrees of extramedullary hemopoiesis. If the hemolytic anemia is longstanding, red cell precursors are often crowded together by nests of phagocytes and numerous basophilic stem cells.

Metastatic Cancer. Metastatic cancer of the spleen is rare. Cancer cells in splenic aspirates usually indicate that the palpable structure that was aspirated was not spleen but tumor. These tumors arise from endothelial tissue. They are more frequent in dogs and may be found in the spleen, liver, heart, and lungs (Theilen and Madewell, 1979). Hemangiosarcoma may be primary or metastatic. The cells of the hemangiosarcoma have indistinct cytoplasmic borders and usually round nuclei. Nuclear pleomorphism may be prominent (Perman et al., 1979) (Figs. 79–32 and 79–33).

SPLENOMEGALY

Hematologic examination should be undertaken when splenomegaly is found unexpectedly on physical examination or during radiologic procedures. The workup of a patient with splenomegaly requires the exercise of careful judgment. The examination can be limited to a history, physical examination, and hemogram or can be extended to the full panoply of modern medicine. Several considerations can be used to guide the extent of the evaluation. It is most important to identify treatable disease precisely and promptly. Infectious causes of splenomegaly must be the focus of such examination. A list of diagnostic possibilities may be found in Table 79–8. In considering the differential diagnosis, the focus should be on history, physical examination, and the blood smear. The clinical exploration includes a survey of recent trauma, recent infections, and joint involvement. Physical examination includes a search for lymphadenopathy. The blood count, reticulocyte count, and peripheral smear provide useful information. The presence of abnormal red cells with reticulocytosis establishes the likely diagnosis of hemolytic anemia or tumor induced malfunction of the spleen. Reactive lymphocytosis focuses on infections. Occasionally leukemia may be diagnosed on the smear (Table 79–9).

SPLENIC RUPTURE

Splenic rupture is a common reason for splenectomy. A normal spleen does not rupture spontaneously but requires considerable trauma. Little trauma may rupture an enlarged spleen, or it may rupture spontaneously with overassiduous palpation. There may or may not be massive intraperitoneal hemorrhage. Paracentesis revealing frank blood may be diagnostic when coupled with decreased hematocrit and lowered total plasma proteins. Shock is an almost invariable component of splenic rupture. Splenic rupture is an emergency requiring surgery and multiple transfusions.

Table 79–8. Mechanisms of Splenic Enlargement and Hypersplenism

Etiology	Mechanism	Disease

Functional	RE hyperplasia or hyperfunction	Hemolytic anemias
		    Immune hemolytic anemia
		    Pyruvate kinase deficiency
		Infection
		    Endocarditis
		    Hepatitis
		Collagen disease
		    Lupus erythematosus

Vascular	Portal hypertension	Cirrhosis Diffusion hepatic disease Chronic active hepatitis
Hemopoietic	Extramedullary hemopoiesis	Myelofibrosis Other myeloproliferative disease
Neoplasm	Malignant proliferations	Acute and chronic leukemias Lymphomas Hemangioma Hemangiosarcoma

Table 79–9. Hemogram Findings Following Splenectomy or With a Nonfunctional Spleen (Tumor Involvement)

Red cells	Increased poikilocytes
	Increased macrocytic reticulocytes
	Increased reticulocytes
	Howell-Jolly bodies
	Heinz bodies
	Increased nucleated red cells
White cells	Increased proportion of 'toxic' granulocytes
	Monocytosis
	Left shift to myelocytes
Platelets	Increased platelet numbers
	Increased megathrombocytes

ACCESSORY SPLEENS

Accessory spleens varying from single nodules to multiple nodules are occasionally found in the small and large intestinal mesentery. They are histologically and functionally similar to the main organ. Occasionally patients who have responded to splenectomy for immune thrombocytopenia or hemolytic anemia have relapses attributable to the presence of accessory spleens.

HYPERSPLENISM

Hypersplenism is defined as reduction in one or more cellular elements in blood associated with splenomegaly and corrected by splenectomy. Clinical signs are referable to the cell line(s) that are depleted. This can be dyspnea associated with anemia, infection associated with leukopenia, and hemorrhage associated with thrombocytopenia (Madewell and Feldman, 1980).

Diagnostic Evaluation. Hemogram findings reveal a decrease in one or more cell lines in peripheral blood associated with abnormal or increased production in bone marrow. Splenomegaly is usually determined by physical examination, but in the large or obese animal it must be confirmed by radiologic studies. If splenectomy is being considered, sites of red cell sequestration by radioactive red cell labeling would be highly desirable to establish that splenectomy will be of value. This type of study is no longer confined to the veterinary institu-

tion and is well within the capabilities of veterinary radiology specialty services. Diagnosis of the underlying cause may require liver tests, blood cultures, and splenic aspiration.

Laboratory Studies. Cellular elements are generally sequestered in the following order: red cells, platelets, and white cells. Normocytic normochromic anemia may be present. Modest to severe thrombocytopenia is seen. Leukocytes are decreased, with a normal distribution. Target cells may be seen in liver disease (congestive splenomegaly). Teardrop-shaped red cells and leukoerythroblastosis are noted when splenomegaly is secondary to bone marrow myelofibrosis (myelophthisis). Bone marrow in primary hypersplenism shows moderate hypercellularity with all cell lines maturing normally.

MYELOFIBROSIS (MYELOPHTHISIS)

Myelofibrosis is a myeloproliferative disorder caused by proliferation of fibrous tissue by reticulum cells that gradually obliterate cell production sites in the marrow. *Myelophthisis* implies a reduction of cell-forming elements in the bone marrow. The reduction of marrow activity is associated with extramedullary hemopoiesis in liver and spleen (myeloid metaplasia), which enlarges both. The extremedullary hemopoiesis may be compensatory to the profound cytopenia or may be, in itself, neoplastic. Lymphadenopathy is uncommon.

Laboratory Studies

Hematology. In myelofibrosis, pancytopenia, leukoerythroblastosis, and poikilocytosis are present. Anemia is often severe and normocytic but may be mildly macrocytic because of reticulocytosis. White cell counts vary, being elevated in early stages and decreased in later stages. A marked left shift to progranulocytes and blasts may be seen. The platelet count is unusually diminished, with giant platelets (megathrombocytes) and megakaryocyte fragments present.

Red cell poikilocytosis is marked. Teardrop forms are said to be diagnostic (Maslow et al., 1980). Polychromasia is marked, owing to the reticulocytosis. Many nucleated red cells and immature granulocytes (leukoerythroblastosis) may be present.

Bone Marrow. Dry aspirates are common in myelofibrosis. If particles can be aspirated they are hypercellular. Biopsy shows variable fibrosis with prominant clusters of megakaryocytes and residual islands of erythroid hyperplasia. More than one area should be biopsied to avoid sampling error if the diagnosis is in doubt. Silver stains reveal an increase in interlacing bands of reticulum fibers.

Other Tests. Liver biopsy, like splenic biopsy may reveal extramedullary hemopoiesis.

REFERENCES

Arseneau, J., and Rosenthal, S.: Hodgkin's Disease. *In* Lichtman, M. A. (ed.): Hematology and Oncology. Grune and Stratton, New York, 1980.

Barcroft, J., and Florey, H. W.: Some factors involved in the concentration of blood by the spleen. J. Physiol. *66*:231, 1928.

Bennett, J. M., and Lichtman, M. A.: Chronic Lymphocyte Leukemia. *In* Lichtman, M. A. (ed.): Hematology and Oncology, Grune and Stratton, New York, 1980, p. 177.

Bernier, G. M., and Lichtman, M. A.: Myeloma. *In* Lichtman, M. A. (ed.): Hematology and Oncology. Grune and Stratton, New York, 1980.

Carr, I., Hancock, B. W., Henry, L., and Ward, A. M.: Lymphoreticular disease. Blackwell Scientific Publications, Oxford, 1977.

Champion, L. A. A.: Platelet Disorders. *In* Hartmann, P. (ed.): Hematologic Disorders. Grune and Stratton, New York, 1980.

Cottier, H., Turk, J., and Sobin, C.: A proposal for a standardized system of reporting human lymph node morphology in relation to immunological function. J. Clin. Pathol. *26*:317, 1973.

Crow, S. E., et al.: Chemoimmunotherapy for canine lymphosarcoma. Cancer *40*:2102, 1977.

David, J.: The Organs and Cells of the Immune System. *In* Rubenstein, E., and Federman, D. D. (eds.): Scientific American Medicine. Scientific American, New York, 1980.

Davie, J. V.: Secondary or symptomatic haemolytic anaemias. I. Haemolytic Anaemia Associated with Hodgkin's Disease, Leukemia, Reticulo-sarcoma and Myelosclerosis. *In* The Haemolytic Anaemias, Part III. Churchill, London, 1967.

Deem, D. A., Traver, D. S., Thacker, H. L., and Perrymen, L. E.: Agammaglobulinemia in a horse. J.A.V.M.A. *1975*:469, 1979.

Epstein, E. H., Leven, D. L., and Croft, J. D.: Mycosis fungoides: survival, prognostic features, response to therapy and autopsy findings. Medicine *15*:61, 1972.

Feldman, B. F.: Clinical Pathology of the Liver. *In* Kirk, R.: Current Veterinary Therapy VII. W. B. Saunders Co., Philadelphia, 1980.

Feldman, B. F., and Kaneko, J. J.: The anemia of inflammatory disease in the dog. The nature of the problem. Vet. Res. Comm. *4*:237, 1981 a.

Feldman, B. F., and Kaneko, J.: The anemia of inflammatory disease in the dog. Clinical characterization. Am. J. Vet. Res. *42*:1109, 1981b.

Feldman, B. F., Kaneko, J. J., and Farver, T. B.: The anemia of inflammatory disease in the dog. Ferrokinetics. Am. J. Vet. Res. *42*:583, 1981c.

Feldman, B. F., and O'Neill, S.: Low ionic strength solution (LISS) and papain to detect incomplete antibody in canine hemolytic anemia. J.A.A.H.A. (in press), 1982.

Garner, F. M., and Lingeman, C. H.: Mast-cell neoplasms in the domestic cat. Pathol. Vet. *7*:517, 1970.

Gilmore, C. E., and Holzworth, J.: Naturally occurring feline leukemia: clinical, pathological and differential diagnostic features. J.A.V.M.A., *158*:1013, 1971.

Gonella, J. S.: Mast cell disease. Prog. Clin. Cancer *3*:281, 1967.

Gunz, F. W.: The epidemiology and genetics of the chronic leukemias. Clin. Haematol. *6*:3, 1977.

Han, T., Stutzman, L., and Rogue, A. L.: Bone marrow biopsy in Hodgkin's disease and other neoplastic diseases. J.A.M.A. *217*:1239, 1971.

Harvey, J. W., Terrell, T. G., Hyde, D. M., Jackson, R. I.: Well-differentiated lymphocytic leukemia in a dog: long-term survival without therapy. Vet. Pathol. *18*:37, 1981.

Havard, C. W. H., and Scott, B. R.: Urticaria pigmentosa with visceral and skeletal lesions. Quart. J. Med. *28*:459, 1959.

Heath, H., Weller, R. E., and Mundy, G. R.: Canine lymphosarcoma: a model for study of hypercalcemia of cancer. Calcif. Tissue Int. *30*:127, 1980.

Henry, K., and Goldman, J. M.: *In* The lymphocyte. Harrison, C. V., and Weinbren, K. (eds.): Recent Advances in Pathology. Churchill Livingston, Edinburgh, 1975.

Hirsh, J., and Brain, E. A.: Hemostasis and thrombosis. Churchill Livingstone, New York, 1979.

Hoerni, B., Legrand, E., and Chauvergne, J.: Les réticulopathies animales de type hodgkinien. Leur intérêt pour l'étude de la maladie humaine. Bull. Canc. (Paris) *57*:37, 1970.

Holzinger, E. A.: Feline cutaneous mastocytomas. Cornell Vet. *63*:87, 1973.

Holzworth, J.: Leukemia and related neoplasms in the cat. I. Lymphoid malignancies. J.A.V.M.A. *136*:47, 1960.

Ihrke, P.: Canine seborrheic disease complex. *In* Muller, G. H. (ed.): Symposium on Skin and Internal Disease. W. B. Saunders Co., Philadelphia. 1979.

Isobe, T., and Osserman, E. F.: Patterns of amyloidosis and their association with plasma cell dyscrasia, monoclonal immunoglobulins, and Bence Jones proteins. N. Eng. J. Med. *290*:473, 1974.

Johnson, R. E., et al.: Comparative, clinical, histologic and radiotherapeutic aspects of canine and human malignant lymphoma. Radiology *93*:395, 1969.

Jones, S. E., and Godden, J. (eds.): Preceedings of the conference on non-Hodgkin's lymphomas. Cancer Treatment Rep. *61*:935, 1977.

Kaufman, L.: Serodiagnosis of Fungal Diseases. *In* Rese, N. R., and Friedman, H. (eds.): Manual of Clinical Immunology. Amer. Soc. Microbiol., Washington, D. C., 1976.

Lichtman, M. A.: Acute Lymphoblastic Leukemia. *In* Lichtman, M. A. (ed.): Hematology and Oncology. Grune and Stratton, New York, 1980.

Lutzner, M., Edelson, R., and Schein, P.: Cutaneous T-cell lymphomas: the Sézary syndrome, mycosis fungoides, and related disorders. Ann. Intern. Med. *83*:534, 1975.

MacEwen, E. G.: Canine Lymphosarcoma. *In* Kirk, R. W. (ed.): Current Veterinary Therapy VII. W. B. Saunders Co., Philadelphia, 1980.

MacEwen, E. G., and Hurvitz, A. I.: Diagnosis and management of monoclonal gammopathies. *In* MacEwen, E. G. (ed.): Clinical Veterinary Oncology. Vet. Clin. North Amer. 7:119, 1977a.

MacEwen, E. G., Patnaik, A. K., and Wilkins, R. J.: Diagnosis and treatment of canine hematopoietic neoplasms. *In* MacEwen, E. G. (ed.): Clinical Veterinary Oncology. Vet. Clin. North Amer. 7:116, 1977b.

Madewell, B. R.: Clinicopathologic aspects of diabetes insipidus in the dog. J.A.A.H.A. *11*:497, 1975.

Madewell, B. R., and Feldman, B. F.: Characterization of anemias associated with neoplasia in small animals. J.A.V.M.A. *176*:419, 1980.

Marshall, A. H. E.: Histiocytic medullary reticulosis. J. Pathol. Bacteriol. *71*:61, 1956.

Maslow, W. L., Beutler, E., Bell, C. A., Hougie, L., and Kieldsberg, C. R.: Hematologic disease. Houghton Mifflin, Boston, 1980.

Mattheeuws, D., DeRick, A., Thoonen, H., and VanderStock, J.: Intestinal lymphangiectasia in a dog. J. Small Anim. Pract. *15*:757, 1974.

Miller, W. H.: Canine Cutaneous Lymphomas. *In* Kirk, R. W. (ed.): Current Veterinary Therapy VII. W. B. Saunders Co., Philadelphia, 1980.

Moore, W. E., and Feldman, B. F.: The use of isoenzymes in small animal medicine. J.A.A.H.A. *10*:420, 1974.

Moulton, J. E., and Dungworth, D. L.: Tumors of the Lymphoid and Hemopoietic Tissues. *In* Moulton, J. E. (ed.): Tumors in Domestic Animals (2nd ed.). University of California Press, Berkeley, 1978.

Munro, D. R.: Rate of protein losing during a model protein losing gastropathy in dogs. Gastroenterology *66*:960, 1974.

Osborne, C. A., Perman, V., and Stevens, J. B.: Needle biopsy of the spleen. *In* Osborne, C. A. (ed.): Biopsy Techniques. Vet. Clin. North Amer. *4*:311, 1974.

Parrott, D. M. V., de Sousa, M. A. B., and East, J.: Thymus-dependent areas in the lymphoid organs of neonatally thymectomized mice. J. Exp. Med. *123*:191, 1966.

Pederson, N. C., and Madewell, B. R.: Feline Leukemia Virus Disease Complex. *In* Kirk, R. W. (ed.): Current Veterinary Therapy VII. W. B. Saunders Co., Philadelphia, 1980.

Perman, V., Alsaker, R. D., and Riis, R. C.: Cytology of Malignant and Nonmalignant Proliferation of Hemic Tissue. *In* Cytology of the Dog and Cat. American Animal Hosp. Assn., South Bend, Indiana, 1979.

Perman, V., Stevens, J. B., Alsaker, R., and Osborne, C.

A.: Lymph node biopsy. Vet. Clin. North Am. *4*:281, 1974.

Priester, W. A.: Canine hemolymphatic neoplasia. Unpublished data, 1972.

Raab, S. O.: The Spleen and the Reticuloendothelial System. *In* Sodeman, W. A., Jr., and Sodeman, W. A. (eds.): Pathologic Pathophysiology. W. B. Saunders Co., Philadelphia, 1974.

Raab, S. O., Athens, J. H., et al.: Granulocytic kinetics in normal dogs. Am. J. Physiol. *200*:83, 1964.

Rappaport, H.: Tumors of the hematopoietic system. Armed Forces Institute of Pathology, Washington, D. C., 1966.

Ree, H., and Fanger, H.: Parocortical alteration in lymphadenopathic and tumor-draining lymph nodes. Histologic study. Hum. Pathol. *6*:363, 1975.

Rosenberg, S. A., Diamond, H. D., Jaslowitz, B., and Craver, L. F.: Lymphosarcoma, a review of 1269 cases. Medicine (Baltimore) *40*:31, 1961.

Rosenthal, S., and Arseneau, J.: Mycosis Fungoides and Sézary Syndrome. *In* Hematology and Oncology. Grune and Stratton, New York, 1980.

Schalm, O. W.: Histiocytic medullary reticulosis. Canine Pract. *5*:42, 1978.

Schalm, O. W., Jain, N. C., and Carroll, E. J.: Veterinary hematology (3rd ed.). Lea and Febiger, Philadelphia, 1975.

Schrier, S.: Hematology. *In* Rubenstein, E. and Federmann, D. P. (eds.): Scientific American Medicine. Scientific American, New York, 1980.

Scott, D. W.: Feline dermatology. J.A.A.H.A. *6*:419, 1980.

Scott, D. W., Miller, W. H., Tasker, J. B., et al.: Lymphoreticular neoplasia in a dog resembling malignant histiocytosis (histiocytic medullary reticulosis) in man. Cornell Vet. *69*:176, 1979.

Shadduck, J. A.: A Canine Cutaneous Lymphoproliferative Disorder Resembling Human Mycosis Fungoides. *In* Muller, G. H. (ed.): Symposium on Skin and Internal Disease. W. B. Saunders Co., Philadelphia, 1979.

Simone, J. V.: Acute leukemia. Clin. Haematol. 7:224, 1978.

Soderstrom, N.: Fine Needle Aspiration Biopsy. Grune and Stratton, New York, 1966.

Strombeck, D. R.: Small Animal Gastroenterology. Stonegate Publishing Co., Davis, Calif., 1979.

Theilen, G. H., and Madewell, B. R.: Leukemia-Sarcoma Disease Complex. *In* Theilen, G. H., and Madewell, B. R. (eds.): Veterinary Cancer Medicine. Lea and Febiger, Philadelphia, 1979.

Theilen, G. H., Worley, M., and Benjamini, E.: Chemoimmunotherapy for canine lymphosarcoma. J.A.VM.A. *170*:607, 1977.

Webster, A. D. B.: Immunodeficiency. Medicine (London) *29*:1707, 1974.

Weiss, L.: The Anatomy of Lymph Nodes. *In* Lichtman, M. A. (ed.): Hematology and Oncology. Grune and Stratton, New York, 1980.

Weiss, L., and Blue, J.: Anatomy of the Spleen. *In* Lichtman, M. A. (ed.): Hematology and Oncology. Grune and Stratton, New York, 1980.

Weller, R. E., Holmberg, C. A., Theilen, G. H., and Madewell, B. R.: Histologic classification as a prognostic criterion for canine lymphosarcoma. Am. J. Vet. Res. *141*:1310, 1980.

Wells, G. A. H.: Hodgkin's disease-like lesions in the dog. J. Pathol. *112*:5, 1974.

Werner, L. L.: Coomb's positive anemias in the dog and the cat. Comp. Cont. Educ. *2*:96, 1980.

Widmann, F. J.: Pathobiology, How Disease Happens. Little Brown and Co., Boston, Mass., 1978.

Wiltshaw, E.: The natural history of extramedullary plasmacytoma and its relationship to solitary myeloma of bone and myelomatosis. Medicine *55*:217, 1976.

Zinkl, J. G., and Keeton, K. S.: Lymph node cytology. I. Cytology of normal lymph nodes. Cal. Vet. *33(1)*:9, 1979a.

Zinkl, J. G., and Keeton, K. S.: Lymph node cytology. II. Cytology of reactive and purulent lymph nodes. Cal. Vet. *33(4)*:6, 1979b.

Zinkl, J. G., and Keeton, K. S.: Lymph node cytology. III. Neoplasia. Cal. Vet. *35(5)*:20, 1981.

CHAPTER **80**

Bleeding Disorders

R. A. GREEN

INTRODUCTION

Hemostasis is the physiologic process that minimizes extravascular blood loss. It is achieved by complex interrelationships between blood flow, vascular endothelium, platelets, and coagulation factors. An appreciation for the pathophysiology of hemostasis is essential for accurate laboratory evaluation, therapy, and prognosis of bleeding patients. Intense investigation into the hemostatic problems of man in recent years has led to an ever widening spectrum of new laboratory approaches and insights into the mechanisms underlying both hemorrhagic and thrombotic disorders. With the knowledge explosion in this field, a variety of new laboratory techniques have become available in veterinary medicine, and subsequently, useful animal models have been confirmed for nearly all the inherited and acquired hemostatic defects of man. Some laboratory tests, however, are available only in laboratories specializing in coagulation research, and consultation is often required in the evaluation of the patient with an atypical or rare bleeding disorder. In this chapter the more common bleeding disorders of dogs and cats will be reviewed with reference to their underlying pathophysiology, laboratory evaluation, and therapy.

Emphasis is placed on those procedures or techniques frequently used by practicing veterinarians in evaluating hemostatic disorders.

THE PHYSIOLOGY OF HEMOSTASIS

THE PLATELET PLUG FORMATION

Formation of the platelet plug following vascular injury is the major physiologic mechanism involved in hemostasis (Fig. 80–1). Immediately following blood vessel injury, blood loss is minimized by local reflex vasoconstriction, which diverts blood flow away from the area of injury. Subendothelial collagen exposure results in platelet adhesion and local release of potent, short-lived biochemical substances that maintain vasoconstriction and further the accumulation of a large mass of aggregated platelets. This complex forms the loose primary platelet plug and is usually sufficient to temporarily arrest bleeding. Simultaneously, activation of the coagulation cascades results in thrombin production and ultimately fibrin formation, which reinforces the primary platelet plug and thereby forms the definitive hemostatic plug. As vasoconstriction diminishes, the definitive hemostatic plug has sufficient stability to maintain hemostasis.

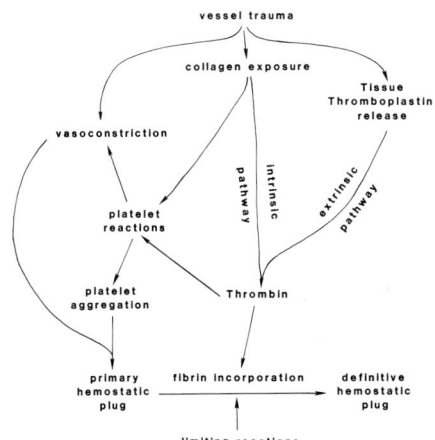

Figure 80–1. Interrelationships of the normal hemostatic mechanism.

The relative importance of vasoconstriction versus hemostatic plug formation depends on the size of the vessel. Although vasoconstriction plays an important role in limiting initial blood loss, the role of the hemostatic plug is more important in sealing the vascular defect of larger vessels. By 24 to 48 hours, the platelets of the hemostatic plug have undergone autolysis and have been replaced by a dense fibrin mass. This mass is slowly digested by the fibrinolytic system, and the vascular defect is covered by endothelial cell proliferation (Sixma and Wester, 1977).

The physiologic responses normally restricting the growth of the hemostatic plug to the site of injury are called limiting reactions. Such limiting reactions include dilution of procoagulant substances by blood flow, endothelial production of prostaglandins causing vasodilatation and inhibition of platelet aggregation, and local inactivation of coagulation factors by natural inhibitors, such as antithrombin III. When these limiting reactions are superimposed on platelet dysfunction or poor fibrin generation, defective hemostasis results.

The Coagulation Cascades

The generation of fibrin occurs by sequential enzymatic activation of coagulation factors occurring as inactive precursor proteins in plasma (Fig. 80–2). Most coagulation factors are synthesized by the liver. Factor VIII is an exception in that endothelial cells are primarily involved in its synthesis. The biologic half-lives of canine coagulation factors appear slightly shorter than those reported for man. In general, the half-lives can be divided into three groups: factor VII with a half-life of four to six hours; factors V, VIII, IX, and X, with half-lives ranging from 0.5 to 1 day; and factors I, II, XI, and XII with half-lives ranging from 1.7 to 3 days. Vitamin K is required for hepatic synthesis of factors II, VII, IX, and X. Little is known about the regulatory mechanisms modulating hepatic synthesis of coagulation factors. Activated coagulation factors (designated by subscript a) that are formed in excess during the coagulation process are rapidly cleared from circulation by the liver.

Factors XII, XI, X, IX, VII, and II have an amino acid, serine, at their active enzymatic site and therefore are called serine proteases. The most important natural inhibitor of coagulation, antithrombin III (AT III), is capable of forming complexes with all serine proteases. Heparin acts as an anticoagulant by markedly enhancing the rate of AT III inhibition of coagulation factors.

The intrinsic coagulation pathway provides a mechanism for fibrin generation initiated by factor XII exposure to subendothelial collagen (*in vivo*) or foreign surfaces (*in vitro*). Two recently discovered factors,

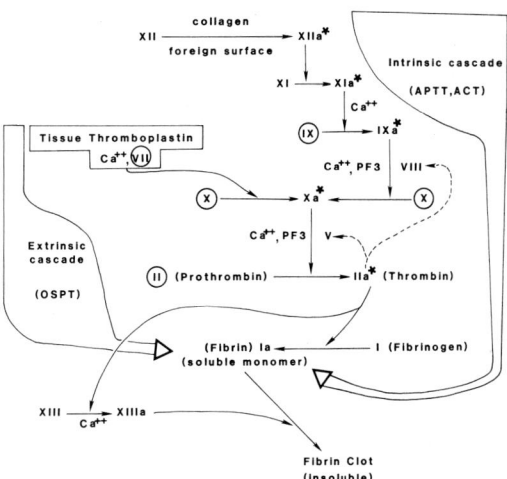

Figure 80–2. Extrinsic and intrinsic coagulation pathways. Circled factors are vitamin K dependent. Subscript a indicates activated form of factor PF3 = platelet phospholipid.

* = sites of antithrombin III inhibition

prekallikrein and high molecular weight kininogen, may play a role by modulating the rate of factor XII activation. In rapid sequence, factor XII_a converts factor XI to XI_a, which converts factor IX to IX_a. Then factor VIII, calcium, platelet phospholipid, and factor IX_a form a complex that converts factor X to X_a. Next, factor X_a with calcium, platelet phospholipid, and factor V convert factor II (prothrombin) to II_a (thrombin). The major role of thrombin is in the conversion of fibrinogen to fibrin; however, it also causes further platelet aggregation, activates factor XIII, potentiates (in trace amounts) factor V and VIII activity, and digests (in high amounts) factor V. Thus, thrombin initially increases and later decreases its own production. The loose fibrin is cross-linked to form a stable fibrin clot by factor XIII_a.

The extrinsic pathway provides an alternate method for factor X activation initiated by a complex interaction between tissue thromboplastin (factor III), calcium, and factor VII. Following production of X_a, the same activation sequence is followed as that given for the intrinsic cascade (the common pathway).

Physiologic fibrinolysis is the process that enzymatically digests the insoluble fibrin clot. Fibrinolysis occurs at a slow rate, which is synchronized with healing of the traumatized tissue. The mediator of fibrinolysis is the serine protease, plasmin, which is formed from an inactive plasma precursor, plasminogen. The rate of plasmin generation is controlled by a delicate balance between plasminogen activators and plasmin inhibitors. Endothelial damage leads to release of plasminogen activator, which in concert with factor XII_a, produces plasmin. Therefore, similar stimuli initiate both clotting and fibrinolysis. In addition to fibrin, other substrates consumed by plasmin include fibrinogen, factor V, and factor VIII. The production of free plasmin in circulation is normally inhibited by a prompt-acting, stable α_2-globulin called antiplasmin. Plasminogen incorporation into the thrombus protects localized plasmin production from circulating antiplasmins. This allows localized fibrin digestion without consumption of circulating fibrinogen and other plasmin substrates (Kwaan, 1977).

PLATELET PRODUCTION AND KINETICS

Platelets are derived from marrow megakaryocytes, which in turn are derived from pleuropotential stem cells similar to other hematopoietic cell lines. The earliest megakaryocyte precursor, the megakaryoblast, is unique, since this cell synthesizes its full complement of DNA before beginning nuclear segmentation and cytoplasmic differentiation. The megakaryoblast also differs from other hematopoietic cells in that it becomes polyploid by repeated nuclear replication within a common cytoplasm (called endomitosis). In most species the ploidy of megakaryocytes can vary from 2 to 128 N, although the majority of megakaryocytes have a ploidy of 8 N or 16 N (Levine et al., 1980). The number of platelets produced per nuclear unit is relatively constant, so the number of the platelets produced per megakaryocyte increases as cell size (or cell ploidy) increases. Although the relationship between ploidy of megakaryocytes and platelet size remains controversial, it is generally accepted that megakaryocytes of lower ploidy produce fewer platelets of larger size and increased density (Tavassoli, 1980; Ebbe, 1979).

Platelet formation commences at the promegakaryocyte stage when specific granules are synthesized in the Golgi region and distributed throughout the cytoplasm. The megakaryocyte's plasma membrane invaginates to form demarcation membranes that define the outer limit of each platelet. Platelet release from the subendothelial marrow megakaryocyte is accomplished by cytoplasmic penetration of endothelial cells. Thus, elongated strands of megakaryocyte cytoplasm, called "proplatelets" extend into the lumen. The mechanism of platelet production from proplatelets is unclear; however, it probably occurs outside the marrow. The finding that more platelets leave the lung than enter it suggests trapping of proplatelets within the pulmonary circulation and subsequent fragmentation at that site. In addition, variable production of platelets can occur from extramedullary distribution of megakaryocytes. Extramedullary megakaryopoiesis is most common in the lung but also may occur in spleen, kidney, liver, and heart tissue. The origin of pulmonary megakaryocytes is thought to be trapping of marrow megakaryocytes that enter the bloodstream. Circulating megakaryocytes may increase in number following surgery, certain forms of neoplasia, and infection.

A poorly characterized humoral substance, called thrombopoietin, is thought to regulate megakaryopoiesis by increasing (1) the rate of megakaryocyte formation from stem cells, (2) the amount of platelet-producing cytoplasm per megakaryocyte, or (3) the rate of cytoplasmic maturation and release of platelets. Thrombopoietin production is assumed to be proportional to platelet count; however, in patients with increased splenic trapping of platelets (hypersplenism) and thrombocytopenia, megakaryopoiesis was proportional to total body platelet mass rather than to the platelet count (Harker, 1974). This has suggested an alternative view that platelet production may be stimulated by a platelet breakdown product released as platelets are destroyed (Ebbe, 1979). Some patients with neoplasia, iron deficiency, immunologic disorders, or chronic inflammation develop platelet counts in excess of 500,000/μl (secondary thrombocytosis). The mechanism of secondary thrombocytosis is unknown but presumably relates to an increased demand for platelets. Rare instances of megakaryocytic neoplasia are observed in animals in which platelet counts exceed $10^6/\mu$l (thrombocythemia or megakaryocytic myelosis). Much remains to be learned about the control of megakaryopoiesis and the role of thrombopoietin in disease states.

In peripheral blood, platelets circulate as tiny discs with an average diameter of about 3 μ, a clear blue peripheral border, and a central area containing azurophilic granules (Wright's strain). The shape of platelets will vary moderately, and this tendency is exaggerated in poorly made blood films or when the smear is not made within 60 minutes of collection. The normal range for platelet count in dogs and cats varies from 2 to 5 × 10^5 and from 3 to 8 × 10^5 platelets/μl, respectively (Schalm et al., 1975). Mature dogs have slightly higher average platelet counts than immature dogs.

Platelet survival has been measured using a variety of radioactive labels (DF^{32}P, ^{14}C-serotonin, ^{51}Cr, and ^{111}In-oxine). Studies with ^{51}Cr-labeled platelets in normal dogs re-vealed an exponential decrease with a ten per cent survival time of 6.8 days (Pierce et al., 1977). When ^{111}In-oxine is used, the sites of destruction and distribution can readily be determined by nuclear medicine imaging techniques. With ^{111}In-oxine, a linear disappearance of platelets was found with a survival time of 124.6 ± 10.5 hr. (Lotter et al., 1980). At zero time about one third of the platelets were located in the spleen and one fifth were found in the liver. These sequestered platelets are in dynamic equilibrium with the peripheral platelet pool, and excitement may induce spurious elevations in platelet count owing to splenic contraction. It is generally assumed that a small percentage of platelets are consumed in "physiologic" hemostasis; however, the spleen is the major site of destruction for senescent platelets. In patients with splenomegaly, splenic platelet sequestration may be markedly increased, resulting in peripheral thrombocytopenia. Platelet turnover can be calculated by dividing the platelet count by the platelet survival time. Therefore, normal platelet turnover in dogs is approximately

$$\frac{300,000/\mu\mathrm{l}}{124.6\ \mathrm{hr}} = 2407\ \mathrm{platelets}/\mu\mathrm{l/hr.}$$

Nuclear medicine studies, particularly with ^{111}In-oxine, appear very promising in attempts to characterize mechanisms of thrombocytopenia, measure responses to therapy, and localize sites of high platelet consumption in spontaneous diseases of animals.

PLATELET FUNCTION

The platelet's central role in hemostasis involves not only its ability to mechanically block the site of vascular injury, but also its provision of a catalytic surface for the coagulation cascade. There are three major platelet reactions: adhesion, release, and aggregation. When platelets are exposed to subendothelial vascular components, such as collagen, the discoid platelets normally adhere to the damaged area and undergo a shape change. Von Willebrand's factor is required for normal platelet adhesion. The adhered platelets release a variety of potent biochemical substances, causing vasoconstriction and furthering platelet aggregation. Greater understanding of the biochemical reactions underlying platelet function has occurred in recent years. During the release reaction, platelets that are adhered to collagen release a variety of chemical mediators including calcium, serotonin, proteolytic enzymes, cationic proteins, and the nucleotide ADP. The released ADP causes other platelets to swell, become "sticky," and adhere to each other. These platelets, in turn, undergo a release reaction, which forms a large platelet syncytium over the area of injury. Another substance playing a central role in platelet function is cyclic AMP. Substances that inhibit aggregation increase platelet cyclic AMP. Prostaglandins produced by endothelial cells, chiefly prostacyclin, stimulate platelet membrane adenylate cyclase, thereby increasing cyclic AMP and inhibiting aggregation. Prostaglandins produced by the platelet, chiefly thromboxane A_2, mobilize calcium from storage sites within the platelet. The mobilized calcium is thought to inhibit adenylate cyclase and stimulate the release of substances contained in platelet dense granules (ADP, serotinin). Thromboxane A_2 is also one of the most potent vasoconstrictors known, but its short half-life limits the duration of its effect (Gingrich and Hoak, 1979). Thus it becomes evident that intricate biochemical relationships between platelets, coagulation factors, and vascular endothelium are necessary for normal hemostasis. These relationships become the basis of the platelet function tests discussed later.

LABORATORY EVALUATION OF HEMOSTASIS

QUALITY CONTROL IN THE COAGULATION LABORATORY

Precise quality control is necessary to detect the subtle differences between normal individuals and those with mild hemostatic defects. At the outset it is conceded that certain screening tests are qualitative. For example, prolongation of activated partial thromboplastin time (APTT) does not occur until a coagulation factor is reduced to less than 30 per cent of normal. It is obvious that all factors that may influence the laboratory coagulation test must be carefully controlled, if one is to correlate coagulation test prolongation with the anticipated severity of the bleeding diathesis in the patient. Improper blood collection techniques are a frequent cause of erratic results from the coagulation laboratory. The sample should be collected with minimum excitement, as this can increase platelet count, platelet aggregation, and factor VIII levels. Ideally, the sample should be obtained with minimal probing for the vessel and minimal venous stasis. Blood samples for coagulation procedures should never be collected through catheters that have been used for heparin therapy. It is important that the surface of any collection, holding, or transfer containers be consistent (all plastic or all siliconized), particularly with reference to platelet function studies (Triplett, 1978).

The preferred anticoagulant for most coagulation tests is 3.8 per cent sodium citrate, owing to its superior preservation of factors V and VIII. The ratio of anticoagulant to blood is 1:9 for most procedures. The sample should be collected in new plastic syringes containing the correct amount of anticoagulant for the volume of blood aspirated. Any deviation from the above ratio can limit calcium availability in the test systems and cause erratic results.

Since many veterinarians submit blood for coagulation tests to nearby hospitals, problems in sample transportation or storage are not uncommon. Although factors V and VIII are particularly labile, losses can be reduced considerably by immediately placing the sample in an ice bath. The sample should be centrifuged and the plasma removed within 30 minutes of blood collection. The plasma is stored in an ice bath and capped to prevent pH changes. If these precautions are followed, the sample should be stable for four hours.

When it is necessary to freeze the sample and mail it to an outside laboratory, the following recommendations should be followed. The blood sample should be centrifuged at high speed (2500 to 3500 rpm) for 15 minutes and the plasma removed with a plastic pipette. Then the plasma should be rapidly frozen (in alcohol and dry ice) in small aliquots (1 ml) to prevent ice crystal formation. Slow freezing or thawing of samples induces cryoprecipitation of coagulation factors, particularly factor VIII, and can be a major source of erratic results in APTT. The sample should subsequently be stored or transported at $-20°C$ or lower.

Packing specimens with a large amount of dry ice (10 to 12 lbs) in a styrofoam container is necessary to maintain this temperature requirement. Similar processing of blood from a normal individual of the same species is imperative to rule out artifacts induced during sample collection and transportation (Dodds, 1975).

Most coagulation tests are enzymatic, and therefore, factors known to influence reaction rates must be controlled. These factors include temperature, ion concentrations, pH, incubation times, and reagent stability. The ability of different technicians to detect the fibrin endpoint varies; however, variation in final results are minimal when controls are assayed by the same technician. Duplicate test determinations should always be performed and tolerance limits for each test should be established. When duplicate results are in agreement, the average result is reported for both the patient and control sample. A graph of laboratory results performed on control samples should be maintained so that shifts or trends are easily recognized. Any changes in reagents, manufacturers, or technical modifications of procedures necessitate that the normal range be reestablished. In general, when results are out of control, the test should be repeated. If the control sample is still abnormal, the sample should be redrawn, usually from an alternate donor.

THE COMMON COAGULATION TESTS

The two tests most commonly used to evaluate the intrinsic coagulation system are activated partial thromboplastin time (APTT) and activated coagulation time (ACT). The ACT test is similar to other whole blood clotting time methods but uses diatomaceous earth as an inert surface-activating agent that shortens the normal clotting time. This results in increased sensitivity of ACT when compared with older whole blood clotting time methods, i.e., the Lee White or capillary tube methods. In the ACT test, two ml of whole blood is injected into the ACT tube, mixed, incubated at 37°C for one min., and then observed at five-second intervals for the first evidence of clotting. The inexpensiveness and simplicity of the ACT test make this test the ideal presurgical or prebiopsy screening test for most veterinary practices. Inexperienced technicians rapidly achieve high precision with ACT. After a diagnosis has been confirmed, ACT provides a convenient test for monitoring response to specific therapy.

Normal values in the dog range from 60 to 90 seconds, with a mean of 75 seconds. The normal range in the cat remains to be established; however, the mean value is approximately 70 seconds. Severe thrombocytopenia ($< 10,000/\mu l$) can prolong the ACT test, owing to reduced platelet phospholipid availability. In addition, some qualitative platelet function defects also prolong ACT, such as the thrombocytopathy of uremia. Severe hypofibrinogenemia is associated with either poor clot quality or formation of only a few small clots. In determining ACT in heparinized patients, the blood must be carefully observed for the first evidence of coagulation, since the normal abrupt production of fibrin clot is inhibited.

In the APTT test, citrated plasma is incubated with an activator of factor XII (kaolin or celite) and cephaloplastins, which substitute for platelet phospholipid requirements. After addition of ionic calcium, the time required to form fibrin is exactly determined. The mean clotting time for dog plasma using different commercial APTT reagents may vary significantly, but the normal range should not be greater than ± three seconds, i.e., a mean clotting time of 17 seconds with a normal range of 14 to 20 seconds.

A variety of acquired and hereditary disorders can reduce one or more factors in the intrinsic coagulation cascade. Usually the availability of a single factor must be reduced below 30 per cent of normal before the APTT test is prolonged. Therefore, most heterozygous carriers (with only 40 to 60 per cent reduction in coagulation factor activity) are not detected by this test. Increased factor VIII levels, which accompany a variety of diseases, may result in an abnormally shortened APTT. Diagnosis of the specific factor deficiency in the intrinsic pathway can be obtained by performing APTT on 1:1 mixtures of patient plasma and known factor deficient plasmas. Factor deficiencies may be differentiated from effects of inhibitors (heparin) by repeating the APTT following dilution of the abnormal plasma 1:1 with normal plasma. Correction of the APTT would suggest factor deficiency, whereas failure to correct would suggest the presence of an inhibitor.

The status of the extrinsic coagulation cascade is evaluated by the one-stage prothrombin time (OSPT). Citrated plasma is added to a thromboplastin-calcium mixture, and the length of time required to form fibrin is exactly determined. Phospholipids contained in the thromboplastin mixture make the test independent of platelet function. If this test is performed by a local hospital laboratory, the patient's sample and the control sample should be transported in an ice bath and performed within four hours of collection. The normal range for most OSPT methods is seven to ten seconds in dogs and 9 to 13 seconds in cats. Duplicate determinations should agree within one second. Abnormal OSPT is associated with liver disease, disseminated intravascular coagulation (DIC), and hereditary or acquired deficiencies of any factors of the extrinsic cascade. Owing to the short half-life of factor VII, the test is very sensitive to vitamin K deficiency or antagonism. It is not as useful in monitoring heparin therapy as are tests assaying the intrinsic cascade.

The thrombin time (TT) test measures the reactivity of fibrinogen to exogenous thrombin. The test is independent of other factors in the intrinsic and extrinsic coagulation cascades. Commerical bovine thrombin is diluted with saline to a concentration that produces a TT of 6.0 to 9.0 seconds when 0.1 ml thrombin is added to 0.2 ml normal canine plasma. Prolonged TT is associated with severe hypofibrinogenemia (< 100 mg/dl) and dysfibrinogenemia. Thrombin inhibitors, such as heparin or fibrinogen degradation products (FDP), may also prolong TT. In a large series of human patients with liver disease, TT was the most frequently abnormal coagulation test (Lewis et al., 1977).

Fibrinogen has the highest concentration of any of the coagulation factors. It is the only factor whose concentration is determined routinely. Fibrinogen concentration is determined by a variety of semiquantitative techniques based on heat precipitation, thrombin time, or ammonium sulfate precipitation. Quantitative fibrinogen determination is performed by converting fibrinogen to fibrin with thrombin. The fibrin clot is dissolved in alkali and a phenol reagent is added, which reacts with tyrosine moieties in the fibrinogen molecule. Subsequent determination of optical density and comparison with a standard curve allows the fibrinogen concentration to be determined. The most common fibrinogen assay is based on the seleective heat precipitation of fibrinogen after incubating plasma at 56°C for three minutes. The accuracy of this technique is improved through use of an ocular micrometer instead of the more common refractometer method (Blaisdell and Dodds, 1977). Discrepancies between methods may be induced by high levels of FDP, which do not clot with thrombin but which can be precipitated by heat. Fibrinogen concentration ranges from 150 to 300 mg/dl in normal dogs and cats using this technique.

Hypofibrinogenemia may be associated with either decreased production (in the late stages of liver failure) or increased consumption (in acute DIC). In chronic DIC syndromes, increased hepatic fibrinogen production may maintain fibrinogen levels within or above the normal range, despite considerable fibrinogen consumption. Hereditary hypofibrinogenemia has been reported in dogs but is very rare. Dysfibrinogenemia has not been reported in animals, although acquired forms may occur in any species secondary to hyperplasminemia.

A variety of techniques are available for detecting FDP. The most commonly used method is the Thrombo-Wellcotest. This test uses antisera to human fibrinogen fragments D and E (which also crossreact with other species' FDP). The specific antibodies are absorbed to latex particles and their concentration is adjusted so that macroscopic agglutination occurs when FDP exceed two μg/ml. By performing the test using different dilutions of the patient's plasma, an approximate concentration of FDP is determined.

The action of plasmin on fibrin or fibrinogen results in an accumulation of FDP in the plasma. The half-life of circulating FDP is about 9 to 12 hours, although clearance may be prolonged by impaired reticuloendothelial cell function. The presence of FDP induces hemostatic abnormalities by impairing thrombin-mediated fibrin formation, fibrin polymerization, and perhaps most importantly, platelet plug formation. Abnormal bleeding is likely to be associated with active fibrinolysis when FDP levels exceed 25 μg/ml (Sherry, 1977).

Another indirect measure of plasmin (or fibrinolytic) activity is the dilute whole blood clot retraction test. In this test, whole blood is diluted 1:10 with cold buffered saline. Two ml of the diluted blood is dispensed into each of two (10 × 75 mm) glass test tubes containing one unit of bovine thrombin. The tubes are capped, mixed, and refrigerated for 30 min. The tubes are then placed in a 37°C water bath, and the degree of clot retraction is compared with that of a control at one and two hours. The tubes are kept in the water bath and checked hourly for clot lysis for six to eight hours. The dilute whole blood clot lysis times ranges from 14 to 22 hours in normal dogs. When marked increases in plasma fibrinolytic activity are present, lysis of the dilute clot may occur within one to two hours. Interpretation of test results can be difficult in conditions wherein small or poorly retracted clots are formed, e.g., marked hypofibrinogenemia or thrombocytopenia. This is noted in certain cases of acute DIC when the blood only forms small clots and the relative role of fibrinolysis may be overestimated.

EVALUATING PLATELETS AND THEIR FUNCTIONS

The laboratory tests for platelet function are primarily used to detect thrombocytopenia and differentiate it from thrombocytopathy.

Platelet Counting. Quantitative platelet counts can be performed by both manual and automated techniques. Standardization of automated techniques is difficult, owing to species differences in platelet size. Therefore, most veterinary clinical laboratories perform platelet counts by manual methods. The preferred manual methodology uses phase microscopy, a standard hemacytometer, and one per cent ammonium oxalate as a diluent. A Unopette system, containing a premeasured amount of diluent, provides a convenient and accurate method for preparing a 1:100 dilution of the blood sample. Platelet clumping may result from poor technique in obtaining the blood sample or from inadequate mixing. Platelet counts can be performed on EDTA blood (preferred) for up to five hours after collection and in citrated blood for four hours after collection. In cases of low platelet count, the feathered edge of the smear should always be reviewed for potential platelet clumping, causing pseudothrombocytopenia.

Since manual platelet counts are time consuming, they are relatively expensive. Several recent studies have shown significant correlation between platelet counts and platelet estimates. Platelet estimates, performed on routine Wright's stained blood films, provide a rapid mechanism for monitoring the platelet count. We have routinely counted the total number of platelets in ten oil immersion fields and compared this value with the platelet count. Again, it is important to count in the area away from the periphery of the smears where red blood cells (RBC) do not overlap. We have found that one platelet per 1000 × field is roughly equivalent to 15,000 platelets per μl (correlation coefficient = .93) Assuming that an "adequate" platelet designation implies a platelet count greater than 100,000, about six to seven platelets per 1000× field should be present. This value is somewhat higher than the three to four platelets per oil immersion field for an "adequate" platelet count given elsewhere (Duncan and Prasse, 1977). Platelet distribution will be influenced by the technique of smear preparation (e.g., "wedge," "cover slip," or slide-spinner techniques), which may necessitate minor modification of these recommendations.

An alternative method for estimating platelet count is the indirect method, which uses the ratio of platelets to white blood cells (WBC) and the WBC count according to the formula

$$\frac{\text{number of platelets}}{\text{number of WBC}} \times$$
$$\text{WBC count}/\mu l = \text{platelets}/\mu l$$

$$Example: \frac{125 \text{ platelets}}{50 \text{ WBC}} \times$$
$$20,000 \text{ WBC}/\mu l = 50,000 \text{ platelets}/\mu l$$

Similar methods using the red blood cell count and a Miller's Disc in the ocular of the microscope are also advocated (Mogadam, 1980).

Platelet Morphology. Microscopic evaluation of erythrocyte size and shape is a well-established laboratory procedure in the differential diagnosis of anemia. Similar use of platelet size and morphology has less acceptance in evaluation of platelet disorders, although recent reports emphasize its relevance. Standarized conditions must be carefully followed if platelet morphology is to be useful in clinical disorders. These conditions include (1) careful collection of the blood specimen to avoid platelet clumping, (2) evaluating platelets away from the periphery of "push" smears where RBC do not overlap, and (3) making smears within 10 to 60 min. of sample collection. Artifactual increase in platelet size has been noted on blood smears prepared from normal people immediately after blood collection. In routine screening of blood smears, platelet size can be approximated by comparing platelet size with that of normal erythrocytes. (Erythrocyte diameters are seven and five μm in dogs and cats, respectively.) The proportion of large platelets, megathrombocytes, as well as their relative granularity should also be determined. The criteria for classifying platelets as megathrombocytes are not well established in dogs and cats. In normal dogs, about one per cent of the platelets were found to exceed a size of ≥ 5 μm and were designated as megathrombocytes. During the thrombocytopenic phase of acute ehrlichiosis, megathrombocytes increased to values approaching ten per cent of the total platelet population (Pierce et al., 1977).

Normal platelet size and morphology are found in thrombocytopenic states associated with reduced platelet production and splenic pooling. Increased numbers of megathrombocytes are found in immune-mediated platelet disorders, particularly those with platelet counts < 50,000/μl. Increased size and hypogranulation of platelets are noted in infiltrated marrows and myeloproliferative disorders, regardless of platelet count. Presumably these changes reflect metabolic abnormalities in megakaryocyte maturation and are occasionally present in cats infected with feline leukovirus. Occasional hypogranular platelets are observed in DIC syndromes in which platelets undergo partial activation but are retained as circulating hyporesponsive platelets.

Platelet Function Tests. A variety of tests are available for evaluating platelet function, but unfortunately they are fairly complex, require specialized equipment, and often must be performed immediately or shortly after blood collection. The most commonly used tests include bleeding time, whole blood clot retraction, platelet aggregation, and platelet factor 3 (PF-3) availability. Although bleeding time is a relatively crude test, careful standardization can make this test an important diagnostic aid. It is generally agreed that bleeding time provides best assessment of ability to form the platelet plug *in vivo* (achieve primary hemostasis). Therefore, the bleeding time tests directly for the adequacy of platelet number and function, von Willebrand's factor, and vascular response. Bleeding time should be one of the first and most useful tests performed on the bleeding patient, but unfortunately, poorly standardized procedures have caused this test to fall into disuse. Older methodologies using random stab wounds are associated with bleeding times of one to five minutes in dogs, depending on the length, depth, and location of the wound. Recently, performance of bleeding times in dogs using a highly standardized protocol allowed detection of several mild platelet function defects induced by drugs (aspirin, low molecular weight dextran) (Thomas et al., 1979). The standard protocol included the following: the dogs were anesthetized, the incision was made in the muscular portion of the lower hind leg that was free of bony prominences and superficial veins, a sphygmomonometer was used to maintain the venous pressure of the limb at 40 mm Hg, a template was used to determine length of incision and a guard controlled the depth of incision. The bleeding time was the length of time from the initial incision to the visual cessation of blood flow onto the filter paper. Normal values for bleeding time in 50 normal dogs ranged from 1.04 to 3.68 minutes, with an average of 1.79 minutes. Although this technique is more cumbersome than others, it is the most accurate technique proposed thus far for dogs and has the potential to disclose subclinical platelet dysfunctions. A disposable bleeding time device is available that standardizes the length and depth of the incision, but it remains to be evaluated in dogs.

Clot retraction is a simple test but has limited usefulness in evaluating platelet function. Clot retraction is dependent upon the contractability of the actomyosin-like protein, thrombosthenin, contained in platelets that are trapped in a fibrin mesh. Factors influencing clot retraction include platelet count, fibrinogen concentration, serum factors, and the nature of container surface. The clot retraction technique consists of incubating one to two ml of whole blood in a clean, dry glass test tube for 24 hours at 37°C. The clot is observed for consistency at one hour and 24 hours by temporarily removing it from the test tube with an applicator stick. Abnormalities in clot retraction are associated with platelet counts less than $100,000/\mu l$, severe hypofibrinogenemia, severe uremia, and a hereditary platelet disorder (thrombasthenia). Most other platelet dysfunctions have normal clot retraction. The rather gross nature of the test and its ability to detect only thrombocytopenia and thrombasthenia have led most investigators to replace this test with other standard tests, such as platelet count and platelet aggregation. The dilute whole blood clot retraction and lysis test has similar limitations with reference to platelet function.

Platelet aggregation is considered the most definitive test in the evaluation of hereditary and acquired platelet dysfunction. Its limitations include the expense of the aggregometer, the numerous variables that must be carefully standardized for each animal species, and the requirement that the test be performed on platelets within two hours of collection. Variables influencing aggregation include citrate concentration, pH, the storage time between preparation of platelet-rich plasma (PRP) and performance of the test, stirring conditions, centrifugation conditions, platelet number, drug effects, and concentrations of aggregating reagents. The impact of species differences on many of these variables usually means that an animal with a suspected platelet function defect must be referred to a veterinary medical center with personnel experienced in platelet aggregation.

Commonly used aggregating reagents include ADP, collagen, epinephrine, thrombin, and recently, prostaglandins. Because erythrocytes contain a rich source of ADP, hemolysis and/or erythrocyte contamination of PRP must be avoided. The antibiotic ristocetin, when used as a platelet aggregating reagent, requires the presence of von Willebrand's factor (VWF) to induce platelet aggregation. This property has been used to identify VWF deficiency in man, but similar studies to identify VWF-deficient dogs have been complicated by a normal plasma protein inhibitor in this species (Johnson et al., 1980). After the addition of aggregating reagents, the aggregometer records changes in light transmission as stirred discrete platelets clump to form large platelet aggregates. Quantitation of the platelet aggregation pattern involves analysis of the aggregation response and consideration of dose-response curves using varying reagent concentrations. Usually the maximal change in light transmission as well as the initial rate of change are compared with control responses (Triplett et al., 1978; Brackett et al., 1976).

A primary platelet function involves supplying phospholipid (PF-3), which is required in the intrinsic coagulation cascade. Several coagulation tests measure the effectiveness of PF-3 generation in shortening the clotting time. These tests include Stypven time and thromboplastin generation time. A modification of this test is also used in identifying the presence of antiplatelet antibodies (see discussion of immune-mediated thrombocytopenia). Following maximal activation of plasma coagulation factors, PF-3 becomes rate limiting, and its relative availability can be assayed by determining the recalcification time. Platelet dysfunctions may therefore produce prolonged clotting times owing to reduced availability of PF-3. Although less sensitive, the ACT:APTT ratio can also reflect a similar deficiency in platelet function. Both tests measure the intrinsic coagulation cascade, but ACT is dependent on endogenous PF-3 release, whereas APTT is independent of PF-3 (it is added exogenously in the test). When ACT is prolonged in the presence of normal APTT, platelet dysfunction accompanying uremia can easily be detected by this combination of tests. The primary advantage of this approach resides in the simplicity of the tests involved and, in combination with a standardized bleeding time, it can provide much useful information about platelet dysfunction with only limited laboratory expertise.

Other platelet function tests that are occasionally used include glass bead adhesiveness and prothrombin consumption time. For the most part, however, these tests are used primarily in research investigations of hemostatic defects.

CLINICAL EVALUATION OF ABNORMAL HEMOSTASIS

EVALUATION OF THE BLEEDING PATIENT

A careful physical examination and detailed medical history are essential to focus the laboratory investigation of bleeding defects. The following questions are particularly applicable in evaluating animals with bleeding problems.

1. What clinical findings suggest an underlying hemostatic abnormality? Investigation of the hemostatic mechanism should be conducted when any of the following are present: (a) spontaneous bleeding into the skin, mucous membranes, or internal tissues; (b) excessive or prolonged bleeding after minor surgery or trauma; and (c) bleeding from multiple sites. The bleeding disorder can range widely in severity. In some cases it is almost inapparent, whereas in others it can rapidly become life threatening, particularly when a superimposed problem also affects the compromised hemostatic mechanism.

2. Does bleeding appear to be associated with an abnormality of primary hemostasis (platelet or vascular disorders) or secondary hemostasis (coagulopathies)? Difficulty in formation of the primary platelet plug (primary bleeding) often results in capillary bleeding that is immediate in onset and is characterized by petechiation or ecchymosis of skin and mucous membranes. Difficulty in formation of the definitive hemostatic plug (secondary bleeding) often results in subcutaneous or deep intramuscular hematomas and delayed onset of bleeding. Significantly prolonged bleeding following minor trauma is often present in patients with secondary bleeding.

3. What historical factors must be considered in hereditary hemostatic defects? The medical history should be reviewed for unexplained lameness, anemia, hematuria, or periodic weakness, which may suggest a subclinical bleeding diathesis. Past instances when therapy was required for bleeding should always be reconsidered in detail. A history of bleeding problems commencing in early life or occurring in related animals (sire, dam, or littermates), as well as the sex of affected animals, may be useful in the diagnosis of hereditary hemostatic defects. A high frequency of neonatal death may be associated with excessive blood loss from the umbilical cords in some hereditary coagulopathies.

4. What other etiologic factors should be evaluated in acquired hemostatic defects? Routine physical examination and laboratory chemistry profiles should be performed to establish the presence of an underlying disorder. Particular attention should be focused on detection of gastrointestinal, renal, hepatic, cardiovascular, splenic, or myelogenous disorders. All drugs being administered to the animal should be carefully reviewed for potential interactions with the hemostatic mechanism. Possible rodenticide exposure should always be considered in animals that are not confined.

THE COAGULOPATHIES

VITAMIN K DEFICIENCY AND ANTAGONISM

Dietary deficiency of vitamin K is virtually nonexistent in dogs or cats fed modern commercial diets. Transient vitamin K deficiency has occasionally been suspected in neonatal puppies; however, malnutrition of the bitch during gestation may also be involved. Long-standing gastrointestinal disorders accompanied by malabsorption of fats may result in mild vitamin K deficiency; only limited amounts are required to sustain adequate synthesis of vitamin K–dependent factors, however. When bleeding is encountered in these patients, other contributing causes of bleeding may be present (liver disease, endotoxemia).

Vitamin K antagonism due to accidental ingestion of anticoagulant rodenticide is a common cause of coagulopathy in dogs (Green et al., 1979). Both commercial exterminators and laymen often place anticoagulant rodenticides in locations that are accessible to pets. The coccidiostat sulfaquinoxaline is also a potent vitamin K antagonist that can produce fatal coagulopathy in dogs. Factors influencing the severity of the induced coagulopathy include the bioavailability of vitamin K, the amount of rodenticide ingested and its rate of metabolism, disappearance rates of vitamin K–dependent coagulation factors, alteration in hepatic receptor affinity for the antagonist, and other coexisting hemostatic abnormalities.

Vitamin K is required for the postribosomal carboxylation of glutamyl residues of coagulation factors II, VII, IX, and X (O'Reilly, 1976). In vitamin K deficiency or antagonism, the liver produces proteins that are antigenically similar to factors II, VII, IX and X; however, they are inactive. The functional forms of factors II, VII, IX and X disappear in accordance with their half-lives of 41, 6, 14, and 16.5 hours, respectively. Their synthesis remains inhibited until the antagonist is metabolized and cleared from the body. The duration of the antagonism is variable, usually lasting from several days to a week following a single ingestion of rodenticide. Warfarin half-life ranges from 15 to 24 hours in the dog. Repeated low doses of warfarin may produce toxicity with a lower total dose than that associated with a massive single exposure.

The spectrum of clinical signs encountered in anticoagulant toxicoses is broad and is generally related to organ dysfunction induced by hypovolemia or by hemorrhage into organ parenchyma, surrounding tissues, or body cavities. The first clinical signs are seen about three days following ingestion of the anticoagulant. Acute death, with no previous signs of illness, may follow hemorrhage into brain, pericardial sac, or thoracic cavity. In less acutely affected animals, anemia, weakness, pallor, dyspnea, hematemesis, epistaxis, or bloody feces are commonly seen. Extensive external hematomas may occur in areas of trauma or at venipuncture sites. Bleeding into joint spaces can lead to acute lameness or hemarthrosis. Neurologic signs may predominate following hemorrhage into brain, spinal cord, or subdural space.

Decreased levels of vitamin K–dependent factors are manifested by abnormalities in laboratory tests of both intrinsic and extrinsic pathways, as indicated in Figure 80–2. In early warfarin toxicosis the rapid disappearance of factor VII may induce prolongation of only the OSPT. After three days' toxicosis, however, bleeding problems become more frequent as APTT is also prolonged with depletion of factors IX, X, and II. Therefore, when an intoxicated patient is presented to the veterinarian, the laboratory findings often include marked prolongation of OSPT with moderate prolongation of APTT or ACT. Platelet count, fibrinogen,

FDP, and thrombin time usually remain within normal limits; however, exceptions do occur (Green et al., 1979).

The three major treatment priorities are, first, correct the hypovolemia; second, correct the coagulopathy; and third, minimize organ dysfunction induced by accumulation of extravascular blood. Patients in shock should be handled with extreme care. Transfusion of fresh whole blood at 20 ml/kg intravenously may be critical to survival in severe cases. Usual guidelines recommend the administration of 50 per cent of this dose rapidly and the remainder slowly by intravenous drip. Correction of the coagulopathy is accomplished by administration of vitamin K_1 (Aquamephyton) parenterally at a dose of ten mg for dogs and two to five mg for cats twice daily. In uncomplicated cases vitamin K therapy alone results in rapid improvement in both clinical signs and laboratory tests within 12 hours. In most cases oral vitamin K therapy is continued for five to seven days in animals making satisfactory progress. If the identity of the rodenticide can be determined, it is well to consult manufacturer's recommendations, as some coumarin analogues have longer half-lives than does warfarin and duration of therapy would need to be extended in such cases. Vitamin K_3 (menadione) is not recommended in treatment toxicoses, as patient response is considerably slower than response to vitamin K_1. Hematomas and most hemorrhagic effusions in the convalescent animal usually resolve without medical intervention. When severe dyspnea is present, a hemorrhagic pleural effusion should be suspected. Careful thoracentesis to remove excess blood is indicated in such cases; however, if coagulation tests are still abnormal, this procedure may only reinitiate bleeding and exaggerate the hypovolemia. Blood obtained from body cavities should not be readministered to the patient, because these effusions often contain procoagulant factors that may initiate thrombosis.

DISSEMINATED INTRAVASCULAR COAGULATION (DIC)

DIC, also known as consumption coagulopathy and defibrination syndrome, is the most common coagulopathy encountered in veterinary medicine and occurs secondary to a wide variety of disease processes (Table 80–1) (Greene, 1975; Moore, 1979). In DIC, simultaneous activation of the coagulation and fibrinolytic system results in microvascular thrombosis or a bleeding tendency as factors and platelets are depleted (Fig. 80–3). Examples of the activating triggers for DIC include vascular damage, bacterial endotoxins, or tissue thromboplastin release from necrotic or malignant tissue. Any disease-producing vascular stasis or vascular endothelial injury favors induction of DIC. The intimal damage associated with severe dirofilariasis in dogs has commonly induced DIC (Kociba and Hathaway, 1974). Alternatively, decreased clearance of procoagulants by impaired reticuloendothelial function may enhance DIC in certain disease states, such as liver failure.

Whether DIC is manifested as an acute or chronic process depends on the activator, its rate of release, duration of exposure, and most importantly, the ability of the liver and bone marrow to replace consumed factors and platelets. Chronic DIC produced experimentally in the dog by infusions of brain thromboplastin revealed varying compensatory ability of the liver and marrow (Owen et al., 1973). In general, the liver's capacity to increase synthesis of coagulation factors was greater than the marrow's ability to increase platelet production. In some cases overcompensation of hepatic produc-

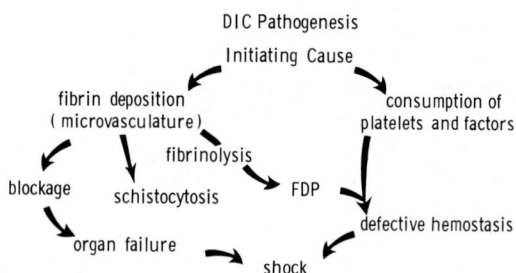

Figure 80–3. Pathogenesis of disseminated intravascular coagulation (DIC).

tion led to elevated levels of fibrinogen and factor V when infusions were continued for longer than one week. Chronic compensated DIC may therefore be characterized solely by elevated FDP, which makes this form of DIC difficult to differentiate from primary fibrinolysis.

The clinical manifestations of DIC are twofold. Fibrin deposition in microvasculature, particularly in the kidney and lung, leads to ischemia and variable organ failure. Simultaneously, the depletion of coagulation factors and platelets in the presence of the anticoagulant effects of FDP leads to a bleeding tendency. Antithrombin III (AT III) complexes with and neutralizes excessive generation of activated serine proteases (VII_a, IX_a, X_a, XI_a). AT III depletion is associated with enhanced thrombosis in some DIC patients (Raymond and Dodds, 1979). Of course, the predominant clinical signs may relate to the primary disease problem causing DIC. Frequently, signs of DIC become more obvious only during the terminal stages of a disease as an animal's ability to compensate deteriorates. The important role of secondary fibrinolysis in minimizing intravascular thrombosis can not be overemphasized, and therapeutic attempts to inhibit fibrinolysis in DIC cases are contraindicated.

DIC can be suspected when the following laboratory findings are present: thrombocytopenia, hypofibrinogenemia, elevated FDP, and prolongation of APTT or ACT. When this constellation of findings is associated with a condition known to induce DIC, further laboratory testing is usually not required. Occasional patients may have disproportionate depletion of specific factors that may merit further tests to rule out other potential diagnoses. For example, a severely depleted factor VIII level and nor-

Table 80–1. Common Initiating Causes of DIC in Animals

Infectious diseases
Bacterial, particularly endotoxin producers
Viral, particularly those causing vascular damage
Dirofilariasis

Neoplasia
Hemangiosarcoma
Tumors causing thromboplastin release

Liver disease
Aflatoxicosis
Sclerosing hepatitis

Miscellaneous
Heat stroke
Massive trauma
Obstetrical complications
Shock-poor vascular perfusion
Intravascular hemolysis
Immune complex disease — amyloidosis
Acute pancreatitis

mal fibrinogen level in a partially compensated DIC patient may be difficult to differentiate from that of a hemophilia A patient without determining factor VIII–related antigen. The most common factors found to be reduced in spontaneous cases of DIC in dogs are factors I, V, and VIII. Other factors may be reduced, depending in part on liver function and the nature of the initiating cause. Intravascular fibrin deposition and intimal proliferation of arterioles may cause fragmentation of erythrocytes that are detected as schistocytes on peripheral blood films (Antman et al., 1979; Madewell and Feldman, 1980). The rapid generation of soluble fibrin monomer can be confirmed by the protamine sulfate or ethanol gelation tests. The latter tests are usually negative in primary fibrinolysis. Favorable response to therapy is most easily determined by documenting an increasing fibrinogen level. Decreasing FDP and ACT also indicate a satisfactory response to therapy. Platelet count is usually the slowest parameter to recover after satisfactory therapy is initiated.

Few cases of DIC have been reported in cats. Experimentally-induced feline infectious peritonitis was characterized by a chronic DIC syndrome that featured elevated fibrinogen and FDP levels, thrombocytopenia, and lowered levels of factors VII, VIII, IX, X, XI, and XII (Weiss et al., 1980).

The therapeutic aspects of DIC remain very controversial (Coleman et al., 1979). Since acute DIC is secondary to severe diseases of high mortality, it is not surprising that when the effects of DIC are superimposed on preexisting disease, a high mortality is anticipated regardless of treatment (Mant and King, 1979). Our present concept of the genesis of DIC dictates that the primary focus of therapy must be on the underlying disease if satisfactory results are to be obtained. Adequate supportive treatment for shock, fluid imbalance, acidosis, systemic infection, or renal failure is often critical to survival of DIC patients.

In DIC patients that are actively hemorrhaging, whole blood should be administered to improve perfusion and to maintain platelet counts and fibrinogen levels. Heparin should not be given to actively bleeding patients that have severe factor depletion and thrombocytopenia, as fatal hemorrhage

may result. Note also that when there is either depletion of AT III or excess of platelet antiheparin factor, heparin is ineffective. For these reasons the author's approach has been to provide sufficient fresh whole blood to maintain platelet counts > $30,000/\mu$l and fibrinogen levels > 50 mg/dl before administering heparin. The goal of heparinization in most DIC patients is to achieve a stable state of anticoagulation approximated by a 1.5- to 2.5-fold increase in normal APTT. If ACT is used similarly to monitor heparinized dogs, it should be about one and a third times normal (i.e., 92 to 108 seconds) (Green, 1980). Initial heparinization is achieved by subcutaneous administration of 500 units/kg three times daily or continuous IV drip at a dose of 50 units/kg/hr. Subsequent patient monitoring with ACT or APTT is necessary to adjust heparin doses according to individual differences in patient response as well as ongoing changes in the primary disease.

When monitoring subcutaneous heparin therapy, ACT should be determined at maximal anticoagulation (two hours) and just prior to the next dose (eight hours). If maximal anticoagulation is too high, the next heparin dose should be reduced. If minimal anticoagulation is too low, the frequency of heparin administration should be increased. When the patient's condition is stable, monitoring once daily is usually considered adequate. Intermittent intravenous bolus administration should be avoided, since it is the least effective method for heparinization. It causes a "roller coaster" effect of transient hypocoagulation to hypercoagulation states, which often results in increased bleeding in DIC patients. No recommendations are currently available concerning heparinization of cats with DIC.

Recent studies in human medicine indicate that heparin therapy is most effective when used prophylactically in syndromes with predisposition for DIC or thrombosis. In such instances, a mini-dose of 75 units/kg heparin subcutaneously at 8- to 12-hour intervals has been found effective in reducing the incidence of thrombotic complications related to DIC. The primary aim of this form of therapy is to enhance effectiveness of AT III and thereby to inhibit the evolution of activated coagulation factors. Certainly, the ongoing AT III consumption that occurs with acute DIC syndromes markedly limits the effectiveness of heparin. This approach may also prove promising in treating diseases prone to thrombosis in veterinary medicine, but recommendations from carefully controlled clinical trials are unavailable at this time.

PRIMARY (PATHOLOGIC) FIBRINOLYSIS

Pathologic fibrinolysis results when either excess activators or decreased plasma inhibitors induce hyperplasminemia (Fig. 80–4). The resultant digestion of fibrinogen modifies the molecule so that it binds thrombin but does not clot, and thereby generates a circulating anticoagulant. As the process continues, depletion of fibrinogen, factor V, and factor VIII ensues, and FDP accumulate. These changes result in a clinical disorder characterized by a bleeding tendency and rapid digestion of blood clots. It most frequently accompanies DIC, in which it is an appropriate response to formation of microthrombi throughout the vascular system (called secondary fibrinolysis). On rare occasions it may occur as a sequel to severe liver disease, when defective synthesis of antiplasmin or reduced clearance of activators leads to hyperplasminemia (called primary fibrinolysis). Other conditions can also lead to primary fibrinolysis by excessive production of plasminogen activators. These include heat stroke, malignancy, genitourinary tract surgery, and progranulocytic leukemia. The existence of primary fibrinolysis as a discrete entity is debated by some, and it may only represent an atypical form of chronic, partially compensated DIC with high fibrinolytic activity.

The laboratory differentiation of primary fibrinolysis from secondary fibrinolysis of DIC is difficult. DIC tends to have thrombocytopenia, hypofibrinogenemia, schistocytosis, and relatively low fibrinolytic activity. In contrast, primary fibrinolysis tends to have more normal platelet counts, no schistocytosis, less severe hypofibrinogenemia, and marked fibrinolytic activity. The relative fibrinolytic activity can easily be obtained by comparing the dilute whole blood clot lysis test in the patient with a control. Occasionally technicians may note the rapid lysis of blood clots in test tubes submitted for other laboratory tests. Other laboratory tests that are used occasionally in differentiation of fibrinolytic states include the euglobulin clot lysis time and paracoagulation tests.

The treatment of primary fibrinolysis tends to be conservative. While epsilon-amino caproic acid (EACA) is an effective inhibitor of fibrinolysis, there is often uncertainty about whether the fibrinolysis is primary or secondary. Certainly in secondary fibrinolysis, one would not want to enhance thrombosis by inhibiting fibrinolysis. Therefore, patients are most often given plasma to replace factor deficiencies and heparin to inhibit consumption of coagulation factors. Dosages for plasma and heparin are similar to those used in DIC.

LIVER DISEASE

Several complex hemostatic abnormalities may accompany severe liver disease; however, the incidence of bleeding is usually low in uncomplicated cases (Lechmer et al., 1977). Platelet dysfunction is usually present when severe bleeding is encountered in liver diseases. Although the compromised liver maintains hemostasis within reasonable limits, it poorly tolerates the added stress of surgical procedures or acute exacerbations of chronic processes. When liver synthetic mechanisms fail, the patient may manifest thrombosis, excessive fibrinolysis, or hemorrhage. The delicate hemostatic balance between activators and inhibitors may be difficult to maintain when the clinician encounters bleeding in severe liver disease.

The common hemostatic defects of liver disease are given in Table 80–2. The diminished synthesis of coagulation factors is primarily manifested in those with shorter half-lives (factors VII, V, IX, X). Only in the late stages of liver disease is hypofibrinogenemia manifested, when it is a poor prognos-

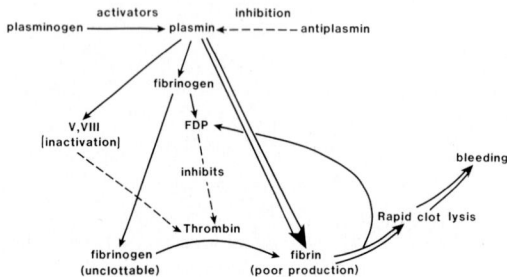

Figure 80–4. Hemostatic alterations induced by hyperplasminemia.

Table 80–2. The Hemostatic Defects in Liver Disease

Diminished Synthesis of Proteins
Coagulation factors
Antiplasmins
Antithrombins

Diminished Clearance Mechanisms
Fibrin degradation products
Activated coagulation factors
Plasminogen activators

Metabolic Abnormalities
Vitamin K deficiency
Platelet dysfunction
Dysfibrinogenemia

tic sign. Although the liver may play some role in factor VIII synthesis, the endothelial cell is considered to be the site of production. Massive hepatic necrosis and cirrhosis are usually associated with elevated levels of factor VIII, which seems to support this concept. In most cases the correlation between immunologic assays and clotting assays of coagulation factors is good, supporting a quantitative rather than a qualitative defect in the synthetic mechanisms. When DIC or hyperplasminemia is present, increased catabolism of factors I, V, and VIII may occur. The reduced synthesis of antiplasmin or reduced clearance of plasminogen activators may enhance the rate of fibrinolysis considerably. The reduced synthesis of AT III and reduced clearance of activated coagulation factors provide a stimulus for thrombosis in liver disease. Renal and pulmonary thrombosis can be a life-threatening sequel of liver disease and must always be considered when a patient's clinical condition suddenly deteriorates.

Several associated metabolic abnormalities may accompany liver disease. As blood is readily converted to ammonia in the gastrointestinal tract, gastrointestinal bleeding can contribute markedly to the production of hyperammonemia and hepatic encephalopathy (Strombeck et al., 1976). Diminished absorption of fat-soluble vitamin K may be associated with chronic biliary obstruction and lead to reduced synthesis of the vitamin K–dependent coagulation factors. For this reason all patients with prolonged prothrombin time should be given vitamin K_1, and its effect should be assayed the following day. Failure to correct the abnormal OSPT confirms decreased protein synthetic ability as the most likely cause of the defect.

Reduced platelet function due to thrombocytopenia may be related to increased splenic sequestration of platelets, particularly in patients with portal hypertension, increased platelet consumption, or poor megakaryocyte production of platelets due to abnormal hepatic metabolism of folic acid or vitamin B_{12}. When hepatic disease is accompanied by underlying DIC, thrombocytopenia due to increased platelet consumption results, as in infectious canine hepatitis and aflatoxicosis (Wigton et al., 1976; Greene et al., 1977). Qualitative defects in platelet function have also been demonstrated in recent studies of patients with chronic liver disease (Rubin et al., 1979). Such defects are infrequently evaluated in hepatopathies, and they may explain the bleeding tendency in some patients having normal coagulation tests and platelet counts. The diminished ability of the diseased liver to clear FDP, in addition to increased production of FDP (due to excessive fibrinolysis) may markedly interfere with platelet function and result in a bleeding tendency.

Laboratory evaluation of liver disease with routine coagulation tests can be misleading. As indicated above, a variety of defects may be present, some of which are not detected with routine coagulation tests (abnormal fibrinolysis or platelet function). In interpreting laboratory results from patients with liver disease, several fundamentals must be considered. The disappearance of coagulation factors reflects not only the liver's ability to synthesize coagulation but also their rate of peripheral consumption. Also, as previously stated, coagulation tests often remain normal until factor depletion approaches 30 per cent of normal, so sudden changes in demand for coagulation factors may rapidly lead to a severe deficiency of coagulation factors and massive hemorrhage. In general, severe, acute canine hepatopathies tend to exhibit prolongation of both OSPT and APTT, whereas the chronic, partially compensated canine hepatopathies tend to induce minor prolongation of APTT with normal OSPT. Determination of relative deficiencies of individual coagulation factors in canine hepatopathies is rarely attempted, with the exception of fibrinogen. When DIC can be excluded, low fibrinogen levels confer an unfavorable prognosis in hepatic disease.

Several of the less commonly requested coagulation tests can give additional insights into the hemostatic defects of liver disease. Thrombin time provides a very useful screening test in hepatopathy, since it can be prolonged by hypofibrinogenemia, dysfibrinogenemia, and increased FDP. Rapid lysis of the clot in the dilute whole blood clot lysis test is indicative of accelerated fibrinolysis and may be useful in screening for disorders of the fibrinolytic system. Although the clot retraction test may give some indication of severe platelet dysfunction, this test is not sensitive to mild platelet abnormalities. Prolonged bleeding time may indicate abnormal platelet function when other causes can be excluded. Platelet aggregation, when available, is the test of choice in evaluating qualitative platelet dysfunction.

Although bleeding is usually not severe in hepatic disease, acute exacerbations of chronic processes may occur, leading to marked bleeding. Often the additional stress and trauma of exploratory surgical procedures may be sufficient to decompensate a mild coagulopathy with delayed bleeding, resulting in a significant post surgical problem. If laboratory tests detect hemostatic abnormalities, these should always be corrected prior to biopsy procedures. Vitamin K$_1$ therapy may result in partial correction of abnormal coagulation tests in occasional patients, although most do not respond. Since the hemostatic defect is multifactorial, fresh whole blood or platelet-rich plasma is the treatment of choice for those animals with active bleeding. If it is concluded that underlying DIC or primary fibrinolysis is present, one needs to be very cautious in treatment with heparin or ε-aminocaproic acid. It may be found that one aspect of the hemostatic defect has been corrected (hemorrhage), only to find that another aspect has markedly worsened (thrombosis). Supportive therapy, with particular emphasis on treatment of shock, is vital to prevent DIC in patients with liver disease.

HEREDITARY COAGULOPATHIES

The hereditary coagulopathies are deficiencies of a single coagulation factor, often noted in highly inbred strains of purebred dogs. Occasional cases are reported in mongrels and cats. Factor VIII deficiency is the most commonly reported hereditary coagulopathy in dogs. Recent studies have also confirmed a high incidence (65 per cent) of von Willebrand's disease (VWD) gene in Doberman pinschers. The current popularity of this breed and the high incidence rate make VWD more common than was previously suspected.

The clinical signs exhibited by affected dogs are influenced by many factors, including severity of the deficiency, size of the dog, concurrent diseases, and organ dysfunction induced by hemorrhage into organ parenchyma or surrounding tissue. In large, frisky breeds, weight-bearing structures such as joints are particularly susceptible to hemorrhagic sequela, leading to hemarthrosis. Hematomas may arise suddenly anywhere on the body. Delayed oozing of blood from poorly formed platelet plugs can eventually lead to life-threatening hypovolemia. Bleeding from mucous membranes of the gastrointestinal or urogenital tract can be difficult to control, since minimal tissue pressure is generated at these sites. Deep, dissecting hematomas may compromise either organ function or associated structures, such as nerve trunks or airways. Spontaneous massive bleeding into body cavities may induce profound hypovolemia and shock. It is not unusual for asymptomatic patients with mild coagulopathies to encounter bleeding problems when platelet dysfunction is also superimposed by a concurrent disease or treatment, such as live virus vaccination or aspirin administration.

Careful consideration of the patient's history and that of related animals may suggest a hereditary defect in hemostasis. The occurrence of the disease in males only suggests the presence of the sex-linked coagulopathies, factor VIII or IX deficency. Breed identification may be useful in suggesting which factor is deficient, although deficiencies in previously unaffected breeds are not unusual (see Table 80–3). Animals with hereditary hemostatic defects do not usually have underlying disease problems, except that of bleeding and its direct sequelae.

The laboratory screening tests, APTT and OSPT, are the most useful in initial classification of the defect. Coagulopathies with normal APTT and abnormal OSPT

Table 80–3. Features of Hereditary Coagulation Disorders in Dogs and Cats

Disease	Factor Deficient	Inheritance Pattern	Severity of Bleeding Diathesis	Affected Breeds	Coagulation Screening Tests				Definitive Tests
					Bleeding T.	OSPT	APTT	ACT	
Hemophilia A (classic hemophilia)	FVIII	Sex-linked recessive	Variable	Reported in many dog breeds, mongrels, and cats	N	N	ABN	ABN	Low FVIII activity; normal to increased FVIII R–Ant
Hemophilia B (Christmas disease)	FIX	Sex-linked recessive	Often severe	Cairn terrier, Alaskan malamute, St. Bernard, Cocker spaniel, French bulldog, British shorthair (cat)	N	N	ABN	ABN	Low FIX activity
Plasma thromboplastin antecedent (PTA) deficiency	FXI	Autosomal	Mild*	Springer spaniel, Great Pyrenees	N	N	ABN	ABN	Low FXI activity
Hageman trait (Hageman factor deficiency)	FXII	Autosomal	Normal hemostatic mechanism†	Domestic cat	N	N	ABN	ABN	Low FXII activity
Hypoproconvertinemia	FVII	Autosomal incomplete dominance	Subclinical to mild†	Beagle, Alaskan malamute	N	ABN	N	N	Low FVII
Stuart factor deficiency	FX	Autosomal	Severe in neonates	Cocker spaniel	N	ABN	ABN	ABN	Low FX activity; abnormal RVVT
Von Willebrand's disease	FVIII	Autosomal incomplete dominance	Mild*	Golden retriever, miniature schnauzer, German shepard, Doberman pinscher, Scottish terrier	ABN	N	V	V	Low FVIII activity; low FVIII R–Ant

*Severe bleeding may occur following major surgical procedures or trauma.
†Usually discovered fortuitously by presurgical screening tests.
Abbreviations: N = Normal   FVIII R–Ant = FVIII related antigen
                ABN = Abnormal   RVTT = Russell's viper venom time
                V = Variable

suggests factor VII deficiency. Coagulopathies with abnormal APTT and normal OSPT suggest VWD, factor VIII, IX, XI, or XII deficiency. Coagulopathies with abnormality of both OSPT and APTT suggest factor X deficiency (factor I, II, or V deficiency is very rare). Based on the above information, specific laboratory studies can be undertaken to further define the defect. In definitive identification of factor VIII deficiency, it is necessary to determine the level of factor VIII–related antigen (F VIII-RA). Low factor VIII activity and normal to increased F VIII-RA indicate factor VIII deficiency (hemophilia A). If factor VIII activity is low and F VIII-RA is also low, this indicates VWD. Diseases inducing DIC often have increased factor VIII consumption and must be excluded by appropriate laboratory tests.

Russell's viper venom time (RVVT) can differentiate between factor VII deficiency, in which RVVT is normal, and factor X deficiency, in which RVVT is prolonged. In most instances, mixing studies with specific factor deficient plasma and the patient's plasma are necessary to confirm a hereditary factor deficiency. Some local hospitals have the expertise and necessary reagents to identify the more common defects. They can also be of assistance in providing information about processing samples for mailing to specialized coagulation laboratories experienced with animal systems.

In addition to those hereditary coagulopathies listed in Table 80–3, hereditary hypofibrinogenemia has been reported in St. Bernards from Germany. Factor II (prothrombin) deficiency has also been found in rare families of boxers and miniature pinschers.

Perhaps the most important obligation of the veterinarian after confirmation of the coagulopathy is to adequately educate the breeder concerning the hereditary nature of the disease. Carrier animals should be removed from breeding programs. Since the normal range for most coagulation factors is quite broad, often ranging from 50 to 150 per cent of normal, and carrier animals have factor activities in the low normal range (40 to 60 per cent of normal), it can be difficult to identify carriers accurately. In the case of factor VIII–deficient carriers, a low normal factor VIII activity by coagulation assays, but a normal F VIII-RA can be useful in screening. In the case of VWD, screening for carrier states should be done on puppies or young adults, since the disorder often diminishes with age and therefore false negatives may be obtained in older animals.

The lifelong treatment of hemophiliacs can be quite difficult in the case of severe deficiencies. As discussed earlier, the half-life of most coagulation factors is quite short and therefore frequent treatment is often necessary. Any condition that increases stress must be minimized in affected animals. In the case of mild or subclinical defects, the animal may live a relatively normal life, only requiring transfusions if it encounters a concurrent disease, or major surgical procedures are required. Animals with hereditary coagulopathies are often referred to research centers where they have proven useful as animal models of human disease. Further information is provided in an excellent review about inherited bleeding disorders (Dodds, 1975).

PLATELET DYSFUNCTION

THROMBOCYTOPENIA

Thrombocytopenia is the most common hemostatic disorder encountered in veterinary practice. Clinical signs of thrombocytopenia relate to inability to form primary plugs, to generate phospholipid for coagulation reactions, and to maintain vascular endothelial integrity. As platelet levels diminish below $40,000/\mu l$, clinical signs of platelet dysfunction become evident. These clinical signs include petechiation, purpura, and ecchymosis in the skin, particularly evident on the ventral abdomen or oral mucous membranes. As the platelet count decreases below $20,000/\mu l$, epistaxis, hematuria, or gastrointestintal bleeding may be manifested. Bleeding episodes due to thrombocytopenia are much more common in dogs than in cats. The bleeding associated with thrombocytopenia is more immediate in onset and of shorter duration than that associated with a coagulation factor deficiency.

The mechanisms of thrombocytopenia include reduced megakaryocyte production, accelerated peripheral destruction, and abnormal distribution (Table 80–4). Reduced megakaryocyte production may occur secondary to marrow stem cell damage in-

Table 80–4. Common Causes of Thrombocytopenia

I. Reduced platelet production (characterized by decreased marrow megakaryopoiesis)
   A. Leukemia leading to myelophthisis
   B. Drug-induced hypoplasia, eg., estrogen toxicity
   C. Radiation/chemotherapy-induced hypoplasia
II. Accelerated platelet destruction (characterized by increased marrow megakaryopoiesis and megathrombocytes)
   A. Associated with disseminated intravascular coagulation
   B. Related to immunologic injury of platelets
      1. Autoantibodies
         a) Immune-mediated thrombocytopenia (IMTP), systemic lupus erythematosis (SLE), autoimmune hemolytic anemia (AIHA)
         b) Drugs
III. Abnormal distribution (characterized by normal marrow megakaryoporesis)
   A. Splenomegaly
   B. Artifact associated with poor venipuncture technique

duced by drugs, radiation, or infectious disease, or may follow displacement by a neoplastic cell population (myelophthisis). Occasionally multiple mechanisms are involved in the genesis of thrombocytopenia. Reduced platelet production is confirmed by finding reduced marrow megakaryopoiesis. A low power (10×) field of a normal bone marrow aspirate smear contains about five megakaryocytes (in or around areas of high cellularity). Often marrows from patients with reduced platelet production have almost no megakaryocytes on the entire smear. Since increased megakaryopoiesis is associated with increased peripheral destruction, and virtual absence of megakaryocytes is associated with reduced production, it is simple to classify thrombocytopenia on the basis of marrow findings.

Decreased platelet production usually follows stem cell damage resulting from myelotoxic drugs (estrogens, chemotherapy) or radiation. Chronic, subclinical canine ehrlichiosis is also associated with pancytopenia and bone marrow hypoplasia. In one series of 30 cases of canine ehrlichiosis in Texas, anemia was present in 90 per cent, leukopenia in 53 per cent, and thrombocytopenia in 100 per cent (Troy et al., 1980). In the same series seven of ten bone marrow aspirates were considered hypoplastic. Bleeding tendencies were seen in less than one half of the cases. It is important to note that *Ehrlichia* organisms were only seen in 5 of the 30 cases, so one must rely primarily on serologic confirmation with the indirect fluorescent antibody test (Ristic et al., 1972). Therapy with tetracycline was found relatively successful, particularly in the earlier stages of ehrlichiosis.

Estrogen therapy for mismating, perianal gland adenomas, prostatic hyperplasia, and urinary incontinence in dogs has often been associated with bone marrow hypoplasia. Leukocyte counts are variable and may be moderately elevated during the early course of toxicity. Marked suppression of erythropoiesis and megakaryopoiesis occurs for 20 days following administration of estrogen (Chiu, 1974). After this time the marrow may recover, depending somewhat on the age of the dog. Older dogs may have an aplastic crisis, whereas younger dogs usually recover. Marked neutropenia following estrogen administration is considered an unfavorable sign, and such cases commonly develop a fatal hemorrhagic diathesis. Obviously, many of the drugs used in chemotherapy suppress mitotic division of both neoplastic and normal hematopoietic cells and must be used judiciously when normal hematopoietic tissue is markedly displaced by a leukemic cell population. When marrow cellularity is increased but megakaryopoiesis is minimal, myelophthesis may be present. In myelophthesis, a relatively homogenous marrow population of leukemic cells is readily observed.

When marrow findings indicate normal to increased megakaryopoiesis, the thrombocytopenia can be due to increased peripheral destruction of platelets, abnormal platelet distribution, or a collection artifact. The primary causes of increased peripheral destruction are DIC and immune-mediated thrombocytopenia (IMTP). The cause of thrombocytopenia of DIC is variable but essentially resides in the intravascular generation of thrombin, which promotes platelet aggregation and platelet plug formation in the microvasculature. In IMTP, an IgG antibody coating of platelets results in premature destruction of platelets by the reticuloendothelial system of the spleen and liver. The diagnosis of IMTP resides in demonstrating a platelet antibody. Unfortunately, most present methodologies are quite complex. The most common test is the platelet factor 3 (PF-3) release test (also known as the PF-3 immunoinjury test) (Wilkins et al., 1973; Pierce et al., 1977). This test is based on the catalytic activity of platelet phospholipid in the intrinsic coagulation cascade. When a factor capable of injuring platelets is added to a platelet rich plasma mixture, the increased availability of PF-3 shortens the clotting time. When controls clot in 60 seconds, a 10-second shortening is considered positive for the presence of platelet immunoinjury. This test was positive in about two thirds of the dogs with a clinical diagnosis of IMTP. About one third of the thrombocytopenic dogs with systemic lupus erythematosus and autoimmune hemolytic anemia were also positive. IMTP is a rare cause of thrombocytopenia in cats (Joshi et al., 1979). In man, positive platelet immunoinjury tests are occasionally noted in individuals that have received multiple blood transfusions or those with rheumatoid arthritis, lymphoma, or chronic hepatitis (Karpatkin, 1980). Platelet antibodies that induce qualitative platelet dysfunction are also described (Clancy et al., 1972). Such antibodies may account for inhibition of the PF-3 immunoinjury test seen in canine ehrlichiosis (Pierce et al., 1977). In some cases antibody-binding to megakaryocytes has been demonstrated by direct and indirect immunofluorescence of bone marrow smears (Joshi et al., 1976). Whether or not these antibodies adversely affect platelet production is unclear at present.

Treatment of IMTP consists of immunosuppressive doses of steroids, usually prednisone at high levels (1 to 3 mg/kg/day) as a divided dose. Increased platelet counts are noted in the majority of patients within 24 to 48 hours, if the dose is effective. Bleeding must be controlled with fresh whole blood or platelet-rich plasma, if available. Platelets stored for more than 12 hours in ACD solution are hemostatically ineffective. After the patient's platelet count returns to safe levels (> 100,000), the steroid therapy may be tapered to a low maintenance dose on an alternate day basis. In some cases the patient's platelet count may not return to normal levels, but increased marrow platelet production achieves a sufficient platelet count to prevent bleeding. In patients failing to respond to steroids, splenectomy and/or chemotherapeutic approaches may be required. As the spleen represents the primary site of platelet destruction and an important site of platelet antibody production, splenectomy is effective in some steroid-resistant IMTP patients.

Occasional patients may develop thrombocytopenia when antibodies are complexed to platelets with adsorbed bacterial, viral, or drug antigens. Subsequent complement fixation can result in direct platelet lysis. Drugs incriminated in IMTP of dogs include sulfonamides and dinitrophenol (Wilkins, 1977). Package inserts should be reviewed carefully for potential drug-platelet interaction when an animal on therapy develops clinical signs of platelet dysfunction.

Because about one third of the total platelet pool resides in the spleen, splenomegaly can result in thrombocytopenia. The term idiopathic thrombocytopenia is reserved for a small percentage of patients in which the cause of thrombocytopenia can not be determined. As stated earlier, collection artifacts should always be considered as a cause of thrombocytopenia, and blood smears should be carefully reviewed to exclude this possibility.

QUALITATIVE DISORDERS OF PLATELET FUNCTION

There is increasing evidence that qualitative disorders of platelets play a role in certain hemostatic disorders, although they are less common than thrombocytopenia. Qualitative disorders of platelets are suspected when coagulation screening tests and platelet count are normal in a patient with a hemostatic problem. The bleeding time is often increased. It is sometimes paradoxical that some patients with thrombocytopenia do not have significant bleeding problems, while others with adequate platelets do have bleeding tendencies. This is often explained on the basis of the relative function of the circulating platelets. Particularly in thrombocytopenia in which megathrombocytes are increased, patients do not bleed because their large platelets are more hemostatically effective. In contrast, some chronic procoagulant stimuli induce degranulation of platelets without necessarily removing them from circulation. Such "ghost" platelets are usually hypogranular, and platelet counts may grossly overestimate the ability of such hypoactive platelets to perform necessary hemostatic functions.

There are both hereditary and acquired causes of qualitative abnormalities in platelet function. Two forms of hereditary platelet dysfunction have been reported in dogs.

A family of otter hounds were noted to have moderate thrombocytopenia and bimodal population of platelets of which about 50 to 80 per cent were bizarre macroplatelets (Dodds, 1967). A clinically apparent hemorrhagic diathesis was characterized by several abnormalities in platelet function tests that included prolonged bleeding times; poor clot retraction; defective platelet aggregation response to ADP, collagen, and thrombin; low platelet retention; reduced PF3 availability; and low prothrombin consumption. The defect was inherited as an autosomal dominant trait with variable expression. Heterozygous carriers were only mildly affected clinically but could be detected by platelet function tests. No abnormalities were detected by coagulation screening tests. The disorder has similarities to two platelet disorders seen in man (Glanzmann's disease and Bernard Soulier syndrome) and subsequently has been termed canine thrombasthenic thrombocytopathia.

A family of basset hounds with a history of recurrent bleeding episodes due to thrombocytopathy were recently described (Johnstone and Lotz, 1979). Although clot retraction, platelet morphology, and platelet count were normal, deficient platelet retention in glass bead columns and defective platelet aggregation responses to ADP and collagen were present. Isolated instances of platelet dysfunction have also been observed in other breeds, namely foxhounds and poodles.

Acquired qualitiative platelet disorders are associated with a broad spectrum of diseases including uremia, myeloproliferative disorders, dysproteinemias, scurvy, and liver disease (Edson, 1979). Perhaps the most common platelet dysfunction is associated with aspirin administration. Platelet dysfunction may be induced by a wide variety of commonly prescribed drugs, including promazine-type tranquilizers, penicillins, phenylbutazone, certain sulfa drugs, estrogens, dextrans, local anesthetics, and antihistamines. The mechanisms of drug-induced platelet dysfunction are poorly understood in many cases. In the case of aspirin, the platelet cyclo-oxygenase system is specifically inhibited, which decreases production of prostaglandin intermediates that are important in platelet aggregation and release. Presently there is much interest in the pharmacologic manipulation of platelet function in order to inhibit the platelet's role in thrombosis but to allow sufficient platelet function to support normal hemostasis. The laboratory evaluation of qualitative platelet disorders was previously discussed and is primarily based on platelet aggregation studies.

REFERENCES

Antman, K. H., Skarin, A. T., Mayer, R. J., Hargreaves, H. K., and Canellos, G. P.: Microangiopathic hemolytic anemia and cancer: A review. Medicine 58:377–384, 1979.

Blaisdell, F. S., and Dodds, W. J.: Evaluation of two microhematocrit methods for quantitating plasma fibrinogen. J.A.V.M.A. 171:340–342, 1977.

Brackett, D. J., Schaefer, C. F., and Gunn, C. G.: Influence of time, temperature and platelet concentration on dog platelet aggregation. Thromb. Res. 8:441–451, 1976.

Chiu, T.: Studies of estrogen-induced proliferative disorders of hematopoietic tissue in dogs. Ph.D. thesis, University of Minnesota, Minneapolis, 1974.

Clancy, R., Jenkins, B., and Firkin, B.: Qualitative platelet abnormalities in idiopathic thrombocytopenic purpura. N. Engl. J. Med. 286:622–626, 1972.

Coleman, R. W., Robboy, S. J., and Minna, J. D.: Disseminated intravascular coagulation: A reappraisal. Ann. Rev. Med. 30:359–374, 1979.

Dodds, W. J.: Familial canine thrombocytopathy. Thromb. Diath. Haemorrh. Supp. 26:241–248, 1967.

Dodds, W. J.: Bleeding Disorders. In Ettinger, S. J.

(ed.): Textbook of Veterinary Internal Medicine. W. B. Saunders Co., Philadelphia, 1975, p. 1679–1698.

Duncan, J. R., and Prasse, K. W.: Veterinary Laboratory Medicine. Ames, Iowa State Press, 1977, p. 74.

Ebbe, S.: Experimental and clinical megakaryocytopoiesis. Clin. Hematol. 8:371–388, 1979.

Edson, J. R.: Acquired Qualitative Abnormalities of Platelet Function. In Schmidt, R. M. (2nd ed.): CRC Handbook Series in Clin. Lab. Science, Section I Hematology, Vol. 1, CRC Press, Inc., Boca Raton, 1979, p. 463–469.

Gingrich, R. D., and Hoak, J. C.: Platelet-endothelial cell interactions. Semin. Hematol. 16:208–220, 1979.

Green, R. A., Roudebush, P., and Barton, C. L.: Laboratory evaluation of coagulopathies due to vitamin K antagonism: Three case reports. J.A.A.H.A. 15:691–697, 1979.

Green, R. A.: Activated coagulation time in monitoring heparinized dogs. Am. J. Vet. Res. 41:1793–1797, 1980.

Greene, C. E., Barsante, J. A., and Jones, B. D.: Disseminated intravascular coagulation complicating aflatoxicosis in dogs. Corn. Vet. 67:29–49, 1977.

Greene, C. E.: Disseminated intravascular coagulation in the dog: A review. J.A.A.H.A. *11*:674–687, 1975.

Harker, L. A.: Hemostasis Manual, 2nd ed., F.A. Davis Co., Philadelphia, 1974, p. 37.

Johnson, G. S., Lees, G. E., Benson, R. E., et al.: A Bleeding Disease (von Willebrand's Disease) in a Chesapeake Bay retriever. J.A.V.M.A. *176*:1261–1263, 1980.

Johnstone, I. B., and Lotz, F.: An inherited platelet function defect in Basset hounds. Can. Vet. J. *20*:211–215, 1979.

Joshi, B. C., and Jain, N. C.: Detection of antiplatelet antibody in serum and megakaryocytes of dogs with autoimmune thrombocytopenia. Am. J. Vet. Res. *37*:681–685, 1976.

Joshi, B. C., Raplee, R. G., Powell, A. L., and Hancock, F.: Autoimmune thrombocytopenia in a cat. J. A. A. H. A. *15*:585–588, 1979.

Karpatkin, S.: Platelet Sizing. *In* Schmidt, R. M. (sec. ed.): CRC Handbook Series in Clinical Laboratory Science Sec. 1: Hematology, Vol. 1, CRC Press, Inc., Boca Raton, p. 409–434, 1979.

Karpatkin, S.: Autoimmune thrombocytopenic purpura. Blood *56*:329–343, 1980.

Kociba, G. J., and Hathaway, J. E.: Disseminated intravascular coagulation associated with heartworm disease in the dog. J.A.A.H.A. *10*:373–378, 1974.

Kwaan, H. C.: Disorders of Fibrinolysis. *In* Ogston, D., and Bennett, B. (eds.): Hemostasis: Biochemistry Physiology and Pathology. John Wiley and Sons, London, 1977, p. 491–510.

Lechner, K., Niessner, H., and Thaler, E.: Coagulation abnormalities in liver disease. Semin. Thromb. Hemost. *4*:40–56, 1977.

Levine, R. F., Bunn, P. A., Hazzard, K. C., and Schlam, M. L.: Flow cytometric analysis of megakaryocyte ploidy. Blood *56*:210–217, 1980.

Lewis, J. H., Spero, J. A., and Hasiba, U.: Coagulopathies. Disease-A-Month *23*(9):1–64, 1977.

Lotter, M. G., Badenhorst, P. N., duP Heyns, A., Van Reenen, O. R., Pieters, H., and Minnaar, P. C.: Kinetics, distribution and sites of destruction of canine blood platelets with In — III oxine. J. Nuc. Med. *21*:36–40, 1980.

Madewell, B. R., and Feldman, B. F.: Characterization of anemias associated neoplasia in small animals. J.A.V.M.A. *176*:419–425, 1980.

Mant, M. J., and King, E. G.: Severe, acute disseminated intravascular coagulation. A reappraisal of its pathophysiology, clinical significance and therapy based on 47 patients. Am. J. Med. *67*:557–563, 1979.

Mielke, C. H., Kaneshiro, M. M., Maher, I. A., et al.: The standardized normal Ivy bleeding time and its prolongation by aspirin. Blood *34*:204–215, 1969.

Mogadam, L.: Application of the Miller's disc for the estimation and quality control of the platelet count. Lab. Med. *11*:131–132, 1980.

Moore, D. J.: Disseminated intravascular coagulation: A review of its pathogenesis, manifestations and treatment. J. S. Afr. Vet. Med. Assoc. *50*:259–264, 1979.

Nosanchuk, J. S., Chang, J., and Bennett, J. M.: The analytic basis for the use of platelet estimates from peripheral blood smears. Am. J. Clin. Pathol. *69*:383–387, 1978.

O'Reilly, R. A.: Vitamin K and the oral anticoagulant drugs. Ann. Rev. Med. *27*:245–261, 1976.

Owen, C. A. Jr., Bowie, E. J. W., and Cooper, H. A.: Turnover of fibrinogen and platelets in dogs undergoing induced intravascular coagulation. Thromb. Res. *2*:251–259, 1973.

Pierce, K. R., Marrs, G. E., and Hightower, D.: Acute canine ehrlichiosis and platelet survival and factor 3 assay. Am. J. Vet. Res. *38*:1821–1825, 1977.

Raymond, S. L. and Dodds, W. J.: Plasma antithrombin activity: A comparative study in normal and diseased animals. Proc. Soc. Exp. Biol. Med. *161*:464–467, 1979.

Ristic, M., Huxsoll, D. L., Weisiger, R. M., Hildebrandt, P. K., and Nyindo, M. B. A.: Serological diagnosis of tropical canine pancytopenia by indirect immunofluorescence. Infect. Immunol. *6*:226–231, 1972.

Rubin, M. H., Weston, M. J., Langley, P. G., et al.: Platelet function in chronic liver disease: Relationship to disease severity. Dig. Dis. Sci. *24*:197–202, 1979.

Schalm, O. W., Jain, N. C., and Carroll, E. J.: Veterinary Hematology, 3rd ed. Lea and Febiger, Philadelphia, 1975.

Sherry, S.: Mechanisms of Fibrinolysis. *In* Williams, W. J., Beutler, E., Erslev, A. J., and Rundles, R. W. (eds.): Hematology, 2nd ed., McGraw Hill Book Co., New York, 1977, p. 1303.

Sixma, J. J., and Wester, J.: The hemostatic plug. Sem. Hematol. *14*:265–299. 1977.

Strombeck, D. R., Krum, S., and Rogers, Q.: Coagulopathy and encephalopathy in a dog with acute hepatic necrosis. J.A.V.M.A. *169*:813–816, 1976.

Tavassoli, M.: Megakaryocyte-platelet axis and the process of platelet formation and release. Blood *55*:537–545, 1980.

Thomas, R., Hessel, E. A., Dillard, D. H., and Harker, L. A.: Standardized template bleeding time in dogs. J. Surg. Res. *27*:244–249, 1979.

Triplett, D. A.: Hemostatic problems encountered in the community hospital. ASCP National Meeting. American Society of Clinical Pathologists, Commission on Continuing Education, Council on Hematology, 1978.

Triplett, D. A., (ed.): Platelet Function Laboratory Evaluation and Clinical Application. Am. Soc. Clin. Path. Educational Products Division, Chicago, 1978.

Troy, G. C., Vulgamott, J. C., and Turnwald, G. H.: Canine ehrlichiosis: A retrospective study of thirty naturally occurring cases. J. A. A. H. A. *16*:181–187, 1980.

Weiss, R. C., Dodds, W. J., and Scott, F. W.: Disseminated intravascular coagulation in experimentally induced feline infectious peritonitis. Am. J. Vet. Res. *41*:663–671, 1980.

Wigton, D. H., Kociba, G. J., and Hoover, E. A.: Infectious canine hepatitis: Animal model of viral-induced disseminated intravascular coagulation Blood *47*:287–296, 1976.

Wilkins, R. J., Hurvitz, A. I., and Dodds, W. J.: Immunologically mediated thrombocytopenia in the dog. J.A.V.M.A. *163*:277–282, 1973.

Wilkins, R. J.: Thrombocytopenic Purpura. *In* Kirk, R. W. (ed.): Current Veterinary Therapy VI. Small Animal Practice, W. B. Saunders Co., Philadelphia, 1977, p. 445–448.

SECTION XV

Immunologic Diseases

CHAPTER 81

ANTHONY SCHWARTZ
and J. MICHAEL KEHOE

Fundamental Principles of Immunology

Much of the significance and appeal of modern immunology resides in its comprehensiveness. It touches many fields, including basic chemistry (structure of humoral mediators of immune reactions), cell biology (origin and nature of cells active in immunity), genetics (transmission and activation of genetic information required in immunologic responses), and clinical medicine (selective induction or suppression of immune reactivity). The application of these principles to clinical problems in veterinary medicine is illustrated in several chapters of this text. The purpose of this chapter is to provide background information necessary to understand the role of immunologic processes in disease.

THE LYMPHOID SYSTEM

CELLULAR INTERACTIONS IN ANTIBODY MEDIATED (HUMORAL) IMMUNITY

Although the ability to mount an immune response has been attributed to cells from lymphoid tissues for some time, only in the past 25 years has it become recognized that a complex division of labor exists between different populations of lymphocytes as well as non-lymphoid cells. From studies performed during the period between the mid-1950s and the mid-1960s it was found that the thymus is involved in both graft rejection and antibody formation, while the bursa of Fabricius in chickens (and its mammalian equivalent) is important only to antibody formation (Good and Gabrielson, 1964). It was later shown that thymus cells and bone marrow cells interact to result in an antibody response (Claman et al., 1966) and that although thymus derived cells do not make antibody (they can proliferate in response to antigen [Davies, 1964; Miller

and Mitchell, 1968]), they somehow "help" the bone marrow cells produce antibody. Cells derived from the thymus were termed T cells, and bone marrow (or the bursal equivalent)–derived cells were referred to as B cells. T cells and B cells will be described in depth later.

A third type of cell has been shown to be required for an effective immune response (Mosier, 1967). These are non-lymphoid, bone marrow–derived "accessory cells," which consist primarily of macrophage-like cells. Since many types adhere to glass or plastic, they have been termed "adherent cells." They include fixed cells in the spleen, lymph nodes, lung alveoli, liver (Kupffer cells), and skin (Langerhans cells), and free cells in the peritoneal cavity and circulation. Accessory cells are important for the production of antibody, the expression of cell-mediated immune (CMI*) responses, and the response of lymphoid cells to mitogens.

Phagocytic cells function by trapping antigenic molecules, most of which are ingested and degraded. Some of this processed antigen is then presented to T lymphocytes. Some, but not all, macrophages can function as accessory cells (bone marrow macrophages cannot), while some adherent cells are nonphagocytic (e.g., dendritic cells of the spleen and lymph nodes) but are excellent antigen presentors (Steinman and Whitmer, 1978). Macrophages can form soluble substances such as lymphocyte activating factor (LAF [Gheri et al., 1972], now termed interleukin I), which can activate certain T cells (Lyt 1 antigen–positive; see following discussion). In addition, macrophages can compose the main component

---

*For the reader's convenience, an Abbreviation Key is provided at the end of this chapter.

of the inflammatory response in CMI reactions and may be the effector cells in such responses, as described in a later section.

LYMPHOCYTE DIFFERENTIATION

Immunologically competent lymphoid cells originate from *pluripotent stem cells* (Wu et al., 1968), which reside first in the fetal yolk sac and then in the bone marrow. By unknown means, stem cells appear to become lymphocyte *progenitor cells,* which are now precommitted to "education" in one of a series of inducing microenvironments called primary or central lymphoid organs (reviewed in Waksman, 1970). One such site is the bursa of Fabricius of birds or its equivalent in mammals (most likely the liver). During their stay in the bursa, or its equivalent, cells progress through a succession of maturational developments leading to B cells, which leave the bursa and produce and secrete one or another of the immunoglobulins (Ig's).

Some precursors become T cells in the other primary lymphoid organ, the thymus. This lymphoepithelial gland, the epithelial portion of which is derived from the third and fourth branchial pouches, is located in the anterior mediastinum. The mouse has been used extensively as a model to study the differentiation and function of T cells, and serves as a prototype for other species. In the mouse, it appears that progenitor cells (prothymocytes) migrate first to the thymus cortex, where they take on T-cell markers but are not yet immunocompetent. These immature thymocytes comprise over 90 per cent of thymic lymphoid cells (see Table 81–1). Under the influence of thymic hormones (thymopoietin) they reproduce repeatedly and somehow become committed to differentiate into T cells that have antigen specificity, with the added ability to recognize self components as self, and nonself components as foreign. Once they migrate to the medulla, immunocompetence is gained. These cells leave the thymus and enter the peripheral functional T lymphocyte pool in the spleen and lymph nodes (secondary lymphoid organs).

The stages of maturation of T cells can be followed by shifts in the surface content of a variety of markers, or differentiation alloantigens, including histocompatibility antigens (H-2 antigens in the mouse), while changes in enzymes such as terminal deoxynucleotidyl transferase (Tdt) and in function (reviewed in McKenzie and Potter, 1979) (Table 81–1) also occur. The quantity of H-2 antigens increases as T lymphocytes mature. In contrast, the major murine T-cell specific antigen (Theta or Thy 1, [Reif and Allen, 1964]) is maximal in immature thymocytes but decreases with maturation (this surface antigen is also found on brain cells, epithelial cells, and fibroblasts). Another T-cell marker, TL, which is found on some leukemia cells and on normal thymocytes, ordinarily disappears in mature T cells (Boyse et al., 1965). The Lyt alloantigens of mice not only are differentiation antigens but also are functional markers. Thus, Lyt 1, 2, and 3 antigens are present on all immature cortical thymocytes (Ly 1, 2, 3 cells), while mature Lyt 1+ 2, 3− (Ly 1) cells contain helper T cells and Lyt 1− 2, 3+ (Ly 2, 3) cells contain suppressor and cytotoxic T cells (to be discussed later).

Differential Effects of Lectins on T cells and B Cells. Other differences between T cells and B cells, which are also used as markers, are their responses to plant lectins. Several lectins are specifically mitogenic for either B cells or T cells (Jannosy and Greaves, 1972). Thus, murine and human B cells, but not T cells, incubated in vitro with lipopolysaccharide (LPS) derived from gram-negative bacteria will undergo blasto-

Table 81–1. Characteristics of Murine T Cells and Their Precursors

Cell Types	Surface Antigens					T-Cell Function
	H-2	*TL*	*Thy 1*	*Lyt*	*Tdt*	
Prothymocytes	+	−	−	−	+	−
Immature thymocytes (cortex)	+	++	+++	123	+	−
Mature thymocytes (medulla) and T cells	+++	−	+	1,2, and 123	−	+

Table 81–2. T Cells and B Cells Compared (Mouse)

Property	B Cell	T Cell
Antigen binding receptor	IgM (heavy concentration) IgD Single idiotype	Unclear and controversial. Idiotype and V_H segment present.
Surface antigens:		
Thy-1	−	+
TL	−	+
Ly	Lyb	Lyt
Pc	+	−
H-2	+	+
Inactivated by		
X-rays	Strongly	Slightly*
Corticosteroids	Moderately	Slightly*
Anti-lymphocyte serum	Slightly	Strongly
Functions:		
Memory	Yes	Yes
Ig secretion	Yes	No
Helper function	No	Yes (Ly 1)
Cell mediated immunity	No	Yes (Ly 2 and Ly 1)
Suppression	Yes	Yes (Ly 23)
Tolerance	Late and transient	Early and long lasting
Differentiation	Bone marrow, then Bursa of Fabricius in birds (liver in mammals), then general circulation	Bone marrow, then thymus, then general circulation
Response to mitogens	Lipopolysaccharide (LPS)	Concanavalin A (Con A) Phytohemagglutinin (PHA)

*Ly 123 cells appear more sensitive.

genesis, synthesize DNA, and divide. In contrast, two other lectins, phytohemagglutinin (PHA) and concanavalin A (Con A), are mitogenic only for T cells. The specificity of T vs. B cell responses to certain lectins varies with the species. Canine T lymphocytes have been shown to respond to both PHA and Con A (Schultz, 1978). These and other characteristics that have proved useful in distinguishing sets of T cells and B cells are collated in Table 81–2.

SECONDARY LYMPHOID ORGANS

Lymph Nodes. Lymphocytes are found in the superficial and the deep cortex of the lymph nodes. In the superficial cortex (or "thymus-independent area") are found follicles that consist mainly of B lymphocytes (Fig. 81–1). Less well organized groups of lymphocytes are found between the follicles. During an immune response the follicles enlarge to become secondary follicles and

Figure 81–1. Basic structure of mammalian lymph node. The sinuses, follicles, and ducts are indicated as well as zones that are especially rich in either T lymphocytes or B lymphocytes.

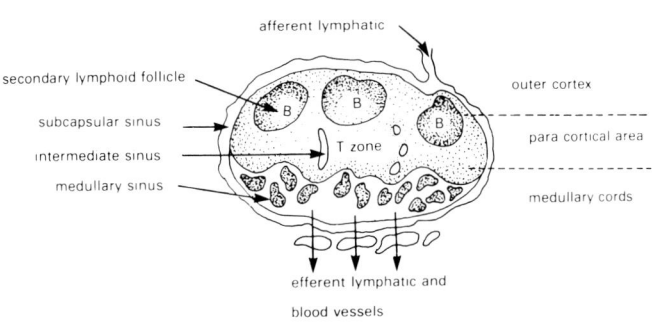

develop a germinal center, which contains proliferating lymphocytes. The deep cortex (or thymus-dependent area) contains three T cells for each B cell. About 95 per cent of lymphocytes that leave an unstimulated lymph node are recirculating cells derived from the blood and not from the node itself. Drainage of recirculating lymphocytes by exteriorizing the thoracic duct will primarily cause depletion of the thymus-dependent areas of the lymph nodes, showing that most recirculating lymphocytes are T cells.

Antigen enters the deep cortex of the lymph node via the afferent lymph and is trapped, partially digested, and presented to T cells by macrophages to initiate the immune response. Trapping of antigen is facilitated if it is already antibody coated. Trapping can also occur in the lymphoid follicles of the superficial cortex, but only when the antigen is bound by antibody and, therefore, only when an immune response has already been initiated. Through secretion of antigen specific and nonspecific factors, T cells *help* B cells, which are also antigen-stimulated, to make antibodies.

Following the entry of antigen into the nodes, the number of lymphocytes leaving the node decreases, while the number of cells found in the deep cortex increases. Within two to five days, more lymphocytes leave the node, but the lymphocytes specific for the antigen in question increase in the node and do not leave. Proliferation of lymphoid cells occurs in the deep cortex, and antibody formation is first seen during this period (see Normal Immune Response). After five days, lymphocytes specific for antigen leave the node, thus disseminating the response. After seven days the superficial cortex develops and germinal centers are seen. Plasma cells, the antibody producing end state of the differentiation of B cells, become abundant.

The Spleen. The spleen is predominantly responsible for responses to blood-born antigens. It is made up of the lymphoid cell rich white pulp and the blood-filled sinuses of the red pulp. The thymus-dependent area of the white pulp surrounds arterioles and is called the periarteriolar lymphoid sheath. The thymus-independent area is made up of the follicular or nodular B-cell regions surrounding the T-cell areas (Waksman, 1970).

THE CONCEPT OF ANTIGENICITY AND THE NORMAL IMMUNE RESPONSE

The notion of antigenicity is fundamental to all of immunology. This property denotes the capacity of given substance (antigen) to induce a state of altered reactivity in an individual such that subsequent encounters with that specific antigen will result in an augmented secondary, or anamnestic, response. This reaction, which can take many forms, is called an *immune response*. The ability to induce an immune response is a function of certain molecular characteristics of the antigen (molecular size, rigidity, net charge, stereospecificity) as well as certain biological characteristics of the host (genetic constitution, species, age). Normally, an antigenic substance will differ from constituents of the responding host's own body. That is, the immune response is capable of distinguishing "self" from "non-self." The loss of this discriminating capacity can lead to disease (autoimmunity).

REQUIREMENT FOR ANTIGENICITY

A *complete* antigen can both induce an immune response and react with the humoral products of the response (antibodies). However, an incomplete antigen, or *hapten* (part of a complete antigen), is unable to induce an immune response but can be bound by already formed specific antibodies previously generated in response to the complete antigen. Haptens (such as metals or small chemical moieties like dinitrophenol) will lead to an immune response only if they are attached to a *carrier* molecule (such as a "self" protein). On a cellular level, it has been shown that while B cells produce the specific anti-hapten antibody, a recognition specificity for the *carrier* molecule is exhibited by T cells (see Thymus-Dependent Antibody Responses). Such hapten-carrier relationships have clinical relevance in certain forms of immunologically mediated *contact hypersensitivity* to various chemicals. These phenomena are only beginning to be identified in dogs, cats and other domesticated animals.

Precise chemical details of the molecular characteristics responsible for antigenic properties of protein molecules have been elucidated. Larger antigens (bacteria or viruses or mammalian cells) are actually mosaics of a number of individual antigens. Even in a single protein molecule, certain local regions, called *antigenic determinants,* stimulate the formation of antibodies whose specificity is directed only against these local regions. Conformational (three dimensional) determinants formed by intramolecular folding are of the greatest importance in proteins, although linear amino acid sequences act as determinants in some cases. Many studies suggest that an antigen is intact when it is recognized as foreign by the immune system, confirming the preeminence of conformational determinants as immunodominant groups in proteins.

Although proteins are the most common antigens known, certain carbohydrates are also very strongly antigenic, as in the case of the bacterial polysaccharides and the blood group substances. Nucleic acids are not strong antigens, but anti-nucleic acid antibodies can be induced by appropriate laboratory manipulations and are seen spontaneously in certain diseases, such as systemic lupus erythematosus. Lipids are normally not antigenic but exceptions do occur.

Adjuvants. The immune response can be enhanced by combining antigens with adjuvants. These substances exert their enhancing effect on the host in several ways, some of which are still unknown. Some adjuvants, such as mineral oil or alum precipitates, retard the destruction of antigen (depot effect), while others, such as Freund's complete adjuvant (which combines a mineral oil depot with killed mycobacteria), cause inflammatory reactions that can permit the recruitment and activation of larger numbers of immunocompetent cells.

THE NORMAL IMMUNE RESPONSE

The immune response is usually very helpful, as, for example, when it is directed against an invading bacterium or virus. The typical humoral immune response to an antigen is graphically illustrated in Figure 81–2. A "primary" response to antigenic stimulation at time zero in a previously unstimulated individual is followed by a lag phase and then an exponential increase in antibody titer to a steady state. The titer then rapidly falls off. Restimulation of a previously sensitized individual leads to a secondary (anamnestic) response. In this case, the lag phase is shorter, the rate of titer increase is greater, a higher final titer is reached at the steady state phase, and the fall off is less rapid than in a primary response. The expansion of antigen-specific clones of T cells and B cells occurs during the primary response. Secondary stimulation with the same antigen can then lead to rapid triggering of these "memory" cells, resulting in an augmented secondary response.

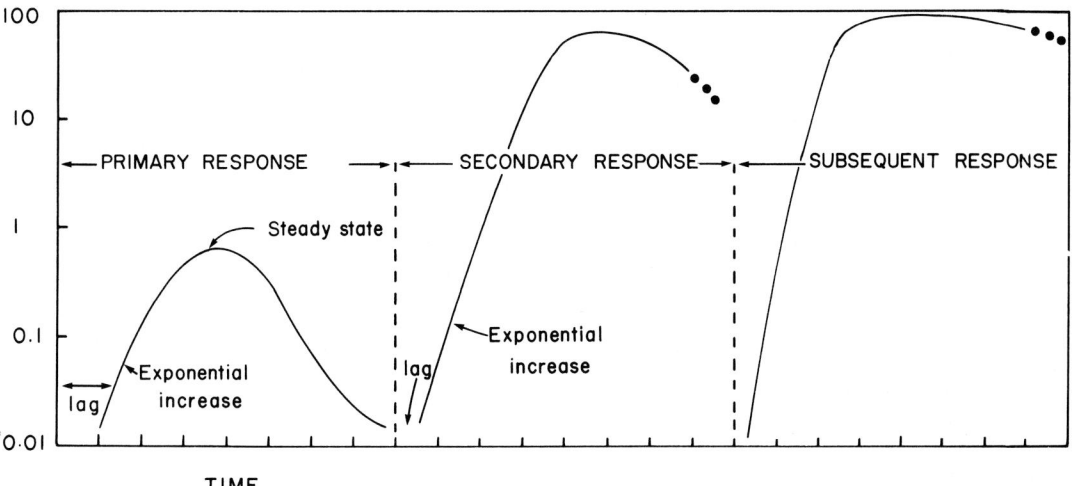

Figure 81–2. Graphic illustration of the normal humoral immune response. The secondary (anamnestic) response is characterized by a greater rate of antibody rise, a higher plateau region, and a more modest titer decrement after challenge. The difference is due primarily to the presence of memory T and B lymphocytes subsequent to an initial antigen sensitization.

Comparable, although diminishing, differences are observed with subsequent stimulations with the same antigen. The appropriate manipulation of this pattern obviously determines such important clinical variables as how often revaccination should be performed, appropriate antigenic dosages, and the like. In practice, a somewhat empirical approach must still be used to determine the extent of antigenic stimulation that is required in given instances.

Thymus-Dependent Antibody Responses

We have noted that an obligatory synergism exists between T and B cells in the antibody response to most antigens. This type of response is called "thymus dependent." T cells *can* respond to the same immunogenic components (determinants) of most antigens, as do B cells. During a response to complex antigens (or to model antigens made up of hapten and carrier), however, T cells generally respond to a different determinant (the carrier) on the same molecule than does the B cell, which is responding to the hapten itself.

T Cell–Independent B-Cell Responses

Optimal specific humoral immune responses to certain antigens can occur without T-cell cooperation (e.g., in neonatally thymectomized mice). The structure of such antigens usually consists of repetitive sequences of identical subunits. Molecules without this structure not only fail to stimulate B cells in the absence of T cells, but may result in a tolerogenic signal upon direct interaction with B-cell receptors. Thymus-independent antigens, such as polysaccharides, often behave as B-cell mitogens (e.g., LPS). The response engendered by these antigens is generally restricted to the IgM class, and little effective memory results (i.e., there is no augmented secondary response on reexposure to the same antigen). It is felt that the special structure of T-cell independent antigens somehow substitutes for the "second signal" given B cells by T cells (antigen is signal 1 and the T-cell signal to the B cell is signal 2) in T cell–dependent responses (Watson et al., 1973). Such responses are of considerable practical significance, since a number of vaccines (e.g., killed bacterial products) contain antigens with repetitive determinants of the sort described previously.

Effect of T Cells on the Class and Affinity of Synthesized Immunoglobulin

Whereas thymus-independent antigens elicit only IgM antibodies, thymus-dependent antigens stimulate all known classes and subclasses of immunoglobulins (refer to Immunoglobulin Structure and Function). There have been recent indications that there are different helper T cells for different Ig classes and subclasses and, perhaps, even for B cells bearing selected idiotypic specificities. There is also evidence that T cells are important regulators of the emergence of cells bearing high-affinity receptors (Gershon and Paul, 1971). Such associations may ultimately be put to clinical use such as when a class-associated phenomenon (e.g., an IgE-mediated allergic response) must be reduced or eliminated.

Control Mechanisms in the Immune Response

Just as in other body systems, the immune apparatus is finely tuned. Thus, in addition to positive (helper) or "on" signals, negative (suppressor) or "off" signals exist as well. The net observed level of the immune response, therefore, is a balance between positive and negative regulatory interactions. Only by comprehending this concept can we understand problems such as why the response to a particular antigen doesn't continually progress to overwhelm the entire lymphoid system, why the fetus as an allotransplant is not rejected by a maternal immune response, and why immune responses to our own tissue antigens are the exception rather than the rule. In a complex system, there are, as might be expected, multiple levels of control.

Antigen. Whether an immune response occurs following exposure to an antigen depends on the dose, timing and nature of the antigen involved. For example, the lethal dose in mice for tetanus toxin is 20 pg (2×10^{-11} gm), while the dose required for immunization is 2 μg (2×10^{-6} gm). Therefore, even though it is a highly immunogenic molecule, tetanus toxin must be detoxified before it can be used. For unknown reasons, certain antigens often have low intrinsic immunogenicity. In this case, adjuvants may be used. Other antigens that have proven immunogenicity do not provoke an immune response, possibly because they fail to reach lymphoid tissues. Thus, ocular lens protein has been considered to be in a privileged state inaccessible to lymphocytes. Some antigens on tumor cells apparently fail to elicit a response because they are covered with sialic acid, which somehow prevents the appropriate cell interaction required for immunity.

Antibody. It has been recognized for many years that the administration or production of antibody results in feedback inhibition of antibody production (Uhr and Möller, 1968). Although the exact mechanism is not known, the appearance of IgG results in a shutoff of IgM antibody production. This might occur because the IgG on B cells is a higher affinity antibody and thus can capture and prevent exposure of antigen to IgM-bearing B cells. Thus, higher affinity antibody-producing B cells are selected for, and antigen contact with IgM-bearing cells decreases. Such a process would also be consistent with the well established trend of increasing antibody affinity as stimulation by a given antigen is continued (Eisen and Siskind, 1964).

Central Effects Mediated by Antigen: Immunologic Tolerance. Immunologic tolerance is operationally defined as a state of specific nonreactivity with respect to a given antigenic determinant (see Benacerraf and Unanue, 1979, and reviews by Möller 1979a, b, and 1980). It may be manifested by diminished or absent cell-mediated or humoral immunity, or both. Specific tolerance is the reason that an animal exists without immunologically attacking its own tissues and cells, while specifically and strongly rejecting everything else that is foreign (e.g., infectious agents, toxins, neoplastic cells, tissue grafts). When something occurs to break this "self-tolerance," the consequences may be minimal or catastrophic, depending on the extent to which the state is lost. When disease occurs, a condition of autoimmunity is said to exist.

In 1945, it was noted that dizygotic bovine twins who share a common vascular supply *in utero*, develop into erythrocyte "chimeras" (i.e., they have a mixture of their own erythrocytes and those of the twin). It was subsequently shown that these twins do not reject each other's skin grafts, although they

are of different sex and color. This natural tolerance can be reproduced in the laboratory by injecting fetuses or neonatal mice with cellular antigens (Billingham et al., 1956). Tolerance of this type can also be induced with more difficulty in adult animals if the histocompatibility differences are weak or if a large and prolonged or repeated exposure to such antigens occurs. Other antigens such as proteins and erythrocytes have been used subsequently to study this phenomenon of acquired tolerance. Adult animals can be rendered essentially immunologically immature and more amenable to tolerance induction by whole body irradiation with x-rays or by the use of immunosuppressive drugs, such as cyclophosphamide. However, even normal adults can be made tolerant if the following conditions obtain:

(1) The antigen is poorly immunogenic in its native state; (2) the antigen is in the proper form; i.e., bovine gamma globulin when in soluble form (monomeric) readily induces tolerance in adult animals, but if it is given with an adjuvant, or if it is in aggregated form, it is immunogenic. This leads to the suggestion that molecules that are in a form not readily phagocytized by macrophages are shifted toward tolerogenicity; (3) either very high or very low doses of antigen are used; and (4) the host is unable to catabolize the substance. High doses of pneumococcal polysaccharides are tolerogenic; such substances can be phagocytized but are resistant to digestion.

Unlike natural tolerance to self antigens, induced tolerance in adult animals spontaneously subsides with time, perhaps, in part, because the level of exposure to antigen decreases in the latter but not in the former case. The rate of recovery generally reflects the generation time of new stem cell precursors specific for the tolerogen plus other factors. Old age or thymectomy will delay loss of tolerance. Acquired tolerance can also be broken by injecting a different but cross-reacting protein; by administering the same B cell–stimulating moiety (hapten) on a different T cell–stimulating component (carrier); or, if the tolerance is to certain self antigens (such as thyroglobulin), by immunizing the animal with the denatured or hapten-conjugated protein. Recently studies of tolerance focusing on both T cells and B cells have rendered some explanations for these phenomena.

The work of Chiller and Weigle (1971) demonstrated that both T cells and B cells can be rendered tolerant. However, the susceptibilities of these two lymphocyte classes differ considerably with respect to the required dose of tolerogen (lower for T than for B cells) and the time required after treatment for tolerance induction (less for T than for B cells). In addition, the duration of tolerance is significantly less in B cells than in T cells. Finally, the specific immune response of the whole animal reflects that of the T-cell population in the case of a thymus-dependent response; i.e., the animal appears tolerant if its T cells are, even when its B cells are not tolerized.

THE MECHANISM OF IMMUNOLOGIC TOLERANCE

Tolerance is a complex of many phenomena manifesting similar or identical functional end-points; that is, the absence of a specific immune response. There is some experimental support for the hypothesis that if little or no helper T-cell function is induced (which would result in an immune response), then more direct interaction with the B cell receptors might occur, thereby somehow generating a tolerogenic signal (e.g., a hapten on a nonimmunogenic carrier or deaggregated protein, which can escape macrophage processing). When B cells from young mice (which display only IgM) are exposed *in vitro* to certain antigens in the absence of T cells, tolerance readily occurs. Recent studies have shown that exposure to antigen causes irreversible modulation (removal) of surface (receptor) Ig in young mice, while comparable modulation is reversible in adult B cells. Burnet (1959) hypothesized that self tolerance is due to clonal deletion (death of responsible clones following exposure to antigen). Tolerance induced to certain antigens early in life (especially self antigens) may be the result of death of clones of B cells ("clonal abortion" of Nossal et al., 1976).

The Role of Specific Suppressor T Cells in Tolerance

Tolerance induced with high doses of antigen (high zone tolerance) was hypothesized to be caused by clonal deletion, as described previously. When Mitchison (1965) found that tolerance could also be induced by extremely low doses of antigen, this explanation seemed untenable. In many cases, this low zone tolerance has been found to be due to suppressor T cells. Suppressor T cells have been shown to play a critical role in both T-cell and B-cell tolerance by acting in a way to actively turn off T-cell or B-cell function (Gershon, 1979). The hallmark of such systems is the ability to transfer tolerance with T cells to normal animals or to normal cells *in vitro,* in what was called infectious tolerance (Gershon and Kondo, 1971). These cells may be required for prevention of excessive or harmful (autoimmune) responses. We have already indicated the occurrence of cellular interactions that lead to an appropriately modulated immune response. To further complicate the situation, the recent work of Gershon, Cantor, and colleagues (Gershon et al., 1981) has indicated that not only can T-cell help for B cells be prevented by suppressor T cells, but the ability of suppressor cells to function also is regulated by other, "contrasuppressor" cells. The induction of all these regulatory functions requires several interacting cell types in each circuit (Fig. 81–3).

Mechanism of Cell Cooperation

Although the possibility cannot be ruled out that lymphoid cells may deliver their signals to one another by direct, intimate contact, there is mounting evidence that T cells generally exert their regulatory influence on other T cells and on B cells by release of biologically active soluble factors. Helper and suppressor factors from T cells have been described and, in fact, virtually all of the components of the regulatory circuits described in Figure 81–3 have been reproduced by using cell-free factors (Gershon, 1980). Some factors are antigen specific, while others are not. Those that are specific contain, in most instances, components coded for by the I region of the major histocompatibility complex (MHC, see below), similar to those found on the cell of origin. Recent evidence indicates that the I region product may determine the functional nature of the factor, while specificity is attributed to a second component which is similar to the variable region of immunoglobulin heavy chain molecules. These molecules do not bear the constant region markers of conventional immunoglobulins

Figure 81–3. Regulatory T cell circuits in B cell responses. *I–J₁ and I–J₂ indicate that at least two different I–J region coded antigens are found on the surface of inducer cells, as determined by differential activities of a variety of anti-I–J sera.

**Whether the Ly 123 acceptor cell acts directly on the effector cell or indirectly through an intermediary cell is not known.

***Presence or absence of I-J antigen on this cell is not defined. TSF-T suppressor factor. CSEF-contrasuppressor effector factor. (Gershon, R. K., personal communiction, 1980.)

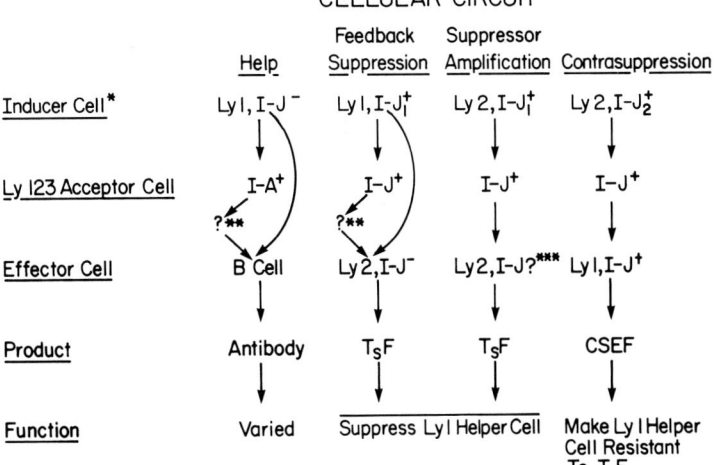

(see below). The molecular weight of such factors is around 50,000 daltons.

Recently it has been discovered that some populations of both helper and suppressor T cells and some of the factors derived from them have specificity not for antigen but for immunoglobulin V_H region determinants themselves. This has led to a resurgence of the concept of idiotype–anti-idiotype regulatory interactions first suggested by Jerne (1971). There is, in fact, some evidence that the first reaction in an immune response results in antibody specific for antigen. The induction of cells bearing these antigen-specific receptors (which have idiotypic determinants as described later) in turn stimulates populations of regulatory cells with anti-idiotypic specificity. The next wave of regulation might then be anti-anti-idiotype, and so on. Some investigators believe that such a system leads to a diminishing ripple effect, eventually reaching a relative steady state response (Kelso and Cerny, 1979). This and the other complex regulatory interactions described heretofore are believed to be operative, with some variations, in all mammalian species and to influence the nature and degree of immune responsiveness that such individuals show.

IMMUNOGLOBULIN STRUCTURE AND FUNCTION

STRUCTURE OF IMMUNOGLOBULIN

Antibodies as Proteins

Antibody molecules are protein products of B cells. Most antibodies are found in the slowly migrating electrophoretic fraction of serum termed the *gamma globulin* region. Since they are elicited in reponse to, and react specifically with, an antigen, antibodies are also termed *immunoglobulins* (Ig). Ig molecules as a whole are now known to compose a heterogenous family of complex but related proteins that differ in their functional properties according to differences in their chemical structure.

Studies of Ig molecules from a wide variety of mammalian species have shown that these proteins can be subcategorized into five distinct classes according to differences in the structure of one of the constituent polypeptide chains termed the *heavy* chain (Fig. 81–4). Structural studies of antibody molecules have been greatly aided by the availability of homogeneous, pure Ig proteins that are produced in large quantities by certain tumors of B lymphocytes called myelomas. Recently, in addition, the technology for fusing normal B cells with malignant B cells (hybridomas) has allowed selective production of homogeneous antibodies of any desired specificity in essentially limitless quantities. Although most of these proteins that have been studied extensively are from the mouse and from man, some myeloma proteins from dogs and cats have been isolated and characterized as well (Hurvitz et al.. 1971; Kehoe et al., 1972a, 1972b). The presence of a characteristic urinary component, termed Bence Jones protein, is often associated with these myeloma tumors *in vivo*. These proteins are now known to be free immunoglobulin "light" chains (Fig. 81–4), which are produced in enormous

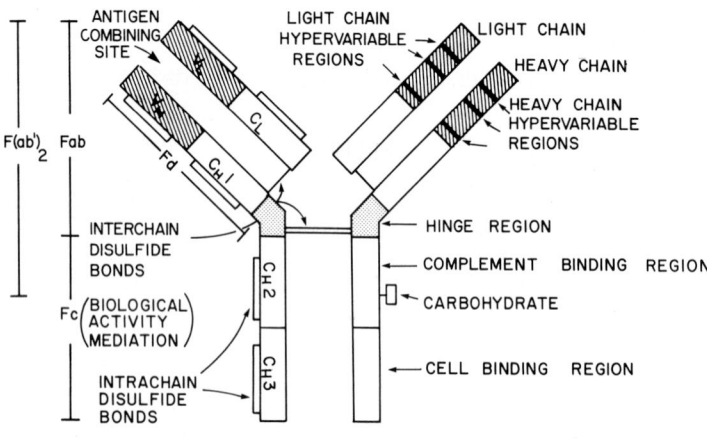

Figure 81–4. A prototype mammalian IgG molecule. The two constituent polypeptide chains — heavy and light — are indicated, as are three major proteolytic fragments that can be produced from this antibody protein [F(ab')₂, Fab, Fc]. The usual locations of the disulfide bonds and the hypervariable (complementarity determining) regions of the variable regions of both the heavy (V_H) and light (V_L) chains are also shown. See text for additional details.

V_L AND V_H : VARIABLE REGIONS

C_L AND C_H : CONSTANT REGIONS

excess by the malignant B lymphocyte clones. Some general characteristics of the five classes of mammalian immunoglobulins are provided in Table 81–3. Additional information, especially concerning additional antigenic and genetic characteristics of this protein family, can be found in the general references cited.

Some further subdivision of certain of these classes, also attributable to differences in heavy chain structure, has been accomplished in numerous species. The IgG class of the dog, for example, is now known to comprise four distinct *subclasses* termed IgG1, IgG2a, IgG2b, and IgG2c. Represen-

tatives of all such subclasses are normally present in the serum of an individual animal. Differences in the structure of the Fc region (Fig. 81–4) of the different subclasses may lead to differing capacities for the expression of important physiologic activities (e.g., complement fixation), as described later in this chapter.

IgG as an Immunoglobulin Prototype

Normal mammalian adult serum contains from 700 to 1500 mg of IgG protein per 100 ml. The great importance of this class is illustrated by the finding that approximately

Table 81–3. Mammalian Immunoglobulin Classes

Characteristics and Functions	IgG	IgA	IgM	IgD	IgE
$S_{20,w}$	7.0	7,10,13,15,16	19	7	8
Molecular weight	150,000	180,000–500,000	850,000	160,000	196,000
Carbohydrate (%)	2.9	7.5	6–10	12	10.7
Approximate concentration in normal serum (mg/100 ml)	700–1500	140–420	50–190	3–40	0:01–0.14
Major biological functions	Principal serum antibody Complement activation, opsonization Passive transfer to fetus or newborn	Secretory antibody, active at mucosal surfaces Polymeric (dimer to higher order polymers)	Initial antibody produced Prominent serum antibody Polymeric (pentamer in serum) Complement activation B lymphocyte antigen receptor as monomer	Important cell surface antibody of developing B lymphocytes	Reagin-humoral mediator of immediate hypersensitivity reactions (e.g., anaphylaxis)

80 per cent of antibacterial, antiviral, and antitoxin antibodies belong to this class. A schematic representation of an intact IgG molecule is shown in Figure 81–4, since the structure of this protein has become the prototype for relating the structural features of antibodies to their functions.

As illustrated, IgG proteins (and antibodies in general) are characterized by a remarkable degree of regional differentiation. At a first level, the IgG molecule can be split by proteolytic cleavage into two segments termed Fab and Fc. The Fab region binds antigen, while the Fc region mediates the biological properties or effector functions such as complement fixation that are such an important aspect of the contribution of antibodies to host resistance to infectious disease and neoplasia. Detailed chemical analysis of antibody proteins has shown further that the light and heavy polypeptide chains of antibodies are folded into discrete but interconnected segments termed *domains*, which possess a certain independence with respect to the expression of the various antibody functions. For example, the antigen binding function is mediated solely by the variable region domains of the antibody molecule (Inbar et al., 1972), while the binding of the first component of the complement cascade by IgG is carried out by the C_H2 domain (Kehoe et al., 1974).

Importance of Amino Acid Sequence of Antibody Proteins

Since 1965, a number of insights concerning antibody function have been obtained through amino acid sequence analysis of selected immunoglobulin molecules, mainly the myeloma paraproteins described previously. Immunoglobulin polypeptide chains contain two distinct regions. One region, termed the variable or V region, shows marked sequence variation from molecule to molecule and participates in antigen binding functions. The other, called the constant or C region, is responsible for many of the other properties of immunoglobulin molecules including cellular binding, fixation of complement, and membrane passage (through gut or placenta). Recent studies have shown that the genes coding for the V and C regions are very widely separated in the embryo and must be brought into closer proximity before the

messenger RNA for the immunoglobulin polypeptide chain is made. In fact, it is now known that *three* separate genetic elements are utilized to form the total stretch of genetic information that is used in coding for a complete immunoglobulin light chain: a *V* segment, a *J* segment (both V and J contribute to the variable region), and a *C* segment for the constant region. Analogous segments plus still another (the *D* segment) are used for the heavy chain. In the lymphocyte, the genes for these regions of the antibody protein are separated by additional DNA. Complex processing events bring these elements together in the mature B lymphocyte, thus contributing to antibody diversity.

Antigen Receptors on B Cells

The immunoglobulins are either attached to the lymphocyte cell membrane or released into the serum to become serum antibody. As shown in Figure 81–4, the antigen receptor of such antibodies (and of a B cell carrying such an antibody) is the combined variable regions of the light and heavy chain and is formed specifically by the *hypervariable* segments that are situated within the variable regions as a whole (Capra and Kehoe, 1975). Thus, the identity of the large variety of antigen specific receptors of the B cell repertoire is clearly antibody itself in the form of the individual cell's own immunoglobulin.

Antigen Receptors on T Cells

T cell–mediated immunologic responses are also highly antigen specific. This implies that these cells must have surface receptors that render them able to recognize and bind specific antigenic determinants. Whether a new class of immunoglobulin is the T-cell receptor has been very controversial (Marchalonis and Moseley, 1979). Conventional IgG, IgA, IgM, IgD, or IgE has not been detectable on T cells (in fact, the presence or absence of surface Ig can serve to distinguish B cells from T cells). Recently, serologically detectable *antigenic determinants* have been found in the variable region of Ig molecules. These markers, called *idiotypes,* are associated with the hypervariable regions that compose an antibody combining site and, when found, are indicative of a certain antigenic specificity of the Ig (Capra and Kehoe, 1975). It is possible to raise antibodies that bind to such idiotypic determinants (i.e., anti-antibodies). Such anti-idiotypic antibodies have been used to show that some T cells and some B cells reactive for a given antigen *share* similar idiotypes (Binz et al., 1979). Therefore, at least a portion of the T-cell receptor is composed of the same variable region found in the Ig produced by B cells. The other portion of the T-cell receptor may comprise a new Ig heavy chain type, as discussed in Marchalonis and Moseley (1979).

BIOLOGICAL PROPERTIES (EFFECTOR FUNCTIONS) OF ANTIBODIES

Immunoglobulin molecules are multi-functional. These functions can be divided into two main categories: antigen binding, mediated by the variable regions of heavy and light chains (part of the Fab fragment), and biological properties, or effector functions, mediated by the Fc region.

The effector functions are very important physiologically, since they often determine exactly what biological consequences follow the union of a given antigen with its antibody. Effector activities, or properties, that have been associated with the Fc region of immunoglobulin include interaction with complement proteins, fixation to skin, reactivity with rheumatoid factors, fixation to macrophages and lymphocytes, membrane passage (placenta, intestine), opsonization, regulation of immunoglobulin catabolism, and interaction with staphylococcal "A" protein. As is evident from this list, these functions are highly varied and reflect the many functional capabilities, other than antigen binding, that immunoglobulin molecules possess. Not all immunoglobulin molecules are capable of all these activities, and some correlations have been made between the class or subclass of given molecules and

their capacity to mediate certain of these functions. For example, certain classes lack certain effector function capabilities (Table 81–4).

These various differences are thought to reflect differences in chemical structure among the Fc regions of the various immunoglobulins, but the exact nature of these differences is not yet known. In fact, for most of the activities shown above, the precise region within Fc that is responsible for the function is not yet known. Evidence has been obtained that the C_H2 homology region (amino-terminal half of Fc) of IgG is responsible for the fixation of the first complement component, as noted previously. The exact amino acid residues involved have not yet been identified with certainty, however.

Some of these activities, such as complement fixation, are expressed by antibodies only after union with antigen has occurred, while others, such as skin fixation, do not require prior antigen union. In those cases in which antigen:antibody interaction is required for the expression of the biological activity, it is presumed that some antigen-induced conformational alteration of the antibody molecule must occur, perhaps exposing a previously buried active site(s). Such conformational alterations, if they do occur, seem to be very subtle, because it has not yet been possible to detect gross alterations of any antibody molecule following antigen:antibody union. An adequate allosteric change would not have to be very large, however, and might well be undetectable by the experimental methods that have been used so far. Alternatively, aggregation alone may lead to the capacity for complement fixation. In fact, much recent experimental evidence supports the view that antigen-induced aggregation may well be adequate to initially activate the complement system.

Another Fc-mediated effector function that is highly important for protection

Table 81–4. Effector Functions of Immunoglobulin Classes

Class	Classical Complement Fixation	Skin Attachment
IgG	+	+
IgM	+	−
IgA	−	−
IgD	−	−
IgE	−	+

against infectious disease is opsonization, the enhancement of the phagocytic process by antibody. It is known that specific IgG immunoglobulins are the major group of antibodies that are involved in the opsonic effects seen in bacterial endocarditis caused by a number of gram-positive organisms, including streptococci or staphylococci. The opsonic effect is dependent on the integrity of the Fc region. Presumably, following interaction of the bacterium and the antibody active site, some part of the Fc region increases the efficiency of phagocytosis by the phagocytic cells. This most likely occurs via an Fc:leukocyte cell membrane interaction, but exact details are not known at present. It does appear that the C_H3 domain of the IgG molecule is important in this process.

THE ANTIGEN-ANTIBODY REACTION

The antigen-antibody reaction itself may be differentiated into two stages. The first is concerned with the actual union (combination), which occurs very rapidly. The second stage (consequences of the antigen-antibody reaction) evolves more slowly following the initial union. Both aspects of the reaction are physiologically significant. Antigen-antibody interactions are relatively weak and reversible. No covalent bonds are formed; rather, several of the weaker types of chemical interaction are involved: hydrophobic, coulombic, van der Waals, hydrogen bonds, and some charge interactions. None of these forces is particularly strong, but when the stereochemical configurations

of the bound molecule and antibody receptor site are in juxtaposition, they form a firm but dissociable union. The consequences comprise those events that follow the union of an antigen with its specific antibody. They can include effects that depend only on the union itself (antitoxin activity, virus neutralization, bacterial agglutination) or those that involve the effector function capabilities of the antibody molecule (complement fixation, opsonic activity). Previously, these distinctions led to the designation of different "kinds" of antibodies (lysins, agglutinins, antitoxins, and so forth). Such categorizations have less meaning now that the structure: function relationships of antibodies are understood in greater detail.

THE PRECIPITIN REACTION AND LATTICE THEORY

A fundamentally important consequence of the union of *soluble* antigens with their specific antibody is the precipitin reaction. This reaction is used in a variety of formats in clinical immunology, especially as a diagnostic tool. In addition, precipitin antibodies play a dominant role in that series of syndromes known as *immune complex* diseases, some examples of which are discussed later. The solution behavior of these antibodies is explained by the lattice hypothesis, which assumes the interaction of multivalent antibody with multivalent antigen. As indicated in Figure 81–4, the most common precipitin antibody, IgG, is divalent. Most

Figure 81–5. The quantitative precipitin reaction characteristic of the interaction of soluble, multivalent antigen with multivalent antibody. The three zones shown can be discerned when antigen is progressively added to a standard aliquot of antibody.

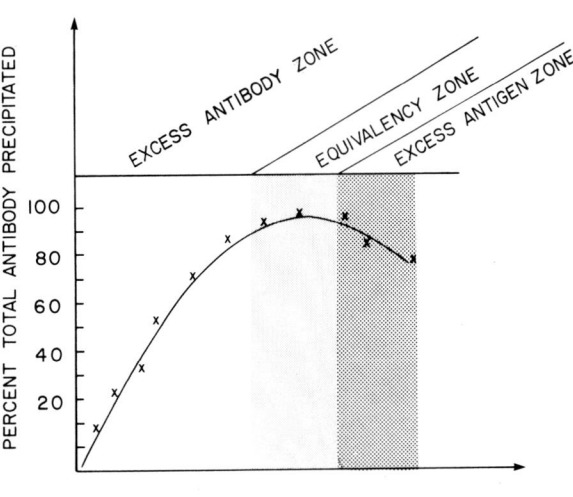

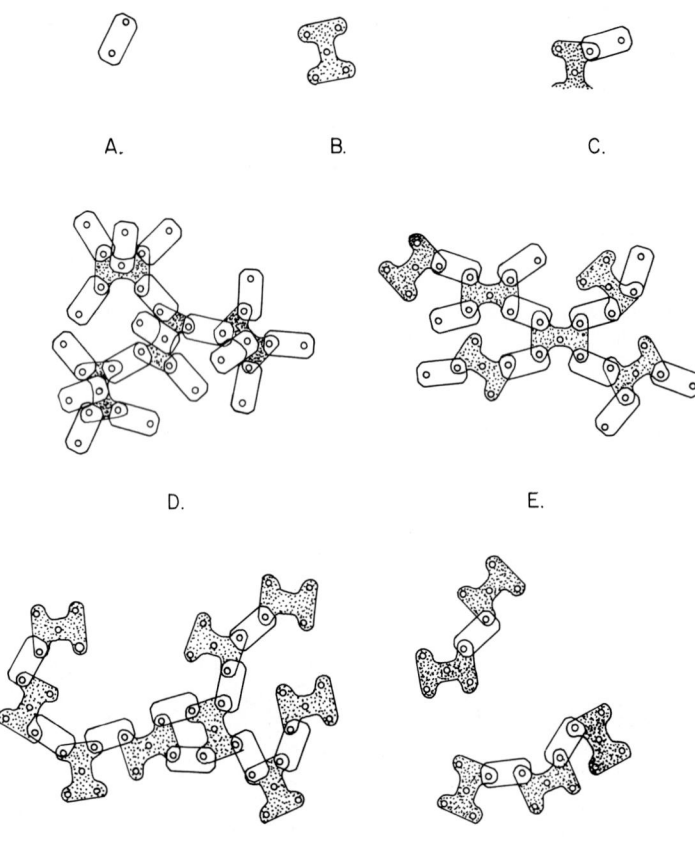

A.

B.

C.

D.

E.

F.

G.

Figure 81–6. Interpretation of the quantitative precipitin reaction in terms of the "lattice" hypothesis. A divalent antibody (IgG) is shown (a) interacting with a pentavalent antigen (B, C). In the excess antibody zone (D), each antigen increment can be incorporated into the lattice, and a progressive buildup of total precipitate is observed. As the equivalence zone is approached (E) and reached (F) there is an optimum (equivalent) proportion of antigen and antibody and the lattice reaches its maximum extent (maximum precipitation). As still more antigen is added, the formation of soluble antigen-antibody complexes (G) becomes possible and the total amount of precipitate declines as the lattice is disassembled to some degree. Significantly for the development of immune complex disease, such "soluble complexes" can retain biological reactivity (e.g., complement fixation).

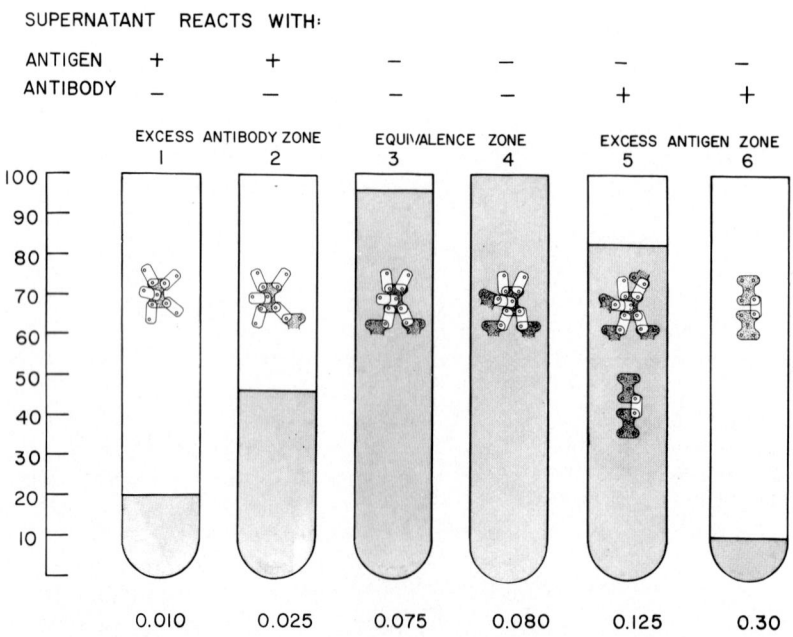

Figure 81–7. Correlation of observations with quantitative precipitin curve and inferred occurrences according to the lattice hypothesis.

antigens involved in the precipitin reaction are highly multivalent with many antigenic determinants that can interact with antibody. The characteristic precipitin curve can be demonstrated in the laboratory by adding increasing increments of antigen to constant aliquots of antibody. The curve itself is located by measuring the *total* amount of precipitate at various points as the ratio of antigen to antibody is increased. This is illustrated schematically in Figure 81–5. The application of the lattice hypothesis to this curve is illustrated in Figures 81–6 and 81–7.

The most important aspect of this curve with respect to disease involves the zone of antigen excess, where soluble complexes of antigen and antibody are formed (Figure 81–7). These complexes can occur in tissue (kidney, joints) and can be biologically active there (by activating the complement cascade, for example). These reactivities are responsible for many aspects of the pathogenesis of immune complex diseases.

The maximum precipitation zone (zone of equivalence, Figures 81–5 and 81–7) is widely used in clinical immunology, especially when antigen/antibody precipitin reactions are allowed to occur in semi-solid media such as gels.

THE COMPLEMENT SYSTEM

The complement system is an interrelated complex of serum proteins that is closely, although not exclusively, associated with the humoral antibody system. While the system, with some variations, is present in all mammals, the most detailed information has been obtained for man and the guinea pig. The general principles are known to hold for other mammalian species, however.

It is now clear that there are two distinct activation schemes for the complement system, one initiated by appropriate antigen-antibody complexes leading to the *classical* cascade and a second, the *alternate* or *properdin* pathway, which occurs because of initiation of the cascade at the C3 level. Both pathways have important *in vivo* implications for the prevention and production of disease.

THE CLASSICAL COMPLEMENT SYSTEM

The classical complement system is composed of 12 serum proteins that interact in a closely ordered and integrated sequence termed the complement cascade (Fig. 81–8,*A*). The reaction sequence is initiated by antibody, produces a series of soluble degradation products (some of which have important physiologic properties), and terminates by generating the capacity to damage a cell membrane.

The classical reaction cascade is initiated by certain Ig molecules that have bound their specific antigen. The IgM class and at least some of the IgG subclasses are active in starting the cascade, while the IgD, IgE, and IgA classes are not. The complement-fixing region of the IgM and IgG molecule has long been known to reside in the Fc portion and involves the C_H2 domain of IgG (Fig. 81–4). The classical complement cascade is activated by an initial interaction between the responsible immunoglobulin site and C1q. An initial regulatory control on the total complement system occurs at this level. Under usual circumstances, an antibody molecule alone will not initiate the cascade; it must be bound to its antigen before its latent potentiality for stimulating the entire cascade can be revealed.

The complement proteins are able to associate with each other in a specific reaction sequence following the initial interaction of antibody with C1q. As indicated in Figure 81–8,*A*), the complement components have been given numbers and in some instances additional letters. A bar over the symbol indicates that an enzymatic activity has been induced, which is common during the cascade. For example, the C1q, C1r, and C1s components exist as a calcium-dependent complex in serum. Following an appropriate association between the antibody and a site on C1q, the C1q molecule undergoes conformational changes, which in turn causes a structural change in the C1r component, resulting in the acquisition of proteolytic activity by C1r. The enzyme complex now cleaves a component of the C1s molecule, resulting in the generation of serine protease activity, referred to as C1s̄. The antibody molecule may thus be envisioned as responsible for activating and directing particular enzyme activities.

The reaction sequence continues (Fig. 81–8,*A*) until the C5b-9 complex is formed. A variety of studies have shown that the C5b-9 complex is the active moiety in producing the damage to the membrane. The available evidence indicates that C8 is primarily re-

Figure 81–8A.

Ag-Ab
↓   + C1 (q,r,s)
Ag-Ab C$\overline{1}$
↓   + C4
Ag-Ab C$\overline{1,4}$
↓   + C2
Ag-Ab C$\overline{1,4,2}$
↓   + C3a,b
Ag-Ab C$\overline{1,4,2,3a,b}$ ↗ 3a cast off
↓   + C5a,b
Ag-Ab C$\overline{1,4,2,3b,5a,b}$ ↗ 5a cast off
↓   + C6
Ag-Ab C$\overline{1,4,2,3b}$,5b,6
↓   + C7
Ag-Ab C$\overline{1,4,2,3b}$,5b,6,7
↓   + C8
Ag-Ab C$\overline{1,4,2,3b}$,5b,6,7,8,
↓   + C9
Ag-Ab C$\overline{1,4,2,3b}$,5b,6,7,8,9
↓
Membrane lysis

Figure 81–8B.

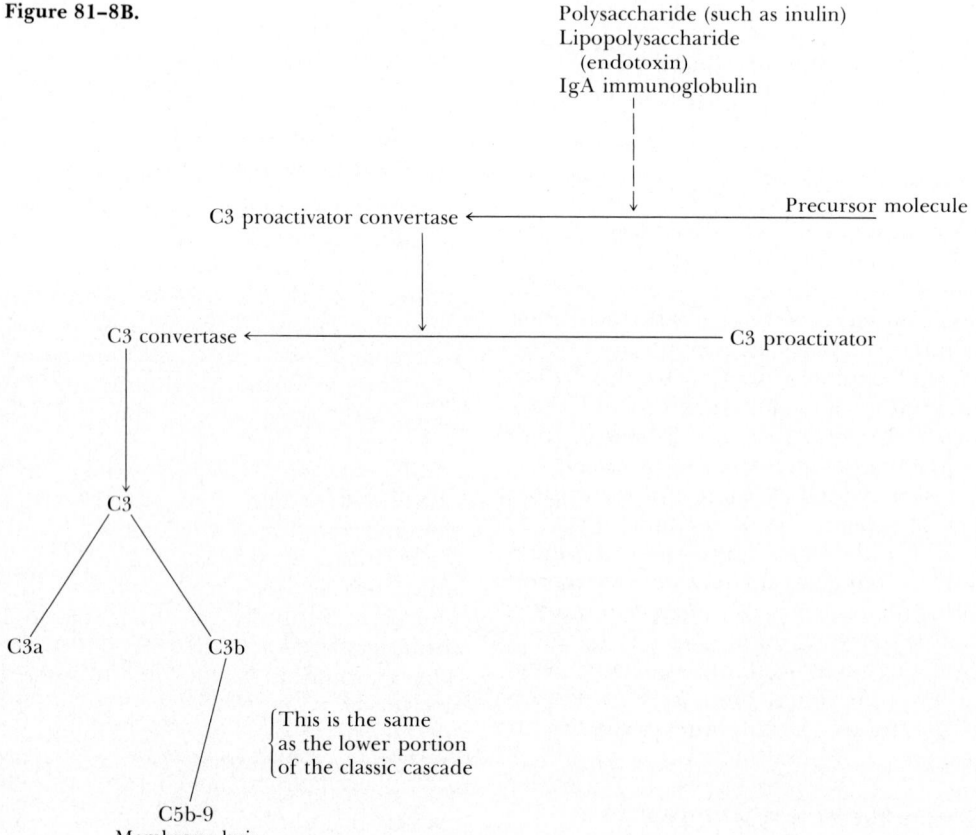

Polysaccharide (such as inulin)
Lipopolysaccharide
  (endotoxin)
IgA immunoglobulin

Precursor molecule

C3 proactivator convertase ←

C3 convertase ←   C3 proactivator

C3

C3a   C3b

This is the same
as the lower portion
of the classic cascade

C5b-9
Membrane lysis

Figure 81–8. *A*, The classical complement cascade. *B*, The alternate complement cascade. See text for detailed discussion.

sponsible for the actual membrane damage, with C9 serving mainly in a potentiating role. *In vivo,* bacterial cell membranes, red blood cell membranes, and, perhaps, tumor cell membranes are the ones most commonly damaged.

THE ALTERNATE (PROPERDIN) PATHWAY OF COMPLEMENT ACTIVATION

A summary of the general features of the alternate pathway is presented in Figure 81-8,*B*. Certain substances — including such polysaccharides as inulin, bacterial endotoxins, and IgA — are capable of activating the precursor of a molecule called C3 proactivator convertase. This causes a sequence of events in which the terminal components of the complement cascade are activated.

As mentioned previously, proteolytic fragmentation of certain complement proteins occurs at several steps in the cascade, leading to the production of small peptides that are released from the cytolysis complex. The fragments C3a and C5a have been shown to have significant physiologic activities, including the capacity to induce the contraction of smooth muscle and the release of histamine from mast cells and basophils. These two molecules, which have different but homologous chemical structures, have similar *in vivo* properties. They both interact with mast cells (leading to histamine release), cause contraction of smooth muscle, and are chemotactic for neutrophils, so they clearly participate in various inflammatory responses. Another important component is formed when C5b binds to C6 and C7 to form a trimolecular complex, which, because it is highly chemotactic for neutrophils, is an important participant in inflammatory reactions. It is likely that additional important biological properties will soon be assigned to other soluble degradation products of the complement cascade.

The description of the complement system presented so far has emphasized the purely positive aspects of the cascade, with activity of one component leading inexorably to effects on the next component in the sequence. The system is also subject to important counterbalancing influences, however. One important control is due to the short life of certain complexes, which will decay to inactivity if the next component in the cascade is not contacted. For example, C2 is known to dissociate itself from the antigen-antibody C1,4,2 complex. This dissociation makes that particular complex incapable of leading to the production of the C5b-9 cytolytic complex and thus has a dampening effect on the overall membrane-destroying role of the entire reaction sequence.

Another important suppressing effect on the complement system is provided by a series of specific inhibitor molecules in serum. For example, a specific inhibitor for C1s, termed the C1 esterase inhibitor, has been described in man and presumably exists in other species as well. Also, a C3b inactivator molecule is capable of cleaving C3b into two components, negating all the functions of C3b. In addition, there is a specific inactivator of the anaphylatoxin C3a. This molecule presumably closely regulates the serum level of the biologically active C3a. As a group, these inhibitors, and probably others still to be identified, are a very important part of the regulation and function of the complement system. Selected genetic deficiencies of either of these inhibitor molecules, or complement components themselves, have been described in some species. These conditions may lead to serious disease, usually involving recurrent infections.

ANTIBODY-MEDIATED HYPERSENSITIVITY

From a clinical perspective, the most significant antibody-mediated hypersensitivity syndromes are acute anaphylaxis or atopy (immediate hypersensitivity) mediated by the specific antibody of the IgE class that is bound to mast cells or basophils, and serum sickness, which is caused by complement-fixing immune complexes that develop following the administration of a large protein dose to a previously sensitized individual (e.g., to an animal that has previously received foreign serum in an attempt to provide passive immunity). The various antibody-mediated hypersensitivity conditions that have been described in a variety of species are tabulated in Table 81-5. Some of those listed are experimentally induced. Immune complex disorders are covered later in the chapter.

While the existence of IgE has not yet

been definitely established in all species, general indications and the existence of acute anaphylaxis in most species imply that this antibody occurs in most mammals. Thus the immunologic component of the IgE-mediated conditions described in Table 81–5 is thought to be comparable in the various species. That is, IgE bound to mast cells of a previously sensitized individual can rapidly trigger the degranulation of this cell when a subsequent encounter with that antigen occurs. This leads to the release by the mast cell of a variety of pharmacologic mediators (which vary from species to species) that cause the subsequent symptomatology. If the antigen exposure is massive, mast cell degranulation can be extensive, rather than just local, and can lead to death from acute anaphylaxis.

CELL-MEDIATED IMMUNE REACTIONS

This section explores those aspects of immune function that are primarily carried out by cellular elements. Sensitized (antigen-specific) T cells are the lymphoid cells that are either the primary effectors of this type of immunity (e.g., cytotoxic T cells) or that induce other cells to be effectors.

DELAYED TYPE HYPERSENSITIVITY REACTIONS (CLASSICAL TYPE IV HYPERSENSITIVITY)

Delayed-type hypersensitivity (DTH) reactions are the prototype of cell-mediated immunity (CMI). An excellent review of the current concepts of DTH has been presented by Askenase (1980). DTH exemplifies

Table 81–5. Antibody Mediated Hypersensitivity Reactions

Reaction	Characteristics	Immunoglobulin Involved	Special Features
Direct Arthus Reaction	Repeated local injection of antigen leads to local erythema, edema, and necrosis at that tissue site, principally as a result of blood vessel reaction. Antibodies are produced by the animal receiving the injections	IgG, IgM (complement fixing)	1. No tissue fixation of antibody 2. Complement participates 3. Polymorphonuclear leukocytes attracted by antigen-antibody-complement complexes leads to tissue injury 4. Antigen-antibody-C' precipitates in tissues 5. Antihistamines have no ameliorating effect
Direct Passive Arthus Reaction	Antigen injected locally, then antibodies injected intravenously	As above	As above
Reverse Passive Arthus Reaction	Antibodies injected into skin, then antigen injected intravenously	As above	As above
Systemic Arthus Reaction	Slow development over several hours of fatal reaction characterized by widespread circulatory changes and hemorrhages. Takes place when antigen exposure occurs in a protracted way (slow absorption from tissue sites) in individuals that already have high levels of circulating antibodies	As above	As above (details depend on where precipitates occur in tissues)
Prausnitz-Küstner (P-K) Reaction	Local injection into skin of antibody-containing serum followed by later (24-hr) injection of antigen (allergen) into same site leads to a reaction at that site (wheal and erythema)	IgE	Mediated solely by reaginic antibodies (IgE), which bind to mast cells in the skin
Systemic Anaphylaxis	Entry of antigen into the systemic circulation of a previously sensitized individual (i.e., one that has antibodies in serum and fixed to cells) leads to a severe general reaction that can be fatal. Details of the general reaction vary with species	IgE	Antigen interaction with specific IgE molecules that have been previously fixed to cells (mast cells) leads to release of pharmacologic mediators (histamine, serotonin), which then results in smooth muscle contraction and increased vascular permeability

Table continued on opposite page

Table 81–5. Antibody Mediated Hypersensitivity Reactions (*Continued*)

Reaction	Characteristics	Immunoglobulin Involved	Special Features
Passive Cutaneous Anaphylaxis	Injection of antibody containing serum into skin of experimental animal of a different species; results in antibody fixation to cells, if they are so capable. After an appropriate waiting period, antigen is injected intravenously together with a marker dye. A circular colored spot develops in a positive reaction	IgG, IgE	Antibodies must fix to cells in skin (probably mast cells); then Ab-Ag reaction leads to release of pharmacologic mediators, circulatory changes, and dye deposition. This is a very sensitive test for antibodies. Antibodies involved are always heterocytotropic
Reverse Passive Cutaneous Anaphylaxis	A test immunoglobulin molecule is injected into the skin. If the molecule is capable of cell fixation, it will be fixed to certain cells (probably mast cells) near the injection site. After a waiting period, an antiserum containing anti-immunoglobulin antibodies is injected intravenously together with a marker dye. The anti-immunoglobulin antibodies will react with the immunoglobulin that has fixed to the cells, and cell degranulation will occur	IgG, IgE	The anti-immunoglobulin antibodies usually react with determinants in the Fc region of the immunoglobulin that is cell fixed. The RPCA reaction is used most to test for the skin fixing property of immunoglobulins
Serum Sickness	Administration of a single injection of antigen is followed by a slowly developing illness characterized by hives, edema, and fever. The reaction peaks 7 to 10 days following the antigen injection and is usually not fatal	IgG (with or without IgE?)	The antibody induced by the antigen(s) reacts with some remaining antigen, often on cell surfaces. The complement system is activated, leading to anaphyla-toxin release, and histamine is released from cells. Serum sickness thus involves several different types of hypersensitivity responses

General comments on cell-fixing antibodies:
1. Cell-fixing antibodies are called "cytotropic" and have been found in both the IgG and IgE classes.
2. Homocytotropic antibodies will fix to cells of the *same* species that synthesized them.
3. Heterocytotropic antibodies will only fix to cells in species *different* from that in which the antibody has been produced.

the ability of T cells to recruit effector leukocytes to a tissue site. The term DTH or, more precisely, *tuberculin-type hypersensitivity,* is now reserved for the classical T cell–dependent reaction associated either with immunization with antigens augmented by a water-in-oil, mycobacteria-containing adjuvant (complete Freund's adjuvant) or with infection with mycobacteria. Therefore, these reactions may be elicited by intradermal challenge either with tuberculin or with antigens administered with the mycobacteria. The development of DTH reactions, in contrast to anaphylactic reactions, requires 24 to 48 hours, probably because it involves interaction of a number of different cell types: *recirculating cells* (antigen specific immune Ly 1 T cells); *resident cells* (vascular endothelial cells, which must be traversed by both recirculating cells and recruited cells, tissue macrophage-like cells,

and mast cells); and *recruited cells* (bone marrow–derived effector leukocytes such as monocytes, basophils and neutrophils, which comprise more than 95 per cent of the cellular infiltrate in a DTH reaction) (Lubaroff and Waksman, 1968; McCluskey et al., 1976). As in humoral immune responses, antigen must be trapped, digested, and presented to T cells by macrophage-like cells (in conjunction with self histocompatibility [Ia] antigens).

The involvement of vasoamines in DTH is presented in Fig. 81–9 (Askenase, 1979). Ly 1 T cells mediating DTH (Huber et al., 1976) are recirculating cells. During normal rounds, they leave the circulation by passing directly through the cytoplasm of high endothelial cells of the post capillary venules, by a process called emperiopolesis (Marchesi and Gowans, 1964). When a rare, passing, specifically immune Ly 1 cell meets the

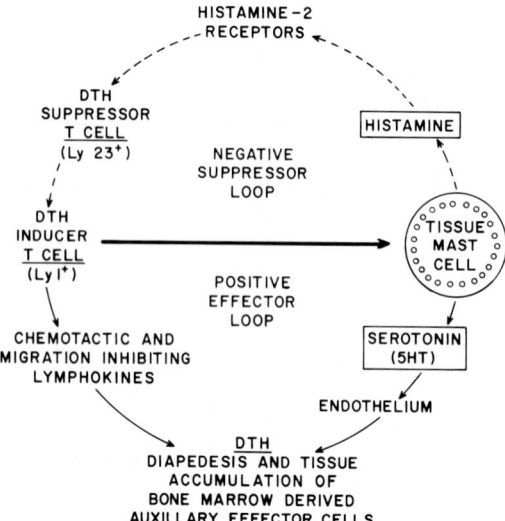

Figure 81–9. The hypothesized vasoactive amine loop in DTH. Inducer (Ly 1) T cell interaction with antigen and consequent release of chemotactic and migration inhibiting lymphokines is viewed as necessary but not sufficient for DTH in mice. In addition, to form a positive effector loop, T cells interact with mast cells, which release vasoactive amines (such as 5-HT in the mouse); these cause endothelial cells to allow the diapedesis of leukocytes in response to the lymphokines. A negative (suppressor) loop is formed by the possibility that mast cells also release histamine, which acts on histamine-2 receptors of suppressor T cells of the Ly 23 phenotype. (From P. W. Askenase, J.: Allergy Clin. Immunol. *64*:79, 1979.)

antigen presenting cell, it stops its migration and becomes activated. In the process of activation, it releases a number of soluble substances called lymphokines (Table 81–6). Some of these substances are chemotactic and may cause recruited cells to be attracted to and to stick to the endothelial wall of blood vessels near the lesion. Recent data imply that T cells may also be responsible for inducing the release of vasoactive amines from local mast cells. These amines (serotonin and/or histamine, depending on the species) cause an increase in the spaces between endothelial cells. The spaces are apparently required for the migration (diapedesis) of recruited cells into the tissues (see Gershon et al., 1975; Schwartz et al., 1977). Once these recruited bone marrow–derived cells enter the tissues, their migration is halted by lymphokines such as macrophage inhibitory factor (MIF, which can be detected *in vitro* in the correlate of DTH, the MIF assay). Some of these bone marrow–derived macrophages also be-

come activated by lymphokines and can then kill the invading pathogen. Although the elicitation of the response is specific at the level of the T cell, the effector arm is not antigenically specific. This is because an activated macrophage can ingest and destroy not only the eliciting antigen (e.g., *Mycobacterium*) but other intracellular bacteria as well (such as *Listeria*). The beneficial aspects of this for host defense are clear.

It is important to note that the lesion of DTH requires antigen presence. Once antigen is removed, the lesion subsides. In the case of a tuberculin skin test, this may take several days, while in chronic diseases in which the pathogen reproduces and cannot be eliminated, systemic or local lesions can last for long periods of time.

OTHER DELAYED-ONSET REACTIONS: CONTACT SENSITIVITY (CS)

In CS, the immunogen is an exogenous, simple haptenic reactive chemical (such as dinitrophenol [DNP] or a metal) or an environmental allergen (such as in poison ivy sensitivity) that becomes covalently linked with host skin components. This complex becomes the complete antigen, which is necessary for the induction of immune T cells and the elicitation of the response as described previously. These lesions are usually rich in basophils in man and guinea pigs and are therefore considered to be a subset of the type of delayed reaction called *cutaneous basophil hypersensitivity* (CBH) Stadeker and Leskowitz, 1973; Askenase, 1979). CBH differs from DTH in that CBH reactions can be induced without mycobacterial adjuvants and that some of these reactions appear antibody mediated. Jones-Mote reactions, for example, are in another subcategory of CBH, induced by injection of protein antigens in saline or with water-in-oil emulsions, without mycobacteria (Richerson et al., 1970). With regard to antibody involvement, some of the antibody-mediated reactions represent a newly recognized late phase of IgE-mediated hypersensitivity and thus have been termed late phase reactions or late cutaneous reactions (reviewed in Askenase, 1977). The antibodies mediating these reactions in man and guinea pigs are homocytotropic IgG_1 and IgE. Antibody attached to tissue mast cells by Fc receptors interacts with antigen

Table 81–6. Representative Lymphokines

Lymphokine	Activity
Affecting Lymphocytes	
Blastogenic or mitogenic factor (BF or MF)	Induces blast cell formation and thymidine incorporation in normal lymphocytes
Potentiating factor (PF)	Augments or enhances ongoing transformation in MLC or antigen-stimulated cultures
Cell cooperation or helper factor	Produced by T cells, increases the number or rate of formation of antibody-producing cells *in vitro*
Suppressor factors	Inhibits activation of and/or antibody production by B cells
Interleukin II (TCGF)	An Ly 1 cell factor that helps T cells, such as CTL precursors, to proliferate
Affecting Macrophages	
Migration-inhibitory factor (MIF)	Inhibits the migration of normal macrophages
Macrophage-aggregation factor (MAF)	Agglutinates macrophages in suspension
Macrophage-spreading inhibition factor (MSIF)	Prevents the flattening and spreading of primary macrophages in culture
Migration-enhancement factor (MEF)	Promotes the migration of macrophages in agarose (antagonistic with MIF)
Affecting Granulocytes	
Inhibitory factor	Inhibits the migration of buffy coat cells or peripheral blood leukocytes from capillary tubes or wells in agar plates
Chemotactic factor	Causes granulocytes to migrate through micropore filter against a gradient
Affecting Cultured Cells	
Lymphotoxin (LT)	Cytotoxic for certain cultured cells, e.g., mouse L cells or HeLa cells
Proliferation inhibitory factor (PIF)	Inhibits proliferation of cultured cells without lysing them
Interferon	Protects cells against virus infection

and leads to release of vasoactive substances. These substances are chemotactic for basophils.

In delayed reactions, the identity of cells recruited into the tissues by T cells varies with the species (monocytes are the principal recruited cell in human DTH reactions, while neutrophils are common in the mouse, the dog, and certain other species); the mode of immunization (basophils are preferentially recruited when the immunization does not involve mycobacteria); and the type of immunogen (eosinophils are recruited to delayed responses to helminthic parasites and basophils to responses to ectoparasites such as ticks). It should be noted that the release of vasoactive mediators by basophils and mast cells may have other functions. For example, they may be protective at sites where reactions are expelling parasites. In addition, there is mounting evidence that at least one of the vasoactive amines — histamine — may have a regulatory role through its ability to interact with functional histamine₂ receptors on various leukocytes. These include cytotoxic T-cell (CTL) precursors or effectors (Plaut et al., 1975; Schwartz et al., 1980) and suppressor T-cell precursors and effectors (Rocklin et al., 1978, Schwartz et al., 1981; Askenase et al., 1981). Along with the effect on lymphocytes, the effect of histamine on other leukocytes leads to a net suppressive and/or anti-inflammatory effect and contributes to the diminution of these reactions (Fig. 81–9) (Askenase, 1977).

CMI AND RESISTANCE TO PATHOGENS

The most convincing proof of the relative importance of the cellular vs. humoral immune mechanisms in protection against pathogens has come from studies of congenital "immunological cripples." Information derived from these human patients and, in selected instances, from other species, is presented in Table 81–7, which sum-

Table 81–7. Defense Mechanisms*

	Bacteria		Viruses†	Fungi	Parasites‡
	Extracellular	*Intracellular*			
CMI	±	+++	+++	+++	+
Antibody	+++	±	++	±	++
Complement	+++	–	++	?	**
NK cells	–	–	++	–	+
Granulocytes	+++	–	+	+	+++§

*From Robert S. Schwartz, personal communication, 1980.

†Depends on nature of virus and stage of infection. Antibody most important for reinfection. Interferon may induce NK cells.

‡Mixed cell mediated response and eosinophils plus antibody.

**Complement may be important in protection against certain blood-borne metazoal parasites via the activation of the alternate pathway.

§Eosinophils, depending on type of parasites.

marizes protective mechanisms known to be operative in infectious diseases.

Bacterial Diseases

The involvement of cell-mediated immunity in resistance to bacterial infections has been the subject of an extensive review (Campbell, 1976). As noted in Table 81–7, the primary immune defense against extracellular bacteria is antibody mediated. This is often by complement-dependent lysis, especially in the case of IgM. The cellular components of these reactions include the phagocytic cells, primarily macrophages and neutrophils. Specific antibody coats and thereby opsonizes bacteria, making them more susceptible to engulfment by phagocytic cells that bear Fc receptors on their surface. Engulfed organisms are subsequently destroyed in phagolysosomes. The antibodies involved in opsonic activity are usually IgG. Complement components, most notably C3b, may aid in this specific opsonization by virtue of C3b receptors on the surface of the phagocyte. Phagocytes can also be specifically *armed* by local antibody, making them more capable of specifically engulfing bacteria.

Intracellular parasites are dealt with primarily or exclusively by DTH-like CMI responses. These include bacteria (such as *Mycobacteria, Salmonellae, Listeria monocytogenes,* and *Brucella*); fungi (e.g., *Coccidioides immitis* [Beaman, et al., 1977] and *Candida*); viruses; and certain protozoal parasites, such as *Toxoplasma,* malaria, *Leishmania,* and various trypanosomes (see Table 81–7). When bacteria are able to invade and grow inside cells, they are safe from antibody mediated attack. The primary defense against such agents is phagocytosis and killing by *activated* macrophages. It appears that less mature macrophages, with few hydrolytic granules, are susceptible to and support the growth of intracellular bacteria. Once influenced by lymphokines in a DTH-like response, the macrophage becomes activated, gains many motile cytoplasmic processes and well-developed intracellular lysosomal granules, and becomes able to kill engulfed bacteria (Mackaness, 1970).

Viral Infections

CMI responses are important to protection against viral diseases as well. Activated macrophages can kill their virus-infected targets by a mechanism that is not totally understood. In addition, through the pioneering work of Zinkernagel and Doherty (1979) it has been demonstrated that CTL are also induced during virus infections and may be the primary mediators of protection. These cells (as well as macrophages) are able to kill infected targets prior to assembly of infectious particles and can therefore break the cycle of viral replication. As with the B-cell response, Ly 1 T cells help (induce) CTL precursors to become killers (Wagner et al., 1980). In order to kill a target cell, in all virus systems tested (in man, mice, rats and chickens), the effectors must recognize not only the relevant virus-associated antigen but self-MHC–coded K or D antigens as well (i.e., virus-modified-self). This contrasts with Ly 1 cells, which recognize antigen in conjunction with MHC Ia antigens. As one might guess, there is evidence that pathologic effects of the immune response may result in host cell destruction in some viral infections, as has been demonstrated in lymphocytic choriomeningitis (LCM) (Doherty and Zinkernagel, 1974).

Other mechanisms of immune protection against virus infections have been described, such as T-cell–dependent antibody formation, which is critical to protection against reinfection with most viruses; IgA secretion at mucosal surfaces; macrophage phagocytosis and killing of certain large viruses and antibody-dependent cell-mediated cytotoxicity (ADCC, see p. 2125).

PARASITIC INFECTIONS

Helminths. Peripheral blood and tissue hypereosinophilia are characteristic of helminth infestations. It has recently been discovered that the eosinophil is a major effector cell in CMI to such parasites, probably by Fc receptor–bound, IgG antibody–dependent destruction of the parasites and their eggs (reviewed in Weller and Goetzl, 1979). Eosinophils produce large quantities of superoxide, which may be a mechanism by which they damage non-phagocytosable parasites. Goetzl and Austen (1977) have presented evidence that eosinophils may also protect the host by regulating histamine release or by breaking down mast cell mediators elaborated during immediate hypersensitivity responses to parasite antigens. Thus, it appears that one major mechanism of protection involves parasite antigen-induced release of eosinophil chemotactic factors both from specifically immune T cells and (by virtue of Fc receptor–bound cytophilic antibody) by degranulation of mast cells. Eosinophils then invade the region and attack the parasite specifically, by antibody-dependent cytotoxic mechanisms. It should be emphasized that other effector mechanisms may also be involved, including complement-dependent antibody-mediated killing, macrophage or neutrophil antibody–dependent killing, and nonspecific inflammatory responses (Table 81–7).

Parasitic disease can be chronic and granulomatous, in many cases associated with an inability of the host to reject the invading parasites. This is because the parasites have evolved to a great variety of mechanisms to survive natural and acquired immune attack by the host (reviewed in Bloom, 1979). For example, although some parasitic larvae, such as schistosomula, are immunogenic and induce a high level of T-cell and antibody responses, as the parasites develop they are no longer recognized as foreign. To avoid destruction, they may lose their ability to activate the alternate complement pathway, abort the ability of activated macrophages to kill them, acquire host antigens, and change the structure of their own surface membrane (Smithers et al., 1977). In addition, activation of suppressor T cells has been demonstrated during certain helminth infections (Attallah et al., 1979; Piessens et al., 1980).

Protozoa. Most intracellular protozoal infections noted above are dealt with in much the same way as intracellular bacteria, i.e., T cell–dependent killing by activated macrophages (McLeod and Remington, 1977). Immunity to the hemoprotozoa such as malaria organisms and *Babezia* is complex (Allison and Clark, 1977). It appears that B cells, T cells, and macrophages are all involved in the recovery from these infections.

It has been demonstrated that protozoan parasites survive by their ability to escape the immune response of the host. Antigenic variation in trypanosomes, for example, is well known (Cross, 1977). This is explained by the sequential expression of alternative cell surface glycoproteins by the parasite. In addition, Jayawardena et al. (1978) recently demonstrated the activation of nonspecific suppressor T cells in experimental trypanosomiasis. The complex immune regulatory mechanisms previously discussed thus apply to protozoal infections as well.

Ectoparasites. There is not a great deal known about immunity to ectoparasites; however, Askenase (1979) has studied the CBH response to ticks. Basophils may play an effector role here, since they comprise up to 90 per cent of the infiltrate, although eosinophils appear to be required as well. Nearly complete resistance can be achieved in guinea pigs (80 to 100 per cent rejection of ticks), which can be transferred to normal animals with sensitized cells and/or immune serum.

TUMOR IMMUNITY

Both normal and malignant cells possess a complex array of molecular entities on the outer surface of the plasma membrane.

Many of these markers are glycoproteins, which differ from one cell type to another. Moreover, when normal cells from one individual are transplanted to an unrelated individual of the same species, these cell-surface markers elicit an immunologic reaction, resulting in an attack by the host's immune cells and rejection of the transplant (allograft rejection, a component of the CMI as discussed later). Therefore, these markers are termed *transplantation antigens.*

Cancer cells possess cell-surface markers that are not normally found on equivalent normal cells of the same individual. These cells often can elicit an immune response within the individual, and a tumor rejection response can be demonstrated in animals that have been previously immunized with the same tumor. These cancer-specific cell-surface molecules are called *tumor-specific transplantation antigens* (TSTA) and include antigens found only in a particular type of tumor, but not in other tumors or normal cells. There are other tumor-associated antigens, which also occur in tumors of various origins and may even occur in normal adult cells in low concentrations. The discovery of cell-surface antigens that distinguish cancer cells from normal cells has been a starting point for attempts to control cancer by immunologic means.

TYPES OF TUMOR-ASSOCIATED ANTIGENS

Four general classes of tumor antigens have been found. The first class comprises those induced by chemical carcinogens. Each carcinogen-induced tumor expresses unique cell-surface antigens that are not found in normal tissue or in another tumor of the same histologic type induced by the same carcinogen in the same or different individuals. For these reasons, each chemically induced tumor can elicit immunity to itself but not to any other tumor.

The second class of tumor-associated antigens comprises those induced by oncogenic DNA viruses. Each of these viruses induces unique nuclear (T) and cell-surface (S) antigens in cells that they transform. For a particular virus these antigens are always the same, regardless of differences in the tissue, the animal, or even the species in which the transformation occurs. The nuclear T antigens of simian virus 40 (SV40)

virus are known to be viral gene products. It is not yet certain whether the surface S antigens are coded by the viral gene or are normal cell-membrane components that are somehow exposed as a result of the transformation process.

The third class of tumor-associated antigens includes those induced by oncornavirus (oncogenic RNA virus) transformation. Like the DNA tumor viruses, each RNA tumor virus induces specific antigens that are the same, regardless of differences in the host cell. By contrast, most, if not all, oncornavirus-specific tumor antigens are viral protein antigens. Some of these proteins represent precursors of virus budding sites on the transformed cell membrane. These antigens may have *group-specific* determinants in common with all viruses of a certain group (e.g., mouse leukemia viruses), *type-specific* determinants shared by only a few closely related viruses (e.g., Gross and Radiation leukemia viruses), and *unique virus-specific* determinants. These determinants may be present on various virion polypeptides, and at least one cell-surface antigen is an internal virion protein. Most of the leukemogenic oncornaviruses induce neoplasms that express normal differentiation antigens as well (e.g., TL antigens of mouse thymocytes).

The fourth class of tumor-associated antigens, called *oncofetal antigens,* is found on cancer cells of various types but also is expressed, normally, during a specific phase of embryonic differentiation. An important example is the *carcinoembryonic antigens* (CEA) of the human colon. This set of antigens is formed on the surface of all tumor cells derived from the gastrointestinal tract, pancreas, liver, and gallbladder. Blood levels of the protein are elevated in most human patients with tumors of the gastrointestinal tract and in about 50 per cent of patients with cancer of breast, lung, and kidney (usually those with metastases). However, elevated levels are frequently seen in patients with alcoholic cirrhosis, pancreatitis, uremia, and occasionally in patients with ulcerative colitis, peptic ulcers, or colonic polyps. Heavy smokers may also show increased levels of these proteins. Thus, oncogenesis is not the only property that gives rise to the expression of such antigens.

Another example of oncofetal antigens is

the *alpha-fetoprotein* (AFP) normally secreted by yolk sac and fetal liver epithelial cells. It is the major protein of fetal serum until mid-gestation, when levels decline gradually and disappear a few weeks after birth. It has also been detected in the sera of human patients with hepatoma, malignant teratomas, or metastases to the liver, and is also present in individuals with acute hepatitis, during pregnancy in which fetuses are malformed, and in some normal subjects. The presence of AFP and CEA is not diagnostic of cancer, and their absence does not rule out a cancer diagnosis.

EFFECTOR MECHANISMS IN TUMOR DESTRUCTION

Several tumor cytotoxic reactions have been demonstrated *in vitro*, but their exact roles in anti-tumor immunity *in vivo* are not known.

Cytolytic Antibodies. In general, tumors of the hematolymphoid system are sensitive to both antibody and cellular immunity, whereas most others are susceptible to cellular immunity only. For tumor cells that have a high density of cell-surface tumor antigens, specific complement-binding IgG antibodies and complement may play important roles in antitumor immunity. IgM-type antibodies are more effective than IgG antibodies in cases wherein tumor cells have a low density of tumor antigens. However, such cytotoxic antibodies of the IgM class are restricted largely to the intravascular compartment and the lymphatic fluid because of their size. They may be unable to reach and penetrate a developing tumor mass. Therefore, most tumors are not susceptible to attack by antibodies alone or by antibodies plus complement, but they are susceptible to attack by killer cells.

Cytotoxic Cells. Three kinds of cytotoxic cells may be involved in cell-mediated immunity to tumors: CTL, cells responsible for antibody-dependent cell-mediated cytotoxicity (ADCC), and natural killer (NK) cells.

CYTOTOXIC T LYMPHOCYTES. Cytotoxic T lymphocytes (CTL), also called T-killer cells or Tc cells, may be the most important T cells that mediate tumor cell cytotoxicity. The action of these cells is antigen specific, and they kill target cells by direct contact.

ANTIBODY-DEPENDENT CELL-MEDIATED

CYTOTOXICITY. Antibody can cooperate with a variety of normal cells to effect immunologically specific target cell destruction *in vitro* without the involvement of the complement system. Antibodies of the IgG class make up the predominant, perhaps exclusive, immunoglobulin type that serves the function of bridging target cells and effector cells. The antibody confers antigenic specificity and provides its Fc portion for linking the target cell at one end and a nonimmune cell at the opposite end. The nonimmune cells involved are of the following types: polymorphonuclear leukocytes, macrophages, platelets, fetal liver cells, and a mononuclear cell of uncertain lineage termed K (for killer) cell. The K cell is also known as a null cell, because it lacks B and T markers. All these cells have Fc receptors, which play a key role in cytolysis.

NATURAL KILLER (NK) CELLS. These are small lymphocytes that also lack the classical markers of T or B cells. These cells can be cytotoxic to neoplastic cells *in vitro* in the apparent absence of antibody or without being specifically sensitized. They are detected in the blood of normal individuals and those with cancer, where their activity is related to tumor burden. Substances that can stimulate levels of NK cells include influenza vaccine (in man), viruses, BCG vaccine, *Clostridium parvum,* polyinosinic-polycytidilic acid, and interferon.

Macrophages. In addition to their phagocytic activity, there are two pathways by which macrophages can be primed to become cytolytically active. One of these, referred to as an "arming" process, may be due to the adsorption of cytophilic antibody onto the macrophage surface or to an acquisition of T-cell receptors. Armed macrophages kill in an immunologically specific manner that depends upon intimate contact between macrophage and target cell. The other pathway by which macrophages acquire cytotoxic potential has been termed "activation." A number of agents (e.g., endotoxin, polyinosinic-polycytidilic acid) can activate macrophages directly *in vitro,* while activation can also occur *in vivo* following immunization with some microbial products, such as BCG. The activated macrophages kill target cells with no immunologic specificity, although they show some selectivity in preferentially killing cells with abnormal growth characteristics (tumor cells). There is evidence that the activated macrophages effect cell destruction by direct secretion of lysosomal enzymes into the cytoplasm of the target cell. Such cells have been described previously in relation to the CMI response and its effect on bacterial infections.

IMMUNOLOGIC ESCAPE MECHANISMS OF TUMORS

By the time a tumor is diagnosed, most affected animals demonstrate both cellular and humoral immunity directed specifically at cell-surface antigens of the tumor cells. How, then, do these tumor cells ever survive in what should be a hostile environment? Several different mechanisms of immunologic escape have been found in studies of experimental tumors.

Immunologic Enhancement. This is a mechanism by which antibody facilitates the growth of a transplant, usually of neoplastic origin, which would otherwise be rejected. There are three forms of enhancement: afferent enhancement, in which the antibodies combine with antigens present on the transplant, preventing immunization; efferent enhancement, in which they bind to and "mask" antigens, which are then not detected by the host's immune cells; and central enhancement, in which they act directly on host lymphoid cells and prevent these from mediating graft rejection. Besides antibodies, other blocking factors (such as antigen-antibody complexes) and free tumor antigens in the sera of individuals bearing tumors can specifically block lymphocyte-mediated cytotoxic reactions to tumor antigens. They do so most commonly by interacting directly with CTL.

Immunosuppression. This can occur in several ways: (1) iatrogenic immunosuppression, caused by agents (ionizing radiation and cytotoxic drugs) used to treat the tumor; (2) immunosuppressive factors released by the tumors (immunosuppressive viruses, alpha-fetal protein); and (3) immunosuppressive factors produced by the host in response to tumor challenge (suppressor T cells, prostaglandins, and many presently unidentified soluble factors and cells).

Other mechanisms of avoiding immune destruction include antigenic modulation, in which tumor antigens are masked or lost in the presence of antibodies and if the anti-bodies disappear, the tumor antigens usually reappear; "sneaking through," in which a small weakly antigenic tumor cell load may not induce immunologic recognition in the early phase of growth, so that by the time the immune system is alerted the cancer is established and too extensive for the host to deal with; tumor growth stimulation, by a weak immune response (mechanism unknown); change to an unrecognized new antigenic variant, which then can selectively grow to dominate the tumor; and immunologic tolerance, in which animals injected very early with tumors or high concentrations of tumor-associated antigens before the development of full immunologic competence maintain a specific unresponsiveness to these tumors if they are transplanted into the same animals later in life.

ROLE OF HOST IMMUNE PROCESSES IN DEFENSE AGAINST CANCER

Immune surveillance is a process by which the immune system is assumed to detect and eliminate nascent tumors. This hypothesis predicts that tumors should sensitize animals against tumor antigens and that immunologically competent individuals should have a lower frequency of spontaneous tumors. However, although most, perhaps all, tumor cells are immunogenic, the growth of small tumors is often progressive. In other cases, termed concomitant immunity, a large primary tumor grows quite well, while antigenic metastases or small doses of the same tumor transplanted distant from the primary tumor site are rejected. One might expect to see a higher incidence of cancer in immunodeficient and immunosuppressed animals. T cell–depleted animals (e.g., congenitally athymic or nude mice, and animals that have been treated with antilymphocyte serum, x-irradiation, and neonatal thymectomy) do have higher incidences of virally induced neoplasms, but the incidence of chemically induced and spontaneous tumors is not greatly elevated. This suggests that the major anti-tumor effect of the immune system *may* be the removal or destruction of oncogenic viruses. Immunodeficiency in man predisposes to only certain types of malignancies, primarily of lymphoreticular origins. This may again be explained by the failure of the immune system to eliminate oncogenic agents, especially viruses, from such individuals.

Immunotherapy. Recent experiments have shown that if the host immune system is properly stimulated, it can cause tumor regression. An approach currently being tested is called adjuvant immunotherapy. For example, the individual bearing a tumor can be inoculated with BCG, an attenuated strain of *Mycobacterium bovis*. BCG may act either as an adjuvant by increasing the immunogenicity of the antigens it is mixed with or by nonspecifically heightening the immune response (most probably via T cells) and increasing the activity of the macrophage system. Thus far, the effect of BCG on human tumors seems limited to those accessible to injection or infection with BCG, since distant metastases and internal tumors are usually unaffected. However, BCG is also potentially dangerous, because it can enhance tumor growth in certain instances, perhaps by increasing the levels of blocking factors or suppressor cells. The varying immunologic regulatory processes discussed above thus must be taken into account to understand, or manipulate, any immunologic influences on tumor growth.

HISTOCOMPATIBILITY REACTIONS AND GRAFT REJECTION

It is well known that tissues and organs do not survive transplantation between two members of the same species, except in the case of identical twins. This phenomenon of allograft rejection primarily involves a CMI response to foreign transplantation antigens on the graft. A firm understanding of transplantation and graft-versus-host (GVH) reactions, the interaction of macrophages and T and B cells, and the genetic control of the immune response and other phenomena requires knowledge of a complex of multiallelic genes coding for the relevant cell surface antigens. The strongest transplantation antigens are coded by a single MHC in all species studied, including the dog (called DLA-dog leukocyte antigens) (Gotze, 1977; Schwartz, 1974). The general structure and function of the MHC of all species studied is similar. Since the mouse MHC (called the H-2 locus) is best known and understood (Klein, 1975; Möller, 1978), it is commonly used as a model system for the other species.

Antibodies that are raised against some MHC-coded antigens can be used to recognize the alloantigens on the surface of cells of a potential graft donor, by employing various serologic techniques (histocompatibility tests), such as complement-dependent antibody-mediated cytotoxicity. Such alloantigens are called serologically defined (SD) antigens. Other antigens, against which antibodies are difficult (but usually not impossible) to raise, more easily induce T-cell responses, such as the mixed leukocyte response (MLR, also used as a histocompatibility test). Therefore, this group of antigens has been called lymphocyte defined (LD).

STRUCTURE OF THE MHC

Table 81–8 summarizes the major traits attributed to specific regions of the H-2 complex of the mouse, a genetic map of which is presented in Fig. 81–10. Each region is large enough from a genetic perspective to contain separate genes for many different traits. More limited, but compara-

Table 81–8. Partial List of Genes Localized to the Mouse MHC (H-2) Region

| Biological Trait | Segment of Mouse H-2 Complex | | | | | |
	K	I-A	I-B	I-C	S	D
H-2 (SD) antigens	+					+
Target antigens for CTL	+					+
Transplantation antigens	+	+				+
Immune response genes		+	+	+		
Ia (LD) antigens		+	+	+		
MLR, GVHR	+	+	+	+		+
Serum proteins					+	

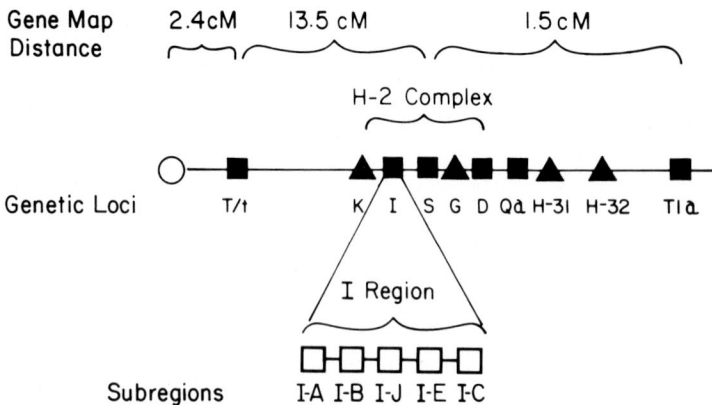

Figure 81–10. A map of the 17th chromosome of the mouse. The positions of the centromere (○), and identified genes (△) and complexes of two or more genes (□) are shown, which code for cell-surface alloantigens. T/t codes for short tail, H-31 and H-32 are minor histocompatibility genes. See the text for descriptions of the other loci. One centimorgan (cM) represents a recombination frequency of 1%; for example, there is approximately a 13.5% recombination rate between T/t and H-2K, and a 1.5% recombination rate between H-2D and Tla.

ble, information is accumulating for other species, but the mouse currently remains the best prototype.

K and D Regions

The K and D regions code for SD antigens. Products of the K and D loci are present separately on the surface of cells. There is structural homology between H-2K and H-2D as well as between the SD antigens of man and mouse and probably other species. SD antigens serve as the targets for allogeneic CTL. They are also involved in the specificity of CTL against tumor, hapten, or virus-modified syngeneic target cells (see p. 2122). K and D region–coded products are the major antigens involved in transplantation reactions.

The I (Immune Response) Region

The I region of the MHC codes for certain I region–associated (Ia) cell surface antigens and for the level of the immune response to certain antigens. In the mouse it is composed of at least five genetic loci: I-A, I-B, I-J, I-E, and I-C. The serologically detected Ia antigens are distinct from the SD antigens. They are selectively expressed on B lymphocytes, some macrophages (I-A and I-E locus coded antigens), and some T-cell subsets (I-J and I-C locus coded antigens). The Ia antigens are the stimulators of MLR and GVH responses. I region genes somehow control cell interactions between the macrophage and T cell, and between T cell and B cell, probably by requiring cellular recognition of conventional antigen in conjunction with Ia antigen.

The I region was originally identified as the site where immune response (Ir) genes map. Ir genes were defined on the basis of the differences in the response levels of different inbred strains of mice and guinea pigs to branched, synthetic polypeptide antigens. The I region also has been found to control the ability to respond to a variety of other thymus-dependent antigens in several species, as described later. The entire MHC is inherited as a package or "haplotype" and is codominantly expressed. That is, genes coding for histocompatibility antigens from one of the paired chromosomes of each parent will be expressed in each offspring.

GRAFT REJECTION

The engraftment of tissues between two nonidentical (allogeneic) members of the same species is termed an allograft. Transplants between two genetically identical members of the same species and sex are termed syngeneic and survive indefinitely.

Skin and tumor allografts usually survive a shorter period (10 to 12 days) than do vascularized organ grafts. This is probably because of the relative ischemia that occurs early in the former exchange. The nonvascularized grafts require lymphatic drainage for sensitization of the host, while this is not required for vascularized organ grafts. Rejection of first allografts ("first set") is associated with a mononuclear infiltrate (primarily lymphocytes and mononuclear phagocytes), which becomes massive by five to seven days after transplantation. Progressive tissue damage and necrosis are seen later, associated with the completion of the rejection process. A second graft from a donor sharing foreign transplantation antigens with the first donor leads to a more rapid "second set" rejection by the same cellular mechanisms. In certain instances, repeated or prolonged contact with foreign grafts leads to the formation of circulating antibody, which, after grafting a fresh organ or skin with similar antigens, leads to hyperacute rejection. In this case the skin is never revascularized and is therefore called a "white graft." A vascularized organ may show immediate rejection at the time of grafting, owing to ischemia. To minimize the chance of rapid rejection, prospective recipients are always tested for preexisting cytotoxic antibody against donor MHC SD antigens, the degree of match of SD antigens (especially to detect antigens in the donor that are absent in the recipient), and MLR for evidence of LD antigen differences. There is evidence that pretransplant histocompatibility matching will increase chances for prolonged survival of a graft from a related living donor, possibly with less intensive and a shorter course of immunosuppressive drug therapy.

Cellular Mechanisms in Rejection of Grafts

Transplantation immunity (allografts) can be transferred to normal animals by T lymphocytes. In contrast, serum may even prolong graft survival (immunologic enhancement; see Tumor Immunity). Specifically precommitted inducer T cells recognize Ia antigens, primarily those that are present on leukocytes (passenger cells) in the vasculature of an organ graft, or, perhaps, on the Langerhans cells of a skin graft. These cells are triggered to undergo blastogenesis (afferent arm of the response) and divide and produce lymphokines. These cells can then help (induce) CTL precursor cells to become activated allospecific CTL (Cantor and Boyse, 1975). CTL recognize and bind to K or D antigens on the surface of cells of the graft and can kill these cells (efferent arm). Killing (cell-mediated lympholysis, or CML) occurs by punching holes similar to those occurring in complement-dependent antibody-mediated lysis. Sensitized inducer T cells can also recruit and activate monocytes and small granulocytes at the site of rejection.

The *in vitro* mixed leukocyte response (MLR) is a correlate of inducer T-cell activation by foreign Ia antigens. Usually, the stimulating cells are x-irradiated or treated with mitomycin C to prevent their response in culture. The MLR is assayed by uptake of tritiated thymidine as a measure of DNA synthesis. Also during the *in vitro* MLR, CTL are induced by K or D antigen stimulator-responder differences. These cell interactions are similar to those indicated previously for the transplantation reaction, and therefore the MLR is used as a predictor of the likelihood of graft rejection between donor and recipient (histocompatibility test).

Graft Versus Host Disease

Bone marrow or other grafts containing immunocompetent T cells can be destructive to the host into which they are injected. This is especially true when the host is immunoincompetent. This response is much like the afferent arm of the transplant response or the MLR in many respects, in that the donor helper (inducer) T cells respond to foreign Ia antigens on the recipient cells. There also appear to be important non-MHC antigen-induced GVH responses. This is a clinically important phenomenon in bone marrow transplantation.

The Biological Role of the MHC

While the MHC is important in graft rejection, it seems clear that nature did not create it to confound the surgeon or the hematologist. We have mentioned not only that CTL are induced by allogeneic stimulator cells, but that syngeneic cells bearing tumor-specific antigens, or cells that are viral or chemically (i.e., hapten) modified, can induce and be the target cells for CTL both *in vivo* and *in vitro*. Zinkernagel and Doherty (1979) discovered that the MHC K or D products appear to be recognition structures by which the host responds to antigens such as viruses (T helper cells and T cells reactive in DTH are also MHC restricted, but for Ia antigens). Recognition is strong enough to lead to rejection of virus-infected cells, which might be recognized in a way similar to that by which foreign MHC antigens are recognized. (This is also one explanation for autoimmune responses. See below.) Certain regulatory T cells have been found to display one or another of the Ia antigens on their surface. For example, suppressor cells often bear I-J antigens. In addition, there is evidence that the presence of I-A and I-C region–coded antigens on macrophages and B cells allows certain T cells to interact preferentially with them.

In all species there are large numbers of alleles for both LD and SD antigens. One explanation for this diversity could be that MHC-coded antigens serve as the binding site for microorganisms, and various microorganisms may have different affinities for different MHC-coded antigens. This variation in viral binding site affinity might render some members of a given animal species more resistant to infection than others, and the population might therefore be protected from annihilation by that infectious agent. In spite of numerous observations of this sort, however, it is not yet totally clear what the general biological role of the MHC may be.

Association of MHC and Disease. In man and in some animal species, an increased predilection for the occurrence of certain infectious, allergic, autoimmune, and other diseases has been associated with individuals bearing one or more specific MHC-coded antigenic specificities on their cell surface. The reason for these associations is not known. The microorganism receptor theory in the preceding paragraph has been invoked as an explanation. Other explanations might include (1) structural similarity of the MHC-coded antigen to the antigens of an infectious agent. The host thus recognizes the agent as self, leading to tolerance, which then increases susceptibility to the infection. Conversely, this could lead to the recognition of a self component as foreign and lead to autoimmunity. (2) "Defective" Ir genes (coding for incorrect responses) might be associated more frequently with one of the genes coding for Ia antigens. Ia antigens might even be directly involved in the pathogenesis of the disordered immune response, perhaps by affecting the events associated with antigen recognition. (3) The genes of the MHC might merely be tightly linked to other genes affecting the pathogenesis of a disease without being directly involved in immune reactivity (linkage disequilibrium).

Immunogenetics and the MHC: Ir Genes. Several autosomal dominant genes have been identified as totally distinct from the structural genes coding for Ig variable regions, which are required for an animal to make a vigorous cellular and/or humoral immune response to a T cell–dependent antigen. Most of these specific immune responses (Ir) genes are located in close proximity to genes coding for MHC antigens, as originally shown in mice and guinea pigs (Benacerraf and McDevitt, 1972). Evidence for MHC linked Ir genes has been found in rats, rhesus monkeys, and man. All species probably have such genes, which may bear heavily on the incidence or severity of a variety of diseases.

IMMUNOLOGIC REACTIONS AND DISEASE

Many specific disease states will be covered in an in-depth manner in Chapters 82 and 83. This section, therefore, will only deal with some general characteristics of some of the disorders as they relate to the fundamental immunologic principles that have been discussed.

AUTOIMMUNITY

Autoimmunity is defined as an immune response to self components and represents a breakdown of self-tolerance. Autoimmune reactions can involve T-cell or antibody-mediated processes. It is important to note that the mere presence of an antibody to a self component is not adequate evidence for the involvement of that antibody in the pathogenesis of an autoimmune disease state. For example, in systemic lupus erythematosus (SLE), there are circulating antibodies to DNA. Such antibodies to intracellular antigens are not known to cause cell damage but could have been the result of an immune response to DNA released following cell death from another cause. (This issue, however, is complicated by recent findings that some putative anti-DNA antibodies also can react with the phosphate moiety of phospholipids, which are constituents of cell membranes.) Autoimmunity to circulating (serum) proteins present in large quantities is not found, possibly because the level of circulating protein maintains both

B-cell and T-cell tolerance (see page 2108). On the other hand, autoimmunity to circulating proteins that are present in small amounts, such as thyroglobulin, does occur, perhaps relating to only T-cell tolerance and not B-cell tolerance. The state of tolerance to intracellular antigens is poor, and autoantibodies are often induced after trauma. Examples are the nonpathogenic antibodies to cytoplasmic antigens of the liver, which are made after chemically induced hepatonecrosis, and the autoantibodies to prostatic antigens, which develop after cryotherapy.

It is possible to induce loss of self-tolerance by immunizing an animal to its own tissues in complete Freund's adjuvant (strong immunization) or by immunizing with antigens cross-reactive with self components (e.g., immunization of rabbits with human thyroglobulin results in autoantibodies to rabbit thyroglobulin). This might stimulate T-cell help for already existent nontolerant B cells. It is possible, therefore, to have either no tolerance (hidden antigens), only B-cell tolerance, or both T-cell and B-cell tolerance to self antigens.

Spontaneous autoimmune diseases in both man and animals have been described. These include Goodpasture's syndrome, in which antibodies are deposited on the glomerular basement membrane (GBM) of the kidney. Such antibodies are occasionally associated with pulmonary damage also. Hashimoto's thyroiditis is a disease associated with the formation of antibodies to thyroglobulin and manifests cellular infiltrates of the thyroid. Other examples of clinically significant autoimmune disease are autoimmune hemolytic anemia, in which autoantibodies to erythrocytes result in premature destruction of the cells; idiopathic thrombocytopenic purpura, in which antibodies destroy circulating platelets; and SLE. A number of factors leading to autoimmune disease have been known for some time and are now discussed.

Viral Infection. Viruses have been postulated to have a role in autoimmune diseases (Schwartz, 1975). Type C RNA viruses (retroviruses) have been shown to regularly induce antinuclear antibodies in experimental animals (Quimby et al., 1977). Viruses are not the exclusive cause of the disease state, however, as is clear from findings that although many strains of mice express retroviral antigens, only NZB and a few other strains develop lesions typical of lupus nephritis.

Disturbance of Immune Regulation. A disturbance of T-cell function has been demonstrated in chickens by the finding of an infectious agammaglobulinemia syndrome (Blaese, 1974). Bursectomy somehow results in the induction of large numbers of suppressor T cells able to cause agammaglobulinemia upon transfer to normal chickens, i.e., this is essentially an autoimmune-induced immunodeficiency disease. These studies imply that the suppressor T-cell defect was secondary to a B-cell lack. Indeed, the existence of a primary B-cell defect (spontaneous production of large quantities of IgM) has been discovered in SLE-prone NZB mice (Manny et al., 1979). In addition, a lack of Ly 123 feedback suppressor cells has been discovered in NZB mice (Cantor et al., 1978). These data imply a possible inverse relationship between suppressor cell activation and the activity or presence of B cells. In this regard, it is noteworthy that spontaneous autoantibodies to T cells have been discovered in NZB mice, humans, and dogs with autoimmune disease (Strelkauskas et al., 1978; Imai et al., 1980; Quimby et al., 1982). In this situation, a lack of suppressor cells has been hypothesized to result in a breakdown of self-tolerance.

Genetics. There is convincing evidence for genetic influences in human SLE, and some strains of mice routinely get autoimmune disorders. In addition, a colony of dogs bred for SLE has been developed at Tufts University. Descendents of these dogs have developed not only SLE but rheumatoid arthritis, autoimmune hemolytic anemia, pernicious anemia, thrombocytopenic purpura hemorrhagica, celiac disease, autoimmune thyroiditis, Sjögren's-like syndrome, and a variety of autoantibodies as well (Quimby et al., 1978). Studies with autoimmune disease–prone mice and dogs have shown that many animals may have autoantibodies without autoimmune disease. This and other data have led to the hypothesis that at least two classes of genes are involved in and required for pathogenesis of autoimmune disorders. Class 1 genes permit a general predisposition to autoimmunity by resulting in disordered lymphocyte function and immunoregulation, and

Class 2 genes determine the phenotypic expression of the disease, by determining the size of immune complexes, participation of the complement system, and other comparable variables.

IMMUNE COMPLEX DISEASES

Immune complex diseases belong to the classical Type III hypersensitivity group (Gell and Coombs, 1974). In such disorders (Table 81–5), which include serum sickness, Arthus reactions, and certain autoimmune diseases, antigen-antibody complexes formed in antigen excess are deposited in tissues and/or blood vessels. The serum complement cascade is activated by the classical or alternative pathway, leading to the formation of chemotactic factors. Neutrophils that are drawn in can cause severe tissue necrosis. They bind to the complexes via C3 receptors, phagocytose the complexes, and release lysosomal enzymes and vasoactive peptides.

IgG is the usual antibody class involved in these reactions. IgM can fix complement also, but is present in considerably smaller concentration in the serum. Any individual capable of making an immune response to conventional foreign antigens (carbohydrate or protein) can produce immune complexes, which, under certain conditions, may produce pathological changes. It is important to understand that most immunologic diseases are of a mixed nature, although one component may predominate. Small amounts of antigen favor delayed-type reactions mediated by T cell–dependent macrophage or other cell infiltrates, while large amounts of antigen favor Arthus-like reactions. In addition, IgE-mediated responses may also occur in responses to the same antigen, especially after skin or mucosal routes of exposure to soluble allergens in genetically predisposed individuals.

The immune complex can be a combination of antibody with antigen circulating in the serum, soluble in the tissue fluid phase, or present on a tissue or a cell. Autoantibodies can either be involved with specificity for fixed tissue components or form circulating immune complexes with unmodified or foreign antigen—modified self immunogens.

Systemic Immune Complex Disease: Serum Sickness

The classical form of this disorder occurs following deposition of circulating immune complexes that are developed by antibodies induced by administration of foreign serum proteins such as horse serum (Dixon, 1963). This circulating antigen is gradually catabolized, and animals remain asymptomatic until an antibody response to the antigen occurs. Later, animals or humans exhibit swollen joints, fever, skin rashes, albuminuria, hematuria, and glomerulonephritis. Early in the response (acute serum sickness), small numbers of antibodies are bound to antigens, so that none can be detected in the circulation. These complexes are small, and are in *antigen excess* (e.g., Ag_2Ab, Ag_3Ab_2, Ag_4Ab_3, and so on), which are taken up poorly by phagocytes and so can circulate. They are deposited in the vessel walls of various organs, especially the kidneys, where they cause endothelial hyperplasia, fibrinoid necrosis of the vessel wall, neutrophilic infiltrates, and increased vascular permeability. In the renal glomerulus, Ig, complement, and antigen are found deposited along the glomerular capillary wall in an irregular ("lumpy-bumpy") pattern characteristic of the lesion. As the immune response progresses, the antibody/antigen ratio increases, the complexes become larger, and they can be taken up by phagocytes in the spleen and liver before causing damage. Once all antigen is cleared from the circulation, free antibody is found and clinical and pathological signs abate. It is evident that there must be a degree of increased vascular permeability to allow immune complexes to penetrate vessel walls, in that antihistamines can decrease complex localization and pathological changes. IgE may lead to release from basophils of a lipid called platelet-activating factor, which may result in the release of platelet vasoamines important to the development of the lesion. Complexes tend to localize in sites at which platelets adhere to endothelium, such as where there is increased blood pressure or turbulence, or in sites such as the kidney. The kidney probably suffers most from immune complex accumulation, because complexes are readily trapped owing to the high blood flow and the fine fenestrated capillary network of this organ, which exposes the glomerular basement membrane. Complexes increase in the circulation when reticuloendothelial mononuclear phagocytes are compromised. Larger, strongly immunogenic antigens that stay in the circulation in quantity for prolonged periods tend to be most capable of inducing serum sickness.

A more chronic form of serum sickness occurs when antigen, often in small quantities, is present in the circulation for prolonged periods. Some animals tend to become tolerant under such circumstances, while others develop a large antibody response that rapidly clears the antigen. Some animals, however, have smaller responses, which favor the formation of immune complexes in slight antigen excess. This results in a more chronic development of immune complex disease, primarily in the kidney, eventually leading to azotemia and renal failure.

Local Immune Complex Disease

Arthus Reactions. The Arthus reaction is an acute immune complex vasculitis produced when antigen is injected intradermally in an animal that has preformed circulating antibodies to that antigen (Table 81–5). The reaction is usually seen later than an immediate response but before a typical DTH response, i.e., at four to ten hours after administration of antigen. The pathogenesis of the reaction is essentially as described for serum sickness, except that the antigen is deposited extravascularly. Damage is therefore restricted to where serum antibody and antigen come in contact. Thus, severe neutrophilic infiltrates are seen along regional vessel walls, occasionally associated with thrombosis and necrosis, and with leakage of proteins and erythrocytes into the extravascular space.

Other. The chronic inflammatory disease of the joints known as rheumatoid arthritis also includes immune complexes as a part of its pathogenesis. Immune complexes are found in joint fluids, together with neutrophils and a low level of complement proteins. Antibodies called rheumatoid factor (which are IgM or IgG) complex with IgG antibodies specific for bound microbial antigens. Another example of a local immune complex disease is Farmer's lung, in which inhaled fungal antigens complex in

the lung with circulating antibodies to that fungus. Other environmental antigens cause similar processes and undoubtedly often produce disease that is not accurately diagnosed.

IMMUNE COMPLEXES ASSOCIATED WITH FIXED TISSUE ANTIGENS

Injection of anti-tissue antibodies (for example, rabbit antibodies to rat GBM) results in immune complex nephritis by means similar to those described for the Arthus reaction. However, the antigen is normal and fixed and the antibody is passively injected. Although much of the early pathological change requires neutrophils, the later stages do not. The second phase is an antibody reaction to the foreign (rabbit) Ig, which serves as a model for how a foreign protein can cause injury by binding to tissue sites.

Examples in man and animals in which immune complexes have been implicated in disease include, in addition to classical serum sickness, (1) post-streptococcal (or other bacterial) glomerulonephritis. This is caused by the acute release of a large amount or continuous slow release of small amounts of bacterial antigen. (2) Malaria. Plasmodial antigens may result in glomerulonephritis. (3) Viruses. In such cases the viruses often circulate for prolonged periods without disease. Animals infected with LCM virus suffer from CTL-mediated damage of virus-modified self–nervous tissue cells. In addition, when neonatal mice are infected with LCM virus and thereby become partially tolerant to the virus, no acute disease develops (Oldstone and Dixon, 1971). Rather, a moderate antibody response gradually develops, resulting in antigen excess immune complex glomerulonephritis. Similar problems occur in Aleutian disease of mink, equine infectious anemia in horses, and possibly hepatitis B virus infection in man. (4) Autoantigens. In a variety of species, antibodies to DNA are developed in association with SLE. Whereas the antibodies themselves are not ordinarily damaging, immune complex glomerulonephritis occurs. Complexes are also deposited in various other tissues (see Chapter 82 and 83). (5) Unknown antigen. In many instances the identity of the antigen is not known; however, Ig with or without complement may be deposited along the GBM with typical pathological changes. Other diseases, such as polyarteritis nodosa, are likely to be immune complex–mediated as well.

Autoantibodies to erythrocytes, platelets, neutrophils, and other cells may bind to such cells and deplete them from the circulation. In some cases, a drug may bind to self components and the complex antigen be recognized as foreign. These drug-induced autoimmune disorders have been brought about by a variety of agents such as quinidine, aspirin, and sulfonamides. The disorder abates once the drug is removed from the system.

TUMORS OF THE IMMUNE SYSTEM

In man and in many domestic species, lymphoid tumors derived from B-cell, T-cell, and stem-cell lineages have been discovered. The characterization of the tumor type often depends on using markers similar to those employed for classifying normal lymphoid cells (see Table 81–2). Such studies have shown, for example, that the majority of leukemias in cats are of the T-cell lineage. Perhaps the most thoroughly studied of the lymphoid tumors, however, is the myeloma or malignant plasma cell tumor. These B-cell tumors are the products of single clones of plasma cells that have escaped regulation. Each cell of the clone secretes an identical immunoglobulin protein. Therefore, the serum of affected animals often contains a large amount of homogeneous Ig, the discovery of which has greatly facilitated studies of the structure and function of immunoglobulins in general. Many of the myeloma proteins have been found to have antigen binding capability. Many others, however, remain "antibodies in search of antigens." The frequency with which different myelomas produce a given immunoglobulin class with a given light chain is a reflection of the frequency of normal Ig producing cells in that species; e.g., the most common human myeloma protein is IgG with kappa light chains, while canine myeloma paraproteins have mainly lambda light chains, and IgE myelomas of *all* species are very rare.

A convenient source of light chains is the urine of animals that suffer from myeloma, since light chains are often secreted in ex-

cess by malignant plasma cells. These proteins have been described in dogs (Hurvitz et al., 1972). Urinary light chains are called Bence Jones proteins. Heating the urine of individuals affected with myeloma to 56° C for 15 minutes results in the formation of a proteinaceous precipitate. Further heating at 100° C for three minutes results in its return to solution. Some tumors make only light chains (light chain disease), while others make only heavy chains (heavy chain disease). The heavy chains are often abnormal in such patients, with variable deletions of amino acids near the amino terminal end of the heavy chain. Recent evidence has shown that the Ig production of plasmacytoma cells can be regulated by anti-idiotypic antibodies (Lynch et al., 1979). In addition, it is becoming apparent that the plasma cell tumor is not homogeneous with regard to the maturation of different cells in the population. That is, cells bearing the characteristics of very immature to fully mature plasma cells are often present in the same neoplasm. In this respect, such lymphoid tumors resemble tumors of other tissues that have been shown to consist of a heterogeneous population of cells.

IMMUNODEFICIENCY STATES

Immunodeficiencies can be classified as congenital or acquired. The congenital immunodeficiency states are often genetic diseases and have been termed experiments of nature. This is because by studying each disease state, the lack of a given component of the immune apparatus may be associated with the absence of a given spectrum of normal functions (see Table 81–7). Although many of these disorders have not been described in domestic animals, many conditions comparable to those described in man have been studied. Only the most important and/or illustrative congenital diseases will be discussed here (for a more complete discussion, see Rosen, 1979).

Congenital Immunodeficiency Diseases

Refer to Figure 81–11, which indicates the cellular location of the defect keyed by the following numbers.

(1) Severe Total Deficiency of Stem Cells. Even under the best conditions, animals that are so affected would live only a few days.

Figure 81–11. Points of defect in some congenital immunodeficiency diseases. SC, stem cell; LP, lymphocyte precursor; MP, myeloid cell precursor; T, T cell; B, B cell; Gr, granulocyte; M, monocyte; PC, plasma cell; Th, T helper cell; Tc, cytotoxic T cell; Ta, Amplifier T cell; Ts, suppressor T cell. Numbers 1–5 relate to text paragraph numbers for defects.

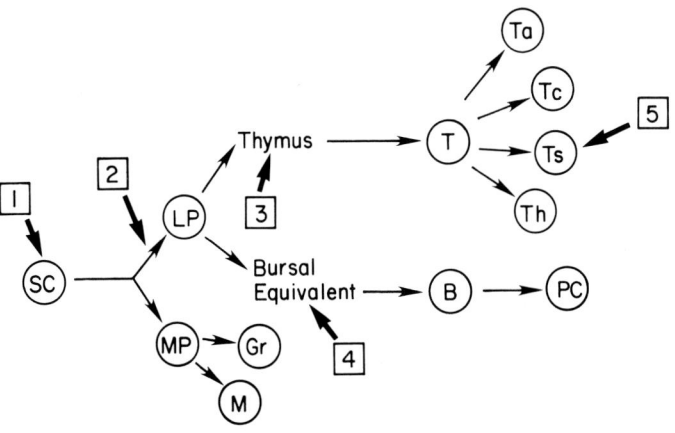

These neonates lack granulocytes, megakaryocytes, erythrocytes, and lymphoid cells, and therefore have no resistance to any microorganism.

(2) Severe Combined Immunodeficiency Disease (SCID) or Swiss-Type Agammaglobulinemia. This X-linked recessive or autosomal recessive trait is due to absence of early committed lymphoid stem cells. There are few or no T cells or B cells. It has recently been noted that some SCIDS (50 per cent of these with the autosomal recessive form) lack either adenosine deaminase, an enzyme required for conversion of adenosine to inosine, or purine nucleoside phosphorylase, which is needed to break down inosine to hypoxanthine. Thus, there is a marked increase in adenosine, ATP, and deoxy ATP that somehow prevents normal maturation of lymphocytes, especially T cells. Since adenosine deaminase is present in normal human erythrocytes, erythrocyte transfusions have been used successfully to treat some human patients. Combined immunodeficiency has been discovered in Arabian foals in association with lymphopenia, thymic aplasia, absent cell-mediated immunity, Ig deficiency, marked decreases in spleen and lymph node lymphocytes, and increased susceptibility to infection. The trait is inherited in an autosomal recessive manner (McGuire et al., 1976a). Interestingly, SCID foals are not lacking an adenosine deaminase or other purine salvage pathway enzymes (McGuire et al., 1976b). Pneumonia is the most common secondary disease and is caused by viral, fungal, bacterial, and protozoal agents. Bone marrow grafts have been employed as a means of treatment of stem-cell defects.

(3) Di George Syndrome. This syndrome is due to congenital (not hereditary in man) lack of the third and fourth branchial pouches. Affected individuals lack both epithelial thymus and parathyroid glands. The disease varies from total absence to severe underdevelopment of the thymus with hypocalcemic tetany. Although the lymphoid cell precursor pool is normal, owing to a lack of a thymic developmental microenvironment and thymic hormones, affected individuals have few or no T cells and marked hypocellularity of T-cell areas of lymphoid organs. Such individuals, in the partial forms, might be likened to a neonatally thymectomized mouse, in that they have a relative lack of T-cell function. Total lack of the thymus is hereditary in the nude mouse, which completely lacks T-cell function. Unless placed in a controlled environment, in complete aplasia, death results from overwhelming viral infection due to herpes viruses, fungi, or often normally nonpathogenic agents such as *Candida albicans* or protozoal infections such as *Pneumocystis carinii*. Fetal thymus transplants have been used for treatment of human patients and might well be applicable to affected animals.

(4) Bruton's Agammaglobulinemia. This condition is an X-linked B-cell deficiency characterized by recurrent pyogenic bacterial infections, no circulating IgM, IgA, IgE, or IgD, and less than ten per cent of the normal level of IgG. Affected individuals make no antibody responses, although they have normal T-cell numbers and function (no increased susceptibility to fungi or most viruses). In man, this condition is usually treated by giving gamma globulin and providing requisite supportive therapy. An exact equivalent has not yet been described in domestic animals.

(5) Common Variable Agammaglobulinemia. This human condition is a late onset disease, often not observed until adulthood in either sex. It is characterized by both hypogammaglobulinemia and a deficiency in cell-mediated immunity. Patients have B cells, but these cells fail to mature into Ig secreting cells in response to antigens. T-cell function decreases with time, especially in patients developing thymomas. The spectrum of disease susceptibility is similar to that in Bruton's disease. Certain forms of this condition are thought to be related to a severe derangement of regulation, particularly suppressor T cells, in that T cells from affected patients can suppress Ig production by normal B cells *in vitro* (Waldmann et al., 1978). Such patients are very susceptible to autoimmune disease. This syndrome probably exists in other mammalian species but is yet to be formally described.

Acquired Immunodeficiencies

Naturally occurring acquired immunodeficiency diseases of the dog and cat have been reviewed by Cockerell (1978).

Viral Infection. In man, nonspecific immunodeficiency associated with measles infection is classical. It has been detected, for example, by a transient lack of response (anergy) to tuberculin in otherwise sensitive individuals. A closely related paramyxovirus of dogs, canine distemper virus, has also been shown to result in immunodeficiency. Lymphopenia is observed in the acute phase, and dogs with active distemper have been shown to reject kidney grafts less well. DTH and T-cell mitogen responses are also decreased. Immunosuppression is probably due to virus replication in cells of the lymphoreticular system and their subsequent destruction or functional alteration.

Feline leukemia virus (oncornavirus)–infected cats also often become immunologic-ally crippled. Affected animals show thymic atrophy and T-cell depletion. Bone marrow cells are also infected and may be a target. T-cell responses are decreased, including allograft rejection and lectin-induced DNA synthesis stimulation. There also appears to be a B-cell functional deficiency. In feline leukemia virus–infected animals that do not develop lymphosarcoma, many animals succumb to secondary infection with other agents such as feline infectious peritonitis virus. A protein constituent of the virus is believed responsible (Olsen and Krakowka, 1979). Feline panleukopenia virus also causes a mild degree of T-cell immunosuppression.

Parasitic Infestations, Chronic Bacterial Diseases, and Malignancy. All these can be nonspecifically immunosuppressive, in some cases involving nonspecific suppressor T-cell activation.

Chemotherapy and Radiotherapy for Cancer. With the increasing use of antimetabolites, alkylating agents, and adrenal corticosteroids, the occurrence of secondary immunodeficiency states is increasing. In many instances there is an increase in susceptibility to herpes viruses, *Candida, Aspergillus, Nocardia,* gram-negative flora, *Pneumocystis,* and other organisms. The primary defect usually is in T cells. In very high doses, however, many of the agents are general bone marrow depressants and general immunosuppressants. As noted previously, the use of immunosuppressive agents in organ transplantation has been associated with a great increase in lymphoreticular neoplasia.

Other Factors. Malnutrition, aging, failure of colostrum transfer, and protein depleting enteropathies and nephropathies are other factors that have been associated with acquired immunodeficiencies.

ACKNOWLEDGMENT: The authors wish to thank Dr. Sidney Leskowitz for concepts presented at lectures at Tufts University, which served as the basis for portions of this chapter.

REFERENCES

Allison, A. C., and Clark, I. A.: Specific and nonspecific immunity to haemoprotozoa. Am. J. Trop. Med. Hyg. 26:216, 1977.

Askenase, P. W.: Effector Cells in Late and Delayed Hypersensitivity Reactions That Are Dependent on Antibodies or T cells. *In* Fougereau, M., and Dausset, J. (eds.): Progress in Immunology IV. Immunology 1980. Academic Press, London, 1980, p. 829.

Askenase, P. W.: Basophil arrival and function in tissue hypersensitivity reactions. J. Allergy Clin. Immunol. 64:79, 1979.

Askenase, P. W.: Role of basophils, mast cells and

vasoamines in hypersensitivity reactions with a delayed time course. Prog. Allergy 23:199, 1977.

Askenase, P. W., Schwartz, A., Siegel, J. N., and Gershon, R. K.: Role of histamine in the regulation of cell–mediated immunity. Int. Arch. Allergy Appl. Immun. 66(suppl. 1):225, 1981.

Attalha, A. M., Smith, A. H., Murrell, K. D., Fleischer, T., Woody, J., Vannier, W. E., Scher, I., Ahmed, A., and Sell, K. W.: Characterization of the immunosuppressive state during Schistosoma mansoni infection. J. Immunol. 122:1413, 1979.

Beaman, L., Pappagianis, D., and Benjamini, E.: Significance of T cells in resistance to experimental murine coccidioidomycosis. Infect. Immun. 17:580, 1977.

Benacerraf, B., and McDevitt, H. O.: Histocompatibility-linked immune response genes. Science 175: 273, 1972.

Benacerraf, B., and Unanue, E. R.: Textbook of Immunology. Williams and Wilkins Co., Baltimore, 1979.

Billingham, R. E., Brent, L., and Medawar, P. B.: Quantitative studies on tissue transplantation immunity. III. Actively acquired tolerance. Philos. Trans. R. Soc. Lond. (Biol.) 239:257, 1956.

Binz, H., Frischknecht, H., Shen, F. W., and Wigzell, H.: Idiotypic determinants on T-cell subpopulations. J. Exp. Med. 149:910, 1979.

Blaese, R. M., Weiden, P. L., Koski, I., and Dooley, J.: Infectious agammaglobulinemia: transmission of immunodeficiency with grafts of agammaglobulinemic cells. J. Exp. Med. 140:1097, 1974.

Bloom, B. R.: Games parasites play: How parasites evade immune surveillance. Nature 279:21, 1979.

Boyse, E. A., Old, L. J., and Stockert, E.: The TL (thymus leukemia) antigen: A review. In P. Grabar and P. A. Miescher (eds.): IV International Symposium on Immunopathology. Schwabe and Co., Basel, 1965.

Burnet, F. M.: The Clonal Selection Theory of Acquired Immunity. Cambridge University Press, Cambridge, 1959.

Campbell, P. A.: Immunocompetent cells in resistance to bacterial infection. Bact. Rev. 40:284, 1976.

Cantor, H., and Boyse, E. A.: Functional subclasses of T lymphocytes bearing different Ly antigens. II Cooperation between subclasses of Ly+ cells in the generation of killer activity. J. Exp. Med. 141:1390, 1975.

Cantor, H., McVay-Boudreau, L., Hugenberger, J., Naidorf, K., Shen, F. W., and Gershon, R. K.: Immunoregulatory circuits among T-cell sets. II. Physiological role in vivo: absence in NZB mice. J. Exp. Med. 147:1116, 1978.

Capra, J. D., and Kehoe, J. M.: Hypervariable regions, idiotypy, and the antibody-combining site. Adv. Immunol. 20:1, 1975.

Chiller, J. M., and Weigle, W. O.: Cellular interactions during induction of immunological unresponsiveness in adult mice. J. Immunol. 106:1647, 1971.

Claman, H. N., Chaperon, E. A., and Triplett, R. F.: Thymus-marrow cell combinations. Synergism in antibody production. Proc. Soc. Exp. Biol. Med. 122:1167, 1966.

Cockerell, G. L.: Naturally acquired immunodeficiency diseases of the dog and cat. Vet. Clin. North Am. 8:613, 1978.

Cross, G. A. M.: Antigenic variation in trypanosomes. Am. J. Trop. Med. Hyg. 26:240, 1977.

Davies, A. J. S.: The failure of thymus derived cells to produce antibody. Transplantation 5:222, 1964.

Dixon, F. J.: The role of antigen-antibody complexes in disease. Harvey Lect. 58:21, 1963.

Doherty, P. C., and Zinkernagel, R. M.: T cell-mediated immunopathology in viral infection. Transplant. Rev. 19:89, 1974.

Eisen, H. N., and Siskind, G. W.: Variations in affinities of antibodies during the immune response. Biochemistry 3:996, 1964.

Gell, P. G. H., Coombs, R. A., and Lachmann, P. (eds.): Clinical Aspects of Immunology. Section IV, 3rd ed. Blackwell Scientific Publications, Oxford, 1974.

Gershon, R. K.: Suppressor T cells: A miniposition paper celebrating a new decade. In Fougereau, M., and Dausset, J. (eds.): Progress in Immunology IV, Immunology 1980. Academic Press, London, 1980, p. 375.

Gershon, R. K.: A disquisition on suppressor T cells. Transplant Rev. 26:170, 1975.

Gershon, R. K., and Kondo, K.: Infectious immunological tolerance, Immunology 21:903, 1971.

Gershon, R. K., and Paul, W. E.: Effect of thymus derived lymphocytes on the amount and affinity of anti-hapten antibody. J. Immunol. 106:872, 1971.

Gershon, R. K., Askenase, P. W., and Gershon, M. D.: Requirement for vasoactive amines for production of delayed type hypersensitivity skin reactions. J. Exp. Med. 143:732, 1975.

Gershon, R. K., Eardley, D. D., Durum, S. K., Green, D. R., Shen, F. W., Yamauchi, K., Cantor, H., and Murphy, D. B.: Contrasuppression: A novel immunoregulatory activity. J. Exp. Med. 153:1533, 1981.

Gheri, I., Gershon, R. K., and Waksman, B. H.: Potentiation of the T-lymphocyte responses to mitogens. I. The responding cells. J. Exp. Med. 136:128, 1972.

Göetze, D. (ed.): The Major Histocompatibility System in Man and Animals. Springer-Verlag, New York, 1977.

Goetzl, E. J., and Austen, K. F.: Cellular characteristics of the eosinophil compatible with a dual role in parasite infections. Am. J. Trop. Med. Hyg. 26:142, 1977.

Good, R. A., and Gabrielson, A. E. (eds.): The Thymus in Immunobiology. Harper and Row, New York, 1964.

Huber, B., Devinsky, O., Gershon, R. K., and Cantor, H.: Cell-mediated immunity. Delayed type hypersensitivity and cytotoxic responses are mediated by different T-cell subclasses. J. Exp. Med. 143:1534, 1976.

Hurvitz, A. I., Kehoe, J. M., and Capra, J. D.: Bence Jones proteinuria associated with canine plasma cell malignancy. J.A.V.M.A. 159:1112, 1972.

Hurvitz, A. I., Kehoe, J. M., and Capra, J. D.: Characterization of three homogeneous canine immunoglobulins. J. Immunol. 107:648, 1971.

Imai, Y., Nakano, T., Sawada, J. I., and Oswawa, T.: Specificity of natural thymocytotoxic autoantibody developed in New Zealand black mice. J. Immunol. 124:1556, 1980.

Inbar, D., Hochman, J., and Givol, D.: Location of antibody combining sites within the variable portions of heavy and light chains. Proc. Nat. Acad. Sci. USA 69:2659, 1972.

Jannosy, G., and Greaves, M. F.: Lymphocyte activation. I. Response of T and B lymphocytes to phytomitogens. Clin. Exp. Immunol. 9:483, 1972.

Jayawardena, A. N., Waksman, B. H., and Eardley, D. D.: Activation of distinct helper and suppressor T cells in experimental trypanosomiasis. J. Immunol. 121:622, 1978.

Jerne, N. K.: The somatic generation of immune recognition. Eur. J. Immunol. *1*:1, 1971.

Kehoe, J. M.: The Structural Basis for the Biological Properties of Immunoglobulins. *In* Good, R. A., and Day, S. B. (eds.): Comprehensive Immunology, Vol. 5, Immunoglobulins. Plenum Press, New York, 1978.

Kehoe, J. M., Bourgois, A., Capra, J. D., and Fougereau, M.: Amino acid sequence of a murine immunoglobulin fragment that possesses complement fixing activity. Biochemistry *13*:2499, 1974.

Kehoe, J. M., Hurvitz, A. I., and Capra, J. D.: Characterization of three feline paraproteins. J. Immunol. *109*:511, 1972a.

Kehoe, J. M., Tomasi, T. B., Ellouz, F., and Capra, J. D.: Identification of "J" chain in a homogeneous canine IgA immunoglobulin. J. Immunol. *109*:59, 1972b.

Kelsoe, G., and Cerny, J.: Reciprocal expansions of idiotypic and anti-idiotypic clones following antigen stimulation. Nature *279*:333, 1979.

Klein, J.: Biology of the Mouse Histocompatibility Complex. Springer-Verlag, New York, 1975.

Lubaroff, D. M., and Waksman, B. H.: Bone marrow as a source of cells in cellular hypersensitivity. I. Passive transfer of tuberculin sensitivity in syngeneic systems. J. Exp. Med. *128*:1425, 1968.

Lynch, R. G., Rohrer, J. W., Odermatt, B., Gebel, H. D., Autry, J. R., and Hoover, R. G.: Immunoregulation of murine myeloma cell growth and differentiation: A monoclonal model of B-cell differentiation. Immunol. Rev. *48*:45, 1979.

Mackaness, G. B.: The Mechanisms of Macrophage Activation. *In* Mudd, S. (ed.): Infectious Agents and Host Reactions. W. B. Saunders Co., Philadelphia, 1970.

Manny, N., Datta, S. K., and Schwartz, R. S.: Synthesis of IgM by B cells of NZB and SWR mice and their crosses. J. Immunol. *122*:1220, 1979.

Marchalonis, J. J., and Moseley, J. M.: The Immunoglobulin-like T-cell Receptor Problem. *In* W. Müeller-Ruchholtz, W., and Muller-Hermelink, H. K. (eds.): Function and Structure of the Immune System. Plenum Press, New York, 1979.

Marchesi, V. T., and Gowans, J. L.: The migration of lymphocytes through the endothelium of venules in lymph nodes. Proc. R. Soc. Lond. (Biol.) *157*:283, 1964.

McCluskey, R. T., Benacerraf, B., and McCluskey, J. W.: Studies on the specificity of the cellular infiltrate in delayed hypersensitivity reactions. J. Immunol. *58*:466, 1976.

McGuire, T. C., Banks, K. L., and Davis, W. C.: Alterations of the thymus and other lymphoid tissues in young horses with combined immunodeficiency. Am. J. Pathol. *84*:39, 1976a.

McGuire, T. C., Polara, B., Moore, J. J., and Poppie, M. J.: Evaluation of adenosine deaminase and other purine salvage pathway enzymes in horses with combined immunodeficiency. Infect. Immun. *13*:995, 1976b.

McLeod, K., and Remington, J. S.: Influence of infection with *Toxoplasma* on macrophage function and the role of macrophages in resistance to *Toxoplasma*. Am. J. Trop. Med. Hyg. *26*:170, 1977.

Miller, J. F. A. P., and Mitchell, G. F.: Immunological activity of thymus and thoracic duct lymphocytes. Proc. Nat. Acad. Sci. U.S.A. *59*:296, 1968.

Mitchison, N. A.: Induction of immunological paralysis in two zones of dosage. Proc. Roy. Soc. Lond. (Biol.) Ser. B. *161*:275, 1965.

Möller, G. (ed.): Unresponsiveness to haptenated self molecules. Immunol. Rev. *50*, 1980.

Möller, G. (ed.): Mechanism of B cell tolerance. Immunol. Rev. *43*, 1979a.

Möller, G. (ed.): Transplantation tolerance. Immunol. Rev. *46*, 1979b.

Möller, G. (ed.): Ir genes and T lymphocytes. Immunol. Rev. *38*, 1978.

Mosier, D. E.: A requirement for two cell types for antibody formation *in vitro*. Science *158*:1573, 1967.

Nossal, G. J. V., Pike, B. L., Stocker, J. W., Layton, J. E., and Goding, J. W.: Cold Springs Harbor Symp. Quant. Biol. *41*:237, 1976.

Oldstone, M. B. A., and Dixon, F. J.: Immune complex disease in chronic viral infections. J. Exp. Med. *134*:325, 1971.

Olsen, R. G., and Krakowka, S. Immunology and Immunopathology of Domestic Animals. Charles C Thomas, Springfield, Ill., 1979.

Piessens, W. F., Ratiwayanto, S., Tuti, S., Palmieri, J. H., Piessens, P. W., Koiman, I., and Dennis, D. T.: Antigen specific suppressor factors in human filariasis with *Bragia malayi*. N. Engl. J. Med. *302*:833, 1980.

Plaut, M., Lichtenstein, L. M., and Henney, C. S.: Properties of a subpopulation of T cells bearing histamine receptors. J. Clin. Invest. *55*:856, 1975.

Quimby, F. W., Jensen, C., Nawrocki, D., and Scollin, P.: Selected autoimmune diseases in the dog. Vet. Clin. North Am. *8*:665, 1978.

Quimby, F. W., Lewis, R. M., and Datta, S.: Characterization of a retrovirus that cross reacts serologically with canine and human systemic lupus erythematosus. Clin. Exp. Immunopathol. *9*:194, 1977.

Quimby, F. W., Mudd, D., and Kaplan, A.: Partial characterization of lymphocytotoxic antibodies in dogs with autoimmune disease. Vet. Immunol. Immunopathol. Submitted for publication, 1982.

Reif, A. E., and Allen, J. M. V.: The AKR thymus antigen and its distribution in leukemias and nervous tissues. J. Exp. Med. *120*:413, 1964.

Richerson, H. B., Dvorak, H. F., and Leskowitz, S.: Cutaneous basophil hypersensitivity. A new look at the Jones Mote reaction. J. Exp. Med. *132*:546, 1970.

Rocklin, R. E., Greineder, D., Littman, B. N., and Melman, K. L.: Modulation of cellular immune function *in vitro* by histamine receptor bearing lymphocytes: mechanism of action. Cell. Immunol. *37*:162, 1978.

Rosen, F. S.: Immunodeficiency Diseases. *In* Benacerraf, B., and Unanue, E. R.: Textbook of Immunology. Williams and Wilkins Co., Baltimore, 1979.

Schultz, R. D. (ed.) Practical immunology. Vet. Clin. North Am. *8*:834, 1978.

Schwartz, A.: Transplantation immunology. Vet. Clin. North Am. *4*:187, 1974.

Schwartz, A., Askenase, P. W., and Gershon, R. K.: Histamine inhibition of the *in vitro* induction of cytotoxic T cell responses. Immunopharmacology *2*:179, 1980.

Schwartz, A., Askenase, P. W., and Gershon, R. K.: The effect of locally injected vasoactive amines on the elicitation of delayed type hypersensitivity. J. Immunol. *118*:159, 1977.

Schwartz, A., Askenase, P. W., and Gershon, R. K.:

Histamine inhibition of Concanavalin A-induced suppressor T cell activation. Cell Immunol., *60*:426, 1981.

Schwartz, R. S.: Viruses and systemic lupus erythematosus. N. Engl. J. Med. *293*:132, 1975.

Smithers, S. R., McLaren, D. J., and Ramalho-Pinto, F. J.: Immunity to schistosomes: the target. Am. J. Trop. Med. Hyg. *26*:11, 1977.

Stadecker, M. J., and Leskowitz, S.: The cutaneous basophil response to particulate antigens. Proc. Soc. Exp. Biol. Med. *142*:150, 1973.

Steinman, R. M., and Witmer, M. D.: Lymphoid dendritic cells are potent stimulators of the primary mixed leukocyte reaction in mice. Proc. Nat. Acad. Sci. U.S.A. *75*:5132, 1978.

Strelkauskas, A. J., Schauf, V., Wilson, B. S., Chess, L., and Schlossman, S. F.: Isolation and characterization of naturally occurring subclasses of human peripheral blood T cells with regulatory functions. J. Immunol. *120*:1278, 1978.

Uhr, J. W., and Möller, G.: Regulatory effect of antibody on the immune response. Adv. Immunol. *8*:81, 1968.

Wagner, H., Rollinghoff, M., Pfizenmiaier, K., Hardt, C., and Jonscher, G.: T-T interactions during *in vitro* cytotoxic T lymphocyte (CTL) responses. J. Immunol. *124*:1058, 1980.

Waksman, B. H.: Atlas of Experimental Immunology and Immunopathology. Yale University Press, New Haven, 1970.

Waldmann, T. A., Blaeze, R. M., Broder, S., and Krakauer, R. S.: Disorders of suppressor immunoregulatory cells in the pathogenesis of immunodeficiency and autoimmunity. Ann. Intern. Med. *88*:226, 1978.

Watson, J., Trenkner, E., and Cohn, M.: The use of bacterial lipopolysaccharides to show that two signals are required for the induction of antibody synthesis. J. Exp. Med. *138*:699, 1973.

Weller, P. F., and Goetzl, E. J.: The regulatory and effector roles of eosinophils. Adv. Immunol. *27*:339, 1979.

Wu, A. M., Till, J. E., Siminovitch, L., and McCulloch, E. A.: Cytological evidence for a relationship between normal colony-forming cells and cells of the lymphoid system. J. Exp. Med. *127*:455, 1968.

Zinkernagel, R. M., and Doherty, P. C.: MHC-restricted cytotoxic T cells: studies on the biological role of polymorphic major transplantation antigens determining T-cell restriction, specificity, function and responsiveness. Adv. Immunol. *27*:51, 1979.

ABBREVIATION KEY

ADCC   Antibody-dependent cell-mediated cytotoxicity

AFP   Alpha-fetoprotein

B cell   Bursal derived lymphocytes

CBH   Cutaneous basophil hypersensitivity

CEA   Carcinoembryonic antigen

CMI   Cell-mediated immunity

CML   Cell-mediated lympholysis-killing by CTL

Con A   Concanavalin A

CTL   Cytotoxic T lymphocyte

DNP   Dinitrophenol

DTH   Delayed-type hypersensitivity

Fab fragment   Antigen binding portion of Ig molecule

Fc fragment   Biological activity (effector function) containing portion of Ig molecule

GBM   Glomerular basement membrane

GVH   Graft versus host

Ia antigen   I region associated antigen

Ig   Immunoglobulin

I region   Genetic region of MHC containing Ir genes and coding for Ia antigens

Ir gene   Immune response gene

K cell   Killer cell of uncertain lineage

LCM   Lymphocytic choriomeningitis

LD   Lymphocyte-defined MHC antigens (Ia in mouse)

LPS   Lipopolysaccharide

Lyt antigens   T lymphocyte differentiation antigens of mice

MHC   Major histocompatibility complex

MIF   Macrophage inhibitory factor

MLR   Allogeneic mixed leukocyte response

NK cells   Natural killer cells

PHA   Phytohemagglutinin

SCID   Severe combined immunodeficiency disease

SD   Serologically defined MHC antigens (K/D in mouse)

SLE   Systemic lupus erythematosus

T cell   Thymus-derived lymphocyte

Tdt   Terminal deoxynucleotidyl transferase

TL antigen   Thymus leukemia antigen of mice

TSTA   Tumor-specific transplantation antigen

CHAPTER 82

Immune-Mediated Diseases of Skin and Mucous Membranes

JAMES D. CONROY

INTRODUCTION

Hypersensitivity has become increasingly important as the essential feature or as a participant in a wide variety of skin and mucous membrane diseases. Historically, the literature contains relatively few references to allergy in the dog and the cat during the first quarter of this century. Some of the earliest incriminations of hypersensitivity as a pathologic mechanism in skin diseases of the dog were made in reference to so-called "grass allergies." At the time, little was known regarding the exact etiology or the pathogenic mechanisms involved. During the second quarter of this century, it was recognized that the dog did indeed develop hypersensitivity to a wide variety of pollens, as well as certain parasitic infestations (flea allergy dermatitis). However, it has only been during the last decade that the true importance of immunologic mechanisms has been recognized for the significant role they play in the pathogenesis of many dermatopathies.

The recognition of many canine and feline diseases that mimic several human disease complexes has created increased interest in the diagnosis and management of animal cutaneous diseases. Widespread use of the skin biopsy combined with more adequate evaluation of histologic lesions, intracutaneous allergy testing, and direct immunofluorescence testing of skin samples have provided an extremely important adjunct in reaching more accurate, meaningful diagnoses.

ALLERGIES TO FOOD (FOOD ALLERGY)

This is an acute or chronic, nonseasonal, cutaneous and/or gastrointestinal disease occurring in pets of all ages. Although the pathogenesis of the signs/lesions is incompletely understood, reagenic antibody (IgE) and secretory intestinal antibody (IgA) are apparently involved in forming complexes with food antigens, which combine with mast cells that release mediators of inflammation. There is no breed, age, or sex predilection (Scott, 1978). Various opinions are held regarding the prevalence of food allergy among dogs and cats. It was estimated by Walton in 1968 that food allergies account for about one per cent of all skin cases. Schreck (1920) provided one of the earliest reports of food allergy in two puppies that developed urticaria and vomiting following ingestion of milk oyster stew (cited by Baker, 1979). Phillips, as early as 1922, provided conclusive evidence that ingested allergens could induce hypersensitivity responses in the dog.

Clinical Signs. Dermal manifestations are usually generalized and include pruritus alone or in conjunction with cutaneous erythema, scaliness, excoriations, hair loss, ulcerations, and urticaria and angioedema. The skin lesions of food allergy in the cat are manifested principally as either a "miliary, eczematous form" with small crusted lesions, or an ulcerative form resembling eosinophilic granuloma complex (Baker, 1975). Ulceration is reported to be the most frequent dermal manifestation of food sensitivity in the cat and must be differentiated from other feline ulcerative dermatoses (Baker, 1975). Gastrointestinal signs of food allergy, mainly watery diarrhea with occasional vomiting, may be preeminent. The manifestations are associated with lesions ranging from mild enteritis to hemorrhagic colitis. Both enteric and dermal signs may be seen concurrently, but usually either the skin or the intestinal tract is involved (Baker, 1974). Other organ systems rarely may be affected in food allergies. Baker (1980) states that most canine and feline food allergies are associated with the feeding of prepared dog and cat foods, biscuits, and rawhide, but virtually any food can produce sensitivity reactions in dogs and cats. Other foodstuffs that have been incriminated in food allergies include milk, wheat, beef, eggs, horse meat, chicken, corn meal, potatoes, salmon, pork, and even rice. Food allergies have been observed in most breeds of dogs and cats; according to Baker (1980), however, the problem appears to be encountered more frequently among German shepherd dogs than other breeds.

Pathology. The histopathologic findings may include mild to moderate acanthosis associated with superficial perivascular infiltrations of mast cells admixed with varying numbers of eosinophils, and scattered plasma cells with or without perivascular edema.

Diagnosis. The differential diagnosis (rule-outs) are chiefly allergic inhalant dermatitis, parasitic dermatitis, flea allergy dermatitis, and seborrheic dermatitis.

The diagnostic plan includes intracutaneous skin testing, skin scrapings for mite infestation, close examination of the skin for fleas or flea excrement, hemogram (eosinophilia of ten per cent or greater is suggestive of hypersensitivity), and blood chemistry profile, including gonad and thyroid endocrine tests to rule out hormone-associated seborrhea.

Diagnosis is based on a good history, the nonseasonal nature of the problem, associated dermal and gastrointestinal signs, and evaluation of the elimination diet. The use of intradermal skin testing in food allergies of the dog and cat is a controversial subject. Baker (1980) has concluded that skin tests are of limited diagnostic value, expensive, and generally not indicated in the diagnosis of food allergy. The use of an elimination diet and/or provocative exposure to suspected foods is a helpful procedure for "confirmation" of food allergies. Baker (1974; 1980) considers the total food elimination diet, or as he names it, "a short-term starvation diet," the most important diagnostic procedure for food allergy in dogs and cats. In this procedure, following a thorough and complete physical examination, a saline cathartic is administered, all

food is withheld for 72 hours, and the patient is placed on bottled spring water only. If improvement occurs before 72 hours, the elimination diet can be stopped and a trial diet begun. Then foods are fed one at a time for a period of five days until a balanced, tolerated, nutritious diet is devised. Baker points out the importance of feeding only fresh foods, free of artificial flavors, colors, or preservatives. Cottage cheese is an excellent choice to start with, since it is nutritious, easily absorbed, and is rarely associated with allergic problems. The objectives of provocative exposure are not only to identify the food products to which the animal is allergic, but also, and of equal importance, to find enough foods to use to formulate a long-term maintenance diet (Knowles, 1966).

Treatment. Therapy includes avoidance of the offending foods and, in some cases, institution of a hypoallergenic diet (mutton and rice). Acute food allergy (angioedema) is responsive to parenteral administration of corticosteroids or antihistamines. Steroids should not be used on a continuous basis for food allergies.

ALLERGY TO INHALED ANTIGENS (ATOPY, ATOPIC DERMATITIS, ALLERGIC INHALANT DERMATITIS)

Atopy or allergic inhalant dermatitis (AID) is a common chronic progressive cutaneous disease with hereditary tendencies associated with inhaled allergens and mediated by skin sensitizing IgE (reaginic) antibody. In the dog, the sensitizing agent may be inhaled or ingested, or it may penetrate the intact skin (Anderson, 1975). Since the most common route of entry is the respiratory tract, Anderson (1975) has named the canine condition allergic inhalant dermatitis. The most common offending antigens in dogs are pollens, molds, and house dust. About ten per cent of all dogs are estimated to be atopic. All breeds may be affected, including mongrels, but it is more common in Dalmations and terrier breeds (Cairn, West Highland, Scottish, and wirehaired fox terriers). Generally there has been no sex predilection reported; however, Halliwell and Schwartzman (1971), and more recently Scott (1981), observed an increased incidence of atopy in females when compared with the general hospital population.

The disorder is rarely seen in dogs less than one year of age. Although the initial signs may be observed at any age, they are most often seen between one and three years of age. Initially, most dogs exhibit *seasonal* manifestations (occasionally nonseasonal from the onset), while chronic patients may show signs throughout the year. Sensitivities, once developed, frequently persist for years or even life.

Clinical Signs. The clinical manifestations relate primarily to pruritus, but also include scaling (secondary seborrhea), face rubbing, foot licking, excoriations, otitis, and occasionally urticaria and hyperhidrosis (excessive sweating). Schwartzman (1968) reported that about ten per cent of canine atopics have a generalized hyperhidrosis that does not appear to be allergic in origin. Curiously, dry skin (xerosis) is reported (Anderson, 1975) to be a common finding in the atopic dog. Lichenified erythematous plaques with or without hyperpigmentation affecting the periocular, axillary, or inguinal skin are often seen in chronic, untreated canines (Conroy, 1979). Anderson (1975) has stated that, "If the allergic dog was prevented from scratching itself, there would be no visible lesions." Inhaled allergens in the dog have been associated with generalized papular reactions (Wittich, 1941) and evidence of generalized skin irritation (Schwartzman, 1967). Nonintegumentary signs such as conjunctivitis, rhinitis, and sneezing also may be present but are uncommon.

Pathology. The pathological findings may be nonspecific — i.e., superficial, subacute, nonsuppurative perivascular dermatitis — or they may be strongly supportive of the allergic disease; that is, they may be characteristic of a superficial, allergic perivascular dermatitis (Type I hypersensitivity) with superficial edema, increased vascularity, and congestion associated with perivascular accumulations of mast cells, eosinophils with or without scattered neutrophils, and plasma cells (Conroy, 1979). The deeper dermis and subcutis are invariably normal. The epidermal changes, although marked in some biopsy specimens, are of little diagnostic value except for the entrapment of clusters of eosinophils within the epidermis (eosinophilic spongiosis), which unfortunately occurs only infrequently. Recently Scott (1981) reported on the histopathologic findings from biopsies of 100 dogs tentatively diagnosed as having atopy, concluding that the presence of a chronic nonsuppurative dermatitis was consistent and supportive of canine atopy but not diagnostic. Surprisingly, eosinophils were seen in only 15 per cent of the cases and increased numbers of mast cells in 35 per cent of the cases (Figs. 82–1 and 82–2).

Diagnosis. The principal rule-outs would include food allergies, flea allergy, scabies, seborrheic dermatitis, and pelodera dermatitis (parasitic dermatitis caused by a free living nematode). Although the characteristic history and clinical signs alone are frequently diagnostic, a diagnostic plan includes intradermal skin testing, skin biopsies, hemogram (usually unremarkable in

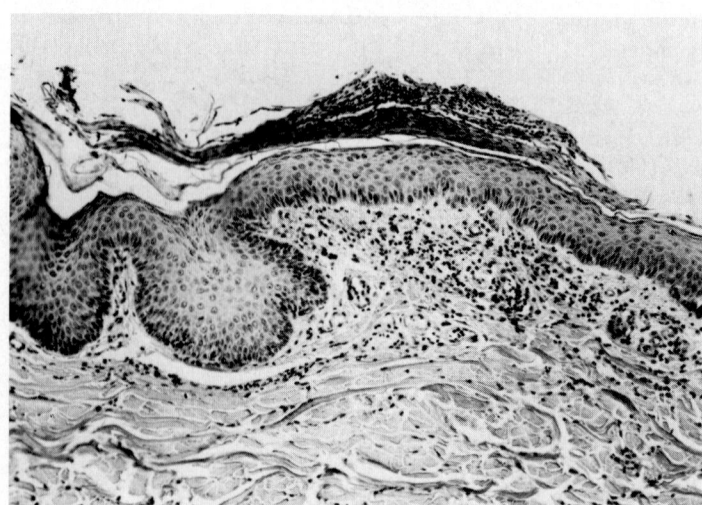

Figure 82–1. Canine atopy. Parakeratotic scale-crust with entrapped leukocytes associated with moderate acanthosis and a patchy superficial perivascular infiltrate.

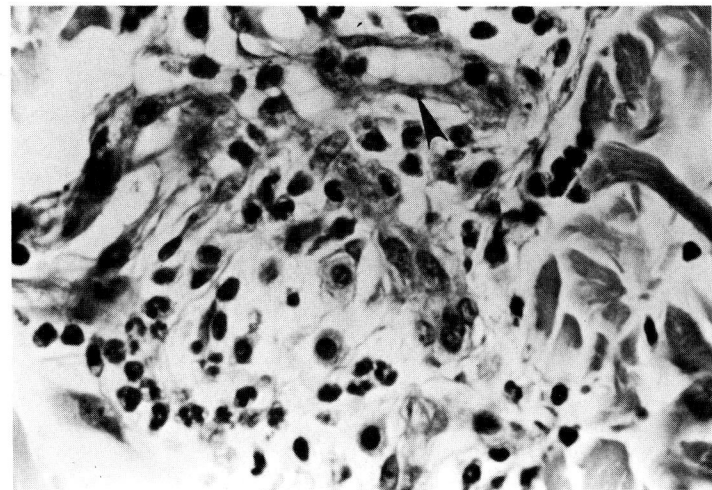

Figure 82–2. Canine atopy. Perivascular infiltration of mast cells, eosinophils, and scattered neutrophils. Vessel seen at arrow.

AID), radioallergosorbent test (RAST), skin scrapings, examination for fleas, and restrictive dieting to exclude food allergy. It is important to be aware that the atopic patient frequently has intercurrent diseases such as superficial pyoderma, hypothyroidism, and secondary seborrhea.

Treatment. Management of the patient naturally requires removal or avoidance of offending allergens whenever possible. Therapy includes the implementation of hyposensitization, if feasible, since this procedure may eliminate the need for prolonged corticosteroid therapy. Intradermal skin testing is not only essential for diagnosis of atopy but is also necessary for identifying specific allergens prior to initiating hyposensitization (Chamberlain, 1977; Chamberlain and Baker, 1974; Halliwell, 1977). It is important to realize that a positive ID skin test is only an indication that the animal has skin sensitizing (IgE) antibodies to the test allergens. It does not necessarily mean that the skin disease is allergic inhalant dermatitis. Indeed, the evaluation of skin testing must be considered in light of the history and clinical signs (Halliwell and Schwartzman, 1971). Although steroid therapy is extremely effective, it sometimes leads to undesirable effects on the canine patient, especially iatrogenic hypercorticism. Steroids, when used, should be given orally on an alternate-day schedule. This regimen minimizes the risk of iatrogenic Cushing's syndrome. Antihistamines are occasionally effective in controlling manifestations of the disease in some dogs, especially

a single dose rather than continuous use (Anderson, 1975). Hyposensitization has been estimated to be 60 to 75 per cent effective in the dog. A third of the dogs hyposensitized will be significantly improved, a third will be moderately benefited, and a third will demonstrate no improvement. Theoretically, hyposensitization results in the formation of circulating IgG blocking antibodies, and hyposensitization may also depress the production of IgE antibodies. Scott (1978) listed the three main hyposensitization techniques used in veterinary medicine as follows: (1) aqueous technique (weekly or biweekly injections, six months to three years for maximum response), (2) pyridine extracts of alum precipitates (eight to twelve injections, three to six months for maximum response), and (3) propylene glycol or glycerin emulsions (four to eight injections, two to four months for maximum response). He indicated that 50 per cent of clinically atopic dogs were controlled by hyposensitization alone.

ALLERGY TO ENDOPARASITES (NEMATODES)

Hypersensitivity to endoparasites (gastrointestinal nematodes) appears to be uncommon in the dog and cat as judged by the infrequency of reports in the literature (Chamberlain, 1974; Scott, 1976, 1978). The pathogenesis involves a Type I hypersensitivity and associated skin-sensitizing (IgE) antibodies.

Clinical Signs. Clinical signs include in-

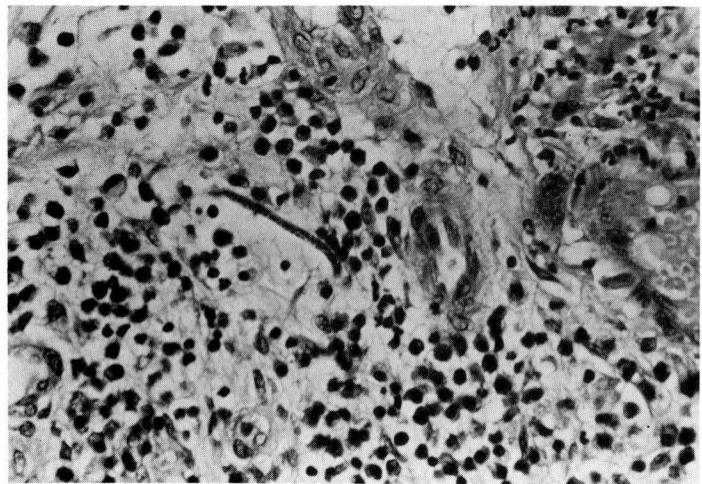

Figure 82–3. Suspected dirofilarial hypersensitivity dermatitis. Extravascular microfilaria associated with a chronic active inflammatory response with abundant plasma cells in the dermis.

tense pruritus without eruptive lesions or a generalized pruritic papulocrustous dermatitis (Scott, 1978).

Diagnosis. Diagnosis is based on history, physical examination, fecal examination, and response to therapy, which includes eliminating the offending nematodes and symptomatic dermatologic treatment. Scott (1979) reported the occurrence of three dogs with dirofilariasis that had dermal disease characterized by pruritus and multifocal nodules that tended to ulcerate. Histologically, the lesions were characterized by angiocentric pyogranulomatous infiltrates with variable numbers of eosinophils. Microfilaria were often seen within vessels at sites of inflammation. The author's limited experience with this uncommon dermal lesion reveals a superficial and deep perivascular dermatitis associated with neovascularity, microhemorrhage with abundant plasma cells, and moderate numbers of neutrophils and eosinophils. Microfilaria were observed within vessels and occasionally extravascularly (Fig. 82–3).

The rule-outs include arthropod injury, acute moist dermatitis, and bacterial and fungal infections. The diagnostic plan includes skin biopsy, examination of blood for microfilaria, and response to antifilarial therapy.

STAPHYLOCOCCAL HYPERSENSITIVITY (BACTERIAL ALLERGY)

Staphylococcal hypersensitivity (SH) appears to be a relatively common canine entity (Baker, 1974; Breen, 1976); it met with initial skepticism but has gained some measure of credibility. Results of skin testing and skin biopsy suggest that staphylococcal hypersensitivity may be a Type III (Arthus) reaction (Scott et al., 1978). Age, breed, and sex predilections have not been recognized. Important historical information in SH dogs includes current or previous pyogenic infections, poor or inconsistent response to steroids, and good to excellent response to appropriate antibiotics.

Clinical Signs. Pruritus is the dominant clinical sign associated with three significant lesion types: (1) erythematous papules, (2) hemorrhagic bulla, and (3) seborrheic plaques (Scott, 1978). Clinical diseases commonly closely associated with staph hypersensitivity include folliculitis, impetigo, seborrheic dermatitis, and interdigital and/or generalized deep pyoderma (furunculosis) (Scott et al., 1978).

Pathology. Histologic lesions will vary with the nature of the clinical lesion but are usually characterized by varying degrees of vascular changes (dilatation, engorgement, endothelial swelling, vasculitis, and hemorrhage) associated with a marked infiltration of neutrophils (Scott, 1978).

Diagnosis. The rule-outs include pyodermas (without hypersensitivity), seborrheic dermatitis, erythema multiforme, toxic epidermal necrolysis of nonallergic nature, arthropod infestations, and other hypersensitivities.

The diagnostic plan should include bacterial culture, skin biopsy, intradermal tests, and response to therapy (antibiotics and/or hyposensitization). However, Halliwell (1981) considers positive skin reactions essentially meaningless, and if the lesion is truly an Arthus reaction as stated, he seriously doubts any benefit could be expected from hyposensitization. Intradermal skin testing for SH is done with a commercial cell wall antigen and toxoid preparation (Baker, 1974). This preparation is diluted with an equal volume of sterile saline, and 0.1 ml of the material is injected intradermally. The results require careful and thoughtful interpretation as specified by Scott (1978). Within twenty minutes, all dogs tested (normal or otherwise) develop an immediate reaction that persists for up to 12 to 18 hours. Normal dogs and those with non-SH skin diseases develop a delayed reaction in 24 to 72 hours; this is an indurated and occasionally erythematous five- to nine-mm lesion. Dogs with SH develop delayed reactions in 24 to 72 hours, characterized by marked erythema, induration, oozing and often purplish discoloration, necrosis, and slough from 9 to 75 mm in diameter. Unfortunately, others have not been able to reproduce these results.

Treatment. Therapy consists of correction of the underlying disease, systemic antibiotics for three to six weeks, and hyposensitization (Baker, 1974; Scott et al., 1978). Many uncertainties exist regarding nature, diagnosis, and treatment of this controversial "entity."

ALLERGIES TO DRUGS AND VACCINES (DRUG ALLERGY, DRUG REACTION, DRUG ERUPTION)

This enigmatic nosologic category remains to be fully characterized in the dog and the cat. Drug allergy and drug reactions are well documented and commonly recognized in the human patient. Indeed, drug reactions frequently are at the very top of the list of rule-outs in the human patient when the physician is confronted with an unexplained cutaneous or mucocutaneous disorder. Immunologic responses associated with drug allergy include Types I, II, III, and IV. Most so-called allergic drug reactions are classified as such mainly on a clinical assessment alone (Scott, 1978). Other than vaccination reactions, penicillin leads the list of those drugs causing undesir-

able reactions in the dog and the cat. There are sporadic reports of other, less common drugs causing cutaneous lesions.

Clinical Signs. In dogs, Scott (1978) has reported eczematous lesions associated with oral triple sulfa, griseofulvin, diethylcarbamazine, 5-fluorocytosine, and sulfisoxazole; exfoliative lesions with quinidine; vesicobullous lesions with diphenylhydantoin; purpuric lesions with chloramphenicol; urticaria-angioedema with tetracycline; pemphigus vulgaris-like lesions with thiabendazole, and a fixed drug eruption with ampicillin. In cats, he has reported eczematous lesions with oral sulfisoxazole, multifocal alopecia with oral hetacillin, and toxic epidermal necrolysis following subcutaneous administration of FeLV antiserum. Calderwood (1980) has observed toxic epidermal necrolysis in a cat with ampicillin.

The clinical manifestations of drug reactions display a wide range of nonspecific morphologic patterns that may mimic diseases with non-drug related etiologies. A drug reaction also may be one of the causes for relatively specific cutaneous lesions that may be produced by widely differing etiologies. Examples of such conditions should be erythema multiforme or toxic epidermal necrolysis, which have specific clinical and morphologic features but have multiple etiologies.

The preceding clinical manifestations display a wide range of morphologic patterns, which include papules; pustules; and bullous, hemorrhagic, erosive and ulcerative, scaly, crusted, or infiltrative lesions.

Diagnosis. It should be apparent that because of the polymorphous nature of drug reactions this disease category could be considered as a rule-out in a majority of cutaneous and mucocutaneous diseases. It is therefore imperative, especially in those cases of a bizarre or refractory nature, that a meticulous history be obtained from the animal owner in regard to any drug, common or uncommon, to which the animal may have been intentionally or accidentally exposed in the several weeks preceding the appearance of the skin lesions. Furthermore, it is frequently impossible to distinguish those drug reactions that are produced by toxicity from those drug reactions that are primarily immunologically mediated.

Treatment. In any case, the therapy and

management of the patient will vary greatly with the severity and nature of the injury produced by the drug reaction. In the case of severe generalized toxic epidermal necrolysis, the prognosis for the patient is poor, often resulting in death.

ALLERGIES TO ARTHROPOD INJURY (ARTHROPOD OR INSECT BITE ALLERGY)

Hypersensitivity to arthropod bites or stings appears to be relatively more common in humans than in animals (with the exception of flea allergy). There are, however, documented cases of cutaneous disease or more serious anaphylactic reactions occurring in animals as a result of arthropod injury. Arthropod injury is further complicated by the fact that both Type I and Type IV hypersensitivities occur. These may interact in the same lesion, thus producing an immediate and relatively short-lived Type I hypersensitivity followed by a more prolonged, insidious, delayed-type response. Certainly the most common and frustrating condition for the animal and for the veterinarian is flea allergy dermatitis (FAD) in dogs and cats. This hypersensitivity disease complex appears to involve both immediate and delayed-type hypersensitivities (Kissileff, 1938; Walton, 1971). Since the flea is so ubiquitous in nature, animals in many parts of the country are plagued by this insect.

Clinical Signs. Clinical signs are usually seasonal but may be nonseasonal, depending on the climate and presence of infestations of the premises. The dominant sign of FAD is intense pruritus. Associated dermal lesions include erythema, papules, pustules, crusts, and acute moist dermatitis. Chronic cases show alopecia, hyperkeratosis, and hyperpigmentation. Lesions usually are confined to the posterior half of the body, especially the base of the tail and the lumbosacral region. The head and neck are also commonly involved in the cat. No breed, sex, or age predilections have been reported (Scott, 1978). Mosquitoes, ticks, fire ants, and chiggers tend to produce single or multiple erythematous, papular, urticarial, and pustular lesions.

Pathology. The pathologic findings vary considerably, depending upon the duration of the lesion. Early lesions are characterized by edema and mast cell hyperplasia with numerous degranulated mast cells. The subacute lesions often become more suppurative in nature and are dominated by neutrophilic leukocytes.

Diagnosis. The rule-outs include pyoderma, food allergies, inhalant allergies, drug reactions, contact irritant dermatitis, and at times, cutaneous neoplasms such as mast cell tumors. The diagnostic plan includes evaluation of the response to short-term corticosteroid therapy, hemogram (eosinophilia), skin biopsies, and careful evaluation of the animal's habits and environment.

Treatment. Treatment and management include elimination or avoidance of the offending agent coupled with short-term corticosteroid and/or antihistaminic therapy. Flea collars are quite effective in some patients, especially cats and small-to-medium-sized dogs; however, they need to be replaced each four to eight weeks. Flea control of the home and yard is essential, since most fleas live off their host most of the time. Hyposensitization of the animal warrants trial when flea control of the animal and environment is impossible. One method employs phenolized glycerine-buffered saline flea extract (1:5,000) and is injected intradermally and/or subcutaneously (0.5 ml) in the flank weekly until an Arthus-like reaction occurs at the injection site(s). After receiving this series, most animals will require one or two injections prior to each (flea) season. However, it must be stated that Halliwell (1981) is dubious of the efficacy of this procedure.

ALLERGIC CONTACT DERMATITIS

Allergic contact dermatitis (ACD) historically appears to be relatively uncommon in companion animals, although Walton (1971) has reported that contact dermatitis (ACD) is responsible for approximately one per cent of dermatologic disease in dogs in two different areas of the United Kingdom. Recently, Nesbitt and Schmitz (1977) reported on 35 cases of canine contact dermatitis (33 ACD and two irritant contact dermatitis) diagnosed among 650 (5.5 per cent) referral dermatologic cases in the Portland, Oregon, and Seattle, Washington area. The pathogenesis usually involves low molecular weight hapten chemicals, which combine with a native protein in either the epidermis or the dermis to produce a complete antigen. The complete antigen initiates and perpetuates a delayed type hypersensitivity response in the host. The offending agent may be any one of a multitude of natural or synthetic chemical compounds (Muller, 1967). It is of interest, but not essential, to differentiate between allergic contact dermatitis and irritant contact dermatitis, the latter being more common and produced by either the physical or chemical irritancy of the offending material. Unfortunately, the clinical lesions of ACD and ICD are often indistinguishable. Many so-called contact dermatoses diagnosed as hypersensitivity to such materials as carpets are in fact due to the irritant effect of the physical property of the fibrous material or the irritating effect of materials such as soaps or detergents. Curiously, virtually all of the 33 cases of ACD reported in dogs by Nesbitt and Schmitz (1977) incriminated synthetic or wool rugs as the allergenic contactant. Experimentally, the author has found that dogs are extremely difficult to sensitize topically, even with potent sensitizers such as dinitrochlorobenzene (DNCB), and once sensitized the hypersensitivity is short lived, usually lasting only a few weeks. Naturally occurring allergic contact dermatitis appears to be rare or nonexistent in the cat (Scott, 1978).

Clinical Signs. Allergic contact dermatitis occurs in the contact areas. These are those areas in which the hair coat is relatively thin and those areas that contact the surface when the animal is sitting or lying, namely, the scrotum; the posterior aspects of the hind limbs, the abdomen, the chest, and the posterior aspects of the forelimbs or the muzzle region that contact feed containers. The acute to subacute lesions often appear as erythematous patches or plaque-like lesions with or without pruritus and exudation. Hyperpigmentation and lichenification are often apparent in chronic lesions.

Pathology. The microscopic findings are variable and may be characterized by epidermal vesiculation or, more commonly, by deeper perivascular and perifollicular dermatitis dominated by histiocytes and lymphoid elements.

Diagnosis. The rule-outs include irritant contact dermatitis, acute moist dermatitis, neurodermatitis, and pelodera dermatitis. The latter condition is in fact a type of parasitic allergic contact dermatitis. The diagnostic plan includes skin scrapings, patch testing, and provocative exposure to a suspected offending material. Scott (1978) has pointed out that patch testing in dogs is fraught with procedural and interpretational pitfalls and is in dire need of standardization.

Treatment. Treatment and management of the patient is essentially symptomatic, since in true allergic contact dermatitis, the antigen becomes part of the native protein in the skin. Therefore, the lesions may persist many days, weeks, or even months. Topical steroid potions or creams are beneficial when oral steroids are contraindicated.

HORMONAL HYPERSENSITIVITY

Hormonal hypersensitivity is thought to be an uncommon Type IV hypersensitivity associated with endogenous progesterone, estrogen, or androgen that has been reported in dogs (Chamberlain, 1974; Scott, 1978) but not reported in cats as yet. The condition appears to be more common in females (19 of 21 cases reported) than in males. Many of the females were atopic and had a history of estral cycle abnormalities (Chamberlain, 1974). Breed and age predilections were not cited.

Clinical Signs. Clinical signs include pruritus, papules, and crusts initially involving the perineal, genital, and posterior thigh regions (bilateral), and progressing cranially. In females, the signs are often associated with estrus or pseudopregnancy and worsen with aging. Histologic findings have not been reported.

Diagnosis. The rule-outs would include ovarian imbalance, seborrheic dermatitis, contact dermatitis, flea allergy dermatitis, atopy, and superficial pyoderma. The diagnostic plan would include intradermal skin testing with aqueous progesterone (0.025 mg), estrogen (0.0125 mg), and testosterone (0.05 mg). A positive (delayed hypersensitivity) response at 24 to 72 hours is diagnostic according to Scott (1978), but no one else has confirmed these results.

Treatment. Ovariohysterectomy or castration is the treatment of choice, and the response is dramatic with marked improvement noted in five to ten days (Scott, 1978).

AUTOIMMUNE DISORDERS

Autoimmunity is associated with the presence of host antibodies and/or immunocompetent lymphocytes that are marked for the host's own specific tissue components. It is important to recognize that the detection of antitissue autoantibodies does not necessarily mean that the clinical and pathological lesions (tissue injury) were produced by the antibodies or immunocytes, since they may have been a result of the disease process or merely associated as a secondary event. Indeed, it is essential to distinguish between *autoimmune response* and *autoimmune disease*. Autoimmune response refers to the detection of autoantibody directed to a "self" antigen or reactivity of lymphocytes sensitized to a "self" antigen. Hence, the autoimmune response may or may not be associated with autoimmune diseases. However, it is essential that autoimmune disease results from tissue damage induced by an autoimmune response. Halliwell (1980) has emphasized that a disease must satisfy a number of criteria before it can be justly called *autoimmune*. Mainly, the autoreactive antibody or cells should be present in all cases of the disease, and their pathogenicity should be demonstrable by *in vitro* or *in vivo* techniques.

Diagnosis of autoimmune disease is based on recognition of typical or suggestive cutaneous, mucocutaneous, and mucosal lesions; immunologic evaluation of the patient; and histopathological evaluation of appropriate tissue specimens. Immunologic evaluation may include direct immunofluorescence, hematologic tests (e.g., LE cell preparation and Coombs test), and serologic tests (e.g., rheumatoid factor). Histopathological interpretation of representative tissue samples may provide confirmation of the clinical diagnosis in a broad or general sense or be nonspecific. Halliwell (1980) correctly stated that the use of histopathology and direct immunofluorescence in combination is more likely to yield a positive diagnosis in autoimmune bullous disorders than is either method used alone (Fig. 82–4).

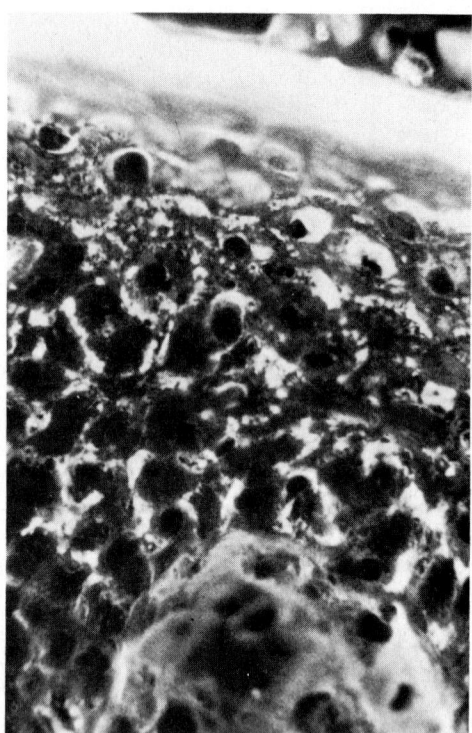

Figure 82–4. Pemphigus variety, direct immunofluorescence. Epidermis showing positive test with an intercellular pattern characteristic of the pemphigus group.

PEMPHIGUS VULGARIS

Pemphigus vulgaris is a progressive vesicular and erosive immune-mediated mucocutaneous disorder associated with circulating autoantibodies. The disease can be classified as a true autoimmune disease, since studies have clearly demonstrated pathogenicity of the autoantibodies even though the precise dysfunction of the immune system remains unclear (Halliwell, 1979). The disease, although relatively rare, is of considerable interest because it was the first immune-mediated vesiculobullous disease recognized in the dog (Hurvitz and Feldman, 1975; Stannard and Gribble, 1975).

Clinical Signs. The clinical lesions consistently occur in the oral cavity and mucocutaneous junctions such as eyelids, lips, and anus. Skin lesions are less common but may be prominent in some cases (Conroy, 1979). Occasionally, the horny portion of the claw is also sloughed secondary to severe paronychia. True vesicles or bullae are rarely recognized, since they are transient owing to the delicate nature of the canine epithelium. The affected dog often shows a positive Nikolsky sign (wrinkling or dislodgment of the epidermis of "normal" skin when sliding pressure is applied). Discrete erythematous erosions and ulcerations are more common findings, often associated with an offensive odor from gingivitis and stomatitis. Middle-aged animals are more commonly affected with no apparent breed predilection (Halliwell, 1979).

Pathology. Microscopically, the classical lesions described in human cases are quite uncommon (Conroy, 1979). When present, they are characterized by intraepidermal or epithelial cleft-like vesicles associated with acantholysis. The residual basal layer frequently has the appearance of a row of tombstones. Fortuitous sections will exhibit acantholytic keratinocytes in the vesicular cavity. The stromal inflammatory reaction is usually minimal. In chronic lesions, however, heavy infiltrations of plasma cells may be seen in the superficial stroma (papillary dermis) (Fig. 82–5).

Diagnosis. The clinical rule-outs include idiopathic ulcerative stomatitis, infectious ulcerative stomatitis (chiefly mucocutaneous candidiasis), chemical irritant stomatitis, and bullous pemphigoid. The diagnostic plan should include histopathologic evaluation of developing lesions and direct immunofluorescence tests for the detection of IgG antibodies, which are characterized by focal immunofluorescence involving the intercellular spaces and possibly cell membrane of the epithelial tissue.

Treatment. Management of the patient requires high levels of corticosteroids, often for a prolonged period. Exacerbation of the lesions is not unexpected after withdrawal from the steroids. Oral prednisone or prednisolone is the drug of choice, initially given at the rate of one to two mg/lb daily. The dose should be *increased* to two to four mg/lb daily if little response is noted during the first five days of therapy. A maintenance dose of 0.25 to 0.5 mg/lb on alternate days should be established as soon as possible. Some canine patients cannot be controlled on steroids alone or are prone to steroid side effects. These animals should be treated with antimetabolites or cytotoxic drugs such as cyclophosphamide (Cytoxan) with 1.0 mg/lb daily for four days each week and monitored with weekly hemograms and urinalysis. Azathioprine (Imuran), 1.5 mg/kg daily, may be preferable because of the undesirable side effects of cyclophosphamide, namely, hemorrhagic cystitis, granulomatous bladder, and possible neoplasia associated with long-term therapy (Halliwell, 1980). Medications may be gradually discontinued after the disease has been in remission for one to two months. Sudden withdrawal of drugs may result in acute exacerbation of clinical disease. Untreated patients usually die because of septicemia associated with overwhelming bacterial in-

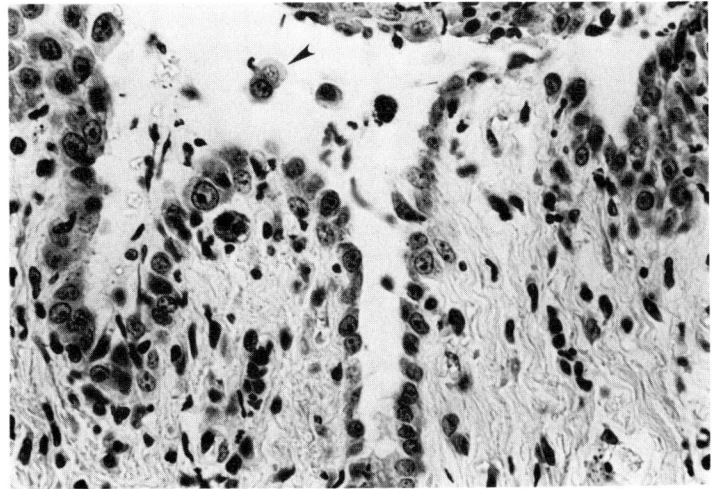

Figure 82–5. Pemphigus vulgaris. Suprabasal vesicle with intact basal cells showing the "tombstone" effect and several acantholytic keratinocytes (example at arrow) floating free in the vesicle.

fection associated with lethargy, cachexia, anorexia, and anemia (Halliwell, 1979).

PEMPHIGUS FOLIACEUS

This less severe but much more prevalent variant of pemphigus vulgaris is characterized by cutaneous and less prominent mucocutaneous lesions, in contrast with the chiefly mucous membrane lesions seen in pemphigus vulgaris. This condition also is associated with circulating autoantibodies directed against the intercellular cement substance of the epithelial tissue. Dogs (Halliwell and Goldschmidt, 1977; Conroy, 1979a, 1979b) and, less commonly, cats and horses are affected. Breed, age, and sex predilections, if any, are not as yet known.

Clinical Signs. Clinical manifestations usually begin on the face, involving the nasal, labial, periocular, and auricular skin, and are characterized by pustules and superficial crusting rather than vesicular and erosive lesions (Conroy, 1979). Progression is expressed by involvement of the feet, especially pads and paronychial skin, and in severe cases the lesions may become generalized. Pruritus of varying degrees occurs. Pemphigus erythematosus is a "bastardized" form that shows clinical and histologic manifestations of pemphigus foliaceus while displaying an immunofluorescence pattern both at the dermoepidermal junction and in the intercellular spaces of the epidermis. Scott et al. (1980) have described pemphigus erythematosus in four dogs and a cat with erythema, alopecia, erosions, ulcerations, epidermal collarettes, leukoderma, oozing, scaling, crusting, and blisters of the nose, face, and ears associated with variable pruritus.

Pathology. Microscopically, pemphigus foliaceus and erythematosus are characterized by moderate acanthosis of the epidermis associated with superficial vesicle-pustules containing predominantly eosinophilic and/or neutrophilic leukocytes associated with acantholytic keratinocytes (Conroy, 1979). Pustular lesions are very superficial, usually occurring at a level of the granular or subcorneal area of the epidermis. The dermal inflammatory response is usually minimal and is often associated with varying numbers of eosinophilic leukocytes (Fig. 82–6).

Diagnosis. The differential diagnosis includes subcorneal pustular dermatosis, superficial pyoderma, pemphigus vegetans, cutaneous (discoid) lupus erythematosus, and facial demodicosis. The diagnostic plan includes histologic evaluation of the tissues, direct immunofluorescent studies, microbiologic cultures, skin scrapings, and hematologic evaluation for LE cells and antinuclear antibody.

Treatment. Therapy and management of the patient require moderately high levels of corticosteroids coupled with initial antibiotics to preclude bacterial infections. Chrysotherapy with aurothioglucose was reported by Manning et al. (1980) to be effective in treating pemphigus foliaceus. Hal-

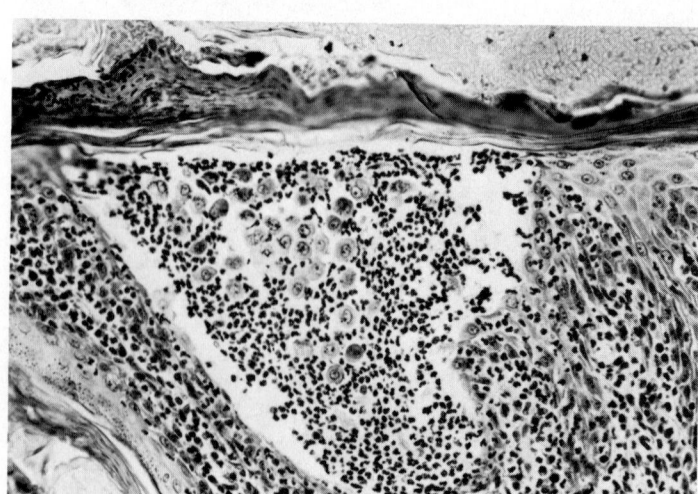

Figure 82–6. Pemphigus foliaceus. Subgranular intraepidermal vesicle-pustule containing numerous acantholytic keratinocytes and granulocytes (neutrophils and eosinophils).

liwell (1980) has achieved good results in both pemphigus foliaceus and vulgaris with aurothioglucose. Weekly test doses of five and ten mg are given, followed by one mg/kg weekly for two to three months, and then a monthly dose as required.

PEMPHIGUS VEGETANS

This autoimmune disorder is closely related to pemphigus foliaceus, occurring in similar locations (face and trunk), without mucosal involvement, and displaying similar histologic and clinical features. The lesions are characterized by thick erythematous, at times verrucous plaque-like lesions that appear more severe and proliferative than the lesions of pemphigus foliaceus. Oral involvement also is not a feature of pemphigus vegetans. First reported by Scott (1977) in a dog, it now appears to be slightly more common than pemphigus vulgaris (which is relatively rare), but much less common than pemphigus foliaceus.

The histologic findings are characterized by hyperplasia of the epidermis and of the outer root sheaths of the hair follicles. Intraepithelial (epidermal and follicular) micropustules containing predominantly eosinophils admixed with acantholytic keratinocytes and scattered neutrophils and associated with a hyperplastic epithelial reaction are characteristic. The dermal inflammatory response is usually superficial and characterized by the presence of varying numbers of eosinophils sometimes admixed with plasma cells (Fig. 82–7). The rule-outs and diagnostic plan are as for pemphigus foliaceus. Therapy and management of the patient requires moderately high levels of corticosteroid therapy, e.g., oral prednisone or the equivalent initially given at 0.5 to 1.0 mg/lb.

BULLOUS PEMPHIGOID (PEMPHIGOID)

As the name "pemphigoid" implies, this condition mimics pemphigus vulgaris in many regards, although it is usually somewhat less severe. It is, however, more common, even though this is not apparent from the paucity of reported cases (Austin and Maibach, 1976; Kunkle and Goldschmidt, 1978). There is a possible breed predilection for collies and collie-related dogs.

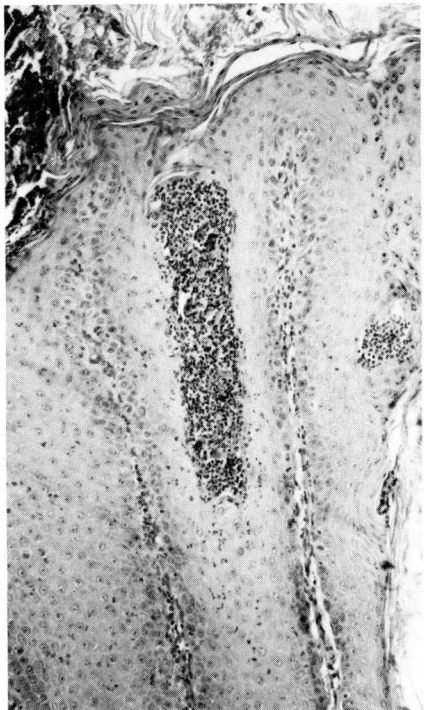

Figure 82–7. Pemphigus vegetans. Marked hyperplasia of the epidermis and hair follicle epithelium associated with deep granulocytic vesico-pustules.

Clinical Signs. The lesions are characterized by sharply circumscribed erythematous erosions and bullous lesions occurring in the oral cavity, mucocutaneous junctions, and skin of the trunk, especially the groin and abdomen. Skin lesions are more common and blisters are more durable than in pemphigus vulgaris (Conroy, 1979).

Pathology. Histologically, the lesions are characterized as subepidermal vesicles showing a fairly clean separation between the dermis and the overlying epithelial layers. Acantholytic cells are not a feature of bullous pemphigoid (Conroy, 1979). The vesicular cavity often contains serum and minimal leukocytes, while the adjacent dermal tissue displays a mild nonspecific inflammatory reaction sometimes associated with scattered eosinophils (Fig. 82–8).

Diagnosis. The rule-outs include chiefly pemphigus vulgaris and, to some extent, toxic epidermal necrolysis. The diagnostic plan should include histopathologic evaluation and immunofluorescence studies. In bullous pemphigoid there is a characteristic linear or globular fluorescence of the base-

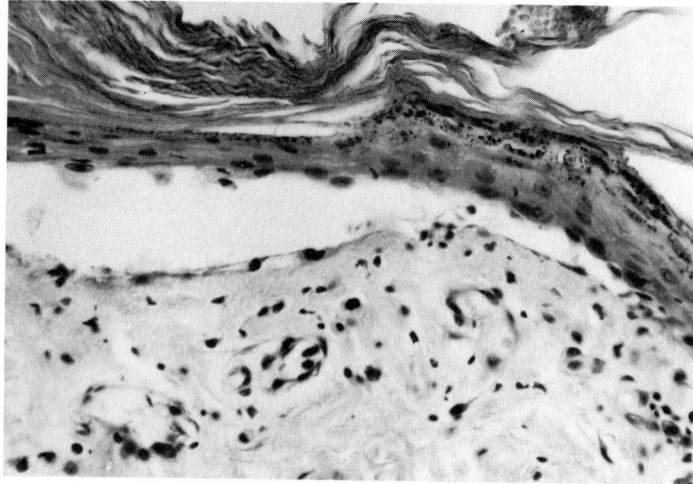

Figure 82–8. Bullous pemphigoid. Subepidermal vesicle with viable epithelium, no acantholysis and minimal inflammatory response.

ment membrane area similar to the fluorescence seen in lupus. The treatment and management of the patient are the same as for pemphigus vulgaris.

DERMATITIS HERPETIFORMIS

Dermatitis herpetiformis is a well recognized, fairly devastating disorder of man, characterized by multifocal or generalized painful vesiculobullous or pustular lesions. If it occurs at all in animals, it is indeed a rare condition. A very few cases have been observed in the dog (Halliwell et al., 1977) that show histologic features and immunofluorescent patterns compatible with human dermatitis herpetiformis. Gluten enteropathy seen in human cases has not been observed in dogs.

Pathology. The histologic characteristics include the presence of subepidermal vesicles associated with dermal papillary necrosis. The immunofluorescent pattern frequently shows immunofluorescence in the papillary dermis adjacent to the lesion site (Fig. 82–9).

Diagnosis. The rule-outs include pustular pyoderma, pemphigus vulgaris, subcorneal pustular dermatosis, bullous pemphigoid, and possibly toxic epidermal necrolysis. The diagnostic plan would include histologic evaluation for the typical lesions and immunofluorescent studies showing the characteristic DH pattern of fluorescence.

Treatment. The treatment of choice is dapsone (Avlosulphon) 0.5 mg per pound given three to four times daily with careful

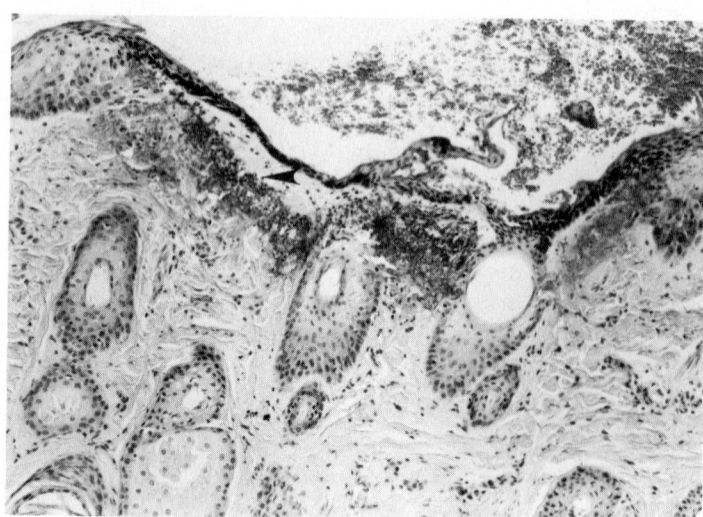

Figure 82–9. Dermatitis herpetiformis-like lesions. Papillary dermal necrosis (arrow) with subepidermal vesicle formation.

monitoring of the patient, since side effects are common (cytopenia and hepatotoxicity). A minimal maintenance dose should be reached as quickly as possible (Scott, 1978).

SYSTEMIC LUPUS ERYTHEMATOSUS (SLE)

SLE is a benchmark for a non–organ specific, multisystemic immune-mediated disease. Although the etiology remains obscure, genetics, viral infections, and aberrant immune response are considered important in the pathogenesis. In man, the disease complex shows an age and sex specificity and a wide range of autoantibodies, and the cardinal signs are a hemolytic anemia, thrombocytopenia, and glomerulonephritis.

Clinical Signs. Canine SLE was first reported by Lewis et al. (1965) as occurring in a variety of breeds, with an age range of four to six years and with equal sex distribution. The canine cases displayed features of autoimmune hemolytic anemia, thrombocytopenic purpura, membranous glomerulonephritis, and/or symmetric (rheumatoid) arthritis. Dermal lesions (alopecia and facial skin eruptions) were inconsistent features. More recently, Scott (1978) described five additional canine cases (two spitz dogs, two Shetland sheepdogs and a collie) with more pronounced skin lesions ranging from seborrheic disorder (alopecia, erythema, scaling, and crusting) to ulcerative mucocutaneous disease. Various other dermal lesions including cellulitis, furunculosis, scarring, and leukoderma observed in the author's clinic indicate the polymorphous nature of canine SLE.

Feline SLE has been reported infrequently (Slauson et al., 1971; Heise et al., 1973). Recently, Scott et al. (1979) reported two additional feline cases that were presented because of a chronic skin disease associated with widespread erythema, vesicobullous eruption, paronychia, and pruritus. In one cat the lesions were localized to the head and feet, while the other cat had more a generalized distribution of lesions.

Pathology. Histologic evaluation of the feline cases were somewhat variable and not diagnostic, according to Scott and co-authors (1979). This is not surprising, since the histologic findings in canine SLE, like the clinical dermal lesions, are quite variable in nature. Apparently this is also true of the dermatohistopathology of human SLE lesions as well.

Diagnosis. The polymorphous nature of the clinical (and· histologic) lesions in the dog and cat creates an endless list of rule-outs that includes bacterial infections, fungal infections, parasitic infestations, neoplasia, toxic dermatoses, drug reactions, other immune-mediated diseases, and many more.

The diagnostic plan for confirmation of SLE includes hemogram, urinalysis, skin biopsy, direct immunofluorescence testing of skin, and tests for LE cells, antinuclear antibody, rheumatoid factor, and antithyroid antibody (if available).

Treatment. Corticosteroid therapy is required for the treatment and control of SLE. Substantial doses (one to two mg per lb per day) are required to produce clinical remission. Thereafter, an alternated daily dose of from 0.5 to 1.0 mg/lb is required as a maintenance level. See Chapter 84 for detailed discussion of other immunosuppressive agents used in SLE.

CUTANEOUS (DISCOID) LUPUS ERYTHEMATOSUS

This relatively newly recognized cutaneous disorder in the dog (Griffin et al., 1979) appears to represent a mild form of systemic lupus erythematosus that lacks the multisystemic effects seen in SLE. The disease is seen most commonly in collies and Shetland sheepdogs and usually is confined to the facial tissues.

Clinical Signs. The initial lesions involve the nasal area, often associated with a focal depigmentation, which leads to extension and enlargement of the lesions associated with erythema, alopecia, scales, and further depigmentation. The eyelids, commissures of the mouth, and auricular tissue may also be involved.

Pathology. Microscopic lesions include epidermal and follicular hyperkeratosis, basement membrane changes (thickening), focal liquefactive necrosis of basal cells, dermal edema, subepidermal vesicles, and band-like inflammatory infiltrate comprised of mononuclear cells (Conroy, 1979). Nodular perifollicular inflammatory foci and pigment incontinence may also be observed.

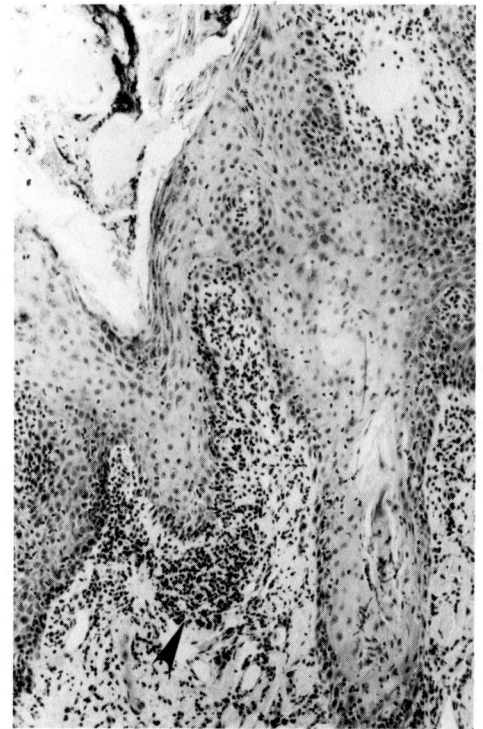

Figure 82–10. Cutaneous ("discoid") lupus erythematosus. Bandlike subepidermal lymphocytic infiltrate (arrow) with penetration of the overlying acanthotic epidermis.

The immunofluorescent pattern is one of fluorescence of the basement membrane zone associated with IgG and C3 (Figs. 82–10 and 82–11).

Diagnosis. The rule-outs include nonimmunologically mediated nasal dermatitis (collie's nose), trauma-induced lesions, early cutaneous neoplasia, pemphigus foliaceus, and pemphigus vegetans. The diagnostic plan should include histopathologic evaluation of the tissue, direct immunofluorescent studies for typical basement membrane pattern, and hematologic evaluation to rule out systemic lupus erythematosus.

Treatment. Successful treatment and management of canine patients have employed topical and systemic corticosteroids and vitamin E.

SUSPECTED IMMUNOLOGIC CONDITIONS

ALOPECIA AREATA

Clinical Signs. Alopecia areata is a condition affecting the hair coat of dogs and cats characterized by focal or multifocal discrete patches of noninflammatory alopecia (Conroy, 1979). The affected sites are usually essentially devoid of all hair and display absence of detectable inflammatory changes. Although the lesions may occur in any haired part, they are most frequently seen on the head, neck, and rear legs.

Pathology. The histologic features are characterized as an acquired noninflammatory alopecia. However, fortuitous sections, especially in early lesions, are characterized by focal accumulations of lymphocytes tending to form a beelike swarm around the hair bulb portion of the hair follicle (Conroy, 1979). Often these hair follicles present a miniature, fetal-like appearance. It is currently proposed that alopecia areata represents an autoimmune disorder. For unknown reasons, the host's immunologic system fails to recognize some of its hair follicles as itself and produces a delayed-type hypersensitivity response to the presumed foreign hair follicles. Human patients with alopecia areata may also exhibit features of immune-mediated thyroiditis,

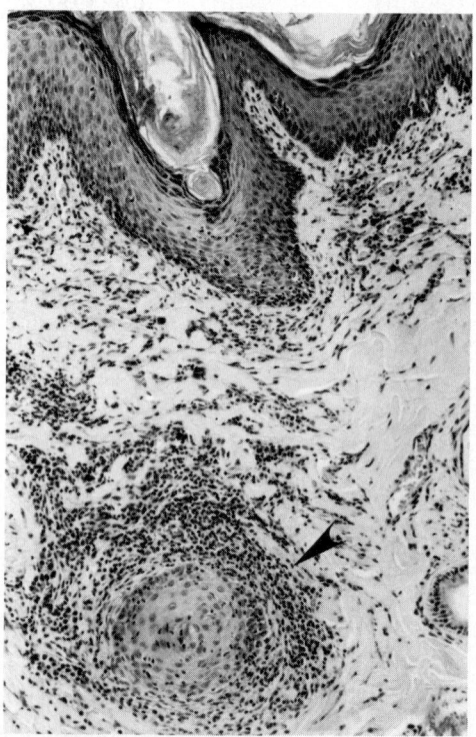

Figure 82–11. Cutaneous ("discoid") lupus erythematosus. Periadnexal (hair follicle) lymphocytic infiltrate (arrow) and follicular hyperkeratosis.

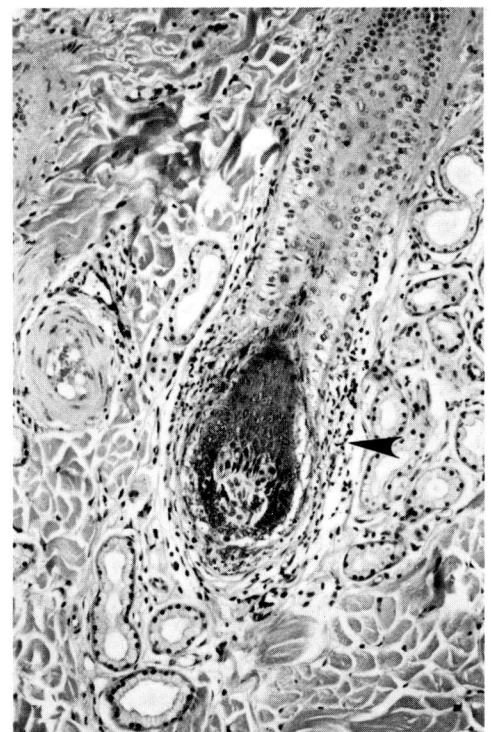

Figure 82–12. Alopecia areata (early lesion). Catagen stage hair follicle with perifollicular (bulb) leukocytic infiltrate (arrow).

although this has not been recognized in the animal cases (Figs. 82–12 and 82–13).

Diagnosis and Treatment. The rule-outs would include acariasis, dermatomycosis, and, less likely, endocrine alopecia or focal steroid atrophy. The diagnostic plan includes histologic evaluation of the alopecic lesions and the assessment of the response to intralesional steroids, which are used as both a diagnostic and therapeutic measure. Local responsiveness (hair growth) to intracutaneous injected soluble steroids is considered to be diagnostic of animal alopecia areata. If the test lesion improves after local injections of steroids, other affected cutaneous sites may also be inoculated. Hair growth usually appears within three to four weeks and may persist for six months or more.

TOXIC EPIDERMAL NECROLYSIS (TEN)

Toxic epidermal necrolysis (Lyell disease) is a curious pathologic response to a variety of underlying conditions or causations. Abnormal immune response is only one of the several causes that have been identified. Additional causes include systemic toxic reactions, drug reactions, visceral neoplasia, and idiopathic disease. TEN is an uncommon, severe mucocutaneous disease of dogs and cats (Scott, 1978; Scott et al., 1979).

Clinical Signs. Regardless of its causation, it is characterized clinically by disseminated, discrete, necrotic erosive and sometimes bullous lesions. Cutaneous pain, cutaneous and mucosal ulcerations, and often a positive Nikolsky sign are significant dermal findings (Conroy, 1979).

Pathology. The microscopic features are essentially diagnostic (Conroy, 1979). The epidermis displays necrosis while often maintaining some structural stability. Subepidermal vesicles also may occur in the affected skin. The dermal inflammatory reaction is usually minimal (Fig. 82–14).

Diagnosis. The differential diagnosis

Figure 82–13. Alopecia areata. Atrophied hair follicle infiltrated with lymphoid cells (arrow).

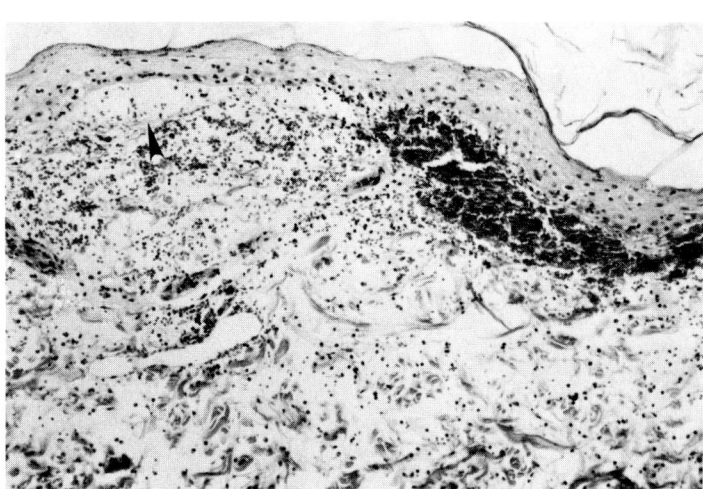

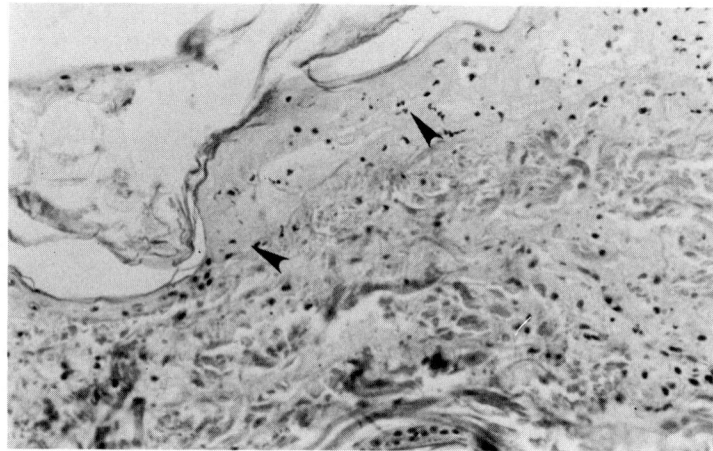

Figure 82–14. Toxic epidermal necrolysis. Necrotic epidermis (arrows) with subepidermal vesicle (between arrows) and minimal dermal inflammatory response.

mainly includes erythema multiforme, bullous pemphigoid, and pemphigus vulgaris. The diagnostic plan should include histologic evaluation of the tissue, immunofluorescent studies to rule out pemphigus and related conditions, and a careful review of the patient information to discover potential drug reactions, as well as a complete physical examination to detect any occult internal disease.

Treatment. Therapy is symptomatic and should include maintenance of fluid, electrolyte, and colloid balance. The prognosis for the patient is guarded to poor, since fatalities do occur.

ERYTHEMA MULTIFORME

Erythema multiforme is recognized in the dog and has for many years been well recognized in man as a disorder or pathologic response involving primarily either the epidermis or the dermis. It often mimics TEN clinically and to some extent pathologically. The etiology may be obscure. Many human cases are associated with a drug reaction or a post-infectious response. The lesions are characterized by erythematous patches or edematous plaques. Histologically, one usually sees marked papillary edema leading to subepidermal vesicle formation. Extravasated erythrocytes may also be observed in the affected dermal papillae (Fig. 82–15). The rule-outs for erythema multiforme include TEN, purpura, and traumatically induced lesions. The diagnostic plan requires critical evaluation of histologic lesions together with a complete physical examination to detect systemic aberrations. Treatment is symptomatic and usually includes corticosteroids. The prognosis depends on the cause but is usually good.

IDIOPATHIC NODULAR AND/OR DIFFUSE GRANULOMATOUS DERMATITIS

Although this enigmatic disease or pathologic response has been recognized clinically

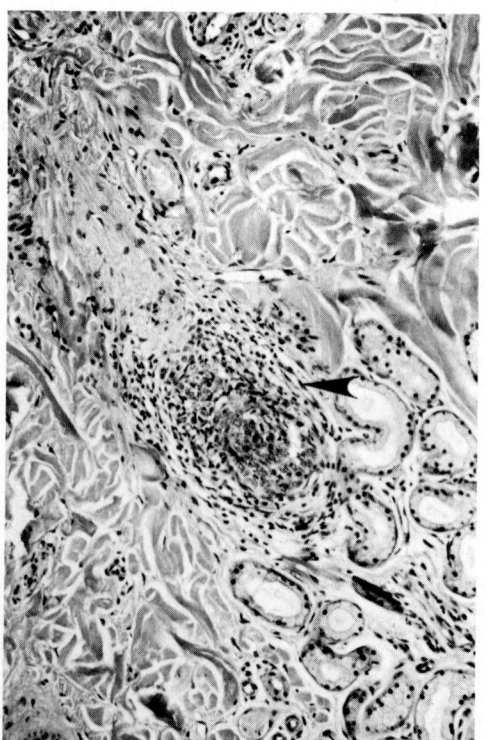

Figure 82–15. Erythema multiforme. Marked interstitial edema, especially in papillary dermis (arrow), associated with hemorrhage and leukocytic infiltration.

and pathologically for several years in both dogs and cats, the etiology is as yet undetermined. This condition occurs in both dogs and cats and is characterized by multiple erythematous nodular and plaque-like lesions that often mimic cutaneous neoplasms. The lesions often affect the head and extremities but are not confined to those locations. Multiple lesions are common and usually range from three to a dozen separate nodular lesions.

Histologically, the lesions are characterized as deep nodular or diffuse perifollicular and perivascular complex granulomatous lesions. Epithelioid macrophages predominate and multinucleated giant cells are rare. Scattered plasma cells, neutrophils, and rare eosinophils may be seen. Exhaustive staining procedures and cultural techniques for microbiologic agents are invariably negative. The rule-outs include cutaneous neoplasia, arthropod hypersensitivity, and deep nonsuppurative folliculitis. Histologic evaluation of a suspected lesion is usually essentially diagnostic. The lesions consistently show a minimal response to antibiotics but will regress during systemic steroid therapy. The prognosis for the patient is good but recurrence of lesions is common.

REFERENCES

Anderson, W. N.: Canine Allergic Inhalant Dermatitis. *In* Drum, S. (ed.): Canine Allergic Inhalant Dermatitis. Ralston Purina Co., Saint Louis, 1975.

Austin, V. H., and Maibach, H. I.: Immunofluorescence testing in a dog. J.A.V.M.A. *168*:322, 1976.

Baker, E.: Food Allergy. Current Views in Veterinary Allergy and Dermatology. Current Views in Veterinary Allergy and Dermatology, Inc., 1979.

Baker, E.: Food allergy in the cat. Feline Pract. May-June, 1975, p. 18.

Baker, E.: Food allergy. Vet. Clin. North Am. *4*:79, 1974.

Baker, E.: Staphylococcal disease. Vet. Clin. North Am. *4*:107, 1974.

Breen, P. T.: Secondary bacterial hypersensitivity reactions in canine skin. Proc. Am. Anim. Hosp. Assoc. *43*:134, 1976.

Calderwood, M.: Personal Communication, 1980.

Chamberlain, K. W.: Inhalant allergic dermatitis. Proc. Am. Anim. Hosp. Assoc. *44*:101, 1977.

Chamberlain, K. W.: Environmental allergens in small animal hypersensitivity disorders. Vet. Clin. North Am. *4*:41, 1974.

Chamberlain, K. W.: Hormonal hypersensitivity in canines. Canine Pract. *4*:18, 1974.

Chamberlain, K. W., and Baker, E.: Diagnostic methods in allergic disease. Vet. Clin. North Am. *4*:47, 1974.

Conroy, J. D.: Dermatopathologic signs of internal causation. Symposium on the Skin and Internal Disease. Vet. Clin. North Am. Small Anim. Pract. *9*:133, 1979.

Gaafar, S. M.: Pathogenesis of Canine Demodicosis. *In* Soulsby, E. J. L. (ed.): Veterinary Medical Review. The Reaction of Host Parasitism. West Lafayette, Ind., 1967, p. 59.

Griffin, C. E., Stannard, A. A., Irke, P. J., Ardans, A. A., Cello, R. M., and Bjorling, D. R.: Canine discoid lupus erythematosus. Vet. Immunol. Immunopath. *1*:79, 1979.

Halliwell, R. E. W.: Skin diseases associated with autoimmunity, Part I. The bullous autoimmune skin diseases. Comp. Cont. Ed. II, 1980, p. 911.

Halliwell, R. E. W.: Skin diseases associated with autoimmunity. Vet. Clin. North Am. *9*:57, 1979.

Halliwell, R. E. W.: Hyposensitization in the Treatment of Atopic Disease. *In* Kirk, R. W. (ed.): Current Veterinary Therapy. VI. W. B. Saunders Co., Philadelphia, 1977.

Halliwell, R. E. W.: Personal communication, 1981.

Halliwell, R. E. W., and Goldschmidt, M. H.: Pemphigus foliaceus in the canine: A case report and discussion. J.A.A.H.A. *13*:431, 1977.

Halliwell, R. E. W., and Schwartzman, R. M.: Atopic disease in the dog. Vet. Rec. *89*:209, 1971.

Halliwell, R. E. W., Schwartzman, R. M., Ihrke, P. J., Goldschmidt, M. H., and Wood, M. G.: Dapsone for treatment of pruritic dermatitis (dermatitis herpetiformis and subcorneal pustular dermatosis) in dogs. J.A.V.M.A. *170*:697, 1977.

Heise, S. C., Smith, R. S., and Schalm, O. W.: Lupus erythematosus with hemolytic anemia in the cat. Feline Pract. *3*:14, 1973.

Hurvitz, A. I., and Feldman, E.: A disease in dogs resembling human pemphigus vulgaris: Case reports. J.A.V.M.A. *166*:585, 1975.

Kissileff, A.: The dog flea as a causative agent in summer eczema. J.A.V.M.A. *93*:21, 1938.

Knowles, J. O.: Provocative exposure for the diagnosis and treatment of certain canine allergies. J.A.V.M.A. *49*:1303, 1966.

Kunkle, G., and Goldschmidt, M. H.: Bullous pemphigoid in a dog: A case report with immunofluorescent findings. J.A.A.H.A. *14*:52, 1978.

Lewis, R. M., Schwartz, R. S., and Henry, W. B.: Canine lupus erythematosus. Blood *55*:143, 1965.

Manning, T. O., Scott, D. W., Kruth, S. A., Sozanski, M., and Lewis, R. M.: Three cases of pemphigus foliaceus and observations on chrysotherapy. J.A.A.H.A. *16*:189, 1980.

Muller, G. H.: Contact dermatitis in animals. Arch. Dermatol. *96*:423, 1967.

Nesbitt, G. H., and Schmitz, J. A.: Contact dermatitis in the dog: A review of 35 cases. J.A.A.H.A. *133*:155, 1977.

Phillips, J. McL.: Angioneurotic edema. J.A.M.A. *78*:497, 1922.

Schreck, O.: Urticaria in the dog. J.A.V.M.A. *15*:83, 1920.

Schwartzman, R. M.: Atopy in the dog. Vet. Cin. North Am. Small Anim. Pract. *63*:1131, 1968.

Schwartzman, R. M.: Atopy in the dog. Arch. Dermatol. *96*:418, 1967.

Scott, D. W.: Observations on canine atopy. J.A.A.H.A. *17*:91, 1981.

Scott, D. W.: Nodular skin disease associated with *Dirofilaria immitis* infection in the dog. Cornell Vet. *69*:233, 1979.

Scott, D. W.: Immunologic skin disorders in the dog and cat. Symposium on Practical Immunology. Vet. Clin. North Am. Small Anim. Pract. *8*:641, 1978.

Scott, D. W.: Pemphigus vegetans in a dog. Cornell Vet. *67*:374, 1977.

Scott, D. W.: Feline dermatology. Proc. Am. Anim. Hosp. Assoc. *43*:99, 1976.

Scott, D. W., Barrett, R. E., and Tangorra, L.: Drug eruption associated with sulfonamide treatment of vertebral osteomyelitis in a dog. J.A.V.M.A. *168*:1111, 1976.

Scott, D. W., Halliwell, R. E. W., Goldschmidt, M. H., and Di Bartola, S.: Toxic epidermal necrolysis in two dogs and a cat. J.A.A.H.A. *15*:271, 1979.

Scott, D. W., Haupt, K. H., Knowlton, B. F., and Lewis, R. M.: A glucocorticoid-responsive dermatitis in cat, resembling systemic lupus erythematosus in man. J.A.A.H.A. *15*:157, 1979.

Scott, D. W., MacDonald, J. M., and Schultz, R. D.: Staphylococcal hypersensitivity in the dog. J.A.A.H.A. *14*:766, 1978.

Scott, D. W., Miller, W. H., Lewis, R. M., Manning, T. O., and Smith, C. A.: Pemphigus erythematosus in the dog and cat. J.A.A.H.A. *16*:815, 1980.

Slauson, D. O., Russell, S. W., and Schechter, R. D.: Naturally occurring immune-complex glomerulonephritis in the cat. J. Pathol. *103*:131, 1971.

Stannard, A. A, and Gribble, D. H.: A mucocutaneous disease in the dog resembling pemphigus in man. J.A.V.M.A. *166*:575, 1975.

Walton, G. S.: Allergic Responses Involving the Skin of Domestic Animals. *In* Brandly, C. A., and Cornelius, E. (ed.): Advances in Veterinary Science and Comparative Medicine. Academic Press 15, 1971, p. 201.

Walton, G. S.: Skin manifestations of allergic responses in domestic animals. Vet. Rec. *82*:204, 1968.

Wittich, F. W.: Spontaneous allergy (atopy) in the lower animals. Seasonal hay fever (Fall type) in the dog. J. Allergy *12*:247, 1941.

CHAPTER **83**

Immunologic Diseases Affecting Internal Organ Systems

LINDA L. WERNER

Clinical immunology, a relatively new discipline in veterinary medicine, has evolved with the rapid expansion of knowledge pertaining to the basic elements of immune function. The past two decades have brought clinically relevant immunologic principles to the forefront with the characterization of a multitude of animal diseases related to defective or inappropriate immune response. Immunologic diseases can be categorized into two basic groups: those which result from failure to mount a protective immune response, the *immunodefi-ciency syndromes*, and those in which the immune response itself causes immunologic injury to the host. This latter group of immunologic disorders is referred to as *hypersensitivity* or *immune-mediated disease*. With the exception of IgE-mediated hypersensitivity, the mechanisms of immune response that cause immunologic injury to the host derive from the same immunologic events that convey protective immunity. However, under certain conditions, such as continuous antigen exposure or failure of precise autoregulation, immunologic injury is perpetuated and immune-mediated disease becomes manifest.

Numerous examples of spontaneous immune-mediated disease exist in veterinary medicine. Allergic hypersensitivity disorders result from IgE-mediated (Type I immunologic injury) degranulation of mast cells and basophils in individuals sensitized to certain antigens (allergens). Systemic Type I hypersensitivity reactions include the fulminant anaphylactic shock syndrome and the less severe urticarial type reactions. More localized, chronic hypersensitivity disorders include allergic rhinitis, allergic bronchitis, inhalant allergic dermatitis, and food allergy.

Autoimmune diseases constitute a major group of immune-mediated disorders in which immune response is directed against self tissue. This failure of self tolerance can invoke either a cytotoxic (Type II) immunologic injury mediated by autoreactive antibody and complement, or a cell-mediated (Type IV) immunologic injury caused by autosensitized T lymphocytes. Numerous autoimmune disorders have been described in dogs and cats (Table 83–1).

While the list of diseases originally classified as autoimmune has diminished, a larger category of immune-mediated disorders has emerged with the recognition that circulating antigen-antibody complexes themselves, under appropriate conditions, are capable of producing immunologic injury (Type III) in conjunction with complement fixation. These so-called immune complex diseases usually result from a vasculitis-type injury, often involving tissues distant from the original site of antigen (whether exogenous or endogenous)-antibody formation. Common examples of immune complex diseases in animals include certain types of glomerulonephritis, myositis, synovitis, uveitis, and dermatitis, though other tissues can be involved as well. Immune complex diseases are found in association with microbial infections, internal parasites, malignancies, drug reactions, and autoimmune disorders such as systemic lupus erythematosus and rheumatoid arthritis. Many are idiopathic, i.e., the antigen source cannot be identified.

Disorders involving cell-mediated (Type IV) immunologic injury are caused by delayed hypersensitivity reactions to self or foreign antigens. Sensitized T lymphocytes, upon antigenic challenge, elaborate constituents called lymphokines, which mediate inflammation by activation and chemotaxis of macrophages, recruitment of additional T lymphocyte participation, and direct cytotoxic effects.

Immune-mediated disorders present a unique challenge to the veterinary clinician, because they often produce signs common to a wide variety of diseases, including infectious, toxic, and neoplastic disorders. Inflammation, fever, pain, and malaise are all common both to the appropriate or protective immune response and to the inappropriate or hypersensitivity perpetuated immune-mediated disease. Furthermore,

Table 83–1.   Autoimmune Diseases of Dogs and Cats

Disease	Tissue Specificity of Autoantibody	Type of Immunologic Injury	Species
Systemic lupus erythematosus	Nuclear antigens, RBC, WBC, platelets	II, III, IV	Canine, feline
Discoid lupus	Unknown	III	Canine
Rheumatoid arthritis	IgG	III, IV	Canine
Autoimmune hemolytic anemia	RBC	II	Canine, feline
Immune mediated thrombocytopenia	Platelets	II	Canine, feline
Autoimmune thyroiditis	Thyroglobulin, thyroid antigen(s)	II, IV	Canine
Pemphigus (varieties)	Intracellular cement substance	II	Canine, feline
Bullous pemphigoid	Dermal-epidermal junction	II	Canine
Myasthenia gravis	Acetylcholine receptor striated skeletal muscle	II	Canine, feline

the clinician must attempt to differentiate true autoimmune disease from the more common immune-mediated disorders that are either secondary to some identifiable agent, such as microbial or chemical, or idiopathic in nature. Thus, a careful and elaborate evaluation of the patient, using a thorough organ systems approach, is mandatory. This chapter reviews first those immunologic diseases commonly associated with polysystemic involvement followed by a discussion aimed at those primarily involving a particular organ system.

SYSTEMIC LUPUS ERYTHEMATOSUS (SLE)

This polysystemic inflammatory disease is perhaps the grandest example of so-called "horror autotoxicus" or autoimmune disease (Ehrlick and Morgenroth, 1900). Recognition of SLE dates as far back as the 13th century, when the term "lupus" was used to describe the wolf-like appearance of human individuals showing characteristic facial erythema (butterfly rash). The association of these cutaneous lesions with other systemic manifestations and the recognition of SLE patients without cutaneous lesions both took place in the late 19th century. Since that time, SLE has been thought to be an immunologic disorder; however, it was not established as an autoimmune disease until the mid 1900s, following the discovery of LE cells and the subsequent identification of circulating antinuclear factors such as immunoglobulin (Lachman, 1961). SLE was first reported in dogs in the early 1960s, and several cases have been reported in cats (Lewis et al., 1963; Scott et al., 1979).

Many types of autoantibodies have been identified in human patients with SLE. Included are autoantibodies with specificity for certain nuclear antigens such as DNA, RNA, histones, and nucleoprotein; cytoplasmic antigens such as mitochondrial, ribosomal, and lysosomal; and cell surface antigens including those of red cells, leukocytes, and platelets. Miscellaneous autoantibodies found in human SLE are rheumatoid factors and antibodies against clotting factors, thyroglobulin, and muscle. Though not all patients show all of these autoantibodies, antinuclear antibodies are nearly always detectable and thus constitute a major diagnostic criteria for SLE. Most of the autoantibodies found in SLE have no particular tissue specificity. Among the autoimmune diseases, therefore, SLE is considered non–organ-specific.

PATHOGENESIS

The precise cause of antoantibody formation in SLE is uncertain. A familial tendency has been demonstrated in human SLE, and the search continues for a viral etiology in conjunction with genetic and environmental factors. The dog and the F_1 hybrid generations from matings of New Zealand Black (NZB) and New Zealand White (NZW) mice have provided important spontaneous models of SLE for the elucidation of these factors. Recently, the discovery of defective immunoregulatory (suppressor T-cell) function in the NZB-NZW mice has led to the association of this activity with the onset of clinical manifestations of the disease, while a number of human SLE patients have been found to have depressed suppressor T-cell function (Horowitz and Coursar, 1975; Krakauer et al., 1976). Thus, the paradoxical concept of *immunologic deficiency* has emerged as a contributing cause of SLE.

Inflammatory lesions in SLE are caused by the Type III immunologic injury, owing to the deposition of soluble circulating immune complexes and subsequent complement fixation in blood vessels and along basement membranes of tissues. Autoantibodies against hematopoietic cells are of course tissue-specific, causing a Type II (cytotoxic) immunologic injury. A role for cell-mediated (Type IV) immunologic injury involving sensitized T lymphocytes has been postulated as well.

Pathologic changes in numerous affected organs are consistent with a vasculitis and generalized destruction of connective tissue. Arterioles undergo an acute necrotizing process followed by fibrinoid deposition and sclerosis. Perivascular lymphocytic and neutrophilic infiltrates are seen adjacent to affected arterioles. Lupus nephritis lesions are characterized by thickening of the glomerular basement membrane (membranous glomerulonephritis), and in severe cases a mesangioproliferative glomerulonephritis is seen, with endothelial swelling and infiltrates of polymorphonuclear cells.

CLINICAL MANIFESTATIONS

Presenting signs of SLE may be acute or chronic and are often cyclic in nature. The more common manifestations of canine SLE include antibiotic nonresponsive fever and malaise, with any of several possible organ systems involved. A stilted gait or shifting leg lameness, with or without obvious joint swelling, is a typical presenting sign of the sterile, nonerosive polyarthritis seen frequently in canine SLE. Polymyositis can occur with similar gait abnormalities, pain, and progressive muscle wasting. A protein-losing glomerulonephritis, a symmetric dermatitis, and hematologic disorders (Coombs-positive anemia, thrombocytopenia purpura, leukopenia) are other possible manifestations. Glomerulonephritis can be either insidious or associated with signs referable to renal failure or the nephrotic syndrome. The dermatologic manifestations of SLE are detailed in Chapter 82 of this text. In the dog, unlike in man, neurologic, cardiopulmonary, and serosal manifestations (pleuritis, pericarditis) are infrequently encountered, although meningitis, myelopathy, myocarditis, and pneumonitis have been recorded (Pedersen et al., 1976; Drazner, 1980). Lymphadenopathy, hepatomegaly, and splenomegaly are common associated findings. Manifestations of probable SLE in cats include fever, lymphadenopathy, dermatologic involvement, glomerulonephritis, hemolytic anemia, leukopenia, thrombocytopenia, and polyarthritis.

CLINICOPATHOLOGIC FINDINGS

Laboratory parameters in SLE vary tremendously, so that no hematologic or biochemical findings are pathognomonic. In the absence of autoantibody-induced hemolytic anemia, thrombocytopenia, or leukopenia, the hemogram is likely to be unremarkable except for evidence of systemic inflammation such as neutrophilic leukocytosis, elevated fibrinogen levels, and increased plasma proteins due to hyperglobulinemia. Biochemical abnormalities vary with the extent of organ involvement. Elevations can occur in liver, muscle, and the non–organ-specific enzymes. BUN and creatinine are sometimes elevated, but they can be normal or mildly elevated even in advanced glomerulonephritis. Low serum albumin signifies probable glomerulonephritis. Globulins can be elevated, and this is characteristically polyclonal in pattern electrophoretically. Urinalysis can be unremarkable or show consistent, moderate to strong protein reactions, proteinaceous and/or cellular casts, and occasionally isosthenuria.

Immunologic Tests

The most important definitive diagnostic criteria for SLE are tests demonstrating the presence of antinuclear antibody (ANA). Classically, the LE cell test was the most widely used until the emergence of the more sensitive ANA test. LE cells are neutrophils or macrophages that have phagocytized a homogeneous mass consisting of nuclear material originating from degenerating leukocytes and opsonized (coated) by anti-deoxyribonucleoprotein antibody (Fig. 83–1, *A*). Though LE cell formation probably occurs to some extent *in vivo*, it is primarily an *in vitro* event. The LE cell test requires five to ten ml of fresh clotted or heparinized blood, depending on the laboratory specification. Briefly, the clot or heparinized sample is incubated for two hours at 37° C and then strained through a wire mesh and centrifuged. Smears made from the buffy coat are stained and examined for the presence of LE cells. The presence of four or more LE cells is considered a positive test and is highly supportive of the diagnosis of SLE. The LE cell test can be negative in ANA-positive lupus patients and is readily suppressed with corticosteroid therapy. Rare or occasional LE cells can accompany other non-SLE inflammatory diseases. The advantages of the LE cell test are that it is simply performed, requires no special or species-specific reagents, and is thus done by many diagnostic laboratories. LE cells have been demonstrated in synovial fluid smears from SLE dogs showing polyarthritis, and in that instance they are highly supportive of the diagnosis. LE cells must, however, be differentiated from a similar cell called a tart cell, which is a phagocyte that has ingested a nucleus showing normal chromatin staining characteristics. Tart cells can be seen in any body fluid accompanying either infection or other causes of inflammation.

The ANA test is the most consistently

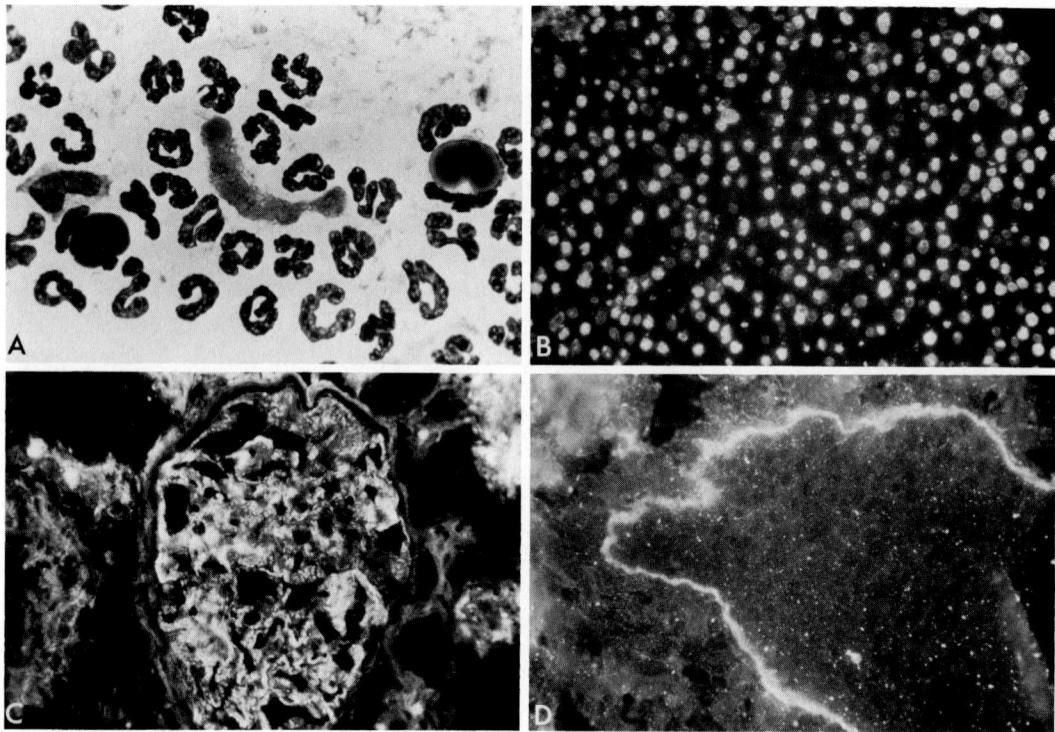

Figure 83–1. *A,* A positive LE cell test. Pictured are two neutrophils showing an eccentrically displaced nucleus and a large homogeneous inclusion body. (From Veterinary Learning Systems and from Halliwell, R. E.: Comp. Cont. Ed. *3*(2):160, 1981. Courtesy of Dr. John W. Harvey.)

B, A postive ANA test (diffuse pattern) using the patient's serum, frozen mouse liver sections, and fluorescein-conjugated rabbit anti-canine IgG.

C, A positive direct immunofluorescent test on frozen sections of renal cortex from an ANA positive dog with protein losing glomerulonephritis and polyarthritis. The granular, discontinuous pattern of fluorescence in the pictured glomerulus is typical of the immunoglobulin deposits (IgG) in immune complex-type glomerulonephritis.

D, A positive direct immunofluorescent test on a skin biopsy from an ANA positive dog who exhibited both dermatologic and hematologic signs of SLE. An irregular linear deposition of IgG along the dermal-epidermal junction is pictured.

reliable test in confirming a diagnosis of SLE. ANA is considered superior to the LE cell test because it is found in a higher percentage of SLE patients, is less transitory over a period of time, and is not as readily influenced by recent steroid therapy. The most widely used ANA test for dogs and cats is the direct immunofluorescent test, using any of a number of accepted cell substrates. Antinuclear antibodies are not species-specific, so that various cell substrates have proved useful, including frozen mouse liver sections, certain tissue culture cell lines, and more recently, a protozoan called *Crithidia lucidae,* which has a unique inclusion body of pure, double-stranded DNA, called a kinetoplast. The ANA test requires one to two ml of serum, best stored frozen if testing is delayed more than a day or two. Dilutions of the patient's serum are incubated on the cell substrate slide, which is then washed and incubated with a fluorescein-conjugated anti-IgG that must be species-specific, rewashed, and examined by fluorescent microscopy. ANA will attach to the nuclei of the cells and react with fluorescein-labeled anti-IgG, producing strong fluorescence (Fig. 83–1, *B*). Since a few normal individuals as well as those with non-SLE inflammatory disease may show low levels of ANA, the level of the ANA titer is extremely important. Titers compatible with SLE will vary according to the laboratory procedure used. The most important pattern of nuclear fluorescence in canine SLE is the speckled pattern, but homogeneous, ring, and nucleolar patterns are also described. A radioimmunoassay for detecting antibodies to double-stranded DNA (DNA binding assay) has proven highly specific for human

SLE. This test has fallen out of favor in canine SLE because of a high incidence of false positives due to a DNA-binding protein (not an anti-DNA antibody) found in dog serum.

Direct immunofluorescent microscopy on renal or skin biopsy specimens from SLE cases showing those organ systems affected often indicates characteristic deposits of IgG and/or complement. In the kidney, a discontinuous, granular deposition along the glomerular capillary loops is characteristic (Fig. 83–1, *C*). In the skin, linear deposits referred to as lupus bands are found in the area of the dermal-epidermal junction (Fig. 83–1, *D*).

THERAPY AND PROGNOSIS

Treatment considerations in SLE include specific and supportive therapy for any concomitant microbial infections or organ dysfunction as well as anti-inflammatory and immunosuppressant therapy. Corticosteroids have been used as the first choice to reduce inflammation and suppress further immunologic injury. When glucocorticoid administration fails to induce satisfactory remission of clinical signs, more potent immunosuppressive therapy is recommended. Cytotoxic drugs such as cyclophosphamide and azathioprine used in combination with moderate glucocorticoid doses have proven beneficial in refractory cases of SLE in dogs (Pedersen et al., 1976). The use of steroids and cytotoxic drugs in SLE is discussed in detail in the final section of this chapter.

The prognosis for longevity in SLE is at best guarded; however, many patients respond favorably to judiciously administered and monitored therapeutic regimens. Severe impairment of vital organ systems, such as the renal system, at the time of presentation yields an unfavorable prognosis. Increased susceptibility to microbial infection often complicates the clinical course of both aggressively and nonaggressively treated lupus patients. In the author's experience pyelonephritis, septicemia, and septic arthritis have all proved ominous signs of advanced, refractory disease.

IMMUNOHEMATOLOGIC DISORDERS

The cells of the hematopoietic system are particularly susceptible to Type II immuno-

logic injury. Anemia, thrombocytopenia, or leukopenia may occur separately or in combination as a result of primary autoimmune- or secondary immune-mediated cytolysis. *Autoimmune hemolytic anemia* (AIHA) and *immune-mediated thrombocytopenia* (IMT) are the most commonly encountered immunohematologic disorders.

PATHOGENESIS

Theories regarding the mechanisms involved in autoimmune disorders are discussed in detail in Chapter 81. Cells of the hematopoietic system can be destroyed by true autoantibodies, cross-reacting antibodies sharing specificity for both self and foreign antigens, or antibodies elicited by drug- or microorganism-induced modification of cell membrane antigens. Some drugs that have been shown to cause AIHA or IMT in man have been similarly incriminated, though not proved. in the dog. Included are penicillins, cephalosporins, sulfas, phenothiazines, and phenytoin. Finally, hematopoietic cells can be destroyed as "innocent bystanders" if circulating immune complexes become adsorbed onto the cell membrane, or if antibody is directed against foreign antigens situated on the cell membrane. The antibody classes involved are most often IgG or IgM. Regardless of the reason for antibody attachment to the cell membrane, cell destruction occurs in two possible ways. Direct cytolysis can occur intravascularly (requiring complement interaction), or the antibody-coated (opsonized) cells are removed from circulation and phagocytized by macrophages of the reticuloendothelial system (RES), a process referred to an extravascular cytolysis.

AUTOIMMUNE HEMOLYTIC ANEMIA (AIHA)

The term autoimmune hemolytic anemia has been applied to a heterogenous group of immunohematologic disorders in which a number of different antibody types and properties have been demonstrated. The antibody-mediated erythrolysis can be *primary* (true AIHA) or *secondary* to underlying disease processes, and either drug induced, infectious, parasitic, or neoplastic. Whether primary or secondary, antibodies or complement (C3) can usually be detected on the red cells by the direct Coombs' antiglobulin test (Coombs et al., 1945). The clinical distinction between primary and secondary AIHA is important from both a therapeutic and a prognostic point of view. For secondary AIHA, specific therapy aimed at elimination of the underlying disease or a suspected drug is mandatory for successful outcome, while the probability of chronic or recurrent hemolytic episodes is reduced. Though Coombs-positive anemias are commonly encountered in cats (in contrast to dogs), the majority are secondary to underlying disease processes. Diseases that have been associated with secondary AIHA in cats include feline leukemia virus infection, hemobartonellosis, and the myelo- or lymphoproliferative disorders (Scott et al., 1973).

Using a classification system for AIHA syndromes in man, five types of AIHA have been reported in dogs (Halliwell, 1978). These differ according to the physicochemical properties of the autoantibody class(es) involved, which to a large extent determine the severity of clinical manifestations. In addition, knowledge of the particular type of AIHA present provides important diagnostic, prognostic, and therapeutic considerations.

Class I. Class I, or *in saline-acting autoagglutinins,* includes those antibodies (IgG or IgM) that result in direct or intravascular hemagglutination. Agglutination can be observed immediately upon withdrawal of blood into a syringe or glass vial or when a drop of blood is deposited onto a glass slide (Fig. 83–2). This must be differentiated from rouleau formation. The two can be distinguished readily by mixing the blood with an equal amount of physiologic saline. Rouleau formation will disperse, whereas true autoagglutination will not. The finding of in saline-acting autoagglutinins is diagnostic for AIHA and precludes the necessity of running a Coombs' test.

Class II. Class II, or *intravascular hemolysins,* consists of antibodies that fix complement in sufficient quantity to result in massive intravascular hemolysis. They are usually of the IgM class but are occasionally of the IgG class.

Class III. Class III, or *incomplete antibody type,* is the most common form of AIHA in the dog. The patient's RBCs are coated with immunoglobulin of insufficient quantity, va-

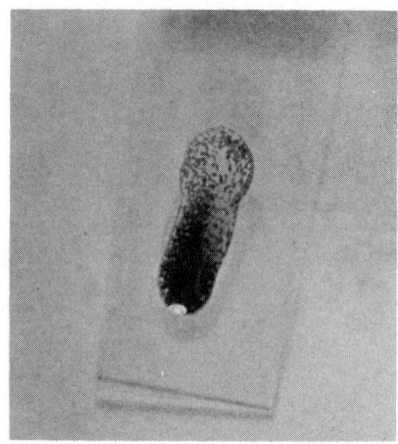

Figure 83–2. Direct agglutination of RBCs in a drop of heparinized blood mixed with a drop of physiologic saline. This finding is virtually diagnostic for AIHA. (Courtesy of Dr. John W. Harvey. From Halliwell, R. E. W., and Werner, L. K.: Canine Medicine and Therapeutics. Blackwell Scientific Publ., LTD., Oxford, England, 1979, p. 215.)

lence, or avidity to cause direct hemagglutination or lysis. In this instance, cell destruction occurs primarily in the RES by phagocytosis of the opsonized RBCs. This antibody is detected only by the Coombs' test.

Class IV. Class IV, or *cold hemagglutinins,* includes agglutinating antibodies that are most active at some degree below body temperature and are most often of the IgM class. Cold hemagglutinins can be detected by the visualization of clumping when blood is allowed to cool to 4° C on a glass slide. The reaction is reversed upon rewarming the blood to body temperature (37° C). As is the case with Class I autoagglutinins, the demonstration of cold agglutinins is diagnostic for AIHA.

Class V. Class V, or *cold-acting nonagglutinating AIHA,* involves antibodies that do not cause direct agglutination but lead to increased RBC destruction by the RES, particularly in cold weather. The Coombs' test, run at 4° C, is necessary to diagnose this form of AIHA.

Clinical Signs

The clinical manifestations of AIHA result from the progressive anemia. Common physical findings include mucous membrane pallor, lethargy, weakness, anorexia, tachypnea, and tachycardia. In the more fulminant cases of massive intravascular hemolysis, icterus, emesis, and fever are often seen. Splenomegaly, hepatomegaly, and lymphadenopathy are occasionally present. Hemoglobinuria is most often seen with intravascular hemolysis, though it may accompany extravascular hemolysis as well. Rarely, cutaneous lesions of the peripheral extremities are a significant presenting sign. Such lesions can occur when the autoantibody has a temperature dependency below that of body temperature. Termed *cold agglutinin disease,* animals showing this type of AIHA may or may not have a significant anemia at the time of presentation. The distal extremity lesions most commonly involve either the ear or tail tips, nose, or feet, and result from ischemic necrosis due to RBC agglutination and obstruction of small vessels (Fig. 83–3). Though periods of cold weather tend to exacerbate these lesions, cold agglutinin disease can be seen in more temperate climates. Transient hemoglobinuria, which may or may not be accompanied by a significant anemia, has been associated with cold-acting AIHA.

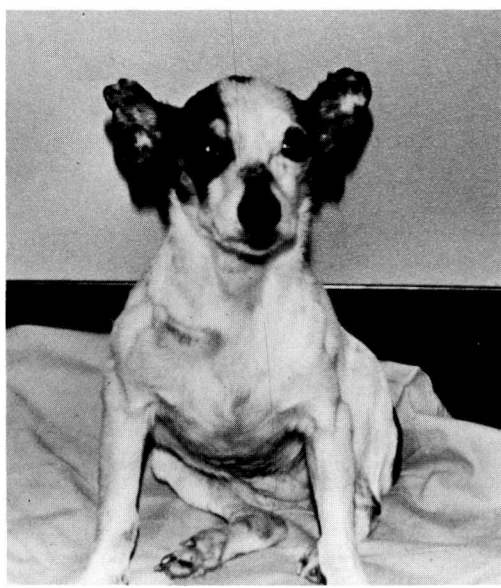

Figure 83–3. Distal extremity lesions involving the pinnae, planum nasale, tail tip and digits of an eleven-year-old female Fox terrier with cold agglutinin disease accompanying a lymphoproliferative disorder. Direct hemagglutination and a positive Coombs' test for IgM (both occurring at 4°C but not at 37°C) were significant diagnostic findings.

Clinicopathologic Findings

Hemogram findings consistent with AIHA generally include evidence of a regenerative anemia and a leukocytosis. Nonregenerative anemias are occasionally encountered in AIHA, particularly during the acute phases of anemia preceding optimal time for bone marrow response. Failure of active erythrogenesis during chronic progressive stages of AIHA has been attributed to autoantibody-mediated damage to red cell precursors in the bone marrow. Though this is not proved in domestic animals, successful immunosuppressive therapy can result in a regenerative response. Recent blood transfusion can also inhibit erythrogenesis (Schalm, 1975).

Spherocytes, when present, are highly suggestive of AIHA. These small, dense RBCs that lack central pallor are thought to result from membrane damage due to antibody and complement fixation. Spherocytes are not consistently found, however. Nucleated RBCs are sometimes found, indicating extramedullary hematopoiesis.

The leukocytosis, often in excess of 25,000/mm³, consists primarily of a neutrophilia, often accompanied by a profound left shift. This so-called leukemoid response accompanies the profound regenerative bone marrow response at the pleuripotential stem cell level and is commonly misinterpreted as a sign of sepsis. Platelet counts are indicated in AIHA to detect those cases that have accompanying IMT.

Bone marrow aspirates usually correspond to the peripheral blood picture, depicting a regenerative response. Increased cellularity dominated by erythrocyte precursors and a normal-to-decreased M:E ratio are typical. Bone marrow aspirates are most indicated when there is continued failure of erythrogenesis, in order to rule out myeloproliferative disease or other bone marrow disorders.

In cats, hemogram findings associated with Coombs-positive anemias are variable, often reflecting the activity of an underlying primary disease such as hemobartonellosis, feline leukemia virus infection, lymphosarcoma, or myeloproliferative disease. The majority of cases exhibit a normal leukogram or a mild-to-moderate leukocytosis. A number of FELV-positive cats showing Coombs-positive hemolytic anemia have accompanying leukopenia, thrombocytopenia, or leukemia. Spherocytosis is difficult to evaluate in feline blood smears, owing to the normally smaller-sized red cells of cats.

Hemoglobinemia, hemoglobinuria, and hyperbilirubinemia usually accompany only those cases of AIHA with significant intravascular hemolysis. Bilirubinuria is common in both intra- and extravascular hemolysis. Hepatic or non–organ-specific enzymes may be elevated as a result of intercurrent disease, hypoxia, or ischemia due to intravascular hemagglutination. Serum haptoglobin determinations can be helpful in differentiating between hemolytic and non-hemolytic causes of anemia in cases in which more routine diagnostic tests yield equivocal results. Haptoglobin values are generally reduced during hemolytic episodes. In the absence of a positive Coombs' test, other causes of hemolytic anemia must be considered as well when serum haptoglobin levels are low.

The Coombs' Test. This test uses specific antiglobulins to detect antibodies or complement attached to the RBC membrane. An effective Coombs' reagent uses species-specific antisera against IgG, IgM, and the third component of complement (C3). The patient's blood sample is collected in heparin or ethylenediaminetetraacetate (EDTA). The RBCs are separated and washed, and a two per cent suspension in buffered saline is added to serial twofold dilutions of the antisera. Ideally, two sets of dilutions are prepared, one for incubation at 37° C and one at 4° C. (If the clinician is particularly interested in a cold Coombs' test, this test should be requested in addition to the routine Coombs' test.) After one hour, the cells are observed macroscopically for agglutination. The Coombs' test is a reliable test when properly done, but false negatives and false positives do occur (Halliwell, 1978).

The indirect Coombs' test detects anti-RBC antibody in the patient's serum. The test serum is incubated with donor RBCs of the same blood type and the Coombs' test is then performed. Presently, there is insufficient knowledge and application of canine and feline red cell antigens and naturally occurring isoantibodies to ensure validity of the indirect Coombs' test for these species.

Differential Diagnosis

Cases of suspected or confirmed AIHA should be thoroughly evaluated to identify the presence of other associated diseases requiring specific therapy. When other hematopoietic cells are decreased, tests for antinuclear antibody, LE cells, or anti-platelet antibody are indicated. Unless there are strong supportive findings for AIHA, including marked spherocytosis, autoagglutination, or a positive Coombs' test, other nonimmunologic causes of regenerative anemia should be considered in the differential diagnosis.

Treatment and Prognosis

The aims in treatment of AIHA are to manage the acute anemic crisis, inhibit the sequestering and phagocytosis of RBCs in the reticuloendothelial system, treat specifically any underlying disease, and lower the production of anti-RBC antibody in lymphoid tissue. Corticosteroids (prednisone or prednisolone), at an initial dose of one to two mg/kg body weight every 12 hours, are used to suppress erythrophagocytosis and antibody production. Blood transfusion should be avoided except in life-threatening anemia, since it may precipitate or accelerate hemolytic crisis, enhance antibody production, or suppress the normal response of bone marrow to anemia. Good supportive care, the elimination of stress factors, and oxygen supplementation, if necessary, will often sustain patients during a hemolytic crisis until steroid therapy takes effect. When blood transfusion is deemed necessary to save the patient during anemic crisis, crossmatched blood should be given, along with immunosuppressant therapy. Tetracycline is usually added to the treatment regime for cats to counter the possibility of an undetected *Haemobartonella* infection. Antibiotic therapy should be instituted in patients with bacterial infections. Corticosteroid therapy in the presence of infection is not recommended unless the anemia is life-threatening.

If significant stabilization or gain in PCV is not achieved during the first 48 to 72 hours of steroid therapy, a more potent immunosuppressant agent, such as cyclophosphamide, should be used. The author prefers to begin cyclophosphamide therapy from the outset in patients showing autoagglutination or intravascular hemolysis, because the prognosis is graver in both instances. Further details on combination immunosuppressant therapy are provided in the final section of this chapter. It is not uncommon, during the first week of therapy, to find an increase in the number of spherocytes due to suppression of erythrophagocytosis by corticosteroids. When clinical remission has occurred, corticosteroid doses should be tapered gradually over a period of one to three months to an alternate day maintenance regime. Alternate day steroid therapy at one fourth to one half the starting dose should be maintained while periodic hemograms are performed to evaluate progress or signs of exacerbation. Although some cases of AIHA tend to recur intermittently, it is worthwhile to withdraw animals in prolonged remission from all therapy and recheck periodic hemograms and a Coombs' test for evidence of exacerbation. Many animals do not manifest recurrent hemolytic disease.

Splenectomy should be considered in those cases that respond inadequately to steroid therapy, tolerate immunosuppressant therapy poorly, or tend to exacerbate frequently in spite of proper medical management. Removal of the spleen eliminates both a concentrated source of antibody-producing lymphocytes and a major portion of the reticuloendothelial system.

In the dog, Classes I and II AIHA have the poorest prognosis and highest percentage of deaths. When AIHA is associated with underlying disease, the course of that disease often determines the ultimate prognosis.

IMMUNE-MEDIATED THROMBOCYTOPENIA (IMT)

Immune-mediated thrombocytopenia can occur as the result of several types of immunologic interactions involving platelets. As in AIHA, there can be autoantibody against platelet membrane antigens, drug- or microorganism-induced antigenic modification of the membrane, cross-reacting antibody, and "innocent bystander" types of immunologic injury. It has been suggested by Wilkins and Hurvitz (1973) that IMT is a more appropriate name for this immunohematologic disorder than the formerly used term, idiopathic thrombocytopenia purpura (ITP). IMT, like AIHA, can occur in conjunction with other immune-mediated disorders, particularly systemic lupus erythematosus.

There is no breed or age predilection, but an increased incidence in female dogs has been reported (Wilkins et al., 1973). Cats can develop IMT, and though there may be an association with feline leukemia virus infection in some instances, the precise etiology is unknown.

Clinical Signs

Petechial and ecchymotic hemorrhages are the hallmarks of thrombocytopenia. Though IMT may be acute, chronic, or cyclic in its course, clinical signs of hemorrhage often do not occur spontaneously until the platelet count falls below 50,000/mm^3. Petechial and ecchymotic hemorrhages can be localized or disseminated. Favored distribution sites include the mucous membranes, pressure points, or areas of excessive trauma. Some patients will present with excessive bleeding following trauma. Retinal hemorrhages, epistaxis, prolonged bleeding during estrus, hematuria, or hemorrhagic diarrhea can be present, sometimes without associated cutaneous petechiae or ecchymoses. Other clinical signs such as neurologic dysfunction and cardiac dysrhythmias can accompany fulminant IMT, presumably as the result of hemorrhage into these tissues.

Clinicopathologic Findings

Hemogram findings compatible with IMT include a decreased platelet count, normal-to-increased neutrophil count, and normal-to-decreased PCV. The platelets seen on blood smears are often abnormally large, denoting recent release from the bone marrow. When anemia is present, it can be either regenerative or nonregenerative, depending on the chronicity of blood loss due to hemorrhage or concomitant autoantibody-mediated erythrolysis, or both. There are no particular biochemical abnormalities associated with IMT, but routine biochemical screening tests are indicated to evaluate possible involvement of other body systems due to hemorrhage, anemic hypoxia, or intercurrent disease.

In most cases, bone marrow aspirates show normal-to-increased megakaryocytes in response to the thrombocytopenia and a normal-to-decreased M:E ratio if active erythrogenesis is occurring. Less commonly,

only rare megakaryocytes are evident, suggesting their involvement in the immunologic injury; however, no appropriate studies have been done to document this. Because the hemostatic defect involves only the platelets, clotting times are normal in uncomplicated cases, while bleeding time is prolonged.

Immunologic Tests. A diagnosis of IMT is confirmed when anti-platelet antibody is demonstrated by the platelet factor 3 (PF-3) test (Wilkins et al., 1973). This test system uses platelets from a normal dog (platelet-rich plasma or PRP), which are incubated with both normal dog globulin (control) and the patient's globulin in the presence of canine contact product (activated clotting factors XI and XII). If anti-platelet antibody is present in the globulin fraction of the test serum, the clotting time of the PRP (initiated by the addition of .025 M CaCl) is shortened by at least ten seconds as compared with the normal control. The anti-platelet antibody injures the platelet membrane, causing release of the procoagulant substance termed platelet factor 3. False negative PF-3 tests have been reported after two to three days of corticosteroid therapy (Wilkins et al., 1973). It is noteworthy that many cases of suspected IMT fail to show a positive PF-3 test. In that instance, and because clinical expediency often demands treatment of the patient before a confirmed diagnosis can be made, a good response to corticosteroid therapy justifies a presumptive diagnosis of IMT. Rickettsial-induced thrombocytopenias should also be ruled out.

Since IMT often co-exists with other autoimmune disorders, a Coombs' test is indicated for patients showing anemia. An LE cell test and ANA are indicated when IMT occurs in association with a Coombs-positive anemia or any other signs of SLE.

Therapy and Prognosis

Treatment of IMT includes the elimination, when possible, of any microbial infection or suspected offending drug. In most cases, underlying contributing factors are not found. Corticosteroid therapy aimed at inhibition of platelet destruction by macrophages of the RES is usually rewarded by return of platelet counts to normal range within a period of days. As in AIHA, pro-longed therapy is recommended, starting at 1 to 2 mg/kg body weight every 12 hours and tapering over a 4- to 12-week period to alternate day doses of 0.5 to 1 mg/kg. Monitoring platelet counts at weekly intervals during the initial stages of therapy is helpful in the early recognition of relapsing thrombocytopenia. Failure to respond adequately to corticosteroids can be seen both in cases that have active megakaryocyte response by the bone marrow and in those that manifest decreased megakaryocyte activity. These steroid refractory cases of IMT can often be managed effectively by adding either cyclophosphamide or vincristine to the therapeutic regime (see final section of this chapter). Splenectomy has been used in the management of chronic relapsing IMT; however, its success as an adjunct to medical therapy has not been evaluated in animals. Fresh whole blood transfusions may be necessary during the acute stages, when systemic signs such as rapidly progressive anemia, CNS disturbances, cardiac dysrhythmias, or gastrointestinal bleeding are indicative of unabated internal hemorrhage. For optimal platelet numbers and function, transfusion with fresh blood stored less than 12 hours at room temperature is recommended. The degree of the thrombocytopenia does not always correspond with the severity of hemorrhage present (Fig. 83–4). Thus, the clinical condition of the patient is the more important factor in the indications for blood (or platelet-rich plasma) transfusion.

In general, the prognosis for IMT is favorable, because the majority of cases are neither critical at the time of presentation nor relapsing once tapered from maintenance therapy. The tendency of some cases to relapse makes periodic monitoring necessary. One author has recommended ovariohysterectomy of intact females with IMT once platelet counts are restored (Wilkins et al., 1973).

DYSPROTEINEMIAS

Abnormalities in serum protein content are found in a variety of diseases. The most common serum protein abnormality is hypoalbuminemia, which may be accompanied by normal, increased, or decreased serum globulin levels. Hypoalbuminemia can result from either inadequate production (chronic

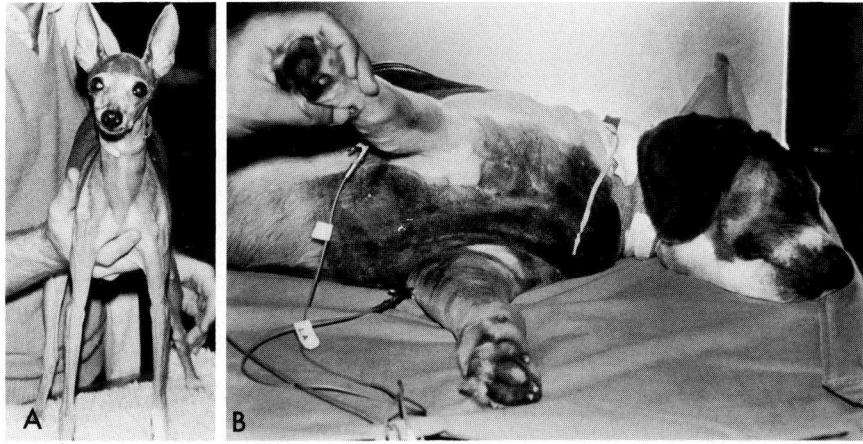

Figure 83–4. *A,* A ten-year-old Italian greyhound with a platelet count of 8,000/mm³ showed no evidence of hemorrhage except for jugular hematomas following venipuncture. In contrast (Fig. 83–4*B*), a four-year-old male beagle with a 32,000/mm³ platelet count presented semicomatose with massive ventral cutaneous ecchymoses, cardiac rhythm disturbance, and neurologic deficits suggestive of internal hemorrhage. Both dogs showed a positive platelet factor 3 test and responded to treatment for IMT. The beagle required fresh blood transfusion to control progressive hemorrhage.

liver disease or protein malnutrition) or increased loss with conditions such as protein-losing nephropathy and enteropathy, chronic external blood loss, and exudative inflammatory diseases. Hypoglobulinemia can accompany these protein-losing states whenever compromise of vascular or lymphatic integrity is great enough to allow larger molecular weight proteins to escape. Hypoglobulinemia associated with normal serum albumin levels is strongly suggestive of immunodeficiency, whether it be congenital or acquired.

Hyperglobulinemia can be seen with a wide variety of underlying diseases, including neoplasia, microbial infections, and chronic inflammatory disorders. The term "gammopathy" has been applied to hyperglobulinemic states, perhaps inappropriately, because the increase in serum globulin levels is not necessarily restricted to those migrating in the gamma distribution on serum protein electrophoresis. This is particularly true in the case of *polyclonal* hyperglobulinemias, so-called because in this instance, multiple classes of immunoglobulins and nonimmunoglobulin proteins can be present in excess. On serum protein electrophoresis, a broad-based or generalized increase in globulin constituents is typical of *polyclonal* hyperglobulinemia and this can be represented in any or all of the globulin fractions (Fig. 83–5). The finding of a polyclonal elevation in serum globulins

has little diagnostic significance per se, except as an indication of some underlying disease resulting in chronic stimulation of the immune system. Common examples in dogs and cats include bacterial, mycotic, and certain internal parasitic infections (such as heartworms or lungworms); persistent virus infections such as feline infectious peritonitis or feline leukemia virus; neoplasia; and a

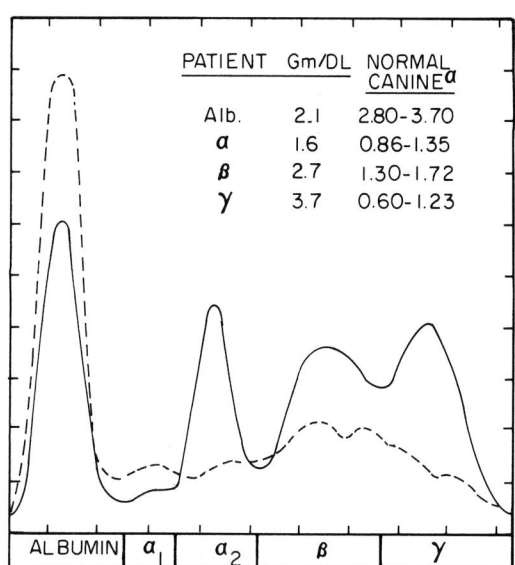

PATIENT	Gm/DL	NORMAL CANINE[a]
Alb.	2.1	2.80–3.70
α	1.6	0.86–1.35
β	2.7	1.30–1.72
γ	3.7	0.60–1.23

ALBUMIN | α₁ | α₂ | β | γ

Figure 83–5. A characteristic polyclonal hyperglobulinemia pattern on a serum protein electrophoresis from a dog with vegetative bacterial endocarditis. (Dotted line depicts a more normal tracing.) (A. Halliwell, 1978.)

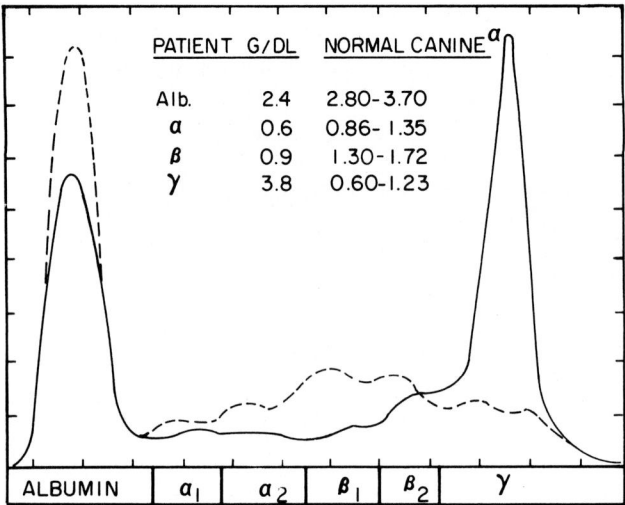

PATIENT G/DL		NORMAL CANINE
Alb.	2.4	2.80-3.70
α	0.6	0.86-1.35
β	0.9	1.30-1.72
γ	3.8	0.60-1.23

Figure 83–6. Electrophoretic tracing from a dog with multiple myeloma. Note the monoclonal spike in the γ distribution. In addition, the albumin and β globulins appear decreased. (Dotted line depicts a normal electrophoretic pattern.) (A. Halliwell, 1978.)

variety of inflammatory disorders such as chronic active liver disease, granulomatous disease, amyloidosis, and other types of immune-mediated disease.

Though polyclonal elevations in serum globulins are fairly nonspecific, they must be differentiated from *monoclonal* elevations, which have more specific diagnostic implications. Monoclonal hyperglobulinemias arise from excessive production of a single type of immunoglobulin. Because the immunoglobulin molecules are all identical, their electrophoretic mobility covers a very distinct, restricted range on protein electrophoresis, a tracing of which resembles a church steeple or pronounced spiking pattern found in either the beta or the gamma region (Fig. 83–6). Excessive production of a single homogenous type of immunoglobulin occurs as the result of proliferation of a population or *clone* of lymphocytes or plasma cells derived from a single parent cell. Monoclonal hyperglobulinemias, therefore, are most likely to accompany lymphoproliferative disorders and plasmacytic neoplasia. It is generally thought that the monoclonal protein, also called a paraprotein or "M" component, is normal immunoglobulin qualitatively, and its presence in excessive amounts is the only abnormal feature. Those paraproteins that are macroglobulins can cause increased serum viscosity, leading to a number of pathophysiologic sequelae, including circulatory disturbances, hemorrhagic tendencies, retinal lesions, neurologic disturbances, and renal or other organ system damage. Multiple myeloma, a dis-

seminated form of plasma cell tumor, is the most commonly seen disorder in dogs associated with a monoclonal hyperglobulinemia. Other causes include lymphosarcoma, lymphocytic leukemia, and benign idiopathic monoclonal hyperglobulinemia. The latter has been reported in the dog as an incidental finding unassociated with any clinical signs or abnormalities (De whirst et al., 1977). Macroglobulinemia with hyperviscosity syndrome has also been reported in dogs (Hurvitz et al., 1977; MacEwen et al., 1977). The macroglobulin consists usually of IgM or polymers of IgA. Macroglobulins that have the characteristic of precipitation or gel formation at temperatures below body temperature are referred to as cryoglobulins. Cryoglobulinemia and monoclonal macroglobulinemia of IgM class has been reported in a ten-year-old female Doberman pinscher with plasma cell tumor invasion of bone marrow (Hurvitz et al., 1977). Approximately ten per cent of human patients with macroglobulinemia have cryoglobulinemia. When clinical signs are associated with the presence of a cryoglobulin, they manifest as cold intolerance with circulatory impairment of peripheral extremities due to cryoprecipitation. Monoclonal hyperglobulinemia has been seen occasionally in cats with lymphocytic or plasmacytic neoplasia.

Multiple Myeloma

Plasmacytoma can occur in both localized and disseminated forms. The disease occurs in middle-aged to older dogs with no documented breed predilection, though Doberman pinschers appear to be overrepresented. Clinical signs are attributed to the distribution of tumor mass and occasionally to the monoclonal immunoglobulin excess produced by the neoplastic cells. This so-called "M" component (monoclonal, macroglobulin, myeloma protein) or paraprotein can cause signs or symptoms related to serum hyperviscosity whenever high molecular weight molecules, such as IgM, or polymers of IgA or IgG are present in large quantity. Signs of hyperviscosity syndrome include a hemorrhagic tendency, retinal vessel tortuosity with "sausage-shaped" dilatations or retinal hemorrhages, and mental dullness or other CNS signs. Because of the tendency of plasmacytoma to invade bone, presenting signs may include skeletal pain, pathologic fracture, or associated compression myelopathy/neuropathy. Multiple myeloma has a variety of possible systemic manifestations, all of which may not be present in every case. Single or multiple highly osteolytic lesions can be found in both the axial and/or appendicular skeleton. Vertebral pain or cord compression can mimic signs of disc disease or vertebral malformation. Solid tumors can occur anywhere in the body, while diffuse infiltration of tumor cells can invade many organs, particularly spleen, liver, bone marrow, and kidney. Signs referable to coagulation defects may accompany the presenting complaint or may develop later. Causes of hemorrhagic tendencies in multiple myeloma patients include platelet function defects resulting from hyperviscosity, thrombocytopenia due to plasma cell infiltration of bone marrow or myelosuppressive chemotherapy, and the formation of clotting factor-paraprotein complexes that result in prolonged clotting time.

Renal damage in multiple myeloma can occur with tumor infiltration, circulatory disturbances, amyloid deposition, tubular obstruction from proteinaceous cast formation, and bacterial infection. Increased susceptibility to infection can be associated with defective immune function acquired with these tumor diseases or with cytotoxic (immunosuppressive) chemotherapy.

Anemia is a common problem in multiple myeloma and other lymphoproliferative disorders accompanied by monoclonal hyperglobulinemia. A number of possible contributing causes can be identified, including blood loss from hemorrhagic diathesis, neoplastic invasion of bone marrow, decreased erythropoietin production with chronic renal involvement, and depression anemia of chronic disease.

Clinicopathologic Tests. Hemogram findings are variable, depending on the extent of bone marrow involvement and whether hemorrhage and/or intercurrent infection are present. Anemia may be regenerative when associated with blood loss, or nonregenerative if caused by either tumor invasion of bone marrow or chronic renal failure with decreased erythropoietin production. Thrombocytopenia and/or leukopenia are strong evidence of neoplastic invasion of bone marrow. Marked elevation in plasma protein content on a routine hemogram is often the first clue to hyperglobulinemia. Serum chemistry findings vary with the extent of organ system involvement. Elevations in liver enzymes are suggestive of hepatic metastasis or circulatory impairment. Elevations in alkaline phosphatase accompany either liver or skeletal involvement. Elevations in BUN and creatinine occur as a result of the aforementioned renal manifestations. Hypoalbuminemia is not an uncommon finding and can result from glomerular damage and/or decreased protein synthesis with hepatic involvement. The globulin fraction is nearly always elevated, resulting in a decreased albumin: globulin (A:G) ratio (<0.6 gm/dl). Protein electrophoresis shows the typical "church steeple" narrow spike in either the β or γ distribution, often accompanied by a decreased albumin content if significant renal glomerular pathology is present.

In rare instances the total protein content and A:G ratio may be normal in a patient with multiple myeloma. However, serum protein electrophoresis may reveal a monoclonal spike indicating the presence of paraprotein insufficient at the time to cause elevation of total serum protein or total globulin content. Several explanations for the absence of a definite monoclonal spike in human multiple myeloma patients are reported (Gordon, 1977). It is possible that no appreciable amount of paraprotein is being produced by the tumor cells. Alternatively, in some instances, the tumor cells produce mainly light chain portions of immunoglobulin that are low in molecular weight and are often not detected on routine serum protein electrophoresis. Finally, it is possible that patients showing elevated serum globulin content may have an electrophoretic pattern that appears polyclonal in nature. Such a finding indicates that the tumor cells may in fact be producing more than one immunoglobulin type (heterogenous), or alternatively, a homogenous or single immunoglobulin type, such as IgA, may be present in several different polymer formations.

Routine urinalysis may show any number of abnormal findings, including proteinuria, isosthenuria, bacteriuria, pyuria, and proteinaceous or cellular cast formation. Strong positive protein reactions on routine urinalysis essentially indicate only the presence of albumin, even though larger molecular weight serum proteins can be present in cases with severe glomerular damage. Twenty-four-hour urine collection and cellulose acetate electrophoresis are used to determine protein loss quantitatively as well as qualitatively. Light chain portions of immunoglobulin, referred to as Bence-Jones proteins, can only be detected in the urine (in some cases), using the heat precipitation test or cellulose acetate electrophoresis. Concentration of the urine specimen at least twenty-fold prior to electrophoresis improves the capability of demonstrating Bence-Jones proteinuria.

Identification of the immunoglobulin class of the paraprotein requires immunoelectrophoresis of the patient's serum using monospecific antisera for each separate class of immunoglobulin. Quantitation of monoclonal as well as other immunoglobulins can be performed using methods such as the radial immunodiffusion (Mancini) test (Fig. 83–7). Patients with monoclonal hyperglobulinemia are often deficient in other immunoglobulin classes.

A bone marrow aspirate or biopsy is recommended in all cases of monoclonal hyperglobulinemia for both diagnostic and prognostic value. Identification of tumor cell infiltrate type has important implications in the therapeutic approach chosen. In addition, the status of myeloid, erythroid, and megakaryocyte production will have significance in both prognosis and modification of chemotherapy regimes that are particularly myelosuppressive.

Therapy and Prognosis. Treatment considerations in multiple myeloma and lymphoproliferative diseases include chemotherapy to reduce the tumor cell mass and reduction of the paraprotein level if severe complications due to hyperviscosity are present. A number of chemotherapy protocols have proven efficacious in the treatment of multiple myeloma. The author's preferred regime includes 0.5 mg/kg body weight prednisone per os divided in two doses daily, a single intravenous injection of cyclophosphamide given at 7 mg/kg at the start of chemotherapy, and 0.1 mg/kg melphalan per os once daily for the first ten days. The melphalan dose is then reduced

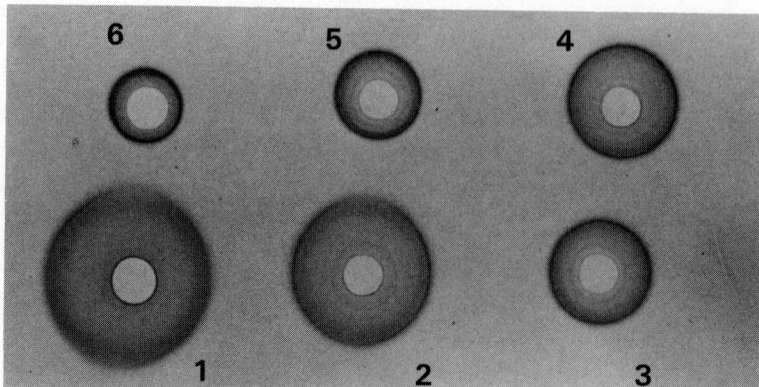

Figure 83–7. Radical immunodiffusion test for quantitation of serum IgG$_{2ab}$ levels in the canine multiple myeloma patient referred to in Fig. 83–6. IgG$_{2ab}$ concentration is determined by measuring the diameters of the precipitant ring using dilutions of the patient's serum (wells 1–3) and a control standard of known IgG$_{2ab}$ content (wells 4–6). Monospecific rabbit antisera to canine IgG$_{2ab}$ is incorporated into the gel agar poured over the glass surface of the slide.

to 0.05 mg/kg daily for one to two weeks followed by alternate day therapy at the same dose. Alterations in the chemotherapy regime are individualized according to the patient's response. Routine patient monitoring should include hemograms, periodic bone marrow aspirates, and assessments of renal, hepatic, and serum protein status. The reader is referred to Chapter 30 in this text for in-depth discussion of chemotherapeutic management.

Plasmapheresis or exchange blood transfusion can be resorted to in the event of life-threatening hyperviscosity syndrome in order to significantly reduce the paraprotein level rapidly. This approach is rarely necessary. Successful chemotherapy will often reduce the serum protein level appreciably within a period of weeks.

The prognosis for multiple myeloma in the dog is often favorable in comparison with other disseminated tumors. Response to chemotherapy can be rewarding even for patients with multisystemic involvement. Longevity in well managed cases can extend up to several years.

IMMUNODEFICIENCY SYNDROMES

Defective immunity can involve single or multiple facets of the *specific* (lymphocytic) or *nonspecific* (phagocytic) immune system. Both congenital (primary) and acquired immunodeficiency syndromes have been recognized. A number of primary immunodeficiency diseases reported in domestic animals (Table 83–2) have been compared with analogous, well characterized syndromes in man (Fudenberg, 1971; McGuire et al., 1974; Stevens and Osburn, 1976). Acquired immunodeficiency may be idiopathic, or secondary to chronic debilitating illness (e.g., neoplasia, microbial infections, and certain autoimmune disorders), failure of passive transfer of maternal antibodies in neonates, myelosuppressive or immunosuppressive drugs, radiation therapy, and malnutrition.

The incidence of primary deficiency of the *specific* immune system in the canine and feline population is unknown. Though there has been sparse documentation in the veterinary literature to date, immunodeficiency syndromes in these animals are currently receiving increased investigative attention. Recently, combined immuno-

deficiency in a line of basset hounds was described by Felsburg (1981). Affected pups were lymphopenic, hypoglobulinemic, stunted, and unthrifty, and succumbed to infectious illness by 16 weeks of age.

Several defects involving nonspecific immunity have been described. A bacteriocidal disorder, *canine granulocytopathy syndrome,* has been documented in an Irish setter showing fever, lymphadenitis, and recurrent bacterial infections associated with profound leukocytosis and defective neutrophil function (Renshaw et al., 1975). *Chediak-Higashi syndrome,* an inherited disorder of granule-containing cells (Table 83–2), has been reported in a number of animal species, including Persian cats (Kramer et al., 1975). Though characteristic eosinophilic cytoplasmic inclusions have been found in the neutrophils of affected cats, no clinical signs of increased susceptibility to infection have been reported thus far. *Cyclic neutropenia* of silver grey collies, the result of an inherited (autosomal recessive) cyclic maturation defect of granulocytes, causes recurrent infections and early death in affected pups (Lund et al., 1967).

Acquired immunodeficiencies are probably more frequently encountered in dogs and cats than the literature would suggest. Canine distemper virus has been shown to cause thymic atrophy, profound lymphoid depletion, lymphopenia, and depressed T-cell function (McCullough et al., 1974; Stevens and Osburn, 1976). Immunosuppression caused by feline leukemia virus infection is also described (Cockerell et al., 1976). Chronic pyogranulomatous infections caused by ubiquitous opportunistic organisms such as *Demodex canis* and a number of mycoses have been associated with depressed T-lymphocyte function *in vitro* (Barrett et al., 1977; Scott et al., 1976). In demodicosis, the degree of lymphocyte suppression seems to correlate with chronicity and dissemination of the infection, while elimination or remission of the infection restores *in vitro* lymphocyte function to normal. It appears that this generalized T-lymphocyte suppression is *acquired* secondary to dissemination of the infection and is associated with the presence of acquired suppressive factors, as yet poorly defined, in the patient's serum. The suggestion has been made that in canine demodicosis, a very specific, inherited T-cell defect limited

Table 83–2. Primary Immunodeficiency in Domestic Animals

Specific Immune System	Animal	Defective Cell Population	Immunopathologic Features	Mode of Inheritance	Analogous Human Disorder
Combined immunodeficiency (CID)	Arabian foals	B and T lymphocytes, pleuripotential stem cells	Thymic hypoplasia, lymphoid panhypoplasia, lymphopenia, hypoglobulinemia	Autosomal recessive	Swiss-type CID
Thymic hypoplasia and T-cell deficiency	Black pied Danish cattle	T Lymphocytes	Thymic hypoplasia, lymphoid hypoplasia, hyperglobulinemia	Autosomal recessive	DiGeorge's syndrome
Agammaglobulinemia	One equine	B Lymphocytes	Absence of germinal centers and primary follicles in spleen and lymph nodes; absence of B cells and immunoglobulins	N.R.*	Bruton's syndrome
Selective immunoglobulin deficiency	Red Danish cattle	B Lymphocytes	Deficient IgG$_2$	N.R.	Selective immunoglobulin deficiency
Transient (selective) hypoglobulinemia	Ovine	B Lymphocytes	Deficient IgG$_2$	N.R.	Transient hypoglobulinemia of infants
Transient hypoglobulinemia	Arabian foals	B Lymphocytes	Deficient IgG(T) and IgG until 4 mo. of age	N.R.	Transient hypoglobulinemia of infants
Nonspecific Immune System					
Canine granulocytopathy syndrome	Irish setters	Neutrophils	Marked neutrophilic leukocytosis with hypersegmentation; bactericidal defect	X-Linked	Granulocytopathy
Chediak-Higashi syndrome	Cattle Persian cats[a]	Neutrophils	Oculocutaneous albinism; platelet defect; eosinophilic (cytoplasmic) inclusions in PMN's	Autosomal recessive	Chediak-Higashi syndrome

a. Not associated with clinical signs
*Not reported

to the offending organism accounts for its pathogenicity, while a more generalized T-cell unresponsiveness is acquired as the organism disseminates (Scott et al., 1976).

Clinical Manifestations

Severe immunodeficiencies usually lead to early neonatal deaths or failure to survive to maturity. Bacterial pneumonia, gastrointestinal infection, and septicemia account for most of the early deaths, while unthriftiness and a variety of recurrent or chronic infections will manifest in animals who survive the neonatal period. Acquired immunodeficiency states can be seen at any age. Immunodeficiency should be considered when any of the following conditions are presented:

1. Early neonatal deaths occurring in litters sharing common parentage.

2. Chronic or recurrent infections that respond poorly to appropriate therapy or recur when therapy is discontinued.

3. Infections caused by organisms that are not usually pathogenic.

4. Instances of modified live vaccines such as those for rabies, canine distemper, or feline upper respiratory viruses that cause signs of those infections.

5. Properly managed wounds or abscesses that fail to heal.

6. Fever spikes or infection in patients receiving potentially myelotoxic or immunosuppressive drugs.

Diagnostic Tests

Increasing availability of laboratory support providing more complete immunodiagnostic capability in a clinical setting will undoubtedly lead to the identification and characterization of previously unrecognized immunodeficiency disorders in dogs and cats. To this end, there are a number of useful, yet practical, screening tests available to the practitioner who suspects a problem with immune competence. Supportive routine clinicopathologic findings include (1) severe, persistent lymphopenia ($<1000/mm^3$); (2) hypoglobulinemia (<2.5 gm/dl); (3) lymphoid depletion (germinal centers, paracortical regions) on lymph node biopsy; (4) decreased β- or γ-globulin fractions on serum protein electrophoresis; (5) persistent neutrophilic leukocytosis with hypersegmentation in young patients refractory to appropriate therapy for infection (phagocytic defects); and (6) failure to mount a neutrophilic leukocytosis in the face of infection (granulocytopenic disorders, chemotactic disorders).

A number of more specific immunodiagnostic tests are available to help elucidate the particular facets of immune response that are inadequate. The three basic categories of immune function tests include evaluation of humoral (B-cell), cell-mediated (T-cell), and nonspecific immunity.

Humoral Immunity. The distribution of immunoglobulins on a serum protein electrophoresis in dogs and cats favors the β and γ regions. A serum protein electrophoresis is not a particularly quantitative test for immunoglobulins, because only about 30 to 60 per cent of the proteins represented in both regions are actually immunoglobulins (Halliwell, 1978). Though hypoglobulinemia may be seen in some cases, in others the total globulin fractions may appear normal or even increased, masking a selective or even multiple immunoglobulin deficiency. More accurate assessment of immunoglobulin content is achieved by immunoelectrophoresis (IEP) and radial immunodiffusion (RID or Mancini).

IEP involves electrophoresis of a drop of serum placed in a well cut into agar gel on a glass slide. A drop of normal control serum is placed in a second well for comparison. A trough is cut across the center of the slide between the two wells and is filled with an antiserum specific for an antibody class or subclass. Following overnight incubation a precipitate will form in an arclike pattern, which is best visualized following staining with amido Schwartz stain. The IEP shows only the presence or absence of a particular antibody class (IgG, IgM, IgA, IgE) or subclass (such as canine IgG_1, IgG_{2ab}, IgG_{2c}), and a comparison of whether the patient's immunoglobulin is roughly equivalent, decreased, or increased compared with the normal control serum (Fig. 83–8).

The Mancini test provides more accurate quantitation of immunoglobulin concentration (Fig. 83–7). Wells are cut into an anti-sera-containing agar gel that has been poured on a glass surface. The anti-sera are again immunoglobulin class-specific. Individual wells are filled with any number

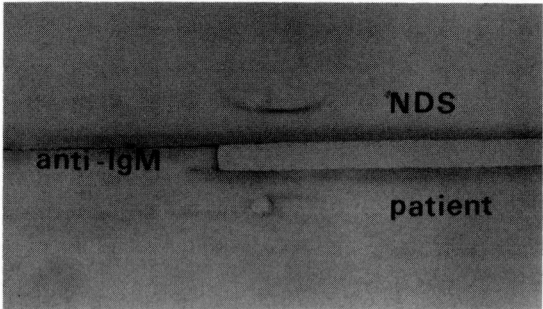

Figure 83–8. Immunoelectrophoresis on serum from the canine multiple myeloma patient referred to in Fig. 83–7 showing deficient levels of IgM compared to the normal dog serum (NDS). Deficiency of nonparaprotein immunoglobulins is not uncommon in multiple myeloma.

of patients' test sera, and the remaining wells are filled with dilutions of a purified immunoglobulin standard of known protein content. A ring of precipitate is formed around the wells, and the protein concentration (which is directly proportional to the square of the precipitant ring diameters) is determined using a curve plotted from measuring the ring diameters of the standard dilutions.

Though lymph node biopsy offers a morphologic evaluation of the presence of adequate or inadequate lymphocyte populations (cortical germinal centers are B-cell regions, while paracortical regions contain T cells), enumeration of peripheral blood lymphocytes (PBL) and lymphocyte function tests offer additional quantitative information. B-cell quantitation using either rosette formation or direct immunofluoresence (IFA) techniques is another method of evaluating humoral immunity. A certain percentage of B cells bear surface receptors for complement. This particular B-cell "surface marker" forms the basis for quantitating circulating B cells by rosette formation with antibody-coated (A) sheep red blood cells in the presence of complement (C). These A-C coated erythrocytes, termed EAC, will attach around the B lymphocyte membrane in rosette fashion (Fig. 83–9). In the cat 24 to 47 per cent, and in the dog 12 to 27 per cent, PBL have been shown to be EAC rosette-forming B cells (Cockerell et al., 1976; Atkinson et al., 1980). Enumeration of circulating B cells by IFA is possible, because all B lymphocytes bear surface immunoglobulin. Therefore, polyspecific antisera (against all immunoglobulin classes) that have been labeled with fluorescein will cause fluorescence of B cells under ultraviolet microscopy. Using this method, Schultz and Adams (1978) have reported B-cell values in the range of 10 to 20 per cent of PBL in dogs.

Lymphocyte stimulation tests (also called lymphocyte transformation [LT], lymphocyte blastogenesis, or lymphocyte blast transformation [LBT]) measure the ability of lymphocytes to undergo increased DNA synthesis and mitosis in response to individual antigens or more general, polyclonal stimulating substances called mitogens. Most mitogens are polysaccharide constituents of plant lectins or certain bacteria, and unlike antigens they have the unique property of being able to stimulate lymphocytes not previously exposed or sensitized to them. Transformed or stimulated lymphocytes will incorporate radiolabeled substrates such as tritiated thymidine during DNA synthesis, thus allowing quantitation of the degree of stimulation by scintillation spectrophotometry. Numerous methods of *in vitro* LT have been applied clinically in dogs and cats using purified peripheral blood lymphocytes (PBL). Pokeweed mitogen, a stimulator of both B cells and T cells, has been used to evaluate humoral immunity; however, some evidence suggests

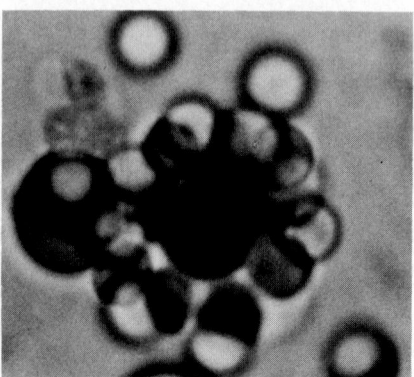

Figure 83–9. Canine EAC (B cell) rosette.

this mitogen is more T-cell–specific in cats (Taylor et al., 1975).

Immunization techniques are less often applied clinically, but they offer the advantage of evaluating *in vivo* antibody response to particular antigens. Antibody titers to distemper vaccine have been used as an indicator of humoral immune response in dogs (Stevens and Osburn, 1976).

Cell-Mediated Immunity. T lymphocytes in peripheral blood can be quantitated by both E rosette and IFA techniques. A small proportion of T cells (11 to 26 per cent of PBL) in cats has been shown to rosette spontaneously with guinea pig red blood cells (Cockerell et al., 1976). E rosette techniques using erythrocytes from various species have failed to provide reliable differentiation between B- and T-lymphocyte populations in dogs. As in other mammalian species, canine T lymphocytes contain a membrane antigen (termed theta) in common with thymic and cerebral cortical tissue (Kongshaven et al., 1973). Fluorescein-conjugated antibody to canine theta antigen has been used to detect T cells in PBL preparations in dogs. One study using this method identified 60 to 75 per cent of canine PBL as T lymphocytes (Schultz and Adams, 1978).

Lymphocyte transformation assays using mitogens specific for T-cell function have been used extensively as research tools in both dogs and cats. Until recently, the large quantities of blood and special requirements for such assays made lymphocyte transformation tests impractical, if not impossible, in a routine clinical setting. The development and standardization of a whole blood microtechnique for LT in small animal patients has minimized the quantity of blood required as well as the technical difficulty and expense, thus bridging the gap between research and clinical application (Felsburg et al., 1980).

Skin testing with antigens or mitogens for evaluation of cell-mediated immunity has received little attention as an applied diagnostic tool in dogs and cats. In one study, delayed hypersensitivity response to intradermal phytomitogens showed positive correlation with ability to survive challenge with virulent canine distemper virus (Krakowka et al., 1977). In general, correlation between *in vivo* and *in vitro* responses to T-cell stimulants is diabolic; nonetheless, this prospect deserves further study in vet-

erinary medicine as a practical screening test in a clinical setting.

Evaluation of the nonspecific immune system consists of neutrophil function tests, complement assays, and various chemotactic evaluations. The nitroblue tetrazolium test (NBT) for detecting neutrophil myeloperoxidase deficiency has been used in the dog, and various bactericidal assays are applicable to veterinary use. Complement and chemotactic assays have had little application in a clinical setting; however, these parameters are being evaluated in certain conditions, such as chronic pyoderma, systemic lupus erythematosus, and rheumatoid arthritis in the dog.

SYSTEMS REVIEW

THE MUSCULOSKELETAL SYSTEM

Immune-mediated diseases that affect the musculoskeletal system include rheumatoid-like arthritis in the dog, chronic progressive polyarthritis in the cat, systemic lupus erythematosus, canine myasthenia gravis, and both polyarthritis and polymyositis conditions of either species thought to be associated with immune complex (Type III) injury. The reader is referred to Chapter 84 for an in-depth review of immunologic joint disease.

Myasthenia Gravis

The immunologic basis for acquired myasthenia gravis in the dog has been a subject of speculation until recently. Convincing evidence exists currently that shows that the acquired form of this disease in dogs shares similar autoimmune etiology with acquired myasthenia gravis in humans (Lennon, 1978). These similarities include deficiency of acetylcholine (ACH) receptors, ACH receptor-antibody (IgG) complexes found in skeletal muscle, serum antibodies (IgG) reactive with soluble ACH receptor preparations, serum anti-striated muscle antibody, and coexistent mediastinal mass (thymoma) in some cases. The reader is referred to Chapter 36 for an in-depth discussion of myasthenia gravis.

Polymyositis

The immunologic basis for myositis conditions in dogs and cats remains conjectural at best. Polymyositis has been found in association with canine SLE and histopathologically resembles the vasculitis-type reactions associated with the Type III (immune complex) immunologic injury. Polymyositis can be cyclic, self-limited, or progressive in its course, and in most cases it is steroid responsive. Early stages of the disease are marked by fever, weakness, gait abnormalities, and occasionally lymphadenopathy. Signs referable to esophageal involvement (megaesophagus) are common, while involvement of pharyngeal and laryngeal muscles is less frequent. Muscles may be tense or swollen, and quite painful. Progressive atrophy often follows the acute stages.

As with any other suspected immune-mediated disease, underlying diseases — particularly of infectious origin — must be ruled out. Toxoplasmosis, usually seen in young dogs, is the most common infectious etiology. Elevations in muscle enzymes, creatine kinase, and aldolase are usually associated. Polymyositis necessitates consideration of SLE, and thus, an ANA test is indicated in addition to careful evaluation for the presence of other organ system manifestations of this disease, such as proteinuria and hematologic abnormalities. Histopathologically, the finding of cellular infiltrates of neutrophilic, lymphocytic-plasmacytic, or eosinophilic composition without evidence of microorganisms is suggestive of immune-mediated polymyositis. Eosinophilic myositis, which occurs most commonly in German shepherds and favors distribution to the muscles of mastication, has also been considered an immune-mediated myositis. Atrophic myositis involving the same muscle groups has been considered both a later sequela of eosinophilic myositis and a separate disease entity. Further study is needed to confirm the immunopathologic nature of these diseases.

RESPIRATORY SYSTEM

Immune-mediated respiratory conditions most frequently involve the Type I immunologic reaction that occurs upon the binding of allergen with IgE linked to the surface of mast cells in sensitized individuals. Species variations in the occurrence of allergic respiratory diseases may be due in part to differences in genetic predisposition and the tissue distribution of both mast cells and receptors for the various biologically active substances released from them.

A diagnosis of allergic rhinitis or bronchitis in dogs and cats is supported by the finding of eosinophils on nasal swabs, expectorated sputum, or tracheal washings. Allergic bronchitis is sometimes accompanied by a peripheral eosinophilia, as is pulmonary infiltrate with eosinophilia (PIE). Cytologic evaluations and culture on specimens obtained from swabs, washings, or biopsy should be routinely done to rule out allergic responses to parasitic, bacterial, or fungal agents. In the case of PIE, further etiologic considerations include visceral larval migrans, heartworm (occult) disease, and lung worms. Therefore, appropriate fecal examinations and heartworm testing are recommended in all cases of PIE. Environmental sources of inhaled allergens should be considered, and exposure minimized whenever possible. The reader is referred to Chapters 39 and 42 for further details on allergic respiratory disorders. Treatment must be individualized (often through trial and error) for each patient according to clinical response, whether or not an inciting agent can be found and eliminated by specific therapy. Adjunct therapy is aimed at minimizing the allergic response through judicious application of short-acting corticosteroids, antihistamines, bronchodilators, and expectorants.

NERVOUS SYSTEM

Distemper demyelinating encephalomyelitis has been linked with the presence of both viral antigen in white matter and anti-myelin antibodies. The role of the autoantibodies is uncertain, but an immune-mediated etiology for this disease has been implicated (Krakowka et al., 1973). It is uncertain whether the demyelination occurs as a result of the autoantibody or a cell-mediated (Type IV) reaction. Two demyelinating diseases in man, multiple sclerosis and subacute sclerosing panencephalitis, have been associated with the finding of measles antigen (a paramyxovirus related to distemper virus) in brain lesions.

Degenerative Myelopathy

Degenerative myelopathy of German shepherds, another demyelinating disease affecting the thoracic cord white matter most severely, has an unknown etiology at present. Recently, studies have shown depressed peripheral blood T-lymphocyte responses to mitogens in dogs with this disease (Waxman et al., 1980). The severity of the neurologic dysfunction correlates with the degree of depressed lymphocyte function. Depressed T-lymphocyte response in severely clinically affected dogs was associated with the presence of suppressor T cells. The significance of these findings is unknown, but the suggestion has been made that increased suppressor T-cell activity occurs as an attempt to suppress an aberrant autoimmune response. Similar abnormalities of suppressor T-cell function have been described in human patients with multiple sclerosis.

Acute Idiopathic Polyradiculoneuritis

Acute idiopathic polyradiculoneuritis (Coonhound paralysis) has been compared with a similar acute demyelinating polyradiculoneuritis (Guillain-Barré) syndrome in man, which is thought to be autoimmune in origin. Demyelination in both instances is associated with inflammatory infiltrates consisting primarily of lymphocytes, plasma cells, and other mononuclear cells.

GASTROINTESTINAL SYSTEM

Immunopathologic mechanisms of gastrointestinal disorders have not been well defined in domestic animals. Atrophic gastritis associated with the presence of anti-parietal cell antibody has been described in progeny from matings of dogs with SLE, suggesting an autoimmune etiology for the disorder (Quimby et al., 1978). Food allergy has been described in dogs and cats when dietary elimination resulted in alleviation of gastrointestinal or dermatologic signs of hypersensitivity. Histologic evidence of eosinophilic, plasmacytic, lymphocytic, or granulomatous type infiltrates tend to support an immunologic basis, in part, for a number of chronic inflammatory bowel disorders. In addition to food allergy, etiologic considerations include hypersensitivity reactions to parasitic, bacterial, protozoan, and mycotic organisms or their products. In most cases, no specific etiologic agent is found. In this instance, corticosteroids and dietary management are sometimes helpful.

Chronic Active Hepatitis

The term chronic active hepatitis refers to a characteristic histologic appearance rather than a particular etiology of liver disease. The histopathologic changes that can be seen include focal hepatocellular necrosis; periportal inflammatory infiltrates consisting of neutrophils, lymphocytes, and plasma cells; varying degrees of fibroplasia; and in some cases, cirrhosis. In man, it is thought that a number of hepatic insults, including hepatitis B virus, can result in a lingering chronic active hepatitis, which is perpetuated by an active and ongoing immunologic response to sequestered (hidden) hepatic antigens released during the initial insult. Immunologic injury, consisting of both cytolytic antibody (Type II) and cell-mediated (Type IV) cytotoxicity, perpetuates a vicious circle of hepatic necrosis, release of more antigen, and replacement of normal architecture with fibrous tissue.

Chronic active hepatitis is not an uncommon liver disease in dogs. It has been diagnosed in a number of cases with no apparent underlying etiology. Experimentally, the disease has been produced by challenging partially immune dogs with virulent canine hepatitis virus (Gocke et al., 1976). Recently, spontaneously occurring chronic active hepatitis was found in five dogs from a kennel infected with *Leptospira interrogans,* and spirochetes were demonstrated in hepatic tissue of four of the dogs (Bishop et al., 1979).

RENAL SYSTEM

The immunologic mechanisms of glomerular injury have been extensively studied experimentally and have provided a basis for our understanding of spontaneously occurring immune complex injury. When antibody reacts with antigen in a state of antigen excess, soluble macromolecular immune complexes circulate and accumulate along glomerular capillary walls. These complexes fix complement, producing increased capillary permeability, influx of neutrophils, endothelial damage, and cellular proliferation. The immune complexes move from their endothelial location to become situated in the subepithelial portion of the glomerulus. They are found as irregular dense deposits on electron microscopy, and on direct immunofluorescent microscopy they appear as granular or "lumpy-bumpy" deposits along the epithelial side of the glomerular basement membrane. When there is a continued source of antigen exposure under certain conditions of antibody response (antigen excess must be maintained), chronic glomerulonephritis results. Chronic glomerulonephritis has been reported extensively in domestic animals (Slauson and Lewis, 1979). In systemic lupus erythematosus, the antigen consists of endogenous nuclear factors, and the antibody is autoantibody against these factors. In cats, chronic immune complex glomerulonephritis has been associated with feline leukemia virus infection. In dogs, immune complex glomerulonephritis has been associated with a variety of underlying diseases, including dirofilariasis, canine adenovirus, neoplasia, pyometra, and systemic lupus erythematosus. Direct immunofluorescent techniques are used to determine the presence of IgG, complement (C3), and antigen in frozen sections of renal cortical tissue using fluorescein-conjugated antisera to each of these portions of the immune complex. Steroids have been used to treat this disease in dogs and cats, but there are no data to show that this therapy is effective. Successful elimination of underlying disease or infection may arrest the inflammatory process but will not reverse renal damage already present.

Autoantibodies with specificity against the glomerular basement membrane are known to cause glomerulonephritis in man. Characteristically, the pattern on direct immunofluorescence is linear or continuous along the glomerular capillary basement membrane. Although this pattern of fluorescence has been reported in canine glomerulonephritis, the presence of anti-basement membrane antibody has never been shown by indirect immunofluorescence using the patient's serum or by elution of autoantibody from renal tissue and reaction with normal canine glomeruli.

Polyarteritis Nodosa. Polyarteritis nodosa is a rare necrotizing inflammatory disease of small and medium-sized arterioles. Renal involvement without other systemic involvement has been described in two cats, while a third cat showed renal, pancreatic, myocardial, and thyroid gland involvement (Lucke, 1968). The disease has also been reported in dogs with associated glomerulonephritis. The exact etiology is unknown, but it is considered an immune complex vasculitis.

ENDOCRINE SYSTEM

Lymphocytic thyroiditis represents the best documented example of endocrine-related autoimmune disease in the dog. It has been studied most extensively in beagles and has been compared with Hashimoto's disease in middle-aged women (Mawdesley-Thomas, 1968; Manning, 1979). Histopathologically, focal clusters of lymphocytes and smaller numbers of plasma cells and macrophages are seen in association with follicular involution. Antibodies to thyroglobulin are detected using the tanned red cell hemagglutination test. Antibodies to thyroid microsomal antigen can be demonstrated using complement fixation or cytotoxicity tests.

The histopathologic finding of lymphocytic thyroiditis in dogs studied from breeding colonies is often unassociated with clinical or biochemical evidence of hypothyroidism. In addition, older dogs with clinical hypothyroidism often show no characteristic histopathology indicating the cause of thyroid atrophy. It is possible that lymphocytic thyroiditis precedes clinical hypothyroidism, making the etiologic diagnosis and incidence in the canine difficult to establish. In a recent survey, 12 of 25 hypothyroid dogs of various breeds had detectable serum antibodies against either thyroglobulin or thyroid microsomal antigen, or both (Gosselin et al., 1980). This survey included a second group of hypothyroid dogs and showed that 7 of 16 had histologic evidence of lymphocytic thyroiditis.

In man, Addison's disease is classified as an autoimmune disease. Studies linking Addison's disease in dogs and cats to autoimmune phenomena are lacking.

PHARMACOLOGIC MODULATION IN IMMUNE MEDIATED DISEASES

The approach to therapy of immunologic hypersensitivity diseases involves two major considerations. First is the elimination of offending exogenous antigens, whether they be environmental allergens, microorganisms, parasites, or chemical compounds. In many instances, no etiologic agent can be identified, while in others, such as viral infection, neoplasia, allergy, or autoimmune disease (endogenous antigens), it is not possible to eliminate the antigen(s) responsible for immunologic hypersensitivity. The second consideration in therapy applies to this latter group of hypersensitivity disorders. Here, pharmacologic modulation can be used to suppress the level of hypersensitivity by decreasing immune responsiveness, inflammation, and sequelae leading to tissue damage.

Approach to the treatment of immune-mediated diseases includes a variety of anti-inflammatory and immunosuppressive measures. Classically, corticosteroids and nonsteroidal anti-inflammatory drugs have been the mainstay. Failure to achieve satisfactory remission of the disease, side effects of prolonged steroid therapy, and tendency to relapse have long been frustrating consequences in the management of patients with immune-mediated disorders. Because exact etiologic mechanisms are at best poorly understood, and because the nature and progression of such diseases tend to vary considerably among individuals, it should be appreciated that there are no "foolproof" therapeutic modalities that allow the outcome for the patient to be predicted with any confidence. This ought not discourage the judicious administration of whatever treatment regime proves beneficial for the patient. It should, however, alert the clinician to become well informed about the indications, actions, and side effects of these drugs, and above all to avoid "cutting corners" (or client expense) by eliminating interim progress checks.

NONSTEROIDAL ANTI-INFLAMMATORY ANALGESICS

Drugs such as salicylates, phenylbutazone, and acetaminophen provide varying degrees of analgesia, antipyretic effect, and anti-inflammatory potency. Properly used, these drugs may be included as adjunct therapy in immune-mediated musculoskeletal disorders in dogs. It is important to remember that these drugs do not alter the underlying immunologic abnormalities or the progression of the disease. They merely suppress the fever, pain, and inflammation that account for many of the clinical signs. Clinical response to these drugs alone is unsatisfactory in many instances. Aspirin is contraindicated in patients with thrombocytopenia or aspirin intolerance (as in gastrointestinal upsets, bleeding tendency, and so forth). Acetaminophen and phenylbutazone are highly toxic in cats and should therefore be avoided. Aspirin administra-

tion in cats should not exceed 10 mg/kg body weight every three days, based on its prolonged half-life in this species (Davis, 1980). Another note of caution regards the use of some of the newer nonsteroidal anti-inflammatory drugs marketed for humans. Indomethacin and tolmetin have both been incriminated in fatal gastrointestinal ulceration and hemorrhage in dogs. Lastly, the nonsteroidal anti-inflammatory drugs all share similar potential side effects, and combination use is not recommended.

CORTICOSTEROIDS

Corticosteroids are the first drug of choice in the treatment of immune-mediated diseases in the absence of bacterial or mycotic infection. Glucocorticoids remain the most potent anti-inflammatory drug class available. In addition to the anti-inflammatory effects, steroids suppress the removal of immunologically "injured" hemopoietic cells by the reticuloendothelial (RE) system. Thus, they are particularly efficacious in AIHA, IMT, and SLE with autoantibodies against RBCs, WBCs, or platelets. The immunosuppressant effects of glucocorticoids are much less potent than those of the antimetabolites and alkylating agents discussed later. However, they produce a pronounced lymphopenia, depress autoantibody formation, and may reduce specific antigen-induced blastogenesis of lymphocytes (Pedersen, 1978). Other beneficial effects of glucocorticoids in immune-mediated diseases include macrophage inhibition, depression of serum complement, and interference with the passage of immune complexes through vascular basement membranes.

The recommended initial dose of short-acting glucocorticoid (prednisone, prednisolone) is 2 to 4 mg/kg body weight divided twice daily. Short-acting preparations are preferred, because the duration of their activity is similar to that of endogenous cortisol, thus allowing stricter dose manipulations (tapering and alternate day therapy) to avoid adrenal suppression and other undesirable effects. Because their effect is less prolonged, the dose can more readily be "titrated" to the minimal effective maintenance level. Duration of therapy must be established for each individual according to clinical response and tolerance to the drug. In general, daily doses at the starting level should be maintained until substantial progressive clinical improvement is seen. At that time, doses should be reduced by gradual decrements until the desired maintenance level is reached (approximately 0.5 to 1.0 mg/kg given as a single dose every other day). It is preferable to maintain steroid therapy (including initial, decremental, and alternate day schedules) over a period of at least 6 to 12 weeks to avoid relapsing clinical signs, which can prove increasingly refractory to treatment.

IMMUNOSUPPRESSIVE DRUGS

Drugs with potent inhibitory effects on immune responsiveness have been used in the treatment of human patients with immune-mediated disease over the past decade. Many of these drugs, which include the cytotoxic antimetabolites and alkylating agents, have become routine in the chemotherapy of a variety of neoplastic diseases in dogs and cats. Using modifications of dose regimes and drug combinations established for cancer patients, many veterinary clinicians are currently employing these drugs in combination with lowered steroid doses in the therapy of immunologic disorders that are poorly responsive to steroid therapy alone, or in cases in which steroid intolerance precludes its successful use in achieving and maintaining clinical remission. Steroid doses are reduced to 1.0 to 2.0 mg/kg body weight daily when used in combination with other immunosuppressive drugs and are tapered following remission as described previously.

Immunosuppressant drugs are not a panacea for the treatment of immune-mediated diseases, because they nonspecifically suppress immune responsiveness in general. Many patients with autoimmune disease are already compromised by inadequate or defective immune responsiveness, and are therefore at increased risk of acquiring infection. This risk is compounded further by the addition of potent immunosuppressants to the therapy regime. In addition, toxic side effects of these drugs make careful patient monitoring (including complete blood counts) mandatory throughout the interval of therapy. The clinician must include in the interim follow-up examinations tests that will quantitate beneficial as well as adverse effects, which include gastrointestinal disturbances, bone marrow suppression,

increased susceptibility to infection, hemorrhagic cystitis (cyclophosphamide), and neuromuscular weakness (vinca akaloids). Other potential side effects include reproductive failure and predisposition to neoplasia due to suppression of immune surveillance mechanisms.

Cyclophosphamide is an alkylating agent that suppresses both humoral and cell-mediated immunity by interfering with cell (lymphocyte) division through crosslinking with DNA. The end result may be cell death, or interference with blast transformation in response to antigenic stimulus. Cyclophosphamide has been used in combination with corticosteroids in the treatment of refractory cases of AIHA, IMT, RA, and SLE in the dog (Pederson, 1976 and 1978), and to a more limited extent in the cat. The dose is based on body surface area rather than weight. Approximate equivalents for the recommended oral dose of 50 mg/m^2 are as follows: >25 kg body weight: 1.5 mg/kg; 5 to 25 kg: 2.0 mg/kg; <5 kg: 2.5 mg/kg. This dose is given once daily for four consecutive days each week. Full dose therapy is continued until good clinical response is achieved (usually one to four weeks) and is then tapered over several weeks prior to discontinuing it altogether. Patients with renal or hepatic dysfunction should receive lower starting doses and be monitored frequently for adverse side effects.

Weekly examination and hemograms (including platelet counts) are recommended while the patient is on full dose therapy. A fall in the white blood cell count to less than 5000/mm^3 is indication for temporary discontinuation until the WBC returns to normal. At that time therapy should be resumed at lower (50 to 75 per cent of starting dose) levels. Platelet counts below 100,000/mm^3 are also cause for temporary withdrawal. Once the starting dose is tapered, examination intervals may be extended to two to three weeks.

Azathioprine is a thiopurine antimetabolite that inhibits immune response by substituting abnormal or "nonsense" bases in DNA synthesis, thus preventing cell division. In addition, it has an inhibitory effect on the inflammatory response. It is used in combination with steroids, with or without cyclophosphamide, most commonly in the treatment of RA and SLE in dogs and chronic progressive polyarthritis in cats. A safe beginning dose is 2 mg/kg body weight per os given once daily. The dose can be tapered in tandem with decreasing doses of corticosteroid, so that the maintenance dose (0.5 to 1.0 mg/kg) is given every other day, on the day that steroid is not given. Hemopoietic side effects are essentially the same as for cyclophosphamide, but it is a relatively safer drug.

The *vinca alkaloids*, vincristine and vinblastine, arrest cell division by inhibiting microtubule formation in the mitotic spindle. They have much less immunosuppressive potency than the alkylating and antimetabolite agents. They do have application, however, in the adjunct therapy of refractory IMT, because of a megakaryocyte stimulating effect on bone marrow. The dose of vincristine is 0.02 mg/kg body weight IV once weekly in combination with steroid therapy. The vincristine should be discontinued when platelet counts return to normal, and no more than six to eight consecutive weekly injections are recommended. This drug has proven beneficial in steroid refractory cases of IMT when bone marrow showed megakaryocyte hypoplasia. Prolonged administration can result in bone marrow suppression, however.

Methotrexate is a folic acid analog that produces a metabolic blockade in thymidine synthesis, thus halting DNA replication and cell proliferation in actively dividing, but not in resting, cells. It has been useful in the treatment of steroid refractory polymyositis, uveitis, pemphigus, and thyroiditis in man. Its use in similar diseases in the dog has not been reported. Side effects include gastrointestinal complaints, which can be severe, and bone marrow suppression. Both of these can be prevented with the use of folinic acid supplementation during the treatment interval. Cost and inexperience make this drug a less favorable choice at present, but the potential for its use should not be overlooked.

TYPE I HYPERSENSITIVITY

Corticosteroids remain prominent in the therapy of allergic diseases. Initial starting doses of shorter-acting steroids such as prednisone or prednisolone are recommended at 2 to 4 mg/kg body weight in two divided doses daily until significant alleviation of clinical signs occurs. At that time gradual tapering to the minimum effective dose given on an alternate-day basis is rec-

ommended. An aerosol corticosteroid preparation related to prednisolone, called betamethasone, has replaced the widespread use of systemic corticosteroids in responding human patients with allergic upper respiratory disease. Although it is absorbed by mucous membranes, the systemic concentrations are considerably less than with oral preparations, while the local concentrations achieved are quite high. Unfortunately, the application of aerosol therapy in dogs and cats is at best limited by the difficulty in administering sprays that require patient cooperation.

Antihistamines have met with varying degrees of clinical response but appear to be unsuccessful when used alone to control allergic symptoms. Blocking of histamine (H_1) receptors is inefficient in the face of ongoing degranulation of mast cells and has no blocking effect whatsoever against other chemical mediators, some of which may be more important in the perpetuation of clinical signs than histamine itself.

Cromolyn sodium and related compounds that prevent the degranulation of mast cells when given prior to allergen exposure have not been investigated for use in small animals. Severe toxic reactions have resulted from the use of intravenous preparations of this drug in dogs. The drug is currently being evaluated in horses with chronic obstructive pulmonary disease.

Hyposensitization techniques have not been investigated in canine or feline allergic respiratory disease. The reader is referred to Chapter 82 for a discussion of hyposensitization therapy in inhalant allergic dermatitis.

IMMUNOSTIMULATION THERAPY

Though a number of chemical and biological compounds are being investigated for their ability to "reconstitute" or stimulate defective immunity, it is premature to make meaningful comment on their clinical application. Compounds such as levamisole and thiobendazole are being investigated for their potential use in immunodeficiency disorders, as well as certain autoimmune diseases, including SLE and RA (levamisole). Lymphocyte-derived substances such as transfer factor and interferon are also a new area of interest in the search for improved therapy modalities for immunodeficiency.

REFERENCES

Atkinson, K., Deeg, H. J., et al.: Canine lymphocyte subpopulations. Exp. Hematol. 8:821–829, 1980.

Barrett, R. E., Hoffer, R. E., and Schultz, R. D.: Treatment and immunological evaluation of three cases of canine aspergillosis. J.A.A.H.A. 13:328–334, 1977.

Bishop, L., Strandberg, J. D., et al.: Chronic active hepatitis in dogs associated with leptospires. Am. J. Vet. Res. 40:839–844, 1979.

Cockerell, G. L., Krakowka, S., et al.: Characterization of feline B- and T-lymphocytes and identification of an experimentally induced cell neoplasm in the cat. J. Natl. Cancer Inst. 57:907–910, 1976a.

Cockerell, G. L., Hoover, E. A., et al.: Lymphocyte mitogen reactivity and enumeration of circulating B- and T- cells during feline leukemia virus infection in the cat. J. Natl. Cancer Inst. 57:1095–1099, 1976b.

Coombs, R. R. A., Mourant, A. E., and Race, R. R.: A new test for the detection of weak and "incomplete" Rh agglutinins. Br. J. Exp. Pathol. 26:255, 1945.

Davis, L. E.: Clinical pharmacology of salicylates. J.A.V.M.A. 176:65–66, 1980.

Dewhirst, M. W., Stamp, G. L., and Hurvitz, A. I.: Idiopathic monoclonal (IgA) gammopathy in a dog. J.A.V.M.A. 170:1313–1316, 1977.

Drazner, F. H.: Systemic lupus erythematosus in the dog. Comp. Cont. Ed. Vol. II, No. 3, pp. 243–253, 1980.

Dubois, E. L.: Lupus Erythematosus II. University of Southern California Press, Los Angeles, 1974.

Ehrlick, P., and Morgenroth, J.: Ueber Haemolysine. Berl. Kin. Wochenschr. 37:453, 1900.

Felsburg, P. J., Reilley, M. T., and Sinnigen, J. K.: A rapid microtechnique for in vitro stimulation of canine lymphocytes using whole blood. Vet. Immunol. Immunopathol. 1:251–262, 1980.

Felsburg, P. J.: Unpublished data, 1981.

Frick, O. L.: Experimental asthma in the dog. Seminar Synopsis, 41st Annual A.A.H.A. Meeting, 1974.

Fudenberg, H., et al.: Primary immunodeficiencies. Report of a World Health Organization Committee. Pediatrics 47:927–946, 1971.

Gell, P. G. H., and Coombs, R. R. A.: Clinical Aspects of Immunology. Blackwell, Oxford, 1968, pp. 575–594.

Gocke, D. J., Morris, T. Q., and Bradley, S. E.: Chronic active hepatitis in a dog. J.A.V.M.A. 169:802–804, 1976.

Gordon, D. S.: Immunoglobulin quantitation and characterization as a diagnostic tool. South. Med. J. 170:236–239, 1977.

Gosselin, S. J., Capen, C. C., and Martin, S. L.: Biochemical and immunological investigation of hypothyroidism in dogs. Can. J. Comp. Med. 44:158–168, 1980.

Halliwell, R. E. W.: Autoimmune disease in the dog. Adv. Vet. Sci. Comp. Med. 22:221–263, 1978.

Halliwell, R. E. W.: The diagnostic value of serum electrophoresis. Small Anim. Vet. Update Ser. 6; Vet. Pub. Inc., Princeton, N. J., 1978.

Horowitz, D. A., and Coursar, J. B.: A relationship between impaired cellular immunity, humoral suppression of lymphocyte function, and severity of systemic lupus erythematosus. Am. J. Med. 58:829–835, 1975.

Hurvitz, A. I., MacEwen, E. G., et al.: Monoclonal cryoglobulinemia with macroglobulinemia in a dog. J.A.V.M.A. 170:511–513, 1977.

Kongshaven, P. A. L., et al.: Ability of anti-brain heteroantisera to distinguish thymus-derived lymphocytes in various species. Clin. Immunol. Immunopathol. 3:1–15, 1974.

Krakauer, R. S., et al.: Loss of suppressor T cells in adult NZB/NZW mice. J. Exp. Med. 144:662–673, 1976.

Krakowka, S., Cockerell, G., and Koestner, A.: Intradermal mitogen response in dogs: Correlation with outcome of infection by canine distemper virus. Am. J. Vet. Res. 38:1539–1542, 1977.

Krakowka, S., McCullough, B., Koestner, A., and Olsen, R.: Myelin-specific autoantibodies associated with CNS demyelination in canine distemper virus infection. Infect. Immunol. 8:819, 1973.

Kramer, J. W., Davis, W. C., et al.: An inherited disorder of persian cats with intracytoplasmic inclusions in neutrophils. J.A.V.M.A. 166:1103–1104, 1975.

Lachman, P. J.: A two-stage indirect L.E. cell test. Immunology 4:153, 1961.

Lennon, V. A.: Myasthenia Gravis in Dogs: Acetylcholine Receptor Deficiency With and Without Antireceptor Autoantibodies. In Rose, N. R., and Bigazzi, P. E. (eds.): Genetic Control of Autoimmune Disease. Elsevier, North Holland, 1978.

Lewis, R. M., and Schwartz, R. S.: Canine systemic lupus erythematosus: genetic analysis of an established breeding colony. J. Exp. Med. 134:417, 1971.

Lewis, R. M., Henry, W. B., Thornton, G. W., et al.: A syndrome of autoimmune hemolytic anemia and thrombocytopenia in the dog. J.A.V.M.A. 1:140, 1963.

Lucke, F. M.: Renal polyarteritis nodosa in the cat. J. Pathol. 95:67–91, 1968.

Lund, J. E., Padgett, G. A., and Ott, R. L.: Cyclic neutropenia in grey collie dogs. Blood 29:452, 1967.

MacEwen, E. G., Hurvitz, A. I., and Hayes, A.: Hyperviscosity syndrome associated with lymphocytic leukemia in three dogs. J.A.V.M.A. 170:1309–1316, 1977.

Manning, P. J.: Thyroid gland and arterial lesions of beagles with familial hyperthyroidism and hyperlipoproteinemia. A.J.V.R. 40:820–828, 1979.

Mawdesley-Thomas, L. E.: Lymphocytic thyroiditis in the dog. J. Small Anim. Pract. 9:539–550, 1968.

McCullough, B., Krakowka, S., and Koestner, A.: Experimental canine distemper virus-induced lymphoid depletion. Am. J. Pathol. 74:155–169, 1974.

McGuire, T. C., Poppie, M. J., and Banks, K. C.: Combined (B- and T-lymphocyte) immunodeficiency: A fatal genetic disease in arabian foals. J.A.V.M.A. 164:70–76, 1974.

Pedersen, N. C.: Immunosuppressive drugs and their role in the treatment of immunologic diseases in the dog. Gaines Symposium, Tuskeegee, Ala., 1978.

Pedersen, N. C., Weisner, K., Castles, J. J., et al.: Noninfectious canine arthritis: the inflammatory, nonerosive arthritides. J.A.V.M.A. 169:304, 1976.

Pedersen, N. C., Pool, R. C., Castles, J. J., et al.:

Noninfectious canine arthritis: rheumatoid arthritis. J.A.V.M.A. *169*:295, 1976.

Renshaw, H. W., Chatburn, C., et al.: Canine granulocytopathy syndrome: Neutrophil dysfunction in a dog with recurrent infections. J.A.V.M.A. *166*:443–447, 1975.

Rogers, T. J., and Balish, E.: Suppression of lymphocyte blastogenesis by *Candida albicans*. Clin. Immunol. Immunopathol. *10*:298–305, 1978.

Schalm, O. W.: Autoimmune hemolytic anemia in the dog. Canine Pract. *2*:37–45, 1975.

Schultz, R. D., and Adams, L. S.: Immunologic detection of humoral and cellular immunity. Vet. Clin. North Am. *8*(No. 4):721–753, 1978.

Scott, D. W., Haupt, K. H., Knowlton, B. F., and Lewis, R. M.: A glucocorticoid responsive dermatitis in cats, resembling systemic lupus erythematosus in man. J.A.A.H.A. *15*:157–171, 1979.

Scott, D. W., Schultz, R. D., and Baker, E.: Further studies on the therapeutic and immunologic aspects of generalized demodectic mange in the dog. J.A.A.H.A. *12*:203–213, 1976.

Scott, D. W., Schultz, R. D., Post, J. E., et al.: Autoimmune hemolytic anemia in the cat. J.A.A.H.A. *9*:530–539, 1973.

Slauson, D. O., and Lewis, R. M.: Comparative pathology of glomerulonephritis in animals. Vet. Pathol. *16*:135–164, 1979.

Stevens, D. R., and Osburn, B. I.: Immune deficiency in a dog with distemper. J.A.V.M.A. *168*:493–498, 1976.

Taylor, D., Hikama, Y., and Perri, S. F.: Differentiating feline T and B lymphocytes by rosette formation. J. Immunol. *115*:862–865, 1975.

Tizzard, I. R.: An Introduction to Veterinary Immunology. W. B. Saunders Co., Philadelphia, 1977, p. 72.

Waxman, F. J., Clemmons, R. M., and Hinrichs, D. J.: Progressive myelopathy in older German shepherd dogs. J. Immunol. *124*:1216–1222, 1980.

Wilkins, R. J., Hurvitz, A. I., and Dodds-Laffin, W. J.: Immunologically mediated thrombocytopenia in the dog. J.A.V.M.A. *163*:277, 1973.

SECTION XVI

Joint and Skeletal Disorders

CHAPTER 84

NIELS C. PEDERSEN,
ROY R. POOL,
and JOE P. MORGAN

Joint Diseases of Dogs and Cats

Disorders involving joints are etiologically diverse, as shown by Table 84–1. The outline of joint disease presented in this table will be used as a basis for the following discussion.

NONINFLAMMATORY JOINT DISEASE

Noninflammatory joint disorders are characterized by normal or near normal synovial fluid, and no systemic signs of illness such as depression, malaise, anorexia, fever, leukocytosis, hyperfibrinogenemia, or elevated erythrocyte sedimentation rate. Included in this group of disorders are degenerative joint disease (primary or secondary), traumatic joint disease, cruciate ligament and meniscal disorders, luxations and subluxations, neuropathic arthropathies, developmental arthropathies, arthropathies secondary to inborn errors of metabolism, dietary arthropathies, and neoplasms involving the joints.

DEGENERATIVE JOINT DISEASE (OSTEOARTHRITIS, OSTEOARTHROSIS)

The term degenerative joint disease has gradually replaced the term osteoarthritis in common usage (Olsson, 1971). The name osteoarthritis implies that the condition is inflammatory in nature; however, degenerative changes occur initially in the cartilage in the absence of inflammation. The term osteoarthrosis, which is widely used in Europe, recognizes the noninflammatory nature of the disorder, yet retains the concept that it is a disease that ultimately involves both cartilage and associated bone.

Degenerative joint disease is the most common noninflammatory arthropathy of man and animals. It is particularly frequent in dogs (Alexander, 1979) but occurs in some older cats. This disorder is more likely, however, to be clinically manifested in the dog than the cat. Degenerative joint disease is mainly a disorder of movable joints. It is characterized grossly by fragmentation and loss of articular cartilage, and radiographically by narrowing of the joint space, sclerosis of subchondral bone, and osteophyte production at the joint margins (Olsson, 1971).

Primary Degenerative Joint Disease

The term "primary" implies that this is a specific disease syndrome that develops in the joints for no precise reason. In this sense, idiopathic degenerative joint disease might be a more correct term, because it is assumed that all cases are due to one or more unrecognized factors. Nevertheless, the term is engrained in usage and in the literature, and it will be used here to describe degenerative joint disease that occurs without readily identifiable cause.

Primary degenerative joint disease becomes increasingly more prevalent with age, usually in dogs and cats aged ten years or older. It is due ultimately to the limited ability of cartilage to regenerate and maintain itself in the face of the cumulative effects of aging, wear and trauma, genetic predisposition, and other unknown factors. Primary degenerative joint disease is not always clinically apparent; discoloration and fibrillation of articular cartilage with lipping are also commonly identified in older dogs and cats even though signs of lameness may not be noticeable. One study of the canine stifle joint revealed that 20 per cent of randomly selected dogs had degenerative joint disease at autopsy; of these dogs, 61 per cent had no identifiable predisposing cause (Tirgari and Vaughn, 1975). Two different studies have also concluded that primary degenerative joint disease is a common entity involving the shoulder joint of old dogs, both large and small in stature (Ljunggren and Olsson, 1975; Tirgari and Vaughan, 1975). A similar, but less frequent, disorder has been observed in the elbow joint of dogs (Ljunggren and Olsson, 1975). The authors have also seen dogs and cats examined because of stiffness or lameness that appeared insidiously with age, tended to involve large weight-bearing joints, and had radiographic signs characteristic of degenerative joint disease. These animals did not have clinical, anatomic, or radiographic evidence of predisposing problems.

Secondary Degenerative Joint Disease

Secondary degenerative joint disease is a more common cause of clinical lameness in dogs and cats than the primary form. In man, it has been recognized that degenerative changes can result basically from either abnormal force on normal joints or from normal force on abnormal joints (Mitchell and Cruess, 1977). With this in mind, Mitchell and Cruess (1977) classified the causes of degenerative joint disease in man, and this classification can be modified somewhat and applied to dogs and cats (Table 84–1). Although oversimplified, such a classification has the advantage of emphasizing the basic pathophysiology of the disease. The net result of the various disorders, listed in Table 84–2, is to hasten the rate of cartilage loss, stimulate marginal bone production, and damage the synovial lining. Because many of these predisposing conditions can themselves be manifested as lameness or gait abnormalities in the early stages before degenerative changes occur, they will be covered in more detail as separate entities.

Table 84–1. Classification of Joint Disorders of the Dog and Cat

I. Noninflammatory Joint Disease
  A. Degenerative joint disease
    1. Primary
    2. Secondary
  B. Traumatic joint disease
    1. Damage of articular cartilage
    2. Damage to soft tissue supporting the joint
  C. Meniscal disorders and cruciate ligament rupture
    1. Rupture of cruciate ligaments
    2. Meniscal problems
      a. Meniscal tears
      b. Meniscal calcification
      c. Discoid meniscus
  D. Luxations and subluxations
  E. Neuropathic arthropathies
  F. Developmental arthropathies
    1. Conformational abnormalities
    2. Chondrodystrophy
    3. Physeal disorders
    4. Limb shortening
    5. Osteochondrosis
    6. Ununited coronoid and anconeal processes
    7. Hypoplasia of the coronoid process
    8. Ectopic ossification centers
    9. Hip dysplasia
    10. Patellar luxations
    11. Aseptic necrosis
  G. Arthropathies due to inborn errors of metabolism
    1. Hemophilia A
    2. Mucopolysaccharidosis
    3. Multicentric periarticular calcinosis
  H. Dietary arthropathies
    1. Secondary hyperparathyroidism
    2. Hypervitaminosis A

  I. Neoplastic arthropathies
    1. Primary
      a. Synovioma
    2. Metastatic
      a. Lymphosarcoma
II. Inflammatory Joint Disease
  A. Infectious arthritis
    1. Bacterial
    2. Mycoplasmal arthritis
    3. Viral arthritis
    4. Fungal arthritis
    5. Protozoal arthritis
  B. Noninfectious
    1. Immunologic
      a. Erosive arthritis
        (1) Canine rheumatoid arthritis
        (2) Polyarthritis of greyhounds
        (3) Feline chronic progressive polyarthritis
      b. Periosteal proliferative arthritis
        (1) Feline chronic progressive polyarthritis
      c. Nonerosive arthritis
        (1) Idiopathic nondeforming polyarthritis
        (2) Nondeforming polyarthritis associated with chronic infectious diseases
        (3) Systemic lupus erythematosus
        (4) Enteropathic arthritis
        (5) Plasmacytic-lymphocytic synovitis
        (6) Polyarteritis nodosa
    2. Crystal-induced arthropathies
      a. Gout
      b. Pseudogout

Table 84–2. Conditions That Predispose to Degenerative Joint Disease

I. Abnormal Concentration or Direction of Force on Normal Articulation
  A. Malalignment (intra-articular cause)
    1. Epiphyseal malformation
      a. Post-traumatic
      b. Congenital
    2. Hip dysplasia
    3. Ligamentous
      a. Ruptured cruciate ligament
      b. Ruptured teres ligament
  B. Malalignment (extra-articular cause)
    1. Inequality of leg length (acquired, congenital)
    2. Achondroplasia
    3. Congenital valgus or varus deformities
    4. Fractures with healing in a malaligned position
    5. Premature epiphyseal closures, e.g., radius curvus
    6. Acquired carpal and tarsal subluxations and luxations
  C. Loss of protective sensory reflexes
    1. Neuroarthropathy
    2. Repeated intra-articular injections of steroids
  D. Miscellaneous
    1. Obesity
    2. Excessive activity (working dogs, e.g., cattle or sheep dogs, hunting dogs, racing dogs, sled dogs)
II. Normal Concentration of Force on Abnormal Articulation
  A. Normal concentration of force on abnormal cartilage
    1. Osteochondrosis
    2. Transchondral fractures
    3. Meniscal tears, discoid menisci, meniscal calcification
    4. Loose bodies in joint
    5. Preexisting arthritis (septic, immunologic, chronic hemarthrosis)
    6. Metabolic abnormalities (chondrocalcinosis, mucopolysaccharidosis, hypervitaminosis A)
  B. Normal concentration of force on normal cartilage supported by weakened subchondral bone
    1. Osteonecrosis (aseptic necrosis, osteomyelitis)
    2. Osteoporosis
    3. Osteomalacia
    4. Osteitis fibrosa (primary or secondary hyperparathyroidism, pseudo-hyperparathyroidism)
  C. Normal concentration of force on normal cartilage supported by stiffened subchondral bone

Clinical Signs of Degenerative Joint Disease

The clinical signs of degenerative joint disease in dogs and cats are similar, regardless of whether the disorder is primary or secondary. In cases that are secondary to some predisposing cause, lameness and gait abnormalities may precede signs referable to degenerative joint disease by months or years. The earliest sign of degenerative joint disease is a reluctance of the animal to perform certain tasks or maneuvers, without more obvious signs of stiffness or lameness. In the next stage, lameness and stiffness may occur following periods of sustained activity or after brief overexer-

tion. After several days of rest, the clinical signs often disappear. As the degeneration becomes more severe, stiffness may be most pronounced following periods of rest, and with movement the animals appear to "warm out" of their lameness or stiffness. Cold and damp weather often increases the severity of clinical signs. In the final stages of the disease, stiffness and lameness are fairly constant features, although the severity of signs may still be influenced by environmental factors. Dogs may show signs of increased irritability and reclusiveness, and may snap or bite when approached or touched. Unfortunately, this type of behavior is often directed against children. The owners may not appreciate that the continuous pain caused by the joint disease is responsible for the abnormal behavior.

Marked gross deformities of the joints are uncommon in primary degenerative joint disease. In contrast, animals with predisposing congenital or acquired deformities often develop pronounced gross joint changes. Gross deformities consist of an increase in the dimensions of the joint due to the marginal new bone formation and thickening of the joint capsule. Destruction of articular surfaces and ankylosis of the joint are uncommon. Palpable swelling of the joints due to effusions can occur in larger dogs with severe arthritis, but are uncommon in smaller dogs and cats. Redness and heat in the area of the joint are not present. Restrictions in the range of motion of the joint can occur, and crepitus can be frequently detected in advanced cases.

Radiographic Signs of Degenerative Joint Disease

Regardless of etiology, the characteristic radiographic features of degenerative joint disease are narrowing of the joint spaces, eburnation of the subchondral bone, formation of subchondral bone cysts, formation of spurs or "lipping" of the joint margins, subluxation, attrition or wearing away of subchondral bone, remodeling of adjacent bones, and intra- or periarticular calcification or ossification, including formation of synovial osteochondromas (Morgan, 1969b) (Fig. 84–1).

The manner of presentation of the radiographic changes is dependent on the joint involved. The hip joint is a ball and socket

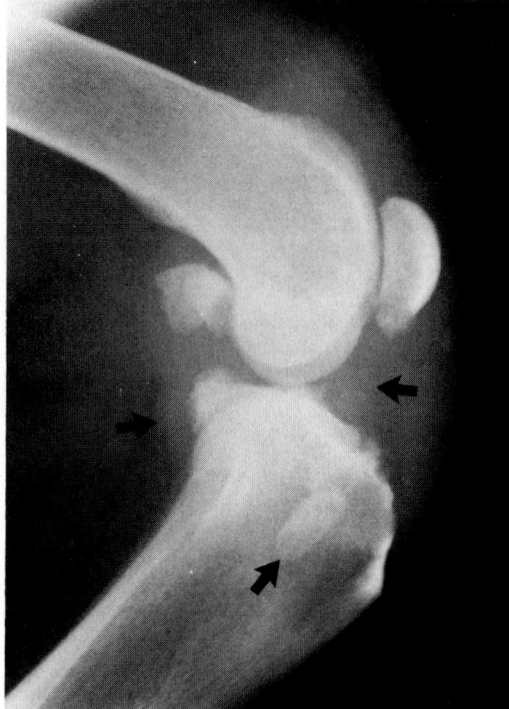

Figure 84–1. A lateral radiograph of the stifle joint of an older dog with secondary joint disease. Radiographic signs seen most clearly are thickening of the joint capsule (arrow) with joint effusion in the area of the fat pad just caudal to the patellar ligament (arrow). Periarticular new bone is noted on the distal patella and tibial plateau. Soft tissue calcification is noted lateral to the proximal tibia (arrow). Subchondral sclerosis is present but difficult to evaluate in this single projection.

that is easily positioned for radiographic examination, and the changes involving the head and acetabulum are easily seen. Because of changes in weight-bearing, the femoral neck becomes involved early in the disease process. In contrast, the radial-carpal joint has motion in only one plane and manifests only limited radiographic changes; the width of the joint space is difficult to evaluate, and changes in the subchondral bone may be minimal. Likewise, other joints have specific patterns of presentation of changes associated with degenerative joint disease.

Eburnation, or increased density of subchondral bone, is a prominent finding of degenerative joint disease and indicates that articular cartilage is wearing thin. Subchondral bone increases in order to assume stress that had previously been absorbed by the cartilage. This change can be visualized irre-

spective of positioning for the radiographic study, and may be uniform in distribution or limited to one part of the subchondral bone.

Narrowing of the joint space is a second finding of importance. Unless the degree of change is severe, however, narrowing may only be noted in dogs on weight-bearing or simulated weight-bearing studies. The joint space may narrow (1) equally throughout the joint or (2) more prominently on one side of the joint. The degree of narrowing can become so severe that there is actual contact between the two opposing surfaces of subchondral bone, with no interposed cartilage present.

Subchondral cysts are frequently noted in degenerative joint disease in horses and other large animals but are infrequently noted in small animals. The cysts vary in size but may reach a centimeter in diameter. The cysts have a very sharp border, and the surrounding subchondral bone is normal in appearance. Frequently the cysts appear to open into the joint space, while in other cases there appears to be a thin layer of subchondral bone between the cyst and the joint space.

Another characteristic feature of degenerative joint disease is periarticular lipping. There is not, however, always a close relationship between the severity of periarticular lipping and articular cartilage damage. It is possible to have periarticular osteophytes without any major joint cartilage damage or change in the subchondral bone (Marshall, 1969).

Another feature of degenerative joint disease, particularly noted in the stifle joint of dogs, is subluxation or joint instability. The degree of instability or subluxation is much more obvious in weight-bearing than nonweight-bearing studies. Different degrees of subluxation can be present. The simplest is a lateral or medial shifting of the bone; a reactive periarticular bone spur forms in an effort to provide some stabilization of the joint. It has been suggested that instability is the initiating factor in osteophyte formation. In addition to a simple lateral or medial displacement, a degree of rotation is often noted. These findings in the stifle joint may be related to concomitant injury to the ligaments or menisci.

Attrition or wearing away of subchondral bone can be seen on the weight-bearing surfaces in cases of severe disease. Attrition of bone is considered to be a radiographic finding indicative of severe degenerative joint disease.

Remodeling of the adjacent bone is infrequent in small animals but a common finding in degenerative joint disease of horses. This results from alterations in the lines of stress in the bones and is usually associated with an increase in width of both subchondral and cortical bone on one side. The shadow of the cortical bone on the opposite side is thinner than usual, indicating a decrease in the lines of stress imposed through that part of the bone.

Intra- or periarticular calcification is a common finding associated with degenerative joint disease of long duration. It is usually associated with the synovial membrane, although it may be within the joint capsule or within intra-articular tendons. The significance of calcified tissues without other radiographic findings of degenerative joint disease is less definite. Many calcified nodules represent foci of cartilaginous metaplasia in the synovium that undergo endochondral ossification to form synovial osteochondromas, while others are possibly chip fractures.

In cases of advanced degenerative joint disease, especially involving the hip joint of the dog, radiographic changes are so extensive that the original cause of the joint disease — e.g., hip dysplasia, aseptic necrosis, or acetabular fracture — is difficult to determine.

Pathologic Findings

The earliest lesions seen in an affected joint present as an area of dullness in the articular cartilage accompanied by a color change from the normal flat-white of mature cartilage to a mottled gray-white or yellow hue. Irregular fissure lines (Fig. 84–2) or a velvety disruption (Fig. 84–3) of the articular surface may be grossly visible. As the articular cartilage deteriorates, the mechanical forces of weight bearing and movement are transferred directly to the underlying subchondral bone. The underlying subchondral bone reacts by becoming thicker and denser (sclerosis) (Fig. 84–4).

Changes in the joint capsule of dogs and cats with degenerative joint disease are stereotyped. There is a generalized increase

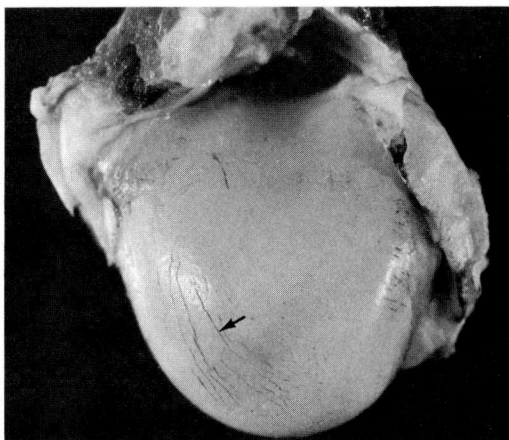

Figure 84–2. Proximal humerus of an older dog with primary degenerative joint disease. Fissures (arrow) in the surface were emphasized by rubbing the articular cartilage with carbon.

in fibrous connective tissue in the synovium. Condensations of collagen occur immediately beneath the surface layer of the synovium, and there is collagenization of the adventitia of the small caliber vessels that form the superficial plexus in the synovium. Hyalinization of the subsynovial connective tissue with chondroid metaplasia and dystrophic calcification are sometimes present. These changes are not necessarily accompanying features of degenerative joint disease; identical changes can also be seen in the joint capsule of aging animals without changes in the joint surfaces. Villous hypertrophy occurs more commonly in larger dogs and mainly in more proximal joints that are severely affected. Inflammation in the synovium is absent or mild. Mild chronic inflammatory changes can be centered around cartilaginous debris in the synovial recesses. Hemorrhage into the deeper tissue, probably resulting from joint instability and microtrauma, can lead to hemosiderosis and a sparse lymphocyte-plasmacyte infiltrate. Joint instability and microtrauma can also lead to sustained edema in the fibrous layer of the joint capsule and increased fibroplasia. This results in a permanent thickening of the joint capsule and contributes to a reduction in range of motion of the joint.

The earliest microscopic change seen in the degenerating articular cartilage is a roughening of the surface fiber layer, followed by the exposure and loss of underly-

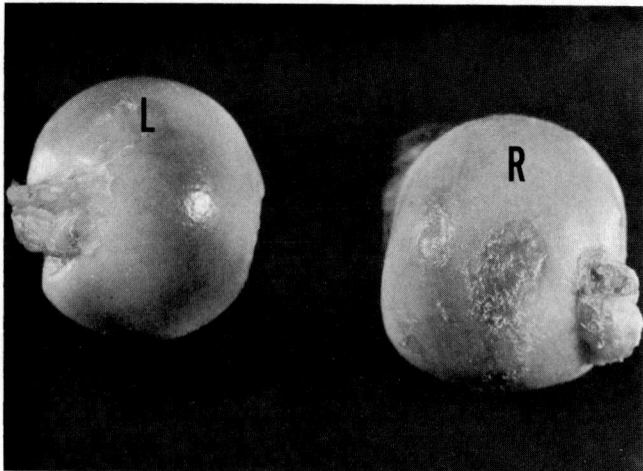

Figure 84–3. Femoral heads of a six-month-old dog two months following fracture of the right acetabulum. The left femoral head (L) is normal. The right femoral head (R) shows effects of secondary degenerative joint disease. Note the alteration in shape and size. Several areas of the articular surface are discolored and have a velvety appearance.

ing chondrocytes (Fig. 84–5). Chondrocytes in these areas appear to have undergone degeneration and death, and there is a generalized loss of normal staining properties of proteoglycan in the surrounding cartilage matrix. As the degenerative process becomes more severe, the most superficial layer of cartilage is worn away, exposing the deeper layer of chondrocytes in the transitional zone. In an attempt at repair, chondrocytes in the area proliferate but are unable to separate and differentiate in the firm chondroid matrix of mature cartilage (Fig. 84–6). These clones of newly formed chondrocytes produce a soft, imperfect matrix that wears more quickly than normal matrix. Fissures develop in the damaged

cartilage, and these fissures may extend through to the subchondral bone (Fig. 84–7). Chondrocytes immediately adjacent to the fissure lines make an abortive attempt at repair (Fig. 84–8). When fissures reach the subchondral bone, a separation of the osteochondral junction occurs along with varying amounts of hemorrhage and necrosis. The resulting osteochondral defect heals with granulation tissue and fibrocartilage, and is visible radiographically as subchondral irregularities or cysts. On occasion, subchondral bone cysts filled with myxoid tissue may be found beneath degenerative articular surfaces. Such cystic changes are uncommon in dogs and cats and are most apt to be seen in larger joints in giant breeds

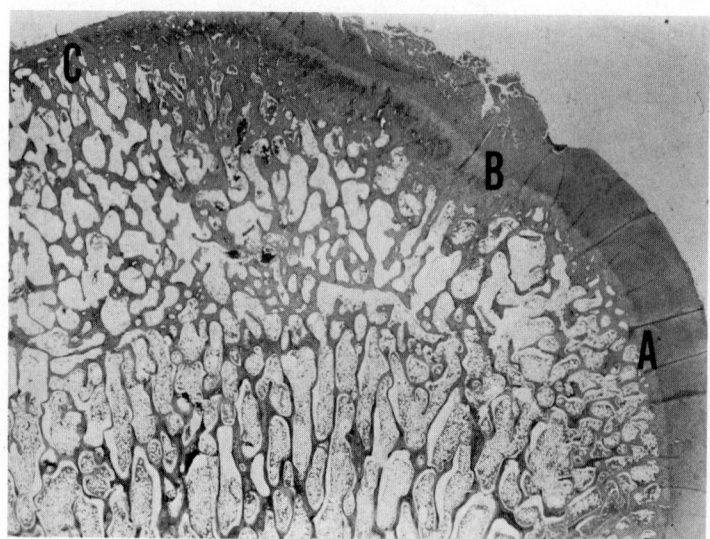

Figure 84–4. Microscopic changes in degenerative joint disease. Observe the loss of normal structure of the joint, beginning at the junction (A) of the normal cartilage and subchondral bone with the area (B) of cartilage degeneration and subchondral bone sclerosis, which becomes progressively more severe until the surface is eburnated (C).

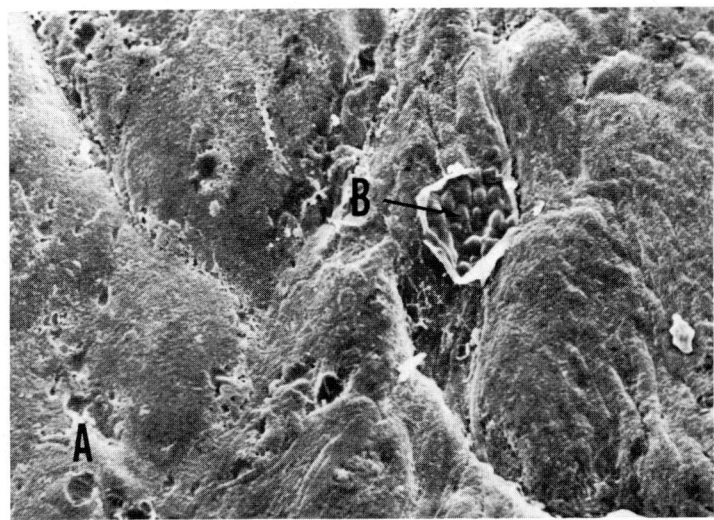

Figure 84–5. Scanning electron micrograph of early changes in a degenerating articular surface. The entire surface shows roughening and irregularity. Microulcerations (A) may be of sufficient depth to expose chondrocytes (B) of the tangential zone to the joint surface.

of dogs. With continued cartilage loss, the sclerotic subchondral bone becomes progressively exposed and is polished by the opposing articular surface, a process called eburnation.

Changes in the articular cartilage and subchondral bone lead to loss of normal contour of the articular surfaces, and this predisposes the joint to further abnormal movement. In an attempt to respond to these new stresses and to contain the abnormal motion, the borders of the articular surfaces undergo remodeling and extend the articular surface area (Fig. 84–9). Typically, this is accompanied by bone proliferation manifested as osteophytes on the periarticular bone surfaces adjacent to or within the insertion line of the joint capsule (Fig. 84–10).

The quantity of synovial fluid found in degenerating joints ranges from normal to copious. Copious effusions are seen mainly in larger joints, particularly the elbows and stifles. Such outpourings of synovial fluid can be more or less persistent, or they can become apparent after a period of overexertion or vigorous exercise. In cases in which the synovial fluid is increased in quantity, it is often thin or watery owing to dilution with edema fluid. The mucin quality remains normal, however, as there is no depolymerization of the hyaluronic acid.

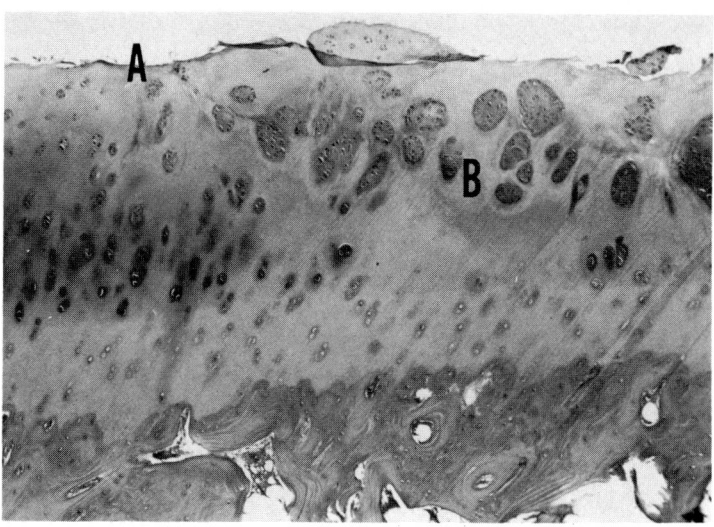

Figure 84–6. Loss of the superficial layer (A) and proliferation of nests of chondrocytes in the transitional and radial zones (B) in an ineffectual attempt at repair.

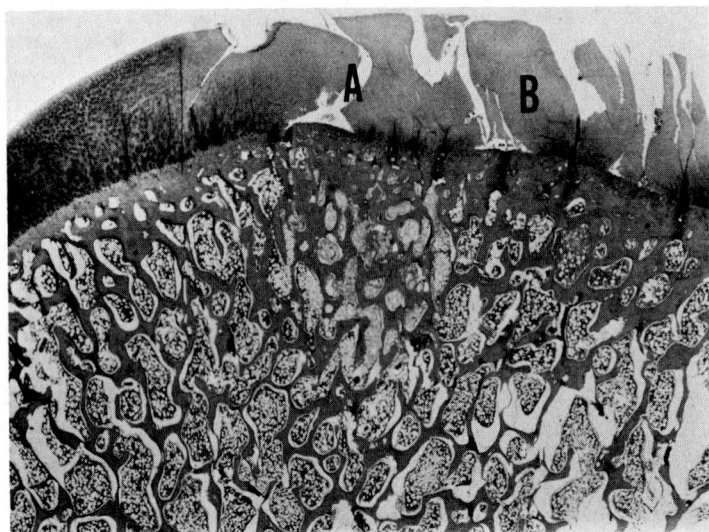

Figure 84–7. Fissures (A) extend completely through the layer of degenerative cartilage (B) and reach the subchondral bone.

Debris from degenerative cartilage matrix and microhemorrhage in soft tissue initiates a sterile synovitis that leads to increased numbers of macrophages in the fluid, although total cell counts rarely exceed 4000 cells/μl. Polymorphonuclear neutrophils are not generally seen in numbers exceeding five per cent. Synovial fluid from degenerative joints is often yellow-tinged, mainly because of hemosiderin pigments originating from microhemorrhage in the deeper layers of the synovium.

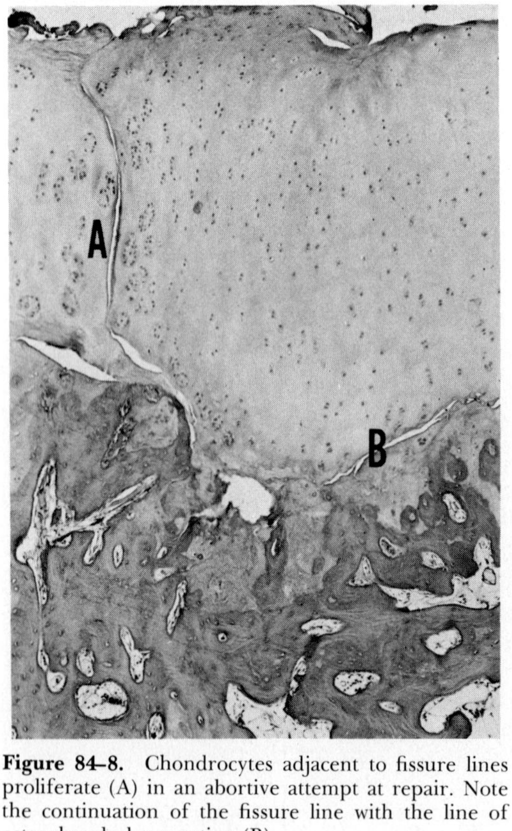

Figure 84–8. Chondrocytes adjacent to fissure lines proliferate (A) in an abortive attempt at repair. Note the continuation of the fissure line with the line of osteochondral separation (B).

Treatment

The treatment of degenerative joint disease involves the following steps: (1) adequate daily periods of rest, (2) avoidance of overexertion of affected joints, (3) reduction of weight if the animal is obese, (4) properly administered exercise, (5) relief of pain by analgesic and anti-inflammatory drugs, and (6) orthopedic operative procedures to relieve pain, regain motion, or correct stressful deformities or instabilities.

Adequate rest of animals with degenerative joint disease is important for several reasons; excessive use of damaged joints can aggravate clinical signs, and more importantly, it can accelerate the joint destruction. Dogs with severe joint disease cannot be expected to function in the same manner as they did before developing the problem. Unfortunately, the amount of rest or exercise that an animal can tolerate is difficult to assess. Many dogs are so eager to please their masters that they will overexert themselves. In addition, some dogs will forego any considerations of pain because of sheer enjoyment of the activity, e.g., hunting, jogging, playing, or hiking with the owner or

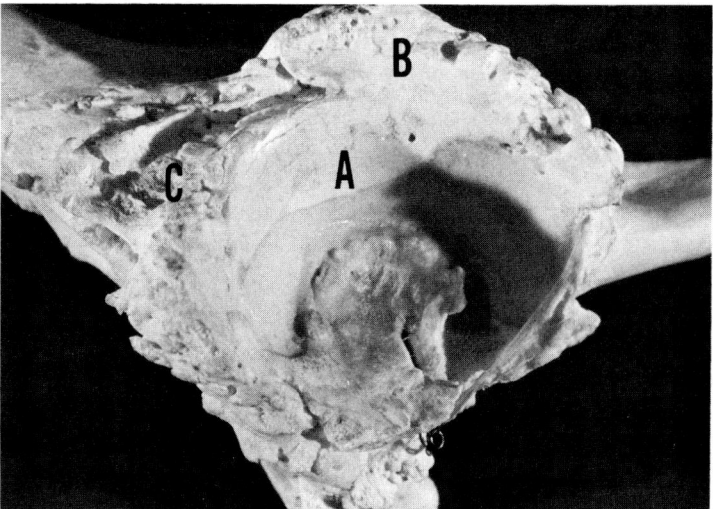

Figure 84-9. Severe secondary degenerative joint disease following chronic luxation of the hip. (A) Eburnated (polished) rim of the acetabulum. Osteophytic bone production is seen at the joint margin (B) and along the joint capsule insertion (C).

working with livestock. As a rule, any activity that causes the animal to become acutely more lame for a period afterward is probably excessive and should be curtailed or cut back.

Although dogs with advanced degenerative joint disease should receive adequate rest and avoid strenuous exercise, they should not be allowed to become complete invalids. Properly administered and controlled exercise is important in maintaining muscle tone and keeping joints limber. Controlled exercise can consist of defined periods of walking with the owner, interspaced with short periods of rest or other controlled periods of play, swimming, or similar activities. As the disease becomes more advanced and less activity is tolerated, the amount of exercise should be reduced.

Analgesic and anti-inflammatory drugs are often necessary to control pain in severely affected dogs. Since cats do not often manifest the disease to the same extent as dogs, drug therapy is usually not needed. Buffered aspirin, at the dose of 25 to 50 mg/kg body weight divided into three daily doses for dogs, and 25 mg/kg once a day for cats, is usually well tolerated (Booth, 1977) and can afford significant relief. It should not be used in individuals in which it causes gastrointestinal upsets. In addition to aspirin, there are several other drugs that are considerably more expensive, have their own side effects, and are not necessarily more efficacious. They should be used only if they provide significantly more relief than aspirin. Ibuprofen (Motrin) has been used to treat degenerative joint disease in man, but there is very little experience with these drugs for dogs. A suggested dosage for dogs is 15 mg/kg divided three times daily and preferably given with meals. Gastrointestinal upsets can be caused by the use of this drug. Indomethacin at a dosage of 1 to 1.25 mg/kg divided two to three times daily to

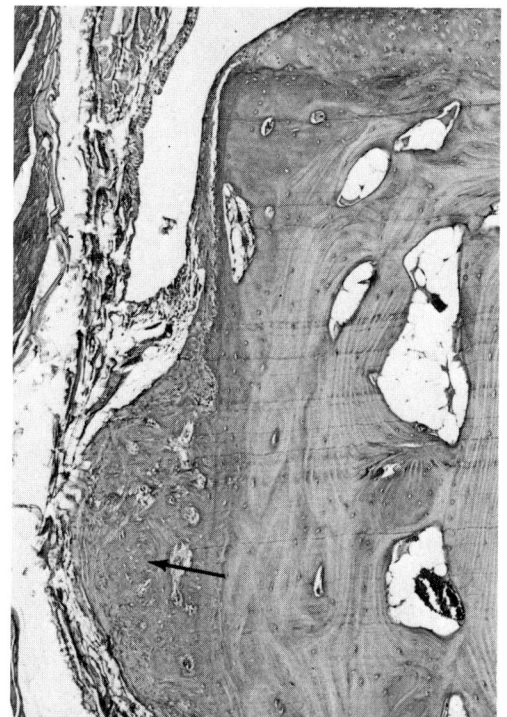

Figure 84-10. Formation of a periarticular osteophyte (arrow).

dogs may also provide some relief. Serious gastrointestinal problems may also result from the use of this drug. Phenylbutazone is widely used by veterinarians to treat dogs with degenerative joint disease, based on the mistaken belief that it is much more effective than aspirin and does not have any side-effects. For chronic use in dogs, the dosage is 40 mg/kg divided three times a day for the first 48 hours, then lowered after that to the lowest effective amount (Booth, 1977). The total daily dosage should not exceed 800 mg, regardless of the size of the animal. Bone marrow suppression is a side effect of prolonged high levels of the drug. Prednisolone or prednisone is given at an initial dosage of 2 mg/kg once daily for several days to either dogs or cats, followed by a chronic maintenance dose that should not exceed 1 mg/kg every other day. There is evidence that corticosteroids may actually hasten the degenerative process, so what is gained in the short term may be lost, and more, in the long term. For this reason they should be restricted to advanced cases that are totally unresponsive to more conservative therapy, especially if the patient is in the terminal phase of life. Intraarticular injections of steroids should be avoided. When instigating chronic drug therapy, owners should be made aware of the fact that the control of signs is only partial and can never be complete.

Surgery should be used very selectively. Fusion of joints such as the elbow, carpus, or hock is occasionally warranted to help relieve pain and restore some use to the limb. Femoral head ostectomy can be effective in selected animals with painful and badly diseased hip joints. Some types of joint instability resulting from ligament damage or rupture can be corrected surgically. Obviously this must be done before secondary degenerative changes become too extensive. In situations wherein pieces of cartilage or osteophytic bone have become free within the joint cavity, surgical intervention is necessary for their removal. Osteophytes should not be excised, except where they break into the joint cavity or impinge on tendons or nerves. If they are excised, further measures are necessary to correct the problems that caused them to occur in the first place. Surgery should be avoided in situations other than the ones mentioned, because surgery without clear objectives and without an understanding of the pathophysiology of the disease can actually add to the joint insult and accelerate degenerative changes.

TRAUMATIC JOINT DISEASE

Joint trauma in dogs and cats is usually accidental, resulting from contact with larger animals or man and his machines. In certain instances, however, distinct types of trauma can be associated with various activities, e.g., skull and scapular fractures in working cattle dogs and various fractures and sprains of the limbs of racing greyhounds (Hickman, 1975; Prole, 1976). Joint trauma can result from fractures of surrounding bones, damage to cartilage, or damage to soft tissue structures supporting the joints. Of these injuries, bone fractures are the easiest to diagnose, and damage to cartilage and soft tissue is more difficult to localize.

Damage to Articular Cartilage

Damage to the articular cartilage can occur as a result of acute or chronic trauma to the joint. In small animals such as the dog and cat, the trauma is usually acutely sustained. The most frequent causes include being hit by automobiles, gunshot wounds (Rendano and Adbinoor, 1977; Renegar and Stoll, 1980), fights with larger animals, or abuse from people. In such instances cartilage damage frequently accompanies bone fractures or luxations. Because the cartilage damage cannot be assessed on radiographs, it may go undetected or be minimized in importance. Even with good bony reconstruction, degenerative joint disease frequently occurs months or years later (Fig. 84–11).

Damage to Soft Tissue Supporting the Joint

Injuries of this sort, usually of traumatic origin, have been termed "sprains." Sprains result from microtrauma to vascular (hemorrhage, edema), ligamentous (separations, tears), bursal, and synovial structures. They are relatively common in dogs, and it is often quite a diagnostic challenge to differentiate them from more serious entities. Careful physical and radiographic analysis to rule out other entities, coupled with time and rest, usually suffice to differentiate sprains from more serious problems.

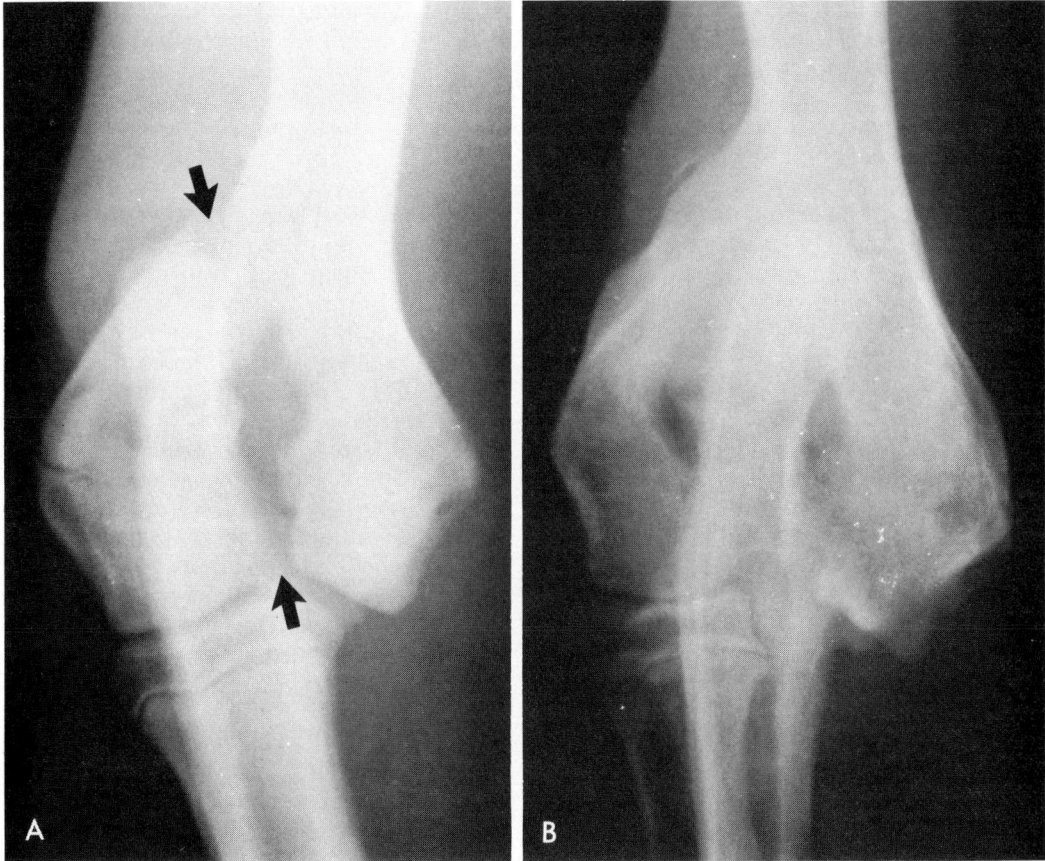

Figure 84–11. Craniocaudal radiographs of the elbow joint of a young dog at the time of intra-articular fracture of the distal humerus (A) (arrows) and later following bony healing (B). Malalignment of the bony fragments is easily seen radiographically along with the new bone formation. The damage to the articular cartilage must be evaluated indirectly.

MENISCAL DISORDERS AND CRUCIATE LIGAMENT RUPTURE

Rupture of the Cruciate Ligaments

An excellent historical review of cruciate ligament rupture in dogs and cats has been written by Knecht (1976). The anterior cruciate ligament of the canine stifle is of particular concern to veterinarians. Anterior cruciate ligament rupture has been also described in cats (Alexander et al., 1977; Cucuel and Frye, 1970; Matis and Kostlin, 1978; McManus, 1967). Rupture of the posterior (caudal) cruciate ligament is much less common but has been reported in both cats and dogs (Dalton, 1979; Knecht, 1976; Johnson, 1978).

Rupture of the cruciate ligaments can result from severe trauma, but more often the rupture follows a progressive degeneration of the ligament that leaves it in a weakened state (Tirgari, 1978; Zahm, 1965). Evidence for such a progressive deterioration includes the findings that most dogs are over five years of age when it occurs, and there is a tendency for both ligaments to eventually rupture. Many of the animals are obese, which puts additional stress on the ligament and contributes to the problem.

Rupture of the anterior cruciate ligament is usually accompanied by clinical signs. Posterior cruciate ligament rupture is more likely to be asymptomatic. Rupture of the anterior cruciate ligament in older dogs often occurs suddenly and is frequently associated with running or jumping. Initially the involved leg is carried off of the ground. After a few days to a month (or more), the dogs will gradually put more and more weight on the leg. On physical examination, there is a noticeable cranial-caudal movement of the tibia in relation to the femur, the "anterior drawer" sign.

Rupture of the anterior cruciate ligament, with its characteristic pattern of joint instability, leads to degenerative joint disease and damage to the medial collateral ligament and medial meniscus (Tirgari, 1978). The rate at which degenerative changes occur will be proportional to the weight and activity of the animal. In very small dogs and cats, degenerative changes may occur rather slowly. It is worth noting that in some studies one half of dogs with ruptured anterior cruciate ligaments regained adequate use of the leg without surgery (Strande, 1967). Because of the high success rate of surgical correction, however, spontaneous recovery should not be relied on to occur.

The treatment for anterior cruciate rupture is surgical, and numerous techniques have evolved since the original procedure for dogs described by Paatsama (1952). A review of these procedures was presented by Hohn and Newton (1975), and by Knecht (1976). More recently, another procedure called the "over the top" technique has been described (Arnoczky et al., 1979). Procedures for correction of the posterior cruciate ligament have been described by DeAngelis and Betts (1973), and by Knecht (1976).

A gradual relaxation of the ligaments of the stifle, associated with "anterior drawer" movement, is often an accompanying feature of plasmacytic-lymphocytic synovitis of the dog (see following section). Such a relationship between cruciate ligament rupture and lymphocytic synovitis has been mentioned in passing by Tigari (1978), although no cause and effect relationship was noted. Upon surgical exploration, the cruciate ligaments are either ruptured, or intact but badly stretched. More importantly, there is an obvious inflammatory synovitis accompanying the cruciate damage. This disorder can be seen in as many as ten per cent of the dogs operated on for "anterior cruciate rupture." For this reason, surgeons should be aware of its existence. If the cruciate is repaired without regard for the underlying disease, the surgery will be unsuccessful.

Meniscal Problems

Meniscal Tears. A tear in the medial meniscus accompanies anterior cruciate ligament rupture in over one half of dogs operated on for this disorder (Flo and DeYoung, 1978). Failure to remove all or part of the damaged meniscus can cause the lameness to persist after cruciate ligament repair (Clamen, 1979; Flo and DeYoung, 1978). Meniscal tears are often manifested by a "click" during walking or on manipulation of the stifle joint in a cranial-caudal direction.

Damage to the medial meniscus, often associated with some degree of collateral ligament damage, can occur infrequently as an isolated event, especially in athletic dogs of the larger breeds. This can be aggravated by genu valgum that is sometimes seen in larger dogs. This disorder can be associated with considerable effusions of fluid into the stifle joint, especially following vigorous exercise. With time there is a thickening of the medial aspect of the stifle joint and radiographic signs of degenerative joint disease.

Meniscal Calcification. Degenerative joint disease associated with calcification of the medial menisci has been seen uncommonly in the stifle joints of dogs and cats. The animals are lame, and there is a pronounced increase in the medial dimensions of the stifle joint. We have seen one feline patient with ossification of the menisci. The pathogenesis of this condition is unknown.

Discoid Meniscus. A discoid meniscus is broad and disclike in appearance, compared with the normal semilunar configuration. The condition occurs in as high as 2.7 per cent of humans (Resnick, 1981). In man it is not known whether it is congenital or acquired. The problem most frequently involves the lateral meniscus, and affected people develop clinical symptoms similar to those produced by meniscal tears. This condition has been identified at autopsy in a dog (Arnoczky and Marshall, 1977). The frequency of this problem in dogs and its clinical significance are both unknown at this time.

LUXATIONS AND SUBLUXATIONS

Luxations and subluxations can involve virtually any joint of the appendicular and axial skeleton. They can be caused by acute trauma, or by developmental or acquired problems that affect the stability of the joint.

The diagnosis of a complete luxation is clinically and radiographically quite easy. Subluxations are most difficult to diagnose and require a knowledge of normal radiographic anatomy. It is important also to consider whether the luxation or subluxation was primary or secondary to preexisting joint disease. The most obvious radiographic change in a dislocation is the failure of two or more opposing articular surfaces to meet normally. It must be remembered, however, that certain normal joints show considerable laxity without pathologic changes. In addition to a determination of whether or not a dislocation has occurred, it is important to note the presence of small fragments originating from the articular surface or periarticular margin. Small avulsion or chip fractures frequently accompany luxation or subluxations of certain joints such as the hip or elbow of the dog.

The duration of a dislocation can only be estimated radiographically. Obvious osteoporosis, muscle atrophy, or bony remodeling leading to formation of pseudoarthrosis suggests a duration in excess of several weeks. A unique change occurs in luxation of the hip, following which the depth of the acetabulum often decreases as it is filled first with soft tissue and later with bone. Any evidence of secondary joint disease, such as periosteal lipping or remodeling, also suggests chronicity. The problem is often that of deciding which came first, the dislocation or the secondary joint disease. Luxation or subluxation due to a congenital anomaly is an important consideration in evaluation of what might otherwise appear to be a simple traumatic event. In these cases the subchondral bone is less dense and the contour of the articular portions of the bone is abnormal. Comparison studies of the opposite leg may be of value in such cases.

Subluxations are more difficult to diagnose than luxations and generally require that the radiographs be taken in weight-bearing, simulated weight-bearing, or in flexed and extended positions. Joints that require such positions include the carpus, tarsus, and stifle joint, and hip joint of animals with hip dysplasia.

Special views can be used to evaluate joint stability in certain joints. Partial luxation of the patella in the dog is best evaluated by a special "skyline" view that determines both the degree of patellar luxation and the depth of the trochlear groove.

Hip Joint

Complete luxation of the hip joint usually involves rupture of the teres ligament and weakening or separation of the joint capsule. Hip dysplasia is probably the greatest predisposing cause in dogs, and possibly in cats also. The inherent laxity of the hip joint in dysplastic animals and shallowness of the acetabulum leads in time to subluxation, followed by luxation in some cases.

Traumatic luxation of the hip joint occurs in both dogs and cats (Boom, 1979). It can occur from ligamentous damage alone or occasionally in association with fractures of the femoral head, neck, or acetabulum. The luxation is usually dorsal and cranial, and results in an acute lameness. The accepted modes for treatment involve closed reduction of the luxation under anesthesia, associated with Ehmer slinging of the limb, DeVita pinning (Fig. 84–12), or transarticular pinning (Bennett and Duff, 1980), to maintain the hip joint in place for several weeks. If there is extensive hemorrhage and soft tissue damage in the area of the joint, closed reduction may be impossible. Surgical exploration of the joint provides an opportunity to visualize and correct the damage.

Acute traumatic subluxations associated with stretching or rupture of the teres ligament and joint capsule have been seen. Owing to the shallowness of the acetabulum, dysplastic dogs are more prone to this than are nondysplastic dogs. Because the joint is still basically intact, these are best treated by a period of rest for two to four weeks.

Even following successful reduction of a luxated or subluxated hip, degenerative changes may ensue with time. Because of the extensive ligamentous damage often associated with dislocation, the hip joint often may retain a degree of instability. In addition, cartilage damage occurs very rapidly after dislocation.

Stifle Joint

Luxations of the stifle joint result most often from severe trauma. They have been described infrequently in the literature (Santi, 1974). Subluxations are common and most frequently involve damage to the anterior cruciate ligaments, medial collateral ligaments, and medial meniscus. A valgoid instability of the stifle has been described in dogs (Cheli et al., 1974). It usually is seen in the recovery stage following repairs of femoral fractures or hip luxations, and involves atrophy of the quadriceps muscle, swelling

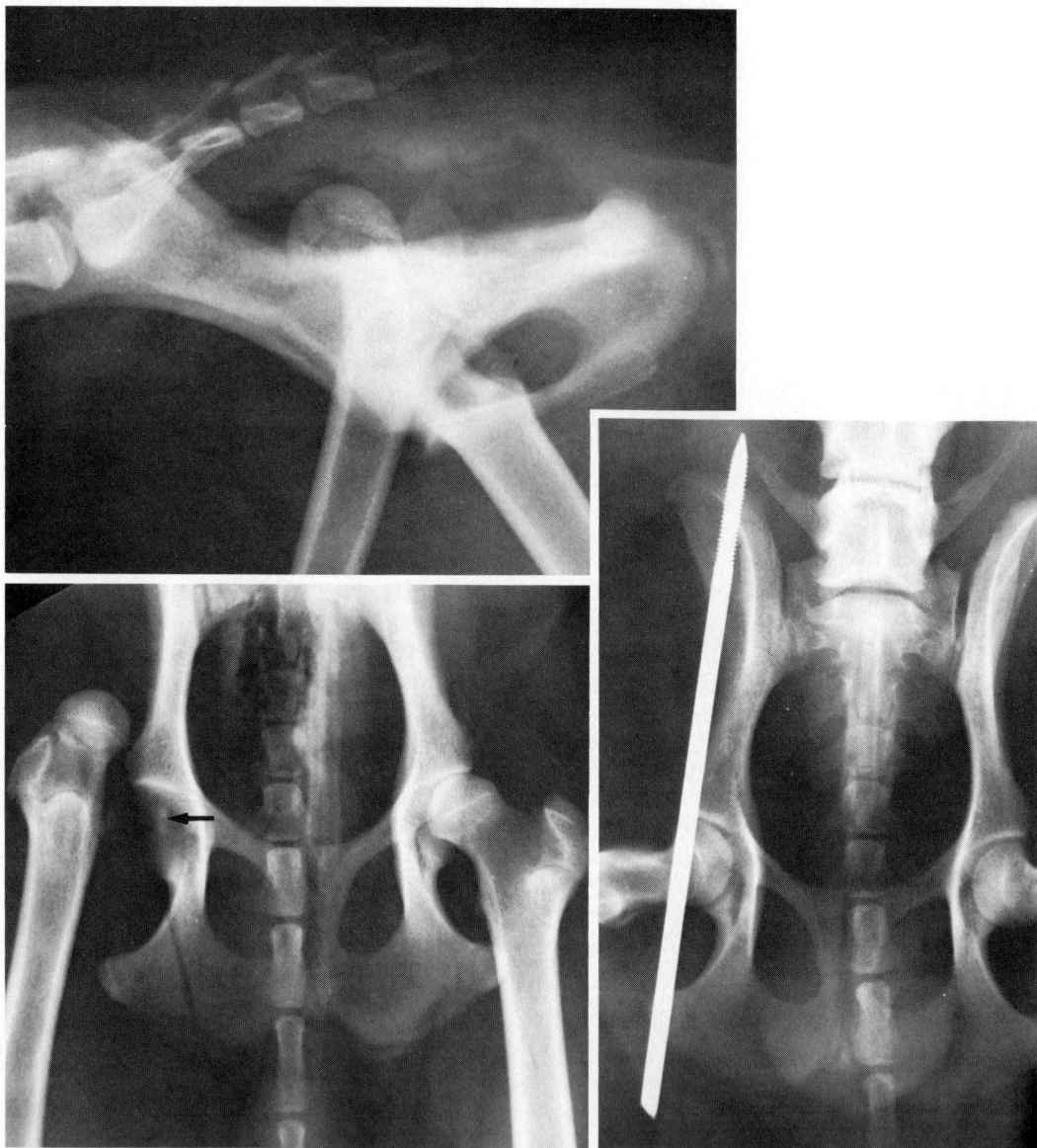

Figure 84–12. Lateral and ventrodorsal radiographs of the pelvis of an immature dog show a femoral head luxation with a free bony fragment within the acetabulum (arrow) that probably represents an avulsion of the attachment on the femoral head of the ligamentum teres. The reduction is stabilized by a deVita pin.

of the anterior cruciate ligament, and weakness of the medial collateral ligaments. The valgoid position of the distal limb can be accentuated by medially directed pressure on the stifle joint, and the distal limb can be excessively rotated by twisting the lower leg while holding the femur in place. The condition responds to cruciate ligament repair procedures.

Tarsal Joint

An extensive review of tarsal subluxations has been compiled by Campbell and coworkers (1976). Other reports have been provided by Arwedsson (1954), Clayton-Jones (1974), Holt (1974), Lawson (1961), Meutstege (1971), and Pettit (1974).

In the report by Campbell and coworkers (1976), only 11 of 44 intertarsal subluxations occurred because of trauma. In most cases the problem was apparently associated with degeneration of the plantar ligaments, borne out by the finding that it most often occurred in dogs over six years of age, in obese dogs, and in Shetland sheepdogs, collies, and Samoyeds. The condition was unilateral in all but five dogs; bilateral involvement is most likely to occur in Shetland sheepdogs.

Clinical signs of intertarsal joint subluxations include a moderate to severe semi–weight-bearing lameness, abnormal dorsiflexion of the tarsal joint, and in chronically affected dogs, a thickening of the joint capsule. Pain can not be elicited in most dogs by manipulation of the joint. Radiographic findings are minimal early in the disorder, but if the condition is left uncorrected, there is a progressive development of degenerative joint disease (Fig. 84–13).

Tarsometatarsal subluxations are less common than intertarsal subluxations (Campbell et al., 1976; Holt, 1974). Unlike intertarsal subluxations, most tarsometatarsal subluxations are traumatic in origin. A separation of the tarsometatarsal joint capsule and overlying plantar attachments are usually associated with the subluxation. The

clinical appearance, except for the frequent signs of accompanying trauma, resemble those of intertarsal joint subluxation.

Tibiotarsal subluxations are slightly more common than tarsometatarsal subluxations in dogs. They may or may not involve malleolar fractures and are generally the result of severe trauma (Holt, 1974).

Tarsal instabilities resulting from degeneration of supporting ligaments are almost always treated with tarsal arthrodesis. The procedure has been described by Campbell and associates (1976), and by Dieterich (1974). Tarsal instabilities of traumatic origin can often be treated by reduction associated with casting, wiring, or temporary intraarticular pinning to maintain the joint in position. If this is unsuccessful, tarsal arthrodesis is performed.

Hyperextension of the tarsal joint has been seen as a developmental problem in

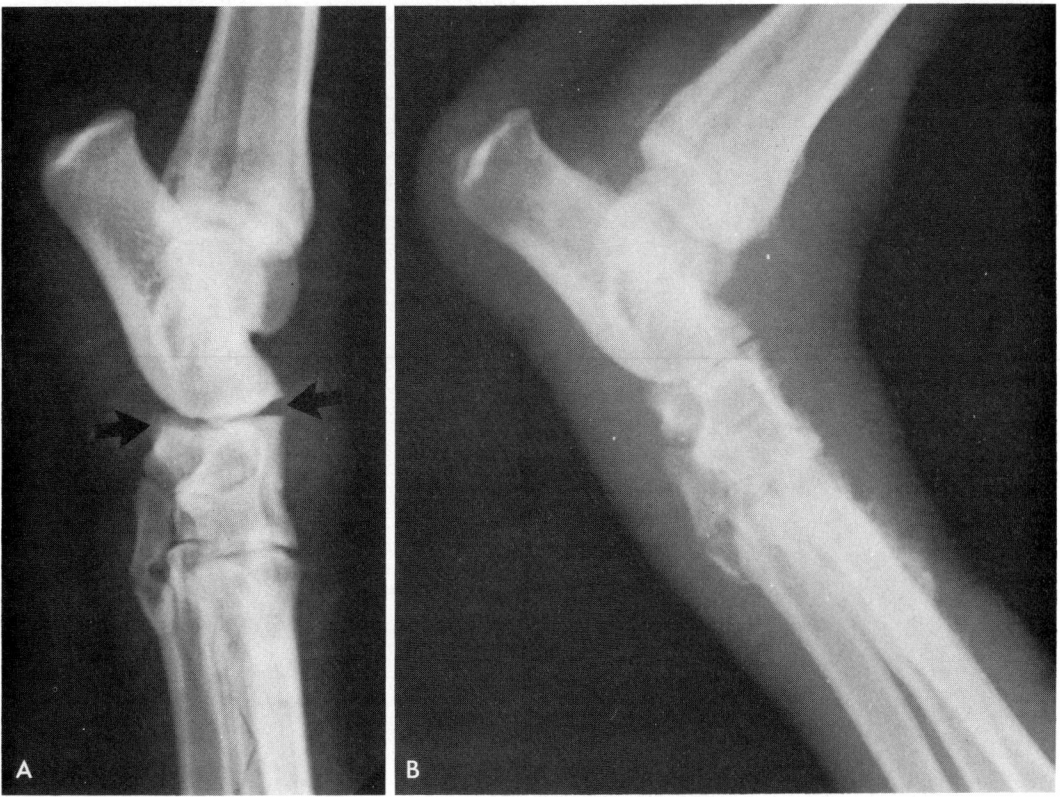

Figure 84–13. Lateral radiographs of the tarsus made at the time of injury (A) and 60 days later (B). The subluxation at the proximal intertarsal joint is seen on the first study (arrows). The second study was made after providing support for the foot for 2 months. Post-traumatic periosteal new bone is noted from the level of the distal tibia to the level of the proximal metatarsal bone. Soft tissue swelling is prominent, and disuse osteoporosis is noted. Radiographic changes involving the joint spaces are difficult to identify, and the degree of cartilage destruction can be estimated only clinically. The foot at the time of the second study was not abnormally warm, the soft tissue swelling was firm, and the foot was without pain. The differential diagnosis radiographically is that of an infectious arthritis.

some puppies. If left untreated, the tarsal joint can be severely traumatized. Smith (1976) treated such problems by shortening the Achilles tendon.

Shoulder Joint

Luxations or subluxations of the shoulder joint are uncommon in both dogs and cats, and when they occur, they are often due to trauma.

Elbow Joint

Luxations or subluxations of the elbow joint can be associated with trauma (Stoyac, 1975) (Fig. 84–14). In some cases, however, they can occur in otherwise normal dogs following fairly routine activity (Lowry and Betts, 1973). The elbow joint can apparently be stressed in such a way as to allow the anconeal process of the ulna to ride up over the humeral condyle. Subluxation of the elbow joint can be associated with deformities of the joint, such as would be associated with radius curvus (Carrig et al., 1975). Luxations of the elbow joint in basset hounds are not infrequent and are often associated with valgus deviation of the manus and radius curvus (Hammerling and Hammerling, 1974).

Congenital luxation of the elbow joint has been seen in puppies (Fig. 84–15). In one case the luxation was corrected by closed reduction and the joint temporarily transfixed with a small Steinmann pin (Winthrow, 1977).

Carpal Joint

Subluxation of the carpal joint, usually in hyperextension, is a frequent problem in

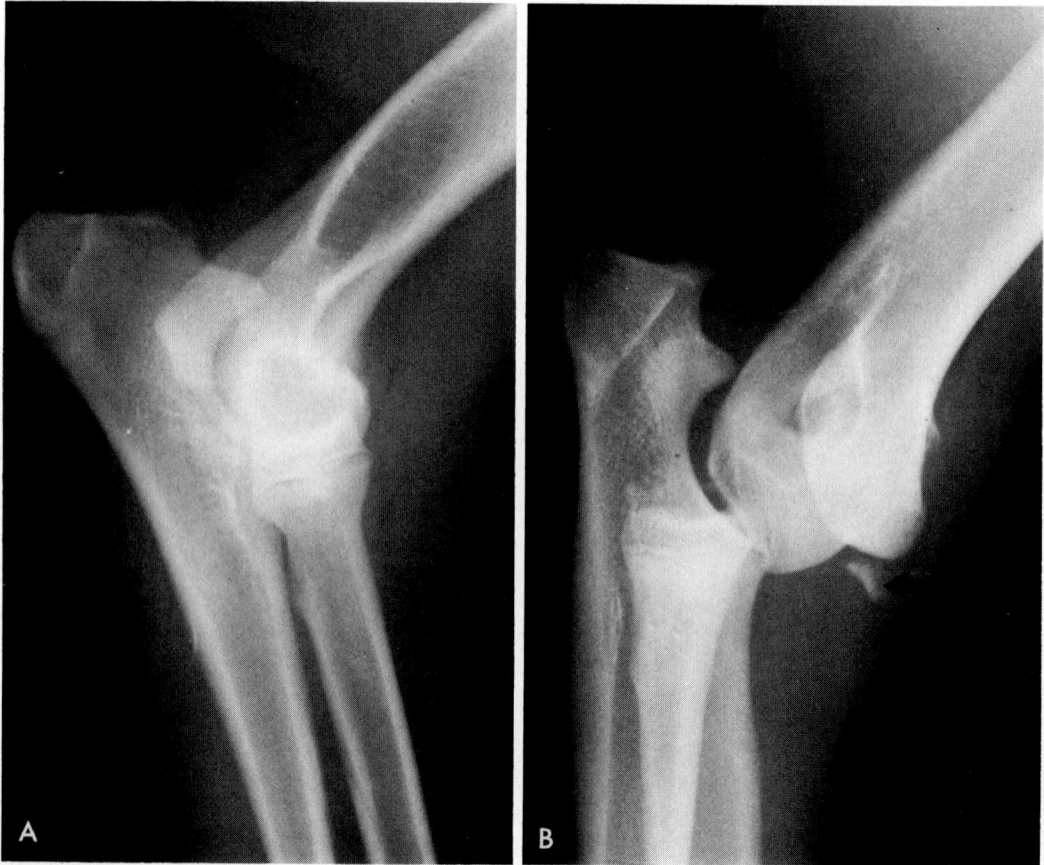

Figure 84–14. Lateral (A) and oblique (B) radiographs of the elbow of an immature dog show a luxation of the elbow joint. The lateral projection shows the bones almost perfectly positioned, and the lesion might be missed. The oblique projection clearly shows the completeness of the luxation and also permits evaluation of a chip or avulsion fragment (arrow) that probably originates from the lateral ulna at the attachment of the lateral collateral ligament.

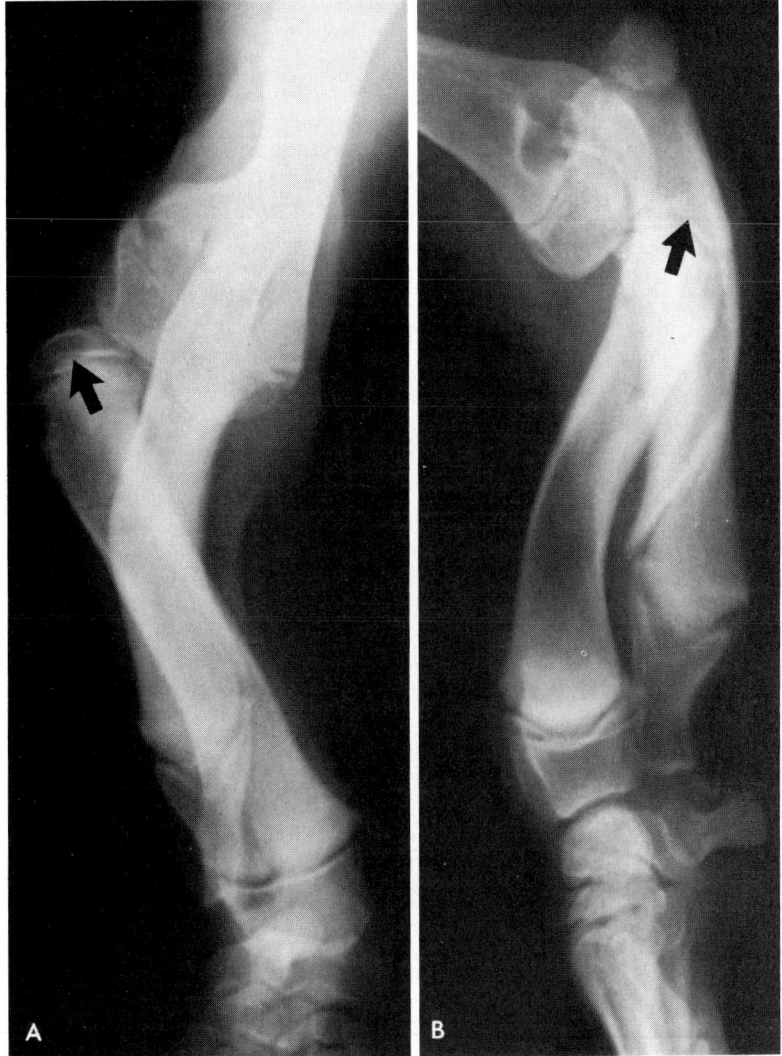

Figure 84–15. Craniocaudal and lateral radiographs of the foreleg of a three-month-old puppy with a congenital luxation of the elbow. The radial head is luxated laterally and caudally (arrows). Note the bowing of the ulna secondary to the luxation. The lucent line within the ulnar diaphysis results from a physeal dysplasia due to abnormal biomechanical forces on the dorsomedial edge of the physeal plate.

dogs. If left uncorrected it can rapidly proceed to complete luxation and to degenerative joint disease. The condition, although sometimes traumatic, is most often associated with a gradual weakening of the suspensory ligaments. This weakening results from deterioration of the ligaments, due to poor carpal configuration or other, unknown causes. A congenital predisposition is seen in collies, Samoyeds, Shetland sheepdogs, and Laborador retrievers. In the first three of these breeds, the condition can also involve the tarsal joints. As with intertarsal subluxations, affected dogs are often older

and obese. The conditon is often bilateral or proceeds from one carpus to the other over a period of time. Complete luxation is frequent and often occurs acutely when a dog runs, plays, or jumps down from something.

As in tarsal subluxations or luxations, dogs or cats with traumatically luxated or subluxated carpal joints can be treated by reducing the joint and keeping it in a slightly flexed position with a splint. In the event that this fails, or in animals with preexisting ligamentous degeneration, the carpus is fused (Leeds, 1978; Wind, 1975).

Temporomandibular Instabilities

Temporomandibular dislocations occur in both dogs and cats (Ticer, 1978). They are usually traumatic in origin and are often associated with fractures. Uncommonly, they can occur without obvious preceding trauma.

Temporomandibular luxations unassociated with trauma can be of two types. In one type, described by White (1949), there is a rostral movement of the mandible. This is manifested by malocclusion of the jaw and some interference with mouth opening. The second type, which is more common, is associated with open mouth "locking" occurring after hyperextension of the jaw, and lasting for several seconds or persisting until manually reduced. Reduction can be achieved by hyperextending the jaw further while placing inward pressure on the displaced mandibular condyle. The condition has been described mainly in young basset hounds (Robins and Grandage, 1977; Thomas, 1979) but has also been seen in Irish setters (Johnson, 1979; Stewart et al., 1975). Prevention of jaw locking in these dogs is accomplished by excising part of the zygomatic arch on the side of the "lock up." This surgery is based on the rationale that the jaw locking occurs because the condyloid process of the mandible is more oblique than is normal, thus allowing for lateral subluxation of the mandible. This allows the coronoid process (usually on the side opposite that of the most involved joint) to slip out of the coronoid fossa and engage the zygomatic arch. The developmental or genetic basis of the underlying deformity is unknown.

Instabilities of the Spinal Articulations

Axial-Atlantal-Occipital Malformations. Malformations of the articulations of the axis, atlas, and occipital bone occur from time to time, most often in small toy breeds of dogs, but occasionally in large dogs as well (Watson, 1979). Such instabilities are usually manifested by cord compression associated with overextension or flexion of these articulations.

Caudal Cervical Instabilities. Caudal cervical instability (spondylolisthesis) has been described in Great Dane and Doberman pinscher dogs (Denny et al., 1977; Trotter et al., 1976). Malformation of the articular facets leads to instability, which in turn causes changes similar to degenerative disease in appendicular joints. These changes include hypertrophy of the ligamentum flavum and dorsal longitudinal ligaments, joint capsular thickening, dorsal enlargement of the anulus fibrosus of the associated intravertebral disc, and osteophytosis. The net result of these changes, plus pressure applied by the vertebral body itself, is to cause chronic cord compression. Signs are therefore mainly neurologic and are referable to damage to the spine at the level of the sixth to seventh cervical vertebrae. Surgical treatment, which generally involves reduction of cord compression and stabilization of the spine, has been described by Trotter and coworkers (1976).

Lumbosacral Joint. Degenerative disease of the lumbosacral articulation is a frequent occurrence in large, usually aged, dogs (Wright, 1980). It is not clear whether this is due to an inherent instability of the true articulation, or to degeneration of the underlying disc (Morgan, 1967). Although often clinically inapparent, disease of this articulation can cause mild to moderately severe lower back pain (Wright, 1980), which can mimic hip lameness in some dogs. Forceful palpation of the lower spine and base of the tail can often help in localizing the lesion.

NEUROPATHIC ARTHROPATHY

Neuropathic arthropathy is uncommon in dogs. When this form of joint disease is identified, it is generally secondary to extensive trauma resulting from diminished pain and proprioceptive reflexes. This leads to a relaxation of supporting structures, chronic hyperflexion and extension, and instability. Animals are frequently destroyed after developing severe neurologic deficits, which may explain why neuropathic arthropathies have a lower incidence in animals than in man.

Chronic steroid injection into a degenerative joint may lead to accelerated and more obvious degenerative changes. The mechanism in part involves diminished pain perception by the animals.

DEVELOPMENTAL ARTHROPATHIES

Conformational Abnormalities

The importance of proper limb conformation, and its influence on soundness, is repeatedly stressed in equine orthopedics but is largely neglected in discussions of small animals. Abnormalities in the angulation of bones of the limbs can put great stress on joints. This stress cannot be normally dissipated by the joint, and the result can be degenerative joint disease and ligamentous degeneration. Conformational abnormalities are also common in small animals and can cause problems, although to a lesser extent than in large animals (cattle or horses). Conformational abnormalities can be acquired or congenital. If they are congenital, the anomaly can be noticeable at birth or will become noticeable only as the animal grows. Straight stifle confirmation, valgus and varus deformities of the elbow, stifles, tarsus, and carpus all occur in dogs, and to a much lesser extent in cats. Excessive plantigrade positions of the distal fore- or hindlimbs are also occasionally seen in both species. Nunamaker and Newton (1975) have described three types of conformational abnormalities that affect only the femoral head and neck: coxa valga, coxa vara, and increased anteversion. Coxa valga can lead to subluxation of the hip, while increased anteversion is associated with gait abnormalities, joint laxity, and pain. Increased anteversion is most often seen in giant breeds such as Saint Bernards, Newfoundlands, and Irish wolfhounds. These hip disorders can be corrected surgically (Nunamaker, 1974; Nunamaker and Newton, 1975).

Chondrodystrophy

Chondrodystrophy is inherent in bulldogs, pugs, Pekinese, basset hounds, dachshunds, and similar breeds. In these breeds the conformational abnormalities associated with chondrodystrophy are considered to be normal. Chondrodystrophy in some breeds such as the Alaskan malamute, however, is considered highly undesirable, probably because enchondral ossification defects in this breed are also associated with defects in other organ systems (Fletch et al., 1975). Chondrodystrophic dwarfism has also been seen in a German shepherd dog (Roberg, 1979).

Chondrodystrophic animals, like chondrodystrophic human dwarfs, demonstrate angular deformities of the limb joints, and the cartilage surfaces vary greatly in structure (Roberg, 1979). These changes predispose the joints to degenerative changes. Fortunately, most chondrodystrophic breeds of dogs are not working animals and often lead rather sedate lives, which slows the progression of joint disease.

Physeal (Growth Plate) Disorders

Conformational abnormalities of the limbs can result from damage to the physes of immature animals. Such damage usually results in the cessation of longitudinal bone growth normally contributed by the injured growth plate. As summarized by Llewellyn (1976), the ultimate outcome is dependent on (1) the particular growth plate involved and its contribution to the total growth of the bone; (2) the age and breed of the animal, which will determine how much the growth will be affected; (3) the method of surgical reduction (if damaged by fracture); (4) the type of injury that caused the damage; and (5) the involvement of infection as a complicating factor.

Growth plate disorders are particularly common in dogs, often result from trauma, and usually involve the radius and ulna (O'Brien et al., 1971). The forearm is vulnerable because it receives a disproportionate amount of stress, its growth comes from several physes, and it is made up of two parallel bones. Growth plate injuries in other bones of the limbs are not usually of clinical significance. The mean age at the time of identifiable trauma is four months, and the angular deformities become apparent five to seven weeks later (O'Brien et al., 1971).

Radioulnar Physeal Disorders. Rudy (1975) describes four possible deformities of the radioulnar segment that can result from premature growth plate closures: retarded or arrested growth of the distal ulnar physis, retarded or arrested growth of the distal radial physis, eccentric lateral premature closure of the distal radial physis, and premature closure of the proximal radial physis. Closure of epiphyses at three months of age will cause greater deformities than will closures at six to seven months of age, by which time most growth has taken place.

Arrested growth of the distal ulnar physis is the most common physeal disorder to occur in young dogs. The condition may or may not result from an identifiable trauma (O'Brien et al., 1971; Ramadan and Vaughan, 1978; Rudy, 1975). It is usually unilateral but can involve both forelimbs in about 15 per cent of the cases (Ramadan and Vaughan, 1978). Because the distal ulnar physis accounts for 70 to 85 per cent of the ulnar growth (Carrig et al., 1975), premature closure of this physis can lead to severe problems. The slow growing ulna can act as a restraining string in the bow formed by the more rapidly growing radius. This leads to a curving of the radius and a lateral angulation of the distal limb with an outward rotation of the paw (Carrig et al., 1975; Rudy, 1975; Skaggs et al., 1973). In addition, deformities often occur in the elbow joint, leading rapidly to a degree of subluxation and eventually to degenerative joint disease (Carrig et al., 1975).

Symmetric closure of the distal radial physis is infrequent, generally unilateral, and often associated with trauma (Rudy, 1975). The condition leads to a medial deformation of the distal limb, accompanied by a slight inward rotation of the paw (Olson et al., 1980; Rudy, 1975) and deformation of the elbow joint leading to subluxation (Wolff, 1975).

Eccentric lateral premature closure of the distal radial physis can occur, leaving the medial portion to continue to grow. This causes mainly an angular deformity of the radial articular surface, manifested by an outward rotation of the paw and carpal valgus deformity (Olson et al., 1980; Rudy, 1975) (Fig. 84–16). Treatment is surgical (Olson et al., 1980).

Premature closure of the proximal radial physis is uncommon. It leads to substantial deformities in the elbow joint (Rudy, 1975).

The treatment of abnormalities resulting from premature growth plate closures requires considerable surgical skill and a knowledge of the normal anatomic relationships. Premature closures of the distal ulnar

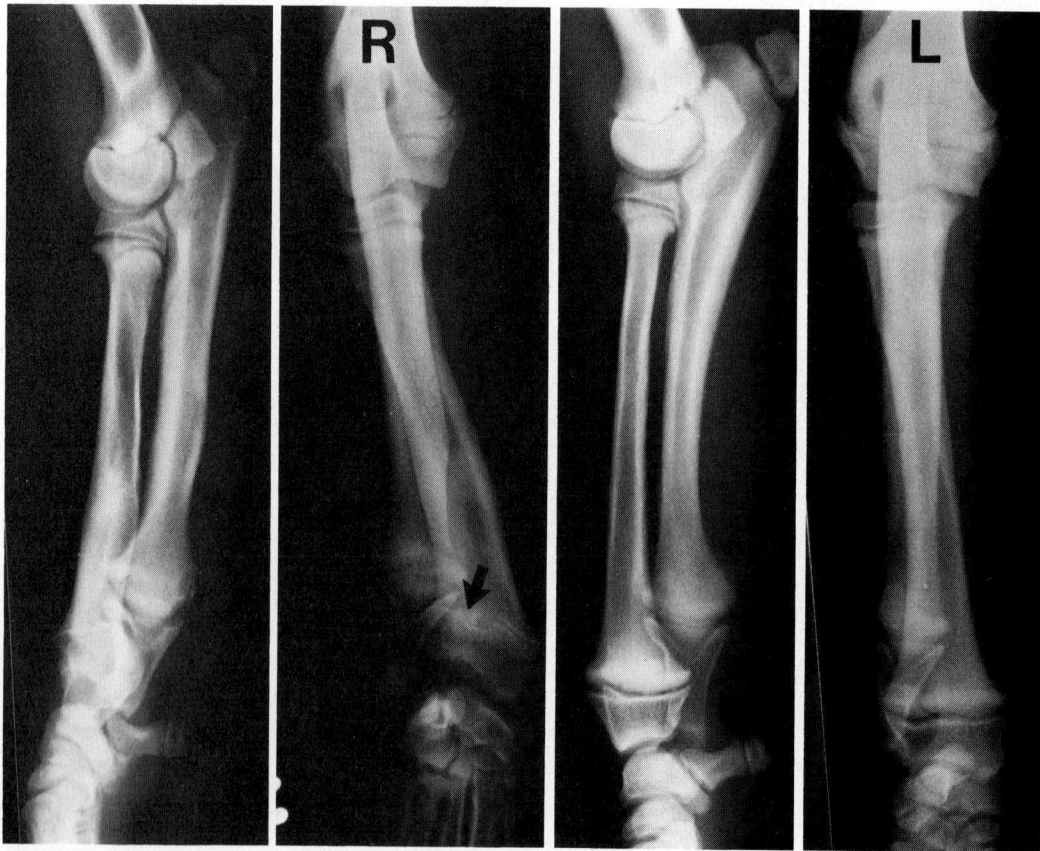

Figure 84–16. Craniocaudal and lateral radiographs of both forelegs of an immature dog with eccentric lateral premature closure of the distal radial physis on the right, leaving the medial portion of the physis continuing to grow. The left foreleg is normal by comparison.

physis can be treated by segmental ostectomies of the ulna if they are detected early enough. This, in effect, cuts the string of the bow, allowing the radius to grow unimpeded. Because the ostectomies can close rapidly, they may need to be repeated before growth ceases. A surgical technique whereby the distal styloid process of the ulna is resected and transposed may circumvent the problem of premature closures of the transected ulna (Egger, 1979). In most cases, the condition is not detected until considerable growth abnormalities have occurred and physeal growth has essentially ceased. Surgery done at this point must be directed at reestablishment of normal angulation and rotational alignment, while maintaining as much of the normal limb length as possible (Rudy, 1975). Loss of too much limb length can create the "longleg-shortleg" syndrome, and predispose the joints of the forelimb to degenerative joint disease. Attention also must be paid to deformities of the elbow joint, which must be surgically corrected (Mason and Baker, 1978).

Epiphysiolysis. Spontaneous lysis of the apophysis of the supraglenoid tuberosity of the humeri has been observed over a eight-month period in a young German wire-haired pointer (Mayrhofer, 1977). This resulted in non-united supraglenoid processes, and radiographic signs of degenerative joint disease in the shoulder joints.

Limb Shortening

Collapsing or folding fractures, if not properly treated, can result in a shortening of the limb upon healing. To compensate for the limb shortening, the angulations of the pelvic or thoracic girdle and distal and proximal joints are altered, which in turn predisposes these joints to degenerative changes. If fractures are repaired so that rotation of the distal segment occurs upon healing, degenerative changes can occur in distal and proximal joints because of abnormal stresses imposed by the resulting malformation.

Osteochondrosis (Osteochondritis)

Osteochondrosis is an important cause of both transient and permanent lameness in dogs (Olsson, 1976). It is not a problem in cats. The clinical, radiographic, etiologic, and pathologic features of this condition in dogs have been extensively reviewed.

Osteochondrosis was originally identified in shoulder joints of dogs, where the lesion occurs on the caudal aspect of the humeral head (Smith and Stowater, 1975). Osteochondrosis affects a number of joints, however, particularly the lateral and medial femoral condyles of the stifle (Punzet et al., 1975; Robins, 1970) (Fig. 84–17), the medial condyle of the humerus (Mason et al., 1980; Wood et al., 1975), femoral trochlea, and the medial ridge of the talus (Alexander, 1980b; Johnson et al., 1980; Mason and Lavelle, 1979; Olson et al., 1980). The condition, regardless of the anatomic location, can be bilateral in one third or more of cases, although the lesion in one limb may clinically predominate.

Osteochondrosis first becomes clinically apparent at six to nine months of age in the dog. It may cause clinical signs of lameness or subtle gait abnormalities, or it may remain inapparent. Clinical signs persist for weeks or months, or permanent lameness may develop over a longer period of time as a result of secondary degenerative joint disease. There is a tendency for the condition to occur more frequently in strains or breeds of dogs that are genetically selected for large size and rapid growth. Whitacre and Harrison (1972) showed that there was a close relationship between size and incidence, with most cases being in dogs over 60 lbs in weight. Males, which tend to grow faster than females, and animals on rapid growth promoting diets are more often affected. There are exceptions, however, such as the high incidence in Brittany spaniels and in some families of bull terriers (Woodard, 1979), Border collies (Knecht et al., 1977), and greyhounds (Johnson and Davis, 1979).

Osteochondrosis is believed to be caused by disturbances in normal enchondral ossification (Olsson, 1976). In osteochondrosis, the articular cartilage in affected sites becomes thicker than normal because enchondral ossification does not keep pace with cartilage growth. Although the etiology is uncertain, the initial lesion is necrosis of chondrocytes in the deeper layers of the articular cartilage. One idea is that the necrosis is due to an inability of these deeply situated chondrocytes to receive adequate

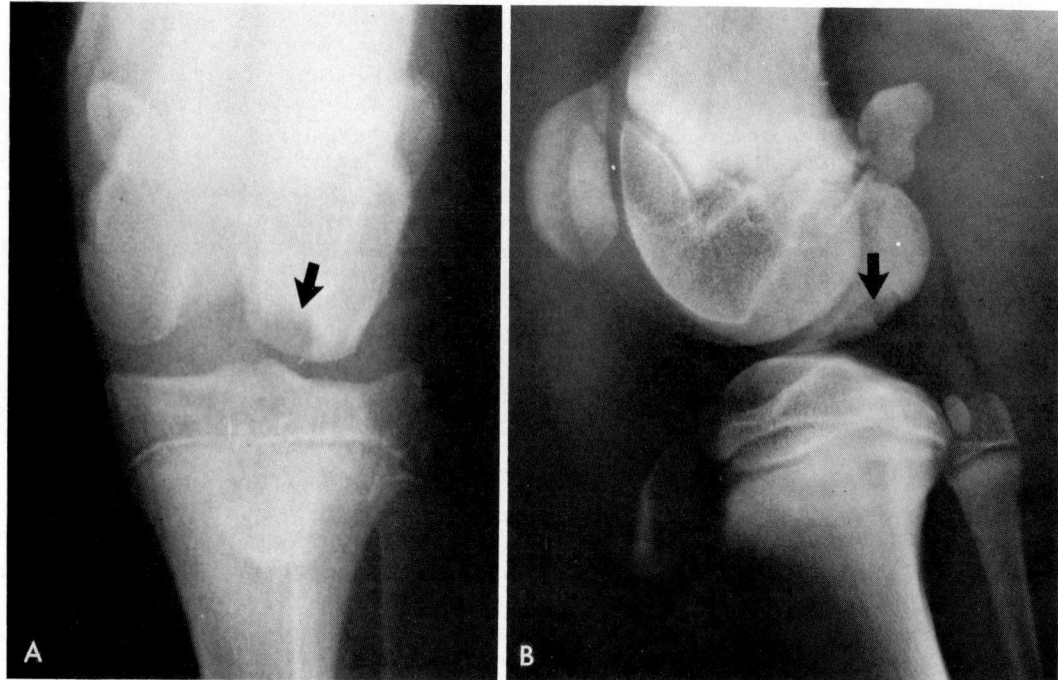

Figure 84–17. Caudocranial and lateral projections of the stifle joint of an immature dog with a large lucent lesion in the lateral condyle of the femur that is characteristic for osteochondrosis in this region.

nutrients by diffusion from the synovial fluid or subchondral capillaries. This cartilage death tends to occur in areas of the joint receiving the greatest stress, and therefore the weight of the animal and type of activity may also be involved in the process. Following death of these deeply situated chondrocytes, the surrounding cartilage matrix fails to mineralize. Blood vessels from the subchondral bone will not invade the area of unmineralized articular cartilage as they normally would. Consequently, the osteogenic mesenchyme that accompanies these vessels does not penetrate the cartilage and normal ossification fails to occur.

All changes in the osteochondritic lesion subsequent to the development of the area of chondromalacia are secondary events. At one extreme in this morphologic spectrum are those animals that are able to resolve the lesion spontaneously. The subchondral capillary bed is able to surround, bridge over, and bypass the area of chondromalacia and reestablish normal enchondral ossification superficial to the lesion. The result is a delay in the modeling of the developing articular surface, seen radiographically as a flattening of the subchondral bone. Grossly, the early lesion in the humoral head is outlined by a discoloration of the cartilage in the affected area (Fig. 84–18). Percussion of the area is normal and indicates that there has been no separation of the cartilage from the subchondral bone. In the advanced lesion, a loosened area of cartilage usually tears partially away from the defective osteochondral junction and forms a flap. Complete separation can occur; in such a case, the detached piece of cartilage becomes a joint body (Fig. 84–18). In either event, the animal is apt to show clinical signs of lameness. Healing of the defect occurs by granulation tissue arising from the subchondral bone, which eventually becomes fibrocartilage.

Synovial fluid from dogs with osteochondrosis resembles that of dogs with degenerative joint disease. If there is a great deal of necrotic cartilage debris, the number of phagocytic synovial mononuclear cells will be increased, and there may be an occasional neutrophil.

The lesion is demonstrated radiographically by an irregularly appearing subchondral surface, a focal defect in the subchondral bone, and varying degrees of increased bone density surrounding the defect (Fig. 84–17). The defect may not have a distinct zone of increased density surrounding it or

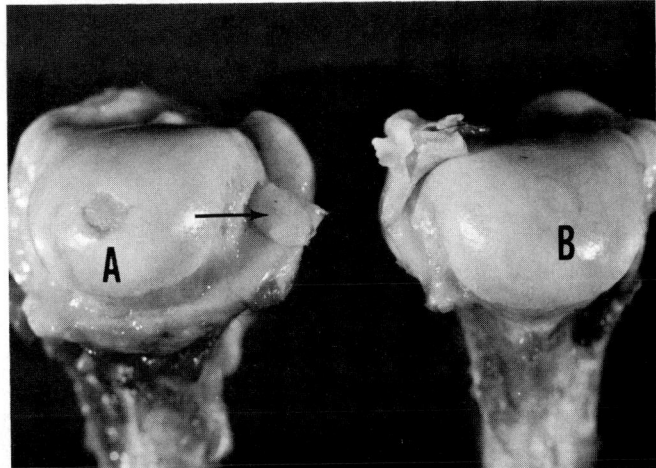

Figure 84–18. Osteochondrosis of the humoral head. Advanced lesion (A) shows a defect that has partially filled with fibrocartilage. Note that the detached piece of cartilage (arrow) has grown to be larger than the original defect. Early lesion (B) has a smooth articular surface but is outlined by discoloration of the cartilage.

may have a zone of one to three mm in thickness. The subchondral defect may have a small distinct opening at the surface of the joint or may appear as a large crater-like lesion. Free fragments are sometimes identified on survey radiographs, while cartilage flaps are more commonly noted on arthrograms. Secondary degenerative joint disease and an abnormal shape of the affected epiphysis are seen in the chronic stages of the clinical disorder.

The treatment of osteochondrosis in the dog involves either rest or rest combined with surgical curettage of the lesion (Berzon, 1979; Clayton-Jones, 1980; Smith and Stowater, 1975; Wissler and Sumner-Smith, 1977). Milder cases can often be successfully managed by strict rest for four to eight weeks, followed by an equal period of limited exercise. Surgery is indicated when the devitalized cartilage defect impedes healing (persistent lameness) or has broken partially or completely free, or if the lesion is extensive. The surgery should be directed at removing mainly loose or devitalized cartilage. Extensive curettage of the crater should be avoided, as it may actually predispose to degenerative joint disease, especially in joints such as the tarsus (Alexander, 1980b). Following surgical removal of the devitalized cartilage and free cartilage debris from the joint cavity, the animal is rested for four to six weeks to allow the defect to undergo fibrocartilaginous repair. Immobilization of the joint for the first week may be helpful. Failure to treat the problem appropriately in the early stages can lead ultimately to debilitating secondary degenerative joint disease.

Ununited Coronoid and Anconeal Processes

These abnormalities may be additional manifestations of osteochondrosis (Olsson, 1976), because the lesions tend to occur in

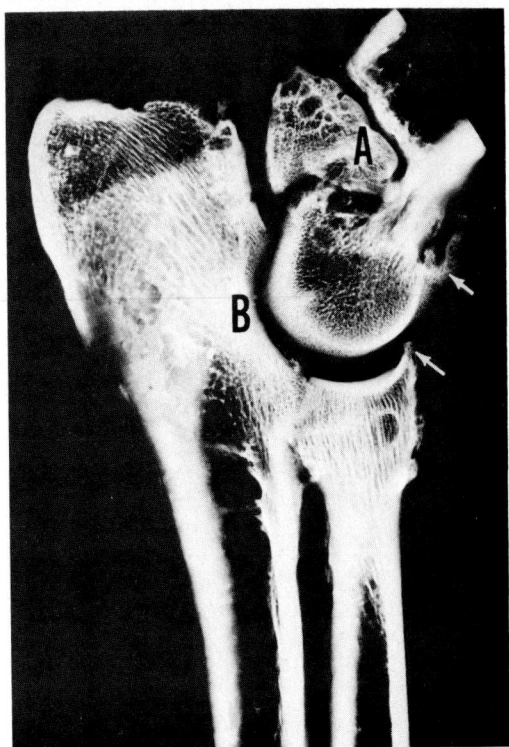

Figure 84–19. Ununited anconeal process (A) is lodged in the olecranon fossa. Secondary degenerative joint disease of the elbow is characterized by subchondral bone sclerosis in the trochlear notch of the ulna (B) and the formation of periarticular osteophytes (arrows).

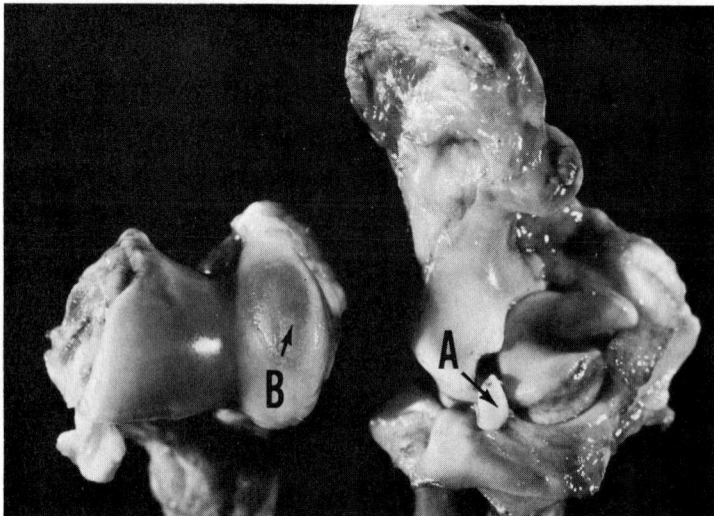

Figure 84-20. Ununited coronoid process (A) has caused secondary degnerative disease in the elbow joint. Note the abraded surface of the medial condyle of the humerus (B) apposing the loose coronoid process.

the same breeds of dogs and under the same conditions of rapid growth and genetic predisposition (Battershell, 1969; Corley et al., 1968). The basic lesion is characterized by degeneration of cartilage along the base of the developing anconeal and coronoid processes. This can delay the bony union of these processes with the shaft of the ulna, and eventual avulsion from the ulnar shaft can occur (Figs. 84–19 and 84–20). After separation, the processes may remain loosely attached *in situ* and retain a blood supply or, in the case of the anconeal process, can become completely detached. In both conditions, the result is joint instability that can lead in time to secondary degenerative joint disease. Early surgical removal of the ununited processes can minimize, but not eliminate, subsequent secondary degenerative changes.

Hypoplasia of the Coronoid Process

Hypoplasia of the coronoid process of the dog is an uncommon clinical disorder. Hypoplasia may result from trauma, loss of contact with the trochlea of the humerus, or sustained pressure to the developing coronoid process. The entire thickness of the articular cartilage over the coronoid process is necrotic, and no germinative cells remain to reinitiate the growth of the process (Fig. 84–21). Radiographically, the lack of development of the coronoid process is readily apparent.

Ectopic Ossification Centers

An ectopic ossification center resembling a sesamoid bone has been observed medial to the head of the radius in the joint capsule of the elbow (Grøndalen and Braut, 1976;

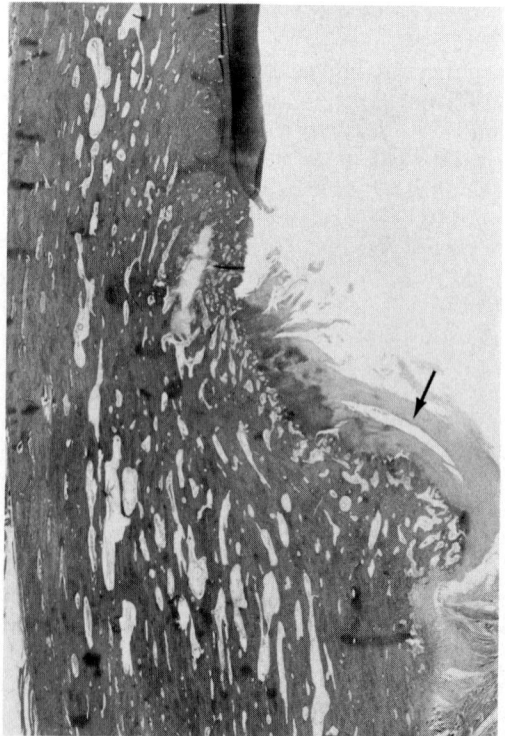

Figure 84–21. Hypoplasia of the coronoid process. Necrosis and fibrillation of the entire layer of articular cartilage (arrow).

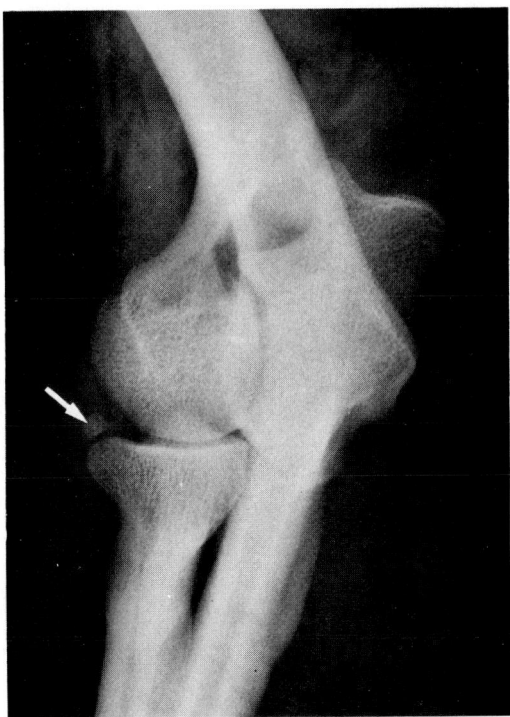

Figure 84–22. Oblique radiograph of the elbow joint of a mature dog with an ectopic ossification center that is craniolateral in location (arrow).

The lameness begins at 8 to 11 months of age and occurs most frequently in certain breeds of dogs, such as Laborador retrievers, German shepherds, Burnese mountain dogs, Newfoundlands, and rottweilers. The elbow disorder can be bilateral or unilateral and may predispose the joint to degenerative changes. The lameness ceases when the ectopic ossification center is surgically removed. A similar ectopic ossification center can occasionally be seen over the dorsocranial aspect of the acetabulum of dogs (Fig. 84–24); this condition does not produce clinical signs, however.

Hip Dysplasia

Hip dysplasia is a developmental disease identified in most breeds of dogs. It tends to occur more frequently, however, in larger, well-fed, faster growing breeds (Lust, 1973; Lust et al., 1973). The development of hip dysplasia is strongly influenced by complex genetic factors (Hedhammer et al., 1979; Fisher, 1979; Leighton et al., 1977) and affects both sexes of dogs with equal frequency. It has also been described in cats (Hayes et al., 1979; Holt, 1978; Kolde, 1974; Peiffer and Blevins, 1978). In cats, purebreds are much more likely to be affected than domestics.

The clinical progression of the disorder has been best documented in the canine, but the evolution of the changes in both dogs and cats appears to be rather stereotyped. Dysplastic dogs are born with normal hip

Price and King, 1977; Vaananen and Skutnabb, 1978) (Figs. 84–22 and 84–23). In some cases, a lameness may result from the presence of the ossification center, and in other cases it is only an incidental radiographic finding in clinically normal animals.

Figure 84–23. Radiograph of a 1-cm thick bone section that shows an ectopic ossification center (A) in the lateral joint capsule of a canine elbow (same case as in Fig. 84–22). This small ossicle has a body of spongy bone that is covered by hyaline cartilage (arrow), which articulates with the head of the radius (B).

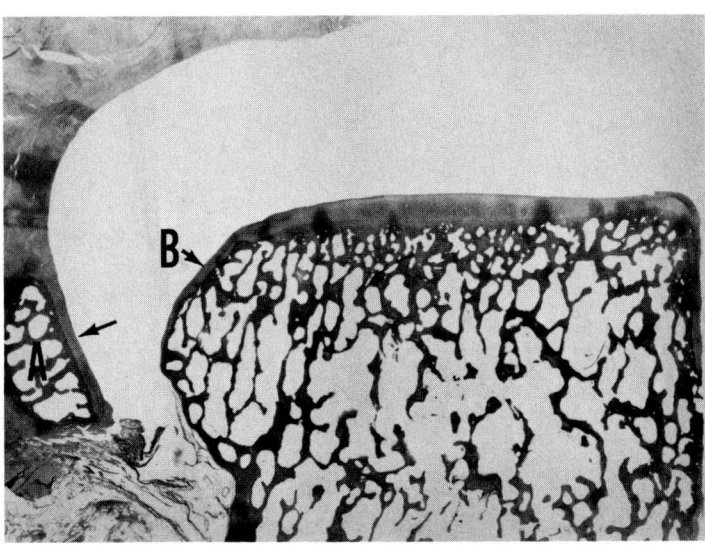

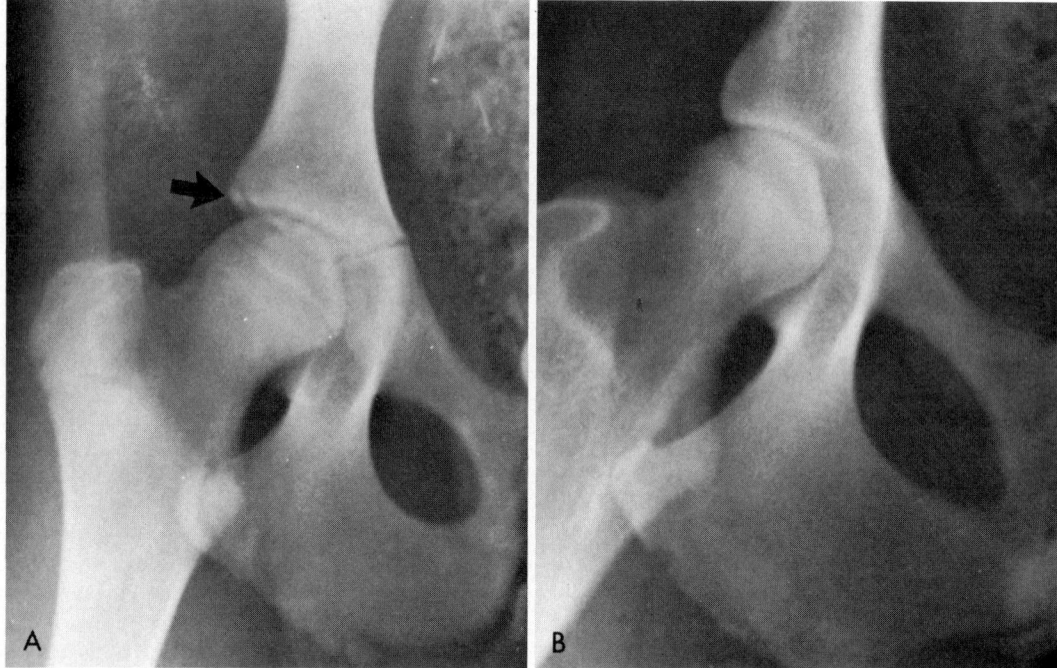

Figure 84–24. Ventrodorsal projections of a hip joint of a Great Dane at six months (A) and two years of age (B) with an ectopic ossification center (arrow) noted on the earlier study. The hip joint at two years of age is felt to be within normal limits.

joints that subsequently undergo progressive structural alterations. The following structural anomalies are identified either pathologically or radiographically: joint laxity; shallow acetabular cavities; subluxation; swelling, fraying, and rupture of the teres ligament; erosion of the articular cartilage, with eburnation of the subchondral bone;

remodeling of the acetabular rim and flattening of the femoral head; and periarticular osteophyte production (Morgan, 1969; Pharr and Morgan, 1976) (Figs. 84–25 and 84–26). There are considerable variations in the severity of the clinical signs, time of onset of structural changes, age at which clinical signs appear, rate of disease pro-

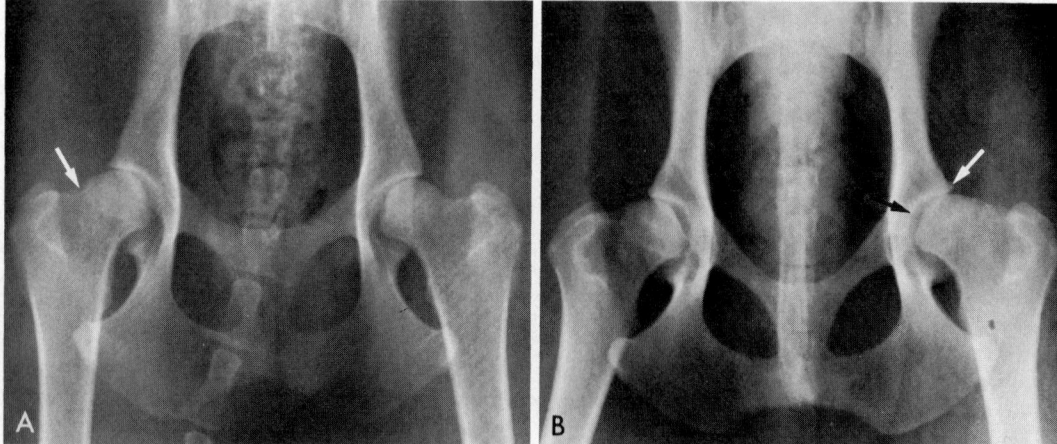

Figure 84–25. Ventrodorsal radiographs of the pelves of two dogs with minimal remodeling of the femoral neck (arrow), lipping of the acetabular rim (arrow), filling of the depths of the acetabulum with bone (black arrow), and subluxation that are characteristic of hip dysplasia.

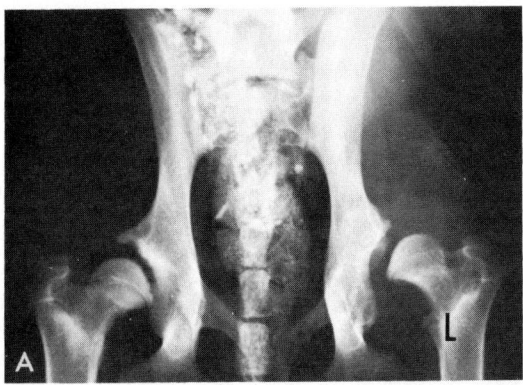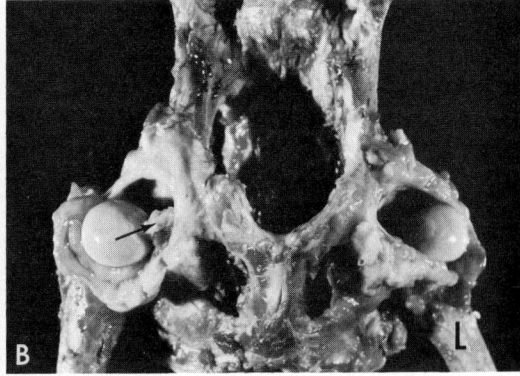

Figure 84–26. Radiograph of a dog with severe bilateral hip dysplasia, as evidenced by lesions characteristic of chronic secondary degenerative joint disease. Severe subluxation of the left hip (L) with an abnormally shallow acetabulum is demonstrated. Note the abnormal contours of the femoral heads and periarticular new bone formation. Gross tissues demonstrate the thickened joint capsules. The ligament of the head of the right femur was thickened and frayed, while the ligament of the left femur (L) was ruptured. Note that the left femoral head has an abnormal shape and that the articular surface is irregular.

gression, and degree of pain and impaired mobility. Since joint laxity is the earliest sign of hip dysplasia (Wright and Mason, 1977), gait abnormalities without overt lameness or stiffness may precede the degenerative joint disease by many months. Degenerative joint disease may occur within the first year of life, but many animals show no clinical and radiographic signs until two to six years of age. There may be a poor correlation between clinical and radiographic signs.

Young dogs with unstable hips are prone to develop bouts of acute lameness following exercise or strenuous activity. This does not mean that degenerative changes have occurred at this stage. Rest, and analgesics for several days, will often be sufficient to treat the condition. It is mentioned only because there is a temptation on such occasions to assume the worst and to initiate more drastic therapeutic measures.

The precise etiology of hip dysplasia in the dog remains in question. As mentioned earlier, genetic factors are important. Environmental and nutritional factors, however, are involved in the expression of the abnormal phenotype (Hedhammer et al., 1974; Kasstrom, 1975). There is debate as to whether the fundamental cause is intrinsic or extrinsic to the hip joint. Proponents of an intrinsic cause believe that the primary change occurs in the development of the coxofemoral joint itself (Larsen, 1973; Lust, 1973). One suggestion is that such structural abnormalities are due to osteochondrosis (Olsson, 1976). Proponents of an extrinsic

cause believe that the hip abnormalities occur secondary to physical anomalies or inadequacies in the muscles that support the coxofemoral joint during development (Cardinet et al., 1972; Riser and Shirer, 1967). Whatever the cause, the end result is a joint that is unstable and predisposed to degeneration.

The treatment of hip dysplasia is mainly palliative and varies with the stage of the disease. In the early stages when there is considerable pain and minimal degenerative changes, rest, restriction of activities that put stress on the hips, and analgesic drugs may prove adequate. In dogs with more advanced disease, restricted activity and analgesics may not be sufficient to provide relief of pain. At this point, most dogs will show signs of degenerative joint disease on radiographs. Sectioning of the pectineus muscle or tendon may afford relief from pain for periods of six months or more (Wallace et al., 1975). The procedure does not prevent the progression of degenerative changes but rather releases painful pressure (and perhaps severs sensory nerves that carry pain sensation) on the capsule of the hip joints. The procedure is not without controversy (Rubin et al., 1979), and while some individual investigators advocate its use wholeheartedly (Wallace et al., 1975), others are more reserved (Nunamaker and Newton, 1975). Some orthopedic surgeons believe that simultaneous sectioning of the adductor magnus muscle gives more relief than if the pectineus muscle alone is sectioned (Nunamaker and Newton, 1975). Pectineal myotomy or tendonectomy has also been used with apparent benefit in cats with hip dysplasia (Kolde, 1974; Peiffer and Blevins, 1974). Surgical repositioning of the acetabulum by pelvic osteotomy has been advocated in young animals with subluxating hips but without signs of degenerative joint disease (Hohn and Janes, 1969). This procedure requires considerable surgical skill and has seen limited application in practice. It does not prevent all subluxation, nor does it prevent degenerative joint disease. It will, however, decrease the rate of progression and severity of such changes. A simpler procedure for acetabular repositioning has been described by Schrader (1981). Short-term evaluation of this surgical procedure has been promising, but whether it will prevent degenerative joint disease in the long term is not yet known.

The treatment of advanced hip dysplasia is essentially directed toward the degenerative joint disease. As such, the treatments listed in the discussion of degenerative joint disease are applicable. Femoral head ostectomies can be very effective in some dogs (Bonneau and Bretton, 1981; Duff and Campbell, 1977; Gendreau and Cawley, 1977). Dogs with intractable hip pain, but without significant disease in other joints or neurologic problems, are the best candidates. Although smaller dogs form more functional false joints, even large dogs can benefit from the surgery (Gendreau and Cawley, 1977). Holt (1978) describes a cat with hip dysplasia that responded favorably to excision arthroplasty after a pectineus myotomy failed to give relief. The most attractive treatment for advanced hip dys-

plasia is total hip replacement (Leighton, 1979; Olmstead and Hohn, 1980). Although this procedure is becoming practical from a technical aspect, the cost of the surgery has limited its use.

Patellar Luxation

Patellar luxation is an orthopedic problem of varied etiology (Harrison, 1975). In cases of extreme valgus or varus deformities of the stifles, pressure by the quadriceps tendon is directed medially or laterally, depending on the character of the deformity. This maldirected tensile force will gradually pull the patella out of the trochlear groove. Such valgus or varus deformities can be congenital or can be acquired by virtue of femoral fractures that have healed with improper alignment. Traumatic luxations of the patella have also been described (Irving, 1979). The most common problem, however, is congenital patellar luxation occurring in small toy breeds of dogs (Harrison, 1975). This condition is less frequently seen in cats (Flecknell and Gruffydd-Jones, 1979; Leighton, 1978).

The basic cause of congenital patellar luxation in small dogs is unknown. The trochlear ridge of the distal femur, which forms the patellar groove, appears unusually flattened. In addition, many of these dogs appear to have a degree of genu valgum.

In toy breeds of dogs, medial patellar luxation is the most common pattern (Fig. 84–27). There is great variation in the disorder in toy dogs. The disorder occurs as a spectrum, depending on the severity of the basic deformities (Harrison, 1975), and the

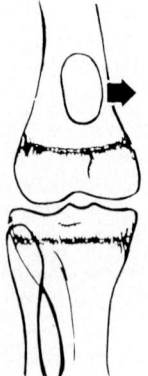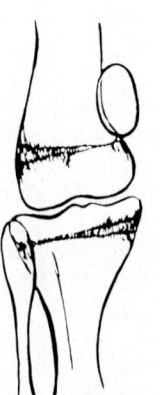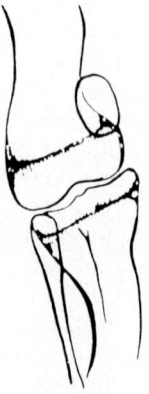

Figure 84–27. Medial patellar luxation in the dog. Medial patellar luxation in the puppy leads to abnormal growth in the physis on either side of the joint. The joint space is more angulated and secondary joint disease with cruciate and collateral ligament damage can result.

deformities will often progress with time. In the mildest form the patella can be luxated with some difficulty by extending the stifle and pushing the patella medially while the pull of the quadriceps tendon remains nearly parallel to the trochlear groove. These dogs will become acutely lame when the patella luxates, but this lameness often lasts for only a few seconds or minutes, until the patella falls back into place. In more severe cases, the patella is pulled progressively more medially, the medial ridge of the trochlear groove becomes flattened, and the pull of the quadriceps tendon is directed more medially. To establish a straight line of motion between the quadriceps tendon and the tibial crest, and to keep the foot in a relatively normal position, the femur and tibia assume an S-shaped deformity. In the most severe cases the patella lies completely without and medial to the hypoplastic trochlear groove, the tibial crest is displaced medially, and there is prominent deformation of the distal femur and proximal tibia (Fig. 84–28).

The treatment of patellar luxation depends mainly on the severity of the condition (Harrison, 1975). Many toy breeds with patellas that dislocate only occasionally can be treated with surgical procedures designed to reinforce the lateral ligamentous attachments to the patella. In more severe cases this is accompanied by procedures for deepening the trochlear groove. In still more severe cases, repositioning of the tibial crest is done. In the worst cases, osteotomies of the femur and tibia may also be needed to help correct malalignments.

Aseptic Necrosis of the Femoral Head

Aseptic necrosis (Legg-Calve-Perthes disease) of the femoral head frequently occurs without an apparent predisposing cause in adolescent dogs of toy and small breeds (Alexander, 1980a). In breeds such as toy poodles, genetic factors may be involved in disease expression (Pidduck and Webbon, 1978). For some undetermined reason, a major portion of the blood supply to the capital epiphysis of the femur is compromised, and the ischemic portion undergoes necrosis (Fig. 84–29). Aseptic necrosis can also occur following fractures through the femoral neck or physis.

Following disruption of the blood supply

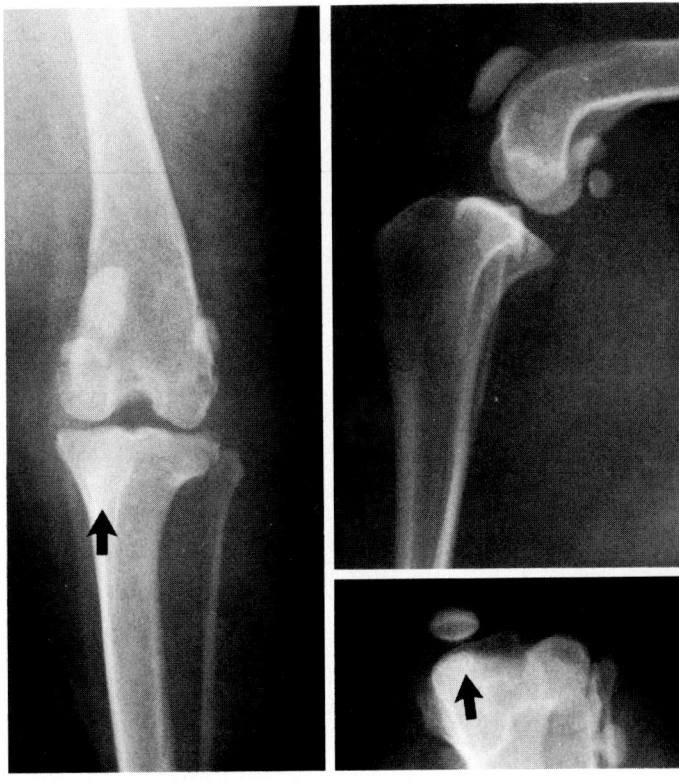

Figure 84–28. Caudocranial, lateral, and "sky-line" projections of the stifle joint that show the medial displacement of the attachment on the tibia of the patellar ligament. The lateral and sky-line projections show the failure of the trochlea to form normally.

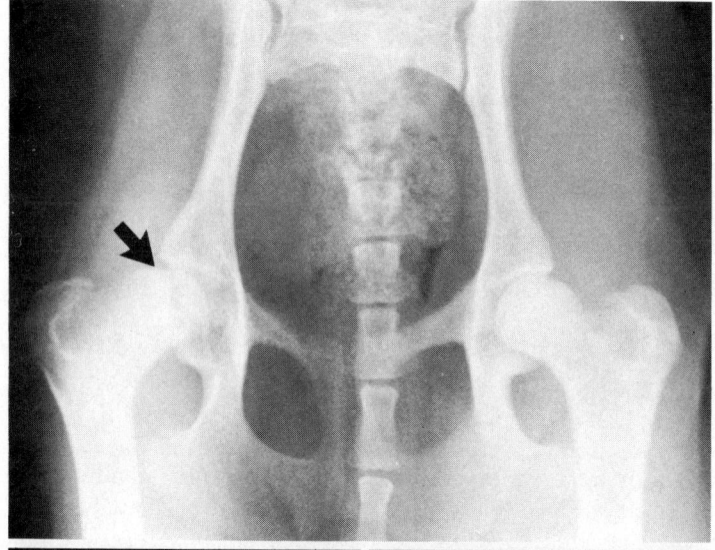

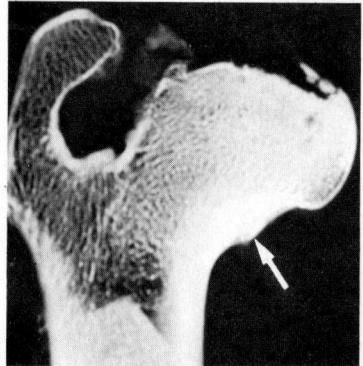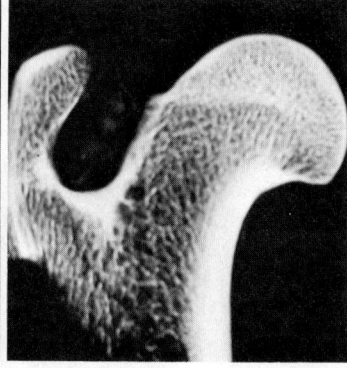

Figure 84–29. Ventrodorsal radiograph of the pelvis and radiographs of thin bone sections show the fragmentation within the femoral head typical of aseptic necrosis or Legg-Calve-Perthes disease. Note the thickened femoral neck (arrow) secondary to the primary bone disease within the femoral head.

to the femoral head, for whatever reason, the affected area of epiphyseal spongiosa undergoes necrosis while the overlying cartilage, which receives its nutrition from the synovial fluid, remains viable. The body tries to repair the defect with granulation tissue and new cancellous bone arising from the resulting fibro-osseus response (Fig. 84–30). Unfortunately, the amount of bony repair is often insignificant or occurs too late to prevent collapse of the unsupported articular cartilage. Collapse of the femoral head affects the congruity of the articular surfaces and predisposes the joint to secondary joint disease.

Necrosis of the femoral head is manifested by slight to severe lameness. Since there is little likelihood of spontaneous resolution, femoral head ostectomy is the accepted treatment (Gendreau and Cawley, 1977; Lee and Fry, 1969; Ljunggren, 1966).

ARTHROPATHIES DUE TO INBORN ERRORS OF METABOLISM

Hemophilia A

Lameness is one of the most common complaints of men and dogs with congenital coagulation defects. In fact, factor 8 deficiency, or hemophilia A, of the dog can lead to an arthropathy indistinguishable from that occurring in hemophiliac humans (Swanton, 1957). Hemophilia A also occurs in cats, but much less is known about associated joint disease in this species.

The arthropathy of hemophilia A is caused by chronic hemorrhage into the joint, which is induced by clinical or subclinical trauma. Obviously, therefore, larger weight-bearing joints such as the elbows and stifles are more likely to be involved, and larger and more active dogs will have more problems than smaller, less active dogs. The

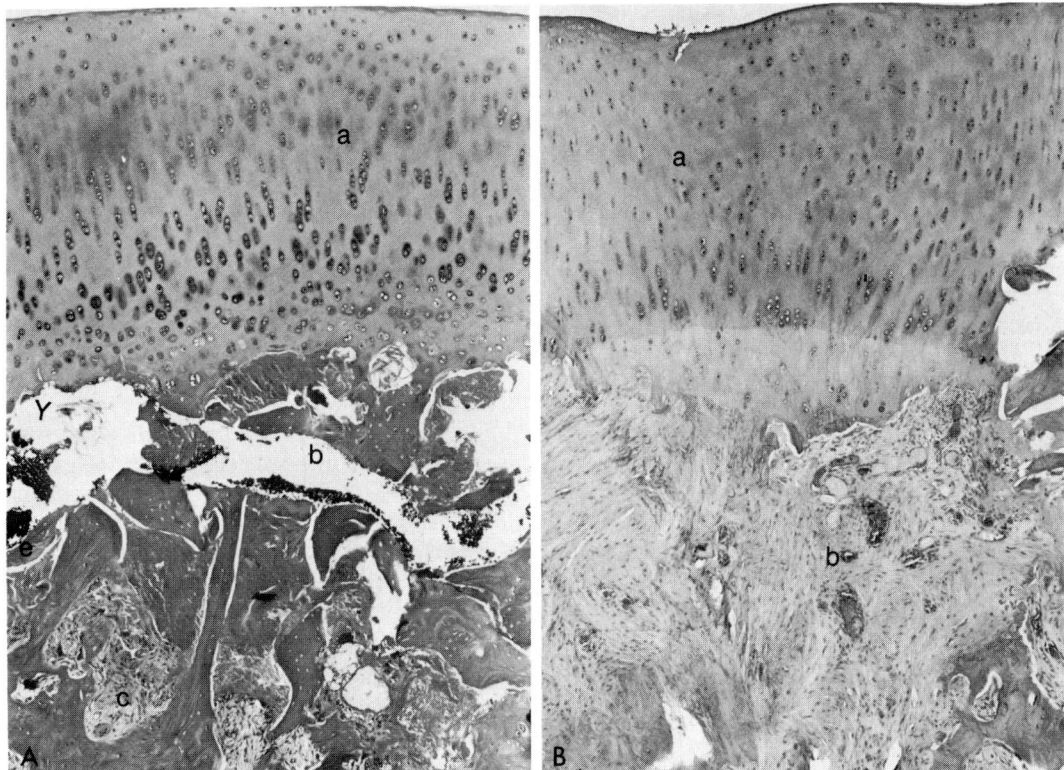

Figure 84–30. Aseptic necrosis of the femoral head. A, Acute lesion shows normal articular cartilage (a), necrosis and hemorrhage in the subchondral bone and adjacent epiphyseal spongiosa (b). Granulation tissue (c) arises in the marrow spaces along the border of the infarct. Healing lesion (B), shows abnormal articular cartilage (a), maturing granulation tissue replacing the area of bone necrosis (b), and attempts at the intramembranous bone formation in the fibrous connective tissue response.

effusion of blood into the joint cavity resulting from synovial or subsynovial hemorrhage provokes an acute inflammatory reaction. The synovial membrane thickens and undergoes villous hypertrophy, and there is hyperplasia of the intimal layer and infiltration of lymphocytes, macrophages, and plasma cells. The reaction subsides after several days to weeks, but each subsequent hemorrhagic episode leads to further synovial fibrosis and hemosiderosis. However, the most significant sites of injury are the articular cartilage and subchondral bone. Injury to the articular cartilage is caused by granulation tissue arising from the synovium and from the subchondral bone. Synovial fluid may be frankly bloody during bouts of hemorrhage or xanthrochromic with excess numbers of macrophages at other times.

Panosteitis

Panosteitis is covered in detail in Chapter 85 and is mentioned here only because it is important in the differential diagnosis of lameness in adolescent dogs. Panosteitis is a disorder of endosteal ossification in the shafts of long bones (Bone, 1980). It tends to occur in the same breeds and in the same age group as osteochondrosis, ununited anconeal and coronoid processes, and hip dysplasia. It is particularly common in German shepherd dogs and Doberman pinschers.

Panosteitis often occurs in dogs with von Willebrand's disease, a blood coagulation defect caused by a deficiency of functional factor 8 and abnormalities in platelet aggregation. This association was first described by Dodds (1978), and about one half of the cases of panosteitis seen by the authors have shown the same relationship. Von Willebrand's disease in dogs is present in 5 to 20 per cent of dogs in some breeds and is often subclinical; the abnormal factor 8 and platelet aggregation tends to disappear with age (Dodds, 1978).

Mucopolysaccharidosis

Arylsulfatase B enzyme deficiency (Maroteaux-Lamy syndrome) has been identified as an autosomal recessive trait in Siamese cats (Jezyk et al., 1977). Hurler's syndrome, caused by a deficiency of alpha-L-iduronidase enzyme, has also been identified in a cat (Haskins et al., 1979). A dog with Morquio's syndrome has been studied by the authors. Animals with these disorders have in common an inability to properly metabolize aminoglycans, such as chondroitin and keratin sulfates. As such, they will often manifest abnormalities in tissues rich in such substances, e.g., cartilage, connective tissue, cornea. Readers are referred to Chapter 85 for detailed descriptions of the cartilage and joint abnormalities in these various disorders.

Multicentric Periarticular Calcinosis

Ellison and Norrdin (1980) described a 12-week-old Vizsla puppy with progressive lameness, and periarticular calcinosis of all diarthrodial joints. Although no definitive data were available, it was suggested that the disorder was due to a renal tubular defect (presumably in calcium-phosphorus transport). A Vizsla with a similar syndrome, and with a proven tubular defect in phosphorous transport, has been seen by the authors.

DIETARY ARTHROPATHIES

Secondary hyperparathyroidism and a rickets-like syndrome has been seen in cats fed diets composed mainly of beef heart (Riser, 1962; Scott et al., 1963). Besides other skeletal lesions, major limb joints may undergo ankylosis of opposing joint surfaces.

Hypervitaminosis A, a condition caused by consuming large amounts of raw liver, has been described as a naturally occurring entity of cats (Seawright et al., 1970). It is characterized by subperiosteal proliferation of new woven bone around the apophyseal joints of the cervical and thoracic vertebrae and proliferation of cartilage from the joint margin. The process can overgrow the synovium and bridge the joint. It is mentioned here because this disorder is frequently misdiagnosed in cats that actually have degenerative joint disease. Dietary problems leading to skeletal abnormalities will be discussed in greater detail in Chapter 85.

NEOPLASTIC ARTHROPATHIES

Primary Neoplastic Arthropathies

Synovial sarcoma, or synovioma, is by far the most common primary joint tumor in animals. These tumors occur most frequently in middle-aged dogs (seven to eight years old) (Lipowitz et al., 1979; Madewell and Pool, 1978). It has also been reported in cats (Gresti, 1975). These tumors in dogs and cats typically involve a major limb joint, usually the stifle or the elbow joint. Radiographic signs include a soft tissue swelling in all cases, and bone destruction with irregular periosteal response from bones on either side of the involved joint in more than one half of the dogs affected. Synovial sarcomas are characterized microscopically by the presence of varying proportions of two intermingled cellular components, a pleomorphic synovioblastic or "epithelioid" component and a spindle-cell or "fibroblastic" cellular component. Synovial sarcomas associated with tendon sheaths are probably just as common but are usually diagnosed as undifferentiated sarcomas of the deeper soft tissue.

The osteogenic sarcoma, or osteosarcoma, is a frequent cause of lameness in large and giant breeds of dogs. It is not technically a joint tumor but is important in the differential diagnosis of lameness in giant breeds of dogs. Osteosarcomas are discussed further in Chapter 85.

Metastatic Neoplastic Arthropathies

Tumors rarely metastasize to the joint, except for the arthropathy that occurs in some cats with lymphosarcoma (Barclay, 1979).

INFLAMMATORY JOINT DISEASE

This major form of joint disease is characterized by inflammatory changes in the synovial membrane and synovial fluid, and by systemic signs of illness such as fever, leukocytosis, malaise, anorexia, and hyperfibrinogenemia. The etiology of inflammatory joint disease of animals is diverse and includes both infectious and noninfectious causes.

INFECTIOUS ARTHRITIS

Bacterial Arthritis

Bacteria may gain entrance to the joint through penetrating wounds (Alexander, 1978) or from contiguous sites of infection in bone or soft tissue. Surgical contamination and nonsterile injections into the synovial cavity are other sources of sepsis. Infection via penetrating wounds is much more frequent in large animals than in dogs and cats. Grass awns, especially from foxtail barley, may penetrate the skin and subcutaneous tissue and enter the joint.

Bacteria may also gain access to the joints from infectious foci within the blood vascular system itself, e.g., heart valves or the umbilical vein. Omphalophlebitis, or umbilical vein infection, is common in both puppies and kittens. In many cases this infection will spread via the bloodstream and is carried to the synovial lining, which has a rich blood supply and contains phagocytic cells that trap the bacteria. Omphalophlebitis in kittens often results when the queen chews off the umbilical cord flush with the abdominal wall. Normally, the umbilical cord is left several centimeters long and dries to form an impenetrable barrier. If it is chewed off too short, infection with direct access to the bloodstream occurs in the umbilical remnant. In kittens, the usual offending organism is *Pasteurella* which normally inhabits the queen's oral cavity.

Bacterial septicemias are seen in puppies and kittens from sources other than omphalophlebitis. Streptococcal pharyngitis with abscessation of the retropharyngeal lymph nodes and septicemia occurs in some puppies during the first two weeks of life. Queens or bitches with post-parturient uterine or mammary gland infections can infect their young shortly after birth. If this leads to systemic infection in the newborn, joint abscessation can be seen.

Subacute bacterial endocarditis occurs in both dogs and cats and is occasionally associated with a septic arthritis (Bennett et al.,

1978; Caywood et al., 1977). It is more common in dogs, probably because dogs have a higher incidence of predisposing congenital or acquired heart problems. Dogs also have a higher incidence of oral, genitourinary, and skin infections, which are frequent sources of bacteria.

Bacterial septicemias are common in older dogs and have been seen in some cats. Such systemic infections are frequently associated with septic arthritis. In older animals, the most common source of infection is the genitourinary tract, followed by the skin, oral cavity, and respiratory tract. Cystitis, pyelonephritis, prostatitis, pneumonia, pyodermas, and tooth infections can all be accompanied by septicemia at times. In dogs, infection of the disc spaces (diskospondylitis) is often associated with septic arthritis, bacteremia, and bacteruria. Systemic spread of infection may be potentiated in older animals by situations brought about by debilitating cancers, immunosuppressive drug therapy, neutropenias, or loss of bowel integrity during fulminating gastrointestinal infection.

Organisms commonly involved in joint infection include staphylococci, streptococci (Bennett et al., 1978), *Erysipelothrix* (Goudswarrd et al., 1973), *Corynebacteria*, coliforms and *Pasteurella* (Bennett et al., 1978), *Salmonella*, and occasionally *Brucella* (Clegg and Rorrison, 1968). The type of organism involved in the joint infection has some clinical significance. *Staphylococci* and some coliforms will cause rapid destruction of articular cartilage, whereas organisms such as *Erysipelothrix* and streptococci may be present in the joint without causing significant cartilage damage. As a rule, organisms that cause severe cartilage damage also cause toxic or degenerative changes in neutrophils present in the synovial fluid.

Septic arthritis, regardless of cause, is more apt to occur in dogs than in cats, and it is more likely to occur in giant or sporting breeds than in smaller dogs. The pattern of joint disease is more likely to be monarticular or pauciarticular (two to five joints) than polyarticular, and larger joints (shoulders, elbows, hips, and stifles) are more apt to be involved than smaller joints. Infection is more likely to localize in joints previously damaged by some other disease process such as osteochondrosis or degenerative joint disease. Septic arthritis will often be painful on palpation, and redness and swelling of the overlying skin and soft tissue may be present.

Synovial fluid from septic joints is frequently bloody, which differentiates it from most noninfectious joint disorders. The fluid contains large numbers of neutrophils, but the absolute count, although high, will overlap with the neutrophil counts in synovial fluid from nonseptic, inflamed joints. The presence of toxic, ruptured, and degranulated neutrophils should make one suspicious of a bacterial infection. As mentioned previously, however, not all types of bacteria are equally proficient at inducing such toxic changes.

The earliest radiographic findings of bacterial arthritis are often missed because of delay in presenting the animal for radiographic examination. These early findings are thickened synovial membrane, distended joint capsule with a displacement of fascial planes, and a slight widening of the joint space. Radiolucent intra-articular shadows due to intra-articular fat pads may disappear, owing to the accumulation of exudate within the joints. Although radiographic changes such as this are often present in the early stages, the diagnosis should not be discarded when radiographic changes are absent. If clinical signs are suggestive, a joint tap should be performed.

A radiographic finding more commonly noted in the later stages is a fine, faintly identifiable, periosteal proliferation on the bones adjacent to the joint space. This type of reactive periostitis is not to be confused with the prominent, better-defined, periarticular bony spurs that develop in degenerative joint disease or following trauma. Aspiration of the joint at this time is still necessary to reach a positive diagnosis. Following the period of early soft tissue swelling and inflammation, and dependent on the organism involved, the process expands with destruction of the articular cartilage and resulting loss of width of the joint space. Narrowing of the joint space is often unappreciated, because of the unwillingness of the animal to bear weight on the leg. If the disease is not controlled, it quickly leads to an osteomyelitis in the adjacent bones and a widening of the joint space as it fills with debris and exudate. It is difficult to attach time intervals from the time of onset for the various stages of bacterial arthritis. This is because of differences in the pathogenicity of the organisms, the manner of inoculation, and the type of superimposed treatment that may delay (inappropriate or inadequate antibiotic therapy) or hasten (immunosuppressive drugs) the development of the pathologic process.

Complications of infectious arthritis include osteomyelitis, fibrous or bony ankylosis, and secondary joint disease. An osteomyelitis is present as soon as the articular plate is breached and the infectious process enters the subchondral bone (Fig. 84–31). This compounds the severity of the disease and makes the prognosis more guarded. If the articular cartilage has been damaged, fibrotic or bony ankylosis can follow. This is a logical consequence, because the destruction of the cartilage exposes the subchondral bone and simulates a condition like that of a fracture. Frequently an abscess forms within the exudate and debris, preventing bony fusion from occurring across the joint space. In these cases, reactive bone bridges the joint, leaving a radiolucent cavity around the abscess.

Dependent on the severity of the arthritis, a certain amount of articular damage is present at the time the infection is brought under control. The rate at which a secondary joint disease develops subsequently depends on the severity of the destructive process, the degree of use of the joint, and other factors such as the weight or conformation of the animal.

The treatment of bacterial arthritis is dependent on the isolation and identification of the organism, and on the determination of antibiotic sensitivities. If bacteria cannot be cultured from the joint, positive isolations from the blood or urine should be considered representative of the infection in the joints. Whenever possible, bactericidal antibiotics should be used. Most antibiotics will penetrate the vascular bed of an inflamed joint, so systemic treatment is usually effective. Local infusions of antibiotics can be used when a single joint is involved. In this situation, antibiotics are most effective if they are infused almost continuously and associated with drainage. Generally, antibiotics are given for periods of two weeks or more after the signs of infection have disappeared. In the case of bacterial endocarditis, antibiotic treatment may have to be continued longer.

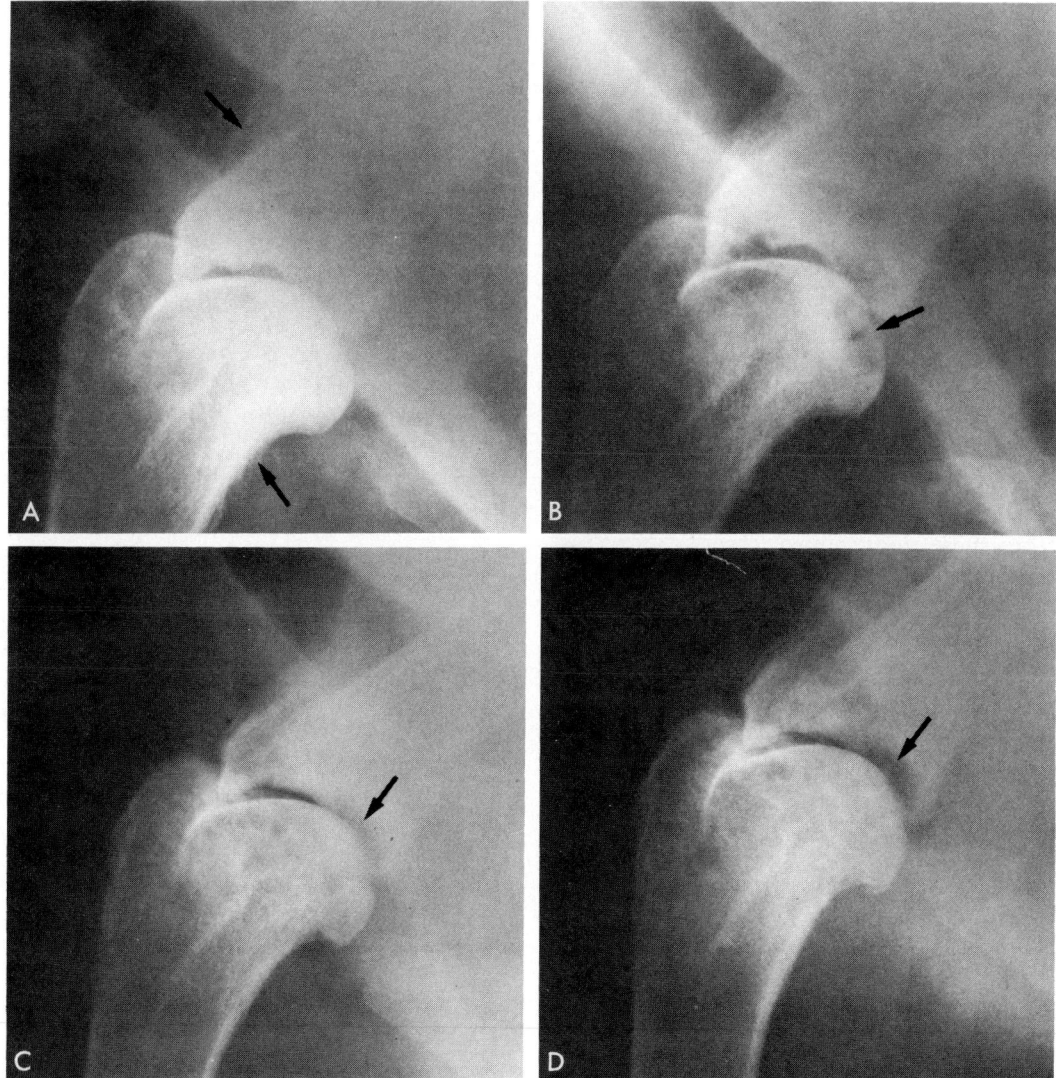

Figure 84–31. Lateral radiographs of the shoulder joint of an eight-year-old male German shepherd dog with progressive infectious arthritis and osteomyelitis, characterized by periosteal new bone response (arrow) and destructive lesions within the humeral head (arrow) and glenoid cavity. Radiographs are made (A) on the day of first examination, (B) 2 months, (C) 1 year, and (D) 16 months after the first examination.

Mycoplasmal Arthritis

A mycoplasmal arthritis can result from the systemic spread of organisms from localized sites of active or latent infection in the respiratory passages, nasal cavity, conjunctival membranes, or urogenital tract. Such a condition is uncommon, however, in dogs and cats. The authors have seen only two such instances in dogs and cats. A generalized mycoplasmal polyarthritis was observed in a dog undergoing chemotherapy for lymphosarcoma. A less widespread joint disease was also observed in an old debilitated cat being treated with surgery and radiation for an oral squamous cell carcinoma.

The synovial fluid in dogs and cats with mycoplasmal arthritis is thin and cloudy, and contains a greatly elevated number of neutrophils. The neutrophils are not toxic, degranulated, or ruptured. The fluid cannot be differentiated from other inflammatory joint fluids except by culture or observation of the organisms using Wright-Leishman or Giemsa stains. Mycoplasmal arthritis can be treated with tylosin, gentamycin, or erythromycin.

Viral Arthritis

A fleeting and sometimes persistent arthropathy is a symptom of many acute viral diseases of man. It usually occurs in the post-convalescent period following mumps, coxsackie virus, or adenovirus infections (Bayer, 1980). Because animals show signs of pain only when the joint inflammation is relatively severe, the degree to which arthropathy complicates acute viral diseases in animals is unknown. A sterile, usually generalized, inflammatory joint disorder is seen commonly in younger dogs from six to ten months of age. The dogs are stiff, lame, and febrile. The arthritis may last for several days or persist for up to a month or more. The pattern and age of disease resembles human post-viral arthritides. Synovial fluid from these dogs is thin, cloudy, and often yellow-tinged, and contains large numbers of normal appearing neutrophils. It is sterile for microorganisms. If the condition persists for more than several days, a week or two on corticosteroids will usually hasten its disappearance.

A fleeting stiffness, soreness, and lameness with high fever has been recognized by the authors in kittens 6 to 12 weeks of age. The kittens will be sick for two to four days and then will recover, and may demonstrate pain when muscles and joints are manipulated. The condition is caused by two or more strains of calicivirus, which can be recovered readily from the blood during the acute phase of illness. At least one strain that has been studied was not neutralized by antibodies produced by the more commonly used vaccine strains. This condition can therefore occur in kittens vaccinated with some calicivirus vaccines. Synovial fluid from kittens with this disease will contain an elevated number of macrophages, many of which contain phagocytosed neutrophils.

A transient, sometimes protracted, sterile inflammatory polyarthritis occurs as an uncommon sequelae to vaccination in both dogs and cats. This postvaccinial reaction has been seen with both killed and live virus vaccines. It has not been possible to say which component of the multivalent vaccines generally used was responsible for the reaction. Postvaccinial arthritis has been described as a rare complication of measles and smallpox immunizations of people (Steere and Malawista, 1979). The arthritis is not usually treated unless it persists for more than five days, in which case corticosteroid therapy is instituted.

Fungal Arthritis

Fungal arthritis is infrequent in dogs and cats. It can occur as an extension of a fungal osteomyelitis or as a primary granulomatous synovitis, with the former occurring more commonly. *Coccidioides immitis, Blastomyces dermatitidis,* and *Filobasidiella (Cryptococcus) neoformans* are the most frequently encountered organisms. Desert rheumatism, an arthropathy that accompanies the primary respiratory stage of coccidioidomycosis of man, has also been seen in dogs.

Protozoal Arthritis

Visceral leishmaniasis, caused by *Leishmania donovani,* is a chronic systemic reticuloendothelial proliferative disease of man and some species of animals. The predominant presenting signs of the disease in dogs are fever, malaise, weight loss, dermatopathy, and polyarthritis. Generalized lymphadenopathy and hepatosplenomegaly are also seen. The synovial membrane is infiltrated by large numbers of macrophages that are filled with *Leishmania* bodies.

NONINFECTIOUS ARTHRITIS

The noninfectious arthritides of animals can be classified into several groups depending on the nature and etiology of the disorder.

Arthritis of Apparent Immunologic Cause

Deforming or Erosive Arthritis

RHEUMATOID ARTHRITIS OF DOGS. Canine rheumatoid arthritis is a well-documented clinical entity (Halliwell et al., 1972; Liu et al., 1969; Newton et al., 1976; Pedersen et al., 1976a). It is an uncommon condition, occurring at an incidence of approximately two per 25,000 dogs examined at the authors' hospital. This disorder occurs mainly in small or toy breeds of dogs as young as eight months and as old as eight years of age.

Canine rheumatoid arthritis is manifested initially as a shifting lameness with soft tissue swelling around involved joints. Within several weeks or months the disease localizes in particular joints and characteristic radiographic signs develop. Joint involvement is more severe in the carpal and tarsal joints, although in individual dogs the elbow, stifle, shoulder, and hip joints may show similar radiographic signs. Involvement of the apophyseal joints and costovertebral articulations rarely progresses to the point of causing radiographic changes. In exceptional cases, however, involvement of the vertebral articulations only can occur. The disease is often accompanied by fever, malaise, anorexia, and lymphadenopathy in the earlier stages.

The earliest radiographic changes consist of soft tissue swelling and a loss of trabecular bone density in the area of the joint. Lucent cystlike areas are frequently seen in the subchondral bone. The prominent lesion is a progressive destruction of subchondral bone in the more central areas as well as marginally at the attachment of the synovium (Biery and Newton, 1975; Pedersen

et al., 1976a). Both narrowing and widening of the joint space are identified radiographically as a result of cartilage erosion and destruction of subchondral bone (Fig. 84–32). Subluxation, luxation, and deformation occur most frequently in the carpal, tarsal, and phalangeal joints and occasionally in the elbow and stifle joints. Fibrous ankylosis can occur in advanced cases, particularly in the intercarpal and intertarsal joint spaces. Soft tissue calcification and atrophy accompany disuse osteoporosis and other radiographic findings.

Hemograms are either normal or reflect the generalized inflammatory process with a leukocytosis, neutrophilia, and hyperfibrinogenemia. Serum electrophoresis will often show hypoalbuminemia and variable elevation in alpha-2 and gamma globulins. Unlike the situation in humans, serologic abnormalities in canine rheumatoid arthritis are often absent. Rheumatoid factor is pres-

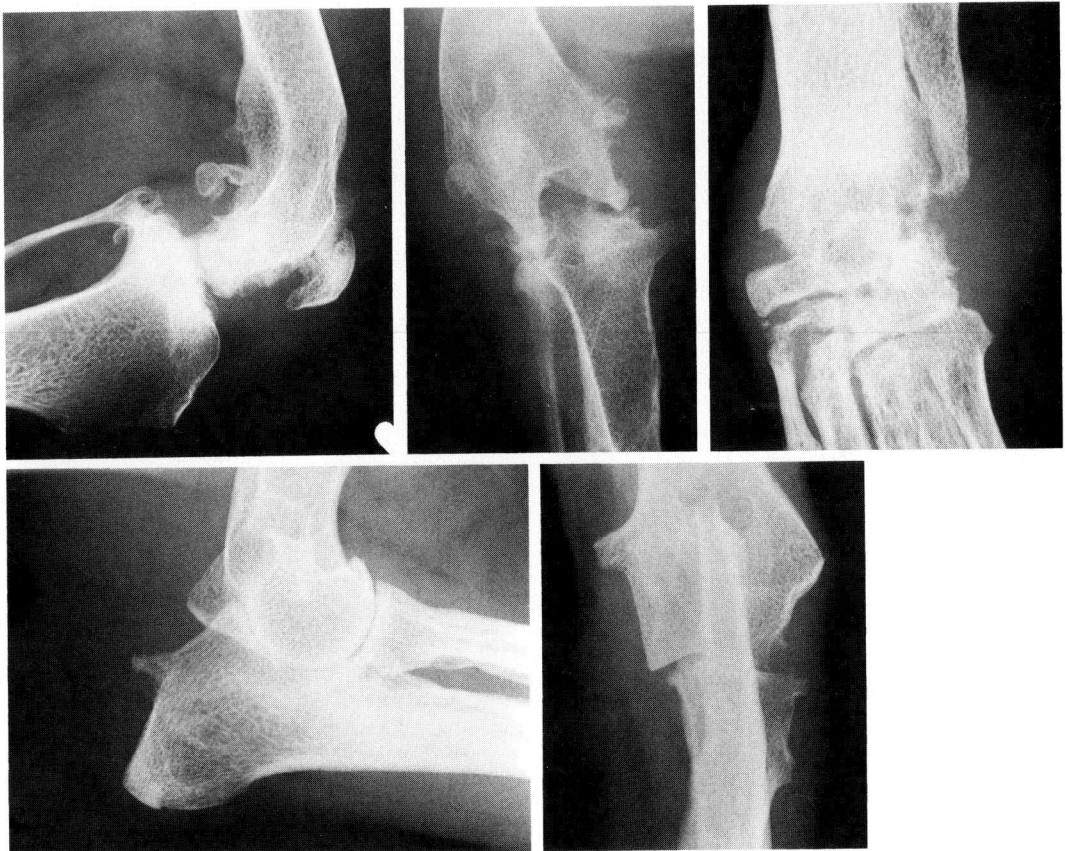

Figure 84–32. Radiographs of multiple joints of a female Welsh corgi with a one-year history of lameness. The soft tissue swelling and formation of cystlike subchondral lucencies cause subluxation and deformity of the joint typical for non-infectious arthritis in the dog (rheumatoid arthritis).

ent in comparatively low titer in about one quarter of the cases. LE cell preparations and fluorescent antinuclear antibody tests are usually negative.

Synovial fluid changes are indicative of an inflammatory synovitis, with an elevated total cell count, a high proportion of neutrophils in the synovial fluid cell population, and a variable decrease in the quality of the mucin clot. Ragocytes (neutrophils that have ingested immune complexes), as described in human rheumatoid arthritis, are not usually seen. A characteristic finding of canine rheumatoid arthritis is the presence in synovial fluid of mononuclear cells containing IgG, with only occasional cells containing C3 protein. These mononuclear cells may be producing the immunoglobulin or ingesting it from the synovial fluid.

The characteristic pathologic lesions consist of a villous hyperplasia of the synovial membrane, lymphoid and plasma cell infiltrates in the synovium, and erosion of articular cartilage at the margins of the joint (Fig. 84–33,A). The dense lymphoid and plasma cell infiltrate in the synovium (Fig. 84–33,B) and the subchondral erosions differentiate this disease from the synovitis seen in the nonerosive types of arthritis, which will be discussed in the following section. The erosion of the articular cartilage at the margins of affected joints occurs as a result of two pathologic processes, i.e., granulation tissue from an inflamed synovium either extends across the articular surface as a pannus or undermines the cartilage and subchondral bone. In the central regions of the joint, cartilage destruction is caused by a pannus arising from granulation tissue in the underlying marrow cavity (Fig. 84–33,C). Ankylosis in advanced lesions is not uncommon in the intercarpal and intertarsal joints (Fig. 84–33,D).

The pathogenesis of this disease in the dog is unknown. It is considered to be immunologic in nature because bacteria, viruses, *Mycoplasma*, or *Chlamydia* cannot be cultured from the affected joints, and because it responds to therapy with potent immunosuppressive drugs. Whether the etiology of the canine disease is identical to that of human rheumatoid arthritis remains to be established.

Canine rheumatoid arthritis responds only temporarily to systemic corticosteroids. There is an initial dramatic response, but this cannot be sustained even with high dosages. Aspirin has no appreciable therapeutic benefits in the authors' hands, probably because the disease is much more severe and rapidly progressive in dogs than in man. If the condition is recognized before severe joint damage occurs, it can usually be arrested with cyclophosphamide and prednisolone given in combination. This type of therapy will be covered in detail in the discussion of drug therapy of immune-mediated arthritides. In dogs with advanced deformities, immunosuppressive drug therapy may have to be combined with arthrodesis of selected joints. Arthrodesis is not warranted if the disease process cannot first be successfully halted with drug therapy.

POLYARTHRITIS OF GREYHOUNDS. An erosive polyarthritis of the greyhound has been described in different parts of the world (Casteli, 1969; Huxtable and Davis, 1976). The disease appears in animals from 3 to 30 months of age and most frequently attacks the proximal interphalangeal, carpal, tarsal, elbow, and stifle joints. The shoulder, hip, and atlanto-occipital joints are less frequently involved. A tenosynovitis may be an accompanying feature. The synovial membrane is edematous and hyperemic in the early course of the disease, and may be covered with a fine layer of fibrin; the synovial fluid is cloudy and yellowish, and often contains fibrin tags. In later stages, a lymphocyte and plasma cell infiltrate is seen in the synovial lining. Peripheral lymph nodes are enlarged and hyperactive. Pannus formation and marginal subchondral erosions are seen to a limited extent. Destruction of articular cartilage is accelerated in some joints but often is not associated with pannus formation. Gross deformities and radiographic changes are not as apparent as those seen in canine rheumatoid arthritis but appear more pronounced than those described for nonerosive joint disease.

Mycoplasmal and bacterial isolation has been unsuccessful, and dogs are serologically negative for *Erysipelothrix* and *Chlamydia*. Although no detailed discussion is available on therapy, it should be treated in the same manner as idiopathic nonerosive polyarthritis of dogs, which it most closely resembles.

FELINE PROGRESSIVE POLYARTHRITIS (EROSIVE FORM). One form of feline chronic progressive polyarthritis is an erosive de-

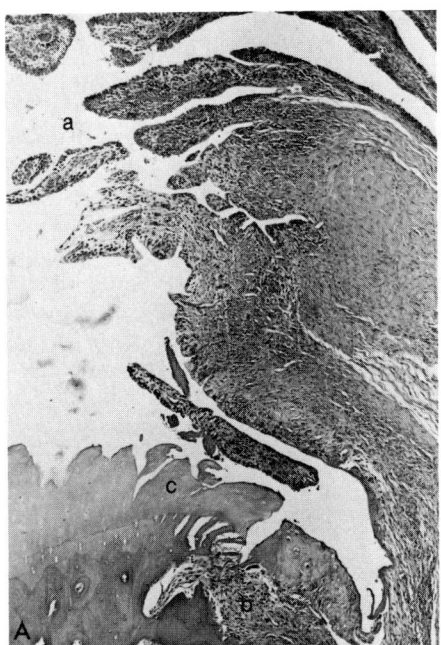

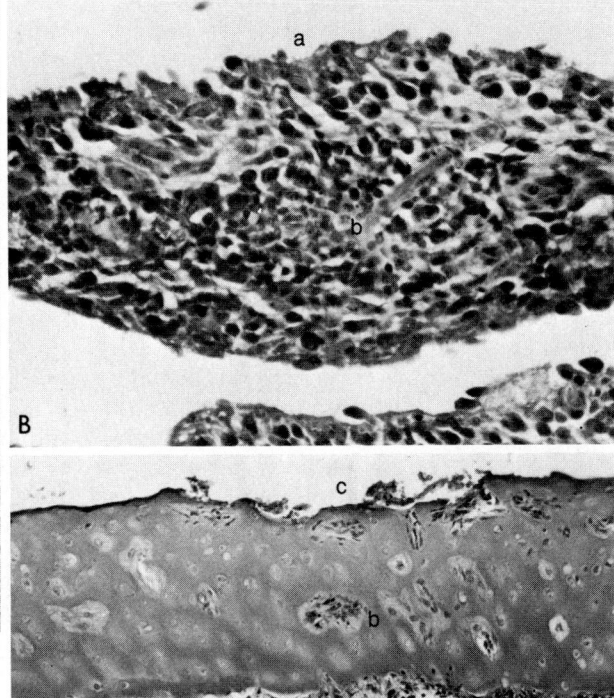

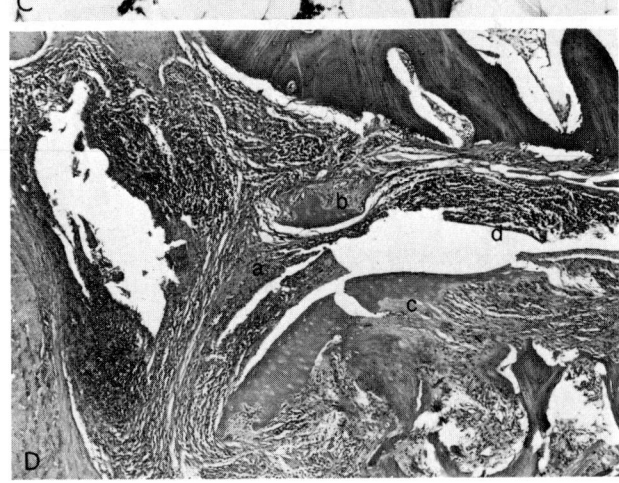

Figure 84–33. A, Joint margin from a dog with rheumatoid-like arthritis. Note the villous hypertrophy (a), destructive of the subchondral bone by granulation tissue arising from the inflamed synovium (b), and fibrillation of the articular cartilage (c). B, Synovial villus from a dog with rheumatoid-like arthritis showing hyperplasia of lining cells (a) and plasma cells and lymphocytes dispersed in the stroma or aggregated around small vessels (b). C, Cartilaginous defect in the trochlear groove of the femur of a dog with canine rheumatoid-like arthritis. Note the destruction of the subchondral bone by granulation tissue arising in the marrow spaces (a), extension of vessels through the articular cartilage (b), and destruction of the articular cartilage by a pannus originating in the marrow spaces of the subchondral bone (c)..

forming arthritis that appears similar to canine and human rheumatoid arthritis (Pedersen et al., 1980). Like the canine disease, the incidence is relatively low. This form of the disease is a less common variant of feline chronic progressive polyarthritis, which will be discussed in the next section.

The disease is insidious in onset, and the first abnormalities noted are often deformities of the carpal, metacarpophalangeal, metatarsophalangeal, and interphalangeal joints. Radiographic signs of erosion of the margins and central parts of the subchondral bone in these joints precede joint instability and deformities. Proliferation of bone adjacent to affected joints can be identified, but proliferative bony findings are minor in degree, while destructive signs are excessive.

Synovial fluid from involved joints is abnormal and demonstrates a slight to moderate elevation of white cells. Neutrophils, lymphocytes, and synovial macrophages are present in varying proportions. There is very little experience with the treatment of this form of arthritis in cats. It appears to respond to immunosuppressive drugs, however. Immunosuppressive drug therapy can be complicated by the presence of an underlying feline leukemia virus infection, which seems to be present in one half or so of the cases (Pedersen et al., 1980).

Periosteal Proliferative Arthritis

FELINE CHRONIC PROGRESSIVE POLY-ARTHRITIS (PERIOSTEAL PROLIFERATIVE FORM). This disorder occurs exclusively in male cats with the common age at onset of 1½ to 4½ years (Pedersen et al., 1980). Histopathologic abnormalities are similar to those occurring in both chronic Reiter's arthritis and rheumatoid arthritis of man.

The disease occurs suddenly with high fever, severe joint pain, and stiffness that usually starts in the tarsal and carpal joints, and lymphadenopathy that is regional to the inflamed joints. Radiographic signs progressing from osteoporosis, periosteal new bone formation, and ankylosis ensue over the next two to eight weeks or so. After the first few weeks, the fever tends to subside, and the disease takes a more chronic progressive course. This is manifested by severe generalized stiffness, emaciation, and gross bony enlargements in the area of the joints. This sequence differs considerably from the erosive or rheumatoid form, which does not begin with any noticeable signs, and tends to progress insidiously over a period of many months.

Chronic progressive polyarthritis of cats is not caused by identifiable bacteria or *Mycoplasma*, but it is etiologically linked to feline leukemia (FeLV) and feline syncytium-forming virus (FeSFV) infections. Feline syncytium-forming virus can be isolated from the blood or detected by serologic means in all of the cats with the disease, while FeLV is isolated from 50 to 70 per cent of the animals. The incidence of FeSFV infection in diseased cats is two to four times greater than age- and sex-matched normal cats living in the same geographic area, while the incidence of FeLV infection is six to ten times greater than expected. The arthritis cannot be reproduced with infectious material from diseased cats, however. It has been postulated, therefore, that the arthritis is an uncommon disease manifestation of FeSFV and FeLV infection that occurs in certain male cats (Pedersen et al., 1980). The actual joint disease is probably immunologically mediated, as evidenced by the dense lymphocytic and plasmacytic synovial infiltrate.

Synovial fluid contains a greatly increased number of neutrophils. The fluid is usually yellow-tinged and very cloudy in appearance. The hemogram is variable, with leukocytosis predominating. Leukopenia and anemia, when present, are usually associated with cats that have an underlying FeLV infection. Immunosuppressive drugs, usually corticosteroids and cyclophosphamide, are used to treat the disease. Corticosteroids alone will lessen the severity of the disease and slow the course, but will rarely halt its progression. Combination immunosuppressive drug therapy has been successful in achieving a remission in about half of the cats treated, but recurrences are common. Because of underlying FeLV-associated bone marrow suppression, cytotoxic drugs cannot be used to full effectiveness in some animals.

Nondeforming or Nonerosive Arthritis.

A nonerosive arthritis is identified in the dog and cat, and though etiologically diverse, it is probably mediated by similar immunopathologic mechanisms. The presenting clinical signs of this type of arthritis are similar, whether it is idiopathic in origin or associated with secondary infectious disease, SLE, or inflammatory bowel disease. The joint disease tends to be cyclic in nature, has a predisposition for smaller distal joints, the carpus and tarsus in particular, and can occur in monarticular, pauciarticular, or polyarticular forms. Radiographic changes, even after many months of joint disease, tend to be minimal or nonexistent. Biopsies of the synovial membranes show a sparse mononuclear cell infiltrate, with moderate to severe superficial inflammation characterized by polymorphonuclear cell infiltrates and fibrin exudation. Villous hyperplasia, marginal erosions, and pannus formation are not prominent features in these diseases. Regardless of the overlying or underlying disease processes that lead to the arthritis, the joint disease is believed to be due to deposition of immune complexes in the synovial membrane with resultant immune-mediated inflammatory reactions. In idiopathic nondeforming arthritis, the origin and nature of the antigen in the complex is unknown; in systemic lupus erythematosus, the antigen is at least in part nucleic acid; in enteropathic arthritis, the antigen probably originates from the bowel contents; and in arthritis secondary to chronic infectious disease, the antigen originates from the microorganism that is causing the infection.

IDIOPATHIC NONDEFORMING ARTHRITIS. Idiopathic nondeforming arthritis is by far the most common disorder of dogs manifesting immune-mediated arthritis (Pedersen et al., 1976b). It is termed idiopathic because there is no evidence of a primary chronic infectious disease process, serologic abnormalities of SLE are absent, and joint disease is often the sole manifestation of the condition. This disorder occurs most commonly in large breeds of dogs, particularly German shepherd dogs, Doberman pinschers, and various breeds of retrievers, spaniels, and pointers. When seen in toy breeds, it most frequently occurs in toy poodles, Lhasa apsos, Yorkshire terriers, and Chihuahuas, and in mixes of these breeds. A similar condition has been less commonly recognized in cats. Females predominate over males in the cases observed by the authors, a pattern that holds true for most immune diseases.

The initial presenting history is one of a cyclic fever, during which malaise, anorexia, lameness, or generalized stiffness are noted. The fever is most pronounced in dogs with polyarticular disease and least pronounced in animals with monarticular involvement. In severely affected dogs, periods of remission are usually incomplete, in which case the disease can be very debilitating. Generalized muscle atrophy and disproportionate atrophy of the temporal and masseter muscles are frequently seen. This atrophy is due in part to disuse, but in many cases the disease process also involves the muscles or nerves.

During the most severe stages of the disease, swelling and heat in distal joints are sometimes detected. Generalized lymphadenopathy is often present in varying degrees. During attacks the dogs run a high fever and demonstrate leukocytosis with neutrophilia and hyperfibrinogenemia. The joint disease can be manifested as a single limb lameness in cases of monarticular or pauciarticular involvement. When the disease is monarticular in presentation, the elbow joint is often involved. Polyarticular involvement is the most common presentation, with the dogs showing generalized stiffness and reluctance to move their spine, tail, or limbs. Toy breeds, which often have severe generalized arthritis, can become virtually immobile, making it difficult to tell whether the joints are the source of the problem, or whether the immobility is due solely to depression.

Radiographic abnormalities are usually not present, except for an increase in the amount of periarticular soft tissue due to inflammation or fibrosis. If the disease is present for many months without treatment, however, some changes can occur in the bone and cartilage. Persistent hyperemia of the synovium can lead to mild, and occasionally severe, periarticular periosteal bone proliferation. In addition, secondary degenerative joint disease can develop, and this may be manifested by some periosteal new bone formation and narrowing of the joint spaces. These radiographic abnormalities can lead to a mistaken diagnosis of primary degenerative joint disease or degenerative joint disease secondary to some other problem. Obviously, this will greatly influence the type of therapy selected. It is important, therefore, to always take a sample of synovial fluid from dogs with periosteal proliferative changes and without obvious disorders that would predispose to degenerative joint disease.

Diagnosis is made by consideration of the clinical history of cyclic fever that is unresponsive to antibiotics, malaise, and anorexia, upon which is superimposed stiffness or lameness. Because of the cyclic nature of the fever and clinical signs, it is often difficult to ascertain whether the condition is responsive to antibiotics or not. Animals will be started on antibiotics when the fever appears and taken off when it disappears. The apparent improvement will frequently be attributed to the antibiotics rather than to the natural cycle of illness. When the fever and signs reappear, veterinarians will often change antibiotics, and the new antibiotics will also appear to work. After numerous cycles of antibiotic therapy using different drugs, it is finally realized that antibiotics are not really effective after all.

Synovial fluid contains from 5000 to 100,000 or more white cells per μl. The predominant cells in the fluid are the neutrophils; these cells appear nontoxic and with normal granulation. The fluid is sterile for bacteria, viruses, *Mycoplasma,* and *Chlamydia.* Serologic abnormalities such as the L.E. cell phenomenon, antinuclear antibody, and rheumatoid factor are absent. Blood cultures are negative for bacteria, and there are no signs of primary infectious processes in other areas of the body.

The treatment of the disorder involves the use of glucocorticoids alone or in combination with more potent immunosuppressive drugs (see following section). A complete remission of signs can usually be achieved. From 30 to 50 per cent of the dogs will have recurrences of illness after the drug therapy is discontinued.

An idiopathic polyarthritis, identical in nature to that seen in dogs, has been seen in cats. It is less frequent, however, and is more common in females. Unlike the dog, the cat exhibits severe fever, malaise, and inappetence less often than the dog. The lameness, as is the case in all lameness in cats, is more subtle and harder to recognize.

NONDEFORMING ARTHRITIS ASSOCIATED WITH CHRONIC INFECTIOUS DISEASES. A nondeforming arthritis associated with chronic infectious diseases has been described in dogs (Pedersen et al., 1976a). Infectious diseases that can be associated with this form of arthritis include chronic bacterial infection, chronic fungal infection, and occasionally parasitic infections such as dirofilariasis. This type of arthritis has been associated with subacute bacterial endocarditis; pyometra; vaginitis; chronic *Actinomyces* infections in the chest, abdomen, or paravertebral musculature; chronic salmonellosis; and severe periodontitis. Since these infections are often difficult to pinpoint, the arthritis may be the main or sole presenting complaint. It is important, therefore, to make a thorough search for secondary infections every time this type of arthritis is found. This is especially important because

immunosuppressive drugs will usually be used to treat cases in which infection is unrecognized.

Joint involvement in this type of disorder is usually monarticular or pauciarticular, and has a predisposition for the carpal and tarsal joints. Since the organisms involved in the primary disease process cannot be identified in the synovial membrane, it is likely that the joint disease is also of immune complex origin. It is also possible that the infection is so low grade that the organism cannot be recovered, or that in the case of bacteria, the organism is present in an "L" form. A similar relationship between a sterile arthritis and chronic infections in other parts of the body was recognized much earlier in man (Coggeshall et al., 1941).

SYSTEMIC LUPUS ERYTHEMATOSUS. Canine systemic lupus erythematosus (SLE) was initially defined as the triad of glomerulonephritis, thrombocytopenia, and hemolytic anemia associated with a salicylate responsive arthralgia in some cases (Lewis et al., 1965). It is apparent, however, that canine SLE is similar in its presentation to SLE of man; that is, articular, dermatologic, renal, and neuromuscular problems seem to be more common than hematologic abnormalities (Krum et al., 1978; Monier et al., 1978; Pedersen et al., 1976, Slappendel et al., 1972). Hematologic abnormalities in the dog, such as thrombocytopenia or hemolytic anemia, occur in only 10 to 20 per cent of the total cases of SLE that the authors have seen. We have seem a similar type of polyarthritis in a cat with SLE. This cat also had meningitis and glomerulonephritis. From what we have seen of SLE in cats, it also resembles SLE in dogs and man. A more detailed description of SLE is given in Chapters 77 and 83.

The arthritis of canine and feline SLE is similar in every detail to that seen in cases of idiopathic nonerosive arthritis. In fact, both conditions predominate in the same breeds, and in these cases, serologic abnormalities such as antinuclear antibodies are the sole basis for classifying the condition as SLE. In cases wherein other systemic manifestations of SLE are present with arthritis, the diagnosis is more easily made. The joint disease is usually polyarticular and, less commonly, pauciarticular.

The arthritis seen in subacute bacterial

endocarditis (SBE), and indeed the entire syndrome of SBE, can mimic SLE. Two dogs described by Bennett and coworkers (1978) best document this point. Chronic bacterial endocarditis can lead to continuous low-grade damage to parenchymal organs, high levels of circulating immune-complexes, and a heightened responsiveness of the host's immune system. In man and animals this may result in the production of numerous auto-antibodies, including anti-nuclear antibody and rheumatoid factors. Anti-nuclear antibodies result from chronic nucleoprotein release and heightened immunologic responsiveness, and rheumatoid factors are made in response to persistent immune-complex production. This phenomenon is important, because if such animals are mistakenly diagnosed as having SLE or rheumatoid arthritis, they will be treated with immunosuppressive drugs, with potentially serious consequences.

ENTEROPATHIC ARTHRITIS. Enteropathic arthritis is frequently associated with diseases like ulcerative colitis and regional enteritis of man. The cause of the arthritis is unknown, but it is thought that either the bowel and joint disease share a common etiology, or antigenic products released into the blood from the inflamed bowel have some effect on the synovium. Hepatopathic arthropathy, which has been seen in several dogs with chronic active hepatitis and cirrhosis, is also a type of enteropathic arthritis. In this disease, antigenic material from the bowel probably gains access to the general bloodstream, because it is not being removed from the portal blood by the reticuloendothelial tissue of the liver.

Polyarthritis in dogs with ulcerative colitis and more fulminating enterocolitis has been recognized (Pedersen et al., 1976b). In addition, a small percentage of the dogs with idiopathic polyarthritis have problems with flatulence, occasional vomiting, and eventual gastric torsion; the latter indicates some degree of preexisting motility problem.

PLASMACYTIC-LYMPHOCYTIC SYNOVITIS. This is a condition that is seen most frequently in the stifle joints of small and medium-sized breeds of dogs. The condition is probably a variant of canine rheumatoid arthritis. It leads to pronounced joint laxity and instability, often manifested by cruciate ligament damage and drawer motion (see also the discussion on ruptured anterior cruciate ligaments). Except for hindlimb lameness, which can be pronounced, the dogs are often not systemically ill. The hemograms, however, may show leukocytosis, elevated gamma globulins, and hyperfibrinogenemia. Many of these dogs will go to surgery for cruciate repairs, and if the abnormal synovium and synovial fluid is not noticed at surgery, an apparently unsuccessful cruciate ligament repair will be the result.

The synovium is grossly thickened and edematous and has a reddish-yellowish tint. The synovial fluid is cloudy, often thin, and yellow-tinged. It contains from 5000 to 20,000 white cells per μl, with only 10 to 40 per cent of these being neutrophils. Unlike other inflammatory joint diseases, the predominant cell is a small mononuclear cell, probably a lymphocyte. The fluid is sterile for known microorganisms.

Radiographic changes, when present, are minimal and include soft tissue swelling and periosteal proliferative changes. Erosive changes are absent or slight. Synovial biopsies show an intense lymphocytic-plasmacytic infiltrate and synovial hypertrophy that is sometimes villous. Subchondral erosions are minimal or absent. The condition can be successfully controlled with immunosuppressive drugs. (See the following discussion.)

POLYARTERITIS NODOSA. An arthritis can be a feature of polyarteritis nodosa, especially in cats (Altera and Bonasch, 1966; Lewis et al., 1965). The arthritis is of the inflammatory type, with profound cellular and fibrinous infiltrates around synovial arterioles. This may be reflected by an increase in neutrophils and macrophages in the synovial fluid. Radiographic signs may be absent or may suggest a rheumatoid-type arthritis. Glucocorticoids are used to treat the condition.

A cat with polyarthritis described by Wilkinson (1979) showed lesions in the synovial vessels. This case probably represented a cat with a similar type of hypersensitivity angiitis.

Treatment of Immune-Mediated Arthritides

Idiopathic Polyarthritis, Systemic Lupus Erythematosus, Plasmacytic-Lymphocytic Sy-

novitis. Disease remission can be achieved with glucocorticoids alone in about 50 per cent of cases. Prednisone or prednisolone at a dosage of 3.0 mg/kg body weight for large dogs and 4.0 mg/kg for small dogs is given orally in divided doses morning and night for the first two days, then reduced to 2.0 mg/kg and 3.0 mg/kg, respectively, and given orally each morning for the next 12 days. By the end of two weeks the signs of joint pain should be improving progressively, and the synovial fluid polymorphonuclear cell count should be greatly decreased. If this is the case, the prednisone or prednisolone dosage is reduced to half of the initial daily dosage for the third week, and then to 1.0 mg/kg per os every other morning for an indefinite period. If remission can be maintained on alternate-day therapy, the glucocorticoids are continued at this same dosage for another one to two months. If the disease is in complete remission after this time, all medication is discontinued. In over half of these dogs, the disease will not recur. If it recurs after drug discontinuation, remission is again induced, but this time the maintenance glucocorticoids are continued for four to six months. At this time a second attempt is made to discontinue drugs. If this fails, remission is again induced with high dosages of glucocorticoids, and the animals are maintained indefinitely on the lowest dosage possible.

In about half of the animals with these types of joint disease, remission cannot be achieved with glucocorticoids alone, or higher levels of glucocorticoids than those aforementioned are needed to maintain remission. Such animals will usually become apparent at the first two-week recheck. If at this time clinical improvement is less than hoped for, the disease starts to recur after the dosages were decreased, and the joints are still considerably inflamed (as determined by synovial fluid analysis), then cytotoxic drug therapy should be added to the glucocorticoid regimen, i.e., glucocorticoids and cyclophosphamide, or glucocorticoids and azathioprine or 6-mercaptopurine.

Of the various cytotoxic drugs, we have found that cyclophosphamide or the thiopurines (azathioprine, 6-mercaptopurine) are the most satisfactory. Cyclophosphamide is preferable to the thiopurines in initiating a remission, but because of the high incidence of sterile hemorrhagic cystitis associated with the chronic (more than four months) use of this drug, the thiopurines are preferable for long-term maintenance in the few cases in which this is necessary. Thiopurines can be used for remission induction therapy but take longer than cyclophosphamide to have the same effect.

The dosage of cyclophosphamide that the authors have found most satisfactory is 2.5 mg/kg body weight for dogs less than 10 kg, and cats 2.0 mg/kg for animals from 10 to 35 kg, and 1.50 mg/kg for animals over 35 kg. This dosage is given orally once daily on four consecutive days of each week. One cycle of therapy consists of four days on and three days off of the drug. Cyclophosphamide is used with glucocorticoids in almost all cases. Glucocorticoids are given as outlined previously or, if necessary, at one-half the dosages listed.

Azathioprine or 6-mercaptopurine are both given at a dosage of 2.0 mg/kg body weight orally daily for the first two to three weeks, then at this dosage every other day (usually on alternating days with the glucocorticoids, so that the glucocorticoids are given one day and the thiopurine the second day). One of the thiopurines can be substituted for cyclophosphamide in cases in which cyclophosphamide therapy is needed for more than four months; in such instances, alternate-day dosing is used.

Complete blood counts are done on all animals receiving cytotoxic drugs beginning two weeks after the initiation of treatment. If the white blood cell count falls below 6000 cells/mm^3, the dosages should be decreased by one fourth; if it falls below 4000 white blood cells/mm^3, the drug should be discontinued for one week, and then reinstituted at one half of the previous dosage.

Cytotoxic drugs, used with the previously described regimen of glucocorticoid therapy, will bring about complete remission in from 2 to 16 weeks. Cytotoxic drugs are discontinued one month after complete remission is achieved. Remission can usually be maintained after this time with 1.0 mg/kg body weight of prednisolone or prednisone every other day. At this point the therapeutic regimen is the same as that described originally for glucocorticoids alone. It is important that cyclophosphamide not be used much longer than four months, because of the potential problems with sterile hemorrhagic cystitis. If cytotoxic drugs are needed for a longer time, one of the thiopurines or chlorambucil should be substituted for the cyclophosphamide.

It is important to use synovial fluid analysis to determine when complete remission is achieved. Drug therapy will often bring about dramatic improvement in clinical signs but will mask the pathological processes that may still be occurring in the joint. If low grade inflammation is allowed to persist, degenerative joint disease will gradually set in and complicate the interpretation of the clinical picture. It is prudent, therefore, to select several joints that initially showed inflammatory changes and to reexamine fluid from these joints periodically during the period of drug therapy. At the opposite extreme, the clinical signs of some animals may be caused in part by some preexisting noninflammatory joint disease, such as degenerative joint disease. If the inflammatory component is removed, some residual lameness may persist. If this residual lameness is blamed on the inflammatory disease, an animal may be subjected to continuous and unnecessary drug therapy.

If, during drug therapy, there is a drastic change in the clinical appearance of the lameness, immediate reevaluation of the status of the joint disease is imperative. The authors have seen dogs that developed septic arthritis or degenerative joint disease months after being treated for immune-mediated arthritis. It is a grave mistake to reinstitute drug therapy in such cases on the presumption that it is the same disorder.

Rheumatoid Arthritis. The experience of the authors is that rheumatoid arthritis should be treated with glucocorticoids used in combination with cytotoxic drugs. Glucocorticoids alone often do not bring about a complete remission, or else they require so long to control the disease that considerable joint damage can occur in the meantime. Gold salt therapy has been used for the treatment of canine rheumatoid arthritis (Newton et al., 1979). It is not nearly as effective in inducing remission as other drugs, but it can be used to advantage in maintaining a remission in cases for which continuous glucocorticoid therapy is undesirable.

Enteropathic Arthritis. The overlying enteric disease should be the primary target of treatment. The arthritis can be controlled with minimal treatment, such as aspirin, provided the bowel disease can be controlled. Immunosuppressive drugs are indicated only in situations wherein the bowel disease can be controlled by their use. In some cases, immunosuppressive drugs can actually worsen the overlying colitis and can make the joint disease worse also.

CRYSTAL-INDUCED ARTHRITIS

Hyperuricemia and gout have been recognized as naturally-occurring entities in chickens, birds, and reptiles. It is rare in mammalian species. The one report of gout in the dog was based on radiographic evidence but was not confirmed by pathologic studies (Miller and Kind, 1966). Many veterinarians believe that the generalized arthropathy in Dalmatian dogs is gout, because this breed metabolizes uric acid differently from all other dogs. This disease in Dalmatians, however, is not gout but rather primary degenerative joint disease. Dalmatians are no more prone to gouty arthritis than other breeds.

Pseudogout, a condition caused by the deposition of calcium phosphate crystals, has been described in a dog (Gibson and Roenigk, 1972). A transient gouty arthritis can uncommonly occur in dogs with lymphosarcoma that have been put on anticancer drugs. A rapid destruction of the tumor results in a large release of nucleic acid, which is metabolized ultimately to uric acid. This will lead to a transient hyperuricemia and gouty arthritis.

REFERENCES

Alexander, J. W.: Legg-Calve-Perthe's-like disease in the dog. Canine Pract. 7(1):32, 1980a.
Alexander, J. W.: Osteochondritis dissecans of the hock in the dog. Calif. Vet. 34:9, 1980b.
Alexander, J. W.: Osteoarthrosis (degenerative joint disease) in the dog. Canine Pract. 6:31, 1979.
Alexander, J. W.: Septic arthritis in the dog. Canine Pract. 5(6):43, 1978.
Alexander, J. W., Shumway, J. D., Lau, R. E., and Westfall, G. J.: Anterior cruciate rupture. Feline Pract. 7:38, 1977.
Altera, K. P., and Bonasch, H.: Periarteritis modosa in a cat. J.A.V.M.A. 149:1307, 1966.
Arnoczky, S. P., and Marshall, J. L.: Discoid meniscus in the dog: a case report. J.A.A.H.A. 13:569, 1977.
Arnoczky, S. P., Tarvin, G. P., Marshall, J. L., and

Saltzman, B.: The over-the-top procedure: a technique for anterior cruciate ligament substitution in the dog. J.A.A.H.A. *15*:283, 1979.

Arwedsson, G.: Arthrodesis in traumatic plantar subluxation of the metatarsal bones of the dog. J.A.V.M.A. *120*:21, 1954.

Barclay, S. M.: Lymphosarcoma in tarsi of a cat. J.A.V.M.A. *175*:582, 1979.

Battershell, D.: Ununited anconeal process. J.A.V.M.A. *155*:35, 1969.

Bayer, A. S.: Arthritis associated with common viral infections. Mumps, coxsackievirus, and adenovirus. Postgrad. Med. *68*:55, 1980.

Bennett, D., and Duff, S. R.: Transarticular planning as a treatment for hip luxation in the dog and cat. J. Small Anim. Pract. *21*:373, 1980.

Bennett, D., Gilbertson, E. M. M., and Grennan, D.: Bacterial endocarditis with polyarthritis in two dogs associated with circulating autoantibodies. J. Small Anim. Pract. *19*:185, 1978.

Berzon, J. L.: Osteochondritis dissecans in the dog: diagnosis and therapy. J.A.V.M.A. *175*:796, 1979.

Biery, D. N., and Newton, C. D.: Radiographic appearance of rheumatoid arthritis in the dog. J.A.A.H.A. *11*:607, 1975.

Bone, D. L.: Canine panosteitis. Canine Pract. 7(4):61, 1980.

Bonneau, N. H., and Breton, L.: Excision arthroplasty of the femoral head. Canine Pract. 8(2):13, 1981.

Boom, J.: Trauma of the hip joint in the dog and the cat. Tijdschr. Diergeneeskd. *104*:934, 1979.

Booth, N. H.: Nonnarcotic analgesics. *In* Jones, L. M., Booth, N. H., and McDonald, L. E. (eds.): Veterinary Pharmacology and Therapeutics. 4th edition. Iowa State Univ. Press, Ames, 1977, p 351.

Campbell, J. R., Bennett, D., and Lee, R.: Intertarsal and tarsometatarsal subluxation in the dog. J. Small Anim. Pract. *17*:427, 1976.

Cardinet, G. H., III, Fedde, M. R., and Tunell, G. L.: Correlates of histochemical and physiologic properties in normal and hypertrophic pectineus muscles of the dog. Lab. Invest. *27*:32, 1972.

Carrig, C. B., and Morgan, J. P.: Asynchronous growth of the canine radius and ulna. Early radiographic changes following experimental retardation of longitudinal growth of the ulna. J. Am. Vet. Rad. Soc. *16*:121, 1975.

Carrig, C. B., Morgan, J. P., and Pool, R. R.: Effects of asynchronous growth of the radius and ulna on the canine elbow joint following experimental retardation of longitudinal growth of the ulna. J.A.A.H.A. *11*:560, 1975.

Castelli, M. J.: Acute periarthritis in a kennel of greyhounds. Vet. Rec. *84*:652, 1969.

Caywood, D. D., Wilson, J. W., and O'Leary, T. P.: Septic polyarthritis associated with bacterial endocarditis in two dogs. J.A.V.M.A. *171*:549, 1977.

Cheli, R., Gresti, A. de, and Addis, F.: Valgoid syndrome resulting from distension of the anterior cruciate ligament in the dog. Folia Vet. Lat. *4*:638, 1974.

Clamen, C.: Lésions méniscales associées aux ruptures du ligament croisé antérieur et ménisctomie. L'Animal de Compagne *14*:311, 1979.

Clayton-Jones, D. G.: Osteochondritis of the canine stifle joint. Kleintierpraxis *25*:441, 1980.

Clayton-Jones, D. G.: Hindleg lameness in the dog. *In* Grunsell, C. S. G., and Hill, F. W. G. (eds.): Veterinary Annual 14th edition. John Wright and Sons Ltd., Bristol, U.K., 1974, p 167.

Clegg, F. G., and Rorrison, J. M.: *Brucella abortus* infection in the dog: A case of polyarthritis. Res. Vet. Sci. *9*:183, 1968.

Coggeshall, H. C., Bennett, G. A., Warren, C. F., and Bauer, W.: Synovial fluid and synovial membrane abnormalities resulting from varying grades of systemic inflammation and edema. Am. J. Med. Sci. *202*:486, 1941.

Corley, E. A., Sutherland, T. M., and Carlson, W. D.: Genetic aspects of canine elbow dysplasia. J.A.V.M.A. *153*:543, 1968.

Cucuel, J. P. E., and Frye, F. L.: Anterior cruciate ligament repair in a cat. A case report. Vet. Med. Small Anim. Clin. *65*:38, 1970.

Dalton, J. R.: Rupture of the posterior cruciate ligament in a cat. Vet. Rec. *104*:319, 1979.

DeAngelis, M. P., and Betts, C. W.: Posterior cruciate ligament rupture. J.A.A.H.A. *9*:447, 1973.

Denny, H. R., Gibbs, C., and Gaskell, C. J.: Cervical spondylopathy in the dog. A review of thirty-five cases. J. Small Anim. Pract. 18:117, 1977.

Dieterich, H. F.: Arthrodesis of the proximal intertarsal joint for repair of rupture of proximal plantar intertarsal ligaments. Vet. Med. Small Anim. Clin. *69*:995, 1974.

Dodds, W. J.: Inherited bleeding disorders. Canine Pract. 6(5):49, 1978.

Duff, R., and Campbell, J. R.: Long-term results of excision arthroplasty of the canine hip. Vet. Rec. *101*:181, 1977.

Egger, E. L., and Stolls, G.: Ulnar styloid transportation as an experimental treatment for premature closure of the distal ulnar physis. J.A.A.H.A. *14*:690, 1979.

Ellison, G. W., and Norrdin, R. W.: Multicentric periarticular calcinosis in a pup. J.A.V.M.A. *177*:542, 1980.

Fisher, T. M.: The inheritance of canine hip dysplasia. Mod. Vet. Pract. *60*:897, 1979.

Flecknell, P. A., and Gruffydd-Jones, T. J.: Congenital luxation of the patella in the cat. Feline Pract. 9(3):18, 1979.

Fletch, S. M., Pinderton, P. H., and Brueckner, P. J.: The Alaskan malamute chondrodysplasia (dwarfism-anemia) syndrome in review. J.A.A.H.A. *11*:353, 1975.

Flo, G. L., and DeYoung, D.: Meniscal injuries and medial meniscectomy in the canine stifle. J.A.A.H.A. *14*:683, 1978.

Gendreau, C., and Cawley, A. J.: Excision of the femoral head and neck: The long-term results of 35 operations. J.A.A.H.A. *13*:605, 1977.

Gibson, J. P., and Roenigk, W. J.: Pseudogout in a dog. J.A.V.M.A. *161*:912, 1972.

Goudswarrd, J., Hartman, E. G., Janmaat, A., and Huisman, G. H.: *Erysipelothrix rhusiopathiae* Strain 7, a causative agent of endocarditis and arthritis in the dog. Tijdschr. Diergeneeskd. *98*:416, 1973.

Gresti, A.: Occurrence of bilateral articular synoviomas in two cats. Clin. Vet. *98*:156, 1975.

Grøndalen, J., and Braut, T.: Lameness in two young dogs caused by a calcified body in the joint capsule of the elbow. J. Small Anim. Pract. *17*:681, 1976.

Halliwell, R. E., Lavelle, R. B., and Butt, K. M.: Canine rheumatoid arthritis. A review and a case report. J. Small Anim. Pract. *13*:239, 1972.

Hammerling, G., and Hammerling, R.: Dislocation of the elbow joint in the basset hound. Tier. Umschau. *29*:622, 1974.

Harrison, J. W.: Patellar Dislocation. *In* Bojrab, M. J.

(ed.): Current Techniques in Small Animal Surgery. Lea and Febiger, Philadelphia, 1975, p. 479.

Haskins, M. E., Jezyk, P. F., Desnick, R. J., McDonough, S. K., and Patterson, D. F.: Mucopolysaccharidosis in a domestic short-haired cat — a disease distinct from that seen in the Siamese cat. J.A.V.M.A. *175*:384, 1979.

Hayes, H. M., Jr., Wilson, G. P., and Burt, J. K.: Feline hip dysplasia. J.A.A.H.A. *14*:447, 1979.

Hedhammer, Å., Olsson, S.-E., Andersson, S.-Å., Persson, L., Pettersson, L., Olausson, A., and Sundgren, P.-E.: Canine hip dysplasia: Study of heritability in 401 litters of German shepherd dogs. J.A.V.M.A. *174*:1012, 1979.

Hedhammer, A., Wu, F. M., Krook, L., Schryver, H. F., Delahunta, A., Whalen, J. P., Kallfelz, F. A., Nunez, E. A., Hintz, H. F., Sheffy, B. E., and Ryan, G. D.: Overnutrition and skeletal disease. An experimental study in growing Great Dane dogs. Cornell Vet. *64*(Suppl 5):5, 1974.

Herron, M. R.: Coxofemoral luxations in small animals. J. Vet. Orthoped. *1*:30, 1979.

Hickman, J.: Greyhound injuries. J. Small Anim. Pract. *16*:455, 1975.

Hohn, R. B., and Janes, J. M.: Pelvic osteotomy in the treatment of canine hip dysplasia. Clin. Orthop. *62*:70, 1969.

Hohn, R. B., and Newton, C. D.: Surgical repairs of ligamentous structures of the stifle joint. *In* Bojrab, M. J. (ed.): Current Techniques in Small Animal Surgery. Lea and Febiger, Philadelphia, 1975, p. 470.

Holt, P. E.: Hip dysplasia in a cat. J. Small Anim. Pract. *19*:273, 1978.

Holt, P. E.: Ligamentous injuries to the canine neck. J. Small Anim. Pract. *15*:457, 1974.

Huztable, C. R., and Davis, P. E.: The pathology of polyarthritis in young greyhounds. J. Comp. Pathol. *86*:11, 1976.

Irving, G. W.: What is your diagnosis? Medial luxation of the right patella. J.A.V.M.A. *175*:845, 1979.

Jezyk, P. F., Haskins, M. E., Patterson, D. F., Mellman, W. J., and Greenstein, M.: Mucopolysaccharidosis in a cat with arylsulfatase B deficiency. A model of Maroteaux-Lamy syndrome. Science *198*:834, 1977.

Johnson, K. A.: Temporomandibular joint dysplasia in an Irish setter. J. Small Anim. Pract. *20*:209, 1979.

Johnson, K. A.: Posterior cruciate ligament rupture in a cat: A case report. J.A.A.H.A. *14*:480, 1978.

Johnson, K. A., and Davis, P. E.: Osteochrondritis dissecans in the greyhound stifle (case report). Aust. Vet. Pract. *9*(4):201, 1979.

Johnson, K. A., Howlett, C. R., and Pettit, G. D.: Osteochondrosis in the hock joints in dogs. J.A.A.H.A. *16*:103, 1980.

Kasstrom, H.: Nutrition, weight gain, and development of hip dysplasia. An experimental investigation in growing dogs with special reference to the effect of feeding intensity. Acta. Radiol. Suppl. *344*:136, 1975.

Knecht, C. D.: Evolution of surgical techniques for cruciate ligament rupture in animals. J.A.A.H.A. *12*:717, 1976.

Knecht, C. D., Stickle, D. C. van, Blevins, W. E., Avolt, M. D., Hughes, R. B., and Cantwell, H. D.: Osteochondrosis of the shoulder and stifle in 3 of 5 Border collie littermates. J.A.V.M.A. *170*:58, 1977.

Kolde, D. L.: Pectineus tenectomy for treatment of hip dysplasia in a domestic cat: A case report. J.A.A.H.A. *10*:564, 1974.

Krum, S. H., Cardinet, G. H., III, Anderson, B. C., and Holliday, T. A.: Polymyositis and polyarthritis associated with systemic lupus erythematosus in a dog. J.A.V.M.A. *170*:61, 1977.

Larsen, J. S. (ed.): Symposium workshop panel reports in canine hip dysplasia. *In* Proceedings of Canine Hip Dysplasia Symposium and Workshop. St. Louis, Missouri, 1973, p 153.

Lawson, D. D.: Intertarsal subluxation in the dog. J. Small Anim. Pract. *1*:179, 1961.

Lee, R.: A study of the radiographic and histological changes occurring in Legg-Calve-Perthe's disease (LCP) in the dog. J. Small Anim. Pract. *11*:621, 1970.

Lee, R. M., and Fry, P. D.: Some observations on the occurrence of Legg-Calve-Perthe's disease (coxa plana) in the dog and an evaluation of excision arthroplasty as a method of treatment. J. Small Anim. Pract. *10*:309, 1969.

Leeds, E. B.: Carpal arthrodesis for overextension of the carpus. Canine Pract. *5*(4):32, 1978.

Leighton, R. L.: The Richard's II canine total hip prosthesis. J.A.A.H.A. *15*:73, 1979.

Leighton, R. L.: Repair of a bilateral medial patellar luxation in a cat. Feline Pract. *8*(2):23, 1978.

Leighton, E. A., Linn, J. M., Wilham, R. L., and Castleberry, M. W.: A genetic study of canine hip dysplasia. Am. J. Vet. Res. *38*:241, 1977.

Lewis, R. M., and Hathaway, J. E.: canine systemic lupus erythematosus presenting with symmetrical polyarthritis. J. Small Anim. Pract. *8*:273, 1967.

Lewis, R. M., Schwartz, R. S., and Henry, W. B., Jr.: Canine systemic lupus erythematosus. Blood *25*:143, 1965.

Lewis, R. M., Schwartz, R. S., and Gilmore, C. E.: Autoimmune diseases in domestic animals. Ann. N.Y. Acad. Sci. *124*:178, 1965.

Lipowitz, A. J., Fetter, A. W., and Walker, M. A.: Synovial sarcoma of the dog. J.A.V.M.A. *174*:76, 1979.

Liu, S. K., Suter, P. F., Fischer, C. A., and Dorfman, H. D.: Rheumatoid arthritis in a dog. J.A.V.M.A. *154*:495, 1969.

Ljunggren, G. L.: Legg-Perthe's disease in the dog. Acta Orthop. Scand. (Suppl.) *95*:1, 1967.

Ljunggren, G. L.: A comparative study of conservative and surgical treatment of Legg-Perthe's disease in the dog. Anim. Hosp. *2*:6, 1966.

Ljunggren, G. L., and Olsson, S-E.: Osteoarthrosis of the shoulder and elbow joints in dogs: A pathologic and radiographic study of a necropsy material. J. Am. Vet. Rad. Soc. *16*:33, 1975.

Llewellyn, H. R.: Growth plate injuries — diagnosis, prognosis and treatment. J.A.A.H.A. *12*:77, 1976.

Lowry, E. C., and Betts, C. W.: Subluxation of the elbow in three dogs. J.A.A.H.A. *9*:458, 1973.

Lust, G.: Pathogenesis of degenerative hip joint disease in young dogs. *In* Proceedings of the Twenty-Third Annual Gaines Veterinary Symposium, Pullman, Wash., 1973, p. 11.

Lust, G., Geary, J. C., and Sheffy, B. E.: Development of hip dysplasia in dogs. Am. J. Vet. Res. *34*:87, 1973.

Madewell, B. R., and Pool, R.: Neoplasms of joints and related structures. Vet. Clin. North Am. *8*:511, 1978.

Marshall, J.: Periarticular osteophytes: Initiation and formation in the knee of the dog. Clin. Orthop. *62*:37, 1969.

Mason, T. A., and Baker, M. J.: The surgical management of elbow joint deformity associated with premature growth plate closure in dogs. J. Small Anim. Pract. *19*:639, 1978.

Mason, T. A., and Lavelle, R. B.: Osteochondritis of the tibial tarsal bone in dogs. J. Small Anim. Pract. *20*:423, 1979.

Mason, T. A., Lavelle, R. B., Skipper, S. C., and Wrigley, W. R.: Osteochondrosis of the elbow joint in young dogs. J. Small Anim. Pract. *21*:641, 1980.

Matis, U., and Kostlin, R.: Cruciate ligament rupture in the cat. Prakt. Tierarzt. *59*:582, 1978.

Mayrhofer, E.: Epiphyseolysis of supra glenoid tuberosity in the dog. Wien. Tierarzt. Monatsschr. *64*:54, 1977.

McManus, J. L., and Nimmons, G. B.: Ruptured anterior cruciate ligament in a cat. Canad. Vet. J. *7*:264, 1967.

Meutstege, F. J.: Die Behandlung der intertarsalen Subluxation beim Hund durch gedeckte Arthrodesis von Os tarsi fibulare und Os tarsale IV. Kleintierpraxis *16*:12, 1971.

Miller, R. M., and Kind, R. E.: A gout-like syndrome in a dog. Vet. Med. Small Anim. Clin. *61*:236, 1966.

Mitchell, N. S., and Cruess, R. L.: Classification of degenerative arthritis. Can. Med. Assoc. J. *117*(7):763, 1977.

Monier, J. C., Schmitt,D., Perraud, M., Gioud, M., and Lapras, M.: Antibody to soluble nuclear antigens in dogs (German shepherd) with a lupus-like syndrome. Develop. Comp. Immun. *2*:161, 1978.

Morgan, J. P.: Radiology of skeletal diseases. Principles of diagnosis in the dog. Vet. Radiol. Associates, Davis, Ca, 1981.

Morgan, J. P.: Radiology in Veterinary Orthopedics. Lea and Febiger, Philadelphia, 1972.

Morgan, J. P.: Hip dysplasia in the beagle: A radiographic survey. J.A.V.M.A. *164*:496, 1969a.

Morgan, J. P.: Radiological pathology and diagnosis of degenerative joint disease in the stifle joint of the dog. J. Small Anim. Pract. *10*:541, 1969b.

Morgan, J. P.: Spondylosis deformans in the dog. Acta Orthop. Scand., Suppl. 96, 1967.

Newton, C. D., Lipowitz, A. J., Halliwell, R. E., Allen, H. L., Biery, D. N., and Schumacher, L.: Rheumatoid arthritis in dogs. J.A.V.M.A. *169*:113, 1976.

Newton, C. D., Schumacher, H. R., Jr., and Halliwell, R. E. W.: Gold salt therapy for rheumatoid arthritis in dogs. J.A.V.M.A. *174*:1308, 1979.

Nunamaker, D. M.: Surgical correction of large femoral anteversion angles in the dog. J.A.V.M.A. *165*:1061, 1974.

Nunamaker, D. M., and Newton, C. D.: Canine hip disorders. In Bojrab, M. J. (ed.): Current Techniques in Small Animal Surgery. Lea and Febiger, Philadelphia, 1975, p. 437.

O'Brien, T. R., Morgan, J. P., and Suter, P. F.: Epiphyseal plate injuries in the dog: A radiographic study of growth disturbance in the forelimbs. J. Small Anim. Pract. *12*:19, 1971.

Olmstead, M. L., and Hohn, R. B.: Total hip replacement in 103 clinical cases at the Ohio State University. Kleintierpraxis *25*:407, 1980.

Olson, N. C., Brinker, W. O., and Carrig, C. B.: Premature closure of the distal radial physis in two dogs. J.A.V.M.A. *176*:906, 1980.

Olson, N. C., Mostosky, U. V., Flo, G. L., and Twedten, H. W.: Osteochondritis dissecans of the tarsocrural joint in three canine siblings. J.A.V.M.A. *176*:635, 1980.

Olsson, S.-E.: Osteochondrosis. A growing problem to dog breeders. Gaines Dog Research Progress, Summer, 1976.

Olsson, S.-E.: Degenerative joint disease (osteoarthrosis): A review with special reference to the dog. J. Small Anim. Pract. *12*:333, 1971.

Paatsama, S.: Ligament injuries of the canine stifle joint: A clinical and experimental study. Thesis, University of Helsinki, Finland, 1952.

Passman, D., and Wolffe, E. F.: Premature closure of the distal radial growth plate in a dog. J.A.V.M.A. *167*:391, 1975.

Pedersen, N. C., Pool, R. R., and O'Brien, T.: Feline chronic progressive polyarthritis. Am. J. Vet. Res. *41*:522, 1980.

Pedersen, N. C., Pool, R. R., Castles, J. J., and Weisner, K.: Noninfectious canine arthritis: Rheumatoid arthritis. J.A.V.M.A. *169*:295, 1976a.

Pedersen, N. C., Weisner, K., Castles, J. J., Ling, G. V., and Weisner, G.: Noninfectious canine arthritis: The inflammatory, nonerosive arthritides. J.A.V.M.A. *169*:304, 1976b.

Peiffer, R. L., Jr., and Blevins, W. E.: Hip dysplasia and pectineus resection in a cat. Feline Pract. *4*(3):40, 1974.

Pettit, G. D.: In Canine Surgery. 2nd Archibald Edition. American Veterinary Publications Inc., Santa Barbara, Calif., 1974.

Pharr, J. W., and Morgan, J. P.: Hip dysplasia in Australian shepherd dogs. J.A.A.H.A. *12*:439, 1976.

Pidduck, H., and Webbon, P. M.: The genetic control of Perthe's disease in toy poodles. A working hypothesis. J. Small Anim. Pract. *19*:729, 1978.

Poulos, P.: Arthrosis of the elbow joint in dogs and cats. Tijdschr. Diergeneeskd. *104*:793, 1979.

Price, C. J., and King, S. C.: Elbow lameness caused by an ossified disc in the joint capsule. Vet. Rec. *100*:566, 1977.

Prole, J. H. B.: Greyhound injuries. (Correspondence.) J. Small Anim. Pract. *17*:197, 1976.

Punzet, G., Walde, J., and Arbesser, E.: Osteochondritis of the stifle joint in the dog. Kleintierpraxis *20*:88, 1975.

Ramadan, R. O., and Vaughan, L. C.: Premature closure of the distal ulnar growth plate in dogs. A review of 58 cases. J. Small Anim. Pract. *19*:647, 1978.

Rendano, V. T., and Adbinoor, D.: Management of intra- and extra-articular extremity gunshot wounds. J.A.A.H.A. *13*:577, 1977.

Renegar, W. R., and Stoll, S. G.: Gunshot wounds involving the canine carpus: Surgical management. J.A.A.H.A. *16*:233, 1980.

Resnick, D.: Arthrography, tenography and bursography. In Resnick, D., and Niwayama, G. (eds.): Diagnosis of Bone and Joint Disorders, Vol. 1. W. B. Saunders Co., Philadelphia, 1981, p. 579.

Riser, W. H.: Juvenile osteoporosis (osteogenesis imperfecta) in the dog and cat. J. Am. Vet. Radiol. Soc. *3*:50, 1962.

Riser, W. H., and Shirer, J. F.: Correlation between canine hip dysplasia and pelvic muscle mass: A study of 95 dogs. Am. J. Vet. Res. *28*:769, 1967.

Roberg, J. W.: Dwarfism in the German shepherd. Canine Pract. *6*(1):42, 1979.

Robins, G. M.: A case of osteochondritis dissecans of the stifle joints in a bitch. J. Small Anim. Pract. *11*:813, 1970.

Robins, G., and Grandage, J.: Temporomandibular joint dysplasia and open-mouth jaw locking in the dog. J.A.V.M.A. *171*:1072, 1977.

Rubin, L. D., Sanders, B. V., Hazlett, J. J., et al.: Panel report. Hip dysplasia in dogs. Mod. Vet. Pract. *60*:255, 1979.

Rudy, R. L.: Correction of growth deformity of the radius and ulna. *In* Bojrab, M. J. (ed.): Current Techniques in Small Animal Surgery. Lea and Febiger, Philadelphia, 1975, p. 535.

Santi, A.: Lateral external luxation of the knee in a dog. Folia Vet. Lat. *4*:581, 1974.

Schalm, O. W., Jain, N. C., and Carrol, E. J.: Veterinary Hematology, 3rd edition. Lea and Febiger, Philadelphia, 1975.

Schrader, S. C.: Triple Osteotomy of the pelvis as a treatment for canine hip dysplasia. J.A.V.M.A. *178*:39, 1981.

Scott, P. P., McKusick, V. A., and McKusick, A. B.: The nature of osteogenesis imperfecta in the cat. J. Bone Joint Surg. *45*:125, 1963.

Seawright, A. H., English, P. B., and Gartner, R. J. W.: Hypervitaminosis A of the cat. Adv. Vet. Sci. Comp. Med. *14*:1, 1970.

Skaggs, S., DeAngelis, M. P., and Rosen, H.: Deformities due to premature closure of the distal ulna in fourteen dogs. A radiographic evaluation. J.A.A.H.A. *9*:496, 1973.

Slappendel, R. J., Kersjes, A. W., and Rijnberk, A.: Canine systemic lupus erythematosus treated with prednisone. Zentralbl. Veterinaermed. *19*:23, 1972.

Smith, C. W., and Stowater, J. L.: Osteochrondritis dissecans of the canine shoulder joint: a review of 35 cases. J.A.A.H.A. *11*:658, 1975.

Smith, K. W.: Achilles tendon surgery for correction of hyperextension of the hock joint. J.A.A.H.A. *12*:848, 1976.

Stewart, W. C., Baker, C. J., and Lee, R.: Temporomandibular subluxation in the dog: a case report. J. Small Anim. Pract. *16*:345, 1975.

Stoyac, J. M.: The elbow: Dislocation of the elbow. *In* Bojrab, M. J. (ed.): Current Techniques in Small Animal Surgery. Lea and Febiger, Philadelphia, 1975, p. 523.

Strande, A.: Repair of the Ruptured Cranial Cruciate Ligament in the Dog. Williams and Wilkins Co., Baltimore, Md., 1967.

Steere, A. C., and Malawista, S. E.: Viral Arthritis. *In* McCarty, D. J. (ed.): Arthritis and Allied Conditions. Lea and Febiger, Philadelphia, 1979, p. 1391.

Swanton, M. C.: The pathology of hemarthrosis in hemophilia. *In* Brinkhaus, K. M. (ed.): Hemophilia and Hemophilioid Diseases. University of N. Carolina Press, Chapel Hill, N. C., 1957, p. 219.

Thomas, R. E.: Temporomandibular joint dysplasia and open-mouth jaw locking in a basset hound: a case report. J. Small Anim. Pract. *20*:697, 1979.

Ticer, J. W., and Spencer, C. P.: Injury of the feline temporomandibular joint: Radiographic signs. J. Am. Vet. Radiol. Soc. *19*:146, 1978.

Tirgari, M.: Changes in the canine stifle joint following rupture of the anterior cruciate ligament. J. Small Anim. Pract. *19*:17, 1978.

Tirgari, M., and Vaughan, M. C.: Arthritis of the canine stifle joint. Vet. Rec. *96*:394, 1975.

Trotter, E. J., Delahunta, A., Geary, J. C., and Brasmer, T. H.: Caudal cervical vertebral malformation-malarticulation in Great Danes and Doberman pinschers. J.A.V.M.A. *168*:917, 1976.

Vaananen, M., and Skutnabb, K.: Elbow lameness in the young dog caused by sesamoidal fragment. J. Small Anim. Pract. *19*:363, 1978.

Wallace, L. J., Guffy, M. M., and Cardinet, G. H., III: Pectineus tendon or muscle surgery for treatment of clinical hip dysplasia in the dog. *In* Bojrab, M. J. (ed.): Current Techniques in Small Animal Surgery. Lea and Febiger, Philadelphia, 1975, p. 443.

Watson, A. G.: Congenital occipitoatlanto-axial malformation (OAAM) in a dog. Anat. Histol. Embryol. *8*:187, 1979.

Whitacre, R., and Harrison, J. W.: Osteochondritis dissecans: A clinical study of morbidity and incidence. The Speculum *25*:14, 1972.

White, C. A.: Bilateral forward mandibular luxation in a dog. North Am. Vet. *50*:777, 1949.

Wilkinson, G. T., and Robins, G. M.: Polyarthritis in a young cat. J. Small Anim. Pract. *20*:293, 1979.

Wind, A.: Surgical Diseases of the Carpal Joints and Methods of Treatment. *In* Bojrab, M. J. (ed.): Techniques in Small Animal Surgery. Lea and Febiger, Philadelphia, 1975, p. 542.

Wissler, J., and Sumner-Smith, G.: Osteochondrosis of the elbow joint of the dog. J.A.A.H.A. *13*:349, 1977.

Withrow, S. J.: Management of a congenital elbow luxation by temporary transarticular pinning. Vet. Med. Small Anim. Clin. *72*:1597, 1977.

Wolff, E. F.: Ununited coronoid process in the dog: a review with two case reports. Vet. Med. Small Anim. Clin. *74*:1299, 1979.

Wood, A. K. W., Bath, M. L., and Mason, T. A.: Osteochondritis dissecans of the distal humerus in a dog. Vet. Rec. *96*:489, 1975.

Woodard, D. C.: Osteochondritis dissecans in a family of bull terriers. Vet. Med. Small Anim. Clin. *74*:936, 1979.

Wright, J. A.: Spondylosis deformans of the lumbosacral joint in dogs. J. Small Anim. Pract. *21*:45, 1980.

Wright, P. J., and Mason, T. A.: Usefulness of palpation of joint laxity in puppies as a predictor of hip dysplasia in a guide dog breeding programme. J. Small Anim. Pract. *18*:513, 1977.

Zahm, H.: Die Ligamenta decessata in gesunden und arthroptischen Kniegelenk des Hundes. Kleintierpraxis *10*:38, 1965

CHAPTER 85

Skeletal Diseases

C. D. NEWTON
and G. SIEMERING

DISEASES OF INFLAMMATION

The most common cause of osteomyelitis in dogs and cats is an infectious inflammation of bone marrow and adjacent bone. While osteomyelitis is caused by suppurative organisms, nonsuppurative osteomyelitis also occurs. Nonsuppurative osteomyelitis results from granulomatous organisms or from metalosis.

SUPPURATIVE OSTEOMYELITIS

Etiology. Suppurative osteomyelitis occurs when bacteria infect bone. Bacteria may reach bone by hematogenous routes, by extension of soft tissue infection into bone, or by direct contact with bone (i.e., open fracture or open surgery). Regardless of the source of contamination, once bacteria are present, bone mounts an inflammatory response that is similar to that of soft tissues.

Bone inflammation results in the infiltration and localization of granulocytic leukocytes. Many of the infiltrating cells are destroyed by the bacteria and release proteolytic enzymes into the bone. Tissue necrosis ensues, and the bacteria and the lytic products of necrosis (the pus cells and debris) are mingled to form a focus of suppuration (Aegerter, 1968).

The severity of osteomyelitis depends on many factors: the occurrence of the process in cortical or metaphyseal bone, the contribution of other disease to bone abnormality, the presence of vascular ischemia, and the animal's age and general health. If the inflammatory process is successful, the osteomyelitis may be contained. If, however, the infection proves overwhelming to the inflammatory process, osteomyelitis will disseminate within the bone (Fig. 85–1).

Infection in metaphyseal bone may break through the thin cortex and spread subperiosteally to most of the diaphysis. Infection in diaphyseal cortical bone spreads through the haversian canals. As infection spreads, vascular thrombosis occurs, resulting in localized areas of cortical bone ischemia. If ischemia is incomplete, the bone may respond by producing new bone around the area of infection. If ischemia is severe, bone death may result. Complete bone death results in cell death, and the resulting area is thus composed only of collagen and mineral. Such dead bone may be slowly revascularized, undergo lysis and subsequent new bone formation, or it may be sloughed. Dead bone is called a sequestrum; it often sits within a granulation tissue–filled bony depression (involucrum) (Fig. 85–2).

Acute osteomyelitis occurs when the early changes herein described are recognized and appropriate treatment is initiated promptly. Chronic osteomyelitis occurs when the process continues for an extended period of time and results in disseminated infection within the bone and the inflammation fails to contain the infection. Chronic infection will usually result in disseminated infection, bone death, and evidence of aborted attempts at containment, i.e., involucrum and suppurating exudate, or pus that drains to the skin.

Diagnosis. Acute or chronic suppurative osteomyelitis usually presents with pain, local swelling, and pyrexia (Caywood, 1978). With chronicity, obvious tracts and drainage may also be present. Most animals do not demonstrate significant hematologic alterations; moderate leukocytosis with a left shift was occasionally found in one study (Caywood, 1978).

Radiographically, bony change associated with suppurative infection is limited to bony lysis, areas of periosteal new bone, or other areas of increased bony density. Typical lytic and periosteal bone changes are not evident for 10 to 14 days following onset of infection (Boland, 1972; Caywood, 1978). Soft tissue changes are visible within 24

47 per cent of the dogs in one study had two or more organisms present simultaneously (Caywood, 1978).

Treatment. The treatment method depends on the type of osteomyelitis, acute or chronic. In acute osteomyelitis, if fluid is present, the first step is to decompress and provide drainage from the area. The drainage should be protected against contamination from its surroundings with a bandage or a Robert Jones dressing.

Systemic antibiotics are used at this time, and although many antibiotics may be considered, a bactericidal drug should be chosen. If fluid is available it is submitted for culture, identification, and sensitivity. Systemic antibiotics are used in the interim before the results of the culture are known. The choice of antibiotic is important, since

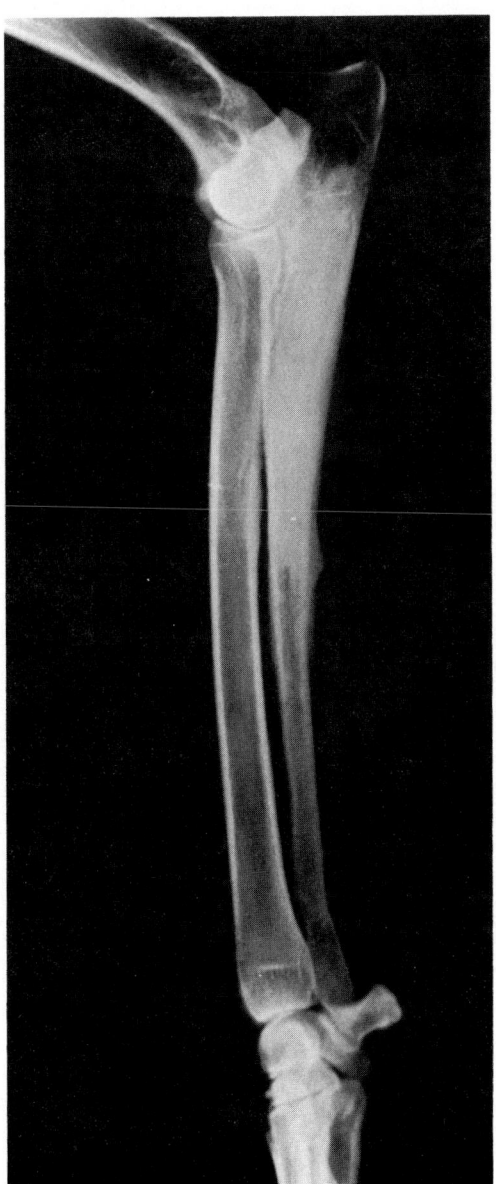

Figure 85–1. Acute bacterial osteomyelitis of the ulna secondary to a dog bite wound.

hours; such changes include soft tissue swelling and loss of fascial planes.

Bacteriologically, the most frequent organism isolated in the dog and cat with osteomyelitis is *Staphylococcus aureus*. *S. aureus* represented 60 per cent of cases in one study (Hirsh and Smith, 1978), 75 per cent of cases in a second study (Caywood, 1978), and 54 per cent in a third study (Smith, 1980). Streptococcal infections follow *S. aureus* in frequency. Of equal importance is the prevalence of mixed infections:

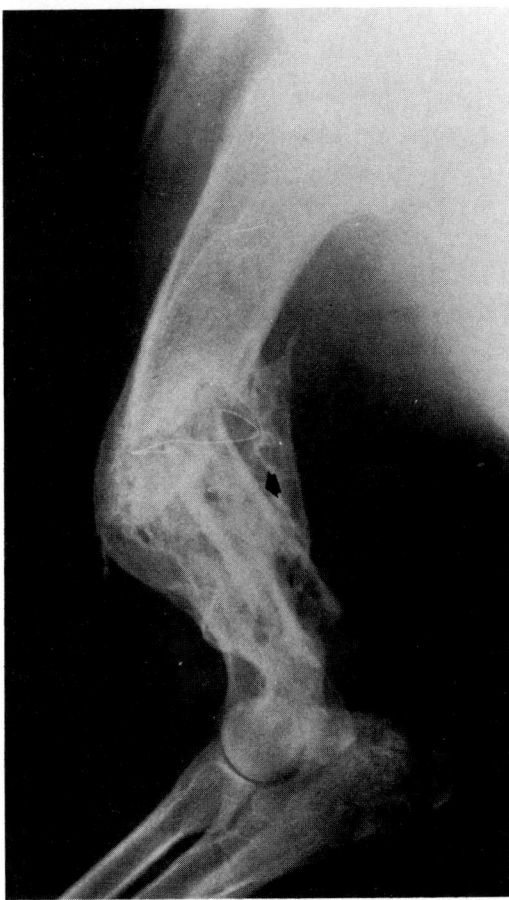

Figure 85–2. Chronic bacterial osteomyelitis of the humerus secondary to fracture repair in a two-year-old male German shepherd dog. Note the bony sequestra (arrow).

the first few days of treatment may determine the course of the infection. The author's experience has shown that the most commonly used drugs (penicillin with streptomycin or chloramphenicol) are often not of value. Most forms of gram-positive cocci and bacilli along with gram-negative cocci respond well to ampicillin and cephaloridine. The remaining gram-negative organisms usually respond to gentamycin or kanamycin. The author prefers cephaloridine or ampicillin empirically until culture and sensitivity results are available, followed by use of one of the four previously mentioned drugs, as determined by sensitivity. Dosage depends on circulation: higher levels of antibiotics are needed when blood perfusion is poor, such as in cases of sequestered bone fragments or soft tissue edema and stasis around the fracture (Nunamaker, 1975).

Immobilization of the limb by bandage or cast may be indicated to prevent swelling, but if used should be checked daily by changing. The area is radiographed at ten-day intervals to evaluate the extent of infection.

The treatment of chronic osteomyelitis may be similar to that of acute osteomyelitis; however, areas of dead bone or sequestra must be surgically removed. Following surgical removal, curettage of dead bone back to healthy bleeding bone is performed. The instillation of drains is often necessary to facilitate removal of blood or other postoperative debris. Culture of the deep wound or bone determines the organism(s) present and their drug sensitivities.

Chronic osteomyelitis is a difficult disease to cure and may persist despite extensive treatment.

NONSUPPURATIVE OSTEOMYELITIS

Systemic Mycoses

Mycotic infections producing systemic disease often have bony manifestations. A nonsuppurative osteomyelitis is the most common bony change. These conditions are discussed at length in Chapter 26.

Coccidioidomycosis. *Coccidioides immitis* is a fungal disease endemic in the southwestern United States. In addition to the primary respiratory disease, bony osteomyelitis often occurs. Bone enlargement and soft tissue enlargement over the bone associated with lameness are common findings. Radiographically the bony lesion is proliferative, with small areas of bony lysis. While the bone appears osteomyelitic, it may be confused with neoplasia of various stages (Reed, 1956; Maddy, 1958; Blake, 1958; Brodey, 1970). Biopsy and culture are necessary for definitive diagnosis and treatment (Fig. 85–3).

Blastomycosis. *Blastomyces dermatitidis* causes a chronic systemic disease of dogs and cats. Skeletal lesions may develop via hematogenous spread or by extension from a subcutaneous nodule. Edema, pain, and occasionally draining tracts are found in the affected area. There is radiographic evidence of bone destruction with resulting periosteal bony reaction. Biopsy and culture are necessary for definitive diagnosis and treatment (Horne, 1964; Dunn, 1977).

Cryptococcus. *Cryptococcus neoformans* causes an upper respiratory disease in cats. Occasionally it may produce lytic bony lesions of the head and sinuses or of the shaft and metaphysis of long bones (Rutman and Chandler, 1975; Small, 1969).

Histoplasmosis. *Histoplasma* capsulation causes a respiratory and gastrointestinal disease most typically resulting in diarrhea or dyspnea (Small, 1969). In two reports, bony lesions of the tarsus or metatarsus resulted in both bony destruction and bony proliferation. The radiographic changes are not unlike those in coccidioidomycosis, cryptococcus, or blastomycosis (Law et al., 1978; Mahaffey et al., 1977).

Other Mycoses. Bony lesions are also reported associated with *Nocardia* (Mitten, 1975; Small, 1969; Skelley and Sauer, 1965; Ditchfield, 1961), *Aspergillus fumigatus* (Lane et al., 1974), adiaspiromycosis (Al-Doory et al., 1971), and *Streptomyces* (Lewis et al., 1972).

Metalosis

A noninfectious, nonsuppurative osteomyelitis often occurs around metal implants, which may result from metal corrosion, use of dissimilar metals, or animal allergy to an implant. Metalosis usually manifests itself clinically by lameness or draining tracts. The tract effluent will be serous and will not grow bacteria. Animals are not febrile and do not have marked hematologic abnormalities. Radiographic

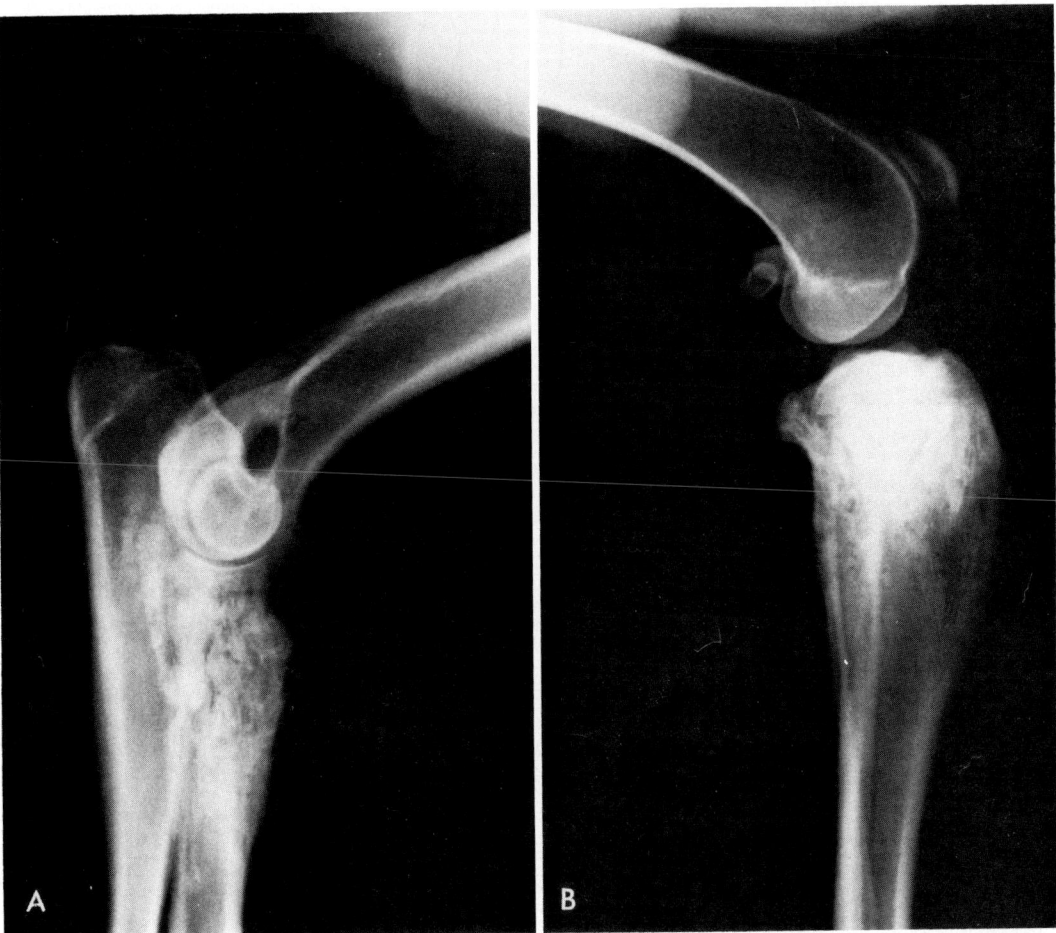

Figure 85–3. Fungal osteomyelitis of the radius (*A*) and tibia (*B*) caused by *Coccidioides immitis* in a five-year-old male Boxer.

evidence of metalosis is bony lysis around the implant. A "halo" effect will be present around a portion or around the entire implant. Treatment will be unsuccessful unless the implant is removed. Following removal recovery is uneventful; antibiotics are unnecessary.

METABOLIC BONE DISEASES

The term "metabolic bone disease" is at best confusing. This term is used to describe a wide range of diseases of bone, including those conditions primarily involving bone, such as panosteitis and hypertrophic osteodystrophy, and those secondarily involving bone, such as secondary nutritional hyperparathyroidism. For the purposes of this chapter, metabolic bone diseases will include osteoporosis, rickets, osteomalacia, primary hyperparathyroidism, secondary

renal hyperparathyroidism, and nutritional hyperparathyroidism. The latter three conditions are covered extensively in Chapter 65, Parathyroid Diseases.

OSTEOPOROSIS

Osteoporosis is a reduction in bone mass due to subnormal osteoid production, subnormal osteoid mineralization, or an excessive rate of deossification. Primary osteoporosis has not been reported in the dog or the cat. In man, primary osteoporosis is a disease of unknown etiology seen in elderly women and men. This is the only type of reduction in bone mass that is properly called osteoporosis, and the term osteoporosis properly refers to no other bone disease (Aegerter and Kirkpatrick, 1968). A reduction in bone mass results from certain anticonvulsive drugs and can be seen in primary hyperparathyroidism, nutritional hyperparathyroidism, secondary renal hyperparathyroidism, pseudohyperparathyroidism, hyperthyroidism, acromegaly, hepatic toxicities, immobilization of a limb, long-term tetraplegia, multiple myeloma, and hyperadrenocorticism. None of these is a primary osteoporosis; therefore, osteoporosis in the dog and cat should be referred to as *secondary* osteoporosis.

The clinical signs of secondary osteoporosis are pathological fractures of the long bones and compression fractures of the vertebrae. A limb immobilized for two to three weeks can develop disuse osteoporosis owing to the lack of stress of the bone. Remineralization occurs after use begins; however, the bone can easily fracture during this remineralization time. Radiographi-

cally, a generalized decrease in bone density is seen. There is resorption of the cortices and folding fractures of the long bones. Compression fractures of vertebral bodies can also be seen.

Histologically, the normal architecture of the bone is preserved; however, there is a decrease in the amount of osteoid present.

The prognosis of osteoporosis depends entirely upon the underlying cause. The prognosis of secondary renal hyperparathyroidism is considerably worse than disuse osteoporosis.

ABNORMAL CALCIUM METABOLISM EFFECTS ON BONE

Calcium metabolism and its pathophysiology is discussed extensively in Chapter 65,

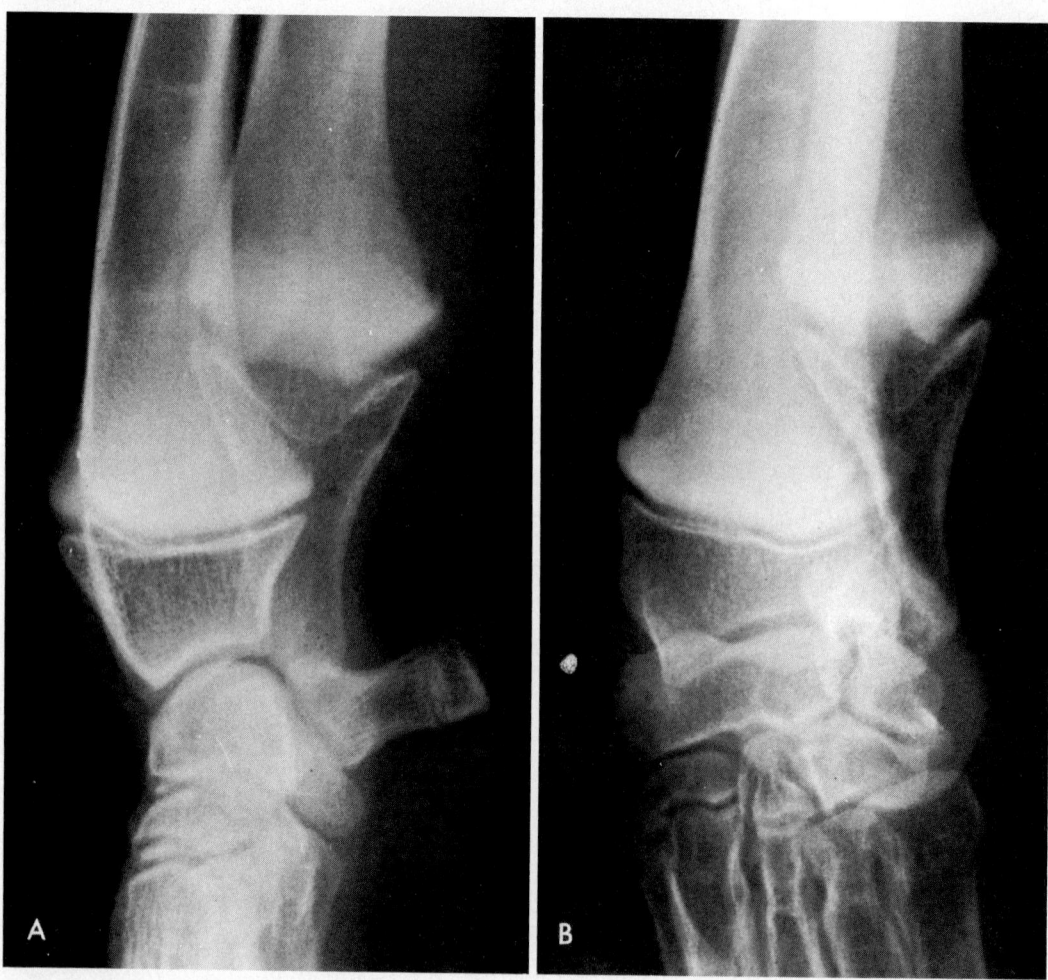

Figure 85–4. *A* and *B*, Retained enchondral core in the distal ulna of a three-month-old male St. Bernard.

as are primary hyperparathyroidism, secondary renal hyperparathyroidism and nutritional hyperparathyroidism.

Retained Enchondral Cores

Retained enchondral cartilage cores are frequently found in the ulnar metaphysis of giant breed dogs. The core can be seen radiographically as a radiolucent inverted cone extending from the epiphysis proximally into the metaphysis. The presence of the core may be associated with forelimb deformity or may be found coincidentally in normal dogs. Deformity, if present, may include forelimb valgus, external rotation, or anterior bowing (Fig. 85–4).

The etiology of the lesion is unknown but may relate to the vasculature of the metaphysis. It is postulated that there is an absence of vascular tissue that would normally penetrate hypertrophied cartilage cells prior to mineralization (Riser and Shirer, 1965). As a result of improper mineralization, the ulna does not lengthen as rapidly as the radius, thus deformity results.

Similarly, retained enchondral cores play a role in the bony deformity of hindlimbs in giant breed dogs called genu valgum. This deformity produces femoral shafts that bow medially ("knock-knees") and lateral patellar luxation. Retained enchondral cores can be seen radiographically and histologically in the lateral femoral condyles (Stone et al., 1969). The slowed growth of the lateral femoral condyle appears to have a primary role in the resultant deformity. The etiology of the retained core is presumed similar to the ulnar core.

Both specific problems that result from retained cores are best handled surgically. Radial and ulnar deformities may be corrected and result in near normal animals (Newton, 1974); genu valgum may be corrected surgically, but the results are less gratifying.

Multiple Cartilaginous Exostoses

Multiple cartilaginous exostoses (MCE) is a benign, proliferative disease of bone and cartilage seen predominantly in young dogs (Gambardella et al.,1975), but it has been reported in cats as well (Pool and Carrig, 1972; Riddle and Leighton, 1970). The disease is also referred to as osteochondromatosis, diaphyseal aclasis, and hereditary multiple exostoses.

Animals are presented for examination with obvious bony enlargements, or musculoskeletal or neurologic dysfunction. The dysfunction results from muscular realignment or compressive neurologic disease. Animals tend to be immature, as the disease occurs during the normal period of enchondral bone formation. Pain is generally not a part of the clinical disease unless neurologic compression occurs. Radiographically, bony exostotic lesions may be seen on any bone except the skull. Lesions tend to have radiopaque bony areas interspersed with more radiolucent areas of cartilage. If lesions originate from long bones, the metaphyseal region is usually involved (Fig. 85–5).

The etiology of MCE is unknown. The disease is hereditary in man, characterized by autosomal dominance with full penetrance (Solomon, 1964). Hereditary aspects of the canine disease have been reported (Gee and Doige, 1970; Chester, 1971) but have not been established.

While the pathogenesis is not entirely known, many aspects of the disease are understood. It is apparent that this is a disease of abnormal chondrocyte differentiation. It has been postulated that chondrocytes in the normal epiphyseal plate are forced out of the plate into surrounding metaphyseal bone (Langenskiold, 1967). Rather than differentiating into osteoblasts, the cells proliferate and continue to produce large islands of cartilage. Eventually the enlarged cartilage islands produce bone, which causes the exostosis (Aegerter and Kirkpatrick, 1964).

Histologically, tissue from an exostosis resembles the epiphysis and metaphysis of growing bone. Normal cortical and cancellous bone is present, usually capped with a layer of hyaline cartilage (Alexander, 1978b). Since the exostoses enlarge by endochondral bone formation, the cartilage cap resembles a normal physis (Gambardella, 1975).

Treatment is usually minimal or unnecessary unless neurologic deficit is present. Without neurologic complications most exostoses mature and remain unchanged. Transformation of cartilaginous exostoses

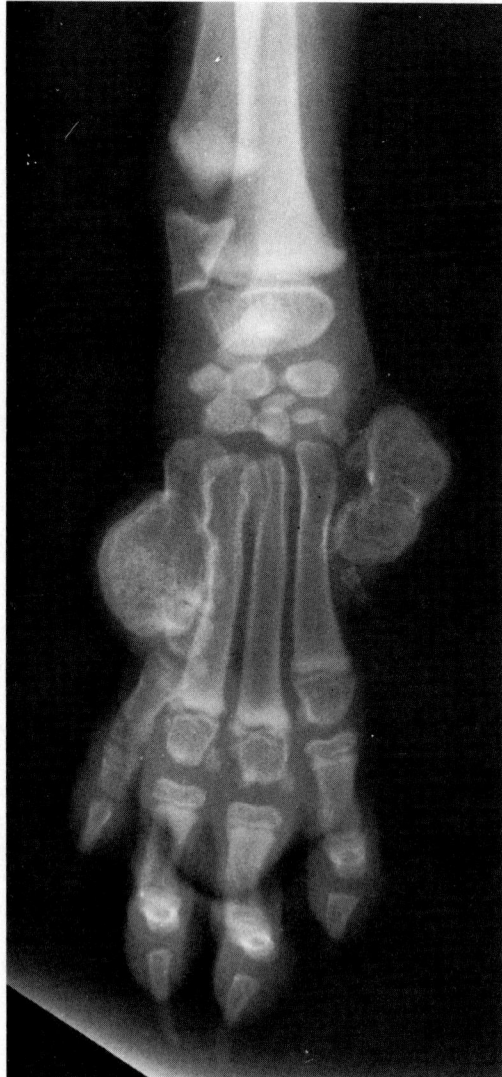

Figure 85–5. Multiple cartilaginous exostoses of metacarpal bones I and V in a four-month-old female mixed-breed dog.

into osteosarcoma (Owen, 1971) and into chondrosarcoma (Banks and Bridges, 1956; Doige et al., 1978) has been reported.

GENETIC DISEASE OF BONE

Mucopolysaccharidosis

Mucopolysaccharidosis (MPS) is a disease primarily of Siamese cats, although three dachshund pups have also been reported with the disease Schalm, 1977). MPS in man has been known as a distinct class of inherited metabolic disease for 60 years (McKusick, 1972). At least seven specific

forms are now recognized, each due to a defect in a different lysosomal enzyme concerned with the degradation of glycosaminoglycase, a general category of lysosomal storage diseases. Prominent features in man include multiple skeletal, neurologic, and ocular abnormalities, usually associated with dwarfism (Pennock and Barnes, 1976).

MPS was first recognized in a female Siamese cat in 1976. The cat exhibited dwarfism, facial abnormalities, severe skeletal deformities, multifocal neurologic deficits, and retinal atrophy (Cowell et al., 1976). Further study revealed metachromatic inclusion bodies in circulating leukocytes and very high urine concentrations of mucopolysaccharide. Subsequent breeding of the affected animal produced kittens with MPS, as well as confirmation of the autosomal recessive transmission of the disease.

Urine samples of the affected cats have high levels of dermatin sulfate. In many animals the level is 90 times that in normal cat urine (Jezyk et al., 1977). Hematologic studies reveal MPS granules in lymphocytes and neutrophils. MPS granules in lymphocytes tend to be larger and to stain more darkly than azurophilic granules (Schalm, 1977). In many cases a clear space or "halo" may surround the granule.

Radiographic evidence of the disease is often confused with hypervitaminosis A. Cats often have severe bony bridging of cervical vertebral bodies with prolonged disease; the thoracic or lumbar spine may fuse. Bony changes in long bone epiphyses occur, resulting in broad irregular epiphyses. Bony proliferation around joints may become severe, resulting in ankylosis as the disease progresses (Fig. 85–6).

This disease is caused by an inheritable defect that specifically results in a deficiency of arylsulfatose B. Treatment of affected animals is nonspecific, but the aim is toward alleviating symptoms. These animals may live comfortably as pets if the disease is treated.

Osteopetrosis

Osteopetrosis is a rare, congenital, familial developmental abnormality of skeletal growth in man and animals (Riser and Frankhauser, 1970). Three cases have been reported; all were dachshund litter mates.

Clinically, the affected dogs are unable to

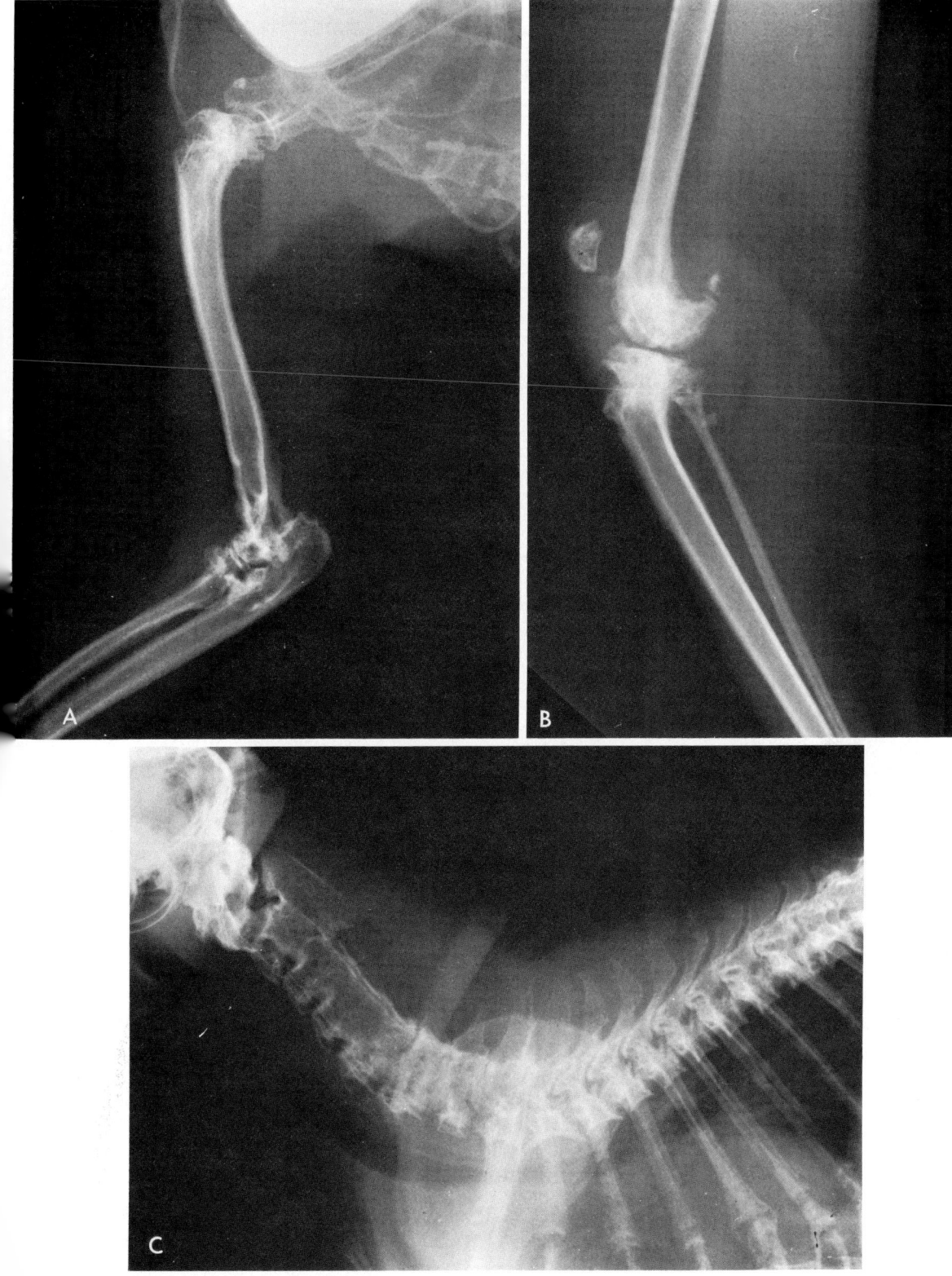

Figure 85–6. Mucopolysaccharidosis affecting the peripheral joints (*A* and *B*) and spine (*C*) in a two-year-old female Siamese cat.

perform normal functions. Radiographically, bones appear over-mineralized, with a uniformly dense and sclerotic bone pattern and a lack of distinction between cortical and cancellous bone in the epiphysis, metaphysis, or diaphysis.

Histologically, the anatomic disturbance is persistent and there is continued deposition of osteoid material and bone on the primary and secondary trabeculae. Normal resorption and remodeling of this new bone to form a cortex of lamellar bone were not present.

The exact mechanism of osteopetrosis is unknown (Aegerter and Kirkpatrick, 1968), but a failure or inhibition of resorption of calcified chondroid and primitive bone appears to be the primary cause. Fractures of affected bone are common; sarcoma has been reported as a late complication in humans surviving to adulthood.

Dwarfism

Pituitary Dwarfism. Pituitary dwarfism results in a proportionate dwarfing of the animal. Growth plates routinely remain open beyond 18 months of age in these dogs. The diagnosis is based on the size of the animal, delayed closure of the epiphyses, or delayed mineralization of the os penis in the male. Normal male dogs show mineralization of the os penis by four to five months of age; if mineralization has not occurred by 15 months, this disease may be suspected (Siegel, 1977) (Fig. 85–7).

The disease is a result of the absence or insufficiency of growth hormone. Growth hormone levels may be determined (Scott, 1978), followed by treatment with bovine growth hormone, 10 I.U. subcutaneously every other day for 30 days (Siegel, 1977).

Achondroplasia. Achondroplasia occurs in Scottish terriers and miniature poodles in which impaired ossification of long bone cartilage produce abnormal, short limbs (Mather, 1956).

Chondrodysplasia. This disease causes stunted forelimbs, lateral deviation of the paw, carpal enlargement, lateral bowing of the forelimbs, and a top-line that slants forward. The disease is seen in malamutes (Fletch, 1973; Subden, 1972).

Achondroplasia in the Cat. This form of dwarfism causes muscular weakness and atrophy primarily in the rear legs. The disease causes death within the first four months of life (Hegreberg, 1974).

NEOPLASTIC DISEASE OF BONE

PRIMARY BONE NEOPLASIA

Osteosarcoma

Osteosarcoma is the most common bone tumor in the dog. The frequency in comparison to other types of bone tumors has been reported as high as 90 per cent (Brodey et al., 1963).

The highest incidence occurs in dogs eight years of age, with a range of 1 to 15 years (Brodey et al., 1963). Males and females are equally affected. Osteosarcoma occurs most frequently in the boxer, Great Dane, Saint Bernard, Irish setter, collie, and German shepherd dogs. Seventy-seven per cent of osteosarcomas originate in long bones and 23 per cent in flat bones (Brodey

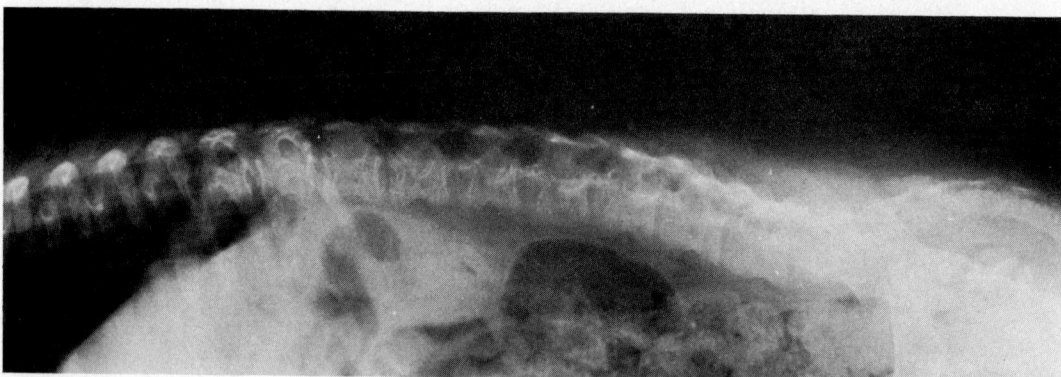

Figure 85–7. Pituitary Dwarfism. Note the immature-appearing vertebral bodies in the spine of a 2½-year-old female German Shepherd Dog.

et al., 1963). This tumor is most prevalent "away from the elbow" (i.e., in the distal radius and proximal humerus) and "around the knee" (in the distal femur and proximal tibia).

Clinical signs include rapid onset of lameness over a two- to five-day period, localized swelling around the lesion, and occasionally fever and anorexia. Metastases occur in the lungs (40 of 45 dogs) (Brodey and Abt, 1976).

Radiographs reveal solitary lesions in the bones with either lytic areas or areas of bony proliferation or both, and an eroded cortex with neoplastic bone extending beyond the cortex. The margin of the lesion is poorly defined. Growth rate is rapid, with a large amount of soft tissue swelling usually present. A pathologic fracture may exist. Pulmonary metastases are not visible in the early stages (Weben, 1978) (Figs. 85–8 and 85–9).

Treatment of osteosarcoma is unrewarding; thus, owner education is important. Owners should be informed that only 10 to 15 per cent of dogs survive longer than nine months following amputation (Brodey and Abt, 1976). Amputation of the involved limb will alleviate pain, although as a clinical

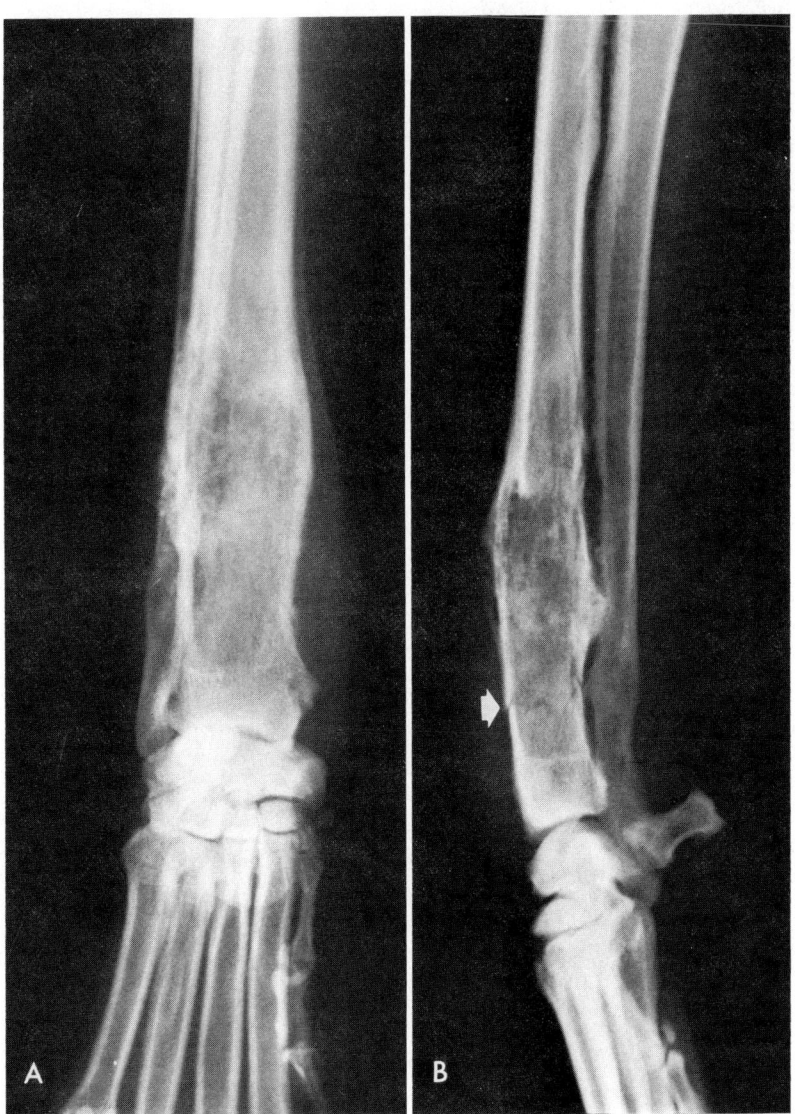

Figure 85–8. *A* and *B*, Osteogenic sarcoma of the distal radial metaphysis in a 10-year-old female mixed breed dog. Note the pathologic fracture (arrow).

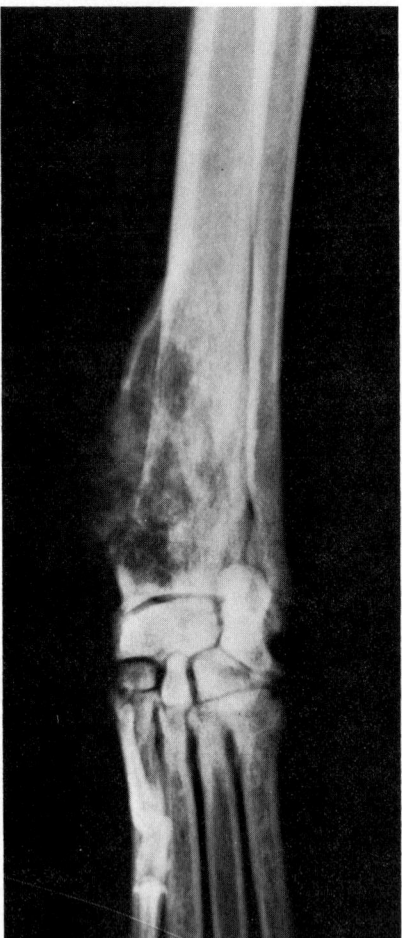

Figure 85–9. Osteogenic sarcoma of the distal radial metaphysis and epiphysis in a nine-year-old female collie. This tumor demonstrates radiographic evidence of both bony lysis and bony proliferation.

impression, it does not necessarily prolong the life of the dog. Large breed dogs tolerate amputation of the limb reasonably well. The owners should be warned that this is a palliative measure.

Recently chemotherapy, immunotherapy, and radiation therapy in various combinations with amputation was reported in 11 cases. Drugs given were cyclophosphamide, methotrexate, calcium leucovorin, vincristine sulfate, and d-oxyrubicin. Immunotherapy consisted of tumor cells modified by acetoacetylation with diketene and given by intramuscular or intradermal injection with Freund's complete adjuvant (Henness et al., 1977). The results of treatment continue to be unrewarding.

Diagnosis is confirmed by biopsy of the lesion. Care must be taken to review radiographs and plan an approach to accurate biopsy. In lieu of biopsy, clinical signs, age, breed, location of lesion, and radiography may be used to formulate a diagnosis.

Histologically, osteosarcoma presents with a wide range of morphologic patterns. This includes a broad range of matrix patterns aligned in a haphazard way with osteonecrosis and/or new bone production (Ling, 1974).

The prognosis is poor. In one report of 65 cases treated with amputation the median survival time was only 18 weeks. In a study by Brodey and Abt (1976), 10.7 per cent survived more than one year. In a study by Henness (1977) 11 dogs were treated with chemotherapy, immunotherapy, and radiation therapy combined with amputation. One dog survived beyond 45 months.

Extraskeletal osteosarcoma does occur in the dog and cat (Bartels, 1975). Osteosarcoma occurs in cats with clinical signs similar to those of the dog. Radiographic signs also resemble those of the dog. Surgical excision of the mass or amputation of the affected limb was performed in five cats. One cat showed pulmonary and renal metastasis five months postoperatively; the remaining cats were alive at 26 months postoperatively (Liu et al., 1974).

Chondrosarcoma

Canine chondrosarcoma is the second most common bone tumor, comprising 10 per cent of all canine bone tumors (Brodey et al., 1974). A review of 35 cases of chondrosarcoma reveals the median age of affected dogs to be six years; there are no sex predilections. Major sites of origin were the ribs, nasal cavity, and pelvis (Brodey et al., 1974).

Clinical signs are related to the location of the lesion: rib involvement — large, hard, painless swelling at the costochondral junction; pelvis — lameness; and nasal cavity — sneezing, epistaxis, and nasal swelling.

Radiographically, chondrosarcoma can produce either osteolysis or reactive periosteum with mineralization of the chondrosarcoma or both. The frequency is greater in flat bones (69 per cent) than in long bones (Brodey et al., 1974).

Histologically, tumors have cartilage cells grouped in chondromas of hyaline cartilage.

Calcification and secondary ossification of neoplastic cartilage is not unusual.

Treatment consists of removal of the tumor. This is difficult in the nasal cavity and the pelvis. The prognosis is good to guarded if complete excision is accomplished.

METASTATIC BONE NEOPLASIA

Metastatic bone tumors occur in both the dog and the cat. These tumors include carcinomas, melanomas, nephroblastomas, aortic body tumors, sarcoma, fibromas, lymphosarcomas, hemangiosarcomas, reticulum cell sarcomas, and meningiomas (Liu et al., 1974; 1977).

DISEASES OF UNDETERMINED ETIOLOGY

PANOSTEITIS

Panosteitis is a spontaneous, self-limiting inflammatory disease of the long bones in immature, large breed dogs. German shepherds have the highest breed incidence, with a ratio of 80 per cent male to 20 per cent female (Bohning et al., 1970; Burt and Wilson, 1972).

Dogs with panosteitis present with an acute onset of lameness unrelated to trauma. The lameness may undergo spontaneous remission, only to reappear in a different limb. The age of onset is between 5 and 12 months; however, older dogs may present with the disease. Physical examination demonstrates pain on deep palpation of affected bone.

Clinical pathologic findings in populations of dogs with panosteitis do not vary significantly from normal animals, and leukocytosis, neutrophilia, and eosinophilia are not characteristic findings (Cotter et al., 1968). Serum values for calcium, phosphorous, and alkaline phosphatase were similar to those for ten German shepherd dogs with active panosteitis and ten age-matched normal control dogs in a study by Cotter and coworkers (1968).

Radiography confirms the presumptive diagnosis; however, often the radiographic appearance lags behind the stage of disease present and may not detect very early lesions. Radioisotopic bone scintigrams using technetium 99m–labeled polyphosphate have been more sensitive in diagnosing early lesions (Turnier, 1978). The radiographic appearance of long bones with panosteitis has been described by Bohning and colleagues (1970). The disease affects primarily the diaphysis of long bones (humerus, radius, ulna, femur, and tibia). Radiographs early in the disease demonstrate a blurring and accentuation of the trabecular pattern of the proximal and distal ends of the diaphysis. An increased density to the medullary cavity and endosteum may be apparent.

In mid-phase the medullary cavity has a pattern characterized as radiodense, patchy, or mottled; these changes often originate in the region about the nutrient foramen (Fig. 85–10). Occasionally the changes may be large enough or may coalesce to fill the entire medullary cavity. The endosteal surface may become roughened. Late in the disease, most previously-mentioned radiographic changes disappear. The residual may be a coarser trabecular pattern or a cortical thickening. Following complete remission of the disease, most long bones will be radiographically normal.

The etiology of panosteitis is unknown; however, theories have been brought forth incriminating bacteria (Evers, 1969), hyperestrinism (Sprinkle, 1970), or hereditary factors (Burt and Wilson, 1972). None of these theories has been conclusively supported.

Histologically marked accentuation of osteoblastic and fibroblastic activity is found throughout the periosteum, endosteum, and marrow cavity. The overall pattern is uniform, and the abundance of osteoblasts and osteoclasts indicates an active bone turnover (Bohning et al., 1970). The processes involved in producing this disease affect periosteal, endosteal, or medullary cells, stimulating them to undergo osteoblastic or fibroblastic differentiation and activity (Cotter et al., 1968).

Treatment is symptomatic, with analgesics serving the primary role. Limitation of activity during the active disease may also be beneficial. The prognosis is complete return to normal; however, the episodes of shifting leg lameness may continue for as long as two to four months.

HYPERTROPHIC OSTEODYSTROPHY

Hypertrophic osteodystrophy (HOD) is a bony disease affecting the metaphysis adja-

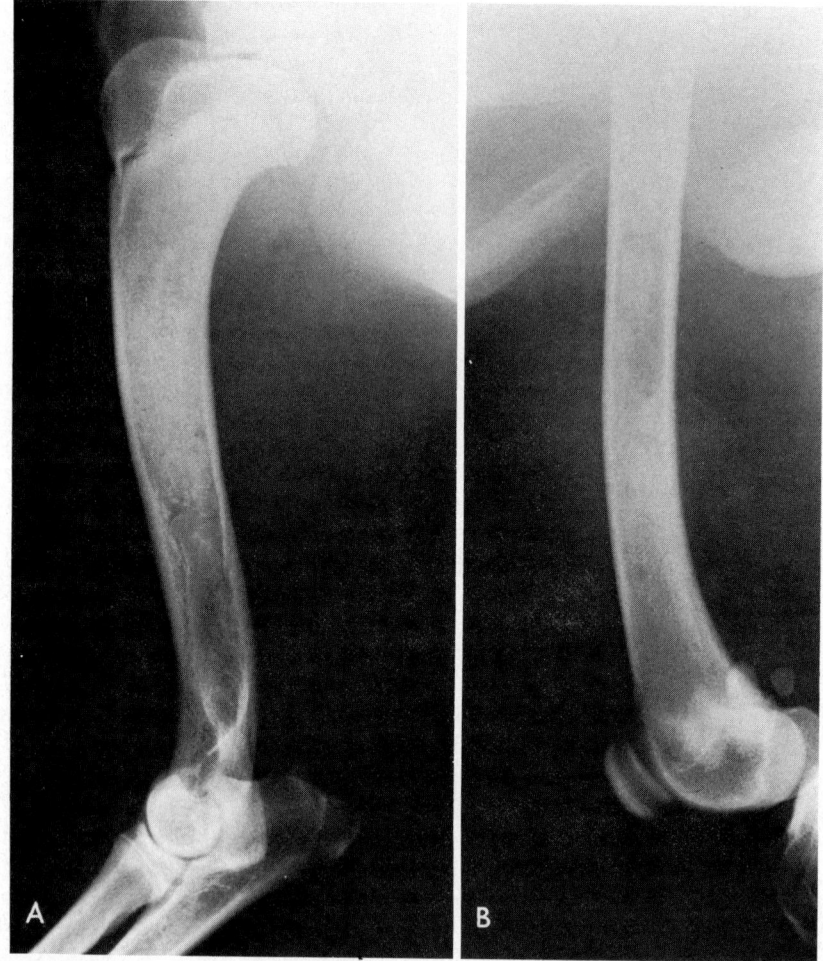

Figures 85–10. Panosteitis. Note the radiodense material occupying the medullary cavity of the humerus (*A*) and femur (*B*) in a six-month-old male German shorthair pointer.

cent to the open growth plate in immature, or large or giant breed dogs. The disease is also known as skeletal scurvy, infantile scurvy, Moeller-Barlow disease, osteodystrophy II, and metaphyseal osteopathy. The etiology, pathophysiology, and appropriate treatment remain unknown.

Dogs with hypertrophic osteodystrophy present clinically with mild to moderate swelling of the metaphyses in the distal radius and ulna or tibia, lameness, fever, lethargy, and often anorexia. Fever may rise as high as 106° F and cycle, or remain high for prolonged periods. The age at onset is between three and seven months; males are more frequently affected than females (Grondalen, 1976). Animals may have spontaneous remission of the disease or may progress to more severe forms of the prob-

lem. Severe disease may lead to bony involvement and enlargement of all metaphyses of long bones, bridging of open growth plates, and limb deformity secondary to epiphyseal plate closure.

Radiographically, early HOD is diagnosed by the presence of a radiolucent line in the metaphysis adjacent to an open growth plate (Fig. 85–11). This finding may be adjacent to distal radial and ulnar growth plates, or it may also include the distal tibial growth plate. As the disease progresses, periosteal new bone forms around the metaphysis. With chronicity the new bone may span the entire diaphysis from proximal to distal metaphysis. Soft tissue swelling over the area of proliferative bone may also be seen radiographically (Olsson, 1972) (Fig. 85–12).

Clinical chemistries and hemograms do not reveal a consistent picture of this disease. Results include elevated sedimentation rates and elevated leukocyte counts as high as 19,000/mm³ (although most will be in the normal range), with calcium, phosphorus, alkaline phosphatase, and serum ascorbic acid levels generally within normal limits (Grondalen, 1976).

Histologically, the areas of abnormality reveal periosteal new bone formation at the perimeter of the lesion. The radiolucent band consists of necrotic bone infiltrated with polymorphonuclear leukocytes and lymphocytes. The necrotic bone band seems to initiate bony resorption by osteoclasts, which is at least temporarily replaced by fibrous tissue. During the course of the disease, rarefaction becomes evident and is followed by periosteal new bone formation along the metaphysis. The periosteal new bone appears to be formed as a reinforcement of the bone that is weakened by the necrotic band. As the animals grow, the band of necrosis and/or fibrous tissue is replaced by bone (Olsson, 1972).

The histologic picture is confusing. Fetter (1980) diagnosed blind slides of HOD as

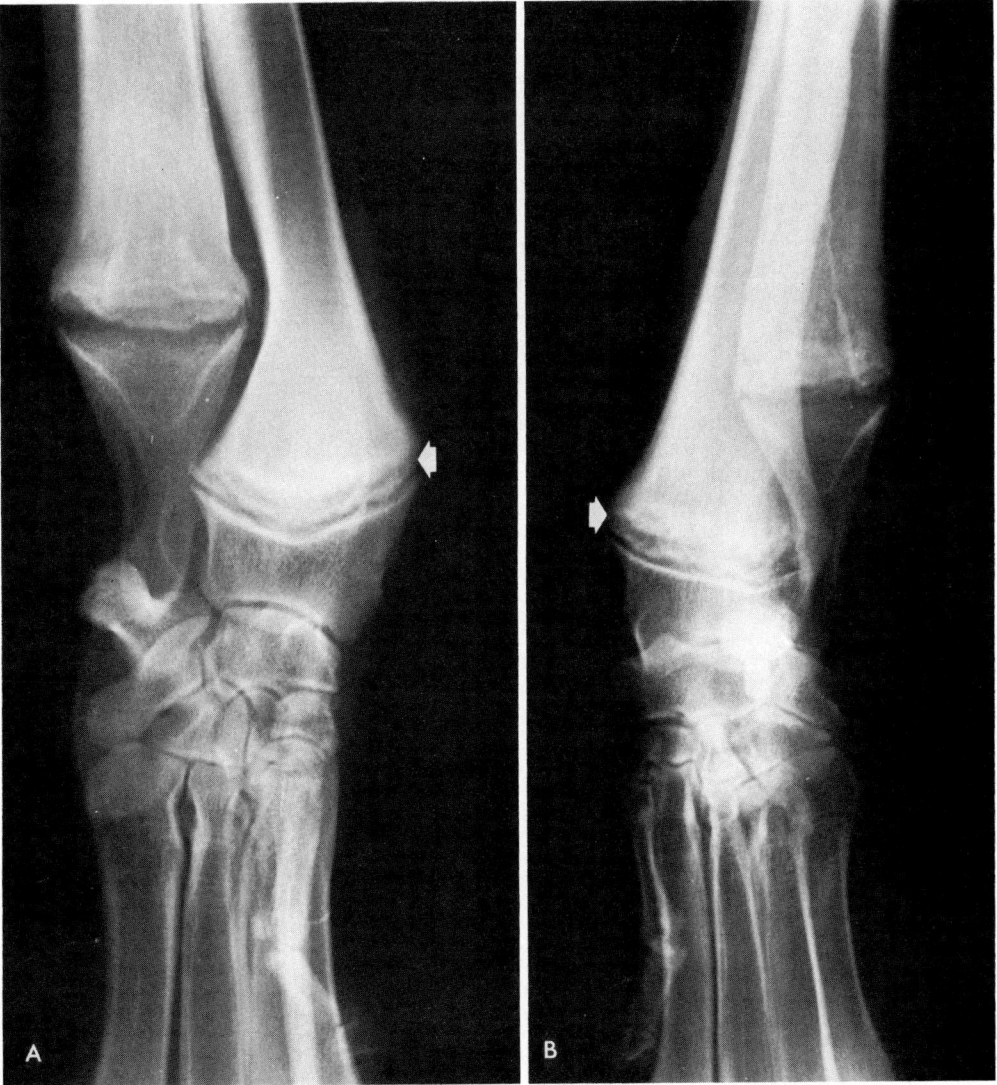

Figure 85–11. *A* and *B*, Acute hypertrophic osteodystrophy. Note the lucent metaphyseal band (arrow) in the radius and ulna seen early in the disease in this five-month-old male Great Dane.

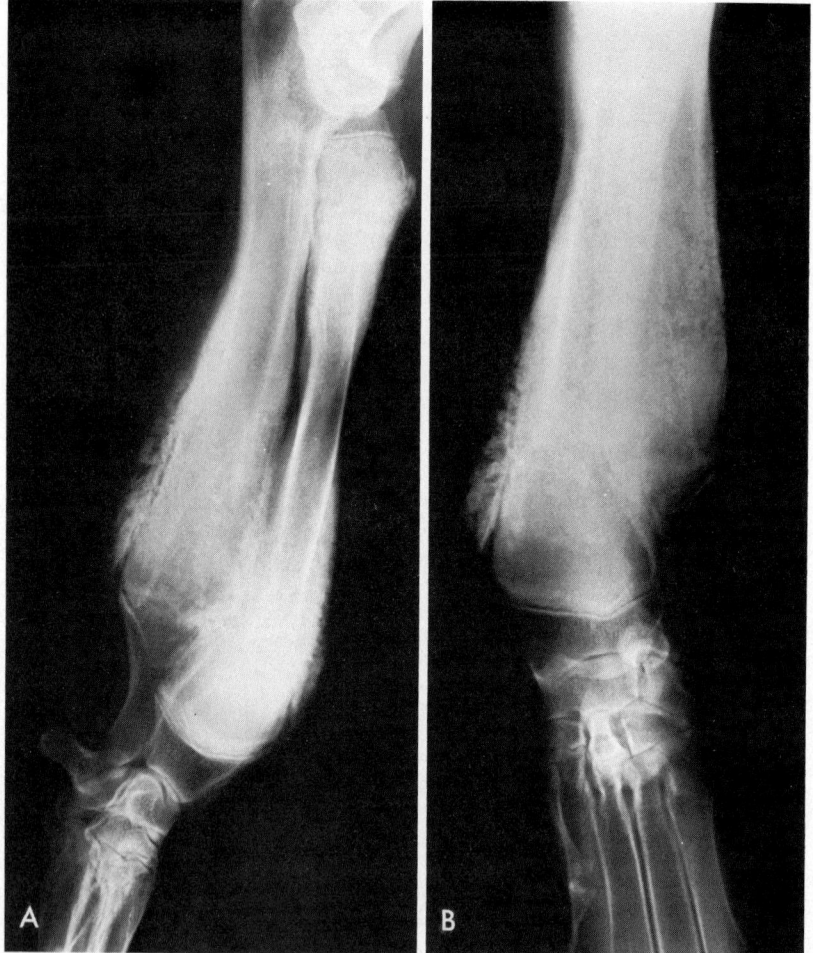

Figure 85–12. *A* and *B,* Chronic hypertrophic osteodystrophy. Note the periosteal new bone around the metaphysis. This is the same dog as in Figure 85–11 at the age of 6½ months.

typical of hypovitaminosis C, hypervitaminosis D, and areas of inflammation, with no clear diagnosis emerging.

The etiology of HOD is undetermined, despite claims of a nutritional disorder (Hedhammar, 1974) or hypovitaminosis C (Holmes, 1962; Vaananen and Wikman, 1979). The claims of hypovitaminosis C as the etiologic factor are substantiated by documenting levels that are slightly lower than normal during clinical disease. Such lowered levels can simply be due to pain and stress during the disease (Bosch, 1971; Teare et al., 1979). Two current studies documented that dogs with HOD had normal or slightly lowered serum ascorbic acid levels, and that the recovery from the disease had no relation to the levels of ascorbic acid (Grondalen, 1976; Teare et al., 1979).

Treatment of HOD is directed toward controlling fever and reducing pain. Rest and analgesics are sufficient; corticosteroids are reserved for severe cases. Most dogs show a spontaneous remission, regardless of treatment modality. In cases of severe disease, the animal may be left with permanent bony deformation or may succumb to the disease owing to hyperthermia.

CRANIOMANDIBULAR OSTEOPATHY

Craniomandibular osteopathy (CMO) is a bony disease of dogs characterized as a noninflammatory, non-neoplastic proliferative disease affecting the mandible, tympanic bullae, and occasionally other bones of the head. The disease predominates in Scottish terriers, West Highland white terriers, and Cairn terriers; however, boxers (Schultz, 1978), Labrador retrievers (Watkins and

Bradley, 1966; Alexander and Ralifela, 1975), Great Danes (Burk, 1976), and Doberman pinschers (Watson et al., 1975) have also been reported in the literature.

Age at onset of the disease is between four and ten months. Presentation may be due to obvious mandibular swelling, drooling, inability to open the mouth, or pain on manipulation of the mouth.

Physical examination demonstrates symmetric swelling of the horizontal and occasionally vertical rami of the mandible. Dogs may be febrile during the period of bony proliferation (Alexander, 1978a). The bony enlargement may be painful on direct palpation of the swelling. Discomfort is elicited when attempting to open the animal's mouth; in advancing disease, the mouth may not open more than 1 to 2 cm.

Radiography demonstrates symmetric bony enlargements of the mandible caudal to the middle mental foramen. The tympanic bullae will often be enlarged. The bone appears woven or as callus bone without a definitive cortex (Riser et al., 1967). Occasionally radiographic evidence of hypertrophic osteodystrophy of long bones will be found simultaneously (Fig. 85–13).

The etiology of CMO is unknown. The pathogenesis, however, seems reproducible. Osteoclastic resorption of mandibular lamellar bone occurs primarily, followed by production of woven bone. The woven bone is sufficiently proliferative to push beyond the normal periosteum. Similar new bone production may fill the medullary cavity. According to Pool and Leighton (1969), "Irregular episodes of bone resorption and osteoblastic proliferation result in a characteristic histologic picture of new fibrous bone deposition separated by blue lines representing stages of metabolic rest from areas of incomplete destruction of older more mature bone." The end result may be maturation of the fibrous bone that remains permanently, although rarely the dog may show a spontaneous reversal of the disease that returns the bone to its normal condition.

Treatment is symptomatic. Most animals can be made comfortable using aspirin or corticosteroids; however, treatment does not result in cure. Most animals stabilize with impaired mouth function but are capable of maintaining normal nutritional status. Surgical intervention to reduce bony mass or to increase temporomandibular joint range of motion has not resulted in improvement.

NUTRITIONAL DISEASES OF BONE

HYPERVITAMINOSIS A (Brown, 1975)

Hypervitaminosis A is caused by the consumption of liver as a consistent diet rich in vitamin A or by the excessive intake of vitamin A concentrates. The disease affects primarily cats (Clark et al., 1970; Seawright and English, 1967), although this condition has been experimentally produced in dogs (Cho et al., 1975).

Clinical signs seen in cats with hypervitaminosis A include lethargy, hyperemia and edema of the gums, anorexia, abdominal distension, lameness, neck stiffness, and evidence of spinal exostoses (Seawright and

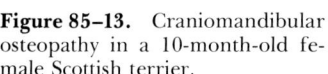

Figure 85–13. Craniomandibular osteopathy in a 10-month-old female Scottish terrier.

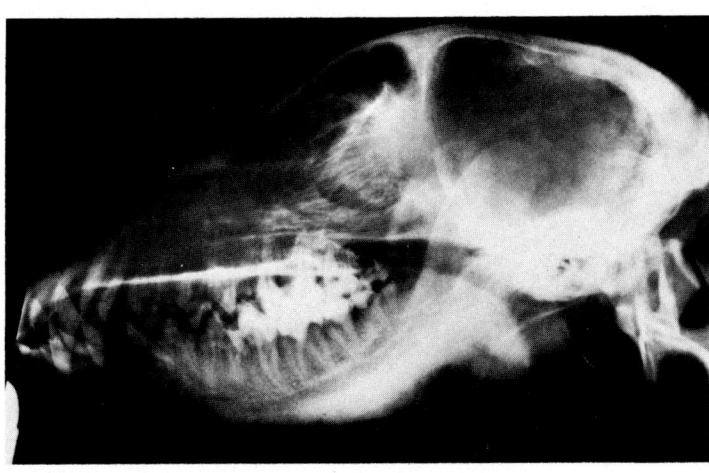

English, 1967). In young animals, bone growth may be severely or permanently retarded, while bony exostoses are the predominant lesions in mature animals.

Radiographically, confluent exostoses are visible bridging cervical vertebral bodies, often over an area as large as C1–T2. In chronic disease, vertebral fusion may occur at other spinal locations. Proliferative bony exostoses are visible on bone metaphyses or surrounding joints. Bony arthrodesis of joints may be seen radiographically if bone proliferation is extensive.

Hypervitaminosis A is caused by ingestion of excessive vitamin A levels; relative proportions of calcium and phosphorus in the diet have little or no influence in the development of exostoses in chronic hypervitaminosis A (Clark, 1970). Vitamin A is essential for the normal production, growth, and maturation of epiphyseal chondroblasts, and in enchondral bone growth. It is also a factor in the remodeling of bone, stimulating osteoblastic activity in areas where changes in conformation of bone mass are occurring (Aegerter, 1968). It is apparent, however, that an excess of vitamin A causes an abnormal subperiosteal bone proliferation, one of the principal findings in chronic vitamin A toxicity (Seawright and English, 1967; Aegerter and Kirkpatrick, 1968; Clark et al., 1970). It has been suggested that chronic ingestion of vitamin A greatly increases the sensitivity of periosteum to the effects of trauma (Seawright and English, 1967). Treatment necessitates removal of the source of vitamin A. Young animals will show permanent retardation of long bone length; however, appositional bone formation will return to normal. Mature cats show clinical improvement and reversal of most signs except those relating to bony arthrodesis. Although plasma concentrations of vitamin A fall to normal limits within a few weeks of dietary change, the liver stores of vitamin A may remain elevated for years (English, 1969).

HYPERVITAMINOSIS D (Brown, 1975)

Hypervitaminosis D is a rare disorder caused by excessive intake of vitamin D, which results in high serum-calcium levels and eventual deossification of the skeleton. The latter usually occurs without symptoms;

however, prolonged high calcium levels produce signs referable to its effect on peripheral nerves, muscles (both skeletal and visceral), and possibly the brain. Metastatic calcification of numerous tissues, particularly the kidneys, may occur (Aegerter and Kirkpatrick, 1968).

The disease is rarely seen, because of general awareness of the toxicity of vitamin D in high levels. When the disease is encountered, it usually results from a high dietary intake of cod liver oil or dietary vitamin supplements. Radiographically, generalized osteoporosis is noted in conjunction with hypervitaminosis D. Serum calcium levels will be elevated, while phosphorus levels are often normal or only slightly elevated.

The pathogenesis of the disease is unknown; however, it is postulated that vitamin D possesses a parathormone-like action that acts directly on bone, causing deossification (Aegerter and Kirkpatrick, 1968).

Proper dietary volumes of vitamin D, calcium, and phosphorus reverse the bony problems.

OTHER BONE DISEASES

BONE CYSTS

Bone cysts are benign lesions not commonly found in the dog or cat. Bone cysts described in dogs are either monostotic, polyostotic, or aneurysmal. One case of an aneurysmal bone cyst in a cat has been reported (Walker et al., 1975).

Polyostotic bone cysts associated with fibrous dysplasia are reported more commonly in dogs than are monostotic cysts (Gourley, 1963; Huff and Brodey, 1964; Carrig and Seawright, 1969; Morgan, 1972). The polyostotic lesion has been reported in five dogs, including four Doberman pinschers and one Bull mastiff. Inheritability of polyostotic cystic fibrous dysplasia in Doberman pinschers has been suggested (Carrig and Seawright, 1969). Its radiographic appearance has been characterized as cystic with trabeculation. The affected bones were expanded with thin cortices. The lesions were limited to the metaphyseal and diaphyseal areas without involvement of the physes or epiphyses. Polyostotic cystic fibrous dysplasia was described in the radius, ulna, femur, and tibia. Subperiosteal cortical defects were seen in several affected bones. Frequently a fracture through the cyst, as well as an associated periosteal reaction, was seen radiographically. All reported dogs presented clinically with lameness and swelling at the lesion site.

Histologic examination was performed in four animals. The findings were similar, consisting of a poorly defined inner lining of probable endothelial origin, an intermediate region of thin osseous trabeculae and/or unmineralized osseous tissue, and an outer fibrous subperiosteal layer. Normal compact bone was absent. No mention is made in the polyostotic case reports of the presence or absence of fluid within the cysts, nor were other clinical or metabolic abnormalities seen.

The four types of treatment reported are benign neglect; splinting; curettage; and bone graft, or en bloc surgical resection of the affected bone. All work equally well.

Monostotic cysts are lesions not commonly found in the dog. The clinical history, radiographic appearance, pathological findings, and clinical course of dogs with monostotic bone cysts appear similar to those for the disease in man (Jaffe and Lichtenstein, 1942; Aegerter and Kirkpatrick, 1968). Most bone cysts do not produce clinical signs of disease unless a pathological fracture occurs through the cyst. The pathological fracture causes lameness with associated pain and/or swelling. The dogs with solitary bone cysts have had both acute and intermittent signs of lameness prior to the diagnosis.

Biery and coworkers (1976) reported in a study of five dogs that three were German shepherds; there does not appear to be a sex predisposition. The age range at time of diagnosis ranged from 4½ months to 2½ years. Three of the dogs presented as puppies prior to closure of the long bone physes. The cysts are most common in the areas of rapid growth, e.g., the proximal femur, the distal femur, and the proximal tibia. The cysts in both dog and man are limited to a single focus in one of the long tubular bones.

Numerous theories of monostotic bone cyst pathogenesis have been proposed (Jaffe and Lichtenstein, 1942, Aegerter and Kirkpatrick, 1968). No definitive evidence of exact cause is known to date. The most popular theory is that a solitary bone cyst results from encapsulation and alteration of a focus of intramedullary hemorrhage.

After encapsulation the affected area becomes distended by the transudation of fluid. Pressure from the cyst causes stagnation of the blood and lymph around it, erosion of the adjacent bone, and finally, expansion of the overlying cortex. Numerous other theories exist regarding the origin of bone cysts, including local disturbance in bone growth.

The radiographic appearance is considered characteristic and enables the correct diagnosis to be made without biopsy in most cases. The radiographic findings are a benign, expansile, cystic (radiolucent) area in a long bone in the metaphysis adjacent to, but not affecting, the physis and epiphysis (Fig. 85–14).

The expansile cystic lesion replaces normal bone and causes thinning of the cortex. As in man, the bone cysts in the dogs were far advanced in evolution before a cyst was diagnosed. Slight trauma to the cyst is frequently followed by a pathological fracture and subsequent clinical signs of lameness. Following fracture, a periosteal reaction and possibly additional fractures produce an active-appearing lesion. Following fracture a bone cyst will usually but not always heal spontaneously.

Although the radiographic signs are rather definitive, a differential diagnosis in the dog should include malignant bone and cartilage neoplasms, enchondroma, bone abscess, nonossifying fibroma, and fibrocystic osseous disease.

Histologically, the lining membrane of a bone cyst consists of flat fibrous connective tissue that may vary greatly in thickness and extent of vascularization. Blood pigment may be present in the lining of the connective tissue either free or within macrophages. Fibrin clot containing erythrocytes may be adherent to the cyst lining. In areas of injury, both osteoblastic and osteoclastic activity will be evident. Callus will be laid down at the sites of pathological fracture. In the dog, histologic appearance of monostotic bone cysts resembles the description of polyostotic cysts associated with fibrous dysplasia.

Some solitary bone cysts in dogs fill spontaneously. This spontaneous healing is probably precipitated by a fracture; however, it is preferable to treat these cysts with surgical exposure, curettage of the walls, filling with cancellous bone, and immobilization of the bone until healing occurs. Surgical intervention expedites healing if frac-

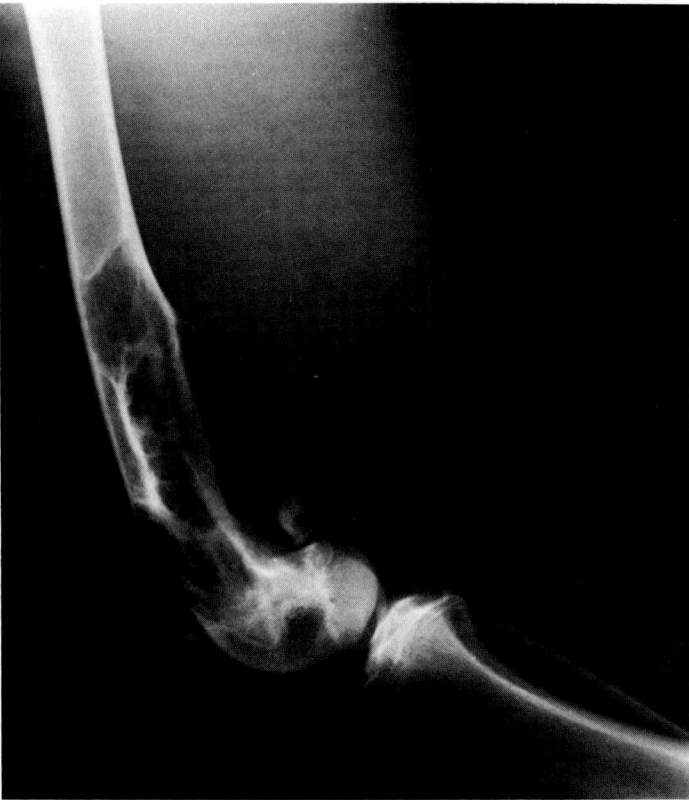

Figure 85–14. Solitary bone cyst affecting the distal femoral metaphysis in a 10-month-old male Afghan hound.

ture has not occurred, and prevents future deformity of the bone due to enlargement of the cyst or pathological fracture.

Aneurysmal bone cysts are far rarer than monostotic or polyostotic cystic lesions. A single canine case was reported in the tibia (Renegar et al., 1979), and a single feline case was reported in the scapula (Walker et al., 1975).

Aneurysmal bone cysts are solitary lesions of bone that bulge through the cortex and resemble the saccular protrusion of an aortic wall aneurysm (Renegar et al., 1979). Aneurysmal bone cysts generally cause pain. The lesion rarely invades a joint but may occur in the end of a long bone near a joint and thus cause joint pain and disability. The affected area is usually swollen because of an expansion of the cortex that overlies the medullary soft tissue mass. It has a remarkable lytic property, because the overlying compact bone is resorbed before it expands. The periosteum is pushed outward and reacts by laying down a thin shell of bone that is continuously replaced as the inner layer is eroded away. A bulky structure soon protrudes beyond the original surface of the uninvolved cortex, pushes soft tissue before it, and erodes other bones on contact.

The pathogenesis of aneurysmal bone cysts is unknown. Evidence from human disease suggests that it is an aggregate of arteriovenous communications that arises consequent to developmental fault or hemorrhage from hemangioma, spontaneous idiopathic hemorrhages in cancellous bone, or secondary to bone injury (Aegerter, 1975). The injury is rarely traumatic; more often it is a primary bone lesion. The destruction of bone appears due to an excessive supply of blood to a localized area. Treatment is directed toward reducing the supply of blood to the area to normal. The lesion may be treated surgically or by irradiation. Even partial curettage with no attempt to remove all the vascular tissue has resulted in cure (Renegar et al., 1979). Malignant transformation has been reported in man (Meschan, 1966).

BONE INFARCT

Bone infarction is a condition of long bones found in association with primary bony neoplasia. It has been reported only in the dog (Riser, 1972; Dubielzig, 1981). Bone infarction is an occupational disease in man caused by exposure to dysbaric conditions (Chryssanthou, 1978). Fat embolization, trauma, hyperviscosity, hyperadrenal corticism, and alcoholism have been implicated (Jacobs, 1978; Jones, 1978).

Bone infarction in dogs rarely presents as a primary disease, since clinical signs are not associated with multifocal osteonecrosis (the term that best describes the bony condition). Usually bone infarcts are found when performing skeletal surveys in association with a bony neoplasia. Occasionally the infarcts are truly coincident to the purpose of the radiograph. Regardless, such infarcts indicate existing or subclinical sarcoma.

Dogs with bone infarcts have been reported to range in age from 6 to 13 years, showing equal sex distribution and affecting mixbreeds as well as purebreeds. In a study of 13 dogs, 5 were miniature schnauzers (Dubielzig et al., 1981).

Radiographically, infarcts are characterized by irregularly demarcated areas of increased radiopacity within the medullary cavity (Riser, 1972). Such areas may be present along the entire medullary cavity of one or multiple bones. In all dogs examined, when bone infarction was diagnosed, an osteosarcoma or fibrosarcoma was also present. Of 17 cases in the literature, only one fibrosarcoma has been found (Fig. 85–15).

Histologically, bone infarcts demonstrate

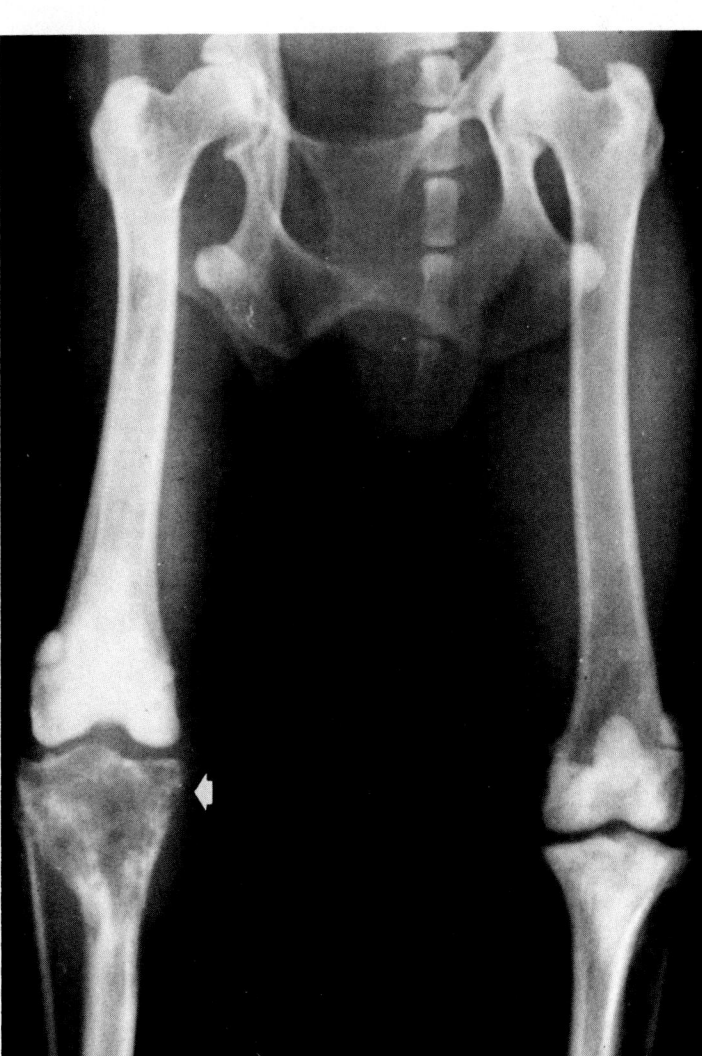

Figure 85–15. Bone infarcts affecting the distal femoral epiphyses and one proximal tibia epiphysis in a 13-year-old female Miniature schnauzer with an osteogenic sarcoma of the tibial metaphysis (arrow).

proliferation of new bone deposited on the endosteum and medullary trabeculae.

The pathogenesis of bone infarction in the dog is unknown. It is possible that metastatic showers of tumor are responsible for such bony necrosis; however, tumor cells have not been found in the infarcted areas. It is also possible that other disease processes (e.g., infection, trauma) cause multifocal bony necrosis, and tumor results from such focus. It is known that sarcoma in man can develop secondary to necrosis (Furney et al., 1960).

Clinical treatment of bone infarction is impossible. Infarction indicates the presence of a primary tumor, which must be found, diagnosed, and treated.

HYPERTROPHIC OSTEOARTHROPATHY

Hypertrophic osteoarthropathy (HOA) is a bony disease of dogs and cats (Carr, 1971). The disease produces periosteal proliferative new bone along the shafts of long bones, often beginning with digits and involving bones as proximal as the humerus or femur. In most cases the disease is associated with an intrathoracic mass (Brodey, 1971).

Dogs with HOA are seen with lameness and swollen, warm distal limbs, and may be reluctant to move. Many animals exhibit pulsatile swellings rather than edematous limbs (Brodey, 1980). There is no breed or sex predisposition noted for HOA; however, most animals are at least middle-aged at the onset of the disease. Radiographically, there is soft tissue swelling of all distal extremities. As the disease progresses periosteal new bone forms and results in extensive osteophyte formation. The osteophytes tend to radiate from cortices at 90 degrees (Brodey, 1980) (Fig. 85–16).

Further clinical tests demonstrate intrathoracic disease or other large, space-occupying tumor. The lung or thoracic disease may be the result of metastatic lung disease, primary tumors of the lung, or esophageal sarcoma following *Spirocerca lupi* infection or thoracic lesions secondary to infections (Brodey, 1958; Leighton, 1967; Brodey, 1980). In a study of 180 dogs (Brodey, 1980), 98 per cent had HOA in association with intrathoracic disease. Of these, 92 per cent had either metastatic lung

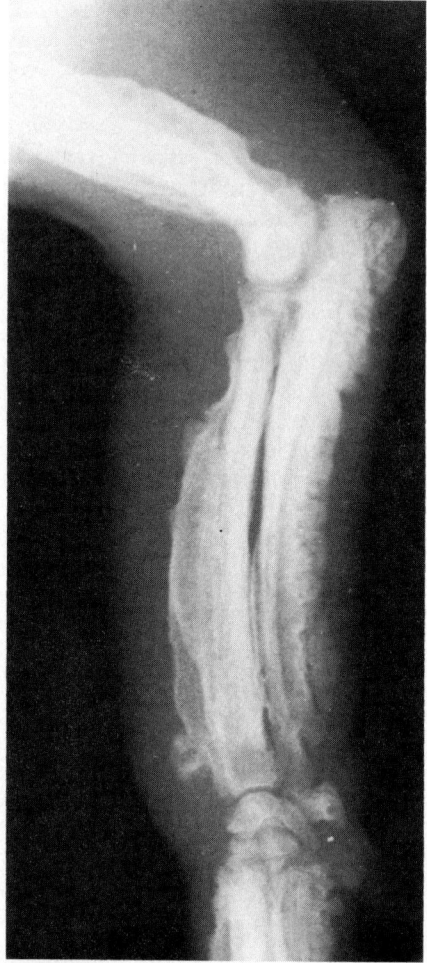

Figure. 85–16. Hypertrophic osteoarthropathy of the forelimb in a nine-year-old female chihuahua with a primary bladder tumor and lung metastasis.

neoplasia or primary tumors of the esophagus or the lung. Only four cases had no intrathoracic involvement.

Gross and histologic examination of affected limbs demonstrated several distinctive features: bone, tendons, and joints are surrounded by highly vascularized connective tissue, and diaphyses of affected bone are covered by irregular osteophytes. Histologically, the vascular connective tissue is composed of many thick-walled arteries. Bony changes are characterized as hypertrophic new bone production from the periosteum.

The etiology of HOA in the dog is unknown. It has been postulated that increased limb blood flow may be indicated.

Treatment is aimed at removal of the

thoracic disease. Removal of solitary intra-thoracic masses may result in regression of the bony changes (Clifford et al., 1967; Madewell et al., 1978). If neoplasia is the cause of the mass, however, many animals die as a result of metastatic disease. While lobectomy or tumor resection are the primary methods of treatment, other treatments may also lead to reversal of HOA, e.g., unilateral intrathoracic vagotomy on the side of the lung lesion, incision through parietal pleura, subperiosteal rib resection, or bilateral cervical vagotomy (Brodey, 1980). Aside from treating the thoracic disease, use of analgesics may make the animal more comfortable while the bony lesions regress.

DISUSE OSTEOPOROSIS

Disuse osteoporosis is a bony loss in an individual bone or limb, or in the entire body caused by lack of normal bony stress. As seen in veterinary medicine, it usually relates to the bone beneath a rigid plate or to the bones immobilized within an external cast.

Radiographically, affected bones will be more radiolucent and may appear obviously different from other bones in the same animal. Care must be taken in such animals to prevent pathologic fractures through the osteoporotic bones.

Animals with this disease show elevated serum calcium and phosphorus levels and may be excreting abnormally large quantities of urinary calcium (Whittick, 1974). The etiology and pathogenesis of disuse osteoporosis are known. With the lack of normal stresses, bones are remodeled by osteoclasts and new bone is not formed to replace it, thus the resulting bony loss. The process is reversible, and normal bone will be replaced when normal stress is reapplied to the affected bones (Aegerter, 1968).

LEAD POISONING

Lead poisoning is a disease of dogs caused by the ingestion of lead paint, linoleum, or other lead-containing materials. Lead toxicity results in gastrointestinal, neurologic, and hematologic abnormalities (Zook et al., 1969). Coincidentally, bony abnormalities also occur if the dog is immature during the time of lead ingestion.

There are no clinical signs specifically referable to the skeletal system occurring following lead toxicity. The bony changes that result may be seen radiographically and suggest the underlying cause of the disease.

Radiographically, lead lines are dense sclerotic bands 2 to 4 mm wide, occasionally seen in the metaphysis of long bones of immature dogs. If present, they will be visible in all long bones; however, they are seen best in the distal radius and ulna. Apparently the more active the growth plate, the more pronounced the effect of lead poisoning (Brown, 1975).

The origin of the bony lesion is presumed to be initiated by lead that is deposited with calcium during endochondral ossification. The lead incorporation stimulates new bone formation, which is seen histologically and radiographically as lead lines. Histologically, the metaphyseal lines are composed of longitudinally oriented trabeculae of new bone on cartilaginous cores containing increased amounts of mineralized cartilage (Schunk, 1978). Chronic toxicity of Vitamin D, phosphorus, or bismuth can cause a similar lesion (Zook, 1973). Bony changes characteristic of lead may be seen radiographically and may aid in the diagnosis of lead poisoning.

ABNORMAL ESTROGEN METABOLISM

The target structures for estrogen in the growing skeleton are the articular cartilage and the osteoblasts. Estrogen arrests the proliferation of cartilage in endochondral ossification and apparently stimulates osteoblastic activity (Krook, 1971). Generally, these compounds will decrease the growth of young animals by producing earlier union of the epiphyses with their shafts. The estrogens will promote a rapid maturation of the skeletal system, although the total bone length may be shorter than normal (Siegel, 1968).

HYPERADRENOCORTICISM

Hyperadrenocorticism can occur when a dog has Cushing's disease or when there is chronic excessive administration of glucocorticoids. The glucocorticoids inhibit absorption of calcium from the gut through an antagonistic effect on vitamin D. The steroids also increase urinary excretion of calcium, although the blood calcium levels are often normal. The development of osteoporosis is believed to be a primary result of the catabolic effect of the glucocorticoid on protein. The protein catabolic effect results in abnormal production of bone matrix. The glucocorticoids also decrease proliferation and differentiation of fibroblasts and osteoblasts, thus affecting the elaboration of collagen and bone matrix. Osteoporosis associated with this disease is usually prominent in the spine and long bones of dog and man (Siegel, 1968). Hyperadrenocorticism is discussed in detail in Chapter 69.

REFERENCES

Aegerter, E., and Kirkpatrick, J. A., Jr.: Orthopaedic Diseases. W. B. Saunders Co., Philadelphia, 1975.

Aegerter, E., and Kirkpatrick, J. A., Jr.: Orthopaedic Diseases. W. B. Saunders Co., Philadelphia, 1968.

Aegerter, E., and Kirkpatrick, J. A., Jr.: Orthopaedic Diseases. W. B. Saunders Co., Philadelphia, 1964.

Al-Doory, Y., Vice, T. E., and Mainster, M. E.: Adiaspiromycosis in a dog. J.A.V.M.A. *159*:87, 1971.

Alexander, J. W.: Craniomandibular osteopathy. Canine Pract. *5*:31, 1978a.

Alexander, J. W.: Solitary and multiple cartilaginous exostoses in the dog. Canine Pract. *5*:43, 1978b.

Alexander, J. W., and Kalifelz, F. A.: A case of craniomandibular osteopathy in a Labrador retriever. VM SAC *70*:560, 1975.

Banks, W. C., and Bridges, C. H.: Multiple cartilaginous extoses in a dog. J.A.V.M.A. *129*:131, 1956.

Bartels, J. E.: Canine extraskeletal osteosarcoma: a clinical communication. J.A.A.H.A. *11*:307, 1975.

Biery, D. N., Goldschmidt, M., Riser, W. H., and Rhodes, W. H.: Bone cysts in the dog. J. Amer. Vet. Rad. Soc. *17*:202, 1976.

Blake, W. P., Hubbard, J. W., and Micuda, J.: Coccidioidomycosis: report of a disseminated case in a dog. J.A.V.M.A. *133*:437, 1958.

Bohning, R. H., Suter, P. F., Hohn, R. B., and Marshall, J.: Clinical and radiological survey of canine panosteitis. J.A.V.M.A. *156*:870, 1970.

Boland, A. L.: Acute hematogenous osteomyelitis. Orthoped. Clin. North A. *3*:225, 1972.

Bosch, F. B., Court, A., and Vivaco, A. C.: Ein Fall von Barlowscher Krankheit beim Hund: erste Beschreibung in Chile. Vet. Med. Nachr. 363, 1971.

Brodey, R. S.: Hypertrophic Osteoarthropathy. *In* Spontaneous Animal Models of Human Disease. Academic Press, Inc., New York, 1980.

Brodey, R. S.: Hypertrophic osteoarthropathy in the dog: a clinical pathologic survey of 60 cases. J.A.V.M.A. *159*:1242, 1971.

Brodey, R. S.: Disseminated coccidioidomycosis in a dog. J.A.V.M.A. *157*:926, 1970.

Brodey, R. S., and Abt, D. A.: Results of surgical treatment in 65 dogs with osteosarcoma. J.A.V.M.A. *168*:1032, 1976.

Brodey, R. S., Craig, P. H., and Rhodes, W. H.: Hypertrophic osteoarthropathy in a dog with pulmonary metastasis from a renal adenocarcinoma. J.A.V.M.A. *132*:231, 1958.

Brodey, R. S., Misdorp, W., and Riser, W. H.: Canine skeletal chondrosarcoma: a clinical pathologic study of 35 cases. J.A.V.M.A. *165*:68, 1974.

Brodey, R. S., Sauer, R. M., and Medway, W.: Canine bone neoplasms. J.A.V.M.A. *143*:471, 1963.

Brown, S. G.: Skeletal Diseases. *In* Ettinger, S. (ed.): Textbook of Veterinary Internal Medicine. W. B. Saunders Co., Philadelphia, 1975.

Burk, R. L., and Broadhurst, J. J.: Craniomandibular osteopathy in a Great Dane. J.A.V.M.A. *169*:635, 1976.

Burt, J. K., and Wilson, G. P.: A study of eosinophilic panosteitis (enostosis) in German shepherd dogs. Acta Radiol. Suppl. *319*:7, 1972.

Carr, S. H.: Secondary hypertrophic pulmonary osteoarthropathy in a cat. Feline Pract. *1*:25, 1971.

Carrig, C. B., and Seawright, A. A.: A familial canine polyostotic fibrous dysplasia with subperiosteal cortical defects. J. Small Anim. Pract. *10*:397, 1969.

Caywood, D. D., Wallace, L. J., and Braden, T. D.: Osteomyelitis in the dog: a review of 67 cases. J.A.V.M.A. *172*:943, 1978.

Chester, D. K.: Multiple cartilaginous exostoses in two generations of dogs. J.A.V.M.A. *159*:895, 1971.

Cho, D. Y., Frey, R. A., Guffy, M. M.: Hypervitaminosis A in the dog. Am. J. Vet. Res. *36*:1597, 1975.

Chryssanthou, C. P.: Dysbaric osteonecrosis. Clin. Orthop. *130*:94, 1978.

Clark, L., Seawright, A., and Hrdlicka, J.: Exostoses in hypervitaminotic A cats with optimal calcium/phosphorus intake. J. Small Anim. Prac. *11*:553, 1970.

Clifford, D. H., Mather, G. W., Sauther, J. H.: Regression of the osseous lesions of hypertrophic pulmonary osteoarthropathy in a dog following lobectomy. Anim. Hosp. *3*:75, 1967.

Cotter, S. M., Griffiths, R. C., and Leav, I.: Enostosis of young dogs. J.A.V.M.A. *153*:401, 1968.

Cowell, K., Jezyk, P. F., and Haskins, M. E.: Mucopolysaccharidosis in a cat. J.A.V.M.A. *169*:334, 1976.

Ditchfield, J.: Nocardiosis in the dog. Mod. Vet. Prac. *42*:43, 1961.

Doige, C. E., Pharr, J. W., and Withrow, S. J.: Chondrosarcoma arising in multiple cartilaginous exostoses in a dog. J.A.A.H.A. *14*:605, 1978.

Dubielzig, R. R., Biery, D. N., and Brodey, R. S.: Bone sarcomas associated with multifocal medullary bone infarction in 13 dogs. J.A.V.M.A., *179*:(1)64, 1981.

Dunn, T. J.: Blastomycosis in a dog. Vet. Med. *72*:1443, 1977.

English, P. B.: Clinical communication: a case of hyperostosis due to hypervitaminosis A in a cat. J. Small Anim. Prac. *10*:207, 1969.

Evers, W. H.: Enostosis in a dog. J.A.V.M.A. *154*:799, 1969.

Fetter, A.: Personal Communication, 1980.

Fletch, S. M., Smart, M. E., Pennock, P. W., and Subden, R. E.: Clinical and pathological features of chondrodysplasia (dwarfism) in the Alaskan Malamute. J.A.V.M.A. *162*:357, 1973.

Furney, J. G., Ferrer-Torells, M., and Reagan, J. W.: Fibrosarcoma arising at the site of bone infarcts. J. Bone Joint Surg. *42A*:802, 1960.

Gambardella, P. C., Osborne, C. A., and Stevens, J. B.: Multiple cartilaginous exostoses in the dog. J.A.V.M.A. *166*:761, 1975.

Gee, B. R., and Doige, C. E.: Multiple cartilagenous exostoses in a litter of dogs. J.A.V.M.A. *156*:53, 1970.

Gourley, J.: Bone cyst in a dog. Vet. Rec. *75*:40, 1963.

Grondalen, J.: Metaphyseal HOD in growing dogs: a clinical study. J. Small Anim. Prac. *17*:721, 1976.

Hedhammar, A.: Overnutrition and skeletal diseases: an experimental study in growing Great Danes. Cornell Vet. Suppl. *5*:64, 1974.

Hegreberg, G. A., Norby D. E., and Hamilton, M. H.: Lysosomal enzyme changes in an inherited dwarfism of cats. Fed. Proc. *33*:598, 1974.

Henness, A. M., Theilen, G. H., and Park, R. D.: Combination therapy for canine osteosarcoma. J.A.V.M.A. *170*:1076, 1977.

Hirsh, D. C., and Smith, T. M.: Osteomyelitis in the dog: microorganisms isolated and susceptibility to antimicrobial agents. J. Small Anim. Prac. *19*:679, 1978.

Holmes, J. R.: Suspected skeletal scurvy in the dog. Vet. Rec. *74*:801, 1962.

Horne, R. D.: Feline systemic mycoses. Mod. Vet. Prac. *45*:45, 1964.

Huff, R. W., and Brodey, R. S.: Multiple bone cysts in a dog: a case report. J. Amer. Vet. Rad. Soc. *5*:40, 1964.

Jacobs, B.: Epidemiology of traumatic and non-traumatic osteonecrosis. Clin. Orthop. *130*:51, 1978.

Jaffe, H. L., and Lichtenstein, L.: Solitary unicameral bone cyst. Arch. Surg. *44*:1004, 1942.

Jezyk, P. F., Haskins, M. E., and Patterson, D. F.: MPS in a cat with arylsuflatose B deficiency: a model of Maroteauz-Lamy syndrome. Science *198*:834, 1977.

Jones, J. P.: Editorial comment. Clin. Orthop. *130*:2, 1978.

Krook, L.: Metabolic bone disease in dogs and cats. Proceedings, 38th Annual Meeting of the Amer. Anim. Hosp. Assn., 1971.

Lane, J. G., Clayton-Jones, D. G., and Thoday, K. L.: The diagnosis and successful treatment of *Aspergillus fumigatus* infection of the frontal sinuses and nasal chambers of the dog. J. Small Anim. Prac. *15*:79, 1974.

Langenskiold, A.: The stages of development of the cartilaginous foci in dyschondroplasia (Olliers Disease). Acta Ortho. Scand. *38*:174, 1967.

Law, R. E., Kim, S. N., and Pirozok, R. P.: *Histoplasma capsulatum* infection in a metatarsal of a dog. J.A.V.M.A. *172*:1414, 1978.

Leighton, R. L., and Olson, S.: Hypertrophic osteoarthropathy in a dog with pulmonary abscess. J.A.V.M.A. *150*:1516, 1967.

Lewis, G. E., Fidler, W. J., and Crumrine, M. H.: Mycetoma in a cat. J.A.V.M.A. *161*:500, 1972.

Ling, G. V., Morgan, J. P., and Pool, R. R.: Primary bone tumors in the dog: a combined clinical, radiographic and histologic approach to early diagnosis. J.A.V.M.A. *165*:55, 1974.

Liu, S. K., Dorfman, H. D., and Hurvitz, A. I.: Primary and secondary bone tumors in the dog. J. Small Anim. Prac. *18*:313, 1977.

Liu, S. K., Dorfman, H. D., and Patnaik, A. K.: Primary and secondary bone tumors in the cat. J. Small Anim. Pract. *15*:141, 1974.

Maddy, K. T.: Disseminated coccidioidomycosis of the dog. J.A.V.M.A. *132*:483, 1958.

Madewell, B. R., Nyland, T. G., and Weigel, J. E.: Regression of hypertrophic osteopathy following pneumonectomy in a dog. J.A.V.M.A. *172*:818, 1978.

Mahaffey, E., Gabbert, N., and Johnson, D.: Disseminated histoplasmosis in 3 cats. J.A.A.H.A. *13*:46, 1977.

Mather, G. W.: Achondroplasia in a litter of pups. J.A.V.M.A. *128*:327, 1956.

McKusick, V. A.: Heritable Disorders of Connective Tissue. C. V. Mosby Company, St. Louis, 1972.

Meschan, I.: Roentgen Signs in Clinical Practice. W. B. Saunders Co., Philadelphia, 1966.

Mitten, R. W.: Nocardial osteomyelitis in dogs. Mod. Vet. Prac. *56*:338, 1975.

Morgan, J. P.: Radiology in Veterinary Orthopedics. Lea and Febiger, Philadelphia, 1972.

Newton, C. D.: Surgical management of distal ulnar physeal growth disturbances in dogs. J.A.V.M.A. *164*:479, 1974.

Nunamaker, D. M.: Management of infected fractures. Vet. Clin. North A. *5*:259, 1975.

Olsson, S. E.: Radiology in veterinary pathology. A review with special reference to HOD and secondary hyperparathyroidism in the dog. Acta Radiol. Supp. *319*:255, 1972.

Owen, L. N.: Bone Tumors in Man and Animals. Butterworth and Company, London, 1969.

Owen, L. N., and Bostock, D. E.: Multiple cartilaginous exostoses with development of a metastasizing osteosarcoma in a Shetland sheepdog. J. Small Anim. Prac. *12*:507, 1971.

Pennock, C. A., and Barnes, I. C.: The mucopolysaccharidoses. J. Med. Genet. Biol. *13*:169, 1976.

Pool, R. R., and Carrig, C. B.: Multiple cartilaginous exostoses in a cat. Vet. Pathol. *9*:350, 1972.

Pool, R. R., and Leighton, R. L.: Craniomandibular osteopathy in a dog. J.A.V.M.A. *154*:657, 1969.

Reed, R. E.: Diagnosis of disseminated canine coccidioidomycosis. J.A.V.M.A. *128*:196, 1956.

Renegar, W. R., Thornburg, L. P., and Burk, R. L.: Aneurysmal bone cyst in the dog: a case report. J.A.A.H.A. *15*:191, 1979.

Riddle, W. E., and Leighton, R. L.: Osteochondromatosis in a cat. J.A.V.M.A. *156*:1428, 1970.

Riser, W. H., and Frankhauser, R.: Osteopetrosis in the dog: a report of 3 cases. J. Amer. Vet. Rad. Soc. *11*:29, 1970.

Riser, W. H., Brodey, R. S., and Biery, D. N.: Bone infarctions associated with malignant bone tumors in dogs. J.A.V.M.A. *160*:411, 1972.

Riser, W. H., Packer, L. J., and Shirer, J. F.: Canine craniomandibular osteopathy. J. Amer. Vet. Rad. Soc. *8*:23, 1967.

Riser, W. H., and Shirer, J. F.: Normal and abnormal growth of the distal foreleg in large and giant dogs. J. Amer. Vet. Rad. Soc. *6*:50, 1965.

Rutman, M. A., and Chandler, F. W.: Feline cryptococcosis. Feline Prac. *5*:36, 1975.

Schalm, O. W.: Mucopolysaccharidosis. Canine Pract. *12*:29, 1977.

Schultz, S.: A case of craniomandibular osteopathy in a Boxer. J. Small Anim. Prac. *19*:749, 1978.

Schunk, K. L.: Lead poisoning in dogs. Small Animal Veterinary Medical Update series *8*:1, 1978.

Scott, D. W., Kirk, R. W., Hampshire, J., and Altszuler, N.: Clinicopathological findings in a German Shepherd with pituitary dwarfism, J.A.A.H.A., *14*(2):183, 1978.

Seawright, A., and English, P.: Spondylosis in cats attributed to hypervitaminosis A. J. Comp. Pathol. *77*:35, 1967.

Siegel, E. T.: Effects of hormones on bone. Cornell Vet. Suppl. *58*:95, 1968.

Siegel, 1.: Endocrine Disease of the Dog. Lea and Febiger, Philadelphia. pp. 23–27, 1977.

Skelley, J. F., and Sauer, R.: Cutaneous nocardiosis. Mod. Vet. Prac. *46*:78, 1965.

Small, E.: Systemic mycoses. J.A.V.M.A. *155*:2002, 1969.

Smith, G.: Unpublished data, University of Pennsylvania, 1980.

Solomon, L.: Hereditary multiple exostoses. Am. J. Hum. Genet. *16*:351, 1964.

Sprinkle, T. A., and Korak, L.: Hip dysplasia, elbow dysplasia and eosinophilic panosteitis: three clinical manifestations of hyperestrinism in the dog? Cornell Vet. *60*:476, 1970.

Stone, J. A., Rogers, M. D., and Riser, W. H.: Clinico-pathologic conference. J.A.V.M.A. *155*:1376, 1969.

Subden, R. E., Fletch, S. M., Smart, M. E., and Brown, R. G.: Genetics of the Alaskan Malamute chondro-dysplasia syndrome. J. Hered. *63*:149, 1972.

Teare, J. A., Krook, L., and Kallfetz, F.: Ascorbic acid deficiency and hypertrophic osteodystrophy in the dog: a rebuttal. Cornell Vet. *69*:384, 1979.

Turnier, J. C., and Silverman, S.: A case study of canine panosteitis: comparison of radiographic and radioisotopic studies. Am. J. Vet. Res. *30*:1550, 1978.

Vaananen, M., and Wikman, L.: Scurvey as a cause of osteodystrophy. J. Small Anim. Pract. *20*:491, 1979.

Walker, M. A., Duncan, J. R., and Shaw, J. W.: Aneurysmal bone cyst in a cat. J.A.V.M.A. *167*:933, 1975.

Watkins, J. D., and Bradley, R.: Craniomandibular osteopathy in a Labrador puppy. Vet. Rec. *79*:262, 1966.

Watson, A. D. J., Hustable, C. R. R., and Farrow, B. R. H.: Craniomandibular osteopathy in a Doberman pinscher. J. Small Anim. Pract. *16*:11, 1975.

Weben, P. M., and Clayton-Jones, D. G.: Bone tumors. J. Small Anim. Prac. *19*:251, 1978.

Whittick, W. G.: Osteopenia due to a stress deficiency. *In* Canine Orthopedics. Lea and Febiger, Philadelphia, 1974.

Zook, B. C.: The pathologic anatomy of lead poisoning. Vet. Pathol. *9*:310, 1973.

Zook, B. C., Carpenter, J. L., and Leeds, E. B.: Lead poisoning in dogs. J.A.V.M.A. *155*:1329, 1969.

Index

Note: Page numbers in *italics* indicate illustrations; those followed by (t) indicate tables.

Achalasia (*Continued*)
esophageal, 1227–1230
Achlorhydria, and chronic
atrophic gastritis, 1257–1258
Achondroplasia, 2244
Acid-base balance
and neurologic disorders, 500
carbon dioxide in, 686–687,
686
determination of, 686–687,
686
Acidophil(s), 1526, *1526*
Acidophil adenoma, of pars
distalis, 1539, *1539*
Acidosis. See *Metabolic acidosis;
Respiratory acidosis.*
Aciduria
paradoxical, in gastric
disorders, 1245
in vomiting, 52
Acne, in Cushing's syndrome,
1677
Acoustic nerve, evaluation of,
441(t), 450. See also *Cranial
nerve(s).*
Acromegaly, iatrogenic,
1544–1547, *1545, 1546,* 1547(t)
ACTH
and leukocytosis, 2016–2018
deficiency of, causes of, 1662
hypersecretion of, in pituitary-
dependent hyperadreno-
corticism, 1673–1674
in aldosterone release, 1658
in glucocorticoid release,
1655–1657, *1656*
plasma levels of, diurnal
variation in, 1656–1657.
1656
in adrenocortical insufficiency, 1666–1669, 1667(t),
1668
normal values for, 1526
tests of, 1666–1668,
1667–1669
radioimmunoassay of,
1667–1668
secretion of, regulation of,
1655–1657, *1656*
ACTH cells, 1527
ACTH-secreting adenomas,
functional, 1535–1538, *1536,
1537*
ACTH-secreting tumors, 1674
ACTH stimulation test, in
Cushing's syndrome,
1686–1687, *1687, 1689*
of plasma cortisol, 1665–1666,
1665(t), *1666*
Actinomycin-D, in cancer
chemotherapy, 377(t), 378–379
Actinomycosis, 264–266
antibiotics for, 359(t), 363
Action potential, electromyographic measurement of,
624–625

Activated coagulation time, 2081,
2085
Activated partial thromboplastin
time, 2081, 2085
Acute. See under nouns; e.g.,
Pancreatitis, acute.
Addison's disease
ACTH deficiency in, 1662
and age, 1659
and breed, 1659
and sex, 1659
anemia in, 1945–1946
blood urea nitrogen in,
1661–1662
causes of, 1658
clinical pathology of,
1661–1663
clinical signs of, 1660, 1660(t),
1661(t)
electrocardiogram in,
1663–1665, *1664*
electrolyte imbalances in,
treatment of, 1670
eosinophilia in, 1661
episodic course in, 1660
erythrocyte parameters in, 1661
glucocorticoids for, 1670
history in, 1660, 1660(t)
hormonal studies in,
1665–1668, 1665(t),
1666–1669, 1667(t)
hypercalcemia in, 1662
hyperkalemia in, 1662–1663
treatment of, 1670
hyperpotassemia in, treatment
of, 1670
hypochloremia in, 1662–1663
hypoglycemia in, 1662
hyponatremia in, 1662–1663
hypovolemia in, treatment of,
1669
leukocyte counts in, 1661
lymphocytosis in, 1661
maintenance therapy for,
1671–1672
metabolic acidosis in, treatment
of, 1670–1671
pathogenesis of, 1659–1660
physical examination in,
1660–1661, 1661(t)
plasma cortisol levels in,
1665–1666, 1665(t), *1666*
plasma endogenous ACTH in,
1666–1669, *1667–1669,*
1667(t), *1668*
prognosis in, 1672
radiography in, 1663
salt supplementation in, 1672
serum carbon dioxide in, 1663
serum electrolytes in,
1662–1663
treatment of, 1667(t),
1669–1671, 1669(t)
urinalysis in, 1661–1662
vascular integrity in,
improvement of, 1670

Addison-like disease,
hypercalcemia in, 1571
Adductor magnus muscle,
sectioning of, in hip dysplasia,
2213–2214
Adenocarcinoma
adnexal, metastasis in, 401(t)
anal, 1512–1513, *1513*
and pseudohyper-
parathyroidism, *1572,
1573, 1573, 1574*
metastasis in, 401(t)
lymph node aspirate in,
2057
colonic, 1367–1369, *1368*
treatment of, 415
gastric, 1267–1269
hormone receptors in, 380
intestinal, 1333–1334, *1334,
1335*
treatment of, 415
nasal, *708,* 709–710, *709*
metastasis in, 400(t)
radioresponsiveness of, 401(t)
pancreatic, 1452–1453
prostatic, 1472–1476, *1473–
1475*
rectal, 1511–1514, *1511, 1512*
and pseudohyperpara-
thyroidism, 1572, 1573
thyroid, and hyperthyroidism,
canine, 1610–1612
feline, 1612–1613
Adenohypophysis, of pituitary
gland, 1525–1527, *1524,
1525, 1528, 1529*
functional corticotroph
adenoma of, 1535–1538,
1536, 1537
Adenoma
chromophobe, endocrino-
logically inactive, 1532–1535,
1534, 1535
corticotroph, functional, with
hypercortisolism, 1535–1538,
1536, 1537
papillary, of colon, 1367
parathyroid, and
hyperparathyroidism,
1566–1567, *1567*
perianal, 1514–1516, *1515,
1516*
metastasis in, 401(t)
radioresponsiveness of, 402(t)
pituitary, corticotroph, of
adenohypophysis,
1535–1538, *1536, 1537*
nonfunctioning, 1532–1535,
1534, 1535
of pars distalis, acidophil,
1539, *1539*
basophil, 1540
of pars intermedia,
1538–1539, *1538*
thyroid, and hyperthyroidism,
canine, 1610–1612

Alveolar edema. See also
Pulmonary edema, alveolar.
Alveolar macrophages
  as pulmonary defense
    mechanism, 765–766
  factors adversely affecting,
    766(t)
Alveolar microlithiasis, 816,
  885–887, *886, 887*
Alveolar oxygen tension, 685,
  685
Alveolar process, structure and
  function of, 1127–1128, *1127,
  1128*
Alveolar transport system, 690
Amblyopia, and quadriplegia, in
  Irish setters, 497
Amebiasis, 1319–1320,
  1353–1354, *1354*
Amikacin, action and use of,
  345–346
Amino acids
  metabolism of, deranged, and
    hepatic coma, 1382
  sequence variations in, 1616(t)
Aminoglycoside(s)
  action and use of, 345–346
  binding of, fecal, 351
    intracellular, 350–351
    to pus, 350–351
  dosage and route of,
    340(t)–341(t), 346
  nephrotoxicity of, 1847–1849
  neuromuscular blockade by,
    356
  ototoxicity of, 630
  toxicity of, 345–346
Aminophylline
  dosage for, 786(t)
  for cardiac disease, 969(t)
  for pulmonary edema, 757
  for tracheitis, 728(t)
Ammonia tolerance test, 1398
Amoxicillin, dosage and route of,
  340(t), 341–342
AMP
  and thyroid-stimulating
    hormone, 1595–1596
  cyclic, and parathyroid action,
    1557, *1558*
  and platelet function, 2080
Amphetamine
  for aggression, 225
  for hyperkinesis, 216
  intoxication with, 216
Amphotericin B
  action and use of, 343
  and hypokalemia, 241
  dosage and route of, 340(t)
  for aspergillosis, 261
  for blastomycosis, 240–242
  for coccidioidomycosis, 247
  for cryptococcosis, 251
  for histoplasmosis, 256
  for sporotrichosis, 258
  for systemic mycoses, 363

Amphotericin B (*Continued*)
  nephrotoxicity of, 241,
    1847–1849
  patient monitoring in, 241–242
Ampicillin
  action and use of, 341–342
  dosage and route of, 340(t),
    342
  for peritoneal lavage, 363
  for pyelonephritis, 1863
  for suppurative osteomyelitis,
    2238
  for wound infection, 363
  prophylactic, for dental
    surgery, 1160
Amputation
  in osteosarcoma, 414
  rectal, *1519,* 1520
Amyloidosis
  hepatic, 1419
  renal, 1830–1833, *1831–1832,*
    1839
  therapy of, 1842–1843
  secondary systemic, 1830
Amylase, serum, in acute
  pancreatitis, 1441–1442, *1444*
Amylorrhea, stool microscopy in,
  1292
Anal reflex, origin of, 538
Anal sac(s)
  abscess of, 1503–1504, *1503*
  adenocarcinoma of, and
    pseudohyperparathyroidism,
    1572, 1573, *1573, 1574*
  anatomy of, 1501
  diseases of, 1501–1504
  excision of, 1504
  impaction of, 1501–1503
Analgesia
  natural, 40–41
  pharmaceutical, 41–45
  pathologic, evaluation of, 439
Analgesics
  classification of, 41–45
  for acute pancreatitis, 1445
  in hepatic failure, 1424
  mild, 44–45, 45(t)
  narcotic, 41–43, 42(t)
  narcotic antagonist, 43–44,
    43(t)
Anaphylaxis
  cutaneous, passive, 2119(t)
    reverse passive, 2119(t)
  systemic, 2118(t)
Anasarca, 67
Anastomosis, bowel, antibiotic
  prophylaxis for, 364
Anconeal and coronoid processes,
  ununited, 2209–2210, *2209,
  2210*
Ancylostoma caninum, 516
  infection with, 1314–1316
  location and detection of, 773(t)
Ancylostoma tubaeforme, infection
  with, 1314–1316
Ancylostomiasis, 1314–1316

Androgen(s)
  defined, 1650
  endogenous, hypersensitivity to,
    2147
  for contraception, 1728
  for renal failure, 1824
  in cancer chemotherapy, 380
Anemia, 102–107, 1972–1985
  anabolic androgenic steroids
    for, 1968(t), 1969
  and exogenous estrogen, 1946
  and feline leukemia virus, 105,
    314–315, 1991
  and hyperphosphatemia, 1940
  and protein deficiency, 1989
  aplastic, 1989–1991
    and feline leukemia virus,
      314–315
    aplastic crisis in, 1977
    drug-induced, 1989
    infectious, 1991–1992
    estrogen-induced, 1990
    therapy of, 1992–1993
  bone marrow evaluation in,
    105, 1959–1962
  chloramphenicol-induced, 1990
  classification of, 1948
  clinical manifestations of, 103,
    1972
  clinical signs of, 1972, 1973(t)
  Coombs-negative, spherocytic,
    steroid-responsive, 1981
  Coombs-positive, autoimmune.
    See *Anemia, hemolytic,
    autoimmune.*
  nonautoimmune, 1983–1985
  defined, 102, 1945
  dyspnea in, 98, 98(t)
  erythrocyte morphologic
    evaluation in, 1952–1958,
    1953, 1955, 1957(t)
  erythrocyte quantitation in,
    1949–1952
  etiology of, 102–103
  evaluation of, clinical, 104
    laboratory, 104–107
  fragmentation, abnormal
    erythrocytes in, *1955,*
    1956–1958
    in disseminated intravascular
      coagulation, 1986–1987
    spherocytes in, 1956–1957
  Heinz body, 104, 1958–1959,
    1985–1986
  hemogram in, 104–107
  hemolytic, 104, 1967–1981. See
    also *Hemolytic disorders.*
    autoimmune, 2163–2167
      as autoimmune disease,
        2159(t)
      blood smear in, *1955*
      classification of, 1980, 2164
      clinical signs of,
        2164–2165, *2165*
      clinicopathologic findings
        in, 2165–2166

Bacterial endocarditis (*Continued*)
  feline, and arterial
    thromboembolism,
    1046–1047, *1047*
  immune factors in, 1056
  incidence of, 1052
  microbiology of, 1052
  organisms causing, 358(t)
  pathogenesis of, 1052–1056
  pathology of, 1056
  pathophysiology of, 1052–1056
  prevention of, 1060
  radiography in, 1057, *1057*
  subacute, and arthritis, 2219
    vs. systemic lupus
      erythematosus arthritis,
      2229
    pathogenesis of, 1053–1054
  treatment of, 1060
Bacterial infections. See also
    Infection(s).
  cell-mediated immunity in,
    2122, 2122(t)
  defense mechanisms in, 2122,
    2122(t)
  neurologic lesions in, 512–513
Bacteriostatic protein synthesis
    inhibitors, 343–346
BAL. See *Dimercaprol*.
Balanoposthitis, organisms
    causing, 358(t)
Balantidiasis, 1319–1320,
    1365–1366, *1365*
  antibiotics for, 361
Balantidium coli, 1319, 1363, *1363*
  fecal examination for, 1291
BALT, functions of, 765
Band neutrophil, *2004*,
    2005–2006, *2009*
Barium enema, 1349–1350
Baruria, 1756–1757
Basenji
  familial anemia of, 1978–1979
  familial renal disease in, 1865
  pyruvate kinase deficiency of,
    106, 1963
Basocytophilia, 2026
Basophil(s), 1526, *1526*,
    2007–2008, 2010
  function of, 2014
  kinetics of, 2014
  production of, 2014
Basophil adenoma of pars distalis,
    1540
Basophilia, 2026
Basophilic leukemia, 2038
Basophilic stippling, in ineffective
    erythropoiesis, 1959
Basset hounds, familial platelet
    disorder in, 2097
BCG, and tumor regression, 2127
BCG test, for tuberculosis, 303
BCG vaccine, in immunotherapy,
    388–389, 389(t)
Beagles, pyruvate kinase
    deficiency of, 1963

Bedlington terriers
  hepatitis in, chronic progressive
    hemolysis in, 1987
  copper-associated,
    1408–1410, *1409*
Behavior. See also *Learning*.
  aggressive. See *Aggression*.
  changes in, 73–76
    classification of, 74
    diagnostic approach to,
      75–76
    etiology of, 74–75
    in brain disease, 461–462
    in rabies, 285
  defined, 208
  extinct, spontaneous recovery
    of, 210
  extinction of, 210
  factors in, 208–209
  predatory, 224
  second order reinforcers of,
    211
Behavior modification, 211–213
  counterconditioning in, 212
  desensitization in, 212
  for aggression, 222–225
  for elimination problems,
    canine, 219
    feline, 219–221
  for fears, of noises, 213–214
    of people, 214–215
  for hyperactivity, 215
  for phobias, 213–215
  for predatory behavior, 224
  for separation anxiety, 217–218
  flooding in, 212
  habituation in, 212–213
  methods of, 208
Behavior problems. See also
    Behavioral disorders.
  and progestogen, 218–219
  aggression as, 221–226
  elimination, canine, 219
    feline, 219–221
  euthanasia in, 228
  fear of noise as, 213–214
  fear of people as, 214–215
  hyperactivity as, 215–216
  masculine, 218
  pathophysiologic, 225–226
  phobias as, 213–215
  predatory behavior as, 224
  separation anxiety as, 216–218
Behavioral disorders, 208–226
  and learning, 209–213
  behavior modification for. See
    Behavior modification.
Behavioral seizures, 88
Bence Jones proteins, 2109, 2134
Bensulide intoxication, 196(t)
Benzydroflumethiazides, for
    congestive heart failure, 924
Benzylpenicillin. See *Penicillin G*.
Benzocaine
  and Heinz body anemia, 1986
  and methemoglobinemia, 1986

Bernese Mountain dogs,
    aggression in, 226
Betamethasone
  for allergic disorders, 2183
  in cancer chemotherapy, 380
Bethanechol chloride, for urinary
    incontinence, 1917
Bicarbonate. See *Sodium
    bicarbonate*.
Biceps reflex, 431–432, 431(t),
    434
Bile
  drug excretion via, 329
  metabolism of, 1373–1374
  reflux of, and gastric mucosal
    injury, 1254
  toxin excretion via, 175
Bile acid(s)
  concentration of, tests of, 1394
  functions of, 1375–1376
  metabolism of, 1375–1377,
    1276
  toxicity of, 1376–1377
Bile ducts, rupture of, 1457
Bile peritonitis, treatment of,
    1458
Bile pigments
  tests of, 1392
  urinary, 1377–1378
Bile pleuritis, 877
Biliary tract disease
  and acute pancreatitis, 1438,
    1440
  jaundice in, 113
Bilirubin
  conjugated, 111(t)
  conjugation of, 1373
  enterohepatic circulation of,
    1374
  in hepatic disease, 1377
  metabolism of, 110, 111–112,
    111
  production and transport of,
    110, 1373–1374, 1375
  renal excretion of, *111*, 112
  serum, measurement of,
    113–114
    antimicrobial interference
      with, 355(t)
  source of, 110
  tests of, 1392
  transport of, 110–111
  unconjugated, 111(t)
  urinary, tests of, 1392
Bilirubinuria, 114, 114(t)
  in anemia, 104
Billing systems, 13–18, *20–22*
Biopsy
  excisional, 407
  in anemia, 105
  in cancer, indications for, 409
    principles of, 410–411
    types of, 407
  in infertility, 1712, *1714*
  in lymphoma, 2064
  incisional, 407

Bone marrow dyscrasias, in
poodles, 2030
Bone marrow function, tests of,
1959–1962
Bone marrow suppression, and
feline leukemia virus, 315
in cancer chemotherapy, 381
phenylbutazone-induced, 1990
Bone resorption factor, 2047
Borate-chlorate herbicide
intoxication, 196(t)
Bordetella bronchiseptica
and canine distemper, 269
and canine respiratory disease,
284, 782
Boston terrier
constipation in, 1516
glial tumors in, 504, 506(t)
mastocytoma in, 155
Botryoid sarcoma, of bladder,
1910
Botulism, 311–312, 643–644
Bowman's capsule
anatomy and physiology of,
1734, 1737, 1737
in urine formation, 1744(t)
Bowel. See *Colon; Intestine.*
Boxer
cancer in, 155–156
cell-mediated immunodeficiency
in, 155–156
glial tumors in, 504, 506(t), *507*
histiocytic ulcerative colitis in,
1355–1359, 1356(t)
inherited polyneuropathy in,
639
mastocytoma in, 155
mycotic diseases in, 155
Brachial plexus
injuries of, body part chewing
in, 533
tumors of, 636–637
Brachial plexus nerve root
avulsion, 634
Brachial plexus neuritis, 640–641
Brachycephalic breeds
airway obstruction in, 696–697
hypoplastic trachea in, 734–736
overlong soft palate in,
698–699, *699*
stenotic nares in, 698, *698*
Bradyarrhythmia(s), 1006–1017
and syncope, 85
Bradycardia, sinus, 1006–1008,
1007–1008
isoproterenol for, 1020(t)
Bradycardia-tachycardia
syndrome, 1008, 1009:
1016–1017
Brain
abscess of, 513, *514*
anatomy of, *464, 465, 467, 468*
contrecoup lesion of, 518
coup lesion of, 518
diseases of, and acid-base
disturbances, 500

Brain (*Continued*)
diseases of, and electrolyte
disturbances, 499–501
and endocrine disturbances,
501–502
and hepatic insufficiency, 501
and hyperthermia, 502
and hypothermia, 501–502
and mineral disturbances,
499–500
and uremia, 501
anoxic, 502–503
behavioral abnormalities in,
75, 461–462
coma in, 462
congenital, 490–493
degenerative, 492–498
developmental, 487–493
diagnosis of,
electrophysiologic,
476–487, *477–486*
radiographic, 470–476,
470–476
epilepsy in, 88
eye movements in, 463
hemiparesis in, 462–463
hypoxic, 502–503
infectious, 508–517
involuntary movement in,
463
lesion localization in,
463–469, 464(t)
to brainstem, 464(t),
466–468
to cerebellum, 464(t), 469
to cerebral cortex,
463–466, 464(t)
to diencephalon, 464(t),
466
to vestibular system, 464(t),
468–469
lethargy in, 462
mental status in, 461–462
metabolic, 498–502
motor dysfunction in,
462–463
neurologic examination in.
See *Neurologic examination.*
nutritional, 498–499
parasitic, 516–517
postural reactions in, 430
proprioceptive dysfunction
in, 462–463
pupillary reflexes in, 446, 463
radiography in, 470–476,
470–476
seizures in, 461, 461(t)
signs of, 461(t)
stupor in, 462
tetraparesis in, 462–463
tremor in, 463
visual abnormalities in, 463
vascular, 503–504
edema of, hypoxic, 502–503
in diabetic ketoacidosis,
1635–1636

Brain (*Continued*)
edema of, traumatic, 518–519,
519
treatment of, 522–523
hemorrhage of, 518
cerebrospinal fluid findings
in, 457(t), 459
herniation of, 519, *519*
tentorial, progressive
bilateral, 522(t)
progressive unilateral, 523(t)
signs of, 522(t), 523(t), 525
treatment of, 525
vs. brainstem hemorrhage,
520–521, *521*, 522(t),
523(t)
infarction of, in feline ischemic
encephalopathy, 503–504
infections of, 508–517
bacterial, 512–513
mycotic, 513–514
of unknown etiology,
515–517
parasitic, 516–517
protozoal, 514–515
viral 508–512
lesions of, localization of, 435(t)
signs of, 463–466, 464(t)
limbic system of, anatomy of,
467
trauma of, 518–525
cerebrospinal fluid
examination in, 521
clinical signs of, 519–521
complications of, 525
diagnosis of, 521–522
differential diagnosis of, 521
eye movements in, 520
motor function assessment in,
520
pathophysiology of, 518–519
pupillary reflexes in, 520
radiography in, 521, *524*
severity of, and level of
consciousness, 519–520
treatment of, 522–525
tumors of, 504–508
arteriography in, 472
behavioral changes in, 75
classification of, 504, 505(t)
clinical signs of, 506, *507*
diagnosis of, 506–507
differential diagnosis of,
506–508
incidence of, 504–505, 506(t)
pathogenesis of, 505–506
treatment of, 508
Brain scanning, 474
in tumor diagnosis, 508
Brainstem
hemorrhage in, signs of, 522(t)
vs. tentorial herniation,
520–521, *521*, 522(t),
523(t)
lesions of, localization of, 435(t)
signs of, 464(t), 466–468

Enzyme(s) *(Continued)*
serum, in hepatic disease, 1394–1398
in renal disease, 1804
Enzyme-linked immunosorbent assay, for feline oncornavirus-associated cell membrane antigen, 313
Eosinopenia, 2025–2026
and corticosteroids, 2015–2028
Eosinophil(s), 2007–2010, *2007, 2009*
function of, 2013–2014
kinetics of, 2014
production of, 2014
pulmonary infiltrates with, 802–803, *803–804*
Eosinophilia, 2025–2026
in Addison's disease, 1661
in lower respiratory disease, 772
Eosinophilic gastritis, 1258
Eosinophilic gastroenteritis, 1258, 1320(t), 1322–1323
Eosinophilic leukemia, feline, 2036–2037
and feline leukemia virus, 314
Eosinophilic pneumonia, 802–803, *803–804*
Eosinophilic ulcerative colitis, 1359–1360
treatment of, 1362–1363, *1362*
Ependymomas, incidence of, 504–505
Ephedrine, 823(t)
for tracheitis, 728(t)
Epidemiology, 163–171
analysis in, 165–166
analytical, 164–171
biostatistical methods in, 165–168, 167(t), 168(t)
case selection in, 16
case-control studies in, 164–168
matched, 168, 168(t)
case selection in, 165
clinical trials in, 170–171
cohort studies in, 168–170
control selection in, 165
descriptive, 163–164
intervention studies in, 170
methods in, 163–171
odds ratio in, 166
prophylactic trials in, 170
relative risk in, 166–168, 167(t), 168(t)
multifactorial, 168, 169(t)
studies in, requirements for, 163
therapeutic trials in, 170
Epidermal necrolysis, toxic, 2155–2156, *2156*
Epididymis, anatomy of, 1698, *1699*
Epidural hemorrhage, 518

Epiglottis
congenital abnormalities of, 715
flaccid, 715
Epilation, in radiotherapy, 403
Epilepsy. See also *Seizure(s)*.
cortical, 87–88
defined, 87
differential diagnosis of, 89–91
grand mal seizures in, 88
idiopathic, 89, 461
inheritance of, 153
management of, 92–94
myoclonic, 494(t), 495
psychomotor, and aggression, 225–226
status epilepticus in, treatment of, 91
symptomatic, 88–89
therapy of, 91–94
Epinephrine, 823(t)
and physiologic leukocytosis, 2015
for traumatic epistaxis, 700
in diabetes pathogenesis, 1621–1622, *1622*
Epiphysiolysis, 2207
Epistaxis, traumatic, 699–700
Epithelial barrier, to toxins, 174
EPTC intoxication, 196(t)
Epulis
acanthomatous, metastasis in, 400(t)
periodontal, 1162, *1164*
Equilibrium, disturbances of, in vestibulocochlear nerve disorders, 630
Erlichiosis, canine, 303, 1984, 1990
thrombocytopenia in, 2023, 2095
Erythema multiforme, 2156, *2156*
Erythremic myelosis, *1953, 2032,* 2035
and feline leukemia virus, 314
blast form of, *2032,* 2035–2036
Erythrocyte(s). See also *Erythron*.
abnormally shaped, 1955, 1956–1959, 1957(t)
and oxidant drugs, 1958–1959
autoimmune defects of, 1963–1964
basophilic stippling in, 1959
crystalloid bodies in, *1953,* 1958
destruction of. See *Hemolysis*.
2,3-diphosphoglycerate concentration in, clinical conditions associated with, 1940, 1940(t)
disorders of. See also *Anemia*.
therapy of, principles of, 1964–1970
enzyme abnormalities of, 1963
evaluation of, 1949–1964
fragmentation of, in systemic disease, 1986–1987

Erythrocyte(s) *(Continued)*
Heinz bodies in, *1953, 1955,* 1958–1959
Howell-Jolly bodies in, *1955,* 1956
hypochromic, 1954, *1955*
immunologic tests for, 1963–1964
indices of, 1950–1952
life span of, measurement of, 1963
macrocytic, 1951, *1953,* 1954
in miniature poodles, 1988
maturation sequence for, 1941–1943, *1941–1944,* 1942(t)
mature, morphology of, 1953
mean corpuscular hemoglobin of, 1950–1952
mean corpuscular hemoglobin concentration of, 1950–1952
mean corpuscular volume of, 1950–1952
metabolism of, defective, 1963
microcytic, 1951, 1954, *1954*
morphology of, 106, 1952–1959, *1953, 1955,* 1957(t)
blood smears for, 1952–1953
normocytic, 1952
nucleated, 1954–1956
packed, for transfusion, preparation of, 1966
packed volume of, in polycythemia, 1970, 1971
measurement of, 1949–1950
physiologic variations in, 1947
Pappenheimer body in, *1955,* 1959
poikilocytic, *1955,* 1956, 1957(t)
polychromatophilic, 1953, *1955*
response test for, 1960–1961, 1960(t), *1961*
potassium concentration in, 1946
precursors of, 1942–1943, 1942(t)
production of. See *Erythropoiesis*.
quantitation of, 1949–1952
regenerative response of, 1961–1962
sodium concentration in, 1946
sphering phenomenon in, 1963–1964
splenic sequestration of, 2069–2070
Erythrocyte antibodies, 1963
Erythrocyte antigens, 1965, 1965(t)
Erythrocyte count, 1950
Erythrocyte refractile bodies, *1953, 1955,* 1958–1959
Erythrocytic islet, 1941
Erythrocytosis-stimulating factor, 1954

Gentamicin (*Continued*)
for burns, 362
for colitis, 1352
for peritoneal lavage, 363–364
for septicemia, 364
nephrotoxicity of, 1847, 1849
optimal pH for, 352(t)
ototoxicity of, 630
toxicity of, 345–346
Genu valgum, and retained
enchondral cores, 2241
Geographic disease distribution,
157–161
Geriatric patients
encephalitis in, 270, 271, 272,
273
hepatic microsomal enzyme
deficiency in, 336
pharmacokinetics in, 335–336
German shepherds
congenital type II muscle fiber
hypertrophy in, 646
degenerative myelopathy of,
562–564, 563(t)
pituitary dwarfism in,
1542–1544, *1543*
and congenital secondary
hypothyroidism, 1608,
1609
Giardia canis, fecal examination
for, 1291
Giardiasis, 1317
antibiotics for, 361
Gila monster poisoning, 201
Gilchrist's disease. See
Blastomycosis.
Gingiva
hyperplasia of, *1160*
in gingivitis, 1148, *1149*
in periodontal disease, 1153,
1155
surgery of, 1159, *1160*
recession of, in periodontal
disease, 1153, *1153, 1155*
structure and function of, 1128,
1129
tumors of, 1173–1175, *1174,*
1174(t), *1175*
metastatic, 400(t)
radiographic staging of, 400
radioresponsiveness of, 401(t)
radiotherapy for, 399
Gingivectomy, 1156, *1156*
Gingivitis, 1148–1153
clinical manifestations of, 1148,
1148, 1149
etiology of, 1148–1150
histopathology of, 1148, *1150*
necrotizing ulcerative,
1152–1153
persistent, and periodontitis,
1155
surgery of, 1159, *1160*
treatment of, 1150–1152, 1156,
1156
Gland. See specific glands.

Glaucoma, signs of, 446
Glial tumors, *507*
incidence of, 504, 506(t)
Globoid cell leukodystrophy,
494(t), 496, 563(t), 638–639
and breed, 155
Globulins, in hepatic disease,
1386
Glomerular basement membrane,
1734, 1735, *1736*
Glomerular capillary endothelial
cells, 1734–1735, *1734, 1735*
Glomerular crescents, 1737
Glomerular disease, 1827–1844.
See also *Glomerulonephritis;*
Glomerulonephropathy;
Glomerulopathy.
types of, 1768(t)
Glomerular filtrate
composition of, 1742, 1742(t)
quantity and quality of,
1741–1742
substances in, molecular
weights of, 1742, 1742(t)
Glomerular filtration
alterations of, localization of,
1738(t)
and tubuloglomerular feedback,
1747
impaired, and azotemia, 1743
and edema, 1743–1744
and hypoalbuminemia, 1743
and proteinuria, 1743
clinical manifestations of,
1743–1744
mechanics of, 1735, *1735,*
1736–1737, 1741–1742
reduced, causes of, 1738(t),
1754
threshold substances in,
1744–1745
Glomerular filtration rate, 1741
evaluation of, 1797–1799, *1798*
normal values for, canine,
1797
reduced, in acute renal failure,
1748
Glomerular filtration slits, 1735
Glomerular function, evaluation
of, 1797–1801, *1798, 1800*
Glomerular injury
immunologic mechanisms of,
2179–2180
response to, 1761
Glomerular mesangial cells, *1734,*
1735–1736
Glomerular visceral epithelial
cells, *1734,* 1735, *1736*
Glomerulonephritis
amyloid deposition in,
1830–1833, *1831–1832,*
1839
therapy of, 1842–1843
and cancer, extrarenal, 1828
and feline leukemia virus, 313,
1828

Glomerulonephritis (*Continued*)
and feline lymphosarcoma,
1828
and hypertension, systemic,
1833
and nephrotic syndrome,
1834–1835
and systemic lupus
erythematosus, 1828
clinical consequences of,
1833–1835
clinical features of, 1835–1839
coagulation disorders in, 1835
diagnosis of, 1835–1836
diet in, 1843
diseases associated with,
1827–1828
edema in, 1743–1744,
1833–1834
therapy of, 1843–1844
etiology of, 1827–1828
glomerular filtration rate
changes in, 1833
hypoalbuminemia in, therapy
of, 1843
immune-complex, 1828–1830,
1837–1838
immune-mediated, 2180
immunologic tests in,
1836–1838
laboratory evaluation in,
1836–1837
membranoproliferative, 1737,
1738, 1839
therapy of, 1842
membranous, *1837,* 1838–1839
pathogenesis of, 1828–1833
poststreptococcal, as immune
complex disease, 2133
prevalence of, 1827
prognosis in, 1844
proliferative, 1839
therapy of, 1842
proteinuria in, 1834, 1836
radiography in, 1836
renal plasma flow alterations in,
1833
sodium retention in, 1833–1834
therapy of, 1843–1844
therapy of, 1839–1844
Glomerulonephropathy,
membranous, reversibility of,
1761
Glomerulopathy, protein-losing,
hypercholesterolemia in, 1781
Glomerulosclerosis, 1839
therapy of, 1842–1843
Glomerulotubular imbalance,
azotemia in, 143
Glomerulus(i)
anatomy and physiology of,
1734–1737, *1734–1738*
function of, 1742
renal, number of, 1733, 1734
vascularization of, 1741
Glossitis, 1169–1170, *1170*

Hageman factor deficiency, 2092–2094, 2093(t)

Hair
color of, and disease, 156
disorders of, in hypothyroidism, 1604
infections of, antibiotics for, 359(t)
loss of. See *Alopecia.*

Halothane, hepatotoxicity of, 1424

Halothane anesthesia, electroencephalogram in, *478–481*

Hamartoma, pulmonary vascular, 898

Hapten, 2104

Hard palate, injuries of, 700, 701, *703*

Harelip, 1165, *1165*

Hashimoto's thyroiditis, 2131, 2159(t), 2180
and primary hypothyroidism, 1603
treatment of, 1607–1608

Haws syndrome, 446

Head injuries, 518–525. See also *Brain, trauma of.*
extracerebral hemorrhage in, diagnosis of, 521–522, *525*

Head tilt, evaluation of, 424
in ataxia, 425, 425(t), 462
in labyrinthine disease, 468
in vestibular disease, 450, 468
paradoxical, 425

Head tremors, in ataxia, 425(t), 462

Hearing tests
brainstem auditory evoked response for, 478–481
impedance audiometry, 481–487
in cochlear disease, 469

Heart. See also *Cardiac.*
electrophysiology of, 981–982, *981, 982*
enlargement of, and cardiovascular reserve, 905, *905*
excitation-contraction coupling in, 981
excitation-contraction-relaxation cycle of, in heart failure, 918
jet lesions of, 972
work performed by, 904

Heartbase tumors, 1087–1088
and tracheal obstruction, *742–743,* 743

Heart block, 1011–1016, *1012–1015*
and syncope, 85
associated cardiac conditions in, 1012–1014
clinical signs of, 1014–1015
complete, 1011–1012, *1014*
isoproterenol for, 1020(t)

Heart block (*Continued*)
partial, 1011, *1012, 1013*
treatment of, 1015–1016

Heart cell(s)
afterdepolarization of, and arrhythmias, 985
automaticity of, 982
electrical activity of, 981–982, *981*
pacemaker, 982
automaticity of, 983
repolarization of, 982
resting membrane potential of, 981
threshold membrane potential of, 981
transmembrane potential of, 982, *982*
triggered impulses in, and arrhythmias, 985

Heart disease
and hyperthyroidism, 1045
and peripheral edema, 71
cardiovascular compensatory mechanisms in, 905–909, *907, 908,* 911–912, *912*
cardiovascular reserve capacity depletion in, 902–905
903–905, *907, 908*
congenital, 933–957
cyanotic, 109
coughing in, 95, 96(t)
drug dosage in, 337
functional response to, 901–910
pharmacokinetics in, 337
uremic, 1784–1785
valvular, 959–979

Heart failure, 901–929
cachexia in, 916
congestive, 910–929
and cardiac tamponade, 1081–1082. See also *Cardiac tamponade.*
and hyperadrenocorticism, 1684–1685
and mitral valvular insufficiency, 959. See also *Mitral valvular insufficiency, chronic.*
and pericardial effusions, 1081–1082
and sex, 152
ascites in, 916
atrial fibrillation in, 1002–1006, *1003–1005*
biochemical changes in, 917–919
calcium binding in, 918
canine vs. feline, 917
cardiac asthma in, 914
treatment of, 928
catecholamine depletion in, 918–919
causes of, 916–917
circulatory dynamics in, 911–912, *912*

Heart failure (*Continued*)
congestive, clinical manifestations of, 913–917
cough in, 914
treatment of, 927
defined, 910
digitalis for, 920–923
digoxin for, 1020(t)
diuretics for, 923–924
dobutamine for, 927
drug dosage in, 337
dyspnea in, exertional, 914
paroxysmal, 914
enzymatic alterations in, 919
excitation-contraction-relaxation cycle in, 918
fluid removal in, 928
hydropericardium in, 916
hydrothorax in, 916
hypoproteinemia in, 916
in heartworm disease, 1101–1102, 1112
incidence of, 933, 934(t)
left-sided, causes of, 916–917
postmortem findings in, 914
signs of, 913–915
liver in, 915–916
low-sodium diet for, 925, 926(t), 927(t)
mechanism of, 910–913, *912*
mitral insufficiency in, 916–917
morphine in, 927
orthopnea in, 914
oxygen therapy in, 928
pharmacokinetics in, 337
phlebotomy in, 928
pulmonary manifestations of, 914–915, *915,* 916
respiratory distress in, 914
rest in, 927
right-sided, and tricuspid insufficiency, 977
causes of, 917
postmortem findings in, 915–916
salbutamol for, 927–928
signs of, 915–916
superficial vein distention in, 916
treatment of, 919–929, 971(t)
ultrastructural changes in, 917–919
vasodilators for, 924–925
visceral congestive lesions in, 915–916
decompensated, 912–913, *912*
fluid retention in, 909–910

Heart murmur(s)
in bacterial endocarditis, 1056
in chordae tendinae rupture, 975
in heartworm disease, 1113
in mitral valvular insufficiency, 962, *962, 963*

Hindlimb
  paralysis of, in canine arterial
    thromboembolism, 1066
  in feline aortic
    thromboembolism,
    1064–1065
  peripheral nerves of, *618,*
    620–621
    lesions of, neurologic
      examination in, 623(t)
Hip
  dysplasia of, 2211–2214, *2212,*
    2213
    and luxation, 2199
  luxations and subluxations of,
    2199, *2200*
Hirschsprung's disease, 65,
  1366–1367
Histamine
  function of, 2121
  in gastric acid secretion, 1238,
    1239
Histamine shock, in mast cell
  tumor excision, 411
Histiocytic leukemia, 2065–2066,
  2066
Histiocytic ulcerative colitis. See
  Colitis, ulcerative, histiocytic.
Histiocytosis, malignant,
  2065–2066, *2066*
Histocompatibility complex, major
  and disease, 2130
    and immunogenicity, 2130
    function of, 2129–2130
    structure of, 2127–2128,
      2127(t), *2128*
Histocompatibility reactions,
  2128–2130
Histoplasma capsulatum, 252
Histoplasmosis, 252–256, 795(t)
  anemia in, 1985
  clinical manifestations of, 254
  cutaneous lesions in, 254
  diagnosis of, 254–256
  epidemiology of, 252–253
  etiology of, 252
  gastrointestinal, 253
  hepatic involvement in, 255
  intestinal, 1329–1330, *1330,*
    1331
    and diarrhea, 1310
    diagnosis and treatment of,
      1320(t)
  ocular lesions in, 254
  osteomyelitis in, 2238
  pathogenesis of, 253
  prognosis in, 256
  pulmonary lesions in, 254, *254,*
    255
  stool microscopy in, 1292, *1293*
  treatment of, 256
Hodgkin's-like disease, 2065,
  2065
Holosystolic murmur
  in chordae tendinae rupture,
    975

Holosystolic murmur (*Continued*)
  in mitral valvular insufficiency,
    962, *963*
Homatropine methylbromide, for
  tracheitis, 728(t)
Hookworms
  infection with, 1314–1316
  location and detection of, 773(t)
Hopping, in neurologic
  examination, 420(t), 427–429,
    428, 430
Hordeum jubatum, as
  tracheobronchial foreign body,
    790, *790*
Horizontal nystagmus, 452
Hormonal abnormalities, and
  diabetes mellitus, 1623, 1624
Hormonal disorders, and
  pruritus, 117
Hormone(s)
  calcium-regulating, 1550–1565
  gastric, 1240–1241, *1240,*
    1241(t), 1242(t)
  hepatic metabolism of, 1385
  hypersensitivity to, 2147–2148
  in cancer chemotherapy, 380
  polypeptide, pathways of,
    1523–1524, *1524*
  releasing, 1527, *1528, 1529*
  renal degradation of, 1746
  stress, in diabetes pathogenesis,
    1621–1622, *1622*
Hormone receptors, functions of,
  1523
Horner's syndrome, 444–446, *444*
Horseshoe kidney, 1864
Hospitalization records, 6–9, *13*
Host resistance, and age, 150
Housebreaking, 219
Household products, intoxication
  with, 201–202
Howell-Jolly bodies, *1955,* 1956
Human chorionic gonadotropin,
  for hypogonadism, 1716–1717
Humoral immunity, tests of,
  2175–2177, *2176*
Hurler's syndrome, joint disease
  in, 2218
Hyaline casts, 1739
Hyalomma spp., as babesiosis
  vector, 310
Hydrancephaly, 490–491
Hydration
  in respiratory disease, 657–658
  respiratory, 819
Hydrocephalus, 487–490
  and breed, 487
  behavioral changes in, 75
  clinical signs of, 487–488
  communicating, 487
  diagnosis of, 488–489, *488, 489*
    cerebral radiography for, 472
    ventriculography for, 473
  etiology of, 487
  neonatal, causes of, 487
  noncommunicating, 487

Hydrocephalus (*Continued*)
  obstructive, 487
  treatment of, 488–490
Hydrochloric acid, gastric
  secretion of, 1237–1238, *1238*
Hydrochlorothiazides, for
  congestive heart failure, 924
Hydrocodone bitartrate
  dosage for, 786(t)
  for cardiac disease, 969(t)
  for tracheitis, 728(t)
Hydrocortisone
  for shock, 523
  in cancer chemotherapy, 380
Hydrogen, in gastric secretions,
  1239
Hydronephrosis, and ureteral
  ectopia, 1881
Hydropericardium, in congestive
  heart failure, 916
Hydrothorax, 865–867, 868(t)
  auscultation findings in, 771(t)
  defined, 854
  in congestive heart failure, 916
  percussion findings in, 771(t)
  treatment of, 872
17-Hydroxycorticosteroids,
  urinary, measurement of,
  antimicrobial interference in,
  355(t)
Hydroxyurea, in cancer
  chemotherapy, 377(t), 379
Hydroxyzine hydrochloride, for
  irritable colon, 1365
Hyoid injury, 715–716
Hypalgesia, evaluation of, 439
Hyperactivity, 215–216
Hyperadrenocorticism,
  1672–1693. See also *Cushing's*
  syndrome.
  adrenal tumor in, surgery of,
    1692–1693
  and osteoporosis, 2257–2258
  and polymyopathy, 646
  and pulmonary
    thromboembolism, 1685
  clinical features of, 1674–1680
  complications of, 1684–1685
  diagnosis of, 1685–1689
  differential diagnosis of, 1684
  etiology of, 1685–1689
  feline, *1679,* 1680
  in-hospital evaluation in,
    1680–1684
  pathogenic mechanisms in,
    1674
  pathophysiology of, 1672–1674,
    1673
  physical examination in,
    1678–1680
  pituitary-adrenocortical axis in,
    direct evaluation of,
    1685–1689
  pituitary-dependent,
    1672–1673
    treatment of, 1690–1692

Infertility (*Continued*)
  physical examination in,
    1711–1712
  psychogenic, male, 1723
  radiography in, 1712–1713
  semen analysis in, 1714–1715
  serologic testing in, 1714
Inflammation
  and coughing, 95, 96(t)
  neutrophil response to,
    2018–2020, *2019*
Inflammatory response,
  glucocorticoid effect on, 1654
Inhalant allergic disorders,
  betamethasone for, 2183
Inhalation pneumonia, 806–807
Inheritance
  sex-influenced, 154
  sex-limited, 154
  sex-linked, 154
Insect bite, allergy to, 2146
Insecticide intoxication, 189–192,
  202
Insulin
  actions of, 1617–1618
  biosynthesis of, 1615–1616
  effect of, on adipose tissue,
    1617–1618, 1618(t)
    on liver, 1618, 1618(t)
    on muscle, 1618, 1618(t)
  exogenous, for diabetes,
    1627–1632. See also under
    Diabetes mellitus.
  for diabetic ketoacidosis,
    1636–1637, 1636(t)
  in adrenocortical insufficiency,
    1670
  metabolism of, in uremia,
    1780–1781
  secretion of, regulation of,
    1616–1617
  structure of, 1615
  transport and binding of,
    1617
Intention tremors
  in brain disease, 463
  in cerebellar ataxia, 462
Interferon, 391, 2047, 2183
Intersex, 1721, *1722*
Interstitial edema. See *Pulmonary
  edema, interstitial.*
Interstitial fluid
  state of, and edema formation,
    67–68, *68*
  viscosity of, 70
Intervertebral disc(s)
  anatomy of, 575, *576*
  calcified, radiography of,
    581–582
  changes in, radiographic
    findings in, 547–548
  protrusion of, in lumbar spinal
    stenosis, 591
  pathogenesis of, 576–578,
    576–580, 582
  traumatic, 584–585, *585*

Intervertebral disc(s) (*Continued*)
  protrusion of, vs. degenerative
    myelopathy of German
    shepherds, 564
Intervertebral disc disease,
  575–584
  clinical features of, 578–583
  diagnosis of, 578
  feline, 584
  myelography in, 549. See also
    Myelography.
  pathogenesis of, 575–578
  prognosis in, 539(t)
  radiology of, 578–583, *579,
    580, 582*
  treatment of, 583–584
  vs. meningitis, 556
Intervertebral foramen,
  radiography of, 548
Intestinal anastomosis, 1514
  antibiotic prophylaxis for, 364
Intestinal motility, disordered,
  and diarrhea, 60–61
Intestinal mucosa, damage to, and
  diarrhea, 60
  enzymes of, tests of, 1298
Intestinal sepsis, preoperative,
  antibiotics for, 361
Intestine(s)
  large. See specific components
    of, e.g., *Cecum; Colon.*
  normal microflora of,
    1302–1303
  small. See also specific
    components of.
  acidification of, in pancreatic
    exocrine insufficiency,
    1447, *1447*
  adenocarcinoma of,
    1333–1334, *1334, 1335*
    treatment of, 415
  anatomy of, 1278–1280,
    1279
  arterial supply of, 1278
  assimilative function of,
    1280–1285, *1281, 1283*
  bacterial overgrowth in, and
    malabsorption, 1331–1332
  biopsy of, 1298–1299
  calcium absorption by,
    1564–1565, *1565*
  carbohydrate assimilation in,
    1282–1284
  carbohydrate digestion in,
    tests of, 1291(t), 1294–1295
  crypt-villus viral predilection
    in, 1279, *1279, 1280*
  disease of, chronic
    inflammatory,
    1320–1321
    diagnosis and treatment
      of, 1320(t)
    diarrhea in, 60
    digestion-absorption tests
      for, 1290(t), 1293–
      1296

Intestine(s) (*Continued*)
  small, disease of, parasitic, 1312–
    1319
    types of, 1322–1324
    vs. colonic disease, 1291(t),
      1347(t)
    vs. large intestinal disease,
      1291(t)
  disorders of. See
    *Malabsorption;
    Malassimilation.*
  endocrine function of, 1286
  epithelial renewal in,
    1278–1279, *1279*
  enterosystemic cycles in, 1285
  fat assimilation by,
    1280–1282, *1281, 1283*
  foreign objects obstructing,
    1335–1340, *1336–1339*
  hypermotility of, and
    diarrhea, 1288–1289
  immune function of,
    1286–1287
  increased transit time in, and
    diarrhea, 1288–1289
  innervation of, 1278
  intussusception of,
    obstructive, *1337*, 1340
  layers of, 1278–1279
  lymphangiectasia of,
    2066–2067
    in protein-losing
      enteropathy, 1320,
      1320(t), 1325–1327,
      1325–1327, 1328(t), *1329*
  lymphoid tissue of,
    1279–1280
  lymphosarcoma of,
    1333–1334, *1334*
  malabsorption in,
    1330–1331, *1331, 1332*
  motor function of,
    1285–1286
  mucosal enzymes in, tests for,
    1298
  obstruction of, 1335–1340,
    1336–1339
  peristalsis in, 1196, 1286
  plasma protein leakage into,
    test for, 1298
  protein assimilation in,
    1284–1285
    tests of, 1295–1296
  sausage loop of, *1337*, 1340
  segmentation in, 1286
  structure and function of,
    1278–1287
  surface area of, 57
  tumors of, 1333–1335, *1334,
    1335*
    and malabsorption,
      1330–1331, *1331, 1332*
  water and electrolyte
    absorption in, 57–58
  water and solute movement
    in, 1285

Lymph node(s) (*Continued*)
hyperplasia of, See
Lymphadenopathy.
hypoplasia of, 2050–2051
lymphocytes in, 2103–2104
metastasis to, *2057–2058*, 2067
aspirate from, 2056,
2056–2058
staging of, in cancer, 369, *370*
structure of, 2046
tumors of, 2052–2056
Lymph node reactions, 2047(t)
Lymphadenitis, 1073
Lymphadenopathy, 2051–2052
diagnostic evaluation of, 2051
hilar, and airway obstruction
and compression, 813–814,
814, 815
laboratory tests for, 2051–2052
tracheobronchial, histoplasma-
induced, 737
Lymphangiectasia, 1074,
2066–2067
and protein-losing enteropathy,
1320, 1320(t), 1325–1327,
1325–1327, 1328(t), *1329*
Lymphangioma, 1077
Lymphangitis, 1073
Lymphatic leukemia, feline,
313–314
Lymphatic system. See also *Lymph
node(s); Lymphatics.*
disorders of, causes of, 1073(t)
inflammatory, 1073
lymphopenia in, 2027
occlusion of, and edema, 69
physiology of, 1072
Lymphatics
aplasia of, 1073–1074
hyperplasia of, 1073–1074
hypoplasia of, 1073–1074
peripheral, diseases of,
1072–1077
Lymphedema, 1073–1077
primary, 70, 1073–1075
secondary, 1075–1077
Lymphoblast(s), *2008*, 2010
defined, 2047
in lymph node aspirate, 2053,
2053
Lymphoblastic leukemia, acute,
2059
Lymphocyte(s), *2008*, 2010,
2046–2047
accessory, 2101
adherent, 2101
B, antigen receptors on, 2111
characteristics of, 2047,
2048(t)
cooperation of with T
lymphocytes, 2108–2109,
2109
EAC rosette–forming, 2176,
2176
immunologic tolerance of,
2108

Lymphocyte(s) (*Continued*)
B, quantitation of, in
immunodeficiency
syndromes, 2176, *2176*
reaction of to antigens, *2048*
vs. T lymphocytes,
2102–2103, 2103(t)
circulation of, 2049–2050
differentiation of, 2102–2103
functions of, 2014–2015
kinetics of, 2014–2015
peripheral blood, enumeration
of, 2176
production of, 2014–2015
recirculation of, 2015,
2049–2050
T, antigen receptors on,
2111–2112
characteristics of, 2047,
2048(t)
cooperation of with B
lymphocytes, 2108–2109,
2109
cytotoxic, in transplantation
immunity, 2129
in tumor immunity, 2125
deficiency of, 2174(t)
E rosette–forming, 2177
effect of on class and affinity
of synthesized
immunoglobulins, 2106
immunologic tolerance of,
2108
maturation of, 2102
murine, characteristics of,
2102(t)
quantitation of, 2177
reaction of to antigens,
2048
suppressor, and immunologic
tolerance, 2108, *2109*
vs. B lymphocytes,
2102–2103,
2103(t)
Lymphocyte blast transformation
tests, 2176–2177
Lymphocyte blastogenesis tests,
2176–2177
Lymphocyte choriomeningitis
virus, 2133
Lymphocyte function tests,
2176–2177
Lymphocyte progenitor cells,
2102
Lymphocyte rosette formation,
2176, *2176*, 2177
Lymphocyte stimulation tests,
2176–2177
Lymphocyte transformation tests,
2176–2177
Lymphocyte transforming factor,
2047
Lymphocytic arthritis, 2229–2231
Lymphocytic leukemia, chronic,
2059–2060
variants of, 2060

Lymphocytic-plasmacytic enteritis,
1320(t), 1323–1324, *1323*
Lymphocytic synovitis, 2229
and cruciate ligament injury,
2198
Lymphocytic thyroiditis, 2131,
2159(t), 2180
and primary hypothyroidism,
1603
treatment of, 1607–1608
Lymphocytosis, 2026–2027
physiologic, 2015
Lymphography, 1074, 1076
Lymphoid organs
primary, 2102
secondary, 2103–2104
Lymphoid system
accessory cells in, 2101
adherent cells in, 2101
development of, *2048*
immunologic functions of,
2101–2104
Lymphoid tissue, bronchus-
associated, 765
Lymphoid tumors, 2134
classification of, 2059(t)
Lymphokines, 2047, 2120, 2121(t)
Lymphoma(s), 2061–2065
alimentary form of, 2062
biochemical investigation in,
2064
classification of, 2062
cutaneous, 2063
defined, 2061
diagnosis of, 2063–2065
hematologic evaluation in,
2063–2064
hematopoietic system in,
2062–2063
hypercalcemia in, 135, 2064
immunologic investigations in,
2064–2065
incidence of, 2062
lymph node aspirate in,
2054–2055, *2055*
of mediastinum, 852–853, *853*
of spleen, *2068*
of thymus, 852
respiratory involvement in,
2062
signs of, 2062–2063
splenic biopsy in, *2068*, 2071
staging of, 2063(t)
treatment of, 2065
with leukemic manifestations,
2060
Lymphomatosis carcinomatosa,
830
Lymphopenia, 2026–2027
in cancer chemotherapy, 381
in uremia, 1797
Lymphoproliferative diseases,
2056–2066
Lymphoreticular carcinoma
feline, 313–314
melphalan for, 376

Mandibular gland (*Continued*)
  injury of, 1183
Mandibular neuropraxia, 1146
Mannitol
  for cerebral edema, 523
  for renal failure, acute,
    1856–1857
  for spinal cord edema, 573
  for urolithiasis, feline, 1929
  in toxicosis, 181
Mannosidase deficiency, 494(t)
Manometry, esophageal, 1201
Manx, spinal malformations in,
  555–556, *555*
Manx calicivirus, and urolithiasis,
  1923
Marine animals, poisoning by,
  201
Maroteaux-Lamy syndrome, joint
  disease in, 2218
Marrow. See *Bone marrow.*
Masseter muscle, atrophy of, in
  trigeminal nerve disease, 629
Mast cells
  function of, 2014
  kinetics of, 2014
  production of, 2014
Mast cell tumors, anaplastic,
    metastasis in, 401(t)
  differentiated, metastasis in,
    401(t)
  excision of, contraindications
    to, 411
  radioresponsiveness of, 402(t)
Mastectomy, 412–413
  BCG vaccine immunotherapy
    for, 389, 389(t)
  hemorrhage in, 412
Master problem list, 6, *13*
  and breed, 155
Mastocytoma
  and gastric ulcers, 1260
  corticosteroids for, 380
  cyclophosphamide for, 374–376
  cytosine arabinoside for, 378
  grading of, 368
  hydroxyurea for, 379
  immunotherapy for, 388(t), 390
  lymph node aspirate in, *2056*
  surgery of, complications of,
    408
  vincristine for, 377(t), 378
Mastocytosis
  lymph node aspirate in, *2056*
  systemic, 2067
Maxilla. See *Jaw(s).*
Mean corpuscular hemoglobin,
  1950–1952
Mean corpuscular hemoglobin
  concentration, 1950–1952
Measles vaccine, for distemper,
  273
Mebendazole
  dosage and efficacy of, 1315(t)
  for trichuriasis, 1351
  hepatotoxicity of, 1407, 1408

Mechanoreceptors, respiratory,
  689
Median nerve
  injury of, 635
  lesions of, neurologic findings
    in, 622(t)
Mediastinal emphysema,
  843–846, *845*
Mediastinal shift, 843, *844*
Mediastinitis, 849–850
Mediastinum
  abnormalities of, 841–854
  abscess of, 847(t), 851
    signs of, 842
  disorders of, examination of,
      clinicopathologic, 843
    physical, 841–842
    radiographic, 842–843
  edema of, 850–851
  granuloma of, 847(t), 851
  hemorrhage in, 851
  infection of, signs of, 842
  lipoma of, 846, 847(t), 852
  regions of, 846
  space-occupying lesions of,
      846–848, *848–850*
    airway obstruction by, 842
    and neurologic deficits, 842
    esophageal obstruction by,
      842
    signs of, 842
    vascular obstruction by, 842
  structure and function of,
    840–841
  tumors of, 847(t), 852–854
  widening of, acute, 848–851
    chronic, 852
Medical record(s) 3–37
  and professional
    communication, 3
  as basis for patient care, 3
  as documentary evidence, 3
  as legal evidence, 4
  as repository of clinical data,
    3–4
  autopsy reports in, 12–13
  color coding of, 24–26, *25*
  consultation reports in, 9–10
  content and structure of, 4–13
  cover for, 5
  diagnostic and procedure
    summary for, 5, *6*
  diagnostic reports in, 12, *17, 18*
  emergency, 12, *19*
  etiologic classification of, 28,
    28(t)
  filling systems for, 18–24
    techniques for improving,
      24–29
  history and examination sheet
    for, 6, *10, 11*
  hospitalization records in, 6–9,
    13
  identification of, 4, *4*
  laboratory reports in, 10–12, *14*
  master problem list for, 6, *13*

Medical record(s) (*Continued*)
  medical-surgical summary for,
    5, *7–8*
  number blocking of, 24–26, *26*
  number index for, 27
  operative procedure
    classification of, 28, 28(t)
  patient index for, 26–27, *26*
  problem-oriented, 29–37
    defined data base for, 31–34,
      32–33
    discharge summary for, 36
    flow chart for, 36–37, *36*
    plans for, 31, 34
    problem list for, 30–31, 34,
      35
    progress notes for, 31,
      34–37, *35*
    vs. standard, 30(t)
    Weed System for, 30–37
  progress notes in, 6, *13, 17, 18*
  purging of, date blocking for,
    26
  purpose of, 3
  radiology reports in, 12, *17*
  registration form for, 5, *9*
  release of, 4
  retrieval and coding of, 27–29,
    27(t), 28(t)
  standard, vs. problem-oriented,
    30(t)
  storage of, 24, *25*
  surgical reports in, 12, *16–17*
  topographic classification of,
    27(t), 28
  vs. billing system, 13–18, *20–22*
Medroxyprogesterone
  for feline spraying, 220
  for intermale aggression, 222
Medullary solute washout, 1751
Megacolon, 64–65, 1366–1367
Megaesophagus, 1227–1230
  in myasthenia gravis, 644
  in polymyositis, 645
  neuropathic, 631
Megakaryoblast, 2078
Megakaryocyte, 2078
Megakaryocytic leukemia,
  2037–2038
Megakaryocytic myelosis, feline,
  2036
Megakaryopoiesis, 2078–2079
Megaloblastic anemia, 1988
  in erythroleukemia, 1988
Megalocyte, 1957(t)
Megathrombocyte, criteria for
  platelet classification as, 2084
Megaureter, 1887
  and ureteral ectopia, 1881
Megestrol acetate
  as contraceptive, 1727–1728
  for aggression, dominance-
    related, 225
    intermale, 222
  for estrus suppression, 1727
  for feline spraying, 220

Tetany
  in hypoparathyroidism,
    1582–1583
  in uremia, 1787
  puerperal, 1584–1586, *1584,
    1585*
Tetracycline(s)
  action and use of, 344–345
  and hepatic lipidosis, 1388
  and polyneuropathy, 644
  and tooth staining, 345,
    1135–1136, *1136*
  as iron chelator, 324
  dosage and route of, 341(t),
    344
  drug interactions with, 345
  for brucellosis, 301, 1715
  for colitis, acute, 1352
  for ehrlichiosis, 304
  for hemobartonellosis, feline,
    1983
  for pyelonephritis, 1863
  for wound infection, 363
  in hepatic failure, 1424
  optimal pH for, 352(t)
  toxicity of, 344–345
  with antacids, 324
  with corticosteroids, 345
  with kaolin preparations,
    354
Tetrahydrozoline, 823(t)
Tetralogy of Fallot, 944–945,
  950–951, *951–953*
L-Tetramisol, for angiostrongylus,
  896
Tetraparesis, in cerebral disease,
  462–463, 466
Thallium intoxication, 184–186
Thenium closylate, 1315(t)
Theophylline
  anhydrous vs. salts, 823, 824(t)
  for cardiac disease, 969(t)
  for tracheitis, 728(t)
  salts vs. anhydrous, 823, 824(t)
Therapy, animal-facilitated,
  231–232
Thermoregulation, 46, *47*
Thiabendazole
  and anorexia, 707
  dosage and efficacy of, 1315(t)
  for aspergillosis, 261
  for immunostimulation, 2183
  for lungworm infection, 728
  for nasal mycoses, 706–707
Thiacetarsamide
  for heartworm disease,
    1114–1115
  for hemobartonellosis, feline,
    1983
  side effects of, 1118–1119
Thiamine deficiency, and cerebral
  disorders, 498–499
Thiazide diuretics, for congestive
  heart failure, 924
6-Thioguanine, in cancer
  chemotherapy, 377(t), 378

Third eyelid
  protrusion of, in ocular
    sympathetic nerve lesions,
    444–445, *444*
  in tetanus, 445–446, *446*
  retraction of, causes of, 446
Thirst
  excessive. See *Polydipsia.*
  physiology of, 133–134
  psychogenic, 136
Thoracentesis
  in feline dilated cardio-
    myopathy, 1042
  in pleural effusion, 857–865,
    864–867, 873
Thoracic duct
  abnormalities of, and
    chylothorax, 874–876
  congenital, 875
Thoracic lavage, 872–873
Thoracic limb reflex
  anatomy of, 431(t)
  evaluation of, 431–435
Thoracic metastases, pleural
  effusions in, triethylene
  thiophosphoramide for, 376
Thoracic vessels, rupture of,
  873–874
Thoracocentesis. See *Thoracentesis.*
Thoracotomy, 873
Thorax
  auscultation of, 659, 660(t)
    in lower respiratory disease,
    769, 770(t),771(t)
  diseases of, 883–898
  empyema of, 868(t), 869–870,
    871, 872
  examination of, in respiratory
    disease, 659
  palpation of, 769
  percussion of, 659–660
    in lower respiratory disease,
    769–771, *771,* 771(t)
  radiography of, 773–776, *774,
    775*
  trauma of, antibiotics in, 363
Threshhold membrane potential,
  981
Thrombin, in coagulation
  cascade, 2078
Thrombin time, 2082
Thrombocytopenia, 2094–2096,
  2095(t)
  causes of, 2094–2095, 2095(t)
  immune-mediated, 2070,
    2159(t), 2167–2168, *2169*
  prognosis in, 2168
  therapy of, 2168
  in cancer chemotherapy, 381
  in hepatic disease, 2091
  mechanisms of, 2094–2095
Thrombocytosis, secondary, 2079
Thromboembolic pneumonia,
  794(t)
Thromboembolism. See also
  Thrombosis.

Thromboembolism (*Continued*)
  aortic, canine, 1066–1068,
    1067
  feline, 1064–1066
  arterial, and cardiomyopathy,
    1064
  canine, 1066–1068
  feline, 1046–1047, *1047,*
    1064–1066
  in bacterial endocarditis,
    1056, 1066, 1068
  in renal disease, 1786
  pathogenesis of, 1064
  pulmonary, 887–890, *888, 890,
    891*
  and hyperadrenocorticism,
    1685
  in heartworm disease, 1101,
    1117
Thromboplastin time, 2085
  activated partial, 2081, 2085
Thrombopoietin, 2079
Thrombosis. See also
  Thromboembolism.
  arterial, 1066–1068, *1067*
  cerebrovascular, 503
  pulmonary, 887–890, *888, 890,
    891*
  venous, 1077
Thrombosthenin, 2084–2085
Thrombo-Wellcotest, 2082
Thromboxane A$_2$, 2080
Thrombus(i)
  formation of, 1064
  pulmonary arterial, in
    heartworm disease, 1101
  saddle, 1064, *1067*
Thrush, 1162, *1163*
Thunderstorms, fear of, 213–214
Thymic lymphocytes. See
  Lymphocyte(s), T.
Thymocytes, 2102
Thymoma, 853–854
Thymopoietin, 2102
Thymus
  as primary lymphoid organ,
    2102
  diseases of, 852, 853–854
  hypoplasia of, 2174(t)
  lymphocyte differentiation in,
    2102
Thymus-dependent antibody
  response, 2106
Thymus-derived cells. See
  Lymphocyte(s), T.
Thyrocalcitonin. See *Calcitonin.*
Thyroglossal duct cyst, 1187
Thyroid
  accesssory, 1593
  anatomy and development of,
    1592–1593
  atrophy of, and primary
    hypothyroidism,
    1603–1604
  in nonfunctioning pituitary
    adenoma, 1535, *1535*